JULY 1995

Diana M Wood

CLINICAL PAEDIATRIC ENDOCRINOLOGY

Clinical Paediatric Endocrinology

Edited by

CHARLES G.D. BROOK

MA MD FRCP DCH

Reader in Paediatric Endocrinology,
University of London;
Consultant Paediatrician,
The Middlesex Hospital,
London

Foreword by

ANDREA PRADER MD

Emeritus Professor of Pediatrics,
University of Zurich,
Switzerland

THIRD EDITION

b

Blackwell
Science

Editorial Offices:
Osney Mead, Oxford OX2 0EL
25 John Street, London WC1N 2BL
23 Ainslie Place, Edinburgh EH3 6AJ
238 Main Street, Cambridge
Massachusetts 02142, USA
54 University Street, Carlton
Victoria 3053, Australia

Other Editorial Offices:
Arnette Blackwell SA
1, rue de Lille, 75007 Paris
France

Blackwell Wissenschafts-Verlag GmbH
Kurfürstendamm 57
10707 Berlin, Germany

Feldgasse 13, A-1238 Wien
Austria

First published 1981
Second edition 1989
Third edition 1995

Set by Excel Typesetters Company, Hong Kong
Printed and bound in Great Britain at
the University Press, Cambridge

DISTRIBUTORS

Marston Book Services Ltd
PO Box 87
Oxford OX2 0DT
(*Orders*: Tel: 01865 791155
Fax: 01865 791927
Telex: 837515)

North America
Blackwell Science, Inc.
238 Main Street
Cambridge, MA 02142
(*Orders*: Tel: 800 215-1000
617 876-7000
Fax: 617 492-5263)

Australia
Blackwell Science Pty Ltd
54 University Street
Carlton, Victoria 3053
(*Orders*: Tel: 03 347-0300
Fax: 03 349-3016)

A catalogue record for this title
is available from the British Library

ISBN 0-632-03632-X

Library of Congress
Cataloging-in-Publication Data

Clinical paediatric endocrinology/
edited by Charles G.D. Brook:
foreword by Andrea Prader – 3rd ed.
p. cm.
Rev. ed. of: Clinical pediatric endocrinology/
edited by Charles G.D. Brook. 2nd ed. 1989.
Includes bibliographical references and index.
ISBN 0-632-03632-X
1. Pediatric endocrinology.
I. Brook, C.G.D. (Charles Groves Darville)
II. Clinical pediatric endocrinology.
[DNLM: 1. Endocrine Diseases –
in infancy & childhood.
2. Endocrine Diseases – in adolescence.
3. Endocrine Diseases – physiopathology.
WS 330 C641 1995]
RJ418. C567 1995
618.92′4 – dc20
DNLM/DLC
for Library of Congress 95-3730

Contents

List of Contributors, vii

Foreword, ix

Preface to the Third Edition, xi

Preface to the First Edition, xiii

1 Gene Structure, Recombinant DNA Technology and its Application in Paediatric Endocrinology, 1
P.E. MULLIS AND P.T. CHEUNG

2 Applications of Molecular Genetics in the Study of Clinical Disorders, 23
R.V. THAKKER

3 Physiology of Sexual Determination and Differentiation, 41
P. SAENGER

4 The Clinical Management of Ambiguous Genitalia, 53
G.L. WARNE AND I.A. HUGHES

5 Growth Factors and Prenatal Development: Recent Lessons from Molecular Biology, 69
D.J. HILL AND A. LOGAN

6 Normal Growth and its Endocrine Control, 85
P.C. HINDMARSH AND C.G.D. BROOK

7 The Insulin-like Growth Factors, 107
R.G. ROSENFELD AND E.K. NEELY

8 Signalling Mechanisms and Hormone Pulsatility, 123
D.R. MATTHEWS AND I.C.A.F. ROBINSON

9 Short Stature, 136
C.T. COWELL

10 The Management of Short Stature, 173
N.A. BRIDGES AND C.G.D. BROOK

11 Growth-hormone-resistant States, 187
A.M. COTTERILL AND M.O. SAVAGE

12 Tall Stature, 195
P.C. HINDMARSH AND C.G.D. BROOK

13 The Fat Child, 210
E.M.E. POSKITT

14 The Physiology of Puberty, 234
D.M. STYNE

15 Disorders of Puberty, 253
N.A. BRIDGES AND C.G.D. BROOK

16 Gynaecology, 274
J.S. SANFILIPPO

17 Reproductive Endocrinology – The Ovary, 288
D.F. WOOD AND S. FRANKS

18 Reproductive Endocrinology – The Testis, 298
E.M. RITZÉN

19 Anatomy and Physiology of the Hypothalamopituitary Axis, 310
S.L. CHEW AND A.B. GROSSMAN

20 Neuroradiology, 320
B.E. KENDALL

21 The Neurosurgical Approach to Hypothalamohypophyseal Tumours, 346
M. POWELL AND D. THOMPSON

22 Thyroid, Adrenal and Pancreatic Surgery, 359
R.C.G. RUSSELL

23 Gynaecological Endocrine Surgery, 364
S.J. STEELE

24 Endocrine-related Urological Surgery, 371
J.M. HUTSON

25 Growth and Endocrine Sequelae Following the Treatment of Childhood Cancer, 383
S.M. SHALET

26 The Thyroid Gland, 397
F. DELANGE AND D.A. FISHER

27 The Adrenal Cortex, 434
J.W. HONOUR

28 Adrenal Steroid Deficiency States, 453
M.G. FOREST

29 Adrenal Steroid Excess, 499
M.G. FOREST

30 Congenital Adrenal Hyperplasia, 536
Z. HUMA, C. CRAWFORD AND M.I. NEW

31 Salt and Water Balance: Sodium-losing States and Endocrine Hypertension, 558
M.J. DILLON

32 The Neurohypophysis and Water Regulation, 580
J. PERHEENTUPA

33 Pathophysiology of Diabetes Mellitus, 616
D.J. BECKER AND B. WEBER

34 The Management of Diabetes Mellitus, 654
J. COURT

35 Hypoglycaemia, 677
P.J. LEE AND J.V. LEONARD

36 Lipid Disorders, 694
D.J. BETTERIDGE

37 Endocrine Control of Calcium and Bone Metabolism, 713
K. KRUSE

38 Disorders of Calcium and Bone Metabolism, 735
K. KRUSE

39 Laboratory Approach to the Child with Suspected Disorders of Calcium and Bone Metabolism, 779
K. KRUSE

40 Tests and Normal Values in Paediatric Endocrinology, 782
J.M. WALKER AND I.A. HUGHES

Index, 799

Colour plates 8.1 and 16.1–16.10 between pp. 290–291; 36.1–36.4 between pp. 706–707.

List of Contributors

D.J. BECKER MB, BCh *Professor of Pediatrics, Children's Hospital of Pittsburgh, One Children's Place, 3705 Avenue at Desoto Street, Pittsburgh, Pennslyvania, USA*

D.J. BETTERIDGE BSc, PHD, MD, FRCP *Reader in Medicine, Department of Medicine, University College London Medical School, 5th Floor, Sir Jules Thorn Institute, The Middlesex Hospital, Mortimer Street, London W1N 8AA*

N.A. BRIDGES BM, MRCP *Lecturer in Paediatric Endocrinology, University College London, The Cobbold Laboratories, The Middlesex Hospital, Mortimer Street, London W1N 8AA*

C.G.D. BROOK MA, MD, FRCP *Professor of Paediatric Endocrinology, University College London, Consultant Paediatric Endocrinology, London Centre for Paediatric Endocrinology & Metabolism, Great Ormond Street Children's Hospital and The Middlesex Hospital, Mortimer Street, London W1N 8AA*

P.T. CHEUNG MD *Department of Paediatric Endocrinology, University Children's Hospital, Inselspital, CH-3010 Bern, Switzerland*

S.L. CHEW BSc, MRCP *MRC Training Fellow and Senior Registrar, Department of Endocrinology, St Bartholomew's Hospital, London EC1A 7BE*

A.M. COTTERILL MBBS, MRCP, MD *Senior Lecturer in Paediatric Endocrinology, Honorary Consultant Paediatrician, Department of Endocrinology, St Bartholmew's Hospital, London EC1A 7BE*

J.M. COURT MD *Senior Physician, Department of Endocrinology and Diabetes, Royal Children's Hospital, Melbourne, Victoria, Australia*

C.T. COWELL MB, PRACP, FRCP(C) *Director, Robert Vines Growth Research Centre, Royal Alexandra Hospital for Children, Camperdown, New South Wales 2050, Australia*

C. CRAWFORD *Academic Research Specialist, Division of Pediatric Endocrinology, The New York Hospital Cornell Medical Center, 525 East 68th Street N-236, NY 10021, USA*

F. DELANGE MD *Department of Paediatrics, Radioisotopes, University Hôpital Saint-Pierre, 322 rue Haute, B-1000 Brussels, Belgium*

M.J. DILLON MB, FRCP, DcM *Consultant Physician and Paediatric Nephrologist, Hospital for Sick Children, NHS Trust, Great Ormond Street, London WC1N 3JH*

D.A. FISHER MD *President, Academic Associates and Chief Science Officer, Corning Nichols Institute, 33605 Ortega Highway, San Juan, Capistrano, CA 92690, USA*

M.G. FOREST MD, PhD *Directeur de Recherchenat INSERM, INSERM U329, Pathologie Hormonale Moléculaire, Hôpital Debrousse, 29, rue Soeur Bouvier, F-69322 Lyon Cedex 05, France*

S. FRANKS MD, FRCP *Professor of Reproductive Endocrinology, Department of Obstetrics and Gynaecology, St Mary's Hospital Medical School, Norfolk Place, London W2 1PG*

P. GLUCKMAN MD *Paediatric and Perinatal Biology, School of Medicine, University of Auckland, Private Bag 92019, Auckland, New Zealand*

A.B. GROSSMAN MD, FRCP *Professor of Neuroendocrinology, Department of Endocrinology, St Bartholomew's Hospital, London EC1A 7BE*

D.J. HILL BSc, DPhil *Health and Development, Lawson Research Institute, University of Western Ontario, London, Ontario N6A 4V2, Canada*

P.C. HINDMARSH MD, FRCP *Senior Lecturer in Paediatric Endocrinology, University College London, The Middlesex Hospital, Mortimer Street, London W1N 8AA*

J.W. HONOUR PhD, FRCPath *Reader in Steroid Endocrinology, Chemical Pathology, University College London Medical School, Rayne Institute 5, University Street, London WC1*

I.A. HUGHES MA, MD, FRCP, FRCP(C) *Professor of Paediatrics, University of Cambridge, Addenbrooke's Hospital, Hills Road, Cambridge, CB2 2QQ*

Z. HUMA MB, BChir, MRCP *Attending Physician, Department of Pediatrics, Division of Pediatric Endocrinology, The New York Hospital Cornell Medical Center, 525 East 68th Street N-236, NY 100021, USA*

J.M. HUTSON MBBS (Monash), MD (Melb), FRACS *Director, Department of General Surgery, Royal Children's Hospital, Melbourne; Professor of Paediatric Surgery, Department of Paediatrics, University of Melbourne, Australia*

B.E. KENDALL FRCR, FRCS, FRCP *Consultant Radiologist, University College London, The Middlesex Hospital, Mortimer Street, London W1N 8AA*

K. KRUSE MD *Professor of Paediatrics, Chairman, Department of Paediatrics, Medical University of Zuebeck, Kahlhorststrasse 31–35, D-23538 Lubeck, Germany*

P.J. LEE MRCP (UK) *Research Fellow, The London Centre for Paediatric Endocrinology and Metabolism, The Institute of Child Health, London*

J.V. LEONARD PhD, FRCP *Professor of Paediatric Metabolic Disease, London Centre for Paediatric Endocrinology and Metabolism, The Institute of Child Health, London WC1N 1EH*

A. LOGAN PhD *Department of Clinical Chemistry, University of Birmingham, Birmingham B15 2TT*

D.R. MATTHEWS MA, DPhil, FRCP *Consultant Physician and Senior Clinical Lecturer, Oxford Diabetes Centre, The Radcliffe Infirmary, Woodstock Road, Oxford OX2 6HE*

P.E. MULLIS PD, MD *Department of Paediatric Endocrinology, University Children's Hospital, Inselspital, CH-3010 Bern, Switzerland*

E.K. NEELY MD *Department of Paediatrics, Room A367, Stanford University Medical Center, Stanford, CA 94305, USA*

M.I. NEW MD *Professor and Chairman, Department of Paediatrics, Chief, Division of Pediatric Endocrinology, Harold and Percy Uris Professor of Pediatric Endocrinology and Metabolism, The New York Hospital Cornell Medical Center, 525 East 68th Street N-236, NY 10021, USA*

J. PERHEENTUPA MD *Professor of Paediatrics, The Children's Hospital, University of Helsinki, SF-22390 Helsinki, Finland*

E.M.E. POSKITT MA, MB, BChir, FRCP *Head of Station and Consultant Paediatrician, Medical Research Council, Dunn Nutrition Group, Keneba, Fajara, PO Box 273, Banjul, The Gambia*

M. POWELL FRCS *National Hospital for Nervous Disorders, Queen Square, London WC1N 3BG*

E.M. RITZÉN MD *Department of Paediatric Endocrinology, Karolinska Hospital, S-17176 Stockholm, Sweden*

I.C.A.F. ROBINSON MA, DPhil *Division of Neurophysiology, National Institute for Medical Research, The Ridgeway, Mill Hill, London NW7 1AA*

R.G. ROSENFELD MD *Professor and Chairman, Department of Pediatrics, Physician-in-Chief, Doernbecher Children's Hospital 3181 S.W. Sam Jackson Road, Portland, Oregon, USA*

R.C.G. RUSSELL MS, FRCS *Consultant Surgeon, University College London, The Middlesex Hospital, Mortimer Street, London W1N 8AA*

P. SAENGER MD *Professor of Pediatrics, Director, Division of Pediatric Endocrinology, Montifoire Medical Center, 111 East 210th Street, Bronx, NY 10407, USA*

J.S. SANFILIPPO MD *Professor of Obstetrics and Gynecology, University of Louisville, School of Medicine, Louisville, Kentucky 40292, USA*

M.O. SAVAGE MA, MD, FRCP *Reader in Paediatric Endocrinology, The Medical College of St Bartholmew's Hospital, London EC1A 7BE*

S.M. SHALET BSc, MD, MB, BS, FRCP *Consultant Endocrinologist, Christie Hospital, Manchester M20 9BX*

S.J. STEELE MA, MB, BChir, FRCS, FRCOE, MFFP *Associate Director, Department of Obstetrics and Gynaecology, 4th Floor, Sir Jules Thorn Institute, University College London, The Middlesex Hospital, Mortimer Street, London W1N 8AA*

D. STYNE MD *Department of Pediatrics, University of California, Davis School of Medicine, Davis, California, USA*

R.V. THAKKER MA, FRCP, *MRC Molecular Medicine Group, Royal Postgraduate Medical School, Hammersmith Hospital, Du Cane Road, London W12 0HS*

D.N.P. THOMPSON MBBS, BSc, FRCS *Department of Neurosurgery, Hospital for Sick Children, NHS Trust, Great Ormond Street, London WC1N 3JA*

J.M. WALKER BA, MB, BS, MRCP *Consultant Paediatrician, Department of Child Health, St Mary's Hospital, Milton Road, Porstmouth, Hants PO3 6AD*

G.L. WARNE MD *Department of Endocrinology, Royal Children's Hospital, Parkville, Victoria 3052, Australia*

B. WEBER MD *Professor of Paediatrics, Kinder Klinik der Freien Universität Berlin, Kaiserin Auguste Victoria Haus, Heubnerweg 6, D-1000 Berlin 19, West Germany*

D.F. WOOD MD, MRCP *Senior Lecturer in Outpatient Medicine and Honorary Consultant, Department of Endocrinology, Royal London Hospital, Whitechapel, London E1 1BB*

Foreword

It gives me great pleasure to write this foreword. The reason is twofold. First, the editor, Professor Charles Brook, started his training in paediatric endocrinology many years ago in our hospital, the Kinderspital in Zurich. He has become a friend and I have followed his professional career with pride and satisfaction. Second, three editions of a book demonstrate that there is a need for it. In a way, the third edition makes it a classical textbook.

To be an editor and to keep all the authors in line is difficult. Charles Brook has succeeded in keeping the size of the book to reasonable limits and in keeping the emphasis on practical clinical aspects. This does not prevent full coverage of the genetic origin and the pathogenesis of the various clinical conditions, including a brief discussion of the newer aspects of molecular biology.

In the preface to the first edition, Charles Brook said that the book had its origins in the friendship of the European Society of Paediatric Endocrinology and its American counterpart the Lawson Wilkins Society of Paediatric Endocrinology. Indeed, practically all contributors are members of these societies. As is to be expected, the majority are from the United Kingdom, but an important number are well-known paediatric endocrinologists from continental Europe and the United States. Thus the book represents a truly international achievement.

The classification follows the tradition of the first two editions. In the first chapters the normal development of the fetus, the child and adolescent and its variations are exposed. This is followed by chapters on the diseases of the various endocrine organs. In the last chapters calcium metabolism, blood glucose regulation, imaging and laboratory tests are discussed. The book is a handy and reliable guide to all those who practise paediatric endocrinology, but also for all those colleagues who need practical information when they are confronted with problems of the physical development of children and their hormonal problems. I hope that the book will find its place in every paediatric and endocrine service.

Andrea Prader

Preface to the Third Edition

I dedicated the first edition of this book to the friendship between the European Society for Paediatric Endocrinology and the Lawson Wilkins Society for Paediatric Endocrinology. Professor Melvin Grumbach was kind enough to write the foreword to the second edition and I am extremely grateful to Professor Andrea Prader, the doyen of European paediatric endocrinology, for writing the foreword to this, the third edition.

Once again, because of the rapid progress of events in endocrinology, the book has been almost completely rewritten. My co-authors and I have tried to reflect the impact of modern technology – specifically molecular biology – on our subject. We have tried to present the newer findings in a way that is as intelligible as possible. No doubt in years to come, physicians will become as familiar with the language of molecular biology as research fellows seem nowadays to be with computer technology. Because we have not reached that time quite yet, the introduction to the language of molecular biology has been written with the non-cognoscenti in mind.

On this occasion, I would like to thank Peter Saugman of Blackwell Science and Rebecca Huxley, who is responsible for getting the book into the shape in which it appears. We owe her a debt of considerable gratitude. We would also like to thank Sarah Rhaiti for her indefatigable pursuit of the missing references.

C.G.D. Brook

Preface to the First Edition

Endocrine problems are not uncommon in paediatric practice and are mostly, *faute de mieux*, rather badly managed by non-specialists. This is especially true in England, where paediatric specialities are relatively newly defined. The same is certainly less true of Europe as a whole and this book has its origins in the friendship of the European Society for Paediatric Endocrinology which has acted as a focus for the subject and which benefits greatly from its transatlantic corresponding members. If the book were to have a dedication, it would be to the health of the Society coupled with a toast to its American counterpart, the Lawson Wilkins Society.

I hope that the book will be of service to general paediatric departments and of help and interest to departments of (adult) endocrinology in their dealings with patients who are still growing. In a book of this size, there may well be sins of omission and commission and for these I alone can take responsibility and I apologize for them in advance. If any readers were to take the trouble to let me know about such sins for future reference, I would be very grateful.

In the completion of my editorial task I have been greatly assisted by Miss Lynette Napper and Mrs Sue Shorvon, my secretaries at The Middlesex Hospital, and by Mr Jony Russell and Mr Peter Saugman at Blackwell Scientific Publications. My co-authors and I thank them for assisting at the birth of our work.

C.G.D. Brook

1: Gene Structure, Recombinant DNA Technology and its Application in Paediatric Endocrinology

P.E. MULLIS and P.T. CHEUNG

INTRODUCTION

Endocrinology is built upon understanding basic scientific principles. It thus comes as no surprise to witness the rapid union of endocrinology and molecular biology. Apart from generating an abundance of new information, this combination also drastically changes the complexity of the scientific questions addressed in clinical endocrinology. Not unexpectedly, new concepts are constantly introduced and the understanding of the language of molecular biology has become a prerequisite to the appreciation of clinical endocrinology.

This chapter is designed to introduce this language, which will be taken for granted in subsequent chapters on more focused subjects.

GENE STRUCTURE AND FUNCTION

A gene is a unit of DNA within a chromosome that provides hereditary information governing the production of a protein (or, in special cases, ribosomal or transfer RNA). For genes encoding proteins, this information determines not only the primary structure of a protein but also when it should be expressed, how much should be produced and where it should be directed, all essential determinants of its functional properties. It is also obvious that proper functionality in proteins composed of different peptide units may require the coordinated expression of more than one gene.

In most eukaryotic genes the DNA sequences encoding the primary sequence of a protein (exons) are interrupted by non-coding DNA sequences (introns) (Fig. 1.1). The number and lengths of these alternating sequences, and consequently the overall lengths of the genes, vary considerably and bear no relation to the actual size of the protein products. The function of the introns is unknown but, at least in some genes, they divide the coding sequence according to the functional domains of the encoded protein. In that case, a gene with multiple exons appears to arise from the coalescence of different fragments of ancestral genes during evolution. On the other hand, transcriptional regulatory elements have been found within these introns, pointing to their potential involvement in gene regulation.

Once a gene has been chosen to be expressed, the information relay from DNA to protein begins with the production of pre-messenger RNA (pre-mRNA, also known as heterogeneous nuclear RNA, hnRNA). An exact nucleotide copy of the DNA template sequence, both exon and intron included, is synthesized, but with the substitution of uridine for thymidine. This pre-mRNA is then processed into a mature RNA by the addition of a methylated structure at the 5′ end, by the removal of the introns and by the addition of a poly-A tail at the 3′ end (Fig. 1.1).

The first post-transcriptional modification of the pre-mRNA, called capping, occurs soon after the initiation of transcription as a guanosine is added to its 5′ end through a triphosphate bond and subsequently methylated in the N-7 position (7-MeGppp) (Figs 1.1 & 1.2). This may facilitate the binding of the mature mRNA to the ribosomes, thereby enhancing translation. Another modification, known as polyadenylation, is the addition of a poly-A tail consisting of repeated adenosine residues to the 3′ end. This is signalled by the presence of a consensus sequence: AAUAAA [1]. Capping and polyadenylation are believed to render mRNA more stable, although the exact function is still unknown.

RNA splicing refers to the removal of the introns and takes place through the joining of the 5′ end of an intron and the 3′ end of the same or another downstream intron, followed by the cleavage of the looped RNA sequence (Fig. 1.1). Once formed, a mature mRNA is translocated to the cytoplasmic compartment where it is translated into protein on ribosomes. Within a mature mRNA the two stretches of nucleotides over the 5′ and 3′ ends are not translated, while the middle translatable protein-coding segment is called an open reading frame (ORF). Protein synthesis begins with the assembly of amino acids into peptide sequences according to the genetic code. Each successive amino acid is chosen by matching the nucleotide triplets of its cognate transfer RNA to the corresponding trinucleotide codon of the mRNA within

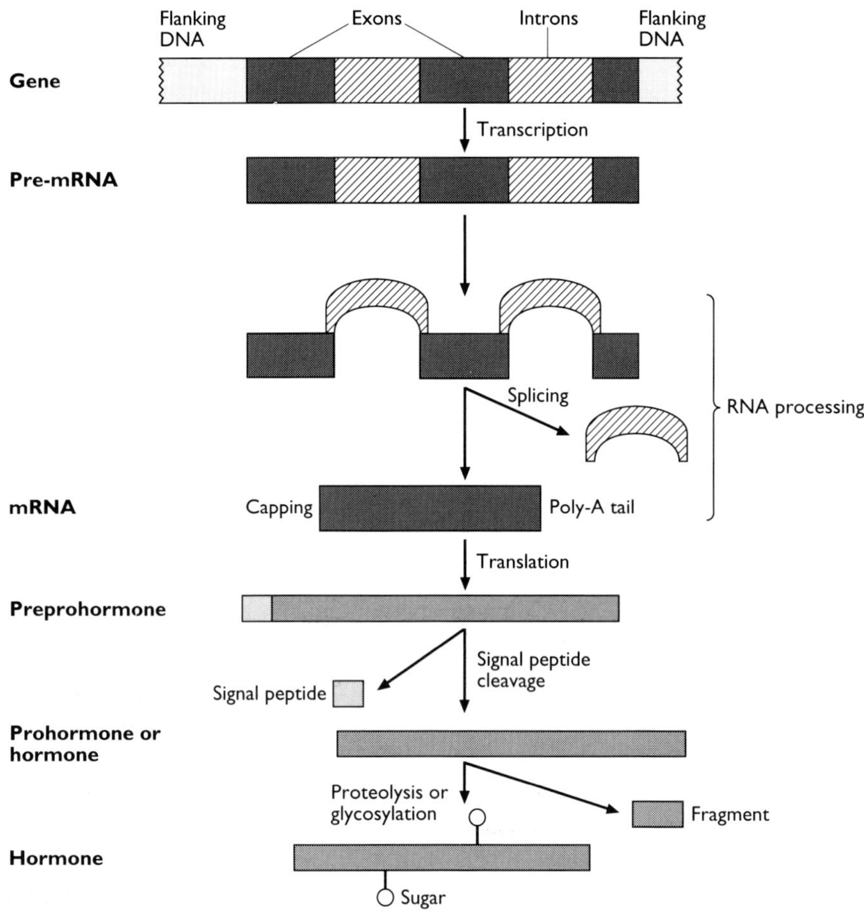

Fig. 1.1 Schematic representation of the pathway of gene expression resulting in peptide hormone synthesis. The gene is first transcribed into pre-mRNA retaining intronic sequences. Thereafter, RNA processing involves splicing of the intron sequences, capping and polyadenylation at the 5′ and 3′ ends respectively. The mature mRNA is translocated to the cytoplasmic compartment and translated into a prepro- or prehormone. The signal peptide is involved in translocating the newly synthesized polypeptide into the endoplasmic reticulum where it is eventually cleaved yielding a prohormone or hormone. Additional post-translational processing of prohormone such as proteolysis and/or glycosylation results in a mature hormone.

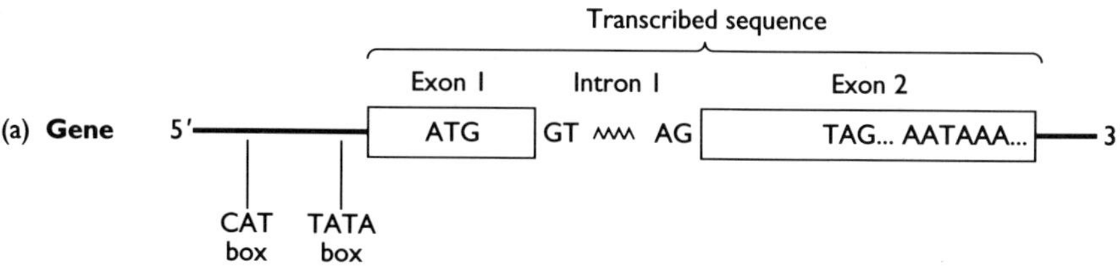

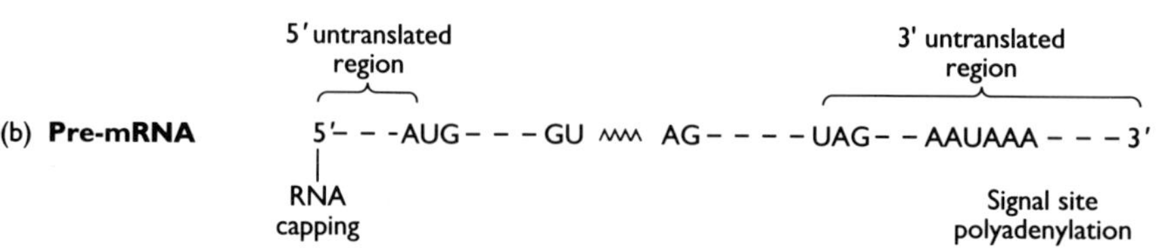

Fig. 1.2 Schematic representation of the structure of a eukaryotic gene. (a) A typical gene is characterized by a putative promoter structure (TATA box), upstream promoter elements such as a CAT box (CAAT, CATAAA) and the presence of introns and exons. Introns generally interrupt the coding sequence (exon) of most eukaryotic genes; the intron splice signals are designated GT at the 5′ end and AG at the 3′ end. The generally transcribed sequence is depicted. (b) The primary RNA transcript is depicted. The CAP site, polyadenylation signal (AAUAAA) and site are indicated and the 5′ and 3′ untranslated regions are shown. (c) Mature mRNA after splicing the introns, addition of the CAP structure (7-MeGppp, 7-methylguanosine residue joined to the mRNA by triphosphate linkage) at the 5′ end and of a poly-A tail (stretch of 100–200 adenosine residues) at the 3′ end is presented. The translation initiation site (AUG) and stop codon (UAG) defining the length of the protein are also shown.

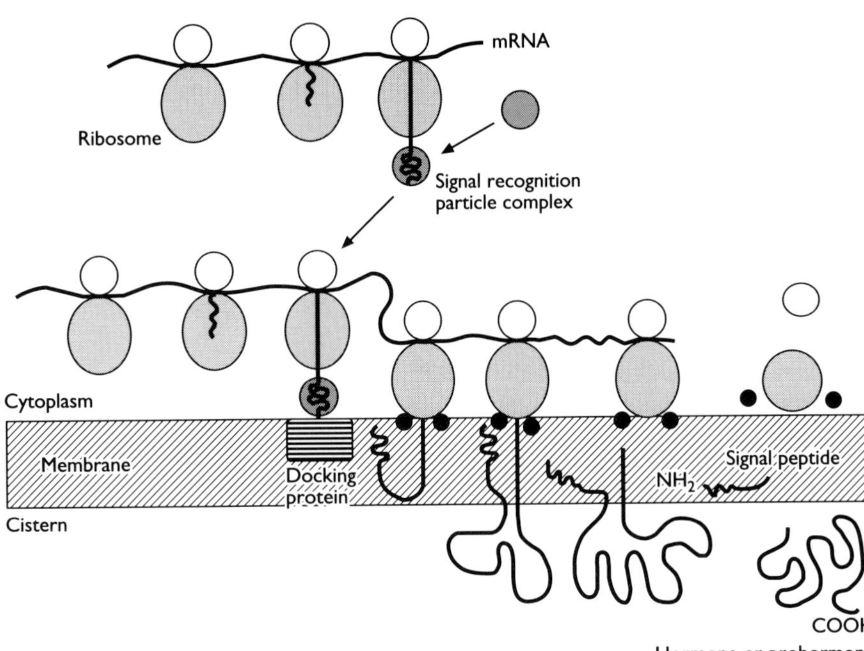

Fig. 1.3 Translation of prehormone or preprohormone mRNA is initiated on free ribosomes. Once the N-terminal sequence of newly synthesized prehormone or preprohormone emerges from the translation complex it is recognized by a signal recognition particle complex composed of protein subunits and 7S RNA molecules. Translation is transiently arrested at this point. The bound signal recognition complex then recognizes a docking protein in the endoplasmic reticulum, thereby resulting in the attachment of the translation complex to the membrane. The peptide synthesis then resumes. The hydrophobic NH_2-terminal signal sequence anchors the protein to the endoplasmic membrane while the extending polypeptide chain extrudes into the cistern of the endoplasmic reticulum. Peptidase then cleaves this signal peptide and the resultant pro- or mature hormone is released into the cistern. Thereafter, the hormone is transferred to the Golgi apparatus for sorting and packaging into vesicles for secretion.

the ORF. Simultaneous peptide syntheses occur on a single mature mRNA and polyribosome complexes are formed (Fig. 1.3).

Peptide hormones are secretory proteins that may be transported to their sites of action by the circulation (endocrine) and/or may remain in their microenvironment (paracrine/autocrine). All secretory proteins are probably synthesized as precursors with sequences called signal peptides at their NH_2 termini (Fig. 1.1). These signal peptides are responsible for the translocation of newly synthesized polypeptides from the cytoplasm into the endoplasmic reticulum (Fig. 1.3). In the cytoplasm there are signal recognition particle complexes each composed of six different proteins and a 7S RNA. This complex binds to the polyribosomes engaged in translation once the signal peptide emerges from the large subunit of the ribosomes (Fig. 1.3). The translational process is temporarily arrested until the signal recognition particle complex binds to a high-affinity binding protein.

Having found a high-affinity binding (docking) protein on the endoplasmic reticulum, protein synthesis resumes. The protein synthesized is then transferred across the membrane of the endoplasmic reticulum. Upon completion of the synthesis, the NH_2-terminal signal sequences are cleaved from the polypeptide by a specific peptidase located on the cisternal surface of the membrane and the prohormone or hormone is freed (Fig. 1.3). The conversion of the prohormone to the mature product takes place in the Golgi apparatus. Subsequently, post-translational processing such as proteolysis and glycosylation results in the mature hormone (Figs 1.1 & 1.3).

Gene regulation

Apart from expression of 'housekeeping' genes, necessary for maintaining general cellular activity, individual gene expression is highly selective and specific, to allow the intricate levels of cellular specialization. Although many have yet to be explored, some basic regulatory mechanisms are outlined in this section. A point of note is that a chromosome forms coils that stack on each other, and thus apparently distant nucleotide segments can be in physical proximity to each other. This may be one of the factors allowing the interactions of distant gene elements. The complexity of the involvement of such physical structure in functional regulation is illustrated by the advance of knowledge of the role of histone–nucleosome–chromosome interaction in transcriptional controls [2].

DORMANT AND ACTIVE GENES

Selective expressions of individual genes, rather than the presence of different genomes in specialized cells, underlie the highly differentiated cellular functions. Just how some genes are maintained active while others stay dormant in various cells is partly related to non-chromosomal structural components of the nucleus. The basic nucleosome structure of the chromatin is maintained during transcription, but there are differences between active genes and inactive chromatin. Active genes are characterized by structural changes, which include undermethylation and looser packing of the nucleosomal DNA. In the case of the heat-shock protein-encoding genes of *Drosophila*, for example, the nucleosomal repeat becomes much less precise following induction and the genes that are being transcribed, or that have the potential to be transcribed, in a particular cell are especially sensitive to attack by DNase I. There is evidence that these DNase I superhypersensitive sequences are involved in regulating gene expression.

TRANSCRIPTIONAL REGULATION

As knowledge of transcriptional regulation has rapidly evolved, part of the terminology used to describe the process has become quite heterogeneous. The glossary provided in this chapter is based on the generally accepted meanings.

It is now known that gene expression is regulated primarily at the transcriptional level. Gene transcription is controlled by sequences located mainly in the 5′-flanking region of the transcriptional unit. These sequences which include promoters, regulatory sequences known as upstream promoter elements (UPEs), regulatory elements and enhancers, are short polynucleotide chains (Figs 1.2 & 1.4).

One common promoter sequence (the TATA or Goldberg–Hogness box), typically found between 25 and 30 nucleotides upstream from the transcription initiation codon, is in fact a binding site for transcriptional factors which form a transcription initiation complex with RNA polymerase II. Another common consensus sequence, the so-called CAT box (a UPE), further upstream from the TATA box also plays a role in initiating transcription. Some genes have neither the TATA nor the CAT boxes, but have a GC-rich sequence – GGGGCGGGGC (another UPE) – known as the Spl box, which is required for transcription. While these basic promoter and UPEs exert the primary control over the expression of many genes, there are additional factors (regulatory elements, enhancers) which regulate transcription through interaction with them [3].

By convention, regulatory sequences residing in the same genomic sequence are known as *cis*-acting elements. *Trans*-acting factors are generally proteins, but may be small nuclear RNA (snRNA). Through interaction with the *cis*-elements they can enhance or repress the binding of RNA polymerase II to regions flanking the TATA box and hence regulate the transcription rate.

Certain groups of genes have common *cis*-acting elements and consequently are thought to be regulated by identical or closely related transcriptional factors. For instance, genes regulated by thyroid hormone (TH) contain the TH-responsive element (TRE) which binds the TH ligand–receptor complex. The formation of the ligand–receptor complex presumably induces conformational changes of the receptor that facilitate the binding of such a complex to the consensus *cis*-acting element. The human growth hormone (hGH) gene (Fig. 1.4) nicely displays such transcriptional organization. It is

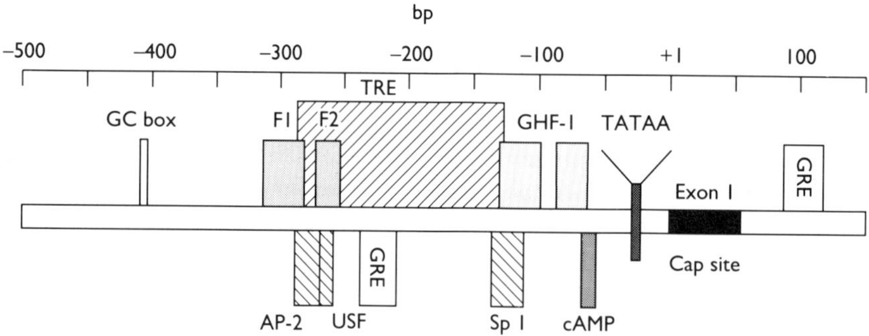

Fig. 1.4 5′ upstream region of the human growth hormone (hGH) gene. The first nucleotide of the start site is designated +1 by convention, while the 5′ nucleotides are counted backwards from −1. Two DNA sequences recognized by glucocorticoid–receptor complex (glucocorticoid response element, GRE) are present, one within the 5′-flanking region and the second within the first intron of the hGH gene (+86 to +115 bp), while the thyroid hormone response element (TRE) is located between −290 and −129 bp. cAMP is the second messenger involved in GH-releasing hormone-induced hGH transcription and the cAMP response element (CRE) has been mapped to lie between the TATAA box and position −100. The tissue-specific expression of hGH is mediated by a protein called pituitary-specific transcription factor (Pit-1) (also called growth hormone factor 1 (GHF-1)) which binds the 5′-flanking DNA at two sites (site I designated −96 to −70 and site II −134 to −106) and promotes hGH gene transcription. Three non-tissue-specific transcriptional factors bind to the sites AP-2, USF and Sp1.

composed of: a TATA box-containing promoter; UPEs (GC-rich region, Spl box); regulatory elements inducing expression in response to glucocorticoid (glucocorticoid regulatory element, GRE), thyroid hormone (TH regulatory element, TRE), cyclic adenosine monophosphate (cAMP regulatory element, CRE), etc.; and other more distant enhancers [4,5].

A particularly intriguing aspect of the regulation of gene expression has been the mechanisms that govern tissue specificity and developmental regulation. In this regard, detailed studies of the regulation of well-characterized genes expressed only in specific cell types have been most informative. For example the transcription factor Pit-1 or GH factor 1 (GHF-1), a *trans*-acting factor present and synthesized only in anterior pituitary cells, activates hGH production by binding to the Pit-1/GHF-1 *cis*-acting element in the upstream part of the hGH promoter [6–8] (Fig. 1.4).

This kind of tissue-specific expression of *trans*-acting factors is a key mechanism involved in tissue-specific gene transcription. However, it is immediately obvious that just how the transcriptional factors and gene products themselves are 'tissue-specifically' expressed is not yet known. Although many of the details of the tissue-specific gene expression remain to be elucidated, it can generally be assumed that it is the expression of the *trans*-acting factors that is tissue-specific. In addition, as nicely shown in limb-pattern formation, the developmental events are not only tissue-specific but also time-dependent ([9] for review). In this case it is thought that the regulation of certain *trans*-acting factors is time-dependently organized and turned on and off at the appropriate time or stage of development [9].

Besides these protein–DNA interactions it is now realized that protein–protein interactions between various transcriptional factors also dramatically affect their functions. Thus while the transcriptional factor *fos–jun* (a heterodimer of two proto-oncogenes *fos* and *jun*) binds the activator protein 1 (AP-1) site with high affinity and induces phorbol-ester-dependent or growth-dependent genes, the *jun–jun* homodimer exhibits a 30-fold lower affinity [10]. Furthermore, *de novo* protein synthesis is often not required in initiation of transcription, suggesting that post-translational modifications of these factors are involved [11].

Enhancers are other transcriptional control elements. They act by increasing the activity of a promoter, although they lack promoter activity themselves and are, therefore, referred to as enhancers. One of the characteristic features of enhancer elements is that they are often located at great distances from the transcription start site, yet they can significantly influence the level of gene expression. These elements can be located upstream, downstream or even within a transcription unit. They can also function in either orientation relative to the start site of transcription.

To recapitulate, four distinct transcriptional control elements are typically present in a eukaryotic gene:

1 the promoter itself;

2 UPEs located close to it, which are required for efficient transcription;

3 regulatory elements adjacent to the promoter that are interdigitated with the UPEs responsible for activating the gene in particular tissues or in response to particular stimuli;

4 enhancer elements that regulate transcriptional activity.

Post-transcriptional regulation and protein synthesis

Although the primary control of gene expression lies at the level of transcription, changes in the rate of synthesis of a particular protein may occur without any changes in the transcription rate of the corresponding gene. In principle, such post-transcriptional regulation can operate at any of the many stages between gene transcription and the translation of the mRNA.

RNA SPLICING

Pre-mRNA transcribed in several tissues may be properly spliced in one tissue and remain unspliced in another tissue [12,13]. Unspliced mRNA is then either degraded within the nucleus or, if transported to the cytoplasm, is unable to produce a functional protein due to the interruption of the protein-coding sequences [13].

ALTERNATIVE SPLICING

Alternative splicing refers to a process whereby the various exons of the pre-mRNA from a single gene are shuffled to yield different functional mRNAs, which are translatable into closely related proteins or even totally different proteins. Numerous examples have been described [14]. The insulin-like growth factor I (IGF-I) gene provides a good example. This gene spans more than 55 Kb of genomic DNA and consists of six exons, five introns and at least two promoters. It encodes the 70 amino acids of a functionally mature IGF-I. However, multiple transcripts of IGF-I mRNAs are present in various fetal and adult tissues and at different developmental stages. This heterogeneity of mRNA transcripts is due to a combination of alternative splicing and the uses of multiple initiation and polyadenylation sites [15–17]. The production of the IGF-IE$_A$ and IGF-IE$_B$ mRNAs, which differ in their E-peptide-coding regions and 3′ untranslated regions, involves exclusive splicing of exon 6 to exon 4 (IGF-IE$_A$) and exon 5 to exon 4 (IGF-IE$_B$) and the respective polyadenylation sites on exons 6 and 5. The signal peptides are cleaved off from prepro-IGF-IE$_A$ and prepro-IGF-IE$_B$, resulting in two different precursors (pro-IGF-IE$_A$ and pro-IGF-IE$_B$) but the same mature IGF- I after cleavage of the E peptide. The E$_A$ and E$_B$ splicing variants of IGF-I mRNAs are differentially regulated by GH and may, therefore, represent the control of the endocrine versus autocrine or paracrine functions of IGF-I [18].

Alternative splicing may also lead to production of different mature proteins in different tissues from a single gene. This is best illustrated in the case of the calcitonin and calcitonin-gene-related peptide (CGRP) gene [19,20]. The pre-mRNA is spliced into two different mature mRNAs with either of the two exons encoding calcitonin (32 amino acids) or CGRP (36 amino acids). Post-translational proteolytic cleavage yields these two structurally unrelated mature proteins. The detailed studies exploring why calcitonin is produced in the thyroid C cells and CGRP in specific neural cells provide evidence that tissue-specific splicing factors are responsible [21].

Yet another example is the switch from the α, β and γ isoforms of cAMP-response element modulator (CREM) to the τ isoform (CREM-τ) by alternative splicing during spermatogenesis [10,22]. The α and β isoforms act as antagonists of the cAMP transcriptional response whereas the τ isoform functions as a transcriptional activator. Though the physiological significance of such a switch has not been fully elucidated, this splicing-dependent reversal in CREM function is a good example of developmental modulation of gene expression. It is thus clear that alternative splicing is a mechanism widely adopted in biological processes as a significant supplement to the regulation of transcription.

REGULATION OF RNA METABOLISM

Changing mRNA stability offers another way of regulating the amount of protein translated from an accumulated population of mRNA [23,24]. For example, prolactin treatment of cultured mammary gland cells increases the half-life of the milk protein casein mRNA from 1 h to over 40 h [25]. The regulation of RNA stability has been demonstrated to involve specific nucleotide sequences within the RNA which, again like DNA sequences involved in transcriptional regulation, are able to interact with other factors [23,26,27]. These sequences can reside in either the 3′ untranslated region (3′-UTR), the 5′-UTR or even in the coding region of the RNA. Interestingly, some of these regulation processes require partial translation of the RNA sequence into protein.

Two observations regarding RNA stability regulation suggest that it constitutes a significant supplement to transcriptional control of a gene where rapid changes in the synthesis of a protein are essential. First, alterations of mRNA stability are very often accompanied by concomitant alterations in the transcription rate of the same genes. Indeed, prolactin treatment of mammary gland cells not only stabilizes casein mRNA but also increases casein gene transcription two- to fourfold [25]. Secondly, RNA stability regulation is often found in genes encoding protein with rapid alteration of rate of synthesis.

REGULATION OF TRANSLATION

The final step in the expression of a gene is the translation of its mRNA into the protein. The regulation of translation such that a particular mRNA is translated into a protein in one situation and not in another occurs in some selected cases. The most important of such cases is fertilization.

In the unfertilized egg, protein synthesis is very slow, but a tremendous increase in the rate of protein synthesis occurs after fertilization [28]. This increase does not involve production of new mRNAs, but is mediated by pre-existing RNAs present in the unfertilized egg which are translated only following fertilization. The RNA populations present before and after fertilization are identical, indicating that translational control processes are operating [28]. Many cases of translational control occur in situations where very rapid responses are required and, like other cases of post-transcriptional regulation, translational control can supplement the regulation of transcription to meet the requirements of particular specialized cases.

POST-TRANSLATIONAL MODIFICATION

Post-translational modifications such as proteolysis, glycosylation and phosphorylation of a protein can profoundly influence its function. Some of these modifications are dictated by the information stored within the specific genetic sequences. Pro-opiomelanocortin (POMC), a precursor of at least seven biologically active peptides, is differentially cleaved by cell-specific proteases to yield different combinations of peptides.

Thus, certain *N*- or *O*-linked glycosylation and phosphorylation sites are determined by specific consensus amino acid sequences. They can be altered resulting in an impairment of its activity. For example, there is evidence that genetic defects (mutations) involving the adenosine triphosphate (ATP)-binding site of the tyrosine kinase domain of the insulin receptor can cause insulin-resistant diabetes mellitus [29].

COMMON METHODS IN MOLECULAR BIOLOGY

The applications of molecular biology to clinical endocrinology extend along several main avenues. First, there are numerous diagnostic tools for endocrine disorders with underlying genetic defects. For instance, the ability to establish early prenatal diagnosis of 21-hydroxylase deficiency has added a new dimension to the therapeutic approach of this form of congenital adrenal hyperplasia [30]. In the area of ambiguous genitalia the advances in the genetics of androgen receptor resistance have made possible more definitive aetiological diagnoses, and hence better genetic counselling for the families involved [31].

A second application is elucidating the pathogenetic basis of disorders of previously unknown aetiology. Thus, a number of point mutations in the sequences encoding different functional domains of insulin receptors have recently been shown to be responsible for hereditary and familial insulin resistance of varying clinical severity [29,32]. This has also led to speculation that milder phenotypic manifestations of similar defects may be responsible for some cases of type II diabetes mellitus.

Another exciting application of molecular biological techniques is illustrated by the study of the aetiology of idiopathic Addison disease [33]. The autoantibodies present in the sera of these patients were used to identify the immunoreactive clones in a human fetal adrenal cDNA expression library (see below). Subsequent sequence analysis revealed that the steroid 17α-hydroxylase encoded by the cytochrome $P450_{c17}$ gene may be the autoantigen involved in the pathogenesis [33]. In addition, Kallman syndrome, a well-known clinical entity associated with hypogonadotrophic hypogonadism, has recently been shown to be related to the potential defect of adhesion molecules affecting the migration of olfactory and gonadotrophin-releasing hormone (GnRH)-synthesizing neurons through identifying the candidate gene responsible for this syndrome [34]. This 'reverse genetics' approach has also been successfully applied in other diseases such as cystic fibrosis with little-known underlying biochemical defects [35]. Since most work in endocrinology has been based on the understanding of the proteins and molecules involved such an approach is certainly rather atypical, but fascinating all the same.

The practical application of recombinant DNA technology has resulted in the production of quantities of polypeptide hormones and growth factors sufficient for therapeutic use. While insulin and human growth hormone (hGH) are the two most outstanding examples, recombinant IGF-I has already been used in treating children with GH resistance [36]. More applications in this direction will certainly emerge.

Last but not least, the constant flux of knowledge regarding cellular and molecular mechanisms of hormonal actions will surely keep opening new concepts in pathogeneses and therapeutic approaches. For instance, the observation of the oncogenic property of mutated G protein subunit [37] has led to the suggestion that the multiple autonomous endocrine hyperfunctions in McCune–Albright syndrome may be due to dysregulated G protein function. Indeed a mutant G protein α-subunit ($G_s\alpha$) causing constitutively active cAMP second-messenger system has been identified in these patients [38,39]. Thus full understanding of such underlying molecular mechanisms may one day lead to intervention tackling the second-messenger system in these patients.

Several commonly used methods in molecular biology will be discussed in the following sections. As with all laboratory methods, the key to applying them successfully depends as much on the technical expertise as on the choice of methods to answer a specific question. Accordingly, unless a new therapeutic alternative was available, establishing the clinical diagnosis of insulin resistance with radioimmunoassay can be as good as having identified the specific molecular defect of the insulin receptor. Nevertheless more of these sophisticated molecular biology methods will find their place in clinical management.

DNA and recombinant DNA techniques

The nucleotide base pairing system gives DNA its exquisite stability and constant reproducibility. Regular phosphodiester bonds between sugar groups (deoxyribose) of nucleotides and phosphate groups of adjacent nucleotides form the backbone of the DNA, which is orientated on the outside of the DNA helix. On the other hand, the purine (adenine (A) or guanine (G)) and pyrimidine (cytosine (C) or thymidine (T)) bases face the inside. With exceptions, such as during transcription or initiation of replication, these nucleotides pair with complementary nucleotides on opposing DNA chains through hydrogen bonds (A=T and G=C), forming very stable double DNA helices. Such physicochemical arrangements allow any combination and length of nucleotide sequences without sacrificing DNA stability. Formation of secondary and tertiary coiling in association with nucleoproteins such as histones further ensures the compactness of DNA molecules, thus enabling the storage of enormous quantities of DNA within the cell nucleus.

However, the technical capability of elucidating the overwhelming amount of information stored within the eukaryotic genome, as well as the elegant mechanism governing genetic regulations, were limited in the early days. Several advances in the 1970s made possible the precise and specific cutting (restriction endonucleases), pasting (ligase) and copying (polymerase) of DNA or RNA (reverse transcriptase or RNA-dependent DNA polymerase) and helped overcome the hurdle. These are the fundamentals of recombinant DNA technologies, which are being constantly refined and perfected and form an

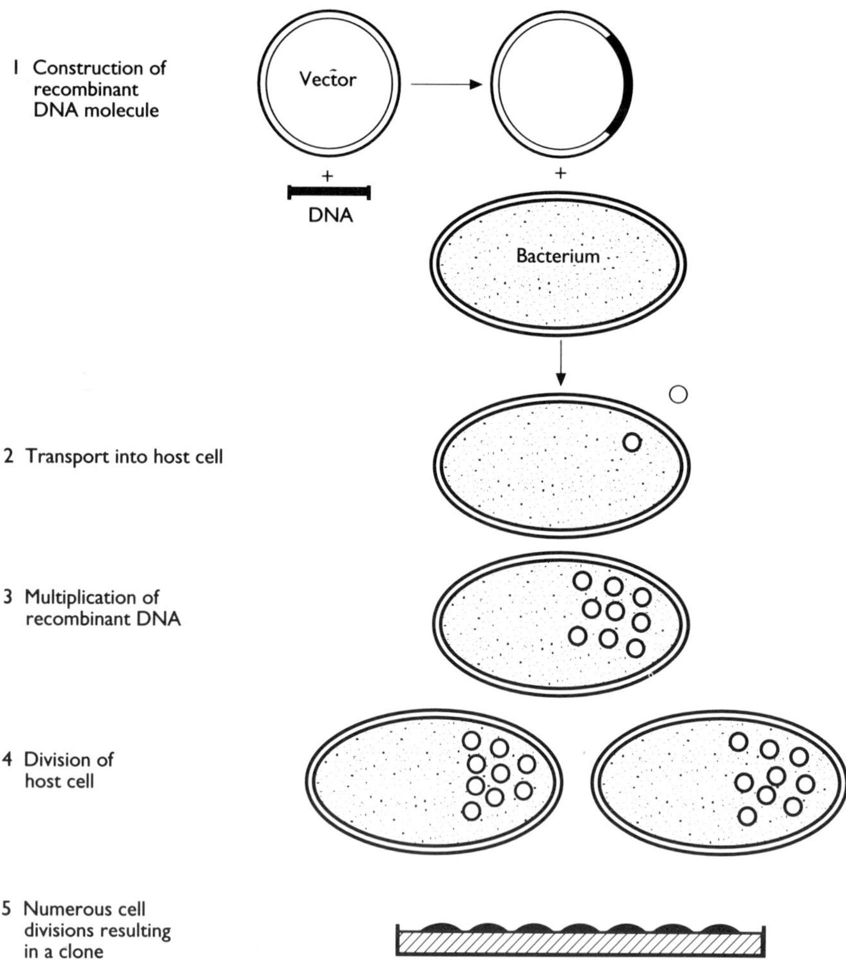

Fig. 1.5 Basic steps in gene cloning. (1) A fragment of DNA containing the gene to be cloned is inserted into a circular DNA molecule called a vector, to produce a recombinant DNA molecule. (2) The vector acts as a vehicle to transport the gene into a host cell, usually a bacterium, although other types of living cell can be used. (3) Within the host cell the vector multiplies, producing numerous identical copies. (4) When the host cell divides, copies of the recombinant DNA are distributed to the daughter cells where further multiplications take place. (5) If plated onto a solid surface such as an agar plate, a colony or clone of cells carrying these DNA copies is produced after a sufficient number of cell divisions.

inseparable component in most molecular biology studies and applications [40].

Gene cloning

While the basic cutting, pasting and copying functions of recombinant DNA technologies make studying genes of suitable sizes possible in principle, the generation of quantities sufficient for practical analyses is equally crucial. To achieve this, DNA sequences of interest are often incorporated into suitable DNA vectors capable of transporting them into host cells for amplification by replication. This is the essence of gene cloning. Lately, the introduction of automated polymerase chain reaction technology has opened up new alternatives to classical gene cloning (see below).

The central component of a gene-cloning experiment is the vector within which the gene to be cloned is inserted. This will then be transported into the host cell where replication of the vehicle, together with the inserted gene, takes place (Fig. 1.5). There are two naturally occurring types of DNA molecule suitable for such functions, plasmids and chromosomes of bacteriophages. Plasmids are small circular extrachromosomal DNA molecules found in bacteria (often in multiple copies) and some other organisms. They are capable of autonomous self-replication in the host cells, thus increasing the final yield. Viral chromosomes, particularly those infecting bacteria (bacteriophage or phage – mainly M13 and λ type), can carry on with replications utilizing the host mechanisms after being injected into the bacteria. Over the years these basic cloning vectors have undergone modification to enhance efficiency for general applications, and also to cater for specific needs. In addition there are special cloning procedures utilizing yeast chromosome as a vector, resulting in yeast artificial chromosomes (YAC), which can handle foreign DNA pieces of megabase size. This technique was used in identifying the candidate gene for Kallman syndrome [34], and has become an indispensable technique in human genomic library projects.

The insertion of any DNA into a cloning vector is

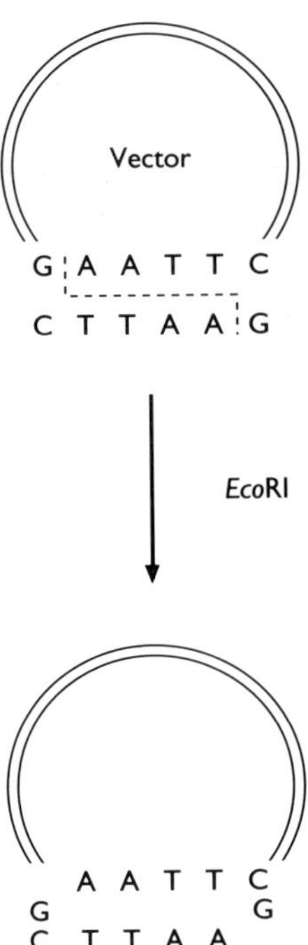

Fig. 1.6 Restriction enzymes in cloning DNA. Most such enzymes recognize four to six bases of DNA which form the same palindromic sequence when read in either direction. The restriction site of *Eco*RI (named after *Escherichia coli* from which it is isolated) is shown. *Eco*RI recognizes and cuts the DNA sequence: 5′ . . . GAATTC . . . 3′; 3′ . . . CTTAAG . . . 5′.

generally accomplished with restriction endonucleases and DNA ligases. Restriction endonucleases are bacterial enzymes which cleave DNA at highly specific sequences of nucleotides, usually 4–6 bp long. They are known as restriction enzymes because they protect the host bacteria against infection and transformation by alien DNA. Many of these enzymes make symmetrical but staggered cuts in the DNA, resulting in DNA fragments with short overhanging single-stranded regions at the cut end (Fig. 1.6). Based on the highly specific base pairing between individual nucleotides, these single-stranded regions will hybridize only to single-stranded ends with complementary nucleotide sequences. These permit the planned assembly of DNA fragments using DNA ligases, which catalyse the formation of a phosphodiester bond between a 5′-phosphate of one nucleotide and the 3′-hydroxyl group of a neighbouring nucleotide.

CLONING OF COMPLEMENTARY DNA

The nucleotide sequence of a mature mRNA contains the essential information governing the primary structure of its encoding protein but it lacks the complexity of the genomic sequence. It is therefore often more direct to begin by working out the mRNA genetic codes of proteins of interest before embarking on establishing the far more complex genomic sequence of the protein. Furthermore, while most genes are represented by single copies in individual cells, mRNAs are often present in high abundance in cells actively synthesizing the proteins. This offers the advantage of having more specific material to work on when tissues expressing high mRNA levels of these proteins are chosen, and hence increases the success rate of getting relevant information.

As most eukaryotic mRNAs have poly-A tails at their 3′ ends (Figs 1.1 & 1.2), it is possible to make DNA copies complementary (cDNA) to these polyadenylated (poly-A) mRNAs with high efficiency and fidelity using poly-dT as primers (which bind to the poly-A sequences) and an RNA-dependent DNA polymerase (reverse transcriptase) to copy. This is a very practical way of generating cDNA copies of mRNA isolated from any specific source without prior knowledge of their sequences (Fig. 1.7).

To facilitate the cloning of the specific cDNA of interest, double-stranded cDNA molecules are generated using DNA polymerase and inserted into vectors for amplification in host bacteria. Bacteria carrying these cDNA inserts will form independent colonies (clones) when grown in permissive media. A carefully constructed set of representative cDNA clones constitutes what is termed a cDNA library. Traditionally a cDNA library is constructed from mRNA extracted from specific tissue and hence is often named after its source tissue; for example liver cDNA library and placental cDNA library. However, it is now possible to make cDNA libraries from single cells using the polymerase chain reaction technique.

CLONING OF GENOMIC DNA

A genomic library, on the other hand, is a set of recombinant clones which contain all of the genomic DNA present in an individual organism. Unlike cloning cDNA it is essential to reduce the genomic DNA molecules to sizes suitable for cloning them into vectors. This is achieved by cutting them in a controlled manner with restriction endonucleases. The number of genomic DNA fragments thereby generated is inversely proportional to the average size of the fragments.

It is immediately obvious that the capacity of the vector used in such cloning procedures is crucial, given the huge amount of genomic DNA present. Thus, λ-bacteriophage-based vectors are used to carry DNA fragments too large to be handled by plasmids or other bacteriophages, such as M13 vectors. For instance, an insertion vector such as λgt10 can carry up to 8 kb of new DNA, while the λEMBL replacement vectors can manage up to 23 kb fragments. This compares with a maximum insert size of 5 kb for most plasmids and less than 3 kb for M13 vectors. On the other hand, cosmids (basically hybrids between λ-phage

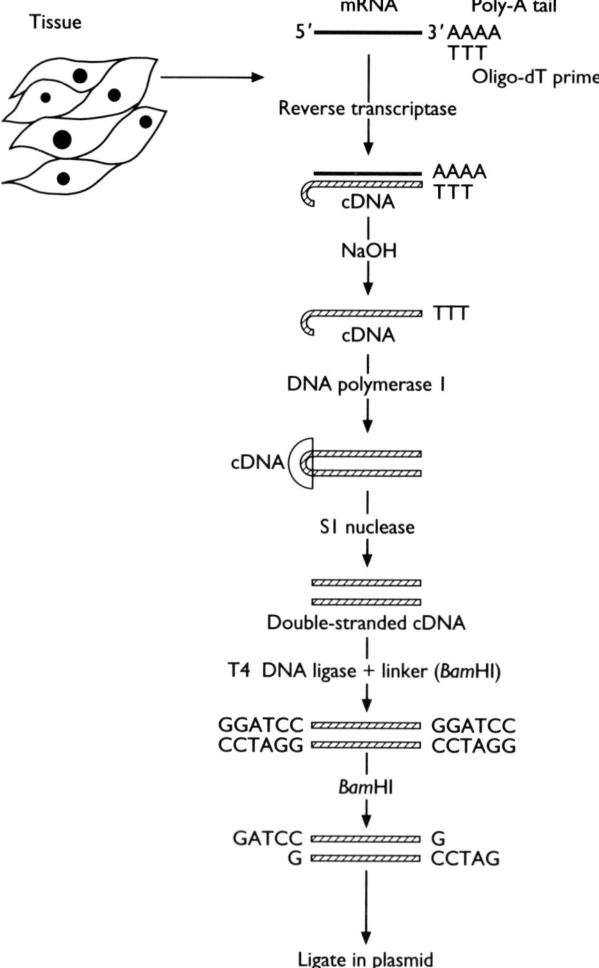

Fig. 1.7 The synthesis of double-stranded cDNA from mRNA. A short oligo-dT chain (typically 16–20 bp) is hybridized to the poly-A tail of an mRNA strand and serves as a primer for the reverse transcriptase. This uses the mRNA as a template for the synthesis of a complementary DNA (cDNA) strand. The resulting cDNA ends in a hairpin loop. Once the mRNA strand is degraded with NaOH, the hairpin loop becomes a primer for DNA polymerase I, which completes the synthesis of a paired DNA strand. The loop is then cleaved by S1 nuclease to produce a double-stranded cDNA molecule. Linkers (synthetic duplex oligonucleotides corresponding to restriction endonuclease (e.g. *Bam*HI) recognition sequences) are added to the ends of the double-stranded cDNA. Thereafter, the linkers are cleaved using *Bam*HI yielding sticky ends. When the same restriction enzyme is used to cut open the plasmid, the ends on the cDNA and the plasmid become complementary, allowing the cDNA to be ligated into the plasmid at the cut site.

DNA which carry the λ *cos* sites and bacterial plasmids) can be used to clone DNA fragments of up to 40 kb in some cases. Recently, the use of YAC has extended the range of the possible insert sizes up to 1000 kb or more.

The principles of genomic DNA cloning are analogous to the cDNA cloning described above (Fig. 1.5). The DNA fragments to be cloned are ligated to pieces of phage DNA and mixed with the bacteriophage proteins, thus 'packing' the DNA into viable phage particles. These λ-phages are then used to infect an *Escherichia coli* (*E. coli*) culture, which will lead to cell lysis as part of the phage infection cycle. Thus, if infected cells are spread on to a solid agar medium immediately after transfection with phage DNA, cell lysis can be visualized as plaques on a lawn of bacteria. Thereafter, the phage DNA containing the genomic DNA of interest can be identified by appropriate methods. These genomic DNA libraries can be retained for many years and propagated so that copies can be sent from research group to research group. Their development, by providing depositories of cloned material, has greatly aided the progress of molecular genetics. In addition, a variety of genomic DNA libraries are commercially available.

METHODS FOR SELECTING CLONES OF INTEREST

Having generated the cDNA or genomic DNA libraries, the next task is to identify which clones contain the information actively sought. The methods employed are dictated largely by the knowledge pertaining to the gene/mRNA/protein under study. For instance, if the partial amino acid sequence of a protein is known, a mixture of short radiolabelled synthetic oligonucleotides complementary to all possible nucleotide sequences inferred from the amino acid sequence could be used as probes for detection by nucleic acid hybridization. Alternatively, a single longer synthetic polynucleotide probe corresponding to the 'best-guess' sequence based on a longer stretch of known amino acid sequence can be used.

For screening cDNA libraries another common method used is to clone the cDNAs into specially designed vectors (cDNA expression vectors) which promote the production of the encoded proteins in the host bacteria and allow immunological detection of the clones. This approach is possible only when an antibody against the protein is available, usually when the protein has been studied long before interest is focused on the genetic information.

CHROMOSOME WALKING

Often the analysis of hundreds of kilobases of contiguous information from a eukaryotic genome is necessary. Although packaging such large stretches of DNA into any single cloning vector (except for the YAC) is often impossible, it is possible sequentially to isolate recombinant plasmids or cosmids which contain overlapping information from the genome. This technique, known as 'chromosome walking', relies on isolating a small segment of DNA from one end of the first recombinant and using this piece of DNA as a probe to rescreen the genomic library. Repeating such screening will eventually yield clones with overlapping sequences and enable the reconstruction of the full sequence of interest.

DNA analyses

The elucidation of information stored in chromosomes has historically been revealed by histological examination of the chromosome structures after appropriate manipulations such as G banding. Structural defects such as gross deletion, formation of ring structure (very often with partial deletion) and translocation of chromosomal segments can often be revealed. While these techniques continue to be a very important part of cytogenetic studies, the integration of some molecular biology techniques (for example *in situ* hybridization of chromosomes with nucleic acid probes) into their repertoire has expanded the capability of identifying finer defects.

Work in traditional molecular biology has been focused on the fundamental components of chromosomes, and has used a totally different range of techniques, which aim at looking at smaller pieces of chromosomal DNA, identifying the individual nucleotides constituting the macromolecules and studying them as functional units. To endocrinologists more familiar with protein analytical work this is in principle similar to studying proteins using tryptic digestion mapping (restriction endonuclease digestion), amino acid sequencing (DNA sequencing), immunological detection of epitopes (nucleic acid probe hybridization) and even functional assays (assessing the rate of RNA/protein end-product productions). In fact a technique such as high-performance liquid chromatography (HPLC), frequently used in protein analysis, has been adapted for DNA sequencing.

SOUTHERN BLOT ANALYSIS

Southern blotting (Fig. 1.8) is the cornerstone of analysing DNA. It combines the high resolution power of gel electrophoresis (which has been further expanded by the refinement of methods such as pulse-field electrophoresis for large genomic DNA fragments) with the fidelity of hybridization between complementary nucleotide sequences. It is possible to detect even a single copy of a specific gene. The method is generally performed by hybridizing a radiolabelled DNA fragment (probe) to restriction-digested DNA (genomic or otherwise) which has been fractionated in an agarose gel and transferred onto a filter membrane. The DNA band patterns on the autoradiogram will reflect the presence or absence of genes, size variation due to partial gene deletion or, when combined with specific restriction enzyme digestion, size variation due to restriction fragment length polymorphisms (see below). Using specific oligonucleotide probes, specific point mutations may be revealed.

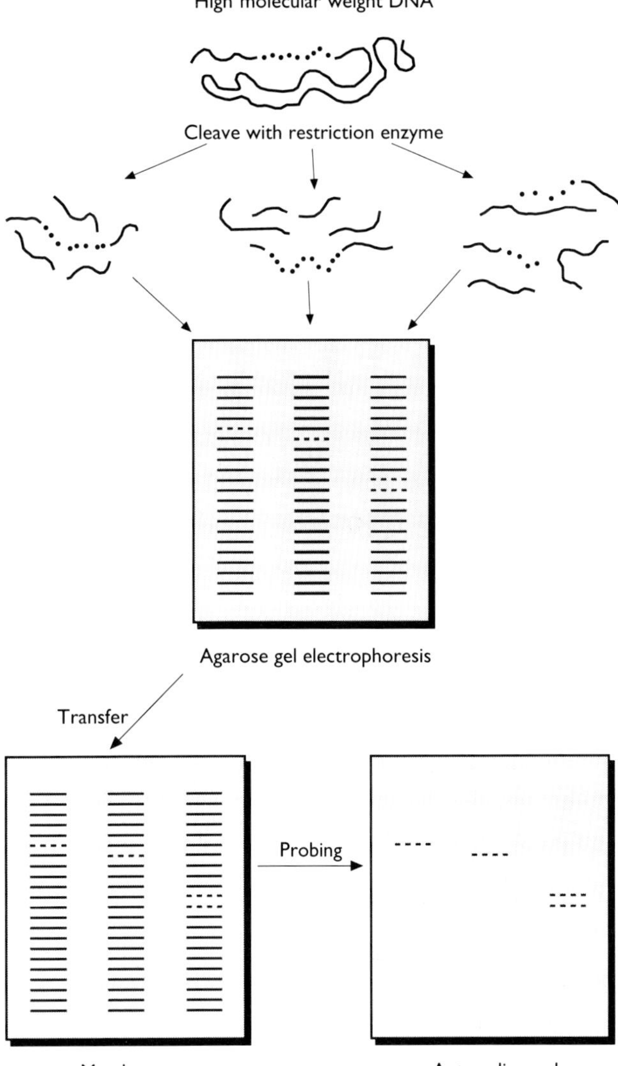

Fig. 1.8 Southern blotting. Eukaryotic high molecular weight DNA is cleaved with one or several restriction enzymes. The cleaved DNA fragments are fractionated by gel electrophoresis according to size. A piece of nitrocellulose/nylon membrane is then laid on the gel, and a flow of buffer is sent through the gel towards the membrane. This drags the DNA fragments out of the gel and binds them to the membrane. A replica of the DNA fragments in the gel is thus created on the membrane, which can be hybridized to a suitable labelled probe. Specific DNA fragments hybridizing to the probe will be identified by autoradiography.

An example of a Southern blot analysis of a kindred with growth hormone deficiency using a probe corresponding to the growth hormone (hGH-1) gene is shown in Fig. 1.9. Here both parents were heterozygous for a 6.7 kb hGH-1 gene deletion while the affected child was

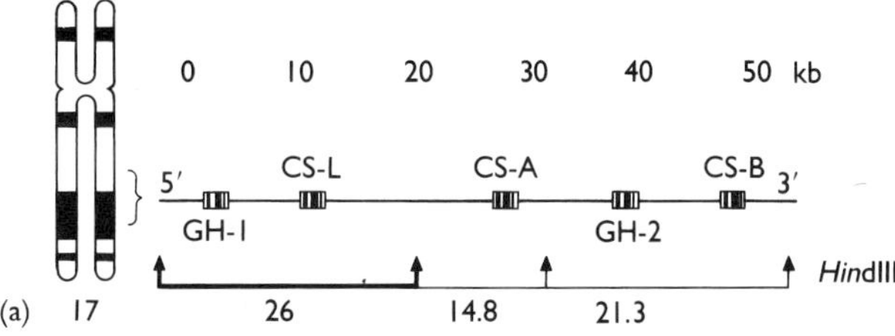

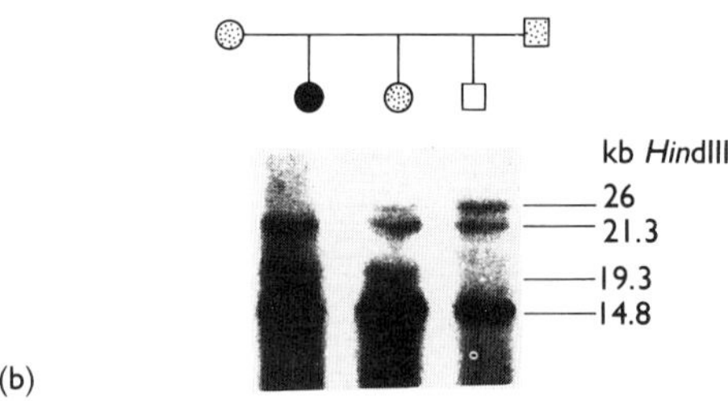

Fig. 1.9 Human growth hormone (hGH) gene deletion of 6.7 kb. (a) The hGH gene locus is on the long arm of chromosome 17, where there is a cluster of five highly sequence conserved genes (GH-1, pituitary GH; CS-L, chorionic somatomammotropin-L, pseudogene; CS-A and CS-B, chorionic somatomammotropin-A and -B; GH-2, placental GH). *Hin*dIII digest of genomic DNA hybridized with the hGH cDNA probe yields three fragments of 26, 21.3 and 14.8 kb respectively. (b) Autoradiograph of a Southern blot of *Hin*dIII digested genomic DNA from three children, hybridized with an α^{32} P-labelled full-length hGH cDNA probe. The 26 kb fragment contains the hGH-1 and the hCS-L genes. In the girl homozygous for the hGH-1 gene deletion the 26 kb fragment is missing. The additional 19.3 kb fragment indicates a 6.7 kb gene deletion of DNA. The combined pattern allows the diagnosis of heterozygotes for the gene deletion. ●, Homozygous affected girl; ◎, girl heterozygous for the hGH-1 gene deletion; □, the boy without any hGH-1 gene deletion.

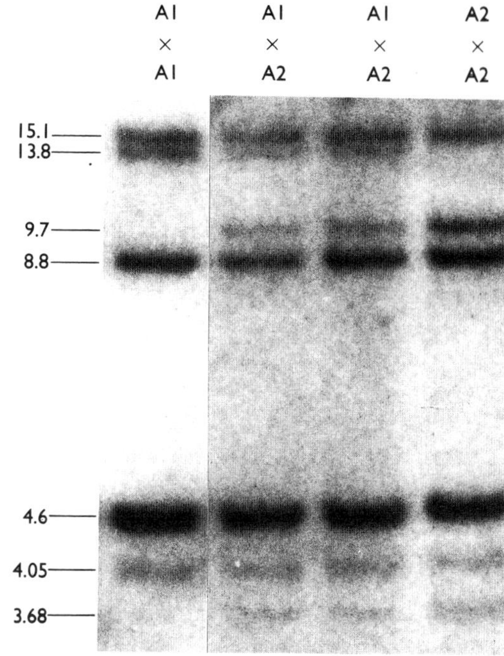

Fig. 1.10 *Bgl*I RFLP for the human erb-Aβ locus. Autoradiograph of Southern-blotted DNA from four individuals after restriction endonuclease digestion with *Bgl*I and hybridization with an erb-Aβ cDNA probe. Fragment sizes in kilobases are indicated on the left. This *Bgl*I digestion identifies a two-allele polymorphism with bands either at 13.8 kb (A1) or 9.7 kb/3.68 kb (A2) and invariant bands at 15.1, 8.8, 4.6 and 4.05 kb.

homozygous for the hGH gene deletion. This is an example of Mendelian autosomal recessive inheritance in which the gene of both chromosomes must be abnormal or absent for the disease to be manifest clinically.

RESTRICTION FRAGMENT LENGTH POLYMORPHISM

The majority of point mutations (change of a single base) occur in the non-coding region of DNA, and do not change the phenotype. They are called silent mutations and constitute part of natural DNA polymorphism. Such mutations may, however, delete or create new restriction enzyme recognition sites, thus leading to the size variation of DNA fragments generated by restriction enzyme digestion of genomic DNA. This is termed restriction fragment length polymorphism (RFLP).

When a disease allele(s) is associated with a particular polymorphism, the recognition of a specific pattern of RFLP may aid the diagnosis of that disease (genetic linkage – see below). Rarely, the mutation may affect the phenotypic expression of the encoded protein, so that the diagnosis may be directly established by the finding of a RFLP. Another type of DNA variation that causes RFLP is the presence of repeated sequences. RFLPs can also result from combined point mutation and repeated sequences.

Although RFLPs do not occur very frequently, sufficient RFLP alleles have been found to be associated with specific disease alleles (for example Huntington chorea, Duchenne muscular dystrophy and cystic fibrosis) that this method has been used with great success. The *Bgl*I (a restriction endonuclease) RFLP for the human thyroid hormone receptor erb-Aβ locus on the chromosome 3p22–3p24.1 is given as an example [41] (Fig. 1.10).

LINKAGE ANALYSIS

During meiosis a reassortment of genes may take place by crossing over, and genomic DNA sequences are therefore randomly shuffled by the process of recombination between sister chromatids. With exceptions the possibility of genes on the same chromosome staying together during the process is inversely related to their proximity; thus, closely situated genes are often inherited together. This forms the basis of linkage analysis.

The most classical of such linkage phenomena are all the known X-linked diseases. For others the linkage is to genes with identifiable phenotypes; for example linkage of 21-hydroxylase deficiency to HLA types. It is possible to identify the chromosomal location of a gene by linkage analysis using DNA sequence variations (RFLPs) at known chromosomal locations. To accomplish this a detailed analysis of the pattern of inheritance of the RFLPs in the family pedigree with special attention to the parental alleles is necessary. The assurance of the degree of genetic penetrance is critical in these studies, and statistical analyses are needed to establish the correlations.

Multilocus linkage analysis of data from informative families can be performed to obtain logarithm of the odds (LOD) scores for linkage [42], which is a statistical index of the certainty in establishing genetic linkage. A score of +3 means that the odds are 1000 to 1 in favour of linkage existence. In humans, genetic linkage is considered established if this score exceeds +3.00 at zero recombination (100% penetrance). As in many inherited disorders, the issue of genetic penetrance is most important in these analyses for scoring a patient as affected or unaffected. Incomplete penetrance, represents a potential source of error in linkage studies.

The application of heritage analysis is illustrated by a study on the genetic linkage of IGF-I to hypochondroplasia, which is one of more than 100 different types of skeletal dysplasias, most of them genetic in origin and associated with growth retardation and short stature [43,44]. This was based on known polymorphism of the IGF-I gene using Southern blot hybridization to reveal two non-polymorphic 8.2 and 3.2 kb fragments and two RFLP alleles of 4.8 and 5.2 kb in *Hin*dIII digests. In *Pvu*II digests two non-polymorphic 8.4 and 2.5 kb fragments and two RFLP alleles of 4.7 and 5.1 kb were found. The *Hin*dIII 5.2 kb and *Pvu*II 5.1 kb RFLP fragments are co-inherited as are the *Hin*dIII 4.8 kb and *Pvu*II 4.7 kb fragments [45].

RFLP analysis for IGF-I gene was performed in a group of patients with hypochondroplasia diagnosed by standard clinical and radiographic criteria [43,44]. Genomic DNA extracted from circulating lymphocytes of these patients was analysed by Southern blot hybridization after either *Hin*dIII or *Pvu*II digestion. The patients with hypochondroplasia had a higher frequency of the 5.2 kb *Hin*dIII/5.1 kb *Pvu*II IGF-I RFLP allele than the control group, suggesting an association between the IGF-I gene and the disease.

This analysis was extended to members of those families with heterozygous affected children (*Hin*dIII 5.2 kb, *Pvu*II 5.1 kb/*Hin*dIII 4.8 kb, *Pvu*II 4.7 kb), who responded to growth hormone therapy with proportionate growth of legs and trunks as opposed to the disproportionate growth response (trunks more than legs) seen in the other subgroup of hypochondroplastic patients. Based on the additional family data, multilocus linkage analysis established significant linkage (LOD score 3.31) between the IGF-I gene and this subgroup of patients, assuming a gene frequency of 1 in 1000 and 100% penetrance (Fig. 1.11).

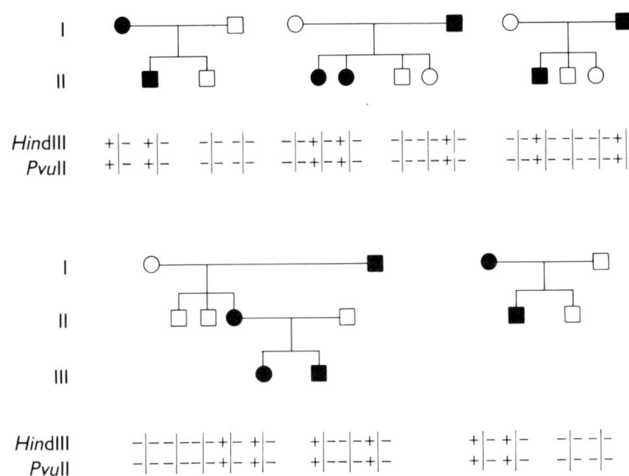

Fig. 1.11 Linkage analysis. Pedigree of five families with short stature presenting with hypochondroplastic features, showing linkage of the IGF-I gene locus at chromosome 12q23. Solid symbols denote affected family members: circles: female; squares: male. The DNA of all the family members was digested with the restriction enzymes *Hin*dIII and *Pvu*II and hybridized with an IGF-I probe. Southern blots of *Hin*dIII and *Pvu*II digests showed non-polymorphic fragments of 8.2 and 3.2 kb and an RFLP with alleles of 4.8 and 5.2 kb, and non-polymorphic fragments of 8.4 and 2.5 kb and an RFLP with alleles of 4.7 and 5.1 kb, respectively. The pattern of inheritance of the *Hin*dIII and *Pvu*II RFLP is shown below each symbol: + indicates the longer fragment of each RFLP (*Hin*dIII: 5.2 kb, *Pvu*II: 5.1 kb), and − indicates the shorter fragment (*Hin*dIII: 4.8 kb, *Pvu*II: 4.7 kb). Multilocus linkage analysis (LOD) scores for linkage between the IGF-I gene locus and short stature with hypochondroplasia were calculated. LOD scores calculated for a range of recombination fractions (theta), using data from five families and assuming 100% penetrance with a disease gene frequency of 1 in 1000, showed a LOD score of 3.311 at zero recombination, which is significant evidence in favour of linkage between the IGF-I gene locus and short stature with hypochondroplasia [44].

POLYMERASE CHAIN REACTION AMPLIFICATION

The polymerase chain reaction (PCR) is an *in vitro* DNA amplification method that can amplify a segment of DNA one million times in 20–30 repetitive cycles [46]. The amplification involves two oligonucleotide primers which complement the opposite strands of the DNA segment to be amplified, repeated cycles of heat denaturation of DNA templates, annealing of the primers to their comple-

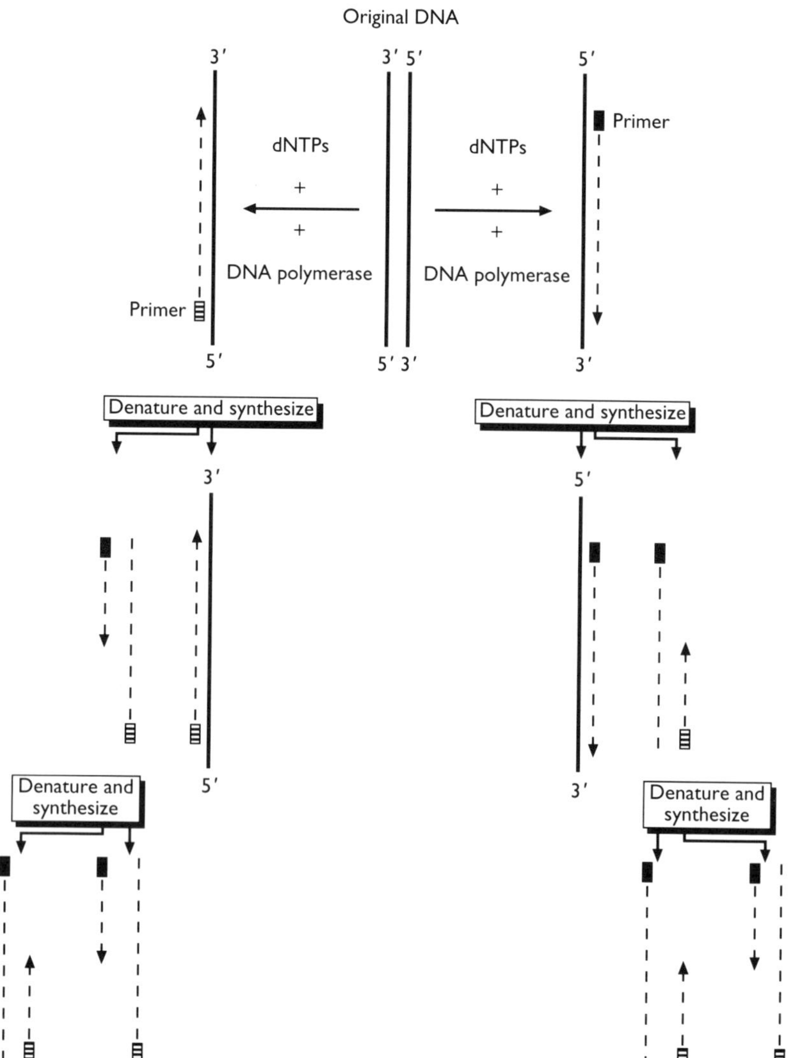

Fig. 1.12 Schematic representation of the DNA amplification by PCR. The first two cycles are shown completely. A double-stranded DNA molecule is denatured by heat; then oligonucleotide primers anneal to specific sequences flanking the segment to be amplified. The primers are then extended by DNA synthesis (dashed arrows) with polymerase and nucleotides which have been added to the reaction mixture. This three-step cycle is repeated up to 40 times. With each cycle the number of PCR products terminating at the end of the oligonucleotides increases exponentially. After 20 cycles of PCR the sequence of interest has been amplified more than a million times.

mentary sequences and extensions of the annealed primers with DNA polymerase (Fig. 1.12).

The discovery of a thermostable DNA polymerase from *Thermus aquaticus* (a bacterial species that grows in hot springs) and Taq polymerase, coupled with the automation of the reactions, have drastically widened the range of applications of this technique. For example, the specific discrete DNA fragment generated by PCR can be used readily for cloning, as well as for direct sequence analysis. The high sensitivity of the method means that single copies of DNA or RNA (following reverse transcription into cDNA) can serve as PCR templates, be amplified and detected. Such a degree of sensitivity justifies the need for extreme care to avoid contamination and hence the possibility of getting false-positive results.

This technique has played a major role in the diagnosis of genetic and endocrine diseases [47,48] and has become a standard procedure in the repertoire of molecular biology techniques. For instance, early prenatal diagnosis is rendered possible using PCR to amplify the scanty DNA obtained by chorionic villus biopsy; thus it is possible to detect the nine most common point mutations of the CYP21B gene causing 21-hydroxylase deficiency after mutation-specific PCR amplification of the functional CYP21B gene [49].

SEQUENCE ANALYSIS

Although chemical methods for DNA sequencing [50] may be used, we will here consider only the more commonly used base-specific chain termination method [51]. The basic reaction is DNA synthesis catalysed by DNA polymerase using a single-strand DNA template. In addition to the four deoxynucleoside triphosphates (dNTPs), usually one of which is radiolabelled for end-product detection (it is possible to use non-radioactive methods), a

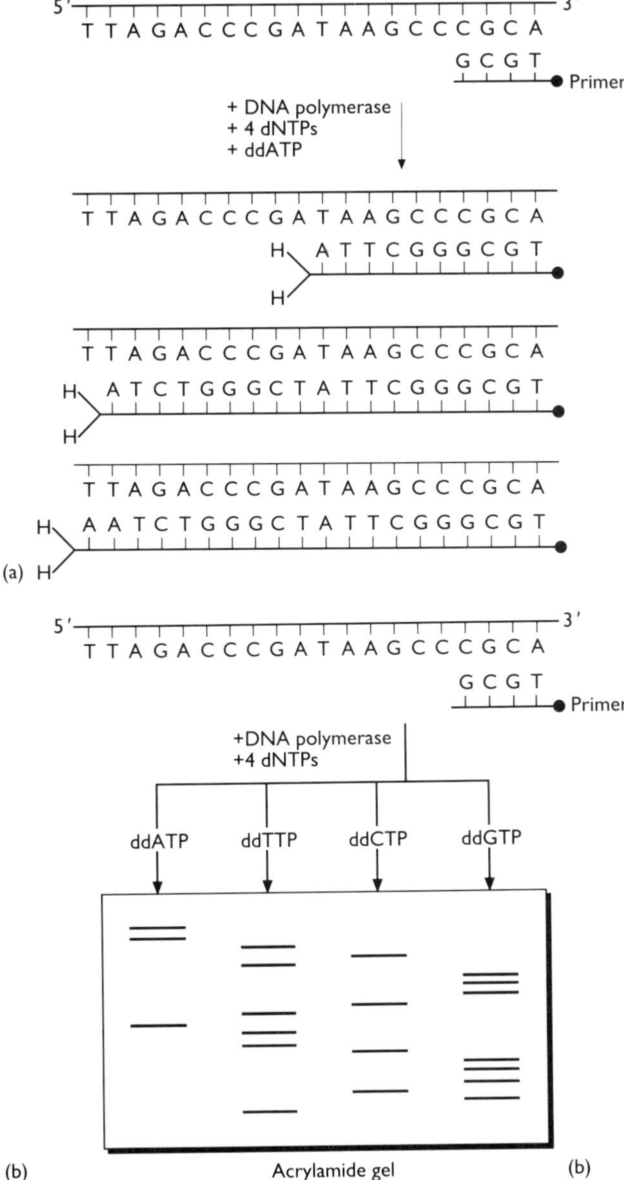

Fig. 1.13 The Sanger DNA sequencing procedure. (a) 2′,3′-dideoxynucleosides triphosphates (ddNTPs) of each of the four bases are used. These ddNTPs can be incorporated onto the growing DNA chain by DNA polymerase because of a normal 5′-triphosphate. However, once any ddNTP is incorporated, elongation of the DNA chain stops as ddNTP cannot form a phosphodiester bond with the next incoming dNTP. Each Sanger sequencing reaction mixture contains a DNA strand to be sequenced, a primer being complementary to one end of the DNA strand to sequence, DNA polymerase and a carefully controlled ratio of one labelled ddNTP (for example ddATP) and all four unlabelled dNTPs. A series of labelled strands, with different lengths but all labelled at their 3′ ends when ddATP are incorporated, among a mixture of unlabelled strands, are generated. (b) Four parallel reactions, each using a different labelled ddNTP, are performed; all of them are then analysed on sequential lanes of the same high-resolution polyacrylamide gel. These labelled strands, separated by size differences of as small as one nucleotide, are identified by autoradiography, and the DNA sequence is deciphered by analysing their relative positions.

small amount of one of the 2′,3′-dideoxynucleoside triphosphates (ddNTPs) is included in the reaction. Due to the lack of 3′-hydroxy groups on the deoxyribose moieties of ddNTPs, no further DNA chain elongation is possible once a ddNTP is incorporated into a growing chain. Thus the addition of, for example, ddATP will give rise to a mixture of DNA fragments all with identical 5′ ends but of varying lengths terminating with ddATP at their 3′ ends. The reaction product can then be fractionated by high-resolution polyacrylamide gel electrophoresis which can separate molecules differing in size by as little as one nucleotide. When four separate DNA synthesis reactions, each with a different ddNTP, are set up (Fig. 1.13), the full DNA sequence can be deciphered by analysing the products in parallel lanes.

Recently, methods for sequencing of PCR-amplified double- or single-stranded DNA without subcloning into plasmids or viral genomes have been developed. This has led to a practical and convenient way to identify specific gene-sequence defects. The recent identification of different mutations of the vasopressin receptor gene responsible for nephrogenic diabetes insipidus illustrates the power of such techniques in this regard [47,52]. It is clear that the importance of knowledge ramified out of precise DNA sequence analyses cannot be overstressed.

RNA quantification/expression studies

As mRNAs guard the gateway linking the information stored in the genome and the phenotypic expressions, much of the present-day understanding of the molecular basis of hormone action stems from meticulous dissection of how RNA expression is regulated. Since both RNA and DNA are basically polynucleotides, many fundamental principles involved in experimental studies of the two are essentially similar; yet there are a number of aspects that underlie their distinctions.

First, due to the 2′-hydroxyl group of ribose, the phosphodiester bonds of RNA molecules are very susceptible to hydrolysis. This means that additional caution is often necessary in handling RNA. Second, while the presence of a normal genomic sequence indicates nothing about its activity, the abundance of the respective mRNA when it is transcribed can give such an indication. It also often, though not invariably, reflects the level of the encoded protein produced. Thus RNA studies, like protein assays, often involve a facet of quantification.

The range of potential approaches in RNA studies is illustrated by those used to analyse the regulation of the hGH receptor by hGH [53]. Here the presence of a specific mRNA species (hGH receptor) in a human hepatoma cell line was first confirmed by Northern blot analysis. Quantitative assessment of the molecular regulation of this receptor by its own ligand, hGH, was achieved by RNase protection analysis. The observed increase in steady-state transcript level by hGH was further demonstrated to be due to an increased rate of transcription.

NORTHERN BLOT ANALYSIS

There are various methods to extract RNA from cells and tissues for analysis, but all have to deal with the same properties of RNA: it is very susceptible to ribonuclease degradation and most RNA exists as RNA–protein complexes.

RNA samples are commonly analysed by Northern blot hybridization, which is analogous to the Southern blot analysis of DNA. Thus the RNA sample is electrophoresed in denaturing agarose gel and transferred to a membrane; hybridization with a radiolabelled probe followed by autoradiography will reveal band(s) corresponding the number and size of mRNA species. Semi-quantification of the relative abundance of mRNA can be done by incorporating the appropriate control and performing densitometric assessment of the autoradiogram.

As mRNA constitutes only 1–2% of total RNA (the majority being ribosomal RNA), it is possible to facilitate analysis of low abundant mRNA species by extracting mRNA from the total RNA, helping to circumvent the problem of overloading of RNA sample for analysis. Figure 1.14 depicts a Northern blot analysis of total RNA prepared from the human hepatoma cell line HuH-7 using a radiolabelled hGH receptor cDNA probe. In contrast to what was found in rat and mouse hepatocytes, only one mRNA species of 4.2 kb was detected. The 1.2–1.5 kb species, which supposedly encodes the GH-binding protein, was not detectable in these hepatoma cells. This is in line with other evidence that GH-binding protein is post-translationally cleaved off the mature GH receptor molecule.

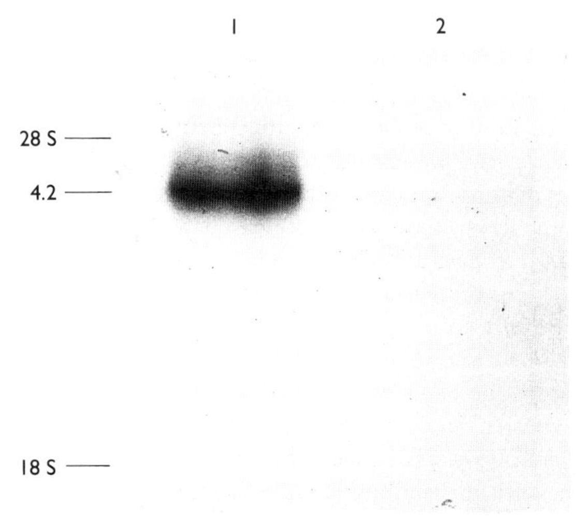

Fig. 1.14 A Northern blot of total RNA isolated from hepatoma cells (track 1) and from colon carcinoma cells (track 2) hybridized with hGH-receptor RNA probe is depicted. The size of the mRNA is shown in kilobases, as estimated by comparison with RNA molecular weight markers. Northern blotting is the term that refers to the transfer of RNA from a gel to a filter, and is analogous to the Southern blotting procedure. An RNA sample is subjected to gel electrophoresis and transferred onto a filter so that the separation achieved on the gel is maintained. Signals obtained after subsequent hybridization with a suitable probe can be compared with control samples in order to obtain information on the abundance (intensity of the signal) or size (distance of migration) of the RNA transcript. In the Northern blot shown the colon carcinoma cells are used as a negative control.

RNase PROTECTION ASSAY

This is a solution hybridization technique using radiolabelled RNA probes which takes advantage of the stability of a RNA–RNA hybrid against RNase digestion. It is more sensitive than Northern blot analysis and allows quantitative assessment of mRNA levels.

In this case a fragment of the hGH receptor cDNA was cloned into a plasmid vector which has specific DNA-dependent RNA polymerase promoter so that an antisense RNA probe can be generated *in vitro* for hybridization with RNA (Fig. 1.15). The protected hybrids at the end of hybridization and RNase digestion were electrophoresed, identified after autoradiography and excised out for scintillation counting. Treatment of these cells with hGH resulted in an increase in mRNA levels.

TRANSCRIPTION ANALYSIS

The two methods mentioned above measure steady-state mRNA levels and cannot differentiate between changes resulting from an altered rate of transcription or altered stability. In order to study transcription itself, a nuclear transcription run-on assay can be performed. The theory behind this experiment is that a RNA polymerase once engaged in a transcription process will remain bound to the DNA template and continue the transcription *in vitro* when provided with the right ingredients; thus in these assays the nuclei are isolated from the studied cells. Transcriptions are then allowed to continue *in vitro* in the presence of radioactive ribonucleoside triphosphates (Fig. 1.16). The newly incorporated radioactive nucleotides in the RNA are quantified by hybridizing to the respective cDNA which have been immobilized on a nylon or nitrocellulose membrane. The hybridization signal is proportional to the ongoing transcriptional activity.

In this study increased transcriptional activity after hGH treatment was demonstrated. In addition, the changes of mRNA observed might be due to the effect of hGH stimulating the transcription of a separate gene, thereby indirectly enhancing the hGH receptor transcription via its

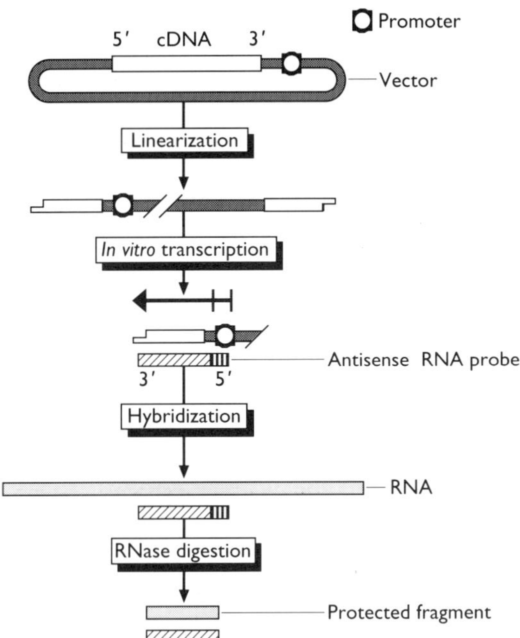

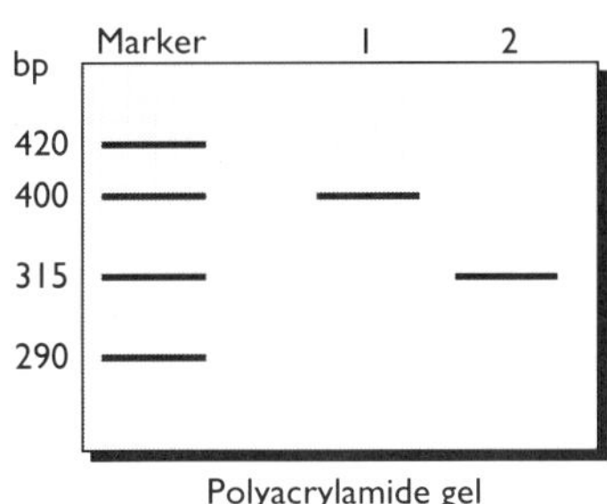

Fig. 1.15 RNase protection assay. cDNA is subcloned into a transcription vector. After linearization of the vector by cutting the DNA with a suitable restriction enzyme, an antisense riboprobe can be synthesized *in vitro* using a DNA-dependent RNA polymerase. The antisense riboprobe is hybridized to the complementary mRNA extracted from the test source. After RNase digestion of single-stranded RNA the undigested (protected, RNase-resistant) double-stranded RNA fragment is detected by gel electrophoresis followed by autoradiography. On the polyacrylamide gel the marker, on track 1 the total antisense RNA probe (including the promoter of vector), and on track 2, the protected fragment, are shown. The quantification of the mRNA can be performed by scanning densitometry of the bands on the autoradiograph.

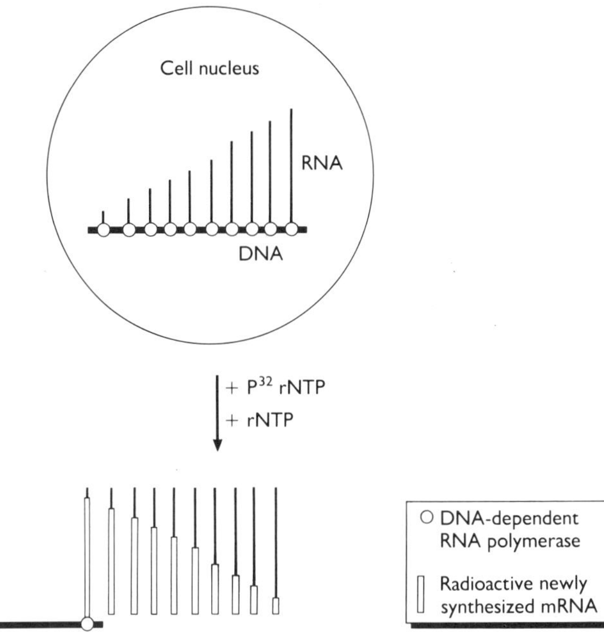

Fig. 1.16 Run-on assay. Nuclei with RNA polymerase attached to DNA and actively engaged in transcription are freshly isolated from live cells. Transcription is allowed to proceed *in vitro* in the presence of radioactive ribonucleoside triphosphates, thus incorporating radioactivity into newly extended mRNA molecules. The amount of incorporated radioactivity of each test condition is thus directly related to the transcription initiated *in vivo*.

protein product. Hence cycloheximide, a protein synthesis inhibitor, was used to show that no new protein synthesis is involved in the observed transcriptional regulation [53].

REVERSE TRANSCRIPTION AND POLYMERASE CHAIN REACTION

Combining the use of reverse transcriptase to synthesize first strand cDNA from mRNA and then amplifying the cDNA sequence of interest with specific sets of primers, it is now possible to design studies analysing mRNA levels of low abundance from a small number of cells or a small amount of tissue. It is also feasible to use this technique to semiquantitate mRNA species of interest, but great care should be taken to incorporate well-designed internal controls [54].

IN SITU HYBRIDIZATION

While the methods described above analyse RNA extracted from cells (or tissues), *in situ* hybridization offers the alternatives of studying mRNA (and also DNA) in fixed cells and tissues. This approach is particularly informative in studying heterogeneous cell populations when extracted RNA will not represent the one subpopulation of interest. The main obstacle to broad application of this technique is the inherent difficulty of preserving the mRNA species, so that freshly prepared or frozen tissues and cells are required for study. The procedures involved otherwise follow the basic principles of solid-phase or solution hybridization, with special attention to protecting mRNA against degradation during the study.

This method lacks the superiority offered by the gel electrophoresis in Northern blot analysis, and the tissues and cells cannot be hybridized many times unlike the filter support used in the latter technique. Thus carefully designed controls are necessary for validating the results obtained by *in situ* hybridization. Once established, it has often proved a major asset in studying gene products when protein detection is either impossible or insensitive; but it should be emphasized that caution is necessary when equating mRNA steady-state levels with active protein synthesis.

Typically, thin cryostat or paraffin tissue sections, or cultured cells, are fixed and used for hybridization with a radiolabelled probe. The tissue histology is preserved during freezing, sectioning and hybridization procedures; cellular identity can be established by histological analysis or combined immunocytochemistry on the same or adjacent section. After hybridization and washing, the radioactive probe remains bound to mRNA within specific cells. The slide is covered with photographic emulsion and developed after a defined period of time, depending on the mRNA abundance and specific activity of the probe. Silver grains will be identified over cells that bound the probe.

Using this technique IGF-I transcripts have been shown to be widely expressed in numerous embryonic tissues, supporting the autocrine/paracrine role of this growth factor [55]. In another study the localization of IGF-II and IGF-binding protein (IGFBP)-2 in adjacent cells across the choroid plexus has led to the suggestion that IGFBP-2 may function as an IGF-II transporter across the blood–brain barrier [56].

Non-radioactive techniques for detecting the specific nucleic acid hybridization have been developed. This offers better cellular localization and resolution, rapidity of detection of results and the distinct advantage of avoiding the use of radioactive agents. The major shortcoming of these techniques at present is the relative insensitivity for detecting mRNA species of low abundance compared to the radioactive methods.

GENE TRANSFER

Of all the progress made in the field of molecular biology over the 40 years since the description of the double helix by Watson and Crick, one sensational topic emerges – human genetic engineering. Important as this is, it is but one important potential application of genetic engineering. Genetic engineering of various sorts has been practised extensively in preclinical research since the introduction of recombinant DNA technology. This has contributed to much of what has been outlined earlier in this chapter. Nonetheless it is interesting to look more closely at some of the techniques involved, and whether they may find applications in clinical endocrinological practice.

It is now possible to introduce genes in a number of ways into cells *in vitro* and *in vivo*. One fundamental application is the *in vitro* introduction of plasmid vectors into bacterial cells (transformation) used in gene-cloning experiments. On the other hand, a gene promoter under study can be linked to a reporter gene, the product of which can be conveniently assessed and introduced into host cells for systematic analysis of the functions of the regulatory elements. Alternatively, a well-characterized promoter from one gene can be joined with the coding sequence of another gene and introduced into suitable host cells. It is then possible to control the expression and study the effects of the gene product *in vitro*.

Furthermore, when the recipient cell is a germ cell, and the vector contains a component which helps the foreign gene to be integrated into the host genome, the effects of the gene expression throughout development *in vivo* can be studied. It is also possible to mutate with precision a component(s) of a normal gene by homologous gene recombination [57,58] to study the consequences. This will help researchers design animal equivalents of known human genetic diseases for evaluating alternative therapeutic approaches, which may well be more realistic than contemplating direct gene therapy in many diseases. The cumulative efforts of research in this direction have already led to the use of designer genes (carrying with them the secret codes for the 'desirable effects' of their products) in clinical research – the beginning of human gene therapy [59,60]. Scrupulous evaluation of our scientific understanding of various aspects involved, and the ethical and socioeconomic implications in human applications, are justified, and successful applications will be realized only by the continual joint efforts of basic and clinical scientists [61].

Gene transfer by physical methods

Physical transfer of DNA (transformation) into bacteria is a standard practice in gene cloning, usually aided by manipulations which increase the efficiency, such as calcium chloride treatment or electroporation (the use of electricity to make the cell permeable to DNA). Transfection describes the same process in the eukaryotic cells (as transformation is historically used to describe changes leading to unrestrained growth of these cells). When electroporation is used in mammalian cells the physical transfer of DNA into these cells is often endocytosis mediated. Calcium chloride treatment can aid the process by precipitating DNA onto the cell surface. Furthermore, although naked DNA (for example DNA cloned into plasmid) *per se* has been successfully introduced into muscle without modification [62], it is usual to modify DNA by putting it into liposome or complexing it to protein recognized by a specific cell surface receptor to enhance efficiency. In addition, DNA-coated microprojectiles have been driven into animal tissues *in vivo* by high-pressure helium gas [63].

In general the exogenous DNA introduced into cells replicates as extrachromosomal DNA particles in the first days. These particles form circular episomes within the nucleus and are subjected to regulatory influences which can closely mimic the regulation of the endogenous gene located within the natural chromosome. In cultured cell systems, although as many as 1–10% of cells transiently take up foreign DNA, it is unstable and often lost from the cells. On further cell divisions the foreign DNA can become stably integrated into the host-cell chromosomes in a small fraction, approximately 1–100/million cells. The cells expressing the foreign gene are often selected by particular markers co-introduced with the foreign gene, for example a gene encoding thymidine kinase or one encoding a protein that inactivates, for example, neomycin.

Transduction of cells with recombinant viral vectors

Retroviral vectors are recombinantly modified viral retroviruses so that no infectious viruses will be produced in host cells. They are highly efficient in introducing gene material into replicating cells. After several cell divisions the recombinant particles are integrated into the host chromosome and stably carry the foreign DNA along with them. Because of these characteristics, retroviral vector is the prime choice in this early phase of preclinical gene therapy trials, especially the *ex vivo* systems [59,60]. Of note, however, is the apparent lack of complete control to prevent resurgence of replication-competent strains on isolated occasions. With similar concern over viral replication, adenovirus vectors offer the advantages of being able to carry large DNA segments, to infect non-replicating cells and also to infect tissues *in situ*. This vector has been used with success in the *in vivo* delivery of cystic fibrosis transmembrane conductance regulator (CFTR) to airway epithelium by intratracheal instillation [61]. Other types of viral vectors have also been studied, but much has to be learned before their use can be safely extended to human beings [61].

Microinjection of genes into cell nuclei

With fine microcapillary pipettes, DNA solutions can be injected directly into the nucleus of a recipient cell. After microinjection the DNA is rapidly integrated into the host genome. When used to insert genomic material into one-cell mammalian embryos which are then allowed to develop, this approach allows analysis of the regulation of defined genes in the context of normal development of a complex organism [62–64]. It is possible to analyse and compare the qualitative and quantitative efficiencies of expression of the genes among various organs.

When the rat GH gene was fused with the mouse metallothionein I gene promoter and injected into the fertilized pronuclei of mouse embryos [65], GH was expressed at high levels in most of the tissues analysed. These mice grew at a rate two to three times faster than normal littermates. In addition, the differential pattern of organ-specific overgrowth they exhibited compared to IGF-I transgenic mice helped to show that GH actions are not all mediated through IGF-I production.

Similar techniques can be used to achieve site-directed mutagenesis of some genes when mutated gene constructs are used to transfect embryonic stem cells [57]. This makes possible the study of a defective gene instead of the added expression of the gene introduced. With this kind of technique some fundamental concepts such as genetic imprinting have been advanced [66,67] which may also find relevance in understanding human disease [68].

Therapy of gene defects

With the ability to manipulate genes in preclinical studies it is reasonable to foresee future success in human applications. Both *in vivo* and *ex vivo* approaches have been actively studied. For the latter one might obtain cells from skin or liver, and use prepared cultured cells into which the appropriate gene can be transferred. These cells may then be transplanted back into the patient. On the other hand the success of introducing CFTR gene into rat respiratory epithelium *in vivo* definitely holds high hopes for similar application in humans [61].

Another, highly speculative, way would be the micro-injection of genes into fertilized ova resulting from the union of germ cells. Oocytes fertilized *in vitro* have already been successfully transplanted back to the uteri of surrogate mothers; therefore an alternative approach could be the development of techniques either to screen for ova and sperms containing normal alleles or to introduce DNA material into the germ cells before fertilization.

Though sensational, gene therapy should be evaluated only as a potential mode of therapy, not losing sight of the rich experiences we have gained in the past using the 'more conventional' methods. This is especially true in clinical endocrinology since superb results have been experienced in many classical endocrine diseases from long-standing treatment. Molecular biology has helped bring forth a very basic and fundamental understanding of biological processes. Although it has already found various applications in clinical endocrinology it will continue to test our abilities to elucidate the molecular details while maintaining the scientific acuity to apply them in the everyday clinical problems we face.

GLOSSARY TO GENE STRUCTURE

CAAT box Consensus sequence commonly interacting with many eukaryotic promoters of the type used by RNA polymerase II, situated at about −70 bp from the initiation site.

CAP structure Gene transcripts are modified at their 5′ end by the addition of a so-called 'cap' structure which may play a role in translation. The cap is an added 5′ terminal guanosine, methylated on the 7 position, and linked to the initiator nucleotide by an unusual 5′–5′-triphosphate linkage. Nucleotides immediately adjacent to the cap structure constitute the complementary transcription initiation site.

***Cis*-acting element** *Cis*-acting elements are short DNA sequences which affect transcription of their cognate genes. They usually act by binding a specific transcription (*trans*-acting) factor.

Consensus sequence Sequence of nucleotides compiled by comparison of homologous regions of many genes, and selecting the one most frequently occurring for each position.

DNA Double-stranded polymeric molecule composed of a chain of deoxyribose residues linked covalently by phosphodiester bonds. One of four bases, adenine (A), thymine (T), cytosine (C) or guanine (G) is connected to each sugar residue.

Enhancer These elements can be located at great distances from the start site of transcription, either upstream, downstream or within a transcriptional unit, and function in either direction. They act by increasing the activity of a promoter, although they lack promoter activity themselves and are therefore referred to as enhancers.

Eukaryote Cells that contain a nucleus are referred to as eukaryotic cells, whereas the nuclei-free bacteria and their close relatives, the blue-green algae, are known as prokaryotic.

Exon Nucleotide sequences encoding the mRNA.

Gene A segment of DNA that codes for an RNA and/or polypeptide molecule.

Initiation site The precise base pair in the DNA at which transcription starts, corresponding to the 5′ end of the mRNA synthesized.

Intron Nucleotide sequences which encode the mature mRNA (exons) are interrupted by intervening non-coding sequences, the introns.

Poly-(A) tail Stretch of 100–200 adenosine residues not encoded by the gene sequence but added after transcription to the mRNA prior to translocation to the cytoplasm.

Polyadenylation signal sequence Most eukaryotic mRNAs contain the sequence AAUAAA just upstream (approximately 20 bp) from the polyadenylation site.

Promoter The region of the gene bracketed by the TATA box and the site of transcriptional initiation (the 'cap' site) has been operationally defined as the gene promoter. It is important in defining the transcriptional start site.

Protein-coding sequence This begins with the codon AUG for methionine and ends with the codon immediately preceding one of the three nonsense, or stop codons (UGA, UAA and UAG).

Regulatory element Sequences involved in regulation of transcription are known as regulatory elements. They are shared by a limited number of genes and are interdigitated with the upstream promoter elements. Hormone response elements (HRE) are an example.

Splice site The sequences at the junctions of introns and exons. The predominant consensus sequences for the 5′ splice 'donor' and the 3′ splice 'acceptor' are: exon/GT–intron–AG/exon.

Stop codon Termination codon which terminates the translation.

TATA box AT-rich sequence common to many eukaryotic promoters of the type used by RNA polymerase II, situated at about −25 bp from the initiation site.

***Trans*-acting factor** *Trans*-acting factors, usually proteins, up- or down-regulate transcription. They are not part of the gene in question.

Transcription factor These are necessary for accurate initiation and rate of transcription but are not integral parts of RNA polymerases.

Upstream promoter element (UPE) The low activity of the promoter itself is dramatically increased by other elements (CAAT box; GC-rich sequences known as the Sp1 box) located upstream of the promoter. These elements are essential for transcription of the genes, and their elimination by deletion or mutation abolishes transcription.

REFERENCES

1 Proudfoot N. Poly(A) signals. *Cell* 1991;64:671–4.

2 Kornberg RD, Lorch Y. Irresistible force meets immovable object: transcription and the nucleosome. *Cell* 1991;67:833–6.

3 Frankel AD, Kim PS. Modular structure of transcriptional factors: implication for gene regulation. *Cell* 1991;65:727–9.

4 Chen EY, Liao YC, Smith DH, Barrera-Saldana HA, Gelinas RE, Seeburg PH. The human growth hormone locus: nucleotide sequence, biology, and evolution. *Genomics* 1989;4:479–97.

5 Phillips JA III. Inherited defects in growth hormone synthesis and action. In: Scriver CR, Beaudet AL, Sly WS, Valle D, eds. *The Metabolic Basis of Inherited Disease*, 6th edn. New York: McGraw-Hill, 1988:1965–83.

6 Bodner M, Castrillo JL, Theill LE, Deerinck T, Ellisman M, Karin M. The pituitary-specific transcription factor GHF-1 is a homeobox-containing protein. *Cell* 1988;55:505–18.

7 Ingraham HA, Chen R, Mangalam HJ *et al.* A tissue specific transcription factor containing a homeodomain specifies a pituitary phenotype. *Cell* 1988;55:519–29.

8 Voss JW, Rosenfeld MG. Anterior pituitary development: short tales from dwarf mice. *Cell* 1992;70:527–30.

9 Eichele G. Retinoids and vertebrate limb pattern formation. *Trends Genet* 1989;5:246–51.

10 Foulkes NS, Sassone-Corsi P. More is better: activators and repressors from the same gene. *Cell* 1992;68:411–14.

11 Hunter T, Karin M. The regulation of transcription by phosporylation. *Cell* 1992;70:375–87.

12 Bingham PM, Chou TB, Mims I, Zachar Z. On/off regulation of gene expression at the level of gene splicing. *Trends Genet* 1988;4:134–8.

13 Sharp PA. Splicing of messenger RNA precursors. *Science* 1987;253:766–71.

14 Leff SE, Rosenfeld MG, Evans RM. Complex transcriptional unit: diversity in gene expression by alternative RNA processing. *Annu Rev Biochem* 1986;55:1091–117.

15 Daughaday WH, Rotwein P. Insulin-like growth factors I and II. Peptide, messenger ribonucleic acid and gene structures, serum, and tissue concentrations. *Endocr Rev* 1989;10:68–91.

16 Giudice LC. Insulin-like growth factors and ovarian follicular development. *Endocr Rev* 1992;13:641–69.

17 Rotwein P, Pollack KM, Didier DK, Krivi GG. Organization and sequence of the human insulin-like growth factor I gene: alternative RNA processing produces two insulin-like growth factor precursor peptides. *J Biol Chem* 1986;261:4828–32.

18 LeRoith D, Roberts CT Jr. Insulin-like growth factor I (IGF-I): a molecular basis for endocrine versus local action? *Mol Cell Endocrinol* 1991;77:C57.

19 Leff SE, Evans RM, Rosenfeld MG. Splice commitment dictates neuron-specific alternative RNA processing in calcitonin-CGRP gene expression. *Cell* 1988;48:517–24.

20 Rosenfeld MG, Amara SG, Evans RM. Alternative RNA processing: determining neuronal phenotype. *Science* 1984; 225:1315–20.

21 Emeson RB, Hedjran F, Yeakley JM, Guise JW, Rosenfeld MG. Alternative production of calcitonin and CGRP mRNA is regulated at the calcitonin-specific splice acceptor. *Nature* 1989;341:76–80.

22 Foulkes NS, Mellström B, Benusigilio E, Sassone-Corsi P. Developmental switch of CREM function during spermatogenesis: from antagonist to activator. *Nature* 1992;355:80–4.

23 Bickel M, Iwai Y, Pluznik DH, Cohen RB. Binding of sequence specific proteins to the adenosine- plus uridine-rich sequences of the murine granulocyte/macrophage colony-stimulating factor mRNA. *Proc Natl Acad Sci USA* 1992;89:10001–5.

24 Brawerman G. Determinants of messenger RNA stability. *Cell* 1987;48:5–6.

25 Guyette WA, Matusik RA, Rosen JM. Prolactin-mediated transcriptional and post-transcriptional control of casein gene expression. *Cell* 1979;17:1013–23.

26 Frankel AD, Mattaj IW, Rio DC. RNA–protein interaction. *Cell* 1991;67:1041–6.

27 Shaw G, Kamen R. A conserved AU sequence from the 3′ untranslated region of GM-CSF mRNA mediates selective mRNA degradation. *Cell* 1986;46:659–67.

28 Rosenthal ET, Hurt T, Rudeman JV. Selective translation of mRNA controls the pattern of protein synthesis during early development of the surf clam *Spisula solidissima*. *Cell* 1980;20:487–94.

29 Odawara M, Kadowaki T, Yamamoto R *et al.* Human diabetes associated with a mutation in the tyrosine kinase domain of the insulin receptor. *Science* 1988;245:66–8.

30 Forest MG, Dörr HG, on behalf of ESPE. Prenatal treatment of congenital adrenal hyperplasia (CAH) due to 21-hydroxylase deficiency: European experience in 223 pregnancies at risk. *Pediatr Res* (Suppl.) 1993;33:S3.

31 McPhaul MJ, Marcelli M, Zoppi S, Griffin JE, Wilson JD. Genetic basis of endocrine disease. 4: The spectrum of mutations in the androgen receptor gene that causes androgen resistance. *J Clin Endocrinol Metab* 1993;76:17–23.

32 Kadowaki T, Bevins CL, Cama A *et al.* Two mutant alleles of the insulin receptor gene in a patient with extreme insulin resistance. *Science* 1988;240:787–90.

33 Krohn K, Uibo R, Aavik E, Peterson P, Savilahti K. Identification by molecular cloning of an autoantigen associated with Addison's disease as steroid 17α-hydroxylase. *Lancet* 1992;339:770–3.

34 Legouis R, Hardelin JP, Levilliers J *et al.* The candidate gene for the X-linked Kallman syndrome encodes a protein related to adhesion molecules. *Cell* 1991;67:423–35.

35 Rommens JM, Iannuzzu MC, Kerem BS *et al.* Identification of the cystic fibrosis gene: chromosome walking and jumping. *Science* 1989;245:1059–65.

36 Savage MO, Wilton P, Ranke MB *et al.* Therapeutic response to recombinant IGF-I in thirty two patients with growth hormone insensitivity. *Pediatr Res* (Suppl.) 1993;33:S5.

37 Lyons J, Landis CA, Harsh G *et al.* Two G protein oncogenes in human endocrine tumors. *Science* 1990;249;655–9.

38 Spiegel AM, Shenker A, Weinstein S. The McCune Albright syndrome: a genetically determined signal transduction disorder. *Pediatr Res* (Suppl.) 1993;33:S6–7.

39 Weinstein LS, Shenker A, Gejman PV, Merino MJ, Friedman E, Spiegel AM. Activating mutations of the stimulatory G protein in the McCune–Albright syndrome. *N Engl J Med* 1991;325:1688–95.

40 Caskey CT. Disease diagnosis by recombinant DNA methods. *Science* 1987;236:1223–9.

41 Kanaka Ch, Eblé A, Mullis PE. *BglI* RFLP for the human erb-Aβ locus on chromosome 3p22-3p24.1 (THRB). *Nucl Acids Res* 1991;19:4574.

42 Ott J. *Linkage Package; Analysis of Human Genetic Linkage.* Baltimore, MD: Johns Hopkins University Press, 1985.

43 Glasgow JFT, Nevin NC, Thomas PS. Hypochondroplasia. *Arch Dis Child* 1978;53:868–72.

44 Mullis PE, Patel MS, Brickell PM, Hindmarsh PC, Brook CGD. Growth characteristics and response to growth hormone therapy in patients with hypochondroplasia: genetic linkage of the insulin-like growth factor I gene at chromosome 12q23 to the disease in a subgroup of these patients. *Clin Endocrinol* 1991;34:265–74.

45 Höppener JWM, dePagter-Holthuizen P, Geurts van Kessel AH *et al.* The human gene encoding insulin-like growth factor I is located on chromosome 12. *Hum Genet* 1985; 69:157–60.

46 Erlich HA, Gelfand D, Sninsky JJ. Recent advances in the polymerase chain reaction. *Science* 1991;252:1643–51.

47 Holtzman EJ, Harris HW Jr, Kolakowski LF Jr, Guay-Woodford LM, Botelho B, Ausiello DA. A molecular defect in the vasopressin V2-receptor gene causing nephrogenic diabetes insipidus. *N Engl J Med* 1993;328:1534–7.

48 Newton CR, Graham A, Heptinstall LE *et al.* Analysis of any point mutation in DNA: the amplification refractory mutation system (ARMS). *Nucl Acids Res* 1989;17:2503–16.

49 Morel Y, Murena M, Forest MG. Prenatal diagnosis of congenital adrenal hyperplasia due to 21-hydroxylase deficiency. *Pediatr Res* 1993;33:S3.

50 Maxam AM, Gilbert W. A new method of sequencing DNA. *Proc Natl Acad Sci USA* 1977;74:560–4.
51 Sanger F, Nicklen S, Coulson AR. DNA sequencing with chain-terminating inhibitors. *Proc Natl Acad Sci USA* 1977; 74:5463–7.
52 Merendino JJ, Spiegel AM, Crawford JD, O'Carroll AM, Brownstein MJ, Lolait SJ. Brief report: a mutation in the vasopressin V2-receptor gene in a kindred with X-linked nephrogenic diabetes insipidus. *N Engl J Med* 1993;328: 1538–41.
53 Mullis PE, Lund T, Patel MS, Brook CGD, Brickell PM. Regulation of human growth hormone receptor gene expression by human growth hormone in a human hepatoma cell line. *Mol Cell Endocrinol* 1991;76:125–33.
54 Chelly J, Kaplan JC, Maire P, Gautron S, Kahn A. Transcription of the distrophin gene in human muscle and non-muscle tissues. *Nature* 1988;332:858–60.
55 Han VK, D'Ercole AJ, Lund PK. Cellular localization of somatomedin (insulin-like growth factor) mRNA in the human fetus. *Science* 1987;286:193–6.
56 Wood TI, Brown AL, Rechler MM, Pintar JE. The expression of an insulin-like growth factor (IGF)-binding protein gene is distinct from IGF-II in the midgestational rat embryo. *Mol Endocrinol* 1990;4:1257–63.
57 Frohman FA, Martin GR. Cut, paste and save: new approaches to altering specific genes in mice. *Cell* 1989;56:145–7.
58 Kuehn MR, Bradley A, Robertson EJ, Evans MJ. A potential animal model for Lesch–Nyhan syndrome through introduction of HPRT mutation into mice. *Nature* 1987;326:295–8.
59 Anderson WF. Human gene therapy. *Science* 1992;256: 808–13.
60 Miller DA. Human gene therapy comes of age. *Nature* 1992; 357:455–7.
61 Mulligan RC. The basic science of gene therapy. *Science* 1993;260:926–32.
62 Ulmer JB, Donnelly JJ, Parker SE *et al.* Heterologous protection against influenza by injection of DNA encoding a viral protein. *Science* 1993;259:1745–54.
63 Williams RS, Johnson SA, Reidy M, DeVit MJ, McElligott SG, Sanford JC. Introduction of foreign genes into tissues of living mice by DNA-coated microprojectiles. *Proc Natl Acad Sci USA* 1991;88:2726–30.
64 Westphal H. Transgenic mammals and biotechnology. *FASEB J* 1989;3:117–20.
65 Palmiter RD, Brinster RL, Hammer RE. Dramatic growth of mice that developed from eggs microinjected with metallothionein–growth hormone fusion genes. *Nature* 1982;300: 611–15.
66 Barlow DP, Stöger R, Herrmann BG, Saito K, Schweifer N. The mouse insulin-like growth factor type-2 receptor is imprinted and closely linked to Tme locus. *Nature* 1991; 349:84–7.
67 DeChiara TM, Robertson EJ, Efstratiadis A. Parental imprinting of the mouse insulin-like growth factor II gene. *Cell* 1991;64;849–59.
68 Nicholls RD, Knoll IHM, Butler MG, Karam S, Lalande M. Genetic imprinting suggested by maternal heterodisomy in non-deletion Prader–Willi syndrome. *Nature* 1989;342: 281–5.

GENERAL READING

Alberts B, Bray D, Lewis J *et al. Molecular Biology of the Cell*, 2nd edn. New York: Garland, 1989.
Davies KE. *Genome Analysis, a Practical Approach.* Oxford: IRL Press, 1988.
Innis MA, Gelfand DH, Sninsky JJ, White TJ. *PCR Protocols. A Guide to Methods and Applications.* San Diego, CA: Academic Press, 1990.
Latchman D. *Gene Regulation, a Eukaryotic Perspective.* London: Unwin Hyman, 1990.
Latchman DS. *Eukaryotic Transcription Factors.* London: Academic Press, 1991.
Sambrook J, Fritsch EF, Maniatis T. *Molecular Cloning.* New York: Cold Spring Harbor Laboratory Press, 1989.
Watson JD, Tooze J, Kurzt DT. *Recombinant DNA – a Short Course.* New York: WH Freeman, 1983.

2: Applications of Molecular Genetics in the Study of Clinical Disorders

R.V. THAKKER

INTRODUCTION

Important advances in endocrinology have resulted from the application of the methods of molecular biology [1]. For example, the molecular basis for mammalian sex development [2–4], for papillary thyroid cancers [5–8], for nephrogenic diabetes insipidus [9,10] and for Kallmann syndrome [11,12] have been elucidated, and some of the susceptibility genes involved in the development of hypertension [13], insulin-dependent diabetes mellitus [14–16] and non-insulin-dependent diabetes mellitus [17] have been identified (Table 2.1). In these studies the first important step towards elucidating the genetic abnormality, and in subsequently characterizing the gene product, that is protein, was represented by the localization of the disease gene locus. This approach has been referred to as 'reverse genetics' [18] or 'positional cloning' [19], and the chromosomal localization of genes, which is also referred to as 'gene mapping', may be accomplished either by the cytogenetic detection of chromosomal abnormalities in affected individuals or by segregation studies in affected families using recombinant DNA genetic markers [20]. The application of these techniques of molecular genetics in the investigation of endocrine and metabolic diseases is reviewed with reference to the study of the hypoparathyroid disorders.

HYPOPARATHYROID DISORDERS

Hypoparathyroidism is an endocrine disorder in which hypocalcaemia and hyperphosphataemia are the result of a deficiency in parathyroid hormone (PTH) secretion. There are a variety of causes [21] of hypoparathyroidism and the disorder may occur as part of a pluriglandular autoimmune disorder or as a complex congenital defect, as for example in the DiGeorge syndrome or in association with other developmental anomalies involving dysmorphic features, nephropathy, sensorineural deafness, lymphoedema and cortical thickening of tubular bones. In addition, hypoparathyroidism may develop as a solitary endocrinopathy and this form has been called isolated or idiopathic hypoparathyroidism. Familial occurrences of isolated hypoparathyroidism have been reported and autosomal dominant [22,23], autosomal recessive [24,25] and X-linked recessive [26–28] inheritances have been established [29] (Table 2.2). The molecular genetic basis for each of these forms of hypoparathyroidism has been investigated either by examining the PTH gene, located on the short arm of chromosome 11 [30], band 11 p15, for abnormalities or by pursuing positional cloning studies in which the chromosomal location of the mutant gene was first elucidated.

PARATHYROID HORMONE GENE ABNORMALITIES IN ISOLATED HYPOPARATHYROIDISM

A deficiency of human PTH, which is an 84 amino acid polypeptide [31] encoded by a single gene located on 11 p15 [30], is the hallmark of hypoparathyroidism, and the PTH gene has been investigated for abnormalities in patients with familial autosomal isolated hypoparathyroidism [22,25,32]. Families with autosomal hypoparathyroidism have been initially investigated for segregation of the disease and PTH gene polymorphisms; families which revealed co-segregation have been further investigated for DNA sequence abnormalities of the PTH gene. The identification of polymorphisms at the PTH locus, together with the ability to amplify and determine the sequence of selected DNA segments by use of the polymerase chain reaction (PCR), has facilitated the investigation of these families for PTH gene abnormalities.

Parathyroid hormone gene polymorphisms

The PTH gene consists of three exons and two introns (Fig. 2.1). Exon 1, which comprises 85 bp, encodes an untranslated region; exon 2 (90 bp) encodes the initiation codon, signal peptide and part of the prohormone sequence; exon 3 (612 bp) encodes the remainder of the prohormone sequence, the 84 amino acid PTH peptide and the 3′ untranslated region. Five polymorphisms of the PTH gene have been reported: two are associated with restriction

Table 2.1 Chromosomal locations of genetic abnormalities associated with some endocrine and metabolic disorders

Disorder	Chromosomal location
Anterior pituitary	
Prolactinomas	11q13
Somatotrophinomas	11q13, 20q13.2
Isolated growth hormone (GH) deficiency	17q22–q24
Isolated thyroid-stimulating hormone (TSH) (β) deficiency	1p13
Isolated luteinizing hormone (LH) deficiency	19q13.3
Isolated follicle-stimulating hormone (FSH) deficiency	11p13.3
Combined deficiency of prolactin (PRL), GH, TSH, due to PIT 1 mutation	3q
Posterior pituitary	
Diabetes insipidus (neurogenic)	20p13
Thyroid	
Papillary thyroid carcinoma	10q11.2
Follicular thyroid carcinoma	3p
Medullary thyroid carcinoma (MTC), MEN2a, MEN2b	10q11.2, (1p)
Goitre associated with thyroglobulin deficiency	8q24
Goitre associated with organification defect	2pter–p24
Adrenal cortex	
Congenital adrenal hyperplasia	6p21.3, 8q21–q22, 10q24–q25, 15q21, 15q23–q24
Congenital adrenal hypoplasia	Xp21.3–p21.2
Adrenoleukodystrophy	Xq28
Adrenal medulla	
Phaeochromocytoma (as part of MEN2)	1p
Phaeochromocytoma (as part of Von Hippel Lindau syndrome)	3p26–p25
Pancreatic islets	
Gastrinomas	11q13
Insulinomas	11q13
Diabetes, mellitus, insulin-dependent (IDDM)	6p21.3, 11p, 11q
Diabetes mellitus, non-insulin-dependent (NIDDM)	7p
Diabetes mellitus, maturity onset diabetes of the young (MODY)	20q
Diabetes mellitus (NIDDM) and deafness	Mitochondrial deletion
Parathyroids	
Multiple endocrine neoplasia type 1 (MEN1)	11q13
Parathyroid tumours (MEN1 and PRAD 1 (BCL 1) genes)	11q13
Isolated hypoparathyroidism, autosomal forms	11p15
X-linked hypoparathyroidism	Xq26–q27
DiGeorge syndrome	22q11.21–q11.23, 10p13
Familal hypocalciuric hypercalcaemia	3q, 19p
Testis	
Testicular cancer	3p21–pter
Azoospermia	Yq11
Gonadal dysgenesis	Yp11.3
Ovary	
Ovarian cancer	3p, 6q
Müllerian persistent duct syndrome	19p13.3
Premature ovarian failure	Xq21.3–q27
Rickets	
X-linked hypophosphataemic rickets	Xp22.2–p22.1
Vitamin D-dependent rickets type I (VDDRI), 1α-hydroxylase deficiency	12q14
Lowe syndrome	Xq25–q26.1
Receptor defects	
Laron syndrome (GH receptor)	5p14–p12
Male precocious puberty (LH receptor)	2p21
Leprechaunism (insulin receptor)	19p13.3–p13.2
Acanthosis nigricans (insulin receptor)	19p13.3–p13.2
Insulin-resistant diabetes (insulin receptor)	19p13.3–p13.2
Polycystic ovarian syndrome (insulin receptor)	19p13.3–p13.2
Polycystic ovarian syndrome, hirsutism with amenorrhoea (E17KS receptor)	17q11–q12
Acromegaly, somatotrophinoma ($G_s\alpha$)	20q13.2
Pseudohypoparathyroidism ($G_s\alpha$)	20q13.2
McCune–Albright syndrome ($G_s\alpha$)	20q13.2
Nephrogenic diabetes insipidus (AVP type II receptor)	Xq28
Vitamin D-dependent rickets type II (VDDRII) (vitamin D receptor)	12q12–q14
Thyroid hormone resistance (thyroid hormone receptor β)	3p24.1–p22
Primary cortisol resistance (glucocorticoid receptor)	5q31–q32
Pseudohypoaldosteronism (mineralocorticoid receptor)	4q31
Testicular feminization (androgen receptor)	Xq12

continued

Table 2.1 *continued*

Disorder	Chromosomal location
Metabolic disorders and syndromes	
Dent disease	Xp11.22
Hypertension (angiotensiogen)	1q42–q43
Kalmann (X-linked)	Xp22.32
Kalmann (autosomal)	7q22 or 12q24
Lesch–Nyhan	Xq26.1
Menke	Xq13.2–q13.3
Phenylketonuria (PKU)	12q22–q24.2
Prader–Willi	15q11.2–q12
Wilson	13q14.2–q21
X-linked recessive nephrolithiasis (XRN)	Xp11.22

fragment length polymorphisms (RFLPs) [33], another two are the result of point mutations [34] and one is due to a variation in the length of a microsatellite repetitive sequence in intron 1 [35]. These polymorphisms are inherited in a Mendelian manner and are thus useful as genetic markers in family studies, so it is useful to consider these polymorphisms in greater detail.

Table 2.2 The hypoparathyroid disorders and their chromosomal localization

Disorder	Inheritance	Chromosomal location
Isolated hypoparathyroidism	Autosomal dominant	11p15*
	Autosomal recessive	11p15*
	X-linked recessive	Xq26–q27
Associated complex congenital syndrome		
DiGeorge	Autosomal dominant	22q11
Kenney–Caffey	Autosomal dominant†	?
Barakat	Autosomal recessive†	?
Lymphoedema	Autosomal recessive†	?
Nephropathy, nerve deafness	Autosomal dominant	?
	Autosomal recessive	?
Dysmorphology, growth failure	Autosomal recessive†	?
Pluriglandular autoimmune syndrome	Autosomal recessive	?
Pseudohypoparathyroidism	Autosomal dominant	20q13.2

* Mutation of PTH gene identified only in some families.
† Most likely inheritance shown.
? Location not known.

RESTRICTION FRAGMENT LENGTH POLYMORPHISMS

Restriction fragment length polymorphisms (RFLPs) are the result of variations in the primary DNA sequence of individuals, and may be due to either single base changes, or deletions or additions or translocation. These changes in DNA sequence occur frequently (approximately once in every 250 bp), usually in the non-coding regions, do not affect gene function and are often at a distance away from the disease gene [37]. Four such mutations are known to be associated with polymorphisms of the PTH gene. Two of these point mutations, designated Mir1 and Mir2, which were respectively due to transition of an adenine (A) to guanine (G) residue in intron 1 and to a transversion of cytosine (C) to adenine (A) in exon 3, were revealed by altered migration of amplified preproPTH gene fragments through denaturing gels [34].

The other two point mutations were detected because they were associated with the presence or absence of a cleavage site for a restriction enzyme [33]. Restriction enzymes are derived from microorganisms and found to cleave DNA in a sequence-specific manner. For example,

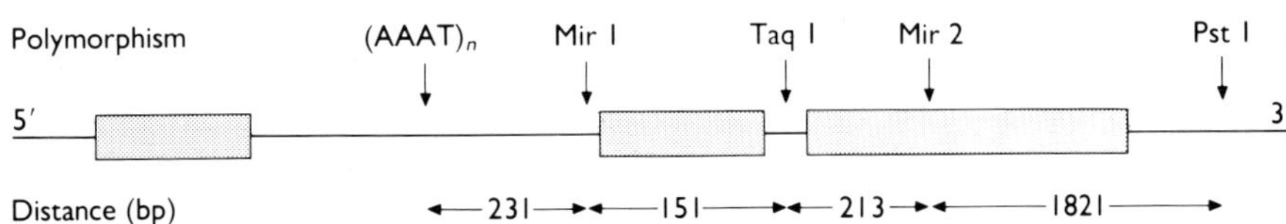

Fig. 2.1 Schematic representation of the PTH gene. The PTH gene consists of three exons and two introns with the order 5′–exon 1–intron 1–exon 2–intron 2–exon 3–3′. The three exons of the PTH gene are shown as shaded boxes and the introns as lines. The polymorphic sites associated with the PTH gene are indicated. Two RFLPs are associated with the PTH gene, and the TaqI polymorphic site is within intron 2 and the PstI polymorphic site is 1.7 Kbp downstream in the 3′ direction of the gene [33]. Two internal polymorphic mutations [34] of the PTH gene designated Mir1 and Mir2 are respectively located in intron 1 and exon 3, and the tetranucleotide $(AAAT)_n$ polymorphism is in intron 1 [35]. The distance between the tetranucleotide $(AAAT)_n$ polymorphism and the polymorphic Mir1 mutation is 231 bp; that between the Mir1 mutation and the TaqI RFLP site is 152 bp, that between the TaqI RFLP site and the polymorphic Mir2 mutation is 213 bp, and that between the Mir2 mutation and the PstI RFLP site is 1821 bp. Linkage disequilibrium between the $(AAAT)_n$, TaqI and PstI polymorphic sites has been established [35] (from Thakker [36]).

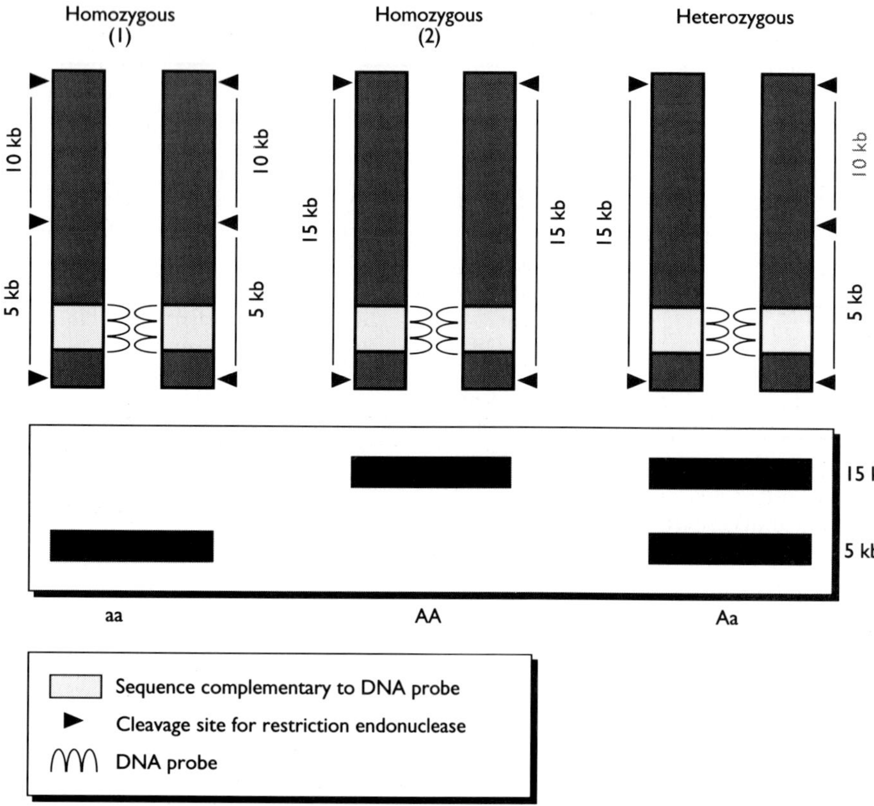

Fig. 2.2 Schematic representation of RFLPs resulting from variations in the number of restriction endonuclease sites. The upper panel represents a pair of chromosomal DNA segments from three individuals – two of whom are homozygous (1) and (2) and one of whom is heterozygous – for the polymorphisms. The lower panel represents the bands, that is RFLPs, revealed on autoradiography and the upper 15 kb RFLP has been designated allele 'A' and the lower 5 kb RFLP has been designated allele 'a' (from Thakker [36]).

the enzyme *Eco*RI, which originated from *Escherichia coli*, will cleave only if the sequence GAATTC is present, and then it will cleave specifically (↓) between the adenine (A) and guanine (G) residues, G ↓ AATTC. A DNA polymorphism, such as a single base change in this sequence, would result in loss of an enzyme cleavage site, and this would be revealed as an RFLP as follows [38].

A restriction enzyme is used to cleave human leukocyte DNA and the resulting DNA fragments are separated according to size by agarose gel electrophoresis, the smaller size fragments migrating furthest away from the cathode. The DNA fragments are then transferred by Southern blotting [39] to a nylon membrane. Digested fragments of single-stranded human DNA are thus immobilized according to size (fragment length) on the membrane, which is next hybridized with a single-stranded, radiolabelled DNA probe. The labelled DNA probe will anneal to any fragments which have a complementary sequence and these restricted fragments of varying lengths are revealed by autoradiography. The exact number and size of RELPs will vary from individual to individual in relation to the number of recognition sites for the restriction enzyme, as shown in Fig. 2.2. In this example the DNA sequence of individual (1) has three restriction enzyme cleavage sites and, following digestion, fragments of two sizes will result. One fragment size will be 5 kb in length and the other fragment size will be 10 kb in length. The labelled DNA probe will hybridize only to the 5 kb fragments, which contain a complementary sequence, and autoradiography will therefore only reveal one band, the RFLP, at 5 kb. However, in individual (2) there has been a loss of one restriction enzyme cleavage site, due to a change in the DNA sequence, and following digestion only restriction fragments of 15 kb will result. A single 15 kb RFLP is observed at autoradiography. The heterozygous individual who has one chromosome with three cleavage sites and another with two cleavage sites, will reveal two RFLPs at autoradiography, one at 15 kb and one at 5 kb.

Alleles can be designated to these RFLPs; for example, individual (1) who has the smaller RFLP is designated as having allele 'aa', individual (2) who has the larger RFLP is designated 'AA', and the heterozygous individual with both the large and smaller RFLPs is 'Aa'. Such RFLPs have been detected at the PTH locus by the two restriction endonucleases TaqI and PstI. The TaqI-derived RFLPs are 2.5 and 2.4 kb in size and the PstI-derived RFLPs are 2.7 and 2.2 kb in size [33]. These RFLPs and the polymorphic point mutations, Mirl and Mir2, are useful genetic markers for linkage studies, as they are inherited in a

Mendelian manner and their inheritance can be followed together with a disease in an affected family.

MICROSATELLITE POLYMORPHISMS

The use of many of the currently available DNA probes used to detect either RFLPs or variable numbers of tandem repeats (VNTRs) in minisatellite sequences by Southern blotting is often limited since they are not highly polymorphic, and information from the marker locus is not obtained for family studies. In order to gain maximal genetic information from the limited number of families with clinical disorders such as hypoparathyroidism, highly polymorphic genetic markers are required. The PCR is useful in the detection of DNA sequence polymorphisms by revealing length variations in microsatellite tandem repeats [40], for example $(CA)_n$, where $n = 10-60$. In addition to tandem repeats in the sequence (CA), microsatellite tandem repeats consisting of $(AT)_n$, $(GA)_n$, $(ATT)_n$, $(ATTT)_n$, $(AAAT)_n$ and the hexanucleotide $[T(Pu)T(Pu)T(Pu)]_n$ have also been reported [35,40]. These tandem repeats, which are highly polymorphic and are inherited in a Mendelian manner, are estimated to occur once in every 50–100 Kbp. Thus, they are a valuable technique in obtaining a detailed genetic map around a disease locus, for example hypoparathyroidism.

In this technique oligonucleotide primers are synthesized on either side of the repeat, and PCR is used to amplify the repeat sequence (Fig. 2.3). The smaller and larger fragment length polymorphisms in these repetitive sequences are detected by separation, either on a polyacrylamide sequencing gel or an agarose gel respectively. The use of one such polymorphic tetranucleotide ($(AAAT)_n$) repetitive sequence from intron 1 of the PTH gene [35] is illustrated in Fig. 2.4.

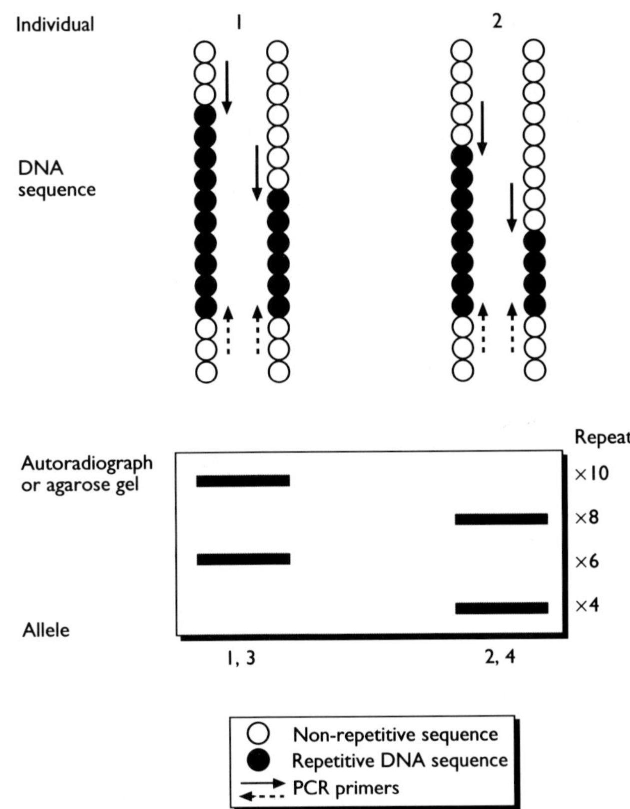

Fig. 2.3 Schematic representation of polymorphisms in microsatellite tandem repetitive DNA sequences, which may consist, for example, of the dinucleotide CA, or the trinucleotide ATT, or the tetranucleotide AAAT, or the hexanucleotide TATATG. Oligonucleotide primers (→, ⇠) corresponding to the nonrepetitive sequences (○) on either side of the repetitive DNA sequence (●) are synthesized and the PCR is utilized to amplify the repeat in genomic DNA obtained from different individuals. The resulting PCR products are separated either by polyacrylamide gel or agarose gel electrophoresis, and the polymorphisms are revealed by autoradiography or by viewing of an ethidium bromide-stained agarose gel under ultraviolet light. Thus, of the pair of chromosomes from individual (1), one has 10 repeats and the other has six repeats, whereas of the pair of chromosomes from individual (2), one has eight repeats and the other has four repeats. Following PCR amplification and separation by gel electrophoresis, these variations in the length of the repeats will be revealed by differences in the size of the bands, which have been designated alleles; for example, the larger band consisting of 10 repeats is designated allele 1, and those consisting of eight, six and four repeats are designated alleles 2, 3 and 4 respectively. These microsatellite tandem repetitive sequences, which are highly polymorphic, show Mendelian inheritance (Fig. 2.4) and can be used as genetic markers in family linkage studies. Such a polymorphic microsatellite consisting of the sequence $(AAAT)_n$ has been identified in intron 1 of the PTH gene [35] (from Thakker [1]).

Family studies

PTH gene polymorphisms have been used in segregation studies of families affected with autosomal dominant and recessive forms of isolated hypoparathyroidism, and abnormalities of the PTH gene were excluded in 50% of the families by demonstrating recombination between the disease and the PTH gene [22,34,35,41]. However, in families which revealed cosegregation of hypoparathyroidism and the PTH locus, restriction endonuclease studies did not reveal an absence of the PTH gene or abnormal restriction patterns, suggesting major structural rearrangements, deletions or insertions in the DNA of affected individuals [22,25,35,42]. Detailed sequence analysis of the PTH gene was therefore undertaken, and the results from patients of four families, two with autosomal dominant [32,43] and two with autosomal recessive isolated hypoparathyroidism, have been reported [25,35].

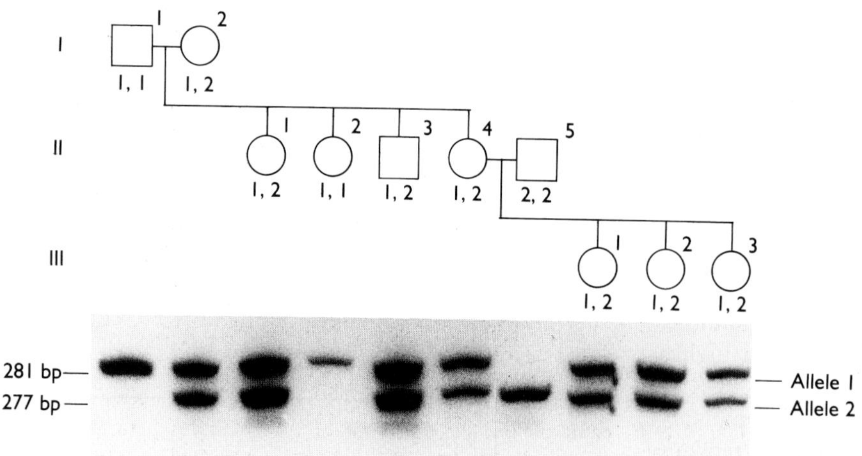

Fig. 2.4 Mendelian inheritance of the tetranucleotide $(AAAT)_n$ polymorphism associated with the PTH gene. The presence of the tandem repeat $(AAAT)_5$ was revealed by the 281 bp fragment (allele 1) and that of $(AAAT)_4$ was revealed by the 277 bp fragment (allele 2). An analysis of the inheritance of these alleles is shown for family 18/92, which is of northern European origin and is not affected with hypoparathyroidism. The family is drawn so that each individual appears above his or her alleles and the genotype is indicated for each individual. The grandmother (I.2) is heterozygous (allele 1,2) and the grandfather (I.1) is homozygous (allele 1,1). An examination of their children and grandchildren reveals Mendelian inheritance of the alleles (from Thakker [36]).

AUTOSOMAL DOMINANT ISOLATED HYPOPARATHYROIDISM

DNA sequence analysis of the PTH gene from one patient with autosomal dominant isolated hypoparathyroidism has revealed a single base substitution (T → C) in exon 2 [32]. This resulted in the substitution of arginine (**CGT**) for cysteine (**TGT**) in the amino acid signal peptide. A mutation involving the signal peptide is of importance since signal sequences, which are present in the precursors of most secreted proteins, are required for correct processing of the protein through the cell's secretory pathway. This entails delivery of the protein to the outer membrane of the endoplasmic reticulum (ER) where the protein undergoes insertion and translocation, during which the signal peptide is cleaved of the protein. In order to facilitate this passage through the ER membrane the signal peptide contains predominantly hydrophobic amino acids. However, the T → C mutation in the patient with hypoparathyroidism would result in the presence of arginine, which is a charged amino acid, in the midst of the hydrophobic core of the signal peptide, and this would impede the translocation of the preproPTH protein.

The processing of this mutant preproPTH has been assessed [32] by *in vitro* translation studies using recombinant plasmids which contained either the normal or mutant form of preproPTH cDNA. The results of this study [32] revealed that RNA was transcribed from the cDNAs, and that both normal and mutant PTH RNA were translated efficiently to the protein. However, the processing of the mutant preproPTH protein to the proPTH protein was greatly impaired, thereby revealing the genetic and cellular basis of hypoparathyroidism in this patient.

The PTH gene sequence has also been investigated in another family with autosomal dominant hypoparathyroidism associated with sensorineural deafness and renal dysplasia [42]. The locations of the PTH gene and a gene encoding renal development, the Wilms tumour gene, in 11p15 and 11p13 respectively, suggested this region as a candidate for genetic abnormalities in the family. A detailed analysis of the PTH gene revealed no abnormalities, and the results of this and other studies indicate that there is likely to be considerable genetic and molecular heterogeneity in autosomal dominant isolated hypoparathyroidism.

AUTOSOMAL RECESSIVE ISOLATED HYPOPARATHYROIDISM

Autosomal recessive hypoparathyroidism has usually arisen in families with consanguineous marriages [25,35, 43]. Abnormalities in the PTH gene have been sought, and a donor splice site mutation at the exon 2/intron 2 boundary has been identified in one such family [25]. This mutation involved a single base substitution (**g** → **c**) at position 1 of intron 1, and this altered the invariant **gt** dinucleotide of the 5′ donor splice site [44] consensus sequence (**gtaagt**) [45] (Fig. 2.5). The mutation resulted in the occurrence of a DdeI restriction enzyme site (**ctaag**), and this facilitated the detection of this donor splice mutation in other members of the family (Fig. 2.6). The donor splice site mutation of the PTH gene, which was found to segregate with hypoparathyroidism in this family, is of importance as it would alter the consensus sequence (**gtaagt**) which is complementary to the sequence of the small ribonucléoprotein (snRNP) designated U1 [46–48]. The U1-snRNP is the 5′ recognition component of the nuclear RNA splicing enzyme, which forms base

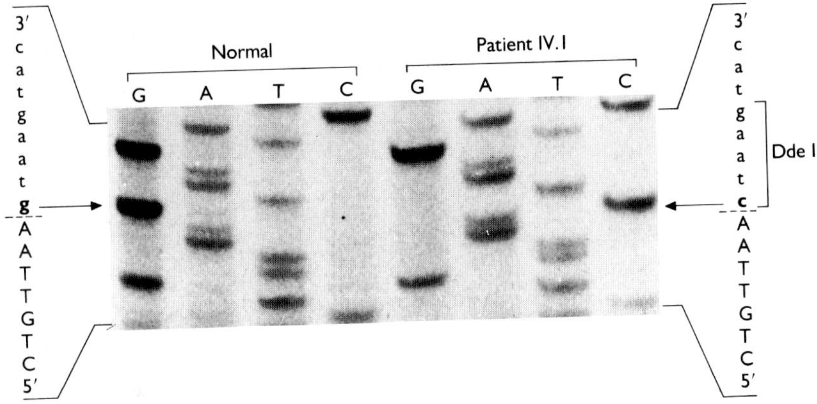

Fig. 2.5 Direct sequence analysis of genomic DNA amplified by the PCR. The autoradiographs show the nucleotide sequences of the PTH exon 2/intron 2 boundary obtained from a normal individual and patient IV.1 (Fig. 2.6) who suffers from autosomal recessive idiopathic hypoparathyroidism. The exon sequence is indicated by upper-case letters, the intron sequence is indicated by lower-case letters and the exon/intron boundary is shown (----). At the first base of intron 2 (indicated by arrow), there is a guanine (g) residue in the DNA sequence of the normal individual. However, in patient IV.1 this g residue is absent and has been replaced by a cytosine (c) residue. Thus, there has been a single base substitution (**g** → **c**), and this has altered the normal consensus 5′ donor splice site sequence (gtaagt). This mutation has resulted in the occurrence of a DdeI restriction enzyme site (**c** ↓ taag) in the DNA of the patient, and this has facilitated the detection of this donor splice mutation in other members of the family (Fig. 2.6). The demonstration of a donor splice site mutation in the PTH gene of the patient indicates that hypoparathyroidism may be associated with an abnormality in PTH mRNA processing (from Parkinson & Thakker [25]).

pairs with the 5′ and 3′ ends of an intron so as to align these terminal regions for cutting and splicing.

Thus, an alteration of the complementary 5′ donor splice site sequence of the intron will affect annealing of the U1-snRNP, and previous studies of β-thalassaemia have demonstrated that such mutations are associated with abnormalities of mRNA processing [49–51] in which there is an accumulation of unspliced precursor mRNA, retention of incompletely spliced precursors, a complete absence of transcripts or the appearance of aberrantly processed mRNA which had resulted from the utilization of alternative normally occurring 5′ splice sites or from the use of cryptic splice sites. *In vitro* studies utilizing the human adenovirus late transcription unit [52] and the rat preprotachykinin gene [53] have additionally demonstrated that alterations at an internal exon/intron boundary result in the splicing out of the exon together with its adjacent introns. This form of abnormal splicing out of the exon has been referred to as 'exon skipping'.

These possibilities were investigated in the hypoparathyroid patient who had inherited a 5′ donor splice site mutation (Fig. 2.6) of the PTH gene by a study of mRNA processing. However, PTH gene expression is usually confined to the parathyroid glands which were not available from these patients. Thus, a novel method which entailed the detection of PTH gene expression by PCR in cultured lymphocytes was utilized (Fig. 2.7).

The detection by PCR of a low level of transcription of a tissue-specific gene in cells that do not exhibit a physiological expression of the gene has been referred to as either 'non-tissue-specific' or 'ectopic' or 'illegitimate' transcription [55–57]. For example, such non-tissue-specific transcription of the Duchenne muscular dystrophy (DMD) gene encoding dystrophin, which is physiologically expressed only in muscle, has been observed to occur in fibroblasts, lymphoblastoid cells, HepG2 hepatoma cell lines and peripheral blood lymphocytes [58,59]. Additional studies have demonstrated that such ectopic transcription with correct splicing of the mRNA also occurs for other highly tissue-specific genes which encode clotting factor VIIIc, β-globin, anti-Müllerian hormone and aldolase A [56]. The extent of the non-tissue-specific expression of these genes has been estimated [55,56,58,] to be one molecule of correctly spliced mRNA per 1000 cells, and the physiological relevance and mechanisms involved in this low level of ectopic transcription are not known.

It has been postulated that the promoter regions of a tissue-specific gene may be activated by some of the ubiquitous transcriptional factors, for example, TATA box factors and CAAT box-binding proteins in the absence of the respective tissue-specific transcriptional factors [56]. The binding of these ubiquitous transcriptional factors to their respective DNA elements would be facilitated by the chromatin disruption that occurs during DNA replication, and non-tissue-specific transcription has been observed to be greater in actively proliferating lymphoblasts than in confluent fibroblasts [56]. The demonstration of non-tissue-specific transcription is of medical importance since it enables the use of easily accessible peripheral blood lymphocytes for the detection of abnormalities in mRNA

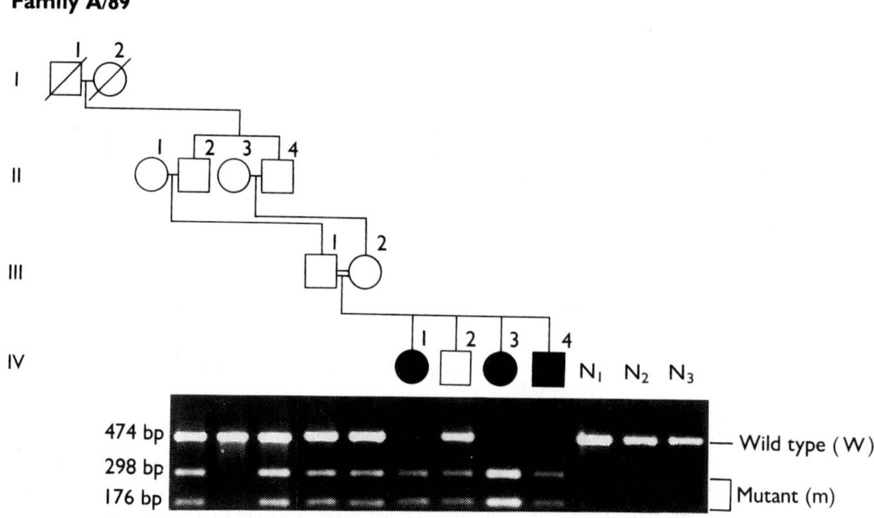

Fig. 2.6 DdeI restriction enzyme analysis in family A/89 detects a donor splice site mutation in the PTH gene. Family A/89, which is of Bangladeshi origin, is shown in the upper panel with each individual appearing above his or her DNA fragments. Nine members from three generations of the family in which the parents (III.1 and III.2) of the affected children (IV.1, IV.3 and IV.4) are consanguineous were investigated, together with 10 unrelated normal (N_n) Bangladeshi individuals. Genomic DNA was prepared using peripheral blood leukocytes from each individual, and the 474 bp PTH gene segment spanning the exon 2/intron 2 region was amplified by PCR. The PCR product was incubated with DdeI and the samples were analysed by electrophoresis on a 1.4% agarose gel stained with ethidium bromide to enable visualization of the DNA fragments, which are shown on the lower panel. The results from all of the 10 normal individuals (results from N_1, N_2 and N_3 are shown) revealed that the 474 bp PCR product was not cleaved with DdeI, and this 474 bp fragment was designated the wild-type (**W**) allele. However, the presence of the DdeI site in the patients (IV.1, IV.3 and IV.4) was revealed as cleavage by DdeI resulted in two fragments of 298 bp and 176 bp, which were designated mutant (**m**) alleles. In the unaffected members (II.2, II.4, III.1, III.2 and IV.2) of the family both the normal 474 bp fragment and the abnormal 298 bp and 176 bp fragments were detected, indicating heterozygosity. Thus, the unrelated normals are homozygous (**WW**) for the wild-type allele, the patients are homozygous (**mm**) for the mutant allele and the unaffected family members heterozygous (**Wm**). These results demonstrate that a g→c donor splice site mutation, which is detected by DdeI, in the PTH gene segregates with hypoparathyroidism (from Parkinson & Thakker [25]).

processing and thereby avoids the requirement for expressing tissue that may only be obtainable by biopsy. Advantage was taken of these methods to demonstrate abnormal processing of PTH mRNA in patients with autosomal recessive isolated hypoparathyroidism, who were shown to have the donor splice site mutation in the PTH gene [25].

The non-tissue-specific transcription of the PTH gene was demonstrated from cultured lymphocytes as illustrated in Fig. 2.7. An analysis of the PTH cDNA obtained from normal and hypoparathyroid individuals (Fig. 2.8) revealed a mutant PTH cDNA from the hypoparathyroid patients which was 90 bp smaller, a size that corresponded to that of exon 2. In addition, DNA sequence analysis of the wild-type or normal PTH cDNA sequence revealed a correctly spliced PTH cDNA with the order exon 1–exon 2–exon 3. However, DNA sequence analysis of the mutant PTH cDNA from the patient with autosomal recessive hypoparathyroidism demonstrated exon skipping, in which exon 2 was lost and exon 1 was spliced to exon 3. Thus, the donor splice site mutation, which is at the exon 2/intron 2 boundary, led to an abnormality of mRNA processing in which the other normally occurring 5′ donor splice site at the exon 1/intron 1 boundary was utilized to splice exon 1 to exon 3. The resulting abnormal mRNA transcript lacked exon 2 and this led to a loss of the initiation codon and the signal peptide sequence which are required respectively for the commencement of PTH mRNA translation [60] and for the translocation [61] of the PTH peptide. These findings thus defined the molecular pathology of the PTH gene which caused autosomal recessive idiopathic hypoparathyroidism in this family. In addition, the demonstration of the non-tissue-specific expression of the PTH gene in cultured lymphocytes avoided the requirement for parathyroid tissue biopsies, and use of this method will help to characterize further defects in the processing of PTH mRNA which may cause disorders of parathyroid activity.

The PTH gene sequence has been similarly investigated [35] in another consanguineous family with autosomal recessive hypoparathyroidism associated with renal insufficiency and developmental delay [43]. Abnormalities of the PTH gene were not found, and other loci at which mutations may affect the embryological development, cell

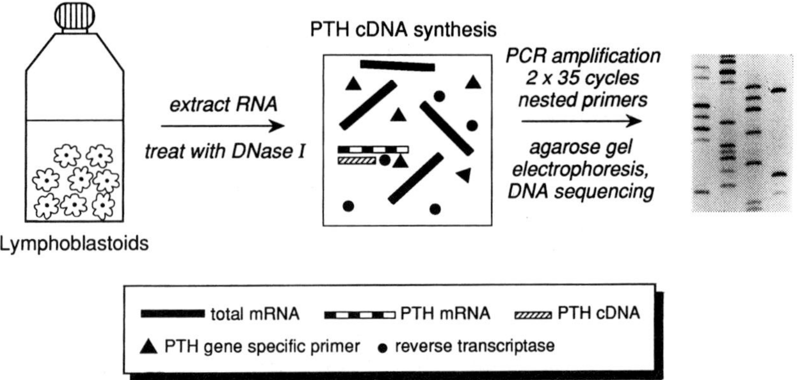

Fig. 2.7 Schematic representation for the detection of 'illegitimate' or 'non-tissue-specific' transcription of the PTH gene by use of PCR. Epstein–Barr virus (EBV) transformed lymphocytes were cultured and total RNA was extracted and treated with DNase I to remove any contaminating DNA. A specific first-strand cDNA copy of the PTH mRNA sequence was made by using a PTH gene-specific oligonucleotide as a primer for the avian myeloblastosis virus (AMV) reverse transcriptase. The yield of the reverse transcribed PTH cDNA was increased by two rounds of PCR amplification in which two pairs of nested primers were used to enhance the sensitivity and specificity of the amplification. On completion the PCR amplification products were analysed by agarose gel electrophoresis (Fig. 2.8) and by direct DNA sequencing [25] (from Parkinson & Thakker [54]).

structure or regulation of the parathyroids need to be elucidated.

X-LINKED RECESSIVE HYPOPARATHYROIDISM

Isolated hypoparathyroidism has been reported to occur as an X-linked recessive disorder in two multigeneration kindreds [26,28] from Missouri, USA. Affected males suffered from infantile onset of epilepsy and hypocalcaemia due to an isolated defect of parathyroid gland development [62]. Linkage studies utilizing X-linked RFLPs in these families have localized [27] the mutant gene to the distal end of the long arm of the X chromosome to band Xq26–Xq27 by establishing linkage between hypoparathyroidism and an MspI-derived RFLP for the probe 4D.8, which defines the locus DXS98. An example of the inheritance of

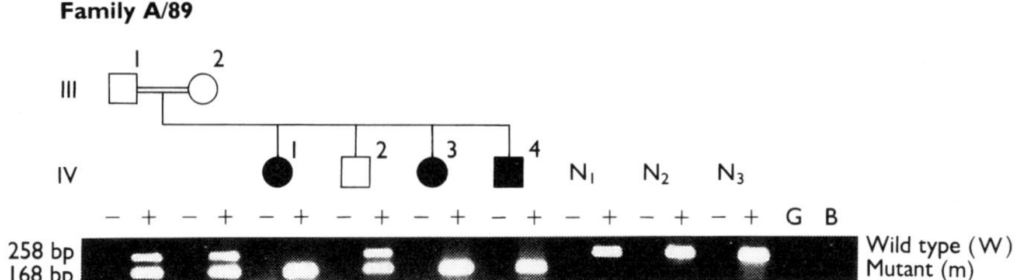

Fig. 2.8 Non-tissue-specific transcription of the PTH gene revealed by detection of PTH cDNA in cultured lymphocytes. The ectopic transcription of the PTH gene in EBV-transformed lymphocytes was detected by PCR amplification of PTH cDNA (Fig. 2.7), which had been synthesized by addition (+) of the enzyme reverse transcriptase to extracts of RNA obtained from Epstein–Barr virus (EBV) transformed lymphocytes of normal and affected individuals. The samples were analysed by electrophoresis on a 1.5% agarose gel stained with ethidium bromide to enable visualization of the PTH cDNA fragments which are shown on the lower panel with the respective family member or control shown above. In 10 normal individuals (N_1 to N_3 shown), the PCR-amplified PTH cDNA was observed at the expected size of 258 bp. This product was not present when reverse transcriptase was omitted (–) from the reaction, or when only genomic DNA (G) or a water blank (B) were used, thereby demonstrating that this product is not due to amplification of a genomic sequence but is RNA specific. Thus, non-tissue-specific transcription of the PTH gene was demonstrated to occur in lymphocytes. In family A/89 the affected individuals (IV.1, IV.3 and IV.4) who were homozygous for the donor splice site mutation (Fig. 2.6) were found to differ from the normals in having an abnormal PTH cDNA of 168 bp in size. Thus, the mutant (m) PTH cDNA differed from the normal or wild type (W) by 90 bp, which corresponds to the size of exon 2. The parents (III.1 and III.2) and the unaffected sibling (IV.2) who are heterozygous for the mutation (Fig. 2.6) have both the mutant and wild-type PTH cDNA. Thus, the donor splice site mutation causing hypoparathyroidism in this family is associated with an abnormal PTH cDNA, which indicates an alteration in the processing of PTH mRNA (from Parkinson & Thakker [25]).

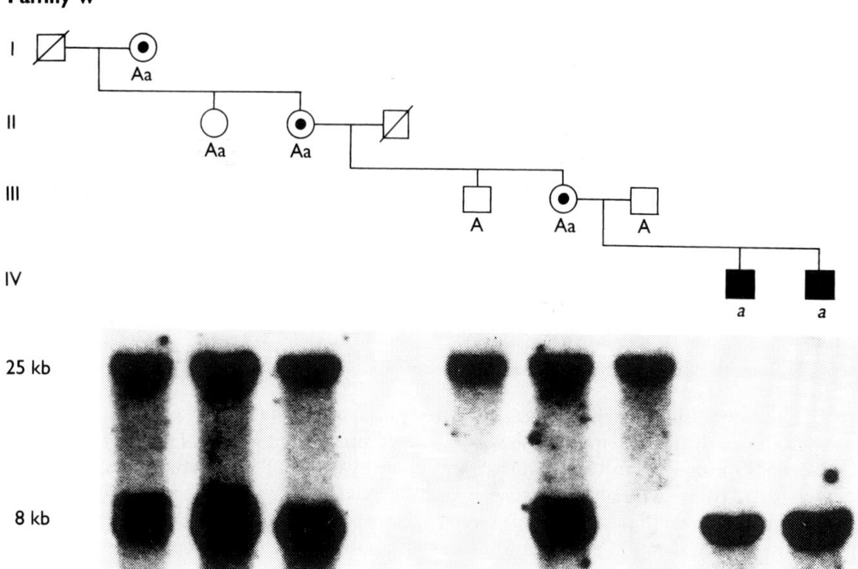

Fig. 2.9 Autoradiograph obtained in eight of the 50 members from family W [28] with X-linked recessive hypoparathyroidism in which the X-linked probe 4D.8 has been hybridized to genomic DNA digested with the enzyme MspI to reveal RFLPs. The detection of RFLPs and the designation of alleles has been described earlier, and illustrated in Fig. 2.2. The 25 kb allele is designated allele 'A' and the 8 kb allele is designated allele 'a'; however, it is important to note that males have one X chromosome only, and are thus hemizygous at this X-linked locus. The family tree is drawn so that each member appears above his or her RFLP pattern. Analysis reveals that the disease is segregating with the 8 kb allele (a). □, Normal male; ■, affected male; ○ normal female; ⊙, carrier female (from Thakker [36]).

hypoparathyroidism and the RFLPs obtained with probe 4D.8 is shown in a portion of one of the families [28] designated family W (Fig. 2.9). In this family, the two sons in generation IV were affected and had allele 'a'. Their mother, grandmother and great-grandmother were all carriers and were heterozygous for allele 'Aa', while their uncle in generation III was unaffected and had allele 'A'. These results indicated that the disease was segregating with the 8 kb allele 'a', and the probability in favour of linkage between hypoparathyroidism and the 4D.8 (DXS98) locus exceeded 6500 to 1. It is useful to consider the results of this linkage analysis in greater detail.

Linkage analysis

RFLPs are inherited in a Mendelian manner, and their inheritance can be followed together with a disease in an affected family. The consistent inheritance of an RFLP allele with the disease indicates that the two genetic loci are close together, i.e. linked. Genes that are far apart do not consistently co-segregate, but show recombination because of the crossing-over during meiosis. By studying recombination events in family studies, the distance between two genes and the probability that they are linked can be ascertained [63,64]. The distance between two genes is expressed as the recombination fraction (θ), which is equal to the number of recombinants divided by the total number of offspring resulting from informative meioses within a family. The value of the recombination fraction can range from 0 to 0.5. A value of zero indicates that the genes are very closely linked, while a value of 0.5 indicates that the genes are far apart and not linked.

The probability that the two loci are linked at these distances is expressed as a LOD score, which is $\log_{10}$ of the odds ratio favouring linkage. The odds ratio favouring linkage is defined as the likelihood that two loci are linked at a specified recombination (θ) versus the likelihood that the two loci are not linked. A LOD score of +3, which indicates a probability in favour of linkage of 1000 to 1, establishes linkage between two loci, and a LOD score of −2, indicating a probability against linkage of 100 to 1, is taken to exclude linkage between two loci. LOD scores are usually evaluated over a range of recombination fractions, thereby enabling the genetic distance and the maximum (or peak) probability favouring linkage between two loci to be ascertained. A fuller description of linkage in families with inherited metabolic and endocrine disorders has been previously described [65].

Location of the X-linked recessive hypoparathyroid gene

The results from linkage analysis in family W [28], in which isolated hypoparathyroidism had been inherited in an X-linked recessive manner for five generations, are shown in Fig. 2.10. A total of 50 members (four affected, seven carriers and 39 unaffected) were studied with 17 X-linked genetic markers of which 11 were informative. Linkage between hypoparathyroidism and the 4D.8 locus was established [27] with a peak LOD score of 3.82 ($\theta = 0.05$), indicating a probability in favour of linkage in excess of 6500 to 1. All the other X-linked RFLP loci gave negative or low (that is < 3) LOD scores, although many of these are also in the distal segment (Xq26–q27) of the long arm of the X chromosome. Thus, the gene causing X-

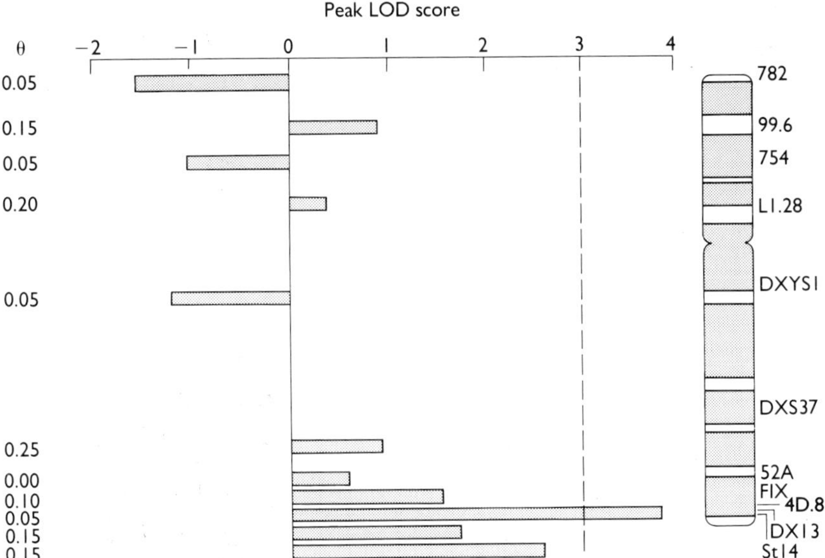

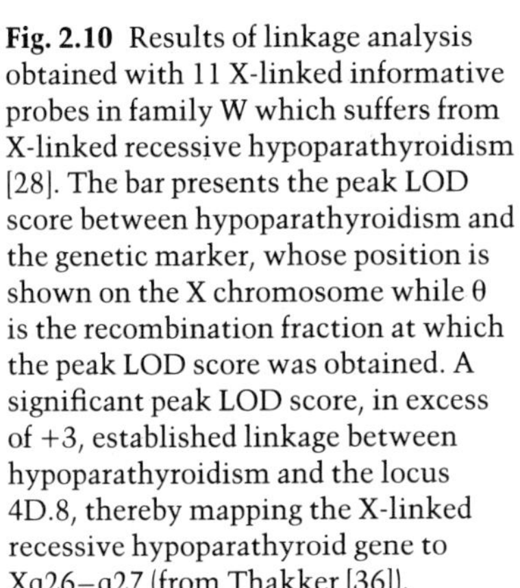
Fig. 2.10 Results of linkage analysis obtained with 11 X-linked informative probes in family W which suffers from X-linked recessive hypoparathyroidism [28]. The bar presents the peak LOD score between hypoparathyroidism and the genetic marker, whose position is shown on the X chromosome while θ is the recombination fraction at which the peak LOD score was obtained. A significant peak LOD score, in excess of +3, established linkage between hypoparathyroidism and the locus 4D.8, thereby mapping the X-linked recessive hypoparathyroid gene to Xq26–q27 (from Thakker [36]).

linked recessive hypoparathyroidism was mapped to the distal region of the long arm of the X chromosome, band Xq26–q27, where the DNA probe 4D.8 had been previously localized. An analysis of recombination events within this distal segment of the long arm of the X chromosome helped to further localize the hypoparathyroid locus [27].

The pedigree in Fig. 2.11 shows 40 members (29 surviving and 11 deceased) in five generations from family W [28] with genetic marker data. The pedigree is informative for five X-linked RFLP loci, whose order in the region Xq25–Xq28 has been established as Xcen–DXS37–F9–DXS98–DXS52–DXS15–Xqter, and multipoint crosses exist. Individual IV.4 is a carrier mother heterozygous for F9, DXS98, DXS52 and DXS15, and the alleles which she has inherited from her mother (III.2) and father (III.1) can be ascertained by examination of her mother's (III.2) and unaffected brother's (IV.1) genotypes. Her affected son (V.2) shows segregation of the disease with the alleles [N, a, 3, t], defined respectively by the polymorphic loci F9, DXS98, DXS52 and DXS15. Her other affected son (V.1) reveals segregation of hypoparathyroidism (HPT) with the distal loci DXS98, DXS52 and DXS15 [alleles a, 3, t], but demonstrates recombination between hypoparathyroidism and the proximal locus F9 [allele n*]. This observation locates hypoparathyroidism distal to the F9 locus.

Analysis of the 11 children of individual II.4 further helps to localize the hypoparathyroid gene. The affected male III.15 shows that, in this branch of the family, hypoparathyroidism is segregating with the alleles [E, a, 3, t]. His carrier sister III.12 is recombinant for hypoparathyroidism and the distal loci DXS52 and DXS15 and for the proximal locus DXS37 but non-recombinant for DXS98. This observation locates hypoparathyroidism proximal to DXS52 and distal to DXS37.

The combined observations of multipoint cross-overs from III.12 and V.1 locate hypoparathyroidism distal to F9 and proximal to DXS52, that is in the vicinity of DXS98. Examination of the multipoint cross in the unaffected male III.6 locates hypoparathyroidism proximal to DXS98; this individual, who has inherited the alleles [a, 3, t] but has not inherited the disease, demonstrates recombination between hypoparathyroidism and the distal loci DXS98 DXS52 and DXS15, and indicates that the location of hypoparathyroidism is not in the chromosome segment distal to DXS98. Thus, the combined observations from all the multipoint crosses suggest that hypoparathyroidism is located distal to F9 and proximal to DXS98.

The likelihood of this location of hypoparathyroidism versus the other possible locations of the disease within the fixed order Xcen–DXS37–F9–DXS98–DXS52–DXS15–Xqter was quantitatively assessed using the LINKMAP program [65] and a location of the hypoparathyroid gene between DXS98 and F9 was favoured above all other locations [27]. The odds favouring the location of the hypoparathyroid gene proximal to DXS98 were 32 to 1, and those favouring a location distal to F9 were 17 to 1. More recent studies have further defined the genetic map around the hypoparathyroid gene and a region of approximately 400 kb containing this mutant gene has been identified [66].

The mapping of the X-linked idiopathic recessive hypoparathyroid gene to Xq26–Xq27 demonstrates that a mutation at a locus distant from the PTH gene, the location of which is on the short arm of chromosome 11 [30], is involved in altering parathyroid gland function. A

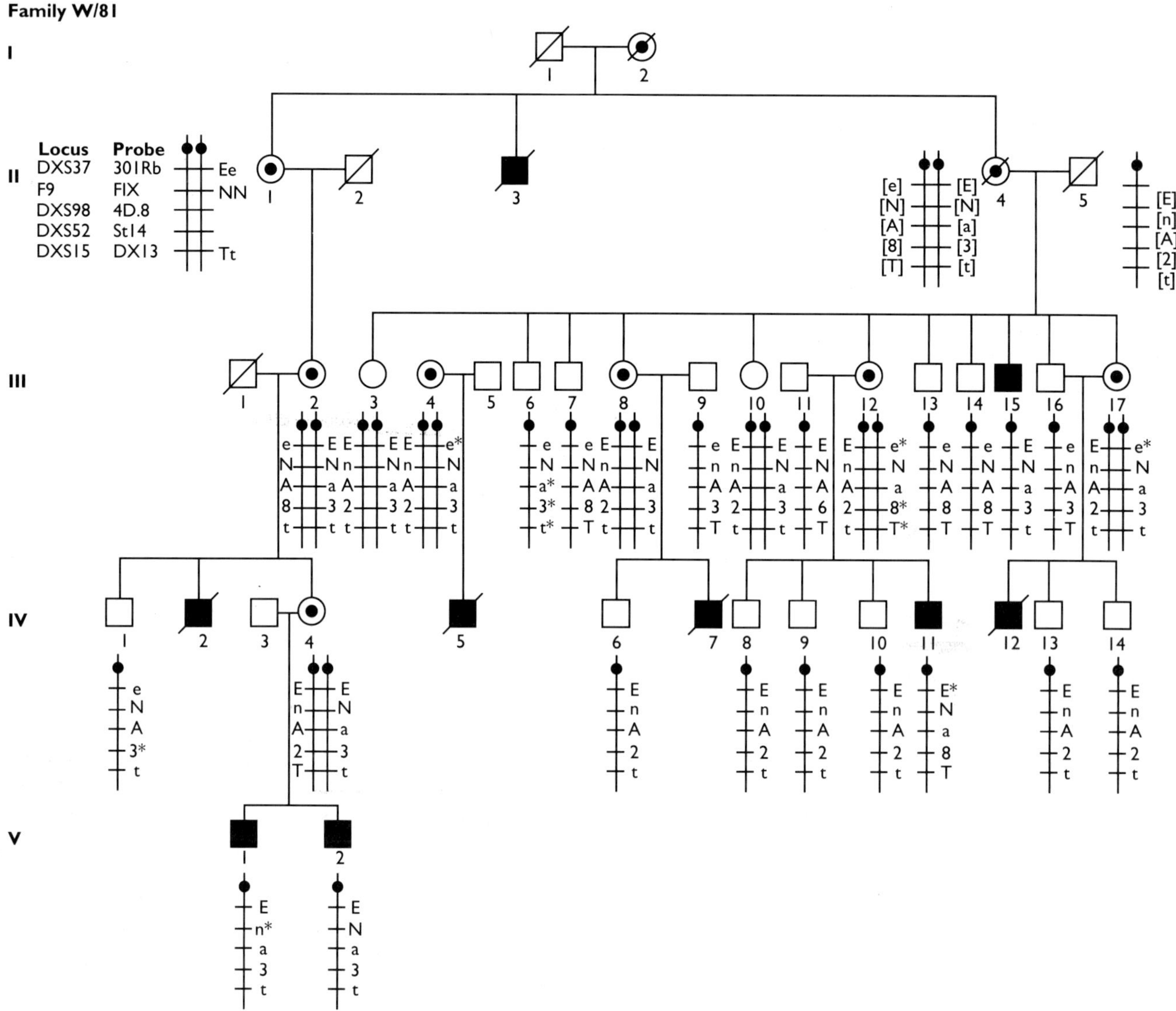

Fig. 2.11 Pedigree from family W, segregating for X-linked recessive idiopathic hypoparathyroidism and distal lòng arm RFLP loci, whose respective alleles are indicated in parentheses: DXS37 (Ee), F9 (Nn), DXS98 (Aa), DXS52 (2,3,6,8) and DXS15 (Tt). The loci are shown in the correct order but not the correct distances apart. Individuals are represented as: unaffected male (□), affected male (■), unaffected female (○) and carrier female (⊙). In some females the inheritance of paternal and maternal alleles can be ascertained, and in these the paternal X chromosome is shown on the left. Recombinants between hypoparathyroidism and each allele are indicated by an asterisk (*). Deduced genotypes are shown in square brackets. Subject IV.4 is a carrier mother who is heterozygous for F9, DXS98, DXS52 and DXS15. Her affected son V.1 is recombinant for hypoparathyroidism and the proximal locus F9 but non-recombinant for DXS98, DXS52 and DXS15. Subject II.4 is a deceased carrier mother whose genotype was deduced from her 11 children. Her carrier daughter III.12 is recombinant for hypoparathyroidism and the distal loci DXS52 and DXS15 and for the proximal locus DXS37, but non-recombinant for F9 and DXS98; whereas the unaffected son III.6 is recombinant for hypoparathyroidism and the distal group of loci DXS98, DXS52 and DXS15, and non-recombinant for the proximal locus DXS37. The minimum number of total recombinants in this pedigree is therefore obtained by locating the hypoparathyroid gene between F9 and DXS98 (from Thakker *et al.* [27]).

possible role for this X-linked gene in parathyroid gland development is suggested by the neonatal or early infantile onset of hypocalcaemic seizures in the two families. This suggests that the disorder may be due to parathyroid agenesis or hypoplasia, and a careful autopsy of a patient from one family has supported this [62]. Thus, the X-linked recessive idiopathic hypoparathyroid gene would appear to be important for the embryological development of the parathyroids, and the situation may be analogous to that occurring in the DiGeorge syndrome. The precise mapping of the X-linked recessive idiopathic hypoparathyroid gene locus to Xq26–Xq27 represents an important step towards understanding this genetic component of parathyroid gland formation, as it has identified the chromosomal segment whose characterization will further elucidate the factors controlling parathyroid development and calcium homeostasis.

COMPLEX SYNDROMES ASSOCIATED WITH HYPOPARATHYROIDISM

Hypoparathyroidism may occur as part of a complex syndrome which may be associated either with a congenital developmental anomaly or with an autoimmune syndrome.

Congenital syndromes

Hypoparathyroidism has been reported to occur in association with the congenital developmental anomalies of the DiGeorge, the Kenney–Caffey and the Barakat syndromes, and also in syndromes associated with either lymphoedema, or renal dysplasia and deafness, or with dysmorphic features and growth failure (see Table 2.2). The inheritance of these congenital disorders, which has been reported in a few patients or a single family, has sometimes not been fully established. However, an autosomal dominant inheritance for the DiGeorge syndrome, which has been investigated by the methods of molecular genetics, is established.

DIGEORGE SYNDROME

Patients with the DiGeorge syndrome suffer from neonatal hypocalcaemic seizures due to PTH deficiency and from severe infections resulting from an immunodeficiency due to thymic aplasia. The disorder arises from a failure of development of the derivatives of the third and fourth pharyngeal pouches, with resulting absence or hypoplasia of the parathyroids and thymus. In addition, deformities of the ear, nose, mouth and aortic arch, and congenital heart defects, may occur. An autosomal dominant inheritance of DiGeorge syndrome has been observed [67] and an association between the syndrome and an unbalanced translocation and deletion involving 22q11 has also been reported in some patients [68,69]; in other patients a deletion of chromosome 10p has been observed in association with the DiGeorge syndrome [70,71]. The 22q11 unbalanced translocation has been further characterized by molecular genetic studies using *in situ* hybridization [72–74] and was found to be proximal to the locus for the immunoglobulin λ-polypeptide constant region, but distal to the locus for the DNA probe D22S9 [75].

Interesting studies of the parental origin or imprinting of the 22q11 unbalanced translocation have revealed that this does not play an important role in the pathogenesis of the DiGeorge syndrome [76]. However, expressed sequences from this region have been isolated; and one of these, T10, encodes a serine/threonine-rich protein of unknown function, which is expressed during early embryogenesis [77]. The other one, ZNF4, encodes a zinc finger DNA-binding motif whose mRNA transcripts are detected in human and mouse embryos but not in adult tissues [78]. The role of these genes in the aetiology of the DiGeorge syndrome, and the embryological development of the parathyroids, is being investigated, together with a mutation involving one of the homeobox genes in the mouse which resulted in a phenotype with shared similarities to the human DiGeorge syndrome [79].

The homeobox genes are a group of genes that specify the body plans of invertebrates such as *Drosophila* and, in all likelihood, vertebrates. In *Drosophila* these homeobox genes specify the identity of cells within each parasegment. The function of the corresponding genes in humans and mice is not known, but as the order of these genes on the chromosomes of *Drosophila*, humans and mice is the same, and because this gene order reflects the order of the anterior boundaries of gene expression along the anteroposterior body axis of the early embryos of all three species, it would appear that these homeobox genes are equally important in mammalian development. In humans and mice this set of 30 or more genes is known collectively as the HOX genes, and they are distributed in the genome in four separate linkage groups, which may have arisen during chordate evolution as the result of two duplications of chromosomal segments [80].

The homeobox genes of *Drosophila* encode transcription factors which share a DNA-binding motif, and these genes act as master switches directing the course of morphogenic development of each segment. As the human and mouse genes share similar homeobox sequences, the HOX proteins are thought to function also as transcriptional factors participating in the specification of regional information in the early mammalian embryo.

In order to determine the genetic function of some of the HOX genes in the mouse, specific mutations have been induced by the use of gene targeting methods in embryo-derived stem (ES) cells. Disruption of the hox 1.5 gene resulted in an abnormal phenotype, which resembled the DiGeorge syndrome [79]. Mice, which were homozygous for the mutation in hox 1.5, died in the neonatal period and were found to be athymic and aparathyroidic, as well as having a wide range of throat abnormalities and a reduction in the mass of the thyroid and submaxillary tissue. In addition, these homozygous mice often suffered from defects of the heart and arteries, as well as craniofacial abnormalities. Mice that were heterozygous were phenotypically normal. Thus, the phenotype of the mice with homozygous mutations of the hox 1.5 gene was very similar to the human DiGeorge syndrome, and this suggests that a HOX gene may be involved in the pathogenesis of the DiGeorge syndrome.

However, the human syndrome is autosomal dominant, whereas the mouse syndrome is autosomal recessive, and the known location of the human hox 1.5 gene to chromosome 7 makes it unlikely that the human hox 1.5 gene is involved in the DiGeorge syndrome, which is associated with deletions and translocations of chromosome 22q11. It is important to note that most patients with the DiGeorge syndrome are karyotypically normal, and it is possible that the DiGeorge syndrome may result from mutations in separate genes. Additional studies of the human and mouse syndromes will help to elucidate this and a possible common developmental pathway.

KENNEY–CAFFEY SYNDROME

Hypoparathyroidism has been reported to occur in over 50% of patients with the Kenney–Caffey syndrome, which is associated with short stature, osteosclerosis and cortical thickening of the long bones, delayed closure of the anterior fontanelle, basal ganglia calcification, nanophthalmus and hyperopia [81,82]. Parathyroid tissue could not be found in a detailed post-mortem examination of one patient [83], and this suggests that hypoparathyroidism may be due to an embryological defect of parathyroid development. A molecular genetic analysis using PTH gene RFLP analysis revealed no abnormalities [84], and mutations at other loci, for example in developmental genes, need to be investigated.

ADDITIONAL FAMILIAL SYNDROMES

Single familial syndromes in which hypoparathyroidism is a component have been reported (see Table 2.2). The inheritance of the disorder in some instances has been established, and molecular genetic analysis of the PTH gene has revealed no abnormalities. Thus, an association of hypoparathyroidism, sensorineural deafness and renal dysplasia has been observed in one British family, in whom an autosomal dominant inheritance of the disorder was established [42]. An analysis of the PTH gene in this family revealed no abnormalities. Autosomal recessive inheritance of hypoparathyroidism in association with renal insufficiency and developmental delay has been reported in one Asian family [43], and a similar analysis of the PTH gene revealed no abnormalities [35]. The occurrence of hypoparathyroidism, nerve deafness and a steroid-resistant nephrosis leading to renal failure, which has been referred to as the Barakat syndrome [85], has been reported in four brothers from one family, and an association of hypoparathyroidism with congenital lymphoedema, nephropathy, mitral valve prolapse and brachytelephalangy has been observed in two brothers from another family [86]. Molecular genetic studies have not been reported from these two families.

A novel syndrome in which hypoparathyroidism was associated with severe growth failure and dysmorphic features has been reported in 12 patients from Saudi Arabia [87]. Consanguinity was noted in 11 of the 12 patients' families, the majority of whom originated from the western province of Saudi Arabia. This syndrome is most likely to be inherited as an autosomal recessive disorder. Molecular genetic investigations of these disorders will help to identify additional genes that regulate the development of the parathyroid glands.

Pluriglandular autoimmune hypoparathyroidism

Hypoparathyroidism may occur in association with moniliasis and autoimmune Addison disease, and the disorder has been referred to either as the autoimmune polyendocrinopathy–candidiasis–ectodermal dystrophy (APECED) syndrome or as the polyglandular autoimmune type 1 syndrome [88]. Additional features of the syndrome include pernicious anaemia, hypothyroidism and occasionally alopecia or vitiligo. A genetic analysis of 58 patients in 42 families indicated autosomal recessive inheritance of the disorder [89], which has a high incidence in Finland. In addition, the disorder has been reported to have a high incidence among Iranian Jews [90], although the occurrence of candidiasis was lower in the Iranian Jews. An association between hypoparathyroidism and the HLA loci, which are located on the short arm of chromosome 6 and which are associated with some autoimmune disorders, has not been established, and the molecular basis of hypoparathyroidism in this syndrome remains to be elucidated.

PSEUDOHYPOPARATHYROIDISM

Patients with pseudohypoparathyroidism are characterized by hypocalcaemia and hyperphosphataemia due to PTH resistance rather than PTH deficiency [91]. The resistance to PTH may be partial or complete, as assessed by the response of urinary cyclic adenosine monophosphate (cAMP) and urinary phosphate excretion to stimulation by intravenous PTH [92]. Patients with complete resistance to PTH demonstrate a lack of increase in urinary cAMP and urinary phosphate excretion, and these patients are referred to as suffering from pseudohypoparathyroidism type I. Patients with a partial resistance to PTH infusion manifested by a marked rise in urinary cAMP, without a phosphaturic response, are referred to as suffering from pseudohypoparathyroidism type II. Some of the patients with pseudohypoparathyroidism type I may also suffer from somatic features, which include short stature, round faces, brachydactyly, mental retardation and subcutaneous ossifications. The association of these abnormal physical features and the biochemical abnormalities is referred to as pseudohypoparathyroidism type Ia, or Albright hereditary osteodystrophy, whereas the sole occurrence of the biochemical features is referred to as pseudohypoparathyroidism type Ib. Patients in whom the somatic features of Albright hereditary osteodystrophy occur without any biochemical abnormalities are referred to as suffering from pseudopseudohypoparathyroidism.

The absence of a normal rise in urinary excretion of cAMP after an injection of PTH in pseudohypoparathyroid patients localized the defect in these patients to the hormone-sensitive adenylate cyclase system which is regulated by at least two G proteins, one of which stimulates ($G_s\alpha$), and another which inhibits ($G_i\alpha$) the activity of the membrane-bound enzyme that catalyses the formation of the intracellular second-messenger cAMP. The G proteins are a family of guanine nucleotide-binding proteins that mediate signal transduction across cell membranes. These proteins couple cell-surface receptors to their second-messenger signal-generation systems and thereby regulate the activity of intracellular effector enzymes and ion channels. The G proteins share a heterotrimeric structure composed of α-, β- and γ-subunits. The β- and γ-subunits are tightly associated with each other as a β–γ complex and appear to be functionally interchangeable among some of the G proteins. The α-subunits are the most diverse and are unique to each G protein. The α-subunit contains the guanine nucleotide-binding site, has intrinsic guanine triphosphatase activity, and is thought to confer specificity on each G protein, thereby allowing it to discriminate among multiple receptors and effectors. A reduced expression or function of the α-subunit of G_s in cells obtained from most patients with pseudohypoparathyroidism type Ia has been demonstrated [93].

Abnormalities in the sequence of the $G_s\alpha$ protein have been demonstrated in patients from one family with pseudohypoparathyroidism type Ia [94]. Immunoblots of erythrocyte membranes from the patients revealed reduced amounts of the normal-sized $G_s\alpha$ protein and the presence of an abnormally larger form of this protein. Restriction endonuclease analysis of the $G_s\alpha$ gene in these patients revealed a mutation in exon 1 of one $G_s\alpha$ allele. PCR amplification of the DNA segment containing exon 1 and direct DNA sequencing revealed that the mutation was associated with an A → G transition at position +1 in one $G_s\alpha$ allele. This mutation alters the initiation codon **A**TG (methionine) to **G**TG (valine), thereby preventing the commencement of translation of the $G_s\alpha$ at the normal site; a translation of the mutant $G_s\alpha$ mRNA would yield a truncated $G_s\alpha$ molecule lacking the amino terminus. Further studies in three other families with pseudohypoparathyroidism type Ia have also identified $G_s\alpha$ mutations [95] in only one allele of the gene, a finding consistent with autosomal dominant inheritance. The $G_s\alpha$ gene has been mapped to the long arm of chromosome 20 [96], and these mutations of the G_s associated with pseudohypoparathyroidism localize this disorder to 20q13.2.

CONCLUSION

Molecular genetics have made it possible to localize, clone and characterize some of the genetic abnormalities which result in endocrine and metabolic disorders, and this has been illustrated by reference to the disorders associated with hypoparathyroidism. The approach outlined in this chapter could be followed in any genetically determined condition, leading to the opportunity to elucidate the pathogenesis of such disorders.

ACKNOWLEDGEMENTS

I am grateful to the Medical Research Council (UK) for support, and to Ms Lesley Sargeant for typing the manuscript.

REFERENCES

1 Thakker RV. The molecular genetics of the multiple endocrine neoplasia syndromes. *Clin Endocrinol* 1993;38:1–14.
2 Gubbay J, Collignon J, Koopman P *et al.* A gene mapping to the sex-determining region of the mouse Y chromosome is a member of a novel family of embryonically expressed genes. *Nature* 1990;346:245–50.
3 Koopman P, Gubbay J, Vivian N, Goodfellow P, Lovell-Badge R. Male development of chromosomally female mice transgenic for *Sry. Nature* 1991;351:117–21.
4 Sinclair AH, Berta P, Palmer MS *et al.* A gene from the human sex-determining region encodes a protein with homology to a conserved DNA-binding motif. *Nature* 1990;346:240–4.
5 Grieco M, Santoro M, Berlingieri MT *et al.* PTC is a novel rearranged form of the ret proto-oncogene and is frequently detected *in vivo* in human thyroid papillary carcinomas. *Cell* 1990;60:557–63.
6 Herrmann MA, Hay ID, Bartelt DH Jr *et al.* Cytogenetic and molecular genetic studies of follicular and papillary thyroid cancers. *J Clin Invest* 1991;88:1596–604.
7 Pierotti MA, Santoro M, Jenkins RB *et al.* Characterization of an inversion on the long arm of chromosome 10 juxtaposing D10S170 and RET and creating the oncogenic sequence RET/PTC. *Proc Natl Acad Sci USA* 1992;89:1616–20.
8 Sozzi G, Bongarzone I, Miozzo M *et al.* Cytogenetic and molecular genetic characterization of papillary thyroid carcinomas. *Genes Chrom Cancer* 1992;5:212–18.
9 Pan Y, Metzenberg A, Das S, Jing B, Gitschier J. Mutations in the V2 vasopressin receptor gene are associated with X-linked nephrogenic diabetes insipidus. *Nature Genet* 1992;2:103–6.
10 van den Ouweland AMW, Dreesen JCFM, Verdijk M *et al.* Mutations in the vasopressin type 2 receptor gene (*AVPR2*) associated with nephrogenic diabetes insipidus. *Nature Genet* 1992;2:99–102.

11 Franco B, Guioli S, Pragliola A *et al.* A gene deleted in Kallmann's syndrome shares homology with neural cell adhesion and axonal path-finding molecules. *Nature* 1991;353:529–36.

12 Legouis R, Hardelin JP, Levilliers J *et al.* The candidate gene for the X-linked Kallman syndrome encodes a protein related to adhesion molecules. *Cell* 1991;67:423–35.

13 Jeunemaitre X, Soubrier F, Kotelevtsev YV *et al.* Molecular basis of human hypertension: role of angiotensinogen. *Cell* 1992;71:7–20.

14 Cornall RJ, Prins J-B, Todd JA *et al.* Type 1 diabetes in mice is linked to the interleukin-1 receptor and *Lsh/Ity/Bcg* genes on chromosome 1. *Nature* 1991;353:262–5.

15 Julier C, Hyer RN, Davies J *et al.* Insulin-IGF2 region on chromosome 11p encodes a gene implicated in HLA-DR4-dependent diabetes susceptibility. *Nature* 1991;354:155–9.

16 Todd JA, Aitman TJ, Cornall RJ *et al.* Genetic analysis of autoimmune type 1 diabetes mellitus in mice. *Nature* 1991; 351:542–7.

17 Froguel Ph, Vaxillaire M, Sun F *et al.* Close linkage of glucokinase locus on chromosome 7p to early-onset non-insulin-dependent diabetes mellitus. *Nature* 1992;356:162–4.

18 Ruddle FH. The William Allan Memorial Award Address: reverse genetics and beyond. *Am J Hum Genet* 1984;36:944–53.

19 Collins FS. Positional cloning: let's not call it reverse any more. *Nature Genet* 1992;1:3–6.

20 Thakker RV, Bouloux P, Wooding C *et al.* Association of parathyroid tumors in multiple endocrine neoplasia type 1 with loss of alleles on chromosome 11. *N Engl J Med* 1989; 321:218–24.

21 Thakker RV. Molecular genetics of mineral metabolic disorders. *J Inher Metab Dis* 1992;15:592–609.

22 Ahn TG, Antonarakis SE, Kronenberg HM, Igarashi T, Levine MA. Familial isolated hypoparathyroidism: a molecular genetic analysis of 8 families with 23 affected persons. *Medicine* 1986;65:73–81.

23 Barr DGD, Prader A, Esper U, Rampini S, Marrian VJ, Forfar JO. Chronic hypoparathyroidism in two generations. *Helv Paediatr Acta* 1971;26:507–21.

24 Bronsky D, Kiamlko RT, Waldstein SS. Familial idiopathic hypoparathyroidism. *J Clin Endocrinol Metab* 1968;28:61–5.

25 Parkinson DB, Thakker RV. A donor splice site mutation in the parathyroid hormone gene is associated with autosomal recessive hypoparathyroidism. *Nature Genet* 1992;1:149–52.

26 Peden VH. True idiopathic hypoparathyroidism as a sex-linked recessive trait. *Am J Hum Genet* 1960;12:323–37.

27 Thakker RV, Davies KE, Whyte MP, Wooding C, O'Riordan JLH. Mapping the gene causing X-linked recessive idiopathic hypoparathyroidism to Xq26–Xq27 by linkage studies. *J Clin Invest* 1990;86:40–5.

28 Whyte MP, Weldon VV. Idiopathic hypoparathyroidism presenting with seizures during infancy: X-linked recessive inheritance in a large Missouri kindred. *J Pediatr* 1981;99: 608–11.

29 McKusick VA. *Mendelian Inheritance in Man.* Baltimore: Johns Hopkins University Press, 1988.

30 Naylor SL, Sakaguchi AY, Szoka P *et al.* Human parathyroid hormone gene (PTH) is on short arm of chromosome 11. *Somatic Cell Genet* 1983;9:609–16.

31 Keutmann HT, Sauer MM, Hendy GN, O'Riordan JLH, Potts JT Jr. Complete amino acid sequence of human parathyroid hormone. *Biochemistry* 1978;12:5723–9.

32 Arnold A, Horst Sa, Gardella TJ, Baba H, Levine MA, Kronenberg HM. Mutation of the signal peptide-encoding region of the preproparathyroid hormone gene in familial isolated hypoparathyroidism. *J Clin Invest* 1990;86:1084–7.

33 Schmidtke J, Pape B, Krengel U *et al.* Restriction fragment length polymorphisms at the human parathyroid hormone gene locus. *Hum Genet* 1984;67:428–31.

34 Miric A, Levine MA. Analysis of the preproPTH gene by denaturing gradient gel electrophoresis in familial isolated hypoparathyroidism. *J Clin Endocrinol Metab* 1992;74:509–16.

35 Parkinson DB, Shaw NJ, Himsworth RL, Thakker RV. Parathyroid hormone gene analysis in autosomal hypoparathyroidism using an intragenic tetranucleotide (AAAT)n polymorphism. *Hum Genet* 1993;91:281–4.

36 Thakker RV. Molecular genetics of hypoparathyroidism. In: Bilezikian JP, Levine M, Marcus R, eds. *The Parathyroids.* New York: Raven Press, 1994 (in press).

37 Cooper DN, Schmidtke J. DNA restriction fragment length polymorphisms and heterozygosity in the human genome. *Hum Genet* 1984;66:1–16.

38 Thakker RV, Ponder BAJ. Multiple endocrine neoplasia. In: Sheppard MC, ed. *Clinical Endocrinology and Metabolism,* Vol. 2, No. 4. London: Baillière Tindall, 1988:1031–67.

39 Southern EM. Detection of specific sequences among DNA fragments separated by gel electrophoresis. *J Mol Biol* 1975; 98:503–17.

40 Weber JL, May PE. Abundant class of human DNA polymorphisms which can be typed using the polymerase chain reaction. *Am J Hum Genet* 1989;44:388–96.

41 Schmidtke J, Kruse K, Pape B, Sippell G. Exclusion of close linkage between parathyroid hormone gene and a mutant gene locus causing idiopathic hypoparathyroidism. *J Med Genet* 1986;23:217–19.

42 Bilous RW, Murty G, Parkinson DB *et al.* Autosomal dominant familial hypoparathyroidism, sensineural deafness and renal dysplasia. *N Engl J Med* 1992;327:1069–84.

43 Shaw NJ, Haigh D, Lealmann GT, Karbani G, Brocklebank JT, Dillon MJ. Autosomal recessive hypoparathyroidism with renal insufficiency and development delay. *Arch Dis Child* 1991;66:1191–4.

44 Breathnach R, Benoist C, O'Hare K, Gannon F, Chambon P. Ovalbumin gene: evidence for a leader sequence in mRNA and DNA sequences at the exon-intron boundaries. *Proc Natl Acad Sci USA* 1978;75:4853–7.

45 Mount SM. A catalogue of splice junction sequences. *Nucl Acids Res* 1982;10:459–72.

46 Lerner MR, Boyle JA, Mount SM, Wolin SL, Steitz JA. Are snRNPs involved in splicing? *Nature* 1980;283:220–4.

47 Lewin B. Alternatives for splicing: recognizing the ends of introns. *Cell* 1980;22:324–6.

48 Rogers J, Wall R. A mechanism for RNA splicing. *Proc Natl Acad Sci USA* 1980;77:1877–9.

49 Treisman R, Proudfoot NJ, Shander M, Maniatis T. A single-base change at a splice site in a β-thalassaemic gene causes abnormal RNA splicing. *Cell* 1982;29:903–11.

50 Weatherall DJ, Clegg JB. Thalassemia revisited. *Cell* 1982; 29:7–9.

51 Wieringa B, Meyer F, Reiser J, Weissmann C. Unusual splice sites revealed by mutagenic inactivation of an authentic splice site of the rabbit β-globin gene. *Nature* 1983;301:38–43.

52 Talerico M, Berget SM. Effect of 5′ splice site mutations on splicing of the preceding intron. *Mol Cell Biol* 1990;10:6299–305.

53 Kuo H-C, Nasim F-UH, Grabowski PJ. Control of alternative

splicing by the differential binding of U1 small nuclear ribonucleoprotein particles. *Science* 1991;251:1045–50.

54 Parkinson DB, Thakker RV. Illegitimate transcription of the parathyroid hormone gene in lymphocytes from normal and hypoparathyroid individuals. In: Cohn DV, Glorieux FH, Martin TJ, eds. *Calcium Regulation and Bone Metabolism. Basic and Clinical Aspects*. London: Elsevier, 1994 (in press).

55 Berg L-P, Wieland K, Millar DS *et al.* Detection of a novel point mutation causing haemophilia A by PCR/direct sequencing of ectopically-transcribed factor VIII mRNA. *Hum Genet* 1990;85:655–8.

56 Chelly J, Concordet J-P, Kaplan J-C, Kahn A. Illegitimate transcription: transcription of any gene in any cell type. *Proc Natl Acad Sci USA* 1989;86:2617–21.

57 Sarkar G, Sommer SS. Access to a messenger RNA sequence or its protein product is not limited by tissue or species specificity. *Science* 1989;244:331–4.

58 Chelly J, Kaplan J-C, Maire P, Gautron S, Kahn A. Transcription of the dystrophin gene in human muscle and non-muscle tissues. *Nature* 1988;333:858–60.

59 Schloesser M, Slomski R, Wagner M *et al.* Characterization of pathological dystrophin transcripts from the lymphocytes of a muscular dystrophy carrier. *Mol Biol Med* 1990;7:519–23.

60 Kozak M. The scanning model for translation: an update. *J Cell Biol* 1989;108:229–41.

61 Emr SD, Hall MN, Silhavy TJ. A mechanism of protein localisation: the signal hypothesis and bacteria. *J Cell Biol* 1980;86:701–11.

62 Whyte MP, Kim GS, Kosanovich M. Absence of parathyroid tissue in sex-linked recessive hypoparathyroidism. *J Pediatr* 1986;109:915.

63 Morton NE. Sequential tests for the detection of linkage. *Am J Hum Genet* 1955;7:277–318.

64 Ott J. Estimation of the recombination fraction in human pedigrees: efficient computation of the likelihood for human linkage studies. *Am J Hum Genet* 1974;26:588–97.

65 Thakker RV, O'Riordan JLH. Inherited forms of rickets and osteomalacia. In: Martin TJ, ed. *Clinical Endocrinology and Metabolism*, Vol. 2, No. 1. London: Baillière Tindall, 1988: 155–71.

66 Thakker RV, Wooding C, Parkinson DB , Blake D, Whyte MP, Davies KE. Linkage analysis of three cloned DNA sequences, DXS294, CDR and DXS105, in X-linked recessive hypoparathyroid families. *Cytogenet Cell Genet* 1992;58:2087.

67 Rohn RD, Leffell MS, Leadem P, Johnson D, Rubio T, Emanuel BS. Familial third-fourth pharyngeal pouch syndrome with apparent autosomal dominant transmission. *J Pediatr* 1984; 105:47–51.

68 de la Chapelle A, Herra R, Koivisto M, Aula P. A deletion in chromosome 22 can cause Di George syndrome. *Hum Genet* 1981;57:253–6.

69 Kelley RI, Zackai FH, Emmanuel BS, Kistenmacher M, Greenberg F, Punnett HH. The association of the Di George anomalad with partial monosomy of chromosome 22. *J Pediatr* 1982;101:197–200.

70 Lai MMR, Scriven PN, Ball C, Berry AC. Simultaneous partial monosomy 10p and trisomy 5q in a case of hypoparathyroidism. *J Med Genet* 1992;29:586–8.

71 Monaco G, Pignata C, Rossi E, Mascellaro O, Cocozza S, Ciccimarra F. DiGeorge anomaly associated with 10p deletion. *Am J Med Genet* 1991;39:215–16.

72 Cannizzarro LA, Emmanuel BS. *In situ* hybridisation and translocation breakpoint mapping. II. Di George syndrome with partial monosomy of chromosome 22. *Cytogenet Cell Genet* 1985;39:179–83.

73 Fibison WJ, Budarf M, McDermid H, Greenberg F, Emanuel BS. Molecular studies of Di George syndrome. *Am J Hum Genet* 1990;46:888–95.

74 Scambler PJ, Carey AH, Wyse RKH *et al.* Microdeletions within 22q11 associated with sporadic and familial Di George syndrome. *Genomics* 1991;10:201–6.

75 Carey AH, Kelly D, Halford S *et al.* Molecular genetic study of the frequency of monosomy 22q11 in DiGeorge syndrome. *Am J Hum Genet* 1992;51:964–70.

76 Driscoll DA, Budarf ML, Emanuel BS. A genetic etiology for DiGeorge syndrome: consistent deletions and microdeletions of 22q11. *Am J Hum Genet* 1992;50:924–33.

77 Halford S, Wilson DI, Daw SCM *et al.* Isolation of a gene expressed during early embryogenesis from the region of 22q11 commonly deleted in DiGeorge syndrome. *Hum Mol Genet* 1993;2:1577–82.

78 Aubry K, Demczuk S, Desmaze C *et al.* Isolation of a zinc finger gene consistently deleted in DiGeorge syndrome. *Hum Mol Genet* 1993;2:1583–7.

79 Chisaka O, Capecchi MR. Regionally restricted developmental defects resulting from targeted disruption of the mouse homeobox gene hox-1.5. *Nature* 1991;350:473–9.

80 Kappen C, Schughart K, Ruddle FH. Two steps in the evolution of *Antennapedia*-class vertebrate homeobox genes. *Proc Natl Acad Sci USA* 1989;86:5459–63.

81 Fanconi S, Fischer JA, Wieland P *et al.* Kenny syndrome: evidence for idiopathic hypoparathyroidism in two patients and for abnormal parathyroid hormone in one. *J Pediatr* 1986;109:469–75.

82 Franceschini P, Testa A, Bogetti G *et al.* Kenny–Caffey syndrome in two sibs born to consanguineous parents: evidence for an autosomal recessive variant. *Am J Med Genet* 1992; 42:112–16.

83 Boynton JR, Pheasant TR, Johnson BL, Levin DB, Streeten BW. Ocular findings in Kenny's syndrome. *Arch Ophthalmol* 1979;97:896–900.

84 Bergada I, Schiffrin A, Abu Srair H *et al.* Kenny syndrome: description of additional abnormalities and molecular studies. *Hum Genet* 1988;80:39–42.

85 Barakat AY, D'Albora JB, Martin MM, Jose PA. Familial nephrosis, nerve deafness, and hypoparathyroidism. *J Pediatr* 1977;91:61–4.

86 Dahlberg PJ, Borer WZ, Newcomer KL, Yutuc WR. Autosomal or X-linked recessive syndrome of congenital lymphedema, hypoparathyroidism, nephropathy, prolapsing mitral valve, and brachytelephalangy. *Am J Med Genet* 1983;16:99–104.

87 Sanjad SA, Sakati NA, Abu-Osba YK, Kaddoura R, Milner RDG. A new syndrome of congenital hypoparathyroidism, severe growth failure, and dysmorphic features. *Arch Dis Child* 1991;66:193–6.

88 Ahonen P, Myllarniemi S, Sipila I, Perheentupa J. Clinical variation of autoimmune polyendocrinopathy–candidiasis–ectodermal dystrophy (APECED) in a series of 68 patients. *N Engl J Med* 1990;322:1829–36.

89 Ahonen P. Autoimmune polyendocrinopathy–candidosis–ectodermal dystrophy (APECED): autosomal recessive inheritance. *Clin Genet* 1985;27:535–2.

90 Zlotogora J, Shapiro MS. Polyglandular autoimmune syndrome type 1 among Iranian Jews. *J Med Genet* 1992;29:824–6.

91 Albright F, Burnett CH, Smith PH, Parson W. Pseudohypoparathyroidism: an example of 'Seabright–Bantam syndrome'. *Endocrinology* 1942;30:922–32.

92 Chase LR, Melson GL, Aurbach GD. Pseudohypoparathyroidism: defective excretion of 3′,5′-AMP in response to parathyroid hormone. *J Clin Invest* 1969;48:1832–44.
93 Farfel Z, Brickman AS, Kaslow HR, Brothers VM, Bourne HR. Defect of receptor–cyclase coupling protein in pseudohypoparathyroidism. *N Engl J Med* 1980;303:237–42.
94 Patten JL, Johns DR, Valle D *et al.* Mutation in the gene encoding the stimulatory G protein of adenylate cyclase in Albright's hereditary osteodystrophy. *N Engl J Med* 1990;322:1412–19.
95 Spiegel AM. Albright's hereditary osteodystrophy and defective G-proteins. *N Engl J Med* 1990;322:1461–2.
96 Blatt C, Eversole-Cire P, Cohn VH *et al.* Chromosomal localization of genes encoding guanine nucleotide-binding protein subunits in mouse and human. *Proc Natl Acad Sci USA* 1988;85:7642–6.

3: Physiology of Sexual Determination and Differentiation

P. SAENGER

INTRODUCTION

In the past 5 years four leaps in our understanding of regulation of sexual differentiation have occurred. It is now realized, after 30 years of work, that the testis-determining factor does not comprise the entire Y chromosome but a region spanning only 14 kb on the short arm (Fig. 3.1) [1]. Secondly, the gene for anti-Müllerian hormone (AMH) has been elucidated, and reliable assays for measurement of AMH have been developed [2–4].

A third breakthrough was the identification of the gene for the androgen receptor, furthering our understanding of complete and partial androgen-resistance syndromes [5–7].

Lastly, the precise identification of the genetic defect which results in 5α-reductase deficiency explains undervirilization in this syndrome. It also extends our understanding of dihydrotestosterone (DHT) action [8,9].

Sex determination and differentiation is a sequential process that involves at least four characteristics that are delineated in various stages. *Genetic sex* is determined at fertilization. *Gonadal sex* is determined by the genetic sex. Sexual differentiation of the gonads leads to the development of internal genital tracts and the external genitalia and hence the *phenotypic sex* during the first half of fetal life.

At puberty the development of secondary sex characteristics provides additional visible phenotypic manifestations. Psychological sexual identity is acquired postnatally by sociological imprinting on the developing personality. This postnatal process, together with prenatal hormonal influences (nature and nurture), then mould gender identity or *psychological sex* [10].

Sex determination is primarily testis determination. The primary event is differentiation of the gonad; all subsequent sexual differentiation is hormonally controlled by testosterone and dihydrotestosterone.

GENETIC SEX: ROLE OF THE SEX-DETERMINING REGION OF THE HUMAN Y CHROMOSOME

The genetic sex is determined by the constitution of the spermatozoid, whether it contains a Y or an X chromosome [11]. The genetic male sex will induce the differentiation of the pluripotential primordial gonad into a testis. Complete female sexual differentiation occurs in the absence of male determinants [12,13]. It is upon this innate female tendency of the genitalia and the gonadal primordium that maleness must be actively imposed [14].

The gonadal primordium, which is common to both sexes, is already visible in the 5 mm human embryo. The development of paired genital ridges shows some proliferation of the coelomic epithelium, and mesenchyme begins to differentiate into gonads at around the fourth week [15,16]. This development is heralded by the appearance of so-called sex cords. During this first step, which is independent from the genetic sex, the gonadal primordium is colonized by primordial germ cells. These germ cells originate from the allantoid sac. When these cells have reached the gonadal primordium they form with the existing epithelium the gonadal ridge. Subsequent differentiation into seminiferous tubules, signalling the first event of male differentiation, is initiated by a 'switch' mechanism brought on by a gene product on the Y chromosome.

The search for this gene product began in earnest more than 30 years ago: in 1959 the Y chromosome was shown to be male-determining in both mice and humans [11]. The search subsequently narrowed the testis-determining factor to the short arm of the Y chromosome. For nearly 10 years H-Y antigen, a male-specific histocompatibility antigen, was widely believed to be the primary testis inducer [17], but when individuals were found with well-formed testes but without the H-Y antigen the hypothesis had to be abandoned [1]. H-Y antigen [18], actually located on the long arm of the Y chromosome, does play a role in spermatogenesis [19]. Attention then turned to the area

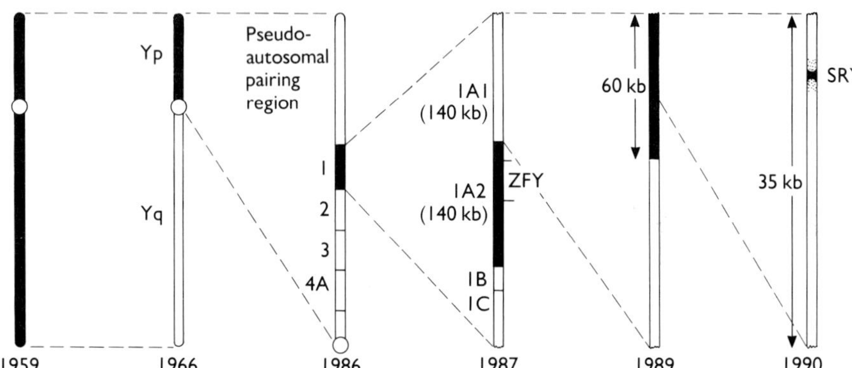

Fig. 3.1 Thirty-one years of hunting the testis-determining factor. The chromosome region thought to include the elusive factor is shaded. The search has narrowed from 30–50 million bases to less than 35 kb of SRY (from McLaren [1]).

near the pairing and exchange region (pseudoautosomal region). This was termed zinc finger Y (ZFY) and seemed an excellent candidate for the testis-determining factor [20,21].

When XX men turned up without ZFY [22,23] this theory also had to be abandoned [24]. With hard work (and a little luck), first a 60 kb and finally a 35 kb area were identified as the areas harbouring the elusive testis-determining factor [25]. Within the 35 kb region a single-copy gene was found that is highly conserved and shows homologies with both the sexual mating protein required for mating in yeast and the non-histone nuclear HMG (high mobility group) proteins thought to function as DNA-binding transcription factor [26].

The testis-determining factor on the Y chromosome which turns the 'switch' has been cloned and designated SRY (sex-determining region of the human Y chromosome) [26]. SRY in humans is a 14 kb region, adjacent to the pseudoautosomal region of the short arm of the Y chromosome (Fig. 3.1) [27].

For SRY to be the testis-determining factor, it had to be located on the very small portion of the short arm of the Y chromosome shown to be testis-determining. It should be conserved on the Y chromosome of all mammals and marsupials (eutherian animals) known to have a Y-determined sex differentiation. Lastly, the gene product should have a structure fully consistent with a regulatory gene [1]. All of these predictions turned out to be correct for SRY, but to prove that SRY is required for sex determination one would need to produce transgenic mice, i.e. insert SRY as a transgene into the genome of an XX mouse.

Further proof would accrue if it could be shown that the expression of SRY in the fetal testis were confined to the somatic-supporting cell lineage, which is believed to be critical for testis determination, rather than to the germ cells [10].

By exploiting detailed maps of the sex-determining region of the human Y chromosome the SRY gene was cloned. As might be predicated for a regulatory gene, SRY encodes a protein containing a DNA-binding motif. SRY also shows a pattern for expression in the mouse which is entirely consistent with a role in testis determination: it is expressed for a short period from about 10.5 to 12 days postcoitum (just before testicular differentiation) and it is expressed in the somatic cells of the genital ridge (Fig. 3.2) [28,29].

In a now-classic experiment the laboratories of Goodfellow and Lovell-Badge [28] succeeded in fertilizing female XX eggs with the 14 kb SRY gene sequence and bred sex-reversed XX phenotypic male mice with gonads demonstrating testicular histology. It is not clear at present how SRY, the 'switch', is turned on. It is quite clear, however, that it is expressed in the critical period when gonadal differentiation takes place in the mouse. SRY is expressed only in the somatic cells of the genital ridge, not in the germ cells [28]. SRY expression in adults is limited to the heads of the spermatids.

The limited time of expression of SRY in the critical period is akin to the time-limited expression of other genes, such as homeobox genes and oncogenes, which are also expressed only at various stages of development [30]. Similarly, SRY is not the only gene causing testis determination; it is, however, the critical initial switch. Other genes on other chromosomes, probably several thousand of them and possibly also regulated by SRY, play as yet unidentified important functions in the completion of orderly sexual differentiation.

The 14 kb fragment of normal mouse DNA containing SRY is thus sufficient to direct the formation of the testes in XX transgenic embryos and subsequently to give rise to full phenotypic sex reversal in an XX transgenic adult mouse. Thus SRY is the only Y-linked gene required to give rise to male development, and it is proposed that it is identical to the testes-determining factor in humans. Furthermore, the outcome of experiments in transgenic mice suggests that the 14 kb fragment contains the entire SRY gene including all the regulatory elements required

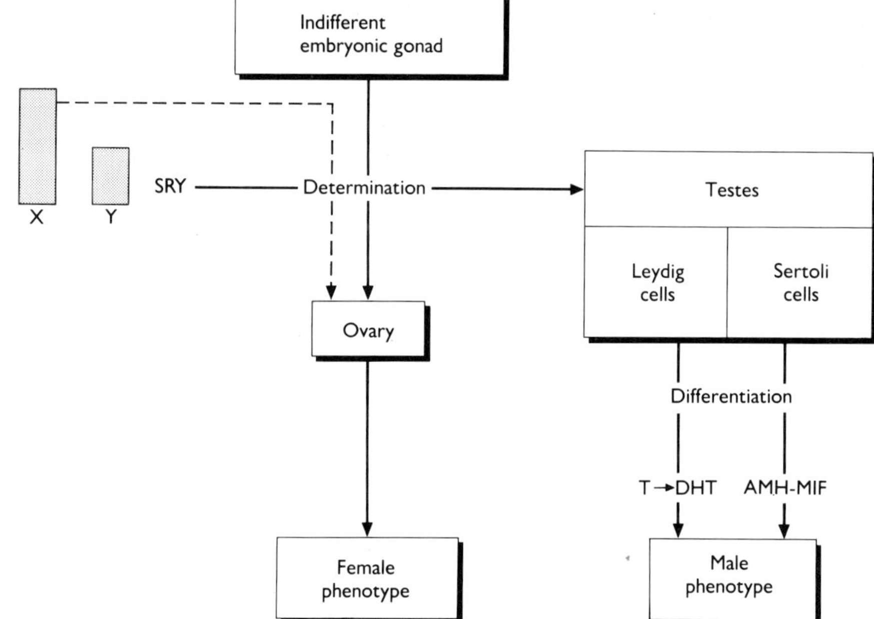

Fig. 3.2 Schematic overview of sex differentation. In XY embryo SRY initiates testis determination and blocks female development. DSS may be the initiator of ovarian development from the short arm of X. All other steps of sex differentiation are hormonally induced. DHT, dihydrotestosterone; DSS, dosage sensitive sex reversal; MIF, Müllerian inhibiting factor or anti- Müllerian hormone; SRY, sex determining region on Y chromosome; T, testosterone.

for appropriate embryonic expression [28]. It is unclear at present whether the fragment also contains the regulatory information required for the 'switch' from expression in the somatic part of the embryogenic gonad to expression in the adult testes associated with germ cells [31].

While SRY alone can promote testicular development in 46XX males in the absence of any other Y-linked genes [28,32], sex reversal does not always occur. SRY-negative males have also been described. The most likely explanation for the first conundrum is that the SRY transgene is sensitive to position effects [30]. It may be affected by adjacent DNA sequences and its new chromosomal location or by the spread of X inactivation curtailing SRY action. SRY initiates testis development through interaction with other genes [33], some of which have been involved in regulation; others will be downstream targets of SRY. In the SRY-negative male, a gain of function mutation downstream of SRY would explain male development in these individuals. Because SRY is shown to be the only Y-linked gene required to bring about male development in the mouse, mutations in some of these genes elsewhere in the genome could explain cases of male development in XX males lacking SRY and XY females where SRY is intact [30,34–36]. Identification of these other genes downstream from SRY will be a goal for the future [31].

The existence of an X-specific gene involved in human sex determination has been postulated for some time. Recently it was discovered that when an individual with a 46,XY karyotype has two active copies of an Xp locus, complete sex reversal or genital ambiguity may occur. This locus has been termed DSS (Dosage Sensitive Sex Reversal). This locus is not required for testis differentiation to take place. DSS may play a key role in ovarian development and/or may function as a link between ovary and testis formation. Two doses of DSS are sufficient to disrupt normal testis development in the presence of SRY. Indeed duplications of the short arm of the X-chromosome have been associated with male to female sex reversal. These data question the old paradigm that the fetus is inherently female. Ovarian development is not therefore simply the 'default' mode. DSS may be a specific gene conferring femaleness [36a].

Several other genes suspected to have roles in developmental decisions in the embryo (for example some homeoboxcontaining genes) also show expression in the adult testis. SRY could have one role in the embryo in testes determination and another, postnatally, in male germ cell development [26,36].

It is very likely that the interactions between the somatic cell matrix and the penetrating germ cell are also important in gametogenesis. In the example of transgenic mice [28], the XX_{SRY} germ cell acts as the switch-on gene in the XX gonadal ridge, initiating the process of testicular differentiation. Since the gonadal ridge is always derived from somatic cells, this implies that in normal differentiation SRY is not normally present in the germ cells.

Taken together these findings suggest that while SRY is the switch gene in the male, the differentiation of the gonads into endocrine organs is controlled by totally different intrinsic gonadal or other factors. Furthermore, the mechanism that converts the gonads from an autonomous endocrine tissue to gonadotrophin-dependent tissue is currently not understood.

GONADAL DIFFERENTIATION AND DEVELOPMENT

The contact between primordial cells and somatic cells in the male under the influence of SRY or some other gene product is made earlier than in the female gonadal ridge, at around 7–8 weeks of gestation [16,37,38]. The differentiation of the gonadal ridge into the testis is a rapid phenomenon, which contrasts with the slowed and delayed development of the ovary. Testicular tissue (particularly seminiferous tubules with germ cells) can be recognized in the human embryo at 7 weeks of fetal age (13–20 mm crown–rump length) [16, 39]. It also coincides with the acquisition of AMH activity by the male gonad, which is secreted by immature Sertoli cells at around 45–50 days [40]. In the mouse the gene for AMH is switched on exactly 1.5 days after SRY is switched off.

SRY, committing the gonad to male development, may also accelerate gonadal development in the male. Since testicular architecture and function is established early (see below), male sex hormones are being produced before the male fetus becomes submerged in a sea of maternally-derived oestrogen. The presence of testosterone and AMH will counteract the danger of the fetus becoming feminized [41,42]. Testes develop faster than ovaries in all mammalian species investigated [43].

Fetal testes, which are localized in the kidney region, begin their descent at the 12th week of fetal age. They reach the inner inguinal ring at midgestation and appear in the scrotum only during the last 12 weeks of gestation. Which mechanical and endocrine factors guide this descent is still unclear, but it is currently believed that the transabdominal descent is not androgen-dependent. It may be due to pressure and pull exerted by the gubernaculum testes, a remnant of Müllerian ductal structures in the male. The transinguinal part of the descent is thought to be androgen-dependent. A role of AMH in the descent has been implied, postulating a bihormonal theory of testicular descent, but this is at present unproven [44,45].

To date, the basic tenet for phenotypic sex differentiation in mammals is a consequence of gonadal differentiation into a testes. All differentiation steps following testicular determination are a direct consequence of further hormonal factors produced by the testes [14]. Although ovarian determining genes are postulated [36a], the ovary does not appear to play an active role in controlling subsequent steps of gonadal development (Fig. 3.3).

Leydig cells formed from interstitial tissue appear at about day 60. By 14–18 weeks gestation Leydig cells take up more than half the volume of the testes [46,47]. By the eighth postfertilization week Leydig cells are actively secreting testosterone and Sertoli cells, still immature, are secreting AMH. A basal membrane is formed, similar to the blood–brain barrier, that separates tubules from mesenchyme and interstitium.

The peak of Leydig cell development closely follows peak placental human chorionic gonadotrophin (hCG) release [48]. The fetal pituitary gland thus controls testicular development only in the second and third trimester. After the 18th week the number of Leydig cells decreases and, by 27 weeks, the seminiferous tubules are separated only by a narrow interstitium containing a few Leydig cells. At 2–3 months after birth Leydig cells are no longer visible. Histologically and functionally they reappear at puberty [15].

Rudimentary ovarian and testicular function begins in the human embryo between 6 and 8 weeks gestation (Fig. 3.4). Both male and female gonads have 3β-hydroxysteroid dehydrogenase enzyme (3β-HSD) at this time [50]. Testes and ovaries acquire the capacity to secrete the characteristic hormones at the same stage of embryonic development, although the activity of 3β-HSD enzyme is 50-fold greater in the fetal testes. In the male, testosterone synthesis coincides with the appearance of Leydig cells and precedes the onset of virilization of the genital ducts. Gonadotrophins are apparently not required for testosterone synthesis until later in embryogenesis [51]. Maximal fetal serum concentrations of testosterone are observed between the 14th and 16th weeks. Levels are compatible

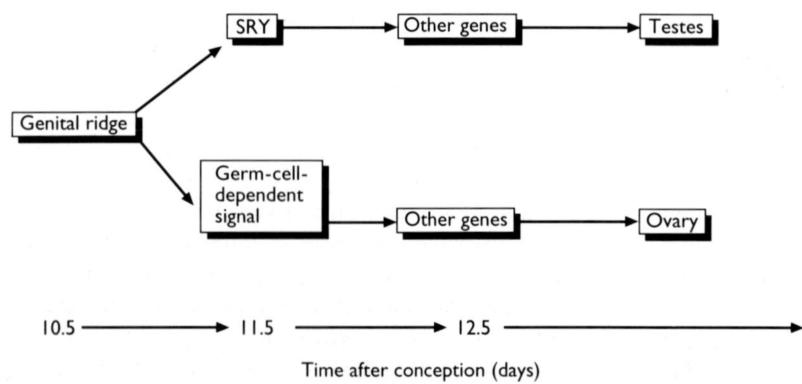

Fig. 3.3 Time sequence of sex differentiation in the mouse. SRY is expressed in the genital ridge only from 10.5–12.5 days postcoitum.

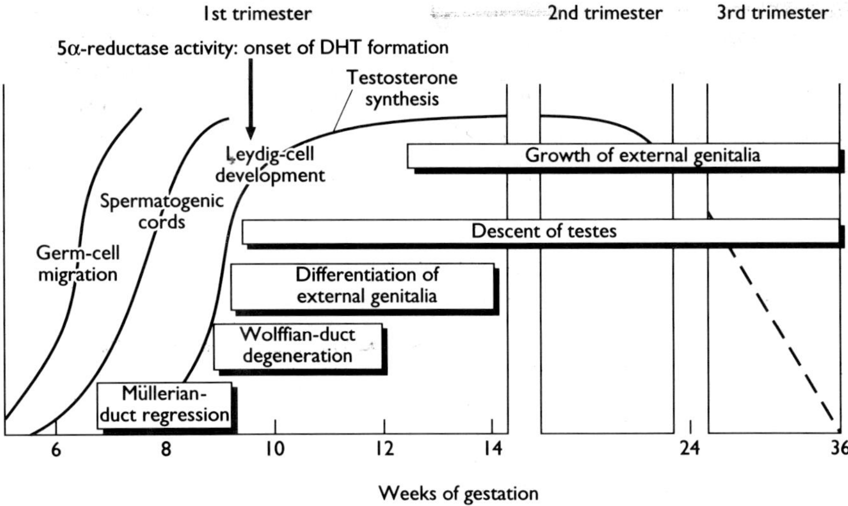

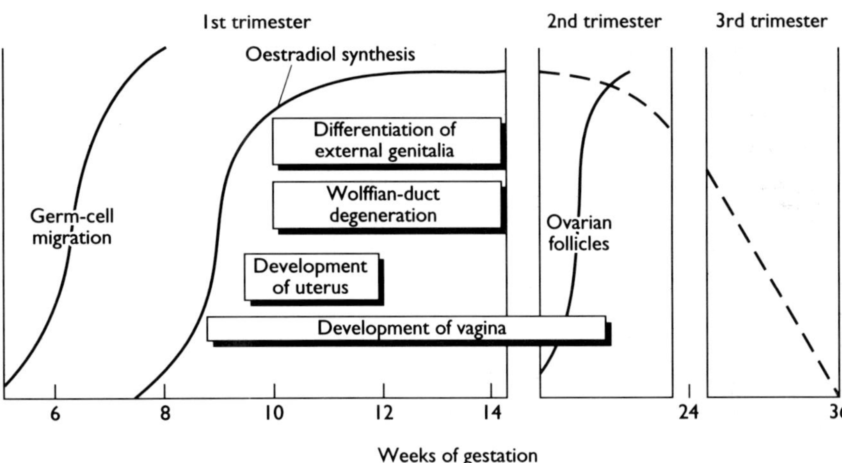

Fig. 3.4 Relationship between the differentiation of gonads and anatomical differentiation of human male and female embryos (redrawn from Saenger [49]).

to those observed in adult males [52–54]. Thereafter levels decline precipitously. Late testosterone-mediated events in male development, such as growth of the male external genitalia, are modulated directly by hormones from the pituitary gland. This explains the association of congenital hypopituitarism and microphallus [55]. At birth cord blood testosterone levels are still somewhat higher in males than in females [56–58].

The ontogeny of hormonal synthesis has been studied in mammalian gonads in detail: in the rabbit embryo testosterone synthesis begins during the 12 h interval between days 17 and 17.5 of gestation; that is approximately 1 day after histological differentiation of the testes. This process is made possible by the appearance of 3β-HSD converting dehydroepiandrosterone (DHEA) to Δ4-androstenedione. The ovary begins to form oestradiol at exactly the same time that the testes begin to synthesize testosterone. This occurs before any histological differentiation of the ovary. The onset of hormonal biosynthesis in the rabbit gonad is thus independent of pituitary control or other hormonal influences [53,54].

At later stages, placental hCG, peaking at 12 weeks of fetal age, may control fetal gonadal steroidogenesis in the human. Indeed $P450_{scc}$ and $P450_{c17}$ genes are expressed in fetal testis, during the 14th–16th weeks. Thereafter hCG concentrations decline and so do mRNA levels for these steroidogenic enzymes, suggesting strongly that expression of steroidogenic enzyme genes is regulated by hCG. The aromatase gene ($P450_{arom}$) is poorly expressed in fetal testes, explaining non-desensitization of fetal Leydig cells in the presence of high hCG [59].

Insulin-like growth factor (IGF)-I concentration is low

in the fetal testis but IGF-II mRNA is abundant, showing an age-dependent rise and fall similar to steroidogenic enzymes in the fetal testis [59].

The morphological development of the fetal ovary is much slower (Fig. 3.4) and the signal for ovarian development has not yet been identified. The human fetal ovary is capable of converting androgens to oestrogens to as early as the eighth week of fetal life [52,54,60–62]. Whether this is of physiological significance is not known, since the ovary lacks other enzymes necessary for synthesis of steroid precursors. $P450_{scc}$ and $P450_{c17}$ gene expression is low [59]. AMH is not detectable in the fetal ovary but IGF-II mRNA can be detected [59].

Ovarian somatic cells, appearing around the 20th week, form granulosa cells, which encircle the oocytes that are blocked at the diplotene state of the first meiosis. They remain arrested at this stage until ovulation commences at puberty [63]. These structures are the first rudimentary ovarian follicles. Whether secretion of oestradiol plays a role in human sex differentiation is not known [53,63].

The ovary may lose its integrity and become a streak without germ cells when the process of oocyte formation is not normal. This may explain streak gonads in many girls with Turner syndrome, who have normal ovaries in the second trimester, but streak ovaries at birth or soon thereafter. A normal 46,XX karyotype is not necessary for induction of ovarian development, but normal meiosis may be necessary for preservation of normal oocyte numbers [64,65].

At the fifth month of fetal age the human fetal ovary contains approximately seven million germ cells. At birth the number has fallen to two million, and at 7 years of age to 300 000 [53]. The difference in development between oogonia and spermatogonia is not explained. In fetal life germ cells may additionally be stimulated by a meiosis-inducing factor secreted by gonads of both sexes [66].

DIFFERENTIATION OF INTERNAL AND EXTERNAL GENITALIA

Two pairs of ducts give rise to the Wolffian and Müllerian ducts. Wolffian ducts, which are initially the excretory ducts of the mesonephros, become androgen-dependent only when renal function of the definitive kidney has been initiated [67]. Wolffian ducts disappear in the absence of androgens. If androgens are present the Wolffian ducts become stabilized and eventually become the vas deferens system (vasa deferentia, seminal vesicles and ejaculatory ducts).

Specifically, the anterior part of the Wolffian ducts communicates with the seminiferous tubules, and the posterior part of each Wolffian duct forms the vas deferens and the seminal vesicle. In the female, Wolffian duct stabilization cannot be maintained by systemic testosterone administration. Therefore, Wolffian ducts are not maintained in female pseudohermaphroditism, even when the virilizing agent reaches the fetus very early in pregnancy [68]. The Wolffian duct is apparently sensitive only to testosterone produced locally by the fetal testis or by a local testosterone crystal [14]. Testosterone is the active hormone in Wolffian duct differentiation and stabilization. The onset of 5α-reductase activity, and thus formation of DHT, begins later (see Fig. 3.4) [69], and the Wolffian duct does not contain 5α-reductase activity at this stage.

The Müllerian ducts serve as the anlagen of the uterus, fallopian tubes, and upper two-thirds of the vagina. Receptors for oestradiol have been found in the Müllerian ducts [70]. Their physiological significance is not known, since oestrogens are not necessary for the differentiation of female internal ducts. Locally implanted fetal testis in female fetuses induces the regression of Müllerian ducts and the development of Wolffian ducts. Local implants of testosterone induce development of the Wolffian ducts but no regression of Müllerian ductal structures. These ground-breaking experiments led Jost to postulate the existence of two hormones, AMH and testosterone, both of which influence the differentiation of the male fetus [14].

In the male fetus, AMH produced by immature Sertoli cells (and surprisingly by postnatal granulosa cells) triggers regression of Müllerian ducts. AMH is a member of the transforming growth factor β (TGF-β) family, and is structurally a glycoprotein [71]. The gene coding for human AMH has been cloned and mapped to chromosome 19 [3,72]. The physiological effects of AMH can be studied in detail, now that human recombinant AMH is available [4,73–75]. The Müllerian duct is sensitive to AMH only during a very early developmental period, which is already over at 8 weeks in the human [76]. This readily explains why postnatal AMH production by granulosa cells has no deleterious effect upon the female internal genital tract.

Unregulated production of AMH by ovaries of transgenic mice leads to Müllerian aplasia [77]. Fetal ovaries exposed to AMH lose their germ cells and develop to resemble seminiferous tubules [76]. Their oestrogen production is diverted to testosterone, as aromatase biosynthesis is inhibited [78]. It is possible that this effect of AMH on aromatase activity plays a role in the human fetal testis at 8–12 weeks gestation when both AMH and testosterone levels are high and aromatase activity is low. Other postnatal extra-Müllerian effects, such as the effect of AMH on female genital tract cancers, is currently still unclear [75].

Müllerian ducts are not affected by testosterone or its derivatives at any developmental stage [73]. When AMH is missing or ineffective, a uterus and fallopian tube develop in otherwise normal males. This condition, termed persistent müllerian duct syndrome, is often detected because the uterus and tubes prolapse into an inguinal hernia. Sometimes both testes are already in the same inguinal canal (transverse testicular ectopia). The molecular basis for persistent müllerian duct syndrome is heterogeneous: AMH-positive patients with an AMH-receptor defect and AMH-negative patients with defects in the AMH gene (e.g. nonsense mutation) [72,79] have been described. Oestrogens are known to oppose AMH effects in chickens, and a similar phenomenon may explain abnormal male differentiation in a mother exposed to diethylstilboestrol [80–82]. This may, however, be solely a pharmacological effect [74,76].

UROGENITAL SINUS AND EXTERNAL GENITALIA: ROLE OF DIHYDROTESTOSTERONE

Until the ninth week of gestation (crown–rump length 30 mm) the external genitalia are capable of differentiation into either sex [81,83]. The common anlagen are the genital tubercle, the urethral folds and the labioscrotal swelling (Fig. 3.5). The paired urethral folds surround a urogenital slit.

Masculinization begins in the male fetus by a lengthening of the anogenital distance. The labioscrotal swellings fuse in midline forming the scrotum. The sinus

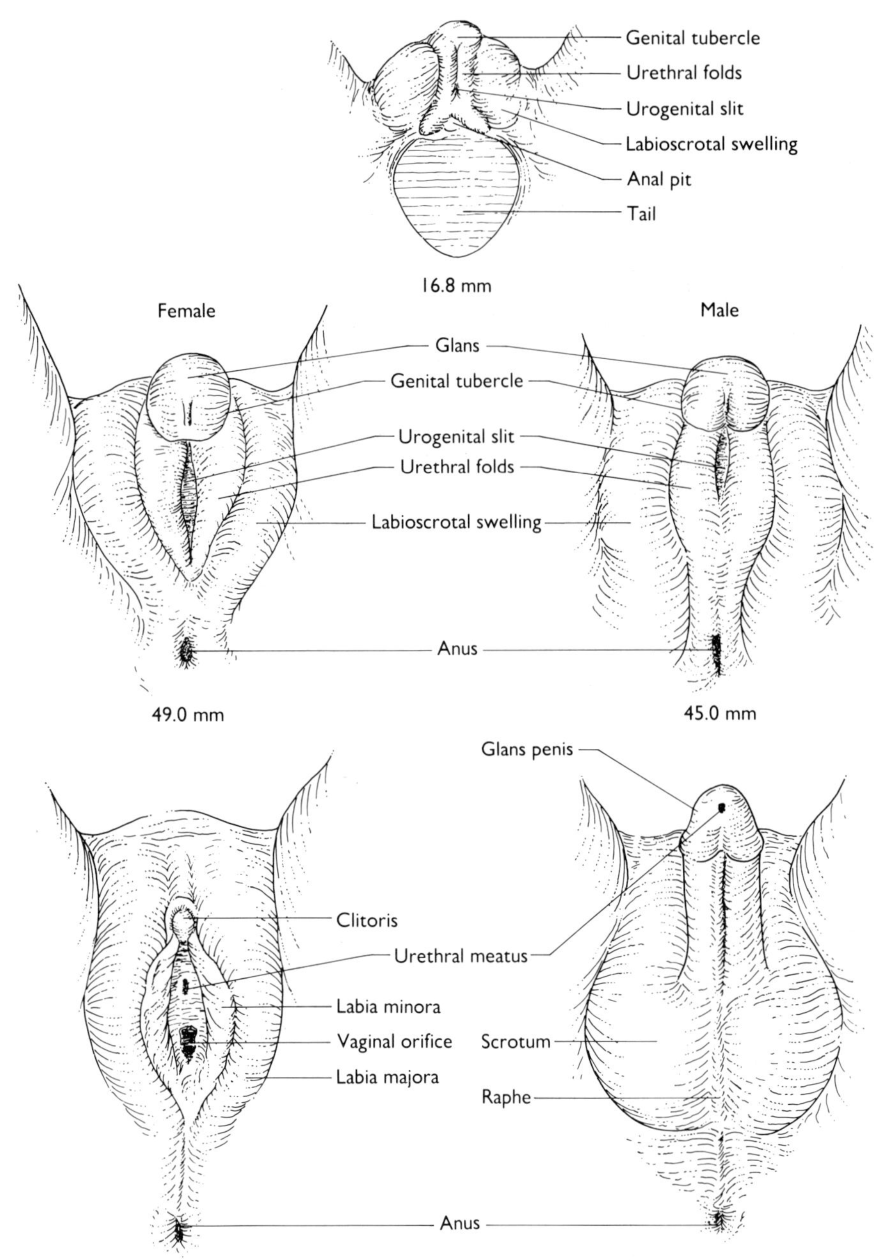

Fig. 3.5 Differentiation of male and female external genitalia from indifferent primordia. Male development will occur only in the presence of androgenic stimulation during the first 12 fetal weeks. Measurements indicate fetal crown-rump length.

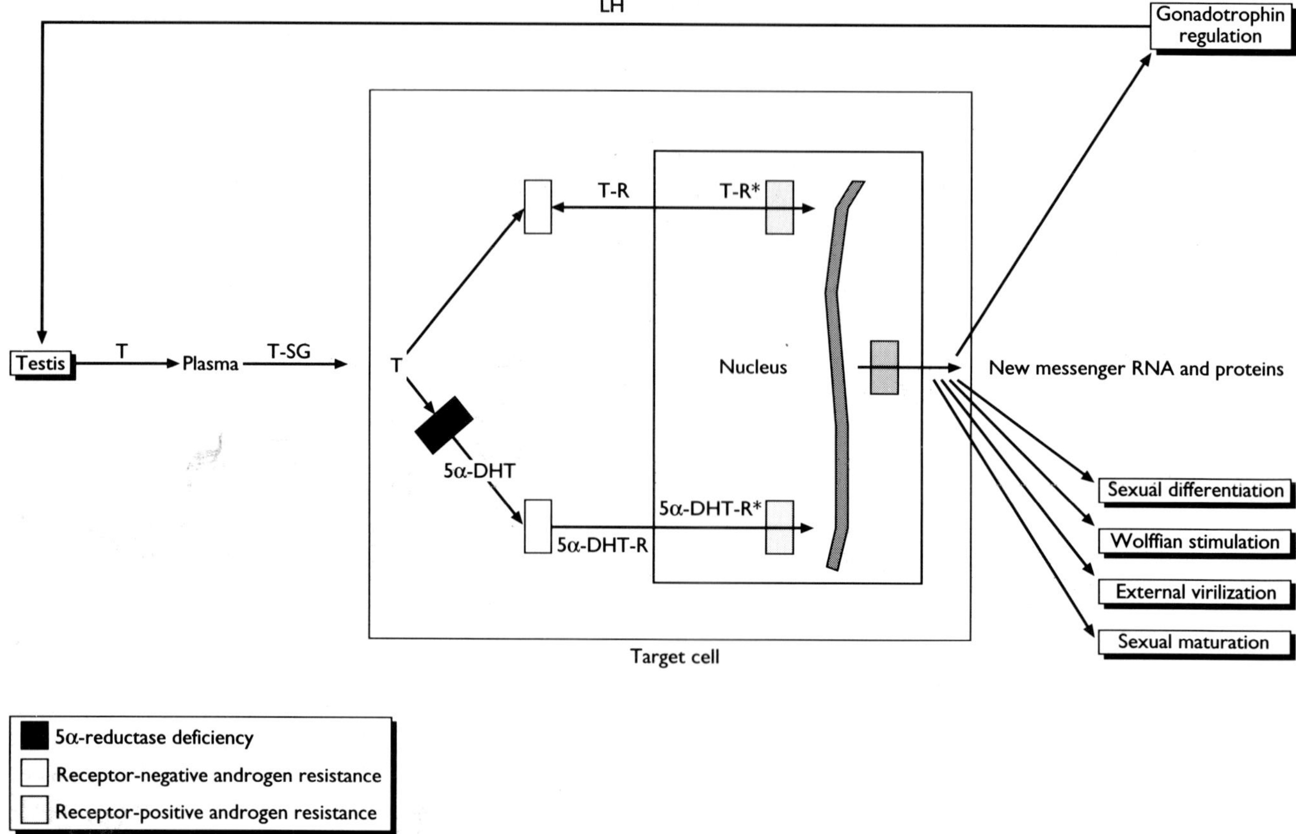

Fig. 3.6 Mechanism by which androgens act to virilize the male embryo. Three types of mutations are particularly informative in proving the clinical applicability of this model: 5α-reductase deficiency and receptor-positive and receptor-negative androgen resistance syndromes. DHT, dihydrotestosterone; LH, luteinizing hormone; R, high-affinity androgen receptor protein; R*, transformed androgen receptor exposing its DNA-binding domain; SG, sex-hormone-binding globulin; T, testosterone.

of the urethral folds close forming the primordium of the cavernous urethra. The genital tubercle becomes the corpora cavernosa and the glans penis. Formation of the penis is complete at 12–14 weeks gestation and labioscrotal fusion cannot be achieved in female fetuses exposed to androgens after this time. Growth of the penis continues throughout gestation and is normally mediated by the pituitary gland-dependent Leydig cell stimulation of the fetal testis. The urogenital sinus increases in length and forms the prostatic and perineal urethra. At 12–14 weeks the penile urethra is formed.

While testosterone is the androgen which differentiates the Wolffian duct, it acts only as a prehormone in other androgen-dependent tissues, notably the urogenital sinus and the external genitalia. In these tissues, testosterone is converted to the more potent 5α-reduced product, 5α-DHT, by a microsomal 5α-reductase. Thus testosterone and DHT play selective roles in embryogenesis. Both testosterone and DHT bind to the same high-affinity androgen receptor protein within the cells of androgendependent target areas [60]. The affinity of the androgen receptor is much greater for DHT than it is for testosterone.

Testosterone enters the target cell by passive diffusion and either binds to the androgen receptor or is metabolized to DHT which then binds to the same receptor. The androgen receptor complex binds to acceptor sites on nuclear chromatin and ultimately initiates transcription of mRNA, starting the complex metabolic processes of androgen action (Fig. 3.6) [84]. The gene for the androgen receptor has been cloned to the long arm of the X chromosome near the centromere [85].

In the urogenital tubercle, high activity of 5α-reductase at the time of sex differentiation provides DHT for preferential binding to the androgen receptor. The reason that testosterone mediates some androgen effects and DHT mediates others is currently not clear, but it may involve subtle differences in the affinity of the receptor for the androgen, some aspect of the metabolism of testosterone, or both [60].

DHT develops the prostate, prostatic utricle, scrotum, penis with male-type urethra and the glans penis. On the

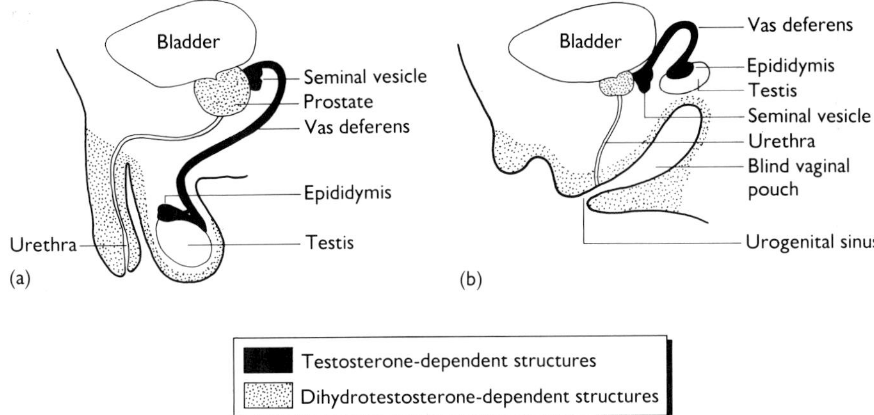

Fig. 3.7 **(a)** Suggested selective role of testosterone and DHT in normal male sexual differentiation. (b) Findings in males who cannot convert testosterone to DHT (5α-reductase deficiency). Testosterone-dependent structures are normal, although testes are not descended. DHT-dependent structures are not developed. Blind vaginal pouch is frequently present (redrawn from Imperato-McGinley *et al.* [87]).

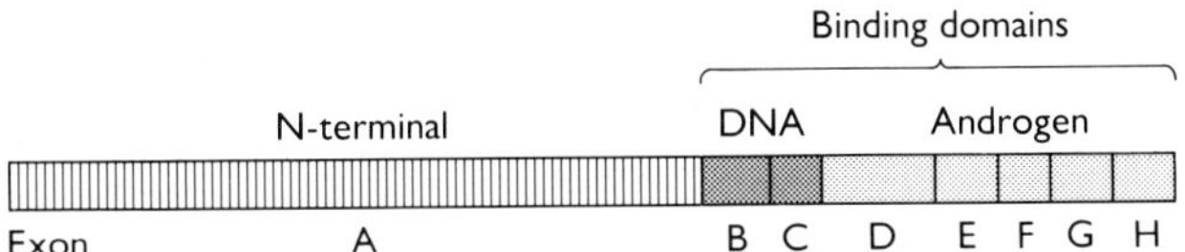

Fig. 3.8 Schematic presentation of androgen receptor. The aminoterminal portion is coded by exon A. Its role is probably modulatory. The DNA-binding domain is coded by exons B and C and the androgen-binding domain is encoded by exons D, E, F, G and H.

other hand, increases in muscle mass and voice changes at puberty appear to be mediated by testosterone. Acne, beard growth, temporal hairline recession, body hair and prostatic growth, however, seem all to mediated by DHT which also plays a role in the negative feedback control of luteinizing hormone (LH). The enzyme 5α-reductase is present in the urogenital sinus and external genital anlagen prior to masculinization (Fig. 3.7) [8,69,84,86–88].

The binding of T and DHT to the receptor complex has been hypothesized to result in a conformational change in the receptor, exposing its DNA-binding domain and enabling it to bind to the nuclear chromatin. The binding of androgen receptor complex to DNA initiates transcription of mRNA and ultimately translation into androgen-specific protein. In humans with complete androgen insensitivity a number of binding abnormalities of the androgen receptor have been described. Absence of high-affinity binding has been demonstrated (receptor negative). Subjects with normal binding and absent androgen receptor complex binding to nuclear chromatin (receptor positive) have also been described. Human androgen receptor DNA has been cloned. The androgen receptor gene belongs to the steroid receptor superfamily, and is composed of eight exons and an androgen, and a DNA-binding domain (Fig. 3.8). Various defects result in synthesis of abnormal androgen receptor. Mutations in the androgen-binding domain result in receptor-negative androgen insensitivity whereas as mutations in the DNA-binding domain result in receptor-positive binding abnormalities to DNA [89–91].

Recently two 5α-reductase genes have been cloned. These genes encode two different isozymes that can be distinguished on the basis of biochemical, pharmacological and genetic criteria. The type 1 isoenzyme is encoded on chromosome 5, and is expressed in low levels in the prostate. High levels are present in scalp hair follicles. Type 1 isoenzyme is relatively insensitive to the 5α-reductase inhibitor finasteride (Proscar, Merck) a 4-azasteroid enzyme inhibitor. The type 2 isoenzyme is encoded on chromosome 2 and is expressed in high levels in the prostate and many other androgen-sensitive tissues. Type 2 isoenzyme is exquisitely sensitive to finasteride [8].

Male pseudohermaphroditism due to 5α-reductase deficiency has been the consequence of mutations in the type 2 gene in all cases studied. Molecular analysis indicates that the majority of patients with steroid 5α-reductase type 2 deficiency have various mutations. One genetic isolate in New Guinea has a deletion of the type 2 gene. Since only the type 2 gene is responsible for 5α reduction of testosterone in genital skin, defects in the type 1 gene would not be expected to be associated with male pseudohermaphroditism [9].

No hormones are necessary for normal female differentiation of external genitalia. In the 8 week female fetus, the genital tubercle becomes the clitoris, the labioscrotal swelling the labia majora and the urethral fold the labia minora. The labioscrotal swellings do not fuse, and the perineal anogenital distance does not increase. Cavitation for vaginal development is first observed at 15 weeks and is complete at 18 weeks. In males, caudal growth of the rudimentary vaginal chord is inhibited, and canalization of this rudimentary structure yields the prostatic utricle, which opens just beneath the bladder neck between the orifices of the vasa deferentia [92].

REFERENCES

1 McLaren A. What makes a man? *Nature* 1990;346:216–17.

2 Josso N, Legeai L, Forest MG *et al.* Enzyme-linked immunoassay for anti-Müllerian hormone: a new tool for the evaluation of testicular function in infants and children. *J Clin Endocrinol Metab* 1990;70:23–7.

3 Cohen-Haguenauer O, Picard JY, Mattei MG *et al.* Mapping of the gene for anti-Müllerian hormone to the short arm of human chromosome 19. *Cytogenet Cell Genet* 1987;44:2–6.

4 Donahoe PK, Cate RL, MacLaughlin DT *et al.* Müllerian-inhibiting substance; gene structure and mechanism of action of a fetal repressor. *Rec Prog Horm Res* 1987;43:431–67.

5 Chang C, Kokontis J, Liao S. Structural analysis of complementary DNA and aminoacid sequences of human and rat androgen receptors. *Proc Natl Acad Sci USA* 1988; 85:7211–15.

6 Lubahn DB, Joseph DR, Sullivan PM *et al.* Cloning of human androgen receptor complementary DNA and localization to the X chromosome. *Science* 1988;240:327–30.

7 Chang C, Kokontis J, Liao S. Molecular cloning of human and rat complementary cDNA encoding androgen receptors. *Science* 1988;240:324–6.

8 Thigpen AE, Davis DL, Milatovich A *et al.* The molecular genetics of steroid 5α-reductase deficiency. *J Clin Invest* 1992;90:799–809.

9 Wilson J *et al.* Androgen resistance syndromes. *Endocr Rev* 1993;14:577–94.

10 Rubin RT, Reinisch JM, Haskett RF. Postnatal gonadal steroid effects on human behavior. *Science* 1981;211:1318–24.

11 Whelsons WJ, Russel LB. The Y chromosome as a bearer of male determining factors in the mouse. *Proc Natl Acad Sci USA* 1959;45:560–6.

12 Mittwoch U. Do genes determine sex. *Nature* 1969;221: 446–8.

13 Polani PE. Abnormal sex development in man. I. Anomalies of sex-determining mechanisms. In: Justin CR, Edwards RG, eds. *Mechanism of Sex Differentiation in Animals and Man.* London: Academic Press, 1981:465–547.

14 Jost A, Vigier B, Prepin J, Perchellet, JP. Studies on sex differentiation in mammals. *Rec Prog Horm Res* 1973;29:1–41.

15 Jirasek JE. Morphogenesis of the genital system in the human. *Birth Defects* 1977;13:13–39.

16 Jirasek JE. Principles of reproductive endocrinology. In: Simpson JL, ed. *Disorders of Sexual Differentiation.* New York: Academic Press, 1976:52–111.

17 Wachtel SS, Ohno S. The immunogenetics of sexual development. *Prog Med Genet* 1979;3:109–42.

18 Simpson E, Chandler P, Goulmý E, Disteche CM, Ferguson-Smith MA, Page DC. Separation of the genetic loci for the H-Y antigen and for testis determination on human Y chromosome. *Nature* 1987;326:876–8.

19 Lau YFC, Chan K. The putative testis-determining factor and related genes are expressed as discrete sized transcripts in adult gonadal and somatic tissues. *Am J Hum Genet* 1990;45: 942–52.

20 Page DC, Mosher R, Simpson EM *et al.* The sex-determining human Y chromosome encodes a finger protein. *Cell* 1987; 51:1091–104.

21 Page DC, Brown LG, de la Chapelle A. Exchange of terminal portions of X and Y chormosomal short arms in human XX males. *Nature* 1987;328:437–40.

22 Palmer MS, Sinclair H, Ellis NA *et al.* Genetic evidence that ZFY is not the testis-determining factor. *Nature* 1989; 342:937–9.

23 Palmer MS, Berta P, Sinclar AH, Pym B, Goodfellow PN. Comparison of human ZFY and ZFY transcripts. *Genetics* 1990;187:1618–85.

24 Burgoyne PS. Thumbs down for the zinc finger? *Nature* 1989;342:860–2.

25 Sinclair, AH, Berta P, Palmer MS *et al.* A gene from the human sex-determining region encodes a protein with homology to a conserved DNA binding motif. *Nature* 1990; 346:240–4.

26 Gubbay J, Collignon J, Koopman P *et al.* A gene mapping to the sex-determining region of the mouse Y chromosome is a member of a novel family of embryonically expressed genes. *Nature* 1990;346:245–50.

27 Shapiro, LJ. X and Y chromosome organization. The pseudo-autosomal region. In: Rosenfeld R, Grumbach M, eds. *Turner Syndrome.* New York: Marcel Dekker, 1990;3–11.

28 Koopman P, Gubbay J, Vivian, N *et al.* Male development of chromosomally female mice transgenic for SRY. *Nature* 1991; 351:117–21.

29 Koopman P, Munsterberg A, Capel B *et al.* Expression of a candidate sex-determining gene during mouse testis determination. *Nature* 1990;348:450–2.

30 Redline, RW, Williams AJ, Patterson P, Collins T. Human *HOX* U.E.: a gene strongly expressed in the adult male and female urogenital tracts. *Genomics* 1992;13:425–30.

31 Hawkins JR, Koopman P, Berta P. Testis-determining factor and Y-linked sex reversal. *Curr Opin Genet Dev* 1991;1:30–4.

32 Jager RJ, Anvret M, Hall K, Scherer SA. Human XY female with a frame shift mutation in the candidate testes determining gene SRY. *Nature* 1990; 348:452–3.

33 Ferrari S, Hartley VR, Pontiggia H *et al.* SRY, like HMG1, recognizes sharp angles in DNA. *EMBO J* 1992;11:497–506.

34 Eccles MR, Wallis LJ, Fidler AE *et al.* Expression of of the *PAX* 2 gene in human fetal kidney and Wilms tumor. *Cell Growth and Diff* 1992;3:279–89.

35 Ohno S. *Major Sex-determining Genes.* New York: Springer Verlag, 1979.

36 Wolgemuth DJ, Viviano CM, Gizang-Ginsberg F *et al.* Differential expression of the mouse homeobox-containing gene HOX-1.4 during male germ cell differentiation and embryonic development. *Proc Natl Acad Sci USA* 1987;50:5815–17.

36a Bardoni P, Zanaria E, Guioli S *et al.* A dosage sensitive locus at chromosome Xp 21 is involved in male to female sex reversal. *Nature Genetics* 1994;7:497–501.

37 Hastie ND. *PAX* in our time. *Curr Biol* 1992;1:324–44.

38 Blyth B, Douchett JAV. Gonadal differentiation: a review of the physiological process and influencing factors based on recent experimental evidence. *J Urol* 1991;145:689–94.

39 Francavilla S, Cordeschi G, Properzi G, Concordia N, Cappa F, Pozzi V. Ultrastructure of fetal human gonad before sexual differentiation and during early testicular and ovarian development. *J Submicrosc Cytol Pathol* 1990;22:389–400.

40 Tran D, Meusy-Dessole N, Josso N. Anti-Müllerian hormone is a functional marker of foetal Sertoli cells. *Nature* 1977; 269:411–12.

41 Sharpe, RM, Skakkebaek NE. Are oestrogens involved in falling sperm counts and disorders of the male reproductive tract? *Lancet* 1992;1:1392–4.

42 Charpentier G, Magre S. Masculinizing effect of testes on

developing rat ovaries in organ culture. *Development* 1990; 110:839–49.
43 Mittwoch U, Burgess AMC, Baker PJ. Male development in a sea of oestrogen. *Lancet* 1993;2:123–4.
44 Saenger P, Reiter EO. Management of cryptorchidism. *Trends Endocrinol Metab* 1992;3:249–53.
45 Fentener van Vlissingen FM, Van Zoelen EJJ, Usem PJF *et al.* *In vitro* model of the first phase of testicular descent: identification of a low molecular weight factor from fetal testis involved in proliferation of gubernaculum testis cells and distinct from specified polypeptide growth factors and fetal gonadal hormones. *Endocrinology* 1988;123:2868–77.
46 Pelliniemi LJ, Niemi M. Fine structure of human foetal testis. I. The interstitial tissue. *Z Zellforsch Mikroskop Anat* 1969;99:507–22.
47 Merchant-Larios H, Taketo T. Testicular differentiation in mammals under normal and experimental conditions. *Electron Microsc Tech* 1991;19:158–71.
48 Clements JA, Reyes RI, Winder JSD *et al.* Studies on human sexual development. III. Fetal pituitary and serum and amniotic fluid concentrations of LH, HCG, FSH. *J Clin Endocrinol Metab* 1976;42:9–19.
49 Saenger P. Abnormal sex differentiation. *J Pediatr* 1984;104: 1–17.
50 Baillie AH, Ferguson MM, Hart DMK. Histochemical evidence of steroid metabolism in the human genital ridge. *J Clin Endocrinol Metab* 1966;26:738–41.
51 Clark SJ, Ellis N, Styne DM *et al.* Hormone ontogeny in the ovine fetus. XVII. Demonstration of pulsatile luteinizing hormone secretion by the fetal pituitary gland. *Endocrinology* 1984;115:1774–9.
52 George FW, Wilson JD. The regulation of androgen and estrogen formation in fetal gonads. *Ann Biol Anim Biochem Biophys* 1979;19:129–306.
53 Baker TG. A quantitative and cytological study of germ cells in human ovaries. *Proc R Soc Lond (Biol)* 1963;158: 417–33.
54 George FW, Simpson ER, Milewich L *et al.* Studies on the regulation of the onset of steroid hormone biosynthesis in fetal rabbit gonads. *Endocrinology* 1979;105:1100–6.
55 Lovinger RD, Kaplan SL, Grumbach MM. Congenital hypopituitarism associated with neonatal hypoglycemia and microphallus: four cases secondary to hypothalamic hormone deficiencies. *J Pediatr* 1975;87:1171–81.
56 Forest MG, Sizonenko PC, Cathiard AM *et al.* Hypophysogonadal function in infants during the first year of life. Evidence of testicular activity in early infancy. *J Clin Invest* 1974;53:819–24.
57 Forest MG. Physiological changes in circulating androgens. In: Forest MG, ed. *Androgens in Childhood. Pediatric and Adolescent Endocrinology*, Vol. 19. Basel: Karger, 1989: 104–29.
58 Forest MG, de Peretti E, Lecoq A *et al.* Concentrations of 14 steroid hormones in human amniotic fluid of midpregnancy. *J Clin Endocrinol Metab* 1980;5:818–22.
59 Voutilainen R. Hormonal development in the fetal gonad. In: Sizonenko PC, Aubert ML, eds. *Developmental Endocrinology*. New York: Raven Press, 1990:27–37.
60 Wilson JD, Griffin JE, Leshin M *et al.* Role of gonadal hormones in development of sexual phenotypes. *Hum Genet* 1981;58:78–84.
61 George FW, Wilson JD. Endocrine differentiation of the foetal rabbit ovary in culture. *Nature* 1980;283:861–3.
62 Payne AH, Jaffe RB. Androgen formation from pregnenolone sulfate by the human fetal ovary. *J Clin Endocrinol Metab* 1974;34:300–4.
63 Pryse-Davies J, Dewhurst CJ. The development of the ovary and uterus in the fetus, newborn and infant: a morphological and enzyme histochemical study. *J Pathol* 1971;103:5–25.
64 Singh PR, Carr DH. The anatomy and histology of XO human embryos and fetuses. *Anat Rec* 1966;155:369–83.
65 Held KR. Turner's syndrome and chromosome Y (editorial). *Lancet* 1993;342:128.
66 Byskov AG, Saxen L. Induction of meiosis in fetal mouse testis *in vitro*. *Dev Biol* 1976;52:193–200.
67 Price D, Zaaijer JJP, Ortiz E, Brinkmann AO. Current views on embryonic sex differentiation in reptiles, birds and mammals. *Am Zool* (Suppl.) 1975;1:173–95.
68 Mürset G, Zachmann M, Prader A, Risher J, Labhart A. Male external genitalia of a girl caused by a virilizing adrenal tumor in the mother: case report and steroid studies. *Acta Endocrinol* 1970;65:627–38.
69 Siiteri PK, Wilson JD. Testosterone formation and metabolism during male sexual differentiation in the human embryo. *J Clin Endocrinol Metab* 1974;38:113–25.
70 Somjen CJ, Kaye AM, Lindner HF. Demonstration of a 8S-cytoplasmic estrogen receptor in rat müllerian duct. *Biochem Biophys Acta* 1976;428:787–91.
71 Pepinsky RB, Sinclair LK, Chow EP *et al.* Proteolytic processing of Müllerian inhibiting substance produces a transforming growth factor-β-like fragment. *J Biol Chem* 1988; 263;961–5.
72 Josso N, Boussin L, Knebelmann B *et al.* Anti-Müllerian hormone and intersex states. *Trends Endocrinol Metab* 1991;2:227–33.
73 Josso N. Anti-müllerian hormone: new perspectives for a sexist molecule. *Endocr Rev* 1986;7:421–33.
74 Cate RL, Mattaliano RJ, Hession C *et al.* Isolation of the bovine and human genes for müllerian inhibiting substance and expression of the human gene in animal cells. *Cell* 1986;45:685–98.
75 Cate RL, Donahoe PK, MacLaughlin DT. Müllerian-inhibiting substance. In Spron MB, Roberts AB, eds. *Handbook of Experimental Pharmacology: Peptide Growth Factors and their Receptors*, 95/II. Berlin: Springer-Verlag, 1990:179–210.
76 Josso N, Picard JY, Tran D. The anti-müllerian hormone. *Rec Prog Horm Res* 1977;33:117–60.
77 Behringer RR, Cate RL, Froelick GJ, Palmiter RD, Brimester RL. Abnormal sexual development in transgenic mice chronically expressing Müllerian inhibiting substance. *Nature* 1990;345:167–70.
78 Vigier B, Forest MG, Eychenne B *et al.* Anti-müllerian hormone produces endocrine sex-reversal of fetal ovaries. *Proc Natl Acad Sci USA* 1989;86:3684–8.
79 Knebelmann B, Boussin L, Guerrier D *et al.* Anti-Müllerian hormone Bruxelles: a nonsense mutation associated in the last exon of the anti-Müllerian hormone gene associated with the persistent Müllerian duct syndrome. *Proc Natl Acad Sci USA* 1991;88:3767–71.
80 Ulfelder H, Robboy SJ. Embryologic development of the vagina. *Am J Obstet Gynecol* 1976;126:769–76.
81 Wilson JD. Testosterone uptake by the urogenital tract of the rabbit embryo. *Endocrinology* 1973;92:1192–9.
82 Henderson BE, Benton B, Cosgrove M *et al.* Urogenital tract abnormalities in sons of women treated with diethylstilbestrol. *Pediatrics* 1976;58:505–7.
83 Grumbach MM, Ducharme JR. The effects of androgens on fetal sexual development: androgen-induced female pseudo-

hermaphroditism. *Fertil Steril* 1960;11:157–80.

84 Griffin KD, Wilson JD. The androgen resistance syndromes: 5α-reductase deficiency, testicular feminization, and related disorders. In: Scriver C, Baudet A, Sly W *et al.*, eds. *The Metabolic Basis of Inherited Disease*, 6th edn. New York: McGraw-Hill, 1989:1919–44.

85 Migeon B, Brown TR, Axelman J *et al.* Studies of the locus for androgen receptor: localization on the human X chromosome and evidence for homology with the Tfm locus in the mouse. *Proc Natl Acad Sci USA* 1981;78:6339–43.

86 Saenger P. Steroid 5α-reductase deficiency. In: Josso N, ed. *The Intersex Child.* Basel: Karger, 1981:156–70.

87 Imperato-McGinley J, Guerrero L, Gautier T, Peterson RE. Steroid 5α-reductase deficiency in man: an inherited form of male pseudohermaphroditism. *Science* 1974;186:213.

88 Peterson RE, Imperato-McGinley J, Gautier T, Sturla E. Male pseudohermaphroditism due to 5α-reductase deficiency. *Am J Med* 1977;62:170–91.

89 McPhaul MJ, Marcelli M, Zoppi S *et al.* The spectrum of mutations in the androgen receptor gene that causes androgen resistance. *J Clin Endocrinol Metab* 1993;76:17–23.

90 Marcelli M, Tilley WD, Wilson JE *et al.* A single nucleotide substitution introduces a premature termination codon into the androgen receptor gene of a patient with receptor-negative androgen resistance. *J Clin Invest* 1990;85:1522–8.

91 Marcelli M, Zoppi S, Grino PB *et al.* A mutation in the DNA-binding domain of the androgen receptor gene causes complete testicular feminization in a patient with receptor-positive androgen resistance. *J Clin Invest* 1991;87:1123–6.

92 O'Rahilly R. The development of the vagina in the human. *Birth Defects* 1977;13:123–36.

4: The Clinical Management of Ambiguous Genitalia

G.L. WARNE and I.A. HUGHES

INTRODUCTION

When a baby is born, the parents are eager to learn whether they have a boy or a girl. The doctor or midwife will often announce the sex before making any comment about the infant's state of health. Gender and identity are closely intertwined, and the parents of a newborn infant will make projections about the child's future identity based on gender. The decision about an infant's sex, with all of the lifelong consequences for that individual, is made by a doctor in no more than a few seconds.

There are situations, however, when the decision is not so straightforward. Once in every 4500 births [1] the genital anatomy is so abnormal that it is extremely difficult, or even impossible, at first to decide the sex. If the doctor hesitates over assigning the sex, the parents will experience intense anxiety. The doctor will therefore be under great pressure to respond quickly. Appropriate investigations should be initiated and expert assistance obtained without delay. At the same time the parents' difficult questions must be answered in a confident and reassuring manner. Well-informed and coordinated counselling will greatly assist the parents to accept the child's problem.

An infant with one of the disorders of sexual differentiation may be born demonstrating a wide spectrum of phenotypic variation – with male, female or ambiguous genitalia. A genotypic female may be completely masculinized, as in congenital adrenal hyperplasia (CAH), and a genotypic male may have a female phenotype, as in complete androgen insensitivity. The term 'ambiguous genitalia' is largely descriptive and does not refer to any single intermediate phenotype. Nearly always, there is the combination of a phallus smaller than a normal penis but larger than a normal clitoris, with a urethral opening either at the base of the phallus or in the perineum. Edmonds' classification (Fig. 4.1) pictorially defines three stages of virilization, and can be used to assess the severity of the virilization.

It is important to realize that a defect which one observer might refer to as 'hypospadias with undescended testes' would possibly be called 'ambiguous genitalia' by another. The two phrases have quite different connotations: the first clearly implies that the observer presumes the infant to be male, while the second implies the infant to have a more fundamental disturbance in sexual differentiation. A process of investigation would be initiated more readily in a child regarded as having ambiguous genitalia than in one regarded as having hypospadias with undescended testes, even though the two descriptions may be referring to the same child.

There are three important reasons why every infant born with ambiguous genitalia should be fully investigated:

1 to diagnose the underlying cause, so that a treatment plan can be prepared;

2 to gather as much information as possible before choosing the sex of rearing;

3 to facilitate genetic counselling.

Malformation of the genitalia may signify the presence of an underlying medical disorder which could threaten future health. Examples include:

1 CAH, which may progress to an adrenal crisis and death from salt loss within 1–2 weeks of birth;

2 other forms of CAH (11β- and 17α-hydroxylase deficiencies), which cause arterial hypertension, sometimes during childhood but particularly in adult life;

3 XY partial gonadal dysgenesis is associated with an increased risk of malignant germinoma (26% by age 30 [3]), Wilms tumour, and a diffuse glomerulopathy;

4 the androgen-insensitivity syndrome is associated with a 9% risk [4] of a malignant gonadal tumour.

A decision about the sex of rearing must be taken without undue delay. The decision is usually based on the results of laboratory investigations, but anatomical and cultural considerations are also involved. A week is as long as most parents can wait. The most useful investigations will therefore be those giving reliable results in less than a week. These include assays of steroid hormones, such as 17-hydroxyprogesterone, karyotyping, radiological investigations and endoscopy. Investigations taking much longer (for example androgen receptor assays or a

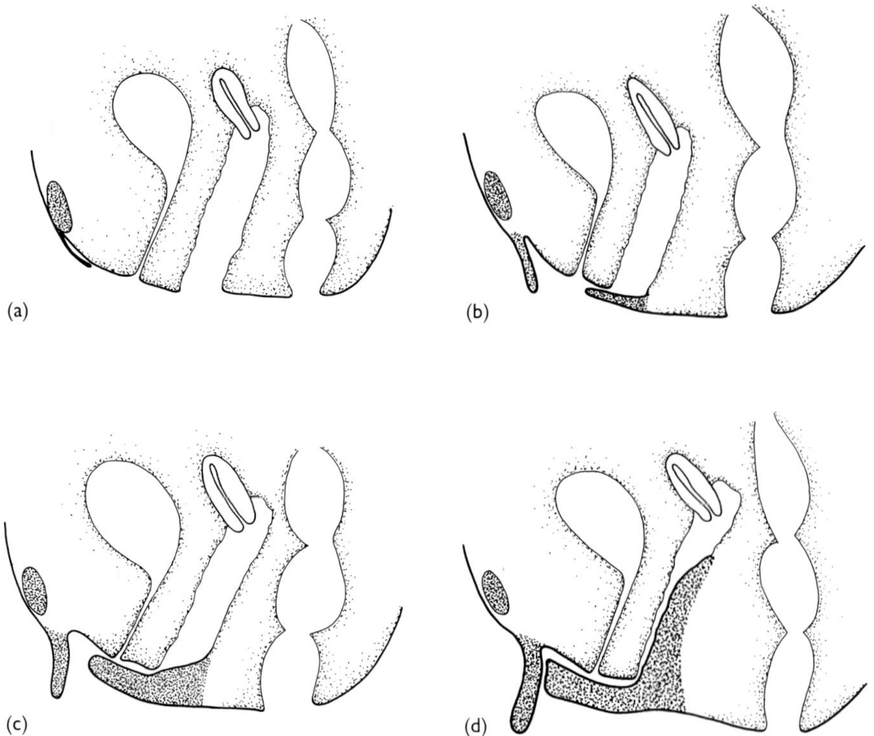

Fig. 4.1 Edmonds' classification of ambiguous genitalia. (a) Normal female; (b) Labial fusion; (c) Cloaca; (d) Urogenital sinus (from Edmonds [2]).

therapeutic trial of testosterone, which take 6–8 weeks) will be used only to confirm the correctness of a clinical diagnosis which has already been used to decide the sex of rearing. They may also give an indication of the genital response to sex hormones at the time of puberty. It is not unusual for even the most extensive investigation to fail to reveal the cause of genital abnormality.

Since a number of the causes of ambiguous genitalia have a genetic basis, more than one member of a family may be affected, and genetic counselling will be needed. CAH is inherited as an autosomal recessive trait. The androgen insensitivity syndrome is X-linked. Direct study by DNA analysis of a number of the key genes involved in sexual differentiation has led to the identification and characterization of many mutations. The mapping of genes through linkage analyses uses indirect techniques to locate disease loci. This usually leads to the development of highly sensitive and specific DNA tests which can be applied in prenatal testing for the mutation in subsequent pregnancies. The identification of carriers among other members of the family may also become possible, thus facilitating genetic counselling.

MANAGEMENT OF THE INFANT WITH AMBIGUOUS GENITALIA

The clinical assessment and investigation of an infant with ambiguous genitalia has to be carried out urgently, so that a decision about the sex of rearing can be made in as few days as possible. In the meantime, every effort must be made to encourage bonding between the parents and child. The parents need counselling about the nature of the baby's abnormality and guidance in how to deal with their friends and relations. Once the sex of rearing has been decided, treatment can be organized. Genetic counselling will need to be deferred until a specific aetiological diagnosis is available.

Counselling the parents before the sex of the infant has been decided

The following points regarding counselling are based on interviews with parents [5]. A positive comment should be made that the baby appears healthy, but that there is a problem concerning the sex. At this point the parents should be shown the genitalia, so that they can see the problem for themselves. They need reassurance that the baby will be definitely either a boy or a girl, and not something 'in between'. They need to know that investigations to determine the true sex are to be initiated immediately and when they will hear the results. The involvement of a trained counsellor may be very helpful during the initial period.

WHILE WAITING FOR RESULTS

1 Avoid referring to the baby as 'it'; say 'your baby'.
2 Say that there are many other babies born with the same kind of problem, and that doctors are familiar with it.
3 Educate other members of staff to follow the same rules. Make it clear that no-one should express an opinion about the baby's sex until a clear decision has been taken.
4 Keep careful notes about communications with the parents, so that all staff will know what has been said.
5 Have a discussion with the parents about how they plan to deal with the questions of friends, relations and other patients. This is often a source of great distress and, although no clear guidelines have been published, it will be helpful if the parents have had the opportunity to think about the alternatives available to them.
6 Advise the parents not to name the baby or to register the birth until the sex has been ascertained.

Essential points about normal sexual differentiation

The clinical assessment and investigation of ambiguous genitalia must be based on an understanding of normal sexual differentiation (summarized in Fig. 4.2). The basic points are as follows.
1 Male and female genitalia differentiate from the same structures.
2 The degree of external masculinization is an expression of the amount of androgen present (regardless of the source), and the ability of the tissues to respond to androgen.
3 The gonadal sex is related to the chromosomal sex through specific genes, such as SRY [7].
4 The internal reproductive organs reflect the presence or absence of testicular anti-Müllerian hormone.

Physical examination of the infant

The features that the clinician should seek when examining an infant with ambiguous genitalia include the following.
1 Palpable gonads: these are likely to be testes, but palpable testes need not be normal, since dysgenetic testes are often palpable. An ovary that has prolapsed into the sac of an inguinal hernia may be palpable. In one series [8], 21% of inguinal hernias in phenotypic females were found to contain an ovary. If both gonads are palpable they are almost certainly testes. The gonads may lie anywhere along the line joining the external inguinal ring and the perineum. It is easy to miss them unless a thorough and systematic search is made.
2 A dysmorphic appearance: features of Turner syndrome (webbed neck, oedema of the hands and feet, characteristic facies) are present in some cases of 45,X/46,XY and 46,XY partial gonadal dysgenesis. Further examination might reveal a cardiac murmur, absent femoral pulses and arterial hypertension, suggesting coarctation of the aorta.

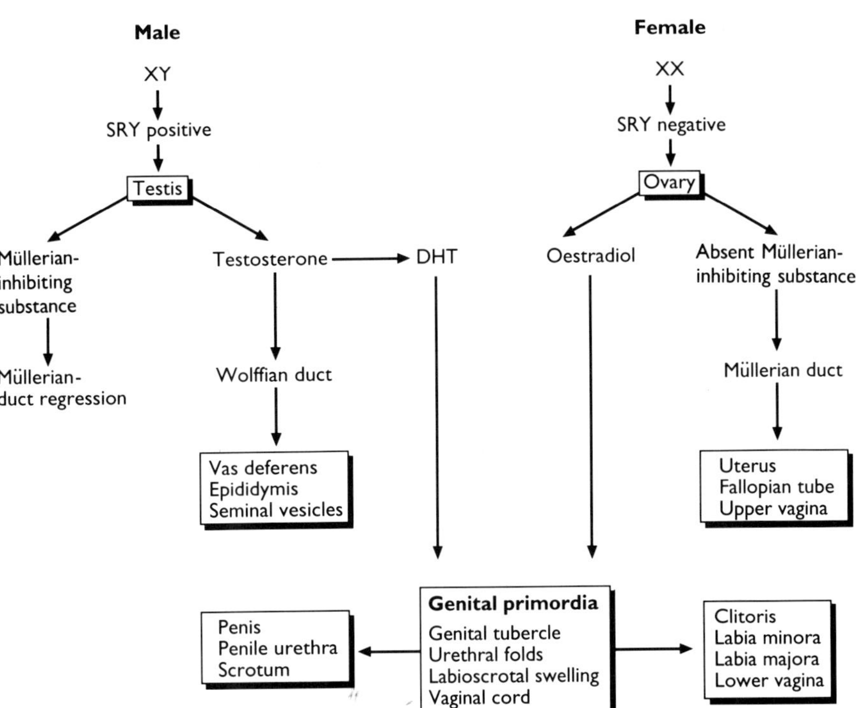

Fig. 4.2 A schematic outline of prenatal events in sexual development (from Batch *et al.* [6]).

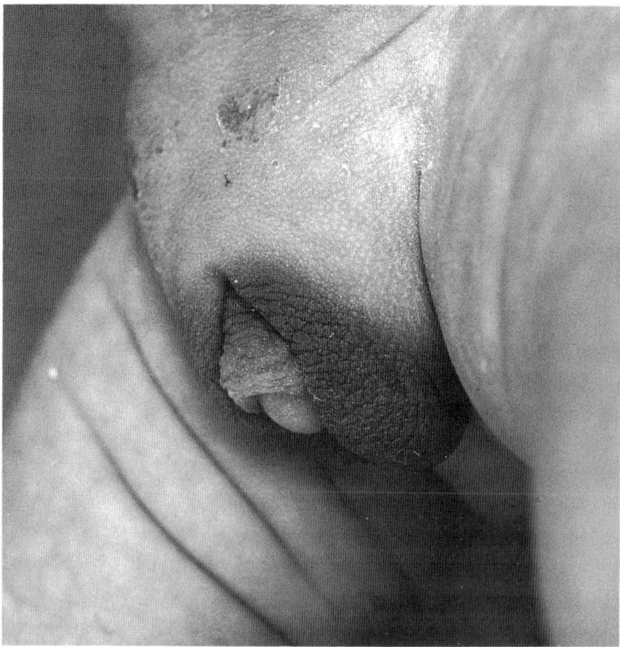

Fig. 4.3 Pigmented ambiguous genitalia in a child with 21-hydroxylase deficiency.

3 Systemic illness: in an infant with ambiguous genitalia the development of severe hypoglycaemia soon after birth suggests adrenocortical insufficiency. Dehydration, salt depletion and vomiting are features of the same condition, but do not usually occur until 1–2 weeks later.

4 Skin pigmentation: an abnormal pigmentation in the genital skin and nipples appears when there is increased secretion of pituitary adrenocorticotrophic hormone (ACTH) and pro-opiomelanocortin. In a child with ambiguous genitalia this would generally point to a diagnosis of CAH. Sometimes the pigmentation is generalized and may even involve the tongue. More commonly the pigmentation is quite hard to see, especially under yellow incandescent light. The infant should ideally be examined in daylight before concluding that hyperpigmentation is absent.

5 Whether or not there is a uterus: the absence of the uterus in an infant with ambiguous genitalia is evidence that functional testicular tissue has been present, since the Müllerian ducts disappear only when MIS has been secreted, and the only source of MIS in the fetus is the testes. With practice the uterine cervix is easy to identify by performing a rectal examination. Only the little finger should be used, and doctors with large fingers should not attempt rectal examinations on small infants, because rectal tears can result. Table 4.1 shows how useful this distinction can be.

Table 4.1 A differential diagnosis based on the presence or absence of the uterus in an infant with ambiguous genitalia

Uterus present	Uterus absent
Genotypic female with CAH	Androgen-insensitivity syndrome
Female virilized by transplacental androgen [9–11] or by endogenous tumour	5α-Reductase deficiency
Partial gonadal dysgenesis	Block in testosterone biosynthesis
	Primary gonadotrophin deficiency
	Absence of Leydig cells [12]
	Drug-induced blockade of androgen action

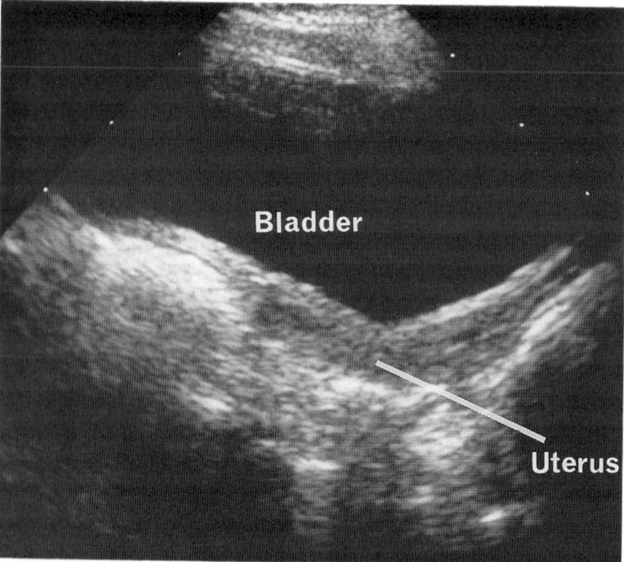

Fig. 4.4 Pelvic ultrasound appearance of the uterus in an infant.

Further investigations to define anatomy

1 Inguinal or intra-abdominal gonads are best located by magnetic resonance imaging (MRI) [13]. Ultrasound is sometimes used to locate inguinal testes, but results are variable. Laparoscopy has been used to locate (and remove) inguinal gonads [14]. Surgical biopsy will be needed to define the histology.

2 The uterus can be located using ultrasonography (Fig. 4.4), MRI [13], urogenital sinus X-rays with contrast, endoscopy, laparoscopy and laparotomy.

3 The presence or absence of a prostate gland (a distinction which may be important if 5α-reductase deficiency is suspected) can be demonstrated with transrectal sonography [15].

Selecting appropriate laboratory investigations

The physical examination of the infant provides the clues needed to formulate a differential diagnosis, and investi-

Table 4.2 Steps in establishing the diagnosis in an infant of uncertain sex

Clinical feature				
Palpable gonad(s)	–	+	+	+
Uterus present*	+	+	–	–
Increased skin pigmentation	+	–	–	–/+
Sick baby	+/–	–	–	–/+
Dysmorphic appearance	–	+/–	–	–
Clinical diagnosis	*21-Hydroxylase deficiency*	*Gonadal dysgenesis with Y chromosome*	*Partial androgen insensitivity*	*Block in testosterone biosynthesis*
Investigation				
Serum 17-OHP	↑	Normal	Normal	Normal
Electrolytes	Abnormal	Normal	Normal	Possibly abnormal
Karyotype	46,XX	45,X/46,XY or other pattern	46,XY	46,XY
Testosterone response to hCG	Not indicated	Definite response	Good response (both T and DHT)	Blunted or absent
Gonadal biopsy	Not indicated	Dysgenetic gonad, +/– tumour	Normal testis (+/– Leydig cell hyperplasia)	Normal testis
Other	Urine steroid profile	–	Genital skin fibroblast culture for AR assay	Measure testosterone precursors

* As determined by ultrasound examination or rectal palpation.
AR, androgen receptor; DHT, dihydrotestosterone; 17-OHP, 17-hydroxyprogesterone; T, testosterone.

gations are then selected so that a final diagnosis may be reached as quickly as possible. Table 4.2 summarizes the processes of clinical and laboratory evaluation in an infant whose initial sex is unclear.

THE KARYOTYPE

Most cytogenetic laboratories can, under favourable circumstances, take peripheral blood and provide a preliminary report on the karyotype within a few days. When it has been established that an infant with ambiguous genitalia is genetically female, the cause of the virilization will be one of those shown in Table 4.3.

If the karyotype proves to be XY, the underlying conditions can be divided into two groups, one in which androgen was insufficient in amount, and one in which there was an impaired response to a sufficient amount of androgen. These are shown in Table 4.4.

Often the karyotype is neither XX nor XY, but a mosaic pattern, such as XO/XY or XX/XY. The two gonads are often different. One may be a streak and the other a testis or an ovotestis, or both may be ovotestes but with different testicular and ovarian components.

Table 4.3 Causes of ambiguous genitalia in infants with a 46,XX karyotype

Problem	Cause	Specific examples
Excessive androgens of fetal origin	Congenital adrenal hyperplasia	21-Hydroxylase deficiency 11β-Hydroxylase deficiency 3β-Hydroxysteroid dehydrogenase deficiency
	Testis or ovotestis present	Partial gonadal dysgenesis*
Androgens crossing the placenta	Maternal ingestion of virilizing drug	Danazol [17], progestogens
	Virilizing disease in the mother	Adrenal tumour [18,19] or hyperplasia [20] Ovarian tumour [21]
	Placental aromatase deficiency [16]	
Non-androgenic	Isolated clitoromegaly due to neurofibromatosis	

* When PGD is associated with a 46,XX karyotype the genitalia are more likely to be female than ambiguous.

Table 4.4 Causes of ambiguous genitalia in infants with a 46,XY karyotype

Problem	Cause	Specific examples
Insufficient androgen	Gonadal dysgenesis	SRY gene mutation
	Block in testosterone biosynthesis	17-Ketosteroid reductase deficiency 3β-Hydroxysteroid dehydrogenase deficiency
	Primary Leydig cell hypoplasia	Unresponsiveness to LH/hCG [22]
Impaired response to androgen	Abnormal androgen receptor	Partial androgen insensitivity syndrome
	Deficient conversion of testosterone to DHT	5α-Reductase deficiency

DHT, dihydotestosterone; hCG, human chorionic gonadotrophin; LH, luteinizing hormone.

Some cautionary remarks about the interpretation of chromosome analyses

A rapid chromosome analysis is extremely useful in many circumstances, but the reader is cautioned to remember the following points.

1 The detection of low levels of chromosomal mosaicism will take the laboratory some extra days, because this may entail the examination of a large number of cells (up to 100).

2 Even if no mosaicism in seen in the peripheral blood, it may still be found in other tissues, such as skin or gonadal tissue.

3 Several sensitive techniques for the detection of small Y chromosome fragments have been reported. These include fluorescent *in situ* hybridization (FISH) using Y chromosome satellite DNA probes [23], Southern blot analysis of amplified DNA [24], and *in situ* hybridization with cosmid clones [25].

The summary of the diagnostic steps taken during the first week are listed below.

1 First 48 hours: family history; physical examination findings; blood glucose series; serum 17-hydroxyprogesterone (if this is measured too soon after birth, the 17-OHP level may be falsely elevated, especially in preterm infants and under conditions of stress (illness); pelvic ultrasound scan and urogenital sinugram or other imaging procedures.

2 Days 2–4: preliminary report taken on chromosome karyotype.

3 Day 7: the result of the hCG stimulation test (rise in serum testosterone) and the result of the urinary steroid gas chromatography.

DECIDING THE SEX OF REARING

The decision about the sex of rearing is one of the most awesome responsibilities faced by any doctor, and it is made under pressure. Many factors need to be considered. The affected person requires the best possible chance of a happy childhood and adolescence, a secure sexual identity and the opportunity to enjoy fulfilling sexual relationships in adult life. The child's future fertility will be an important issue to the parents.

The chromosome result is an important piece of information which helps the physician to understand better the patient's underlying problem, but the sex of rearing is not dictated by the chromosomes and infants who are 46,XY are often raised as females.

In general, genetic females with virilizing congenital adrenal hyperplasia should have corrective surgery to create female genitalia, because they have normal female internal reproductive organs and are capable of being fertile. Long-term follow-up studies [26,27] indicate that this policy is successful for most cases, but the incidence of sexual dysfunction in this group of women is significantly higher than for the rest of the population [28,29].

In boys with partial androgen insensitivity, puberty may be associated not only with poor penile growth but also with marked gynaecomastia. It is hazardous to advise male sex of rearing if virilization is likely to be deficient at puberty. Boys are expected to be able to micturate standing. Furthermore, comparisons of penile size occur between boys of primary-school age, and a boy with a very small penis may be made to feel inadequate. This will adversely affect adolescent self-esteem and social relationships. Normal sexual function requires the penis to be capable of sustained erection. The doctor examining an infant with ambiguous genitalia must check that erectile tissues are present and try also to predict whether the penis will grow sufficiently under testosterone stimulation, to be adequate for intercourse. If androgen insensitivity is suspected, a poor penile growth response to testosterone would be predicted.

Infertility is highly likely in an adult who was born with ambiguous genitalia and was raised as a male, for the following reasons:

1 the testes may have to be removed to prevent cancer if they prove to be dysgenetic;

2 there will be no prostate gland if there is a vagina, and therefore no ejaculate.

Prostheses may possibly be inserted to overcome the cosmetic problem of anorchia, although the safety of silicone gel prostheses is in question. Long-term hormone replacement therapy with one of the forms of testosterone will be needed to maintain libido, sexual function, muscle and bone mass. Infertile men can become fathers, either through the adoption of children or by artificial insemination of the partner using donated semen.

Assignment to female sex of rearing also carries problems. At puberty the girl will require further surgery followed by dilation to enlarge the vaginal introitus. Oestrogen replacement therapy will be needed by girls whose gonads have been removed. Despite this treatment, some girls will never menstruate because they lack a uterus. Infertility is the usual outcome, either because the gonads were removed or because there was no uterus. Many people with gonadal dysgenesis have the phenotype of Turner syndrome, and can be expected to have short stature as children and adults, a point which may influence the decision about the sex of rearing. Good treatment can, however, reduce the burden. A girl with a uterus may be a candidate for *in vitro* fertilization using a donated egg, even if she has had her gonads removed [30,31]. Supportive therapy may provide some extra height for a girl with the Turner phenotype [32].

Cultural factors may have a strong bearing on the decision about sex of rearing. In many developing countries there is a strong preference for sons over daughters, and the much lower ratio of females to males in these societies is evidence that even normal females have a lower chance of survival than males. For this reason it is inadvisable to ignore the cultural background of the parents when a decision about the sex of rearing is being taken. An infertile male may be considered preferable even to a fertile female in some cultures [33].

COUNSELLING PARENTS ABOUT THE RECOMMENDED SEX OF REARING

The clinician should:

1 be prepared to discuss all results openly with the parents, but take into account their cultural background and level of education;

2 be careful about the terminology he or she chooses to use. It is not helpful for parents to hear terms such as 'male pseudohermaphrodite' (meaning an undervirilized male) or 'female pseudohermaphrodite' (meaning a virilized female). Similarly, terms such as 'testicular feminization' and 'hermaphrodite' should be scrupulously avoided;

3 state very clearly what is the recommended sex of rearing, with reasons;

4 listen to the parents' views carefully, and try to reflect their attitudes in any subsequent discussion. This will make them feel more confident;

5 start using the baby's given name and the word 'he' or 'she' as soon as the sex of rearing has been decided. Ask all staff to follow suit.

SURGERY TO CORRECT AMBIGUOUS GENITALIA AND ITS TIMING

Once the sex of rearing has been decided, surgery can be planned. The usual operation is clitoral reduction and vaginoplasty, which will make the genitalia female. The operation can be performed safely when the infant is 2–3 months old, and as a single-stage procedure. The operation described by Hutson *et al.* [34] preserves the blood supply and nerves to the glans clitoris, and reduces the girth of the shaft, so that the clitoris can be folded on itself and recessed back. In the vaginoplasty the fused labia are divided in the midline. The skin is then used to fashion the labia minora and a flap of skin is stitched into the posterior wall of the vagina.

Steroid cover will be required when this operation is to be performed on an infant with CAH. An injection of hydrocortisone (25–50 mg) before the induction of anaesthesia is usually sufficient cover for the operation itself, and a further dose of 25 mg in the recovery room may be given. Hydrocortisone should be injected 6-hourly until the infant is feeding well again, and can be given oral steroid replacement therapy.

In a girl who is expected to menstruate, the vaginal orifice should be reassessed when she reaches 12–13 years of age, to ensure that menstruation will not be obstructed. At a later stage the need for surgery or dilation of the vagina to permit sexual intercourse will arise. This is best left until after the genital tissues have become oestrogenized.

DESCRIPTIONS OF INDIVIDUAL CONDITIONS

The frequency of different causes of ambiguous genitalia is shown in Table 4.6.

Table 4.6 An 8-year surgical experience of intersex disorders (J.M. Hutson, Royal Children's Hospital, Melbourne, personal communication)

XX karyotype (n = 22)	
Congenital adrenal hyperplasia	20
Exogenous androgens	2
46,XY karyotype, or mosaic containing 46 XY (n = 53)	
Gonadal dysgenesis: complete and partial	30
Androgen insensitivity: complete	5
Androgen insensitivity: partial	5
Persistent Müllerian duct syndrome	4
Severe hypospadias, bifid scrotum	3
5α-Reductase deficiency	2
17-Ketosteroid reductase deficiency	2
Urogenital sinus (cause undiagnosed)	2

Congenital adrenal hyperplasia

The cause of 90–95% of neonatally diagnosed CAH is 21-hydroxylase deficiency, which has an incidence of about 1:12 000 [35–37]. 11β-Hydroxylase deficiency causes 5–8% of CAH in the newborn (incidence 1:100 000). The other forms of CAH that may cause ambiguous genitalia, which include 3β-hydroxysteroid dehydrogenase deficiency, $P450_{scc}$ (20,22-desmolase deficiency) and 17α-hydroxylase deficiency, are all rare.

An infant with ambiguous genitalia, pigmented genital skin, a uterus and no palpable gonads is likely to be a virilized genotypic female with 21-hydroxylase deficiency. With this diagnosis two in three are salt-losers [38]. The extent of clitoral enlargement and labial fusion is quite variable, even between affected members of the same family. Within a particular family, nevertheless, the affected members would be expected to be all salt-losers or all non-salt-losers. The diagnosis of 21-hydroxylase deficiency is strengthened by an assay of serum 17-hydroxyprogesterone (17-OHP). The serum 17-OHP level 24 h after birth would be expected to be >100 nmol/l (normal <5 nmol/l) in a salt-loser. Non-salt-losers generally have lower levels than salt-losers. Plasma renin activity will also become grossly elevated in salt-losers, but care should be taken not to overinterpret levels that appear only moderately raised, since plasma renin levels in normal infants are up to 10-fold higher during the first year of life than in adults and older children [39]. If the infant is a salt-loser, a rise in serum potassium will be first seen at about 7 days after birth, slightly preceding a fall in serum sodium. The infant will usually start to feed poorly and to vomit after 1–2 weeks of life.

The severity of genital changes may vary considerably between different members of one family, for reasons that are not clearly understood. Family studies have shown that, in some families, more than one allele for 21-hydroxylase deficiency is present [40]. One allele may be for a severe form of the deficiency, and the other for a milder form. Affected individuals within such families may be compound heterozygotes (that is they inherit two abnormal alleles, but the two alleles are different), and so clinical or biochemical differences between different individuals may be because they have inherited different combinations of the two alleles.

PRENATAL DIAGNOSIS AND TREATMENT OF 21-HYDROXYLASE DEFICIENCY CAH

The 21-hydroxylase gene is located on chromosome 6, adjacent to the genes for complement and the major histocompatibility loci. The close linkage between the 21-hydroxylase gene and the HLA haplotype can be used in the prenatal diagnosis of CAH provided that there has previously been an affected child and that the HLA types for the index case and both parents have been established. Alternatively, it is possible to use DNA probes directed at parts of the 21-hydroxylase B gene to make a prenatal diagnosis in a chorionic villus biopsy. The accuracy of prenatal diagnosis using this method is high. Another highly sensitive and specific analytic technique is amplification of the active gene by polymerase chain reaction (PCR), followed by direct sequencing [41]. This technique identifies all mutations.

A mother who has previously given birth to a child with CAH may elect to take dexamethasone in subsequent pregnancies, because this treatment may ameliorate or completely prevent genital virilization in an affected female fetus [42–44]. The treatment must be started before the eighth week of gestation to be effective, and a dexamethasone dose of 10–20 μg/kg body weight, divided into three doses a day, is recommended. Suppression of the mother's urinary oestriol excretion provides evidence of fetal adrenal suppression.

In a series of 38 pregnancies in which the fetus was an affected female, dexamethasone treatment completely prevented virilization of the genitalia in 10, and a fairly good result was obtained in another 20 [38]. A disappointing result was obtained in the other eight cases. Whether dexamethasone treatment has any adverse effects on fetal development is uncertain [45]; generally, no abnormality has been observed. The maternal complications of dexamethasone treatment during pregnancy, however, do warrant attention; they include gastric irritation, excessive weight gain, oedema of the feet, increased facial hair, acne, depression and hyperglycaemia. Abrupt cessation of dexamethasone during pregnancy may cause steroid withdrawal symptoms; therefore gradual withdrawal over 3–4 weeks is recommended.

Gonadal dysgenesis

CLASSIFICATION

One system of classification [46] defines individual cases on two features, the karyotype and the gonadal histology. Gonadal dysgenesis is described as 'partial' when the gonads contain recognizable testicular or ovarian elements and 'complete' when the gonads are purely streaks. Examples are: 46,XY complete gonadal dysgenesis; 46,XY partial gonadal dysgenesis; 46,XY/45,X partial gonadal dysgenesis.

The presence of even a small part of a Y chromosome greatly increases the risk of gonadal malignancy in a person with dysgenetic gonads [47]. In such gonads three stages in the evolution of germ-cell tumours have been observed. The first is represented by the presence of carcinoma-*in-situ* (CIS) cells [48]. These are large, glycogen-rich cells with pleomorphic nuclei. The second stage is the formation of a gonadoblastoma [49,50]. These tumours are sometimes present at birth, and they may be bilateral. If a gonadoblastoma is not treated it will inexorably develop into a malignant germinoma. Some pathologists contend that all patients with CIS will eventually develop invasive malignancy, unless preventive treatment is given.

The gonads in partial gonadal dysgenesis are usually asymmetrical. Usually one gonad is a streak and the other a dysplastic testis or ovotestis capable of secreting some testosterone. The gonads appear to secrete little or no MIS, since most children with XY gonadal dysgenesis are found to have a uterus [51]. The uterus, however, is often hypoplastic.

Associated renal anomalies are not uncommon in patients with genital malformations. One such example is the Denys–Drash syndrome, which comprises the clinical triad of nephropathy, Wilms tumour and genital abnormalities [52–55]. The nephropathy is a consistent feature of the syndrome and characteristically presents with early-onset proteinuria. Renal histology shows mesangial sclerosis, which may be diffuse or focal. The nephrotic syndrome and subsequent progression to end-stage renal failure is the usual outcome of this nephropathy. Wilms tumour may precede, coincide with or follow the onset of nephropathy, and is often bilateral. The onset of tumour is invariably earlier than sporadic Wilms. The external genitalia are usually ambiguous in the presence of a 46,XY karyotype, but they may be normal female with either a 46,XY or 46,XX karyotype. The testes in this syndrome may be normal, dysgenetic or frankly streak in appearance. There is therefore an additional risk of gonadoblastoma formation.

A related disorder forming an expanded syndrome is the WAGR complex, comprising Wilms tumour, aniridia, genital abnormalities and mental retardation. Individuals with this syndrome have a constitutional deletion of the short arm (11p13) of chromosome 11 [56]. Further studies to map this area of the chromosome led to the identification and cloning of a Wilms tumour suppressor candidate gene, named WT1 [57,58]. WT1 encodes a transcription factor and is expressed in the genital ridge and fetal gonad, as well as in the fetal kidney. When examined as a candidate gene in the Denys–Drash syndrome, point mutations were found in one copy of the WT1 gene [59, 60]. The Denys–Drash syndrome is rare, but should be considered when a male infant presents with severe genital abnormalities. Proteinuria is a simple screen for nephropathy and, if present, renal ultrasound will detect the early signs of Wilms tumour. If there is a high index of suspicion it is possible to screen directly for a mutation in the WT1 gene. Genital abnormalities alone, with no evidence to suggest one of the abnormalities listed in Table 4.3, do not appear to be associated with a WT1 gene mutation [61].

Features of Turner syndrome, particularly short stature, are present in 15% of patients with prenatal gonadal dysgenesis. Cardiac anomalies seen in Turner syndrome (bicuspid aortic valve, coarctation, aberrant left subclavian artery, right aortic arch with a retro-oesophageal arch segment) have also been documented [62].

The chromosomal patterns found in association with partial gonadal dysgenesis include 45,X/46,XY (35%), 46,XY (31%), and other karyotypes (24%) [63]. The gonadal karyotype may differ from that in the blood. Since the risk of malignancy increases markedly when a Y chromosome is present, it is important that small marker chromosomes are examined by the technique of FISH, using Y-specific satellite probes to detect Y chromosomal material [64,65]. There is some evidence from studies on Y chromosome deletions that the gene(s) associated with the development of gonadal malignancy in XY gonadal dysgenesis is located on the long arm of the Y chromosome.

Although 45,X/46,XY mosaicism is commonly found in patients with partial gonadal dysgenesis, an outcome study in 76 prenatally ascertained cases of 45,X/46,XY mosaicism showed that 95% had normal male genitalia [66]. Three of 11 in whom testicular histology was studied had gonadal dysgenesis. The risk of gonadal malignancy in phenotypic males with 45,X/46,XY mosaicism has yet to be determined. Long-term follow-up is recommended.

Speculation on the role of SRY gene mutations in the pathogenesis of complete gonadal dysgenesis has stimulated a number of clinical studies. Altogether, 60 XY females with complete gonadal dysgenesis have so far been studied [3]. Only seven *de novo* SRY mutations have been detected in DNA from peripheral leukocytes. All of them were in the so-called HMG box domain (part of the coding region) of SRY. A small number of inherited mutations were also found, including a conditional mutation shared by a father and his two XY daughters; expression of the mutation was conditional upon the activities of other genes in the make-up of the affected individual, so that one individual with the mutation became male, while the others became female [67]. Other familial forms of XY gonadal dysgenesis have been reported where no SRY gene mutations could be found in blood. These could, in theory, be explained if the mutation was either in the promoter region of SRY (a region that has not yet been identified), or in a putative testis-determining gene other than SRY. There is, however, another explanation, which is that the genetic mutation may be confined to the gonad. The existence of a postzygotic SRY mutation that was present only in the dysgenic gonad and not present in the blood, has been recently demonstrated in a case of 46,XY partial gonadal dysgenesis [68].

TREATMENT OF COMPLETE AND PARTIAL GONADAL DYSGENESIS WHEN A Y CHROMOSOME IS PRESENT

The risk of gonadal malignancy is high in both the streak gonad and the better-differentiated gonad, and the only way of eliminating this risk is to remove both gonads as soon as the diagnosis has been established. There will be no argument about this when the decision has been made to raise the child as a female. Quite frequently, however, the genital abnormality is no more than penile hypospadias associated with an undescended testis, and the parents' perception will be that the child is a boy. This may remove any choice about the sex of rearing. Commonly, in this situation, the undescended testis is brought down, or a streak gonad is removed, while the scrotal testis is left. None of these procedures provides a satisfactory protection from the development of a malignant tumour. It is important to recognize that if the gonads are dysgenetic, but to unequal degrees, the risk of malignancy in the better-differentiated testis is similar to that in the less-differentiated one. Surgery to bring down an undescended testis has not been proved to reduce the risk of malignant change in that testis later on. A testis that failed to descend may have done so because it was dysgenetic.

The following procedures are therefore recommended when the male sex of rearing has been selected.

1 Always biopsy both testes and request a careful histological examination for CIS. If CIS is found during infancy or childhood, the testis should be removed. Testicular irradiation is an inadvisable alternative because inadvertent irradiation of the penis is likely to impair its growth.

2 If no CIS cells are found, a repeat testicular biopsy should be obtained after puberty. In postpubertal specimens CIS has been shown to be evenly distributed [69], and a single biopsy can therefore be assumed to be representative. If the result is negative after puberty there is no need to biopsy the testis again.

3 If the patient is first seen as an adult or adolescent with a functioning testis, the testis should be scanned ultrasonographically or by MRI and lesions looked for.

4 If a lesion is found either by palpation or by an imaging technique, blood should also be tested for the presence of β-human chorionic gonadotrophin (β-hCG) subunit and α-fetoprotein (α-FP), two cancer markers. These markers are not found in patients who have only CIS. If either is present, the patient should be investigated for the presence of metastases before orchidectomy is considered.

5 If the blood tests for β-hCG and α-FP are negative, a biopsy for histological examination should be taken from any testicular lesions found. If no lesion is seen, a wedge biopsy from the lower pole will be satisfactory.

6 If one testis in an adolescent or adult is found to contain CIS and the other does not, the affected testis should be excised.

7 If both testes show CIS, or if the patient's only remaining testis has CIS, external radiotherapy (given incrementally to a total dose of 20 Gy) can be given [70]. A patient who has CIS in one or both of his testes would be infertile with or without radiotherapy. The irradiated testis might, however, be capable of testosterone secretion, and therefore be worthy of preservation.

8 If there is any histological or clinical evidence of invasive carcinoma the patient will require radical orchidectomy and chemotherapy. Radiotherapy is given in some cases.

REVIEW OF SURGICAL PATIENTS TO DETECT GONADAL DYSGENESIS

Some males who have been treated for hypospadias or microphallus may, in fact, have gonadal dysgenesis and be at considerable risk of germ-cell cancer. Investigations to exclude gonadal dysgenesis should be recommended in boys born with hypospadias who also have:

1 short stature (height below the third centile);

2 microphallus (stretched penile length below the 10th centile);

3 undescended testis, especially if associated with a bifid scrotum;

4 small testes;

5 delayed puberty.

The investigations needed are: (i) chromosome analysis; (ii) serum follicle-stimulating hormone and luteinizing hormone (elevated levels indicate primary gonadal failure); (iii) pelvic ultrasound; and (iv) micturating cystourethrogram. Investigations (iii) and (iv) are to identify urogenital or Müllerian duct remnants. If these are present, or if there is a sex chromosome abnormality, the likely diagnosis is gonadal dysgenesis, and testicular biopsies should be performed to assess the risk of cancer.

Severe perineal hypospadias may also be due to partial androgen insensitivity [71] or to 5α-reductase deficiency [72]. A positive family history increases the likelihood of one of these diagnoses.

Partial androgen insensitivity syndrome

The androgen insensitivity syndrome is associated with mutations in the androgen receptor which maps in the region Xq11–12 on the long arm of the X chromosome. The phenotypic expression of such mutations is variable but can be subdivided into complete and partial forms [6]. The latter is probably the commonest cause of ambiguous genitalia associated with a 46,XY karyotype. However, there is a spectrum of genital abnormality ranging from isolated clitoromegaly with mild rugosity of the labial

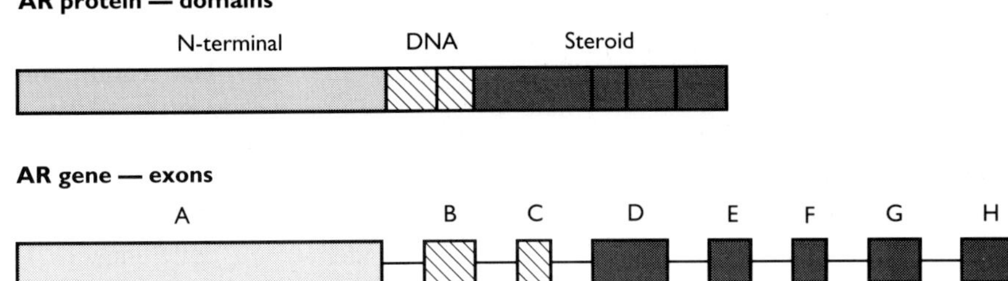

Fig. 4.5 Diagram of the functional domains of the androgen receptor (AR), and the exonic structure of the androgen receptor gene.

folds to an otherwise normal male with oligospermia. The typical genital abnormality in the partial form of androgen insensitivity is severe perineoscrotal hypospadias with micropenis, chordee, a bifid scrotum and undescended testes. The uterus is invariably absent but a vaginal remnant is common. In the partial form the vas deferens is often normally formed, whereas this is not the case in complete androgen insensitivity.

The androgen receptor forms part of a large superfamily of nuclear receptor transcription factors which include receptors for all classes of steroid hormones, thyroid hormones and retinoic acid [73]. The receptor comprises three functional domains (Fig. 4.5). The central domain is involved with the binding of the hormone–receptor complex to chromosomal DNA target sites; a carboxy-terminal domain is required for hormone binding; an amino-terminal domain, the function of which is least well characterized, is somehow involved with the regulation of gene transcription. The function of the hormone-binding domain has been studied using cultured genital skin fibroblasts in a binding assay and incubation with a radiolabelled androgen such as dihydrotestosterone (DHT) or the synthetic androgen, mibolerone [74]. A genital skin biopsy intended for androgen receptor studies may be taken under local anaesthetic from an area of pubic skin that is normally androgen-responsive. Alternatively, a small piece of skin from the prepuce or labioscrotal folds can be obtained at the time of surgery. The biopsy should be kept sterile and placed in cell-culture medium for transport to the laboratory at room temperature (freezing will kill the cells).

The majority of patients with the complete form demonstrate no binding in a fibroblast-binding assay; by contrast, the amount of binding is often within the normal range in the partial form but a subgroup of these have a qualitative defect in androgen binding. These results suggest some defect in the hormone-binding domain of the receptor. Patients with normal binding may have a defect in the DNA-binding domain of the receptor, particularly when the phenotype is complete [75]. The androgen-binding assay currently takes a minimum of 6–8 weeks to perform because of the requirement to culture sufficient numbers of fibroblasts. This may not be a practical proposition in early infancy when collecting sufficient information to make a decision about the sex of rearing. However, the results of androgen-binding studies have been relevant in predicting the genital response to high-dose androgen treatment when a qualitative receptor defect is present [76,77].

The concentration of sex-hormone-binding globulin (SHBG) is hormone-dependent. Androgens, in particular, cause a decrease in levels. The absence of such a response in androgen-insensitive patients given a short course of androgens has been proposed as a useful biological indicator of androgen responsiveness in male infants with features of the partial androgen insensitivity syndrome [78].

There are many data on the variety of androgen receptor gene mutations found in complete and partial forms of androgen insensitivity [79–89]. Complete gene deletions are uncommon and are associated with a complete phenotype [90,91]. The role of the central domain of the receptor, which contains zinc fingers involved in binding in the major groove of DNA, is vividly illustrated by two siblings who have the complete phenotype and high levels on the binding assay [87], but in whom there has been a complete in-frame deletion of the exon encoding the second zinc finger of the androgen receptor [92]. Most mutations occur in one of the five exons which encode the hormone-binding domain and are point mutations involving a single nucleotide substitution. Splice site and premature stop-codon mutations generally result in marked loss of receptor function and a complete phenotype.

The substitution of one amino acid for another can give rise to either form of phenotype but it is difficult to understand the phenotypic variability which can arise within a family whose affected members all carry the same mutation. This is especially the case in the partial form of androgen insensitivity [93].

Experiments that recreate a mutant receptor to study both the binding characteristics *in vitro* and the capacity to stimulate an androgen-responsive reporter gene may be useful to test the biological potency of various androgens, and possibly to predict if high-dose treatment will be effective in causing virilization. Many infants with clinical and biochemical features consistent with partial androgen insensitivity do not have an identifiable mutation of the androgen receptor gene. Such cases illustrate the requirement of other genes, currently unidentified, for the complete differentiation of the male external genital phenotype.

Prenatal diagnosis and carrier detection is possible in both the complete and partial forms of androgen insensitivity if the mutation in the index case has been identified. Prenatal diagnosis can also be corroborated by the use of fetal ultrasound, particularly for the complete form. When the mutation has not yet been identified, information for genetic counselling can still reliably be sought by the study of polymorphisms in the androgen receptor gene. This is especially applicable to the complete form, where there is usually little doubt about the diagnosis based on clinical findings and the karyotype. More caution is needed in the partial form because of the other disorders which can present with the same genital abnormalities. The amino-terminal domain of the androgen receptor contains a hypervariable stretch of repeat glutamine residues which can be used to detect carriers [94]. A dramatic expansion of the polyglutamine region is a consistent feature in the X-linked syndrome of spinal and bulbar muscular atrophy [95,96]. Such tandem repeat loci are also a feature of other genetic disorders such as myotonic dystrophy, Huntington disease and fragile-X syndrome.

TRIAL OF TESTOSTERONE THERAPY

If male sex of rearing is being considered for a 46,XY infant with ambiguous genitalia and no uterus, it is extremely important to demonstrate that the genital tissues can respond to androgen. To do this a therapeutic trial of testosterone [97] is given. The purpose of the treatment is to test whether the penis will be capable of growth at puberty; a poor response leads to the recommendation against raising the child as a male. The phallus should be measured and photographed and then 25 mg testosterone (enanthate or esters) administered by intramuscular injection every 4 weeks for up to three injections. An adequate response is an increase in stretched penile length into the normal range. Androgen receptor assays on cultured fibroblasts take 6–8 weeks to provide a result; the same time as will be taken to complete the trial of testosterone therapy.

INTERSEX DISORDERS NOT ASSOCIATED WITH GENITAL AMBIGUITY

Not all disorders of sexual differentiation give rise to confusion about gender at birth. The external genitalia may be entirely unambiguous but discordant with the internal genital organs. In the absence of a strong family history, discovery of the abnormality may be delayed, sometimes for decades.

The female phenotype will be found in the following disorders: (i) XY complete gonadal dysgenesis, in which the gonads show complete lack of function as well as complete histological disorganization; (ii) XY females with a complete block in testosterone biosynthesis due to a deficiency of 17α-hydroxylase, cholesterol side-chain cleavage enzyme, 20,22-desmolase or 17β-ketosteroid reductase; and (iii) complete androgen insensitivity.

The male phenotype may be seen in CAH, persistent Müllerian duct syndrome, partial androgen insensitivity syndrome, the XX male syndrome, and in some cases of XO/XY mosaicism.

Clinical features

FEMALE PHENOTYPE

1 Girls with 46,XY complete gonadal dysgenesis often present with the features of Turner syndrome (failure of pubertal development, short stature, dysmorphic features) but may present with a malignant tumour in one of the streak gonads.
2 Deficiencies of cholesterol side-chain cleavage enzyme and 20,22-desmolase are recognized in the neonate with pigmentation, dehydration, vomiting, shock, an absent uterus and palpable testes.
3 Girls with complete androgen insensitivity usually present with inguinal herniae containing testes, but in some the diagnosis is not made until puberty, when breast development occurs without the development of any pubic or axillary hair and there is primary amenorrhoea due to absence of the uterus. Girls with androgen insensitivity syndrome (AIS) are usually tall.

MALE PHENOTYPE

1 A female with complete virilization due to CAH will have pigmentation of the skin, absent testes and a palpable uterus. Most CAH patients with this degree of virilization would be salt-losers, so dehydration, vomiting and electrolyte disturbance would be expected. Early sexual development might be another presenting feature. A rare presentation is cyclical haematuria (which on investigation is found to be due to uterine bleeding) in an adolescent male.
2 Persistent müllerian duct syndrome [98–100] is usually diagnosed during surgery for undescended testis, when a uterus or fallopian tube is discovered. The testes are essentially normal, but fertility may be threatened by inadvertent surgical division of the vasa deferentia, which are located in or near the lateral wall of the uterus.
3 Boys with the XX male syndrome [101,102] may be

entirely normal, or may have small testes because germ cells are lacking. XX males may have the features of Klinefelter syndrome. The XX male syndrome is rare (1:20 000 male births) [103].

Management of girls with complete androgen insensitivity syndrome

There is an increased risk of germ-cell cancer in complete AIS [3,104], and it is generally agreed that the testes should be removed. The main controversy centres on the timing of this surgery. In many centres, particularly in the USA, the accepted practice is to leave the testes in until after puberty has been completed. It is argued that this allows more normal emotional development, since breast development occurs spontaneously and the need to take hormone replacement therapy is deferred. The risk of cancer in the first two decades is also reported to be low (1%). In other centres the testes are removed during childhood, because it is considered simpler for the parents to make the decision than to obtain consent from a young adult for the removal of her gonads. An argument which supports the policy of early excision of the gonads is that there is a high incidence of CIS in the testes of patients with complete AIS [105].

Oestrogen treatment is needed after excision of the gonads in girls with complete AIS. Since the uterus is absent, the addition of a progestogen is unnecessary. Oestrogen replacement therapy in low doses should begin at 11 years of age or at 150 cm in height, whichever is the sooner, and should progress to normal adult replacement.

COUNSELLING FOR A GIRL WITH AIS AND HER PARENTS

One of the greatest challenges for any paediatric endocrinologist is to find acceptable words for explaining AIS to a family. The essential message to convey is that the girl with AIS is healthy, but destined to be infertile because she has no uterus. In addition the gonads are abnormal. Because of these differences in her body she will require some medical treatment, consisting of an operation to remove the abnormal tissues, followed at the age of 11 years or so by lifelong treatment with female hormone. The hormonal treatment will induce puberty.

Parents will want to know why the girl's internal reproductive organs developed this way, and a truthful explanation about chromosomes, the role of hormones in sexual development and the girl's androgen receptor status can be given to them. The nature of the inheritance of AIS will need to be explained, so that a survey of other family members can be performed. Parents will find it reassuring to be told that sex chromosome abnormalities are very common (1:600 in the newborn [1]) and that a person's gender is not dictated by his or her chromosomes. Other examples of conditions caused by sex chromosome abnormalities, such as Turner syndrome and Klinefelter syndrome, can be discussed to reinforce this concept and broaden the discussion.

It is much more difficult to find an acceptable way of providing the same information to the patient. The best approach will be one which gradually builds up the picture for the girl, and which provides her with information at a pace matched to that of her development. A useful developmental framework for such an explanation has been described by Goodall [106].

ACKNOWLEDGEMENT

The authors thank Drs J.A. Batch, G. Price, M. Zacharin, H. Slater and J.M. Hutson for their helpful criticism of the manuscript during its preparation.

REFERENCES

1 Hamerton JL, Canning N, Ray M *et al.* A cytogenetic survey of 14,069 newborn infants. *Clin Genet* 1975;8:223–43.
2 Edmonds DK. *Dewhurst's Practical Paediatric and Adolescent Gynaecology*, 2nd edn. London: Butterworths, 1989.
3 Scully RE. Neoplasia associated with anomalous sexual development and abnormal sex chromosomes. In: Josso N, ed. *The Intersex Child. Pediatric and Adolescent Endocrinology*, Vol. 8. Basel: Karger, 1981:203–17.
4 Rutgers JL, Scully RE. The androgen insensitivity syndrome (testicular feminization): a clinicopathologic study of 43 cases. *Int J Gynaecol Pathol* 1991;10:126–44.
5 Warne GL, Sahhar M, Hutson J. *Tell me doctor, boy or girl?* (video). Department of Endocrinology and Diabetes, Royal Children's Hospital, Parkville Victoria 3052, Australia, 1988.
6 Batch JA, Patterson MN, Hughes IA. Androgen insensitivity syndrome. *Reprod Med Rev* 1992;1:131–50.
7 Sinclair AH. The cloning of SRY. In: Wachtel S, ed. *Molecular Genetics of Sex Determination.* San Diego, CA: Academic Press, 1994:23–41.
8 Rowe MI, Lloyd DA. Inguinal hernia. In: Welch KJ, Randolph JG, Ravitch MM, O'Neill JA Jr, Rowe MI, eds. *Pediatric Surgery*, 4th edn. Chicago, IL: Year Book Medical Publishers, 1986:779–93.
9 Grumbach MM, Ducharme JR, Moloshok RE. On the fetal masculinizing action of certain oral progestins. *J Clin Endocrinol Metab* 1959;19:1369–80.
10 Murset G, Zachmann M, Prader A *et al.* Male external genitalia of a girl caused by a virilizing adrenal tumour in the mother. *Acta Endocrinol* 1970;65:627–38.
11 Duck SC, Katayama KP. Danazol may cause female pseudohermaphroditsm. *Fertil Steril* 1981;35:230–31.
12 Martinez-More J, Saez JM, Toran N *et al.* Male pseudohermaphroditism due to Leydig cell agenesis and absence of testicular LH receptors. *Clin Endocrinol (Oxf)* 1991;34:485–91.
13 Gambino J, Caldwell B, Dietrich R *et al.* Congenital disorders of sexual differentiation: MR findings. *AJR* 1992;158:363–7.
14 Kristiansen SB, Doody KJ. Laparoscopic removal of 46XY

gonads located within the inguinal canals. *Fertil Steril* 1992; 58:1076–7.
15 Imperato-McGinley J, Gautier T, Zirinsky K *et al.* Prostate visualization studies in males homozygous and heterozygous for 5-alpha-reductase deficiency. *J Clin Endocrinol Metab* 1992;75:1022–6.
16 Shozu M, Akasofu K, Harada T *et al.* A new cause of female pseudohermaphroditism: placental aromatase deficiency. *J Clin Endocrinol Metab* 1991;72:560–6.
17 Brunskill PJ. The effects of fetal exposure to danazol. *Br J Obstet Gynaecol* 1992;99:212–14.
18 Kirk JM, Perry LA, Shard WS. Female pseudohermaphroditism due to a maternal adrenocortical tumour. *J Clin Endocrinol Metab* 1990;70:1280–4.
19 Fuller PJ, Pettigrew IG, Pike JW *et al.* An adrenal adenoma causing virilization of mother and infant. *Clin Endocrinol* 1983;18:143–53.
20 Kai H, Nose O, Iida Y *et al.* Female pseudohermaphroditism caused by maternal congenital adrenal hyperplasia. *J Pediatr* 1979;95:418–20.
21 Malinak LR, Miller GV. Bilateral multicentric ovarian luteomas associated with masculinization of a female infant. *Am J Obstet Gynecol* 1965;91:251–9.
22 Saldanha PH, Arnhold AJP, Mendonca BB *et al.* A clinico-genetic investigation of Leydig cell hypoplasia. *Am J Med Genet* 1987;26:337–44.
23 Laversha MA. FISH and the technicolour revolution. Molecular cytogenetics and its application in chromosome analysis today. *Med J Aust* 1993;158:545–51.
24 Kocova M, Siegel SF, Wenger SL *et al.* Detection of Y chromosome sequences in Turner's syndrome by Southern blot analysis of amplified DNA. *Lancet* 1993;342:140–3.
25 Lichter P, Tang C-JC, Call K *et al.* High-resolution mapping of human chromosome 11 by *in situ* hybridization with cosmid clones. *Science* 1990;247:64–9.
26 Dittmann RW, Kappes MH, Kappes ME *et al.* Congenital adrenal hyperplasia I: gender-related behaviour and attitudes in female patients and sisters. *Psychoneuroendocrinology* 1990;15:401–20.
27 Nass R, Baker S. Androgen effects on cognition: congenital adrenal hyperplasia. *Psychoneuroendocrinology* 1991;16· 189–201.
28 Money J, Schwart M, Lewis VG. Adult herotosexual status and fetal hormonal masculinization and demasculinization: 46XX congenital adrenal hyperplasia and 46XY androgen insensitivity syndrome compared. *Psychoneuroendocrinology* 1984;9:405–14.
29 Azziz R, Mulaikal RM, Migeon CJ *et al.* Congenital adrenal hyperplasia: long term results following vaginal reconstruction. *Fertil Steril* 1986;46:1011–14.
30 Cornet D, Alvarez S, Antoine JM *et al.* Pregnancies following ovum donation in gonadal dysgenesis. *Hum Reprod* 1990;5: 291–3.
31 Serhal PF, Craft IL. Oocyte donation in 61 patients. *Lancet* 1989;1:1185–7.
32 Rosenfeld RG and the Genentech Collaborative Study of GH in Turner syndrome. Long-term effects of growth hormone and oxandrolone on height in Turner syndrome: five year result. In: Ranke MB, Rosenfeld RG, eds. *Turner Syndrome: Growth Promoting Therapies.* Amsterdam: Elsevier, 1991: 221–4.
33 Abdullah MA, Katugampola M, Al-Habib S *et al.* Ambiguous genitalia: medical, socio-cultural and religious factors affecting management in Saudi Arabia. *Ann Trop Paediatr* 1991; 11:343–8.
34 Hutson JM, Voigt RW, Kelly JM *et al.* Girth reduction clitoroplasty: a new technique with 15 years' experience in 38 patients. *Pediatr Surg Int* 1991;6:336–40.
35 White PC, New MI, Dupont B. Congenital adrenal hyperplasia. Part 1. *N Engl J Med* 1987;316:1519–24.
36 White PC, New MI, Dupont B. Congenital adrenal hyperplasia. Part 2. *N Engl J Med* 1987;316:1580–6.
37 Miller WL. Congenital adrenal hyperplasias. *Endocrinol Metab Clin N Am* 1991;20:721–49.
38 Forest MG, Dörr HG on behalf of ESPE. Prenatal treatment of congenital adrenal hyperplasia due to 21-hydroxylase deficiency: European experience in 223 pregnancies at risk. *Horm Res* (Suppl.) 1993;33:S3 (Abstr.).
39 Siegler RL, Crouch RH, Hackett TN *et al.* Potassium–renin–aldosterone relationships during the first year of life. *J Pediatr* 1977;91:52–5.
40 Speiser PW, Dupont J, Zhu D *et al.* Disease expression and molecular genotype in congenital adrenal hyperplasia due to 21-hydroxylase deficiency. *J Clin Invest* 1992;90:584–95.
41 Wedell A, Ritzen EM, Harglund-Stengler B, Luthman H. Steroid 21-hydroxylase deficiency: three additional mutated alleles and establishment of phenotype-genotype relationships of common mutations. *Proc Natl Acad Sci USA* 1992; 89:7232–6.
42 David M, Forest MG. Prenatal treatment of congenital adrenal hyperplasia resulting from 21-hydroxylase deficiency. *J Pediatr* 1984;105:799–803.
43 Karaviti LP, Mercado AB, Maercado MB *et al.* Prenatal diagnosis/treatment in families at risk for infants with steroid 21-hydroxylase deficiency (congenital adrenal hyperplasia). *J Steroid Biochem Mol Biol* 1992;41:445–51.
44 Forest MG, Bétuel H, David M. Prenatal treatment in congenital adrenal hyperplasia due to 21-hydroxylase deficiency: update 88 of the French multicentric study. *Endocr Res* 1989;15:277–301.
45 Couper JC, Hutson JE, Warne GL. Hydrometrocolpos following prenatal dexamethasone treatment. *Eur J Pediatr* 1993;152:9–11.
46 Berkovitz GD, Fechner PY, Zacur HW *et al.* Clinical and pathologic spectrum of 46,XY gonadal dysgenesis: its relevance to the understanding of sex differentiation. *Medicine (Balt)* 1991;70:375–83.
47 Simpson JL, Photopulos G. The relationship of neoplasia to disorders to abnormal sexual differentiation. *Birth Defects: Original Article Series* 1976;XII(1):15–50.
48 Jorgensen N, Muller J, Giwercman A *et al.* Clinical and biological significance of carcinoma *in situ* of the testis. *Cancer Surv* 1990;9:287–302.
49 Muller J, Skakkebaek NE, Ritzen M, Ploen L, Peterson KE. Carcinoma *in situ* of the testis in children with 45,X/46,XY gonadal dysgenesis. *J Pediatr* 1985;106:431–6.
50 Scully RE. Gonadoblastoma. A review of 74 cases. *Cancer* 1970;25:1340–56.
51 Morishima A, Grumbach MM. The interelationship of sex chromosome constitution and phenotype in the syndrome of gonadal dysgenesis and its variants. *Ann NY Acad Sci* 1968; 155:695–715.
52 Denys P, Malvaux P, Van den Bergh H *et al.* Association d'un syndrome anatomo-pathologique de pseudohermaphrodisme masculin, d'une tumeur de Wilms, d'une néphropathie parenchymateuse et d'un mosaicism XX/XY. *Arch Fr Pédiatr* 1967;24:729–39.
53 Drash A, Sherman F, Hartmann WH *et al.* A syndrome of pseudohermaphroditism, Wilms' tumor, hypertension, and degenerative renal disease. *J Pediatr* 1970;76:585–93.

54 Jadresic L, Leake J, Gordon I *et al.* Clinicopathologic review of twelve children with nephropathy, Wilms' tumour and genital abnormalities (Drash syndrome). *J Pediatr* 1990;117: 717–25.

55 Coppes MJ, Huff V, Pelletier J. Denys–Drash syndrome: relating a clinical disorder to genetic alterations in the tumor suppressor gene *WT1. J Pediatr* 1993;123:673–8.

56 Riccardi VM, Sujansky E, Smith AC *et al.* Chromosome imbalance in the aniridia–Wilms' tumour association: 11p interstitial deletion. *Pediatrics* 1978;61:604–10.

57 Call K, Glaser T, Ito CY *et al.* Isolation and characterisation of a zinc finger polypeptide gene at the chromosome 11 Wilms' tumour locus. *Cell* 1990;60:509–20.

58 Gessler M, Poutska A, Cavenee W *et al.* Homozygous deletion in Wilms' tumours of a zinc finger gene identified by chromosome jumping. *Nature* 1990;343:774–8.

59 Pelletier J, Bruening W, Kashtan C. Germline mutations in the Wilms' tumour suppressor gene are associated with abnormal urogenital development in the Denys–Drash syndrome. *Cell* 1991;67:437–47.

60 Bruening W, Bardeesy N, Silverman B. Germline intronic and exonic mutations in the Wilms' tumour gene (WT1) affecting urogenital development. *Nature Genet* 1992;1: 144–8.

61 Clarkson PA, Davies HR, Williams DM *et al.* Mutational screening of the Wilms' tumour gene, WT1, in males with genital abnormalities. *J Med Genet* 1993:30:767–72.

62 Wallace TM, Levin HS. Mixed gonadal dysgenesis. A review of 15 patients reporting single cases of malignant intratubular germ cell neoplasia of the testis, endometrial adenocarcinoma, and a complex vascular abnormality. *Arch Pathol Lab Med* 1990;114:679–88.

63 Nonomura N, Nakamura M, Namiki M *et al.* Mixed gonadal dysgenesis: case reports and a review of 65 Japanese cases. *Arch Androl* 1991;26:15–19.

64 Diekmann L, Palm K, Pfeiffer RA *et al.* Multiple minute marker chromosomes derived from Y identified by FISH in an intersexual infant. *Hum Genet* 1992;90:181–3.

65 Emanuel BS. The use of fluorescence *in situ* hybridization to identify human chromosomal abnormalities. *Growth Genet Horm* 1993;9:6–12.

66 Chang HJ, Clark RD, Bachman H. The phenotype of 45,X/46,XY mosaicism: an analysis of 92 prenatally diagnosed cases. *Am J Hum Genet* 1990;46:156–67.

67 Jager RJ, Harley VR, Pfeiffer RA *et al.* A familial mutation in the testis-determining gene SRY shared by both sexes. *Hum Genet* 1992;90:350–5.

68 Braun A, Kammere S, Cleve H *et al.* True hermaphroditism in a 46,XY individual, caused by a postzygotic somatic point mutation in the male gonadal sex-determing locus (SRY): molecular genetics and histological findings in a sporadic case. *Am J Hum Genet* 1993;52:578–85.

69 Giwercman A, Skakkebaek N. Cryptorchidism and testicular cancer. In: Oshima H, Burger HG, eds. *Current Topics in Andrology*. Tokyo: Japan Society of Andrology and TOYO Shobou Co. Ltd., 1993:230–5.

70 Giwercman A, von der Maase H, Berthelsen JG *et al.* Localized irradiation of testes with carcinoma *in situ*: effects on Leydig cell function and eradication of malignant germ cells in 20 patients. *J Clin Endocrinol Metab* 1991;73:596–603.

71 Batch JA, Evans BAJ, Hughes IA *et al.* Mutations of the androgen receptor gene identified in perineal hypospadias. *J Med Genet* 1993;30:198–201.

72 Imperato-McGinley J, Gautier T. Inherited 5α-reductase deficiency in man. *Trends Genet* 1986;2:130–3.

73 King RJB. Effects of steroid hormones and related compounds on gene transcription. *Clin Endocrinol* 1988;36:1–14.

74 Hughes IA, Evans BAJ. The fibroblast as a model for androgen resistant states. *Clin Endocrinol* 1988;28:565–79.

75 Hughes IA, Evans BAJ. Complete androgen insensitivity syndrome characterised by increased concentration of a normal androgen receptor in genital skin fibroblasts. *J Clin Endocrinol Metab* 1986;63:309–15.

76 Price R, Wass JAH, Griffin JE *et al.* High dose androgen therapy in male pseudohermaphroditism due to 5 alpha reductase deficiency and disorders of the androgen receptor. *J Clin Invest* 1984;74:1496–508.

77 Grino PB, Isidro-Guttierrez RF, Griffin JE *et al.* Androgen resistance associated with a qualitative abnormality of the androgen receptor and responsive to high dose androgen therapy. *J Clin Endocrinol Metab* 1989;68:578–84.

78 Sinnecker G, Köhler S. Sex hormone-binding globulin response to the anabolic steroid stanozol: evidence for its suitability as a biological androgen insensitivity test. *J Clin Endocrinol Metab* 1989;68:1195–200.

79 French FS, Lubahn DB, Brown TR *et al.* Molecular basis of androgen insensitivity. *Rec Prog Horm Res* 1990;46:1–42.

80 Brown TR, Lubahn DB, Wilson EM *et al.* Functional characterisation of naturally occurring mutant androgen receptors from subjects with complete androgen insensitivity. *Mol Endocrinol* 1990;4:1759–72.

81 Dihauro SL, Betizadia A, Tho SPT *et al.* Probing genomic deoxyribonucleic acid for gene rearrangement in 14 patients with androgen insensitivity syndrome. *Fertil Steril* 1991;55: 481–5.

82 Zoppi S, Marcelli M, Deslypere J-P *et al.* Amino acid substitutions in the DNA-binding domain of the human androgen receptor are a frequent cause of receptor-binding positive androgen resistance. *Mol Endocrinol* 1992;6:409–15.

83 Batch JA, Williams DM, Davies HR *et al.* Androgen receptor gene mutations identified by SSCP in fourteen subjects with androgen insensitivity syndrome. *Hum Mol Genet* 1992;1: 497–503.

84 DeBellis A, Quigley CA, Cariello NF *et al.* Single base mutations in the human androgen receptor gene causing complete androgen insensitivity: rapid detection by a modified denaturing gradient gel electrophoresis technique. *Mol Endocrinol* 1992;6:1909–20.

85 McPhaul MJ, Marcelli M, Zoppi S *et al.* Mutations in the ligand-binding domain of the androgen receptor gene cluster in two regions of the gene. *J Clin Invest* 1992;90:2097–101.

86 Saunders PTK, Padayachi T, Tincello DG *et al.* Point mutations detected in the androgen receptor gene of three men with partial androgen insensitivity syndrome. *Clin Endocrinol* 1992;37:214–20.

87 Lobaccaro JM, Belon C, Chaussain JL *et al.* Molecular analysis of the androgen-receptor gene in 52 patients with complete or partial androgen insensitivity: a collaborative study. *Horm Res* 1992;37:54–9.

88 Pinsky L, Trifiro M, Kaufman M *et al.* Androgen resistance due to mutation of the androgen receptor. *Clin Invest Med* 1992;15:456–72.

89 Sultan C, Lumbroso S, Poujol N *et al.* Mutations of androgen receptor gene in androgen insensitivity syndromes. *J Steroid Biochem Mol Biol* 1993;46:519–30.

90 Quigley CA, Friedman KJ, Johnson A *et al.* Complete deletion of the androgen receptor gene: definition of the null phenotype of the androgen insensitivity syndrome and

determination of carrier status. *J Clin Endocrinol Metab* 1992;74:927–33.

91 MacLean HE, Chu S, Warne GL *et al.* Related individuals with different androgen receptor gene deletions. *J Clin Invest* 1993;91:1123–8.

92 Quigley CA, Evans BAJ, Simental JA *et al.* Complete androgen insensitivity due to deletion of exon C of the androgen receptor gene highlights the functional importance of the second zinc finger of the androgen receptor *in vivo*. *Mol Endocrinol* 1992;6:1103–12.

93 Batch JA, Davies HR, Evans BAJ *et al.* Phenotypic variation and detection of carrier status in the partial androgen insensitivity syndrome. *Arch Dis Child* 1993;68:453–7.

94 Edwards A, Hammond HA, Jin L *et al.* Genetic variation at five trimeric and tetrameric tandem repeat loci in four human population groups. *Genomics* 1992;12:241–53.

95 La Spada A, Wilson E, Lubahn D *et al.* Androgen receptor gene mutations in X-linked spinal and bulbar muscular atrophy. *Nature* 1991;352:77–9.

96 Choi W-T, MacLean HE, Chu S *et al.* Kennedy's disease: genetic diagnosis of an inherited form of motor neuron disease. *Aust NZ J Med* 1993;23:187–92.

97 Burstein S, Grumbach MM, Kaplan S. Early determination of androgen responsiveness is important in the management of microphallus. *Lancet* 1979;2:983–6.

98 Brook CGD. Persistent Müllerian duct syndrome. In: Josso N, ed. *The Intersex Child. Pediatric and Adolescent Endocrinology*, Vol. 8. Basel: Karger, 1981:100–4.

99 Lee MM, Donohue PK. Müllerian inhibiting substance: a gonadal hormone with multiple functions. *Endocr Rev* 1993; 14:152–64.

100 Harbison MB, Magid ML, Joss N *et al.* Anti-Müllerian hormone in three intersex conditions. *Ann Genet* 1991;34:226–32.

101 Chapelle A de la, Hortling H, Niemi M *et al.* XX chromosomes in a human male. First case. *Acta Med Scand* (Suppl.) 1964;412:25–8.

102 Abbas NE, Toublanc JE, Boucekkine C *et al.* A possible common origin of 'Y-negative' human XX males and XX true hermaphrodites. *Hum Genet* 1990;84:356–60.

103 Chapelle A de la. Analytic review: nature and origin of males with XX sex chromosomes. *Am J Hum Genet* 1972;24:71–105.

104 Cassio A, Cacciari E, D'Errico A *et al.* Incidence of intratubular germ cell neoplasia in androgen insensitivity syndrome. *Acta Endocrinol (Copenh)* 1990;123:416–22.

105 Bangsbøll S, Qvist I, Lebech PE *et al.* Testicular feminization syndrome and associated gonadal tumours in Denmark. *Acta Obstet Gynecol Scand* 1992;71:63–6.

106 Goodall J. Helping a girl to understand her own testicular feminization. *Lancet* 1991;337;33–5.

5: Growth Factors and Prenatal Development: Recent Lessons from Molecular Biology

D.J. HILL and A. LOGAN

INTRODUCTION

Embryonic and fetal growth is an interactive process of intercellular signalling which facilitates early morphogenic events, the condensation and differentiation of organ systems and, in the third trimester, the maturation of those organs for the transition to postnatal life. In the embryo many of these cellular interactions are direct and involve the deposition and subsequent modification of extracellular matrix and the temporal expression of cellular recognition molecules. However, the coordination of these processes and the primary stimulus to mitogenesis is provided by a phylogenetically ancient and ubiquitous intercellular communication system generically termed peptide growth factors.

Growth factors are among the first products of the embryonic genome and continue to direct growth and differentiation until birth and beyond, their actions becoming coordinated with, and in some instances subservient to, a developing endocrine system. Other reviews, including the previous edition of the present chapter [1], have emphasized the interactions between peptide growth factors and hormones such as insulin, thyroid hormones and glucocorticoids. While disorders in these axes may contribute to many clinically relevant fetal and newborn disorders, including micro- and macrosomia, respiratory distress syndrome and neuronal maturation, the evidence has previously been predominantly association-based: for example circulating insulin-like growth factor I (IGF-I) is reduced in small for gestational age infants; IGF-I is a potent mitogen for isolated fetal cell types; therefore growth retardation may be causally related to IGF-I deficiency. In the past few years it has been possible, through molecular biological techniques, to test such assumptions directly in animal models.

This chapter will review the emerging evidence which suggests that peptide growth factors are far more fundamental determinants of morphogenic events, organ maturation and birth size than was previously considered.

PEPTIDE GROWTH FACTORS

As a class of messenger molecules, peptide growth factors share a number of characteristics which separate them from classical endocrine hormones. They are widely expressed at both messenger (m)RNA and peptide levels in developing tissues; they have limited access to target tissues for much of the time due to an ability to bind to extracellular matrix, specific binding proteins or cell surface molecules other than high-affinity receptors. They often rely on proteolytic processing from the target tissue to become bioavailable and they mostly interact with high-affinity cell membrane receptors which signal to the nucleus via tyrosine kinase phosphorylation events and the *ras* proto-oncogene signalling pathway [2].

The IGFs have the structural configuration of A and B chains connected by a C peptide and share about a 40% homology with insulin. Two types, IGF-I and -II, have been purified from serum with molecular sizes of approximately 7.6 kD. Liver is a major site of expression, although almost all tissues express these peptides in the human and animal fetus [3,4], suggesting a predominantly autocrine or paracrine role. In the fetus the most abundant isomer is IGF-II, but in some species, such as the rat (but not in humans), IGF-II is absent from adult serum having been replaced by IGF-I. In humans, IGF-II persists throughout life, although the relative abundance of IGF-I increases postnatally. A high-affinity type 1 IGF receptor, which recognizes IGF-I with an order of magnitude greater binding affinity than it does IGF-II, is ubiquitous in developing tissues. Consequently, IGF-I is the more potent mitogen, but the IGFs are although relatively inefficient compared to the mitogenic properties of other growth factors such as the fibroblast growth factors (FGFs) and epidermal growth factor (EGF).

The role of IGFs may not be prédominantly mitogenic. They have been shown to support the differentiated function of many cell types, including the synthesis of extracellular matrix molecules such as fibronectin, collagens and glycosaminoglycans. In postnatal life, synergy between endogenous IGF-I and trophic endocrine hormones facilitates endocrine glandular function. For instance, thyroid-stimulating hormone synergizes with IGF-I to support thyroxine synthesis, while a synergy of IGFs with follicle-stimulating hormone allows sex steroid production in the ovary [2]. The type 1 IGF receptor has an intracellular tyrosine kinase domain which is capable of phosphorylating the insulin receptor substrate protein. Coupling by *src* homology 2 (SH2) and SH3 domains to adaptor molecules, such as *Grb-2* and *sos*, allows activation of the proto-oncogene *ras*, which subsequently signals gene transcriptional changes in cell nuclei by a MAP kinase pathway, culminating in the activation of the transcriptional factors, *fos* and *jun*. An additional high-affinity receptor, which specifically binds IGF-II, the type II or cation-independent mannose-6-phosphate receptor, is ubiquitous but has no clear intracellular signalling pathway or biological endpoint.

The IGFs are seldom found in free form but are complexed to one of six distinct classes of specific binding protein, termed IGFBP-1 to -6. These are found both in serum and in extracellular fluids, and serve not only as carrier proteins to extend the biological half-life of the ligands but also modulate their biological actions by either interacting or competing with the type 1 IGF receptors. While all six IGFBPs have a conserved core structure, differences in their amino and carboxy termini confer individual relative binding affinities for IGF-I and -II, and an ability to interact with both extracellular matrix and the cell surface [5]. Two of these IGFBPs, IGFBP-1 and -2, contain an integrin-binding motif which allows binding to the cell surface $\alpha_5\beta_1$ integrin, which is the fibronectin receptor. The ability of the IGFBPs to potentiate IGF action is related to their integrin-binding activity, which may facilitate an advantageous presentation of the ligand to its high-affinity receptor.

All IGFs except IGFBP-1 contain heparin-binding domains, allowing binding to sulphated glycosaminoglycans in the extracellular matrix and on the cell membrane. The majority of IGF-I and -II in blood is carried on IGFBP-3. From the second half of fetal development, IGFBP-3 is associated, together with an IGF molecule, with an acid-labile subunit in the circulation to generate a tertiary complex of 150 kD. IGFs cannot leave the circulation in this form, the fraction being accessible to extracellular fluids being carried by IGFBP-1 or -2.

A large proportion of the IGF–IGFBP complexes in extracellular fluids and stored within the extracellular matrix are probably inaccessible to the cell surface receptors. Their availability depends on modification of the IGFBPs by specific proteases resulting in a reduced binding affinity for IGFs. Such proteases have been identified for IGFBP-2 to -5. An IGFBP-3-degrading protease appears in maternal serum from the second trimester of human pregnancy until term, which reduces the amount of IGFs carried by IGFBP-3 and increases its transcapillary passage in association with other IGFBPs [6]. A naturally occurring tissue protease can also remove the three amino terminal amino acids from IGF-I, resulting in a much-reduced binding affinity for IGFs. Thus, while IGF-I and -II are present in the circulation, they are serving predominantly as an extracellular store. Controlled proteolysis of IGFBPs and extracellular matrix molecules is likely to be the key regulatory step in the bioavailability and subsequent actions of IGF-I and -II.

The FGFs are a family of at least nine structurally related heparin-binding growth factors which are mitogenic for many different cell types. They are potent mitogens for vascular endothelial cells and are angiogenic *in vivo* [7]. The two most studied of these growth factors are FGF1 (acidic FGF) and FGF2 (basic FGF). Both are unusual in that their translated products have no signal sequence peptide necessary for conventional secretion via the endoplasmic reticulum. Despite this, both FGF1 and 2 are released to the cell membrane where they bind strongly to glycosaminoglycans such as heparan sulphate or to extracellular matrix-associated glycosaminoglycans.

The actions of FGFs are mediated by a family of at least four high-affinity receptors which are single-chain peptides of 110–150 kD. These are designated FGFR1–4, and all have intracellular tyrosine kinase domains which signal via *ras* activation and *fos* and *myc* induction. Alternate exon splicing of the FGFR genes yields a variety of subtypes with differing ligand-binding affinities and the potential for some to act as secreted binding proteins. Binding of FGFs to heparan sulphate on the cell surface greatly enhances the ability of the ligands to interact with high-affinity receptors, and this can be reproduced by addition of heparin during tissue culture. Since most FGFs are probably bound to extracellular glycosaminoglycans in an insoluble form, proteolysis is necessary to form small, soluble glycosaminoglycan–FGF complexes which can activate the receptor. Binding to glycosaminoglycans itself protects the FGFs from proteolytic degradation.

The EGF family includes EGF, transforming growth factor α (TGF-α), heparin-binding EGF and amphiregulin. All share structural homology and an ability to bind and activate a single type of high-affinity EGF receptor. Mature EGF has 53 amino acids and a molecular weight of 6 kD, but is derived from a much larger precursor molecule of 130 kD. The C terminus of the precursor represents mature EGF and is followed by eight EGF-like repeat sequences before containing a hydrophobic region which may represent a cellular transmembrane domain. This suggests that the EGF precursor is a membrane-bound molecule from which EGF may be liberated by extracellular proteolysis. Alternatively, the precursor may exert EGF-like activity in its own right as a 'juxtacrine' molecule interacting directly with EGF receptors on adjacent cells. The EGF precursor may also have distinct, non-mitogenic actions, including the regulation of sodium and chloride ion transport at the proximal convoluted tubular epithelium of the kidney, where it is abundant.

Although mature TGF-α is of similar size to EGF, its precursor is much smaller without EGF repeat sequences. However a transmembranal hydrophobic region is present, suggesting a possible juxtacrine mode of action. While TGF-α is expressed by many embryonic and fetal tissues and persists in some postnatally, EGF expression is seen in predominantly epithelial tissues in postnatal life. The EGF receptor is a glycoprotein of 170 kD with a single high-affinity binding site for all EGF family members. It is expressed in almost all adult tissues with the exception of the haemopoietic system. Alternate exon splicing can give rise to a mRNA transcript encoding a truncated form of the receptor which lacks an intracellular domain, and may be secreted as an EGF-binding protein.

Platelet-derived growth factor (PDGF) consists of two separate peptide chains, an A and a B chain, which are encoded by genes on separate chromosomes. This allows the construction of three isomers, AA, AB and BB, giving molecular weights between 28 and 35 kD. Platelets are a rich source of PDGF, of which 70% is in an AB configuration. Most other tissues express the BB isomer in normal development, while AA is a product of many neoplasias. The high-affinity PDGF receptor is a dimer representing separate pools of 'a' subunits which can bind either PDGF-A or -B chains, or 'b' subunits which can bind only PDGF-B chains. In the absence of PDGF the subunits exist as separate monomers, but upon ligand binding they dimerize to undertake mitogenic signalling via the autophosphorylation of tyrosine residues on the intracellular domain and the activation of *ras* protein.

The transforming growth factor β (TGF-β) family is extensive and includes at least five isomers of TGF-β designated TGF-β1–5, the inhibins, activins and bone morphometric proteins (BMPs). In mammals the predominant forms of TGF-β are TGF-β1 and TGF-β2, which are of about 25 kD molecular size, and are widely distributed among tissues. TGF-β3 mRNA transcripts have been identified in placenta, ovary and cartilage. All TGF-βs share a well-conserved amino acid sequence, are translated as much larger precursor molecules which require proteolytic activation extracellularly to liberate the bioactive molecule and have integrin-binding domains. Three classes of high-affinity receptor have been identified. The class 1 receptor is of 65 kD and is not itself an intracellular signalling receptor. However, binding of TGF-β to this receptor allows its further recognition by a 85–95 kD class 2 receptor which has an intracellular threonine kinase domain and signals changes in cell growth and differentiation. A class 3 receptor is the cell surface proteoglycan, betaglycan, which binds TGF-βs with high affinity and appears to present the ligand to the signalling receptor in an advantageous configuration. All three binding components need to complex for optimal signalling by TGF-β. TGF-β acts predominantly as a growth inhibitor for epithelial cell types and some mesenchymal cells, but has widespread effects on cell differentiation and morphogenesis.

The neurotrophic growth factors represent a diverse group of homologous peptides which include nerve growth factor (NGF), brain-derived neurotrophic factor (BDNF) and the neurotrophins. Variable regions of the molecular structures give specificity to the different family members, and it is evident that all have unique biological activities and may cooperate to support the development of the nervous system. The high-affinity NGF receptor is a heterodimer comprising a member of the 140 kD proto-oncogene tyrosine kinase *trk* family (*trk*A) and a low-affinity membrane-binding protein known as p75. BDNF and neurotrophin 4 interact with the related receptor, *trk*B, while *trk*C mediates the actions of neurotrophin 3. Each of the neurotrophins has a different ontogeny and spatial distribution in the brain, and different tropic effects on various neuronal phenotypes. The predominant effect of NGF is to promote the survival, differentiation, maintenance and axonal outgrowth of sensory and sympathetic ganglia. NGF is selectively produced by peripheral tissues, to which the neurites of the developing sensory and sympathetic neurons are attracted by chemotaxis. After receptor binding, NGF is transported retrogradely to the neuronal cell bodies where it initiates the cellular response.

GROWTH FACTOR INTERACTIONS

Stimulation of DNA synthesis and mitogenesis are common functions of many of the growth factors. This does not imply a simple duplication of function, since each growth factor may play a precise role within the cell replication cycle, as first elucidated for fibroblast cells [8]. The G_1 phase of the cycle is a period when the cell acquires the necessary nutrients, proteins and enzymes to begin the preparation for DNA synthesis in the subsequent S phase. Some growth factors, such as the FGFs and PDGF, have a major role at the beginning of G_1 and are called competence factors, rendering the cell capable of entering the cell cycle. Once within G_1, growth factor requirements change and epidermal growth factor becomes necessary for the initial period and the IGFs for the latter half of G_1 progression. Since these peptides allow the cells to progress to the S phase they are known as progression factors. When present together competence and progression factors are synergistic, and a change in the number of cells involved in active proliferation within any tissue can be modulated by altering the relative abundance of growth factors in the microenvironment. This allows for precise growth control without the need for *de novo* expression or suppression of individual growth factors. Following DNA synthesis during the S phase, cells are driven by the sequential expression of cyclin genes to mitosis without further external stimulation.

Growth factors also interact during cellular differentiation, as seen during the differentiation of immortalized myoblast cell lines, such as rat L6 cells, into postmitotic, contractile myotubes. This will occur spontaneously as the myoblasts grow to high density, but can be precipitated prematurely by incubation with IGF-I, or high concentrations of IGF-II or insulin [9]. While IGF-I will initially induce cell proliferation, a commitment to terminal differentiation is mediated by an IGF-dependent activation of specific genes controlling differentiation such as myogenin [10]. Conversely, incubation with FGF2 will potentiate the proliferation of myoblasts and prevent commitment to terminal differentiation [11]. TGF-β also prevents terminal differentiation, but has little effect on proliferative rate. Control of the onset of differentiation can therefore be finely controlled by relative changes in the abundance of particular growth factors in the microenvironment. These growth factor signals derive, in part, from the cells themselves. Proliferating myoblasts synthesize FGFs and high-affinity FGF receptors, but synthesize little IGF-I or -II. Upon muscle differentiation, the synthesis of FGF(s) and its receptor(s) declines while the expression of IGF-II increases dramatically [12]. This results in a down-regulation of the type 1 IGF receptor.

GROWTH FACTOR INTERACTIONS WITH EXTRACELLULAR MATRIX

Extracellular matrix contains proteinaceous material such as collagens, fibronectin and laminin, and mucopolysaccharides, such as hyaluronic acid, heparan sulphate, and chondroitin and keratin sulphates. Most epithelia are tightly attached to a basement membrane rich in type IV collagen, which forms a connection with the fibrillar forms of collagen within the connective tissue stroma. Basement membranes are also rich in laminin, which forms a connecting bridge between matrix components and the cell membranes. Laminin has a high binding affinity for type IV collagen, heparan sulphate and cell surface integrins, and matrix pathways rich in laminin are thought necessary for the migration of dendritic and axonal projections of neurites during the development of the central nervous system. In the extracellular matrix of connective tissues the role of laminin is served by fibronectin which forms a bridge between the cell surface, through integrins, and other matrix components such as type I collagen. Integrins, in turn, are linked to actin within the intracellular cytoskeleton by the connecting peptides vinculin and talin.

A continuum is thus formed between the cells via matrix molecules, which is able to determine cell shape and migration properties. An example of this is the migration of neural crest cells during embryogenesis. Cells leave the area of the neural tube to become the peripheral nervous system, the adrenal medulla and the melanocytes of skin; the migration routes are defined by tracts of fibronectin-rich mesenchymal matrix. These tracts are also rich in hyaluronic acid, a hydrophilic molecule which creates a gel through which cells can easily migrate. Hyaluronic acid binds to the plasma membranes of migrating cells and can inhibit intercellular adhesion.

Matrix molecules not only provide an enormous extracellular store of growth factors, due to specific binding domains within the growth factor molecules or their specific binding proteins, but the formation and subsequent remodelling of the extracellular matrix is ultimately controlled by growth factor actions. In this way, extracellular matrix is a key player in the regulation of early development.

Matrix molecule synthesis is first differentially controlled by growth factors. Type IV collagen, a major component of basement membranes, and type I collagen are synthesized in response to TGF-β. Type I collagen forms a complex with decorin, a dermatan sulphate within the extracellular matrix which has a high binding affinity for TGF-β [13]. Thus, TGF-β can theoretically increase its own extracellular storage capacity. Other growth factors also potentiate extracellular matrix formation, the IGFs being potent inducers of type I and II collagen synthesis and of sulphated glycosaminoglycans. Since most IGFBPs will bind to highly sulphated glycosaminoglycans, ligand action on the cell will again favour the regeneration of the extracellular store. The FGFs have a tissue-specific effect on hyaluronic acid synthesis, which has been documented for muscle cell precursors migrating from trunk somites into the limb buds, and prevents muscle cell adhesion and terminal differentiation.

Tissue remodelling is dependent on the production of matrix-specific proteases and glyconases. One such ubiquitous protease is the neutral protease, plasminogen, which is enabled by plasminogen activator. FGF2 is a potent initiator of plasminogen activator expression in mesenchymal tissues, while this is suppressed by TGF-β. Since such proteases can activate and/or release growth factors during extracellular matrix reconstruction, growth factor availability can be controlled interactively by other growth factors via modulation of the extracellular matrix composition.

GROWTH FACTOR DISTRIBUTION IN DEVELOPMENT

Growth factors are widely expressed at mRNA and protein levels throughout the embryo and fetus; but gene transcription may not be a primary level at which biological control is exerted. Growth factors such as IGF-II, FGF2 and TGF-β are expressed in almost every tissue of the rat and mouse embryo [14–16]. In the human fetus in late first and early second trimester, IGF-II and much lower levels of IGF-I mRNAs are widely expressed, but are mostly localized to mesenchymal cells [17]. However, immunohistochemical localization of the IGF peptides showed that they are predominantly associated with epithelia of the lung, gut, kidney, liver parenchymal cells and adrenal cortex and with differentiated muscle [18], suggesting disparate sites of synthesis and action. The sites of IGF peptide presence agree with the localization of mRNA or protein for IGFBPs [19–21], and suggest that the growth factors are present *in vivo* complexed with their specific binding proteins.

At a cellular level the IGF–IGFBP complexes are associated with the plasma membranes and/or extracellular matrix [20], suggesting that the specific binding of IGFBPs to matrix components demonstrated *in vitro* is also widespread *in vivo*. Similarly, TGF-β1 mRNA is found throughout the mouse embryo and is particularly abundant in bone and megakaryocytes of liver, which are also sites of TGF-β1 peptide synthesis [22]. Elsewhere in the embryo, TGF-β1 mRNA is associated predominantly with epithelia, while the peptide is localized to adjacent mesenchymal cells. This growth factor is particularly abundant at sites of mesenchymal/epithelial interaction during morphogenesis, such as in secondary palate formation and hair follicles. TGF-β1, -β2 and -β3 have distinct spatial and temporal patterns of expression in the human fetus [23] which predominate during morphogenic events. The translocation of TGF-β1 peptide from epithelia to mesenchymal tissues suggests binding to extracellular matrix molecules such as the cell surface proteoglycan, betaglycan, and the extracellular matrix molecule decorin, which is a dermatan sulphate.

Messenger RNA for FGF2 increases steadily in the mouse embryo during development until day 16, expression being greatest in the tail, face and developing limbs [24]. Conversely, FGF3 is expressed in parietal endoderm, primitive mesoderm, the pharyngeal pouches and neuroepithelium of the hindbrain between 7.5 and 9.5 days of gestation. Different members of the FGF family appear to have distinct anatomical and ontological patterns of expression, which together cover almost every embryonic and fetal tissue. However, outside the central nervous system, FGF peptides are predominantly associated with extracellular matrix, especially the basement membranes underlying epithelia, and in this form may be inaccessible to target tissues without liberation due to proteolysis.

GROWTH FACTORS AND EMBRYOGENESIS

Peptide growth factors appear very early in development. In the oocyte and fertilized egg, mRNAs for TGF-α, FGF2 and PDGF-A chain are present as products of the maternal genome [25]. However, shortly after fertilization these maternally encoded transcripts are rapidly degraded so that products of the embryonic genome may predominate. In the mouse embryo the fetal genomic products are first apparent at the two- to four-cell stage, and mRNAs encoding TGF-α, TGF-β, activin and IGF-II are immediately detectable following amplification by reverse transcriptase polymerase chain reaction. Two members of the FGF family, FGF3 and FGF4, are also present at the four-cell stage, and are maximally expressed prior to organogenesis. Platelet-derived growth factor A was detected as an embryonic mRNA transcript in the eight-cell embryo. Some of the first products of the activated fetal genome are therefore peptide growth factors, suggesting fundamental roles in morphogenesis.

One of the best-studied morphogenic events is the induction of mesoderm in the *Xenopus* embryo, and both FGF2 and members of the TGF-β family have been implicated. Mesoderm induction occurs from the embryonic animal pole ectoderm in response to diffusible morphogenic signals from the vegetal pole ectoderm. Basic FGF was able to induce the development of elements of the ventral mesoderm in explanted animal pole ectoderm from *Xenopus* embryos [26]. mRNA encoding FGF2 was identified in the embryo at the time of mesoderm induction [27], while endogenous mesoderm-inducing activity could be neutralized with antiserum against FGF2 [28]. Proof that the endogenous members of the FGF family were responsible for the induction of ventral mesoderm was provided by Amaya *et al.* [29], who expressed a dominant negative mutant of a high-affinity FGF receptor in the *Xenopus* embryo, which would bind FGFs, interfered with intracellular signalling, and down-regulated the endogenous receptors. Serious defects in gastrulation and in ventral mesoderm formation resulted, including a developmental failure of ventral somites leading to an absence of a tail.

FGF2 action is coordinated with other factors which regulate dorsal mesoderm formation, members of the TGF-β family being pre-eminent. Exogenous TGF-β2 was able to induce dorsal mesoderm formation in isolated animal pole ectoderm from the *Xenopus* embryo, while the actions of the endogenous morphogen(s) could be blocked by exposure to TGF-β2 antiserum [30]. Despite these results the failure of the *Xenopus* embryo to express endogenous TGF-β at the appropriate time suggested that other members of the TGF-β-related family were biologically relevant. Both activin B_A and B_B chain mRNAs are expressed, the B_B form first appearing in late blastulation, increasing in abundance during gastrulation, and being present in greatest amounts in the tadpole [31]. The B_A form of activin mRNA did not appear until late gastrulation. Despite this, analysis of the endogenous dorsal mesoderm-inducing activity in conditioned medium from embryonal ectodermal cells revealed this to be related to mammalian activin B_A. Clearly, one of the activins is responsible for dorsal mesoderm formation in amphibians, and parallel studies suggest that this is also so in the chick and mouse [32,33].

Platelet-derived growth factor has also been implicated directly in embryonic morphogenesis. The Ph/+ mutant mouse is viable in the heterozygous condition but the homozygous state gives rise to grossly malformed fetuses consistent with a failure of neural crest cell migration [34]. Embryos can exhibit an open neural tube, clubbed limbs, a lack of thymus, no dermal layer to the skin, a lack of connective tissue within the organs and a failure of craniofacial development. The condition has been linked to a deletion of one of the PDGF receptors, PDGF-α, suggesting an important role for PDGF in neural crest cell migration [35]. Both PDGF-A and the PDGF-α receptor are known to be expressed within the neural crest area in amphibian embryos.

SELECTIVE DELETIONS OF GROWTH FACTOR GENES

Gene deletion by the process of homologous recombination is a powerful way of examining the morphological and anatomical implications of growth factor deficiency. Some of the most dramatic findings from gene targeting have been obtained with the IGF family and their receptors. Homologous recombination has been used to disrupt either the IGF-I, the IGF-II, or the type 1 IGF receptor gene locuses in mice. By interbreeding, combination gene 'knockouts' have then been obtained.

Deletion of the IGF-I gene yielded homozygotes with a birth weight about 60% that of normal; some died within 6 h of birth [36]. Some of the mutant mice survived to adulthood but females were infertile due to a failure of ovarian follicular development. A similar strategy revealed that the IGF-II gene was parentally imprinted and transmitted only from the male allele in the majority of tissues, exceptions being the choroid plexus and meninges where the gene is active on both alleles [37]. IGF-II-deficient homozygotes had a similar growth deficiency at birth to animals lacking IGF-I, demonstrating that both isomers have a role in prenatal growth. However, IGF-II-deficient mice were fertile.

Deletion of the type 1 IGF receptor, which is primarily responsible for the signalling of both mitogenic and differentiation by both IGF-I and IGF-II, yielded homozygous animals only 45% of normal weight at delivery which died within minutes of birth [38] due to a failure to breathe and probably resulting from a widespread muscle hypoplasia, including that of the respiratory muscles. There was an increase in neuronal cell density in the spinal cord and brainstem of the mutant animals, while the skin was thinner due to a reduction in the stratum spinosum. Bone ossification was delayed by about two fetal days.

Double gene knockout, involving both the IGF-I and type 1 receptor genes, resulted in a phenotype similar to that found after deletion of the receptor alone but co-deletion of IGF-II and the type 1 receptor yielded a subgroup of animals with only 30% of normal birth weight at term and grossly retarded skeletal development. This suggests that an additional receptor to the type 1 form may also contribute to IGF-II signalling. The type II/mannose-6-phosphate receptor is deleted in a naturally occurring gene deletion identified by the lack of the imprinted locus '*Tme*', and results in lethality at the embryonic stage [39]. Whether this receptor can contribute to IGF-II signalling *in vivo* is not clear.

Thus neither IGF-I nor IGF-II is crucial for key morphological events in early development but they act as 'true' growth factors, contributing to the expansion of stem cell populations and the progression of cell differentiation. While both IGF-I and -II contribute to fetal growth, the size of the placenta was normal following deletion of the IGF-I and type-1 receptor genes but reduced after deletion of IGF-II [38]. This suggests that a high expression of IGF-II in the placenta may contribute to its development as an autocrine or paracrine agent. Other attempts to delete the TGF-α gene and that for TGF-β1, which might be predicted to severely influence early embryonic development due to their early ontological expression, resulted in essentially normal mice at birth, although postnatal pathologies do exist. The lack of effects of these gene deletions suggests considerable support by other related gene products which are able to compensate for the missing ligands. In the case of TGF-β1 this redundancy may be covered by other TGF-β isomers, while a compensatory upregulation of EGF or amphiregulin may occur for TGF-α.

LIMB DEVELOPMENT

Formation of the limb buds and the subsequent skeletal structure of the limbs has been well studied in the chick embryo and is tightly controlled by peptide growth factors. The limb buds first develop as a thickening of the body wall mesenchyme, the surface ectoderm of which is induced by the underlying mesenchyme to form a specialized structure called the apical ectodermal ridge. The mesenchyme beneath the apical ectodermal ridge is maintained in an undifferentiated, rapidly proliferating state and enables outgrowth of the limb to occur. Limb outgrowth is promptly arrested following removal of the apical ectodermal ridge. As mesenchyme moves distally to the progress zone, so it undergoes a condensation and morphogenic change to become cartilage. Subperiosteal bone then develops on the surface of the cartilage immediately below the perichondrium to give rise to primary ossification structures. Increase in length of the long bones continues by epiphyseal chondrogenesis and subsequent ossification.

Superimposed upon this sequence of outgrowth and differentiation is the formation of the pentadactyl pattern of the limb in the dorsoventral plane. This is controlled by a diffusible morphogen released within a specialized area of mesenchyme on the ventral aspect of the progress zone called the polarizing region, the actions of which include the sequential activation of homeobox genes.

In the rat embryo, Beck *et al.* [40] localized IGF-II mRNA to precartilaginous mesenchymal condensations, perichondrium and immature chondrocytes, in addition to the periosteum and centres of intramembraneous ossification. Both IGF-I and -II mRNAs were also localized to limb bud mesenchyme in the rat fetus by Streck *et al.* [41], who additionally showed that while IGF-II expression was strongest in the presumptive skeleton and muscle at the centre of the limbs, IGF-I mRNA was absent from these areas but strongly expressed in the peripheral mesenchyme beneath the epithelium. Neither IGF isomer was strongly expressed in the rapidly dividing mesenchymal cells of the progress zone.

While IGF-II is a potent mitogen for isolated limb bud mesenchyme from the rat *in vitro* [42], these findings suggest that the role of IGFs is not primarily mitogenic, but involves the initiation or progression of differentiation pathways for skeletal and muscular elements. In the first trimester human fetus IGF-II mRNA was abundant in perichondrial areas [17]. We localized IGF peptides by immunocytochemistry in the chick embryo limb buds [43]. At stages 20–24 a uniform presence of IGFs was seen in undifferentiated mesenchyme, but this disappeared in the prechondrogenic areas of condensation. As chondrocytes appeared around stage 28, immunoreactive staining for IGFs returned. By stage 36 endochondrial calcification had begun and intense IGF staining was associated with hypertrophic chondrocytes, as well as osteoblasts in the subperiosteum of the membranous bone.

During the early development of the limb bud, IGFBP-2 expression is seen within the anterior–posterior strip of ectoderm which will become the apical ectodermal ridge, and IGFBP-2 continues to be expressed here until outgrowth is complete [41]. It is possible that the function of IGFBP-2 in the apical ectodermal ridge is to negate an IGF-II-dependent drive towards differentiation in the underlying progress zone mesenchyme, and to maintain a stem cell population.

TGF-β1, -β2 and -β3 isomers are all expressed within the developing skeleton of the mouse embryo. Heine *et al.* [44] observed the distribution of TGF-β1 peptide by immunocytochemistry from 11 to 18 days gestation. Strong staining was seen in all mesenchyme undergoing condensation and cartilage formation; it persisted during ossification within the newly formed osteoblasts. Analysis of TGF-β1 mRNA distribution by *in situ* hybridization revealed a high expression in perichondrial osteocytes involved with membranous calcification [45]. However, differentiated cartilage contained little TGF-β1 mRNA, although this is a site of peptide synthesis. A similar pattern has been described for TGF-β2 and -β3 in developing skeletal tissues [22].

In the human embryo of 32–57 days gestation, TGF-β2 and -β3 mRNAs were localized to chondrogenic areas [23]. TGF-β2 mRNA was located within the precartilaginous blastoma of limb bud mesenchyme and, in later development, in actively proliferating chondroblasts at the epiphyseal/diaphyseal boundary. Messenger RNA for TGF-β3 was first seen in the developing intervertebral discs and in the perichondrium of cartilage associated wih the vertebral column, but not with long bones. An intense site of TGF-β1 abundance was in areas of membranous bone formation and in osteogenic cells at sites of endochondrial calcification in the long bones of fetuses of 10–12 weeks gestation. No TGF-β mRNA was located in the hypertrophic chondrocytes which immediately precede the area of provisional calcification.

A divergent expression of TGF-β isoforms in skeletal primordia suggests distinct biological roles, and that of TGF-β2 would support a role in cartilaginous induction. Evidence for this is provided by the observations that mammalian TGF-β1 and -β2 induced the appearance of phenotypic chondrocytes associated with increased sulphated mucopolysaccharide and type II collagen synthesis in chick embryo mesenchyme cultures. Other members of the TGF-β family, namely bone morphometric proteins 2B and 3 (osteogenin), will also induce cartilage formation from embryonic mesoderm in the chick [46,47], making the identity of the endogenous active ligand unclear. When TGF-β1 or -β2 was injected into the subperiosteal region of the femurs from newborn rats, local intramembranous bone and cartilage formation resulted [48]. After injections were terminated, the new cartilage underwent endochondrial calcification. These results strongly suggest that TGF-β isomers are key players in the formation of cartilage from undifferentiated mesenchyme and in the subsequent primary ossification process.

FGF2 was present at both mRNA and protein levels during limb bud formation in the chick and mouse [24,49], peptide levels in the chick limb being greatest on day 3 of gestation (stage 18) when the cell proliferation rate was highest. During this rapid proliferation, mesenchymal cells secrete an extracellular matrix rich in hyaluronic acid. Using isolated chick limb bud cells, FGF2 was shown to potentiate hyaluronic acid release to form pericellular coats [50]. A loss of hyaluronic acid synthesis *in vitro* coincided with the timing of condensation of mesoderm into the chondrogenic and myogenic regions of the limb bud and a decline in FGF2 abundance at stages 22–26. Within the mouse embryo, Gonzalez *et al.* [14] used immunocytochemistry to localize FGF2 at 18 days gestation. Positive staining was apparent in chondrocytes of the hyaline cartilage and in the perichondrium. Within ossification centres FGF2 was absent from hypertrophic cells but present within the extracellular matrix, osteoblasts and vascular endothelial cells.

A different experimental approach was that of Liu and Nichol [51], who transplanted fetal rat paws, harvested on day 10 of gestation, under the kidney capsule of adult hosts which were then infused with FGF2 or anti-FGF2 antiserum via the renal artery. Infusion of FGF2 antiserum significantly retarded the growth of the explants and their ossification. Conversely, paw size was increased by administration of FGF2. Other isomers of FGF may also be involved in limb development, FGF5 mRNA appearing within the limb mesenchyme between embryonic days 12.5 and 14.5 in the mouse [52]. Expression was limited to a patch of cells ventral to the presumptive femur which was undergoing cartilage formation. The above evidence suggests a mitogenic role for FGF2 in mesenchyme proliferation and a possible morphogenic role for FGF5 during cartilage induction. However, the strongest evidence linking FGFs to limb formation does not involve the mesenchyme but the apical ectodermal ridge.

As soon as the apical ectodermal ridge is formed, at day 10 of gestation in the mouse, a high expression of FGF4 mRNA is seen in the posterior half, and expression persists until day 12 [53]. Several members of the FGF family can substitute for the apical ectodermal ridge and maintain limb bud outgrowth *in vitro* in both the mouse and chick [53,54], suggesting that an FGF is involved in the endogenous signalling between the epithelium and the underlying mesenchyme. Recently, Niswander *et al.* [55] demonstrated that recombinant FGF4 could substitute for the ridge *in ovo*, and not only maintain limb bud outgrowth but signal the correct spatial information to achieve normal pattern formation. This would imply that FGF4 is capable of regulating an appropriate release of morphogens from the polarizing zone within the mesenchyme. Contradictory evidence was provided by Fallon *et al.* [56], who showed that only FGF2 was detectable in the chick limb, and that exogenous FGF2 could substitute for the apical ectodermal ridge.

It is now possible to predict which receptor types are involved in FGF signalling within both mesenchyme and ectoderm in the developing limbs. In the mouse embryo the FGFR2 receptor was first expressed on day 9.5 in limb bud mesenchyme, with a concentration gradient increasing in a posterior and proximal direction. At this time the expression of FGFR1 was more diffuse than that of FGFR2 within the limb bud mesenchyme, the somites and organ rudiments [57]. By day 11.5 FGFR2 mRNA was localized to mesenchymal aggregates corresponding to the future bones, and in the surface ectoderm of the limb being strongest in the interdigital web. At day 12.5 gestation, FGFR2 mRNA located to chondrification centres, and at day 14.5 to the bodies of the distal bones. This temporal pattern of expression strongly suggests that FGFR2 mediates FGF actions on the chondrogenic pathways, while FGFR1 may mediate FGF actions on the surrounding undifferentiated mesenchyme. The FGFR4 receptor mRNA was found by *in situ* hybridization to map to areas of cartilage condensation, while FGFR3 mRNA was abundant in the resting cartilage during the subsequent process of endochondrial calcification [58,59].

EPIPHYSEAL CHONDROGENESIS

We have studied the regulation of epiphyseal chondrogenesis in the fetus as a model of peptide growth factor interaction during cell proliferation and differentiation. Within the growth plates of the long bones, chondrocytes arise from a rapidly proliferating stem cell population. Following several rounds of cell replication, chondrocytes begin to hypertrophy and demonstrate an increased synthesis of cartilage-specific matrix molecules such as type II collagen and chondroitin sulphates. As matrix synthesis increases, the cells become postmitotic and terminally differentiated, with an accompanying activation of alkaline phosphatase and type X collagen expression. Mineralization then occurs between the columns of chondrocytes, and the chondrocytes are replaced by macrophages and osteocytes.

The proximal tibia of the ovine fetus can be used as an experimental model for expression of peptide growth factor mRNAs and peptides. We found that FGF2 and its high-affinity receptor, FGFR1, were strongly expressed in the proliferative chondrocyte zone, decreased during cell differentiation, and were absent from the hypertrophic chondrocytes. No IGF-I mRNA was observed in the fetal growth plate, but IGF-II mRNA and peptide was associated predominantly with the differentiating, but still mitotically active, chondrocytes. An associated expression of IGFBP-2 and IGFBP-3 was found. As chondrocytes began to hypertrophy, mRNA for IGF-II declined and that encoding TGF-β1 appeared.

In summary, as chondrocytes passed from proliferation

to differentiation to hypertrophy, they sequentially expressed FGF2, then IGF-II, and finally TGF-β1. This anatomical distribution allowed testable hypotheses to be formulated with regard to growth factor contribution to epiphyseal chondrogenesis.

The expression of FGF2 and its receptor in stem and proliferating chondrocyte populations suggests a role as an autocrine mitogen. Using isolated chondrocyte cultures, FGF2 was found to be released and to contribute to DNA synthesis, being 100–500 times more potent than IGF-I, IGF-II or insulin [60,61]. A neutralizing antibody against FGF2 decreased endogenous DNA synthesis in cells by 50% [62]. Conversely, IGF-II, which was expressed by differentiating chondrocytes, was a relatively weak mitogen but a potent stimulator of glycosaminoglycan and collagen synthesis [63]. Finally, TGF-β1, which was located in terminally differentiated cells, inhibited chondrocyte replication in response to other mitogens but potentiated extracellular matrix molecule production. Many of the biochemical features of epiphyseal chondrogenesis might therefore be explained by interactions between endogenously produced peptide growth factors. It seems likely that mineralization involves the further interaction with thyroxine, which was found to reverse the mitogenic actions of IGFs on chondrocytes while inducing alkaline phosphatase production, a marker of terminal differentiation.

The skeletal muscles of the trunk and limbs arise in the somites, which in turn derive from segmentation of mesoderm in an anterior to posterior sequence, beginning in the mouse embryo on day 8. Limb muscle precursor cells migrate out from the newly formed myotome in the trunk and enter the limb buds on days 9 and 10. Several FGF isomers are expressed during muscle development, and may together coordinate both the proliferation of precursors and the programmed differentiation of the myotome. FGF2 peptide, detected by immunocytochemistry, is located throughout cardiac muscle, somite myotome and limb bud muscle in the developing chick and rat [24,64].

When applied to myogenic cell lines *in vivo*, FGF2 enhances proliferation and prevents differentiation [65]. Further, FGF2 can suppress transcription of at least two of the myogenic regulatory genes, myogenin and *Myo*D1 [66,67], suggesting that a widespread presence *in vivo* serves to prevent a premature differentiation of muscle. However, a specific expression of FGF4 mRNA occurs in embryonic mouse muscle immediately prior to activation of myogenin and *Myo*D in the developing myotome [53]. FGF5 is also expressed in developing muscle, appearing in the myotomes of the trunk on day 10 of mouse gestation following expression of muscle-specific genes such as actin [52], but never appearing in tail region myotomes. As trunk myotomal cells migrate ventrally and laterally, including those entering the limb buds, expression of FGF5 continues.

One explanation for this pattern is that FGF5 selectively suppresses the differentiation of these cell lineages while migrating. Thus different FGF species may coordinate the amplification of myoblast populations, their migration schedules and their eventual differentiation. This is unlikely to depend on any one class of growth factor in isolation. As has already been described, deletion of the IGF signalling pathways in transgenic mice resulted in a severe deficiency in muscle mass, while TGF-β isomers are expressed within developing muscle and are thought especially to contribute to cardiogenesis [68].

ADRENAL GLAND

Growth factors have key functions in the maturation of organ systems before birth. Of the steroidogenic tissues, most information exists for the fetal adrenal gland. Adrenocorticotrophic hormone (ACTH) is a major trophic factor for the fetal adrenal cortex, in addition to regulating steroidogenesis. Much research on growth factors has focused on whether these might mediate or complement ACTH action.

Human fetal adrenal expresses mRNA for FGF2 [69], and this is mitogenic for cells of the fetal and adult zones of the human fetal gland [70]. Additionally the expression of FGF2 mRNA is increased by ACTH [71], suggesting that FGF2 may act as an autocrine mediator of the trophic actions of the pituitary hormone. EGF is also a potent mitogen for adrenal cells, but an adrenal source of EGF has not been identified. Han *et al.* [17] showed that the capsule and definitive zone of the human fetal adrenal expressed abundant IGF-II mRNA, and some IGF-I from at least 16–20 weeks gestation. The IGF type 1 receptor has been localized by autoradiography to the fetal zone and medulla of the adrenal gland of human fetuses at 26–33 weeks gestation [72].

Direct evidence that IGFs exert effects on functional maturation of the adrenal have come mainly from studies *in vitro*. Pretreatment of ovine fetal adrenocortical cells with IGF-I for 4 days increased the accumulation of cyclic adenosine monophosphate (cAMP) and corticosterone output in response to ACTH stimulation [73]. The effects of IGF-I were exerted not only on the ACTH-dependent adenylate cyclase pathway, but at steps beyond this, since cAMP metabolites and IGF-I together also synergized to increase corticosterone release. It has been suggested that the primary action of IGF-I is to increase the uptake of cholesterol by adrenal cortical cells. However, work using cultured bovine adrenocortical cells has also shown that IGF-I can increase the activity of 3β-hydroxysteroid dehydrogenase [74].

In cultured human adrenal cells, IGF-II mRNA increased in association with increases in mRNA for steroidogenic enzymes such as $P450_{scc}$ and $P450_{c17}$ in response to ACTH stimulation [75,76]. However, the addition of IGFs to human adrenocortical cell cultures did not affect the mRNA levels of these enzymes. It is therefore unclear whether IGFs influence multiple enzymatic processes in the steroidogenic pathways or simply maintain cholesterol uptake by the cells.

An increase in the levels of IGF-II mRNA in response to ACTH by cultured human fetal zone adrenal cells in the second trimester suggests that IGF-II may mediate ACTH effects on adrenal growth [76]. However, infusion of ACTH into the adult rat caused a decrease in adrenal IGF-II mRNA content [77], while infusion of either ACTH or cortisol into the ovine fetus also reduced IGF-II mRNA and peptide content in the adrenals. These discrepancies may be explained by the effects of glucocorticoids on IGF-II expression.

In human tissue, fetal zone adrenal cells were used which lack 3β-dehydroxysteroid dehydrogenase and cannot, therefore, synthesize cortisol. Glucocorticoids were also blocked *in vivo* by infusion of metyrapone into the fetal rhesus monkey [78]. In this experiment ACTH levels would have increased, and an increase in IGF-II mRNA levels resulted. Thus, ACTH and glucocorticoids are likely to have opposing actions on IGF-II expression in the fetal adrenal. The rise in free cortisol levels which precedes parturition in fetal sheep may precipitate a reduction in tissue IGF-II mRNA levels and circulating IGF-II, since infusion of cortisol to the fetus during the last third of pregnancy was able to reproduce this phenomenon [79].

By contrast, TGF-β had an inhibitory effect on both basal and ACTH-stimulated growth and steroidogenesis by adrenal cortical cells. The effects on steroidogenesis appear to result from an inhibition of the enzyme responsible for converting cholesterol precursor to cholesterol, although more distal pathways may also be involved since Rainey *et al.* [80] showed that TGF-β blocked stimulation of P450 17α-hydroxylase mRNA and protein in ovine fetal adrenocortical cells.

PITUITARY GLAND

The pituitary is a rich source of growth factors and/or their receptors, including the IGFs, EGF, TGF-α, FGFs and TGF-β. While many of these are mitogens for pituitary cells when applied *in vitro*, few have been demonstrated to have a role in the control of pituitary hormone release. An exception is EGF, which was found to increase ACTH secretion when infused into fetal sheep or rhesus monkey [81,82]. Immunoreactivity for EGF was seen in both the lactotrophs and corticotroph cells. Bondy *et al.* [83] showed that IGF-II mRNA was present in the pituitary primordia, and in Rathke's pouch in the rat embryo. Using cultures of human and ovine fetal pituitary, IGF-I or -II were shown to decrease both basal and theophyllinestimulated growth hormone release [84,85] and this is likely to result from a direct effect on growth hormone gene transcription. No effects of IGFs on ACTH release from pituitary cultures were found [85].

LUNG

During the embryonic development of the rat, mRNA transcripts for IGF-I and -II are detectable from at least day 16 of gestation (term 22 days) [86], with the latter being more abundant. Levels of IGF-II fall in late gestation and IGF-II is almost entirely replaced postnatally by an expression of IGF-I. The sites of expression of IGF-II were examined by *in situ* hybridization in mid-trimester human fetal lung [74]. The cells containing IGF-II mRNA included the pleura, interlobular septa and fibroblast cells around the pulmonary vessels. This implies a mesenchymal source of IGF-II. However, immunocytochemistry showed a strong co-localization of IGF peptides with IGFBP mRNA and peptide distribution on or within the pulmonary epithelium of the developing airways [19,21]. This would imply a sequestration of IGF-II by IGFBPs and the identification of the lung epithelium as a likely target site of IGF action. IGFBP-2 peptide was localized to the apical membrane of the lung epithelium in fetal rat lung [87].

A biological role for IGFs on pulmonary epithelium is supported by the identification of IGF receptors on membrane preparations from fetal porcine lungs [87] and the synthesis of functional type 1 IGF receptors by canine tracheal epithelial cells *in vitro*. Members of the FGF family are potent mitogens for isolated lung pneumonocytes, and both FGF2 and its receptor have been localized by immunocytochemistry to the airway epithelia of fetal rat lung [89]. A morphogenic role for the FGF family in lung development was shown in studies of functional ablation of the FGFR2 gene [90]. In homozygous mice no branching of the central airway occurs, and animals die at birth with an absence of lung development.

Fetal lung is rich in high-affinity EGF receptors, and exogenous EGF given in the rabbit or lamb induced lung epithelial maturation and surfactant production [91,92]. Studies with fetal rat lung explants showed that EGF increased phospholipid biosynthesis, thereby increasing surfactant production. Conversely, TGF-β inhibited pneumonocyte development in explants of fetal rabbit lung, the mechanism of which was postulated to involve a reduced synthesis of fibroblast–pneumonocyte factor, a lung fibroblast-derived factor which regulates the maturation of the adjacent epithelial cells [93].

CENTRAL NERVOUS SYSTEM

The adult nervous system contains approximately 10^{12} neurons, each of which makes hundreds of synapses with other neurons. Each part of the system has a characteristic structure and function, with its cellular components organized into distinct patterns of nuclei and/or lamellae. Understanding what regulates the complex differentiation pathways in this tissue requires analysis in terms of the characteristics of constitutive cells and their interactions with the mechanochemical environment. Some of the trophic signals that determine the cellular events of development and differentiation of the neural tube are beginning to be defined and specific neurotrophic factors identified. These trophins permit selective limitation of the neuronal death that occurs during development. Developing neurons may derive trophic support from innervated cells (retrograde influences), from afferent neurons (anterograde influences), from glial cells (paracrine influences) to enhance their survival and differentiation.

These trophic factors include the classical 'neurotrophins', such as nerve growth factor (NGF), brain derived neurotrophine factor (BDNF), and neurotrophins 3, 4 and 5 (NT-3, NT-4, NT-5). Other growth factors (which include the FGFs, EGF, the TGFs and the IGFs) are also strongly implicated as regulators of neuronal development and function and are also considered to be 'neurotrophic factors'. Although information is being accumulated mostly from animal studies concerning patterns of expression and activity of individual neurotrophic factors, it seems that an extremely complex pattern of trophic interaction determines the highly specific connectivity of the nervous system. Understanding how this network of factors interacts to determine the developmental events in this tissue is a formidable challenge.

During embryogenesis, neuroepithelial cells of the neural tube proliferate and give rise to different populations of neurons, astrocytes and oligodendrocytes. Glial and neuronal cell lineages diverge at an early stage of development (for example days 10–12 for mouse cortex) in response to paracrine/autocrine factors. The pathways of glial cells have been well studied [94]. Growth factors are known to regulate the differentiation of astrocyes from glioblasts. For example, type 1 astrocytes secrete PDGF which keeps 0-2A progenitor cells proliferating, thereby preventing their premature differentiation [95]. Ciliary neurotrophic factor (CNTF) promotes the differentiation of bipotential 0-2A cells into type 2 astrocytes [96].

The roles of growth factors in the proliferation and differentiation of neuronal cells are not well defined. FGF2 is expressed during early embryo development and may play a role in embryogenesis [14]. The expression of high-affinity FGFR1 receptor in the central nervous system (CNS) is developmentally regulated, and it is primarily localized to the ependymal layer of the CNS, which contains mitotic precursor cells in embryos [97]. The complexity of the system *in vivo* makes definition of the precise role of growth factors in early neuroblast proliferation and differentiation difficult. Short-term proliferative effects of growth factors, including FGF2, IGFs and EGF, on cultured rat and mouse neuroblasts have been reported [98–100] and these factors have been shown to be interactive [101]. FGF2 was also reported to stimulate a longer-term proliferation of embryonic hippocampal cells [102]. EGF was found to have similar proliferative and differentiation effects on cultured striatum neuroblasts [103]. A number of growth factors, including the neurotrophins and FGF2, are known to enhance neuron survival in cultured neurons [4,104–106].

The patterns of expression of the neurotrophin family and their receptors change during development, and each has been implicated in the later development of various subsets of neurons. The prototype neurotrophin, NGF, stands as a good example of the influence of these peptides in the maturing CNS, since the principles of their actions hold good for most neurotrophins. Maisonpierre *et al.* [107] demonstrated low levels of NGF mRNA in the fetal rat brain, which increase postnatally approximately 20-fold until 3 weeks after birth, when adult levels are attained. This expression correlates with the period of neuronal migration, maturation and innervation. Highest levels of NGF mRNA and protein were found in the hippocampus, neocortex and olfactory bulb of the newborn and adult rat brain. Each of these regions serves as a target of basal forebrain cholinergic neurons. It seems that NGF is an essential survival factor during maturation of sympathetic neurons and possibly cholinergic neurons of the basal forebrain. NGF and its mRNA have also been localized to other CNS regions, including the caudate, putamen, cerebellum, hypothalamus and spinal cord, each with a distinct developmental regulation, which suggests that NGF also acts on other cholinergic neuronal populations.

Only recently has it been possible to assess directly the roles of NGF in development by targeted mutation of its receptors as described earlier. The common low-affinity receptor (p75) is widely expressed, both on cells that respond to neurotrophins and others that do not. Mice homozygous for a mutation in the p75 gene survive with only mild defects to their peripheral sensory nervous system [108].

It is likely that p75 plays only an accessory role in mediating neurotrophin function. Both NGF and *trk*A gene knockouts result in dramatic phenotypes in which animals are born viable but die within a month of delivery [109,110]. Neurons are depleted in the dorsal root ganglia and trigeminal nerves and there are almost no sympathetic ganglia in either by 10 days after birth. The loss of neurons in the dorsal root ganglia involves only a subset of peptidergic neurons which mediate pain and thermoreceptor functions, while neurons which express receptors for other neurotrophins remain viable.

The influence of the neurotrophin receptors, *trk*B, on the embryonic and fetal development of mice has been investigated by targeted disruption of the gene [111]. A mutant receptor carrying a non-functional tyrosine kinase catalytic domain was inserted into the mouse germ line. Since *in situ* hybridization to localize *trk*B mRNA had shown a wide expression in multiple structures of the central and peripheral nervous systems, including cerebral cortex, hippocampus, thalamus, brainstem and spinal cord [112], it could be anticipated that gene disruption would have widespread behavioural and motor deficits. Homozygous animals developed to birth, but did not feed, and quickly died. Neuroanatomical examination showed a deficiency of neurons in the facial motor nucleus and spinal cord, and in the trigeminal and dorsal root ganglia. The loss of neurons in the facial motor nucleus probably disables the mastication muscles so that suckling is not possible.

Destruction of the *trk*C gene caused a loss of neurons in the superior cervical ganglion, the trigeminal ganglion, and motor neurons in the CNS [113]. This led to abnormalities of proprioception and abnormal posture and movements. While the NGF family may play a primary role in directing axonal projections to targets, it seems that the other side of NGF activity during development pertains to the rescue of neurons from the programmed cell death that occurs during development. Competition between specific populations of neurons for target-derived NGF leads to the selection of a subset of neurons for survival. Although the actions of NGF are restricted to a few populations of neurons, the generality of the phenomenon of programmed cell death in the nervous system suggests that most neurons are regulated by growth factors via a target-derived mechanism.

Hence, the principles of retrograde NGF influences during maturation of neurons are broadly applicable across this family of neurotrophins. For example, BDNF demonstrates a pattern of expression in the developing brain very similar to NGF, and has retrograde effects like NGF in promoting survival, differentiation and maintenance of septal cholinergic neurons, suggesting that they may have overlapping effects. Elucidation of the biology of NT-3 is preliminary, but it seems that this neurotrophin may act like BDNF and NGF as a target tissue-derived survival factor. By contrast to NGF and BDNF, the expression of NT-3 is much higher in the brain during development than in the adult. In particular, NT-3 levels are very high in the cerebellum and hippocampus during the peak rate of proliferation of the granule cells that populate these structures. These reciprocal patterns may suggest a major role for NT-3 as a target-derived mitogenic factor during development, whereas NGF and BDNF may be more important in the regulation of guidance, selection, maintenance and differentiated function of maturing and mature neurons.

GROWTH FACTORS AND FETAL GROWTH DISORDERS

Since, of the major growth factor classes, only the IGFs are found to any extent within the fetal circulation, it is only within this field that an extensive literature exists with regard to changes associated with fetal pathology. In the human infant subject to intrauterine growth retardation, IGF-I concentrations are lower than in age-matched control infants, while levels of IGF-II are unaltered [114]. Conversely, in macrosomic infants of diabetic mothers, circulating levels of IGF-I are elevated [115]. While this suggests that fetal IGF-I expression may be closely related to growth rate in the last trimester, this association may not be the determining biological parameter since circulating levels of IGFBP-1 are substantially elevated in the circulation of the growth-retarded infant [116]. This may limit IGF availability to its high-affinity IGF receptors.

The observations in human pregnancy have been reproduced and extended in animal studies. When fetal growth in the rat is restricted, either by uterine vessel ligation or by maternal fasting, there is a reproducible reduction in IGF-I mRNA levels in fetal liver and other tissues, an increase in IGF-II mRNA, a reduction in IGF-I but an increase in IGF-II in plasma, and an increase in the hepatic expression and circulating levels of IGFBP-1 and -2 [117–120]. Acute hypoxia in the ovine fetus induces a rapid but selective reduction in DNA synthetic rate in a number of tissues including adrenal and lung [121]. This is associated with only small changes in the circulating levels of IGF-I or -II, but substantial and prompt increases in circulating levels of IGFBP-1 and its levels of steady-state mRNA in the liver and kidney [122,123]. Collectively these data suggest that tissue growth rate can be altered rapidly by a local or widespread change in IGFBP synthesis or by a limitation of the bioavailability of IGF-I and -II. A more sustained insult to the fetus may induce a down-regulation of IGF-I synthesis, such as is seen in fetal rats following prolonged ethanol exposure of the mother [124].

FUTURE DEVELOPMENTS

Messenger RNA detection, quantitation and localization and gene manipulation have already had an enormous impact in revealing the biological roles of growth factors in development. Gene deletions throughout the body of the embryo demonstrate critical cell populations which are growth factor-dependent, while deletion of specific receptor molecules can reveal growth factor signalling pathways. Existing technology will allow such deletions to be targeted to specific tissues at particular times of development. This can be achieved by the coupling of gene constructs to the promoter regions of tissue and developmentally specific genes; for instance, expression can be targeted to skin by the use of a keratin sulphate promoter, to cartilage by using the type II collagen promoter, and to lung by using surfactant protein promoter regions. Expression of the transgene will then be activated in a tissue- and time-specific manner.

The most promising method of disrupting growth factor action appears to be the transgenesis of the dominant-negative receptor mutant. By overexpression of mutated receptor species no longer capable of dimerization and intracellular signalling, the influence of a single growth factor can be selectively ablated. The same strategy, making use of a functional receptor gene, would provide for gene therapy where the endogenous receptor population was abnormal. These are, indeed, exciting times.

ACKNOWLEDGEMENTS

Those studies performed in the authors' laboratories were made possible by funding from the Wellcome Trust and the Medical Research Council of Canada.

REFERENCES

1 Hill DJ, Milner RDG. Mechanisms of fetal growth. In: Brook CGD, ed. *Clinical Paediatric Endocrinology*, 2nd edn. Oxford: Blackwell Scientific Publications, 1989:3–31.

2 Hill DJ, Hogg J. Growth factors and the regulation of pre- and postnatal growth. In: Jones CT, ed. *Clinical Endocrinology and Metabolism, Perinatal Endocrinology*, Vol. 3, No. 3. London: Baillière Tindall, 1989:579–625.

3 Brown AL, Graham DE, Nissley SP, Hill DJ, Strain AJ, Rechler MM. Developmental regulation of insulin-like growth factor II mRNA in different rat tissues. *J Biol Chem* 1986;261:13144–50.

4 Hatikka J, Hefti F. Comparison of nerve growth factor effects on development of septum, striatum and nucleus basalis cholinergic neurons *in vitro*. *J Neurosci Res* 1988;21:352–64.

5 McCusker RH, Clemmons DR. The insulin-like growth factor binding proteins: structure and biological functions. In: Schofield PN, ed. *The Insulin-like Growth Factors, Structure and Biological Functions*. Oxford: Oxford University Press, 1992:110–50.

6 Giudice LC, Farrell EM, Pham H, Lamson G, Rosenfeld RG. Insulin-like growth factor binding proteins in maternal serum throughout gestation and in the puerperium: effects of a pregnancy-associated serum protease activity. *J Clin Endocrinol Metab* 1990;71:806–16.

7 Baird A, Bohlen P. Fibroblast growth factors. In: Sporn MB, Roberts AB, eds. *Peptide Growth Factors and their Receptors*. Berlin: Springer Verlag, 1990:369–418.

8 Van Wyk JJ, Underwood LE, D'Ercole AJ *et al.* Role of somatomedin in cellular proliferation. In: Ritzen M, Aperia A, Hall K *et al.*, eds. *Biology of Normal Human Growth*. New York: Raven Press, 1981:223–39.

9 Ewton DZ, Florini JR. Effects of somatomedins and insulin on myoblast differentiation *in vitro*. *Dev Biol* 1981;56:31–9.

10 Florini JR, Ewton DZ, Roof SL. Insulin-like growth factor I stimulates terminal myogenic differentiation by induction of myogenin gene expression. *Mol Endocrinol* 1991;5:718–24.

11 Linkhart TA, Clegg CH, Hauscha SD. Myogenic differentiation in permanent clonal mouse myoblast cell lines: regulation by macromolecular growth factors in the culture medium. *Dev Biol* 1981;86:19–30.

12 Florini JR, Magri KA, Ewton DZ, James PL, Grindstaff K, Rotwein PS. 'Spontaneous' differentiation of skeletal myoblasts is dependent upon autocrine secretion of insulin-like growth factor II. *J Biol Chem* 1991;266:15917–23.

13 Yamaguchi Y, Mann DM, Ruoslahti E. Negative regulation of transforming growth factor-β by the proteoglycan decorin. *Nature* 1990;346:281–4.

14 Gonzalez A-M, Buscaglia M, Ong M, Baird A. Distribution of basic fibroblast growth factor in the 18-day rat fetus: localization in the basement membranes of diverse tissues. *J Cell Biol* 1990;110:753–65.

15 Han VKM, Lund PK, Lee DC, D'Ercole AJ. Expression of somatomedin/insulin-like growth factor messenger ribonucleic acids in the human fetus: identification, characterization and tissue distribution. *J Clin Endocrinol Metab* 1988; 66:422–9.

16 Roberts AB, Sporn MB. The transforming growth factor-βs. In: Sporn MB, Roberts AB, eds. *Peptide Growth Factors and their Receptors*. Berlin: Springer Verlag, 1990:419–72.

17 Han VKM, D'Ercole AJ, Lund PK. Cellular localization of somatomedin (insulin-like growth factor) messenger RNA in the human fetus. *Science* 1987;236:193–7.

18 Han VKM, Hill DJ, Strain AJ, Towle AC, Lauder JM, Underwood LE, D'Ercole AJ. Identification of somatomedin/insulin-like growth factor immunoreactive cells in the human fetus. *Pediatr Res* 1987;22:245–9.

19 Delhanty PJD, Hill DJ, Shimasaki S, Han VKM. Insulin-like growth factor binding protein-4, -5 and -6 mRNAs in the human fetus: localization to sites of growth and differentiation? *Growth Regul* 1993;3:8–11.

20 Hill DJ, Clemmons DR. Similar immunological distribution of insulin-like growth factor binding proteins-1, -2, and -3 in human fetal tissues. *Growth Factors* 1992;6:315–26.

21 Hill DJ, Clemmons DR, Wilson S, Han VKM, Strain AJ, Milner RDG. Immunological distribution of one form of insulin-like growth factor (IGF) binding protein and IGF peptides in human fetal tissues. *J Mol Endocrinol* 1989;2: 31–8.

22 Pelton RW, Dickinson ME, Moses HL, Hogan BLM. *In situ* hybridization analysis of $TGF\beta_3$ RNA expression during mouse development: comparative studies with $TGF\beta_1$ and β_2. *Development* 1990;110:609–20.

23 Gatherer D, TenDijke P, Baird DT, Akhurst RJ. Expression of TGF-β isoforms during first trimester human embryogenesis. *Development* 1990;110:445–60.

24 Herbert JM, Basilico C, Goldfarb M, Haub O, Martin GR. Isolation of cDNAs encoding four mouse FGF family members and characterization of their expression patterns during embryogenesis. *Dev Biol* 1990;138:454–63.

25 Rappolee DA, Brenner CA, Schultz R, Werb Z. Developmental expression of PDGF, TGF-α, and TGF-β genes in preimplantation mouse embryos. *Science* 1988;241: 1823–5.

26 Kimelman D, Kirschner M. Synergistic induction of mesoderm by FGF and TGF-beta and the identification of an mRNA coding for FGF in the early *Xenopus* embryo. *Cell* 1987;51:869–71.
27 Kimelman D, Abraham JA, Haarparanta T, Palisi TM, Kirschner MW. The presence of fibroblast growth factor in the frog egg: its role as a natural mesoderm inducer. *Science* 1988;242:1053–6.
28 Slack JMW, Isaacs HV. Presence of basic fibroblast growth factor in the early *Xenopus* embryo. *Development* 1989; 105:147–53.
29 Amaya E, Musci TJ, Kirschner MW. Expression of a dominant negative mutant of the FGF receptor disrupts mesoderm formation in *Xenopus* embryos. *Cell* 1991;66:257–70.
30 Rosa F, Roberts AB, Danielpour D, Dart LL, Sporn MB, Dawid IB. Mesoderm induction in amphibians: the role of TGF-β_2-like factors. *Science* 1988;239:783–5.
31 Thomsen G, Woolf T, Whitman M *et al.* Activins are expressed early in *Xenopus* embryogenesis and can induce axial mesoderm and anterior structures. *Cell* 1990;63:485–91.
32 Mitrani E, Ziu T, Thomsen G, Shimoni Y, Melton DA, Bril A. Activin can induce the formation of axial structures and is expressed in the hypoblast of the chick. *Cell* 1990;63: 495–501.
33 Smith JC, Price BMJ, Van Nimmen K, Huylebroeck D. Identification of a potent *Xenopus* mesodern-inducing factor as a homologue of activin A. *Nature* 1990;345:729–31.
34 Morrison Graham K, Schatteman GC, Bork T, Bowenpope DF, Weston JA. A PDGF receptor mutation in the mouse (patch) perturbs the development of a non-neuronal subset of neural crest-derived cells. *Development* 1992;115:133–42.
35 Orrurtreger A, Bedford MT, Do MS, Eisenbach L, Lonai P. Developmental expression of the alpha receptor for platelet-derived growth factor, which is deleted in the embryonic lethal patch mutation. *Development* 1992;115:289–97.
36 Liu J-P, Baker J, Perkins AS, Robertson EJ, Efstratiadis A. Mice carrying null mutations of the genes encoding insulin-like growth factor I (*Igf*-1) and type 1 IGF receptor (*Igf*1r). *Cell* 1993;75:59–72.
37 De Chiara TM, Efstratiadis A, Robertson EJ. A growth-deficiency phenotype in heterozygous mice carrying an insulin-like growth factor II gene disrupted by targeting. *Nature* 1990;345:78–80.
38 Baker J, Liu J-P, Robertson EJ, Efstratiadis A. Role of insulin-like growth factors in embryonic and postnatal growth. *Cell* 1993;75:73–82.
39 Barlow DP, Stoger R, Herrmann BG, Saito K, Schweifer N. The mouse insulin-like growth factor type-2 receptor is imprinted and closely linked to the Tme locus. *Nature* 1991;349:84–7.
40 Beck F, Samani NJ, Penschow JD, Thorley B, Tregear GW, Coghlan JP. Histochemical localization of IGF-I and -II mRNA in the developing rat embryo. *Development* 1987; 101:175–84.
41 Streck RD, Wood TL, Hsu M-S, Pintar JE. Insulin-like growth factor I and II and insulin-like growth factor binding protein-2 RNAs are expressed in adjacent tissues within rat embryonic and fetal limbs. *Dev Biol* 1992;151:586–96.
42 Bhaumick B, Bala RM. Differential effects of insulin-like growth factors I and II on growth, differentiation and glucoregulation in differentiating chondrocyte cells in culture. *Acta Endocrinol* 1991;125:201–11.
43 Ralphs J, Wylie L, Hill DJ. Distribution of insulin-like growth factor peptides in the developing chick embryo. *Development* 1990;109:51–8.
44 Heine UI, Munoz EF, Flanders KC *et al.* Role of transforming growth factor-β in the development of the mouse embryo. *J Cell Biol* 1987;105:2861–76.
45 Lehnert SA, Akhurst RJ. Embryonic expression pattern of TGF beta type-1 RNA suggests both paracrine and autocrine mechanisms of action. *Development* 1988;104:263–73.
46 Carrington JL, Chen P, Yanagishita M, Reddi AH. Osteogenin (bone morphometric protein-3) stimulates cartilage formation by chick limb bud cells *in vitro*. *Dev Biol* 1991; 146:406–15.
47 Chen P, Carrington JL, Hammonds RG, Reddi AH. Stimulation of chondrogenesis in limb bud mesoderm cells by recombinant human bone morphometric protein 2B (BMP-2B) and modulation by transforming growth factor β_1 and β_2. *Exp Cell Res* 1991;195:509–15.
48 Joyce ME, Roberts AB, Sporn MB, Bolander ME. Transforming growth factor-β and the initiation of chondrogenesis and osteogenesis in the rat femur. *J Cell Biol* 1990;110: 2195–207.
49 Munaim SI, Klagsbrun M, Toole BP. Developmental changes in fibroblast growth factor in the chicken embryo limb bud. *Proc Natl Acad Sci USA* 1988;85:8091–3.
50 Munaim SI, Klagsbrun M, Toole BP. Hyaluronan-dependent pericellular coats of chick embryo limb mesoderm cells: induction by basic fibroblast growth factor. *Dev Biol* 1991; 143:297–302.
51 Liu L, Nicoll CS. Evidence for a role of basic fibroblast growth factor in rat embryonic growth and differentiation. *Endocrinology* 1988;123:2027–31.
52 Haub O, Goldfarb M. Expression of fibroblast growth factor-5 gene in the mouse embryo. *Development* 1991;112: 397–406.
53 Niswander L, Martin GR. *Fgf-4* expression during gastrulation, myogenesis, limb and tooth development in the mouse. *Development* 1992;114:755–68.
54 Niswander L, Martin GR. FGF-4 and BMP-2 have opposite effects on limb growth. *Nature* 1993;361:68–71.
55 Niswander L, Tickle C, Vogel A, Booth I, Martin GR. FGF-4 replaces the apical ectodermal ridge and directs outgrowth and patterning of the limb. *Cell* 1993;75:579–87.
56 Fallon JF, Lopez A, Ros MA, Savage MP, Olwin BB, Simandl BK. FGF-2: apical ectodermal ridge growth signal for chick limb development. *Science* 1994;264:104–6.
57 Peters KG, Werner S, Chen G, Williams LT. Two FGF receptor genes are differentially expressed in epithelial and mesenchymal tissues during limb formation and organogenesis in the mouse. *Development* 1992;114:233–43.
58 Peters K, Ornitz D, Werner S, Williams L. Unique expression pattern of the FGF receptor 3 gene during mouse organogenesis. *Dev Biol* 1993;155;423–30.
59 Stark KL, McMahon JA, McMahon AP. FGFR-4, a new member of the fibroblast growth factor receptor family, expressed in the definitive endoderm and skeletal muscle lineages of the mouse. *Development* 1991;113:641–51.
60 Hill DJ, Logan A. Interactions of peptide growth factors during DNA synthesis in isolated ovine fetal growth plate chondrocytes. *Growth Regul* 1992;2:122–32.
61 Hill DJ, Logan A, Ong M, DeSousa D, Gonzalez AM. Basic fibroblast growth factor is synthesized and released by isolated ovine fetal growth plate chondrocytes: potential role as an autocrine mitogen. *Growth Factors* 1992;6:277–94.
62 Hill DJ, Logan A. Cell cycle-dependent localization of

immunoreactive basic fibroblast growth factor to cytoplasm and nucleus of isolated ovine fetal growth plate chondrocytes. *Growth Factors* 1992;7:215–31.

63 Hill DJ, Logan A, McGarry M, DeSousa D. Control of protein and matrix molecule synthesis in isolated ovine growth plate chondrocytes by the interactions of basic fibroblast growth factor, insulin-like growth factor I, insulin and transforming growth factor β. *J Endocrinol* 1992;133:363–73.

64 Joseph-Silverstein J, Consigli SA, Lyser KM, Ver Pault C. Basic fibroblast growth factor in the chick embryo: immunolocalization to striated muscle cells and their precursors. *J Cell Biol* 1989;108:2459–66.

65 Clegg CH, Linkhart TA, Olwin BB, Hauschka SD. Growth factor control of skeletal muscle differentiation: commitment to terminal differentiation occurs in G_1 phase and is repressed by fibroblast growth factor. *J Cell Biol* 1987; 105:949–56.

66 Brunetti A, Goldfine ID. Role of myogenin in myoblast differentiation and its regulation by fibroblast growth factor. *J Biol Chem* 1990;265:5960–3.

67 Vaidya TB, Rhodes SJ, Taparowsky EJ, Konieczny SF. Fibroblast growth factor and transforming growth factor β repress transcription of the myogenic regulatory gene MyoD1. *Mol Cell Biol* 1989;9:3576–9.

68 Akhurst RJ, Lehnert SA, Faissner A, Duffie E. TGF beta in murine morphogenetic processes: the early embryo and cardiogenesis. *Development* 1990;108:645–56.

69 DiBlasio AM, Voutilainen R, Jaffe RB, Miller WL. Hormonal regulation of messenger ribonucleic acids for P450scc (cholesterol side-chain cleavage enzyme) and P450c17 (17 alpha-hydroxylase/17,20-lyase) in cultured human fetal adrenal cells. *J Clin Endocrinol Metab* 1987;65:170–5.

70 Crickard K, Ill CR, Jaffe RB. Control of proliferation of human fetal adrenal cells *in vitro*. *J Clin Endocrinol Metab* 1981;53:790–8.

71 Mesiano S, Mellon SH, Gospodarowicz D, DiBlasio AM, Jaffe RB. Basic fibroblast growth factor expression is regulated by corticotropin in the human fetal adrenal: a model for adrenal growth regulation. *Proc Natl Acad Sci USA* 1991;88: 5428–32.

72 Shigematsu K, Niwa M, Kurihara M, Yamashita K, Kawai K, Tsuchiyama H. Receptor autoradiographic localization of insulin-like growth factor-I (IGF-I) binding sites in human fetal and adult adrenal glands. *Life Sci* 1989;45:383–9.

73 Naamen E, Chatelain P, Saez JM, Durand P. *In vitro* effect of insulin and insulin-like growth factor-I on cell multiplication and adrenocorticotropin responsiveness of fetal adrenal cells. *Biol Reprod* 1989;40:570–7.

74 Chatelain P, Penhoat A, Perrard-Sapori MH, Jaillard C, Naville D, Saex J. Maturation of steroidogenic cells: a target for IGF-I. *Acta Paediatr Scand* 1988;Suppl.347:104–9.

75 Voutilainen R, Miller WL. Coordinate tropic hormone regulation of mRNAs for insulin-like growth factor II and the cholesterol side-chain-cleavage enzyme, $P450_{ssc}$, in human steroidogenic tissues. *Proc Natl Acad Sci USA* 1987;84: 1590–4.

76 Voutilainen R, Miller WL. Developmental and hormonal regulation of mRNAs for insulin-like growth factor II and steroidogenic enzymes in human fetal adrenals and gonads. *DNA* 1987;7:9–15.

77 Townsend SF, Dallman MF, Miller WL. Rat insulin-like growth factor-I and -II mRNAs are unchanged during compensatory adrenal growth but decrease during ACTH-induced adrenal growth. *J Biol Chem* 1990;265:22117–22.

78 Coulter CL, Goldsmith PC, Mesiano S, Voytek CC, Martin MC, Jaffe RB. *In vivo* regulation of growth and expression of IGF-II and steroidogenic enzymes in the rhesus monkey fetal adrenal. In: *40th Annual Meeting Soc Gynecol Invest, Toronto, Canada* 1993 (Abstr. S144).

79 Li J, Saunders JC, Gilmour RS, Silver M, Fowden AL. Insulin-like growth factor-II messenger ribonucleic acid expression in fetal tissues of the sheep during late gestation: effects of cortisol. *Endocrinology* 1993;132:2083–9.

80 Rainey WE, Oka K, Magness RR, Mason JI. Ovine fetal adrenal synthesis of cortisol: regulation by adrenocorticotropin, angiotensin II and transforming growth factor-β. *Endocrinology* 1991;129:1784–90.

81 Luger A, Calogero AE, Kalogeras K *et al.* Interaction of epidermal growth factor with the hypothalamic-pituitary-adrenal axis: potential physiologic relevance. *J Clin Endocrinol Metab* 1988;66:334–7.

82 Polk DH, Ervin MG, Padbury JF, Lam RN, Reviczky AL, Fisher DA. Epidermal growth factor acts as a corticotropin-releasing factor in chronically catheterized fetal lambs. *J Clin Invest* 1987;79:984–8.

83 Bondy CA, Werner H, Roberts CT, LeRoith D. Cellular pattern of insulin-like growth factor-I (IGF-I) and type I IGF receptor gene expression in early organogenesis: comparison with IGF-II gene expression. *Mol Endocrinol* 1990;4:1386–98.

84 Blanchard MM, Goodyer CG, Charrier J, Barenton B. *In vitro* regulation of growth hormone (GH) release from ovine pituitary cells during fetal and neonatal development: effects of GH-releasing factor, somatostatin, and insulin-like growth factor-I. *Endocrinology* 1988;122:2114–20.

85 Goodyer CG, Marcovitz S, Hardy J, Lefebvre Y, Guyda HJ, Posner BI. Effect of insulin-like growth factors on human foetal, adult normal and tumour pituitary function in tissue culture. *Acta Endocrinol (Copenh)* 1986;112:49–57.

86 Davenport JL, D'Ercole AJ, Azizkhan JC, Lund PK. Somatomedin-C/insulin-like growth factor I (SM-C/IGF-I) and insulin-like growth factor II (IGF-II) mRNAs during lung development in the rat. *Exp Lung Res* 1987;14:607–18.

87 Klempt M, Hutchins A-M, Gluckman PD, Skinner SJM. IGF binding protein-2 gene expression and the location of IGF-I and IGF-II in fetal rat lung. *Development* 1992;115:765–72.

88 D'Ercole AJ, Foushee DB, Underwood LE. Somatomedin C receptor ontogeny and levels in porcine fetal and human cord serum. *J Clin Endocrinol Metab* 1976;43:1069–77.

89 Han RNN, Liu J, Tanswell AK, Post M. Expression of basic fibroblast growth factor and receptor: immunolocalization studies in developing rat fetal lung. *Pediatr Res* 1992;31: 435–40.

90 Williams LT, Peters KG, Kikuchi A *et al.* Signalling molecules that mediate the actions of fibroblast growth factors. In: *Embo Workshop on Molecular and Cellular Aspects of Fibroblast Growth Factors and their Receptors, Capri, Italy*, 1994 (Abstr.).

91 Catterton WZ, Escobedo MB, Sexson WR, Gray ME, Sundell HW, Stahlman MT. Effect of epidermal growth factor on lung maturation in fetal rabbits. *Pediatr Res* 1979;13: 104–8.

92 Sundell HW, Gray ME, Serenius FS, Escobedo MB, Stahlman MT. Effects of epidermal growth factor on lung maturation in fetal lambs. *Am J Pathol* 1980;100:707–25.

93 Nielson HC, Kellogg CK, Doyle CA. Development of fibroblast type-II cell communications in fetal rabbit lung organ culture. *Biochem Biophys Acta* 1992;1175:95–9.

94 Raff MC. Glial cell diversification in the rat optic nerve. *Science* 1989;243:1450–5.
95 Noble M, Murray K. Purified astrocytes promote the *in vitro* division of bipotential glial progenitor cells. *EMBO J* 1984; 3:2243–7.
96 Hughes SM, Lillien LE, Raff MC, Rohrer H, Sendter M. Ciliary neurotrophic factor induced type 2 astrocyte differentiation in culture. *Nature* 1988;335:70–3.
97 Wanaka A, Milbrandt J, Johnson EM. Expression of FGF receptor gene in rat development. *Development* 1991;111: 455–61.
98 Deloulme JC, Baudier J, Sensenbrenner M. Establishment of pure neuronal cultures from the fetal rat spinal cord and proliferation of the neuronal precursor cells in the presence of fibroblast growth factor. *J Neurosci Res* 1991;29:499–509.
99 Gensenburger C, Labourdette G, Sensenbrenner M. Brain fibroblast growth factor stimulates the proliferation of rat neuronal precursor cells *in vitro*. *FEBS Lett* 1987;217:1–5.
100 Murphy M, Drago J, Bartlett PF. Fibroblast growth factor stimulates the proliferation and differentiation of neuronal precursor cells *in vitro*. *J Neurosci Res* 1990;25:463–75.
101 Drago J, Murphy M, Carroll SM, Harvey RP, Bartlett PF. Fibroblast growth factor-mediated proliferation of central nervous system precursors depends on endogenous production of insulin-like growth factor. *Proc Natl Acad Sci USA* 1991;88:2199–203.
102 Ray J, Peterson DA, Schinstine M, Gage FH. Proliferation, differentiation and long-term culture of primary hippocampal neurons. *Proc Natl Acad Sci USA* 1993;90:3602–6.
103 Reynolds BA, Tetzlaff W, Weiss S. A multipotent EGF-responsive striatal embryonic progenitor cell produces neurons and astrocytes. *J Neurosci* 1992;12:4565–74.
104 Alderson RF, Alterman AL, Barde Y-A, Lindsay RM. Brain-derived neurotrophic factor increases survival and differentiation of rat septal cholinergic neurons in culture. *Neuron* 1990;5:297–306.
105 Ip NY, Li Y, Yancopoulos GD, Lindsay RM. Cultured hippocampal neurons show responses to BDNF, NT-3 and NT-4, but not NGF. *J Neurosci* 1993;13:3394–405.
106 Walicke PA. Basic and acidic fibroblast growth factors have trophic effects on neurons from multiple CNS regions. *J Neurosci* 1988;8:2618–27.
107 Maisonpierre PC, Belluscio L, Friedman B *et al*. NT-3, BDNF, and NGF in the developing rat nervous system: parallel as well as reciprocal patterns of expression. *Neuron* 1990;5: 501–9.
108 Davies AM, Lee KF, Jaenisch R. p75-Deficient trigeminal sensory neurons have an altered response to NGF but not to other neurotrophins. *Neuron* 1993;11:565–75.
109 Crowley C, Spencer SD, Nishimura MC *et al*. Mice lacking nerve growth factor display perinatal loss of sensory and sympathetic neurons yet develop basal forebrain cholinergic neurons. *Cell* 1994;76:1001–12.
110 Smeyne RJ, Klein R, Schapp A *et al*. Severe sensory and sympathetic neuropathies in mice carrying a disrupted trk/ NGF receptor gene. *Nature* 1994;368:246–9.
111 Klein R, Smeyne RJ, Wurst W *et al*. Targeted disruption of the *trkB* neurotrophin receptor gene results in nervous system lesions and neonatal death. *Cell* 1993;75:113–22.
112 Klein R, Parada LF, Coulier F, Barbacid M. *trkB*, a novel tyrosine protein kinase receptor expressed during mouse neural development. *EMBO J* 1989;8:3701–9.
113 Klein R, Silos-Santiago I, Smeyne RJ *et al*. Disruption of the neurotrophin-3 receptor gene *trkC* eliminates 1a muscle afferents and results in abnormal movements. *Nature* 1994; 368:249–51.
114 Lassarre C, Hardouin S, Daffos F, Forestier F, Frankenne F, Binoux M. Serum insulin-like growth factor binding proteins in the human fetus. Relationships with growth in normal subjects and in subjects with intrauterine growth retardation. *Pediatr Res* 1991;29:219–21.
115 Delmis J, Drazancic A, Ivanisevic M, Suchanek E. Glucose, insulin, HGH and IGF-I levels in maternal serum, amniotic fluid and umbilical venous serum: a comparison between late normal pregnancy and pregnancies complicated with diabetes and fetal growth retardation. *J Perinat Med* 1992; 20:47–56.
116 Wang HS, Lim J, English J, Irvine L, Chard T. The concentration of insulin-like growth factor-I and insulin-like growth factor binding protein-1 in human umbilical cord serum at delivery: relationship to birth weight. *J Endocrinol* 1991;129:459–64.
117 Price WA, Rong L, Stiles AD, D'Ercole AJ. Changes in IGF-I and -II, IGF binding protein, and IGF receptor transcript abundance after uterine artery ligation. *Pediatr Res* 1992; 32:291–5.
118 Straus DS, Ooi GT, Orlowski CC, Rechler MM. Expression of the genes for insulin-like growth factor-I (IGF-I), IGF-II, and IGF-binding proteins-1 and -2 in fetal rat under conditions of intrauterine growth retardation caused by maternal fasting. *Endocrinology* 1991;128:518–25.
119 Unterman T, Lascon R, Golway MB *et al*. Circulating levels of insulin-like growth factor binding protein-1 (IGFBP-1) and hepatic mRNA are increased in the small for gestational age (SGA) fetal rat. *Endocrinology* 1990;127:2035–7.
120 Vileisis R, D'Ercole AJ. Tissue and serum concentrations of somatomedin-C/insulin-like growth factor I in fetal rats made growth retarded by uterine artery ligation. *Pediatr Res* 1986;20:126–30.
121 Hooper SB, Bocking AD, White S, Challis JRG, Han VKM. DNA synthesis is reduced in selected fetal tissues during prolonged hypoxemia. *Am J Physiol* 1991;261:R508–14.
122 Iwamoto HS, Murray MA, Chernausek SD. Effects of acute hypoxia on insulin-like growth factors and their binding proteins in fetal sheep. *Am J Physiol* 1992;263:E1151–6.
123 McLellan KC, Hooper SB, Bocking AD *et al*. Prolonged hypoxia induced by the reduction of maternal uterine blood flow alters insulin-like growth factor-binding protein-1 (IGFBP-1) and IGFBP-2 gene expression in the ovine fetus. *Endocrinology* 1992;131:1619–28.
124 Breese CR, D'Costa A, Ingram RL, Lenham J, Sonntag WE. Long-term suppression of insulin-like growth factor-1 in rats after in utero ethanol exposure: relationship to somatic growth. *J Pharmacol Exp Ther* 1993;264:448–56.

6: Normal Growth and its Endocrine Control

P.C. HINDMARSH and C.G.D. BROOK

INTRODUCTION

The growth process is a complicated one, but its measurement is necessary for monitoring child health generally, and for the management of endocrine disorders particularly. The study of growth is a basic discipline of paediatrics, and as understanding growth and how to measure it is so crucial to the diagnosis and management of endocrine conditions in childhood a brief practical resumé is included as background against which to read the clinical sections of this book.

GENERAL PRINCIPLES

Growth begins at conception, and influences on prenatal growth are covered in detail in other chapters of this book. Environmental influences on the growth process are at their maximum when growth is at its fastest. This is during the prenatal period and the consequences of intrauterine growth disturbance are profound in postnatal life. It is important to remember that these influences are not simply confined to disorders of stature. There is increasing evidence to suggest that poor nutrition in early life may be an important factor in cardiovascular morbidity and mortality in later life [1].

In terms of describing postnatal growth the chart of the growth of the son of Count Phillip DeMontbeillard, between the years of 1759 and 1777, cannot be surpassed (Fig. 6.1). The top half of the figure shows the increase in height plotted every 6 months, year by year – a distance chart. In the bottom half the increment in height every 6 months has been converted into an annual figure (by doubling) and is plotted against chronological age – a velocity chart. From this figure one can readily discern the three principal phases of growth in childhood: the rapid and rapidly decelerating growth of the first 3 years, the steady and slowly decelerating growth of midchildhood and, finally, growth of adolescence. In the lower panel the midchildhood growth spurt is clearly demonstrated. This feature of children's growth is more pronounced in boys [2,3], but not, as was first thought, absent in girls [4].

In Fig. 6.2 the standard centile distance chart for the population coupled with pubertal staging for girls is shown. This description of height at any age is a necessary instrument for the management of endocrine disorders. It is worth reiterating that centiles mean nothing more than the proportion of children who had reached given heights at given ages when they, the standardizing population, were measured. The centile position, of itself, is of no consequence in the diagnosis or management of an individual child. The number of children below the third centile is approximately 3%, regardless of whether or not there is anything the matter with them. Children can be equally ill irrespective of whether they have a height within or without the centile. Although it is generally true that the further away the child is from the average height of the population, the more likely there is to be an abnormality, the truism does not serve the clinician well.

The majority of children who present because of concern regarding their stature have heights close to the third height centile. Simply screening for stature and investigating those with heights below the third centile may identify a number of children whose growth is abnormal, but it will miss those whose height is, for the present, above the third centile. The financial implications are immense. To investigate all children with height below the third centile means investigating 2000 individuals each year in the UK, which has a birth rate of 600 000 per year. The majority of these individuals will be normal.

Although this truth is obvious, and appreciated intellectually by most health visitors and physicians, it is still common to find children investigated, quite unjustifiably, for 'failure to thrive' when in fact at the time of investigation they are actually thriving. Children who are growing abnormally need investigation: normal children do not. What then defines normality?

Velocity measurements

To estimate the rate at which a child is growing, it is necessary to measure height on more than one occasion over a period of time, and divide the increment in height

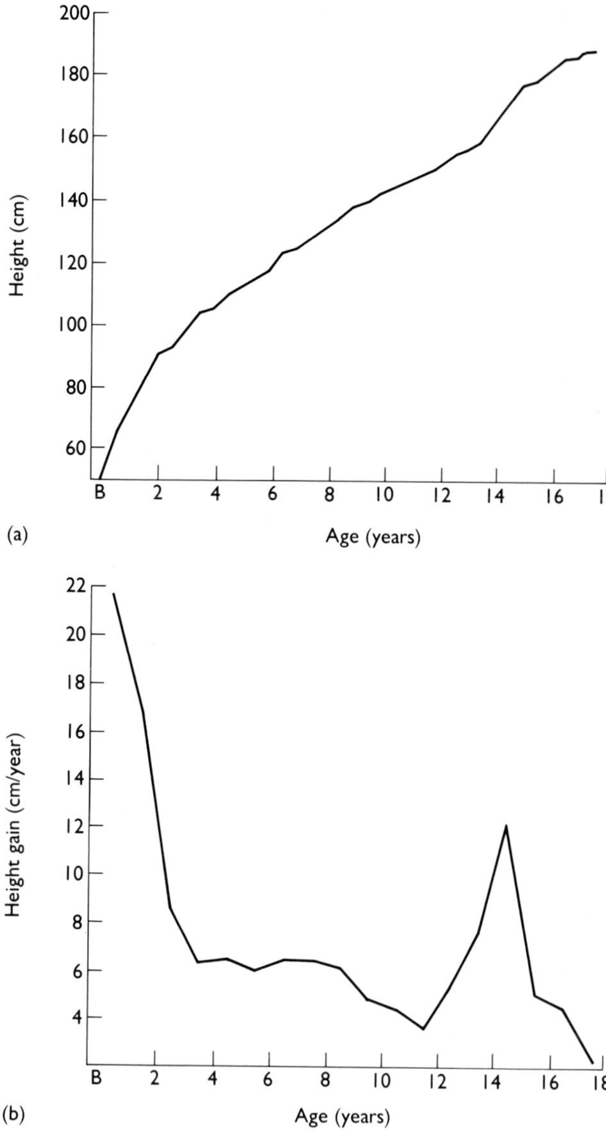

Fig. 6.1 Growth charts of the son of Count Phillip de Montbeillard: (a) distance plot; (b) velocity plot.

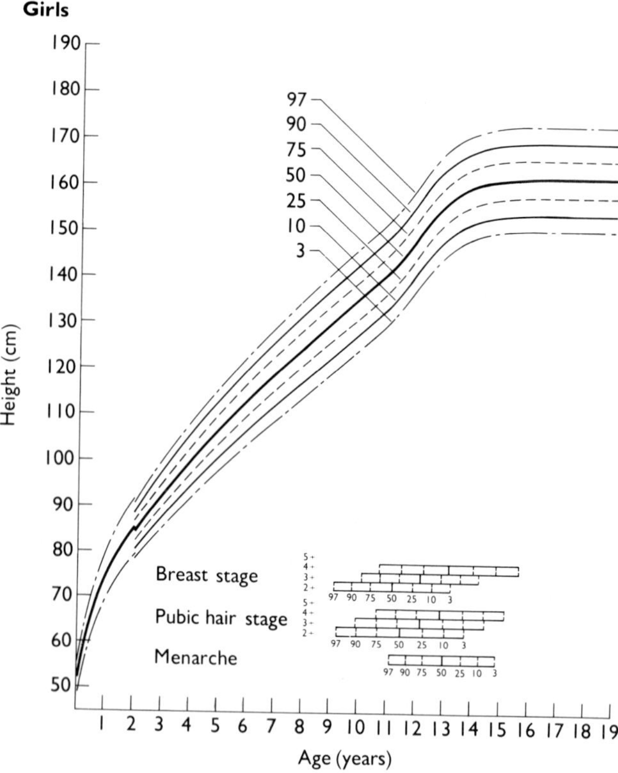

Fig. 6.2 Standard distance centile chart for girls showing age at attainment of different pubertal stages.

Table 6.1 Effect of short intervals of time between measurements on calculated growth velocity

Time (months)	Height (cm)	Annualized growth velocity (cm/year)
0	120.2	–
3(a)	121.4	4.8
(b)	121.5	5.2

(a) and (b) represent two measurements at 3 months which produce a difference in annualized growth velocity of 0.4 cm/year.

by the time elapsed. The amount of time which has to pass before a reliable estimate of growth velocity can be calculated depends upon the accuracy with which the measurement is made. Sufficient time must pass for the increment in height to exceed considerably the cumulative errors on each of the two measurements. Quite apart from changes in growth rates over short periods of time [5], errors of 1 mm on measurements of height at either end of a 3-month period amount to an error of at least 1.6 cm/year if the results are converted to an annual rate.

Great caution is therefore needed in interpreting measurements of velocity over short periods of time (Table 6.1).

Particular use of purpose-built standard equipment by the same measurer minimizes errors, but does not eliminate them. Great emphasis has been placed on accuracy of measurements, but the precision with which the measurements are made is of equal if not more importance. Clinicians long ago learned to live with inaccuracy. Anyone who has followed the saga of the measurement of growth hormone (GH) by radioimmunoassay knows that it is impossible to measure the serum concentration of GH with any degree of accuracy. What we are prepared to accept is that there is an inaccuracy in the measurement of GH, but as long as the measurements are precise then

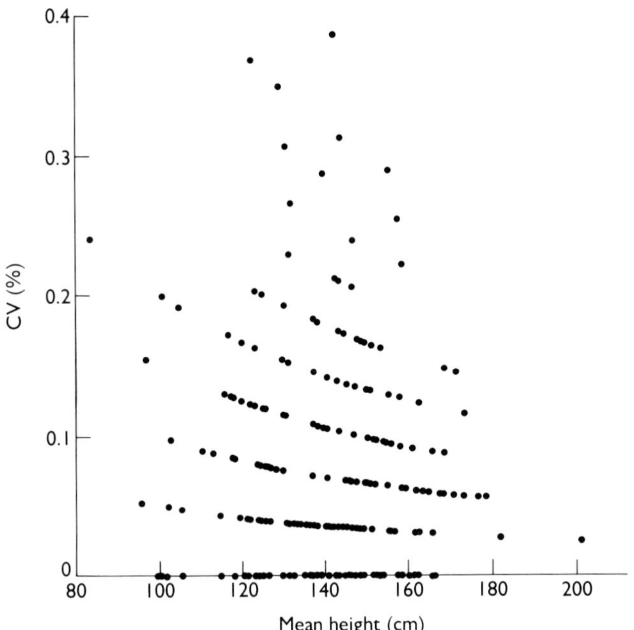

Fig. 6.3 Precision profiles for height measurements. CV, coefficient of variation.

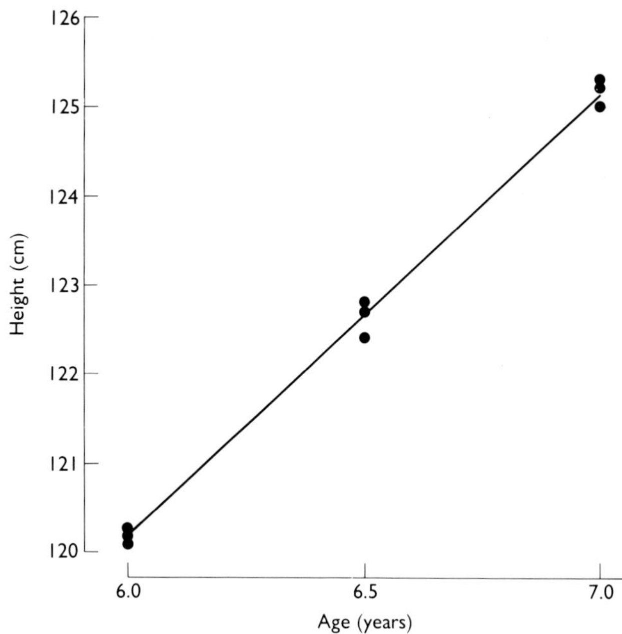

Fig. 6.4 Linear regression of age and height in order to determine growth velocity. Gradient of the line (growth velocity) 5.0 cm/year with standard error of ±0.12 cm/year.

decision-making is permissible. Each centre needs to consider its own precision profile for height and other anthropometric measures. Figure 6.3 shows precision profiles obtained in our clinical practice. The protocol for obtaining these measurements has been described elsewhere [6]. Since the coefficient of variation of measurements of height is considerably less than 1%, this clinical tool has an order of sensitivity which very considerably exceeds that of most biochemical measurements.

Calculation of velocity needs to take into account the errors inherent in measurement of stature. Frequent measures made at 3-monthly intervals over a period of 1 year are extremely helpful in determining the overall growth velocity over that time period. Growth velocity can be calculated to give a rough clinical guide by dividing the difference in height measurements over a period of time by the time that has elapsed between the two measurements.

The use of a table of decimals of year (Table 6.2) is a useful aid. The calculation of velocity in this manner gives a guide to the clinician, but is subject to measurement errors (Table 6.3). However, a more formal assessment of velocity, and one upon which decision-making can then be made, needs the estimation of growth rate by linear regression analysis (Fig. 6.4). This method uses all height measurements made over a period of time. For example, if two measurements are made on each occasion, and the process is repeated at 3-monthly intervals for a whole year, then a total of 10 measurements are available for linear regression analysis. The plot is simple to construct; namely the height measurements at the particular decimal age. The slope of the regression line gives the estimated growth rate over that year, along with an estimate of the error incurred in making that velocity estimation.

Successive points on a distance chart are highly correlated. The child who is small on one occasion is almost certain to be small on a subsequent one. The growth of a normal child tends to follow a particular centile. Only if the child is growing extremely slowly, or if growth continues at a slightly diminished rate for a long time, will deviation from the centile lines become apparent. This is why the calculation of velocity in the clinic becomes important, because there is a difference when successive points are plotted on a velocity chart. Successive velocities hardly correlate at all, and indeed must oscillate about the 50th centile if the child is not to lose or gain in respect to his or her peers (Fig. 6.5).

The child whose velocity over successive years was consistently at the 25th centile will become short, whereas one with a 75th centile velocity will grow tall. We can use these observations to calculate the probability of two successive annual velocities falling on the 25th centile in a normal child, and this is only about $0.25 \times 0.25 = 6.25$. In other words, only 6.25% of healthy children will grow as slowly as this over the whole of a 2-year period.

Growth velocity centiles may better be regarded as probability charts: if treatment were to be administered to all children growing at the third centile velocity for 1 year,

Table 6.2 Table of decimals of year

	1 Jan	2 Feb	3 Mar	4 Apr	5 May	6 June	7 July	8 Aug	9 Sept	10 Oct	11 Nov	12 Dec
1	000	085	162	247	329	414	496	581	666	748	833	915
2	003	088	164	249	332	416	499	584	668	751	836	918
3	005	090	167	252	334	419	501	586	671	753	838	921
4	008	093	170	255	337	422	504	589	674	756	841	923
5	011	096	173	258	340	425	507	592	677	759	844	926
6	014	099	175	260	342	427	510	595	679	762	847	929
7	016	101	178	263	345	430	512	597	682	764	849	932
8	019	104	181	266	348	433	515	600	685	767	852	934
9	022	107	184	268	351	436	518	603	688	770	855	937
10	025	110	186	271	353	438	521	605	690	773	858	940
11	027	112	189	274	356	441	523	608	693	775	860	942
12	030	115	192	277	359	444	526	611	696	778	863	945
13	033	118	195	279	362	447	529	614	699	781	866	948
14	036	121	197	282	364	449	532	616	701	784	868	951
15	038	123	200	285	367	452	534	619	704	786	871	953
16	041	126	203	288	370	455	537	622	707	789	874	956
17	044	129	205	290	373	458	540	625	710	792	877	959
18	047	132	208	293	375	460	542	627	712	795	879	962
19	049	134	211	296	378	463	545	630	715	797	882	964
20	052	137	214	299	381	466	548	633	718	800	885	967
21	055	140	216	301	384	468	551	636	721	803	888	970
22	058	142	219	304	386	471	553	638	723	805	890	973
23	060	145	222	307	389	474	556	641	726	808	893	975
24	063	148	225	310	392	477	559	644	729	811	896	978
25	066	151	227	312	395	479	562	647	731	814	899	981
26	068	153	230	315	397	482	564	649	734	816	901	984
27	071	156	233	318	400	485	567	652	737	819	904	986
28	074	159	236	321	403	488	570	655	740	822	907	989
29	077		238	323	405	490	573	658	742	825	910	992
30	079		241	326	408	493	575	660	745	827	912	995
31	082		244		411		578	663		830		997

Table 6.3 Effect of measurement error on height velocity derived from measurements taken at the beginning and end of 1 year in one individual

Beginning of year measurements (cm)	Measurements 1 year later (cm)
120.1	125.0
120.2	125.2
120.3	125.3

Nine combinations that yield median growth velocity of 5.0 cm/ year (range 4.7–5.2) are possible.

3% of the children treated would actually be normal children who would have been expected to catch up in the following year; 97% of the children needed the treatment.

These observations have been graphically depicted in the paper by Butler *et al.* [8] demonstrating the oscillatory nature of growth in children (Fig. 6.6). Oscillations in growth are not a new phenomenon. In the original description of growth velocity, by Tanner and Whitehouse, clear oscillatory events could be demonstrated in the growth velocity charts of the original Harpenden cohort [7].

Knemometry measurements have also demonstrated oscillatory cycles taking place on average every 3 weeks [9]. Seasonal growth in children has been well described, and the presence of the midchildhood growth spurt has already been mentioned. The data from Butler *et al.* [8] have extended these observations to the longer term, demonstrating that the midchildhood growth is not the only oscillatory event in the child's growth curve, but that similar oscillatory events take place on average every 2 years. These observations support the probability concepts put forward above, and demonstrate the need in therapeutic intervention studies for careful consideration of probability theory in the construction of the treatment

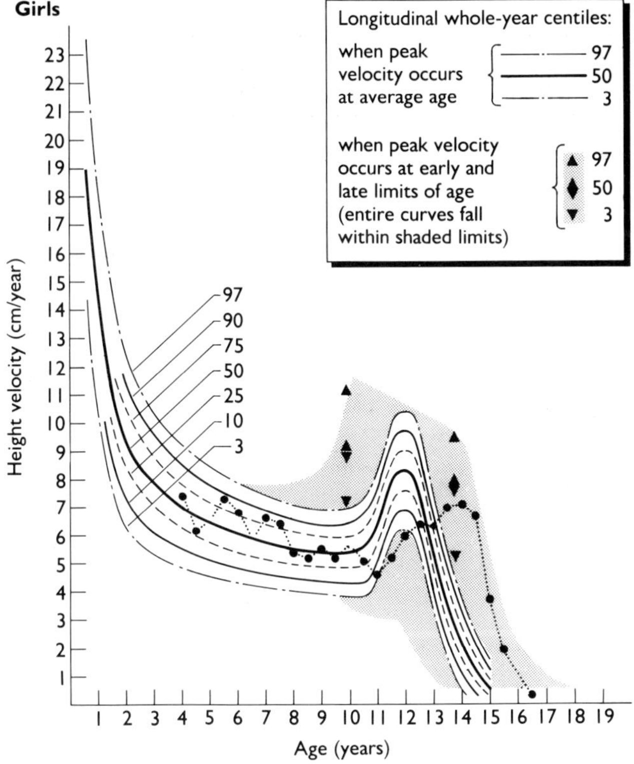

Fig. 6.5 Oscillation of growth velocity around the 50th height velocity centile (from Tanner & Whitehouse [7]).

groups, and also the inclusion of a placebo or observation group.

In practice, because velocity is independent of height achieved, it can be used as a measure of good health in childhood, and a chart which is designed to be used for screening purposes is shown in Fig. 6.7. The advantage of using velocity as a criterion of normality is that it detects abnormal growth regardless of stature achieved, and is thus to be preferred to a distance screening chart. Velocity measurements are also of much more value than distance measurements for the assessment of response to therapy, not least because velocity is the only parameter which can be altered.

At puberty the situation becomes more difficult. The 50th centile in Fig. 6.8 represents a flattening of a number of individual peaked curves occurring at different times, denoted by the shaded zone. The effect of smoothing a succession of individual curves is to flatten the main curve. Calculations of velocity in puberty require interpreting in the light of clinical findings.

Little help is gained either from reference to the standard charts or from standard deviation scores calculated for pubertal-age subjects. Without knowledge of pubertal staging inappropriate conclusions may be reached in children with delayed puberty. Because the puberty growth spurt is delayed the normal childhood velocity (50th centile) continues to decline, so that a child not entering a puberty growth spurt until the 16th year may grow exceedingly slowly, or may even stop growing and yet have a normal growth spurt in the end. Standards are now available to describe this problem precisely [10]. For practical purposes if a growth spurt of 5 cm/year is normal for a prepubertal 12-year-old of either sex then this value can be expected to fall in a child continuing to show no signs of puberty by 1 cm/year for every year that elapses so that, by the age of 17–18, growth will be at a standstill

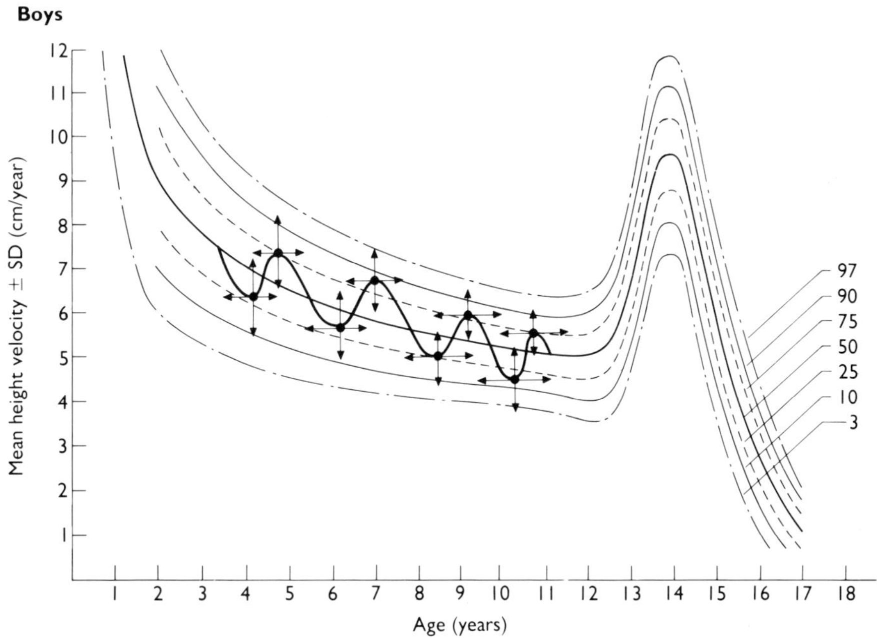

Fig. 6.6 Oscillation of growth velocity in the Edinburgh Growth Study [8] (from Butler *et al.* [8]).

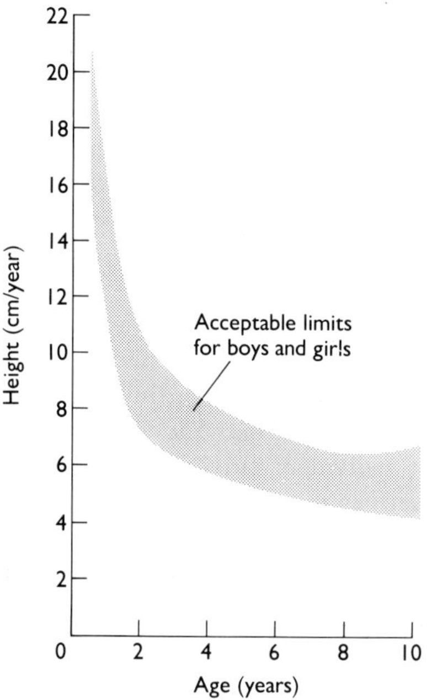

Fig. 6.7 Middlesex height velocity assessment chart, 1–10 years (based on Tanner–Whitehouse Standards (1976)) suggested for the screening of growth disorders using the estimation of height velocity. To use this chart: (a) measure height on two occasions; (b) plot the rate of growth (cm/year) against the median age of the two measurements, for example if heights measured at ages 4 and 6 years show a difference of 6 cm/year they should be plotted at age 5; (c) height velocities persistantly outside the tinted area should be referred for the opinion of a paediatric endocrinologist.

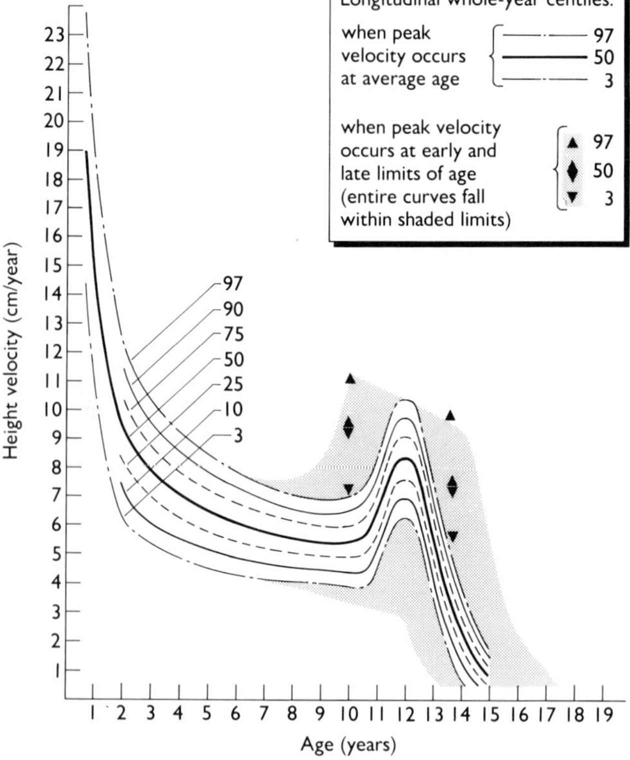

Fig. 6.8 Standard height velocity chart with shaded zone in the pubertal years representing the variations in timing and magnitude of the pubertal growth spurt.

until sex steroids are introduced. A normal lower limit of velocity can be taken as 1 cm/year less than these figures.

Bone age

Throughout this book reference will be made to estimates of bone age. It is important to understand just what bone age means in growth terms and just as important, if not more important, to understand what it does not mean. The maturation of the epiphyseal centres in the skeleton proceeds in an orderly fashion, each centre going through relatively easily definable stages of radiographic change from the first appearance of the epiphyseal centre to its fusion with the appropriate long bone. Bone age can be estimated by the time of appearance at different epiphyseal centres or, when all are present, by the stage of maturity. Conventionally we use X-rays of the hands and wrists for the estimation of skeletal maturity, simply because there is a large aggregation of long and round bones in one readily available area. Standards can, however, be made for estimation of bone age at other centres. When using the hand and wrist there are two principal systems in use.

The Greulich and Pyle system [11] depends upon using a series of radiographic standards to estimate the maturity of each epiphyseal centre in the hand and wrist. These standards were compiled by taking hand radiographs in many children at different ages. The 8-year-old male standard was achieved by taking the radiographs of all the 8-year-old boys, and by progressively eliminating the most skeletally advanced and retarded films until a single representative film remained. Since centres do not mature in individual cases at exactly the same rate, or in the same order, it is not good enough to compare an individual hand radiograph with a whole standard. Each epiphyseal centre must be compared with the standard radiographs and allotted a bone age. The sum of the bone ages of each of the centres is divided by the number of centres rated, and an overall bone age is computed.

Done in this way, estimates of bone age using the atlas of Greulich and Pyle are extremely accurate and reproducible, and they predict a value for adult stature using the tables of Bayley and Pinneau [12]. The problem with the method is that it is frequently abused by comparing an individual X-ray with the whole X-ray standard in the book, and coming up with the best approximation of bone

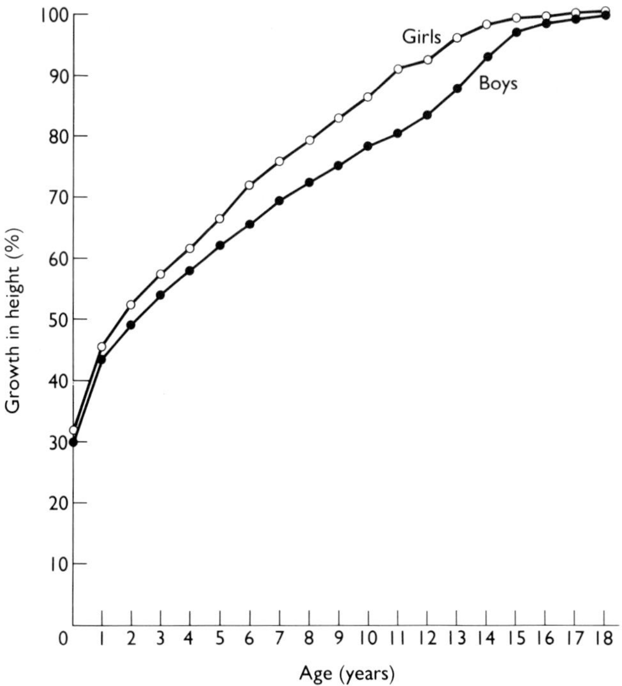

Fig. 6.9 Proportion of adult height attained at any given bone age.

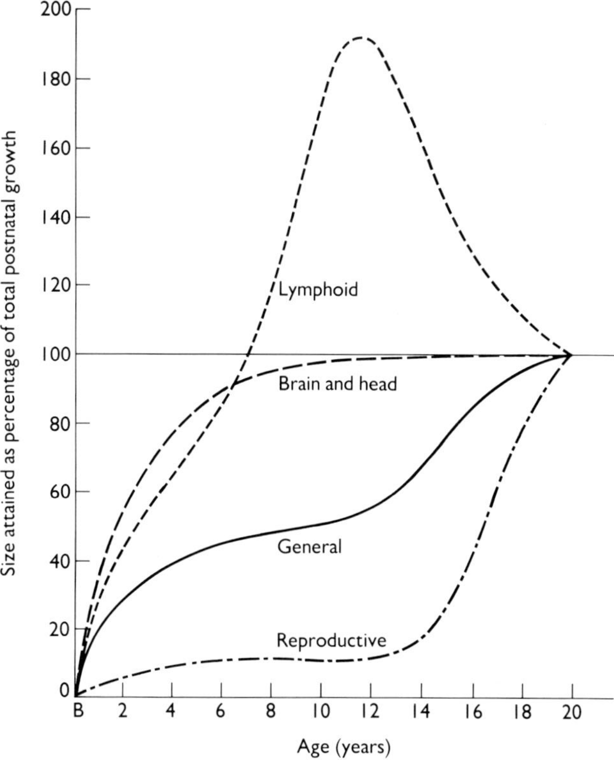

Fig. 6.10 Growth of different parts of the body (redrawn from Tanner [14]).

age, which may be very misleading in the management of endocrine disorders.

For this reason a system was devised by Tanner *et al.* [13] which forces the consideration of each epiphyseal centre in turn, and the attribution to each of a score which, when added together, leads to a bone maturity score. Examination of hand radiographs of many children of both sexes at different ages, from birth to maturity, permitted the calculation of centile charts for bone maturity scores against chronological age. The 50th centile values represent the average bone age of an individual. Bone age is an acceptable measure of maturity, since all adults possess the same (adult) bone age. By the same token, 'height age' and 'weight age' are not acceptable, since all adults manifestly do not have the same height and weight.

An estimate of bone age defines the amount of growth which has already taken place and the amount of growth which is to come. These proportions are shown in Fig. 6.9. An 11-year-old boy has completed approximately 80% of his growth and an 11-year-old girl approximately 90% of hers. A boy of 13 with a bone age of 11 has equally completed 80% of his growth. If, therefore, he is small in comparison to 'standard' 11-year-olds at the age of 13, one can confidently predict that his final adult stature will also be short. This is as far as bone age goes in helping the assessment of endocrine disorders. It does not help, except in the most general way, to indicate a diagnosis.

Once a diagnosis has been made, repeated measurements of bone age are crucial to the management of endocrine disorders: a bone age which is advancing more rapidly than increments in height (however small these may be) leads inevitably to a decrease in growth prognosis. Once the height of a child at a given chronological age related to a given bone age has been attained, the height prognosis of that child cannot be improved, since history cannot be retraced. The prediction can be damaged considerably by inappropriate treatment, but the growth prognosis at the time of commencing treatment is a fixed quantum. This is why early treatment of endocrine disorders is a prerequisite for a successful outcome in terms of growth, and is a reason for the continual emphasis on measurements of height and bone age in this book.

Growth in different organs

Different parts of the body grow at different rates at different times, and different organs certainly have very different patterns of growth from others. Figure 6.10 shows the acquisition of adult size of various different organs, to illustrate just a few of the growth curves in normal growth and development. Body fat has a growth curve all of its own (Fig. 6.11) and individual skinfolds

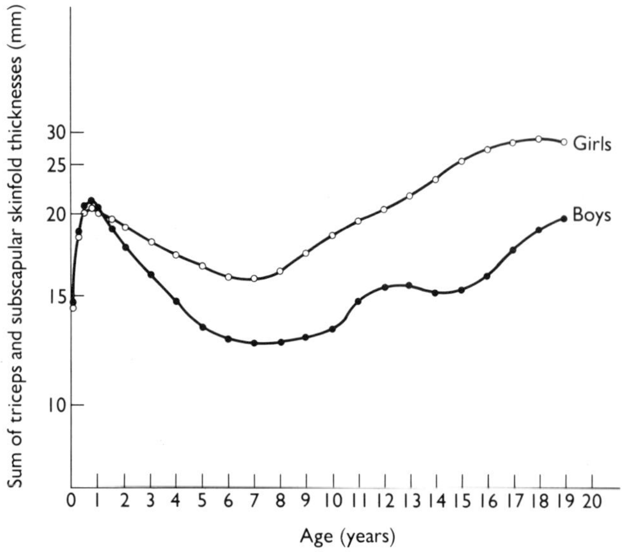

Fig. 6.11 Growth of body fat.

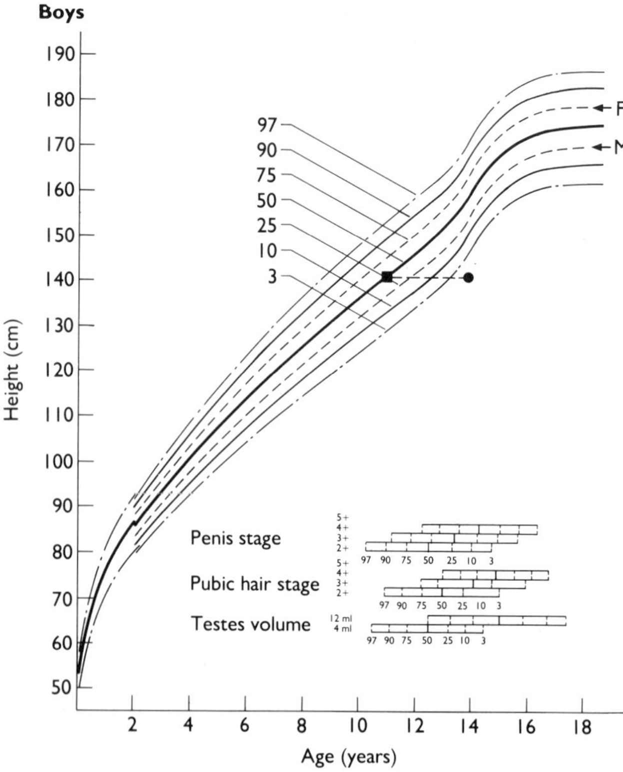

Fig. 6.12 Height plotted for chronological (●) and bone (■) ages of a boy. F, Father; M, Mother. For more details, see text.

behave quite differently from each other, so that changes in different skinfold thicknesses alone can be helpful in estimating maturity. A boy heralds his entry into puberty, for example, by change in the distribution of fat; trunk fat increasing at the expense of limb fat.

INFLUENCES ON THE GROWTH PROCESS

As the growth process is influenced by each and every endocrine disorder covered in this book, it is necessary here only briefly to mention influences which will not be highlighted in other sections.

Genetic influences

Height in normal individuals is a strongly genetically determined characteristic [14,15]. This means that parental heights can give a good indication of the target height to which a child is aiming. Parental heights must be measured, not reported; but when they have been so measured, distribution of heights of the children of parents of given heights is reduced by about one-third compared to the population [16].

The physician should inscribe the centile positions of parents on the height chart of every child, to obtain an idea of whether the present situation is 'on line' for final expected height. Obviously the height centile of a child at any age does not translate directly into the final height centile, since differences in the duration of the growing period (growth advance or growth delay as reflected in bone age) considerably influence the picture. An example is shown in Fig. 6.12. Here the height of a prepubertal boy of 14 is shown at 140 cm. His bone age of 11 years is shown by the solid square connected by a dotted line to the measurement of height. The boy's height prognosis may be assessed from his height for chronological age compared to his height for bone age. Since he is already late entering puberty his growth spurt in puberty will not achieve the magnitude of an early spurt. The later a child goes into puberty, the lower his growth at adolescence. The final height of this child will be somewhere between the centile positions of his height for chronological age and height for bone age, but at present this is within the target limits for the parents. Whether or not he will achieve it depends on whether there is anything wrong with him, how that affects his growth in height and skeletal maturation and whether anything can be done to treat him. Without a knowledge of how he is growing we can infer nothing from the facts we presently have. This is the practical implication of bone age, and of the genetic contribution to final height.

The genetic contribution to the timing of the events of growth and of the determination of adult size is, as yet, poorly researched, and therefore not of much practical relevance to the management of growth disorders. For example, although it is frequently stated that growth delay is a familiar characteristic, and we feel reassured when there is a positive family history in an individual case, the actual documented evidence for the statement is not yet available, so the presence or absence of such a history is of no scientific relevance.

The precise way in which these descriptions of genetic influences are translated into endocrine manifestations, and what the underlying genetic mechanism is, are unclear. A number of levels of genetic influence could be postulated, ranging from the generation of the hypothalamic factors growth-hormone-releasing hormone (GHRH) and somatostatin (SS) right down to the distribution and number of receptors for GH and insulin-like growth factor (IGF) I. It is quite clear that the situation is extremely complex because we are considering not simply the GH axis but the influence of factors such as the IGFs, insulin and the hypothalamopituitary–gonadal–adrenal axis.

Nutrition

Students of animal husbandry have long known that the overfeeding of animals before weaning can profoundly influence the course of growth, leading to early increase in size and early maturation [17]. It appears that the same process can apply to humans, in whom early overfeeding leads to tall stature and growth advance which implies the early acquisition of normal adult stature. It is the early acquisition of adult dimensions which benefits the farmer who, by overfeeding, achieves an adult animal earlier than his neighbour. Such an advance is not necessarily advantageous to children, although it is generally true that physically advanced children fare better at school than children of comparable ability who are physically less mature, always assuming that the advanced child is not too advanced. When this happens, or when children are physically very immature, the psychological consequences may be considerable and school performance compromised.

The effects of overnutrition in humans are shown in Fig. 6.13. This distribution of heights dependent on the time at which obesity became manifest depicts the important role of nutrition-related growth factors in the growth of the human in the first and second years of life. Obesity during this time period leads to tall stature, whereas obesity, or rather overfeeding, in later years leads to an increase in body fat and weight but no increment in stature. This means that intensive regimens to improve growth in childhood by increasing calorie intake are destined to fail because the food intake is introduced during the wrong component of growth. Table 6.4 illustrates this point. It shows the effects of increasing the energy intake of children with asthma in order to promote growth. Weight increased nicely but no effect was observed on height.

Undernutrition, particularly at a period of especially rapid growth such as *in utero*, has equally long-standing effects [19]. However, it is not just in the areas of postnatal growth and neurodevelopmental outcome that there are implications arising from *in utero* undernutrition. Important as these are, it is only now that we are becoming aware of the effects of undernutrition *in utero* on long-term health. A recent series of publications from Barker and colleagues [1] have demonstrated an increased risk of cardiovascular morbidity and mortality in children who were born small for dates as a result of undernutrition *in utero*. Further, the data demonstrated evidence for an increased predisposition to the development of type 2 diabetes mellitus. These observations, coupled with the pioneering work of Fancourt *et al.* [19], mean that the obstetrician, paediatrician and paediatric endocrinologist need to consider very carefully the approach to the question of intrauterine growth, and the small time window

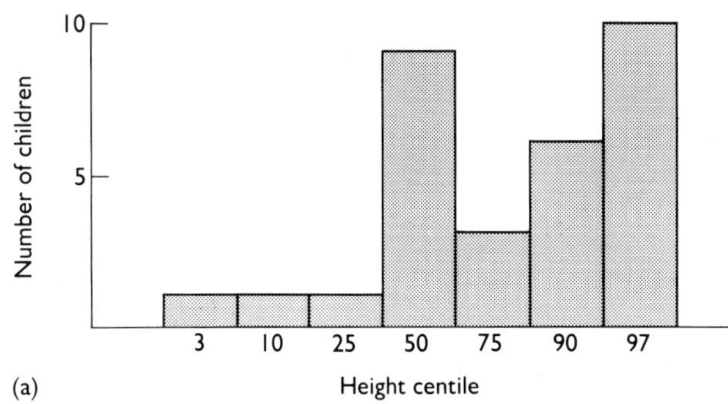

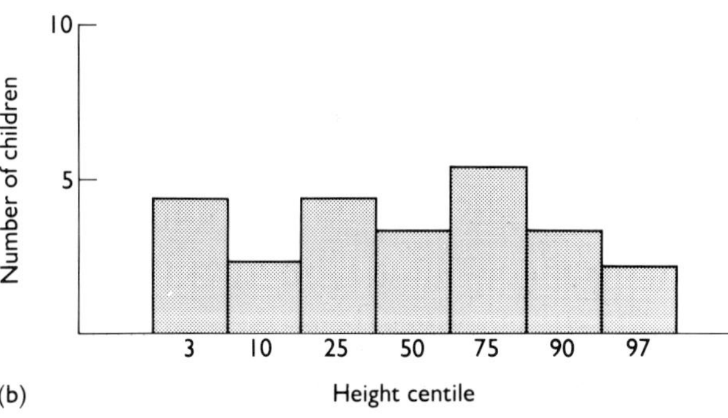

Fig. 6.13 Distributions of height depending on whether obesity was experienced: (a) during, or (b) after the first year of life.

Table 6.4 Effects of altering nutritional intake on growth of asthmatic children (from Cogswell & El-Bishti [18])

	Preintervention	Intervention
Total energy supplement (% RDA)	81.9 ± 6.2	99.1 ± 3.2
Height velocity SDS	−0.6 ± 0.4	−1.1 ± 0.4
Weight velocity (kg/year)	1.7 ± 0.2	2.2 ± 0.5

RDA, recommended daily allowance; SDS, standard deviation score.

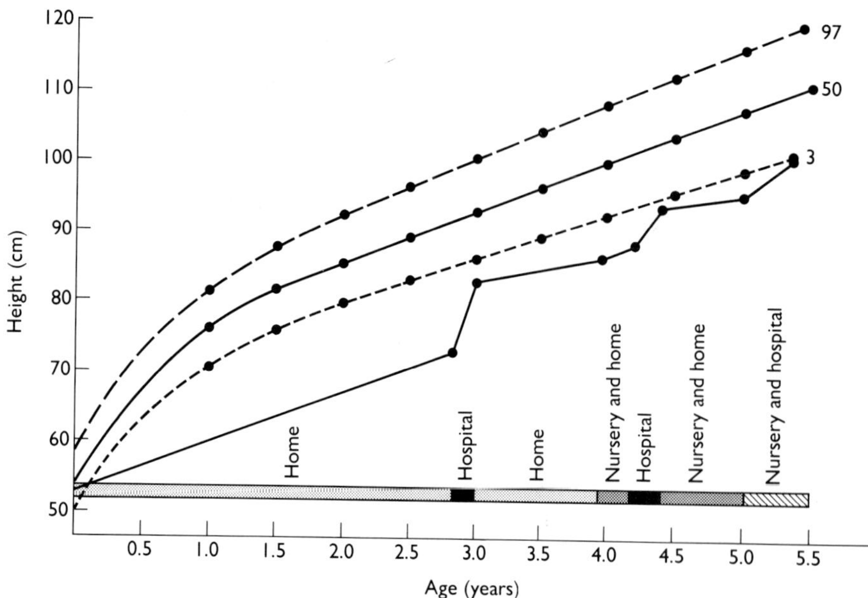

Fig. 6.14 Emotional deprivation. Note the changes in height velocity compared to the changes of environmental circumstances.

available for altering growth prognosis in these children, namely the first and second years of life.

The influence of undernutrition later in childhood is a complicated interaction of quality and quantity of diet with duration of dietary inadequacy. Although many studies attest the effect of such events on postnatal growth, they are not sufficiently quantitated to offer an encapsulated view of the situation.

Emotional deprivation also has a profound influence on the growth process and may interact with the provision of food. Children need a good emotional climate to thrive, and the observant paediatrician can document disturbances of growth in association with emotional disturbances. Figure 6.14 is a case in point: the mechanism of the effects of emotional deprivation on growth is still far from clear, probably reflecting the heterogeneous nature of the complaint. There are, however, a number of studies which have implicated GH in the growth failure associated with this particular problem. The original observations of Powell *et al.* [20] documented recovery of apparent GH insufficiency once the individual was placed in a caring environment, and the recent work of Stanhope and colleagues [21] suggests that this recovery takes place very rapidly within 1–3 weeks of admission to a hospital. Figure 6.15 shows the improvement in GH secretion resulting from hospitalization in one of these cases.

Ethnic differences

Populations differ not only in size and physique but also in the timing of events in the growth process. Children of African origin mature earlier in all respects than children of Caucasian origin. There is a substantial literature on the growth differences between races [22] and, in an ideal world, all populations would have their own growth standard. In fact the variation of growth between races is not very large in comparison to the variation within races. Height standards constructed from, say, British children can be used to look at the children of Asian parents, if one bears in mind the principles of growth assessment, particularly reliance on measurements of growth velocity. It is interesting to note that, in population studies where growth velocities have been calculated, growth rate is remarkably constant between all studies in the childhood years.

Much the largest difference between races are those of shape. Africans, for example, have longer legs than Caucasians, and Europeans have wider shoulders in relation to their hips. For the overall management of growth in endocrine problems these differences are relatively unimportant.

HUMAN GROWTH CURVE

The human growth curve has been described by several mathematical functions [23,24]. The major criticism of these models is that they do not cover the whole of postnatal growth and, more importantly, the majority are descriptive in nature. Little attempt has been made to discern different facets of growth which have important biological connotations. This is why the observations of Butler and colleagues [8] are so important, because they concentrate on explaining a number of different components of childhood growth. A description of the endocrine control of growth requires a model which embodies a number of principles. Important changes occur at crucial

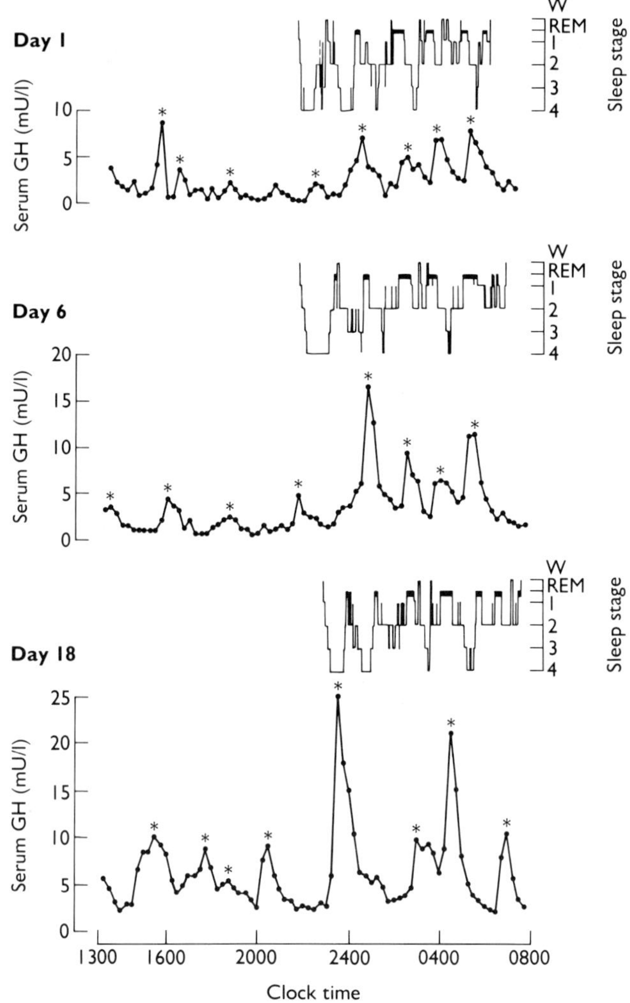

Fig. 6.15 Changes in serum GH concentration profiles during hospitalization in a child with psychosocial deprivation. Note the increase in GH pulse amplitude and the shift in stage 4 sleep to the earlier part of the night (from Stanhope *et al.* [21]).

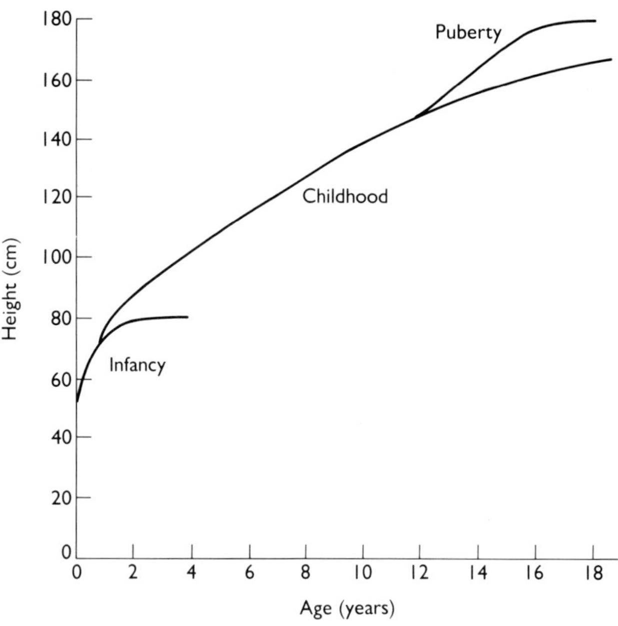

Fig. 6.16 The infancy–childhood–puberty (ICP) model of growth for boys. Data shown are the mean values for age.

points in a child's development, for example when the velocity changes in the third year of life. This change probably represents a switch to dependency on GH for growth. Important clinical clues to the aetiology of the growth problem in an individual child can easily be lost from the rather static approach suggested by some of the descriptive models.

The human growth curve comprises at least three distinct functions, and our understanding of the hormonal regulation of growth concurs with this. The infancy–childhood–puberty (ICP) model proposed by Karlberg *et al.* presents clinicians with an account of growth which places the assessment of growth disorders in a dynamic context, and one which easily lends itself to the application of our understanding of the endocrinology of growth [25]. Figure 6.16 illustrates the three components of the model. Like many growth charts the midchildhood growth spurt has been smoothed. The model presents growth as the additive effect of various biological processes.

The rapid, but rapidly decelerating, growth of the first 2–3 years of life is described by an exponential function representing factors important in fetal growth (see Chapter 5). This is the infancy component, which appears to be largely nutritionally determined. Long-term effects on growth are seen following overnutrition or undernutrition at this stage of life, as mentioned earlier in this chapter.

The childhood component is represented by a second-degree polynomial regression, the earliest onset of which could be recognized at 6 months of age. The impact of the different factors in influencing growth has been highlighted by the study of growth of children in developing countries [26,27]. In a study conducted in the Highlands of Nepal [26] poor growth alternating with rapid growth was documented in infants after weaning, and correlated with the availability of food. Once the childhood component of growth became predominant, age 3 years, then growth proceeded at a normal rate. Short stature in this population arose as a result of inadequate nutrition during the infancy component. The implication for child health-care programmes in this context must be to concentrate resources on improving nutrition during the first 2–3 years of life.

Until the age of 3 years, growth is an additive combination of the infancy and childhood components. Such a statement is supported by these studies of children in

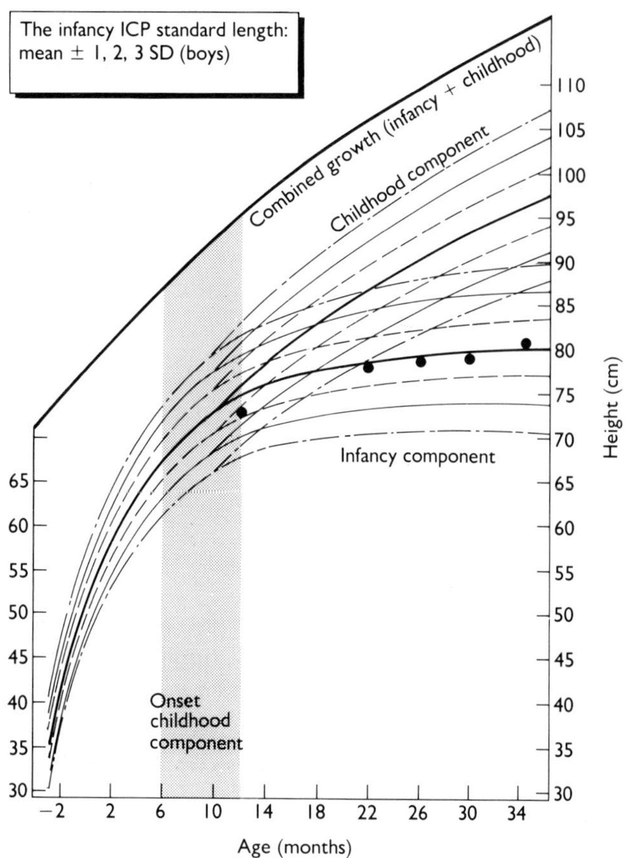

Fig. 6.17 Growth of a boy with growth hormone insufficiency (peak GH to Insulin tolerance test (ITT) < 2 mU/l) plotted on the ICP standard.

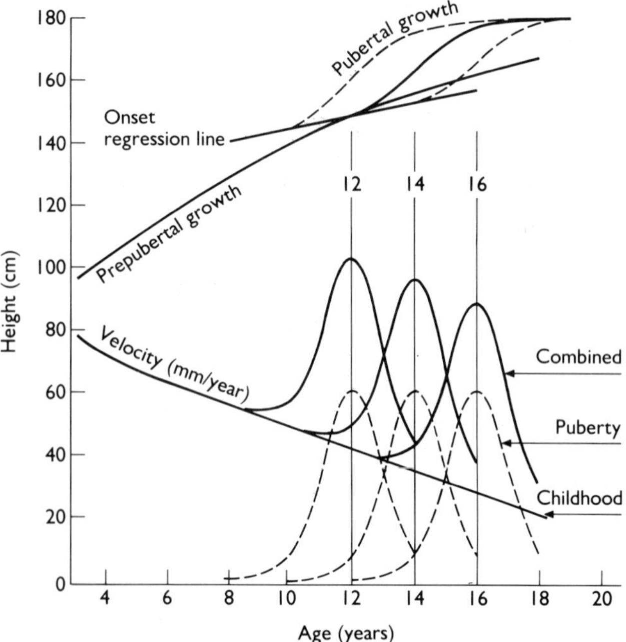

Fig. 6.18 Velocity chart from the ICP model showing the contribution of the pubertal component (from Karlberg [27]).

the developing world, and by the study of children with GH deficiency (particularly where there is a gene deletion) who show a growth pattern compatible with a continuation of the infancy component (Fig. 6.17). Large studies from the Netherlands largely support this general thesis [28] although other reports [29], where detailed anthropometric measurements have not been so readily available as in the Netherlands, have produced rather contradictory findings. The childhood component is largely determined by GH secretion, and the regulation of GH secretion and synthesis and the relationship with growth are described further below.

Of the infants studied by Karlberg *et al.*, 76% showed an abrupt increase in growth rate at the onset of the childhood component. Those children with an early onset had a smoother transition, and these children had a smaller infancy component. No relationship was found with cessation of breast-feeding, season of the year, social group or midparental height [25]. Statistical analysis suggested that an onset of the childhood component after the age of 12 months was extremely unlikely, and should therefore be a cause for concern leading to clinical investigation.

The final component of the model concerns puberty, when growth is described by a logistic function dependent endocrinologically on a combination of GH and sex steroids. This is superimposed on the decelerating childhood component, which explains the well-known fact that the magnitude of the adolescent growth spurt is inversely related to the age at peak height velocity (Fig. 6.18). The contribution of the pubertal component is independent of time. What constitutes the difference is the point at which it is superimposed on the (decelerating) childhood component. The puberty component depends on sex steroids which have a direct anabolic action and a modulating effect on GH secretion.

A clear rise in GH secretion occurs during puberty [30–32]. Growth acceleration takes place in girls during stages 2 and 3 of puberty, whereas in boys the growth spurt takes place later at a testicular volume of 10 or 12 ml or genitalia stage 4. Cross-sectional and longitudinal studies have demonstrated that changes in serum GH concentrations parallel these anthropometric events [30,33,34]. The change in GH secretion is brought about by an alteration in GH pulse amplitude with pulse periodicity remaining unchanged at 180–200 min [33,35].

Children with gonadotrophin-dependent precocious puberty have similar GH secretory profiles to pubertal children [36,37]. Treatment with gonadotrophin-releasing hormone agonists switches off gonadotrophin secretion and thereby sex steroid concentrations are reduced. With this reduction in sex steroid concentration there is a decrease in both GH and IGF-I levels [37,38]. Further evidence for the role of sex steroids in mediating these changes comes from studies of IGF-I levels in children with GH deficiency and precocious puberty, in whom the rise in IGF-I is blunted [39]. Short courses of testosterone (approximately 6 weeks) increase GH pulse amplitude [40,41].

The difference in the timing of the pubertal growth spurt between boys and girls is interesting, particularly when it is recalled that the timing of the onset of puberty differs little between the sexes. Longitudinal studies suggest that serum testosterone concentrations need to be elevated towards the normal adult male range for a considerable proportion of the 24-h period before an increase in serum GH concentrations can be recorded [34]. Acute intervention studies of testosterone administration suggest a concentration and duration of exposure effect in altering GH secretory dynamics [42]. Aromatization of testosterone, rather than conversion to dihydrotestosterone, appears to be the important step for testosterone action.

ENDOCRINOLOGY OF GROWTH IN CHILDHOOD

Conventional accounts of the endocrinology of growth and development usually start with an account of the hormones which are known to be involved, and then an examination of their respective actions. This pattern is followed in the majority of this book. However, from what has been written about normal growth it is evident that any endocrine account must explain the three phases of that process, and must view hormone action as an integrative effect rather than the contribution of distinct entities.

As indicated, the infancy component probably represents the persistence of the effects of factors operative during fetal growth. The principal hormone influencing midchildhood growth is GH, the secretion of which is regulated by two hypothalamic peptides, GHRH and SS. GHRH controls synthesis and release of GH, while SS modulates its pulsatile secretion. The effects of GHRH on GH synthesis are independent of those on GH release and on extracellular calcium mobilization [43]. GHRH acts as a mitogen via cyclic adenosine monophosphate (cAMP) on somatotrophs, as evidenced by increases in thymidine incorporation, stimulation of proto-oncogene (c-*fos*) expression and an increase in somatotroph number [44–47]. The proposed interrelationships in the GH axis are shown in Fig. 6.19.

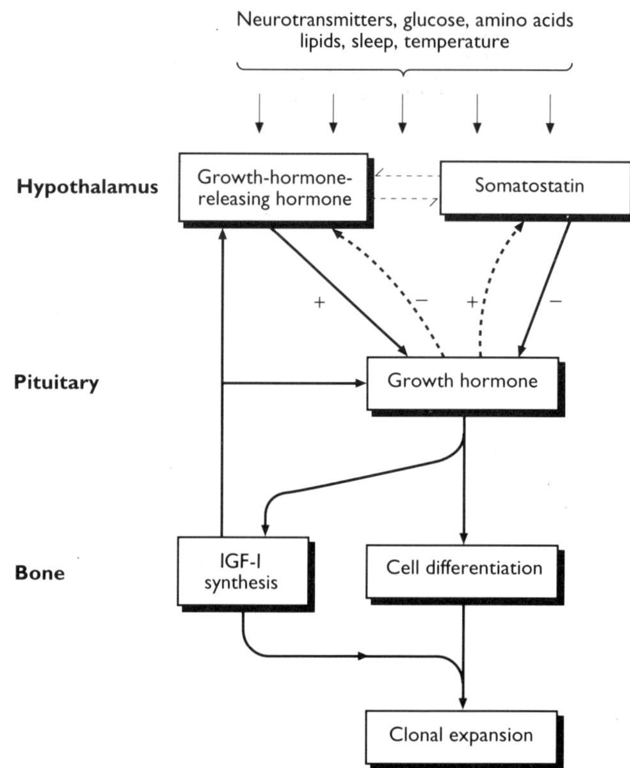

Fig. 6.19 The growth hormone axis.

Effects of growth-hormone-releasing hormone and somatostatin on the somatotroph

GHRH selectively stimulates pituitary somatotrophs, and its effects are initiated by its binding to a specific receptor on the cell membrane [48,49]. Recent work has demonstrated that the receptor is identical to other adenylate cyclase-linked peptide receptors and bears all the hallmarks of a G protein-coupled receptor [49]. Only 30% receptor occupancy is required for full biological activity [50], which means that the system is less prone to receptor down-regulation than has been otherwise thought.

The mechanisms involved in GHRH signal transaction have not been completely elucidated, but a number of secondary messenger systems are likely to be involved. The adenylate cyclase/cAMP system appears to be the most important, and is activated via G_s regulatory protein linked to the GHRH receptor [51–53]. The guanine-nucleotide-binding proteins (G proteins) are involved in peptide hormone signal transduction. There are a number of members of this family, G_s, G_i, G_q and G_t. They may be stimulatory or inhibitory and are heterotrimers consisting of α-, β- and subunits; a schematic representation is shown in Fig. 6.20. Activation takes place by the interaction of the hormone receptor complex with the heterotrimer. Guanine diphosphate (GDP) bound to the α-subunit is replaced by guanine triphosphate (GTP) upon activation and the α-subunit is released from the heterotrimer to interact with and stimulate membrane-bound adenylate

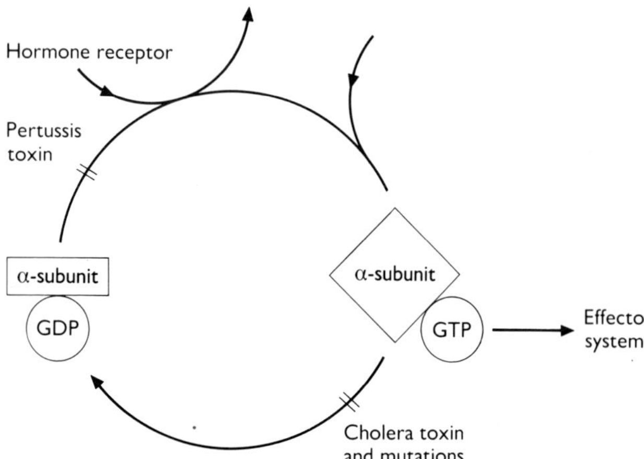

Fig. 6.20 Schematic representation of the G protein system showing points of action of agents in the cycle.

cyclase. Intrinsic GTPase activity in the α-subunit converts GTP to GDP; the subunit rejoins to form the heterodimer, and adenylate cyclase activity is switched off.

There are a number of clinical situations where inappropriate prolongation of G_s regulatory protein action leads to uncontrolled hormone synthesis and release (for example pituitary somatotroph tumour cells [54,55] and the McCune–Albright syndrome [56]).

GHRH also stimulates the phosphatidylinositol–protein kinase C pathway and calcium mobilization events which lead also to GH release [57,58].

There are a number of naturally occurring animal models which are the consequence of spontaneous mutations suggesting impaired GHRH secretion or action. These animal models may prove of value in understanding GH deficiency states in humans. There are a number of strains of GH-deficient mice and in one (little (lit/lit)) there are identifiable somatotrophs which only contain 10% of the normal GH content and reduced levels of GH mRNA. These somatotrophs are resistant to GHRH stimulation and the homozygous animals are growth-retarded [59]. There appears to be an impairment in intracellular signal transduction as a result of a mutation in the GHRH receptor [60]. Analysis of the anterior pitutary in these animals suggests a requirement for sequential growth factors in the regulation of cell proliferation. In a group of dwarf rats (dw) the somatotrophs secrete GH in response to exogenous GHRH *in vitro*, but *in vivo* administration of GHRH fails to stimulate growth. A disturbance of GHRH signal transaction in thought to be the cause [61].

The clinical counterpart to these animal models is seen in some patients with idiopathic isolated GH deficiency. Although many of these children do respond to GHRH, suggesting a problem with GHRH secretion rather than action, some do not respond at all, even with supramaximal doses, and many show a reduced response. The problem does not appear to lie within the GHRH gene, which in the majority of GH-deficient children is intact [62].

SS suppresses GH secretion by a number of mechanisms. There is a specific SS membrane receptor which is linked to the catalytic subunit through a separate, inhibitory G_i protein [63]. SS exerts only a partial inhibitory effect on cAMP accumulation. Other routes of action of SS include an inhibitory effect via a calcium-dependent step in the GH release pathway [64]. In addition, there is also a cAMP-independent route via the phosphatidylinositol – protein kinase C system [65,66]. SS does not have any effect on GH synthesis as GHRH-stimulated GH gene transcription is not blocked by SS. Rather, any effects SS might have on reducing GH gene transcription appear to be mediated at the hypothalamic level by a suppression in GHRH release.

Gene regulation of growth hormone secretion

The human GH (hGH) gene is present on the long arm of chromosome 17 and is part of the hGH gene cluster which consists of five very similar genes spanning approximately 66.5 Kbp. The nomenclature of the hGH gene has changed considerably over the years, and Fig. 6.21 shows the current classification. The hGH 1 (LGHN) gene and its mRNA transcripts have five exons separated by five introns [67]. Transcription of this gene leads to the synthesis of 22 kD hGH, which accounts for 90% of the GH synthesized.

The excision of the second intron of the hGH-1 gene leads to an alternative splicing site, resulting in deletion of the message for amino acid residues 32–46 leading to a smaller molecule termed the 20 kD hGH variant; it forms 10% of the GH synthesized. Translation occurs as a two-step process with the final events being coordinated in the rough endoplasmic reticulum. The importance of the hGH-1 gene can be seen in children with deletion of this gene, most commonly a 6.7 kb deletion. This leads to severe postnatal growth failure, which is characterized by a response to exogenous GH with rapid subsequent attenuation of growth due to formation of high-affinity-binding antibodies to the GH molecule [68–70] for which these children have no immunological tolerance.

An increasing number of patients have been reported in whom immune intolerance after GH treatment has not developed [71,72]. This has led to the idea that familial isolated GH deficiency type 1a cannot be simply identified on the basis of anti-hGH antibodies causing growth arrest. A second autosomal recessive type of familial isolated GH deficiency (type 1b) is characterized by the production of insufficient amounts of hGH to provocative stimuli; in

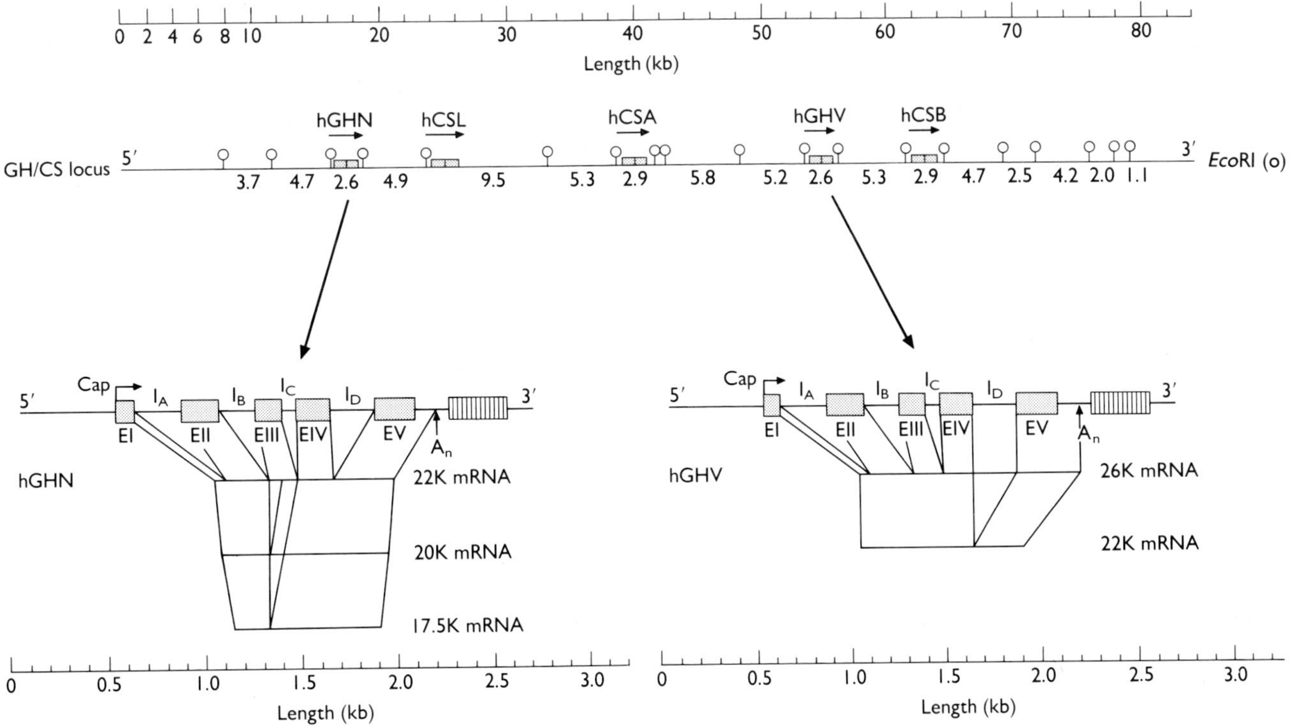

Fig. 6.21 Representation of the GH gene family with alternate splice sites shown.

contrast to type 1a no detectable hGH gene deletions have been described. A third form (type 2) has an autosomal dominant mode of inheritance, whereas the fourth form is X-linked. The same criteria used to diagnose type 1b applies to types 2 and type 3 [73].

These conditions are rare causes of milder forms of GH deficiency [62]; however, in children with severe isolated GH deficiency with heights less than 4.5 standard deviation scores from the mean a number of studies have reported a high prevalence for hGH-1 gene deletion (Table 6.5).

The hGH-2 (LGHV) gene appears to express a GH in the placenta. The polypeptide produced differs from pituitary hGH at 15 positions. Cross-reaction with hGH antibody in a number of immunoassays is poor. Nonetheless there is now an impressive body of evidence to suggest that a complete copy of the hypothalamopituitary growth hormone–insulin-like growth factor 1 axis also exists in the placenta with the demonstration of placental GHRH mRNA/peptide [79]. Insulin-like growth factors are synthesized and secreted by placental tissues, and probably influence placental function in either an autocrine or paracrine fashion [80].

Although the hGH gene is present in all cells in the human body it is only in the pituitary somatotrophs that full expression takes place. Our understanding of the specificity of this expression has increased with the recognition that there are genes present in the human that govern embryonic development and gene expression. These genes were first demonstrated in *Drosophila* and are a family of genes known as the homeobox group. These genes share a common DNA-binding domain. With respect to the pituitary, interest has centred on the homeobox gene Pit-1, which governs pituitary cell differentiation and function [81,82].

In 1989 Wit *et al.* [83] reported a form of hypopituitarism in two Dutch families in which each family contained two affected siblings with GH deficiency and partial deficiency of thyrotrophin. Coincident with this report was the description of the product of the Pit-1 gene

Table 6.5 Prevalence of hGH-1 gene deletion in children with height standard deviation scores less than four from different populations

Population	Number affected/ total studied	Percentage affected	Reference
Japanese	0/10	1.0	[74]
North European	3/32	9.4	[75]
Chinese	3/26	11.5	[76]
Mediterranean	3/22	13.6	[75]
Saudi Arabian	2/13	15.4	[77]
Turkish	4/24	16.6	[75]
Oriental Jewish	5/13	38.4	[78]

which was a protein necessary for embryonic development, proliferation and specialized function of GH-, prolactin- and thyrotrophin-producing cells [81,82]. Animal counterparts exist: the Snell dwarf mouse has a point mutation in Pit-1 and has served developmental biologists over many years as an example of GH deficiency [84]. The cDNA from affected family members of the Dutch families contained a single base difference from the normal Pit-1 cDNA sequence [85]. The two affected children were homozygous for the mutation.

The consequences of this mutation in humans were different from those seen in the Snell mouse. The Snell mutation eliminated binding to DNA, whereas the mutation in the Dutch children, although it allowed binding to GH and prolactin promoter sites with nearly the same affinity as that of the wild-type protein, completely lacked the ability to activate transcription from the site. The loss of proline as a result of this mutation altered the Pit-1 protein structurally so that it could not dimerize. Dimerization is important for Pit-1 binding and activation of DNA.

Other proteins involved in signalling cascades may also be important in hormone production and cell proliferation. Expression of a transgene for cholera toxin, stimulating the cAMP pathway, results in somatotroph proliferation, pituitary hyperplasia and gigantism [86]. Loss of function mutations of the cAMP response element binding protein transcription factor results in somatotroph hypoplasia [87]. These observations, coupled with reports of other families with Pit-1 problems [88], suggest that there are likely to be a number of abnormalities yielding a number of different effects on pituitary cell differentiation and proliferation. Although these observations explain how Pit-1 defines cell types they still do not explain how cell specificity is conferred. Other factors must be operative.

In the rat the promoter region of the GH gene is influenced by Pit-1 which binds to two sites on the promoter. More tissue-general factors are also important, including the thyroid hormone receptor [89], SP1 [90] and GHF-3 [91]. Synergy between Pit-1 and the thyroid hormone receptor has been demonstrated in a series of experiments in which Pit-1 was relatively inactive in isolation from the thyroid hormone receptor. Protein kinases also appeared to have an important role, underlining the dependence of Pit-1 action on other transcription factors and implicating Pit-1 as a cofactor, rather than the dominant factor, influencing the tissue-specific expression of the rat GH promoter [92] (Fig. 6.22). The role of protein kinase A in Pit-1 action is significant given that GHRH activates adenylate cyclase with subsequent activation of protein kinase A [51].

The GH gene probably represents the final pathway for the expression of many of the factors important in GH control. The role of GHRH and SS has already been discussed above. The insulin-like growth factors are important in regulating GH release. IGF-I inhibits basal GH gene transcription [93], suggesting a feedback role for IGF-I in GH regulation. This is probably unlikely to be mediated through small changes in plasma concentration of IGF-I, which is principally a paracrine hormone, especially as mRNA for IGF-I has been demonstrated within the pituitary of adult rats [94]. The situation is complicated further by the demonstration of somatotroph populations which are differentially responsive to IGF-I and SS. SS is a much more effective inhibitor of total GH release than IGF-I, and appears to affect most, if not all, somatotrophs [95]. At the cellular level it would appear that IGF-I inhibits only the secretion of newly synthesized GH, while SS inhibits both stored and newly synthesized GH pools [96].

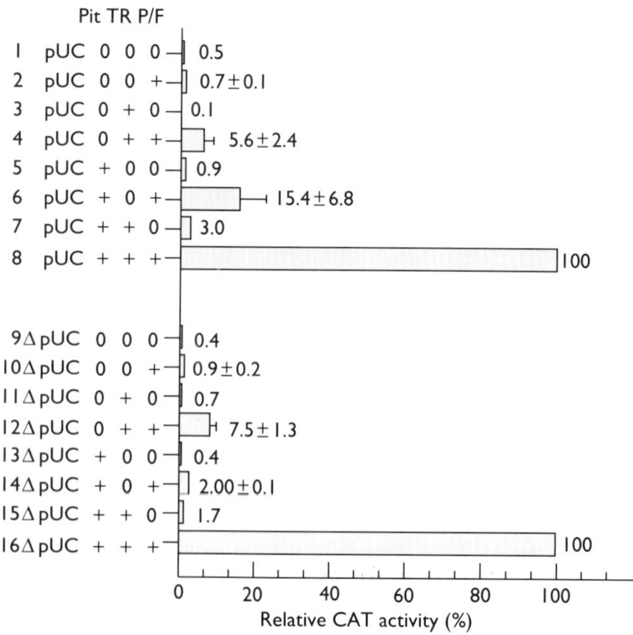

Fig. 6.22 Chloramphenicol acetyltransferase (CAT) activity derived from the rat GH237 promoter electroporated into U937 cells in the presence and absence of vectors expressing rat Pit-1, human thyroid hormone receptor and the presence or absence of forskolin and phorbol ester (from Schaufele *et al.* [92]).

The effect of thyroid hormone on GH gene expression has provided a detailed analysis of the regulation of the GH gene. Poor growth in children with hypothyroidism is well known, and blunting of GH responses to a variety of stimuli have been documented [97–99]. On replacement therapy these responses return to normal, and catch-up growth is observed.

Hypothyroidism is associated with a fall in pituitary GH mRNA levels which is accompanied by a decrease in pituitary GH content. Treatment of hypothyroid rats with triiodothyronine (T_3) rapidly increased GH mRNA levels with a gradual restoration of pituitary GH content and serum GH concentrations [100]. Stimulation of GH gene transcription appears to be mediated by a thyroid hormone nuclear receptor which is a DNA-binding protein [101]. Two areas exist for binding on the 5′-flanking DNA of the GH gene: the first is important for basal expression and the second for the full expression of the stimulatory effect of thyroid hormone [102,103]. The interactions with Pit-1 are described above.

Glucocorticoids appear to regulate the gene at sites different to that of thyroxine (T_4) [104]. The sites are probably contained in the structural portion of the gene and/or the 3′-flanking sequence [102]. Other steroids such as oestrogen are also effective in stimulating transcription of the gene. Testosterone has little effect, which may be important for explaining some of the sex differences in growth patterns seen at puberty.

Finally, insulin regulation of the rat GH gene has also been demonstrated, but the effect can be either positive or negative and is critically dependent on the metabolic state of the cells and the incubation medium used [105]. At physiological concentrations in the rat, insulin inhibits transcription of the GH gene [106] and has a suppressive effect on T_3-stimulated GH mRNA levels [107]. The mechanism appears to operate at the transcriptional and post-transcriptional levels.

Circulating forms of growth hormone

The molecular forms of hGH secreted *in vivo* are independent of the secretory stimuli applied to the somatotroph. GHRH, exercise and sleep-related GH-secretory bursts all produce monomeric hGH forms (22 kD, 20 kD and acidic hGH), of which 22 kD is the predominant fraction [108,109]. In plasma, large forms of GH can be detected with molecular weights in the order of 40–70 kD. The precise origin and function of these larger forms is unclear, but they probably represent the interaction of GH with a circulating binding protein. The precise role which these binding proteins play in the regulation of GH action is unclear, but is discussed to a certain extent in the section on growth hormone resistance states (Chapter 11).

Presentation of growth hormone to the target cells

In common with other pituitary hormones GH secretion occurs in a pulsatile fashion [110]. The importance of this pulsatile secretion is less clear in humans than it is in other animals, such as rodents. The studies in adult rats showed that male rats exhibit regular bursts of GH every 3 h 20 min, whereas female rats have a different pattern of secretion. A highly variable GH secretory pattern occurs in female rats with sustained periods of low, almost continuous, secretion followed by a very rapid high-amplitude burst of short duration occurring mostly at night [111]. The pattern of pulsatile secretion in this group of animals is important in the modulation of several metabolic enzymes in the liver [112,113] and for stimulating growth [114,115].

In the human, major alterations in the frequency component of pulsatile secretion have not been demonstrated to any great extent. High GH levels have been noted in the umbilical cord of premature infants and, in situations where cordocentesis has been performed, high GH levels have also been documented. Pulsatile GH release can be observed in premature infants (32–33 weeks) with values rarely reaching the undetectable concentrations seen in childhood [116,117]. Circulating IGF-I levels are low in these infants, but the elevated levels may result from a lack of SS, the secretion of which is not fully developed at this stage of gestation. Sleep-related peaks of GH appear in the first year of life in relation to the organization of sleep–awake cycles [118]. Faster frequencies have been demonstrated in pubertal boys compared to adults [119], and changes in GH pulse amplitude with age are well documented, with an increase occurring around the time of puberty coincident with the pubertal growth spurt. A subsequent decrease in pulse amplitude occurs as time progresses [31,35].

The only situation where the frequency of GH secretion appears to be altered is during starvation. Experiments in which fasting has been conducted over a 7-day period demonstrate an increase in GH pulse frequency along with an elevation in the baseline of GH concentrations measured. These changes appear over a 56 h period and as serum IGF-I concentrations were unchanged during the study period it has been suggested that starvation-induced enhancement of GH secretion is mediated by an increased frequency of GHRH release, and longer and more pronounced periods of SS withdrawal [120].

The use of 24 h profiles to investigate the physiology of GH secretion has increased our awareness of the importance of the relationship between growth and GH secretion. The techniques for evaluating such pulsatile patterns of hormone secretion are discussed in Chapter 8 of this book.

During childhood, stature is determined by the size that an infant has reached by the end of the first year of life, which is partly determined by genetic circumstances and influenced greatly by nutrition, and the rate at which the child grows henceforward. The rate is related in an asymptotic fashion to the amount of GH secreted [121] (Fig. 6.23). Similar findings have been reported by other groups [122,123]. These are cross-sectional studies, and as longitudinal studies of GH secretion in children have not been reported we can only infer from the examinations of profiles of children with the same height standard deviation score at different ages what happens to GH secretion in an individual child.

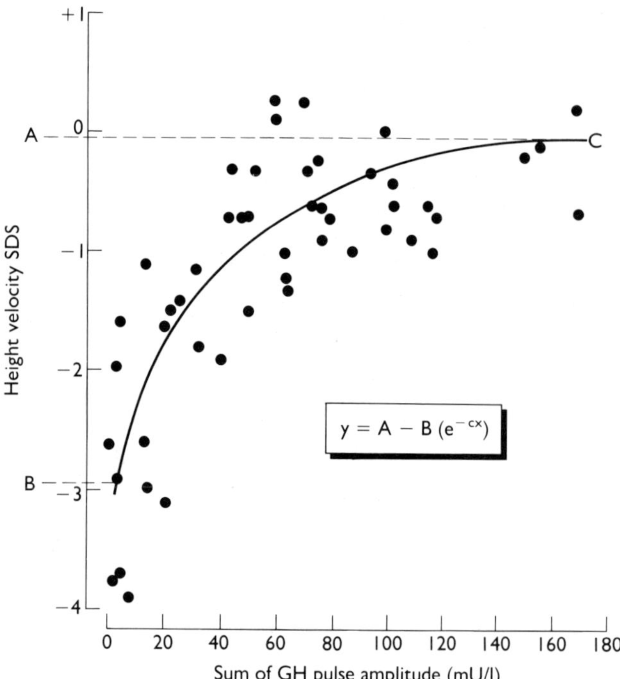

Fig. 6.23 Relationship between GH secretion and growth velocity expressed as a standard deviation score (SDS) [121].

Childhood growth would appear to be a GH pulse amplitude-modulated process, and the frequency of secretion remains unchanged during childhood at a dominant periodicity of 200 min [33]. This does not appear to change much until late adolescence. This dominant GH periodicity appears around the age of 7 years; before this there appears to be no clear dominant periodicity that can be determined [33]. At this age a rise in GH pulse amplitude can also be documented. The most likely explanation for these changes in midchildhood is that they occur concurrently with the midchildhood growth spurt, which probably reflects the processes taking place within the hypothalamopituitary–adrenal axis, and known loosely as adrenarche. Testosterone and oestrogen change GH pulse amplitude in puberty [35,40]. It is probable that adrenal androgens can do the same, and there is some evidence to suggest that androgens are important in determining the pulsatile nature of GH secretion [124]. It is axiomatic that, at this stage of development, any other factors operating do so through the GH axis. As shown already, thyroid hormones are important in mediating GH gene expression, although a direct effect of thyroxine on cartilage (IGF-I-independent) also exists [125].

CONCLUSION

Growth assessment forms the basis of the management of endocrine disorders in childhood. It is more important than a biochemical measurement, because its precision has a different order of magnitude and because it has long-term predictive relevance at every stage of development.

Children growing at a normal rate are normal children; when they are not growing at a normal rate something is wrong. A diagnosis, or at least an explanation, is needed and the environment needs to be changed (usually in terms of starting treatment) if ultimate damage to growth prognosis is to be avoided.

The importance of the infancy–childhood–puberty model is that it allows the clinician to target investigations to the various components of human growth. The corollary of this is that it also allows the clinician to target effective treatment. For growth failure during infancy nutritional factors should be addressed, whereas during childhood an abnormality within the GH axis, either primary or secondary, is likely to be the explanation for the poor growth observed. In the primary instance then GH treatment is clearly indicated.

It is apparent that advances in molecular biology are going to lead to a better understanding of somatotroph function. This area has advanced considerably from simply demonstrating gene deletions and point mutations to a new area where investigation is centred on the genes which control proteins, which in turn regulate the expression of the hormone gene of interest. These observations have important implications because they open up a whole new area for understanding physiological and pathological processes; in particular the embryology of the anterior pituitary gland. Not all genetic diseases are inherited, and mutations in somatic cells may prove to be important causes for a number of situations where hormone products are overexpressed or underexpressed.

REFERENCES

1 Barker DJP. *Fetal and Infant Origins of Adult Disease.* London: British Medical Journal, 1992.
2 Berkey CS, Reed RB, Baladian I. Midgrowth spurt in height of Boston children. *Ann Hum Biol* 1983;10:25–30.
3 Tanner JM, Cameron N. Investigation of the mid-growth spurt in height, weight and limb circumferences in single-year velocity data from the London 1966–76 growth survey. *Ann Hum Biol* 1980;7:565–77.
4 Gasser T, Kohler W, Muller HG, Largo R, Molinari L, Prader A. Human height growth: correlational and multivariate structure of velocity and acceleration. *Ann Hum Biol* 1985; 12:501–15.
5 Marshall WA. Evaluation of growth rate in height over periods of less than a year. *Arch Dis Child* 1971;46:414–20.
6 Voss LD, Wilkin TJ, Bailey BJR, Betts PR. The reliability of height and height velocity in the assessment of growth (the Wessex growth study). *Arch Dis Child* 1991;66:833–7.
7 Tanner JM, Whitehouse RH. *Atlas of Children's Growth.* London: Academic Press, 1982.
8 Butler GE, McKie M, Ratcliffe SG. The cyclical nature of prepubertal growth. *Ann Hum Biol* 1990;17:177–98.

9 Hermanussen M, Sippell WG. Changes of short term growth velocity (mini-growth-spurts) in 36 healthy children, measured twice weekly by knemometry. *Ann Hum Biol* (Suppl.) 1985:79A.

10 Rikken B, Wit JM. Prepubertal height velocity references over a wide age range. *Arch Dis Child* 1992;67:1277–80.

11 Greulich WW, Pyle ST. *Radiographic Atlas of Skeletal Development of Hand and Wrist.* Stanford, CA: Stanford University Press, 1959.

12 Bayley N, Pinneau SR. Tables predicting adult height from skeletal age revised for use with the Greulich–Pyle hand standards. *J Pediatr* 1952;40:423–41 (erratum 1952;41:371).

13 Tanner JM, Whitehouse RJ, Cameron N *et al. Assessment of Skeletal Maturity and Prediction of Adult Height.* London: Academic Press, 1983.

14 Tanner JM. *Growth at Adolescence.* Oxford: Blackwell Scientific Publications, 1961.

15 Hawk LJ, Brook CGD. Family resemblances of height, weight and body fatness. *Arch Dis Child* 1979;54:877–9.

16 Tanner JM, Goldstein H, Whitehouse RH. Standards for children's height at ages 2–9 years allowing for heights of parents. *Arch Dis Child* 1970;45:755–62.

17 Widdowson EM, McCance RA. Some effects of accelerating growth. *Proc R Soc Lond (Biol)* 1960;152:188–206.

18 Cogswell JJ, El-Bishti MM. Growth retardation in asthma: role of calorie deficiency. *Arch Dis Child* 1982;57:473–5.

19 Fancourt R, Campbell S, Harvey D. Follow up study of small-for-dates babies. *Br Med J* 1976;i:1435–7.

20 Powell GT, Brasel JA, Raiti S, Blizzard RM. Emotional deprivation and growth retardation stimulating idiopathic hypopituitarism. II. Endocrinologic evaluation of the syndrome. *N Engl J Med* 1967;276:1279–83.

21 Stanhope R, Adlard P, Hamill G, Jones J, Skuse D, Preece MA. Physiological growth hormone secretion during the recovery from psychosocial dwarfism: a case report. *Clin Endocrinol* 1988;28:335–9.

22 Eveleth PB, Tanner JM. *Worldwide Variation in Human Growth.* London: Cambridge University Press, 1976.

23 Preece MA, Hendrich I. Mathematical modelling of individual growth curves. *Br Med Bull* 1981;37:247–52.

24 Stuetzle W, Gasser TH, Molinari L, Largo RH, Prader A, Huber PJ. Shape-invariant modelling of human growth. *Ann Hum Biol* 1980;7:507–28.

25 Karlberg J, Engstron I, Karlberg P, Fryer JG. Analyses of linear growth using a mathematical model. *Acta Paediatr Scand* 1987;Suppl.76:478–88.

26 Costello AM. Growth velocity and stunting in rural Nepal. *Arch Dis Child* 1989;64:1478–82.

27 Karlberg J, Jalil F, Lindblad BS. Longitudinal analysis of infantile growth in an urban area of Lahore, Pakistan. In: Karlberg J, ed. *Modelling of Human Growth.* Goteborg: University of Goteborg, 1987 (PhD thesis).

28 Wit JM, Van Unen H. Growth of infants with neonatal growth hormone deficiency. *Arch Dis Child* 1992;67:920–5.

29 Gluckman PD, Gunn AG, Wray A *et al.* Congenital idiopathic growth hormone deficiency associated with prenatal and early postnatal growth failure. *J Pediatr* 1992;212:920–3.

30 Dunger DB, Matthews DR, Edge JA *et al.* Evidence for temporal coupling of growth hormone, prolactin, LH and FSH pulsatility overnight during normal puberty. *J Endocrinol* 1991;130:141–9.

31 Finkelstein JW, Roffwarg HP, Boyer RM *et al.* Age-related change in the twenty four hour spontaneous secretion of growth hormone. *J Clin Endocrinol Metab* 1972;35:665–70.

32 Miller JD, Tannenbaum GS, Colle F *et al.* Daytime pulsatile growth hormone secretion during childhood and adolescence. *J Clin Endocrinol Metab* 1982;55:989–94.

33 Hindmarsh PC, Matthews DR, Brook CGD. Growth hormone secretion in children determined by time series analysis. *Clin Endocrinol* 1988;29:35–44.

34 Stanhope R, Pringle PJ, Brook CGD. The mechanism of the adolescent growth spurt induced by low dose pulsatile GnRH treatment. *Clin Endocrinol* 1988;28:83–91.

35 Mauras N, Blizzard RM, Link K, Johnson ML, Rogol AD, Veldhuis JD. Augmentation of growth hormone secretion during puberty: evidence for a pulse amplitude modulated phenomenon. *J Clin Endocrinol Metab* 1987;64:596–601.

36 Ross JL, Pescovitz DH, Barnes K *et al.* Growth hormone secretory dynamics in children with precocious puberty. *J Pediatr* 1987;110:369–72.

37 Stanhope R, Pringle PJ, Brook CGD. Growth, growth hormone and sex steroid secretion in girls with central precocious puberty treated with gonadotrophin releasing hormone analogue. *Acta Paediatr Scand* 1988;Suppl.77:525–30.

38 Mansfield MJ, Rudlin CR, Crigler JR *et al.* Changes in growth and serum growth hormone and plasma somatomedin-C levels during suppression of gonadal sex steroids secretion in girls with central precocious puberty. *J Clin Endocrinol Metab* 1988;66:3–8.

39 Cara JF, Burstein S, Cuttler L *et al.* Growth hormone deficiency impedes the rise of plasma insulin-like growth factor 1 levels associated with precocious puberty. *J Pediatr* 1989; 115:64–8.

40 Link K, Blizzard RM, Evans WS *et al.* The effect of androgens on the pulsatile release and the twenty four hour mean concentrations of growth hormone in peripubertal males. *J Clin Endocrinol Metab* 1986;62:159–64.

41 Ulloa-Aguirre A, Blizzard RM, Garcia-Rubi E *et al.* Testosterone and oxandrolone, a non-aromatizable androgen, specifically amplify the mass and rate of growth hormone (GH) secreted per burst without altering GH secretory burst duration or frequency of the GH half-life. *J Clin Endocrinol Metab* 1990;71:846–54.

42 Foster CM, Hopwood NJ, Hassing JM *et al.* Nocturnal serum growth hormone concentration is not augmented by short term testosterone infusion in pubertal boys. *Pediatr Res* 1989;26:320–4.

43 Barinaga M, Bilezikjian LM, Vale WW, Rosenfeld MG, Evans RM. Independent effects of growth hormone releasing factor on growth hormone release and gene transcription. *Nature* 1985;314:279–81.

44 Barinaga M, Yamamoto G, Rivier C, Vale W, Evans R, Rosenfeld MG. Transcriptional regulation of growth hormone gene expression by growth hormone-releasing factor. *Nature* 1983;306:84–5.

45 Billestrup N, Swanson LW, Vale W. Growth hormone-releasing factor stimulates proliferation of somatotrophs *in vitro. Proc Natl Acad Sci USA* 1986;83:6854–7.

46 Billestrup N, Mitchell R, Vale W, Verma I. Growth hormone-releasing factor induces c-fos expression in cultured primary pituitary cells. *Mol Endocrinol* 1987;1:300–5.

47 Glick GG, Zeytin F, Brazeau P, Ling NC, Esch F, Bancroft FC. Growth hormone-releasing factor regulates growth hormone mRNA in primary cultures of rat pituitary cells. *Proc Natl Acad Sci USA* 1984;81:1553–5.

48 Gaylinn BD, Harrison JK, Zysk JR, Lyons CE, Lynch KR, Thorner MO. Molecular cloning expression of a human anterior pituitary receptor for growth hormone-releasing

hormone. *Mol Endocrinol* 1993;7:77–84.
49 Mayo KE. Molecular cloning and expression of a pituitary-specific receptor receptor for growth hormone-releasing hormone. *Mol Endocrinol* 1992;6:1734–44.
50 Bilezikjian LM, Vale W. Chronic exposure of cultured rat anterior pituitary cells to GRF causes partial loss of responsiveness to GRF. *Endocrinology* 1984;115:2032–4.
51 Bilezikjian L, Vale W. Stimulation of adenosine 3′,5′-monophosphate production by growth hormone-releasing factor and its inhibition by somatostatin in anterior pituitary cells in vitro. *Endocrinology* 1983;113:1726–31.
52 Labrie F, Gagne B, Lefevre G. Growth hormone-releasing factor stimulates adenylate cyclase activity in the anterior pituitary gland. *Life Sci* 1983;33:2229–33.
53 Struthers R, Perrin M, Vale W. Nucleotide regulation of growth hormone-releasing factor binding to rat pituitary receptors. *Endocrinology* 1989;124:24–9.
54 Landis C, Masters S, Spada A, Pace A, Bourne H, Vallar L. GTPase inhibiting mutations activate the α chain of G_s and stimulate adenyl cyclase in human pituitary tumors. *Nature* 1989;340:692–6.
55 Vallar L, Spada A, Giannattasio G. Altered G_s and adenylate cyclase activity in human GH-secreting pituitary adenomas. *Nature* 1987;330:566–8.
56 Weinstein LS, Shenker A, Gejman PV, Merino MJ, Friedman E, Spiegel AM. Activating mutations of the stimulatory G protein in the McCune–Albright Syndrome. *N Engl J Med* 1991;325:1688–95.
57 Canonico PL, Cronin MJ, Thorner MD, MacLeod RM. Human pancreatic GRF stimulates phosphotidylinositol labeling in cultured anterior pituitary cells. *Am J Physiol* 1983;245:E587–90.
58 Login IS, Judd AM, MacLeod RM. Association of $^{45}Ca^{2+}$ mobilization with stimulation of growth hormone (GH) release by GH-releasing factor in dispersed normal male rat pituitary cells. *Endocrinology* 1986;118:239–43.
59 Jansson JO, Downs T, Beamer W, Frohman L. Receptor-associated resistance to growth hormone-releasing factor in dwarf 'little' mice. *Science* 1986;232:511–12.
60 Lin S-C, Lin CR, Gukovsky I, Lusis AJ, Sawchenko PE, Rosenfeld MG. Molecular basis of the little mouse phenotype and implications for cell type-specific growth. *Nature* 1993;364:208–13.
61 Downs T, Frohman L. Evidence for a defect in growth hormone-releasing factor signal transduction in the dwarf (dw/dw) rat pituitary. *Endocrinology* 1991;129:58–67.
62 Mullis P, Patel M, Brickell PM, Brook CGD. Isolated growth hormone deficiency: analysis of the growth hormone (GH) releasing hormone gene and the GH gene cluster. *J Clin Endocrinol Metab* 1990;70:187–91.
63 Yamada Y, Post S, Wang K, Tager H, Bell G, Seino S. Cloning and functional characterisation of a family of human and mouse somatostatin receptors expressed in brain, gastrointestinal tract and kidney. *Proc Natl Acad Sci USA* 1992; 89:251–5.
64 Ray KP, Hart GR, Wallis M. Effects of dopamine and somatostatin on phorbolester-stimulated prolactin and growth hormone secretion. *Mol Cell Endocrinol* 1986; 48:205–12.
65 Cronin MJ, Hewitt EL, Evans WS, Thorner MO, Rogol AD. Human pancreatic tumour growth hormone-releasing factor and cyclic adenosine 3′,5′-monophosphate evoke GH release from anterior pituitary cells: the effects of pertussis toxin, cholera toxin, forskolin and cycloheximide. *Endocrinology* 1984;114:904.
66 Simard J, Lefevre G, Labrie F. Somatostatin prevents the desensitizing action of growth hormone-releasing factor on growth hormone release. *Peptides* 1987;8:199–205.
67 Moore D, Walker MD, Diamond DJ *et al.* Structure, expression and evolution of growth hormone genes. *Rec Prog Horm Res* 1982;39:197–225.
68 Illig R, Prader A, Ferrandez A, Zacghmann M. Hereditary prenatal growth hormone deficiency with increased tendency to growth hormone antibody formation. *Synp Deutsch Ges Endokrinol* 1970;16:246–7.
69 Phillips JA, Hjell BL, Seeburg PH *et al.* Molecular basis for familial isolated growth hormone deficiency. *Proc Natl Acad Sci USA* 1981;78:6372–5.
70 Schwartz S, Berger P, Frisch H, Mancayo R, Phillips JA, Wick G. Growth hormoone blocking antibodies in a patient with deletion of the GH-N gene. *Clin Endocrinol* 1987;27:213–24.
71 Braga S, Phillips III JA, Joss E, Schwarz H, Zuppinger K. Familial growth hormone deficiency resulting from a 7.6 kb deletion within the growth hormone gene cluster. *Am J Med Genet* 1986;25:443–52.
72 Laron Z, Kelijman M, Pertzelan A, Keret R, Shoffner IM, Parks JS. Human growth hormone gene deletion without antibody formation or growth arrest during treatment: a new disease entity? *Isr J Med Sci* 1985;21:999–1006.
73 Phillips III JA. The growth hormone (hGH) genes and human disease. In: Caskey CT, White R, eds. *Banbury Report 14. Recombinant DNA: Application to Human Disease.* Cold Spring Harbor, NY: Cold Spring Harbor Press, 1983:305–15.
74 Kamijo T, Phillips III JA, Ogawa M, Yuan L, Shi Y, Bao XI. Screening for growth hormone gene deletions in patients with isolated growth hormone deficiency. *J Pediatr* 1991; 118:245–8.
75 Mullis PE, Akinci A, Kanaka CH, Eble A, Brook CGD. Prevalence of human growth hormone-1 gene deletions among patients with isolated growth hormone deficiency from different populations. *Pediatr Res* 1992;31:532–4.
76 Vnencak-Jones CL, Phillips III JA, DeFen W. Use of polymerase chain reaction in detection of growth hormone gene deletions. *J Clin Endocrinol Metab* 1990;70:1550–3.
77 Miller-Davis S, Cogan J, Phillips III JA, Milner RDG, Al-Ashwal A, Sakati NA. Detection of heterogenous growth hormone (GH) gene splicing by DNA analysis of dried blood spots from GH deficient subjects. *Pediatr Res* 1993;33:137 (Abstr.).
78 Parks JS, Meacham LR, McKean MC, Keret R, Josefsberg Z, Laron Z. Growth hormone (GH) gene deletion is the most common cause of severe GH deficiency among Oriental Jewish children. *Pediatr Res* 1989;25:90 (Abstr.).
79 Margioris AN, Brockman G, Bohler HLC, Grino M, Vamvakopoulos N, Chrousos GP. Expression and localization of growth hormone-releasing hormone messenger ribonucleic acid in the rat placenta: in vitro secretion and regulation of its peptide product. *Endocrinology* 1990; 126:151–8.
80 Fant M, Munro H, Moses AC. An autocrine/paracrine role for insulin-like growth factors in the regulation of human placental growth. *J Clin Endocrinol Metab* 1986;63:499–505.
81 Bodner M, Castrillo JL, Theill L, Deerinck T, Ellisman M, Karin M. The pituitary-specific transcription factor GHF-1 is a homeobox-containing protein. *Cell* 1988;55:505–18.
82 Ingraham H, Chew R, Mangalam H *et al.* A tissue specific transcription factor containing a homeobox domain specifies a pituitary phenotype. *Cell* 1988;55:519–29.
83 Wit JM, Drayer NM, Jansen M *et al.* Total deficiency of growth hormone and prolaction and partial deficiency of

thyroid stimulating hormone in two Dutch families: a new variant of hereditary pituitary deficiency. *Horm Res* 1989;32:170–7.

84 Li S, Crenshaw III EB, Rawson EJ, Simmons DM, Swanson LW, Rosenfeld MG. Dwarf locus mutants lacking three pituitary cell types result from mutations in the POU-domain gene pit-1. *Nature* 1990;347:528–33.

85 Pfaffle RW, Di Mattia GE, Parks JS *et al.* Mutation of the POU-specific domain of Pit-1 and hypopituitarism without pituitary hypoplasia. *Science* 1992;257:1118–21.

86 Burton FH, Hasel KW, Bloom FE, Sutcliffe JG. Pituitary hyperplasia and gigantism in mice caused by a cholera toxin transgene. *Nature* 1991;350:74–7.

87 Struthers RS, Vale WW, Arias C, Sawchenko PE, Montminy MR. Somatotroph hypoplasia and dwarfism in transgenic mice expressing a non-phosphorylatable CREB mutant. *Nature* 1991;350:622–4.

88 Ohta K, Nobukani Y, Mitsubuchi H *et al.* Mutations in the pit-1 gene in children with combined pituitary hormone deficiency. *Biochem Biophys Res Commun* 1992;189:851–5.

89 Ye ZS, Forman BM, Aranda A *et al.* Rat growth hormone gene expression: both cell-specific and thyroid hormone response elements are required for thyroid hormone regulation. *J Biol Chem* 1988;263:7821–9.

90 Schaufele F, West BL, Reudelhuber TL. Overlapping Pit-1 and Sp 1 binding sites are both essential to full rat growth hormone gene promoter activity despite mutally exclusive Pit-1 and Sp 1 binding. *J Biol Chem* 1990;265:17189–96.

91 Schaufele F, Cassill JA, West BL, Reudelhuber TL. Resolution by diagonal gel mobility shift assays of multisubunit complexes binding to a functionally important element of the rat growth hormone gene promoter. *J Biol Chem*1990; 265:14592–8.

92 Schaufele F, West BL, Baxter JD. Synergistic activation of the rat growth hormone promote by Pit-1 and the thyroid hormone receptor. *Mol Endocrinol* 1992;6:656–65.

93 Yamashita S, Melmed S. Insulin-like growth factor 1 regulation of growth hormone gene transcription in primary rat pituitary cells. *J Clin Invest* 1987;79:449–52.

94 Lund PK. Regulation and expression of genes for insulin-like growth factors as studied with *in situ* hybridisation. In: *Growth Hormone: Basic and Clinical Aspects*. Nordisk Insulin Symposium No. 1, Stockholm, Sweden, 1987; 397–414.

95 Hoeffler JP, Hicks SA, Frawley S. Existence of somatotroph subpopulations which are differentially responsive to insulin-like growth factor 1 and somatostatin. *Endocrinology* 1987;1205:1936–41.

96 Sheppard MS, Bala M. Cyclohexamide blocks insulin-like growth factor 1 but not somatostatin inhibition of growth hormone secretion. *Can J Physiol Pharmacol* 1987;65: 515–19.

97 Katakami H, Downs TR, Frohman LA. Decreased hypothalamic growth hormone-releasing hormone content and pituitary responsiveness in hypothyroidism. *J Clin Invest* 1986;77:1704–11.

98 Katz HP, Youlton R, Kaplan SL *et al.* Growth and growth hormone. III. Growth hormone release in children with primary hypothyroidism and thyrotoxicosis. *J Clin Endocrinol Metab* 1969;29:346–52.

99 Valcavi R, Jordan V, Dieguez C *et al.* Growth hormone responses to GRF 1–29 in patients with primary hypothyroidism before and during replacement therapy with thyroxine. *Clin Endocrinol* 1986;24:693–8.

100 Franklyn JA, Cynam T, Docherty K, Ramsden DB, Sheppard MC. Effect of hypothyroidism on pituitary cytoplasmic concentrations of messenger RNA encoding thyrotrophin β and α subunits, prolaction and growth hormone. *J Endocrinol* 1986;108:43–7.

101 Ye ZS, Samuels HH. Cell and sequence specific binding of nuclear proteins to 5′-flanking DNA of the rat growth hormone gene. *J Biol Chem* 1987;262;6313–17.

102 Flug F, Copp RP, Casanova J *et al.* *Cis*-acting element of the rat growth hormone gene which mediates basal and regulated expression by thyroid hormone. *J Biol Chem* 1987;262: 6373–82.

103 Wight RA, Crew MD, Spindler SR. Discrete positive and negative thyroid hormone-responsive transcription regulatory elements by the rat growth hormone gene. *J Biol Chem* 1987;262:5659–63.

104 Birnbaum MH, Baxter JD. Glucocorticoids regulate the expression of a rat growth hormone gene lacking 5′ flanking sequences. *J Biol Chem* 1986;261:291–7.

105 Issacs RE, Gardner DG, Baxter JD. Insulin regulation of rat growth hormone gene expression. *Endocrinology* 1987; 120:2022–8.

106 Yamashita S, Melmed S. Insulin regulation of rat growth hormone gene transcription. *J Clin Invest* 1986;48:1008–14.

107 Prager D, Weber MM, Gebremedhin S, Melmed S. Interaction between insulin and thyroid hormone in rat pituitary tumour cells: insulin attenuates tri-iodothyroxine-induced growth hormone mRNA levels. *J Endocrinol* 1993;137: 107–14.

108 Baumann G, Stolar MW. Molecular forms of human growth hormone secreted *in vivo*: non-specificity of secretory stimuli. *J Clin Endocrinol Metab* 1986;62:789–90.

109 Wehrenberg WB, Chatelain P, Baird A. The molecular weight forms of rat growth hormone secreted in response to growth hormone-releasing factor. *Proc Soc Exp Biol Med* 1986; 182:107–11.

110 Hunter WM, Rigal WM. The diurnal pattern of plasma growth hormone concentration in children and adolescents. *J Endocrinol* 1966;34:147–53.

111 Clark RG, Carlsson LMS, Robinson ICAF. Growth hormone secretory profiles in conscious female rats. *J Endocrinol* 1987;114:399–407.

112 Mode A, Gustafsson JA, Jansson JO, Eden S, Isaksson O. Association between plasma levels of growth hormone and sex differentiation of hepatic steroid metabolism in the rat. *Endocrinology* 1982;111:1692–7.

113 Norstedt G, Palmiter R. Secretory rhythm of growth hormone regulates sexual differentiation of mouse liver. *Cell* 1984;36:805–12.

114 Clark RG, Jansson JO, Isaksson O, Robinson ICAF. Intravenous growth hormone: growth responses to patterned infusion in hypophysectomised rats. *J Endocrinol* 1985; 104:53–61.

115 Jansson JO, Albertsson-Wikland K, Eden S, Thorngren KG, Isaksson O. Circumstantial evidence for a role of the secretory pattern of growth hormone in control of body growth. *Acta Endocrinol* 1982;99:24–30.

116 Miller JD, Wright NM, Esparza A *et al.* Spontaneous pulsatile growth hormone release in male and female premature infants. *J Clin Endocrinol Metab* 1992;75:1508–13.

117 Miller JD, Esparza A, Wright NM *et al.* Spontaneous growth hormone release in term infants: changes during the first four days of life. *J Clin Endocrinol Metab* 1993;76:1058–62.

118 Vigneri R, D'Agata R. Growth hormone release during the first year of life in relation to sleep-wake periods. *J Clin Endocrinol Metab* 1971;33:561–3.

119 Parker DC, Rossman LG, Kripke DF, Gibson W, Wilson K. Rhythmicities in human growth hormone concentrations in plasma. In: Krieger DT, ed. *Endocrine Rhythms*. New York: Raven Press, 1979:143–73.
120 Hartman ML, Veldhuis JD, Johnson ML *et al*. Augmented growth hormone (GH) secretory burst frequency and amplitude mediate enhanced GH secretion during a two-day fast in normal men. *J Clin Endocrinol Metab* 1992;74:757–65.
121 Hindmarsh PC, Smith PJ, Brook CGD, Matthews DR. The relationship between growth velocity and growth hormone secretion in short prepubertal children. *Clin Endocrinol* 1987;27:581–91.
122 Albertsson-Wikland K, Rosberg S. Analyses of 24-hour growth hormone profiles in children: relation to growth. *J Clin Endocrinol Metab* 1988;67:493–500.
123 Kerrigan JR, Martha PM, Blizzard RM, Christie CM, Rogol AD. Variations of pulsatile growth hormone release in healthy short prepubertal boys. *Pediatr Res* 1990;28:11–14.
124 Millard WJ, Politch JA, Martin JB, Fox T. Growth hormone secretory patterns in androgen resistant (testicular feminised) rats. *Endocrinology* 1986;119:2655–60.
125 Burch WM, Van Wyk JJ. Triiodothyromine stimulates cartilage growth and maturation by different mechanisms. *Endocrinol Metab* 1987;15:176–82.

7: The Insulin-like Growth Factors

R.G. ROSENFELD and E.K. NEELY

INTRODUCTION

The insulin-like growth factors (IGF-I and IGF-II) are related growth hormone (GH)-dependent peptide factors which are believed to mediate many of the anabolic and mitogenic actions of GH. They were originally identified by their ability to stimulate [^{35}S]sulphate incorporation into rat cartilage. The IGFs were so named because of their evolutionary and structural relationship with proinsulin, correlating with their weak insulin-like metabolic activity. It has been well documented that IGF-I and IGF-II possess mitogenic and metabolic activities in diverse tissues and cells; reduced levels of IGF associated with GH deficiency or GH receptor defects result in profound growth failure.

BASIC ASPECTS

Historical background

Salmon & Daughaday [1] demonstrated in 1957 that the capacity of serum from hypophysectomized rats to stimulate [^{35}S]sulphate incorporation into rat chondrocyte proteoglycans *in vitro* was not restored by the addition of GH. By contrast, [^{35}S]sulphate incorporation could be restored by the addition of serum from hypophysectomized rats which had been treated with GH, thereby demonstrating the existence of a GH-dependent 'sulphation factor'. Separate investigations on insulin activity in rat muscle and adipose tissue indicated that only a fraction of the apparent insulin-like activity of normal serum could be blocked by the addition of anti-insulin antibodies. The remaining activity was termed 'non-suppressible insulin-like activity (NSILA)' and was later demonstrated to contain two soluble, low molecular weight (7 kD) forms [2–4].

A parallel line of investigation originated in studies by Dulak & Temin [5] on the mitogenic nature of bovine serum. Serum-free medium conditioned by fetal Buffalo rat liver cells (BRL-3A) was found to support the growth of other cultured cells. The mitogenic factor in the medium was termed 'multiplication stimulating activity (MSA)' and was thought to share metabolic and mitogenic activities with both sulphation factor and NSILA. As a result, the term 'somatomedin' [6] was coined to describe the diverse GH-dependent actions of the factors, including: (i) GH dependence of serum concentrations, (ii) insulin-like activity in extraskeletal tissues, (iii) promotion of the incorporation of sulphate into cartilage, and (iv) stimulation of DNA synthesis and cell multiplication. Purification efforts yielded two somatomedin peptides, a basic peptide (SM-C) and a neutral peptide (SM-A) [7,8]. In 1978 Rinderknecht & Humbel [9,10] isolated two active somatomedins from human plasma. Both peptides demonstrated a striking structural resemblance to proinsulin and were renamed 'insulin-like growth factor' -I and -II (collectively, the IGFs), which ultimately supplanted the more physiologically descriptive somatomedin.

IGF structure

IGF-I, a basic peptide of 70 amino acids, is the same as SM-C; IGF-II is a slightly acidic peptide of 67 amino acids. The peptides share 45 of 73 possible amino acid positions and have approximately 50% amino acid homology with insulin [11,12] (Fig. 7.1). Like insulin, both IGFs have A and B chains connected by disulphide bonds. The connecting C-peptide region, which bears no homology with the C-peptide region cleaved from proinsulin in peptide processing, is 12 amino acids long in IGF-I and eight amino acids in IGF-II. IGF-I and IGF-II also differ from proinsulin in possessing carboxy-terminal extensions, or D peptides, of eight and six amino acids, respectively. The structural homology with proinsulin explains the ability of both IGFs to bind with low affinity to the insulin receptor, and for insulin to bind to the type 1 IGF receptor. On the other hand, structural differences contribute to the failure of insulin to bind to the IGF-binding proteins.

Synthetic analogues of both IGF-I and IGF-II have been developed in an effort to elucidate key amino acids and molecular features important in binding to IGF receptors and IGF-binding proteins. Des(1–3)IGF-I, a naturally occurring form of IGF-I with a truncated amino terminus,

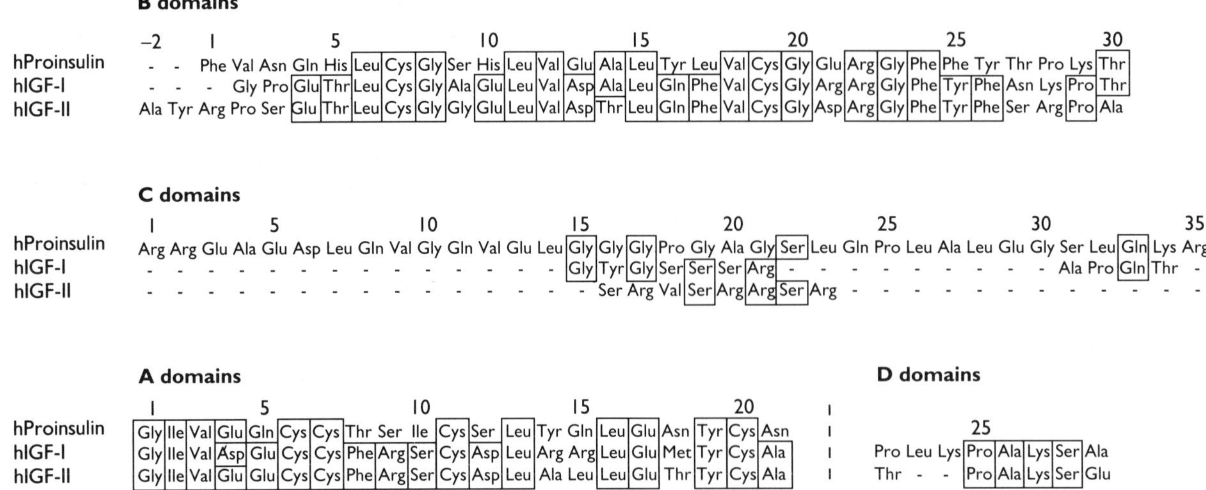

Fig. 7.1 Amino-acid sequence homologies between human proinsulin, IGF-I, and IGF-II, demonstrating conservation in the B and A domains (from Underwood & Van Wyk [13]).

exhibits increased biological potency attributable to reduced affinity for IGF-binding proteins (IGFBPs) [14]. Cascieri and colleagues have used site-directed mutagenesis of synthetic IGF-I to produce various IGF-I analogues. Multiple substitutions at Gln^3, Ala^4, Tyr^{15}, Leu^{16} result in markedly diminished affinity for IGFBPs without reducing IGF receptor affinities [15]. On the other hand, mutation of tyrosine residues at positions 24 and 31 markedly reduces binding to the type 1 IGF receptor, and substitution at position 60 interferes with binding to both the type 1 and type 2 IGF receptors [16]. Substitution of leucine for Tyr^{27} in IGF-II (Fig. 7.2) reduces affinity for the type 1 IGF receptor [17]. These and other synthetic IGF analogues have become important probes of IGF actions via IGF receptors and of IGF interactions with IGFBPs.

IGF expression

The human IGF-I gene (Fig. 7.3) spans approximately 95 kb of genomic DNA on the long arm of chromosome 12 [19,20]. The gene contains at least six exons. Exons 1 and 2 encode alternative signal peptides, each containing multiple transcription start sites. Exons 3 and 4 encode the remaining signal peptide, the mature IGF-I molecule and part of the trailer peptide. Exons 5 and 6 encode alternative segments of the trailer peptide, as well as untranslated 3′ sequences with multiple polyadenylation sites. Two different forms of IGF-I precursor molecules have been identified [12,21]. The first 134 amino acids of each are identical, comprising the signal peptide (48 amino acids), the mature IGF-I molecule (70 amino acids), and the first 16 amino acids of the E domain of the precursor. IGF-IA has an additional 19 amino acids (total 153 residues), while IGF-IB has an additional 61 amino acids (total 195 residues). Alternative splicing from exons 5 and 6 of the IGF-I gene presumably generates the two alternative mRNAs.

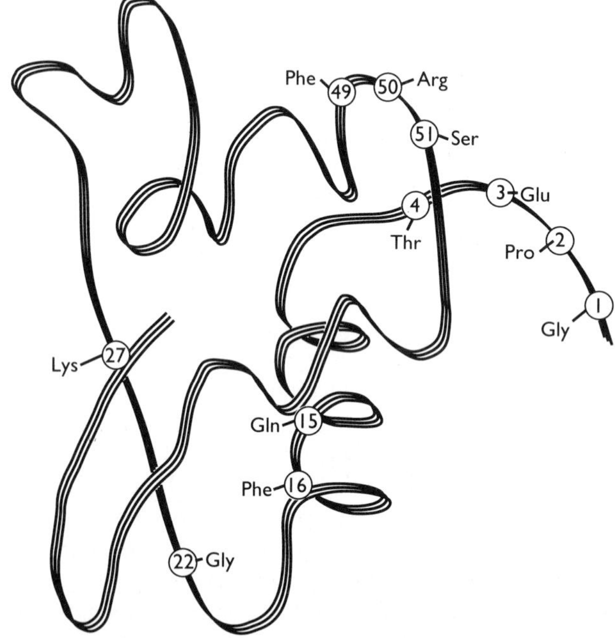

Fig. 7.2 Schematic representation of the tertiary structure of IGF-I showing amino-acid substitutions present in synthetic IGF-I analogues (from Cascieri *et al.* [15]).

The human IGF-II gene (Fig. 7.4) is located on the short arm of chromosome 11 [21,22], immediately adjacent to the insulin gene, and spans 35 kb of genomic DNA con-

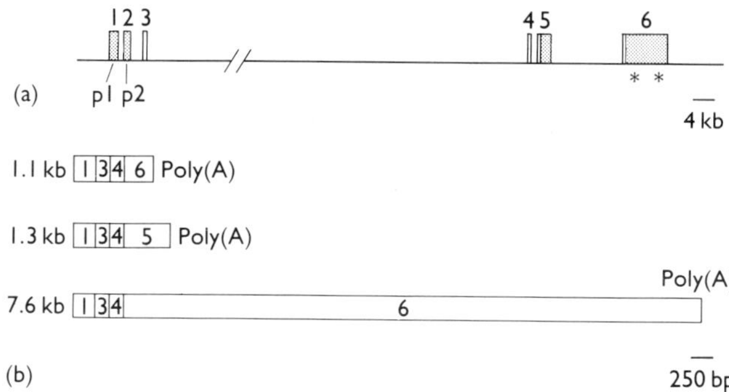

Fig. 7.3 Schematic structure of the IGF-I gene. (a) Exons 1 to 6, where exons 3, 4, 5 and 6 (open boxes) designate the protein-encoding regions, p1 and p2 are alternate promoters, and asterisks indicate polyadenylation sites. (b) The three major mRNA species encoded by the indicated exons (from Sussenbach *et al.* [18]).

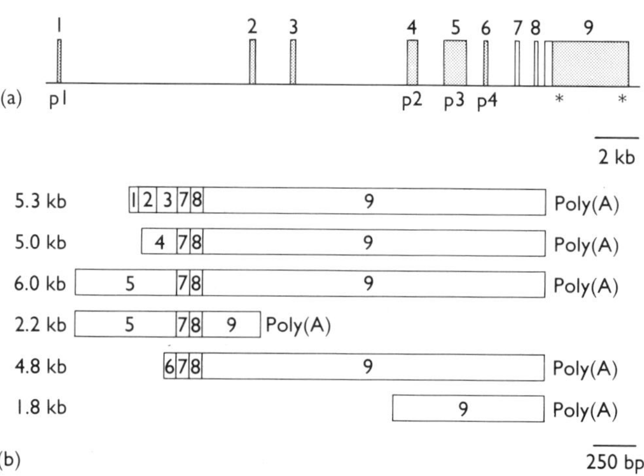

Fig. 7.4 Schematic structure of the IGF-II gene. (a) Exons 1 to 9, where exons 7, 8 and 9 (open boxes) represent the protein-encoding regions, p1 to p4 are alternate promoters, and asterisks indicate polyadylation sites. (b) Six IGF-II mRNA forms encoded by the indicated exons (from Sussenbach *et al.* [18]).

taining nine exons. Exons 1–6 encode untranslated 5′ RNA, including multiple promoter sites. Exon 7 encodes the signal peptide and most of the mature protein, while exon 8 encodes the carboxy-terminal portion of the protein, plus the trailer peptide, the coding of which is completed in exon 9. The primary IGF-II translation product in the human, rat and mouse contains 180 amino acids, including a 24-residue signal peptide, the 67 amino acid mature IGF-II sequence, and a carboxy-terminal E peptide of 89 amino acids.

Complex control of IGF gene expression contributes to variability in tissue expression and changing developmental expression [12,18,23–25]. Liver is a major site of IGF production, but expression has also been detected in many other tissues. IGF-I is considered an important postnatal growth factor because of rising levels at term in humans. By contrast, IGF-II is abundantly expressed in diverse tissues throughout gestation in both the human and rat, and has thus been regarded as an essential fetal growth factor. This argument is certainly supported by the dramatic reduction in body size when an IGF-II gene is 'knocked out' by homologous recombination [26]. However, serum IGF-II levels remain significant and constant during the human lifespan (compared with the low levels found in rats), and the postnatal role of IGF-II in humans is unresolved.

Expression of IGF-II messenger (m)RNA, perhaps representing a process of cellular dedifferentiation, has been demonstrated in diverse primary tumours and malignant cell lines, including many sarcomas, Wilms tumour, phaeochromocytoma, neuroblastoma and hepatoma [27, 28]. Secretion of high levels of IGF-II peptides, following rigorous exclusion of potential assay interference from IGFBPs, has also been documented in several tumour cell lines. Many investigators speculate that tumour growth is stimulated by IGF-II autocrine action. Daughaday and others have reported the presence of large forms of IGF-II (10–20 kD) in the serum of patients with tumours associated with symptomatic hypoglycaemia, particularly sarcomas [29]. The non-islet cell tumour hypoglycaemia (NICTH) attributable to tumour production of 'big IGF-II', resolves following tumour resection. It is thought that the incompletely processed pro-IGF-II may have greater insulin-like metabolic activity than mature IGF-II due to impaired formation of the normal 150 kD serum IGFBP-3 complex [30,31].

IGF receptors

In the early 1970s it became apparent that the IGFs could bind with low affinity to insulin receptors, providing an explanation for their insulin-like activity [32]. Subsequently, Megyesi *et al.* [33] identified distinct receptors for insulin and IGF in rat hepatic membranes. Specificity studies employing radiolabelled IGF preparations demonstrated two classes of IGF receptors (in addition to the insulin receptor), which were distinguished by the competitive binding of insulin at high concentrations to one form of IGF receptor, compared to effectively no insulin affinity for the second form of IGF receptor.

In the late 1970s and early 1980s, development of methodologies for structural characterization of these receptors enabled the clear discrimination of two IGF receptor forms [34–37]. Affinity cross-linking studies demonstrated the similarity of the type 1 IGF receptor and the insulin receptor (Fig. 7.5), since both are heterotetramers composed of two IGF-binding α-subunits of apparent molecular weight of 130 000 and two intracellular β-subunits of apparent molecular weight of 90 000. The

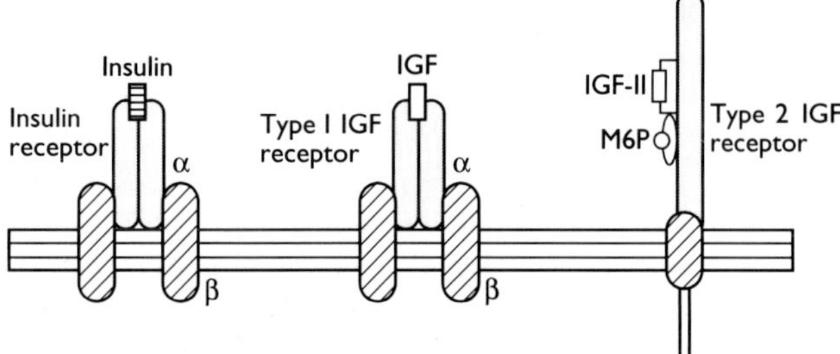

Fig. 7.5 Depiction of the insulin, type 1 IGF, and type 2 IGF-II receptors (from Oh *et al.* [37]).

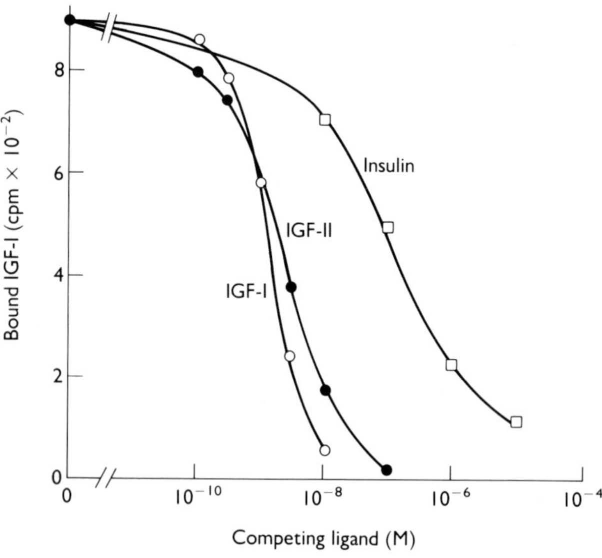

Fig. 7.6 Competitive binding to type 1 IGF receptors isolated by immunoadsorption from CHO cells overexpressing the receptor. The figure shows IGF-I binding in the presence of increasing concentrations of IGF-I, IGF-II, and insulin, demonstrating the high affinity of the type 1 IGF receptor for both IGF-I and IGF-II (from Steele-Perkins *et al.* [39]).

membrane-spanning α-subunits are linked by disulphide bonds. While each αβ-heterodimer appears capable of binding one molecule of IGF ligand, it also appears that one mole of the full heterotetrameric receptor binds only one mole of ligand in apparent negative cooperativity.

Ullrich *et al.* [38] later deduced the complete primary structure of the human type 1 IGF receptor from cDNA cloned from a human placental library. The mature peptide consists of 1337 amino acids, with a predicted molecular mass of 151 869. The translated αβ-heterodimer is cleaved at the Arg–Lys–Arg–Arg sequence at positions 707–710. As is the case with the insulin receptor, the β-subunit has the expected hydrophobic transmembrane domain, as well as the intracellular tyrosine kinase domain and adenosine triphosphate (ATP) binding site. Although it is reasonable to presume that both receptors have evolved from a common ancestor protein, the type 1 IGF receptor is encoded on chromosome 15 and the insulin receptor on chromosome 19.

Although the type 1 IGF receptor has been commonly thought of as the 'IGF-I receptor', more recent studies have emphasized that the receptor is capable of binding both IGF-I and IGF-II with high affinity (Fig. 7.6). Furthermore, both IGF peptides appear capable of activating tyrosine kinase by binding to this receptor. Studies in which Chinese hamster ovary cells overexpressed human type 1 receptor cDNA indicated that intact cells bound IGF-I with a dissociation constant (K_d) of 1.5×10^{-9} and IGF-II with a K_d of 3×10^{-9} [39]. Affinity of the type 1 receptor for insulin is approximately 100-fold less, thereby providing a mechanism for the relatively weak mitogenic effect commonly observed with insulin.

The occasional observation of seemingly anomalous competitive binding results [40,41] has led to the suggestion that variant or atypical insulin and IGF receptors might exist [42]. One possible explanation for such findings is the existence of hybrid receptors comprising one α–β dimer of the insulin receptor and one α–β dimer of the type 1 IGF receptor [43]. Ligand-dependent formation of hybrid IGF/insulin receptors has been reported by Treadway *et al.* [44], and studies with monoclonal antibodies specific for the insulin or type 1 IGF receptor have suggested that such receptors may develop spontaneously in cells with abundant native receptors [45]. The physiological significance of such hybrid receptors is speculative.

The type 2 IGF receptor is entirely distinct from the insulin and type 1 IGF receptors and bears no structural similarity to them. By sucrose density separation (SDS) polyacrylamide gel electrophoresis the type 2 IGF receptor migrates at an apparent molecular weight of 220 000 under non-reducing conditions and 250 000 following reduction, indicating that it is monomeric protein. The cloned human type 2 receptor has a predicted molecular mass of 270 294 and is characterized by a lengthy extracellular domain containing 15 repeat sequences of 147 residues each [46]. This is followed by a 23-residue transmembrane domain and a small cytoplasmic domain consisting of only 164 residues. The receptor does not contain an intrinsic tyrosine kinase domain or any other recognizable signal transduction mechanism.

When the sequence of the type 2 IGF receptor gene was determined, the most striking finding was its identity with the earlier sequence found for the cation-independent mannose-6-phosphate (CIM6P) receptor, a protein involved in the intracellular lysosomal targeting of a variety of acid hydrolases and other mannosylated proteins [47–49]. IGF-II/M6P receptors are located on plasma membranes, but predominantly on intracellular membranes [50]. Why this receptor binds both IGF-II and M6P-containing lysosomal enzymes remains unresolved [51]. Unlike the type 1 IGF receptor, which binds both IGF peptides with high affinity and insulin with lower affinity, the type 2 receptor binds IGF-II with high affinity, IGF-I with vastly reduced affinity, and insulin not at all [52]. One mole of IGF-II binds per mole of receptor, and the binding sites for IGF-II and M6P appear to reside in different portions of the receptor [53]. Nevertheless, the two classes of ligand do show some reciprocal inhibitory effects upon receptor binding, suggesting a potential effect of IGF-II on the sorting of lysosomal enzymes. Binding of IGF-II to type 2 receptors in bovine liver [54], rat receptor preparations [55] and mouse L cells expressing type 2 IGF receptors [56] can be inhibited by M6P-bearing ligands, such as β-galactosidase and β-glucuronidase. Conversely, IGF-II can inhibit the binding of β-galactosidase [57]. Several other ligands not known to be related to lysosomal enzymes, including proliferin [58], transforming growth factor β_1 precursor [59] and thyroglobulin [60] also appear to bind to M6P recognition sites on the type 2 IGF/M6P receptor.

Physiological actions of the IGFs mediated by each receptor

Most studies have indicated that the classic mitogenic and metabolic actions of both IGF-I and IGF-II are mediated through the type 1 IGF receptor, presumably via its tyrosine kinase signal transduction mechanism. This evidence has accumulated from comparisons of physiologically effective ligand concentrations, from inhibition by receptor antibodies and, recently, by the use of synthetic IGF analogues. Both Conover *et al.* [61] and Furlanetto *et al.* [62] have demonstrated that monoclonal antibodies directed against the IGF-I binding site on the type 1 IGF receptor (αIR-3) inhibit the ability of both IGF-I and IGF-II to stimulate thymidine incorporation and cell replication. Similarly, several groups have shown that polyclonal antibodies capable of blocking IGF-II binding to the type 2 IGF/M6P receptor do not block IGF-II actions [63–65].

Direct evidence for the role of the type 1 IGF receptor in mediating classical IGF actions of IGF-II comes from the use of IGF-II analogues as probes of receptor function, as mentioned above. IGF-II analogues with decreased affinity for the type 1 receptor and conserved affinity for the type 2 receptor have been markedly less potent than IGF-II in stimulating DNA synthesis [66]. In indirect support of the concept that the type 2 IGF receptor does not mediate the mitogenic actions of IGF-II, it has been demonstrated that hepatic M6P receptors from the chicken [67] or frog [68] do not bind IGF-II at all. IGF-II mitogenic actions in these species must therefore be mediated solely through the type 1 IGF receptor.

Several experimental observations are consistent with IGF-II actions mediated by the IGF-II/M6P receptor. Tally *et al.* [69] reported that IGF-II, but neither IGF-I nor insulin, stimulated the growth of a subclone of the K562 human erythroleukaemia cell line. In primary cultures of human placental cytotrophoblasts, IGF-II alone diminished the ability of cells to convert androstenedione to oestrogen [70]. Rogers & Hammerman [71] have suggested that the type 2 receptor is involved in production of inositol triphosphate and diacylglycerol in proximal tubule preparations and canine kidney membranes. Minniti *et al.* reported that IGF-II appears capable of acting as an autocrine growth factor and cell motility factor for human rhabdomyosarcoma cells, actions apparently mediated through the type 2 receptor [72]. Studies in epidermal growth factor (EGF)-primed Balb/c3T3 cells [73] have suggested that IGF-II can activate a calcium-permeable cation channel via the type 2 IGF receptor, perhaps through coupling to a pertussis toxin-sensitive guanine nucleotide-binding protein (G_i protein) [74]. Functional coupling between the type 2 IGF receptor and G_i2 has been demonstrated in phospholipid vesicles constructed with purified type 2 IGF receptors and G_i2 [75]. These studies provide a potential mechanism for signal transduction through the type 2 IGF receptor, but it is still generally assumed that most actions of IGF-II are mediated by the type 1 IGF receptor.

The elegant gene-targeting work of Efstradiatis, Robertson, and colleagues has provided definitive evidence concerning the actions of IGF-I and IGF-II through the type 1 IGF receptor [26,76,77]. Their initial work demonstrated that mice homozygous for the mutated IGF-II gene were 55% of wild-type birth weight, but otherwise normal [26]. Additionally, analysis of heterozygote animals revealed that the IGF-II gene undergoes 'imprinting' and is expressed only from the paternal allele, in surprising contrast with the IGF-II/M6P gene, which is expressed only from the maternal allele. 'Knockouts' of IGF-I and the type 1 IGF receptor have been reported recently, and neither of these genes is imprinted. Mice with IGF-I mutations demonstrated a high incidence of neonatal lethality and birth weight 60% of normal, whereas animals homozygous for a mutated type 1 IGF receptor were completely non-viable, dying of asphyxia, and exhibited muscle, skin, gonadal, and neural histopathology, and a birth weight 45% of controls, more severe than that seen with knockout of either IGF-I or IGF-II alone [77]. Analysis of double mutants suggested that IGF-I, as expected, acts only via the type 1 IGF receptor, that IGF-II may act via a second receptor (thought not to be the IGF-II/M6P receptor), and IGF-I and IGF-II have overlapping but distinct physiological roles. IGF-II and IGF-I have significant fetal growth effects in the mouse beginning at days 11.5 and 13.5 of gestation, respectively, but only IGF-I is a significant postnatal growth factor [76].

IGF-binding proteins

Although insulin and the IGFs share significant structural homology and overlapping receptor affinities, the IGFs differ from insulin in one important respect. In contrast to insulin, the IGFs circulate in plasma complexed to a family of binding proteins [78–80]. These carrier proteins extend the serum half-life of the IGF peptides, transport IGFs to target cells and modulate the interaction of the IGFs with their cell surface receptors.

The existence of IGFBPs was inferred 20 years ago from chromatographic studies describing the size distribution of IGF peptides in serum [81]. However, it was only following the development of the Western ligand blotting technique in the late 1980s [82,83] that the number of IGFBPs and the complexity of IGF/IGFBP interactions began to be appreciated. The characterization of IGFBPs in body fluids and in conditioned media from cultured cells has been facilitated by the application of additional techniques, including gel chromatography, radioreceptor assays, affinity cross-linking, immunoblotting, specific radioimmunoassays (RIAs) and molecular identification.

Six distinct human and rat IGFBPs have been cloned and sequenced [84–90]. The amino acid homologies between human and rat IGFBPs exceed 70%, indicating that these proteins are well conserved from an evolutionary perspective. Amino acid conservation within species is in the 30–50% range, consistent with the hypothesis that they share a common genetic origin and have diverged structurally in order to permit specific functional roles (Table 7.1 & Fig. 7.7). Determination of the primary amino acid sequences from the cloned cDNAs of the IGFBPs has revealed impressive sequence homologies and structural similarities related to conservation of cysteine residues among the six IGFBPs. The total number of cysteines varies from 16 to 20, and each of the IGFBPs has a cysteine-rich region in both the amino and C-terminal. Since secondary structure of the IGFBPs is dependent upon disulphide bonding of cysteines (reduction of IGFBPs results in loss of IGF binding), their highly conserved order indicates strict conservation of IGF binding sites among all of the IGFBPs.

Analysis of the structure of the IGFBPs also reveals the presence of an RGD (arginine–glycine–aspartic acid), amino acid sequence near the C-terminal of IGFBP-1 and -2 [91]. This sequence is the minimum required in many extracellular matrix proteins for their binding by membrane receptors of the integrin protein family. It has been suggested that IGFBPs may associate with the cell surface through such amino acid sequences. On the other hand, IGFBP-3 and IGFBP-5, which lack an RGD sequence, appear to associate with the cell surface and extracellular matrix, respectively [92,93].

Under most experimental conditions the IGFBPs appear to inhibit IGF action, presumably by competing with IGF receptors for IGF peptides [94]. This is supported by observations that IGF analogues with decreased affinity for IGFBPs generally have increased biological potency [95–97]. Under specific conditions, however, several of the IGFBPs appear capable of enhancing IGF action, perhaps by facilitating IGF delivery to target receptors [98]. Furthermore, evidence exists for a possible direct inhibitory role of IGFBPs in certain cell systems. In studies involving transfection of the human IGFBP-3 gene into Balb/c

Table 7.1 Structure of IGF-binding proteins

IGFBP	Molecular weight	Amino acids	Cysteines	RGD	Glycosylation sites	mRNA (kb)
rIGFBP-1	26919	247	18	+	0	1.5–1.6
hIGFBP-1	25271	234	18	+	0	1.6
rIGFBP-2	29561	270	18	+	0	1.5
hIGFBP-2	31355	289	18	+	0	1.5
rIGFBP-3	28856	265	18	–	4	2.5
hIGFBP-3	28717	264	18	–	3	2.4
rIGFBP-4	25681	233	20	–	1	1.7
hIGFBP-4	25957	237	20	–	1	1.7
rIGFBP-5	28428	252	18	–	0	6.0
hIGFBP-5	28553	252	18	–	0	6.0
rIGFBP-6	21461	201	16	–	0	1.3
hIGFBP-6	22847	216	14	–	0	1.1

h, human; r, rat.

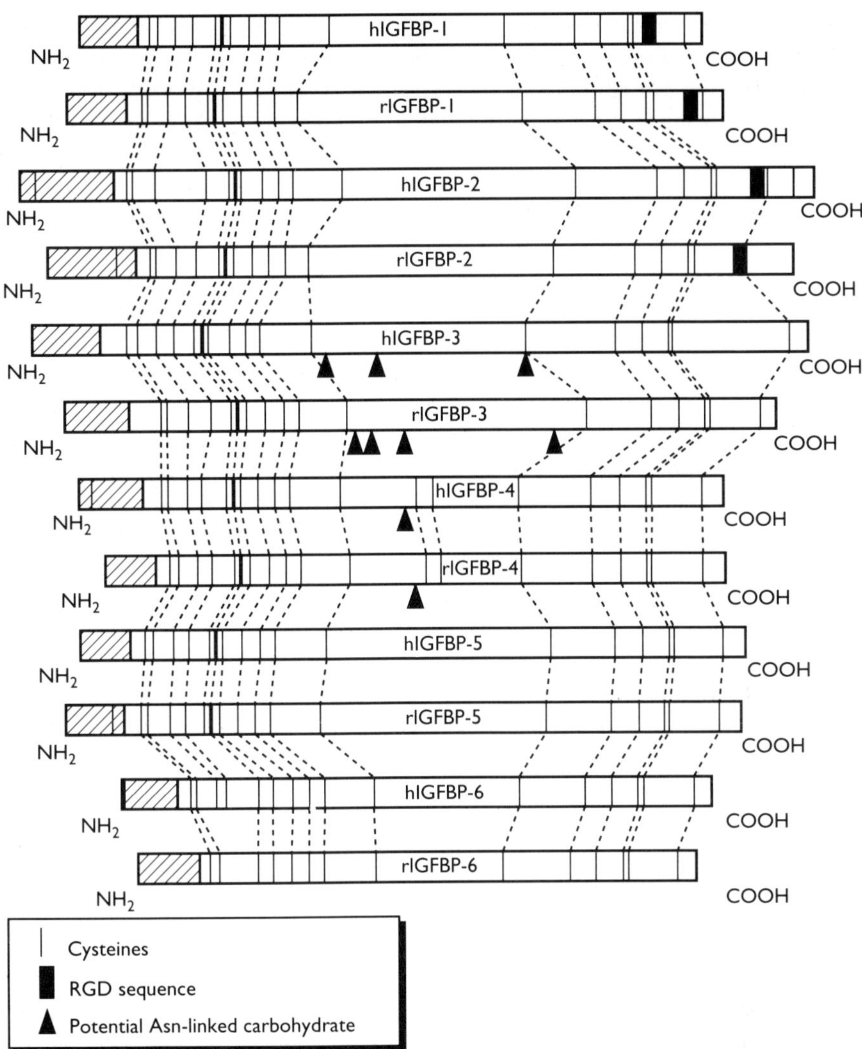

Fig. 7.7 Schematic representation of the protein sequences of human (h) and rat (r) IGFBP-1 through IGFBP-6, showing the marked conservation of cysteine residues.

fibroblasts, expression of IGFBP-3 resulted in an inhibition of cell growth in the absence of either endogenous or exogenous IGFs [99].

Analysis of IGFBPs has been further complicated by the discovery of IGFBP proteases capable of various levels of IGFBP degradation. Proteases for IGFBP-3, -4 and -5, initially reported in the serum of pregnant women [100,101], have been demonstrated in serum, seminal plasma [102], cerebrospinal fluid [103] and urine [104]. Proteolysis of IGFBPs potentially eliminates their detection by both Western ligand blotting and RIA methodologies, although IGFBP fragments may continue to be detected by affinity cross-linking or some RIAs. This phenomenon must be considered when concentrations of the various IGFBPs in biological fluids are reported [105]. The physiological significance of limited proteolysis of IGFBPs remains to be determined, although evidence suggests that protease activity results in decreased affinity of the IGFBP for IGF peptides.

CLINICAL ASPECTS

IGF serum concentrations

The IGF peptides have been remarkably difficult to measure accurately and easily. Bioassay methods were often complicated by the effect of a variety of serum factors capable of mimicking or inhibiting IGF action. Virtually all assays were influenced by the presence of IGFBPs, which have been found in all biological fluids tested to date. Early bioassay methods included stimulation of [^{35}S]-sulphate incorporation, using various modifications of the original method described by Salmon & Daughaday [1, 106–108]. A wide variety of other bioassays included stimulation of DNA synthesis [109], RNA synthesis [110], protein synthesis and glucose uptake [111]. In general, however, such assays were cumbersome, were subject to interference by IGFBPs, and could not distinguish between IGF-I and IGF-II. When SM-C and MSA were identified and purified it became possible to radiolabel and employ them in a variety of radioreceptor assays (RRAs) [112–114] and competitive protein-binding assays [115,116]. However, it was not until the development of specific antibodies that it became possible to distinguish IGF-I and IGF-II and to measure each peptide accurately [117–123].

Interference from the presence of IGFBPs has been a problem [124]. Powell *et al.* [125], for example, have demonstrated that the discrepant results found in uraemic sera assayed for IGF by bioassay, RRA and RIA could be entirely attributed to the interference of IGFBPs. Even antibodies with high affinity and specificity will exhibit interference by IGFBPs; this is particularly true in conditions where there is a relatively high IGFBP/IGF peptide ratio or at the clinical extremes of the assay (that is growth hormone deficiency or acromegaly). The most effective and reliable method to manipulate IGFBPs is their separation from IGF peptides by sizing chromatography under acidic conditions [31,40]. Both IGF-I and IGF-II, with molecular weights of approximately 7000, can be readily separated from the IGFBPs, the molecular weights of which range from about 25 000 to 45 000. This is a labour-intensive procedure and has been replaced by the more rapid acid-ethanol extraction process [126]. While this method may be reasonably effective for many serum samples, it has problems when IGFBP/IGF peptide ratios are elevated, as in conditioned media from cell lines, and in sera from newborns, GH deficiency, uraemia and other conditions.

Other methods include the use of antibodies generated against synthetic peptides, such as the C-peptide region of IGF-I [127] or IGF-II [128]. In general, such antibodies have high specificity and relatively low affinity, but interference from IGFBPs is eliminated. An alternative approach, developed by Blum *et al.* [129], has been the use of an antibody with high specificity for IGF-II, which permits the addition of excess unlabelled IGF-I to saturate endogenous IGFBPs. Bang *et al.* [130] have employed truncated IGF-I, which has decreased affinity for IGFBPs, as radioligand.

In human fetal serum, IGF-I levels increase with gestational age [131–134]. A positive correlation of fetal cord serum IGF-I levels with birth weight has been reported by some groups [49–51,135], but others have reported no correlation [136,137]. IGF-I levels in human newborn serum are generally 30–50% of adult levels. Serum concentrations rise gradually during childhood, attaining adult levels by the onset of sexual maturation [138,139]. During puberty, IGF-I concentrations rise to levels 2–3 times those seen in adults [56,57,140,141]. Accordingly, IGF-I levels during adolescence correlate better with stages of puberty than with chronological age. The failure of girls with gonadal dysgenesis to exhibit the normal adolescent increase in serum IGF-I argues for their dependence upon sex steroid stimulation [142,143]. It has been suggested that the pubertal rise in sex steroids stimulates IGF-I production indirectly, through an initial rise in GH secretion. However, this argument is contradicted in patients with GH receptor defects who show a pubertal rise in serum IGF-I despite a decline in GH levels, thereby implying a direct effect of sex steroids upon IGF-I [144].

Serum IGF-I levels demonstrate a progressive age-associated decline in adults [145,146]. Several investigators have suggested that this may be responsible for the negative nitrogen balance, decrease in body musculature and osteoporosis characteristic of ageing [147]. While this provocative hypothesis remains to be proved, it has generated considerable interest in the use of GH and/or IGF-I therapy in normal ageing (see below) [66,148].

Serum IGF-II levels do not follow the developmental pattern of IGF-I levels. Human newborn concentrations of IGF-II are approximately 50% of adult levels [149]. Adult concentrations are attained by 1 year of age, without the marked pubertal rise seen with IGF-I. There is little, if any, subsequent decline. The developmental pattern of IGF-II in humans is quite different from that seen in the rat or mouse, where serum IGF-II levels are highest in the fetus and decline rapidly postnatally to low levels in the adult [149–151].

IGF levels in growth disorders

The relationship of serum IGF levels to GH status has been established [152,153]. Measurement of each IGF peptide offers particular advantages. Determination of serum IGF-II concentrations has the advantage of diminished age dependency, but IGF-II exhibits a blunted responsiveness to GH. IGF-I levels exhibit more pronounced GH dependency and are thus more likely to identify differences in GH secretory patterns. Construction of age-defined normal values is necessary, but still may be misleading due to the influence of sexual maturation, nutritional status and other factors. Low IGF-I levels in young children overlap with values seen in GH insufficiency.

To test the use of serum IGF-I levels in predicting GH secretion, Moore *et al.* [154] performed GH stimulation tests in 78 children with heights below the fifth percentile and serum IGF-I levels $< 0.5\,U/ml$. While 19 of these children were subsequently diagnosed as GH deficient on the basis of standard provocative tests, significant overlap of serum IGF-I levels existed between GH-deficient patients and children with other forms of short stature and normal provocative GH levels. It was only in children with bone ages beyond 12 years that serum IGF-I levels permitted accurate discrimination beween GH deficiency and normal short children.

Similarly, Reiter & Lovinger [155] found that four of 16

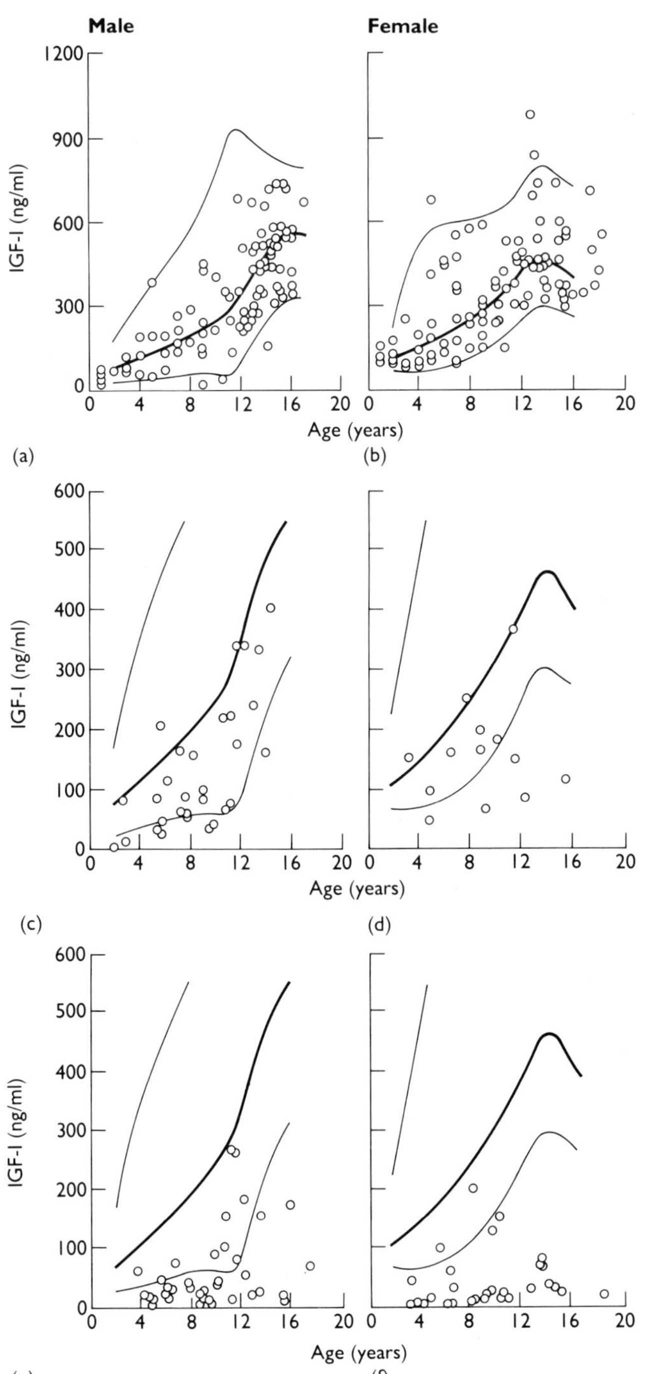

Fig. 7.8 Plasma IGF-I values by age in male and female (a, b) normal subjects, (c, d) short GH-sufficient subjects, and (e, f) GH-deficient subjects, where lines represent the 95th, 50th and 5th percentiles (from Rosenfeld *et al.* [153]).

children with low provocative GH levels had normal serum IGF-I concentrations while seven of 25 children with normal provocative GH levels had low serum IGF-I concentrations. Rosenfeld *et al.* [153] evaluated the efficacy of IGF-I and IGF-II RIAs in 68 GH-deficient children, 197 normal-statured children, and 44 normal short children. Overlap in serum IGF-I levels was evident (Fig. 7.8). Eighteen per cent of the GH-deficient children had serum IGF-I levels within the normal range, whereas 32% of normal short children exhibited low IGF-I concentrations. Low IGF-II levels were found in 52% of GH-deficient children, but also in 35% of normal short children. Assay of both IGF-I and IGF-II provided better discrimination than either IGF alone. Only 4% of GH-deficient children had normal plasma levels of both IGF-I and IGF-II but only 0.5% of normal children and 11% of normal short children had reduced serum concentrations of both IGF-I and IGF-II. Nevetheless, many paediatric endocrinologists routinely measure only serum IGF-I levels in evaluation of short stature, reserving measurement of serum IGF-II for special circumstances.

The observation that many short children without classically defined GH deficiency have low serum levels of either IGF-I or IGF-II calls into question the criteria by which the diagnosis of GH deficiency is currently made. Given that provocative GH testing is both arbitrary and non-physiological, and that inherent variability in GH RIAs exists, it is not surprising that the correlation between IGF-I levels and provocative GH levels is imperfect. Because both provocative GH testing and overnight GH secretion are considered imperfect discriminators of GH deficiency from normal short stature, IGF levels continue to be used for screening for GH deficiency.

Clinical utility of IGFBP measurements

The concentrations of IGFBPs vary among biological fluids. IGFBP-1 is the major IGFBP in human amniotic fluid [156], and IGFBP-2 is prominent in cerebrospinal fluid [157] and seminal plasma [158]. IGFBP-3 is clearly the major IGFBP in normal human serum, and demonstrates clear GH dependence [159]. On Western ligand blots of serum this binding protein appears as a doublet of approximately 40–44 kD. However, in neutral sizing chromatography of adult serum the majority of IGFBP-3 is detected in the 140–150 kD range. IGFBP-3, uniquely among the IGFBPs, normally circulates in adult serum as part of a ternary complex, consisting of IGFBP-3, an IGF peptide, and an acid-labile subunit [160,161] with an approximate molecular weight of 90 000.

Specific RIAs have been developed for several of the IGFBPs, including IGFBP-1 [150,162,163] IGFPB-2 [164], and IGFBP-3 [149,165,166]. Currently, measurement of IGFBP-3 appears to have the greatest potential clinical value, since it appears to be directly GH-dependent. Blum *et al.* [166] have argued that RIA determination of serum IGFBP-3 levels may be superior to IGF-I assays in the diagnosis of GH deficiency, because normal levels of IGF-I are so low in young children, and many 'normal' short children have low levels of IGF-I. Since IGFBP-3 determinations reflect combined IGF-I and IGF-II concentrations, IGFBP-3 agedependency is not nearly as striking as that of IGF-I alone. Even in young children, IGFBP-3 levels are normally above 500 ng/ml.

Further analysis of the usefulness of IGFBP-3 assays in the diagnosis of GH deficiency is clearly warranted, since evidence suggests that IGFBP-3 levels correlate with spontaneous GH secretion [167]. In GH receptor deficiency (GHRD) over 60 patients from the Ecuador cohort have all been found to have strikingly low serum concentrations of IGFBP-3, clearly reflecting the insensitivity to GH expected from this mutation of the GH receptor gene [168]. Savage *et al.* [169] have reported similar results in determinations of serum IGFBP-3 concentrations in a heterogeneous group of GH-insensitive patients from Europe, Asia and Australia.

It is unclear whether IGFBP-3 levels will reliably segregate with other measures of GH secretion in patients without GH insensitivity syndromes. In this context, Blum *et al* [166] have reported that 128/132 children with GH deficiency had serum IGFBP-3 levels below the fifth percentile (Fig. 7.9). By contrast, 124/130 'normal' short children had concentrations above the fifth percentile. These results led to immediate optimism regarding the clinical utility of IGFBP-3 levels in the diagnosis of GH deficiency. However, the percentage of GH-deficient children with low IGFBP-3 serum concentrations by our IGFBP-3 assay (R.G. Rosenfeld *et al.*, unpublished data) is substantially lower than that reported by Blum *et al.*, whereas the normal ranges are comparable. Since our reported IGFBP-3 levels in children with GHRD [63] are similar to those reported by Savage *et al.* in GHRD [169] employing the Blum IGFBP-3 RIA, it appears likely that the discrepancy in IGFBP-3 levels seen in GH deficiency reflects differences in use of provocative GH test results in diagnosing GH deficiency.

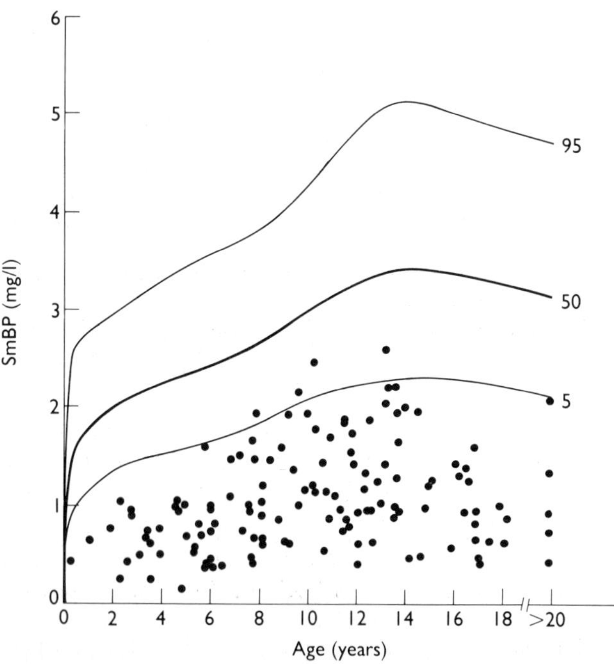

Fig. 7.9 IGFBP-3 levels by age in patients with GH deficiency, superimposed on the normal range bounded by the 5th and 95th percentiles (from Blum *et al.* [166]).

IGF therapy

The recent introduction of recombinant IGF peptides has provided the opportunity for clinical trials of IGF therapy. The initial trial of IGF-I in normal adult male volunteers examined the effect of a single intravenous injection of 100 μg/kg; hypoglycaemia occurred within 15 min, with a nadir at 30 min and a return to normal serum levels within 2 h [170]. IGF-I was estimated to have approximately 6% of the hypoglycaemic potency of insulin on a molar basis. Subsequently, intravenous infusions of IGF-I at a continuous rate of 20 $\mu g/kg\,h^{-1}$ in normal men normalized serum IGF-I levels without producing significant hypoglycaemia. Serum GH levels were suppressed, creatinine clearance increased, and plasma urea decreased [171] in these brief trials. Subcutaneous administration of 100 $\mu g/kg\,day^{-1}$ in healthy adults for 7 days resulted in a 250% increase in serum IGF-I levels, with only a slight drop in glucose levels [172].

An immediately apparent clinical use of recombinant IGF-I therapy was in patients with GH insensitivity. In initial trials of IGF-I in patients with GHRD, acute and symptomatic hypoglycaemia resulted from a single intravenous bolus of 75 μg/kg [173]. When IGF-I was administered subcutaneously to eight GHRD patients in a dosage of 150 $\mu g/kg\,day^{-1}$ for 7 days, no symptomatic hypoglycaemia was noted [174]. Vaccarello *et al.* [144] administered IGF-I subcutaneously for 7 days to six Ecuadorian adults with GHRD. Because the marked deficiency of IGFBP-3 in GHRD subjects leads to a more rapid turnover of IGF-I, a dose of 40 μg/kg was administered twice daily in this study. No symptomatic hypoglycaemia was observed. Mean 24 h GH levels were suppressed and urinary calcium increased two-fold.

At this dose a mean peak serum IGF-I level of 253 ± 11 ng/ml was achieved 2–6 h after injection, with a mean trough level of 137 ± 8 ng/ml. Serum IGF-II levels fell reciprocally, and the total serum IGF levels (IGF-I + IGF-II) did not change significantly. Surprisingly, serum IGFBP-3 levels did not increase despite the known GH dependence of IGFBP-3 [175]. The relatively lower serum IGF-I levels attained in IGF-I therapy in GH-deficient subjects probably reflects a GH-dependent deficiency in serum IGFBPs or the acid-labile subunit. These findings demonstrated the importance of IGFBPs in modulating the serum half-life of either endogenous or administered IGF peptides.

In longer-term studies in GHRD patients, Walker *et al.* [176] reported an increase in growth rate to 11.4 cm/year in a boy treated with twice daily subcutaneous injections of 120 μg/kg. Laron *et al.* [177] reported significant growth acceleration (to 8.8–13.6 cm/year) in five children treated for 3–10 months with a single daily injection of 150 μg/kg. In the European population Wilton *et al.* [178] have reported preliminary results in 30 children with GH insensitivity attributable to either GHRD or GH deficiency IA with anti-GH antibodies. The dosage of IGF-I varied from 40 to 120 μg/kg twice daily, and observed side-effects included hypoglycaemia, headache, convulsions, possible urolithiasis and papilloedema, which resolved spontaneously. With the exception of the two oldest patients the growth velocity of all subjects increased by at least 2 cm/year. In recent reports on these European children and adolescents [179] five children treated with 40 μg/kg twice daily for 9 months exhibited a mean growth rate of 7.8 cm/year, while nine subjects treated with 120 μg/kg twice daily had a mean growth rate of 11.0 cm/year.

None of these studies was controlled, but the data demonstrate a potent anabolic and growth-promoting action of IGF-I in children with GHRD. Prospective, placebo-controlled trials are currently in progress in Ecuador, and should provide answers about the growth-promoting actions of the IGF peptides. The failure of serum levels of IGFBP-3 to rise with IGF-I administration underscores the relevance of complex GH–IGF–IGFBP–IGF receptor interactions to potential IGF therapeutic response [168,169]. While the early studies have been promising, little is known about the long-term anabolic effect of IGF-I, nor about the optimal dosage and frequency of administration. Nonetheless, the early clinical findings indicate that the IGF peptides, long considered to function primarily as autocrine or paracrine growth factors, are capable of acting as classical endocrine hormones. The studies in normal volunteers and in patients with GH insensitivity have established a foundation for current and future studies of IGF therapy in a wide variety of growth-related, catabolic and metabolic disorders (Table 7.2).

Table 7.2 Potential IGF therapies

Growth failure
Syndromes of GH insensitivity
Chronic renal failure
Glucocorticoid treatment
Intrauterine growth retardation
Ageing: nitrogen balance, body composition, osteoporosis
Catabolic states
Malnutrition, hyperalimentation
Surgical
Burns
Sepsis
Cachexia: cancer, AIDS
Diabetes mellitus: type 1, type 2

REFERENCES

1 Salmon WD Jr, Daughaday WH. A hormonally controlled serum factor which stimulates sulfate incorporation by cartilage *in vitro*. *J Lab Clin Med* 1957;49:825–36.

2 Burgi H, Muller WA, Humbel RE, Labhart A, Froesch ER. Non-suppressible insulin-like activity of human serum. I. Physicochemical properties, extraction and partial purification. *Biochim Biophys Acta* 1966;121:349–59.

3 Froesch RE, Zapf J, Meuli C *et al.* Biological properties of NSILA-S. *Adv Metab Disord* 1975;8:211–35.

4 Froesch ER, Muller WA, Burgi H, Waldvogel M, Labhart A. Non-suppressible insulin-like activity of human serum. II. Biological properties of plasma extracts with non-suppressible insulin-like activity. *Biochim Biophys Acta* 1966;121:360–74.

5 Dulak NC, Temin HM. A partially purified polypeptide fraction from rat liver cell conditioned medium with multiplication-stimulating activity for embryo fibroblasts. *J Cell Physiol* 1973;81:153–60.

6 Daughaday WH, Hall K, Raben MS, Salmon WD Jr, Van den Brande JL, Van Wyk JJ. Somatomedin: proposed designation for sulphation factor. *Nature* 1972;235:107.

7 Hall K, Takano K, Fryklund L, Sievertsson H. Somatomedins. *Adv Metab Disord* 1975;8:19–46.

8 Van Wyk JJ, Underwood LE, Hintz RL, Clemmons DR, Voina SJ, Weaver RP. The somatomedins: a family of insulin like hormones under growth hormone control. *Rec Prog Horm Res* 1974;30:259–318.

9 Rinderknecht E, Humbel RE. The amino acid sequence of human insulin-like growth factor I and its structural homology with proinsulin. *J Biol Chem* 1978;253:2769–76.

10 Rinderknecht E, Humbel RE. Primary Structure of human insulin-like growth factor II. *FEBS Lett* 1978;89:283–6.

11 Daughaday WH, Rotwein P. Insulin-like growth factors I and II. Peptide, messenger ribonucleic acid and gene structures, serum, and tissue concentrations. *Endocr Rev* 1989;10:68–91.

12 Humbel RE. Insulin-like growth factors I and II. *Eur J Biochem* 1990;190:445–62.

13 Underwood LE, Van Wyk JJ. Normal and aberrant growth. In: Wilson JD, Foster DW, eds. *Williams Textbook of Endocrinology*, 8th edn. Philadelphia, PA: WB Saunders, 1992: 1079–138.

14 Ross M, Francis GL, Szabo L, Wallace JC, Ballard FJ. Insulin-like growth factor binding proteins inhibit the biological activities of IGF-I and IGF-II but not des-(1-3)-IGF-I. *Biochem J* 1989;258:267–72.

15 Cascieri MA, Saperstein R, Hayes NS *et al.* Serum half-life and biological activity of mutants of human insulin-like growth factor I which do not bind to serum binding proteins. *Endocrinology* 1988;123:373–81.

16 Bayne ML, Applebaum J, Chicchi GG, Hayes NS, Green BG, Cascieri MA. Structural analogs of human insulin-like growth factor I with reduced affinity for serum binding proteins and the type 2 insulin-like receptor. *J Biol Chem* 1988;263:6233–9.

17 Beukers MW, Oh Y, Zhang H, Ling N, Rosenfeld RG. Leu 27 insulin-like growth factor II is highly selective for the type II IGF receptor in binding, cross-linking and thymidine incorporation experiments. *Endocrinology* 1991;128:1201–3.
18 Sussenbach JS, Steenbergh PH, Holthuizen P. Structure of the human insulin-like growth factor genes. *Growth Regul* 1992;2:1–9.
19 Brissenden JE, Ullrich A, Francke U. Human chromosomal mapping of genes for insulin-like growth factors I and II and epidermal growth factor. *Nature* 1984;310:781–4.
20 Tricoli JV, Rall LB, Scott J, Bell GI, Shows TB. Localization of insulin-like growth factor genes to human chromosomes 11 and 12. *Nature* 1984;310:784–6.
21 Jansen M, van Schaik FMA, Ricker AT *et al.* Sequence of cDNA encoding human insulin-like growth factor I precursor. *Nature* 1983;306:609–11.
22 Bell GI, Gerhard DS, Fong NM, Sanchez-Pescador R, Rall LB. Isolation of the human insulin-like growth factor genes. Insulin-like growth factor II and insulin genes are contiguous. *Proc Natl Acad Sci USA* 1985;82:6450–4.
23 Roberts CT, Lasky SR, Lowe WL, LeRoith D. Rat IGF-I cDNAs contain multiple 5′ untranslated regions. *Biochem Biophys Res Commun* 1987;146:1154–8.
24 Lund PK, Moats-Staats BM, Hynes MA *et al.* Somatomedin-C/insulin-like growth factor-I and insulin-like growth factor-II mRNAs in rat fetal and adult tissues. *J Biol Chem* 1986;261:14539–44.
25 Brown AL, Graham DE, Nissley SP, Hill DJ, Strain AJ, Rechler MM. Developmental regulation of insulin-like growth factor II mRNA in different rat tissues. *J Biol Chem* 1986;261:13144–50.
26 DeChiara TM, Efstradiatis A, Robertson EJ. A growth deficiency phenotype in heterozygous mice carrying an insulin-like growth factor II gene disrupted by targeting. *Nature* 1990;345:78.
27 Reeve AE, Eccles MR, Wilkins RJ, Bell GI, Millow LJ. Expressions of insulin-like growth factor II transcripts in Wilms' tumor. *Nature* 1985;317:258.
28 Daughaday WH, Deuel TF. Tumor secretion of growth factors. *Endocrinol Metab Clin N Am* 1991;20:539–63.
29 Daughaday WH, Kapadia M. Significance of abnormal serum binding of insulin-like growth factor II in the development of hypoglycemia in patients with non-islet cell tumors. *Proc Natl Acad Sci USA* 198;86:6778–82.
30 DeChiara TM, Efstradiatis A, Robertson EJ. A growth deficiency phenotype in heterozygous mice carrying an insulin-like growth factor II gene disrupted by targeting. *Nature* 1990;345:78.
31 Zapf J, Futo E, Peter M, Froesch ER. Can 'big' insulin-like growth factor II in serum of tumor patients account for the development of extrapancreatic tumor hypoglycemia? *J Clin Invest* 1992;90:2574–84.
32 Hintz RL, Clemmons DR, Underwood LE, Van Wyk JJ. Competitive binding of somatomedin to the insulin receptors of adipocytes, chondrocytes, and liver membranes. *Proc Natl Acad Sci USA* 1972;69:2351–3.
33 Megyesi K, Kahn CR, Roth J *et al.* Insulin and non-suppressible insulin-like activity (NSILA-s): evidence for separate plasma membrane receptor sites. *Biochem Biophys Res Commun* 1974;57:307–15.
34 Massague J, Czech MP. The subunit structures of two distinct receptors for insulin-like growth factors I and II and their relationship to the insulin receptor. *J Biol Chem* 1982; 257:5038–45.
35 Kasuga M, Van Obberghen E, Nissley SP, Rechler MM. Demonstration of two subtypes of insulin-like growth factor receptors by affinity crosslinking. *J Biol Chem* 1981;256: 5305–8.
36 Chernausek SD, Jacobs S, Van Wyk JJ. Structural similarities between human receptors for somatomedin C and insulin: analysis by affinity labeling. *Biochemistry* 1981;20:7345–50.
37 Oh Y, Muller H, Neely EK, Rosenfeld RG. New concepts in insulin-like growth factor receptor physiology. *Growth Regul* 1993;3:113–23.
38 Ullrich A, Gray A, Tam AW *et al.* Insulin-like growth factor I receptor primary structure: comparison with insulin receptor suggests structural determinants that define functional specificity. *EMBO J* 1986;5:2503–12.
39 Steele-Perkins G, Turner J, Edman JC *et al.* Expression and characterization of a functional human insulin-like growth factor I receptor. *J Biol Chem* 1988;236:11486–92.
40 Hintz RL, Thorsson AV, Enberg G, Hall K. IGF-II binding on human lymphoid cells: demonstration of a common high affinity receptor for insulin peptides. *Biochem Biophys Res Commun* 1984;118:774–82.
41 Misra P, Hintz RL, Rosenfeld RG. Structural and immunological characterization of insulin-like growth factor II binding to IM-9 cells. *J Clin Endocrinol Metab* 1986;63:1400–5.
42 Jonas HA, Cox AJ. Insulin-like growth factor binding to the atypical insulin receptors of a human lymphoid-derived cell line (IM-9). *Biochem J* 1990;266:737–42.
43 Feltz SM, Swanson SM, Wemmie JA, Pessin JE. Functional properties of an isolated heterodimeric human placenta insulin-like growth factor I complex. *Biochemistry* 1988; 27:3234–42.
44 Treadway JL, Morrison BD, Goldfine ID, Pessin JE. Assembly of insulin/insulin-like growth factor-1 hybrid receptors in vitro. *J Biol Chem* 1989;264:21450–3.
45 Soos MA, Siddle K. Immunological relationships between receptors for insulin and insulin-like growth factor I. *Biochem J* 1989;263:553–63.
46 Morgan DO, Edman JC, Standring DN *et al.* Insulin-like growth factor II receptor as a multifunctional binding protein. *Nature* 1987;329:301–7.
47 Lobel P, Dahms NM, Kornfeld S. Cloning and sequence analysis of the cation-independent mannose-6-phosphate receptor. *J Biol Chem* 1988;263:2563–70.
48 Roth RA, Stover C, Hari J *et al.* Interactions of the receptor for insulin-like growth factor II with mannose-6-phosphate and antibodies to the mannose-6-phosphate receptor. *Biochem Biophys Res Commun* 1987;149:600–6.
49 MacDonald R, Pfeffer SR, Coussens L *et al.* A single receptor binds both insulin-like growth factor II and mannose-6-phosphate. *Science* 1988;239:1134–7.
50 Kornfeld S. Trafficking of lysosomal enzymes. *FASEB J* 1987;1:462–8.
51 Tong PY, Tollefsen SE, Kornfeld S. The cation-independent mannose-6-phosphate receptor binds insulin-like growth factor II. *J Biol Chem* 1988;239:2585–8.
52 Rosenfeld RG, Conover CA, Hodges D *et al.* Heterogeneity of insulin-like growth factor-I affinity for the insulin-like growth factor-II receptor: comparison of natural, synthetic and recombinant DNA-derived insulin-like growth factor-I. *Biochem Biophys Res Commun* 1987;143:199–205.
53 Braulke T, Causin C, Waheed A *et al.* Mannose 6-phosphate/insulin-like growth factor II receptor: distinct binding sites for mannose 6-phosphate and insulin-like growth factor II. *Biochem Biophys Res Commun* 1988;150:1287–93.

54 Kiess W, Blickenstaff GD, Sklar MM *et al.* Biochemical evidence that the type II insulin-like growth factor receptor is identical to the cation-independent mannose 6-phosphate receptor. *J Biol Chem* 1988;263:9339–44.

55 Kiess W, Thomas CL, Sklar MM, Nissley SP. Beta-galactosidase decreases the binding affinity of the insulin-like growth factor II/mannose 6-phosphate receptor for insulin-like growth factor II. *Eur J Biochem* 1990;190:71–7.

56 Nolan CM, Kyle JW, Watanabe H, Sly WS. Binding of insulin-like growth factor II (IGF-II) by human cation-independent mannose 6-phosphate receptor/IGF-II receptor expressed in receptor-deficient mouse L cells. *Cell Regul* 1990;1:197–213.

57 Kiess W, Thomas CL, Greenstein LA *et al.* Insulin-like growth factor-II (IGF-II) inhibits both the cellular uptake of beta-galactosidase and the binding of beta-galactosidase to purified IGF-II/mannose 6-phosphate receptor. *J Biol Chem* 1989;264:4710–14.

58 Lee SJ, Nathans D. Proliferin secreted by cultured cells binds to mannose 6-phosphate receptors. *J Biol Chem* 1988;263: 3521–7.

59 Kovacina KS, Steele-Perkins G, Purchio F *et al.* Interactions of recombinant and platelet transforming growth factor beta-1 precursor with the insulin-like growth factor II/ mannose 6-phosphate receptor. *Biochem Biophys Res Commun* 1989;160:393–403.

60 Herzog V, Neumuller W, Holzmann B. Thyroglobulin, the major and obligatory exportable protein of thyroid follicle cells, carries the lysosomal recognition marker mannose 6-phosphate. *EMBO J* 1987;6:555–60.

61 Conover CA, Misra P, Hintz RL, Rosenfeld RG. Effect of an anti-insulin-like growth factor I receptor antibody on insulin-like growth factor II stimulation of DNA synthesis in human fibroblasts. *Biochem Biophys Res Commun* 1987;139:501–8.

62 Furlanetto RW, DiCarlo JN, Wisehart C. The type II insulin-like growth factor receptor does not mediate deoxyribonucleic acid synthesis in human fibroblasts. *J Clin Endocrinol Metab* 1987;64:1142–9.

63 Mottola C, Czech MP. The type II insulin-like growth factor receptor does not mediate DNA synthesis in H-35 hepatoma cells. *J Biol Chem* 1984;25:12705–13.

64 Kiess W, Haskell JF, Lee L *et al.* An antibody that blocks insulin-like growth factor (IGF) binding to the type II IGF receptor is neither an agonist nor an inhibitor of IGF-stimulated biologic response in L6 myoblasts. *J Biol Chem* 1987;262:12745–51.

65 Adashi EY, Resnick CE, Rosenfeld RG. Insulin-like growth factor-I (IGF-I) hormonal action in cultured rat granulosa cells: mediation via type I but not type II IGF receptors. *Endocrinology* 1989;126:216–22.

66 Beukers M, Oh Y, Zhang H, Ling N, Rosenfeld RG. [Leu27] insulin-like growth factor II is highly selective for the type II IGF receptor in binding, cross-linking and thymidine incorporation experiments. *Endocrinology* 1991;128:1201–3.

67 Canfield WM, Kornfeld S. The chicken liver cation-independent mannose 6-phosphate receptor lacks the high affinity binding site for insulin-like growth factor II. *J Biol Chem* 1989;264:7100–3.

68 Clairmont KB, Czech MP. Chicken and *Xenopus* mannose 6-phosphate receptors fail to bind insulin-like growth factor II. *J Biol Chem* 1989;264:16390–2.

69 Tally M, Li CH, Hall K. IGF-2 stimulated growth mediated by the somatomedin type 2 receptor. *Biochem Biophys Res Commun* 1987;148:811–16.

70 Nestler JE. Insulin-like growth factor II is a potent inhibitor of the aromatase activity of human placental cytotrophoblasts. *Endocrinology* 1990;127:2064–70.

71 Rogers SA, Hammerman MR. Insulin-like growth factor II stimulates production of inositol triphosphate in proximal tubular basolateral membranes from canine kidney. *Proc Natl Acad Sci USA* 1988;85:4037–41.

72 Minniti CP, Kohn EC, Grubb JH *et al.* The insulin-like growth factor II (IGF-II)/mannose 6-phosphate receptor mediates IGF-II-induced motility in human rhabdomyosarcoma cells. *J Biol Chem* 1992;267:9000–4.

73 Kojima I, Nishimoto I, Iiri T, Ogata E, Rosenfeld RG. Evidence that type II insulin-like growth factor receptor is coupled to calcium gating system. *Biochem Biophys Res Commun* 1988;154:9–19.

74 Nishimoto I, Murayama Y, Katada T, Ui M, Ogata E. Possible direct linkage of insulin-like growth factor-II receptor with guanine nucleotide-binding proteins. *J Biol Chem* 1989; 264:14029–38.

75 Murayama Y, Okamoto T, Ogata E *et al.* Distinctive regulation of the functional linkage between human cation-independent mannose 6-phosphate receptor and GTP-binding proteins by insulin-like growth factor-II and mannose 6-phosphate. *J Biol Chem* 1990;265:17456–62.

76 Baker J, Liu J-P, Robertson EJ, Efstradiatis A. Role of insulin-like growth factors in embryonic and postnatal growth. *Cell* 1993;75:73–82.

77 Liu J-P, Baker J, Perkins AS, Robertson EJ, Efstradiatis A. Mice carrying null mutations of the genes encoding insulin-like growth factor I and type 1 IGF receptor. *Cell* 1993;75: 59–72.

78 Rosenfeld RG, Lamson G, Pham H *et al.* Insulin-like growth factor binding proteins. *Rec Prog Horm Res* 1990;46:99–163.

79 Lamson G, Giudice L, Rosenfeld RG. The insulin-like growth factor binding proteins: structural and molecular relationships. *Growth Factors* 1991;5:19–28.

80 Rechler MM. Insulin-like growth factor binding proteins. *Vitamins Horm* 1993;47:1–114.

81 Hintz RL, Liu F. Demonstration of specific plasma protein binding sites for somatomedin. *J Clin Endocrinol Metab* 1977;45:988–95.

82 Hossenlopp P, Surin D, Segovia-Quinson B, Hardouin S, Binoux M. Analysis of serum insulin-like growth factor binding proteins using western blotting: use of the method for titration of the binding proteins and competitive binding studies. *Anal Biochem* 1986;154:138–43.

83 Hardouin S, Hossenlopp P, Segovia B *et al.* Heterogeneity of insulin-like growth factor binding proteins and relationships between structure and affinity. 1. Circulating forms in man. *Eur J Biochem* 1987;170:121–32.

84 Lee Y-L, Hintz RL, James PM, Lee PDK, Shively JE, Powell DR. Insulin-like growth factor (IGF) binding protein complementary deoxyribonucleic acid from human HEP G2 hepatoma cells: predicted protein sequence suggests an IGF binding domain different from those of the IGF-I and IGF-II receptors. *Mol Endocrinol* 1988;2:404–11.

85 Binkert C, Landwehr J, Mary J-L, Schwander J, Heinrich G. Cloning, sequence analysis and expression of a cDNA encoding a novel insulin-like growth factor binding protein (IGFBP-2). *EMBO J* 1989;8:2497–502.

86 Wood WI, Cachianes G, Henzel WJ *et al.* Cloning and expression of the growth hormone-dependent insulin-like growth factor-binding protein. *Mol Endocrinol* 1989;3:1176–85.

87 LaTour D, Mohan S, Linkhart TA, Baylink DJ, Strong DD. Inhibitory insulin-like growth factor binding protein

(hIGFBP-4): cloning, complete sequence and physiological regulation. *Mol Endocrinol* 1990;4:1806–14.
88 Kiefer MC, Ioh RS, Bauer DM, Zapf J. Molecular cloning of a new human insulin-like growth factor binding protein. *Biochem Biophys Res Commun* 1991;176:219–25.
89 Kiefer MC, Masiarz FR, Bauer DM, Zapf J. Identification and molecular cloning of two new 30-kDa insulin-like growth factor binding proteins isolated from adult human serum. *J Biol Chem* 1991;266;9043–9.
90 Shimasaki S, Shimonaka M, Zhang H-P, Ling N. Identification of five different insulin-like growth factor binding proteins (IGFBPs) from adult rat serum and molecular cloning of a novel IGFBP-5 in rat and human. *J Biol Chem* 1991; 266:10646–53.
91 Brewer MT, Stetler GL, Squires CH, Thompson RC, Busby WH, Clemmons DR. Cloning, characterization, and expression of a human insulin-like growth factor binding protein. *Biochem Biophys Res Commun* 1988;152:1289–97.
92 Oh Y, Muller HL, Pham H, Lamson G, Rosenfeld RG. Non-receptor mediated, post-transcriptional regulation of insulin-like growth factor binding protein (IGFBP)-3 in Hs578T human breast cancer cells. *Endocrinology* 1992;131:3123–5.
93 Oh Y, Muller H, Lamson G, Rosenfeld RG. Insulin-like growth factor (IGF)-independent action of IGF binding protein (BP)-3 in Hs578T human breast cancer cells. Cell surface binding and growth inhibition. *J Biol Chem* 1993;268: 14964–71.
94 Ritvos O, Ranta T, Julkanen J *et al.* Insulin-like growth factor (IGF) binding protein from human decidua inhibits the binding and biological action of IGF-I in cultured choriocarcinoma cells. *Endocrinology* 1988;122:2150–7.
95 Ross M, Francis GL, Szabo L, Wallace JC, Ballard J. Insulin-like growth factor (IGF)-binding proteins inhibit the biological activities of IGF-1 and IGF-2 but not des-(1-3)-IGF-1. *Biochem J* 1989;258:267–72.
96 Clemmons DR, Cascieri MA, Camacho-Hubner C, McCusker RH, Bayne ML. Discrete alterations of the insulin-like growth factor I molecule which alter its affinity for insulin-like growth factor-binding proteins result in changes in bioactivity. *J Biol Chem* 1990;265:12210–16.
97 Okajima T, Nakamura K, Zhang H *et al.* Sensitive colorimetric bioassays for insulin-like growth factor (IGF) stimulation of cell proliferation and glucose consumption: use in studies of IGF analogs. *Endocrinology* 1992;130:2201–12.
98 Elgin RC, Busby WH, Clemmons DR. An insulin-like growth factor (IGF) binding protein enhances the biologic response to IGF-I. *Proc Natl Acad Sci USA* 1987;84:3254–8.
99 Cohen P, Lamson G, Okajima T, Rosenfeld RG. Transfection of the human insulin-like growth factor binding protein-3 gene into Balb/c fibroblasts inhibits cellular growth. *Mol Endocrinol* 1993;7:380–6.
100 Giudice LC, Farrell EM, Pham H, Lamson G, Rosenfeld RG. Insulin-like growth factor binding proteins in the maternal serum throughout gestation and in the puerperium: effects of a pregnancy-associated serum protease activity. *J Clin Endocrinol Metab* 1990;71:1330–8.
101 Hossenlopp P, Segovia B, Lassarre C, Roghani M, Bredon M, Binoux M. Evidence of enzymatic degradation of insulin-like growth factor binding proteins in the 150K complex during pregnancy. *J Clin Endocrinol Metab* 1990;71:797–805.
102 Cohen P, Graves HCB, Peehl DM, Kamarei ME, Giudice LC, Rosenfeld RG. Prostate specific antigen (PSA) is an IGF binding protein-3 (IGFBP-3) protease found in seminal plasma. *J Clin Endocrinol Metab* 1992;75:1046–53.
103 Muller HL, Oh Y, Gargosky SE, Hintz RL, Rosenfeld RG. Concentrations of insulin-like growth factor binding protein-3, insulin-like growth factors and IGFBP-3 protease activity in cerebrospinal fluid (CSF) of children with leukemia, brain tumors, or meningitis. *J Clin Endocrinol Metab* 1993 (in press).
104 Lee D-Y, Cohen P, Krensky AM, Rosenfeld RG, Yorgin PD. Insulin-like growth factor binding protein-3 (IGFBP-3) protease activity in the urine of children with chronic renal failure. *Pediatr Nephrol* 1993;7:416–23.
105 Gargosky SE, Pham HM, Wilson KF, Liu F, Giudice LC, Rosenfeld RG. Measurement and characterization of insulin-like growth factor binding protein-3 in human biological fluids: discrepancies between radioimmunoassay and ligand blotting. *Endocrinology* 1992;131:3051–60.
106 Salmon WD, DuVall MR. A serum fraction with 'sulfation factor activity' stimulates in vitro incorporation of leucine and sulfate into protein-polysccharide complexes, uridine into RNA, and thymidine into DNA of costal cartilage from hypophysectomized rats. *Endocrinology* 1970;86:721–7.
107 Hall K. Quantitative determination of the sulphation factor activity in human serum. *Acta Endocrinol (Copenh)* 1970; 63:338–50.
108 Phillips LS, Herington AC, Daughaday WH. Somatomedin stimulation of sulfate incorporation in porcine costal cartilage discs. *Endocrinology* 1974;94:856–63.
109 Garland JT, Lottes ME, Kozak S, Daughaday WH. Stimulation of DNA synthesis in isolated chondrocytes by sulfation factor. *Endocrinology* 1972;90:1086–90.
110 Garland JT, Buchanan F. Stimulation of RNA and protein synthesis in isolated chondroctyes by human serum. *J Clin Endocrinol Metab* 1976;43:842–6.
111 Meuli C, Froesch ER. Effects of insulin and of NSILA-S on the perfused rat heart: glucose uptake, lactate production and efflux of 3-*O*-methyl glucose. *Eur J Clin Invest* 1975;5: 93–9.
112 Hall K, Takano K, Fryklund L. Radioreceptor assay for somatomedin A. *J Clin Endocrinol Metab* 1974;39:973–6.
113 Van Wyk JJ, Underwood LE, Baseman JB, Hintz RL, Clemmons DR, Marshall RN. Explorations of the insulin-like and growth-promoting properties of somatomedin C by membrane receptor assays. *Adv Metab Disord* 1975;8:128–50.
114 Horner JM, Liu F, Hintz RL. Comparison of (125I) somatomedin-A and (125I) somatomedin C radioreceptor assays for somatomedin peptide content in whole and acid-chromatographed plasma. *J Clin Endocrinol Metab* 1978; 47:1287–95.
115 Zapf J, Kaufmann U, Eigenmann EJ, Froesch ER. Determination of nonsupressible insulin-like activity in human serum by a sensitive protein-binding assay. *Clin Chem* 1977;23: 677–82.
116 Schalch DS, Heinrich UE, Koch JG, Johnson CJ, Schlueter RJ. Nonsuppressible insulin-like activity (NSILA). Development of a new sensitive competitive protein-binding assay for determination of serum levels. *J Clin Endocrinol Metab* 1978;46:664–71.
117 Furlanetto RW, Underwood LE, Van Wyk JJ, D'Ercole AJ. Estimation of somatomedin-C levels in normals and patients with pituitary disease by radioimmunoassay. *J Clin Invest* 1977;60:648–57.
118 Zapf J, Rinderknecht ER, Humbel RE, Froesch ER. Nonsuppressible insulin-like activity (NSILA) from human serum: recent accomplishments and their physiologic implications.

Metabolism 1978;27:1803–28.

119 Zapf J, Walter H, Froesch ER. Radioimmunological determination of insulin-like growth factors I and II in normal subjects and in patients with growth disorders and extrapancreatic tumor hypoglycemia. *J Clin Invest* 1981;68:1321–30.

120 Bala RM, Bhaumick B. Radioimmunoassay of a basic somatomedin: comparison of various assay techniques and somatomedin levels in various sera. *J Clin Endocrinol Metab* 1979;49:770–7.

121 Baxter RC, Axiak S, Raison RL. Monoclonal antibody against human somatomedin-C/insulin-like growth factor I. *J Clin Endocrinol Metab* 1982;54:474–6.

122 Rosenfeld RG, Wilson DM, Lee PDK, Hintz RL. Insulin-like growth factors I and II in the evaluation of growth retardation. *J Pediatr* 1986;109:428–33.

123 Tanaka H, Asami O, Hayano T, Sasaki I, Yoshitake Y, Nishikawa K. Identification of a family of insulin-like growth factor II secreted by cultured rat epithelial cell line 18,54-SF. Application of a monoclonal antibody. *Endocrinology* 1989; 124:870–7.

124 Daughaday WH, Kapadia M, Mariz I. Serum somatomedin binding proteins: physiologic significance and interference in radioligand assay. *J Lab Clin Med* 1986;109:355–63.

125 Powell DR, Rosenfeld RG, Baker BK, Hintz RL. Serum somatomedin levels in adults with chronic renal failure: the importance of measuring insulin-like growth factor (IGF)-1 and IGF-2 in acid chromatographed uremic serum. *J Clin Endocrinol Metab* 1986;63:1186–92.

126 Daughaday WH, Mariz IK, Blethen SL. Inhibition of access of bound somatomedin to membrane receptor and immunobinding sites: a comparison of radioreceptor and radioimmunoassay of somatomedin in native and acid-ethanol-extracted serum. *J Clin Endocrinol Metab* 1980;51:781–8.

127 Hintz RL, Liu F, Seegan G. Characterization of an insulin-like growth factor-I/somatomedin-C radioimmunoassay specific for the C-peptide region. *J Clin Endocrinol Metab* 1982;55:927–30.

128 Hintz RL, Liu F. A radioimmunoassay for insulin-like growth factor II specific for the C-peptide region. *J Clin Endocrinol Metab* 1982;54:442–6.

129 Blum WF, Ranke MB, Bierich JR. A specific radioimmunoassay for IGF-II: the interference of IGF binding proteins can be blocked by excess IGF-I. *Acta Endocrinol (Copenh)* 1988; 118:374–80.

130 Bang P, Eriksson U, Sara V, Wivall I-L, Hall K. Comparison of acid ethanol extraction and acid gel filtration prior to IGF-I and IGF-II radioimmunoassays: improvement of determinations in acid ethanol extracts by the use of truncated IGF-I as radioligand. *Acta Endocrinol (Copenh)* 1991;124:620–9.

131 Ashton IK, Vessey J. Somatomedin activity in human cord plasma and relationship to birth size, growth hormone, and prolactin. *Early Hum Dev* 1978;2:115–21.

132 Bennett A, Wilson DM, Liu F, Nagashima R, Rosenfeld RG, Hintz RL. Levels of insulin-like growth factor-I and -II in human cord blood. *J Clin Endocrinol Metab* 1983;57:609–12.

133 Gluckman PD, Barrett-Johnson JJ, Butler JH, Edgar B, Gunn TR. Studies of insulin-like growth factor I and II by specific radioligand assays in umbilical cord blood. *Clin Endocrinol* 1983;19:405–13.

134 D'Ercole AJ. Somatomedin/insulin-like growth factors and fetal growth. *J Devel Physiol* 1987;9:481–5.

135 Lassare C, Hardouin S, Daffos F, Forestier F, Frankenne F, Binoux M. Serum insulin-like growth factors and their binding proteins in the human fetus. Relationships with growth in normal subjects and in subjects with intrauterine growth retardation. *Pediatr Res* 1991;29:219–25.

136 Hall K, Hansson U, Lundin G *et al.* Serum levels of somatomedins and somatomedin-binding protein in pregnant women with type I or gestational diabetes and their infants. *J Clin Endocrinol Metab* 1986;63:1300–5.

137 Wang HS, Lim J, English J, Irvine L, Chard T. The concentration of insulin-like growth factor-I and insulin-like growth factor binding protein-1 in human umbilical cord serum at delivery: relation to fetal weight. *J Endocrinol* 1991;129: 459–64.

138 Bala RM, Lopatka J, Leung A, McCoy E, McArthur RG. Serum immunoreactive somatomedin levels in normal adults, pregnant women at term, children at various ages, and children with constitutionally delayed growth. *J Clin Endocrinol Metab* 1981;52:508–12.

139 Luna AM, Wilson DM, Wibbelsman CJ *et al.* Somatomedins in adolescence: a cross-sectional study of the effect of puberty on plasma insulin-like growth factor I and II levels. *J Clin Endocrinol Metab* 1983;57:258–71.

140 Rosenfield RL, Furlanetto R, Bock D. Relationship of somatomedin-C concentrations to pubertal changes. *J Pediatr* 1983;103:723–8.

141 Cara JF, Rosenfield RL, Furlanetto RW. A longitudinal study of the relationship of plasma somatomedin-C concentration to the pubertal growth spurt. *Am J Dis Child* 1987;141: 562–4.

142 Cuttler L, Van Vliet G, Conte FA, Kaplan SL, Grumbach MM. Somatomedin-C levels in children and adolescents with gonadal dysgenesis: differences from age-matched normal females and effect of chronic estrogen replacement therapy. *J Clin Endocrinol Metab* 1985;60:1087–91.

143 Rosenfeld RG, Hintz RL, Johanson AJ *et al.* Methionyl human growth hormone and oxandrolone in Turner syndrome: preliminary results of a prospective randomized trial. *J Pediatr* 1986;109:936–40.

144 Vaccarello MA, Diamond FB Jr, Guevara-Aguirre J *et al.* Hormonal and metabolic effects and pharmacokinetics of recombinant human insulin-like growth factor-I in growth hormone receptor deficiency (GHRD)/Laron syndrome. *J Clin Endocrinol Metab* 1993;77:273–80.

145 Rudman D, Kutner MH, Rogers CM *et al.* Impaired growth hormone secretion in the adult population. *J Clin Invest* 1981;67:1361–9.

146 Johanson AJ, Blizzard RM. Low somatomedin-C levels in older men rise in response to growth hormone administration. *Johns Hopkins Med J* 1981;149:115–17.

147 Rudman D, Feller AG, Nagraj HS *et al.* Effects of human growth hormone in men over 60 years old. *N Engl J Med* 1990;323:1–6.

148 Froesch ER, Guler H-P, Schmid C, Binz K, Zapf J. Therapeutic potential of insulinlike growth factor I. *Trends Endocrinol Metab* 1990;1:254–60.

149 Gluckman P, Harding J. The regulation of fetal growth. In: Hernandez M, Argente J, eds. *Human Growth: Basic and Clinical Aspects*. New York: Elsevier, 1992:253–9.

150 Donovan SM, Oh Y, Pham H, Rosenfeld RG. Ontogeny of serum insulin-like growth factor binding proteins in the rat. *Endocrinology* 1989;125:2621–7.

151 Glasscock GF, Gelber SE, Lamson G, McGee-Tekula R, Rosenfeld RG. Pituitary control of growth in the neonatal rat: effects of neonatal hypophysectomy on somatic and organ growth, serum insulin-like growth factors (IGF)-I and

-II levels, and expression of IGF binding proteins. *Endocrinology* 1990;127:1792–803.
152 Underwood LE, Van Wyk JJ. Somatomedin-C and the assessment of growth. *Pediatr Clin N Am* 1980;27:771–82.
153 Rosenfeld RG, Wilson DM, Lee PDK, Hintz RL. Insulin-like growth factors I and II in the evaluation of growth retardation. *J Pediatr* 1986;109:428–33.
154 Moore DC, Ruvalcaba RHA, Smith EK *et al.* Plasma somatomedin-C as a screening test for growth hormone deficiency in children and adolescents. *Horm Res* 1982;16: 49–55.
155 Reiter EO, Lovinger RD. The use of a comercially available somatomedin-C radioimmunoassay in patients with disorders of growth. *J Pediatr* 1981;99:720–4.
156 Drop SLS, Valiquette G, Guyda HJ, Corvol MT, Posner BI. Partial purification and characterization of a binding protein for insulin-like activity (ILAs) in human amniotic fluid: a possible inhibitor of insulin-like activity. *Acta Endocrinol* 1979;90:505–18.
157 Rosenfeld RG, Pham H, Conover CA, Hintz RL, Baxter RC. Structural and immunological comparison of insulin-like growth factor (IGF) binding proteins of cerebrospinal and amniotic fluids. *J Clin Endocrinol* 1989;68:636–46.
158 Rosenfeld RG, Pham H, Oh Y, Lamson G, Giudice LC. Identification of insulin-like growth factor-binding protein-2 (IGF-BP-2) and a low molecular weight IGF-BP in human seminal plasma. *J Clin Endocrinol Metab* 1989;69:963–5.
159 Martin JL, Baxter RC. Insulin-like growth factor binding protein from human plasma purification and characterization. *J Biol Chem* 1986;261:8754–60.
160 Furlanetto RW. The somatomedin C binding protein: evidence for a heterologous subunit structure. *J Clin Endocrinol Metab* 1980;51:12–19.
161 Baxter RC. Characterization of the acid-labile subunit of the growth hormone-dependent insulin-like growth factor binding protein complex. *J Clin Endocrinol Metab* 1988;67: 265–72.
162 Povoa G, Roovete A, Hall K. Cross-reaction of a serum somatomedin-binding protein in a radioimmunoassay developed for somatomedin-binding protein isolated from human amniotic fluid. *Acta Endocrinol* 1984;107:563–70.
163 Baxter RC, Cowell CT. Diurnal variation of growth hormone-independent binding protein for insulin-like growth factors in human plasma. *J Clin Endocrinol Metab* 1987;65: 432–40.
164 Cohen P, Peehl DM, Stamey TA, Wilson KF, Clemmons DR, Rosenfeld RG. Elevated levels of insulin-like growth factor binding protein-2 in the serum of prostate cancer patients. *J Clin Endocrinol Metab* 1993;76:1031–5.
165 Baxter RC, Martin JL. Radioimmunoassay of growth hormone dependent insulin-like growth factor binding protein in human plasma. *J Clin Invest* 1986;78:1504–12.
166 Blum WF, Ranke MB, Kietzmann K, Gauggel E, Ziesel HJ, Bierich JR. A specific radioimmunoassay for the growth hormone-dependent somatomedin-binding protein: its use for diagnosis of GH deficiency. *J Clin Endocrinol Metab* 1990;70:1292–8.
167 Hasegawa Y, Hasegawa T, Aso T *et al.* Comparison between insulin-like growth factor-I (IGF-I) and IGF binding protein-3 (IGFBP-3) measurement in the diagnosis of growth hormone deficiency. *Endocr J* 1993;40:185–90.
168 Rosenfeld RG, Rosenbloom AL, Guevara-Aguirre J. Growth hormone (GH) insensitivity due to primary GH receptor deficiency. *Endocr Rev* 1994;15:369–90.
169 Savage MO, Blum WF, Ranke MB *et al.* Clinical features and endocrine status in patients with growth hormone insensitivity (Laron syndrome). *J Clin Endocrinol Metab* 1993 (in press).
170 Guler HP, Zapf J, Froesch ER. Short-term metabolic effects and half-lives of intravenously administered insulinlike growth factor I in healthy adults. *N Engl J Med* 1987;317: 137–40.
171 Guler HP, Schmid C, Zapf J, Froesch R. Effects of recombinant insulin-like growth factor-I on insulin secretion and renal function in normal human subjects. *Proc Natl Acad Sci USA* 1989;86:2868–72.
172 Takano K, Hizuka N, Shizume K, Asakawa K, Fujuda I, Demura H. Repeated sc administration of recombinant human insulin-like growth factor-I (IGF-I) to human subjects for seven days. *Growth Regul* 1991;1:23–8.
173 Laron Z, Erster B, Klinger B, Anin S. Effect of acute administration of insulin-like growth factor-I in patients with Laron-type dwarfism. *Lancet* 1988;2:1170–72.
174 Laron Z, Klinger B, Jensen JT, Erster B. Biochemical and hormonal changes induced by one week of administration of rIGF-I to patients with Laron type dwarfism. *Clin Endocrinol* 1991;35:145–50.
175 Grahnen A, Kåstrup K, Gourmelen M *et al.* Pharmacokinetics of recombinant human insulin-like growth factor I given subcutaneously to healthy volunteers and to patients with growth hormone receptor deficiency. *Acta Paediatr Scand* 1993;Suppl.391:9–13.
176 Walker J, Van Wyk JJ, Underwood LE. Stimulation of statural growth by recombinant insulin-like growth factor-I in a child with growth hormone insensitivity syndrome (Laron type). *J Pediatr* 1992;121:641–6.
177 Laron Z, Anin S, Klipper-Auerbach Y, Klinger B. Effects of insulin-like growth factor-I on linear growth, head circumference, and body fat in patients with Laron-type dwarfism. *Lancet* 1992;339:1258–61.
178 Wilton P (on behalf of the Kabi Pharmacia Study Group). Treatment with recombinant insulin-like growth factor-I of children with growth hormone receptor deficiency (Laron syndrome). *Acta Paediatr Scand* 1992;Suppl.282:137–41.
179 Savage MO, Wilton O, Ranke MB *et al.* Therapeutic response to recombinant IGF-I in thirty-two patients with growth hormone insensitivity. *Pediatr Res* 1993A;33(5) Suppl. Abs 17.

8: Signalling Mechanisms and Hormone Pulsatility

D.R. MATTHEWS and I.C.A.F. ROBINSON

INTRODUCTION

The concept of hormone pulsatility implies a specific regulation of both the amount and the rate of hormone released. Measurements of most hormone concentrations with sufficient frequency show that pulsatility is the rule rather than the exception, and that endocrine rhythms can range over an enormous time-scale, ranging from seasons to seconds. Pulsatility has been described for insulin, glucagon, cortisol, luteinizing hormone (LH) (see reviews in [1]), somatostatin [2], growth hormone (GH), thyroid-stimulating hormone (TSH) and prolactin. The phenomenon of oscillatory secretion is so widely found in animal physiology that it can be regarded as fundamental [3]. The pulsatile nature of the endocrine system is either so important, so efficient, so economical or so sensitive that evolution has dictated that hormones should preferentially adopt this method of signalling. Why should this be so? There are now emerging new principles and insights. We discuss here some of the theory and experimental evidence relating to endocrine pulsatility, and draw some conclusions which reflect that pulsatility may be one of the most important features of endocrinological signalling.

SIGNALLING IN A NOISY SYSTEM

It is self-evident that endocrine signals should be reliable, but less obvious that precision of any individual signal is severely limited by biological 'noise'. For example, insulin is secreted in response to a glycaemic stimulus to the pancreas, but cannot achieve euglycaemia by any simple single response. Insulin is secreted into the circulation and is subject to signal degradation immediately. The hormone is diluted; it is bound onto cells by receptors (for example erythrocytes); it is variably excreted; it is variably bound onto target organs where receptor numbers and receptor affinity may change; it is degraded intracellularly and the final signal depends on variable postreceptor mechanisms. The signal may be generally qualitative, for example an instruction to switch on hexokinase and glycolysis, but it can scarcely be quantitative. Thus, between the endocrine signal production and the body's action on the signal, lies a fog of uncertainty.

Chirp systems

One mechanism that endocrine systems have evolved to overcome the fog of uncertainty utilizes a mechanism similar to the navigation system of bats. Bats navigate by emitting high-frequency audio signals (around 22 kHz) and detecting the time delay on such signals. However, physicists were initially puzzled that it was very difficult to 'jam' bat signals. One would think that an oscillator producing a 22 kHz tone should cause the bats to crash: it had no effect. It emerged that this was because the signal was a frequency-modulated burst of sound (a 'chirp') whose reflection could be matched with the emitting chirp. Insulin is similarly secreted in chirps. The signal of such a burst is much more likely to penetrate the noise of the periphery.

Down-regulation

Down-regulation is the modern term for a phenomenon well recognized by classical physiology and called 'adaptation' or 'tachyphylaxis'. If the effect of a drug diminishes when it is given repeatedly, so that larger and larger doses have to be given to produce an equal therapeutic or pharmacological effect, the effect is described as *tolerance* in humans, and as *tachyphylaxis* in experimental animals and isolated tissues. Down-regulation would be an annoyance to a telephone engineer! The uncertainty that any signal will have the same quantifiable effect when given a second or a third time seems, at first thought, to be a mistake of biological systems. Indeed our language reflects this attitude when we speak of a system 'recovering' from down-regulation. An analogy would be the shooting of arrows at a target which diminished in size the more successful the archery. There are, however, aspects of down- and up-regulation that are adaptive and protective.

In the case of insulin, there is a wide range of basal concentrations in humans, some of the variation being related to obesity. The range is explained on the basis of varying insulin sensitivity, and can be quantified in any individual using techniques such as glucose clamping or mathematical modelling. This gives a general measure of the overall response of subjects' tissues to insulin – and some individuals are more sensitive than others. But how do individual cells 'know' whether the rest of the body is thin or fat, resistant or sensitive? The answer is simply that cells cannot know, except from the signal itself. If the mean concentration reflects the state of resistance or sensitivity, it cannot be used at the same time as a signal for 'on' (glucose uptake) or 'off' (no glucose uptake). Under these circumstances a *change* of concentration can be the signal, and the message is in the pulse and not in the mean background level. Thus down-regulation (at the receptor or postreceptor level) is probably an adaptive process, which we know works well in normal humans, for example, health is compatible with a basal insulin of 2 or 20 mU/l concentration. At the extremes of the adaptation, one observes pathological changes: resistance exacerbates non-insulin-dependent diabetes, despite high insulin concentrations, and low insulin concentrations also cause high glucose levels. Between the extremes the body is highly and successfully adaptive.

In addition to the amplitude of the signal, its pattern can have a major influence on the sensitivity of the system via down-regulation mechanisms either of the specific receptor or of postreceptor mechanisms. The classical endocrine example is the response of the gonadotroph to gonadotrophin-releasing hormone (GnRH). Intermittent pulses of GnRH induce priming and facilitate a large output of gonadotrophins, whereas continuous stimulation of the GnRH receptors by GnRH superagonists leads to a subsequent down-regulation of the gonadotroph. Induction of fertility in men and women with primary GnRH insufficiency by intermittent pulsatile infusion has a fairly narrow optimal range for both frequency and dose of GnRH [4,5], whereas down-regulation merely requires long-term maintenance of overstimulation and is always preceded by a transient stimulation. Despite suppression of feedback from gonadal hormones, which would enhance endogenous GnRH output, the system is completely refractory – the target has vanished – to re-emerge slowly as the flood of exogenous GnRH subsides.

Unfortunately, not all pituitary cells show this protective adaptation. Cushing syndrome due to ectopic adrenocorticotrophic hormone (ACTH) secretion and acromegaly with somatotroph hyperplasia in patients with continuous ectopic growth-hormone-releasing hormone (GHRH) production testify to the powerful and damaging up-regulation that these systems manifest in response to a prolonged signal [6]. For the gonadotrophs, the pituitary sensitivity to the pattern of stimulation is markedly affected by temporal changes in gonadal steroids [7]; this probably reflects changes in intracellular pathways, in addition to changes in GnRH receptor expression at the cell surface.

MAXIMIZING SIGNAL EFFICIENCY

Endocrine signalling is non-specific and inefficient in its delivery. For example, erythrocytes bind insulin without such a mechanism having any known useful effect. On the other hand, the chemical signalling of the endocrine system is a useful way of passing a simultaneous message to millions of cells. The signal efficiency may be less with slow changes of steady states than with pulsatile delivery.

Dose–response curves

A practical advantage of pulsatile hormone delivery is that higher concentrations of hormone for short periods of time achieve greater end-organ response than an identical total concentration spread over a longer time period. One such demonstrated effect is that insulin is more efficient as a hypoglycaemic agent when delivered in pulses than as a steady infusion (Fig. 8.1) [8]. The reason for this is the sigmoidal nature of the dose–response curve of receptor systems. At the low end of a dose–response curve, moderate hormonal stimuli have little effect. Doubling the dose of hormone with the same exposure time will achieve more response than doubling the exposure time. An initial midrange dose that signals at the sharply rising part of the of the curve near the EC_{50} will confer a huge increase in efficiency of signalling. So signalling is more efficient with pulses of higher concentration than continuing low-level activity. Non-physiological delivery of hormones in high doses near the top asymptote of the dose–response curve is also ineffective in its ability to change signalling. This dynamic signal characteristic is demonstrated in the observation that GH rate-of-change (modulation) is a more important factor in determining growth than duration of exposure [9]. Physiological pulsatile dosage is economical, but high pulsatile dose is wasteful.

FREQUENCY AND AMPLITUDE MODULATION

The classical concept of an endocrine signal is focused on the concentration of the hormone in the blood. In this view the receptors in target tissues are assumed to respond simply in proportion to the concentration of hormone to which they are exposed, and the task of an endocrine gland is simply to control the plasma concentration by varying the amount secreted. In other words, the system signals by detection of concentration. However, as soon as there are episodic signals, the system may signal by a variety of differing mechanisms. The amplitude of the signals may change (amplitude modulation (AM)) or the frequency

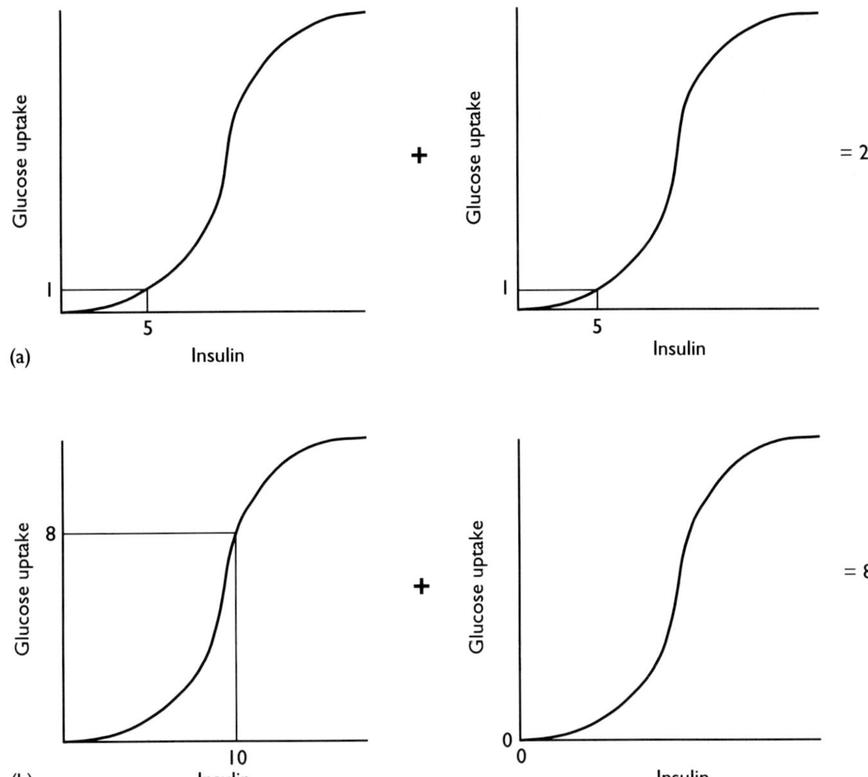

Fig. 8.1 An illustration of one reason why pulsations may be more efficient than steady insulin infusions: (a) shows how a dose of 10 insulin units can give a signal to achieve 2 units of glucose uptake if given as 5 + 5 units; (b) shows how 10 units given as a pulse (followed by zero) achieves 8 units of uptake.

may change (frequency modulation (FM)) or there may be complex combinations of both these phenomena to alter the baseline, peaks or even shape of signal pulse.

It is certain that biological signals can use both FM or AM. The classic example of FM signalling is the nervous system. All neuronal signals for transmission are frequency-coded and reamplified by nodes of Ranvier to prevent signal loss. In myelinated nerve fibres there is no component of amplitude in the signal (other than its presence or absence): all the data transmission is binary FM. By contrast, the oxytocin response for milk 'let-down' is related to the size of the hormone stimulus amplitude and is an AM signal. What is now emerging is that no biological system utilizes pure AM or pure FM. The nervous system uses synapses for integration of amplitude-based signals, and the endocrine system uses FM as a tuning superimposed on otherwise generally AM-mediated signals. For example, secretion of both insulin and GH is highly pulsatile. Frequency domains can be easily demonstrated, but signalling changes are often related predominantly to AM. The task of the endocrine system can be perceived as ensuring that the pattern and timing of hormone release is optimized.

Peaks and troughs

Amplitude modulation may not depend for its signalling on peak concentrations alone. The trough concentrations in pulsatile signalling may be equally important – to maintain tone or to prevent down-regulation. One may characterize these aspects by use of calculated 5% or 95% concentration domains – OC_5 and OC_{95} [10]; GH data demonstrate an evolution of an OC_5 which increases into puberty and then declines to a low adult value. The change in the OC_5 is one of the dominant differences detectable in GH profiles. OC_{95} alters at the same time, but the changes appear not to be equally distributed since a 10-fold decrease in trough concentrations has been observed in contrast to only a 4-fold reduction in OC_{95} values.

Secretion – reaction time lags

Feedback principles apply to many hormone systems. One of the shortest feedback loops studied is that of insulin and glucose. Glucose rises in the body; insulin rises to clear the glucose; the glucose falls; insulin secretion falls. This feedback loop, or limit cycle, settles to a point predictable from the non-linearities of the system [11]. But the body does not function in such a straightforward way. There are significant time lags in the system. Insulin

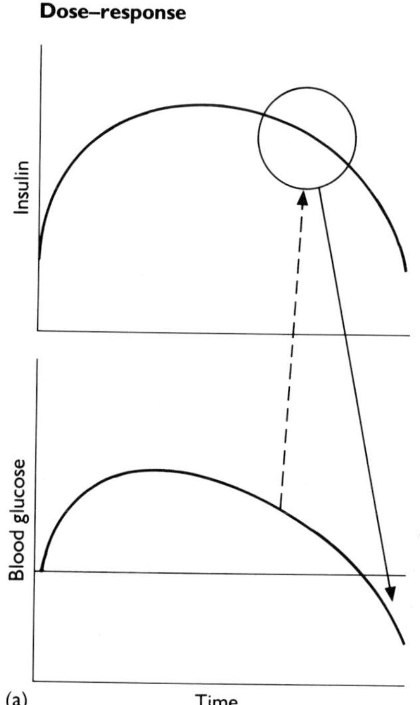

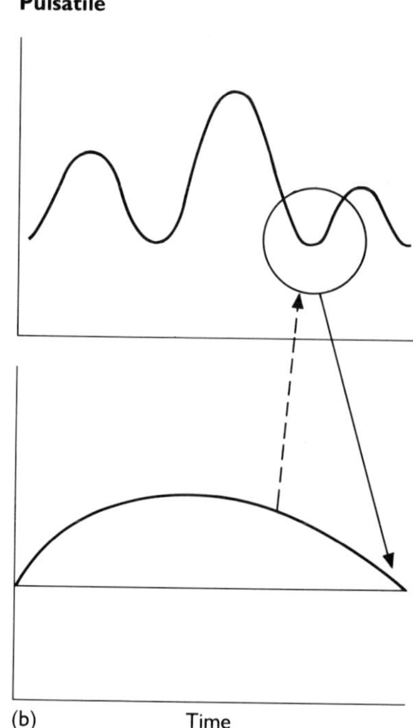

Fig. 8.2 (a) Demonstrates how reactive hypoglycaemia occurs if insulin is secreted as a direct function (dashed line) of glucose concentration. Because of the delay in insulin action the insulin circled causes later hypoglycaemia (solid line). (b) With pulsatile secretion hypoglycaemia is less likely as insulin secretion moves through refractory phases (circle).

is secreted by the β cells within 1 min of the glucose concentration rising; on the other hand glucose takes a significant time to clear in the presence of hyperinsulinaemia, so that it takes about 15 min to observe the maximal rate of decline of glucose and about 45 min before the nadir of glucose occurs (Fig. 8.2) [12]. In addition, insulin continues to act for some time after the peripheral concentrations have returned to normal. With time lags inherent in the system it becomes important that the control loop does not function solely on the basis of β cell secretion, being a moment-by-moment 'reading' of a glucose insulin dose–response curve. If this were to occur, major problems of insulin excess would be encountered.

By analogy, one can take the case of a patient admitted to hospital with a high blood glucose, for whom insulin treatment is a necessity. The attending physician would measure the glucose concentration and might give a single dose of insulin. It would be unwise immediately to measure the glucose again, find it high and give another injection, measure it again, find it high, and give a third! The knowledgeable physician departs for an interval and returns at some suitable time with expectations of limited success. At this point more insulin might be prescribed on the basis of both the current glucose concentration and the rate of fall of glucose.

Pulsatile insulin secretion from the pancreas follows much the same strategy. Hyperglycaemia triggers insulin secretion, but *not* simply on the basis of a dose–response curve. The secretion is in the form of a finite 'package' (which gives rise to a pulse), and the pancreas then becomes quiescent for about 13 min (a time course analogous to the time lag of 15 min for maximal declination of glucose). The evidence is that secretion actually switches off for this time period [13] and then recommences depending on the new glucose level. Under these conditions the total secretion is less, and the glucose has an opportunity to react before the advent of the next pulse. The result is a more precise achievement of normoglycaemia.

Differential signalling

Differential signalling becomes a possibility where receptor dose–response curves are different in differing tissues. An example of such a system in humans is the differential sensitivity of the hepatocyte and peripheral cells to insulin concentration change. In the fasting state there needs to be enough insulin to allow glucose clearance into peripheral tissues (an 'on' signal) while the hepatocytes should be allowed to continue gluconeogenesis (an 'off' signal). The amplitude of the insulin signal may be a factor which achieves this. At the same time double hormone signalling may be a crucial mechanism for mediating successful differential effects. Using the same example of gluconeogenesis it may be that glucagon secretion is the prime mechanism for allowing different hepatic and peripheral messages.

Principles of pattern recognition

In principle, the ability to detect different hormonal patterns of exposure could be a property of the receptor protein itself, for example of its turnover kinetics. On the other hand, pattern sensitivity could also be a property of the many different intracellular systems, to which the receptor is biochemically coupled. It is also possible that receptors may couple to more than one transducing system with differing abilities to respond to transient stimuli. Hormone binding may induce a rapid membrane event (such as opening an ion channel), a slower biochemical change (for example phosphorylation of rate-limiting enzymes which stimulate other proteins) and a long-term signal (such as a switch on of gene expression). In extreme cases the latter could even involve a non-reversible change in the differentiation of a cell or cell system (for example central nervous system differentiation during critical periods of exposure to androgens or thyroid hormone). It is clear that the difference between a pulsatile or continuous exposure of a hormone at different concentrations can be transduced into different cellular responses in several systems, but how this is achieved remains obscure.

MAXIMIZING SIGNAL PRODUCTION EFFICIENCY

Pulsatile signals may optimize receptor functions, but they may also simply be a way in which endocrine organs can most efficiently create the signal.

Pulsatility as an efficient release mechanism

Secretion from neuronal cells depends on electrophysiological activation to induce a rise in intracellular calcium; the amount of neurotransmitter released is increased over a certain range by increasing the frequency of firing, a process known as frequency facilitation. Oxytocin, vasopressin and all of the hypothalamic hypophysiotropic hormones are products of neuroendocrine cells, and the output of these hormones has also been shown to exhibit frequency facilitation. For an individual neuroendocrine cell, hormone secretion is determined largely by the frequency of action potentials invading the terminals, which contain hormone stored in granules; release is by a process of exocytosis. The timing of these impulses is determined by the afferent neural input to the cells. On the other hand, the amount of hormone released from a cell in response to a single depolarization event will be determined also by the amount of biosynthesis, transport and storage of the hormone in a releasable pool. The 'fullness' of this pool will of course depend on the recent history of secretory activity, and the balance between the rate of depletion and the ability of synthetic mechanisms to refill the stores.

Single and multiple cellular reactions

It is important to distinguish between the properties of a single cell and those of the population as a whole, since it is the population response that determines the overall pattern of hormone release into the bloodstream. This is well illustrated by the posterior pituitary hormones, oxytocin and vasopressin. These are released into the blood-stream in response to specific stimuli (suckling, dehydration) and stimulate specific receptors in peripheral target tissues (mammary myoepithelial cells, renal collecting duct cells) to elicit their biological responses (milk ejection, antidiuresis). However, the pattern of plasma hormone release is very different between the two hormone systems.

During suckling, oxytocin is released in a highly episodic pattern, and the large sharp increase of oxytocin is necessary to elicit a sharp rise in intramammary pressure causing milk 'let-down' to the suckling infant. In marked contrast, dehydration induces a much more modest and gradual rise in plasma vasopressin concentration, but this is maintained over a longer time period to promote water reabsorption at the kidneys. Thus these closely related neuroendocrine systems with very similar peptide structures and similar anatomical and cellular organization show a completely different pattern of activation.

Control of pulsatile hormone release: neural mechanisms

The size and location of hypothalamic cell bodies and the projection of their axons to the posterior pituitary has made it possible to record electrically from identified oxytocin or vasopressin cells to see how the electrophysiological activation brings about these different release patterns (Fig. 8.3). Such recordings from oxytocin cells during spontaneous milk ejection in experimental animals have shown that the oxytocin pulse is preceded by an intense short burst of action potentials. However, if this occurred at different times in different cells, there would be no coordinated pulse of oxytocin in the blood. It seems that all of the oxytocin cells capable of firing in this pattern are somehow synchronized to fire over 1 or 2 s, and it is this synchrony of the population of cells that causes the large brief pulse of oxytocin to be released from the pituitary gland.

Using the same techniques to record from vasopressin cells, it has been shown that the individual cells increase their firing rate in a phasic fashion and do not show synchrony. The result is that vasopressin is increased much more gradually from the posterior pituitary, and it is this relatively small but prolonged change in plasma vasopressin concentration which increases water reabsorption at the kidney to counteract the osmotic stimulus of dehydration.

The hypothalamic-releasing factors are also products of neuronal terminals at the median eminence, whence they are carried by the hypophyseal portal circulation to the anterior pituitary gland to stimulate or inhibit hormone

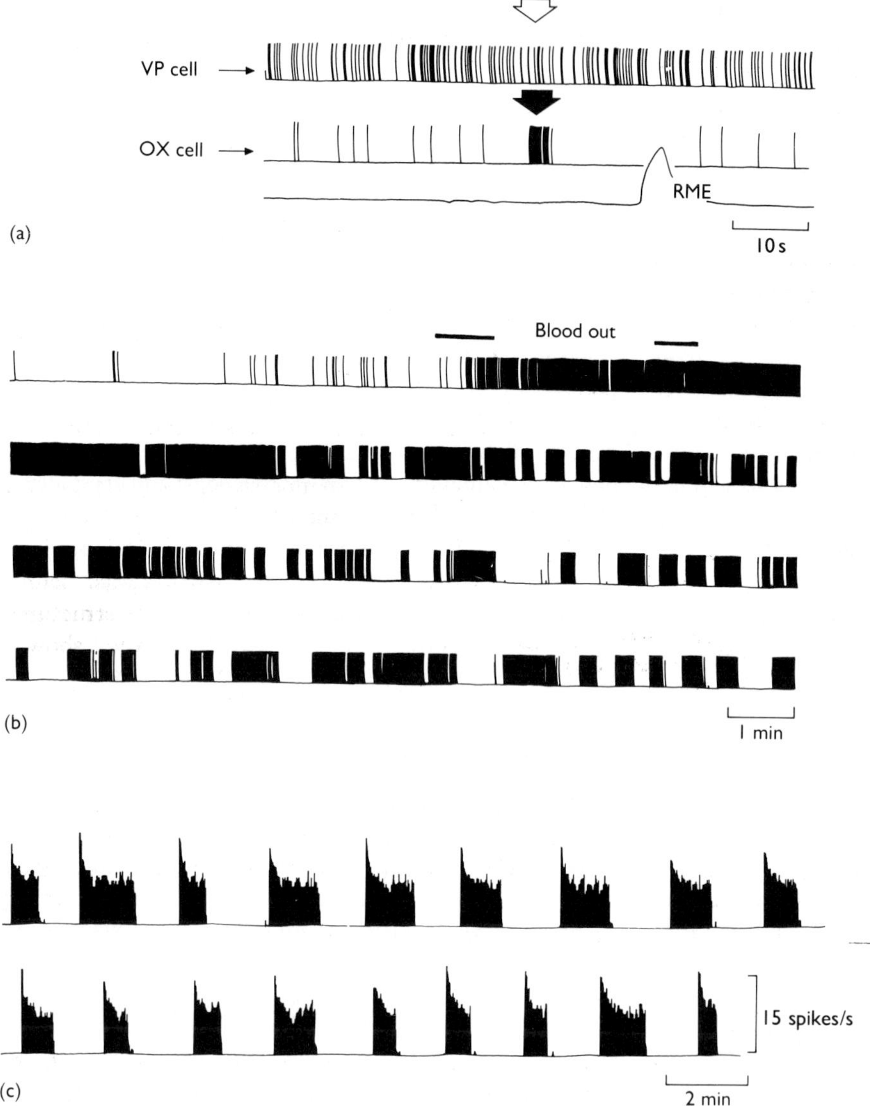

Fig. 8.3 Although very similar in many ways, oxytocin (OX) and vasopressin (VP) cells show very different firing patterns when activated. (a) During suckling, oxytocin cells in the supraoptic nucleus show a spontaneous high-frequency discharge (solid arrow), followed 15 s later by a rise in intramammary pressure as the released oxytocin reaches the mammary gland to cause reflex milk ejection (RME). Recordings from vasopressin cells show no change in activity at this time (open arrow). (b) Haemorrhage is a selective stimulus for vasopressin release. Recordings from vasopressin neurons in the supraoptic nucleus show that blood withdrawal induces neuronal firing which then develops into a phasic firing pattern. (c) Phasic activity can also be observed in such neurons *in vitro* when they are activated by a stimulus such as glutamate (from Wakerley [14]).

output from the different pituitary cell types. When sufficiently rapid sampling methods have been applied, all anterior pituitary hormones have been shown to be secreted in an episodic fashion, although the frequency of pulsatility varies from system to system. While *in vitro* studies of isolated pituitary cells have shown that spontaneous basal hormone release can also show oscillatory behaviour, and this could be enhanced *in vivo* by a degree of cell–cell communication within the pituitary gland, it appears that the major determinant of the pattern of pulsatile secretion of anterior pituitary hormones is the pattern and amount of hypothalamic-releasing hormones. Where it has been possible to measure these directly in hypophyseal portal blood, the pulsatile nature of their output has also been confirmed. It has proved more difficult to obtain electrophysiological recordings from releasing factor neurons, but it is likely that the sizeable pulses of GnRH, thyrotrophin-releasing hormone (TRH) or corticotrophin-releasing hormone (CRH) measured in portal blood imply some degree of synchronization of pulsatile output of many individual neurons, as shown for the oxytocin system.

The search for the anatomical location of the 'pulse generators' in these systems has been under way for several years, but has not yet borne fruit. It is possible that they are driven by a more generalized biological clock, such as is thought to arise from the circadian activity of the suprachiasmatic nucleus, and it is also possible that rhythmicity arises from the interconnections of the releasing factor neurons themselves, perhaps being triggered by an external input. There is intriguing evidence for intrinsic rhythmicity in the suprachiasmatic nucleus which can be observed *in vitro*, and there is evidence in a variety of species that these rhythms may be specified by particular genes. However, it is still poorly understood how neural mechanisms which vary over the millisecond to minute time-scale, can accurately determine endocrine rhythms, the cycle lengths of which may vary from days to months. Paracrine feedback has been suggested as one mechanism whereby insulin secretion can be turned on and off with a periodicity of 13 min (for example by somatostatin), and there is evidence from cellular studies that internal biochemical mechanisms can generate phasic events – for example the glycolytic oscillator.

CONTROL OF PULSATILE RELEASE: INTEGRATIVE MECHANISMS AT THE PITUITARY

It should be borne in mind, however, that it is frequently the case that there may be no tight link between releasing factor pulses and hormone pulses, and that other factors modify the pattern of output for any given pattern of input. This non-linearity is seen in the pituitary secretory response to hypothalamic input, and is well illustrated by the gonadotroph and somatotroph systems. In the GnRH/gonadotrophin system LH output is pulsatile, and pulses of GnRH induce pulses of LH. Yet, as has been described, continuous exposure of the same cells to GnRH produces a dramatic down-regulation of GnRH receptors and a reduced LH output. In this extreme case a GnRH agonist given in pulses can stimulate LH and induce ovulation, whereas the same compound given continuously will suppress LH output and block ovulation. The cellular basis of this response in the gonadotroph has not yet been fully explained, and may be relatively specific in that a similar dramatic down-regulation in receptors has not been observed in other releasing factor systems. For example, growth-hormone-releasing factor (GHRF) is also secreted in a pulsatile fashion, and stimulates pulsatile GH output (provided somatostatin secretion is low) but prolonged continuous GHRF exposure also causes an increased GH output and does not induce significant pituitary desensitization.

The GH system illustrates another aspect of the response of the pituitary gland to conflicting inputs. In addition to the GHRH, GH release is also controlled by the secretion of somatostatin, which inhibits both basal GH output and GH release induced by GHRF. Episodic GH release can be achieved both by a pulsatile secretion of GHRF and by a continuous exposure to GHRF in the presence of a varying somatostatin tone. Indeed, rapid removal of somatostatin can induce a rebound release of GH, although the magnitude of this may be smaller in humans than in experimental animals. These observations show that the balance and pattern of GHRF and somatostatin is an important determinant of the resultant secretory pattern of GH (Fig. 8.4). A similar interaction, this time resulting in a synergy

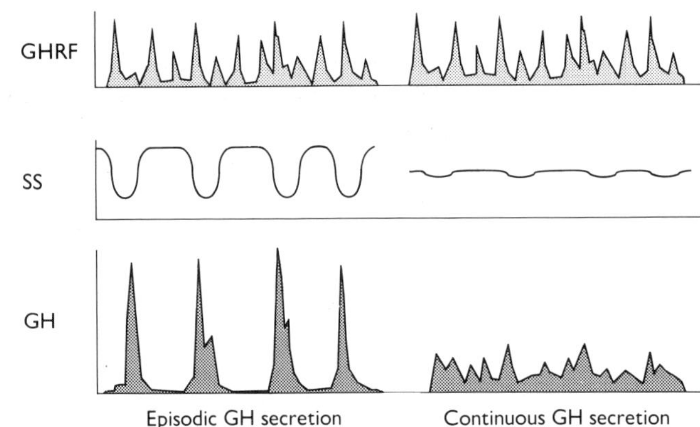

Fig. 8.4 The pattern of GH secretion is determined by the interactions between somatostatin (SS) and GH-releasing factor (GHRF). GHRF pulses are necessary for GH pulses to occur, but the GH output is ultimately determined by variations in somatostatin tone. Not all GHRF pulses cause GH release, and these may be important in building up GH stores, so that higher GH peaks eventually result when the SS blockade is removed. The figure shows schematically how the same GHRF pattern can produce all the features of either episodic (high peaks, low baseline) or continuous (multiple irregular peaks, high baseline) GH secretion simply by interacting with different patterns of SS release.

rather than antagonistic effect, is seen in the control of pulsatile ACTH release where the releasing effect of corticotrophin-releasing factor (CRF) is markedly enhanced by concentrations of vasopressin which have little ACTH-releasing activity in their own right.

SIGNAL RECEPTION

In the foregoing we have discussed the signalling inherent in the concentration and temporal profiles of circulating hormones. Implicit in this discussion is the notion that there are receptors in peripheral target tissues which can detect these patterns and produce an appropriate response. There are many clinical examples of the failure to detect or to respond to a normal hormonal signal (for example testicular feminization, Laron syndrome and nephrogenic diabetes insipidus). There are also examples of relative insensitivity of the cellular system to the signal, the most well known being that of so-called insulin resistance. In general, protein and polypeptide hormones act by binding to receptors expressed on the cell surface, and this stimulation is transmitted by activation of a variety of second-messenger systems coupled to the receptor. By contrast, steroid and thyroid hormone receptors are essentially transcription factors that bind to and activate the expression of particular genes (that is those that have specific sequences of DNA called response elements which, when bound by hormone/receptor complexes, mediate a change in the rate of transcription of the gene). This does not exclude other possible signal transduction mechanisms, such as membrane effects of steroids or their metabolites, or nuclear effects of translocated protein hormone receptor complexes after internalization.

A common feature of endocrine signalling mechanisms is the triggering of biochemical response cascades, each with their own kinetics and rate-limiting steps. This has several important implications when comparing the output signal with the input signal. First, two responses to the same signal can have a very different time-course (compare the few seconds required to achieve a maximal secretory response in an anterior pituitary cell, with the hours or even days for the maximal rise in protein synthesis in response to gene transcription stimulated by the same signal). Second, the response to repeated endocrine signals will be governed by the overall kinetics of all the elements in the biochemical cascade between receptor binding and cellular response, which includes such diverse parameters as rate of calcium release and subsequent uptake, rates of phosphorylation or dephosphorylation of protein kinase substrates and the half-lives of messenger (m)RNAs following activated gene expression. A biochemical response which has a half-time of up to a maximum of 6 h may well be stimulated most effectively by stimuli repeated every hour rather than by a continuous stimulus (because of the properties of the receptor), but the kinetics of the response mechanism dictates that it can be manifest only by an increased amplitude, rather than frequency, of the output response.

The peripheral filter

Hormones have to traverse a number of diffusion barriers *en route* from secretory cell to target cell, while travelling in a fluid which does its best to clear small molecules at a very rapid rate. This is a positive advantage to pulsatile signalling since the decay from a pulse peak is rapid. The compartments and distribution volumes differ substantially between peptide and protein hormones compared with steroid and thyroid hormones, which must also traverse the target cell membrane to act in the nucleus. Tissue uptake and enzymatic degradation processes compete with receptor binding for the signalling molecules, and their rates are also proportional to hormone concentration in the plasma. Variations in clearance mechanisms will also alter the net hormone bioavailability, whether by tissue damage, as in diseases which limit renal or hepatic clearance function, or by alterations in the amount or binding capacity of circulating proteins which can hold a reservoir of hormone in the circulation.

Circulating binding proteins have long been recognized as a part of steroid and thyroid endocrine signalling, the equilibrium between free and bound forms altering the kinetics of any induced change in endogenous or exogenous hormone [15]. In extreme cases a circulating reservoir of bound hormone can constitute the major endocrine 'tissue', as for example with the insulin-like growth factors (IGFs). Far from being an uninteresting pharmacokinetic nuisance, the circulating IGF-binding protein complexes seem to offer a major site for control of IGF action [16,17]. Exogenous IGF is rapidly complexed and its half-life greatly prolonged when protein-bound [18]. Shifts of IGF between different binding protein complexes can serve to control the bioavailability of circulating IGF to the tissues, and this in turn is affected by related hormones, such as GH and insulin.

Binding protein production is separately regulated by hormones and nutrition, and probably occurs in the vicinity of many sites of IGF action, to regulate local bioavailability of the hormones. Steroid-binding proteins may be produced locally in some tissue compartments (for example the testes) to regulate the access and bioavailability of both paracrine and endocrine steroids. To complete the circle some binding proteins may themselves be regulated by the concentration or timing of the hormone signal, and could even provide some guide as to hormonal responsiveness under some circumstances [19].

Plasma-binding proteins are usually regarded as bridesmaids, readily relinquishing their cargo to the waiting receptor grooms who show much greater avidity for their hormonal brides. However, this is not always the case. For example, one of the circulating binding proteins for GH derives from the extracellular domain of the GH receptor, has only slightly lower binding affinity than the membrane-bound receptor and can compete with receptors for GH action [20]. The specific GH-binding protein (GHBP) has a profound effect on GH clearance, and acts like a high-pass filter on the GH signal. Large pulses rapidly saturate the limited binding capacity and most of an endogenous pulse escapes circulating GHBP. On the other hand, low concentrations of GH on the waning edge of a GH pulse are retained in the circulation, and may act as a slow-release reservoir of GH [21]. Curiously, GH upregulates both GH receptors and GHBP, but only when given in a prolonged continuous infusion and not as discrete pulses, so there appears to be some sort of autoregulatory system linking secretory signal pattern, receptor responsiveness and hormone clearance mechanisms. Furthermore it is primarily one GH target tissue, the liver, that pours this protein into the circulation to modulate the GH signal to other GH targets.

All these peripheral influences on concentration, distribution and elimination of hormones have a major impact on the endocrine signal so that interpretation of signals by simple measurements of hormone concentration in serial samples of peripheral blood can be very difficult. Methods have been devised, both to describe pulsatility more objectively and to attempt to 'deconvolute' the secretory signal from the hormone's concentration/time profile in blood [22,23]. While this yields much useful information about the secretory behaviour of the endocrine tissue originating the signal, one should remember that it is the fully convoluted signal that is presented to the receptor.

SIGNAL RECOGNITION

Receptor-binding constraints

The first stage of signal recognition invariably involves ligand binding, and this is conventionally studied using radiolabelled ligands, although in the years to come it is likely that this will also be studied directly using physical, optical and electronic methods. Although a cell without an appropriate receptor will not be able to receive the hormone signal, the converse does not hold true. The presence of a receptor protein does not guarantee that ligand binding will signal to that cell; for example, many circulating blood cells express hormone receptors without obvious functional significance. Nor is it always the case that the intrinsic ligand-binding specificity of receptors will prevent cross-talk of other related ligands. For example, aldosterone signalling via the mineralocorticoid receptor in some tissues would be swamped by glucocorticoid binding without the protection of 11-hydroxysteroid dehydrogenase, which is a receptor-independent method of sharpening specificity in mineralocorticoid signalling [24].

Information in an FM signal also places demands on the kinetics of receptor response. Determination of association and dissociation rate constants and receptor concentrations is essential to be able to estimate the signalling power of any given receptor to detect a change in hormone concentration with time. There are conflicting requirements for receptors to detect frequent hormone pulses. Rapid responses require rapid association rates, but high-affinity binding requires slower dissociation rates. Surface receptors generally internalize their ligands either as part of the signalling process or in a degradation cycle, and this receptor turnover process will limit the ability of a receptor system to follow frequent hormone signals. Binding studies are performed at long incubation times approaching equilibrium kinetics, and calculations are made to determine the extent of receptor occupancy. This is very different from the *in vivo* situation. For pulsatile hormone secretion, binding is always in non-equilibrium conditions, the hormone concentrations are subject to partition between several compartments as well as differing rates of elimination reactions and the fractional occupancy of receptors is invariably low. It will be the rate of association or dissociation, as well as the occupancies achieved over a few seconds, that transduces a pulsatile (as opposed to continuous) hormone signal.

Molecular basis of signalling

Until recently the structural information about how receptors meet this challenge has been relatively scant. Receptors are usually large and complicated proteins, frequently glycosylated and sometimes with multiple subunits, not readily amenable to experimental manipulation. This has changed dramatically in the past few years with the application of molecular biology. From a minimal amount of protein sequence information, cDNA libraries can be screened with specific probes to identify clones containing all or part of the nucleotide sequence coding for the receptor of interest. Translation of this sequence gives the sequence of the protein and from analysis of this, structural predictions about the receptor can be made. For example, potential glycosylation sites can be identified, predictions of the regions most likely to be intracellular or extracellular, and the number of transmembrane domains can be estimated, although these are predictions – they still require experimental verification.

Similar considerations for the steroid receptors have enabled the delineation of several different domains which are homologous across wide classes of receptors. These include domains involved in ligand binding, binding of accessory proteins, nuclear translocation signals, DNA binding and transcriptional activation [25]. This has led in turn to the detailed definition of the hormone response elements in DNA, which are the short stretches of DNA through which the receptors enhance or repress expression of their target genes. Progress in this field has been astonishing, and many receptors are now cloned purely by functional assays or by homologies in common domains without requiring any initial protein sequence data.

It has long been known that it is possible to group together structurally similar 'families' of hormones, based on their amino acid sequences. Biochemical studies on the mechanism of action of many hormones have identified similar 'family' groupings in terms of the type of signalling mechanisms involved (such as activation or inhibition of adenylate or guanylate cyclases, protein or tyrosine kinases or phosphoinositol turnover). One feature emerging from the avalanche of sequence data on new hormone receptors is that these receptors can also be grouped in similar families on the basis of structural homologies and common signal transduction mechanisms [26,27]. This can be extended to include superfamilies, the members of which represent many different signalling systems other than endocrine (cytokines, tissue growth factors, sensory signalling systems, neurotransmitters, developmental regulators). Some members of the GH/prolactin/cytokine receptor superfamily are shown in Fig 8.5 and this family is still enlarging [26].

The appearance of conserved regions of sequence which correspond with functional 'domains' in the receptor may

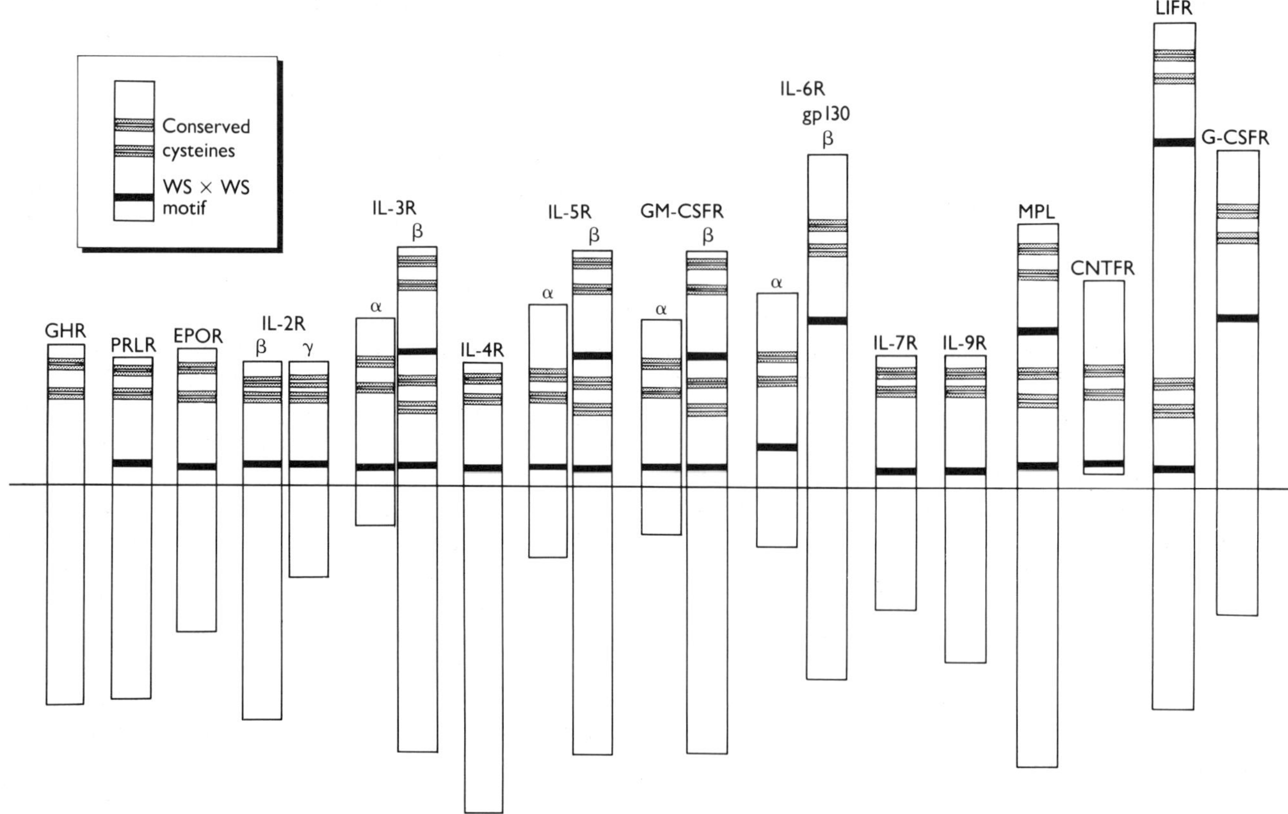

Fig. 8.5 The GH and prolactin (PRL) receptors are now recognized to be members of a much larger family of receptors sharing similar structural features, including many cytokine receptors. A conserved cysteine-rich domain, and a pentapeptide WS × WS motif can be recognized in most members of the family. The intracellular domains may vary dramatically in length both within and between receptor families, while the extracellular domains provide ligand-binding specificity and undergo homo-, or hetero-oligomerization (updated from Kelly *et al.* [26]).

also shed light on the evolutionary relationship between the different hormone and non-hormonal receptor systems. As a generalization the concept that 'similarity in structure equals similarity in signalling mechanism' has proved of value, although, as more details emerge within each superfamily of receptors, it turns out that differences in the proteins involved in the intracellular transduction of the hormone/receptor signal are emerging. In future, it is likely that receptor transduction families will also be recognized, which share the same key intracellular enzymes across each superfamily structural lineage [28].

One of the most elegant experimental verifications of key signalling regions is to form chimaeric receptors by 'domain swapping', which allows one ligand to signal through a different receptor. The success of this process in several systems suggests that the domain functions are surprisingly independent of the structure of the ligand. It is also clear that nature can use the same interactions between related families of receptors [29].

Receptor diversity allows signal diversity or differential recognition of different components of a complex signal waveform. One hormone may have several distinct receptors activating different intracellular pathways which may be expressed on the same or different cell types. For example, vasopressin has at least two receptor types (V1 and V2 types) activating different biochemical mechanisms (phospholipase or adenylate cyclase activities), with dose–response curves over quite different concentration ranges: antidiuresis occurs maximally at a 10–20-fold lower circulating vasopressin concentration than that necessary to cause a rise in blood pressure. Somatostatin provides another example: both binding studies and bioassays with hundreds of different analogues have shown that it is possible to separate many of the biological activities of this pleiotropic peptide, which could best be explained by different receptor subtypes. Currently, at least five distinct somatostatin receptors have been cloned, not counting post-translational modifications which could alter the properties of each one further. Given the widespread distribution of somatostatin and its effects in many different tissues, it will be of great interest to discover which receptor subtype subserves which function of somatostatin, since analogues already exist which will be able to target each of these subtypes specifically, and provide new opportunities for more specific diagnosis and therapeutic intervention [30].

By 'choosing' which receptor subtype to express, different tissues can determine which type of intracellular signal is activated by the same extracellular ligand. Even for the same transduction mechanism, the expression of multiple receptors with different affinity states for ligand binding may explain how different hormone concentrations at 'peak' or 'trough' levels are able to send different signals to one cell and its neighbour. This requires both complex encoding of the signal broadcast by the secretory cell and a 'decision' taken by the receiving cell as to which part(s) of the signal it wishes to receive.

It is difficult to overstate the impact that developments in molecular biology have already had in our understanding of hormone/receptor signalling. Probes can be designed to localize mRNAs for hormones or their receptors in different tissues by *in situ* hybridization, which can indicate hitherto unrecognized hormonal targets (for example GH receptor mRNA in fetal tissues [31]); many hormonal peptides and receptors are found in lymphocytes, with scant idea as to their functions. Molecular techniques have also identified variants of hormones or their receptors in different tissues [32]. These methods make it possible to identify and determine the sequence of mutations in hormones or receptors in individual patients which can then shed considerable light on the importance of particular amino acids in the signalling mechanisms in either ligand or its receptor [33]. While knowledge of the exact molecular mutation in an endocrine disease rarely enables us to correct the defect therapeutically, it makes it possible to model it experimentally *in vitro*, or even *in vivo*, by transgenesis or homologous recombination in mice. Not only will this enable us to study the consequences of this failure in signal transmission, it will also provide relevant models with which to test new therapeutic strategies. For example, the knowledge that a particular receptor mutation leads to impaired but residual thyroid signalling function provides a rational basis for attempts to overcome incomplete end-organ resistance with much-increased doses of hormone replacement therapy [34].

There are many points in the receptor signalling mechanism which are susceptible to mutational disruption and can vary from deletions of all or parts of the binding domains, down to single amino acid residues which are critical for transduction [35]. There are examples in the nuclear receptor systems which can lead to relative or complete insensitivity by changes in steroid or DNA binding, leading to partial or complete inactivation or even dominant inhibitory mutations [36]. A common theme across a wide variety of receptors is a secondary multimeric interaction following initial ligand binding. Steroid receptors, like other transcription factors, appear to function as dimers in complex with other proteins, binding to hormone response elements which contain direct or palindromic repeat motifs. Many polypeptide hormone receptors also assemble as homomeric or heteromeric oligomers. Ligand induces dimer or tetramer formation, or oligomers with other proteins to form activated complexes. Inactivating mutations can then occur which leave ligand binding intact, but block formation of multimers or prevent the binding or activation of other proteins in these oligomeric assemblies. These will also disrupt cell signalling and may be recognized as clinical end-organ resistance states.

A landmark in this field was the establishment of the first crystallographic structural analysis of a protein hormone/receptor binding site (Plate 8.1, facing p. 290) [37]. This involved binding of the extracellular domain of the human GH receptor (GHR) and human GH, both produced by recombinant DNA technology [38]. A major surprise was that GH could bind in both a 1 : 1 and a 1 : 2 stoichiometry, using two different faces of the GH molecule to bind to the equivalent site in two receptor molecules. Kinetic studies showed clearly that GH can indeed bind to one or two molecules of GH receptor in a concentrationdependent fashion, that the binding was sequential, that the dimerization of the GH receptor was important in signal transduction in several cell-based assays, and that it was possible to design GH analogues that bound tightly to one site on the GH receptor but failed to induce dimer formation; these acted as GH antagonists [39].

As already mentioned, the GH and PRL receptors belong to a superfamily of receptors which includes cytokine and haematopoietic factor receptors, and binding of the hormone/receptor complex as heterodimers or trimers with accessory proteins is an important signalling mechanism in these systems. It is not yet clear whether other accessory proteins are involved in additional binding to the GH/GH receptor complex, but some of the intracellular signalling steps are beginning to be unravelled [40], and it is possible to begin modelling the first steps in the signalling process.

One intriguing finding for GH is that the dimer complex is dissociated in the presence of large amounts of GH, which is thus self-inhibitory. While this might be seen as a self-protective mechanism, the concentrations required are vast, and high GH self-evidently causes acromegaly, so it is unlikely that a self-inhibitory mechanism operates over the physiological range of GH concentrations. However, it is still unclear whether the monomer/dimer interchange is important in discriminating pulsatile vs. continuous hormone exposure, nor whether it influences receptor internalization and turnover, which has an important bearing on the kinetics of GH signalling [41]. Is dimerization necessary for all signalling via the GH receptor or can a different set of signals be produced by GH receptor monomers? Is it possible to eliminate GH entirely and induce dimerization of the receptors by some other mechanism (antibodies can act as hormone agonists by inducing dimerization of hormone receptors in the absence of the hormone signal), or can cells reduce the effects of GH by other factors which interfere with receptor dimerization? These are not simply theoretical questions: there are reported examples of normal or even excessive growth in the presence of little or no circulating GH, which could be explained by autoimmunity to GH receptors causing dimer formation, or point mutations in the receptors which lead to constitutive dimer formation. These questions are relevant for all hormone/receptor signalling systems which show oligomerization, and can be addressed at the molecular level once equivalent structural information becomes available.

One way to affect the reception of a complex hormone signal is to alter the threshold for detection, or the gain of the receiver. In endocrine terms this is commonly achieved by varying the amount of receptor expressed in different cells, either long term, as during development, or short term in response to changes in the physiological environment, such as nutrition, temperature or stress. When one considers a 'normal range' of hormone concentration, implicit in this assumption is an equivalent 'normal range' for receptor sensitivity. A change in receptor sensitivity will have a dramatic effect on the efficacy of a hormone, with no change in its blood hormone concentration. This is difficult to study in isolation and impossible in every patient, for whom we would ideally like individual data on responsiveness. Yet in practice that is what the diabetologist does to assess individual insulin requirements, and all diabetic patients recognize when their responses to the prescribed insulin dose vary with exercise, stress or infection. Whilst the information content of any endocrine signal can be assessed by an accurate measure of the hormone concentration–time profile, its physiological meaning will be clarified only when the mechanisms of signal reception and transduction in the target tissues are more fully understood. Since we already know that receptor signalling is complex and subject to a variety of non-linear inputs, and that most endocrine signals also regulate their own reception directly or indirectly by feedforward or feedback loops, our understanding of the receptor side of hormone signalling is also somewhat foggy!

REFERENCES

1 Krieger DT. Rhythms in CRF, ACTH, and corticosteroids. In: Krieger DT, ed. *Endocrine Rhythms*. New York: Raven Press, 1979:123–42.

2 Stagner JI, Samols E, Weir GC. Sustained oscillations of insulin, glucagon and somatostatin from the isolated canine pancreas during exposure to a constant glucose concentration. *J Clin Invest* 1980;65:939–42.

3 DiStefano JJ, Stubberud AR, Williams IJ. *Theory and Problems of Feedback Control Systems*. New York: McGraw Hill, 1976.

4 Whitcomb R, Crowley W. Diagnosis and treatment of isolated gonadotropin-releasing hormone deficiency in men. *J Clin Endocrinol Metab* 1990;70:3–7.

5 Martin K, Santoro N, Hall J, Filicori M, Wierman M, Crowley W. Management of ovulatory disorders with pulsatile gonadotropin-releasing hormone. *J Clin Endocrinol Metab* 1990;71:1081A–G.

6 Sano T, Asa SL, Kovacs K. Growth hormone-releasing hormone-producing tumors: clinical, biochemical, and morphological manifestations. *Endocr Rev* 1988;9:357–73.

7 Kalra SP. Mandatory neuropeptide-steroid signaling for the preovulatory luteinizing-hormone-releasing hormone discharge. *Endocr Rev* 1993;14:507–38.

8 Matthews DR, Naylor BA, Jones RG, Ward GM, Turner RC. Pulsatile insulin has greater hypoglycaemic effect than continuous delivery. *Diabetes* 1983;32:617–21.

9 Hindmarsh PC, Matthews DR, Stratton I, Pringle PJ, Brook CGD. Rate of change (modulation) of serum growth hormone concentration is a more important factor in determining growth rate than duration of exposure. *Clin Endocrinol* 1992; 36:165–70.

10 Matthews DR, Hindmarsh PC, Pringle PJ, Brook CGD. A distribution method for analysing the baseline of pulsatile endocrine signals as exemplified by 24H growth hormone profiles. *Clin Endocrinol* 1991;35:245–52.

11 Matthews DR, Holman RR, Turner RC. Physiology of insulin secretion; problems of quantity and timing. *Neth J Med* 1985;28:20–4.

12 Matthews DR. Physiological implications of pulsatile hormone secretion. *Ann NY Acad* Sci 1991;618:28–37.

13 Matthews DR. Insulin: the physiological basis of its administration. In: Radder JK, Lemkes HHPJ, Krans HMJ, eds. *Pathogenesis and Treatment of Diabetes Mellitus*. Dordrecht: Martinus Nijhoff, 1986:131–41.

14 Wakerley JB. Electrophysiology of the central vasopressin system. In: Gash DM, Boer GJ, eds. *Vasopressin: Principles and Properties*. New York: Plenum Press, 1987:211–56.

15 Rosner W. Plasma steroid binding proteins. *Endocrinol Metab Clin N Am* 1991;20:697–720.

16 Oh Y, Muller HL, Neely EK, Lamson G, Rosenfeld RG. New concepts in insulin-like growth-factor receptor physiology. *Growth Regul* 1993;3:113–23.

17 Cohick WS, Clemmons DR. The insulin-like growth-factors. *Annu Rev Physiol* 1993;55:131–53.

18 Grahnen A, Kastrup K, Heinrich U *et al.* Pharmacokinetics of recombinant human insulin-like growth factor I given subcutaneously to healthy volunteers and to patients with growth hormone receptor deficiency. *Acta Paediatr Int J Paediatr* (Suppl.) 1993;82:9–13.

19 Martha PJ, Reiter EO, Davila N, Shaw MA, Holcombe JH, Baumann G. Serum growth hormone (GH)-binding protein/receptor: an important determinant of GH responsiveness. *J Clin Endocrinol Metab* 1992;75:1464–9.

20 Baumann G. Growth hormone-binding proteins. *Proc Soc Exp Biol Med* 1993;202:392–400.

21 Veldhuis JD, Johnson ML, Faunt LM, Mercado M, Baumann G. Influence of the high-affinity growth hormone (GH)-binding protein on plasma profiles of free and bound GH and on the apparent half-life of GH. Modeling analysis and clinical applications. *J Clin Invest* 1993;91:629–41.

22 Pal BR, Matthews DR, Edge JA, Mullis PE, Hindmarsh PC, Dunger DB. The frequency and amplitudes of growth hormone secretory episodes as determined by deconvolution analysis are increased in adolescents with insulin dependent diabetes mellitus and are unaffected by short-term euglycaemia. *Clin Endocrinol* 1993;38:93–100.

23 Albertsson-Wikland K, Rosberg S, Libre E, Lundberg LO, Groth T. Growth hormone secretory rates in children as estimated by deconvolution analysis of 24-H plasma concentration profiles. *Am J Physiol* 1989:257(6).

24 Funder JW. Aldosterone action. *Annu Rev Physiol* 1993;55: 115–30.

25 Smith DF, Toft DO. Steroid-receptors and their associated proteins. *Mol Endocrinol* 1993;7:4–11.

26 Kelly PA, Djiane J, Postelvinay MC, Edery M. The prolactin growth-hormone receptor family. *Endocr Rev* 1991;12:235–51.

27 Stahl N, Yancopoulos GD. The alphas, betas, and kinases of cytokine receptor complexes. *Cell* 1993;74:587–90.

28 Rui H, Djeu JY, Evans GA, Kelly PA, Farrar WL. Prolactin receptor triggering – evidence for rapid tyrosine kinase activation. *J Biol Chem* 1992;267:24076–81.

29 Zhang XK, Pfahl M. Regulation of retinoid and thyroid-hormone action through homodimeric and heterodimeric receptors. *Trends Endocrinol Metab* 1993;4:156–62.

30 Lamberts S, Hofland LJ, Deherder WW, Kwekkeboom DJ, Reubi JC, Krenning EP. Octreotide and related somatostatin analogs in the diagnosis and treatment of pituitary disease and somatostatin receptor scintigraphy. *Front Neuroendocrinol* 1993;14:27–55.

31 Werther GA, Hayes K, Waters MJ. Growth hormone (GH) receptors are expressed on human fetal mesenchymal tissues – identification of messenger ribonucleic acid and GH-binding protein. *J Clin Endocrinol Metab* 1993;76: 1638–46.

32 Urbanek M, Macleod JN, Cooke NE, Liebhaber SA. Expression of a human growth hormone (hGH) receptor isoform is predicted by tissue-specific alternative splicing of exon 3 of the hGH receptor transcript. *Mol Endocrinol* 1992;6: 279–87.

33 Jameson J, Arnold A. Recombinant DNA strategies for determining the molecular basis of endocrine disorders. *J Clin Endocrinol Metab* 1990;70:301–7.

34 Gharib H, Nagaya T, Stelter A *et al.* Characterization of the c-erbAb R438H mutant in generalized thyroid hormone resistance. *Endocr J* 1993;1:193–201.

35 Taylor SI, Cama A, Accili D *et al.* Mutations in the insulin-receptor gene. *Endocr Rev* 1992;13:566–95.

36 McDermott MT, Ridgway EC. Thyroid-hormone resistance syndromes. *Am J Med* 1993;94:424–32.

37 De Vos AM, Ultsch M, Kossiakoff AA. Human growth hormone and the extracellular domain of its receptor: crystal structure of the complex. *Science* 1992;255:306–12.

38 Cunningham BC, Ultsch M, Devos AM, Mulkerrin MG, Clauser KR, Wells JA. Dimerization of the extracellular domain of the human growth-hormone receptor by a single hormone molecule. *Science* 1991;254:821–5.

39 Wells J, Cunningham B, Fuh G *et al.* The molecular basis for growth hormone–receptor interactions. *Rec Prog Horm Res* 1993;48:253–75.

40 Argetsinger LS, Campbell GS, Yang X *et al.* Identification of JAK2 as a growth hormone receptor-associated tyrosine kinase. *Cell* 1993;74:237–44.

41 Roupas P, Herington AC. Cellular mechanisms in the processing of growth hormone and its receptor. *Mol Cell Endocrinol* 1989;61:1–12.

9: Short Stature

C.T. COWELL

INTRODUCTION

Growth is a sensitive indicator of a child's state of health, nutrition and genetic background. Deviations from the normal range both for height and for rate of growth may indicate an underlying congenital or acquired problem. Fortunately, most individuals who present to paediatricians and paediatric endocrinologists with concern about their growth do not have a significant disorder, but a thorough understanding of the process of growth and how to assess growth disorders is essential if one is to provide the reassurance that most families are seeking. This chapter focuses on the diagnostic possibilities and their evaluation when confronted with a short child.

REFERENCE STANDARDS

Short stature is usually defined in an individual whose height is less than the third centile for the reference range, i.e. 1.88 standard deviation scores (SDS) below the population mean. It needs to be emphasized that most children who are less than the third centile are part of the continuum of a normal distribution curve and only a minority will have a defined abnormality. This definition is arbitrary and other centiles may be used, the fifth (−1.6 SDS) often in the USA. Reference ranges have been developed in many countries based on cross-sectional data for their population [1–4]. An international reference range has been recommended by the World Health Organization (WHO) based on the growth standards developed within the United States during the 1970s [1,5]. This may not be appropriate for populations with ethnicity different from the reference population, for example the mean final height of the Japanese male is 6 cm less than the mean final height for the WHO reference range (Table 9.1). Population standards may also be subject to secular change. The mean final height for males in Japan has increased 8 cm since 1950, whereas it is believed that little changes has occurred in Western countries such as the USA or UK.

Disease-specific cross-sectional standards are available for a variety of growth disorders including the Noonan syndrome, Russell Silver syndrome, Turner syndrome, skeletal dysplasias, Down syndrome, Laron-type dwarfism and others [6–10]. Once a diagnosis of such a disorder is established, these charts are helpful in demonstrating the natural history of growth for individuals within their own disorder. They may also be useful to monitor the effect of an interventional therapy.

Many other cross-sectional standards are available which may be useful when assessing a child with possibly disproportionate growth. These include reference ranges for head circumference, sitting height, hand and foot lengths, as well as other body segments [11].

There are clinical situations for which the population cross-sectional definition of short stature (less than the third centile) may be at variance with the circumstances of an individual's family. An individual may be on the 10th centile but can be perceived to be short by the family if the parents are tall. To determine the significance of this, the midparental height (MPH), alternatively known as the target height, should be calculated with the 10th to 90th centile range being determined using the following formulae:

MPH if male = (father's height + (mother's height + 13))/2 ± 7.5 cm

MPH if female = ((father's height − 13) + mother's height)/2 ± 6 cm.

If the individual falls outside this range, a reason should be sought. Standards may be helpful to assess a child's height in relation the height of the parents [12].

A further example where population cross-sectional standards may not be appropriate is for an individual who is short (less than the third centile), who has a short family background, but who has just emigrated from a country where the population reference standards differ from the local standards. In this situation it is useful to assess the individual in relation to his or her own growth standard, if available, in addition to the local standard.

Cross-sectional standards provide a reference for an individual at a point in time which is the summation of

Table 9.1 Adult mean final height (cm) in different countries

Country	Male	Female
Thailand	165	154
Japan	170	158
UK	175	162
USA	177	164

genetic potential and past health. For children with a potential growth disorder we need to know their rate of growth by longitudinal observation. Longitudinal growth standards are available for several reference populations [13–15] and those that are recommended for use in association with the WHO cross-sectional standards were published by Tanner and colleagues in 1985 [15]. These standards demonstrate the variation in peak growth velocity (GV) which is dependent on the age of onset of puberty, early maturers having a greater peak GV in comparison to average or late maturers (Figs 9.1–9.4). A

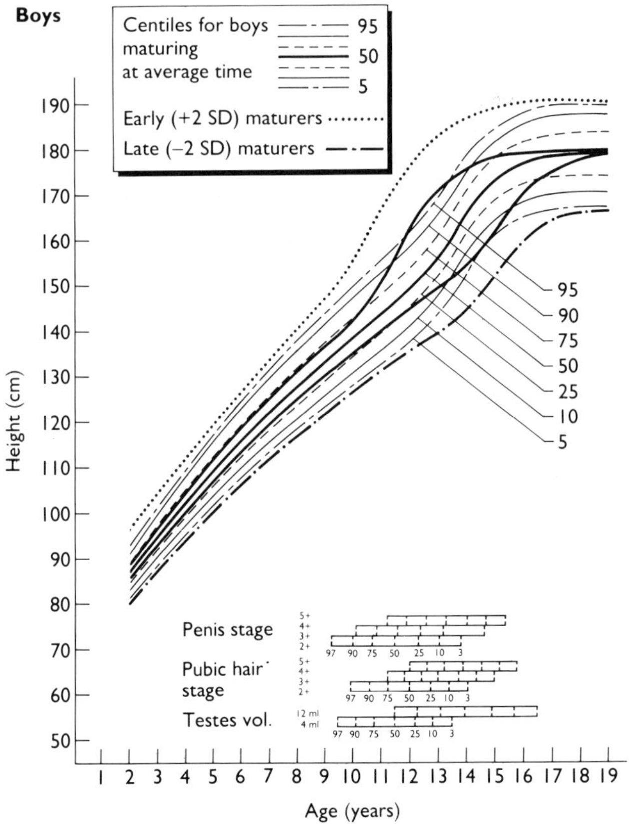

Fig. 9.1 Height attained for males from the USA. The 50th and 95th centile are demonstrated for early maturers and for late maturers defined as puberty commencing −2 SDS and +2 SDS respectively (from Tanner *et al.* [15]).

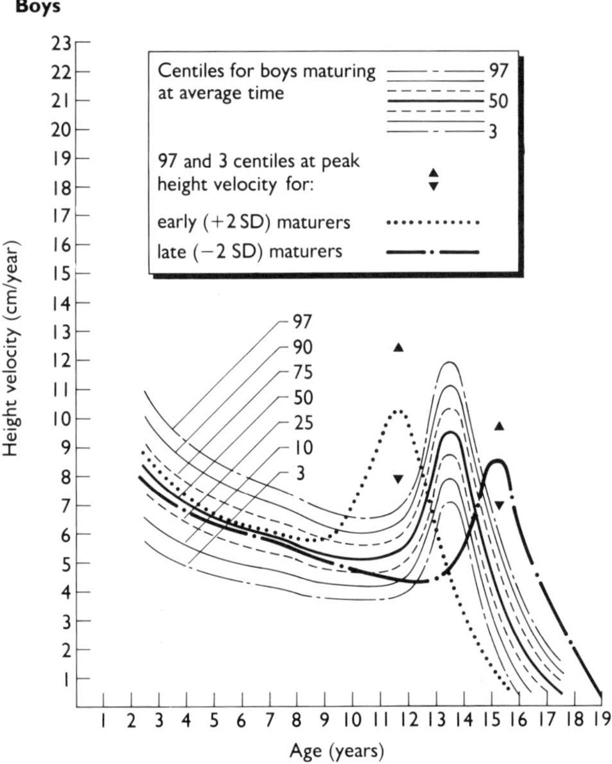

Fig. 9.2 Height velocity for boys from the USA. This demonstrates a peak growth velocity at age 13.5 years for average maturers. The 50th centile and third and 97th centiles are demonstrated for early maturers with peak growth velocity occurring at age 11.5, and also for late maturers with their peak growth velocity occurring just after age 15. Note that the magnitude of the peak growth velocity is inversely related to the age of onset of puberty (from Tanner *et al.* [15]).

further longitudinal standard has been developed which demonstrates the prepubertal GV of individuals with delayed maturation [16] – this may be useful if assessing an individual with delayed puberty. It is based on the extrapolation of the mathematical models which divide postnatal growth into three phases: infantile, childhood and pubertal, named the infancy–childhood–pubertal (ICP) model (see Figs 9.5 & 9.6) [17,18]. Each phase is described mathematically, and possibly relates to differing biological processes, fetal growth factors and nutrition, growth hormone (GH) and sex steroids, respectively, for the three phases [17].

Longitudinal observations should be plotted on longitudinal standards, but they are all too frequently plotted on the cross-sectional charts which may give a false impression of an individual's growth [19]. Cross-sectional charts demonstrate a splaying of the third to 97th centile with age as the population variance increases. At age 4 for males the ±2 SDS is 16 cm and at adult height the ±2 SDS has reached 25 cm using the WHO standard [5]. For this to

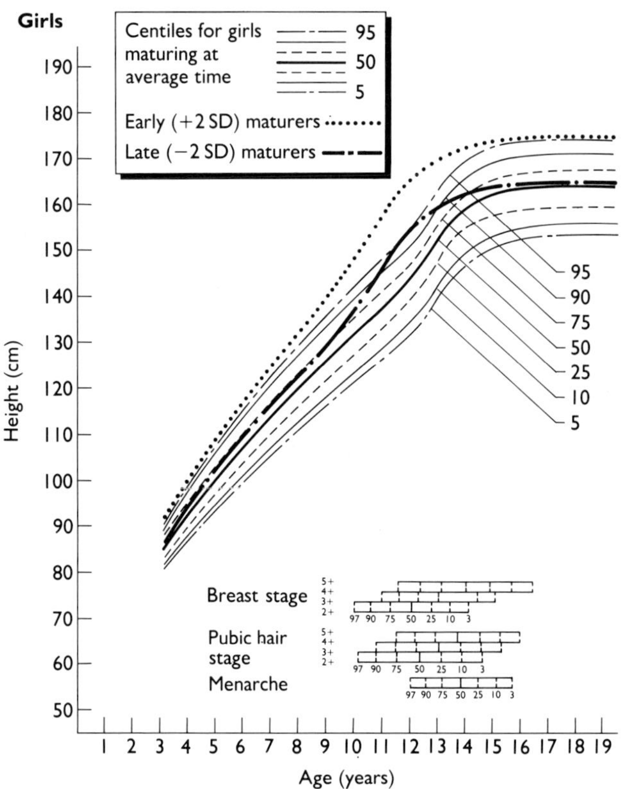

Fig. 9.3 Height attained for females from the USA. The 50th and 95th centile are demonstrated for early maturers and for late maturers defined as puberty commencing −2 SDS and +2 SDS respectively (from Tanner *et al.* [15]).

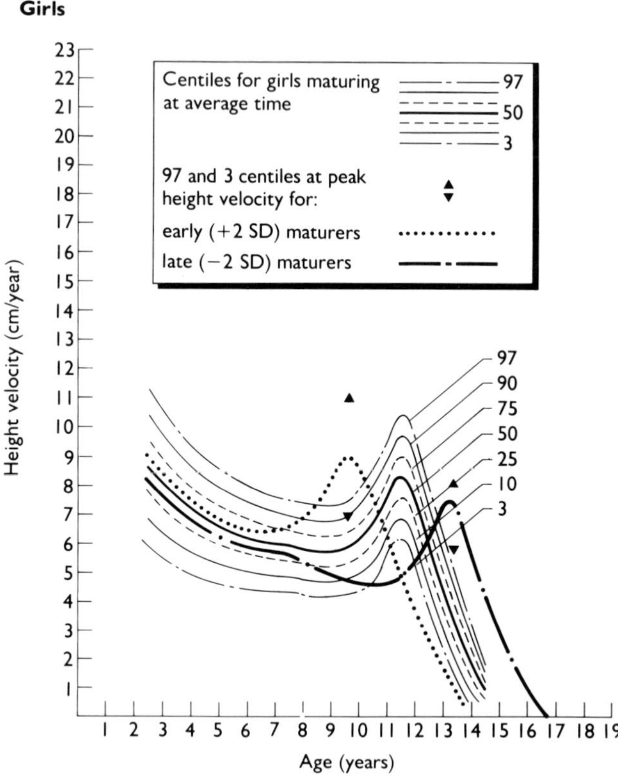

Fig. 9.4 Height velocity for females from the USA. This demonstrates a peak growth velocity at age 11.5 years for average maturers. The 50th centile and third and 97th centiles are demonstrated for early maturers with peak growth velocity occurring at age 9.5, and also for late maturers with their peak growth velocity occurring just after age 13. Note that the magnitude of the peak growth velocity is inversely related to the age of onset of puberty (from Tanner *et al.* [15]).

occur, the extremes of the population are growing at significantly different growth velocities with means above and below the 50th centile for age respectively for tall and short individuals. Thus growing on or parallel to the third centile does not imply that such children have a GV on the 50th centile for age; it will actually be slightly less. This becomes more apparent at the time of puberty when growth on the third centile of a cross-sectional chart is equivalent to a GV of 6–7 cm/year, which is suboptimal when plotted on a longitudinal chart (see Figs 9.2 & 9.4). This blunting of the growth spurt on the cross-sectional standards occurs because they incorporate both the variation in tempo and the magnitude of the growth spurt.

Voss *et al.* have made useful observations regarding GV in healthy normal and short stature children when followed for 1–2 years [20]. They found no relationship between the GV measured during successive time periods; that is, the GV varies from one time period to the next for an individual. Among the healthy short children, 44% had a GV less than the 25th centile for age over 1 year and 18% had a GV less than the 25th centile for age during 2 consecutive years. Some of this variation can be explained by seasonal changes in GV, at least in the northern hemisphere, slower growth rates being experienced in winter months [21].

MEASUREMENT OF GROWTH

The limitations of height measurement and determining GV have been addressed in recent years and deserve mention because of their relevance to the clinical management of a short child [20,22]. Using trained observers, the accuracy of height is within ±0.2–0.3 cm. This is perfectly acceptable for a single assessment of height, but this error will have an impact on the calculation of GV, particularly if successive heights are measured over a few months. As an example, if an individual has grown 1.3 cm in 3 months and the error of measurement is 0.3 cm, then the range of height change will be 0.7–1.9 cm – the range for annualized GV will be 2.8–7.6 cm/year! Thus, it is important to develop an accurate, reproducible technique,

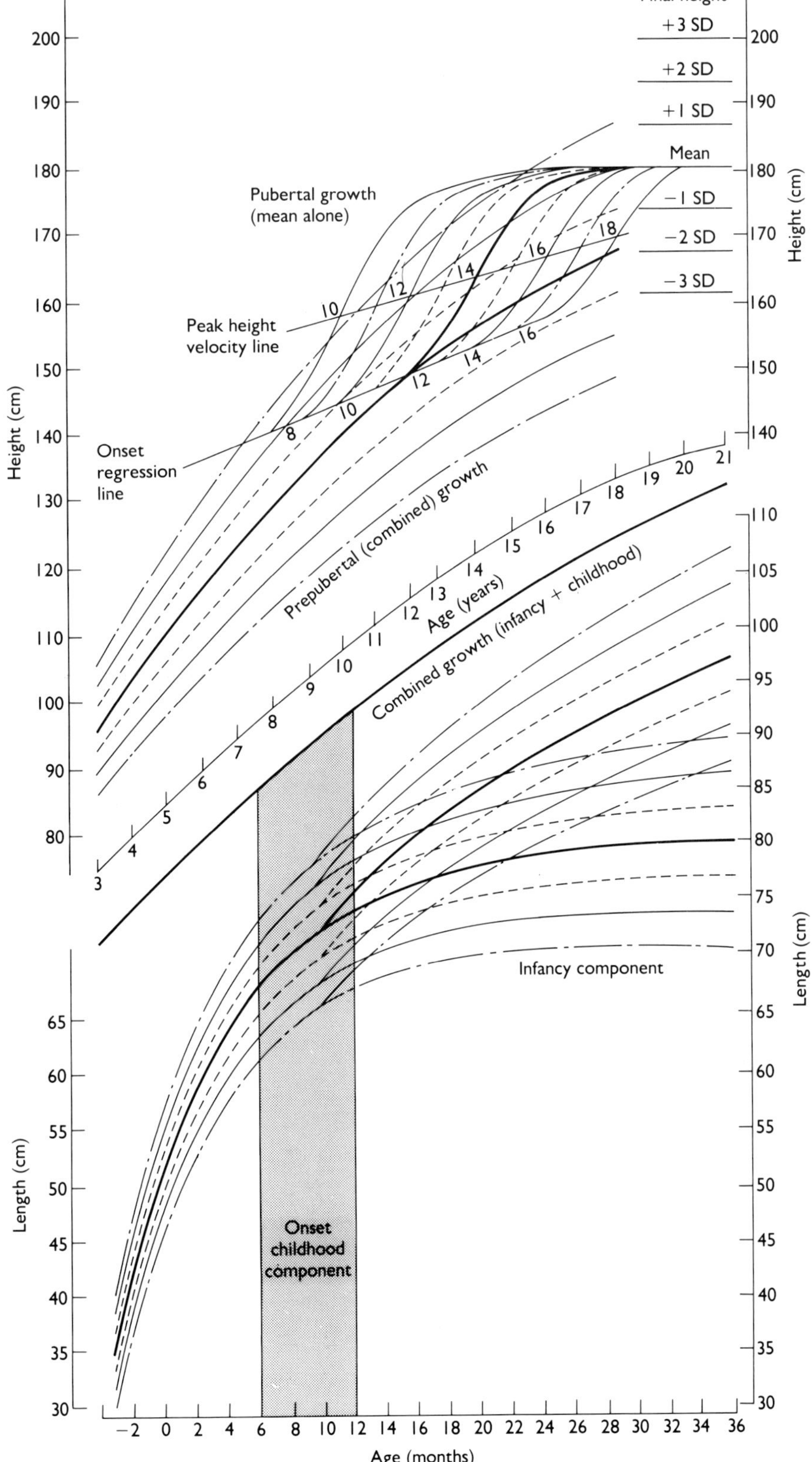

Fig. 9.5 ICP growth standard for males, demonstrating the pattern of growth in attained height for the three main components of the ICP model, the infancy, childhood and pubertal components. The sum of these components is demonstrated as the combined growth. The contribution of the mean childhood component is added to this sum at about 9 months of age, and the mean pubertal component is added at the average age of peak height velocity. The mean increase in length for the infancy component is 79 cm, the increase in height for the childhood component is 85.2 cm and 15.4 cm for the pubertal component, giving a combined mean attained height of 179.6 cm. The discontinuity at 3 years of age reflects the change in measuring position from lying down to standing up (from Kalberg [17]).

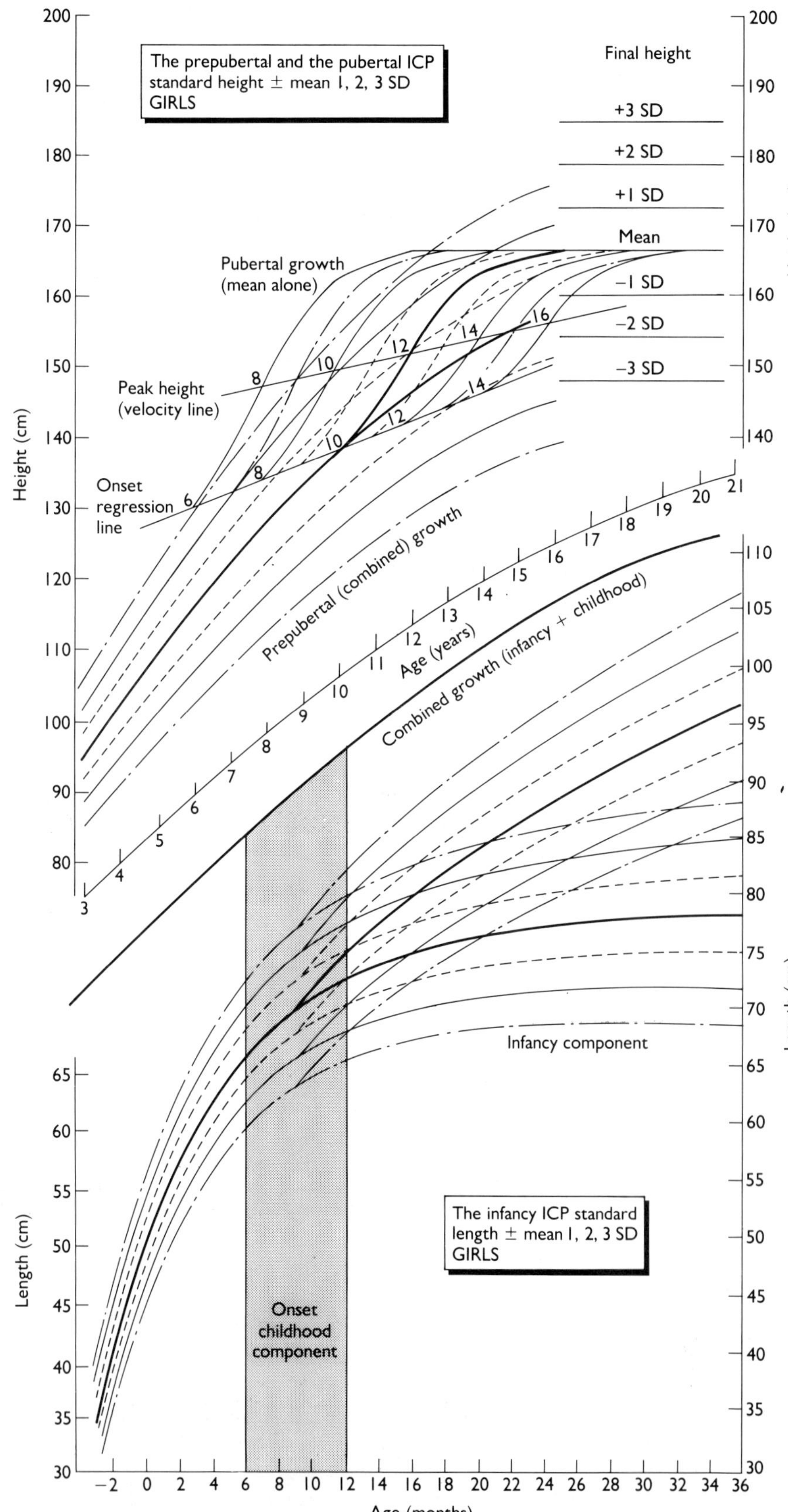

Fig. 9.6 ICP growth standard for females, demonstrating the pattern of growth in attained height for the three main components of the ICP model, the infancy, childhood and pubertal components. The sum of these components is demonstrated as the combined growth. The contribution of the mean childhood component is added to this sum at about 9 months of age and the mean pubertal component is added at the average age of peak height velocity. The mean increase in length for the infancy component is 76.8 cm, the increase in height for the childhood component is 78.4 cm and 10.9 cm for the pubertal component, giving a combined mean attained height of 166.1 cm. The discontinuity at 3 years of age reflects the change in measuring position from lying down to standing up (from Kalberg [17]).

and assessment of an individual's GV should be made over intervals of at least 4–6 months, preferably longer [21].

Comments on techniques for measuring height, arm span and lower segment follow.

Standing height

1 Recommended for children over the age of 2–3 years.
2 Remove shoes and socks (baggy socks may disguise the lifting of heels).
3 Ask the child to stand straight and tall (like a soldier) with heels firmly on the floor, shoulders relaxed and looking straight ahead.
4 The eyes and outer ears should be in the same horizontal plane (Frankfurt plane).
5 Ask the child to breathe in whilst applying gentle pressure on the mastoid process, then out, and observe the height.
6 Read to the nearest millimetre and plot on the appropriate chart.

Sitting height

1 Useful for assessing proportions and/or non-ambulatory patients.
2 Ask the patient to sit as tall and straight as possible.
3 Thighs should be at right angles to the lower limbs.
4 Ask the patient to breathe in and out, maintaining pressure on the mastoid process, and read the height to the nearest millimetre.

Arm span

1 Stand the child against a flat surface (for example a wall).
2 Measure the distance between the tip of the middle fingers when the arms are held horizontally.
3 It is usually within 5 cm of the child's height.
4 Important when assessing disproportionate growth.

Lower segment

1 Ask the patient to stand straight and tall, looking over the top of your head.
2 Palpate the top of the pubic symphysis and measure from that point vertically to the ground.
3 Accuracy is often compromised in obese patients.
4 Important in assessing disproportionate growth.
5 Upper to lower segment ratio: babies, 1.6/1; 8 years, 1/1; adults: male, 0.92/1 female, 0.95/1.

Weight

1 Weigh with minimal clothing.
2 Use scale with accuracy to nearest 100 g.

EPIDEMIOLOGY OF SHORT STATURE

Despite the frequency of short stature as a presenting problem to medical practitioners, little information exists regarding epidemiology. Vimpani *et al.* [23] examined all children < −2.5 SDS in a region of southern Scotland (n = 449). They determined the following causes of short stature: organic, 24%; familial and/or constitutional growth delay, 41%; small for gestational age (SGA), 7.5%; GH deficiency, 8%; not determined, 19%. GH deficiency was defined by a peak GH response < 15 mU/l following an exercise test and a pharmacological test. The prevalence of GH deficiency was 1/4000. A lower frequency has been suggested from a further study [24]. The case-mix of

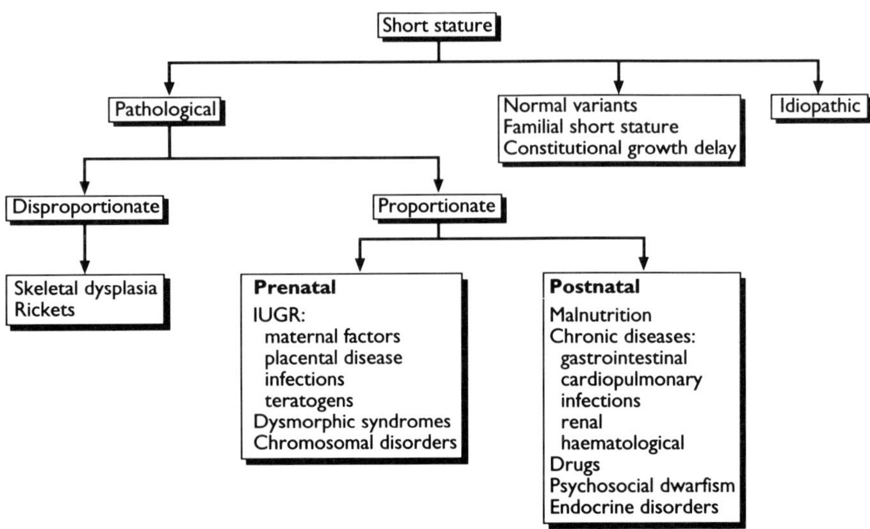

Fig. 9.7 Classification of short stature. IUGR, intrauterine growth regulation.

280 consecutive new referrals presenting to our endocrinology clinic is very similar except that we found that skeletal dysplasias were less represented (presumably referred to an alternative clinic such as Genetics) and that 19% were actually more than the third centile (unpublished observations).

CAUSES OF SHORT STATURE

A scheme for disorders presenting with short stature is shown in Fig. 9.7. This is one of many potential classifications for short stature with the basic groupings being variations of normal, skeletal abnormalities (primary cause), prenatal and postnatal onset of growth failure. A brief description of the more common diagnoses follows.

Familial short stature

This is the most common diagnosis encountered in clinical practice. Although it is usual to find an immediate family member who is short, the diagnosis should still be considered if the short family member is more distant, such as an aunt, uncle or grandparent. It is important to remember that the affected family members may have underlying pathology which should be excluded; examples include skeletal dysplasias. We can also look forward to understanding more about this disorder when the gene(s) for growth are determined. It is possible that some individuals may have a subtle abnormality of the GH/GH receptor axis or of the growth plate/skeleton, and more research is required to ascertain causes of familial short stature [25,26]. Clearly defined abnormalities of GH secretion have not been determined in individuals with familial short stature (FSS) but pulsatile secretion may be diminished as part of the continuum of GH secretion between short, normal and tall stature [27].

In this disorder the bone age is not greatly delayed, usually within 2 years of the chronological age and/or within 2 SDS of the radiological assessment method and the height SDS falls within the target range for the family. The target range is calculated as the MPH with the range being the 10th to 90th centile for MPH, which is sex-dependent (see above). Alternatively, the MPH can be expressed as a SDS with the target range being ±1.28 SDS. An example follows:

Father's height 170 cm = −1.0 SDS
Mother's height 154 cm = −1.9 SDS
MPH SDS = −1.45, target range −2.73 to −0.17 SDS
For male child, MPH = 168.5 cm, target range 161–176 cm
For female child, MPH = 155.5 cm, target range 149.5–161.5 cm

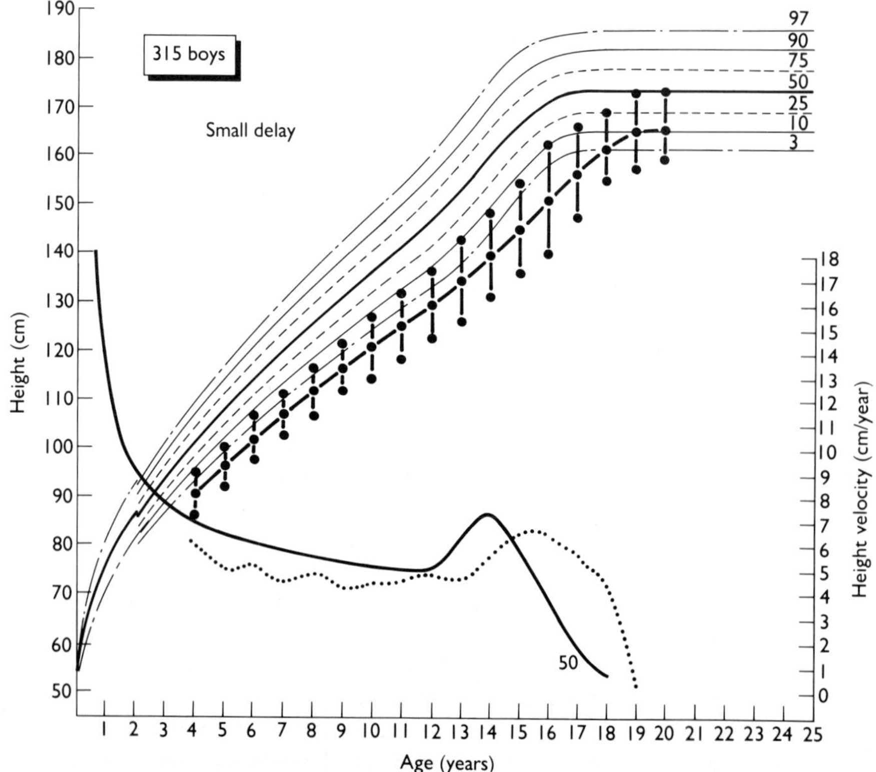

Fig. 9.8 Mean heights of 315 boys with growth delay and short stature. Their mean growth velocity is also shown (lower dotted line), with a delayed and diminished peak growth velocity. Data are taken from males attending the growth disorder clinic at the Hospital for Sick Children in London (from Preece *et al.* [28]).

Maturational (or constitutional growth) delay

This diagnosis is considered in individuals with a late onset of puberty where there is a family history of delayed puberty and absence of systemic symptoms or signs. Characteristically, individuals present between the ages of 10 to 16 years with a history of slow growth manifest by a decrease in height percentiles since early to midchildhood (see Fig. 9.8) and delay in their pubertal development [28]. Males are much more frequently seen, which is a reflection of their different biology and possibly a societal bias. They may be significantly disadvantaged by their short stature and immature physique compared to their peers, and some will present with behavioural disturbances.

At presentation, their height SDS may fall outside the parental target range. Their weight is appropriate for their height although many look slim. Pubertal signs may be absent or, in males, they may have commenced puberty (G2–G3) but still have a low GV. This finding relates to the timing of the growth spurt during puberty; in males not commencing until stage 3–4 puberty after attaining at least 10 ml testes, whereas in females the growth spurt occurs relatively early at stage 2–3. Their GV prior to the growth spurt may be very slow, 3–4.5 cm/year, and it is inversely related to the age of their growth spurt [16]. The bone age will usually be delayed > 2 years and/or > 2 SDS for the radiological assessment. The estimated mature height (EMH), which is calculated from the height and bone age (see later), should fall within the parental target range (MPH SDS ± 1.28 SDS). It is not unusual for characteristics of both maturational delay and familial short stature to be present in the same individual.

Absence of a positive family history makes it important that other diagnostic possibilities are excluded. Examples include nutritional disorders including anorexia and inflammatory bowel disease, brain tumours, growth hormone deficiency, hypothyroidism, Noonan syndrome and Turner syndrome in girls. For children who are seen prior to the pubertal years, a tentative diagnosis of maturational delay can be made if there is a strong family history – longitudinal observation of these individuals will be required. Although it is accepted that maturational delay is programmed by as yet unidentified genetic factors, nutrition may play a role, especially in the early childhood years. In comparison to individuals with familial short stature, differences have been found in weight for length and height and in biochemical parameters of nutrition [29].

The long-term outcome of individuals with maturational delay has recently been reviewed [30–32]. Final height is on average 3–5 cm less than predicted by the EMH during the teenage years or their target height. There is evidence to suggest that this attenuated outcome may relate to disproportionate growth secondary to decreased growth of the spine [33]. Another possibility is that the transient GH deficiency (GHD) that has been previously noted may affect long-term outcome [34,35].

Idiopathic short stature

This is a diagnosis made after exclusion of the other causes of short stature. By definition there will not be any evidence of short family members or family history of delayed puberty and systemic, endocrine and prenatal factors should have been excluded.

Some of these children have been described as having GH neurosecretory dysfunction [36]. This term denoted children who are short, had slow GV but who had at least one GH value > 15 to 20 mU/l after a stimulation test. Their GH secretion profile showed low GH secretion overlapping those individuals with GHD. The implication was that children with neurosecretory dysfunction are similar to children with GHD, and thus may respond to GH as a therapy. Preliminary analysis of the 4-year experience of GH treatment of short children in Australia supports this concept. The mean increase in height SDS and EMH for individuals with peak GH between 10 and 20 mU/l is similar to the gain in height SDS and EMH for those with either familial short stature or idiopathic short stature, both these groups having peak GH >20 mU/l. The group with GHD and peak GH < 10 mU/l, however, have a much greater response (unpublished data).

Skeletal dysplasias

Most of the skeletal dysplasias may be associated with short stature, and it is beyond the scope of this chapter to discuss either their pathology or clinical manifestations. Interested readers may like to refer to reviews [37,38] and to their growth patterns [11]. Clues that suggest a diagnosis of a skeletal dysplasia include the following: extreme short stature, strong family history (many dysplasias are dominant disorders), abnormal body proportions and abnormalities of the limbs or trunk. Examples include decreased arm span and short spine seen in spondyloepiphyseal dysplasia, and abnormal position of the shoulders in cleidocranial dysostosis. A skeletal survey will be required to confirm the clinical diagnosis, and these X-rays usually require interpretation by a radiologist who has an interest in genetic bone disease.

Special mention is made of individuals with hypochondroplasia as this condition may only present at the time of puberty with failure of the normal growth spurt, despite appropriate genital development. Patients have an increased head circumference and relatively short lower segment. An anteroposterior view of the lumbar spine should be requested (often only lateral films of the spine are taken) which demonstrates a failure of the normal increase in interpeduncular distance from the first to the fifth lumbar vertebrae in individuals with hypochondroplasia [39].

Hypophosphataemic rickets is a metabolic bone disease that may present with short stature and signs of rickets. The latter includes frontal bossing, rachitic rosary, splaying of the wrists and bowing of the legs. It is an X-linked dominant disorder. Medical therapy with phosphate and vitamin D improves the rickets and usually the stature [40], although the increase in height SDS may be restricted to those with less severe disease [41].

Children born small for gestational age

The definition for children born SGA can involve measurement of weight, length or a combination of both. Weight less than the 10th centile for gestation is most commonly used but lower percentiles including the fifth or third centile are also employed. Length less than the 10th centile or a lower centile, although less frequently quoted, may be more relevant as it is a stronger predictor of subsequent short stature than weight. A combination of weight and length, called the ponderal index, has been established [42,43]. The formula for the ponderal index is (weight (g)/length $(cm)^3$) × 100. The ponderal index is helpful to classify intratuterine growth retardation as one of the following.

1 Symmetric – length, weight and head circumference all fall within a similar centile range. The ponderal index for these individuals will be in the normal range, defined either as the 10th–90th centile for the reference range or within the values of 2.3–3 according to the standards of Miller & Merritt [43]. These infants have intrauterine growth failure commencing early in gestation. Examples include chromosomal disorders, dysmorphic syndromes, teratogens and intrauterine infections.

2 Asymmetric – weight is on a lower centile than length or head circumference, consequently the ponderal index will be low. Poor weight gain in the last trimester will cause asymmetric growth retardation in disorders such as nutritional insufficiency and hypertension in the mother.

3 Combination of symmetric and asymmetric growth retardation.

In the short term, a low ponderal index is a better predictor of perinatal morbidity than low birth weight or short birth length [44], whereas birth length is a stronger predictor of future growth [45].

Birth size, weight or length, is the culmination of many factors, including maternal nutrition, size, and diseases, especially hypertension; placental factors include vascular anomalies, hypoxia and placental GH; fetal factors include nutrition, infection, chromosomal anomalies and syndromes; environmental factors include teratogens such as alcohol, smoking and drugs, including narcotics and anticonvulsants. A full list of all the potential causes of SGA is beyond the scope of this chapter, and the reader is referred to a review [46].

The long-term outcome of children born SGA is highly relevant, and information is available from several studies [45,47–49]. Follow-up during childhood and to adult height has determined four different postnatal growth patterns in SGA children:

1 catch-up growth before 6 months of age in approximately 40%,

2 catch-up growth before 3 years in a further 25%,

3 catch-up after 3 years in 20%, and

4 no catch-up growth in approximately 15%.

The latter two groups never achieve their genetic potential. The growth patterns of low birth weight preterm infants may differ from those born SGA at term. Catch-up growth for length is found during the first postnatal year, but during the next 2 years no further catch-up to the normal centiles occurs [48]. Their size at 3 years is directly related to size at birth.

Albertsson-Wikland and Karlberg have been able retrospectively to review the birth data and longitudinal growth of individuals born full term who have now reached final height, to determine the relationship between birth size and final height in Goteborg, Sweden [50,51]. They found that children with low birth length were overrepresented in the population of short teenagers at age 18 – specifically, 20% of the teenagers who were less than the third centile at age 18 had a birth length < -2 SDS [51]. Viewed from the perspective of being born with birth length < -2 SDS, catch-up growth to achieve a height more than the third centile occurred in 87% by age 2 years, and in 90% by age 8 years. The mean final height of those who demonstrated catch-up growth was -0.7 SDS whereas it was -1.8 SDS for those without catch-up growth at 2 years of age [50].

Little is known of the endocrinology of SGA children perinatally. Placental GH, which is produced by the syncytiotrophoblast, and maternal IGF-I are lower in the third trimester in growth-retarded infants when compared to normal-weight infants. Whether this is a primary defect or secondary to reduced placental size and function is not clear. In a study done on day 4 of life, GH-releasing hormone was given to SGA infants and normal-weight infants [52]. The GH response and insulin-like growth factor I (IGF-I) was increased in the SGA infants, suggesting either that there was resistance to GH/IGF-I or that they were overcompensating in an attempt to catch up postnatally. Studies in older children have demonstrated no consistent abnormalities of GH secretion, although mean pulsatile GH tends to be lower than anticipated for age [53].

Recent data from epidemiological studies in the UK

Table 9.2 Common syndromes that present with short stature

Syndrome	Genetics	Common manifestations
Noonan	Dominant or sporadic	Moderate short stature, delayed puberty, mild intellectual impairment, ptosis, low-set ears, occasional neck webbing, pectus carinatum, cubitus valgus, right-sided heart lesions, left axis deviation on electrocardiography, cryptorchidism
Russell–Silver	Dominant, X-linked dominant or sporadic	Small for gestational age, skinny phenotype, clinodactyly, triangular face with prominent forehead, body asymmetry, increased naevi
Aarskog	X-linked dominant or sporadic	Hypertelorism, short nose with anteverted nares, maxillary hypoplasia, crease below the lower lip, mild interdigital webbing with short and broad hands, short fifth finger with clinodactyly, shawl scrotum
Shprintzen	Dominant or sporadic	Dysmorphic face – long nose with narrow alveolar base, small mandible, myopathic facies, cleft palate (overt or submucous); congenital heart disease; hypotonia; intellectual impairment; moderate short stature; hypernasal speech

demonstrate an inverse relationship between size at birth and adult outcomes including hypertension, coronary vascular disease and impaired glucose tolerance [54]. The data are tantalizing, but a causal relationship has not been established. It requires prospective evaluation to examine hypotheses which may be able to explain these observations [55].

Dysmorphic syndromes

There are many syndromes of which short stature is a feature [56–60]. For most clinicians, characteristic features of only a few syndromes can be easily recognized. For other dysmorphic children who present with short stature, a consultation with a geneticist, use of textbooks and computer databases are necessary to identify the individual's pattern of dysmorphism. Characteristic features of some of the more common syndromes which present with short stature are shown in Table 9.2 and Figs 9.9–9.14.

RUSSELL–SILVER SYNDROME

The prenatal growth failure in Russell–Silver syndrome (Fig. 9.9) is striking and is a prerequisite for the diagnosis. Birth weights at term are 1.2–2.5 kg. Patients do not show catch-up growth after birth, and their mean height SDS during childhood years is −3.6 [61]. The pattern of pubertal growth is essentially normal, although it commences marginally early and has a slightly reduced peak pubertal growth spurt [62]. The mean final height is 151 cm for males and 142 cm for females, approximately −3.6 SDS. Changes in nocturnal pulse frequency for GH have been demonstrated during childhood [53] as well as occasional cases of GHD, but consistent abnormalities of the GH/IGF-I axis are not present. Although most cases are

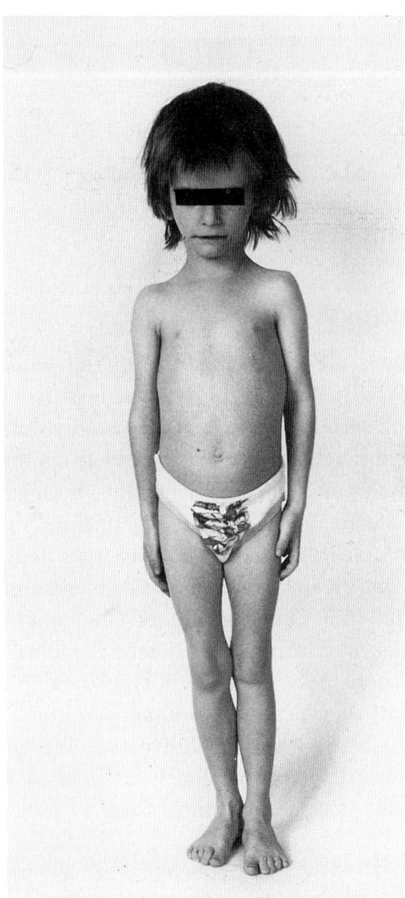

Fig. 9.9 Four-year-old male with Russell–Silver syndrome. His birth weight was 1.68 kg at term and at age 4 his height SDS is −5.3 and weight SDS is −4.5. A triangular face is present with a broad forehead and narrow point to the mandible. There is obvious body asymmetry with the right arm and right leg greater than the respective left side.

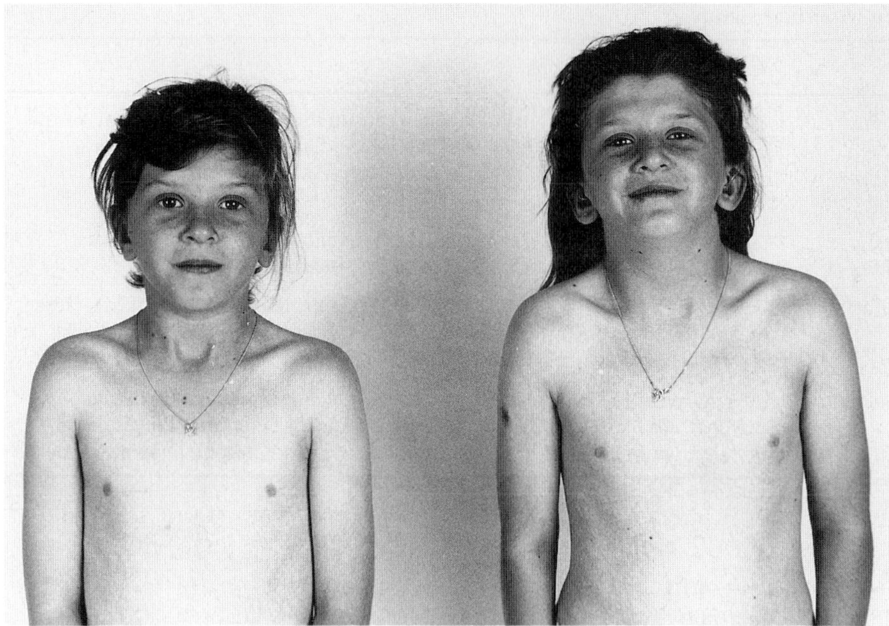

Fig. 9.10 Sisters, aged 10 and 12, with Noonan syndrome are shown. Both have short stature, −2.4 SDS, and no evidence of puberty. Phenotypic features include increased carrying angle (not shown in photograph), low-set posteriorly rotated ears and broad chest. The younger girl has mild pulmonary stenosis.

sporadic, familial cases have been described with various forms of inheritance proposed, dominant and X-linked dominant being favoured [63,64].

NOONAN SYNDROME

Short stature is a common feature of the Noonan syndrome (Fig. 9.10), 83% of children being less than the third centile in one series [65]. Puberty is usually delayed and the mean final height has been reported as approximately 162 cm for males and 153 cm for females, both equivalent to the third centile [66]. The aetiology of the short stature has not been clarified. IGF-I values are reportedly low or low normal, but mean GH and peak GH to stimulation are usually normal [67]. Dominant inheritance may be found in the Noonan syndrome [68]. A recent report has suggested that there may be a phenotype overlap between neurofibromatosis type 1 and Noonan syndrome in some patients. This raises the possibility that the gene(s) for Noonan syndrome may be closely associated with the neurofibromatosis gene on chromosome 17 [69].

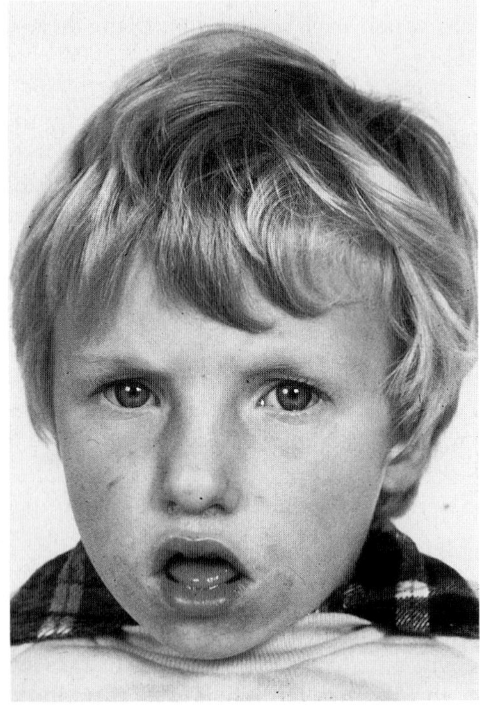

Fig. 9.11 A 5-year-old male with Shprintzen syndrome. He was referred because of hypotonia, undescended testes, mild intellectual impairment and hypernasal speech. His height is on the 10th centile. Note the myopathic facies, almond-shaped palpebral fissures, deficient nasal alae, long narrow nose, prominent nasal bridge and apparent micrognathia.

AARSKOG SYNDROME

The clinical features of Aarskog syndrome are not as striking as those of individuals with the Noonan and Russell–Silver syndromes; nor is their short stature. Most reports describe their stature as being less than the third centile. GH deficiency has also been found [70].

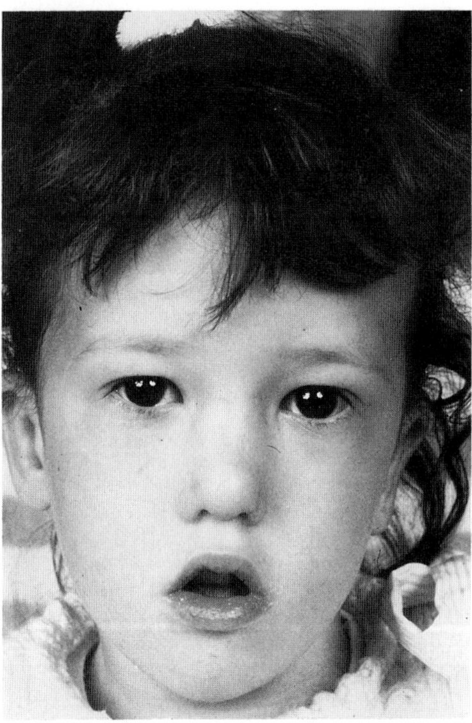

Fig. 9.12 A 4-year-old girl with Shprintzen syndrome. A cleft of the palate was noted at birth and repaired at 9 months. Hypotonia and learning difficulties had been experienced. Her height is on the third centile. Note the myopathic facies, almond-shaped palpebral fissures, deficient nasal alae, long narrow nose, prominent nasal bridge and apparent maxillary and mandibular hypoplasia.

Table 9.3 Phenotypic features of Turner syndrome

Feature	Frequency (%)
Short stature	88–100
Amenorrhoea	87–96
Lymphatic abnormalities	
Neck webbing	23–65
Low posterior hairline	40–80
Lymphoedema	21–47
Nail convexity/dysplasia	43–83
Skeletal abnormalities	
Micrognathia	60
High arch palate	35–84
Short fourth/fifth metacarpals	35–77
Increased carrying angles	27–82
Madelung deformity	7
Kyphoscoliosis	12–16
Broad chest	33–75
Abnormal upper–lower segment	90
Recurrent middle-ear infections	53
Decreased hearing	93*
Cardiac – coarctation or aortic stenosis	16–23
Renal anomaly	11–37
Naevi	22–78
Metabolic	
Thyroiditis	21
Carbohydrate intolerance	34

* Documented in only one study (Palmer *et al.* [78]) in which 17 children were studied.
Information summarized from: Lippe [75]; Hall *et al.* [76]; Nielsen *et al.* [77]; Padilla CD, personal communication (93 patients studied), Royal Alexandra Hospital for Children, Sydney; Palmer CG *et al.* [78]; Park *et al.* [79]; Suwa [80].

SHPRINTZEN SYNDROME

Shprintzen (velocardiofacial) syndrome (Figs 9.11 & 9.12) is not usually mentioned as a diagnosis to consider among individuals with short stature and dysmorphism. It is now believed to be a disorder of relatively high prevalence [71]. Approximately 60% will have an overt or submucous cleft palate, and it is the commonest recognizable disorder in cleft palate clinics, 5–10% of cases [72,73]. Short stature is found in more than 60% of cases [72]. Representative facial features are shown in Figs 9.11 & 9.12. The Di George anomaly may coexist. A diagnostic test has become available with the finding that it is caused by a small deletion of chromosome 22 – fluorescent *in situ* hybridization (FISH) using a specific probe can be diagnostic for the deletion [74].

TURNER SYNDROME

This diagnosis should be thought of in any girl who presents with unexplained short stature. Some common phenotypic features are noted (Table 9.3 and Fig. 9.13) but in many girls, these characteristics are not obvious (Fig. 9.14). Thus it is important to have a high index of suspicion for this chromosomal disorder, and we currently recommend a karyotype for any girl under the third centile who does not have an obvious explanation for short stature.

Turner syndrome occurs at a frequency of approximately 1 in 2500 live births [75]. The frequency of abnormalities of the X chromosome varies between series but 45,X is usually found in 50–60% of cases. 46,X,i(Xq) and 45,X/46,XX are the next most frequent with a variety of structural rearrangements and partial deletions of the X chromosome also found. Non-dysjunction of chromosomes is the suggested mode of development of 45,X individuals with a loss of paternal X being the common situation [81].

The relationship between chromosomal loss and short stature has been examined in several series. Although the results are conflicting, no one region of the X chromosome has been determined as the major regulator of stature. A recent report on a girl without Turner syndrome but with significant short stature demonstrated a loss of chromosome material at the terminal end of Xp in the pseudoautosomal region [82]. The authors suggested that

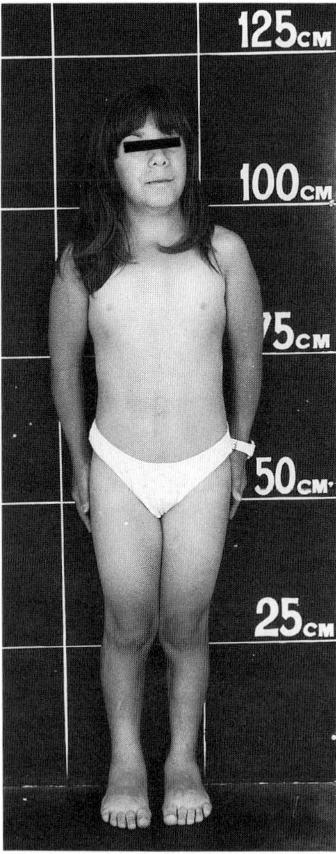

Fig. 9.13 An 11-year-old girl with Turner syndrome. Her birth weight was 2 kg at 37 weeks and she presented to the paediatrician at age 10 because of concerns about short stature and slow growth velocity. She had a past history of recurrent ear infections. Her height SDS at presentation was −3.3 and weight SDS was −1.5. Her karyotype was 45,XO. Note the rather solid appearance with a broad chest. Mild webbing of the neck was present, as was an increased carrying angle of the elbows and hyperconvex nails. Lymphoedema of the fourth and fifth toes was present in the first few months of life.

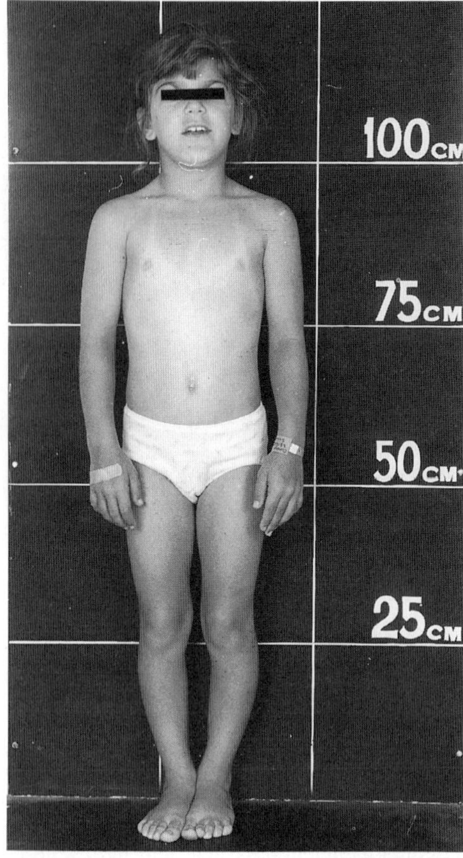

Fig. 9.14 A 9-year-old girl with Turner syndrome. She had normal birth weight at term, 3.6 kg, and presented at age 9 because of slow growth in the preceding 2 years. Her height SDS was −2.1 and weight SDS −1.0. Her karyotype is 45,XO/46,XX. Note the almost complete absence of phenotypic features of Turner syndrome. A broad chest is suggested, and hyperconvex nails were present but are not shown. Recurrent middle-ear infections had been a feature of her first 6 years of life.

there may be a gene(s) regulating growth in this region. If this were the case, Turner syndrome with monosomy for Xp may be expected to be significantly short and those with disomy for Xp, that is those with karyotype 46,X,i(Xp), to be taller – this has not been found [83]. Thus it seems reasonable to conclude that the major genes for stature are autosomal.

The mean final height of women with Turner syndrome is in the region of 143–146 cm in Western societies, which is approximately 20 cm less than the average final height for normal adult females [6,84,85]. In Japan a similar relationship exists, with the mean final height of Turner syndrome women being 140 cm which is 18 cm less than the average for adult women [86]. The final height is related to the genetic background. No difference in final height is observed between those with and without spontaneous onset of puberty [86,87]. However, those with spontaneous menarche are taller during the teen years as they experience a small growth spurt [86,87].

The growth pattern of girls and women with Turner syndrome has been characterized from cross-sectional data in several countries [6,84,85] (Fig. 9.15). There are four phases [88].

1 There is mild prenatal growth failure with mean birth weight and birth length 1 SDS below the mean, approximately 2.85 kg and 47 cm respectively.

2 The growth rate during infancy is close to normal in the majority.

3 After age 3 the GV is slow and the height SDS decreases. Most of the difference in final height between Turner syndrome and normal females arises during the childhood years.

4 Pubertal growth is similarly slow and does not have the normal growth spurt even if signs of puberty are present.

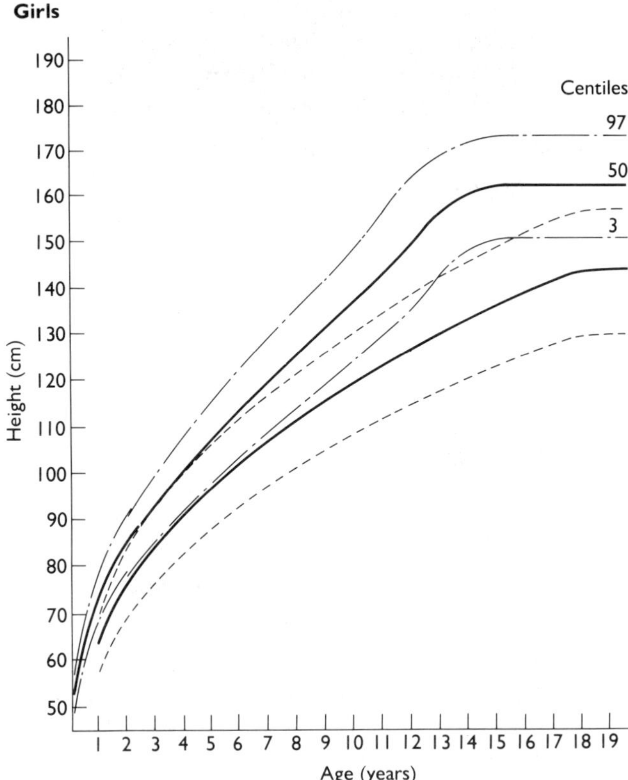

Fig. 9.15 Growth curve for girls with Turner syndrome. Cross-sectional data from girls within Europe with Turner syndrome was used for the construction of these percentiles. The cross-sectional standard has been demonstrated to be useful for the observation of longitudinal growth in girls with Turner syndrome. The majority of girls with Turner syndrome grow along their percentile; thus an estimate of their projected adult height can be made from the plotting of their height on this cross-sectional standard (from Lyon *et al.* [6]).

However the total pubertal growth from age 11 to the final height, if untreated, has been calculated as being similar to the growth achieved during puberty in normal females.

The bone age is delayed approximately 1 year until age 10–11 but thereafter, bone maturation is less than 1 year for each chronological year unless spontaneous puberty occurs [84]. This slow bone maturation between ages 10 and 16 may allow the EMH to increase in girls with Turner syndrome undergoing GH therapy.

The evidence for an abnormality of the skeleton and/or growth plate as a cause of the short stature is compelling. Defects of the skeleton are commonly found in Turner syndrome; examples include short fourth and fifth metacarpals, Madelung deformity, kyphoscoliosis in approximately 10%, but with the exception of the latter, these defects do not limit growth. The abnormal upper-to-lower segment ratio indicates that long bone growth may be impaired, but X-rays do not show convincing evidence of a skeletal dysplasia. Skeletal surveys may demonstrate increased trabeculation and mild osteopenia even before the pubertal years. Furthermore the response to GH using a conventional dose ($14\,IU/m^2\,week^{-1}$) is disappointing, and higher doses are required, suggesting that there is a relative resistance to GH at the growth plate.

An endocrine cause for the short stature has been sought by several investigators. Pulsatile GH secretion (and stimulated GH) prior to age 10 is not different from age-matched controls [89–91]. Thereafter, the usual rises in GH secretion and IGF-I are blunted [90,91]. This is in part secondary to their lack of pubertal development but growth hormone secretion is also attenuated in association with the relative obesity that occurs in teenage years in many girls with Turner syndrome [89,90]. IGF-I is at the lower end of the pubertal range [90]. These abnormalities, however, do not explain the low GV which occurs in midchildhood. Other causes of slow GV, such as hypothyroidism, should be sought in an individual, since thyroiditis is more common in Turner syndrome [75].

The other major feature of Turner syndrome is ovarian dysgenesis; 10–20% will show evidence of spontaneous puberty, spontaneous menarche occurs in 5–10% and approximately 1% will be fertile [75,86,87]. Spontaneous puberty is most frequent in those disomic for Xp, but may occur with any karyotype [75]. Evidence of ovarian dysgenesis may be found during the first few years of life with elevated luteinizing hormone (LH) and follicle-stimulating hormone (FSH), but from age 3 to 10 most females with Turner syndrome will have normal gonadotrophins. Elevated gonadotrophins after age 10 suggest impairment of ovarian function such that secondary sex characteristics will not develop, but this is not always the case. Induction of puberty with low-dose oestrogen should be age-appropriate and considered in relation to GH therapy if it is being used to promote growth (see Chapter 10).

Other phenotypic aspects of Turner syndrome are shown in Table 9.3 and have been recently reviewed [75]. In view of the high frequency of cardiac defects, cardiac ultrasound is a useful test at the time of diagnosis of Turner syndrome. Routine ultrasounds of the kidney and pelvis are of questionable value.

Ear infections and hearing loss are often not appreciated as being a major concern. Recurrent middle-ear infection, and glue ear requiring ventilation tubes, are a frequent problem in the first 10 years of life. Many women with Turner syndrome are left with a significant hearing loss, some of which may have been avoidable with appropriate intervention during childhood years.

Intelligence is within the normal spectrum. However, specific difficulties with learning may be encountered, particularly in the areas of arithmetic and reasoning. Formal testing reveals specific impairments in visuospatial and memory areas [92,93]. Lower social competence is also reported.

NUTRITIONAL INSUFFICIENCY

On a global scale, malnutrition is the most common cause of poor growth and short stature [94,95]. Kwashiorkor and marasmus are the classical conditions describing protein–calorie and calorie insufficiency respectively, but the distinction between them is rarely made clinically. Linear growth is very sensitive to the effect of protein–calorie insufficiency, and individuals will present with dramatic growth failure, weight usually being more affected than height with head size relatively preserved. Severe wasting, poor subcutaneous tissue, abdominal distension, chronic diarrhoea secondary to mucosal flattening, and infectious diseases are all part of the picture of individuals with marasmus. In kwashiorkor, where there may be more selective or qualitative defects of protein, the clinical picture may include oedema and ascites.

In addition to the biochemical abnormalities associated with nutritional insufficiency, including anaemia and liver function disturbances, the GH/IGF-I axis will be impaired. IGF-I will be low, as will be IGF-binding protein 3 (IGFBP-3). Mean GH secretion may be increased or blunted. Increased pulse amplitude and also higher trough values, often not returning to the usual undetectable values that are characteristic of normal pulse profiles, can be found especially if protein deficient [96]. Refeeding will gradually reverse these findings. It can be argued that the changes in GH and IGF-I are important homeostatic mechanisms, with the increased GH providing an alternative source of fuel by its action on adipocytes and the lower IGF-I restricting anabolism when energy is required for survival rather than tissue growth.

Deficiency of minerals and/or vitamins may also affect growth, particularly the vitamin B complex, iron and zinc. These deficiencies are usually in association with either chronic disease or caloric insufficiency. Zinc deficiency may be associated with decreased appetite and taste, low GV, delayed puberty and decreased resistance to infection [97]. Several reports have described abnormalities of growth with low zinc levels measured in hair or plasma, or by zinc clearance studies [98,99]. Transient GH deficiency has been found [100,101] but others have shown normal GH secretion. Zinc supplementation improves GV [99,101,102] and increases IGF-I [99]. These studies indicate a possible role for zinc as a cause of slow GV, particularly if nutrition may be suboptimal, but there remain questions about how to define this entity and whether the responses witnessed are primarily related to the zinc supplementation or changes in caloric intake [103].

Nutritional insufficiency as a cause of low GV and short stature is also found in countries where adequate nutrition is easily obtained. Infants during the first 2–3 years of life may present with non-organic failure to thrive, demonstrating poor weight gain and linear growth. Nutritional insufficiency in these children is secondary to abnormal feeding practices and/or disturbed parent/child interaction (see below). Improving the feeding or removing the child from the environment will lead to rapid weight gain and growth. In older children and teenagers, anorexia nervosa and/or fear of obesity is a cause of low GV and short stature [104,105]. Features of anorexia nervosa may be subtle when an individual first presents with short stature, but it is an important diagnosis to consider, particularly if there are no clues to alternative diagnoses. Detailed history enquiring about eating habits, exercise pattern, body image and alternative behaviours such as laxative abuse or self-induced vomiting is required. Anorexia nervosa is much more common in females, and before establishing the diagnosis in males one needs to exclude organic disorders including intracranial lesions, especially germinomas and gastrointestinal disease such as Crohn disease. Features on examination are important, weight being more affected than height – this is unusual for most disorders presenting with short stature. There will be little subcutaneous tissue, there may be increased body hair (lanugo) and puberty will be delayed for age.

Abnormalities of the hypothalamopituitary axis are common in anorexia nervosa. IGF-I and IGFBP-3 will be low for age and GH may be low, normal or elevated, reflecting nutritional and emotional status [106]. Blunted GH responses to provocation may be found [107]. The sick euthyroid state may be found with a decrease in thyroxine (T_4), normal triiodothyronine (T_3) and thyroid-stimulating hormone (TSH). Gonadotrophins will be low for their age, but consistent with their pubertal status. These abnormalities are all reversible with refeeding.

Other chronic diseases may have low GH and IGF-I during active phases of their disease processes; an example includes juvenile chronic arthritis, the low GH and IGF-I being reversible if disease remission is possible [108].

Psychosocial deprivation

Two types of psychosocial deprivation (PSD) are described: type 1 refers to children presenting in the first 2–3 years of life with failure to thrive on a non-organic basis; type 2 describes children after the age of 2–3 who present with short stature and low GV [109]. Type 1 is primarily caused by nutritional insufficiency whereas GH deficiency will be found in type 2, which is reversible with removal of the child from the environment [109,110]. The abnormal growth patterns of both type 1 and type 2 PSD are dramatically reversed if appropriate changes are made to the child's environment, so it is important that the historical features that suggest this disorder are recognized and appropriate investigations are performed to rule out an organic disorder. Although the final mechanism for growth failure may be different for type 1 and type 2 PSD, it is the poor quality of the relationship between the infant and child and their carers which is common to both, whether they be the biological parents, extended family or foster parents. Rejection by parents is characteristic of older patients with type 2 PSD. The parent may exhibit a variety of psychopathologies; alcoholism is common, and fathers are frequently absent or not involved. Parental punishment is often severe, and the children display a variety of regressive behaviours. In a series by Sah *et al.* [111] all the children demanded affection, the majority were ignored by their mother, 54% manifested anxiety, 25% were aggressive and 46% had delayed language development. Extreme behavioural abnormalities, such as enuresis, encopresis, difficulty in sleeping, hyperphagia and polydipsia, were found in a minority. The parent/child distrubance is less obvious in type 1 PSD, but may become apparent under close observation in a hospital setting.

Boys are more commonly affected than girls and may present at any age until the early teen years. Delayed adolescence may be a feature in the older children and hence the differential diagnosis will include boys with maturational delay. The bone age will be delayed and this may be dramatic if the deprivation has been present for a long time. Growth arrest lines in the metaphysis are frequently observed, and may be a clue to the diagnosis of psychosocial deprivation. In type 1 PSD it is unusual to find abnormal laboratory values, whereas in type 2 decreased GH secretion and IGF-I is frequently found [109]. If the child is removed from the offending environment, pulsatile GH secretion will return to normal over a period of 2–3 weeks [110]. Concomitant electroencephalogram (EEG) profiles with GH secretion studies have been performed, but no consistent abnormalities have been obtained.

Treatment requires changing the child's psychological environment. This may be possible by working with the families but, in severe cases, it will usually require removal of the child from the current environment. This is not always easy, and requires the help of the Child Protection Agencies. Treatment with GH for the slow GV has not been of any value [112–114].

Chronic medical conditions

Chronic diseases may affect growth by a variety of mechanisms: decreased caloric intake and increased energy expenditure affect children with congenital heart disease, cystic fibrosis and other forms of chronic lung disease [115,116]; decreased caloric intake occurs in gastrointestinal disease and/or increased caloric loss; decreased caloric intake and disturbed fuel metabolism are frequent in chronic renal failure. Most cases present in the first few years of life with failure to thrive, weight being more affected than length. If nutrition is the major cause of growth failure, IGF-I will be low unless measured in an assay where the IGF-binding proteins are not extracted before measurement of IGF-I, in which case a variety of IGF-I levels will be obtained.

Coeliac disease

Symptomatic coeliac disease presenting as an irritable infant/toddler with diarrhoea, abdominal distension and failure to thrive will frequently be associated with a length under the third centile. There are several reports attesting to the diagnosis of asymptomatic coeliac disease in children presenting with short stature [117–119]. Antigliadin antibody, which is usually strongly positive in individuals with coeliac disease, is a simple method to screen for coeliac disease, and is a recommended test for children with short stature without an obvious cause [119]. Confirmation of an abnormal result will require a small bowel biopsy. In our clinic in Sydney, Australia, we have not detected coeliac disease presenting asymptomatically in children with short stature in over 300 sequential new referrals. The explanation for the difference between the published series [117–119] and this experience may relate to the varying prevalence rates for coeliac diasease, or to the diagnosis of coeliac disease being established before referral is made to an endocrinology clinic in Sydney.

Inflammatory bowel disease

Approximately 20% of individuals diagnosed with Crohn disease have height under the third centile at the time of their presentation [120,121]. The mean height SDS of 100 patients at presentation was −1.11 for males, −1.05 for females [120]. Thus it is important to have a high index of suspicion for this disorder, particularly in countries or ethnic populations where the incidence is high. Historical and physical clues that may lead one to consider inflammatory bowel disease will usually be present, including vague abdominal pain/mass/tenderness, finger clubbing, anal skin tags, arthropathy and anaemia – appropriate investigations to rule out inflammatory bowel disease need to be instigated. The GV of children with inflammatory bowel disease will be low because of inflammation, drug therapy, especially steroids, and nutritional insufficiency. In the study of Griffith *et al.* [120] 49 of 100 children followed for a mean of 4.9 years had a GV of $\leq$4 cm/year for 2 or more years of follow-up during treatment. In this context IGF-I is low, but there is little information about GH secretion [122]. Improving nutrition or causing disease remission with either medical therapy or surgery will reverse the growth failure [120–122]. The overall prognosis for growth after diagnosis is good, with a modest increase in mean final height SDS compared to height SDS at diagnosis [120].

Chronic renal failure

Nutritional, metabolic and therapeutic factors all contribute to slow GV in children with chronic renal failure (CRF). Depending on the renal function there may be significant attenuation of prepubertal growth [123]. Puberty is delayed and the pubertal growth spurt is attenuated [124,125]. The mean final height of individuals with CRF is −3 SDS [125]. Optimizing nutrition and medical therapy can normalize GV [126] but catch-up growth has been difficult to maintain with conventional treatment regimes. GH replacement in a high dose has shown promise in the short term to enhance catch-up growth [125].

Significant perturbations of the GH/IGF-I axis exist in CRF, which can be summarized as increased mean pulsatile GH, normal to increased plasma IGF-I for age and increased IGFBP-3 [127,128]. This picture suggests that there is relative resistance to the GH/IGF-I axis. The increase in IGFBP-3 has been shown to be secondary to decreased renal clearance and probably contributes to the IGF-I resistance by binding IGF-I [128]. Disturbances of IGF-I action are also quite possible in the context of the metabolic abnormalities of CRF. GH therapy in pharmacological doses causes a further increase in IGF-I but no significant change in IGFBP-3 [129].

Other renal diseases without evidence of CRF may be associated with short stature. Renal tubular disorders including renal tubular acidosis, Bartter syndrome and calcium-losing tubulopathy (neonatal Bartter syndrome) may present with short stature with or without accompanying symptoms [130]. Polyuria and polydipsia are especially features of calcium-losing tubulopathy; tetany is occasionally found in either disorder. Hypokalaemic alkalosis is the biochemical feature that alerts the clinician to these diagnoses. Further tests are required to establish the exact cause of the hypokalaemic alkalosis, including urine electrolytes, urine calcium to creatinine ratio which is elevated in calcium-losing tubulopathy, urinary prostaglandins if possible, plasma renin and aldosterone, and a renal ultrasound – nephrocalcinosis is seen in calcium-losing tubulopathy. Treatment with either prostaglandin inhibitors (indomethacin or aspirin) or replacement of the mineral deficiencies with potassium and magnesium supplementation in Bartter syndrome should normalize the metabolic abnormalities and improve growth. GHD has been infrequently reported in association with Bartter syndrome [131].

Chronic chest disease

The most frequently seen chronic medical disorder in children is asthma. Linear growth may be affected by the disease if severe, with hypoxaemia and nutrition being important factors [132,133], as well as by the therapy, particularly oral or inhaled steroids and possibly other factors including changes to the endocrine axis. The growth pattern has been described in several studies; growth is usually normal in the first few years of life [134–135] followed by a period of slower growth during childhood and the prepubertal years similar to individuals with maturational delay. Growth delay is not seen in those with mild disease, and is more common in boys, those with severe disease, in those who require oral steroids and if asthma occurred before the age of 3 [136–139]. The pubertal growth spurt was delayed by 1.3 years in one study [137]. The bone age was consistently delayed in these children. In another study those individuals requiring oral steroids were shorter at age 14 than those not requiring steroids, suggesting the prepubertal growth attenuation was greater in the steroid-treated group [138]. Final height has not been reported to be compromised by asthma, even in those individuals who have had severe disease requiring oral or inhaled steroids [138–140].

The relationship between disease severity, use of steroids and delayed growth is difficult to unravel. In a longitudinal study where disease severity was graded, oral steroids did have a significant effect on growth delay in comparison to those with the same grade of asthma severity but who were not treated with steroids [138]. Growth attenuation with oral steroids is dependent on the dose, the duration of therapy and frequency of administration. A dose as low as 2.5 mg/day has been reported to suppress short-term linear growth over 5 weeks [141]. In other longer-term studies, daily doses of $\leqslant 3\,\mathrm{mg/m^2}$ [142] have been reported not to inhibit growth. Doses approximately double these may be safe for alternate-day therapy. Treatment for periods of 1 week on two or three occasions a year will not affect growth, but more frequent administration of oral steroids for short time periods may slow growth velocity [138].

Despite the widespread use of inhaled steroids, it is not clear at what dose and in whom growth may become a problem. In children <6 years old, doses of 200–400 μg/day of budesonide have been demonstrated not to affect growth [136]. In older children, doses of up to 1600 μg of budesonide did not affect growth in another study [143]. In contrast, in an 8 week study examining the growth of the lower limb, 800 μg/day of budesonide reduced growth velocity by one-third in prepubertal children [144]. In another study using 600 μg/day of budesonide, age may be important, with a decrease in GV found in the immediate prepubertal years whereas GV was normal in midchildhood [145]. Further studies are required to determine the relationship between GV and dose of inhaled steroid, at it is clear from studies examining cortisol secretion that there is significant systemic absorption of inhaled steroid in doses as low as 400 μg/m^2 day^{-1} [146]. For an individual with slow GV it may be difficult to determine if the slow GV is secondary to the disease (chronic hypoxia or nutritional insufficiency), to the steroid therapy or to maturational delay. Clinical signs of steroid excess should be keenly sought and estimation of plasma adrenocorticotrophin (ACTH) and cortisol may be required to exclude suppression of the pituitary–adrenal axis.

It is widely believed that the steroids inhibit growth by a direct action on the growth plate – by decreasing either IGF-I synthesis or IGF-I action [147,148]. Involvement of the hypothalamopituitary axis is also possible, as in short-term studies both attenuated and exaggerated GH responses to stimuli have been found [149].

Hypoxia and nutritional insufficiency, if present in children with other forms of chronic lung disease including cystic fibrosis and the chronic lung disease of prematurity, will cause attenuated growth and delayed puberty. IGF-I will be low for age in these children.

Thalassaemia major

Secondary haemochromatosis can cause a mixed endocrinopathy in thalassaemia. Primary end-organ failure is the usual cause of hypothyroidism and diabetes mellitus, whereas hypothalamic involvement may lead to relative insufficiency of gonadotrophins especially, GH and ACTH less often being affected. Growth retardation is a common concern in teenage years and its origins are multifactorial. Chronic anaemia will cause slow growth, and may contribute to short stature at an early age if an individual is transfused to only maintain a low haemoglobin – this is rarely seen today. Present management with regular transfusions to maintain a normal haemoglobin and intensive chelation therapy to reduce the effects of iron overload has improved the growth pattern of thalassaemic patients, especially in prepubertal years [150]. A decline in GV and height SDS may become apparent only in late childhood or teenage years. Delayed puberty and/or failure to progress through puberty occurs, the origin being decreased gonadotrophin secretion; primary gonadal disease is less frequently seen [150]. In one series, 36% of males and 14% of females over age 15 were under the third centile for height [150]. Abnormalities of GH secretion and of GH action can be found, and are presumed to be secondary to iron deposition which occurs despite desferrioxamine therapy. When investigated at the time of slow GV, normal GH values following stimulation are usually found, but low values can occur. The IGF-I is low for age and does not increase significantly after GH [151]. This implies that there is relative resistance to GH in peripheral tissues which is reflected by suboptimal growth response to GH therapy.

GROWTH HORMONE DEFICIENCY

Considerable heterogeneity exists amongst children who are classified as having GHD. This heterogeneity exists partly because of the variety of causes of GHD (Tables 9.4 & 9.5) but also because of the difficulties in defining what constitutes GHD. GHD can be defined by clinical features which include *auxology*, phenotype and associated abnormalities, by *biochemical abnormalities* and more recently by *genetic mutations* of the hypothalamo-pituitary axis.

Children with GHD present with short stature and a low GV for age, but age at presentation can vary from the first few months of life to early teenage years. It has been previously described that there is a bimodal presentation, and when one examines the age of commencement of GH therapy in children with non-organic GHD, the median age is approximately 9 years [152]. The variability and age of presentation may relate to a variety of factors, including access to medical services, but the major contribution is likely to be the severity of GHD.

Individuals with undetectable GH secretion and/or a gene deletion present under age 3 years with a height SDS

Table 9.4 Causes of GHD

Genetic (see Table 9.5)
Idiopathic
Congenital
Associated with structural defects
Agenesis of corpus callosum
Septo-optic dysplasia
Holoprosencephaly
Encephalocele
Hydrocephalus
Arachnoid cyst
Associated with midline facial defects
Single central incisor
Cleft lip/palate
Nasal dimple
Acquired
Perinatal trauma
Postnatal trauma
Central nervous system infection
Primary tumours of hypothalamus or pituitary
Craniopharyngioma
Glioma/astrocytoma
Germinoma
Secondary tumours of hypothalamus or pituitary
Histiocytosis
Lymphoma
Cranial irradiation
Autoimmune hypophysitis
Transient – prepubertal, psychosocial deprivation

Table 9.5 Genetic causes of phenotypic GHD

	Inheritance	Plasma GH	Plasma IGF-I	Associated abnormalities
Primary defect: growth hormone				
Type IA	AR	Absent	↓	Gene deletion/mutation of hGH
Type IB	AR	↓	↓	Multiple pituitary hormone deficiency
Type II	AD	↓	↓	
Type III	X-linked	↓	↓	Hypogammaglobulinaemia
Multiple pituitary hormones				
Type I: Pit-1 gene deletion	AR	↓	↓	TSH, prolactin usually low
Type II	X-linked	↓	↓	Gonadotrophin deficiency present
Growth hormone receptor				
GH insensitivity syndrome	AR	↑	↓	Mutation of GH receptor
IGF-I resistance				
IGF-I receptor abnormality	?AR	↑	↑	
IGF-I binding protein	?AR	↑	↑	

AD, autodominant; AR, autorecessive.

< −3 and a GV under the third centile for their age. It is now recognized that, in these individuals, GH plays a minor role in fetal growth, as their mean birth weight and length are significantly less than the mean for the population [153]. At the other end of the spectrum, individuals who have detectable levels of GH but still considered to be low will present at an older age with less significant growth retardation, height SDS < −2.5 and a GV less than the 25th centile for their age. The auxology of these individuals does not differ from that of many other children with short stature, including those with familial short stature, children with short stature secondary to chronic diseases and those with maturational delay. Thus auxology is helpful in defining a population in whom GHD needs to be considered amongst other causes of short stature, but it does not clearly differentiate children with GHD from other causes of short stature.

Phenotypic features of GHD relate to the action of GH on facial structure and body composition. The face is characteristically immature for the individual's age and will have a prominent forehead and depressed midface development – this is related to the lack of GH effect on endochondral growth at the base of the skull, occiput and the sphenoid bone. Dentition is significantly delayed. Body composition is characterized by low muscle bulk and increased subcutaneous fat, especially around the trunk, but children with GHD are not usually obese. In males a small phallus may be present. Associated abnormalities may also be present, including midline defects of the face, optic nerve hypoplasia or signs of acquired brain lesions such as optic atrophy or raised intracranial pressure.

It has been standard practice since the late 1960s to confirm the clinical impression of GHD by evaluating GH secretion. Because of the pulsatile nature of GH secretion, known stimulants of GH secretion have been used to evaluate potential abnormalities of GH (Table 9.6) [154–160]. These tests are potentially hazardous, especially insulin-induced hypoglycaemia, during which two deaths have been reported [161]. The stimulation tests should be carried out only in a centre where appropriate expertise is available.

GHD has been variously defined with the use of these tests, initially as peak value < 7–10 mU/l and in subsequent years a value of < 15–20 mU/l has been used. Individuals with values > 7–10 but < 15–20 mU/l have been described as having partial GHD. Many difficulties arise with these definitions of GHD [162,163]. These include the lack of data from children with normal stature, variability between the different commercial assays of GH [164–166], lack of reproducibility within an individual [167,168], false-negative responses in individuals prior to puberty and associated with obesity [34,35,90]. Furthermore, when individuals classified as having GHD are reinvestigated during teenage or early adult years, approximately 30% will now have normal GH values following stimulation [169,170]. To overcome these difficulties most centres still recommend the use of two stimulation tests, but there will remain a degree of uncertainty about the results of these tests if they are in contrast to the clinical picture. The 'normal' cut-off value needs to be defined in each laboratory by relating the peak GH response to the auxology [163].

In recent years, because of the uncertainties with the GH stimulation tests, sampling every 15–30 min for 12–24 h has been investigated. The advantage of this methodology is that it provides clear information about the pulsatility of GH secretion, the mean GH level can be

Table 9.6 GH stimulation tests: uses and side-effects

Test	Administration	Timing of peak GH	Side-effects
Insulin-induced hypoglycaemia	0.05–0.1 IU/kg, i.v. bolus 50% fall in blood glucose	30–60 min	Severe hypoglycaemia; requires glucose i.v.
Clonidine	0.125 mg/m^2, oral	60–120 min	Drowsiness, hypotension
L-Dopa	125 mg if body weight < 15 kg 250 mg if body weight 15–30 kg 500 mg if body weight > 30 kg oral	30–60 min	Nausea, vomiting, headache
Glucagon–propranolol	Propranolol: 0.75 mg/kg, oral Glucagon; 1 mg, s.c. or i.m.	120–180 min	Vomiting, fatigue, late hypoglycaemia
Arginine	Arginine hydrochloride 0.5 g/kg, i.v. over 20 min	45–70 min	Late hypoglycaemia
GHRH	1 or 2 µg/kg, i.v. bolus	30–60 min	Flushes
Exercise	15 min exercise with heart rate > 150/min	0–20 min post-exercise	Exhaustion, exercise-induced asthma

calculated and, for research studies, considerable information is gained about the physiology of GH secretion in relation to biological events [171,172]. It has been demonstrated that there is a continuum of GH secretion from children with very low GV to normal GV for age, as well as between children with short stature and tall stature [27]. It is apparent from the studies that at the extremes of GH secretion, such as in severe GHD or in acromegaly, individual results can be clearly differentiated, but thereafter there is considerable overlap in GH secretion in children with short stature demonstrated to have or not have GHD [173]. Thus pulsatile GH profiles currently remain in the province of research rather than as a conventional diagnostic tool to evaluate children with short stature, which was thought possibly to be due to GHD.

GH is excreted in the urine in small amounts corresponding to approximately 0.05% of the total daily circulation. Assays have been developed which are sensitive enough to measure GH in the urine, and studies have demonstrated that urinary GH reflects mean plasma GH secretion [174]. Urinary GH increases during puberty and thus reference ranges taking into account age and sex and possibly pubertal status are required for meaningful results [174]. Similar to difficulties with plasma GH following pharmacological stimulation or by pulsatile studies, there is considerable day-to-day variation in urinary GH within an individual; it has thus been suggested that, to reduce this intra-individual variation, urine samples on three or four consecutive nights should be collected to provide a mean [174]. This will decrease the variation from 60–80% to approximately 20%. Additional limitations to this method include the reliability of collecting urine either overnight or for 24 h – ideally, an estimate of the completeness of collection is required. The benefits of urinary GH are obvious if it was able to discriminate between individuals with GHD and normal GH secretion. As with pulsatile GH, there is considerable overlap between individuals with GH insufficiency and GH sufficiency such that urinary GH does not offer significant diagnostic advantages over established pharmacological tests.

During the past few years major progress has been achieved in our understanding of the physiology of growth and GH secretion but, despite this knowledge, we have not made major advances in defining children who may be relatively growth hormone insufficient. Delineating the end of the spectrum where GH secretion is absent is relatively easy, but confidently delineating those with relative GHD remains a challenge. It is hoped that, in these individuals, the response to GH therapy may be a useful indicator of their GH secretion status, but we need to wait for results of long-term studies examining this question. Defining GHD, however, remains important, as there are further diagnostic tests which are required to rule out organic causes of GHD and there are also the implications of GHD in adult life to consider [175]. At present, pharmacological tests in association with the clinical picture and neuroradiological imaging remain the benchmark for defining GHD.

CAUSES OF GROWTH HORMONE DEFICIENCY

The frequency of GHD in the community is estimated to be 1 in 4000 in one study [23], although other authors suggest a lower frequency [24,176]. An outline of the causes is shown in Table 9.4. The frequency of these various causes has been estimated in a large database of children commencing GH therapy in North America [152]

Table 9.7 Frequency of causes of GHD

Cause	Male	Female	Total	Percentage of total
Idiopathic	978	388	1366	72
Organic	291	133	424	23
Septo-optic dysplasia	57	43	100	5
n	1326	564	1890	100

Adapted from August *et al.* [152].

and is shown in Table 9.7. Similar data are available from Europe and Japan for children commencing GH treatment [177]; 2691 of 3557 were described as having idiopathic GHD, 729 with acquired GHD and 137 were classified as having congenital GHD. Of these, 35 had septo-optic dysplasia and 34 the empty sella syndrome.

Genetic causes of growth hormone deficiency

Autosomal recessive, autosomal dominant and X-linked recessive forms of GHD are described, and are shown in Table 9.5. At the time of writing (1993), molecular defects are known for GH, GH receptor genes as well as an embryological development factor, the Pit-I gene. It is likely there will be further rapid progress in determining gene deletions as a cause of GHD as more laboratories develop the expertise to explore for mutations.

Type 1A growth hormone deficiency

The human GH (hGH) gene is located on chromosome 17 in a cluster of five genes – hGH-N encodes the gene for pituitary GH, hGH-V encodes the gene for placental GH and three genes for human chorionic somatomammotrophin (hCS).

Children with gene mutations or deletions of hGH-N present with severe short stature beginning in early infancy, often with associated hypoglycaemia and, in males, microgenitalia. They have the characteristic phenotypic features of GHD. The biochemical features are demonstrated in Table 9.5 with no GH detectable and low IGF-I. Two common mutations that have been described are large deletions of the hGH-N gene of either 6.7 kb or 7.6 kb [178]. Additional deletions have been described which include the hCS and hGH-V gene [179]. A recent study examined for hGH-N deletions in 78 subjects with severe short stature and height SDS <−4.5 [180]; 10 deletions were found with a similar prevalence among families of European, Mediterranean and Turkish origin. A higher frequency of gene deletions as a cause of GHD was found in this study than had previously been suspected, and indicates that further studies are required to examine for gene mutations, particularly if extreme short stature is present. In these individuals there is an initial good response to GH therapy, but this response is usually attenuated after 6–12 months because of the development of antibodies to GH. A potential future therapy for these children in such situations will be the administration of IGF-I.

Other genetic causes of GHD, both recessive and dominant, have been described in a few cases, sometimes associated with multiple pituitary hormone deficiency. GH may be detectable in these individuals and their growth failure is not usually as extreme as in type 1A individuals. An X-linked form of GHD is found which is associated with hypogammaglobulinaemia [181]. GHD has also been described with combined immunodeficiency [182]. A further form of familial GHD with associated gonadotrophin deficiency has been described in several families [183]. The inheritance is X-linked but the aetiology is unclear. It is speculated that some of these genetic abnormalities may be caused by defects in the hypothalamic growth-hormone-releasing factor (GHRF) but no definitive mutations have been described.

Several families have now been described with deletion of the Pit-1 gene [184,185]. The Pit-1 gene was first described in the mouse and is a pituitary transcription factor which is important for cell differentiation of somatotrophs and lactotrophs. Additionally it may be important for thyrotroph development especially in humans [185, 187]. A mutation of the Pit-1 gene in the mouse leads to the Snell dwarf mouse [186]. Mutations of the human Pit-1 gene have now been demonstrated. These families have an autosomal recessive form of GH deficiency with associated TSH and prolactin deficiency although the latter deficiencies are variable [184,185].

Mutations of the GH receptor have been well characterized to be the aetiology of the GH insensitivity syndrome [188–190]. Individuals with this disorder present with severe growth failure, phenotypic features of absent GH action but high plasma levels of GH, low levels of IGF-I and usually low levels of GH-binding proteins. This disorder is described in detail in Chapter 7.

To date there have only been a few reports of possible resistance to IGF-I [191–195]. The individuals in these reports usually have the phenotypic features of absent GH action but dysmorphism has also been noted in some. Biochemistry is characterized by high plasma GH and high plasma IGF-I levels. It has been postulated that this disorder may represent abnormalities of either the IGF-I molecule, IGF-I receptor or binding proteins for IGF-I. Tollesfsen and coworkers recently reported an individual with high levels of IGFBPs and excess production of binding proteins from fibroblast culture, suggesting that there may be a primary abnormality of regulation of the IGFBPs [191].

The African pygmy

Pygmy adults are recognized as being the shortest ethnic group in the world, the mean adult male height being 128 cm [196]. Children are born smaller than comparable African communities and show a steady decrease in height SDS during the first 5 years, mean length SDS of −2.71 at 6 months, −4.16 SDS at age 5 [197]. At the time of puberty there is no major growth spurt, and this further accounts for their decrease in total height [196,198].

IGF-I values are in the low end of the normal range until the age of 10, and significantly lower during pubertal and adult years [198]. GH values are not as clearly different from normal, but hyperresponsiveness to stimuli such as arginine suggests that they may have a mild GH insensitivity. GH-binding proteins, which in normal subjects tend to rise during childhood years to reach peak values after puberty, are clearly different in African pygmies. Values of GH-binding protein in the first few years of life are similar to the reference range, but thereafter the values are lower and there is no rise at the time of puberty [199]. This evidence suggests that there may be an abnormality of the GH receptor, affecting possibly its transcription. Consistent with this, the expected IGF-I and metabolic responses to GH are not seen in African pygmies. An alternative explanation has been suggested with *in vitro* evidence of IGF-I resistance using a transformed T cell line [200]. Further elucidation of the endocrine defect in the African pygmy is keenly awaited.

The Mountain Ok people of Papua New Guinea are also extremely short, and may have a similar defect with low IGF-I and GH-binding protein [201].

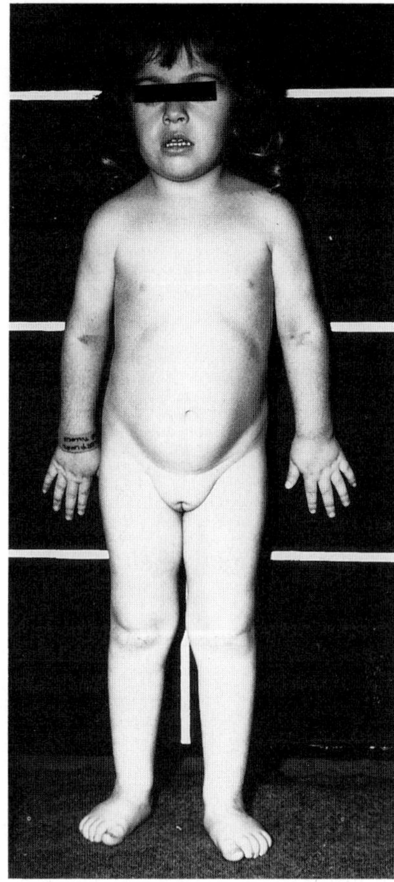

Fig. 9.16 A 4-year-old girl with multiple pituitary hormone deficiency. She had a birth weight of 4 kg at term but had early-onset growth failure. At age 4 her height SDS was −4 and weight SDS −2.7. Features noted include a young face for her chronological age and increased subcutaneous tissue, especially around the abdomen.

Idiopathic growth hormone deficiency

This accounts for the majority of individuals with GHD (Table 9.7). The presentation can be in early childhood with severe growth failure and typical phenotypic features of GHD (Figs 9.16 & 9.17). The history provides clues to the diagnosis. There is often a history of a difficult delivery, breech presentation being overrepresented [202]. Hypoglycaemia is often present in the neonatal period. It is important that, at the time of hypoglycaemia, plasma is obtained for assay of GH, ACTH and cortisol, as it is difficult evaluating the hypothalamopituitary axis during the first year of life. If evaluation is required, this author uses arginine stimulation, which may be combined with thyrotrophin-releasing hormone (TRH) (200 μg/m^2 as a single dose) and synacthen stimulation (250 μg/m^2 as a single dose).

Prolonged jaundice is occasionally a feature – it is cholestatic in nature and the characteristic which helps to differentiate GHD as the cause is that the liver transaminases are only mildly elevated [203]. The aetiology of the cholestatic jaundice is not clear. Receptors for GH are present in liver hepatocytes and the small bowel, but the action of GH in relation to biliary clearance has not been determined [204]. Neonates presenting with a history of hypoglycaemia and cholestatic jaundice will usually have deficiencies of other pituitary hormones, particularly ACTH and TSH. The jaundice improves soon after commencement of any of these hormones.

Many individuals present beyond the first few years of life. Their clinical features may be more subtle and a history of neonatal hypoglycaemia and prolonged jaundice is less frequently encountered. Their specific enquiry is usually uneventful other than the fact that their parents may comment that they have less energy than their peers or siblings. Investigations will show a delayed bone age, plasma urea may be at the upper end of the normal range because of the lack of GH effect on the glomerular filtration rate and IGF-I and IGFBP-3 will be low, consistent

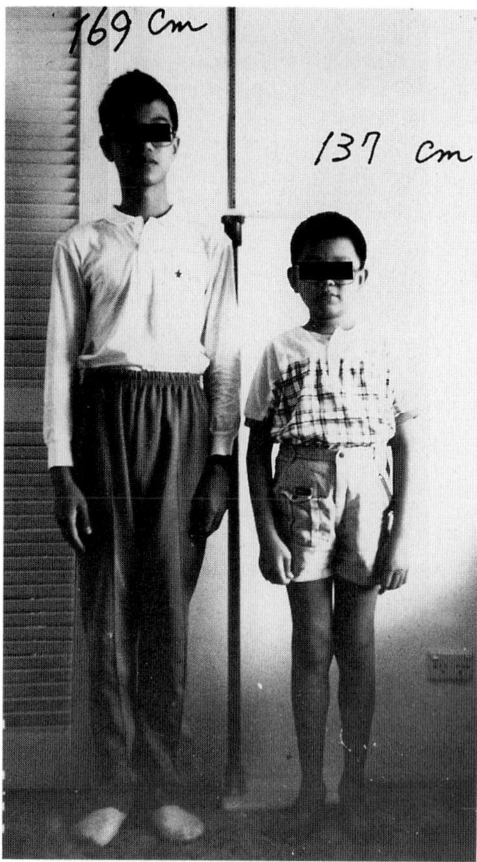

Fig. 9.17 A 15-year-old male with multiple pituitary hormone deficiency, along side his identical twin. At age 15 his height SDS was −4.8, weight SDS −2.9 and the height deficit between the identical twins is noted. He is prepubertal, his face is young for his age and he has increased subcutaneous tissue in his face, neck and trunk (the latter not shown). Four years of replacement therapy has corrected the deficit.

with the low GH response to pharmacological stimulation. In this situation it is important to rule out, by history, examination and imaging, the possibility of an intracranial lesion causing the GHD.

Transient GHD needs also to be considered, particularly if the patient is in the years preceding puberty, when the GH stimulation tests may need to be repeated after priming with sex steroids (see later).

Idiopathic GHD (IGHD) is associated with other hypothalamopituitary deficiencies in approximately 30%, TSH and ACTH being the most frequent but also gonadotrophin-releasing hormone (GnRH). Posterior pituitary deficiencies are uncommon unless secondary to an intracranial lesion or in association with septo-optic dysplasia (SOD).

The aetiology of IGHD has not been clearly established. Perinatal trauma is often associated, and may cause a disruption of the pituitary stalk [202]. There is often evidence of hypothalamic abnormalities including mild elevation of prolactin, a prolonged TSH response to TRH suggesting hypothalamic deficiency of TRH, and GH response to growth-hormone-releasing hormone (GHRH) indicating an intact pituitary. Magnetic resonance imaging (MRI) of the pituitary has provided further information relating to the aetiology of IGHD in recent years [205–208]. In children with IGHD there are three groups of findings. The first is that the posterior pituitary lies ectopically superior to the pituitary fossa, the pituitary fossa is small and no anterior pituitary tissue is seen. The second is where the posterior pituitary similarly lies ectopically superior to the pituitary fossa but a small amount of anterior pituitary tissue can be seen in the fossa. The third finding is where both posterior and anterior pituitary tissue are present in the fossa. The first group is nearly always associated with a multiple pituitary hormone deficiency, the second group is heterogeneous with either multiple pituitary hormone deficiency being present or isolated GHD, whereas in the last group the clinical picture is nearly always IGHD. These anatomical findings are discussed further in Chapter 20.

The male-to-female ratio for IGHD is approximately 2 : 1 in most series [152,177]. It is tempting to believe this is secondary to societal selection bias with more males being referred for evaluation. However, in the community study of Vimpani *et al.* [23], the same ratio was observed, suggesting that there is a true biological variation between males and females, possibly at the hypothalamic level.

Children with severe IGHD, if untreated, will achieve approximately 70% of their postnatal growth, thus GH accounts for approximately 38 cm of postnatal growth if male, and 33 cm if female. It is this deficit that GH therapy will hopefully correct if commenced early in life. Biological maturation demonstrated by maturation of teeth, growth plate and development of puberty is delayed in IGHD. The bone age is commonly 2–4 years younger than chronological age; more extreme values are occasionally seen. GH receptors are present in teeth [209] and thus it is not surprising that teeth development may also be delayed. The average age of onset of puberty in individuals with IGHD while undergoing therapy is delayed by approximately 1.5 years. There is always the possibility that this delayed puberty may be a manifestation of GnRH deficiency and require evaluation. GnRH stimulation tests should be performed for females who have no signs of puberty after the age of 13, and males after the age of 15, in the context of IGHD.

The outcome of children with IGHD as young adults is the focus of current research [175]. Adults with GHD have been shown to have decreased energy, decreased zest for living, increased body fat (especially truncal), decreased muscle bulk and muscle power. Metabolic consequences of adult GHD include increased low-density lipoprotein, decreased glomerular filtration rate, and decreased bone mineral density, all of which may be partially corrected by replacement therapy [175]. These issues are relevant to the diagnosis and management of children with GHD, as studies have demonstrated that adult morbidity is high, and there is an early mortality [210].

The long-term management of children with GHD may require re-evaluation of the hypothalamopituitary axis. Secondary hypothyroidism has been encountered during GH therapy [211,212]. This may be in part due to the direct affect of GH on deiodinase with increased conversion of T_4 to T_3. In human volunteers, GH has been demonstrated in the short term to decrease free T_4, maintain or slightly increase T_3 and decrease TSH [213]. Previous clinical studies in children with IGHD in which low T_4 has been demonstrated may not have evaluated T_3, so it is difficult to determine the frequency of subclinical hypothyroidism developing during therapy. Clinical hypothyroidism is rarely encountered during GH therapy. Progression of suboptimal ACTH/cortisol secretion may occur after the initial assessment, and it should be thought of if a child with IGHD has an illness which is not responding to appropriate therapy.

Growth hormone deficiency with midline defects

Children with midline defects commonly, though not exclusively, have multiple pituitary hormone deficiencies and may present with hypothyroidism, cortisol deficiency, short stature or a combination of these. The most common abnormality is SOD [214]. In SOD there is absence or partial absence of the septum pellucidum, optic nerve hypoplasia and variable dysfunction of the hypothalamo-pituitary axis. Children usually present in the first year of life with visual abnormalities including nystagmus, decreased visual acuity and optic nerve hypoplasia, but they may also present with endocrine symptoms of poor growth or diabetes insipidus. Whatever their presentation, children with SOD should have an evaluation of their hypothalamopituitary axis so that appropriate replacement therapy or observation can be instituted. In some children with SOD, despite demonstrating low GH secretion and low IGF-I, the GV may remain acceptable for several years before a declining rate requires intervention. The diagnosis of SOD is suggested by the visual findings and confirmed by imaging, cranial ultrasound if an infant, computerized tomography (CT) scan or MRI in an older individual.

Agenesis of the corpus callosum is also associated with GHD and deficiencies of other pituitary hormones. These children present with signs of multiple pituitary hormone deficiency, and the diagnosis of agenesis of the corpus callosum is made only after the appropriate imaging studies.

Other less frequent structural abnormalities which are associated with GHD include holoprosencephaly (diabetes insipidus is common in this disorder) and arachnoid cysts [215]. Children with hydrocephalus may occasionally have deficiencies of GH and other pituitary hormones. The empty sella syndrome is a radiological diagnosis in which the pituitary fossa is filled with cerebrospinal fluid due to an incompetent sella diaphragm. Anterior pituitary tissue may not be seen. This radiological abnormality may be associated with deficiencies of anterior pituitary hormones but, if found as an incidental finding, it is most likely that normal pituitary function will be demonstrated [216].

GHD has been found with a variety of midline facial defects including nasal encephalocele, single central incisor, nasal dimple, cleft lip and palate [217–219]. The latter is a common congenital malformation but only rarely is associated with GHD [217]. Growth failure in the first year of life in children with a cleft lip and/or palate is more commonly secondary to feeding difficulties – if no catch-up growth occurs after surgical correction, and there are other features to suggest GHD, then investigations may be required to exclude GHD.

Craniopharyngioma

Craniopharyngioma is a congenital squamous-cell tumour which arises from remnants of Rathke's pouch, an invagination of the epithelium within the third pharyngeal pouch from which the anterior pituitary evolves. It can present in children and adults, and may arise within the pituitary fossa or more frequently in the suprasellar region. Although it is a benign tumour, it is locally invasive and involves juxta-anatomical tissues, especially the optic tracts, base of the third ventricle and posteriorally towards the brainstem. It usually has a solid and cystic component, the latter containing a thick cholesterol-rich fluid which may be described as similar to machinery oil.

The presenting symptoms are usually visual disturbances or raised intracranial pressure (morning headaches, vomiting). Visual field defects are common and include homonymous hemianopia, bitemporal hemianopia, decreased visual acuity and optic atrophy. Neurological defects may be present; particularly long tract signs. Approximately 10% of individuals diagnosed with craniopharyngioma seek medical attention because of endocrine symptoms, typically diabetes insipidus or short stature but secondary hypothyroidism and delayed puberty may occur. Endocrine abnormalities prior to any treatment for the craniopharyngioma have been demonstrated at a higher frequency when formally evaluated; short stature in 53%, GHD in 72%. ADH, ACTH and TSH deficiencies were found in approximately 25% of assessments [220]. Cortisol and T_4 deficiency, as well as the possibility of diabetes insipidus, should be assessed in any child with craniopharyngioma prior to surgical intervention, as these hormone deficiencies require replacement prior to anaesthesia.

Treatment varies from centre to centre with the options including surgery, total removal; surgery, partial removal; irradiation; installation of radioactive substances yttrium or gold to the cystic component; or a combination of these options. Management of this tumour and the results vary from centre to centre, and it seems reasonable to summarize that an ideal therapy for the cure of a craniopharyngioma has not been attained, and morbidity remains high [221].

For those that have undergone surgery, endocrine deficiencies of antidiuretic hormone (ADH), ACTH, TSH, GH, LH and FSH are highly likely. There is often a characteristic triphasic response of ADH following surgery – initially water conservation with high urine specific gravity for 6–24 h followed by mild ADH deficiency with increased urine output and low urine specific gravity, followed by partial recovery of ADH. The final status of the individual may be ADH-sufficient or ADH-insufficient, the latter requiring replacement deamino-D-arginine vasopressin.

Hypothyroidism usually manifests biochemically within the first 7–14 days postoperatively and will require permanent replacement. ACTH and cortisol deficiency may be difficult to assess immediately because it is common for dexamethasone to be used for the purpose of reducing cerebral oedema – it is reasonable to continue such patients on hypopituitary replacement doses of hydrocortisone ($8–10\,mg/m^2\,day^{-1}$) until a formal evaluation of the hypothalamopituitary axis is performed.

The growth of children following surgery for craniopharyngioma is an area of great interest, as many children continue to grow with a normal GV despite documentation of low GH and low IGF-I [222–224]. Several possibilities exist which may help explain this phenomenon, including the remarkable weight gain and hyperphagia that occur in some children – this is associated with hyperinsulinism, itself a possible growth stimulant [223]. Hyperprolactinaemia is also found in some children, and has been suggested as a possible growth stimulant; however, it more likely reflects the fact that there is some functioning pituitary tissue with an as-yet-unidentified pituitary trophic factor. Friesen *et al.* have found a novel pituitary peptide which stimulates growth *in vitro*, which may be of relevance to the phenomenon of growth without GH in children with craniopharyngiomas [225].

Other postoperative issues are important. The weight gain many children experience suggests a metabolic/hypothalamic cause. It has its own morbidity, which compounds some of the other difficulties that confront these children. Poor short-term memory may also be a problem [226] and needs to be recognized, especially in relation to schooling.

Other intracranial tumours

Gliomas, astrocytomas and germinomas may all have hypothalamic involvement [227,228]. Gliomas and astrocytomas usually present with raised intracranial pressure, but germinomas can present in a variety of ways including anorexia and weight loss in older boys and mild diabetes insipidus with normal imaging studies. In such cases imaging should be repeated at least on an annual basis.

Histiocytosis

Diabetes insipidus may be a presenting feature of this reticulosis, or it may occur during follow-up of an individual being observed or treated. Tumours are usually seen in the pituitary stalk as circumscribed lesions and may resolve with chemotherapy. Diabetes insipidus, however, is usually permanent. Anterior pituitary dysfunction is associated in approximately 30% of cases with diabetes insipidus [229].

Cranial irradiation

Cranial irradiation is used for therapy of solid brain tumours and as prophylactic therapy in children with leukaemia in which the central nervous system may act as a sanctuary site for recurrence of leukaemia. The sensitivity of the hypothalamopituitary axis to radiation-induced damage is dependent on a number of factors including the total dose, fractionation of the irradiation, tissue location and age of the patient.

For children with solid brain tumours in the hypothalamic region (examples include glioma, germinoma and occasionally craniopharyngioma), radiation may be used as adjunctive therapy to surgery and/or chemotherapy, or it may be the primary therapy. The dose of radiation for these tumours is generally in excess of 30 Gy, and attenuation of hypothalamic function can be anticipated which is time-dependent [230–232]. GH secretion is typically the most sensitive, followed by involvement of TSH and ACTH secretion, gonadotrophin secretion being the most resistant to radiation. Within 5 years of receiving >30 Gy, 85% of children will demonstrate GHD [232]. Clinically this will manifest by slow GV, but precaution is required for an individual at the time of puberty. Puberty may occur earlier in individuals with a history of cranial irradiation [232], and although their GV may be suboptimal compared to the normal pubertal growth spurt [233], this may be overlooked.

In children treated for leukaemia, cranial irradiation with doses of 24 Gy has been demonstrated to cause GHD in frequencies of 30–60% [234,235]. The younger the age at irradiation, the more sensitive is the hypothalamus to damage, as are other cerebral functions, particularly cognition [234]. The number of fractions may also be important, reduced morbidity occurring with increased fractions and smaller doses. Intensive chemotherapy has been speculated as being a possible contributing factor to development of GHD [235], and this may be relevant to modern treatment regimes for leukaemia which frequently use more intensive regimes than those used in previous years.

Doses of 18 Gy have not been associated with a significant risk of GHD, at least in the first few years after therapy, but attenuation of GH secretion in the long term needs to be considered, particularly at time of puberty [233,236]. Crowne *et al.* have described an abnormality of GH pulse periodicity and a reduction in GH secretion in pubertal individuals, whereas normal GH secretion was found for pre- and postpubertal individuals [236].

Radiation damage to body tissues is a major contributor to slow GV following treatment of posterior fossa tumours, including medulloblastoma and ependymoma. The spinal irradiation severely impairs subsequent growth, so that growth becomes disproportionate with increased arm span and increased lower segment. In these individuals GHD is also usually present, and it is important to intervene early with GH in order to decrease the loss of height potential that inevitably occurs [232].

Conditioning regimes for bone marrow transplant include chemotherapy and total-body irradiation (TBI). The dose of TBI, approximately 12 Gy, may affect GH secretion, and growth may additionally be attenuated because of an irradiation effect on cell growth [237]. A single dose of 12 Gy has a much greater toxicity both acutely and in the long term than when the same amount is divided into three or four doses. Blunting of GH responses to insulin-induced hypoglycaemia 6–12 months after fractionated TBI has been found in 23 individuals treated for leukaemia irrespective of whether they had previous cranial radiation [238]. Ogilvy-Stuart *et al.* found 15/29 with GH insufficiency 1–5 years post-TBI [239]. Other aspects of the hypothalamopituitary axis are usually normal, but the risk of primary hypothyroidism and germ-cell failure is significant.

Other acquired causes of GHD include trauma [240] and complications of medical illnesses such as meningitis or diabetes ketoacidosis [241].

Transient growth hormone deficiency

Prior to an individual commencing puberty, particularly if it commences later than average, their GV may reach a nadir of 3–4.5 cm/year, which is similar to individuals with GHD. Peak GH secretion to stimulation tests in this age group may fall into the diagnostic range of children with GHD, but priming with sex steroids will unmask this transient attenuation of GH secretion [34–35,242–244]. Various regimens have been suggested for males in the past, including intramuscular testosterone esters, but it would now be reasonable to use oral testosterone undecanoate in a dose of 40 mg b.d. for 1 week if available. For females a dose of ethinyloestradiol 10 μg/day for 1 week can be used.

If GH secretion remains low after priming, then IGHD is much more likely as the cause, and should be treated with GH rather than sex steroids, which is the treatment of choice for maturational delay. Many individuals who are commenced on GH with a diagnosis of GHD in this group do have transient GHD. Follow-up studies of GH secretion in individuals who have completed GH therapy demonstrate normal GH secretion in approximately 30% [169].

Low GH secretion and IGF-I are found in individuals with psychosocial deprivation. Removal of the child from the environment to a more nurturing situation reverses the poor GV and the attenuated GH secretion [110]. Obesity is recognized as a cause of attenuated GH secretion with decrease in pulse frequency in some studies as well as mean GH secretion and/or peak GH secretion to pharmacological stimuli [90]. Most of these children do not present with short stature, nor will their GV be low; thus they are not considered in the differential diagnosis for IGHD. Plasma IGF-I is in the normal range for their age, which is in contrast to individuals with IGHD. Some children with hypothalamic obesity syndromes such as Prader–Willi syndrome or Lawrence–Moon–Biedl syndrome may warrant investigation of their GH axis because of extreme short stature. Their GH results need to be interpreted with caution, especially if IGF-I values are normal.

Autoimmune hypophysitis

Hypophysitis is a cause of postpartum hypopituitarism. It is possible that some individuals with IGHD have pituitary dysfunction on the basis of an autoimmune hypophysitis [245], and studies to examine this hypothesis are under way.

OTHER ENDOCRINE CAUSES OF SHORT STATURE

Hypothyroidism

One of the first signs of primary hypothyroidism may be a low GV which, if undiagnosed, will cause short stature. Children born with congenital hypothyroidism will have a decrease in their length percentiles following birth if they remain untreated, and will present with weight disproportionate to their length as well as symptoms and signs of hypothyroidism. Children with lingual hypothyroidism may present with slow GV and/or short stature after the age of 2. Clinical signs of hypothyroidism will be present, and the lingual gland is often visible.

In countries where screening for congenital hypothyroidism is performed, primary hypothyroidism in childhood is rare. Acquired cases of primary hypothyroidism, thyroiditis being the most common, may have as a feature a decline in GV, increase in weight plus other symptoms or signs of hypothyroidism. Most of these individuals will present in late childhood or in the teenage years. Puberty is late in the majority but can also arise early [246].

The mechanism of slow growth in hypothyroidism is well understood, as T_4 is an important regulator of GH secretion. Consequently, low GH pulsatility is found at the time of biochemical hypothyroidism, which returns to normal when T_4 replacement occurs [246]. Bone age delay of at least 2–4 years will be present, but remarkable delay is sometimes seen. It is not unusual to be able to time the onset of the acquired hypothyroidism to be coincident with the bone age at the time of presentation even if symptoms have been present for more than 4 years. Other radiological findings include an increased size of the pituitary fossa, which is presumed secondary to an increased thyrotrope volume, and a slipped epiphysis may be observed in teenagers presenting with hypothyroidism.

Replacement therapy with T_4 leads to a rapid normalization of GH secretion and catch-up growth. Underlying the importance of T_4 in epiphyseal maturation, replacement therapy may lead to an excessive rate of skeletal maturation so that an individual's genetic height potential may not be attained despite the excellent GV [247].

Cushing syndrome

Cushing syndrome is discussed fully in Chapter 29. Glucocorticoid excess, whether it be endogenous or iatrogenic, has a profound effect on GV. Thus in a child who presents with a low GV and increasing weight, the diagnosis of Cushing syndrome has to be entertained, although it is an unusual disorder in childhood. The growth attenuation of glucocorticoids is predominantly a direct effect at the growth plate [147,148]. Abnormalities of the GH/IGF-I axis are also possible, but investigations in the past are conflicting with both normal GH [248] and IGF-I values [249] being found, as well as low GH values to stimulation tests [250]. The dose of exogenous glucocorticoid that will suppress growth is equivalent to approximately double normal requirements, viz. 7.5–10 $mg/m^2\,day^{-1}$ of prednisone or 30–40 $mg/m^2\,day^{-1}$ of hydrocortisone. Alternative-dose steroid regimens do allow the opportunity for continuing normal growth, while a reasonable dose of steroid is being used. Growth suppression is still seen, but the range is 10–40 mg/m^2 of prednisone on alternate days [251].

For children who have had a long period of suppressed growth because of either Cushing syndrome or exogenous steroids, catch-up growth does occur on removal of the steroids or a decrease in the therapeutic dose to less than the threshold mentioned above, but catch-up is often incomplete. Important determinants for catch-up growth are the duration and dose of glucocorticoids and the age that the individual is treated, the peripubertal years having the most significant effect [252].

Pseudohypoparathyroidism

Short stature is a feature of this disorder, and may be its presenting feature. Clinical characteristics of pseudohypoparathyroidism are described in detail in Chapter 38. The aetiology of the short stature is presumed to be secondary to skeletal abnormalities, but abnormalities of the GH/IGF-I axis should be considered. Stirling *et al.* have described a 4-year-old boy with pseudohypoparathyroidism who had features consistent with a deficiency of GHRH and who responded in the short term to GH replacement therapy [253].

CLINICAL ASSESSMENT OF THE SHORT CHILD

The main historical and physical features that need to be elicited when seeing a short child are shown in Table 9.8. Additional history and examination should be targeted to any additional symptom or sign that may be found during the consultation. An assessment of the child's appreciation of the problem is an important component of the initial and subsequent consultations. For children with normal variations it is difficult to demonstrate in formal studies that they perceive their short stature as a significant handicap – the parents' perception frequently differs [254].

Investigations for short children

An important question is to decide in which children investigations should be performed, and how extensive these investigations should be. In general, the shorter the child and/or the slower the GV, the more likely it is that an underlying disorder will be detected [255]. Children with height SDS <-3 and/or GV under the third centile for age generally require extensive investigations, as well as longitudinal observation, whereas many children >-3 SDS will require only a minimum of investigations but do need longitudinal observation of growth rate. Suggested investigations are shown in Table 9.9. It is appropriate to

Table 9.8 Historical and physical features for clinical assessment of the short child

History	
Nature of growth problem	Duration; extent; emotional involvement
Psychological factors	
Birth size	Weight, length, gestation
Perinatal events	Delivery; drugs, infections; hypoglycaemia; cholestatic jaundice; oedema of hands and feet
Family history	Stature; puberty; heritable disease
Systemic symptoms	Raised intracranial pressure; visual field defects and acuity; chest: chronic infections, asthma; abdominal: pain, vomiting and diarrhoea; renal: polyuria, polydipsia and infections
Nutritional review	
Development history	
Examination	
Auxology/proportions	
Body composition:	Broad chest; truncal obesity/poor musle bulk
Dysmorphism	Facial features, midline defect, ears and palate
Hands/feet	Short metacarpals; clinodactyly; palmar creases; lymphoedema; clubbing
Visual	Field/acuity defects; optic atrophy/papilloedema; optic nerve hypoplasia, nystagmus
Genitalia	Small penis; pubertal staging
Systemic signs	Chest; cardiac; abdomen: distension, masses and anal skin tag; renal: hypertension, anaemia and renal masses

perform tests in a stepwise scheme, as outlined in Fig. 9.18, if there are no clues to the diagnosis after the history and examination. Full blood count, renal function, liver function, calcium homeostasis, thyroid function and anti-gliadin antibody are measured to exclude occult disorders such as anaemia, chronic renal failure, Bartter syndrome, hypophosphataemic rickets, hypothyroidism and coeliac disease.

A routine investigation in most children is a bone age assessment. Several methods are available to interpret bone age [256–258]. Although there are advantages and disadvantages for each method, this author does not believe that any method should be recommended in

Table 9.9 Suggested investigations for assessing the short child

Investigations	Clinical disorders
Bone age	
Karyotype (if female)	Turner syndrome
Systemic screen	
Full blood count	Anaemia, neutropenia of Schwachmann syndrome
ESR	Inflammatory bowel disease
Renal	Chronic renal failure, Bartter syndrome, renal tubular acidosis
Thyroid function	Hypothyroidism
Calcium, phosphorus, alkaline phosphatase	Vitamin D-deficient rickets, hypophosphataemic rickets
Gliadin antibody	Coeliac disease
Urine microscopy, culture and sensitivity	Renal infections
GH/IGF-I axis	
IGF-I and IGFBP-3	Nutritional insufficiency, chronic inflammatory disorders, GHD, transient GHD
GH provocation tests	GHD
Pulsatile GH secretion	GH insensitivity
Other imaging	
Skeletal survey	Skeletal dysplasias
Cranial ultrasound	Structural defects associated with GHD in infants
CT scan and MRI	Aetiology of GHD

ESR, erythrocyte sedimentation rate.

preference to the others; rather an observer should become proficient with one method. The clinical value of the bone age is threefold; first, it provides an estimation of an individual's remaining growth potential, remembering that girls reach skeletal maturity at a bone age of 15 years and boys reach a skeletal maturity at a bone age of 17 years. Secondly, it may provide a clue to an underlying diagnosis. An example of the latter is if a short fourth or fifth metacarpal is found, then Turner syndrome or pseudohypoparathyroidism should be considered. Thirdly, it is useful as a predictor of adult height which can be used to monitor a patient's progress longitudinally. Knowledge of an individual's bone age, chronological age and height allows one to calculate their EMH using either the tables of Bailey–Pinneau, Tanner–Whitehouse or Roche–Wainer–Thissen [257,259,260]. There is a significant standard deviation for the EMH which varies inversely with age; details are available in tables in various reference books. It is important to recognize the limitations in bone age assessment and, consequently, the EMH calculations. Various pathologies have different effects on the EMH calculated by the three methods [261–263]. In our clinic, using trained observers, the standard deviation for a measurement of bone age is 0.5 years (unpublished observ-

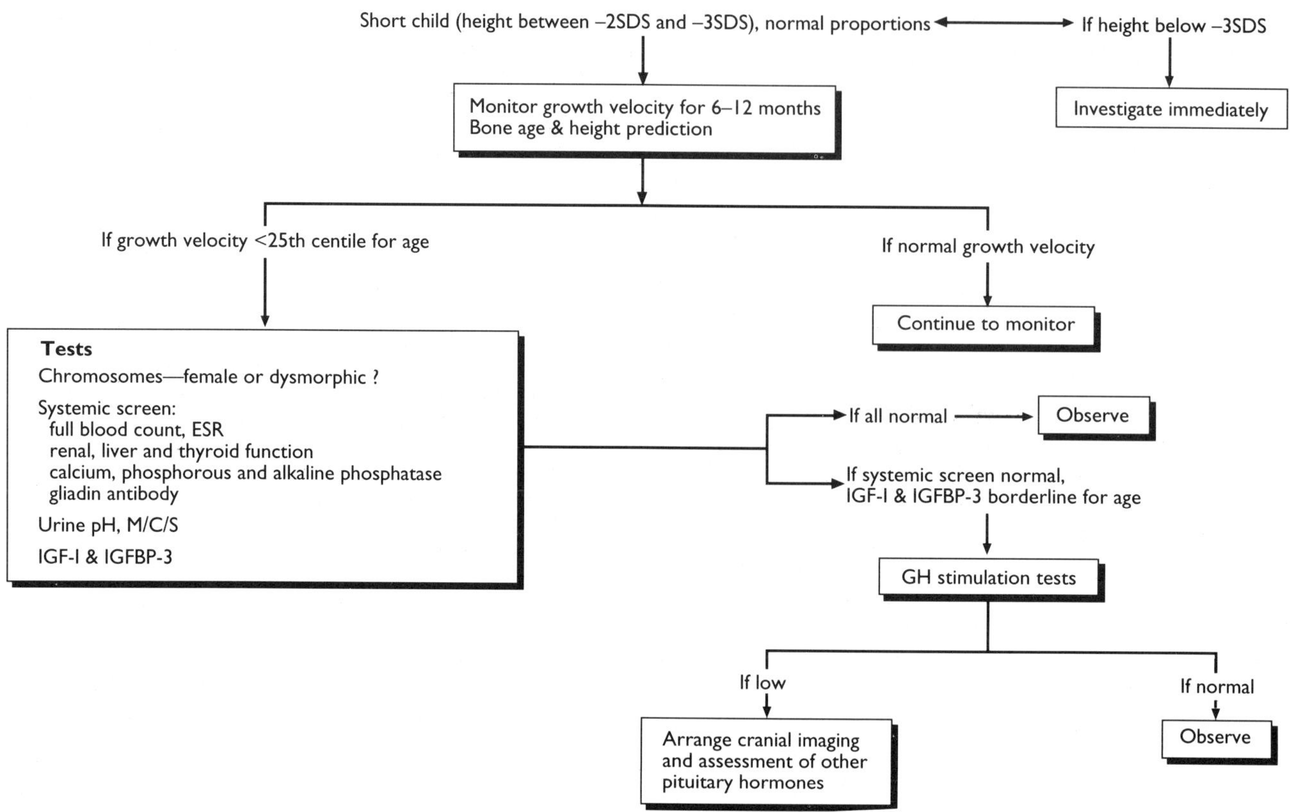

Fig. 9.18 Schema for short stature investigation. ESR, erythrocyte sedimentation rate; M/C/S, urine microscopy, culture and sensitivity.

ation) when assessed by the method of Greulich and Pyle or Tanner–Whitehouse. Thus, repeated assessment of bone age should be performed no more frequently than yearly.

Determining the GH status of an individual is not easy despite nearly 20 years experience of radioimmunoassays for GH. The debate about the interpretation of the provocation tests and the usefulness of determining pulsatile GH secretion has already been discussed. Random GH is of no value except in the neonatal period if GHD is suspected. Despite this, it is important to determine if an individual does have GHD, and the lower the values that are obtained, the more confident one can feel about the diagnosis. The importance is twofold: there may be an underlying acquired disorder which requires treatment and, the more convincing the GHD, the stronger is the rationale for GH replacement therapy. Until a better method of defining GHD is developed, the use of stimulation tests with all their limitations is currently recommended.

The tissue effects of IGF-I can be regarded as the final component of the endocrine/growth axis. Plasma IGF-I levels are age-dependent, rising during childhood years to peak during puberty similar to GH secretion, and this is followed by a gradual decline, especially during late adult years. Important regulators of IGF-I are GH, sex steroids and nutrition, low plasma values being seen with GHD and inadequate nutrition, high values being found with acromegaly and modest elevation with obesity. Measurement of plasma IGF-I is thus theoretically useful as a screening test for GHD, but consideration of the individual's age, pubertal and nutritional status is required [264,265]. For children under 6 years, the lower limit of the normal range is often close to the sensitivity of most assays; thus discriminating the child with GHD on the basis of a low IGF-I is particularly difficult in this age group. Some of the variability in the assay for IGF-I is probably consequent on interference by the binding proteins in the assay; thus most assays for IGF-I now require an extraction process to free IGF-I from these binding proteins [266].

IGF-I (and IGF-II) are tightly bound in the circulation by at least six binding proteins. IGFBP-3 is the major carrier protein for the insulin-like growth factors, and its concentration in the circulation is equimolar to the sum of IGF-I and IGF-II [267]. The regulation of IGFBP-3 is similar to IGF-I; that is age, nutrition and GH being important [268]. Blum *et al.* have demonstrated that measurement of IGFBP-3 may be more sensitive for diagnosing GHD than

IGF-I, but larger studies are needed to confirm this [268]. The other binding proteins for the insulin-like growth factors have not been demonstrated to be clinically useful as tests for growth problems [269].

The GH receptor through which GH stimulates IGF-I was identified only in 1987, and this receptor is widely distributed throughout human tissues [204]. It is now well established that there is a binding protein for growth hormone (GHBP) which circulates in the plasma, and probably in the human this is a proteolytic cleavage product of the GH receptor [204]. It has been proposed that measurement of plasma GHBP reflects tissue GH receptor concentrations, and while this is broadly the case, there is evidence for differential regulation of the two. It has been demonstrated that GHBP levels rise gradually during childhood years to reach a plateau at the time of puberty. Other important regulators appear to be sex steroids, but it is not as dependent upon GH as IGF-I [204]. Abnormalities of GHBP have been described: absent or low values in GH insensitivity, pygmies, Mountain Ok people, and high values in Alagille syndrome [270] and in some individuals with familial short stature [271].

Imaging of the hypothalamopituitary region is required if GHD is found. MRI is more sensitive than CT scans, both in detecting congenital abnormalities and defining organic disorders [272]. Investigations such as a CT scan or skull X-ray may be indicated early in the investigations if there are any symptoms or signs of an intracranial lesion. Cranial ultrasound is useful in infants suspected of hypopituitarism.

Management

For most individuals and families, knowledge that they do not have an underlying disorder, coupled with an understanding of their 'normal' growth potential, is reassuring. Future infrequent observation may be all that is required. For some, therapy of an underlying non-endocrine disorder will be needed, and for the remainder, intervention with a growth-promoting agent (either GH or sex steroid) may be considered (see Chapter 10).

ACKNOWLEDGEMENTS

The author wishes to thank Dr Geoff Ambler and Dr Peiwen Peggy Lu for their constructive comments and assistance with the production of figures. Ms Robyn Frater has provided invaluable secretarial assistance.

REFERENCES

1 Hammill PVV, Drizid TA, Johnson TL *et al.* Physical growth: National Center for Health Statistics percentiles. *Am J Clin Nutr* 1979;32:607–29.

2 Chavalittamrong B, Tantiwongse P. Height and weight of Thai children: update. *J Med Assoc Thailand* 1987;70:1–40.

3 Suwa S, Tachibana K, Tanaka T *et al.* Longitudinal growth and growth velocity of normal Japanese children from birth through 18 years old. *Clin Paediatr Endocrinol* 1992;1:5–13.

4 Tanner JM, White RH, Takaishi M. Standards from birth to maturity for height, weight, height velocity, and weight velocity: British children, 1965. *Arch Dis Child* 1966;41: 454–71.

5 WHO. *Measuring Change in Nutritional Status.* World Health Organization, 1983.

6 Lyon AJ, Preece MA, Grant DB. Growth curve for girls with Turner syndrome. *Arch Dis Child* 1985;60:932–5.

7 Horton WA, Rotter JI, Rimoin DL. Standard growth curve for achondroplasia. *J Pediatr* 1978;93:435–8.

8 Laron Z, Lilos P, Klinger B. Growth curves for Laron syndrome. *Arch Dis Child* 1993;68:768–70.

9 Witt DR, Keena BA, Hall JG, Allanson JE. Growth curves for height in Noonan syndrome. *Clin Genet* 1986;30:15–53.

10 Cronk C, Crocker AC, Pueschel SM *et al.* Growth charts for children with Down syndrome: 1 month to 18 years of age. *Pediatrics* 1988;81:102–10.

11 Growth references from conception to adulthood. *Proceedings of the Greenwood Genetic Centre* (Suppl. 1). Clinton, South Carolina: Jacobs Press, 1988.

12 Tanner JM, Goldstein H, Whitehouse RH. Standards for children's height at ages 2–9 years allowing for height of parents. *Arch Dis Child* 1970;45:755–62.

13 Tanner JM, Whitehouse RH. Clinical longitudinal stndards for height, weight, height velocity, weight velocity and stages of puberty. *Arch Dis Child* 1976;51:170–9.

14 Prader A, Largo RH, Molinari L, Issler C. Physical growth of Swiss children from birth to 20 years of age. First Zurich longitudinal study of growth and development. *Helv Paediatr Acta* (Suppl.) 1989;52:1–125.

15 Tanner JM, Davies PSW. Clinical longitudinal standards for American children. *J Pediatr* 1985;107:317–29.

16 Riken B, Wit JM. Prepubertal height velocity reference ranges over a wide age range. *Arch Dis Child* 1992;67: 1277–80.

17 Karlberg J. On the construction of the infancy–childhood–puberty growth standard. *Acta Paediatr Scand* (Suppl.) 1989; 356:26–37.

18 Karlberg J. A biologically oriented mathematical model (ICP) for human growth. *Acta Paediatr Scand* 1989;Suppl.350: 70–94.

19 Tanner JM. Use and abuse of growth standards. In: Falkner F, Tanner JM, eds. *Human Growth, a Comprehensive Treatise,* Vol. 3, 2nd edn. New York: Plenum Press, 1986:95–109.

20 Voss LD, Wilkin TJ, Bailey BJR, Betts PR. The reliability of height and height velocity in the assessment of growth (the Wessex Growth Study). *Arch Dis Child* 1991;66:833–7.

21 Marshall WA. Evaluation of growth rate in height over periods of less than one year. *Arch Dis Child* 1971;46: 414–20.

22 Voss LD, Bailey BJ, Cumming K, Wilkin TJ, Betts PR. The reliability of height measurement (the Wessex Growth Study). *Arch Dis Child* 1990;65:1340–4.

23 Vimpani GV, Vimpani AF, Lidgard GP, Cameron EHD, Farqhuar JW. Prevalence of severe growth hormone deficiency. *Br Med J* 1977;2:427–30.

24 Parkin JM. Incidence of growth hormone deficiency. *Arch Dis Child* 1974;49:904–5.

25 Mullis PE, Patel MS, Brickell PM, Brook CG. Constitution-

ally short stature: analysis of the insulin like growth factor I gene and the human growth hormone gene cluster. *Pediatr Res* 1991;29:412–15.

26 Thompson K, Dempsher DP, Bier DM, Tollefsen SE. Low prevalence of autoantibodies to the insulin-like growth factor I receptor in children with short stature. *Pediatr Res* 1992;32:455–9.

27 Albertsson-Wikland K, Rosberg S, Libre E, Lundberg LO, Groth T. Growth hormone secretory rates in children as estimated by deconvolution analysis of 24-h plasma concentration profiles. *Am J Physiol* 1989;257:E809–14.

28 Preece MA, Greco L, Savage MO *et al.* The auxology of growth delay. *Pediatr Res* 1980;15:76–7.

29 Solans CV, Lifshitz F. Body weight progression and nutritional status of patients with familial short stature with and without constitutional delay in growth. *Am J Dis Child* 1992;146:296–302.

30 Crowne EC, Shalet SM, Wallace WH, Eminson DM, Price DA. Final height in girls with untreated constitutional delay in growth and puberty. *Eur J Pediatr* 1991;150:708–10.

31 Crowne EC, Shalet SM, Wallace WH, Eminson DM, Price DA. Final height in boys with untreated constitutional delay in growth and puberty. *Arch Dis Child* 1990;65:1109–12.

32 LaFranchi S, Hanna C, Mandel SH. Constitutional delay of growth: expected versus final adult height. *Paediatrics* 1991;87:82–7.

33 Albanese A, Stanhope R. Does constitutional delayed puberty cause segmental disproportion and short stature? *Eur J Pediatr* 1993;152:293–6.

34 Gourmelen M, Pham Huu Trung MT, Girard F. Transient partial hGH deficiency in prepubertal children with delay of growth. *Pediatr Res* 1979;13:221.

35 Eastman CJ, Lazarus L, Stewart MC, Casey JH. The effect of puberty on growth hormone secretion in boys with short stature and delayed adolescence. *Austr NZ J Med* 1971;1: 154–9.

36 Spiliotis BE, August GP, Hung W, Sonis W, Mendelson W, Bercu BB. Growth hormone neurosecretory dysfunction. *J Am Med Assoc* 1984;251:2223–30.

37 Stanescu V, Stanescu R, Maroteaux P. Pathogenic mechanisms in osteochondrodysplasias. *J Bone Jt Surg* 1984;66A: 435–8.

38 Maroteaux P. International nomenclature of constitutional disorders of bones with bibliography. *Birth Defects* (original article series) 1986;XXII(4):1–54.

39 Mullis PE, Patel MS, Brickell PM, Hindmarsh PC, Brook CG. Growth characteristics and response to growth hormone therapy in patients with hypochondroplasia: genetic linkage of the insulin like growth factor I gene at chromosome 12q23 to the disease in a subgroup of these patients. *Clin Endocrinol (Oxf)* 1991;34:265–74.

40 Verge CF, Cowell CT, Howard NJ, Donaghue KC, Silink M. Growth in children with X-linked hypophosphataemic rickets. *Acta Paediatr Scand* 1993;Suppl.388:70–5.

41 Friedman NE, Lobaugh B, Drezner MK. Effects of calcitriol and phosphorus therapy on the growth of patients with X-linked hypophosphatemia. *J Clin Endocrinol Metab* 1993;76:839–44.

42 Lubchenco LO, Hansman C, Boyd E. Intrauterine growth in length and head circumference as estimated from live births at gestational ages from 26 to 42 weeks. *Paediatrics* 1966;37: 403–8.

43 Miller HC, Merritt TA. *Fetal Growth in Humans.* Chicago, IL: Year Book Medical Publishers, 1979:37–40.

44 Fay RA, Dey PL, Saadie MJ, Buhl JA, Gebski VJ. Ponderal index: a better definition of the 'at-risk' group with intrauterine growth problems than birthweight for gestational age in term infants. *Aust NZ J Obstet Gynaecol* 1991;31:17–19.

45 Paz I, Seidman DS, Danon Yl, Laor A, Stevenson DK, Gale R. Are children born small for gestational age at increased risk of short stature? *Am J Dis Child* 1993;147:337–9.

46 Heinrich UE. Intrauterine growth retardation and familial short stature. *Baillières Clin Endocrinol Metab* 1992;6: 589–601.

47 Tenovuo A, Kero P, Piekkala P, Korvenranta H, Sillanpaa M, Erkkola R. Growth of 519 small for gestational age infants during the first two years of life. *Acta Paediatr Scand* 1987;Suppl.76:636–46.

48 Sung I, Vohr B, Oh W. Growth and neurodevelopmental outcome of very low birth weight infants with intrauterine growth retardation: comparison with control subjects matched by birth weight and gestational age. *J Pediatr* 1993;123:618–24.

49 Fitzhardinge PM, Inwood S. Long-term growth in small-for-date children. *Acta Paediatr Scand* 1989;349:2–33.

50 Albertsson-Wikland K, Karlberg J. Natural growth in children born small-for-gestational-age (SGA) with and without catch-up. *Acta Paediatr Scand* 1994;Suppl.399: 64–70.

51 Karlberg J, Albertsson-Wikland K. Spontaneous growth and final height in SGA infants. *Pediatr Research* 1993;33:5.

52 Deiber M, Chatelain P, Naville D, Putet G, Salle B. Functional hypersomatotrophism in small for gestational age (SGA) newborn infants. *J Clin Endocrinol Metab* 1989; 68:232–4.

53 Ackland FM, Stanhope R, Eyre C, Hammill G, Jones J, Preece M. Physiological growth hormone secretion in children with short stature and intra-uterine growth retardation. *Horm Res* 1988;30:241–5.

54 Barker DJP, Fall CDH. Fetal and infant origins of cardiovascular disease. *Arch Dis Child* 1993;68:797–9.

55 Barker DJ, Gluckman PD, Godfrey KM, Harding JE, Owens JA, Robinson JS. Fetal nutrition and cardiovascular disease in adult life. *Lancet* 1993;341:931–2.

56 Buyse ML (ed.) *Birth Defects Encyclopedia.* Dover, MA: Center for Birth Defects Information Services, 1990.

57 Winter RM, Baraitser M (eds) *Multiple Congenital Anomalies; a Diagnostic Compendium.* London: Chapman & Hall Medical, 1991.

58 Jones KL (ed.) *Smith's Recognisable Patterns of Human Malformation.* Philadelphia, PA: WB Saunders, 1988.

59 McKusick VA. *Mendelian Inheritance in Man. Catalogues of Autosomal Dominant Recessive and X-linked Phenotypes*, 9th edn. Baltimore: Johns Hopkins University Press, 1990.

60 Enders H. Chromosomal and genetic forms of growth failure. *Baillières Clin Endocrinol Metab* 1992;6(3):621–43.

61 Tanner JM, Lejarraga H, Cameron N. The natural history of the Silver–Russell syndrome: a longitudinal study of thirty-nine cases. *Pediatr Res* 1975;9:611–23.

62 Davies PSW, Valley R, Preece MA. Adolescent growth and pubertal progression in the Silver–Russell syndrome. *Arch Dis Child* 1988;63:130–5.

63 Patton MA. Russell–Silver syndrome. *J Med Genet* 1988;25: 557–60.

64 Duncan PA, Hall JG, Shapiro LR, Vibert BK. Three-generation dominant transmission of the Silver–Russell syndrome. *Am J Med Genet* 1990;35:245–50.

65 Nora JJ, Nora AH, Sinha AK, Spangler RD, Lubs HA. The Ullrich–Noonan syndrome (Turner phenotype). *Am J Dis Child* 1974;127:48–55.
66 Ranke MB, Heidemann P, Knupfer C, Enders H, Schmaltz AA, Bierich JR. Noonan syndrome: growth and clinical manifestations in 144 cases. *Eur J Pediatr* 1988;148:220–7.
67 Ahmed ML, Foot ABM, Edge JA, Lamkin VA, Savage MO, Dunger DB. Noonan's syndrome: abnormalities of the growth hormone/IGF-I axis and the response to treatment with human biosynthetic growth hormone. *Acta Paediatr Scand* 1991;Suppl.80:446–50.
68 Mendez HMM, Opitz JM. Noonan syndrome: a review. *Am J Med Genet* 1985;21:493–506.
69 Stern HJ, Saal HM, Lee JS *et al.* Clinical variability of type 1 neurofibromatosis: is there a neurofibromatosis–Noonan syndrome? *J Med Genet* 1992;29:184–7.
70 Teebi AS, Rucquoi JK, Meyn MS. Aarskog syndrome: report of a family with review and discussion of nosology. *Am J Med Genet* 1993;46:501–9.
71 Hall JG. Catch 22. *J Med Genet* 1993;30:801–2.
72 Lipson AH, Yuille D, Angel M, Thompson PG, Vandervoord JG, Beckenham EJ. Velocardiofacial (Shprintzen) syndrome: an important syndrome for the dysmorphologist to recognise. *J Med Genet* 1991;28:596–604.
73 Shprintzen RJ, Goldberg RB, Lewin ML *et al.* A new syndrome involving cleft palate, cardiac anomalies, typical facies and learning disabilities. Velo-cardiofacial syndrome. *Cleft Palate J* 1978;15:56–62.
74 Driscoll DA, Salvin J, Sellinger B *et al.* Prevalence of 22q11 microdeletions in DiGeorge and velocardiofacial syndromes: implications for genetic counselling and prenatal diagnosis. *J Med Genet* 1993;30:813–7.
75 Lippe B. Turner syndrome. *Endocrinol Metab Clin N Am*, 1991;20:121–52.
76 Hall JG *et al. West J Med* 1982;137:32–44.
77 Nielsen J *et al. Acta Jutlandica Liv Med Ser* 22, *Arttus.*
78 Palmer CG *et al. Hum Genet* 1976;35:35–49.
79 Park E *et al. Paediatr Res* 1983;17:1–7.
80 Suwa S. *Acta Paediatr Jpn* 1992;34:206–21.
81 Connor JM, Loughlin SAR. Molecular genetics of Turner's syndrome. *Acta Paediatr Scand* (Suppl.) 1989;356:77–80.
82 Henke A, Wapenaar M, van Ommen GJ, Maraschio P, Camerino G, Rappold G. Deletions within the pseudoautosomal region help map three new markers and indicate a possible role of this region in linear growth. *Am J Hum Genet* 1991;49:811–19.
83 Ranke MB. Growth disorder in the Ullrich–Turner syndrome. *Baillière's Clin Endocrinol Metab* 1993;6:603–19.
84 Massa G, Malvaux P, Vanderschueren-Lodeweyckx M. Spontaneous growth in Turner syndrome: the Belgian experience. In: Ranke MB, Rosenfeld RG, eds. *Turner's Syndrome and Growth Promoting Therapies*. Amsterdam: Excerpta Medica, 1991:95–9.
85 Ranke MB, Chavez-Meyer H, Blank B, Frisch H, Hausler G. Spontaneous growth and bone age development in Turner syndrome: results of a multicentre study, 1990. In: Ranke MB, Rosenfeld RG, eds. *Turner Syndrome and Growth Promoting Therapies*. Amsterdam: Excerpta Medica, 1991: 101–6.
86 Tachibana K, Suwa S. The longitudinal natural growth of Turner syndrome and normal Japanese children. In: Cowell CT, Werther G, Ho K, eds. *Growth and Sexual Development*. Harwood Academic Publishers, Chur, Switzerland,1993: 117–29.
87 Massa G, Vanderschueren-Lodeweyckx M, Malvaux P. Linear growth in patients with Turner syndrome: influence of spontaneous puberty and parental height. *Eur J Pediatr* 1990;149:246–50.
88 Karlberg J, Albertsson-Wikland K, Naeraa RW. The infancy–childhood–puberty (ICP) model of growth for Turner girls. In: Ranke MB, Rosenfeld RG, eds. *Turner Syndrome: Growth Promoting Therapies*. Amsterdam: Excerpta Medica, 1991: 89–94.
89 Reiter JC, Craen M, Van Vliet G. Decreased growth hormone response to growth hormone releasing hormone in Turner's syndrome: relation to body weight and adiposity. *Acta Endocrinol (Copenh)* 1991;125:38–42.
90 Lu PW, Cowell CT, Jimenez M, Simpson JM, Silink M. Effects of obesity on endogenous growth hormone secretion in Turner syndrome. *Arch Dis Child* 1991;66:1184–90.
91 Wit JM, Massarano AA, Kamp GA *et al.* Growth hormone secretion in patient's with Turner's syndrome as determined by time series analysis. *Acta Endocrinol (Copenh)* 1992;127: 7–12.
92 Rovet JF. The psychoeducational characteristics of children with Turner syndrome. *J Learn Disabil* 1993;26:333–41.
93 Downey J, Elkin EJ, Ehrhardt AA, Meyer Bahlburg HF, Bell JJ, Morishima A. Cognitive ability and everyday functioning in women with Turner syndrome. *J Learn Disabil* 1991;24(1):32–9.
94 Latham MC. Protein–energy malnutrition. Its epidemiology and control. *J Environ Pathol Toxicol Oncol* 1990;10: 168–80.
95 Meredith HV. Research between 1960 and 1970 on the standing height of young children in different parts of the world. *Adv Child Dev Behav* 1978;12:1–59.
96 Lifshitz F, Moses N. Nutritional growth retardation. In: Lifshitz F, ed. *Pediatric Endocrinology, a Clinical Guide.* New York: Marcel Dekker, 1985:111–32.
97 Laitinen R, Vouri E, Dahlstrom S, Akerblom HK. Zinc, copper, and growth status in children and adolescents. *Pediatr Res* 1988;25:323–6.
98 Gibson RS, Smit Vanderkooy PD, MacDonald AC, Goldman A, Ryan BA, Berry M. A growth-limiting, mild zinc deficiency syndrome in some southern Ontario boys with low height percentiles. *Am J Clin Nutr* 1989;49:1266–73.
99 Nakamura T, Nishiyama S, Futagoishi-Suginohara Y, Matsuda I, Higashi A. Mild to moderate zinc deficiency in short children: effect of zinc supplementation on linear growth velocity. *J Pediatr* 1993;123:65–9.
100 Nishi Y, Hatano S, Aihara K, Fujie A, Kihara M. Transient partial growth hormone deficiency due to zinc deficiency. *J Am Coll Nutr* 1989;8:93–7.
101 Collip PJ, Castro-Magana M, Petrovic M *et al.* Zinc deficiency: improvement in growth and growth hormone levels with oral zinc therapy. *Ann Nutr Metab* 1982;26: 287–90.
102 Walravens PA, Hambidge KM, Koepfer DM. Zinc supplementation in infants with a nutritional pattern of failure to thrive: a double-blind, controlled study. *Pediatrics* 1989; 83:532–8.
103 Payne-Robinson HM, Golden MHN, Golden BE, Simeon OT. The zinc sandwich and growth. *Lancet* 1991;337:925–6.
104 Herzog DB, Copeland PM. Eating disorders. *N Engl J Med* 1985;313:295–303.
105 Fosson A, Knibbs J, Bryant-Waugh R, Lask B. Early onset anorexia nervosa. *Arch Dis Child* 1987;62:114–18.
106 Abdenur JE, Pugliese MT, Cervantes C, Fort P, Lifshitz F.

Alterations in spontaneous growth hormone (GH) secretion and the response to GH-releasing hormone in children with non organic nutritional dwarfing. *J Clin Endocrinol Metab* 1992;75:930–4.

107 Rappoport R, Prevot C, Czernichow P. Somathormone et activite somatomedine plasmatique au cours amaigrissements graves de l'anorexie mentale chez l'enfant. *Ann Endocrinol* 1978;39:259–60.

108 Allen RC, Jimenez M, Cowell CT. Insulin like growth factor and GH secretion in juvenile chronic arthritis. *Ann Rheum Dis* 1991;50:602–6.

109 Blizzard RM, Bulatovic A. Psychosocial short stature: a syndrome with many variables. *Baillières Clin Endocrinol Metab* 1992;6:687–712.

110 Stanhope R, Adlard P, Hammill G, Jones J, Skuse D, Preece MA. Physiological growth hormone (GH) secretion during recovery from psychosocial dwarfism: a case report. *Clin Endocrinol* 1988;28:335–9.

111 Sarr M, Job JC, Chaussain JL, Golse B. Les retardes de croissance psychogenes. Etude critique des elements de diagnostic. *Arch Fr Pediatre* 1987;44:331–8.

112 Tanner JH. Resistance to exogenous human growth hormone in psychosocial short stature (emotional deprivation). *J Pediatr* 1973:82:171–2.

113 Frazier SD, Rallison O. Growth retardation and emotional deprivation: relative resistance to treatment with human growth hormone. *J Pediatr* 1972;80:603–9.

114 Boulton TJ, Smith R, Single T. Psychosocial growth failure: a positive response to growth hormone and placebo. *Acta Paediatr Scand* 1992;Suppl.81:322–5.

115 Salzer HR, Haschke F, Wimmer M, Heil M, Schilling R. Growth and nutritional intake of infants with congenital heart disease. *Pediatr Cardiol* 1989;10:17–23.

116 Byard PJ. Early childhood growth in patients with cystic fibrosis. *Ann Hum Biol* 1990;17:483–99.

117 Verkasalo M, Kuitunen P, Leistri JS, Perheentupa J. Growth failure from symptomless coeliac disease. *Helv Paediatr Acta* 1978;33:489–95.

118 Groll A, Preece MA, Candy DCA, Tanner JM. Short stature as the primary manifestation of coeliac disease. *Lancet* 1980;2:1097–9.

119 Knudtzon J, Fluge G, Aksnes L. Routine measurements of gluten antibodies in children of short stature. *J Pediatr Gastroenterol Nutr* 1991;12:190–4.

120 Griffiths AM, Nguyen P, Smith C, Macmillan JH, Sherman PM. Growth and clinical course of children with Crohn's disease. *Gut* 1993;34:939–43.

121 Kanof ME, Lake AM, Bayless TM. Decreased height velocity in children and adolescents before the diagnosis of Crohn's disease. *Gastroenterology* 1988;95:1523–7.

122 Kirschner BS. Growth and development in chronic inflammatory bowel disease. *Acta Paediatr Scand* 1990;Suppl.366: 98–104.

123 Ray PE, Holliday MA. Growth rate in infants with impaired renal function. *J Pediatr* 1988;113:594–600.

124 Van Diemen-Steenvoorde R, Donckerwolcke RA, Brackel H, Wolff ED, De Jong MCJW. Growth and sexual maturation in children after kidney transplantation. *J Pediatr* 1987;110: 351–6.

125 Scharer K, Mehls O, Schaefer F, Tonshoff B. Growth retardation in chronic renal failure. In: Cowell CT, Werther G, Ho K, eds. *Growth and Sexual Development*. Harwood Academic Publishers, Chur, Switzerland 1993:103–16.

126 Jureidini KF, Hogg RJ, van-Renen MJ *et al.* Evaluation of long-term aggressive dietary management of chronic renal failure in children. *Pediatr Nephrol* 1990;4:1–10.

127 Hokken-Koelega ACS, Hackeng WHL *et al.* 24-hour plasma GH profiles, urinary GH excretion and plasma IGF-I and -II levels in prepubertal children with chronic renal insufficiency and severe growth retardation. *J Clin Endocrinol Metab* 1990;71:688–95.

128 Blum WF, Ranke MB, Kietzmann K, Ganggel EM, Zeisel HJ, Bierich JR. A specific radioimmunoassay for the growth hormone-dependent somatomedin binding protein: its use for diagnosis of GH deficiency. *J Clin Endocrinol Metab* 1990;70:1292–8.

129 Cowell CT, Loke Y, Baxter RC. The response of insulin-like growth factor binding protein-3 complex to growth hormone. *Clin Pediatr Endocrinol* 1993;2(Suppl. 2):45–50.

130 Bettinelli A, Bianchetti MG, Girardin E *et al.* Use of calcium excretion values to distinguish two forms of primary renal tubular hypokalemic alkalosis: Bartter and Gitelman syndromes. *J Pediatr* 1992;120:38–43.

131 Ruvalcaba RH, Martinez FE. Case report: familial growth hormone deficiency associated with Bartter's syndrome. *Am J Med Sci* 1992;303:411–14.

132 Murray AB, Fraser BM, Hardwick DF, Pirie GE. Chronic asthma and growth failure in children. *Lancet* 1976;2: 197–8.

133 Cogswell JJ, El-Bishiti MM. Growth retardation in asthma: role of calorie deficiency. *Arch Dis Child* 1982;57:473–80.

134 Hauspie R, Susanne C, Alexander F. A mixed longitudinal study of the growth in height and weight in asthmatic children. *Hum Biol* 1976;48:271–83.

135 Chang KC, Miklich DR, Barwise G *et al.* Linear growth of asthmatic children: the effects of the disease and various forms of steroid therapy. *Clin Allergy* 1982;12:369–78.

136 Volovitz B, Amir J, Malik H, Kauschansky A, Varsano I. Growth and pituitary function in children with severe asthma treated with inhaled budesonide. *N Engl J Med* 1993;329:1703–8.

137 Hauspie R, Susanne C, Alexander F. Maturational delay and temporal growth retardation in asthmatic boys. *J Allergy Clin Immunol* 1977;59:200–6.

138 Martin AJ, Landau LI, Phelan PD. The effect on growth of childhood asthma. *Acta Paediatr Scand* 1981;70:683–8.

139 Shohat M, Shohat T, Kedem R *et al.* Childhood asthma and growth outcome. *Arch Dis Child* 1987;62:63–5.

140 Oberger E, Engstrom I, Karlberg J. Long-term treatment with glucocorticoids/ACTH in asthmatic children. III. Effects on growth and adult height. *Acta Paediatr Scand* 1990; Suppl.79:77–83.

141 Wolthers OD, Pedersen S. Short term linear growth in asthmatic children during treatment with prednisolone. *Br Med J* 1990;301:145–8.

142 Kerrebjin KF, de Kroon JPM. Effect on height of corticosteroid therapy in asthmatic children. *Arch Dis Child* 1968; 43:556–61.

143 Ninan T, Russell G. Asthma, inhaled corticosteroid treatment and growth. *Arch Dis Child* 1992;67:703–5.

144 Wolthers OD, Pedersen S. Controlled study of linear growth in asthmatic children during treatment with inhaled glucocorticosteroids. *Pediatrics* 1992;89:839–42.

145 Balfour-Lynn L. Growth and childhood asthma. *Arch Dis Child* 1986;61:1049–55.

146 Tabachnik E, Zadik Z. Diurnal cortisol secretion during therapy with inhaled beclomethasone dipropionate in children with asthma. *J Paediatr* 1991;118:294–7.

147 Hill DJ. Effects of cortisol on cell proliferation and proteoglycan synthesis and degradation in cartilage zones of the calf costochondral growth plate *in vitro* with and without plasma somatomedin activity. *J Endocrinol* 1981;88: 425–30.
148 Mosier HD Jr, Jansons RA, Hill RR *et al.* Cartilage sulfation and serum somatomedin in rats during and after cortisone-induced growth arrest. *Endocrinology* 1976;99:580–9.
149 Miell JP, Corder R, Pralong FP, Gaillard RC. Effects of dexamethasone on growth hormone (GH)-releasing hormone, arginine- and dopaminergic-stimulated GH secretion, and total plasma insulin-like growth factor-I concentrations in normal male volunteers. *J Clin Endocrinol Metab* 1991;72: 675–81.
150 Kattamis C, Liakopoulou T, Kattamis A. Growth and development in children with thalassemia major. *Acta Paediatr Scand* 1990;Suppl.366:111–17.
151 Postel-Vinay MC, Giro R, Leger J *et al.* No evidence for a defect in growth hormone binding to liver membranes in thalassemia major. *J Clin Endocrinol Metab* 1989;68:94–8.
152 August GP, Lippe BM, Blethen L *et al.* Growth hormone treatment in the United States: demographic and diagnostic features of 2331 children. *J Pediatr* 1990;116:899–903.
153 Gluckman PD, Gunn AJ, Wray A *et al.* Congenital idiopathic growth hormone deficiency associated with prenatal and early postnatal growth failure. *J Pediatr* 1992;121:920–3.
154 Root AW, Rosenfield RL, Bongiovanni AM, Eberlein WR. The plasma growth hormone response to insulin-induced hypoglycaemia in children. *Pediatrics* 1967;39:844–52.
155 Penny R, Blizzard RM, Davis WT. Sequential arginine and insulin tolerance test on the same day. *J Clin Endocrinol Metab* 1968;29:1499–501.
156 Gil-Ad I, Topper E, Laron Z. Oral clonidine as a growth hormone stimulation test. *Lancet* 1979;2:278–9.
157 Weldon VV, Gupta SK, Haymond MW, Pagliara AS, Jacobs LS, Daughaday WH. The use of L-dopa in the diagnosis of hyposomatotropism in children. *J Clin Endocrinol Metab* 1973;36:42–6.
158 Mitchell ML, Suvunrungsi P, Sawin CT. Effect of propranolol on the response of serum growth hormone to glucagon. *J Clin Endocrinol Metab* 1971;32:470–5.
159 Gelato MC, Malazowski S, Caruso-Nocoletti M *et al.* Growth hormone (GH) response to GH-releasing hormone during pubertal development in normal boys and girls: comparison to idiopathic short stature and GH deficiency. *J Clin Endocrinol Metab* 1986;63:174–9.
160 Ranke MB, Gruhleer M, Rosskamp R *et al.* Testing with growth hormone-releasing factor ((GRF)(1–29)NH2) and somatomedin C measurements for the evaluation of growth hormone deficiency. *Eur J Pediatr* 1986;145:465–92.
161 Shah A, Stanhope R, Matthew D. Hazards of pharmacological tests of growth hormone secretion in childhood. *Br Med J* 1992;304:173–4.
162 Silink M. Alternative methods of diagnosis of growth hormone deficiency. *J Paediatr Endocrinol* 1992;5:43–52.
163 Dattani MT, Pringle PJ, Hindmarsh PC, Brook CG. What is a normal stimulated growth hormone concentration? *J Endocrinol* 1992;133:447–50.
164 Reiter EO, Morris AH, McGillvray MH, Weber D. Variable estimates of serum growth hormone concentrations by different radioassay systems. *J Clin Endocrinol Metab* 1988;66:68–71.
165 Celniker AC, Chen AB, Wert RM, Sherman B. Variability in the quantitation of circulating growth hormone using commercial immunoassays. *J Clin Endocrinol Metab* 1989;68:469–76.
166 Chatelain P, Bouillat B, Cohen R *et al.* Assay of growth hormone levels in human plasma using commercial kits: analysis of some factors influencing the results. *Acta Paediatr Scand* (Suppl.) 1990;370:56–61.
167 Zadik A, Stuart AC, Gukula X, Kowarski AA. Reproducibility of growth hormone testing procedures: a comparison between 24-hour integrated concentration and pharmacological stimulation. *J Clin Endocrinol Metab* 1990;71: 1127–30.
168 Saini S, Hindmarsh PC, Matthews DR *et al.* Reproducibility of 24-hour serum growth hormone profiles in man. *Clin Endocrinol (Oxf)* 1991;34:455–62.
169 Cacciari E, Tassoni P, Parisi G *et al.* Pitfalls in diagnosing impaired growth hormone (GH) secretion: retesting after replacement therapy of 63 patients defined as GH deficient. *J Clin Endocrinol Metab* 1992;74:1284–9.
170 Buchanan CR. Growth hormone deficiency: lessons from the past. In: Cowell CT, Werther G, Ho K, eds. *Growth and Sexual Development*. Harwood Academic Publishers, Chur, Switzerland 1993:73–90.
171 Rose ST, Municchi G, Barnes KM *et al.* Spontaneous growth hormone secretion increases during puberty in normal girls and boys. *J Clin Endocrinol Metab* 1991;73:428–35.
172 Mauras N, Blizzard RM, Link K, Johnson MC, Rogol AD, Veldhius JD. Augmentation of growth hormone secretion during puberty: evidence for a pulse amplitude-modulated phenomenon. *J Clin Endocrinol Metab* 1987;64:596–601.
173 Rose SR, Ross JL, Uriatre M, Barnes KM, Cassorla FG, Cutler GB. The advantage of measuring stimulated as compared with spontaneous growth hormone levels in diagnosis of growth hormone deficiency. *N Engl J Med* 1988;31:201–7.
174 Girard J, Celniker A, Price A *et al.* Urinary measurement of growth hormone secretion. *Acta Paediatr Scand* (Suppl.) 1990;366:149–54.
175 Christiansen JS, Jorgensen JO, Muller J *et al.* Growth hormone deficiency in adults. Clinical, metabolic and pharmacological aspects. In: Cowell CT, Werther G, Ho K, eds. *Growth and Sexual Development*. Harwood Academic Publishers, Chur, Switzerland 1993:63–70.
176 Rona RJ, Tanner JM. Aetiology of idiopathic growth hormone deficiency in England and Wales. *Arch Dis Child* 1977;52:197–208.
177 Wilton P, Wallstrom A. An overview of the diagnoses in the Kabi Pharmacia International Growth Study. *Acta Paediatr Scand* 1991;Suppl.379:93–8.
178 Goossens M, Brauner R, Czernichow P, Duquesnoy P, Rappaport R. Isolated growth (GH) deficiency type 1A associated with a double deletion in the human GH gene cluster. *J Clin Endocrinol Metab* 1986;62:712–16.
179 Rivarola MA, Phillips JA III, Migeon CJ, Heinrich JJ, Hjelle BL. Phenotypic heterogeneity in familial isolated growth hormone deficiency type 1-A. *J Clin Endocrinol Metab* 1984;59:34–40.
180 Mullis PE, Akinci A, Kanaka C, Eble A, Brook CG. Prevalence of human growth hormone-1 gene deletions among patients with isolated growth hormone deficiency from different populations. *Pediatr Res* 1992;31:532–4.
181 Fleisher TA, White RM, Broder S. X-linked hypogammaglobulinemia and isolated growth hormone deficiency. *N Eng J Med* 1980;302:1429–34.
182 Tang Mimi LK, Kemp AS. Growth hormone deficiency and

combined immunodeficiency. *Arch Dis Child* 1993;68: 231–2.

183 McArthur RG, Morgan K, Phillips JA III, Bala M, Klassen J. The natural history of familial hypopituitarism. *Am J Med Genet* 1985;22:553–66.

184 Wit JM, Drayer NM, Jansen M *et al.* Total deficiency of growth hormone and prolactin and partial deficiency of thyroid stimulating hormone in two Dutch families: a new variant of hereditary pituitary deficiency. *Horm Res* 1989; 32:170–7.

185 Yoshimoto M, Kinoshita E, Baba T *et al.* Growth hormone, prolactin and thyroid stimulating hormone deficiencies with hypoplasia of the anterior pituitary gland: a new type of primary multiple pituitary hormone deficiency. *Act Pediatr Scand* 1990;Suppl.79:1247–51.

186 Li S, Creshaw EB, Rawson EJ, Simmons DM, Swanson LW, Rosenfeld MG. Dwarf locus mutants lacking three pituitary cell types result from mutations in the POU-domain gene pit-1. *Nature* 1990;347:528–33.

187 Simmons DM, Voss JW, Ingraham HA *et al.* Pituitary cell phenotypes involve cell-specific pit-I mRNA translation and synergistic interactions with other classes of transcription factors. *Genes Dev* 1990;4:695–711.

188 Laron Z, Petzelan A, Mannheimer S. Genetic pituitary dwarfism with high serum concentration of growth hormone. A new inborn error of metabolism? *Isr J Med Sci* 1966;323:1367–74.

189 Rosenbloom AL, Aguirre JG, Rosenfeld RG, Fielder PJ. The little women of Loja – growth hormone-receptor deficiency in an inbred population of southern Ecuador. *N Engl J Med* 1990;323:1367–74.

190 Amselem S, Duquesnoy P, Goossens M. Molecular basis of Laron dwarfism. *Trends Endocrinol Metab* 1991;2:35–40.

191 Tollesfsen SE, Heath-Moning E, Cascieri MA, Bagne ML, Daughaday WH. Endogenous insulin-like growth factor (IGF) binding proteins cause IGF-1 resistance in cultured fibroblasts from a patient with short stature. *J Clin Invest* 1991; 87:1241–50.

192 Lanes R, Plotnick LP, Spencer EM, Daughaday WH, Kowarski AA. Dwarfism associated with normal serum growth hormone and increased bioassayable, receptorassayable, and immunoassayable somatomedin. *J Clin Endocrinol Metab* 1980;50:485–8.

193 Bierich JR, Moeller H, Ranke MB, Rosenfeld RG. Pseudopituitary dwarfism due to resistance to somatomedin: a new syndrome. *Eur J Pediatr* 1984;142:186–8.

194 Pintor C, Loche S, Cella SG, Muller EE, Baumannn G. A child
with phenotypic Laron dwarfism and normal somatomedin levels. *N Engl J Med* 1989;320:376–96.

195 Momoi T, Yamanaka C, Kobayashi M *et al.* Short stature with normal growth hormone and elevated IGF-I. *Eur J Pediatr* 1992;151:321–5.

196 Bailey RC, Devore I. Research on Efe and Less populations of the Tituri forest. *Am J Phys Anthropol* 1989;78:459–71.

197 Bailey RC. The comparative growth of Efe pygmies and African farmers from birth to age 5 years. *Ann Hum Biol* 1991;18:113–20.

198 Baumann G, Shaw MA, Merimee TJ. Low levels of high-affinity growth hormone-binding protein in African pygmies. *N Engl J Med* 1989;120:1705–9.

199 Merimee TJ, Baumann G, Daughaday W. Growth hormone-binding protein. II. Studies in pygmies and normal statured subjects. *J Clin Endocrinol Metab* 1990;71:175–80.

200 Geffner ME, Bailey RC, Bersch N, Vera JC, Golde DW. Insulin-like growth factor-I unresponsiveness in an Efe pygmy. *Biochem Biophys Res Commun* 1993;193:1216–23.

201 Baumann G, Shaw MA, Brumbaugh RC, Schwartz J. Short stature and decreased serum growth hormone-binding protein in the Mountain Ok people of Papua New Guinea. *J Clin Endocrinol Metab* 1991;72:1346–9.

202 Craft WH, Underwood LE, Van Wyk JJ. High incidence of perinatal insult in children with idiopathic hypopituitarism. *J Pediatr* 1980;96:397–402.

203 Sheehan AG, Martin SR, Stephure D, Scott RB. Neonatal cholestasis, hypoglycemia and congenital hypopituitarism. *J Paediatr Gastr Nutr* 1992;14:426–30.

204 Waters MJ, Lokie PE, Garcia-Aragon J *et al.* Structure, location and role of the growth hormone receptor. In: Cowell CT, Werther G, Ho K, eds. *Growth and Sexual Development*. Harwood Academic Publishers, Chur, Switzerland 1993: 3–27.

205 Root AW, Martinez CR, Muroff LR. Sub-hypothalamic high-quality signals identified by magnetic resonance imaging in children with idiopathic anterior hypopituitarism. Evidence suggestive of an 'ectopic' posterior gland. *Am J Dis Child* 1989;143:366–7.

206 Kikuchi K, Fujisawa I, Momoi, T *et al.* Hypothalamic–pituitary function in growth hormone-deficiency patients with pituitary stalk transection. *J Clin Endocrinol Metab* 1988;67:817–23.

207 Argropoulou M, Perignon F, Brunelle F, Brauner R, Rappaport R. Height of normal pituitary gland as a function of age evaluated by magnetic resonance imaging in children. *Pediatr Radiol* 1991;22:247–9.

208 Marwaha R, Menon PSN, Jena A, Pant C, Wethi AK, Sapra ML. Hypothalamic–pituitary axis by magnetic resonance in isolated growth hormone deficiency patients born by normal delivery. *J Clin Endocrinol Metab* 1992;74:654–9.

209 Zhang CZ, Young WG, Waters MJ. Immunocytochemical localization of growth hormone receptor in rat maxillary teeth. *Arch Oral Biol* 1992;37:77–84.

210 Rosen T, Bengtsson BA. Premature cardiovascular mortality in hypopituitarism – a study of 333 consecutive patients. *Lancet* 1990;336:285–8.

211 Lippe BM, Van Herle AJ, Lafranchi SH, Uller RP *et al.* Reversible hypothyroidism in growth hormone-deficient children treated with human growth hormone. *J Clin Endocrinol Metab* 1975;40:612–18.

212 Suter SN, Kaplan SL, Aubert ML, Grumbach MM. Plasma prolactin and thyrotropin-releasing factor in children with primary and hypothalamic hypothyroidism. *J Clin Endocrinol Metab* 1978;47:1015–20.

213 Ho KY, Weissberger AJ, Stuart MC, Day RO, Lazarus L. The pharmacokinetics, safety and endocrine effects of authentic biosynthetic human growth hormone in normal subjects. *Clin Endocrinol* 1989;30:335–45.

214 Hoyt WF, Kaplan SL, Grumbach MM. Hypothalamic–pituitary function in children with optic nerve hypoplasia. *Am J Dis Child* 1985;1:893–4.

215 Pierre-Kahn A, Capelle L, Brauner R *et al.* Presentation and management of suprasellar arachnoid cysts. Review of 20 cases. *J Neurosurg* 1990;73:355–9.

216 Shulman DI, Martinez CR, Bercu BB, Root AW. Hypothalamic–pituitary dysfunction in primary empty sella syndrome in childhood. *J Pediatr* 1986;108:540–54.

217 Rudman D, Davis T, Priest JH *et al.* Prevalence of growth hormone deficiency in children with cleft lip or palate. *J*

Pediatr 1978;91:378–28.
218 Rappaport EB, Ulstrom RA, Gorlin RJ, Lucky AW, Collie E, Miser J. Solitary maxillary central incisor and short stature. *J Pediatr* 1977;91:924–8.
219 Sadeghi-Nejad A, Senoir B. Autosomal transmission of isolated GH deficiency in iris-dental dysplasia. *J Pediatr* 1974;85:644–8.
220 Thomsett MJ, Conte FA, Kaplan SL, Grumbach MD. Endocrine and neurologic outcome in childhood craniopharyngioma: review of effect of treatment in 42 patients. *J Pediatr* 1980;97:728–35.
221 Laws ER Jr. Craniopharyngioma: diagnosis and treatment. *Endocrinologist* 1992;2:184–8.
222 Bistritzer T, Chalwe SA, Lovechik JC, Kowardk AA. Growth without growth hormone, the 'invisible' GH syndrome. *Lancet* 1988;i:321–3.
223 Sorva R. Children with craniopharyngioma. Early growth failure and rapid postoperative weight gain. *Acta Paediatr Scand* 1988;Suppl.77:587–92.
224 Bucher H, Zapf J, Torresani T, Prader A, Froesch R, Illig R. Insulin-like growth factors I and II, prolactin, and insulin in 19 growth hormone-deficient children with excessive, normal, or decreased longitudinal growth after operation for craniopharyngioma. *N Engl J Med* 1983;309:1142–6.
225 Yamamoto T, Katsumata N, Tachibana K, Friesen HG, Nagy JI. Distribution of a novel peptide in the anterior pituitary, gastric pyloric gland, and pancreatic islets of rat. *J Histochem Cytochem* 1992;40:221–9.
226 Dennis M, Spiegler BJ, Obonsawin MC *et al.* Brain tumours in children and adolescents – III. Effects of radiation and hormone status on intelligence and on working, associative and serial-order memory. *Neuropsychologia* 1992;30:257–75.
227 Brauner R, Malandry F, Rappaport R *et al.* Growth and endocrine disorders in optic glioma. *Eur J Pediatr* 1990;149: 825–8.
228 Sklar C, Grumbach MM, Kaplan SL, Conte FA. Hormonal and metabolic abnormalities associated with central nervous system germinoma in children and adolescents and the effect of therapy: report of 10 patients. *J Clin Endocrinol Metab* 1981;52:9–16.
229 Braunstein GD, Kohler PO. Endocrine manifestations of histiocytosis. *Am J Paed Haem Oncol* 1981;3:67–75.
230 Darendeliler F, Livesey EA, Hindmarsh PC, Brook CG. Growth and growth hormone secretion in children following treatment of brain tumours with radiotherapy. *Acta Pediatr Scand* 1990;Suppl.79:950–6.
231 Rappaport R, Brauner R. Growth and endocrine disorders secondary to cranial irradiation. *Pediatr Res* 1989;25:561–7.
232 Shalet SM, Crowne EC, Didi MA, Ogilvy-Stuart AL, Wallace WH. Irradiation-induced growth failure. *Baillières Clin Endocrinol Metab* 1992;6:513–26.
233 Moell C. Disturbed pubertal growth in girls after acute leukemia: a relative growth hormone sufficiency with late presentation. *Acta Paediatr Scand* 1988;Suppl.343:162–6.
234 Kirk JA, Raghupathy P, Stevens MM *et al.* Growth failure and growth hormone deficiency after treatment for acute lymphoblastic leukemia. *Lancet* 1987;1:190–3.
235 Clayton PE, Shalet SM, Morris-Jones PH, Price DA. Growth in children treated for acute lymphoblastic leukaemia. *Lancet* 1988;1:460–2.
236 Crowne EC, Moore C, Wallace WH *et al.* A novel variant of growth hormone (GH) insufficiency following low dose cranial irradiation. *Clin Endocrinol* 1992;36:59–68.
237 Sanders JE, Pritchard S, Mahoney P *et al.* Growth and development following marrow transplantation for leukemia. *Blood* 1986;68:1129–35.
238 Ryalls M, Spoudeas HA, Hindmarsh PC *et al.* Short-term endocrine consequences of total body irradiation and bone marrow transplantation in children treated for leukemia. *J Endocrinol* 1993;136:331–8.
239 Ogilvy-Stuart AL, Clark DJ, Wallace WH *et al.* Endocrine deficit after fractionated total body irradiation. *Arch Dis Child* 1992;67:1107–10.
240 Girard J, Marelli R. Posttraumatic hypothalamopituitary insufficiency. *J Pediatr* 1977;90:241–2.
241 Keller RJ, Wolfsdorf JI. Isolated growth hormone deficiency after cerebral edema complicating diabetic ketoacidosis. *N Engl J Med* 1987;61:857–9.
242 Martin LG, Grossman MS, Connor TB, Levitsky LL, Clark JJW, Carnitta FD. Effect of androgen on growth hormone secretion and growth in boys with short stature. *Acta Endocrinol* 1979;91:201–12.
243 Illig R, Prader A. Effect of testosterone on growth hormone secretion in patients with anorchia and delayed puberty. *J Clin Endocrinol Metab* 1979;30:615–18.
244 Link K, Blizzard RM, Evans WS, Kaiser DL, Parker MW, Rogol AD. The effect of androgens on the pulsatile release and the twenty-four mean concentration of growth hormone in peripubertal males. *J Clin Endocrinol Metab* 1986;62: 159–64.
245 Crock P, Salvi M, Miller A, Wall J, Guyda H. Detection of anti-pituitary autoantibodies by immunoblotting. *J Immunol Methods* 1993;162:31–40.
246 Buchanan CR, Stanhope R, Adlard P, Jones J, Grant DB, Preece MA. Gonadotrophin, growth hormone and prolactin secretion in children with primary hypothyroidism. *Clin Endocrinol* 1988;29:427–36.
247 Rivkees SA, Bode HH, Crawford JD. Long-term growth in juvenile acquired hypothyroidism. *N Engl J Med* 1988;318: 599–602.
248 Morris HG, Jorgensen JR, Jenkins SA. Plasma growth hormone concentrations in corticosteroid-treated children. *J Clin Invest* 1968;47:427–35.
249 Gourmelen M, Girard F, Binoux M. Serum somatomedin/insulin-like growth factor (IGF) and IGF carrier levels in patients with Cushing's syndrome or receiving glucocorticoid therapy. *J Clin Endocrinol Metab* 1982;54:885–91.
250 Hokken-Koelega ACS, Stijnen T, Keizer-Schrama SMPF de M, Blum WF, Drop SLS. Levels of growth hormone, insulin-like growth factor-I (IGF-I) and -II, IGF-binding protein-1 and -3, and cortisol in prednisone-treated children with growth retardation after renal transplantation. *J Clin Endocrinol Metab* 1993;77:932–8.
251 Sadeghi-Nejad A, Senior B. Adrenal function, growth, and insulin in patients treated with corticoids on alternate days. *Pediatrics* 1969;443:277–83.
252 Mosier SD, Smith FG, Schulz MA. Failure of catch-up growth after Cushing's syndrome in childhood. *Am J Dis Child* 1967;113:693–701.
253 Stirling HF, Barr DGD, Kelnar CJH. Familial growth hormone releasing factor deficiency in pseudopseudohypoparathyroidism. *Arch Dis Child* 1991;66:533–5.
254 Voss LD, Bailey BJ, Mulligan J, Wilkin TJ, Betts PR. Short stature and school performance – the Wessex Growth Study. *Acta Paediatr Scand* 1991;Suppl.377:29–31.
255 Voss LD, Mulligan J, Betts PR, Wilkin TJ. Poor growth in school entrants as an index of organic disease: the Wessex

growth study. *Br Med J* 1992;305:1400–2.

256 Greulich WW, Pyle SI. *Radiographic Atlas of Skeletal Development of the Hand and the Wrist*, 2nd edn. Stanford, CA: Stanford University Press, 1959.

257 Tanner JM, Whitehouse RH, Cameron N, Marshall WA, Healy MJR, Godstein H. *Assessment of Skeletal Maturation and Prediction of Adult Height (TW2 Method)*. New York: Academic Press, 1983.

258 Roche AF, Wainer H, Thissen D. *Skeletal Maturity. The Knee Joint as a Biological Indicator*. New York: Plenum Press, 1975.

259 Bailey N, Pinneau SR. Tables for predicting adult height from skeletal age: revised for use with the Greulich–Pyle hand standard. *J Pediatr* 1952;40:423–41.

260 Roche AF, Wainer H, Thissen D. The RWT method for the prediction of adult stature. *Pediatrics* 1975;56:1026–33.

261 Zachmann M, Solzadillo B, Frank M, Frisch H, Prader A. Bayley–Pinneau, Roche–Wainer–Thissen and Tanner height prediction in normal children and in patients with various pathological conditions. *J Pediatr* 1978;93:749–55.

262 Lenko HL. Prediction of adult height with various methods in Finnish children. *Acta Paediatr Scand* 1979;Suppl.68: 85–92.

263 Naeraa RW, Eiken M, Legarth EG, Nielsen J. Prediction of final height in Turner syndrome – a comparative study. *Acta Paediatr Scand* 1990;Suppl.79:776–83.

264 Rosenfeld RG, Wilson DM, Lee PDK. Insulin-like growth factors I and II in evaluation of growth retardation. *J Pediatr* 1986;109:428–33.

265 Lee PDK, Wilson DM, Rountree L, Hintz RL, Rosenfeld RG. Efficacy of insulin-like growth factor 1 levels in predicting the response to provocative growth hormone testing. *Pediatr Res* 1990;27:45–51.

266 Breier BH, Gallagher BW, Gluckman PD. Radioimmunoassay for insulin-like growth factor I: solutions to some potential problems and pitfalls. *J Endocrinol* 1991;128:347–57.

267 Baxter RC, Martin JL. Radioimmunoassay of growth hormone-dependent insulin-like growth factor binding protein in human plasma. *J Clin Invest* 1986;78:1504–12.

268 Blum WF, Rank MB, Keitzmann K, Gauggel E, Zeisel HJ, Beirich JR. A specific radioimmunoassay for the growth hormone (GH)-somatomedin-binding protein: its use for diagnosis of GH deficiency. *J Clin Endocrinol Metab* 1990; 70:1292–8.

269 Cohen P, Fielder PH, Hasegawa Y, Frisch H, Gludice LC, Rosenfeld RG. Clinical aspects of insulin-like growth factor binding proteins. *Acta Endocrinol* 1991;124:74–85.

270 Bucuvalas JC, Horn JA, Carlsson L, Balistreri WF, Chernausek SD. Growth hormone insensitivity associated with elevated circulating growth hormone-binding protein in children with Alagille syndrome and short stature. *J Clin Endocrinol Metab* 1993;76:1477–82.

271 Rieu M, Le-Bouc Y, Villares SM, Postel-Vinay MC. Familial short stature with very high levels of growth hormone binding protein. *J Clin Endocrinol Metab* 1993;76:857–60.

272 Vannelli S, Avataneo T, Benso I *et al.* Magnetic resonance and the diagnosis of short stature of hypothalamic–hypophyseal origin. *Acta Paediatr Scand* 1993;Suppl.82:155–61.

10: The Management of Short Stature

N.A. BRIDGES and C.G.D. BROOK

INTRODUCTION

The preceding chapter covered the differential diagnosis of short stature: this chapter deals with its management. Although management of short stature can be approached logically only with a knowledge of the cause, the situation as regards growth hormone (GH) treatment may be far from clear, even when the diagnosis is known.

MAKING A DIAGNOSIS

Many paediatric diseases interfere with the rate of growth; for example renal disease, heart disease, inflammatory bowel disease and malabsorption [1,2]. This does not necessarily mean that the affected child is short; a relatively tall child developing a disorder which results in abnormally slow growth may take years before stature falls below the third centile. The initial consideration of a short child should include a search for non-endocrine causes of short stature.

The pattern of growth, and the factors controlling it, change as the child grows older. Karlberg *et al.* demonstrated through mathematical models that the human growth curve divided itself into three phases [3]. Each is controlled by different mechanisms. The first period occurs between birth and 3 years of age. The curve can be described by an exponential equation which is a continuation of intrauterine growth. It is mediated by the action of insulin and other fetal growth factors. In individuals who lack the effect of GH (for example children with GH insensitivity [4]), this pattern of growth continues into childhood.

The second period of growth can be described by a second-degree polynomial which commences at 0.6 years, reaches a peak by 8 years and gradually declines thereafter. This period of growth appears to be GH-dependent. The final portion of the growth curve can be described by a logistic expression. This accounts for the pubertal growth spurt which is sex steroid- and GH-dependent [3].

An understanding of this pattern is the basis for the logical investigation of growth disorders. Once a diagnosis has been made, it must not be automatically assumed that this is the cause of the entire growth problem – thyroid disease develops more commonly in girls with Turner syndrome, and hypochondroplasia is a cause of poor response to treatment in children with GH insufficiency.

HOW TO INVESTIGATE

Baseline investigations

At least two accurate measurements of height are required. Most children will require about a year of observation, but exceptionally slow growth may be manifest over a shorter period. Measurements of sitting height are of value in assessing disproportionate growth, but also in checking the accuracy of height estimation. The child should be weighed and an assessment of nutrition, such as limb circumference or skinfold thickness, is also useful. Bone age assessment is a way of estimating the potential for height. Puberty should be staged [5,6]. The heights of the parents should be measured. The birth weight and current height of siblings can be useful information. When assessing the children of short parents it should be borne in mind that the parents may be short because they have the same disorder (such as hypochondroplasia), or may have failed to reach their genetic potential because of adverse conditions in their childhood.

A measurement of serum thyroxine (T_4) concentration (or some other index of thyroid hormone status, such as free T_4 or free triiodothyronine (T_3)) and thyroid-stimulating hormone (TSH) should be performed in all short or slowly growing children. The possibility of Turner syndrome should be considered in all short girls, and a karyotype performed if there is suspicion. Not all girls with Turner syndrome have a characteristic appearance, and pubertal progress and even regular periods do not rule out the diagnosis.

The assessment of other hormone concentrations is complicated by the pulsatile pattern of secretion. Random GH or cortisol levels are likely to be low if taken during an outpatient clinic, and are not informative as to the sub-

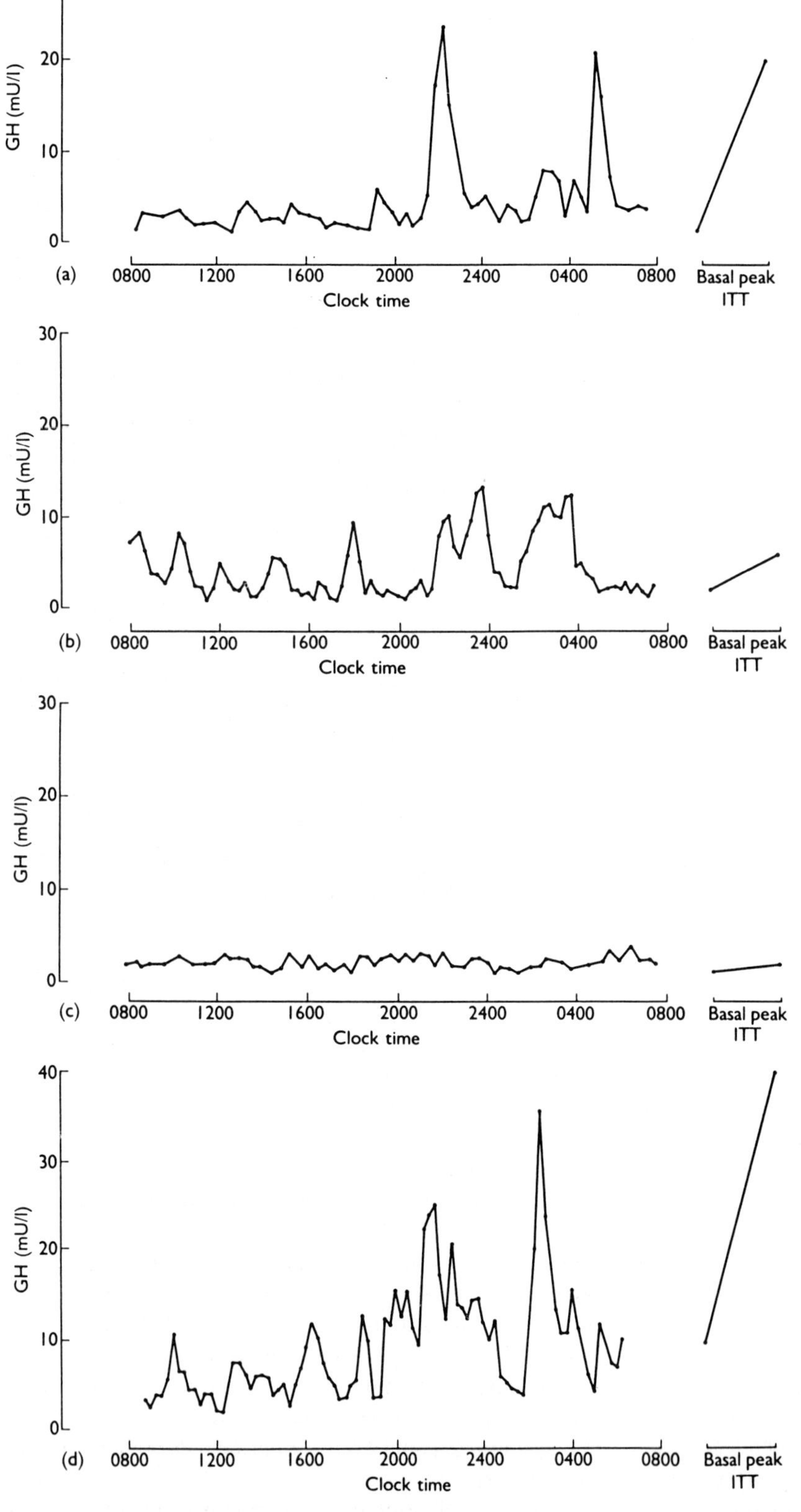

Fig. 10.1 Twenty-four-hour GH profiles in four children with comparison to peak GH response after insulin-induced hypoglycaemia. (a) Third centile child growing at normal velocity. (b) Short child growing at a height velocity SDS −2.0 (moderate insufficiency). (c) Short child growing at a height velocity SDS −4.0 (severe insufficiency). (d) Short child growing at a height velocity SDS −2.5 (dysfunctional). ITT, insulin tolerance test.

ject's overall secretory status. Midnight and 0800 h samples for cortisol are needed to demonstrate a normal diurnal rhythm. Because of the pulsatile pattern of cortisol secretion a single sample may still be unrepresentative, and serial samples taken every 15 min for 1 h may be more informative.

Assessment of growth hormone status
(see Chapter 34)

GH insufficiency should be suspected in any child who is consistently growing abnormally slowly. The term GH deficiency should be reserved for the very rare individuals with a deletion of the GH gene. However short they may be, a child whose growth rate is normal is likely to have normal GH secretion and another cause should be sought for the short stature. There is an asymptotic relationship between growth rate and GH secretion [7], and there is no sharp cut-off between children who are GH insufficient and those who are sufficient (Fig. 10.1). The cut-off point for a given pharmacological test should be assessed in terms of the relationship of the GH response to the growth rate. The characteristics of the assay used must also be taken into account [8].

The pattern of GH secretion is an important factor in its action [9]. In some individuals there is an abnormal pattern of GH secretion which has a diminished growth-promoting effect, even though the 24-h mean GH concentration may be normal. The GH response to an insulin tolerance test may even be elevated (Fig. 10.1d); this is termed neurosecretory dysfunction.

Other investigations

A radiological skeletal survey should be performed in any child whose short stature is disproportionate [10]. Many skeletal dysplasias, of which hypochondroplasia is the prototype, may not result in disproportion until the end of puberty. Such a diagnosis should be considered in children whose pubertal growth is poor, or who are surprisingly short compared to their parents. In hypochondroplasia there is loss of the normal widening of the interpedicular distance going down the lumbar spine, as well as a number of other defects of the long bones (Fig. 10.2) [11,12].

Radiographs for bone dysplasias should be assessed by an expert, even in children who appear obviously to have achondroplasia. We have not infrequently found these children to have a number of other skeletal dysplasias such as pseudoachondroplasia and Jeune thoracic dystrophy. This distinction is important for prognosis, and also in terms of the psychological effect on the family if the diagnosis is changed at a later date.

A thyrotrophin-releasing hormone (TRH) test is useful in assessing primary, secondary or tertiary hypothyroidism. Prolactin should be measured, as well as TSH. A modestly elevated prolactin level is suggestive of a pituitary stalk or hypothalamic problem, and a massively elevated level is suggestive of a prolactinoma. A low prolactin level or an absent response of TSH and prolactin to TRH is suggestive of a pituitary tumour.

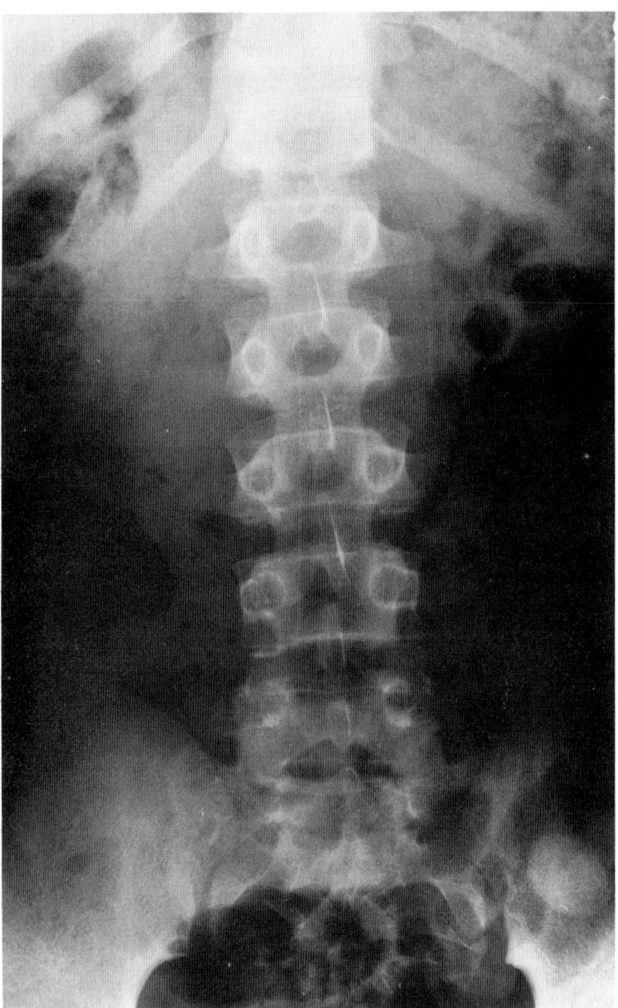

Fig. 10.2 Anteroposterior lumbar spine X-rays in an individual with hypochondroplasia. The normal spine shows a gradual widening of the interpedicular distances from L1 to L5. This dose not occur in hypochondroplasia and the distance at L1 is the same as at L5.

There is gonadotrophin secretion in children of all ages, but during most of childhood and early puberty this occurs at night, and daytime gonadotrophin concentrations are very low [13]. Elevated gonadotrophins in a child in prepuberty or early puberty are suggestive of gonadal failure (for example Turner syndrome) [14]. Sex steroid levels are at their highest in the early hours of the morning and are likely to be low during the day. The response to gonadotrophin-releasing hormone (GnRH) is exaggerated in gonadal failure and absent when the pituitary is damaged. Between these extremes the response is difficult to assess, and is not helpful in distinguishing hypogonadotrophic hypogonadism from pubertal delay in children. The cortisol response to insulin-induced hypoglycaemia is helpful in assessing the response to severe stress. Recent studies have reported the use of physiological doses of adrenocorticotrophin (ACTH) as a means of assessing more subtle abnormalities in adrenal function [15].

PSYCHOLOGICAL PROBLEMS OF SHORT STATURE

Underwood, in a study involving mothers and male university students, found that both groups attached negative attributes to short individuals (toddlers in the case of the mothers and adult men for the university students) when given no more information than pictures of the same individuals altered to change their apparent height [16]. Given the picture of a man, students would estimate a taller height if told he was a professor than if they were told he was a student [17]. It appears that society has a bias towards taller individuals, and parents are often concerned that their child's height will be a disadvantage in adult life.

Several studies have reported the effect of short stature on the child. Voss *et al.*, in a study of Wessex schoolchildren aged 7–9 years, found that there were no difference in ratings of self-esteem and behaviour between short children and controls. Although IQ was not different the short children were underachieving at school, but this difference was mostly due to the effect of socioeconomic class on school performance [18]. While adults perceive problems with short children, it appears that short children themselves do not feel disadvantaged until they reach adolescence [19].

Long-term follow-up studies of growth hormone-insufficient adults have found that these individuals have a poorer than normal quality of life. They are more likely to live still with their parents, to be unemployed or unmarried and to have a poor social life [20].

TREATMENT OF SHORT STATURE

Growth hormone

Almost all children grow faster if given GH [21]. The rate of growth achieved with treatment depends on the diagnosis, the pretreatment height velocity and the GH secretory status. Experience has confirmed that the treatment of GH-insufficient children with GH will result in improved final height, but cannot correct the deficit already incurred at the start of treatment [22]. There is a growing body of data concerning the treatment of girls with Turner syndrome with GH, but there remain many areas of uncertainty, about the time to administer GH and its dose. Trials of GH are under way for a number of other causes of short stature, but so far final outcome is uncertain. Short-term increases in height velocity and increases in height prediction may not result in worthwhile increases in final height. This leaves us with considerable problems concerning the management of children presenting now, and who will probably have stopped growing when firm data are available. While the situation is so uncertain it would be a mistake to embark on the widespread one-off prescription of GH for these 'wider indications'.

The dose of GH must be tailored to the size of the child (calculated by weight or surface area) and the diagnosis. The dose should be altered to keep pace with growth. Although it would appear logical to increase the dose at puberty, there are no data confirming this, and the increase in the pace of pubertal development seen with GH treatment means that this strategy could decrease final height [23]. Most authorities suggest giving the injections in the evening, although there is no evidence to confirm that this is better.

There are a range of devices available to help with injections [24]. Good initial teaching and subsequent support are important in ensuring compliance with the treatment. Lack of compliance and poor injection technique are very common reasons for poor growth on treatment [25]. These can usually be overcome if the situation is recognized. Giving regular injections to toddlers and children too young to understand the reason for them presents particular problems.

THE SAFETY OF GROWTH HORMONE

GH was prepared from human cadavers until 1985 when Creutzfeldt–Jakob disease was diagnosed in patients in the USA who had received this GH [26]. Treatment with pituitary GH was then stopped in most countries. The disorder has since developed in a number of patients in different countries, and the link between human pituitary GH and Creutzfeldt–Jakob disease is indisputable. The disorder has shown a different natural history to the sporadic naturally occurring cases, with predominance of cerebellar signs and a more rapid progression. The apparent incubation period has varied – an average of 15 years in the US cases, 11 years in the UK and 6 years in the cases seen in France. There is no predictive test, and the impossibility of predicting the natural history of this outbreak puts individuals who have received human GH in an extremely uncertain situation. They may also find problems with jobs, insurance and mortgages. They are advised that they should not donate blood or organs [27].

The introduction of recombinant GH has removed the

threat of infection. Recombinant GH has proved extremely safe, and there is to date no evidence of serious adverse effect in the treatment of short stature. Cell cultures expressing GH and employing fetal calf serum, the origin of which cannot be guaranteed to come from a source free of bovine spongiform encephalopathy (BSE), remains an anxiety. Concern about the potential problems of GH treatment now centres on two aspects – the potential mitogenic properties of GH and its metabolic effects.

Watanabe *et al.* reported in 1988 that patients who had received GH were at increased risk of developing leukaemia [28]. Subsequent studies outside Japan have not confirmed this finding. A survey of GH-treated individuals who had developed leukaemia, by Gunnarsson & Wilton, found 40 cases; of these, 15 had additional risk factors (Fanconi anaemia, Bloom syndrome, myelodysplastic syndrome, previous radiotherapy). The remaining patients did not exceed the number to be expected in the population [29]. Other follow-up studies have not found an increased risk of leukaemia [30], or an increased risk of recurrence in patients who have been treated for leukaemia and later received GH [31]. A follow-up study of patients treated for brain tumours who received GH treatment did not find an excess risk of recurrence over those who were untreated [31]. There are no data as to whether brain tumours grow faster with GH treatment, but most clinicians would be advised not to treat children who have active malignancy.

A decrease in body fat and a change in its distribution from central to peripheral adiposity has been noted with GH treatment [32,33] and a reverse of this effect is seen when treatment is stopped in GH-insufficient individuals [34]. Relative insulin insensitivity has been demonstrated in individuals treated with GH, but they have not developed diabetes [35]. GH has an effect on protein kinetics, increasing amino acid utilization and improving nitrogen balance in cachectic and postsurgical patients [36,37]. GH increases glomerular filtration rate (GFR) in individuals with normal renal function, and the initiation of therapy has been found to affect the renin–angiotensin system [38,39]. Fluid retention has not been a problem in children [40], but has been a significant side-effect (resulting in carpal tunnel syndrome) in elderly individuals on trials of GH [41]. None of these effects is a contraindication to the use of GH, but they serve as a reminder that GH receptors are found on many different cell lines and the administration of GH results in widespread metabolic changes as well as linear growth.

In many GH-insufficient children antibodies in low titre to GH develop during the course of treatment. With the new recombinant preparations there is no evidence that these low levels decrease the response to treatment [42]. However, in GH-deficient children (who have had no prior exposure to GH), antibodies develop which effectively prevent treatment.

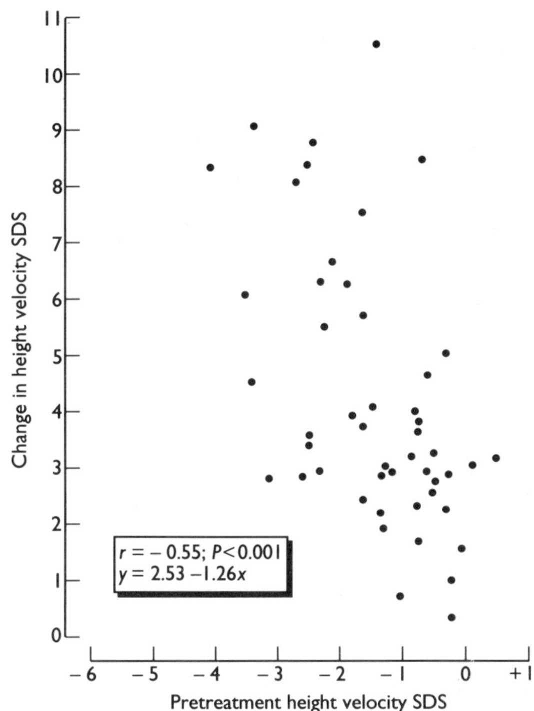

Fig. 10.3 Change in height velocity standard deviation score (SDS) plotted against pretreatment height velocity SDS.

GROWTH HORMONE TREATMENT

Growth hormone insufficiency

The effect of GH treatment on growth rate in GH insufficiency depends on the pretreatment velocity, the GH status of the subject and the dose used. Figure 10.3 shows the change in height velocity standard deviation score (SDS) over the first year of treatment for 50 children, plotted against their pretreatment velocity SDS. Those with the slowest pretreatment height velocity demonstrated the greatest increase on treatment.

The height velocity of children is related to their GH secretion in an asymptotic manner, and the response to treatment is similarly related [7]. Figure 10.4a shows the increase in height velocity SDS in the first year of treatment plotted against a measure of physiological GH secretion, the sum of pulse amplitude from a 24-h profile, and Fig. 10.4b shows the change in height velocity SDS in the first year for a group of children treated with a similar dose of GH, divided according to their pretreatment response to an insulin tolerance test. The nearer to normal the GH secretion, the smaller was the increment in growth rate. This means that the faster a child is growing, the greater will be the dose of GH required to produce the same increase in height velocity.

Dose–response curves can be derived for GH treatment,

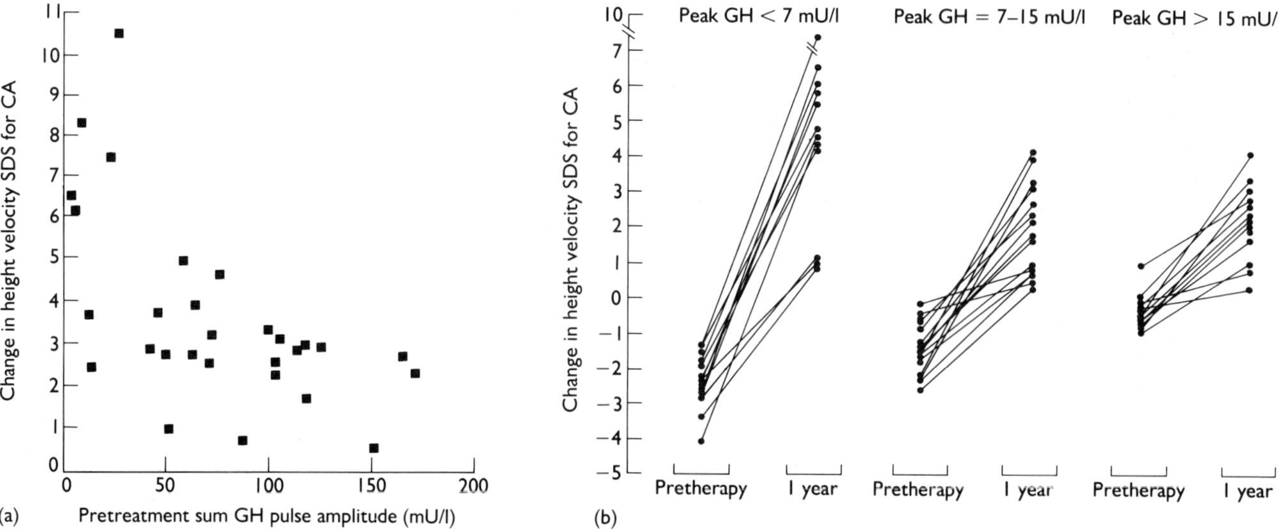

Fig. 10.4 The effect of pretreatment GH secretory status on the response to GH treatment. (a) A measure of physiological GH secretion, the pretreatment GH amplitude measured by 24-h profile, plotted agairst the change in height velocity SDS (for chronological age, CA) over the first year of treatment. The increase in height velocity is greatest in those with the lowest GH secretion. (b) The change in height velocity SDS (for chronological age) in the first year of treatment divided into three groups according to the response to insulin-induced hypoglycaemia; the individuals with the lowest GH response demonstrated the greatest increase in height velocity.

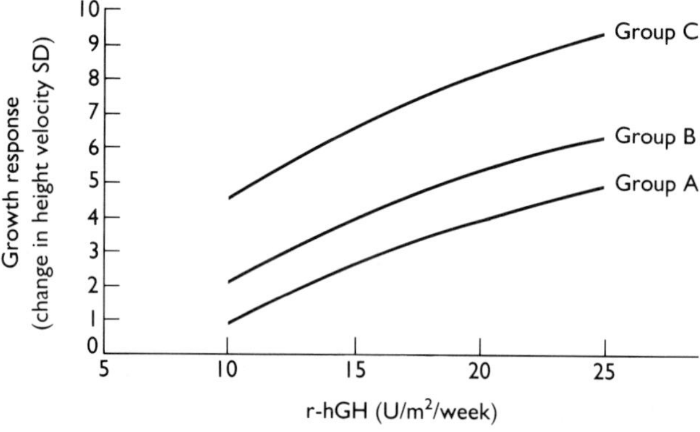

Fig. 10.5 Relationship between dose of GH and response (the difference between pretreatment and the first year's height velocity SDS) for a group of 90 short prepubertal children. Group A ($n = 27$) had a pretreatment height velocity SDS between +1.3 and −0.8, group B ($n = 35$) a pretreatment height velocity SDS between −0.9 and −2.0, and group C ($n = 28$) had a pretreatment height velcity SDS less than −2.0. The faster the child was growing pretreatment, the greater the dose of GH needed to produce a given increment in growth rate [43]. r-hGH, recombinant human growth hormone.

but they vary according to the pretreatment height velocity [43]. This has implications for the treatment of so-called 'short normal' children, whose height velocity and GH secretion is normal, because they will require a larger dose of GH to produce increments in height velocity comparable to those seen in GH-insufficient children (Fig. 10.5). The other factor important in the response to GH is the frequency of administration. Several studies have confirmed that, for a given overall dose of GH, a better increment in height velocity will result if given as a daily dose instead of three or four times a week [44]. The same observation is true for Turner syndrome [45].

Apart from monitoring of height, it is standard practice to perform bone age estimation approximately every year. This is a useful guide to the potential for growth, but it must be remembered that there is a considerable degree of variation in estimates of bone age, even with experienced observers, and height predictions based on the growth pattern of normal individuals may not hold true for those with an abnormal growth pattern. Height predictions based on bone age do not hold true for those with abnormal skeletons, for example in hypochondroplasia. Studies of the effect of GH fasting on insulin and blood sugar in children suggest that monitoring these parameters would not be helpful [35].

Turner syndrome

The success of GH in the treatment of GH insufficiency meant that trials of GH treatment for a range of causes of short stature, other than GH insufficiency, were commenced before 1985 [46]. The increase in GH supplies that came with the introduction of recombinant GH increased this trend. Turner syndrome has received the most attention, and is now a recognized indication for GH therapy in many countries. GH secretion in Turner syndrome is

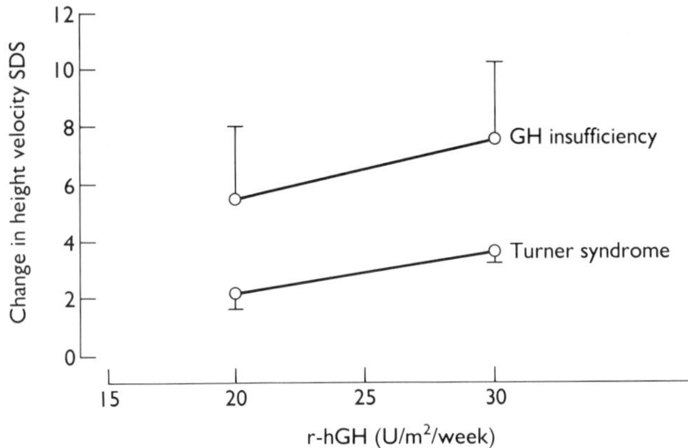

Fig. 10.6 Dose–response relationship for girls with Turner syndrome compared with children with GH insufficiency growing with the same pretreatment height velocity.

normal, and the poor growth is secondary to a skeletal dysplasia which is part of the syndrome. Short-term studies of the use of GH in Turner syndrome demonstrated that treatment resulted in an increase in height velocity [47].

The dose–response curve is different for Turner syndrome and more GH is required than for GH-insufficient individuals to give the same increment in height velocity (Fig. 10.6). Long-term studies have demonstrated that GH treatment results in an increase in height relative to Turner standards and an increase in height prediction, but the actual amount is not yet established because the number of girls who have reached final height remains small. The adult height of most of these girls is greater than their height predicted at the start of treatment. In his long-term study Rosenfeld compared the effect of GH alone with GH and oxandrolone. Combination treatment resulted in increased height velocity in the short term, but bone age advancement was greater in the long term and final heights were not significantly different [48,49].

While these results are encouraging, the role of GH in the management of Turner syndrome is not completely clear. An improvement in stature in childhood can be of great psychological benefit to girls with Turner syndrome, but low-dose steroids can achieve this at a fraction of the cost, and using the oral route [50]. Despite treatment the final height of most Turner syndrome girls remains very short, and many are disappointed. It may be possible to improve matters when more information is gained about the best time to start GH treatment, and whether combining the treatment with other growth-promoting agents (or using these before starting GH), improves final height. There are no data to suggest that height can be 'bought in advance' by starting GH early, and it is far from certain that every girl with Turner syndrome should start GH as early as possible.

Short normal children

A 'short normal' child is one who is genetically short, with normal GH secretion and growing at a normal velocity; that is, a child at the extreme of the normal range of height. Because growth rate is related to GH secretion these children secrete less GH than their taller peers. A number of trials have tested the hypothesis that giving these children extra GH will increase their final height. In the short term these studies have confirmed that (as one would predict) these individuals show an increase in height velocity, but more GH is required to produce a given increment than for GH-insufficient individuals, and those growing fastest show the least increment [51,52]. There are so far few data concerning final height. It appears that the effect of exogeneous GH in accelerating the progress of puberty diminishes the increase in height prediction that occurs prepubertally, and final height is very little greater than predicted height at the start of treatment. Many trials are still in progress. So far it appears that the small gain in height does not justify the cost (years of injections and hospital visits for the family, as well as the cost of the drug), and GH is not routinely indicated for short normally growing children.

For the physician who wished to resist instituting treatment it is as well to remember that GH increases blood pressure, increases free fatty acids and increases serum insulin concentrations. This must be regarded as a recipe for accelerated atherosclerosis [53].

Low birth weight

In a study of 24 children with intrauterine growth retardation, Stanhope *et al.* found that there was an increase in height velocity with GH treatment, but that this did not result in a long-term improvement in height prediction over 2 years of the study. There are no data on final height, but it appears that GH treatment is not of benefit to children whose short stature is due to intrauterine growth retardation [54]. These children anyway have a tendency towards early pubertal development. The action of GH is to accelerate pubertal progress [23], and such treatment would in theory decrease final height.

Skeletal dysplasia

Most of the skeletal dysplasias result in short stature, and many in disproportionate growth. The gene defect is known in very few, and little is known of the processes that result in abnormal or disproportionate bone growth [10]. GH secretion is normal, and previously it was assumed that treatment with GH would have little to offer. A number of studies have now demonstrated that short-term GH treatment results in an acceleration in

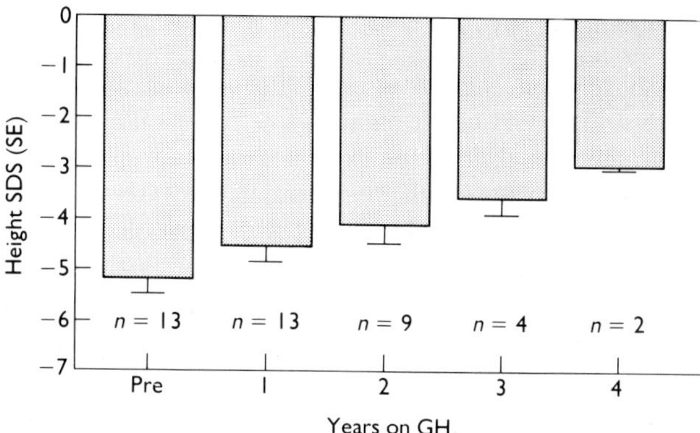

Fig. 10.7 The height SDS scores for a group of children with achondroplasia treated with GH at a dose of 20–30 units/m² per week for up to 4 years.

growth rate in achondroplasia [55,56] and hypochondroplasia [57].

In a long-term study of GH treatment in achondroplasia there has been an increase in height velocity and an increase in height relative to both achondroplastic and normal standards (Fig. 10.7). This improvement has been maintained for up to 6 years in one of our subjects. It is not certain whether there will be an increase in final height, and in particular the growth pattern in puberty remains to be seen. There is no evidence that GH improves the disproportion of achondroplasia, and there is a suggestion that it may worsen with treatment. However, this does mean that GH treatment does not rule out the possibility of leg-lengthening operations.

Hypochondroplasia is a variable condition, which may present with short stature in childhood or poor growth in puberty. Disproportion varies, and may be obvious in childhood or only manifest at puberty. Trials of GH have demonstrated a variable response and the genetic heterogeneity of the condition may be responsible for this [58]. Trials of GH treatment of hypochondroplasia at the Middlesex Hospital have used two approaches; the first to treat with GH as soon as possible, and the second to wait for puberty (the loss of pubertal growth being a prominent feature of hypochondroplasia). The results of these trials to date are shown in Fig. 10.8, with the subjects divided according to whether they had physical signs of puberty at the start of treatment. Those treated in puberty have demonstrated the greatest improvement (Fig. 10.9), and this may turn out to be the best strategy for treating these individuals. This observation is the basis for our postulation that GH therapy might be most effective if started at puberty to restore the spurt which is characteristically absent in girls with Turner syndrome.

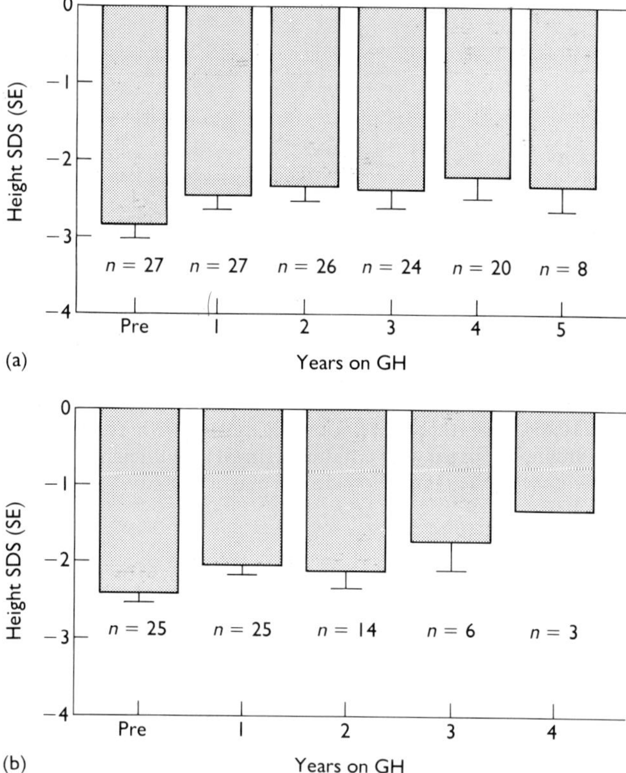

Fig. 10.8 (a) Height SDS scores for a group of children with hypochondroplasia treated with GH at a dose of 15–25 units/m² per week, starting their treatment before showing any physical signs of puberty. (b) Height SDS scores for a group of children with hypochondroplasia treated with GH at a dose of 15–40 units/m² per week, starting their treatment with physical signs of puberty (testicular volume over 4 ml or breast stage 2).

Renal disease

In chronic renal failure, serum GH concentrations are elevated. The clearance of GH is reduced in dialysed and non-dialysed individuals, and deconvolution analysis has demonstrated that GH secretion is normal. GH-binding protein levels are reduced. There is a reduction in insulin-like growth factor I (IGF-I) bioactivity and an increase in IGF-binding protein 3 (IGFBP-3). These factors all contribute to GH resistance, and even with optimal biochemical management and nutritional advice, height velocity is reduced. Pubertal development is delayed and the pubertal growth spurt is attenuated. In children with renal allografts, highdose steroids result in suppression of GH secretion and reduced height velocity [59,60].

A number of studies have commenced which examine whether GH therapy can improve the growth of children with renal disease. GH results in an increase in GFR in humans and animals [38], and there has been concern that GH therapy may adversely affect renal function in chronic

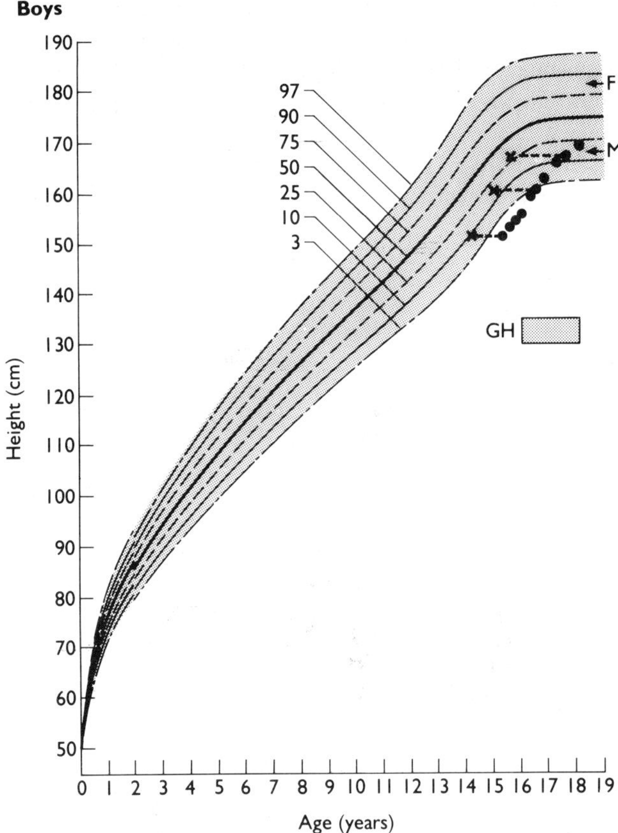

Fig. 10.9 GH treatment in hypochondroplasia. This boy was seen at 15.4 years because of short stature. At that time his testicular volume was 8 ml. A skeletal survey was performed because of his poor growth, and a diagnosis of hypochondroplasia was made. He commenced a trial of GH at 16.1 years (testicular volume 12 ml) and stopped at 18.1 years. Treatment with GH in puberty has restored the pubertal growth spurt, and his final height was 171.3 cm. F, Father's height centile; M, Mother's height centile.

renal failure. Studies in treated children have found no increase in GFR and no deterioration in renal function which could be related to GH treatment [2]. Children with chronic renal failure treated for several years with GH demonstrated increased height velocity [59]. In children with functioning allografts, similar good results have been reported in the short term, without any apparent increase in the number of rejection episodes [61,62].

Studies of growth hormone in other indications

Trials of the use of GH are under way in a wide range of other causes of short stature, such as Noonan syndrome, Prader–Willi syndrome, Bloom syndrome, Down syndrome [63] and hypophosphataemic rickets. There are no data concerning final height. These diagnoses are not indications for GH treatment unless the child also has GH insufficiency. In Prader–Willi syndrome GH has been found to have beneficial effects on muscle strength.

Other growth-promoting agents

SEX STEROIDS AND ANABOLIC STEROIDS

In 1941, McCullagh & Rossmiller demonstrated that testosterone acetate increased the height velocity of boys, but it was found that this also resulted in an advance in bone age and reduced final height [64]. Steroids structurally related to testosterone, but devoid of androgenic activity, were developed; the first was fluoxymesterone, and later oxandrolone was developed, which was anabolically very potent but had less than 1% of the androgenic activity of testosterone.

The effect of oxandrolone in increasing height velocity has been demonstrated in a number of groups of short children. Early studies demonstrated its effect in Down syndrome [65]. Low doses of oxandrolone and fluoxymesterone have both been demonstrated to increase height velocity in younger children with constituitional delay [66,67]. Oxandrolone, alone and in combination with both GH and low-dose oestrogen, has been demonstrated to increase growth rate in Turner syndrome [48,50,68]. Table 10.1 shows the growth-stimulating effect of oxandrolone on six slowly growing children treated for 6 months. These children received oxandrolone in lieu of GH in the period after the withdrawal of pituitary GH in 1985.

Table 10.1 Effects of treatment with oxandrolone 1.25 mg/day in six prepubertal children during a treatment period of 6 months

Age (years)	Sex	Pretreatment height velocity SDS	Treatment height velocity SDS	Post-treatment height velocity SDS	Change in height SDS for bone age
3.044	M	−3.81	+1.55	–	+0.75
3.413	F	−1.19	+2.06	−0.80	+1.80
4.482	M	−1.40	+2.25	−0.61	+1.14
5.638	M	−1.10	+3.86	+0.45	+0.24
5.836	M	−0.41	+0.01	–	−0.50
9.209	M	−1.15	+4.10	–	−0.24

SDS, standard deviation score.

The greatest value of oxandrolone is in treating individuals whose short stature is secondary to pubertal delay. A dose of oxandrolone of 1.25 or 2.5 mg daily for 3 months will result in an increase in growth rate without adverse advancement of bone age. For boys with a testicular volume over 5 ml this increase in growth rate normally continues after the treatment stops. The alternative to oxandrolone in treating pubertal delay is low-dose sex steroids [69]. The use of oxandrolone and sex steroids is discussed in Chapter 15. There is no evidence that GH treatment confers any advantage over sex steroids or oxandrolone in the management of short stature secondary to pubertal delay, and there is a risk of GH accelerating the progress of puberty and thus limiting final height [23,70].

GROWTH-HORMONE-STIMULATING AGENTS

Growth-hormone-releasing hormone

Interest in the use of GH-releasing hormone (GHRH) was stimulated when pituitary GH was withdrawn. GHRH has proved effective when given as overnight pulsatile infusions [71,72], as overnight continuous infusions [73] and as twice-daily injections [74]. The response is not as good as that with GH, and the fact that not all patients respond has meant that this treatment has not progressed beyond clinical trials. However, GHRH may eventually prove to have a place in the treatment of short stature. In particular the demonstration that a continuous infusion does not result in down-regulation [75] and stimulates growth [73] suggests that the use of GHRH as a depot preparation would be possible. A GH depot would probably not work, because the pulsatile pattern of GH secretion is important to its action [9].

Growth-hormone-releasing peptide

GH-releasing peptide is a hexapeptide which specifically stimulates GH secretion by way of non-opiate, non-GHRH receptors. This peptide enhances GH secretion in adults and in children following both intravenous and oral administration [76,77]. There are no data as to its effect on growth, but this substance may offer the prospect of an effective oral growth-promoting agent.

Clonidine

Several investigators have examined the effect of long-term clonidine treatment on GH secretion and growth. There is an increase in GH secretion in the short term [78]. Accounts of the long-term effect on growth have varied. An increase in growth rate in children with constituitional delay and short stature treated with clonidine has been documented [79,80]; another group found that 35% did not respond, and Allen, in a group of 10 short children, found no increase in growth rate [81]. The result was in all cases inferior to that to be expected from GH. The effect of clonidine on final height is not known. The disappointing and patchy effect on short-term growth makes its use justified only if GH is not available, and its potent hypotensive effect can result in side-effects.

Leg lengthening

Surgical leg lengthening can result in increases in height of between 7 and 14 cm [82]. Modern orthopaedic techniques, and in particular the external fixator method developed by Ilizarov, have made this a relatively safe

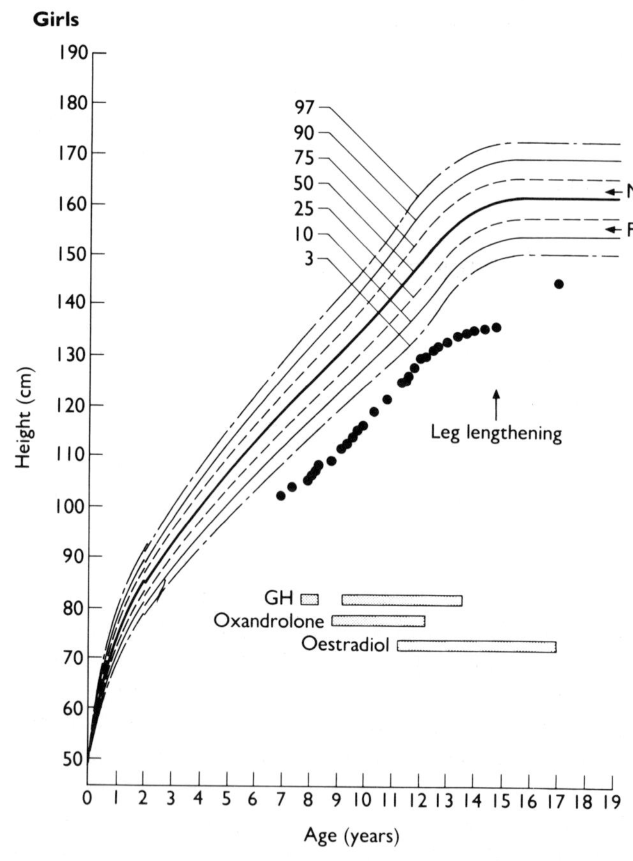

Fig. 10.10 Effect of leg lengthening on final height. The growth pattern of this girl with Turner syndrome exemplifies many of the problems of treating this syndrome. GH treatment was given for a short while from 7.8 years, but stopped when GH was withdrawn in 1985. Low-dose oxandrolone was started at 8.7 years and GH restarted at 9.2 years. Both treatments resulted in an increase in growth rate. Poor growth in puberty has meant that this girl's position on stopping growth hormone at 13.6 years is relatively much worse than it was prepubertally. She decided to have leg lengthening and returned 2 years later having gained 9 cm in height. F, Father's height centile; M, Mother's height centile.

operation, but the process remains extremely time-consuming (up to 2 years) and still involves discomfort, prolonged lack of mobility and disruption of schooling. It can, however, confer a useful increment in height (Fig. 10.10). The majority of those operated on have achondroplasia (in which the operation acts to improve the proportions, and the lax muscles make stretching easier). Some individuals have orthopaedic problems which make leg lengthening impossible, such as joint laxity or joint deformity. There are continuing concerns about the long-term effect on joint stability. Availability is limited because of the cost, and the fact that there are not many centres with the necessary surgical skills and facilities.

Insulin-like growth factor I

Recombinant human IGF-I is now being used for clinical trials in children with GH insensitivity (Laron dwarfism). Administration has proved more of a problem than for GH, partly because of the insulin-like properties of IGF-I which have resulted in hypoglycaemia and electrolyte problems. In short-term studies these children have demonstrated an increase in growth rate. Recombinant IGF-I (and other recombinant growth factors) may eventually prove to have a role in the management of short stature due to causes other than GH insensitivity.

Holding up puberty

Several investigators have examined whether holding up puberty will result in improved final height. This strategy is particularly tempting in children whose puberty is early. Lindner *et al.* and Municchi *et al.* [83,84] have demonstrated that there is an increase in height prediction with treatment. Followed to final height, the patients in Lindner's study did not reach actual heights greater than their initial predicition. No final heights are available for the latter study. This is a similar pattern to that seen in true precocious puberty, where improvements in height prediction during treatment are lost after stopping treatment [85]. There is no evidence that holding up puberty in short individuals, or delaying its induction in those who will not enter puberty spontaneously, confers any advantage in terms of final height, and it cannot be worth the considerable psychological price to pay for holding up puberty in children who already feel at a disadvantage because of their short stature [83].

LONG-TERM FOLLOW-UP

Most adolescents with GH insufficiency can stop their treatment without apparent ill-effect. However, studies of fat and muscle distribution have demonstrated changes with stopping GH treatment in young adults [34]. The long-term follow-up of patients with hypopituitarism has found that, despite adequate replacement of all hormones except GH, these individuals have an increased mortality. Studies of GH-insufficient adults have found that they have an increased incidence of obesity and psychological problems [86]. This has suggested that there may be some merit in continuing GH replacement in adult life in some cases. Benefit has been reported in individual adult patients with severe GH insufficiency (for example after craniopharyngioma). There have been a number of short-term studies which have demonstrated increased muscle bulk, decreased fat and increased psychological well-being on GH treatment [87]. These effects have so far proved to be fairly short lived. The situation with regard to treating GH-insufficient children with GH in adult life remains uncertain, and our current knowledge does not allow us to clearly identify which individuals would benefit.

REFERENCES

1 Griffiths AM, Nguyen P, Smith C, MacMillan JH, Sherman PM. Growth and clinical course of children with Crohn's disease. *Gut* 1993;34:939–43.

2 Tönshoff B, Tönshoff C, Mehls O *et al.* Growth hormone treatment in children with preterminal renal failure: no adverse effect on glomerular filtration rate. *Eur J Pediatr* 1992;151:601–7.

3 Karlberg J, Engstrom I, Karlberg P, Fryer JC. Analysis of linear growth using a mathematical model. *Acta Paediatr Scand* 1987; Suppl.76:478–88.

4 Laron Z, Lilos P, Klinger B. Growth curves for Laron syndrome. *Arch Dis Child* 1993;68:768–70.

5 Marshall WA, Tanner JM. Variations in the pattern of pubertal changes in boys. *Arch Dis Child* 1970;45:13–23.

6 Marshall WA, Tanner JM. Variations in the pattern of pubertal changes in girls. *Arch Dis Child* 1969;44:291–303.

7 Hindmarsh P, Smith PJ, Brook CGD, Matthews DR. The relationship between height velocity and GH secretion in short prepubertal children. *Clin Endocrinol* 1987;27:581–91.

8 Dattani MT, Pringle PJ, Hindmarsh PC, Brook CGD. What is a normal stimulated growth hormone concentration? *J Endocrinol* 1992;133:447–50.

9 Hindmarsh PC, Matthews DR, Stratton I, Pringle PJ, Brook CGD. Rate of change (modulation) of serum growth hormone concentrations is a more important factor in determining growth rate than duration of exposure. *Clin Endocrinol* 1992; 36:165–70.

10 Spranger J. Classification of skeletal dysplasias. *Acta Paediatr Scand* 1991;Suppl.377:138–42.

11 Maroteux R, Falzon P. Hypochondroplasie. *Arch Fr Pediatr* 1988;45:105–9.

12 Hall BD, Spranger J. Hypochondroplasia: clinical and radiological aspects in 39 cases. *Radiology* 1979;133:95–100.

13 Dunkel L, Afthan UH, Selstam G, Rosberg S, Albertsson Wikland K. Developmental changes in 24 hour profiles of luteinising hormone and follicle stimulating hormone from prepuberty to midstages of puberty in boys. *J Clin Endocrinol Metab* 1992;74:890–7.

14 Conte FA, Grumbach MM, Kaplan SL, Reiter EO. Correlation of LHR factor induced LH and FSH release from infancy to 19

years with the changing pattern of gonadotrophin secretion in agonadal patients: relation to the restraint of puberty. *J Clin Endocrinol Metab* 1980;50:163–8.

15 Crowley S, Hindmarsh PC, Honour JW, Brook CDG. Reproducibility of the cortisol response to stimulation with a low dose of ACTH(1–24): the effect of basal cortisol levels and comparison of low dose with high dose secretory dynamics. *J Endocrinol* 1993;136:167–72.

16 Underwood IE. The social cost of being short: societal perceptions and biases. *Acta Paediatr Scand* 1991;Suppl.377: 3–8.

17 Wilson PR. Perceptual distortion of height as a function of ascribed academic status. *J Social Psychol* 1968;74:97–102.

18 Voss LD, Bailey BJR, Mulligan J, Wilkin TJ, Betts PR. Short stature and school performance – the Wessex growth study. *Acta Paediatr Scand* 1991;Suppl.377:29–31.

19 Gordon M, Crouthamel C, Post EM, Richman RA. Psychosocial aspects of constitutional short stature: social competence, behaviour problems, self esteem and family functioning. *J Pediatr* 1982;101:477–80.

20 Stabler B. Growth hormone insufficiency during childhood has implications for later life. *Acta Paediatr Scand* 1991; Suppl.377:9–13.

21 Moore KC, Donaldson DL, Ideus PL, Gifford RA, Moore WV. Clinical diagnoses of children with extremely short stature and their response to growth hormone. *J Pediatr* 1993;122: 687–92.

22 Bundak R, Hindmarsh PC, Smith PJ, Brook CDG. Long term auxological effects of human growth hormone. *J Pediatr* 1988; 112:875–9.

23 Darendelier F, Hindmarsh PC, Preece MA, Cox L, Brook CGD. Growth hormone increases rate of pubertal maturation. *Acta Endocrinol* 1990;122:414–16.

24 Stanhope R, Albanese A, Moyle L, Hamill G. Optimum method for administration of biosynthetic growth hormone: a randomised crossover trial of an autoinjector and a pen injection device. *Arch Dis Child* 1992;67:994–7.

25 Smith SL, Hindmarsh PC, Brook CDG. Compliance with growth hormone treatment – are they getting it? *Arch Dis Child* 1993;68:91–3.

26 Koch TK, Berg BO, Armond SJ, Gravina RF. Creutzfeldt–Jakob disease in a young adult with idiopathic hypopituitarism: possible relation to the administration of cadaveric human growth hormone. *N Engl J Med* 1985;313:731–4.

27 Preece M. Human pituitary growth hormone and Creutzfeldt–Jakob disease. *Horm Res* 1993;39:95–8.

28 Watanabe S, Tsunematus Y, Fujimoto J, Komiyama A. Leukaemia in patients treated with growth hormone. *Lancet* 1988;1:159.

29 Gunnarsson R, Wilton P. *Haematological Malignancies in Growth Hormone Treated Children. Kabi Pharmacia Report.* Stockholm: Kabi Pharmacia, 1992.

30 Stahnke N. Leukaemia in growth hormone treated patients: an update. *Horm Res* (Suppl.) 1992;38:56–62.

31 Ogilvy Stuart AL, Ryder WD, Gattamaneni HR, Clayton PE, Shalet SM. Growth hormone and tumour recurrence. *Br Med J* 1992;304:1601–5.

32 Walker JM, Bond SA, Voss LD, Betts PR, Wootton SA, Jackson AA. Treatment of short normal children with GH – a cautionary tale? *Lancet* 1990;336:1331–4.

33 Bengtsson BA, Brummer RJ, Eden S, Rosen T, Sjostrom L. Effects of growth hormone on fat mass and fat distribution. *Acta Paediatr Scand* 1992;Suppl.383:62–5.

34 Rutherford OM, Jones DA, Round JM, Buchanan CR, Preece MA. Changes in skeletal muscle and body composition after discontinuation of growth hormone treatment in growth hormone deficient young adults. *Clin Endocrinol* 1991;34: 469–75.

35 Hindmarsh PC, Pringle PJ, Di Silvio L, Brook CGD. Effects of 3 years of GH therapy in short normal children. *Acta Paediatr Scand* 1990;Suppl.366:6–12.

36 Pacitti AJ, Inoue Y, Plumley DA, Copeland EM, Souba WW. Growth hormone regulates amino acid transport in human and rat liver. *Ann Surg* 1992;216:353–61.

37 Wolf RF, Pearlstone DB, Newman E *et al.* Growth hormone and insulin reverse net whole body and skeletal muscle protein catabolism in cancer patients. *Ann Surg* 1992;216:280–8.

38 Ogle GD, Rosenberg AR, Kainer G. Renal effects of growth hormone. I. Renal function and kidney growth. *Pediatr Nephrol* 1992;6:394–8.

39 Barton JS, Hindmarsh PC, Preece MA, Brook CGD. Blood pressure and the renin angiotensin system in children recieving recombinant human growth hormone. *Clin Endocrinol* 1993;38:245–51.

40 Di Martino Nardi J, Wesoly S, Schwartz L, Saenger P. Lack of clinical evidence of sodium retention in children with idiopathic short stature treated with recombinant human growth hormone. *Metabolism* 1993;42:730–4.

41 Rudman D, Feller AG, Cohn L, Shetty KR, Rudman IW, Draper MW. Effects of human growth hormone on body composition in elderly men. *Horm Res* 1991;36(Suppl. 1):73–81.

42 Pringle PJ, Hindmarsh PC, Di Silvio L, Teale JD, Kurtz AB, Brook CGD. The measurement and effect of growth hormone in the presence of growth hormone binding antibodies. *J Endocrinol* 1989;121:193–9.

43 Darendelier F, Hindmarsh PC, Brook CGD. Dose response curves for treatment with biosynthetic GH. *J Endocrinol* 1990;125:311–16.

44 Hindmarsh PC, Stanhope R, Preece MA, Brook CGD. Frequency of administration of GH – an important factor in determining growth response to exogenous GH. *Horm Res* 1990;33(Suppl. 4):83–9.

45 Rongen-Westerlaken C, van Es A, Wit J-M *et al.* Growth hormone therapy in Turner syndrome. Impact of injection frequency and initial bone age. *Am J Dis Child* 1992:146:817–20.

46 Tanner J, Whitehouse RH, Hughes PCR, Vince FP. Effect of growth hormone treatment for 1 to 7 years on growth of 100 children with GH deficiency, low birthweight, inherited smallness, Turner's syndrome and other complaints. *Arch Dis Child* 1971;46:745–82.

47 Takano K, Hizuka N, Shizume K. Treatment of Turner syndrome with methionyl human growth hormone for six months. *Acta Endocrinol (Copenh)* 1986;112:130–7.

48 Rosenfeld RG, Frane J, Attle KM *et al.* Six year results of a randomised prospective trial of human growth hormone and oxandrolone in Turner syndrome. *J Pediatr* 1992;121:49–55.

49 Rosenfeld RG. Growth hormone therapy in Turner's syndrome: an update on final height. Genentech National cooperative study group. *Acta Pediatr Scand* 1992;Suppl. 383:3–6.

50 Bainbridge JWB, Spoudeas HA, Massarano AA *et al.* The application of the infancy childhood puberty model of growth to the management of the Turner syndrome. In: *Turner's Syndrome and Growth Promoting Therapies.* Proceedings of an International Workshop, Frankfurt. Amsterdam: Excerpta Medica, 1990:159–67.

51 Moore WV, Moore KC, Gifford R, Hollowell JG, Donaldson DL. Long term treatment with growth hormone of children with short stature and normal growth hormone secretion. *J Pediatr* 1992;120:702–8.

52 Hindmarsh PC, Pringle PJ, Di Silvio L, Brook CGD. Effects of 3 years of GH therapy in short normal children. *Acta Paediatr Scand* 1990;Suppl.366:6–12.

53 Reaven GM. Role of insulin resistence in human disease (syndrome X): an expanded definition. *Ann Rev Med* 1993;44: 121–31.

54 Stanhope R, Preece MA, Hamill G. Does growth hormone improve final height attainment of children with intrauterine growth retardation? *Arch Dis Child* 1991;66:1180–3.

55 Horton WA, Hecht JT, Hood OJ, Marshall RN, Moore WV, Hollowell JG. Growth hormone therapy in achondroplasia. *Am J Med Genet* 1992;42:667–70.

56 Okabe T, Nishikawa K, Chiaki M, Sato T. Growth promoting effect of human growth hormone on patients with achondroplasia. *Acta Paediatr Jpn* 1991;33:357–62.

57 Appan S, Laurent S, Chapman M, Hindmarsh PC, Brook CGD. Growth and GH therapy in hypochondroplasia. *Acta Paediatr Scand* 1990;Suppl.79:760–803.

58 Mullis PE, Patel MS, Brickell PM, Hindmarsh PC, Brook CGD. Growth characteristics and response to GH therapy in patients with hypochondroplasia: genetic linkage of the IGF 1 gene at chromosome 12q23 to the disease in a subgroup of these patients. *Clin Endocrinol* 1991;34:265–74.

59 Mehls O, Tönshoff B, Tönshoff C, Haffner D, Blum WF. Therapeutic values of recombinant growth hormone in children with chronic renal failure. *Miner Electrolyte Metab* 1992; 18:320–4.

60 Schaefer F, Schärer K, Mehls O. Pathogenic mechanisms of pubertal growth failure in chronic renal failure. *Acta Paediatr Scand* 1991;Suppl.379:3–10.

61 Benfield MK, Parker KL, Waldo FB, Overstreet SL, Kohaut EC. Treatment of growth failure in children after renal transplantation. *Transplantation* 1993;55:305–8.

62 Tönshoff B, Haffner D, Mehls O *et al.* Efficacy and safety of growth hormone treatment in short children with renal allografts: three year experience. *Kidney Int* 1993;44:199–207.

63 Allen DB, Frasier SD, Foley TP, Pescovitz OH. Growth hormone for children with Down syndrome. *J Pediatr* 1993;123: 742–3.

64 McCullagh EP, Rossmiller HR. Methyltestosterone. II. Calorigenic activity. *J Clin Endocrinol* 1941;1:195–200.

65 Ray CG, Kirshwink JF, Waxman SH, Kelley VC. Studies of anabolic steroids. III. The effect of oxandrolone on height and skeletal maturation in mongoloid children. *Am J Dis Child* 1965;110:618–23.

66 Papadimitriou A, Wacharasindhu S, Pearl K, Preece MA, Stanhope R. Treatment of constituitional growth delay in prepubertal boys with a prolonged course of low dose oxandrolone. *Arch Dis Child* 1991;66:841–3.

67 Strickland AL. Long term results of treatment with low dose fluoxymesterone in constituitional delay of growth and puberty and in genetic short stature. *Pediatrics* 1993;91:716–20.

68 Massarano AA, Brook CGD, Hindmarsh PC *et al.* Growth hormone secretion in Turner's syndrome and influence of oxandrolone and ethinyloestradiol. *Arch Dis Child* 1989;64: 587–92.

69 Tse WY, Buyukgebiz A, Hindmarsh PC, Stanhope R, Preece MA, Brook CGD. Long term outcome of oxandrolone treatment in boys with constitutional delay of growth and puberty. *J Pediatr* 1990;117:588–91.

70 Bierich JR, Nolte K, Drews K, Brügmann G. Constitutional delay of growth and adolescence. Results of short term and long term treatment with GH. *Acta Endocrinol* 1992;127: 392–6.

71 Smith PJ, Brook CGD, Rivier J, Vale W, Thorner MO. Nocturnal pusatile growth hormone releasing hormone treatment in growth hormone deficiency. *Clin Endocrinol* 1986; 25:35–44.

72 Low LC, Wang C, Cheung PT *et al.* Long term pulsatile growth hormone (GH) releasing hormone therapy in children with GH deficiency. *J Clin Endocrinol Metab* 1988;66:611–17.

73 Brain CE, Hindmarsh PC, Brook CGD. Continuous subcutaneous GHRH(1–29)NH2 promotes growth over 1 year in short slowly growing children. *Clin Endocrinol* 1990;32:153–63.

74 Duck SC, Schwartz HP, Costin G *et al.* Subcutaneous growth hormone releasing hormone therapy in growth hormone deficient children: first year of therapy. *J Clin Endocrinol Metab* 1992;75:1115–20.

75 Vance ML, Kaiser DL, Martha PM *et al.* Lack of *in vivo* somatotroph desensitisation or depletion after 14 days of continuous growth hormone (GH) releasing hormone administration in normal men and a GH deficient boy. *J Clin Endocrinol Metab* 1989;68:22–8.

76 Bowers CY, Alster DK, Frentz JM. The growth hormone releasing activity of a synthetic hexapeptide in normal men and short statured children after oral administration. *J Clin Endocrinol* 1992;74:292–8.

77 Huhn WC, Hartman ML, Pezzoli SS, Thorner MO. Twenty four hour growth hormone (GH) releasing peptide (GHRP) infusion enhances pulsatile GH secretion and specifically attenuates the response to a subsequent GHRP bolus. *J Clin Endocrinol Metab* 1993;76:1202–8.

78 Ghigo E, Arval E, Nicolosi M *et al.* Acute clonidine administration potentiates spontaneous diurnal, but not nocturnal, growth hormone secretion in short normal children. *J Clin Endocrinol Metab* 1990:71:433–5.

79 Loche S, Puggioni R, Fanni T, Cella SG, Muller EE, Pintor C. Augmentation of growth hormone secretion in children with constitutional delay by short term clonidine administration: a pulse amplitude mediated phenomenon. *J Clin Endocrinol Metab* 1989;68:426–30.

80 Castromorgana M, Augulo M, Fuentes B, Castelar ME, Canas A, Espinoza B. Effect of prolonged clonidine administration on GH concentrations and rate of linear growth in children with constitutional delay. *J Pediatr* 1986;109:784–7.

81 Allen DB. Effects of nightly clonidine administration on growth velocity in short children without growth hormone deficiency: a double blind cross over study. *J Pediatr* 1993; 122:32–6.

82 Correll J. Surgical correction of short stature in the skeletal dysplasias. *Acta Paediatr Scand* 1991;Suppl.377:143–8.

83 Lindner D, Job JC, Chaussain JL. Failure to improve height prediction in short stature pubertal adolescents by inhibiting puberty with luteinising hormone releasing hormone analogue. *Eur J Pediatr* 1993;152:393–6.

84 Municchi G, Rose SR, Pescovitz OH, Barnes KM, Cassorla FG, Cutler GB. Effect of deslorelin induced pubertal delay on the growth of adolescents with short stature and normally timed puberty: preliminary results. *J Clin Endocrinol Metab* 1993;77:1334–9.

85 Oerter KE, Manasco P, Barnes KM, Jones J, Hill S, Cutler GB. Adult height in precocious puberty after long term treatment with deslorelin. *J Clin Endocrinol Metab* 1991;73: 1235–40.

86 Lamberts SW, Valk NK, Binnerts A. The use of growth hormone in adults: a changing scene. *Clin Endocrinol* 1992;37: 111–15.

87 Bengtsson BA, Eden S, Lonn L *et al.* Treatment of adults with growth hormone (GH) deficiency with recombinant human GH. *J Clin Endocrinol Metab* 1993;76:309–17.

11: Growth-hormone-resistant States

A.M. COTTERILL and M.O. SAVAGE

INTRODUCTION

Growth hormone (GH) resistance is a pathological state, characterized by a disturbance of the physiological relationships between GH secretion, insulin-like growth factor (IGF)-I synthesis and the biological actions of GH. Endocrine characteristics include high circulating GH levels, low IGF-I levels and, in children, impaired growth. The extreme form of GH resistance or insensitivity, Laron syndrome, may be further defined by the IGF-I generation test, during which there is no increase of serum IGF-I after stimulation with exogenous human GH (hGH).

Insensitivity to GH is usually thought of as a rare cause of short stature, represented only by conditions such as Laron syndrome, but this may not be the case. Rare as such syndromes may be, they may represent only the extreme form of a spectrum of congenital and acquired conditions associated with variable degrees of resistance to the actions of GH (Table 11.1). Malnutrition leading to stunted growth is, for example, a common form of reversible GH insensitivity. Others include parenchymal hepatic disease and severe illness associated with catabolic states.

The investigation and treatment of rare conditions such as Laron syndrome have led to a major expansion in the understanding of the physiological actions of GH, its receptor and the IGFs since this condition is a model for the absence of biological action of GH.

GROWTH HORMONE INSENSITIVITY SYNDROME (LARON SYNDROME)

In 1966, Laron described the appearance of three siblings of Israeli origin with an apparently new inborn error of metabolism [2]. Laron syndrome is an autosomal recessive condition caused by a variable defect in the GH receptor gene [3,4], which leads to resistance to the actions of both endogenous and exogenous GH with the inability to generate normal quantities of IGF-I [5,6]. GH bioactivity, when assessed *in vitro*, is normal [7]. The pathogenesis of Laron syndrome is shown in Fig. 11.1.

Three large series of patients with Laron syndrome have been reported. The first two comprised patients of specific ethnic backgrounds, oriental Jews [8] and Ecuadorian subjects of Spanish descent [6,9]. A European series [10] is genetically heterogeneous and was assembled for potential treatment with recombinant human IGF-I.

Molecular genetics

The GH receptor is a member of the cytokine receptor superfamily, which also includes the receptors for prolactin, interleukins IL-2, IL-3, IL-4, IL-6, IL-7, interferon, granulocyte/macrophage colony-stimulating factor and erythropoietin [11]. The gene for the human GH receptor is localized on chromosome 5p13.1–p12 and contains 10 exons, spanning 87 kb. The receptor consists of an extracellular ligand-binding domain containing 246 amino acids, encoded by exons 3–7, a transmembrane domain encoded by exon 8 and a cytoplasmic domain of 350 amino acids encoded by exons 9 and 10 along with a 3′ untranslated region.

Following the characterization of the genetic sequence of the GH receptor a number of Laron syndrome families were screened for major gene deletions. Four of the 12 Israeli subjects have been shown to have major gene deletions with loss of exons 3, 5 and 6 together with an abnormality of exon 4 [12]. This pattern of deletion leads to the appearance of a translational stop signal in exon 7, hence the loss of the cytoplasmic and transmembrane domains with deletions in the extracellular domain. The subsequent search for point mutations in the gene led to Amselem *et al.* [4] reporting the first family from Tunisia, in which all four affected siblings had a T to C substitution which resulted in a significant amino acid concession at position 96 of the extracellular domain of the GH receptor. GH binding. A number of additional mutations in the GH receptor gene have been identified [3].

The findings in the Ecuador population are unusual in that all but one of the subjects is homozygous for an A to G substitution in exon 6 creating a preferentially used alternative splice site at this position which results in the

Table 11.1 Classification of GH insensitivity

1 Primary GH insensitivity syndromes (Laron syndrome; hereditary/congenital defects)
  (a) GH receptor deficiency (quantitative and qualitative)
  (b) Abnormalities of GH signal transduction (postreceptor)
  (c) Primary defect of IGF-I synthesis

2 Secondary (acquired) GH insensitivity syndromes
  (a) Circulating GH-inhibiting antibodies
  (b) GH receptor antibodies
  (c) Malnutrition
  (d) Liver disease
  (e) Other causes, e.g. catabolic states, adolescent diabetes, etc.

From Laron *et al.* [1].

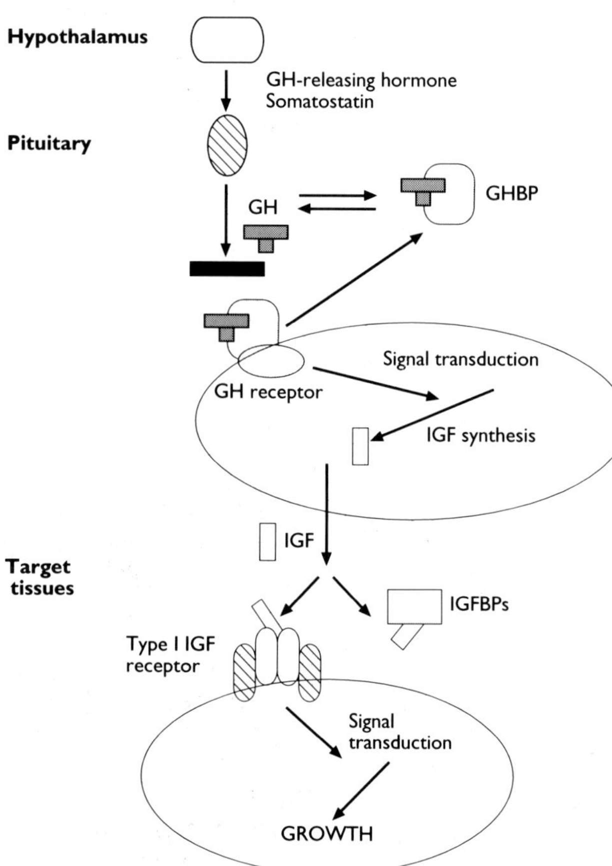

Fig. 11.1 The GH–IGF axis, indicating the site (solid bar) of the defect of GH binding to the extracellular domain of its receptor (redrawn from Rosenfeld *et al.* [2]).

deletion of eight amino acids from the extracellular domain of the GH receptor [13].

Amselem's group, studying Laron syndrome patients with normal GH-binding protein (GHBP) [10], has identified another mutation in exon 6 which results in an amino acid substitution at a site known to be involved in receptor dimerization [14a].

The 18 separate point mutations reported to date [3] indicate the considerable heterogeneity of this syndrome. It is possible that there may also be defects in the GH receptor gene which cause partial defects of GH binding resulting in short stature, but not to the profound degree seen in Laron syndrome.

Clinical features

The clinical features of Laron syndrome are shown in Table 11.2. Patients have a characteristic phenotype with severe postnatal growth failure (Fig. 11.2) and markedly reduced adult height [6,8,10]. The condition is recognizable at birth [9] and birth weight and length have been below average [10]. Facial appearance is similar to GH deficiency type 1A with a prominent forehead, an underdeveloped midface with a small nose and depressed nasal bridge. There is significant shortening of facial height and width compared to the vault of the skull [3]. Other similarities with GH deficiency are the relative excess of body fat and recurrent hypoglycaemia, particularly in infancy [10].

Nutritional status is difficult to assess since the lack of GH action leads to fat accumulation and failure of lipolysis during fasting but hyperalimentation may improve linear growth [14]. This suggests that relative malnutrition may be present in some of these children. Subjects with Laron syndrome are usually of normal intelligence [6,10].

There is significant delay in bone maturation, but the height for bone age is severely impaired [9]. Pubertal development is generally but not universally delayed and the adolescent growth spurt significantly attenuated. Fertility appears to be normal, with offspring recorded

Table 11.2 Clinical features of Laron syndrome

Genetic
Consanguinity
Family history

Fetal, neonatal
Low birth weight
Low birth length
Abnormal facies at birth
Hypoglycaemia
Micropenis
Blue sclerae

Auxological
Extreme short stature
Parental short stature
Abnormal craniofacial growth
Small hands and feet
Excess subcutaneous fat
Increased weight/height index
Delayed skeletal maturation
Delayed puberty

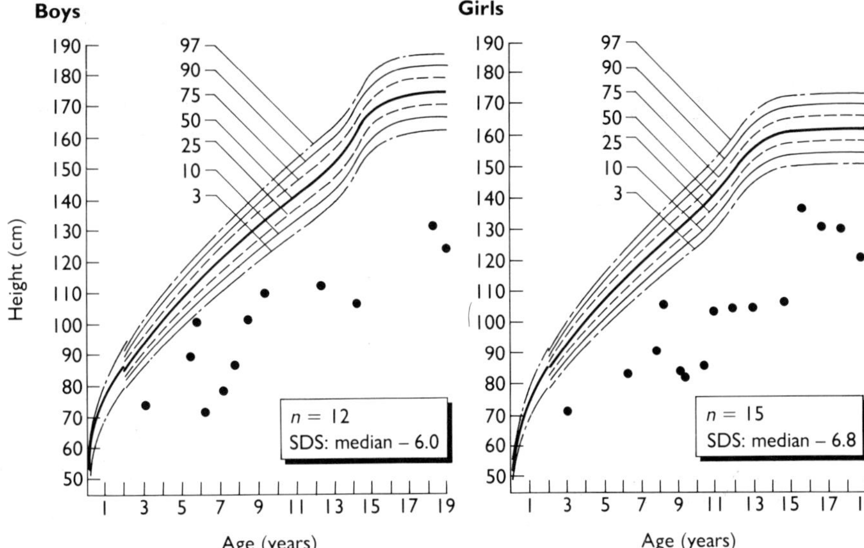

Fig. 11.2 Individual heights of patients with Laron syndrome. The 27 patients form a heterogeneous multi-ethnic population of patients with classical Laron syndrome (from Savage *et al.* [10]).

from both male and female subjects. Final adult height in the Ecuadorian population varied from −7.4 to −8.2 SDS (standard deviation score) [9].

Endocrine features

GH–IGF AXIS

Endocrine function is normal apart from the disruption of the GH–IGF axis. GH secretion is increased because of the failure of normal feedback regulation mediated by IGF-I. The secretory pattern of GH is normally pulsatile with three major pulses occurring overnight [15] (Fig. 11.3). GH levels are elevated between pulses and fail to fall to normal undetectable values [15]. The normal hypothalamic control mechanisms of GH-releasing hormone (GHRH) and somatostatin are therefore preserved and their interaction seems not to be influenced by lack of GH feedback control.

GH-BINDING PROTEIN

The extracellular portion of the GH receptor can be cleaved by proteolytic enzymes and shed into the circulation, where it is known as GH-binding protein. The physiological role of GHBP is not clear but it has been important in the diagnosis of Laron syndrome. If a mutation is present in the GH-receptor gene disrupting the GH-binding domain, GHBP will also be affected, and will therefore not be detectable in qualitative assays relying on GH binding [16]. Several Laron patients with detectable GHBP have now been reported [10,17]. This finding, together with the demonstration of the gene defect in the receptor dimerization site of some subjects, indicates that the absence of GHBP in the plasma is no longer a requirement for the diagnosis of Laron syndrome.

IGF-I, IGF-II AND IGF-BINDING PROTEINS

The majority of the anabolic actions of GH are mediated by IGF-I. IGF-I and IGF-II are structurally related to proinsulin and stimulate metabolic activities in a way similar to insulin, as well as having anabolic effects [18]. In the circulation both IGFs are handled in a complex manner by a group of specific IGF-binding proteins (IGFBP-1–6) [19]. IGFBP-3 is the major circulating IGFBP and is GH-dependent [19]. In Laron syndrome, circulating concentrations of IGF-I [6,10], IGF-II [3,6,10] and IGFBP-3 [9,10] are reduced (Fig. 11.4). IGFBP-1 is increased, possibly related to suppressed insulin secretion, but shows the normal physiological fall with age during childhood [10]. IGFBP-2 concentrations are normal [10].

The GH receptor defect is demonstrated by impaired short-term responses of serum IGF-I and IGFBP-3 levels to stimulation by exogenous hGH (hGH 0.1 U/kg subcutaneously daily for 4 days) in the so-called *IGF-I generation test* [10,19,20]. Using a combination of clinical and endocrine parameters, diagnostic criteria for the diagnosis of Laron syndrome, and its differentiation from growth hormone insufficiency, have been established [21] (Table 11.3).

TREATMENT OF LARON SYNDROME WITH RECOMBINANT IGF-I

Linear growth

IGF-I has metabolic and anabolic effects in short-term

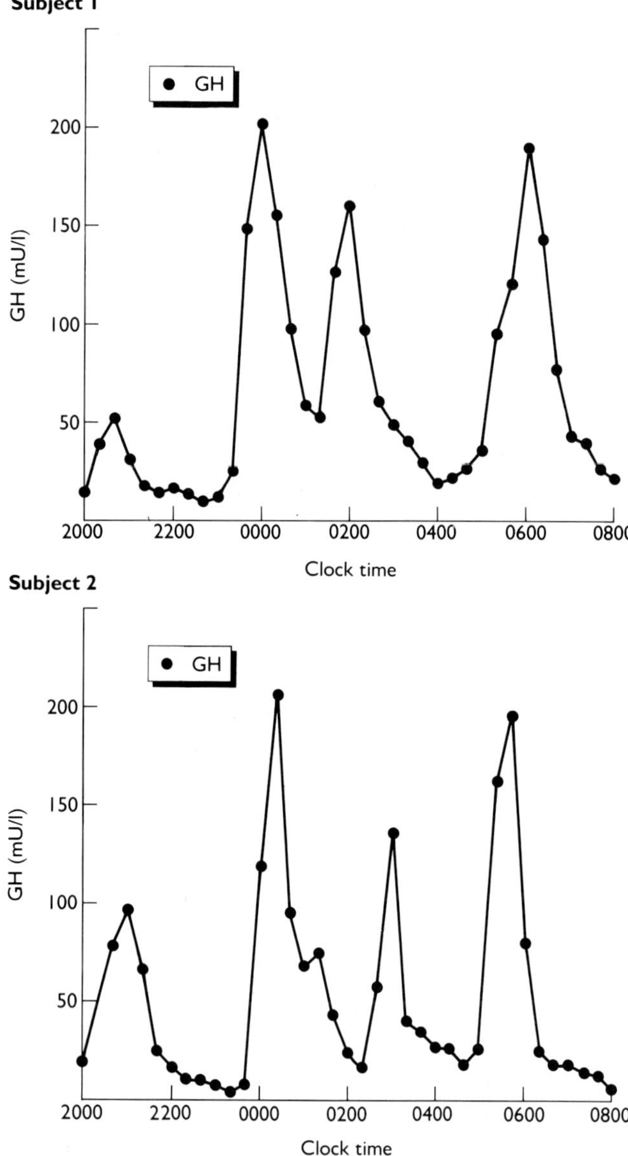

Fig. 11.3 Patterns of overnight serum GH levels in two patients with Laron syndrome, showing increased GH pulse amplitude and failure of GH to fall to undetectable values between pulses (from Crosnier *et al.* [14]).

treatment of Laron syndrome [22,23]. The dose used in long-term therapy has varied from 40 μg/kg twice daily given by subcutaneous injection [24] to over 120 μg/kg once daily [25]. The linear growth response has been greater when the higher dose has been used. With a dose of 40 μg/kg twice daily, growth rates in two patients returned to pretreatment values after 18 months of therapy [24].

In a cohort of patients from the heterogeneous, predominantly European, series [26], height velocity increased from a mean pretreatment value of 4.2 cm/year to 8.8 cm/year at 12 months of therapy (Fig. 11.5). Height velocity was inversely related to bone age at start of treatment. The lack of IGFBP-3 in subjects with Laron syndrome significantly alters the handling of exogenous IGF-I, reducing the plasma half-life from 16–20 h to 4–8 h [27]. Exogenous IGF-I suppresses GH secretion in Laron syndrome [28] but a study of GH pulsatile secretion following IGF-I administration to two patients showed a short-lived biological effect with a return of GH secretion [29] within 4 and 7 h respectively (Fig. 11.6).

Lipolytic and anabolic effects

Clear lipolytic and anabolic effects also occur during IGF-I therapy. Laron reported a reduction of skinfold thickness values in his patients [25], and similar findings accompanied by maintenance of mid-arm circumference measurements and weight gain, indicating a net anabolic effect, were demonstrated in the multi-ethnic 'European' series of patients [30]. Increase in head circumference has also been demonstrated [25].

Change in facial appearance

A striking change in facial appearance in children and adolescents with Laron syndrome has been described during treatment with IGF-I (Fig. 11.7). Although difficult to quantitate, the face becomes more mature, there is a loss of subcutaneous fat and a dramatic increase in quantity and thickness of hair is seen, most strikingly in the eyebrows. It has been said that these patients are starting to look 'acromegalic', but time will tell if this is the case. It is possible that the normal facial maturation which occurs at puberty may be induced by physiological changes in circulating IGF-I (R. Rosenfeld, personal communication).

Adverse effects of recombinant IGF-I

Treatment with IGF-I in Laron syndrome has hitherto been associated with few serious side-effects. Hypoglycaemia occurred in some of the younger patients, although this was generally preventable by ensuring calorie intake before the IGF-I injection. Hypokalaemia normally occurs transiently during the first 48 h of therapy. Mild and transient papilloedema has been documented. It is important to remember that, at the time of writing, the combined world experience of IGF-I therapy amounts to a little more than 2 years. Consequently a great deal remains to be learnt from this new form of therapy.

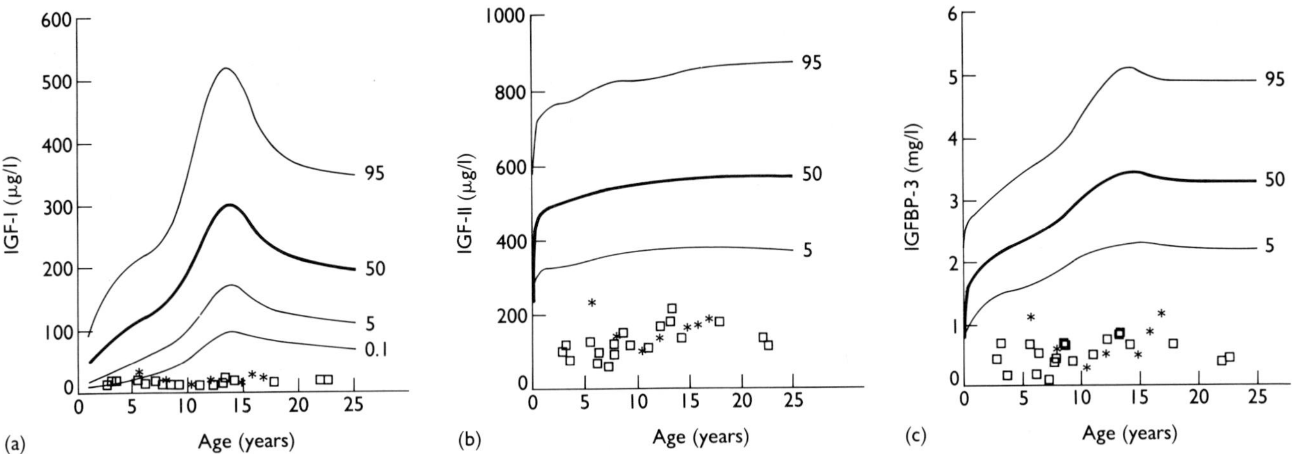

Fig. 11.4 Serum concentrations of (a) IGF-I, (b) IGF-II, and (c) IGFBP-3 in patients with Laron syndrome [10]. Assays were performed by Dr W.F. Blum, Tübingen, Germany, and values are plotted against normal ranges for age [19]. *, patients with normal GHBP; □, patients with extremely low or undetectable GHBP.

Table 11.3 Diagnostic criteria for Laron syndrome

1 GH: basal or stimulated > 20 mU/l
2 IGF-I: very low or absent
3 IGFBP-3: very low
4 IGF-I generation test (GH 0.1 U/kg subcutaneously daily for 4 days)
  (a) IGF-I: absolute increment of < 20 μg/l
  (b) IGFBP-3: absolute increment of < 300 μg/l
5 Height: < −3 SDS

Collect for analysis
1 GHBP
2 DNA for molecular analysis

From Blum *et al.* [21].

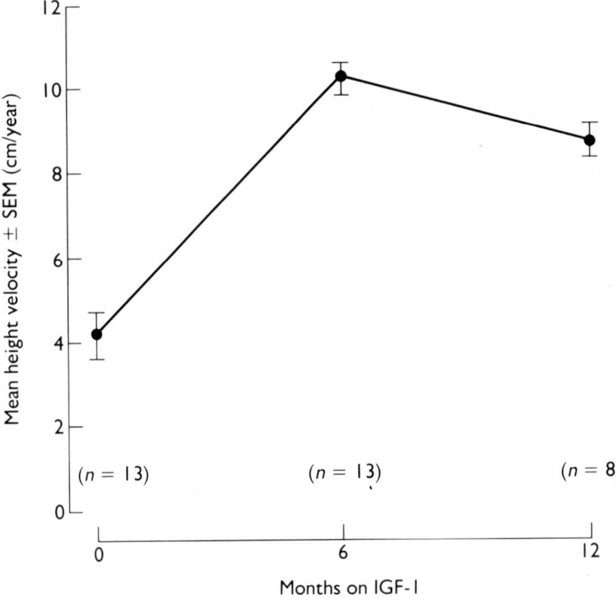

Fig. 11.5 Height velocity during treatment with recombinant IGF-I 120 μg/kg twice daily in patients with Laron syndrome. SEM, standard error mean.

OTHER GROWTH-HORMONE-RESISTANT STATES

Pygmies

The best-characterized pygmy group lives in central Africa. These subjects have a stable genetic defect, which presumably confers advantages to survival and does not significantly affect fertility. Prepubertal growth appears to be normal, the condition becoming apparent at puberty when there is a failure of the pubertal growth spurt associated with an impaired rise of IGF-I and GHBP levels [32]. A defect of the GH receptor has been suggested since pygmies are insensitive to exogenous hGH in terms of growth, as well as in IGF-I generation [33]. GH secretion is increased during provocation tests compared with normal subjects.

Catabolic states

Severely ill, catabolic subjects may be GH-resistant with high GH and low IGF-I levels [34,35]. hGH therapy, except in pharmacological doses, appears not to be effective in improving outcome, even in the presence of adequate nutrition [36]. IGF-I therapy, although still experimental, may contribute to the conversion of these patients to an anabolic state with an increase in both muscle mass and strength. IGF-I is a logical treatment since associated

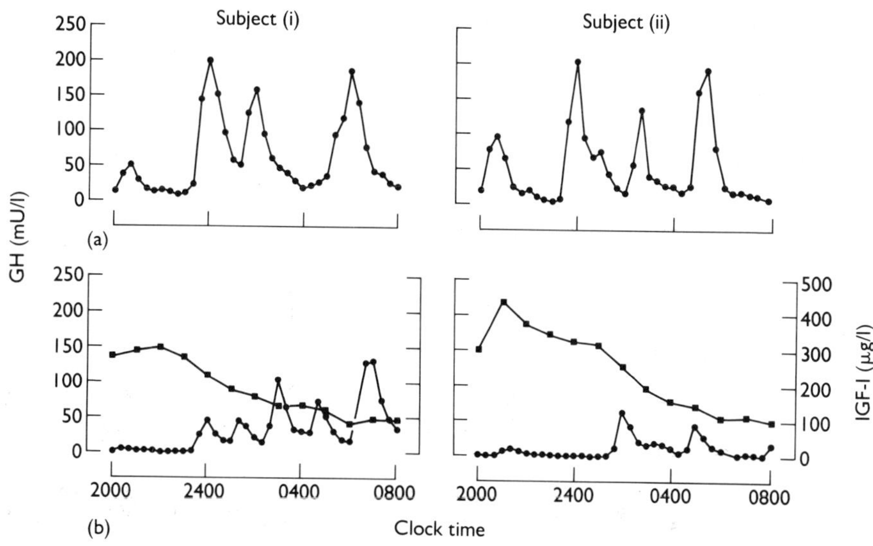

Fig. 11.6 (a) Serum GH levels in two subjects with Laron syndrome before commencement of IGF-I therapy; (b) serum GH (●) and IGF-I (■) levels following administration of IGF-I (120 μg/kg subcutaneously) after 6 months of IGF-I therapy.

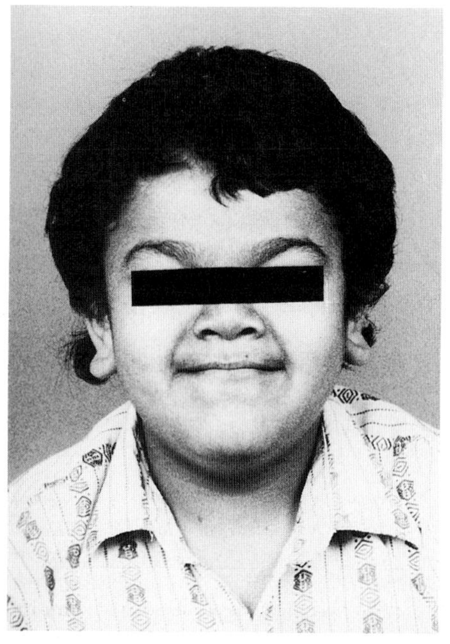

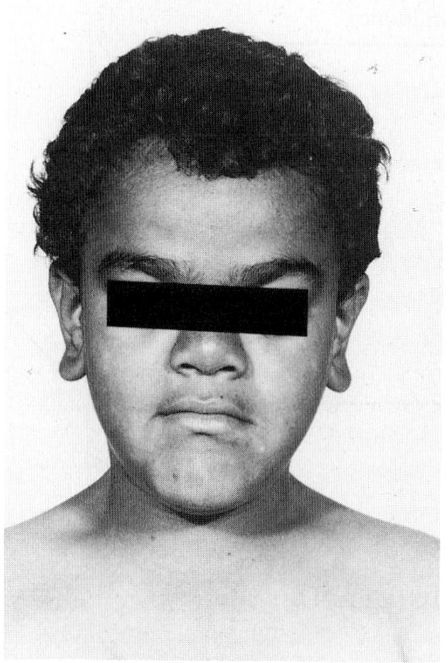

Fig. 11.7 Change in facial appearance before (left) and after 12 months (right) IGF-I treatment (120 μg/kg subcutaneously twice daily) in a 14-year-old child with Laron syndrome. Note progression of maturity, loss of fat and increased hair growth (from Leonard *et al.* [31]).

insulin resistance is common and its insulin-like effect may facilitate the utilization of parenteral nutrients.

Malnutrition

Nutritional status has a profound effect on GH secretion and IGF-I levels. Malnutrition is a well-recognized form of reversible GH resistance. Growth hormone levels may be elevated and associated with low IGF-I concentrations. These parameters are normalized in response to nutritional supplementation [37]. Serum IGF-I shows a close correlation with nitrogen balance in sick and malnourished patients, and is a sensitive indicator of nutritional status. The pathophysiology of malnutrition-induced GH resistance is complex and precise mechanisms remain poorly understood [38].

Adolescent diabetes

In adolescent patients with type 1 diabetes mellitus there is abnormally high GH secretion and relative IGF-I deficiency [39,40]. The abnormal increase in GH secretion correlates with marked insulin resistance, hence increasing insulin requirements [41]. Recombinant IGF-I therapy has recently been shown to reduce both pulsatile GH secretion and insulin requirements [42]. The value of this new and promising form of therapy remains to be confirmed in long-term therapeutic trials.

REFERENCES

1 Laron Z, Blum WF, Chatelain PG *et al.* Classification of growth hormone insensitivity syndrome. *J Pediatr* 1993; 122:241.

2 Laron Z, Pertzelan A, Mannheimer S. Genetic pituitary dwarfism with high serum concentration of growth hormone – a new inborn error of metabolism? *Isr J Med Sci* 1966; 2:152–5.

3 Rosenfeld RG, Rosenbloom AL, Guevara-Aguirre J. Growth hormone insensitivity due to primary GH receptor deficiency. *Endocr Rev* 1994;15:369–90.

4 Amselem S, Sobrier ML, Duquesnoy P *et al.* Recurrent nonsense mutations in the GH receptor from patients with Laron dwarfism. *J Clin Invest* 1991;87:1098–102.

5 Laron Z, Pertzelan A, Karp M, Kowadlo-Silbergeld A, Daughaday WH. Administration of growth hormone to patients with familiar dwarfism with high plasma immunoreactive growth hormone. Measurement of sulphation factor, metabolic and linear growth responses. *J Clin Endocrinol Metab* 1971;64:1042–6.

6 Rosenbloom AL, Aguirre JG, Rosenfeld RG, Fielder PJ. The little women of Loja – growth hormone-receptor deficiency in an inbred population of Southern Ecuador. *N Engl J Med* 1990;323:1367–74.

7 Eshet R, Laron Z, Pertzelan A, Arnon R, Dintzman M. Defects of human growth hormone receptors in the liver of two patients with Laron-type dwarfism. *Isr J Med Sci* 1984; 20:8–11.

8 Laron Z, Pertzelan A, Karp M, Kauli R, Keret R, Doron M. The syndrome of familial dwarfism and high plasma immunoreactive growth hormone (IR-hGH). In: Pecile A, Muller EE, eds. *Growth and Growth Hormone.* Amsterdam: Excerpta Medica, 1972:458–82.

9 Guevera-Aguirre J, Rosenbloom AL, Fielder PJ, Diamond FB, Rosenfeld RG. Growth hormone receptor deficiency in Ecuador: clinical and biochemical phenotype in two populations. *J Clin Endocrinol Metab* 1993;76:414–23.

10 Savage MO, Blum WF, Ranke MB *et al.* Clinical features and endocrine status in patients with growth hormone insensitivity (Laron syndrome). *J Clin Endocrinol Metab* 1993;77:1465–71.

11 Kelly PA, Dijane J, Postel-Vinay MC, Edery M. The prolactin/growth hormone receptor family. *Endocr Rev* 1991;12:235–51.

12 Godowski PJ, Leung DW, Meacham LR *et al.* Characterisation of the human growth hormone receptor gene and demonstration of a partial gene deletion in two patients with Laron-type dwarfism. *Proc Natl Acad Sci USA* 1989;86:8083–7.

13 Berg MA, Guevarra-Aguirre J, Rosenbloom AL, Rosenfeld RG, Francke U. Mutation creating a new splice site in the growth hormone receptor genes of 37 Ecuadorian patients with Laron syndrome. *Hum Mutat* 1992;1:24–34.

14 Crosnier H, Gourmelen M, Prevot C, Rappaport R. Effects of nutrient intake on growth, insulin-like growth factors and their binding proteins in a Laron-type dwarf. *J Clin Endocrinol Metab* 1993;76:248–50.

14a Duquesnoy P, Sobrier M-L, Duriez B *et al.* A single amino acid substitution in the exoplasmic domain of the human growth hormone receptor confess familial GH resistance (Laron Syndrome) with positive GH binding activity by abolishing receptor homodimerization. *EMBO J* 1994;13:1386–95.

15 Cotterill AM, Holly JMP, Taylor AM *et al.* The insulin-like growth factor (IGF)-binding proteins and IGF bioactivity in Laron-type dwarfism. *J Clin Endocrinol Metab* 1992;74: 56–63.

16 Baumann G, Shaw MA, Winter RJ. Absence of the growth hormone-binding protein in Laron-type dwarfism. *J Clin Endocrinol Metab* 1987;65:814–16.

17 Buchanan CR, Maheshwari HG, Norma MR, Morrell DJ, Preece MA. Laron-type dwarfism with apparently normal high affinity serum growth hormone binding protein. *Clin Endocrinol* 1991;35:179–85.

18 Sara VR, Hall K. Insulin-like growth factors and their binding proteins. *Physiol Rev* 1990;70:591–614.

19 Blum WF. Insulin-like growth factors and their binding proteins. In: Ranke MB, ed. *Functional Endocrinological Diagnostics in Children and Adolescent.* J & J Verlag, 1992: 102–17.

20 Ranke MB, Blum WF, Bierich JR. Clinical relevance of serum measurements of insulin-like growth factors and somatomedin binding proteins. *Acta Paediatr Scand* 1988; Suppl.347:114–26.

21 Blum WF, Ranke MB, Savage MO, Hall K. Insulin-like growth factors and their binding proteins in patients with growth hormone receptor deficiency: suggestions for new diagnostic criteria. *Acta Paediatr Scand* 1992;Suppl.383:125–6.

22 Laron Z, Klinger B, Jensen LT, Erster B. Biochemical and hormonal changes induced by one week of administration of IGF-I to patients with Laron type dwarfism. *Clin Endocrinol* 1991;35:145–50.

23 Walker JL, Ginalska-Malinowska M, Romer TE, Pucilowska JB, Underwood LE. Effects of the infusion of insulin-like growth factor I in a child with growth hormone insensitivity syndrome (Laron dwarfism). *N Engl J Med* 1991;324:1483–8.

24 Heinrichs C, Vis HL, Bergmann P, Wilton P, Bourguignon JP. Effects of 17 months treatment using recombinant insulin-like growth factor-I in two children with growth hormone insensitivity (Laron) syndrome. *Clin Endocrinol* 1993;38: 647–51.

25 Laron Z, Anin S, Klipper-Aurbach Y, Klinger B. Effects of insulin-like growth factor on linear growth, head circumference and body fat in patients with Laron-type dwarfism. *Lancet* 1992;339:1256–61.

26 Wilton P. Treatment with recombinant human insulin-like growth factor-I of children with growth hormone receptor deficiency (Laron syndrome). *Acta Paediatr Scand* 1992; Suppl.1992;383:137–41.

27 Grahnen A, Kastrup K, Heinrich U *et al.* Pharmacokinetics of recombinant human insulin-like growth factor-I given subcutaneously to healthy volunteers and to patients with growth hormone receptor deficiency. *Acta Paediatr Scand* 1992;Suppl.391:9–13.

28 Rosenfeld RG, Hoffman AR, Adashi EY, Fielder PJ, Ocrant I, Ceda GP. Effects of insulin-like growth factors on neuroendocrine function. In: Savage MO, Bourguignon JP, Grossman A, eds. *Frontiers of Paediatric Neuroendocrinology.* Oxford: Blackwell Scientific Publications, 1994:156–60.

29 Cotterill AM, Camacho-Hübner C, Holly JMP, Savage MO. The effect of recombinant human insulin-like growth factor-I treatment on growth hormone secretion in two subjects with growth hormone insensitivity (Laron syndrome). *Clin Endocrinol* 1993;39:119–22.

30 Savage MO, Wilton P, Ranke MB *et al.* Therapeutic response to recombinant IGF-I in patients with growth hormone insensitivity syndrome (GHIS). *Paediatr Res* (Suppl.) 1993; 33:abstract 7.
31 Leonard J, Samuës M, Cotterill AM, Savage MO. Effects of recombinant IGF-I on cranio-facial morphology in growth hormone insensitivity syndrome. *Acta Paediatr Scand* 1994; Suppl.399:140–1.
32 Baumann G, Shaw MA, Merimee TJ. Low levels of high-affinity growth hormone-binding protein in African pygmies. *N Engl J Med* 1989;320:1705–9.
33 Merimee TJ. Similarities and dissimilarities between pygmies and Laron-type dwarfs. In: Laron Z, Parks JS, eds. *Lessons from Laron Syndrome 1966–1992. Pediatric and Adolescent Endocrinology*, Vol. 24. Basel: Karger, 1993:266–81.
34 Ross RJM, Miell J, Jones J, Matthews D, Preece MA, Buchanan C. Critically ill patients have high basal growth hormone levels with attenuated oscillatory activity associated with low levels of insulin-like growth factor-I. *Clin Endocrinol* 1991;35:47–54.
35 Ross RJM, Miell JP, Holly JMP *et al.* Levels of GH binding activity, IGF BP-1, insulin, blood glucose and cortisol in intensive care patients. *Clin Endocrinol* 1991;35:361–7.
36 Wilmore DW. Catabolic illness, strategies for enhancing recovery. *N Engl J Med* 1991;325:695–702.
37 Clemmons DR, Underwood LE, Dickerson RN *et al.* Use of plasma somatomedin-c/insulin-like growth factor-I measurements to monitor the response to nutritional depletion in malnourished patients. *Am J Clin Nutr* 1985;41:191–8.
38 Ross RJM, Buchanan CR. Growth hormone secretion: its regulation and the influence of nutritional factors. *Nutr Res Rev* 1990;3:143–62.
39 Tambourlane WV, Hintz RL, Bergman M, Genel M, Felig P, Sherwin RS. Insulin infusion pump treatment of diabetics, influence of improved metabolic control on plasma somatomedin levels. *N Engl J Med* 1981;305:303–7.
40 Edge JA, Matthews DR. Overnight concentrations of growth hormone in diabetic and normal adolescents. *J Clin Endocrinol Metab* 1990;71:1356–9.
41 Amiel SA, Sherwin RS, Simonson DC, Lauritano AA, Tambourlane WV. Impaired insulin action in puberty. A contribution factor to poor glycaemic control in adolescents with diabetes. *N Engl J Med* 1986;315:215–19.
42 Cheetham TD, Jones J, Taylor AM, Holly JMP, Matthews D, Dunger DB. The effects of recombinant insulin-like growth factor I administration on growth hormone levels and insulin requirements in adolescents with Type 1 (insulin-dependent) diabetes mellitus. *Diabetologia* 1993;36:678–81.

12: Tall Stature

P.C. HINDMARSH and C.G.D. BROOK

INTRODUCTION

Tall stature in childhood usually generates less anxiety initially than shortness and, consequently, less is known of the auxology of tall children, although many have received treatment to limit final height. The concept of treating tall adolescents to reduce final height developed from the work of Albright and co-workers who were using oestrogens in adult patients with acromegaly [1]. Since then, hormonal treatment using oestrogens in girls has become a standard mode of therapy following the observations of Goldzieher [2].

The endocrinology of tall stature has received little attention. However, with recent advances in the understanding of neuroendocrinology, different treatment modalities may become available for the management of the tall child. Whatever treatment modality is chosen its efficiency has to be considered in the light of the known growth patterns of tall children and the important contribution made by the pubertal growth spurt to final height. This chapter reviews the auxology and endocrinology of tall stature and the therapeutic armamentarium available for the management of the tall individual.

CLINICAL ASPECTS OF TALL STATURE

Auxology of tall stature

Apart from the growth curves of Tanner & Whitehouse [3], there has been little documentation of the growth of children with constitutional tall stature. A comprehensive study was provided by Dickerman *et al.* [4], who studied 65 tall non-obese patients. Mean birth length of both girls and boys was the 75th centile and birth weight was also above the mean. Maximal growth velocity was achieved from birth to 6 months of age but, although there was a gradual decrease in velocity after this time, it still remained above the 50th centile to 9 years of age. In both sexes a prominent midchildhood growth spurt was observed. The result of this pattern of growth was a stature consistently above the 97th height centile in all cases. The means of the growth velocity data are shown in Fig. 12.1. This figure highlights two important points. First, the midchildhood growth spurt can be easily defined in both sexes, and this period of rapid growth may often be the precipitating reason for concern of parents or health workers. Second, the growth velocity of tall children is never normal; in other words they never grow at a 50th-centile height velocity, and so, year by year, they gain height compared to their peers. This is the reason why the height centiles widen with age.

Figure 12.2 illustrates the growth patterns of two sisters attending our clinic. Both displayed a midchildhood growth spurt, but patient A entered puberty slightly earlier than her sister and consequently continued growing at a rapid rate while her sister displayed prepubertal deceleration. The important point to note, however, is not so much that the discrepancy in stature became more marked during the early part of the second decade of life (which it clearly does), but that the magnitude of the pubertal growth spurt in both individuals was similar, approximately 30 cm. In other words the most important factor in determining the differences in height in these two individuals was the difference in their heights when the pubertal growth spurt began.

Height prediction

The use of skeletal maturity to predict height is important to the management of tall stature. It bears on the decision whether or when to embark on therapy, and helps in assessing the effects of therapy. The prediction depends on the adequacy of assessment of skeletal maturity, which is probably best obtained from the clinician in charge of the case. Radiologists' assessment of skeletal maturity can be very capricious. Height prediction is discussed in Chapter 6 on normal growth.

Table 12.1 shows comparisons of actual heights attained in tall children with the heights predicted using three methods. Overall, it appears that there is no superiority for any method, although only Sorgo *et al.* [8] and Reeser

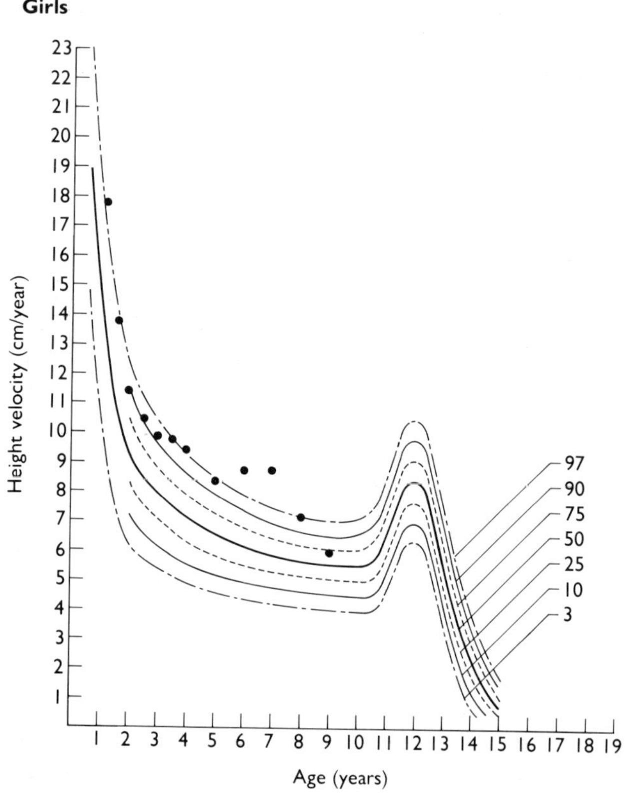

Fig. 12.1 Mean height velocity measurements of 29 prepubertal girls (from Dickerman *et al.* [4].

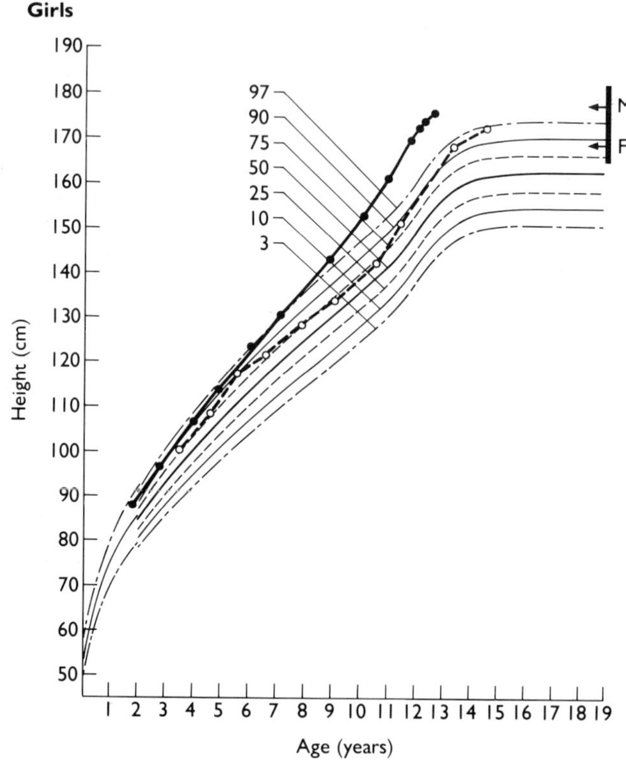

Fig. 12.2 Distance charts of two sisters showing different patterns of growth due to early puberty at the age of 9 years (A, closed circles) and normal onset of puberty at the age of 10 years (B, open circles). F, Father's height centile; M, Mother's height centile.

et al. [6] compared all methods in the same individuals. There is a bias in some of these figures, however, as the untreated patients in some groups selected themselves on the basis of their original height prediction [7]. Other authors who have avoided this bias have suggested that prediction methods can overestimate final height by anything between 0.4 and 1.2 cm, but that an underestimation of 0.7 cm can be observed when the bone age of the child is below 12.5 years [9,10]. Joss *et al.* [5] have also suggested that height-prediction scores may be related to the sex and height of the individuals, an observation which warrants further consideration.

The accuracy of prediction is judged by the size of the residual standard deviation. The standard deviation of predicted adult height in girls with a bone age of 12 years is approximately 2.5 cm according to Bayley & Pinneau

Table 12.1 Differences of height predicted from actual final height in untreated tall children

Number of children	Age (years)	BP–FH (cm)	RWT–FH (cm)	TW–FH (cm)	Study reference
6*	12.13		+1.3	+0.9	Joss *et al.* [5]
26†	12.13	−0.8		+1.8	Joss *et al.* [5]
14	10.7	−0.8	−3.7	+0.1	Reeser *et al.* [6]
17	12.1	+0.3			Schoen *et al.* [7]
7	13.5	+2.3	+2.3	+3.4	Sorgo *et al.* [8]

* Boys with bone ages between 12 and 13 years.
† Girls with bone ages beween 12 and 13 years.
BP–FH, Bayley–Pinneau, final height; RWT–FH, Roche–Wainer–Thissen, final height; TW–FH, Tanner–Whitehouse, final height (parents corrected for).

[11], which is confirmed by other groups who described a nearly similar standard deviation with all three methods [6,12]. The TW method [13] has a standard deviation of 3.5 cm for a 12-year-old boy, 2.7 cm for a premenarcheal girl and 2.1 cm for a postmenarcheal 12-year-old girl. This means that 95% of values of final heights in premenarcheal girls falls within a range of 10.8 cm which, although it is a wide margin, is certainly less than the 95% adult range for women, which spans 23 cm, but not much less than the 14 cm span when parents' heights are allowed for. Similar results have been observed using a number of height prediction methods [5].

The newer equations (TW mark 2) [14] have improved on the original Tanner predictions because very tall and very short individuals were included in the data. The situation has been further improved by the inclusion in these prediction equations of more than one measurement of height or bone age where these are available. When these are included the 12-year-old boys' height prediction standard deviation reduces to 3.2 cm and for postmenarcheal girls it is 1.1 cm.

Diagnosis

The diagnoses with which tall stature may be associated, although rare, are in some respects more sinister than those associated with short stature. It is conventional when considering differential diagnoses to list them in order of incidence, but such an approach offers little to the clinician faced with an individual and his or her parents and the question of what to do. Clinical algorithms can be useful in dealing with this problem, and one devised for the management of tall stature is shown in Fig. 12.3. The principles of growth assessment are the means to making a diagnosis. The height of child should be compared to the measured heights of the parents in the same way as it is for short stature. The questions which then arise are whether the child is tall for the heights of the parents, whether the appearance is normal and whether the growth velocity is normal. Additional information at the first examination may come from the child showing signs of puberty.

The question of what is a normal growth velocity for the tall child is complex but, as we have pointed out in the work of Dickerman *et al.* [4], growth rates are seldom less than the 50th percentile; a height velocity persistently above the 95th centile would be a matter of course. A similar formula to that employed for managing short children can be used. Children with a height velocity greater than the 97th centile over 1 year should be considered for immediate investigation. Children with height velocities between the 75th and 97th centile should be

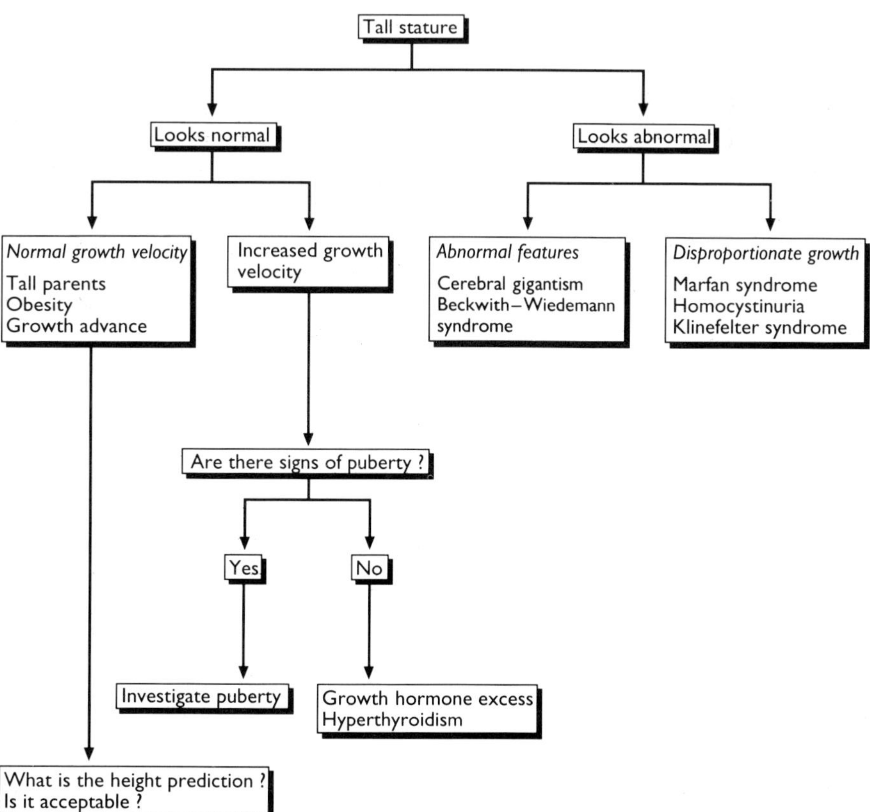

Fig. 12.3 Clinical algorithm for the management of tall stature (redrawn from Roche & Wettenhall [15]).

observed; if 2 years pass with this growth velocity the chances of being normal decrease to about 5%. Special care is required in the management of children who are growing fast without signs of puberty.

Growth hormone (GH) excess and hyperthyroidism are suggested diagnoses in the algorithm, but it is important to realize that, although adrenal disease usually presents with the appearance of pubic hair and growth of the phallus, increased growth velocity may be the only complaint initially. A more common problem is the accentuation of the midchildhood growth spurt (adrenarche) which may cause concern in some tall children. This acceleration in growth is self-limiting and is usually associated with an advance in skeletal maturation over this time period, which effectively cancels out the short-term height increment. In other words the height for bone age remains unchanged, or may decrease slightly.

One final point is worth making in the anthropometric assessment of the tall child. The physician needs to be aware of the effect of overnutrition in the first year of life. Figure 12.4 shows the distribution of heights for children who became obese in their first year compared to children whose obesity postdated this time period. Overnutrition in the first year of life leads to tall stature, and it is not uncommon to see these individuals in the growth clinic. Their growth usually continues parallel to the 97th centile for height with or without further excessive increments in weight. Of note in these individuals is an advancement in skeletal maturation.

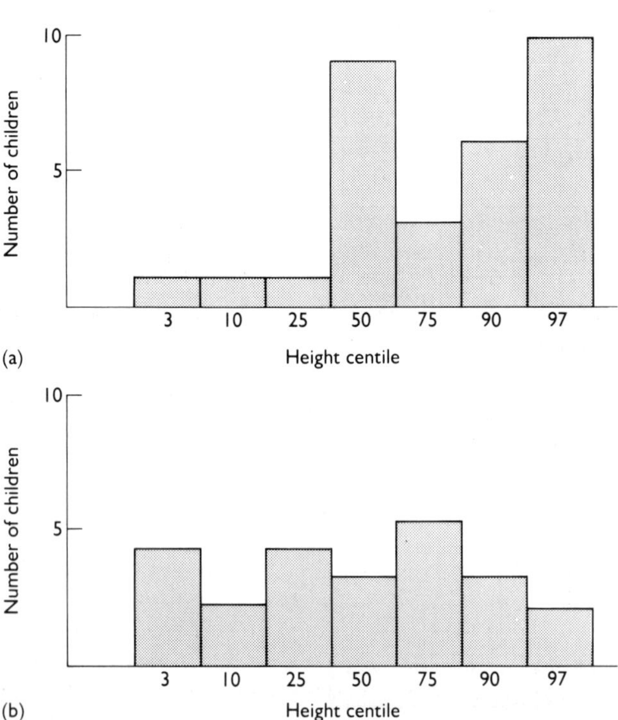

Fig. 12.4 Distributions of height depending on whether obesity was experienced (a) during or (b) after the first year of life.

Tall stature with abnormal features

Cerebral gigantism (Sotos syndrome) and Beckwith–Wiedemann syndrome are both rare [16–18]. In both syndromes mental retardation is common, and rapid growth occurs in the first few years of life, probably as a continuation of the rapid intrauterine growth leading to the large birth weights and lengths recorded in these children. The pattern of growth in a girl with Sotos syndrome is shown in Fig. 12.5, and a full description of the pattern of growth of these children is given in the paper by Karlberg & Wit [19]. The underlying defect in patients with Sotos syndrome is still unclear. Genetic studies have suggested mutations or translocations on the short arm of chromosome 3 [20,21] but a balanced reciprocal translocation involving chromosome 2 has also been described [22] and the situation is made more complicated by the description of a dominantly inherited childhood gigantism resembling Sotos syndrome.

The growth of children with Beckwith–Wiedemann syndrome is very similar to that observed in Sotos syn-

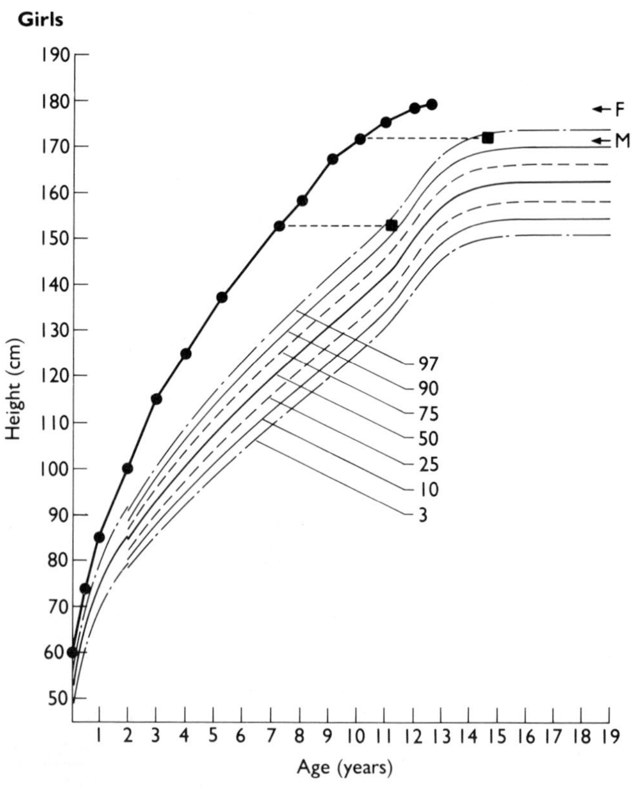

Fig. 12.5 Distance chart of a girl with Sotos syndrome. F, Father's height centile (adjusted for girls' chart); M, Mother's height centile; ■, bone age.

drome. The rapid early growth could be due to the effect of an excess of fetal growth factor. For example, hyperinsulinism is a feature of Beckwith–Wiedemann syndrome and insulin is an important fetal growth factor [23]. Abnormalities in insulin and insulin-like growth factor (IGF)-I genes have not as yet been clearly defined [24] but the association of Wilms tumour in these cases, coupled with the knowledge that the gene product of the Wilms tumour gene is a DNA regulatory protein which also influences the expression of IGFs, could prove a link in the understanding of the growth disorder and the potential for malignancy seen in this condition [25].

IGF-II has also been considered a candidate gene for Beckwith–Wiedemann syndrome. Constitutional paternal isodisomy of chromosome 11 found in some of these patients might lead to an increased gene dosage of the active IGF-II allele [26]. In sporadic cases the frequency of chromosome 11p restriction fragment length polymorphism (RFLP) markers is highest at the insulin–IGF-II locus [27]. IGF-II imprinting is altered in some Wilms tumours, indicating that this event might also occur in Beckwith–Wiedemann syndrome [28]. The argument would then develop along the line that defective imprinting of the inherited maternal IGF-II allele would lead to biallelic IGF-II expression functionally similar to the paternal chromosome 11p duplications and isodisomies seen in some patients. In this case the magnitude and pattern of growth abnormalities and the risk of tumour development would be determined, in part, by the extent to which imprinting of the IGF-II maternal allele was defective. Relaxation of imprinting could be an important factor in understanding growth disorders and cancer development.

In both conditions the endocrinology is normal when investigated later in childhood. In particular in Sotos syndrome the presence of obesity often leads to blunted GH secretion when assessed by physiological or pharmacological means.

Tall stature with disproportionate growth

Marfan syndrome is a genetic disorder inherited as an autosomal dominant trait. Patients may arise as a result of fresh mutations, and so a positive family history is not a prerequisite for a diagnosis. The syndrome consists of the clinical triad of excessively long limbs, ocular abnormalities and cardiovascular problems. In childhood the commonest cardiovascular problem is prolapse of the mitral valve; aneurysm rarely occurs in childhood, although an increased aortic diameter can be demonstrated in 56% of children by the age of 18 years [29]. Homocystinuria is the differential diagnosis, but mental retardation is a feature of this condition and homocystine is detectable in the urine.

Marfan syndrome has been linked to a polymorphic marker on chromosome 15 [30,31] and further detailed studies have demonstrated that the syndrome appears to be caused by mutations in a single fibrillin gene on chromosome 15 [32]. Studies have also demonstrated that fibrillin gene defects do cause familial Marfan syndrome, but that mutations in the epidermal growth factor-like motif of the fibrillin gene are not uniformly associated with severe disease, so it would appear that the fibrillin genotype is not the sole determinant of the Marfan phenotype [33].

Klinefelter syndrome is another cause of being tall for parental height. The clinical features include small testes, poor school performance and excessively long legs. Many cases, however, are not diagnosed until adult life when they present with hypogonadism, infertility or gynaecomastia. Mental retardation is not a necessary concomitant. Tall stature results not only from the presence of additional chromosomal material but also from inadequate sexual development, which allows growth to continue at a normal rate far beyond its usual age of cessation [34]. The explanation about additional X-chromosomal abnormality to patients and their parents requires special care to prevent the misapprehension that psychosexual problems might ensue from the presence of 'female' chromosomes.

Gigantism

In 1886 Marie described acromegaly in adult patients [35]. Hutchinson noted 14 years late that acromegaly and gigantism were similar diseases occurring in different age groups [36]. Experience of the management of gigantism is limited as no clinician has extensive experience of the condition [37–40]. Endocrinological investigations have revealed features characteristic of acromegaly.

Figure 12.6 shows the 24-h growth hormone profile of a boy with pituitary gigantism compared to that obtained from an age-matched tall control. A diagnosis of gigantism should be considered if a child is tall for his parents, is prepubertal and grows excessively fast. Making the diagnosis in the pubertal years can be difficult (see below). Diagnosis and management is considered below.

ENDOCRINOLOGY OF TALL STATURE

In children growing rapidly, investigation of the hypothalamopituitary axis, the thyroid and adrenal glands is required. Hyperthyroidism is relatively unusual in countries with low iodine intake and is easily identified by measuring free levels of triiodothyronine (T_3) and thyroxine (T_4) as well as serum thyroid-stimulating hormone (TSH) concentration. Adrenal disorders may present with increased growth velocity before virilization

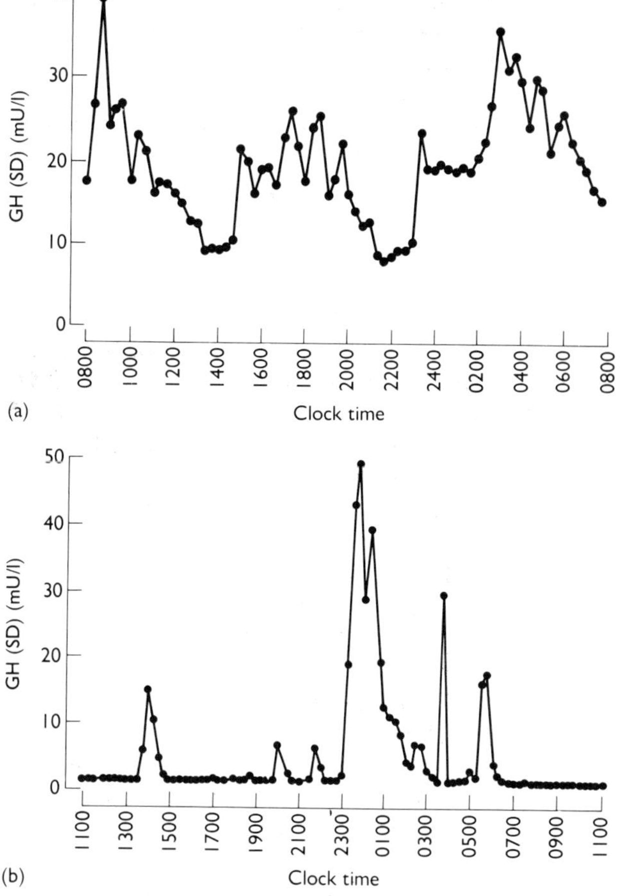

Fig. 12.6 The 24-h serum GH concentration profiles from two 7-year-old boys, one with pituitary gigantism (a) and the other constitutional tall stature (b).

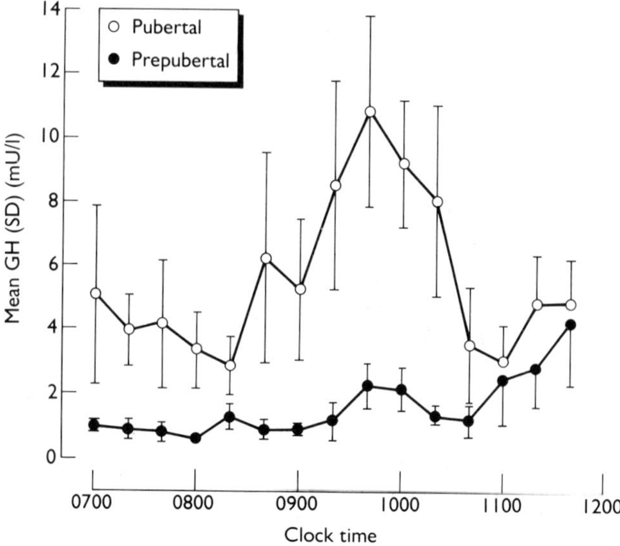

Fig. 12.7 Pooled serum GH concentrations obtained during a morning sampling period in 10 prepubertal (closed circles) and 15 pubertal (open circles) tall children illustrating significant increments in serum GH concentrations during puberty.

becomes obvious, and congenital or acquired adrenal hyperplasia, or a functioning adrenal tumour, can manifest thus. The tall stature and rapid growth of precocious puberty has also to be considered. The differential diagnosis in investigation of such children is detailed in Chapter 15. The final stature of children with obesity does not ultimately become excessive because of advanced epiphyseal maturation.

Growth hormone

Midchildhood growth is GH-dependent and, during this period, tall children grow with a height velocity greater than their peers by secreting a greater concentration of GH over a 24-h period [41]. These findings are not simply confined to physiological profiles, as tall children have a greater GH response to exercise [42] and to GH-releasing hormone [43] than controls of normal stature. Investigation of GH secretory patterns in genetically large and small rats has reached similar conclusions [44].

The majority of GH secretory episodes in childhood occur during the night, but increasing GH secretory activity with age can also be observed during the day [45]. The increase in GH-pulse amplitude with age is probably due to sex steroid secretion, first from the adrenal glands and then from the gonads. Daytime GH secretion is more marked in tall than in small children and Fig. 12.7 shows the pooled serum GH concentration measured over the morning period in prepubertal and pubertal tall children. The presence of morning peaks makes it difficult to interpret results of pharmacological tests of GH secretion in tall children, as these are performed against a background of GH secretory activity. This may partly explain the poor association between measures of physiological secretion (stage 4 sleep) and pharmacological tests seen in tall children [46] and why tall children may have elevated unstimulated GH levels.

Although it is accepted that gigantism and acromegaly are diseases of GH hypersecretion occurring respectively before and after epiphyseal fusion, it has been observed that some constitutionally tall children have biochemical findings reminiscent of acromegaly [47]. Acromegaly is a condition characterized by elevated unstimulated GH levels, a paradoxical rise in GH to an oral glucose load [48,49] and GH release in response to exogenous thyrotrophin-releasing hormone (TRH) [50].

In tall children who have frequent GH pulses it is difficult to separate abnormal responses from the endogenous secretory pattern. This point is illustrated in Fig. 12.8. Here the spontaneous GH secretion of a patient is compared to that following glucose administration: it is

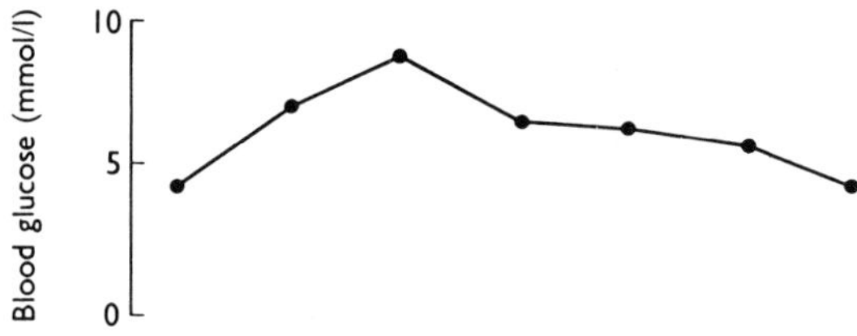

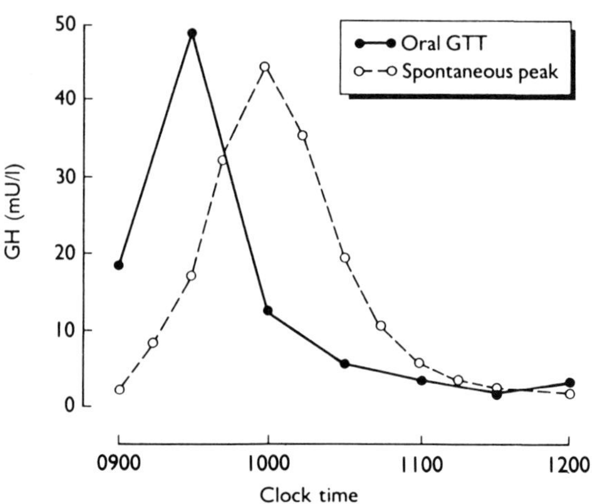

Fig. 12.8 Spontaneous GH peak and GH peak recorded during oral glucose loading in a 14-year-old tall pubertal boy. Glucose tolerance test (GTT).

difficult to make a strong case in the patient for this to be 'paradoxical'. It has also been reported that paradoxical GH responses to an oral glucose load are common in adolescence [51,52] and return to normal suppression in adult life. This could simply be an effect of puberty.

Similar arguments can be advanced against the likelihood that the paradoxical GH response to TRH is a pathological disturbance in tall adolescents. This abnormality lacks specificity: it is seen in acromegaly [50], anorexia nervosa [53], diabetes mellitus [54] and chronic renal failure [55], conditions all associated with elevated GH concentrations. In depressed patients, paradoxical responses are probably more related to frequent spontaneous circadian GH release than to a pathological process [56]. We and others have analysed GH responses to TRH in prepubertal and pubertal children: a paradoxical response was a common feature only in pubertal children and occurred whether the child was tall or short (Table 12.2). Similar conclusions have been observed by other workers [57] and several groups have demonstrated mathematically that paradoxical responses to TRH can be predicted by prior knowledge of the GH secretory status of an individual [58].

Table 12.2 Number of tall and short children with a GH response to exogenous TRH above and below 15 mU/l

	GH < 15 mU/l	GH > 15 mU/l
Tall prepubertal	5	0
Tall pubertal	9	4
Short pubertal	10	5

Insulin-like growth factor I and insulin

The most extensive study of serum IGF-I concentrations in tall stature has been performed by Gourmelen *et al.* [59]. Serum IGF-I concentrations rise with age in tall children in a manner similar to that in normal subjects, although the values are higher. During puberty, tall children have much higher values than controls but values tend to return to the normal range following epiphyseal fusion.

Insulin is implicated in the biosynthesis of IGF-I [60], and recent work has demonstrated that insulin is important in diabetic rats for full expression of IGF-I synthesis [61]. There are significant increases in the circulating concentration of insulin during oral glucose loading in tall pubertal children compared to tall prepubertal individuals [62].

IMAGING IN THE MANAGEMENT OF TALL STATURE

Plain skull radiographs in tall children are unhelpful in the majority of cases, although evidence of the effects of an expanding lesion of the pituitary gland may be seen in children suffering from gigantism. Based on our findings in the high-resolution computerized tomography (CT) scans of tall children we do not recommend routine CT scanning of the pituitary gland in children with constitutional tall stature. This is because radiological abnor-

Table 12.3 Pubertal status in 31 tall children related to findings on CT scan imaging of the pituitary gland

	Breast stage		
Girls	1	2/3	4/5
Normal gland	3	1	1
Large homogeneous gland			3
Large gland with space-occupying lesion		2	10
	Testicular volume (ml)		
Boys	<2	2–12	>12
Normal gland	1	3	1
Large homogeneous gland			1
Large gland with space-occupying lesion		1	4

malities suggestive of microadenomas are frequently found in tall pubertal children [46] and because puberty complicates the issue.

In puberty, large homogeneous glands may be normal [63] and large glands containing low-density lesions with all the radiological appearances of microadenomas may be seen then, as well as in the puerperium [64]. Of the tall children we have studied by high-resolution CT scan those with the lesions suggestive of the presence of the microadenomas were all pubertal and predominantly in late puberty (Table 12.3). In 14 of the 18 in whom a radiological lesion was observed, resolution of the lesion has been seen in all cases.

Radiology of tall children (like the endocrinology) is often difficult to interpret, and unexpected findings do not necessarily reflect pathology.

MANAGEMENT

A height that is acceptable in adult life must necessarily be a matter of opinion and, as there is still a secular trend in height in many countries, will vary from generation to generation. For boys heights up to 200 cm are increasingly acceptable, whereas for many girls and their families heights greater than 180 cm are unacceptable. The first consideration that needs to be given to the question 'who needs treatment' is whether a predicted height is acceptable considering the heights of other members of the family and of the child's peer group. In the case of girls it is mainly the experience of the tall mother that counts.

There are several reasons for treatment. The psychological problems expressed by tall children include difficulties with self-image and rejection from their peer group. A considerable number, particularly girls, express concern about how a tall person is treated by the opposite sex. Tall children may experience problems at school. It is difficult to remember that a 6-year-old with a stature of a 9-year-old is actually 6. The inappropriate behavioural expectations required of such children may lead to retrogressive behaviour, and such children may be labelled as infantile, aggressive, clumsy or accident-prone simply because they cannot cope either with the physical handicap of being large or the emotional problem of being treated as their height-age dictates. On a more practical level, tall children, especially tall teenage children, find that they are unable to wear current fashions in clothes, and that fashionable shoes are hard to find.

From the medical point of view a common problem is kyphoscoliosis. In our practice approximately 15% of tall adolescents have some degree of kyphoscoliosis, many having been referred from orthopaedic colleagues because of concern over spinal curvature. These children deserve medical treatment since the pubertal growth spurt is likely to make kyphoscoliosis worse. More important, the observation of abnormal patterns of ventilation in adolescents with a mild asymptomatic scoliosis may lead to cardiorespiratory problems at an older age [65].

General principles

Like any disorder of growth, the earlier that therapy is introduced, the better the outcome; this is true also of tall stature, where numerous studies have demonstrated that, for example, the earlier that oestrogen treatment is introduced, the better the reduction in final height. It is an often-forgotten fact that the magnitude of the pubertal growth spurt is relatively resistant to any form of manipulation. As children gain between 25 and 30 cm during the pubertal growth spurt it is self-evident that, unless therapy is commenced at a height 25–30 cm less than that desired, little impact on final height will be achieved. Thus, if a child is seen who is prepubertal at the age of 9 years, and has a height of 150 cm, the clinician can be fairly sure that the final height will be in the region of 175–180 cm, assuming that the child enters puberty within the year.

The practice of giving oestrogens to tall girls to reduce their stature was based on two clinical observations. First, children with precocious puberty did not become tall adults if premature epiphyseal closure occurred. Second, in the absence of gonadal steroids, epiphyseal closure was delayed. Although both statements are true the over-emphasis on the effects of sex steroids on bone maturation has led to a less than critical evaluation of these modes of therapy, since the fact that little can be done to manipulate the magnitude of the pubertal growth spurt has not been fully appreciated.

Observational studies of the effects of GH deficiency on the pubertal growth spurt have suggested that pubertal growth is made up of two components, GH and sex steroids [66,67]. Although it might be tempting merely to reduce GH secretion during puberty, and leave or increase sex steroid concentrations, this is unlikely to make a major difference to final height. The only way in which this can be achieved in tall children is to slow the childhood component of growth so that puberty starts from a lower height, or to terminate that component prematurely by inducing puberty. It is possible to combine these two approaches.

Few of the treatment regimens proposed so far have taken account of these observations, and this probably explains the generally disappointing results obtained with treatments, which are usually given too late to improve the situation. For example, commencing oestrogen treatment in a girl with a skeletal maturation of 12 years, when 92–94% of the growth has already taken place, is unlikely to have a significant impact on final height.

Table 12.4 Reduction in final height as a result of using varying doses of ethinyloestradiol in tall girls

Study	Dose of ethinyloestradiol (μg)		
	300–500	250	100
Bartsch *et al.* [9]	4.4	–	4.2
Gruters *et al.* [68]	4.9	–	5.1
Normann *et al.* [69]	5.9	5.3	4.4
Svan *et al.* [10]	5.9	5.5	–

Sex steroid treatment

The use of oestrogens to treat tall girls was first introduced into clinical practice in the 1950s [2]. Various oestrogen preparations have been available and most have been used, but most practitioners now use ethinyl oestradiol continuously, together with progesterone for 5–7 days at the end of each monthly cycle to promote endometrial shedding. Intermittent therapy has been used [7] with an average reduction of predicted height only 50% of that achieved by groups using continuous treatment.

In the initial reports, doses up to 300 or 500 μg of ethinyl oestradiol per day were used. Nausea is often encountered with these doses, and Table 12.4 shows that height reductions comparable to those observed using very high doses of ethinyl oestradiol can be achieved using 100 μg/day. Doses such as those used in the contraceptive pill are probably adequate, and there is now no justification for the prescription of high-dose oestrogen treatment. Studies are now required to determine whether early induction of puberty with conventional doses of oestrogen (Chapter 15) is as effective as the low-dose regimens.

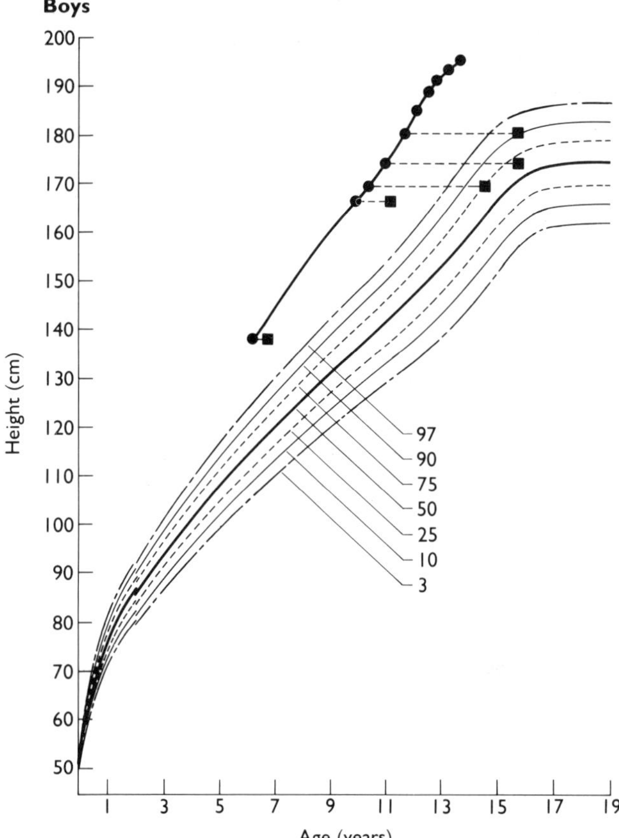

Fig. 12.10 Growth of a boy with tall stature, demonstrating how easily height is accumulated during childhood and how little effect testosterone therapy (commenced age 12 years) had on the pubertal growth spurt (×, bone age).

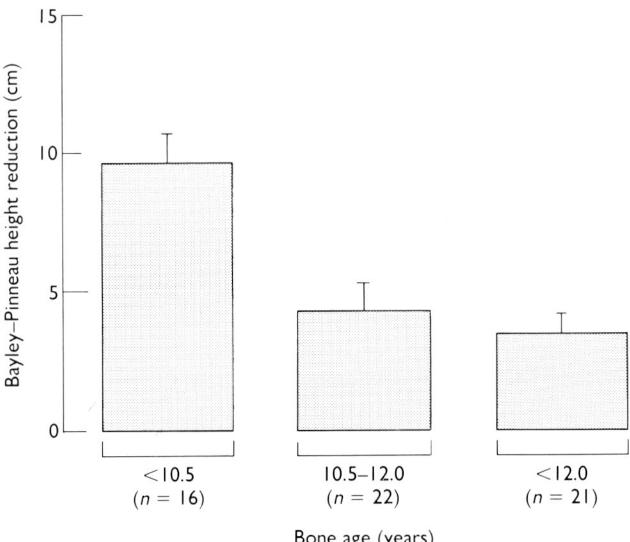

Fig. 12.9 Effects of oestrogen treatment of tall girls on height reduction with respect to the skeletal maturation at commencement of therapy. Data from Ignatius *et al.* [71] and shown as mean and standard error mean.

The major factor affecting the response to treatment is chronological age. The earlier treatment is started, the greater the reduction in final height [70–74] (Fig. 12.9). These observations simply echo the points made above regarding the timing of pubertal induction in tall children. The fixed gain in stature during puberty cannot be overemphasized. It is easy for a tall child to reach heights of 150 cm or more during childhood without much attention being drawn to the changes. By then hormonal manipulations are probably too late; the pubertal growth spurt is going to add 30 cm, so little can be done to seriously limit height. Figure 12.10 highlights this point.

In the management of tall girls, auxology should be performed every 3 months. Blood pressure should be recorded fortnightly for the first 3 months and thereafter at each 3-monthly clinic visit. When the height has remained unchanged for two successive measurements, radiography can be performed to check epiphyseal fusion.

A hand X-ray may not be ideal for this purpose, since epiphyseal fusion here is not necessarily reflected in fusion at other sites. A better marker is fusion of the ilial apophyses assessed on an anteroposterior view of the pelvis. Until these fuse, withdrawal of therapy may lead to a further increase in spinal height. Some groups have suggested stopping therapy when 99% of adult growth has been reached, but simple arithmetic suggests that such an approach defeats the object of the exercise [73]. When related to a stature of 190 cm, 1% is still a lot of growth to the individual, who at that stage is often concerned about any growth. Measurement of sitting heights can be useful in this respect in giving the clinician an idea of how much further growth is likely to come from the spine. Spinal growth comes to an end after long-bone growth, so estimating the rate of deceleration of spinal height velocity gives a useful index of how things are progressing.

It is remarkable that very few serious side-effects have been reported using high doses of oestrogen. Headaches and nausea, particularly on starting treatment, have been frequently observed. Post-therapeutic amenorrhoea is less common than it is following withdrawal of the contraceptive pill. This is because the majority of patients with amenorrhoea have it before treatment commences [75,76]. Obviously the treatment does not affect the underlying problem. Such a problem does not usually pre-exist in tall girls.

Fertility has been assessed in a detailed fashion only in a large Australian study. The treatment of tall girls with high-dose oestrogen did not seem to affect reproductive capacity [77].

Thromboembolism, which is a source of concern in patients receiving the contraceptive pill, has only been reported occasionally, but can be devastating when it does [78]. It must be remembered that the numbers of women suffering from thrombotic complications from the combined contraceptive pill is very similar to the incidence of clotting disorders, such as antithrombin 3 deficiency. It is probable, therefore, that oestrogens may simply unmask a previously undiagnosed condition by reducing antithrombin 3 levels rather than causing thrombosis *per se*.

Long-term side-effects such as diabetes mellitus, hyperlipidaemia, hypertension and carcinomas, especially of the breast and uterus, are more difficult to assess, and it is in the area of increased risk of carcinoma that there is least information and most concern [79].

Experience with testosterone therapy in boys is limited because fewer boys complain of tall stature than girls. Intramuscular injection of 250 mg testosterone oenanthate, fortnightly, led to a mean reduction height of 5.4 cm in one study [73]. There is a theoretical hazard of long-term impairment of Leydig cell function, and recent reports suggest that this may not just be of theoretical concern. In addition, there is no doubt of the profound psychological upsets that can be associated with testosterone therapy. These are most commonly outbursts of temper, but rarely, frank psychosis can occur. Again, the approach of gently inducing puberty at an appropriate height and age (Chapter 15) is probably the way forward.

Because of the anxiety about side-effects, a search has long been made for alternative remedies. In the context of our thesis, namely to induce puberty at a height 30 cm below that ultimately desired, the above-mentioned agents have a limited role because the need to start at a young age makes the induction of puberty unacceptable. A way has therefore to be found in those destined to be very tall to slow down the childhood component of growth.

Bromocriptine

Bromocriptine is a semisynthetic derivative of ergor which decreases growth hormone levels in the majority of patients with acromegaly [80]. It is a dopamine agonist, so its effects in acromegaly are in marked contrast to those seen in normal subjects. L-Dopa stimulates GH secretion in humans and has been used as a test of GH secretion in children [81]. Because of a misunderstanding over the endocrinology of tall stature [47], it was suggested that bromocriptine might be of value in the management of tall children. Although in one study a reduction in height prediction of between 1.1 and 10.3 cm was observed [82], this was only over a very short period of time (6 months). More carefully constructed studies [83,84] have failed to confirm these findings, and Fig. 12.11 illustrates the height reduction experienced by one of the groups from Switzerland. By and large bromocriptine therapy made little difference to height prediction in either of the Swiss studies.

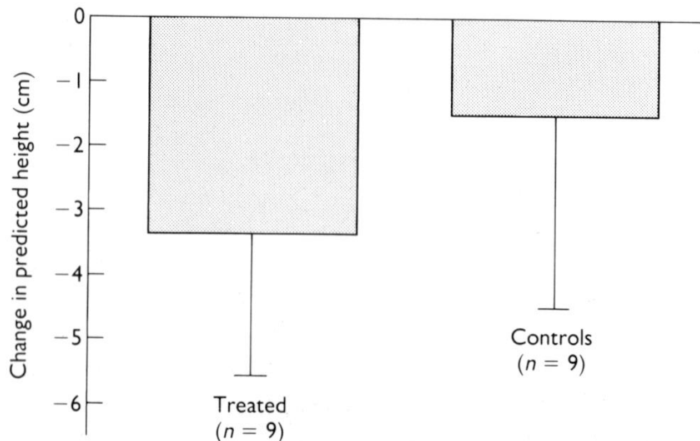

Fig. 12.11 Effects of bromocriptine treatment on height prediction of tall girls compared to a control group (data from Schwarz *et al.* [84]).

Anticholinergic therapy

Acetylcholine is a neurotransmitter involved in the control of GH secretion [85–87]. Its precise mechanism of action is unclear, although there is a suggestion, and it is certainly true in rodents, that it acts by altering somatostatin tone.

As the growth spurt in puberty has two endocrine components, sex steroids and GH, it should in theory be possible to block GH secretion, reduce growth and leave sex steroids free to advance skeletal maturation. The main advantage of this therapy would be that prepubertal children, who were too young to receive sex steroids, could receive this form of therapy.

One of the main problems with anticholinergic therapy is that rebound GH secretion takes place, and when agents such as atropine are used, impairment of short-term memory can result. Both of these problems can be overcome to some extent by using preparations with a longer half-life, such as pirenzepine, which needs to be administered in a dose of 50 mg twice a day to be effective, and possibly three times a day in some individuals. Studies with this drug show that it is well tolerated, with none of the side-effects associated with atropine. We reported mean reductions in final height of −3.5 cm using the Tanner–Whitehouse height prediction method, but although the changes were statistically significant it is questionable how clinically relevant such a reduction in stature actually is [88].

Somatostatin

Intravenous infusion of native somatostatin suppresses GH secretion in normal subjects and in patients with acromegaly [89,90]. However, cessation of infusion induces rebound GH secretion. The short half-life limits the use of native somatostatin for the treatment of patients with acromegaly. With the introduction of long-acting analogues of somatostatin [91] it is now possible to administer the medication as a subcutaneous injection which suppresses GH secretion with little or no rebound [92]. Somatostatin analogues have proved successful in reducing the excessive GH secretion seen in acromegaly with resolution of some of the clinical features [93,94].

At present two studies have investigated the role of subcutaneous administration of somatostatin analogues in the management of children with tall stature. The short-term studies of Tauber *et al.* have suggested that twice-daily injections of 250 µg somatostatin analogue produced GH suppression and a mean reduction in height prediction over a period of 1 year of 4.9 cm [95]. We have observed reductions in height prediction of between 3 and 5 cm following treatment of seven tall children to final height using doses of 37.5–50 µg once or twice a day [96].

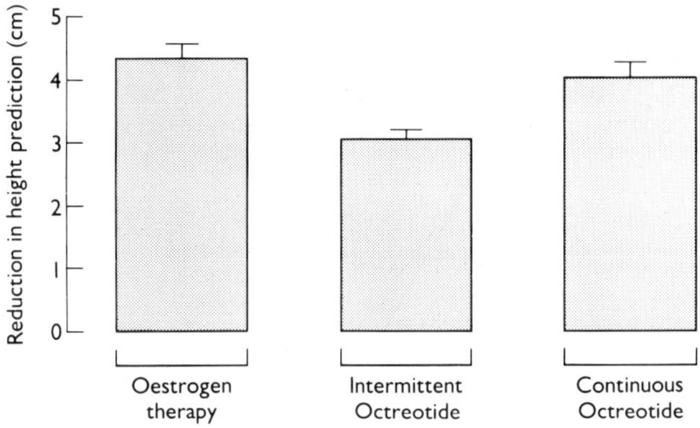

Fig. 12.12 Effects of treating tall girls with somatostatin analogues (Octreotide, Sandoz) given as a once- or twice-daily subcutaneous injection compared to a 12-h overnight infusion. Standard treatment with oestrogens is shown for comparison. Data shown as mean and standard error mean.

The somatostatin analogue appeared to suppress both GH and insulin secretion, with the major effect observed on GH.

In the management of acromegaly, several groups have demonstrated that better overall control of serum GH concentration is achieved by administering the somatostatin analogue as a continuous infusion. We have developed this theme further in the management of tall children, infusing somatostatin analogue for 12 h overnight in a total dose of 50–100 µg. The effects of this intensive regimen did not appear to lead to a greater reduction in final height than that observed using the subcutaneous injection method given once or twice daily (Fig. 12.12).

It is unlikely that there will be a single mode of treatment that will be helpful for the individual with tall stature. Somatostatin analogues themselves are unlikely to lead to significant reductions in final height, because they only influence GH secretion. The asymptotic relationship between growth rate and GH secretion described in Chapter 6 (Fig. 6.23) predicts that reducing GH secretion to zero will lead only to a 50–60% reduction in growth velocity, which is precisely the value observed during the course of treatment with the somatostatin analogues (Fig. 12.13). Therefore, the more promising approach to the management of the tall child is to use somatostatin analogues or anticholinergic therapy in the prepubertal years to a point where puberty can be induced. Whether these modulators of GH secretion should be continued during the pubertal induction process in order to blunt the pubertal growth spurt remains open. The major factor limiting the use of somatostatin analogues is the gastrointestinal side-effects of diarrhoea, fat intoler-

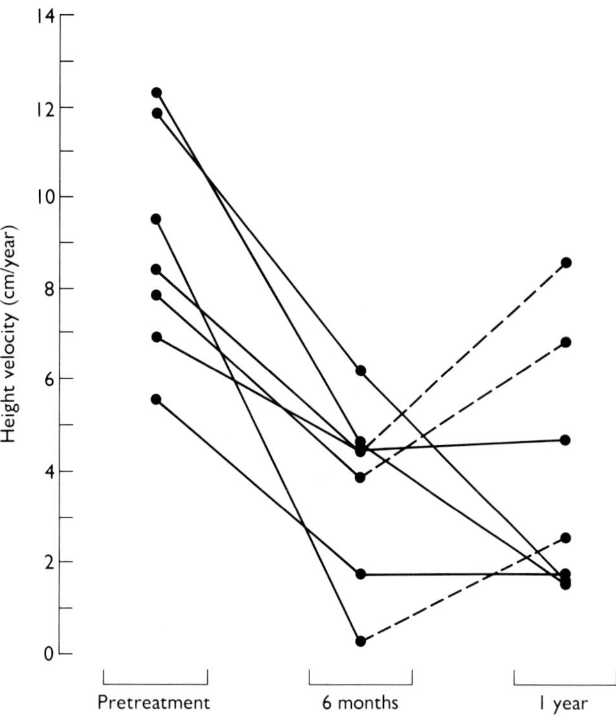

Fig. 12.13 Effect of somatostatin analogue (Octreotide (SMS 201-995), Sandoz) given as a once- or twice-daily subcutaneous injection in a dose of 37.5–50 μg on growth rate in seven tall children (from Hindmarsh *et al.* [96]).

ance and gallstone formation, all of which we have seen, and which have actually prevented the treatment being employed in one tall boy.

Surgery

The surgical correction of tall stature cannot be recommended. It is a high-risk procedure which leads inevitabiy to skeletal disproportion. Major complications are those accompanying the fracture necessary to produce limb shortening. Infection is an important problem, but the major concern is non-union at the fracture site with the generation of a pseudoarthrosis.

Pituitary surgery is indicated for tall children with gigantism. It needs to be remembered that high-resolution CT scans or magnetic resonance imaging studies of pituitary gland performed in tall normal children may show lesions with all the radiological appearances of microadenoma. We advise a conservative approach, especially in pubertal children. If GH secretory profiles reminiscent of acromegaly are obtained in a child with an excessive growth rate, transphenoidal hypophyseal exploration may be appropriate. Further consideration is given to this topic in Chapter 21.

CONCLUSION

In the majority of children, tall stature is constitutional and merely an exaggeration of the normal growth curve. Endocrinological evaluation of tall normal children has demonstrated that they secrete more GH than their peers of normal stature. In puberty they display endocrinological and radiological findings reminiscent of acromegaly, which resolve in later adolescence.

Gigantism is a rare but disabling condition and should be suspected in a tall prepubertal child growing excessively quickly. As it is often difficult to dissect the endocrinology of the normal tall pubertal child from that of a pituitary giant using conventional investigative techniques, clearer insight may be gained by the performance of 12- or 24-h GH profiles. An aggressive approach to therapy is advocated in children with gigantism, and hypophyseal exploration should be considered as a first line of therapy.

Tall children and their parents may seek treatment because of psychological, social and/or physical complications. Treatment should be employed only when height prediction is excessive. A variety of therapeutic regimens is available, but the overall aim should be to try to reduce growth rate using neurotransmitter agents in the prepubertal years with a view to the induction of puberty at a height that is 30 cm below the desired height. Unfortunately, as the majority of children actually present in puberty with concern over their excessive growth, such an option is unlikely to be available in the majority of individuals. Caution should be exercised in the management of such children and expectations should not be raised inadvertently. The results of using sex steroids to treat pubertal children who have a bone age greater than 12 years are poor, and there is nothing to be gained in treating a child with a skeletal maturation greater than 13 years with sex steroids. At this point any potential beneficial reduction in height prognosis, which is very low, is offset by the rare but real complications associated with sex steroid usage.

REFERENCES

1 Albright F, Reifenstein EC Jr, Forbes AP *et al.* Effect of oestrogens in acromegaly. In: *Conference on Metabolic Aspects of Convalescence: Transactions of the 14th Meeting.* New York: Josia H May Jnr Foundation, 1946:102.
2 Goldzieher MA. Treatment of excessive growth in the adolescent female. *J Clin Endocrinol Metab* 1956;16:249–52.
3 Tanner JM, Whitehouse RH. Clinical longitudinal standards for height, weight, height velocity, weight velocity, and stages of puberty. *Arch Dis Child* 1976;51:170–9.
4 Dickerman Z, Loewinger J, Laron Z. The pattern of growth in children with constitutional tall stature from birth to age 9 years. A longitudinal study. *Acta Paediatr Scand* 1984;Suppl. 73:530–6.

5 Joss EE, Temperli R, Mullis PE. Adult height in constitutionally tall stature: accuracy of five different height prediction methods. *Arch Dis Child* 1992;67:1357–62.

6 Reeser HM, Heremans GFP, Van Geldren HH. Reduction of adult height in tall girls. *Eur J Pediatr* 1979;132:37–41.

7 Schoen EJ, Solomon IL, Warner O, Winegerd J. Estrogen treatment of tall girls. *Am J Dis Child* 1983;125:71–4.

8 Sorgo W, Scholler K, Heinze F, Heinze E, Teller WM. Critical analysis of height reduction in oestrogen-treated tall girls. *Eur J Pediatr* 1984;142:260–5.

9 Bartsch O, Weschke B, Weber B. Oestrogen treatment of constitutionally tall girls with 0.1 mg/day ethinyloestradiol. *Eur J Pediatr* 1988;147:59–63.

10 Svan H, Ritzen EM, Hall K, Johansson L. Estrogen treatment of tall girls: dose dependency of effects on subsequent growth and IGF-1 levels in blood. *Acta Paediatr Scand* 1991;Suppl. 80:328–32.

11 Bayley N, Pinneau SR. Tables for predicting adult height from skeletal age. Revised for use with the Greulich–Pyle hand standards. *J Pediatr* 1952;40:463–9.

12 Roche AF, Wettenhall HNB. The prediction of adult stature in tall girls. *Aust J Paediatr* 1969;5:13–22.

13 Tanner JM, Whitehouse RH, Cameron N, Marshall WA, Healy MJR, Goldstein H. *Assessment of Skeletal Maturation and Prediction of Adult Height (TW2 Method)*. New York: Academic Press, 1983.

14 Tanner JM, Landt KW, Cameron N, Carter BS, Patel J. Prediction of adult height from height and bone age in childhood. *Arch Dis Child* 1983;58:767–76.

15 Brook CGD, ed. *A Guide to the Practice of Paediatric Endocrinology*. Cambridge: Cambridge University Press, 1993.

16 Beckwith JB. Macroglossia, omphalocoele, adrenal cytomegaly, gigantism and hyperplastic visceromegaly. *Birth Defects* 1969;5:186–8.

17 Sotos JF, Dodge PR, Muirhead D *et al.* Cerebral gigantism in childhood: a syndrome of excessively rapid growth with acromegalic features and non-progressive neurologic disorder. *N Engl J Med* 1964;271:109–16.

18 Wiedemann HR. Complexe malformation familial avec hernie ombilicale et macroglossie. *J Genet Hum* 1964;13: 223–32.

19 Karlberg J, Wit JM. Linear growth in Sotos syndrome. *Acta Paediatr Scand* 1991;80:956–7.

20 Cole TRP, Hughes HE, Jeffreys MJ, Williams GT, Arnold MM. Small cell lung carcinoma in a patient with Sotos syndrome: are genes at 3p21 involved in both conditions? *J Med Genet* 1992;29:338–41.

21 Schrander-Stumpel CTRM, Fryns JP, Hamers GG. Sotos syndrome and *de novo* balanced autosomal translocation (t(3;6)(p21p21)). *Clin Genet* 1990;37:226–9.

22 Tamaki K, Horie K, Go T *et al.* Sotos syndrome with a balanced reciprocol translocation t(2;12)(q33.3;q15). *Ann Genet (Paris)* 1989;32:244–6.

23 Milner RDG. Fetal growth control: the role of insulin and related peptides. In: Aynsley-Green A, ed. *Paediatric Endocrinology in Clinical Practice*. Lancaster: MTP Press, 1983.

24 Spritz RA, Magger D, Pauli RM, Laxova R. Normal dosage of the insulin and insulin-like growth factor II genes in patients with the Beckwith–Wiedemann syndrome. *Am J Hum Genet* 1986;39:265–73.

25 Drummond IA, Madden SL, Rohwer-Nutter P, Bell GI, Sukhatme VP, Rauscher FJ. Repression of the insulin-like growth factor II gene by the Wilms tumour suppressor WT1. *Science* 1992;257:674–7.

26 DeChiara TM, Robertson EJ, Efstratiadig A. Parental imprinting of the mouse insulin-like growth factor II gene. *Cell* 1991;64:849–59.

27 Henry I, Bonaiti-Pellie C, Chehensse V *et al.* Uniparental disomy in a genetic cancer predisposing syndrome. *Nature* 1991;351:665–7.

28 Ogawa O, Eccles MR, Szeto J *et al.* Relaxation of insulin-like growth factor II gene imprinting implicated in Wilm's tumour. *Nature* 1993;362:749–51.

29 Vetter U, Mayerhofer R, Lang D, von Bernuth G, Ranke MB, Schmaltz AA. The Marfan syndrome – analysis of growth and cardiovascular manifestations. *Eur J Pediatr* 1990;149:452–6.

30 Dietz HC, Pyeritz RE, Hall BD *et al.* The Marfan syndrome locus: confirmation of assignment to chromosome 15 and identification of tightly linked markers at 15q15–q21.3. *Genomics* 1991;9:355–61.

31 Kainulainen K, Steinmann B, Collins F *et al.* Marfan syndrome: no evidence for heterogeneity in different populations, and more precise mapping of the gene. *Am J Hum Genet* 1991;49:662–7.

32 Tsipouras P, Del-Mastro R, Sarfarazi M *et al.* Genetic linkage of the Marfan syndrome, ectopia lentis, and congenital contractual arachnodactyly to the fibrillin genes on chromosomes 15 and 5. The International Marfan Syndrome Collaborative Study. *N Engl J Med* 1992;326:905–9.

33 Dietz HC, Pyeritz RE, Puffenberger EG *et al.* Marfan phenotype variability in a family segregating a missense mutation in the epidermal growth factor-like motif of the fibrillin gene. *J Clin Invest* 1992;89:1674–80.

34 Schibler D, Brook CGD, Kind HP *et al.* Growth and body proportions in 54 boys and men with Klinefelter syndrome. *Helv Paediatr Acta* 1974;29:325–33.

35 Marie P. Hypertrophie singuliere non congenitale des extremities superieures, inferieures et cephalique. *Rev Med Paris* 1886;6:297–333.

36 Hutchinson W. The pituitary gland as a factor in acromegaly and gigantism. *NY Med J* 1900;72:89–100.

37 Anniko M, Ritzen EM. Pituitary tumour causing gigantism. *ORL* 1986;48:180–90.

38 Favre L, Rogers LM, Cobb CA, Rabin D. Gigantism associated with a pituitary tumour secreting GH and prolactin and cured by transphenoidal hypophysectomy. *Acta Endocrinol* 1979; 91:193–200.

39 Frasier SD, Kogut MD. Adolescent acromegaly: studies of growth hormone and insulin metabolism. *J Pediatr* 1967;71: 832–9.

40 Guyda H, Robert F, Colle E, Hardy J. Histologic, ultrastructural and hormonal characterisation of a pituitary tumour secreting both hGH and prolactin. *J Clin Endocrinol Metab* 1973;36:531–47.

41 Albertsson-Wikland K, Rosberg S. Analysis of 24-hour growth hormone profiles in children: relation to growth. *J Clin Endocrinol Metab* 1988;67:493–500.

42 Greene SA, Torresani T, Prader A. Growth hormone response to a standardised exercise test in relation to puberty and stature. *Arch Dis Child* 1987;62:53–6.

43 Batrinos M, Georgiadis E, Panitsa-Faflia C, Sratigopoulos S. Increased GH response to GHRH in normal tall men. *Clin Endocrinol* 1989;30:13–17.

44 O'Sullivan D, Millard WJ, Badger TM, Martin JB, Martin RJ. Growth hormone secretion in genetic large and small rats. *Endocrinology* 1986;119:1948–53.

45 Miller JD, Tannenbaum GS, Colle F *et al.* Daytime pulsatile growth hormone secretion during childhood and adolescence. *J Clin Endocrinol Metab* 1982;99:161–5.

46 Hindmarsh PC, Stanhope R, Kendall BE, Brook CGD. Tall stature. A clinical, endocrinological and radiological study. *Clin Endocrinol* 1986;25:223–31.

47 Evain-Brion D, Garnier P, Schimpff RM, Chaussain JL, Job JC. Growth hormone responses to thyrotrophin-releasing hormone and oral glucose loading tests in tall children and adolescents. *J Clin Endocrinol Metab* 1983;56:429–32.

48 Beck P, Parker ML, Daughaday WH. Paradoxical hypersecretion of growth hormone in response to glucose. *J Clin Endocrinol Metab* 1966;26:463–9.

49 Roth J, Glick SM, Yalow RS, Berson SA. Secretion of human growth hormone: physiologic and experimental modification. *Metabolism* 1963:12:577–9.

50 Irie I, Tshushima T. Increase of serum GH concentrations following TRH injection in patients with acromegaly or gigantism. *J Clin Endocrinol Metab* 1972;35:97–100.

51 Eiholzer V, Torresani T, Bucher H, Prader A, Illig R. Paradoxical rise of growth hormone after oral glucose in tall girls: a physiological finding in puberty. *Pediatr Res* 1985;19:633.

52 Pieters GFFM, Smals AG, Kloppenberg PWC. Defective suppression of GH after oral glucose loading in adolescents. *J Clin Endocrinol Metab* 1980;51:256–70.

53 Maeda K, Kato Y, Yamaguchi N *et al.* Growth hormone release following thyrotrophin releasing hormone injection into patients with anorexia nervosa. *Acta Endocrinol* 1976; 81:1–8.

54 Ceda GP, Speroni G, Dall'Aglio E, Valenti G, Butturi V. Nonspecific growth hormone response to thyrotrophin releasing hormone in insulin-dependent diabetics: sex and age related pituitary responsiveness. *J Clin Endocrinol Metab* 1982;55: 170–4.

55 Gonzalez-Barcena D, Kastin AJ, Schalch DS *et al.* Responses to thyrotrophin releasing hormone in patients with renal failure and after infusion in normal men. *J Clin Endocrinol Metab* 1973;35:117–20.

56 Hsiao JM, Garbutt JC, Loosen PT, Mason GA, Prance AJ. Is there paradoxical growth hormone response to thyrotropin-releasing hormone in depression? *Biol Psychiatry* 1986;21: 595–600.

57 Theintz GE, Tang ZJ, Marti C, Dayer-Metroz MD, Sizonenko P. Growth hormone response to thyrotropin-releasing hormone during puberty: a reappraisal. *Pediatr Res* 1986;20: 1181.

58 Edge JA, Human DH, Matthews DR *et al.* Spontaneous growth hormone (GH) pulsatility is the major determinant of GH release after thyrotrophin-releasing hormone in adolescent diabetics. *Clin Endocrinol* 1989;30:397–404.

59 Gourmelen M, Le Bouc Y, Girard F, Binoux M. Serum levels of insulin-like growth factor (IGF) and IGF binding protein in constitutionally tall children and adolescents. *J Clin Endocrinol Metab* 1984;59:1197–203.

60 Binoux M, Lassarre C, Hardouin N. Somatomedin production by rat liver in organ culture. III studies on the release of insulin-like growth factor and its carrier protein measured by radiological assays. *Acta Endocrinol* 1982;99:422–32.

61 Scheiwiller E, Guler HP, Merryweather J *et al.* Growth restoration of insulin-deficient diabetic rats by recombinant insulin-like growth factor I. *Nature* 1986;323:169–71.

62 Hindmarsh P, Di Silvio L, Pringle PJ, Kurtz AB, Brook CGD. Changes in serum insulin concentration during puberty and their relationship to growth hormone. *Clin Endocrinol* 1988; 28:381–8.

63 Peyster RG, Hoover ED, Viscarello RR, Moshang T, Haskin ME. CT appearance of adolescent and preadolescent pituitary gland. *Am J Neuroradiol* 1983;4:411–14.

64 Hinshaw DB, Hasso AN, Thompson JR, Davidson BJ. High resolution computerised tomography of the post partum pituitary gland. *Neuroradiology* 1984;26:299–301.

65 Smyth RJ, Chapman KR, Wright TA, Crawford JS, Rebuck AS. Ventilatory patterns during hypoxia, hypercapnia and exercise in adolescents with mild scoliosis. *Pediatrics* 1986;77:692–7.

66 Aynsley-Green A, Zachmann M, Prader A. Interrelation of the therapeutic effects of growth hormone and testosterone on growth in hypopituitarism. *J Pediatr* 1976;89:992–9.

67 Tanner JM, Whitehouse RH, Hughes PCR *et al.* Relative importance of growth hormone and sex steroids for the growth at puberty of trunk length, limb length and muscle width in growth hormone deficient children. *J Pediatr* 1976; 89:1000–8.

68 Gruters A, Heidemann P, Schluter H, Stubbe P, Weber B, Helge H. Effect of different oestrogen doses on final height reduction in girls with constitutional tall stature. *Eur J Pediatr* 1989;149:11–13.

69 Normann EK, Trygstad O, Larsen S, Dahl-Jorgensen H. Height reduction in 539 tall girls treated with three different dosages of ethinyloestradiol. *Arch Dis Child* 1991;66:1275–8.

70 Bierich JD, Schoenberg D. Hormonal treatment of familial tall stature. *Acta Paediatr Scand* 1973;62:90–5.

71 Crawford JD. Treatment of tall girls with oestrogen. *Pediatrics* 1978;62:1202–10.

72 Ignatius A, Lenko HL, Perheentupa J. Oestrogen treatment of tall girls: effect decreases with age. *Acta Paediatr Scand* 1991;Suppl.80:712–17.

73 Prader A, Zachmann M. Treatment of excessively tall girls and boys with sex hormones. *Pediatrics* 1978;62:1189–95.

74 Wettenhall HNB, Cahill C, Roche AF. Tall girls: a survey of 15 years of management and treatment. *J Pediatr* 1975;86: 602–10.

75 Jacobs HS, Knuth VA, Hull MGR *et al.* Post-pill amenorrhoea – cause or coincidence? *Br Med J* 1972;2:940–2.

76 Kaiser R, Kloppenburg W, Ehmake H, Schwenk H. Menstruationszyklus nach hormonaler Wachstumshemmung bei Madchen. *Geburtshilfe-Frauenheilkd* 1987;47:410–13.

77 Wettenhall HNB. The tall child. In: Brook CGD, ed. *Clinical Paediatric Endocrinology*. Oxford: Blackwell Scientific Publications, 1981:134–40.

78 Werder EA, Waibel P, Sege D, Flury R. Severe thrombosis during oestrogen treatment for tall stature. *Eur J Pediatr* 1990;149:389–90.

79 WHO. WHO collaborative study of neoplasia and steroid contraceptives, invasive cervical cancer and combined oral contraceptives. *Br Med J* 1986;290:961–5.

80 Wass JAH, Thorner MO, Morris DV *et al.* Long term treatment of acromegaly with bromocriptine. *Br Med J* 1977; 1:875–8.

81 Collu R, Leboeuf G, Letarte J *et al.* Stimulation of growth hormone secretion by levodopa-propranolol in children and adolescents. *Pediatrics* 1975;56:262–6.

82 Evain-Brion D, Garnier P, Blanco-Carcia M, Job JC. Studies of constitutionally tall adolescents. II. Effects of bromocriptine on growth hormone secretion and adult height prediction. *J Clin Endocrinol Metab* 1983;58:1022–6.

83 Schoenle E, Thieintz G, Torresani T, Muritano M, Sizonenko P, Illig R. Lack of bromocriptine-induced reduction of predicted height in tall adolescents. *J Clin Endocrinol Metab* 1987;65:355–8.

84 Schwarz HP, Joss E, Zuppinger K. Bromocriptine treatment in adolescent boys with familial tall stature. A pair-matched controlled study. *J Clin Endocrinol Metab* 1987;65:136–40.

85 Casanueva FF, Villanueva L, Cabranes JA, Cabezas-Cerrato J,

Fernandez-Cruz A. Cholinergic mediation of growth hormone secretion elicited by arginine, clonidine and physical exercise in man. *J Clin Endocrinol Metab* 1984;59:526–30.

86 Mendelson WB, Lantigua RA, Wyatt RJ, Gillin JC, Jacobs LS. Piperidine enhances sleep-related and insulin-induced growth hormone secretion: further evidence for a cholinergic secretory mechanism. *J Clin Endocrinol Metab* 1981;52:409–15.

87 Taylor BJ, Smith PJ, Brook CGD. Inhibition of physiological growth hormone secretion by atropine. *Clin Endocrinol* 1985;22:497–501.

88 Hindmarsh PC, Pringle PJ, Brook CGD. Cholinergic muscarinic blockade produces short-term suppression of growth hormone secretion in children with tall stature. *Clin Endocrinol* 1988;29:289–96.

89 Besser GM, Mortimer CH, Carr D *et al.* Growth hormone release inhibiting hormone in acromegaly. *Br Med J* 1974;1: 352–5.

90 Hall R, Besser GM, Schally AV *et al.* Action of growth hormone release inhibiting hormone in healthy men and in acromegaly. *Lancet* 1973;2:581–6.

91 Bauer W, Brimer V, Doepfner W *et al.* SMS 201-995: a very potent and selective octapeptide analogue of somatostatin with prolonged action. *Life Sci* 1982;31:1133–41

92 Del Pozo E, Neufeld M, Schluter K *et al.* Endocrine profile of a long-acting somatostatin derivative SMS 201-995. *Acta Endocrinol* 1986;111:433–9.

93 Lamberts SWJ, Oosterom R, Neufeld M, del Pozo E. The somatostatin analogue SMS 201-995 induces long-acting inhibition of GH secretion without rebound hypersecretion in acromegalic patients. *J Clin Endocrinol Metab* 1985;60: 1161–5.

94 Lamberts SWJ, Vitterlinden P, Verschoor L, Van Donken KJ, del Pozo E. Long-term treatment of acromegaly with the somatostatin analogue SMS 201-995. *N Engl J Med* 1985; 313:1576–80.

95 Tauber MT, Tauber JP, Vigoni F, Harris AG, Rochicchioli P. Effect of the long-acting somatostatin analogue SMS 201-995 on growth rate and reduction of predicted adult height in ten tall adolescents. *Acta Paediatr Scand* 1990;Suppl.79:176–81.

96 Hindmarsh PC, Pringle PJ, Di Silvio L, Brook CGD. A preliminary report on the role of somatostatin analogue (SMS 201-995) in the management of children with tall stature. *Clin Endocrinol* 1990;32:83–91.

13: The Fat Child

E.M.E. POSKITT

INTRODUCTION

Recent surveys of overweight and obesity amongst adults in the United Kingdom suggest that there will be few of the adult population who are not at least overweight at the end of the twentieth century if present trends continue [1]. This is despite the target set by *The Health of the Nation* to reduce the incidence of obesity back to 1980 levels of less than 6% for men and less than 8% for women by 2005 [2].

There are no good data on the incidence of obesity among children in Britain. Lack of data is partly due to lack of a widely accepted definition of obesity. A number of studies show children in most Westernized countries to be getting steadily fatter [3–6]. Since many obese children progress to obesity in adult life, and estimates have suggested that one-third of adult obesity has its origins in childhood obesity [7], the fat child has an important problem, with implications not only for present nutritional status but also for long-term health and longevity.

When obesity was relatively uncommon it was often considered an endocrine problem, particularly as some endocrine disorders have obesity as a clinical feature. The vast majority of obese individuals, including most grossly obese individuals, have no recognizable endocrine or other medical problem underlying their obesity, although they may have some biochemical endocrine disturbance consequent upon their abnormal body composition. These obese people with no obvious causative pathophysiology can be described as having 'simple' obesity. Those individuals who have underlying medical problems to their obesity can be categorized as having 'pathological' obesity. A few of these children have endocrine disorders.

ADIPOSE TISSUE GROWTH AND DEVELOPMENT

One of the problems in discussing obesity in childhood is the definition of normal fatness. There are physiological changes in body composition through childhood, so fatness varies with age, sex and pubertal development. This, apart from the lack of good methods for determining body composition, complicates the definition of obesity.

Body fat consists of essential and non-essential (storage) fat [8]. Essential fat is that in the nervous system, bone marrow, cell membranes and deposited in association with the female reproductive organs. Storage fat consists of adipose tissue deposited subcutaneously, intra- and retroperitoneally, around the heart and within muscle. In normal men and women, essential fat comprises about 3% and 9% of body weight, respectively. Storage fat is the most variable tissue in the body in terms of amount, but non-obese men and women have approximately 12% and 18% body weight respectively [8].

Before 26 weeks gestation, the fetus has very little fat and what fat is present is essential. At 26 weeks about 1% of the body weight is fat [9]. There is vigorous fat deposition in the third trimester, both as essential fat, with development and myelinization of the central nervous system, and as subcutaneous storage fat. At birth the infant has about 11–16% body weight as fat [9,10]. In the next 4 months the weight of fat in the body trebles, whilst total body weight only doubles. At 4 months 26% body weight is fat [10]. It is relevant that this is achieved on a diet in which >50% energy is derived from fat.

In the second 6 months of life there is a gradual slimming process as fat deposition slows and infants become physically more active and mobile. The nutritional uncertainties of changing to solid foods and the increase in infectious illnesses as maternally acquired immunity is lost contribute to the slimming process. It is natural for young children to appear to slim (although they may not have actual loss of fat) as they grow, so that around the age of 5 or 6 years they have lower percentage body weight as fat than perhaps at any time in the rest of their lives [10,11].

The prepubertal years are marked by some increase in fat deposition. The growth spurt of puberty is usually associated with reduction in fatness, but in girls the spurt is relatively short, and slimming may not be noticed as it is quickly followed by vigorous fat deposition, particularly around the breasts and hips to give the characteristic

Table 13.1 Some published estimates of the fat component of body weight at different ages

Age (years)	Fat component of body weight (%) Males	Females	Reference
Birth	11.0	—	[10]
0.25	26.3	—	[10]
1	23.9	—	[10]
2	20.6	—	[10]
3	18.3	—	[10]
4.5	14.3	14.3	[14]
5	16.5	15.4	[11]
10	17.6	16.0	[15]
14	18.4	27.0	[3]
15	11.4	23.3	[15]
Young adults*	18.3	23.7	[16]*

* There is wide variation in quoted results in adults, depending on method used and age of subjects.

Table 13.2 Some estimates of the prevalence of obesity in the UK

Age (years)	Prevalence (%)	Reference	Year of publication
0.125	59	[19]	1971
0–1	35	[20]	1970
	28 overweight	[21]	1972
	16 obese	[21]	1972
2–5	0.5	[22]	1971
4–6	2.5	[11]	1977
10	2	[23]	1977
13	12.1 boys	[24]	1969
	16.5 girls	[24]	1969
14	3.6 boys	[25]	1974
	32.4 girls	[25]	1974
All school-children	3.1	[24]	1969
	3.5	[22]	1971

physique of adult women. In boys the growth spurt is more prolonged. Boys with delayed puberty may become quite obese, but the vigorous growth of lean tissue at puberty often results in spontaneous slimming with actual loss of fat and return to normal fatness by the end of puberty [12,13].

These changes in body fatness are reflected not only in estimates of body fatness (Table 13.1) but also in the shape of skinfold thickness centiles [17,18] and the relation of weight to height at different ages in childhood. Ages associated with rapid fat deposition are ages when the prevalence of obesity in childhood tends to be high. Some children seem to escape the normal controls of fat deposition at times of physiological fattening and become significantly obese. If they do not slim in the following lean tissue deposition phase, they are likely to develop obesity which persists into adult life. Table 13.2 shows how estimates of the prevalence of obesity in childhood tend to rise and fall with the relative fatness of children at different ages.

In adults the significance of obesity for health is now recognized as relating not only to relative fatness, but also to fat distribution. Realization that central fat is more likely to be associated with hypertension [26], diabetes mellitus [27] and hyperlipidaemia [28] than peripheral fat has clarified into appreciating that it is the intra-abdominal fat which is most concerning in adult obesity [29,30]. In children, amounts of intra-abdominal fat vary (as in adults) but most storage fat is subcutaneous [30].

DEFINITION OF OBESITY

There are few conditions which can be diagnosed so easily by the layman when severe and can present such difficulties in definition for the clinician when mild. Obesity is defined as an excess of body fat either in the total weight of fat in the body or as a proportion of whole body mass. There are no totally satisfactory methods of determining body composition, and consequently there are no recognized normal ranges for fatness.

BODY COMPOSITION IN OBESITY

The body consists of fat and lean tissue. Body water is confined to the lean tissue compartment but adipose tissue is more than just fat. It contains adipocytes, which may or may not be stuffed full of triglyceride, and supporting stroma of connective tissue and blood vessels. Thus 'body fat' could indicate total lipid in the body, the number of fat cells, total adipose tissue or superficial adipose tissue. It is not surprising that estimates of 'body fat' vary widely using different methodologies in the same individual.

The fat content and physiological responsiveness of adipose cells vary in different parts of the body. Even within the same area of subcutaneous adipose tissue there may be differing responses to nutritional and metabolic stimuli, with superficial layers of subcutaneous fat being more resistant to mobilization, thus resembling essential fat [31].

Estimation of body fatness

Body fat cannot be measured directly, although skinfold calipers provide a measure of the thickness of the skin and subcutaneous fat layer [32]. Estimation of total body fat is thus derived from estimations of body composition, usually using a two-compartment model of fat and lean body mass (LBM), although greater accuracy can be achieved from methods which use more compartments, for example fat, bone, extracellular water and body cell mass. Two-compartment modelling tends to assume that the only tissue affected in amount and composition in obesity is adipose tissue. This is not the case. For every 1 kg increase in fat there is an increase in approximately 300 g of LBM due to increased circulating blood volume, supporting stroma and perhaps muscle bulk and bone density [33]. Extracellular water is also commonly increased in the obese. Total body water and LBM fall with loss of fat mass. The physiological properties (density, impedance, water content) of lean tissue are altered in obesity. Thus interpreting changes in these properties as totally due to changes in the amount of fat can lead to misleading results.

Since obesity is a common problem, an ideal method of estimating obesity will be cheap, safe, easily repeatable, able to be practised by untutored investigators and able to interpret changes accurately. Such a method does not exist. The most widely used techniques are anthropometric techniques, particularly those involving weight and height.

ANTHROPOMETRY: WEIGHT AND HEIGHT

Standards for expected weight and height for age exist for many populations. From these values percentage expected weight or percentage expected weight for height can be determined, but the method of determining expected weight or weight for height can vary, so methodologies should always be precisely defined. Although there is considerable variation in weight for height, the more excessive weight is for height and/or age, the more likely is the excess due to excessive amounts of fat.

The relationship between weight and height is not the same at all ages, nor at any height for age. Children with simple obesity are usually above average stature in the prepubertal years at least [34,35], and consequently estimating obesity in terms of excessive weight for age compared with average weight for age, or excessive weight for height using standardized weight for height tables, can bias towards making all tall children overweight and most fat children more 'overweight' than justified.

In adults, overweight and obesity are widely classified clinically by the body mass index (BMI) or Quetelet index [36]. This index,

Body weight in kilograms/(height in metres)^2,

is unsatisfactory for assessment of obesity in children since the average values for BMI vary with age, being low in early infancy, rising, falling in early childhood years and then rising again after about 8 years [37,38]. The variation in average BMI can be controlled by relating BMI to that of an average child of the same age. Overweight and obesity are then a relative BMI expressed as percentage expected from centiles for age [37], centile value from published standards [38] or Z score from published standard deviations for age [39]. Clinically this relative BMI is the most practical way of assessing childhood obesity even though correlations with skinfold measurements are not particularly good.

SKINFOLD THICKNESS

Skinfolds provide a direct estimate of fatness in one site, by measuring the layer of fat under the skin (together with overlying skin). Measurement of a few skinfolds does not necessarily represent the depth of subcutaneous fat throughout the body. Skinfolds also take no account of fat stored internally, which increases in children towards adolescence. Some children are so fat that it is not possible to grasp skinfolds with the calipers, or the folds form peaks and slip through the calipers whilst being measured. In fat individuals it may also be impossible to elevate skinfolds. It seems more uncomfortable to measure the folds in fat than in slim individuals, even though calipers are meant to provide even pressure on the fold, however thick. Thus with many obese children the measurement of skinfolds is frequently either impossible or declined by the subjects.

Regression equations for estimating fatness as a clinical procedure have been developed from summed skinfold thicknesses (usually expressed as the log sum of skinfolds because of skew distribution) and an experimental method of assessing lean body and total fat mass, such as body water by deuterium oxide space, or body density by underwater weighing [40,41]. These indirect estimates are not accurate. Although appropriate for the children among whom the equations were developed, they do not allow for individual variations in fat distribution.

PHYSICAL PROPERTIES OF LEAN AND FAT TISSUE: BIOELECTRICAL IMPEDANCE

The resistance and conductance of tissues reflect their water content [42]. Bioelectrical impedance (BEI) has become a popular method of assessing body composition in terms of the percentage of body weight that is fat. However, resistance alters with changes in body water content of LBM as well as with excess fat. In young children measurements are unreliable because of the need for a certain distance between the electrodes on the wrist and ankle, and because of the high total body water of children under 3 years. Body fat estimated by BEI is probably no more accurate than estimated by well-performed anthropometry, particularly when used to estimate changes in fatness.

Table 13.3 Advantages and disadvantages of some methods of determining body composition in obesity

Method	Cost	Measures intra-abdominal fat	Comments
Weight, height especially relative BMI	Low	No	Clinically practical, ? best clinical method. Repeatable; does not measure *fatness*
Skinfolds	Low	No	May be impossible and may yield inconsistent results
BEI	Moderate	No	Not useful in very young; poor at showing change accurately
Underwater weighing	High	No	Measures density. Often considered 'gold standard'. Not useful clinically nor in very young
Ultrasound	High	To some extent	Requires experienced technician. Gives accurate skinfold measurement
CT	Very high	Yes	Excellent but involves radiation. Not useful clinically
MRI	Very high	Yes	Excellent images. Not practical

IMAGING TECHNIQUES

Ultrasound, computerized tomography (CT) and magnetic resonance imaging (MRI) can all be used to distinguish intra-abdominal and subcutaneous fat [43]. Ultrasound is the least useful in this respect, but will provide accurate measurements of skinfolds and, by estimating the depth of the abdomen from the back of the anterior muscle layer to the abdominal aorta, can be used to provide an estimate of intra-abdominal fat. It involves no radiation, is painless, non-invasive, and relatively cheap. CT can provide good images of body fat distribution but involves a considerable dose of radiation and is thus unsuitable for children. It also requires children to lie still for a protracted period, which may necessitate sedation. MRI measurements are also time-consuming. Whilst providing excellent images of fat distribution, MRI is not a realistic method of assessing body fatness routinely.

Table 13.3 lists some of the issues relating to methods of assessing body fat in children in the above methods and with other techniques. For providing some assessment of relative fatness, and for demonstrating changes in body fat, relative BMI is probably the most satisfactory method. BEI has become very popular but may be relatively poor at indicating changes in body fat accurately.

FAT CELL SIZE AND NUMBER

In the late 1960s there was much interest in the number of fat cells in children. Work in rats had suggested that maximum fat cell numbers might be reached early in life, and might have a determining effect on relative fatness later. Since that time it has become clear that fat cells may develop throughout life, and the size and number of fat cells is largely a reflection of the fatness of an individual, since adipocytes are recruited when existing fat cells reach a certain size and lipid content. Fat cell size varies with different areas of the body and even within a tissue, so estimations of fat cell size in one area of the body can be very misleading in relation to adipose tissue as a whole [44].

Adipocytes are recognizable, although very small, at 24 weeks gestation [45]. At term, adipose cells are 45–75 μm in diameter and contain approximately 0.12 μg lipid per cell. During the first year of life the mass of each adipose cell increases to a mean content of about 0.5 μg lipid per cell [46]. Cell size and lipid content are then about the same as in non-obese adults. Most, if not all, of the increase in the amount of stored fat can be accommodated by this increase in fat cell size. There is relatively little fat cell multiplication in the first year of life. Fat cell numbers in infancy are not a major determinant of later obesity.

Studies by Knittle *et al.* [46] show that fat cell size decreases in normal children between 1 and 4 years before increasing only very slowly until puberty, when there is rapid multiplication of fat cells along with multiplication of many cells in the body. The lack of progressive increase in the size of fat cells, despite increase in total amount of fat in the body, is accommodated by an increase in the number of fat-containing adipocytes and recruitment of adipocyte precursors.

In obese infants who do not lose their obesity after about 6 months of age, adipose cell size does not diminish. At age 2 years adipose cell size is much the same as in adults. Adipose cell numbers are higher than in non-obese children and increase steadily throughout childhood, unless there is a period of slimming [46].

The young infant is unique in the relatively large proportion of fat which is brown fat. Brown fat (brown adipose tissue, BAT) consists of fat cells with many large mitochondria and lipid distributed in small locules instead of the large single lipid droplet of white adipose tissue (WAT) cells. BAT is highly active metabolically, and cells respond to sympathomimetic stimuli and to noradrenaline and glucagon by rapid hydrolysis of triglyceride to glycerol and fatty acids with the generation of heat. BAT is important in maintaining body temperature in the neonate. Its distribution, particularly in the neck, mediastinum and retroperitoneally, may be important in maintaining the function of internal organs under cold stress. The volume of BAT diminishes rapidly in the first months of life. As the cells mature they store more fat, which coalesces to form one large globule, so cells assume the appearance of white adipose cells. BAT has little role in metabolism in the adult, and seems independent of nutritional state in that cells change little in appearance, even in the presence of severe lipid depletion [47].

Fat distribution

There has been growing interest in the distribution of fat in adults, with emphasis on the proportion of central to peripheral fat [48,49]. The ratio of waist to hip circumference (WHR) has been widely used to assess fat distribution. This is not a very satisfactory ratio since definitions of waist and hips have often been vague, but it does seem to have a significant relationship with adult morbidity from the complications of obesity. The waist is now defined as the horizontal circumference in a standing subject at a position half-way between the lower border of the ribs and the iliac crest in the midaxillary line. Hips are the widest horizontal circumference around the buttocks below the iliac crest [28]. Imaging techniques are now used wherever possible to assess intraabdominal fat in adults [43]. In children WHR values are high compared with adults, for whom the ratio of 0.85 may be taken as the division between central and peripheral fat distribution.

Mean WHR decreases from about 1.1 in very young children to about 0.8 in pubertal children [50]. Levels are higher in boys than in girls at all ages. The high WHR may be as much an indication of the narrow pelvis of childhood as an indication of central fat, although it is noticeable that subcutaneous abdominal fat is very pronounced in many young children. Imaging suggests that this is largely external with little intra-abdominal fat [30]. As children mature and the pelvis grows in girls, WHRs change and the adult distribution develops. WHR has been reported to be associated with levels of total cholesterol, low-density lipoprotein cholesterol, apo-B lipoprotein and with the apo-A_1/apo-B lipoprotein ratio in 10-year-old girls, when results were controlled for body fatness [51]. Other studies have shown low correlations of high WHR with weight loss in 10-year-old boys [52] and 15-year-old girls [53].

It is difficult to understand why the distribution of body fat could be so significant for morbidity in adult life. Gluteal fat is recognized as particularly characteristic of females and is more resistant to slimming procedures. It is characterized by high lipoprotein lipase (LPL: the main regulatory hormone for uptake of lipid by adipose tissue) activity but slow overall mobilization of lipid, except in pregnancy and lactation. Progesterone may enhance LPL activity through expression of glucocorticoid receptors in WAT.

Bjorntorp [54] has suggested that lipid is trapped in the gluteofemoral region by being taken up readily but released only slowly. By contrast intra-abdominal fat (omental and mesenteric) is highly sensitive to lipolytic stimuli. Lipid uptake is high so fat is turned over quickly. The tissue has many glucocorticoid receptors inducing high LPL activity and fat uptake. The glucocorticoid stimulation of these receptors is inhibited by testosterone, which tends to be low in many abdominally obese men. Testosterone enables expression of β-adrenergic receptors present in abundance in the mesenteric and periportal adipose tissue in men, and may allow amplification of lipolytic glucocorticoid effects. Fatty acids from intra-abdominal fat enter the liver via the portal vein and lead to secretion of very low-density lipoproteins and LPL by the liver. They may also decrease insulin binding and degradation by liver cells, thereby contributing to hyperinsulinaemia [54].

CAUSES OF OBESITY

Obesity is an excess of fat and is associated in normal children with normal or increased lean tissue mass. Thus it must arise from an excess of energy intake over energy expenditure. It is not clear how far to attribute the excess to excessive energy intake, deficiency in energy expenditure or underlying greater efficiency of metabolism in individuals with a propensity to obesity. All these factors are probably relevant, although precipitating factors may vary between individuals.

In the risk factors for obesity (Table 13.4), a family history of obesity predominates. About 80% of signifi-

Table 13.4 Risk factors for childhood obesity

Risk factors
Family history of obesity
Low social class
Deprived home environment
High-fat diet
Single child
Single parent
Excessive television viewing
Short sleep duration
? Low intelligence
? High birth weight

cantly obese children have one or both parents obese and around 30% have both parents obese [55–58]. This finding does not of itself decide whether obesity is genetically or environmentally determined, but there is now accumulating evidence to suggest that obesity usually results from environmental factors acting on genetically predisposed individuals.

Twin and adoption studies

Borjeson [59] demonstrated that the physiques of identical twins of obese parents were more likely to be obese than those of non-identical twins, suggesting a genetic factor to obesity. Identical twins, as adults, even though separated from one another in childhood, have greater similarity in body mass index than non-identical twin pairs [60]. Adopted children as adults also have greater similarity in fatness and BMI with their natural parents and siblings than with their adopting families [61]. Studies such as these suggest strong genetic elements in the predisposition to obesity. Bouchard [62] has suggested that genotype accounts for more than 40% of individual differences in resting metabolic rates, the thermic effects of food and the energy costs of light exercise.

Recognition of a genetic predisposition to obesity opens a new area for metabolic investigation. In the future the role of hormones in intracellular metabolism in the obese may be better understood but, currently, mechanisms explaining genetic predisposition to obesity are unknown. Obesity is so common and so varied in presentation that several genetic mechanisms seem likely. Thus there may be subtle differences in metabolism in some individuals leading to obesity, while others have inherited tendencies for large appetite, poor appetite control or relative physical inertia. Those individuals with a strong predisposition to obesity will tend to obesity in only mildly adipogenic environments. Those with less strong predisposition will become obese only in environments which readily lead to excess energy intake over expenditure.

Energy intakes in obesity

It is a widespread view that the obese are greedy, have excessive energy intakes of energy-dense foods and are consequently fat. Although some obese children undoubtedly eat excessively, and thus have an obvious cause for excess fat, this is not always the case. There is an enormous range in 7-day energy intakes by children of the same age, and a lack of correlation between intakes for age and weight or height for age [63]. Within the same age group some normal-weight children eat twice as much energy as others, and yet do not get fat. There has been a gradual decline in the average energy intakes of children in the developed world, despite steady increases in weight for age, height for age, and fatness [64]. Energy intakes cannot alone account for the rise in obesity prevalence.

Because the obese, for whatever reason, eat more than they individually require in terms of energy, there have been many searches for abnormalities in their appetite control. These have succeeded in demonstrating a number of differences between obese and non-obese people, but none which is found so consistently that it seems to explain the development of obesity [65]. Appetite, if regarded as the perceived desire to eat, is probably influenced more by external than internal stimuli in the developed world today. The pressures on children to eat, and the opportunities for them to eat, are greater than ever before.

Appetite is affected by the quality of the food consumed. Foods with a relatively high fat content seem more appetizing to children in modern Western society than those with lower fat content [66]. If the fat content is high, the food is likely to be dense in energy. Wholefoods (fresh fruit and vegetables), because they usually require more chewing, take longer to eat and may thus increase satiety, as well as possibly creating prolonged satiety due to gradual digestion and absorption of food. Food that is rapidly absorbed, particularly carbohydrate, leads to rapid rise in blood glucose and insulin, and subsequent reactive hypoglycaemia, resulting in a craving for more food.

The environment in which eating takes place is important to the amount of food eaten. Food eaten alone is often consumed rapidly, preventing satiety developing before the end of the meal. Food eaten in company may be eaten more slowly. Speed of eating, and the pleasure of the company, contribute to stronger feelings of satisfaction.

Changes in eating habits relevant to the increase in obesity

There is considerable evidence that in Europe and North America children and adults consume less energy per 24 h than 40 or 50 years ago, yet they are significantly fatter. Diets and patterns of eating are very different from 40 years ago. Children consume higher proportions of total daily food intake as snacks outside their homes. Snacks tend to be energy-dense and high in fat; they come in a great variety of flavours and presentations. Satiety is thus minimized by the possibility of trying new flavours or new shapes. Television and other advertising, and peer pressures, encourage children to think about and eat snacks and prepared-before-purchase foods.

One of the main differences between the typical Western diet and the diet of most of the developing world is the fat content. It is the recommendation in many Western countries that the fat content of the diet should provide no more than 30–35% of total energy. Diets in much of the developing world, where obesity is rare, have only 20–25% total energy derived from fat. The low fat content of a diet means foods are usually of low energy density and have to be consumed in large volumes to meet requirements. This has until recently been seen as an explanation for differences in the adipogenic effects between Westernized and traditional diets.

Evidence is now accumulating that the fat content of the diet may relate directly to the ease and efficiency of fat deposition [67]. Pre- and post-obese adults have reduced capacity for oxidation of fat. It is possible that the genetic propensity to weight gain is caused by impaired capacity to increase lipid/carbohydrate oxidation when fed high-fat/low-carbohydrate diets [68]. Lipid storage is thus promoted with diets of high fat content compared with isoenergetic diets of low fat content. The high fat content rather than the overall energy content may be the critical adipogenic factor in the Western diet.

Energy expenditure in obesity

Energy is expended in basal metabolism, growth, thermogenesis, resistance to infection and tissue repair, as well as in activity. Except in the unusually active, the majority of energy expenditure is expended in basal metabolism. Do the obese have reduced basal metabolic rates (BMR)?

BASAL METABOLISM

There is no strong evidence that the obese have lower BMR than the non-obese. It is difficult to determine expected energy expenditure per kilogram LBM since methods of determining body composition in the obese are less reliable than in the non-obese. BMRs vary widely between individuals, and members of the same family tend to have levels that are similar in terms of relatively high or low rates [69]. Families with genetic predisposition to obesity do not predominate below the average ıange of BMR.

Obesity might be explained by reduced energy expenditure in processes other than BMR. The above-average height of obese children makes it unlikely that the energy expended in growth is *less* than average. Reduced need for thermogenesis because of much wider use of central heating in Europe and North America may have contributed to a greater prevalence of obesity among children than in the past, but seems inadequate to account for the degree of change in the prevalence of obesity. Children with obesity are usually remarkably healthy, suggesting that they have had less illness which might have drained energy reserves, but again this seems inadequate to explain the difference in nutrition between them and other children.

Although there is some evidence that those with established obesity are less physically active than those who are not obese, this may be secondary to the physical handicap of obesity [70,71]. Comparative energy expenditure in activity by obese and non-obese people is not easy to assess because the heavier bodies of obese individuals require more energy to move than those of lighter individuals. As with energy intakes, there are some obese children whose abnormally low level of activity seems sufficient to explain their obesity, but this does not explain all obesity in children.

The explanation for obesity is thus complex. Energy intakes exceed expenditures. Energy excess may arise in some because of the availability of energy, because the energy is ingested as fat and as such is efficiently stored or because energy expenditure is relatively low due to low levels of activity and/or relatively low BMR. There may be genetic determinants to all these aspects of energy balance. It seems unlikely that one explanation or one gene will account for all obesity. There are opportunities for a variety of environmental precipitating factors.

Environmental associations

Lissau-Lund-Sorensen & Sorensen [72] showed that in Copenhagen obesity persisted or developed in adult life in those who had been reared in deprived urban circumstances, irrespective of the level of education of the parents or their income. This is perhaps understandable. If children are in deprived circumstances they are unlikely to have much opportunity to play outside in safe circumstances. They remain indoors and watch television and, in boredom and frustration, reach for food to provide interest and comfort. Home circumstances are unlikely to be associated with shops providing fresh fruit and vegetables at reasonable prices. The children consume snack foods, often high in fat, which provide little satisfaction. Parents, because of the difficulty or expense of cooking in poor housing, may buy prepared meals which again are usually high in fat energy. The parents become bored and depressed by their circumstances and unable to alter their way of life, or to encourage their children to disciplined eating or activity.

Dietz & Gortmaker [73] showed that the percentage over-weight of adolescents boys in the USA was proportional to the average number of hours a week spent watching television. Klesges *et al.* [74] recorded metabolic rates close to basal levels during television viewing, and surmised that children relapsed into torpor when viewing. Video games may be a more hopeful development, since they induce metabolic rates equivalent to mild exercise [75]. A recent study of schoolchildren in Northern Ireland [76] showed that, although at 11 years old boys and girls both expressed interest in participatory sport, by the age of 16 sporting interests had declined and more sedentary occupations were preferred. Girls' favourite leisure activities were listening to records and talking with friends.

CLINICAL RISK FACTORS FOR OBESITY IN CHILDHOOD

Table 13.4 lists known risk factors for obesity. The effect of social class seems likely to act through deprivation [72]. Social class may also influence the fat content of food, those foods high in fat often being cheaper than high-protein foods and fruit and vegetables. The tendency for single children [77,78] to become obese is difficult to explain unless we postulate either that these children are overindulged or that they grow optimally due to the absence of rivals within the family. Since single children are often taller than children with parents of similar heights but from families of several children, the second suggestion might have some relevance.

Locard *et al.* [79] found short sleep duration was a highly significant risk factor for obesity in 5-year-old children. This association persisted even when duration of television viewing was taken into account. Why short sleep duration should be associated with obesity is not clear, unless it is a reflection of a disorganized household where sleeping is as undisciplined as eating. The authors suggest decreased physical activity could lead to overweight and a shortage of slow-wave sleep which is increased by exercise. Lipolytic activity is maximal at night and reduction in sleep may reduce overall lipolysis.

THE OBESE INFANT

Obesity in infancy is common, but this is the one age group in which the incidence of obesity has fallen. Twenty-five years ago about 40% of infants in the UK were overweight [19,20]. The prevalence of overweight was attributed to the predominance of bottle-feeding and the introduction of weaning solids at a few weeks of age [19]. Changes to later weaning and/or reduction in the salt, protein and saturated fat content of infant formulas and weaning foods have been associated with a fall in the incidence of overweight in infancy [80]. The high salt and protein content of infant formulas at that time led to critical hyperosmolality even in healthy infants. This was thought to induce thirst, greater formula intake and thus excessive energy intake. Breast-feeding was a minority practice. Breast-feeding does not prevent obesity in infancy or later, but it is associated with less obesity in infancy and the breast-feeding mother's approach to weaning and weaning practices may be very different from that of many bottle-feeding mothers [81].

The majority of obese infants do not stay obese [11], and thus obesity occurring in infancy is perhaps less disturbing than that occuring later in childhood. However, this statement needs qualification in that obesity occurring when all infants are fattening rapidly, that is in the first 4 months of life, is likely to resolve. Obesity developing in the second 6 months of life suggests a different aetiology than an overexuberant fattening phase. Since it is occurring at an age when fat infants often begin to slim, obesity beginning in the second 6 months of life is worrying. Obesity developing in the infants of obese parents should always be viewed seriously, and the parents should be advised on appropriate feeding and ways of exercising their young children. Growth progress should be monitored.

Overanxiety about creating fat children has led some mothers to be overcautious about weaning their infants on to appropriate highish-fat, high-carbohydrate diets, with the result their infants receive low-fat, high-fibre diets and may develop malnutrition. Infants have high energy requirements per kilogram body weight which can only be achieved on relatively high fat intakes fed frequently. Guidance concerning obesity in infancy must be tempered with understanding of the high energy needs of young children.

Unlike older children with simple obesity, obese infants are not above average length [21]. They show no particular diagnostic features.

Obesity in infancy presents few problems. There are studies suggesting that obese infants are more prone to respiratory tract infections with wheezing than are non-obese infants [20,82]. These studies date largely from a time when obesity or overweight affected about 40% of 4–6-month-old infants. Infants of that age quite frequently develop wheezing due to an asthma/wheezy bronchitis-type response to viral upper respiratory tract infections. As they usually respond poorly to bronchodilators these infants remain wheezy, although not particularly distressed, for prolonged periods. Whether the obesity of infancy predisposes to wheezing, or whether wheezing tends to be obvious at an age when infants are at their fattest, is thus uncertain. The latter seems a likely explanation.

How much does obesity in infancy predispose to obesity later?

It is not surprising that obesity at one age predisposes to obesity at another age. Yet when obesity amongst infants was very common, only one in five obese infants was still overweight or obese at the age of 5 years. Eighty per cent had returned to normal weight for height and normal fatness [11]. Studies from Sweden at around the same time as the studies quoted above showed similar incidence of obesity at age 7 as in the UK, although incidence of obesity in infancy had been much less [83]. Obesity in infancy does not seem a very important determinant for obesity later.

These studies of obese infants are now quite old. With the increased incidence of obesity in childhood and a relatively less fat infant population, it might be interesting to know the present relationship of obesity in infancy and obesity in childhood. The greater incidence of obesity in childhood seems – by its rapid increase – to be determined by environmental factors. The tendency for fat infants to stay fat may be greater than in the past since, with more balanced infant feeding, infants with a strong genetic predisposition to obesity may form a larger proportion of obese infants. If the factors influencing the genetic predisposition to obesity in infancy are different from those acting later, this would not be so.

Rolland Cachera *et al.* [38] have demonstrated the changing relationship of weight to height in BMI centiles for age. Following individual children along these curves demonstrated that children who had an early rebound in adiposity (that is they had increasing BMI values before the age of 6), were more likely to stay obese [84]. This reiterates what has been said earlier: children who fatten at ages when other children are not fattening, or who do not show signs of lessening fatness at ages when other children are slimming, are most at risk of developing persistent obesity.

THE OBESE CHILD

Clinical features

The majority of children who are obese have no underlying medical problem which is recognized as contributing to their obesity. They have simple obesity. Most of them are symptom-free and well. Occasional children have vague complaints of tiredness, breathlessness and aches and pains in their limbs. Appetite is usually good but not necessarily enormous. Some have fussy appetites and disorganized eating patterns. Reliable dietary histories are very difficult to obtain, but children commonly report high intakes of sweets and snack foods and chips. Many are very reluctant vegetable and fruit eaters and may even eat meat only when prepared as hamburgers, sausages or in bought precooked meals. This reluctance with fruit and vegetables could be a feature of the cultural environment in which the children live or indicative that they have been overindulged but, by encouraging diets that can be consumed quickly without satiety, fussiness probably contributes to the development of obesity.

Birth weight

Correlations between birth weight and relative weight in infancy are to be expected, since birth weight and weight in later infancy are not truly independent variables. Most, although not all, studies of older obese children show mean birth weight not different from average [21,34,85]. There is perhaps a group of children who are long and heavy from birth, thus inflating the upper centiles in some studies. Wilkinson *et al.* [23] found 21% of a community sample of obese children had had birth weights over the 90th centile for gestation. Locard *et al.* [79] found birth weight a predisposing factor for obesity in 5-year-old children. Mossberg [85] found obese children with a birth weight >4500 g were significantly more likely than other obese children to be overweight 40 years later.

Linear growth and puberty

Obese children are commonly tall for their age prepubertally [34]. Stature is quite frequently above the 97th centile and virtually all obese prepubertal children with simple obesity have stature above the 25th centile for age.

Studies have suggested that obese children have early puberty, early cessation of growth and below-average stature in adult life [86]. It is unusual to be able to follow obese children through puberty to review mature height. It is the author's experience that at least 50% of the obese children seen over 14 years of age have been above average adult height when last reviewed, although many of them had not stopped growing. Some of these have been children with notably tall and usually very obese parents. Review of parental height is likely to provide some indication of whether a child's tall stature will persist through puberty. Some of the children with shorter stature and obesity in adolescence seem to be those (often girls) with early menarche who have developed obesity during and after puberty.

A hospital clinic population is not necessarily typical of the obese child population. Delayed puberty is not uncommon in obese boys, and does not seem particularly advanced in most obese girls. This is in contrast to the findings of others. Boys with obesity and delayed puberty can become very disturbed. Pubertal delay is very obvious due to the contrast between small immature genitalia hidden in abdominal fat and the boy's large size.

Why obese children are tall is not clear but, in view of the above, it cannot be explained merely by advanced growth due to overnutrition. Secular trends in stature in most Westernized countries have been attributed to better diets. It is difficult to feel that diets have improved in the UK in recent decades and energy intakes are, in population terms, less than before. Although Forbes [87] described children with acceleration in height velocity in association with periods of rapid weight increase, this is not widely recognized. Strict dieting may be associated with slowing in linear growth, but this is not inevitable. Increase in stature and a propensity to obesity seem to go together, so that obese Asians in the UK tend to have tall stature similar to obese Caucasian children [88]. Children from the affluent countries of the Pacific rim show disturbingly rapid increases in incidence of obesity, and very impressive changes in height compared with previous generations [6].

Obesity and tall stature could be a reflection of a genetic predisposition to overall florid growth undisturbed by adverse circumstances. Even when there is no obesity, tall stature tends to be accompanied by increased lean body mass for height and above-average skinfold thickness.

Successful slimming may result in some slowing of height velocity and slight crossing of height centiles downwards, but this is not true for all successful slimmers.

Classification of simple obesity

There have been many attempts to categorize different forms of childhood obesity. None is satisfactory. Forbes [35] separated obese children on the basis of whether LBM was increased for height and age. He found children with increased LBM for age were of above average stature with advanced bone age, and had usually been obese since infancy. The composition of their excess weight was 29% LBM and 71% fat. These percentages are very similar to the stated increases in LBM in all adults with simple obesity and, given the difficulties of measuring LBM, the increases may characterize the majority of obese children also.

Griffiths *et al.* [89] classified 4-year-old boys who were overweight or overfat as fat and heavy, fat but not heavy and heavy but not fat. They did not elucidate particular aetiological features despite making speculations about the relation of physique to overeating. The boys were not followed to review persistence or otherwise of their obesity. We have not found many obese children fit into the group of 'fat but not heavy'. Significant obesity in short but otherwise normal children seems to us rare prior to puberty. Most short children are noticeably lean.

Court & Dunlop [90] separated obese children according to age at onset of obesity and height for age. Children obese from infancy were usually tall with increased weight for height and advanced bone age. Lipid profiles were normal. Weight, although excessive, increased in proportion to height so that percentage expected weight remained the same. The authors concluded that children obese from infancy were prenatally primed for obesity, and their weight was following a normal pattern of growth subject to normal physiological control. By contrast, the children who became obese after infancy gained weight out of proportion to height, were less tall for age and had abnormal lipid profiles. These children had a better response to dieting than those whose excess weight was thought to be part of their physiological growth pattern.

These classifications are now historic. That they have not been widely accepted suggests that, although they may be appropriate for the populations studied, the clinical features of obese children range widely and do not fit easily into these classifications. Nevertheless there is an underlying impression that there are some children whose obesity seems almost inevitable in modern Westernized society, and who commonly have parents who have been obese since childhood. These children have fewer medical complications than those whose obesity may be more related to extremes of energy imbalance imposed by their environment, and may be those with very strong genetic predisposition to obesity. Whether they have a discrete familial defect leading to severe obesity or whether they just reflect one extreme of the wide range of possible fatness requires detailed genetic studies.

There has been considerable research into antenatal factors affecting later nutrition and health. These studies are largely concerned with the effects of poor intrauterine growth and later health outcomes. The consequences of poor intrauterine growth tend to be poor postnatal growth and thus detracting from, rather than causing, obesity [91].

Complications of childhood obesity

The medical complications of obesity in childhood are few and minor, although there is increasing evidence of complications such as hyperinsulinaemia [92], impaired glucose tolerance [93] and hypertension [94] with increasing age. Many older obese children show quite marked knock-knee. Why this should occur is not clear, but there is sometimes an impression that it develops from rotation of the legs to try and minimize rubbing together grossly obese thighs. Tibia vara [95] is also a problem in some obese. Here inhibition of growth of the medial tibial epiphysis leads to discrepant growth in the tibia and gradual bowing of the legs. Possibly this begins from abnormal pressures on the tibial growth plate. Discomfort from these deformities is uncommon, but many obese children do have difficult and ungainly running.

Slipped capital femoral epiphysis occasionally occurs in adolescence. This can easily be dismissed as insignificant aches and pains (possibly referred to the knees) in an obese child. The problem may be bilateral. Treatment to contain the slipping is needed. If children require bed rest in association with correction, it is important that they are given a suitable diet, since inactivity is otherwise likely to exacerbate their obesity.

INSULIN AND GLUCOSE TOLERANCE

All obese children have hyperinsulinaemia. The relation of glucose tolerance to the degree of hyperinsulinaemia is very variable. Hyperinsulinaemia is more marked in girls, older children and those with obesity of prolonged duration, but is unrelated to adipose cell size [96,97]. Hyperinsulinaemia is due to peripheral resistance to uptake of glucose, sometimes made worse by a high-carbohydrate diet. Voluntary overfeeding induces hyperinsulinaemia in adults and this resolves when normal diets are resumed. In obese children plasma insulin levels fall with low-energy diets. Overt insulin-resistant diabetes mellitus is not very common in our experience. However, 40% of children studied by Drash [92] had chemical diabetes mellitus. The risk of developing diabetes mellitus increases with age and increasing obesity. It is not clear to what extent a family history of diabetes influences glucose intolerance in obesity. It seems wise to recommend slimming to those overweight with a family history of non-insulin-dependent diabetes mellitus. The hyperinsulinaemia of obesity is frequently associated with the polycystic ovarian syndrome.

LIPIDS

Serum cholesterol and fasting triglycerides are generally within normal limits in obese children, although a higher proportion of children than expected have total cholesterol mildly above the normal range. High-density lipoprotein (HDL) cholesterol may be low, and low-density lipoprotein (LDL) cholesterol elevated. Fasting triglyceride levels may be higher than normal as a result of increased hepatic production together with decreased uptake by non-adipose tissues. Uptake of triglycerides by adipose tissue is increased [98]. Fasting non-esterified fatty acids are also frequently elevated in obese children. The fall following a glucose load is less than in normal children even when glucose tolerance is retained. This effect seems unrelated to the degree of obesity or fat cell size. Exercise has a beneficial effect by increasing the HDL/LDL cholesterol ratio, possibly independent of any weight loss [99,100]. Court & Dunlop [90] found normal fasting glycerol, triglyceride and fasting free fatty acid change (a measure of the variability of free fatty acid levels) in children obese since infancy, but abnormal values for these lipids in children developing obesity after infancy.

STEROIDS

Excretions of metabolites of cortisol and corticosterone are increased in obese children [101]. Results are normal when related to body weight, although not when related to surface area. Increased cortisol excretion may be a function of increased body weight. Alternatively, high energy intakes in obese children may potentiate liver metabolism of cortisol. Normal or low plasma cortisol with shortened cortisol half-life in obese children could then be explained by an increased turnover of cortisol. There is some evidence suggesting that increased turnover of free triiodothyronine (T_3) stimulates cortisol metabolism in obese adult women [102]. However, in many obese children, cortisol levels are above expected. Usually these levels show normal diurnal rhythm with falls late in the day. If there is concern about underlying Cushing syndrome, a dexamethasone suppression test should show normal suppression. Mantero *et al.* [103] found cortisol secretion rate and urinary free cortisol the most helpful investigations for distinguishing Cushing syndrome from simple obesity.

Adipose tissue is important in the aromatization of oestrogens. Obesity may therefore have some bearing on the development of the steroidal abnormalities in polycystic ovarian syndrome where there is obesity, amenorrhoea and hirsutism [104,105].

GROWTH HORMONE

Growth hormone (GH) output in response to hypoglycaemia, exercise, sleep and arginine tolerance testing is diminished in obese children [106]. Administration of GH stimulates lipolysis but the results are not long-lasting [107]. Binet *et al.* [108] found serum somatomedin activity of obese children not significantly different from that of a control group. They found no correlation between serum somatomedin activity and GH response or between this and deviation of height from the mean. Loche *et al.* [109], in contrast, found plasma somatomedin C levels significantly higher in obese children than in non-obese controls. GH responses to GH-releasing hormone (GHRH) were low compared with non-obese controls. Non-esterified fatty acids and insulin levels were higher in the obese but did not relate to the GH response. These authors felt there was feedback inhibition of the GH response operated by the elevated levels of somatomedin C. Obesity in childhood thus presents a conundrum. GH output seems subnormal, yet the children have above-average stature and excellent growth velocity.

THYROID FUNCTION

Serum thyroxine levels are usually normal in simple obesity. However, the response to increased body weight may be a relative increase in thyroid hormone production in order to sustain normal thyroid function despite increased body mass [110]. Thyroid-stimulating hormone responses in obese adults are greater than for non-obese following thyroid-releasing hormone stimulation [111]. Some adult studies suggest serum T_3 levels correlate with carbohydrate and total energy intakes. Fasting falls in T_3, for example, are reversed by oral but not by intravenous glucose, suggesting control through gastroenterological factors [110].

WORKING CAPACITY AND THE EFFECTS OF EXERCISE

The decreased activity of many obese children may be partly related to the increased energy cost of activity due to extra weight. Physically fit normal-weight individuals show a rapid rise in serum cortisol and glucose, and a lowering of plasma insulin levels with exercise. Training lowers plasma insulin and seems to lessen the exercise required to mobilize glucose reserves. The inability of the unfit obese child to mobilize reserves means, presumably, that energy is conserved during activity. A meaningful and permanent reduction in body weight is likely to be achieved only if the obese are retrained sufficiently to mobilize energy reserves rapidly in response to stress and activity. If fitness is defined from maximum oxygen uptake (Vo_2 max) with exertion, obese adolescents have reduced maximum exercise capacity Vo_2 max when compared with that expected for height and age. We found respiratory minute volume did not increase in relation to mean oxygen uptake as much as expected. Thoracic or abdominal fat may reduce expiratory reserve volume and the normal ventilatory response to aerobic metabolism, although data on this are conflicting [112,113].

Sasaki *et al.* [99] found HDL cholesterol increased and triglycerides decreased slightly in obese children after 1 year's regular aerobic exercise without dietary advice. There was weight reduction and it is not clear whether improved fitness or reduced weight was responsible for the changed lipid levels. Exercise could benefit obese children independent of fat loss if improved fitness led to improved self-esteem.

HYPERTENSION AND CARDIOVASCULAR PROBLEMS

When taking blood pressures in obese children correct procedures should be followed or falsely high levels are likely [114]. The inflatable cuff of the sphygmomanometer should encircle the arm. The depth of the cuff should be two-thirds the length of the upper arm. It may be necessary to use a folded leg cuff on the arm of the larger adolescent obese in order to encircle the arm with inflatable cuff.

Hypertension is not very common in childhood obesity although distribution of blood pressure is shifted upwards within the normal range [94]. Obesity-associated hypertension forms a significant proportion of all hypertension in childhood. Hypertensive obese children had higher serum insulin levels than normotensive obese, but blood pressure did not correlate with WHR.

Clinical signs of cardiac disease are unusual, but grossly obese children may show an increased cardiac diameter on chest X-ray, and cardiac wall thickening is not unusual on ultrasound in more severely affected children. Obesity increases the circulatory blood volume and thus the afterload on the heart [115], so cardiac enlargement is not unexpected.

PICKWICK SYNDROME

Gross obesity can lead to severe respiratory inadequacy with somnolence, hypercapnia, hypoxia and congestive cardiac failure secondary to pulmonary hypertension [116]. Ventilatory response to carbon dioxide is decreased in obese children in proportion to their excess weight. This seems to be due to the thickness of the chest wall and abdominal girth as much as due to primary hyposensitivity of the respiratory centres [117]. Respiratory drive becomes determined by hypoxia rather than hypercapnia. Weight reduction, as well as treatment of congestive cardiac failure, is urgent. Oxygen must be used very cautiously, if at all, with close monitoring of arterial oxygen levels.

PSYCHIATRIC DISTURBANCE

Significantly disturbed obese children are relatively uncommon. Some children use eating as a manipulative weapon or as a substitute for parental love. Some become reclusive and solitary as a result of teasing over their obesity. Wilkinson *et al.* [118] found no difference in intelligence or personality score between obese and non-obese 10-year-olds matched for social class. Using a Rutter behaviour inventory obese girls had a higher total score, suggesting that they had more behaviour disturbance of a non-specific kind than did non-obese girls. Obese and non-obese boys showed no such difference.

Borjeson [119] found moderate degrees of obesity were not a cause of low popularity rating among classmates except when choosing companions for physical activities such as cross-country running!

Some obese children may try to set themselves over-ambitious and unattainable goals. They compensate for failure to achieve their aims by overeating so that at least they are bigger and more special than their peers [120]. Perhaps this is true of a few obese children but many develop poor body images for themselves in adolescence, having previously seemed unconcerned about their appearance.

Where there does seem psychological difficulty underlying obesity, it is important to determine the functional significance of obesity to the child's whole development. It is our impression that psychological problems commonly antedate obesity associated with psychological disturbance. Children and their families use the obesity to excuse lack of friends, poor school performance and low achievement. Low achievement may have been present before obesity was apparent, with lack of friends and self-pity contributing to, rather than causing, obesity. Low persistence, low tolerance of discomfort, and frequently reluctance to be independent and to do things for themselves, seem to characterize many obese children.

The process of successful slimming may improve children's self-esteem and change previously introverted children into more confident outgoing personalities, who achieve better at school. For some the process of dieting uncovers, or exaggerates, personality disorder. Preadolescent boys particularly may become aggressive and deceitful over dieting. Adolescents also may become uncooperative and quite unpleasant with their parents over attempts to help them diet, but children of this age group are so independent that they are more likely to be openly uncooperative anyway. Disruptive behaviour is most likely when children have inadequate help over dieting and yet are blamed by their parents and siblings for not cooperating with a slimming regime. Often they are the children with obese parents who themselves make no attempts to slim. Under these circumstances the prognosis for slimming is poor, and there is little sense in pursuing slimming regimes with children who have no wish to cooperate.

PATHOLOGICAL OBESITY

In the author's experience of a hospital-based obesity clinic accepting referrals from both hospital and community, fewer than one in ten referrals from hospital and community have pathological obesity. In these cases by far the commonest recognized pathology was mild to moderate mental retardation. Perhaps our clinic was biased, since a study of non-institutionalized mentally retarded children showed no increase in adiposity when compared with a non-institutionalized group of non-mentally retarded children of the same age [121].

It is important to distinguish those children with pathology underlying their obesity, so they can be investigated and managed appropriately. Table 13.5 lists the main causes of pathological obesity. It will be apparent from the list that clinical features such as short stature, low intelligence and dysmorphic features raise the possibility of pathological obesity, and further investigation should be considered.

Table 13.5 Some causes of pathological obesity in childhood

Congenital	
Chromosomal defects	Down syndrome, Klinefelter sydrome, Prader–Willi syndrome
Genetic defect	Laurence – Moon syndrome, growth problems: achondroplasia, some GH deficiency, etc.
Acquired	
Endocrine problems	Hypothyroidism, growth hormone deficiency, Cushing syndrome
'Hypothalamic' damage	Craniopharyngioma, pseudohypoparathyroidism, cerebral trauma, postencephalitis
Immobility	Spina bifida
Poor linear growth	Skeletal causes
Drugs	Corticosteroids, antithyroid drugs, sodium valproate

These categories are not self-limiting – conditions overlap.

Endocrine problems

HYPOTHYROIDISM

Energy requirements for basal metabolism, growth and activity are low in hypothyroidism. Energy intake readily exceeds energy expenditure, and low levels of thyroid hormone encourage fat deposition. Gross obesity is fairly rare. Most affected children are short and only moderately overweight for height. Some of the plump features of hypothyroidism are due to deposition of myxoedematous tissue, not fat. Fluid mobilization from this tissue produces dramatic initial loss of weight when thyroid treatment begins.

GROWTH HORMONE DEFICIENCY

Infants or toddlers with GH deficiency may be quite thin, but older children usually show some increase in fat, particularly around the trunk, suggesting centrally distributed fat cells may be more sensitive to GH-stimulated lipolysis than elsewhere in the body. Adipose cell numbers are below the mean for age, although cell size and lipid content of the cells are increased. Treatment with GH produces multiplication or recruitment of adipose cells, but diminution of cell size and skinfold thickness [107]. Loss of adipose tissue is one of the first detectable responses to GH treatment in deficient children [122]. There is rapid reduction in limb fat in the first month of treatment and little change thereafter. Fat is also redistributed with decrease in size of abdominal adipose cells and no change in more peripherally distributed adipose cells. GH appears to promote site-specific changes in tissue responses to insulin-induced antilipolysis. GH treatment is also associated with a fall in the previously elevated unsaturated fatty acid fraction of serum lipids.

GH is important in mediating hepatic LDL receptor expression. Increase in receptors will accelerate elimination of LDL particles and lower plasma LDL cholesterol [123].

CUSHING SYNDROME

Obesity, although frequently only mild, is characteristic of Cushing syndrome. Usually short stature and the typical truncal deposition of fat distinguish this condition from simple obesity. Confusion may occasionally occur between these children and relatively short pubertal children with simple obesity, particularly when the latter develop the pale pink striae of rapid fat accretion. Plasma corticosteroids tend to be increased in simple obesity, making differentiation from Cushing syndrome difficult, although in simple obesity corticosteroids should show normal diurnal variation and suppression with dexamethasone.

Explanation of obesity in Cushing syndrome is complicated [124]. Glucocorticoids inhibit glucose uptake in adipose tissue and promote lipolysis through enhancing the effect of catecholamines and GH on adipose tissue. Adrenocorticotrophin (ACTH) also has a direct fat-mobilizing effect unrelated to its effect on glucocorticoid production. These direct effects of glucocorticoids and ACTH are lipolytic and antilipogenic; yet clinically corticosteroids cause obesity. The explanation for this seems to be that glucocorticoids induce gluconeogenesis which stimulates insulin secretion and fat deposition. High levels of steroids due to extrapituitary causes also depress ACTH production. The direct effects of glucocorticoid excess on adipose tissue appear to be overridden by these indirect effects of enhanced lipogenesis and inhibition of lipolysis secondary to high levels of circulating insulin. When steroids are used therapeutically the sense of well-being they induce enhances appetite and further encourages fat deposition.

As in GH deficiency, the characteristic truncal distribution of obesity in Cushing syndrome may be due to variations in the response to hormones by adipose tissue at different sites. Glucocorticoid administration to rodents causes deposition of more brown than white fat. Perhaps in humans the adipose tissue of the trunk and face is particularly susceptible to hyperinsulinaemia, and that of the limbs more susceptibile to the direct effect of glucocorticoids and ACTH.

CRANIOPHARYNGIOMA

The child with craniopharyngioma may be obese for a variety of reasons. Unfortunately obesity often increases with treatment. Hypothalamic or pituitary damage may cause deficiency of growth hormone or thyroid-stimulating hormone (TSH). Irradiation of the lesions or spread of the tumour may destroy hypothalamic centres associated with appetite and weight control. Poor vision limits activity. Blindness and the poor prognosis may encourage friends and relatives to indulge affected children with sweets and other unnecessary food.

HYPOTHALAMIC SYNDROMES

Large bilateral lesions in the ventromedial hypothalamus of experimental animals lead to a characteristic syndrome of voracious appetite and obesity provided food is easily available, but the searching instinct is reduced if food is not easily available. Lesions in the lateral hypothalamus cause refusal to feed, and death from starvation. A feeding centre in the lateral hypothalamus and a satiety centre in the ventromedial hypothalamus have been postulated to explain these results.

In humans, obesity, which may or may not be associated with hyperphagia, can occur in association with brain damage from cerebral tumours, meningitis, encephalitis or other severe brain trauma. In these conditions obesity may develop without detectable hormone abnormality.

Eponymous hypothalamic syndromes

'FROHLICH SYNDROME'

As clinical descriptions gradually acquire pathophysiological bases, definitions change and some diseases even disappear, in name at least. Frohlich described a boy with a cyst in the region of the sella turcica with blindness, short stature, obesity and pubertal failure. The syndrome should therefore refer to this group of signs alone. Referrals as Frohlich syndrome never, in our experience, fulfil these criteria. Most relate to boys with simple obesity and pubertal delay in whom the contrast between immature genitalia and overall large size suggests, incorrectly, hypogonadism. In our view the term Frohlich syndrome is best avoided.

LAURENCE-MOON-BIEDL SYNDROME

In 1865 Laurence and Moon desribed a syndrome complex of mental retardation, obesity, retinitis pigmentosa polydactyly and genital hypoplasia. Other features described since in association with this syndrome include renal abnormalities, diabetes insipidus, strabismus, clinodactyly of the fifth finger and moderately short stature. Perhaps one-quarter of described cases show the full pentad, and the wide variety of clinical manifestations have led to attempts to separate groups of signs into Laurence–Moon–Biedl and other syndromes. This does not advance understanding or diagnosis. Moreover, subdivision of the syndrome may overlook the possibility that the condition is inherited through one autosomal gene with pleiotropic effect and variable expression. Certainly the condition usually follows an autosomal recessive pattern of inheritance. Polydactyly is the only manifestation of the pentad recognizable at birth, and is the least common of the five cardinal signs [125].

Obesity in Laurence–Moon syndrome does not present until after infancy. Most affected children show marked obesity by the age of 4 years. Previously modest obesity often becomes gross in adolescence when the growth spurt is poor or absent. Short stature is a common feature that may be apparent from early childhood, but becomes more noticeable in adolescence. Hypogonadism and pubertal failure are secondary to pituitary gonadotrophin deficiency. Both Laurence–Moon and Prader–Willi syndromes (see below) may have congenital cerebral abnormalities involving the hypothalamus as primary defects, but pathological studies have so far failed to show any consistent histological or biochemical abnormalities in the brain. Developments in molecular biology may change this.

PRADER–WILLI SYNDROME

This is the commonest pathological obesity syndrome presenting at paediatric obesity or endocrine clinics. For many years its aetiology was unknown, although an association with mothers who were relatively elderly at the time of the children's births suggested similarities with Down syndrome and a possible chromosomal abnormality. About 50% of children with Prader–Willi syndrome have a 15q11–13 deletion on chromosome 15 [126]. Deletion is always on the paternally derived section of the chromosome. Recently it has been shown that Prader–Willi syndrome can be an example of uniparental disomy, where parts of both arms of one of a pair of chromosomes are derived from the same parent. In Prader–Willi syndrome both sections of chromosome 15, when uniparental disomy is present, are derived from the mother. A very different syndrome – Angelman syndrome – characterized by failure to thrive and thinness, although also with mental retardation, has very similar uniparental disomy for chromosome 15, but in this condition the existing sections of the chromosome have a paternal origin [126]. Uniparental disomy accounts for almost all the children presenting with definite Prader–Willi syndrome who do not have deletions on chromosome 15. Recognition of the chromosomal abnormalities in this syndrome gives hope that a biochemical explanation for the problem, and even genetic therapy, will ultimately be forthcoming.

Table 13.6 lists the main clinical features. Birth weight is normal or low. Hypotonia is marked at birth and may result in infants being considered less mature than estimated from mothers' dates. Feeding difficulties and characteristic facies make the syndrome recognizable at birth, although with difficulty for those unfamiliar with the facies. Failure to thrive is a common early presentation.

Obesity develops usually in the second year of life and is most marked around thighs, buttocks, abdomen and shoulders. Appetite may be enormous and undescriminating [127]. Children may develop curious habits in order to obtain food. They stay up late or get up early in order to raid biscuit tins or refrigerators. They steal from shops or complain to neighbours that their parents do not feed them. Even those children without excessive appetite gain weight rapidly. Energy requirements are low because activity levels are low and growth rates slow. Holm & Pipes [128] studied energy balance in children with Prader–Willi syndrome and found mean resting energy requirements for expected normal growth velocity were below the 10th centile for age. Others have not found significantly lower resting energy requirements.

Table 13.6 Clinical features of Prader–Willi syndrome

Facial	Narrow forehead, olive-shaped eyes, antimongoloid slant, epicanthus, strabismus, carp mouth, micrognathia, abnormal ear lobes
Skeletal	Small hands and feet, tapering fingers, flat ulnar border to hand, clinodactyly, syndactyly, scoliosis, congenital dislocation of hips, retarded bone age
Neuromuscular	IQ 40–70, hypotonia in infancy, feeding difficulties in infancy and failure to thrive, normal EMG and motor conduction velocity in muscle, insatiable appetite, uncontrollable rage
Endocrine	Hypogonadism: micropenis, hypoplastic scrotum, bilateral cryptorchidism; poor secondary sexual development; delayed menarche; normal or increased gonadotrophins; gross obesity; insulin-resistant diabetes mellitus

The short stature of Prader–Willi syndrome, as with Laurence–Moon syndrome, is not necessarily very marked until puberty, when the absence of a normal pubertal growth spurt makes these children noticeably short. Adult height is usually below the third centile. In boys cryptorchidism and poorly developed genitalia are expected. In girls menarche may or may not be delayed. Pituitary gonadotrophin secretion is variable, but hormonal studies show no consistent difference from those of children with simple obesity.

Eventual intelligence quotient (IQ) in these children is between 40 and 70 in the majority of cases. The early hypotonia may cause a lot of concern. Slow motor development and the severity of the mental retardation are often overlooked until early childhood. Extrovert cheerfulness or garrulous personality may disguise the low IQ, but a more typical affect is much more negative. The children can be aggressive, vicious and bad-tempered, particularly when food intake is restricted. Battles over dieting, together with the distress at the prognosis for the child, place great strain on families. Parents may respond to advice about management and prognosis by despair over the apparent impossibility of controlling their child, and may fail to exert any dietary discipline. This is unfortunate because not all children have uncontrollable appetites and occasional children are kept within normal weight for height through wise dietetic management.

Children with Prader–Willi syndrome are depressing to treat. They have low energy requirements for their height and age either because of low basal metabolism or because of slow growth, apathy and indolence. Energy intakes must be strictly controlled if obesity is to be prevented, but children are unable to understand the need for dietary control. Holm & Pipes [128] estimated these children only required daily energy intakes of 7–8 kcal (28–33 kJ) per centimetre of height to maintain growth in height and normal increments in weight. Once obesity develops the progress may be inexorable despite vigorous efforts to control intakes.

Ultimately severe obesity in Prader–Willi syndrome lead to complications such as genu valgum, intertrigo, cellulitis precipitated by postural oedema and self-mutiliation. Non-insulin-dependent diabetes mellitus and Pickwick syndrome may occur in adolescence or early adult life. Death from septicaemia, bronchopneumonia, the complications of diabetes or cor pulmonale is common around the age of 30 [129].

OBESITY ASSOCIATED WITH PHYSICAL AND MENTAL HANDICAP

Any condition which leads to reduction in energy requirements for growth and/or activity has the potential for encouraging the development of obesity. Since growth utilizes only a small proportion of total energy after the first few months of life, children with skeletal causes for short stature are quite frequently overweight, but not often grossly obese. In contrast, children with some specific forms of mental retardation seem at particular risk of obesity, although not all studies show this. In Down syndrome and Klinefelter syndrome there may be a genetic or metabolic component to the development of obesity. In other mentally handicapped children obesity may develop from disorganized eating due to lack of self-discipline and 'spoiling' from parents and friends who indulge the children from misguided kindness. Apathy and lack of peer friendships may contribute to children becoming sedentary and reclusive.

Activity forms a high proportion of the non-basal energy requirements of normal children. Some physically handicapped children will use little energy in activity, and if they eat for their age rather than their needs they may become obese. Guy [130] found 69% of physically handicapped schoolchildren were overweight for height. When grouped according to cause of the handicap, 100% of the children with spina bifida and 30% of the children with muscular dystrophy were overweight. Virtually all handicapped children ate between meals.

Increasing the activity of the physically handicapped is difficult. Some children give up making efforts to mobilize themselves. Spina bifida children who have been taught to walk with calipers may decide it is easier to lead wheelchair existences than struggle with calipers and discomfort. Energy expenditure in activity drops. Children with muscular dystrophy are now kept mobile for longer, through a variety of aids, and these increase interest, morale and energy expenditure in activity, thus helping control the tendency to develop obesity shown by some.

Increasing activity is unlikely to have major effects on energy expenditure, and dietary control is almost always necessary in handicapped children who are becoming obese. In conditions where there is well-recognized risk, dietary advice should be given from the time of recognition of the syndrome and progress monitored. One of the main aims of diets in younger children may be to give normal balanced and organized diets. Handicapped children, perhaps because of early feeding difficulties, often have faddy appetites. Parental concerns may have allowed disorganized eating. Children who will not eat vegetables or fruit, and who tend to exist on diets of snack foods, are extremely difficult to slim successfully.

MANAGEMENT OF THE OBESE CHILD

Management of obesity includes deciding whether children should be investigated for underlying pathology, and whether slimming should be attempted or not. If slimming is not attempted, it is wise at least to curb further fattening. For some children help in coping with their obesity may be more useful than further futile attempts at slimming.

We routinely examine all children referred for possible complications of obesity, paying particular attention to blood pressure, cardiorespiratory and neurological signs and orthopaedic problems. Children who are short and fat, have low intelligence or who have physical abnormalities or dysmorphism should be checked for underlying pathology causing obesity. Children who appear to be cases of simple obesity but who have symptoms or signs suggestive of complications – for example hypertension, breathlessness, abnormal somnolence or glycosuria – deserve cardiovascular and respiratory investigation, evaluation of glucose tolerance and determination of lipid profile. It is our practice to check lipid profile, random blood glucose, plasma cortisol and thyroid function tests in all grossly obese children with apparently simple obesity – if they consent to the investigations. However, we rarely find abnormality except slightly raised total cholesterol levels (separation into HDL and LDL cholesterol is not routine).

Who should be slimmed?

INFANTS

Young infants are naturally fat, sometimes very fat, and they tend to slim spontaneously as they change to mixed diets and develop weight-bearing activities. It is probably inappropriate in most cases to advise any slimming regimen, although it is important to check that feeding practices are appropriate to infants' needs. Parents should be advised on weaning practices which do not encourage obesity and on giving young children space and opportunity to be active safely.

If there is parental obesity a fat infant is more worrying. Infants' weight for length progress should be monitored closely, and parents should be advised on weaning practices which do not encourage overfeeding. Adding sugars and fats to foods should be avoided. Low-energy margarines may be more suitable than butter. Snacks should be limited in number, so obese weanlings are fed three or four times a day with two small snacks. Sweets, chocolate, biscuits, crisps and chips should be discouraged. As infants move on to solid foods milk intakes should be reduced to around 500 ml/day.

It is often queried whetther infants and young children who are overfat should be fed skimmed or semiskimmed milk. Recommendations in the UK are that infants who are not breast-fed are fed infant formulas until the age of 1 year [131]. We support that recommendation. Skimmed milk should be fed only to children over the age of 5 years, and semiskimmed milk fed to children over 2 years if they are receiving a 'balanced' diet. However, when milk is still a major part of the nutrient intake, reducing the amount of fat in the milk can be a useful way of reducing energy intakes without reducing the volumes of food consumed. Skimmed milk has approximately half the energy content of whole milk, and semiskimmed milk approximately two-thirds the energy content. These milks lack the fat-soluble vitamins A and D, and are low in polyunsaturated fatty acids.

Use of low-energy milks in young children must be accompanied by vitamin supplements (children's vitamin drops: vitamin A 214 μg; vitamin C 21 mg; vitamin D 7 μg). Growth in length should be closely monitored. It may be wise to introduce low-energy versions of yoghurt, cheese and margarine before reducing the fat in milk itself. If these and other dietary interventions do not control fattening, introducing low-energy milks can then be tried.

Increasing the fibre content of the diet reduces energy density of foods and may be helpful with slimming regimens. Fibre can be provided through fresh fruits and vegetables puréed, and these should be encouraged. High-fibre cereals may inhibit absorption of some important nutrients such as iron.

The aims of slimming in the first few years of life should be to control weight gain and fatness gain rather than to induce weight loss. Normal infant weight gain velocity is so rapid that restriction sufficient to induce weight loss may risk essential nutrient deficiency or restriction of linear growth. Increasing activity may be accomplished by providing play areas or playpens in which infants can practise weight-bearing activities. Baby walkers and similar apparatus should be discouraged.

Management of older children with obesity

It is often said that the outlook for the obese is so poor that it is not worth trying to control obesity; this is probably unjustified. Children presenting for medical help for their obesity have often tried dieting and failed, either due to lack of compliance or because the regimen was not strict enough. Following other children's growth suggests that many children slip in and out of obesity during periods of childhood without obvious intervention, or with only slight modification of activity or diet. Children with persistent obesity thus seem likely to be those with a great propensity to obesity, excessively adipogenic habits, or lack of self-control.

One of the problems with the treatment of obesity is that total cure is often considered the only desirable end-point. Many conditions in paediatrics are managed by palliative control rather than cure (for example diabetes mellitus). If the obese can reduce their fatness, even if not return to totally normal fatness, they may have improved morale, greater ease with daily life, and improved long-term outlook in terms of minimizing later complications. Thus to try to control fatness, or to reduce fatness, should be as much the aim of the management of obesity as total cure.

It has been suggested that it is dangerous to slim obese schoolchildren and adolescents because of the danger of inducing anorexia nervosa, and the real and immediate risks to mortality of that condition. It is our experience that obese children themselves do not seem to have the personality, physiology or perhaps persistence, to progress to anorexia nervosa. However, there is a risk that their schoolmates, watching their dieting, may be inspired to slim when they have no need to do so, and become anorexic. It is therefore important that children who are advised on slimming are children who have significant excess fat, not just children who perceive a need to be slimmer. Advice should be for energy-reduced but balanced diets with proper meals and regulated snacks, and crash dieting should be deplored. Slimming advice should be accompanied by general nutritional eduction.

Emphasis should be on the development of healthy lifestyles rather than on weight loss.

Our policy is to advise all those who are overfat and who request help; but we are more concerned with changes in lifestyles that should reduce the risks of morbidity later and may, in the long run, lead to gradual control of weight, than with rapid return to normal weight and fatness. It is also important that the children who are obese develop more positive affects so that, even if obesity remains, they are not psychologically handicapped by their size.

Motivation

This is perhaps the most important but most difficult aspect in the management of obesity. Possibly lack of drive is so inherent to obesity that these children cannot see that the solution to their problem is in themselves and their lifestyle. Some children respond well to frank explanation about the difficulties, the likely achievements and the slow progress with slimming. Other children want to slim in a fortnight and are not prepared to struggle over a long period of time. Where actual loss of fat and weight loss is the aim, around 500 g/week weight loss is the maximum that should be expected after the first week (when loss of glycogen stores results in shifts of body water and sometimes higher losses). It is not unusual for obese children to be 15–20 kg heavier than expected from growth centiles. Loss of this excess weight will take 6 months even if progress is steady and maintained. Usually there are falters in the slimming process and slimming takes longer. As children grow, expected weight for age increases, so weight excess diminishes.

General principles for slimming obese children

DIET

1 Find out the normal dietary pattern and intake of the child.
2 Confine eating to mealtimes and regulated snack times.
3 Encourage family meals at a table and spend time in socialization.
4 Avoid fried foods and added fats and sugars.
5 Encourage wholemeal cereals, whole fruits and vegetables.
6 Limit intake of bread, and advise a staple such as potatoes, rice or pasta only once a day.
7 Aviod carbonated drinks, even if low-energy versions, as their sweet taste can encourage a craving for sweetness.
8 Use low-energy margarines, yoghurts, cheeses, soups and fruit squashes (encourage water rather than flavoured drinks if possible).
9 Avoid food rewards.
10 Avoid chewing gum as, even if low energy density, it encourages children to be always chewing.
11 Modify school dinners. It may appear less interfering and discriminating if the child is allowed to eat a normal school dinner and kept on a strict diet at home. It is much easier to diet children when they are at school. At home food is easily available and can be used to combat boredom. At school minds are occupied most of the day, and food is available only at lunch and break times. School dinners tend to be very rich in fat and other energy. Recommendations should be that the child either eats a salad without salad dressing, or potatoes or bread followed by fresh fruit, low-energy yoghurt, or no pudding; or has meat (no pastry), no potatoes but a good helping of vegetables with the same 'sweet' course. If neither of these is possible, parents can send the child to school with a box of salad with cold meat, chicken, cheese or hard-boiled egg and fresh fruit. If it is felt necessary to provide something hot, a flask of low-energy soup can be added.

ACTIVITY

1 Encourage walking rather than taking buses and cars. Get up early enough to walk to school if possible.
2 Encourage participation in sport even if obesity makes the child self-conscious. Non-participation only increases the sense of isolation.
3 Encourage teachers to be supportive rather than derogatory of obese children's participation in physical activity.
4 Encourage activities outside school hours, both formal and around the home. Children should be encouraged to fetch and carry and help with the housework, and to do things for themselves rather than expect to be 'waited on' by parents.
5 Limit television viewing.
6 Encourage interests and hobbies, active or less active, so boredom is diminished.
7 Encourage positive interest in health and fitness through school health education programmes.

Activity not only increases energy consumption in the obese, but also improves insulin sensitivity and increases the HPL/LPL cholesterol ratio. It may therefore benefit individuals even without loss of fat. Theoretically, very vigorous activity could increase muscle bulk, resulting in loss of fat but no loss of weight.

DRUGS

The author does not recommend the use of drugs in the management of childhood obesity. The effect of most of these drugs on fatness is questionable. Many induce nausea, with the result that those who might benefit most refuse to take the drugs. Those who persist with drugs and lose weight seem to be those who have the persistence to lose weight equally well without the drugs. Several of the drugs which have been used are liable to induce addiction, and this is undesirable.

D-Fenfluramine is probably the drug of choice if it is felt appropriate to try drug therapy in adolescent obese patients. The effects of fenfluramine on growth and GH production have been questioned [132] and for this reason it may be advisable to restrict use for children who have more or less completed their growth. Courses should be short, and limited to only a few weeks.

SURGERY

The enthusiasm for treating obese children with surgical techniques has diminished. Jejunoileal bypass has too many complications to be recommended for adolescents and children. Gastric plication, effective in reducing stomach capacity, may be very rarely suitable in adolescence, but it would seem more appropriate to leave this sort of intervention until children have matured and have had opportunities to attempt more traditional slimming, independent of their parents. Jaw wiring has been used in obese adolescents but is a very interfering procedure and most children (and probably most adults) have difficulty coping with a lifestyle which prevents all except fluid diet. It is very difficult to maintain dental hygiene.

Children for whom any surgical procedure is planned should have formal psychiatric assessment beforehand. Most obese children with behaviour disturbances will not have their behaviour improved by radical measures to control their obesity. They are likely to be intolerant of the effects of the procedures. If the intervention is for a limited period, such as the case with jaw wiring, any weight loss is likely to be restored rapidly once the intervention ceases. Currently there are no criteria for delineating a group of children or adolescents who might benefit from these procedures.

Psychiatric management

Interest and encouragement from the clinical team are an important part of management of obesity. Frequent clinic visits help reinforce dietary and other advice, and provide evidence of progress. Support of this kind is the only psychological support needed by most obese children. Severely disturbed children require more formal psychiatric assessment, but it is our experience that this rarely aids weight loss, although child and family may end up more balanced and able to cope with the obesity.

Group therapy is often seen as the approach for obese children. Summer camps may be quite successful in producing fat loss which is or is not retained, but the success is probably due to the strict regimen of camp life. Some children do benefit from commercial groups such as Weight Watchers but these tend to be the more mature adolescent girls. Younger children may be confused by these groups, since concepts of 'ideal' weight are often based on age rather than height for age and may thus be unnecessarily low. Target weights are unlikely to take account of the time taken for children to reach targets and the growth that takes place meanwhile. Stress on weight loss may also be inappropriate for rapidly growing children, since growth may cause static weights to hide considerable fat loss. Sooner or later children's weights are likely to increase from starting weights unless they are grossly above expected mature weight at presentation. Thus motivation may be achieved by these groups, but there is a risk of incorrect diagnosis and advice.

Group therapy for children led by child psychologists or paediatric dieticians, or even paediatricians, can be helpful, but is very dependent on the time and enthusiasm of leaders. Many groups seem successful at improving self-esteem among the children and their parents, but have little effect on the degree of obesity. Group activities which try to educate about nutrition, healthy lifestyles and cooking, and which encourage trying new foods and recipes, sports and general activity on the principle that these are 'fun', can have considerable success. The man/womanpower needed to organize and run such groups makes them expensive procedures.

Follow-up

However obese children are managed or advised there should be follow-up of their progress. Without this advisers cannot learn whether their advice is helpful, and children are left without obvious goals or endpoint. To be useful follow-up needs to be frequent, particularly initially. Children should be weighed and measured. They should be questioned about their diet and advice should be given where there are lapses. There should also be enquiries about physical activity. Every possible encouragement should be given to those who are trying, even if not very effectively, to slim. Those who clearly are making no effort should probably be advised to cease attendance. There is little point, when treating the enthusiastic is so difficult, in filling clinic spaces with those who use clinic attendance as a pretence that they are slimming.

Many children who attend obesity clinics attend only once or twice. This is particularly likely if they do not succeed in losing weight. Some stop coming when they have lost a couple of kilograms because they perceive themselves as having slimmed, although they may still be grossly overfat.

Most children who persist in attending do achieve some fat loss. In many this is most successful in spring and early summer, with lapses in autumn and winter. Second half of the year lapses are probably due to less activity with dark cold evenings (in the northern hemisphere) and a tendency to eat more energy-dense foods in colder weather. Christmas undoubtedly has a disastrous effect on most children's dieting. Whether the shortening days also lead to a change in human metabolism, which encourages fat deposition, has never been satisfactorily decided.

Long-term outlook

In the intermediate term some reduction in fat can be achieved in a high proportion of those who persist with slimming regimens. Sadly too few persist long and successfully enough to achieve normal fatness. Nuutinen & Knip [133] found, irrespective of the method of encouraging slimming used, a 2-year slimming programme resulted in 49% of children losing at least 10% relative weight. The majority of these children maintained relative weight loss 5 years from starting slimming.

Most children who are referred to obesity clinics do remain obese to a greater or lesser extent. Lloyd *et al.* [86], many years ago, found 75% of those attending a hospital-based obesity clinic were still obese in adult life. Persistence of obesity is most likely for girls past menarche. Boys, even in adolescence, may slim quite dramatically, particularly those with genetic predisposition to very tall stature.

Abraham *et al.* [134] found 60% of obese teenagers were still obese 40 years later, and 84% were at least moderately overweight; yet over a wider age range, skinfold thickness in childhood seems to provide only a poor degree of accuracy for predicting skinfold thickness in adult life. By contrast, Mossberg [85], reviewing overweight children (> +1 SDS (standard deviation score) weight for height) admitted to hospital for treatment of obesity 40 years before, found weight for height had deviated from the normal most at adolescence, but 47% of the individuals still had weight for height > +1 SDS in adulthood. Excessive overweight (> +3 SDS weight for height) at puberty was associated with greater than expected morbidity and mortality. The overall trend in weight for height over the years was towards normal and diminishing overweight for height.

What is not clear is how much childhood obesity contributes to the complications of obesity seen in adult life. Mossberg [85] found cardiovascular, neurological and gastrointestinal disease appeared at a younger age in the obese than in the population as a whole. Those with chronic diseases had mean weight for height +1.25 SDS compared with +0.5 SDS, suggesting adult weight for height may have been more important than childhood weight for height. In the study by Abrahams *et al.* [134] those developing the most severe hypertension were those who had been on the lowest weight for height centiles in adolescence and had become obese in adult life. It may be that the children who have been obese since infancy, and who have strong genetic predisposition to obesity, are less at risk than those suddenly becoming obese as they cease the activities of youth and take to eating 'business lunches'. The speed with which fat accumulates seems a likely risk factor for adverse prognosis.

PREVENTION

In view of the data presented at the beginning of this chapter the prevention of obesity is an urgent problem. Unfortunately there are no successful programmes for the prevention of obesity, and recommendations can be made only from an understanding of the factors which may have contributed to the epidemic of obesity today.

With a condition as prevalent as obesity in Western Europe, prevention probably needs to be directed at the whole population rather than to target specific groups. Although reducing the mean fatness of the whole populations would not return the very fat to normality, such an effort would probably have a greater impact on morbidity and mortality than simply trying to prevent gross obesity. Mild obesity may carry little health risk *per se* but – if associated with conditions such as hypertension, heart disease, diabetes mellitus, osteoarthritis or even pregnancy – it increases the risk of adverse outcome in these conditions.

It is important that preventive messages are free from harm to those who are not obese, as well as likely to benefit those with risk of obesity. Prevention should be directed towards developing healthy lifestyles. Children should be encouraged to be active and to be independent at levels appropriate to their age. Physical activity should be encouraged in schools, and local councils should make safe play areas for formal and informal activities available at no cost to users. There should be efforts directed towards reducing the dependency of so many children on television for their entertainment. Hobbies and interests, whether involving physical activity or not, should be encouraged so as to prevent the boredom that so often leads to eating. Television advertising (during hours when children are watching at least) should reduce the amount of advertising of novel foods, and particularly avoid emphasis on 'it's good for you'. Industry should be persuaded to divert some of the money it spends on television advertising of snack foods to supporting sporting activities and play areas. Are these proposals so unrealistic?

Ideally families should be encouraged to return to traditional eating practices with family meals and time taken eating. This may be difficult with modern lifestyles, fast foods and microwave oven availability; many people are no longer prepared to spend time in the kitchen preparing family meals from basic ingredients.

Those preparing meals should be encouraged to reduce the fat content of meals by avoiding frying and using more low-fat versions of foods. Sugar should not be added unnecessarily to foods. Whole fruit and vegetables should be encouraged from early childhood. Wholemeal cereals may also help slimming by inducing satiety more readily. Snacks should be infrequent and consist of relatively low-energy-density foods. Eating should be seen as an intermittent activity, not one which takes place whenever food is within reach.

One action that could be most rewarding in helping to prevent obesity is more widespread development of quality school lunches. If healthy foods in the form of fruit, vegetables and relatively low-fat meals could be served in environments that lead to relaxed eating and enjoyment from meals, children might be encouraged to follow healthier methods of eating. Good school meals need support from a nutrition education curriculum which encourages children to be adventurous in eating.

Prevention of obesity also requires supervision of children's growth, and action to help those who seem to be progressing towards obesity. Children whose weight is crossing centiles upwards unrelated to changes in linear growth centile seem likely to be getting undesirably fat. Too often they are told 'nothing can be done' or 'it's just puppy fat'. Dietary history and details of physical activity and lifestyle may indicate action which can be advised. Those responsible for school health should regard developing obesity as a concerning issue, although at the same time be discerning about the significance of obesity at different ages. Thus boys with delayed puberty who are putting on fat rapidly should be advised and watched closely, but may not require strict slimming regimens. Five-year-olds who are getting progressively fatter need close dietary supervision and encouragement to pursue high levels of activity.

One of the problems with the treatment of obesity seems to be the severity of obesity at presentation. Children who are 100 kg at the age of 13 may have an irreversible predisposition to become obese; but it is possible that, had they taken advice at an earlier stage in their obesity, control could have been achieved. Monitoring growth needs to be linked with active intervention when weight velocity is excessive. Only by trying to intervene with obesity at early stages will we discover what action is ultimately effective.

Prevention of obesity is not a medical issue. It is a social, economic and political issue. In order to effect necessary changes in school meals, sports facilities, food availability and costs, and self-esteem in at-risk groups, financial backing is needed. It is futile to make grandiose statements on targets for obesity reduction without considering what is needed to fund the facilities which will enable change for those locked into deprivation, depression and unhealthy lifestyles.

We now know much more about the nature of the excess in obesity, and about its associated risks and complications. Among adults it is possible to recognize high-risk and low-risk obesity. Yet, having recognized the problem, we are rarely able to specify why it occurred. Even less can we guarantee successful treatment. Where familial obesity is all too obvious our advice on prevention remains rudimentary. These are sad reflections for a condition which is in danger of affecting the majority of the population in the developed world.

REFERENCES

1 White A, Nicholaas G, Foster K, Browne F, Carey S. *Health Survey for England 1991*. London: HMSO, 1993.

2 Department of Health. *The Health of the Nation; a Strategy for Health in England*. London: HMSO, 1992.

3 Durnin JGVA, Lonergan ME, Good J, Ewan AA. Cross-sectional nutritional and anthropometric study with an interval of seven years on 611 young adolescent schoolchildren. *Br J Nutr* 1974;32:169–79.

4 Chinn S, Rona RT. Secular trends in weight, height, weight for height and triceps skinfold thickness in primary schoolchildren in England and Scotland from 1972 to 1980. *Ann Hum Biol* 1987;14:311–19.

5 Gortmaker SL, Dietz WH, Sobol AM, Wehler CA. Increasing pediatric obesity in the United States. *Am J Dis Child* 1992;141:535–40.

6 Ho JF, Yip WC, Tay JS, Rajan U. Social class distribution of obese Chinese children. *J Singapore Paediatr Soc* 1991;33: 55–8.

7 Mullins AG. The prognosis in juvenile obesity. *Arch Dis Child* 1958;33:307–14.

8 Gibson R. *The Principles of Nutritional Assessment*. Oxford: Oxford University Press, 1990:187–208.

9 Widdowson EM. Changes in body proportions and body composition during growth. In: Davis JA, Dobbing J, eds. *Scientific Foundations of Paediatrics*. London: Heinemann, 1974:153–63.

10 Fomon SJ. *Infant Nutrition*, 2nd edn. Philadelphia, PA: W.B. Saunders, 1974.

11 Poskitt EME, Cole TJ. Do fat babies stay fat? *Br Med J* 1977;1:7–9.

12 Forbes GB. Relation of lean body mass to height in children and adolescents. *Pediatr Res* 1972;6:32–7.

13 Amador M, Bacallao J, Hermelo M. Adiposity and growth: relationship of stature at fourteen years with relative body weight at different ages and several measurements of adiposity and body bulk. *Eur J Clin.Nutr* 1992;46:213–19.

14 Griffiths M, Payne PR. Energy expenditure in small children of obese and non-obese parents. *Nature* 1976;260:698–700.

15 Rauh JL, Schumsky DA. Lean and non-lean body mass estimates in urban schoolchildren. In: Cheek DB, ed. *Human Growth*. Philadelphia, PA: Lea & Febiger, 1968:242–52.

16 Lesser GT, Deutsch S, Makofsky J. Use of independent measurements of body fat to evaluate overweight and under-

weight. *Metabolism* 1974;20:792–804.

17 Tanner JM, Whitehouse RH. Standards for subcutaneous fat in British children. Percentiles for thickness of skinfolds over triceps and below scapula. *Br Med J* 1962;1:446–50.

18 Tanner JM, Whitehouse RA. Revised standards for triceps and subscapular skinfold in British children. *Arch Dis Child* 1975;50:142–5.

19 Taitz LS. Infantile overnutrition among artificially fed infants in the Sheffield region. *Br Med J* 1971;2:315–16.

20 Hutchinson-Smith B. The relationship between the weight of an infant and lower respiratory tract infection. *Med Off* 1970;123:257–62.

21 Shukla AP, Forsyth HA, Anderson CM, Marwah SM. Infantile overnutrition in the first year of life. A field study in Dudley, Worcestershire. *Br Med J* 1972;4:507–15.

22 Howard AN, Dub I, McMahon M. The incidence, cause and treatment of obesity in Leicester schoolchildren. *Practitioner* 1971;207:662–8.

23 Wilkinson PW, Pearlson J, Parkin JM, Philips PR, Sykes P. Obesity in childhood. A community study in Newcastle-upon-Tyne. *Lancet* 1977;1:350–2.

24 McLaughlin GP. Obesity in schoolchildren. *Med Off* 1969; 121:327–31.

25 Colley JRT. Obesity in schoolchildren. *Br J Prev Soc Med* 1974;28:221–5.

26 Terry RB, Page WF, Haskell WL. Waist–hip ratio, body mass index and premature cardiovascular disease mortality in US Army veterans during a twenty three year follow-up study. *Int J Obes* 1992;16:417–24.

27 Vague J. The degree of masculine differentiation of obesity: a factor determining predisposition to diabetes, gout and uric calculus disease. *Am J Clin Nutr* 1956;4:20–34.

28 Jakicic JM, Donnelly JE, Jawad AF, Jacobsen DJ, Gunderson SC, Pascale R. Association between blood lipids and different measurements of body fat distribution: effects of body mass index and age. *Int J Obes* 1993;17:131–7.

29 Bjorntorp P. 'Portal' adipose tissue as a generator of risk factors for cardiovascular disease and diabetes. *Arteriosclerosis* 1990;10:493–6.

30 Fox K, Peters D, Armstrong N, Sharpe P, Bell M. Abdominal fat deposition in 11-year-old children. *Int J Obes* 1993;17: 11–16.

31 Alexander HG, Dugdale AE. Fascial planes within subcutaneous fat in humans. *Eur J Clin Nutr* 1992;46:903–6.

32 Edwards DA, Hammond WH, Heely MJR, Tanner JM, Whitehouse RH. Design and accuracy of calipers for measuring subcutaneous fat thickness. *Br J Nutr* 1955;12:133–43.

33 Garrow JS. *Obesity and Related Diseases*. Edinburgh: Churchill-Livingstone, 1988.

34 Wolff OH. Obesity in childhood. *Q J Med* 1955;24:109–23.

35 Forbes GB, Lean body mass and fat in obese children. *Pediatries* 1964;34:308–14.

36 Quetelet LAJ. *Physique Sociale*, Vol. 2. Brussels: Muquardt, 92.

37 Cole TJ. A method for assessing age standardised weight for height in children seen cross sectionally. *Ann Hum Biol* 1979;7:457–73.

38 Rolland-Cachera M-F, Cole TJ, Sempe M, Tichet J, Rossignol C, Charraud A. Body mass index variations: centile from birth to 87 years. *Eur J Clin Nutr* 1991;45:13–21.

39 Frisancho AR. *Anthropometric Standards for the Assessment of Growth and Nutritional Status*. Ann Arbor, MI: University of Michigan Press, 1990.

40 Durnin JVGA, Rahaman MM. The assessment of the amount of fat in the human body from measurements of skinfold thickness. *Br J Nutr* 1967;21:681–9.

41 Brook CGD. Determination of body composition in children from skinfold measurements. *Arch Dis Child* 1971;48: 725–8.

42 Duerenberg P, van der Kooy K, Leenan R, Schouten FJM. Body impedance is largely dependent on the intra- and extra-cellular water distribution. *Eur J Clin Nutr* 1989;43: 845–53.

43 van der Kooy K, Seidell JC. Techniques for the measurement of visceral fat: a practical guide. *Int J Obes* 1993;17:187–96.

44 Widdowson EM, Shaw J. Full and empty fat cells. *Lancet* 1973;2:905.

45 Enzi G, Ingelman EM, Caretta F, Rubatelli F, Grella P, Barithussio A. Adipose tissue development *in utero*. *Diabetologia* 1980;18:135–40.

46 Knittle JL, Timmers K, Ginsberg-Fellner F, Brown RE, Katz DP. The growth of adipose tissue in children and adolescents. *J Clin Invest* 1979;63:239–46.

47 Bonnet FP. White and brown adipose tissue – main histological features and physiological role. In: Bonnet FP, ed. *Adipose Tissue in Childhood*. Boca Raton, FL: CRC Press, 1981:1–8.

48 Vague J. The degree of masculine differentiation of obesity: a factor determining predisposition to diabetes, gout, and uric calculus disease. *Am J Clin Nutr* 1956;4:20–34.

49 Ashwell M, Chinn S, Garrow JS. Female fat distribution – a simple classification based on two circumference measurements. *Int J Obes* 1982;6:143–52.

50 Westrate JA, Deurenberg P, van Tinteren H. Indices of body fat distribution and adiposity in Dutch children from birth to 18 years of age. *Int J Obes* 1989;13:465–78.

51 Zonderland ML, Erich WBM, Erkelens DW *et al.* Plasma lipids and apoproteins, body fat distribution and body fatness in early pubertal children. *Int J Obes* 1990;14:1039–46.

52 Zwiauer K, Widhalm K, Kerbi B. Body fat distribution in children and adolescents: influence on blood lipids, glucose and weight reduction. *Int J Obes* 1989;13(Suppl. 1):89.

53 Wabitsch M, Hauner H, Beckman A *et al.* The relationship between body fat distribution and weight loss in 51 obese adolescent girls during a weight reduction program. *Int J Obes* 1991;15(Suppl. 1):89.

54 Bjorntorp P. Regional obesity. In: Bjorntorp P, Brodoff BN, eds. *Obesity*. Philadelphia, PA: J.B. Lippincott, 1992: 579–86.

55 Gurney R. Hereditary factor in obesity. *Arch Intern Med* 1934;57:557–61.

56 Garn SM, Clark DC. Trends in fatness and the origins of obesity. *Pediatrics* 1976;57:443–56.

57 Poskitt EME, Cole TJ. Overfeeding and overweight in infancy and their relation to body size in early childhood. *Nutr Metab* 1977;21(Suppl. 1):54–5.

58 Poskitt EME, Cole TJ. Nature, nurture and childhood overweight. *Br Med J* 1978;1:603–5.

59 Borjeson M. The aetiology of obesity in children. A study of 101 twin pairs. *Acta Paediatr Scand* 1976;Suppl.65:279–87.

60 Stunkard AJ, Harris JR, Pedersen NL, McClearn GE. The body mass index of twins who have been reared apart. *N Engl J Med* 1990;322:1483–7.

61 Stunkard A, Sorensen TIA, Harris C *et al.* An adoption study of human obesity. *N Engl J Med* 1986;314:193–8.

62 Bouchard C. Genetic aspects of human obesity. In: Bjorntorp P, Brodoff BN, eds. *Obesity*. Philadelphia, PA: J.B. Lippincott, 1992:343–51.

63 Widdowson EMA. *Study of Individual Children's Diets*. MRC special reports series, no. 257. London: HMSO, 1947.

64 Whitehead RG, Paul AA, Cole TJ. Trends in food energy intakes throughout childhood from one to 18 years. *Hum Nutr Appl Nutr* 1982;36A:57–62.

65 Poskitt EME. The control of appetite and food intake in the obese child. In: Giorgi PL, Suskind RM, Catassi C, eds. *The Obese Child. Paediatric and Adolescent Medicine*, Vol. 2. Basel: Karger, 1992:172–80.

66 Birch LL. Children's preference for high fat foods. *Nutr Rev* 1993;9:249–55.

67 Garby L, Astrup A. A simple hypothesis for the development of obesity. *Eur J Clin Nutr* 1992;93:685–6.

68 Astrup A, Raben A. Obesity: an inherited metabolic deficiency in the control of macronutrient balance? *Eur J Clin Nutr* 1992;9:611–20.

69 Bogardus C, Lillioja S, Ravussen E, Abbott W, Zawadzki JK, Young A. Familial dependence of the resting metabolic rate. *N Engl J Med* 1986;315:96–100.

70 Bullen BA, Reed RB, Mayer J. Physical activity of obese and non-obsese adolescent girls appraised by motion picture sampling. *Am J Clin Nutr* 1964;24:211–23.

71 Bradfield RB, Chan H, Bradfield NR, Payne PR. Energy expenditure and heart rates of Cambridge boys at school. *Am J Clin Nutr* 1971;24:1461–6.

72 Lissau-Lund-Sorensen I, Sorensen TIA. Prospective study of the influence of social factors in childhood on risk of overweight in young adulthood. *Int J Obes* 1992;16:169–76.

73 Dietz WH, Gortmaker SL. Do we fatten our children at the television set? Obesity and television viewing in children and adolescents. *Pediatrics* 1985;75:807–12

74 Klesges RC, Shelton ML, Klesges LM. Effects of television on metabolic rate: potential implications for childhood obesity. *Pediatrics* 1993;91:281–6.

75 Segal KR, Dietz WH. Physiological responses to playing a video game. *Am J Clin Nutr* 1991;145:115–24.

76 Riddoch C, Savage JM, Murphy N, Cran GW, Boreham C. Longterm health implications of fatness and physical activity patterns *Arch Dis Child* 1991;66:1426–33.

77 Bruch H. Obesity in childhood. III. Physiological and psychological aspects of the food intake of obese children. *Am J Dis Child* 1940;59:739–81.

78 Jacoby A, Altman DG, Cook J, Holland WW, Elliott A. Influence of some social and environmental factors on the nutrient intake and nutritional status of school children. *Br J Prev Soc Med* 1975;29:116–20.

79 Locard E, Mamelle N, Billette A, Miginiac M, Munoz, F, Rey S. Risk factors of obesity in a five year old population. Parental versus environmental factors. *Int J Obes* 1992;16: 721–30.

80 Taitz LS, Lukmanji Z. Alteration in feeding patterns and rates of weight gain in south Yorkshire infants 1971–1977. *Hum Biol* 1981;53:313–20.

81 Dewey K, Heinig MJ, Nommsen LA, Peerson JM, Lonnerdal B. Breast-fed infants are leaner than formula-fed infants at 1 y of age: the DARLING study. *Am J Clin Nutr* 1993;57: 140–5.

82 Tracey VV, De NC, Harper JR. Obesity and respiratory infection in infants and young children. *Br Med J* 1971;1: 16–18.

83 Mellbin T, Vuille J-C. Physical development at 7 years of age in relation to velocity of weight gain in infancy with special reference to incidence of overweight. *Br J Prev Soc Med* 1973;27:225–35.

84 Rolland-Cachera M-F, Deheeger M, Bellisle F, Sempe M, Guilloud-Bataille M, Patois E. Adiposity rebound in children: a simple indicator for predicting obesity. *Am J Clin Nutr* 1984;39:129–35.

85 Mossberg H-O. 40-year follow-up of obese children. *Lancet* 1989;2:491–3.

86 Lloyd JK, Wolff OH, Whelan WS. Childhood obesity – a longterm study of height and weight. *Br Med J* 1961;2:145–8.

87 Forbes GB. Nutrition and growth. *J Pediatr* 1977;91:40–2.

88 Poskitt EME. Marasmus and kwashiorkor. Detection, treatment and prevention. In: Wilkinson AW, ed. *Early Nutrition and Later Development*. London: Pitman Medical, 1976; 164–74.

89 Griffiths M, Rivers JPW, Hoinville EA. Obesity in boys: the distinction between fatness and heaviness. *Hum Nutr Clin Nutr* 1985;39C:259–70.

90 Court JM, Dunlop M. Obese from infancy: a clinical entity. In Howard A, ed. *Recent Advances in Obesity Research*, Vol. I. London: Newman, 1975;34–6.

91 Barker DJP, Osmond C, Golding J, Kuh D, Wadsworth MEJ. Growth *in utero*, blood pressure in childhood and adult life, and mortality from cardiovascular disease. *Br Med J* 1989; 298:564–7.

92 Drash A. Relationship between diabetes mellitus and obesity in the child. *Metabolism* 1973;22:337–44.

93 Chiumello G, Guercio MJ, Do I, Carnelutti M, Bidone G. Relationship between obesity, chemical diabetes and pancreatic function in children. *Diabetologia* 1969;18:238–43.

94 Rames LK, Clarke WR, Cannon WE. Normal blood pressures and the evaluation of sustained blood pressure elevation in childhood: the Muscatine study. *Pediatrics* 1978;61:245–51.

95 Henderson RC. Tibia vara: a complication of adolescent obesity. *J Pediatr* 1992;121:482–6.

96 Brook CGD, Lloyd JK. Adipose cell size and glucose tolerance in children. *Arch Dis Child* 1973;48:301–4.

97 Lestradet H, Deschamps I, Giron B, Ostrowski ZL. Relation between the size of the adipocytes, blood glucose, plasma insulin, NEFA and the degree of obesity in children. In: Howard A, ed. *Recent Advances in Obesity Research*, Vol. I. London: Newman, 1975:167–9.

98 Forget PP, Fernandes J, Haverkamp-Bergemann P. Plasma triglyceride clearing in obese children. *Am J Clin Nutr* 1975; 28:858–65.

99 Sasaki J, Shindo M, Tanaka H, Ando M, Arakawa K. A longterm aerobic exercise program decreases the obesity index and increases the high density lipoprotein cholesterol concentration in obese children. *Int J Obes* 1987;11:339–46.

100 Widhalm K, Maxa E, Zyman H, Effect of diet and exercise upon the cholesterol and triglyceride content of plasma lipoproteins in overweight children. *Eur J Pediatr* 1978; 127:121–6.

101 Savage DL, Forsyth CC, Cameron J. Excretion of individual adreno-cortical steroids in obese children. *Arch Dis Child* 1974;49:946–54.

102 Stockholm KH. Serum free tri-iodo-thyronine: determinant of the pseudohypercortisolism in obesity. *Int J Obes* 1982; 6:211–15.

103 Mantero F, Boscaro M, Sonino N, Ridolfi P, Benato M. Obesity and Cushing's syndrome in childhood: problems of differential diagnosis. In: Cacciari E, Laron Z, Raiti S, eds. *Obesity in Childhood*. London: Academic Press, 1978: 197–205.

104 McKenna TJ. Pathogenesis of polycystic ovary syndrome. *N Engl J Med* 1988;318:558–62.

105 Kopelman PG, White N, Pilkington TE. The effort of

weight loss on sex steroid secretion and binding in massively obese women. *Clin Endocrinol* 1981;14:113–16.

106 Wilkinson PW, Parkin JM. Growth hormone response to exercise in obese children. *Lancet* 1974;2:55.

107 Bengtsson B-A, Brummer RJM, Eden S, Rosen T, Sjostrom L. Effects of growth hormone on fat mass and fat distribution. *Acta Paediatr Scand* 1992;Suppl.(1)383:62–5.

108 Binet E, Schlumberger A, Chaussain JL, Job JC. Serum somatomedin activity in obese children. In: Laron Z, ed. *The Obese Child. Pediatric and Adolescent Endocrinology*, Vol. 1. Basel: Karger, 1976;153–6.

109 Loche S, Cappa M, Borrelli A *et al.* Reduced growth hormone response to growth hormone releasing hormone in children with simple obesity and evidence for somatomedin C inhibition. *Clin Endocrinol* 1987;27:145–53.

110 Stockholm KH, Lindgreen P. Serum free tri-iodothyronine in obesity. *Int J Obes* 1982;6:573–8.

111 Ford MJ, Cameron EHD, Ratcliffe WA, Horn DB, Toft AD, Munro JE. TSH response to TRH in substantial obesity. *Int J Obes* 1980;4:122–5.

112 Gleispach H, Fischbacher F, Hofler G, Rainer H, Silli S. The influence of physical training on plasma cortisol and other plasma parameters in adipose and normal persons. In: Laron Z, ed. *The Adipose Child. Pediatric and Adolescent Endocrinology*, Vol. 1. Basel: Karger, 1976:167–73.

113 Linder CW, DuRant RH. Exercise, serum lipids and cardiovascular disease – risk factors in children. *Ped Clin N Am* 1982;29:1341–54.

114 Conceicao S, Ward MK, Kerr DNS. Defects in sphygmomanometers: an important source of error in blood pressure recording. *Br Med J* 1976;1:886–8.

115 Messerli FH, Sundgaard-Riise K, Reisin ED *et al.* Dimorphic adaptation to obesity and arterial hypertension. *Ann Intern Med* 1983;99:757–61.

116 Ward WA, Kelsey WM. The Pickwickian syndrome. *J Pediatr* 1962;61:745–50.

117 Chaussain M, Gamain B, Latorre A-M, Chaussain JL. Respiratory function in obese children. In: Laron Z, ed. *The Adipse Child. Pediatric and Adolescent Endocrinology*, Vol. 1. Basel: Karger, 1976:174–6.

118 Wilkinson PW. *Obesity in Childhood: A Community Study*. MD thesis, University of Leeds, 1976.

119 Borjeson M. Overweight children. *Acta Paediatr Scand* 1962;51(Suppl. 132):1–76.

120 Bruch H. Psychological aspects of obesity in adolescence. *Am J Public Hlth* 1958;48:1349–53.

121 Murphy CM, Allison DB, Babbitt RL, Patterson HL. Adiposity in children: is mental retardation a critical variable? *Int J Obes* 1992;16:633–8.

122 Tanner JM, Hughes PCR, Whitehouse RH. Comparative rapidity of response of height, limb muscle and limb fat to treatment with human growth hormone in patients with and without growth hormone deficiency. *Acta Endocrinol* 1977;84:681–96.

123 Angelin B, Ruding M, Olivecrona H, Ericsson S. Effects of growth hormone on low-density lipoprotein metabolism. *Acta Paediat Scand* 1992;Suppl.383:67–8.

124 Myles AB, Daley JR. *Corticosteroid and ACTH Treatment: Principles and Problems*. London: Edward Arnold, 1974.

125 Warkany J. *Congenital Malformations*. Chicago, IL: Year Book Publishers, 1971.

126 Hall JG. Genomic imprinting and its clinical implications. *N Engl J Med* 1992;326:827–9.

127 Laurance BM. The Prader–Willi syndrome. *Mat Child Hlth* 1985;10:106–9.

128 Holm VA, Pipes PL. Food and children with Prader–Willi syndrome. *Am J Dis Child* 1976;130:1063–7.

129 Laurance BM, Brito A, Wilkinson J. Prader–Willi syndrome after 15 years. *Arch Dis Child* 1981;56:181–6.

130 Guy R. The growth of physically handicapped children with special emphasis on appetite and activity. *Publ Hlth (Lond)* 1978;92:1485–54.

131 Department of Health. *Present-day Practice in Infant Feeding*. Third report, 1988. Report on health and social subjects no 32. London: HMSO.

132 Poskitt EME, Rayner PHW. Fenfluramine and growth hormone release. *Br Med J* 1973;3:348.

133 Nuutinen O, Knip M. Long-term weight control in obese children: persistence of treatment outcome and metabolic changes. *Int J Obes* 1992;16:279–88.

134 Abraham S, Collins G, Nordsieck M. Relationship of childhood weight status to morbidity in adults. *Publ Hlth Rep* 1960;86:273–84.

14: The Physiology of Puberty

D.M. STYNE

INTRODUCTION

The remarkable physical and psychological changes of pubertal development emanate from sequential changes in endocrine activity. Far from being a *de novo* event in the second decade of life, puberty is in many ways a recapitulation of changes that occurred during the fetal and neonate period [1]. Puberty is thus viewed as a process that is restrained until the appropriate time in development for secondary sexual development to occur.

SECULAR TRENDS IN PUBERTY

The age of puberty today is earlier than in past centuries, as demonstrated by the fact that the age of menarche in industrialized European countries and in the United States decreased 2–3 months per decade over the past 150–100 years, respectively (Fig. 14.1) [2,3]. This positive secular trend ceased in the USA in approximately 1940, probably due to the increasing stability in socioeconomic conditions, nutritional status and states of health. This is contrasted to the nomadic Lapp culture, in which the standard of living had changed little between 1870 and 1930 and no trend towards earlier menarche was documented. According to the most recent survey by the US National Center for Health Statistics the age of menarche in the USA is 12.8 years [5].

The interaction of nutritional status and puberty is extremely important in areas of the world where nutrition is suboptimal. Moderate obesity (up to 30% above normal weight for age) is associated with earlier menarche, although pathological obesity is associated with delayed menarche [6]. Delayed puberty is a feature of chronic disease and malnutrition; strenuous physical activity in girls can delay or arrest puberty, especially when associated with thin habitus [7]. Inactive, bedridden children with mental retardation reach menarche at an earlier age and at a lower body fat than do similarly retarded children who are more active.

Genetic factors play an important role in the onset of puberty, as illustrated by the similar age of menarche between members of an ethnic population and within mother–daughter pairs. Secondary sexual development occurs earlier in black girls compared with white girls, but there is no apparent effect of social or economic factors on this relationship. Thus, when socioeconomic and environmental factors lead to good nutrition, general health and infant care, the age of onset of puberty in normal children is determined largely by genetic factors.

PHYSICAL CHANGES OF PUBERTY

The physical changes in individuals are described by an objective method developed by Tanner [8–12] to describe the maturation of secondary sexual characteristics.

Female

TANNER STAGING

The development of the breast is primarily controlled by oestrogen secreted by the ovaries while the growth of pubic and axillary hair is mainly under the influence of androgens secreted by the adrenal gland (Fig. 14.2) [8]. Initially breast development may be unilateral for several months, and may be cause for unfounded concern by girls or parents. Indeed, surgical biopsies have been performed inappropriately in girls in whom it was not appreciated that the asymmetrical development is normal. Changes in the diameter of the papilla of the nipple are linked to stages of pubertal development [10]. Nipple papilla diameter does not increase much during pubic hair stage (PH)1–3 or breast stage (B)1–3 (diameter 3–4 mm) but does increase after stage B3, providing an objective method of differentiating stage 4 from 5 (final diameter approximately 9 mm) (Table 14.1). The stage of breast development is usually equal to the stage of pubic hair development in normal girls (Fig. 14.3), but as different endocrine organs control these two processes, stages of each phenomenon should be classified separately. Although rarely evident in individual girls, increase in height velocity rather than breast development is actually the

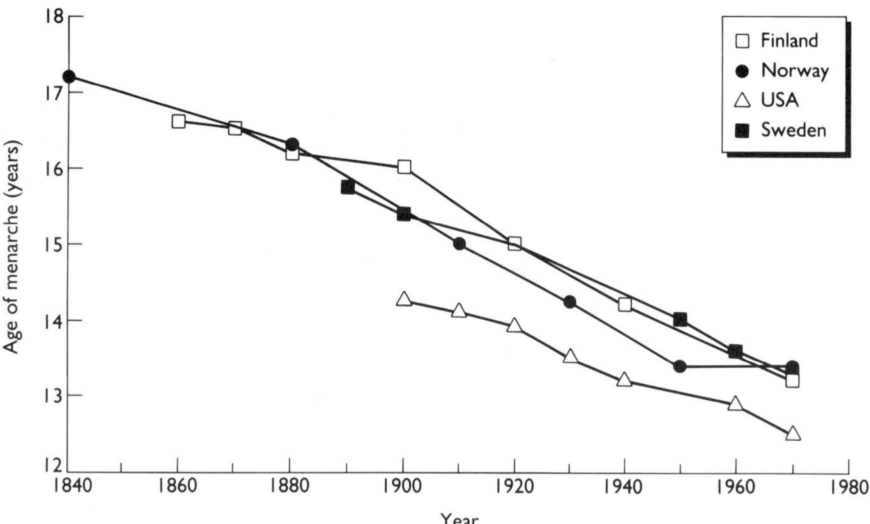

Fig. 14.1 Changes in age at menarche, 1840–1978 (redrawn and modified from data in Tanner & Eveleth [4]).

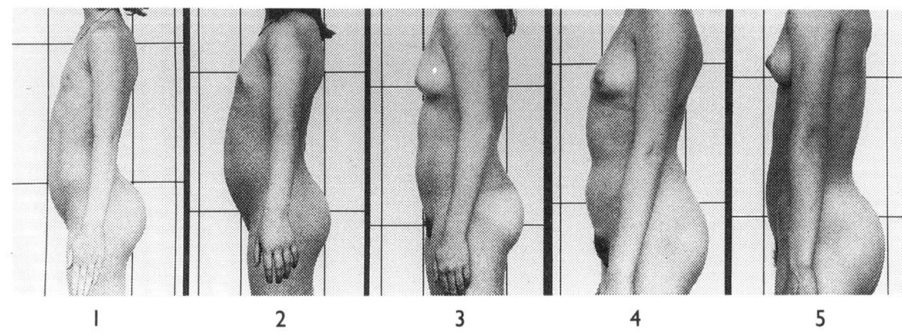

Fig. 14.2 Stages of breast development, according to Marshall & Tanner [8] and Reynolds & Wines [9]. Stage 1: preadolescent; elevation of papilla only. Stage 2: breast bud stage; elevation of breast and papilla as a small mound, enlargement of areolar diameter. Stage 3: further enlargement of breast and areola, with no separation of their contours. Stage 4: projection of areola and papilla to form a secondary mound above the level of the breast. Stage 5: mature stage; projection of papilla only, resulting from recession of the areola to the general contour of the breast.

Table 14.1 Nipple diameter versus breast (B) and pubic hair (PH) stages: comparison of longitudinal and cross-sectional data*

	Nipple size (mm)	
Stage	Cross-sectional data	Longitudinal data
B1	2.89 (0.81)	3.0 (0.77)
B2	3.28 (0.89)	3.37 (0.96)
B3	4.07 (1.32)	4.72 (1.40)†
B4	7.74 (1.64)†	7.25 (1.46)†
B5	9.94 (1.38)†	9.41 (1.45)†
PH1	2.95 (1.02)	3.14 (1.31)
PH2	3.32 (0.91)	3.69 (1.34)
PH3	4.11 (1.54)	4.44 (1.17)†
PH4	7.15 (1.81)†	6.54 (1.47)†
PH5	9.66 (1.59)†	8.98 (1.56)†

* Results are means ± SD (in parentheses).
† Significantly different from previous stage, $P < 0.05$.
From Rohn [10].

first sign of puberty in girls as determined by surveys of populations (Fig. 14.4).

OVARIAN DEVELOPMENT IN PUBERTY

Oogonia arise from the primordial germ cells in the wall of the yolk sac near the caudal end of the embryo [14]. By the sixth month of fetal life the cells have migrated to the genital ridge and progressed through sufficient mitoses to reach a complement of 6–7 million oogonia, which represents the maximal number of primordial follicles the individual will have throughout life. Meiosis begins but is not completed as the nucleus and chromosomes persist in prophase to mark the conversion of the oogonia to primary oocytes. Primordial follicles are composed of the primary oocyte surrounded by a single layer of spindle-shaped cells that will develop into granulosa cells and a basal lamina which will later in development be the boundary of the

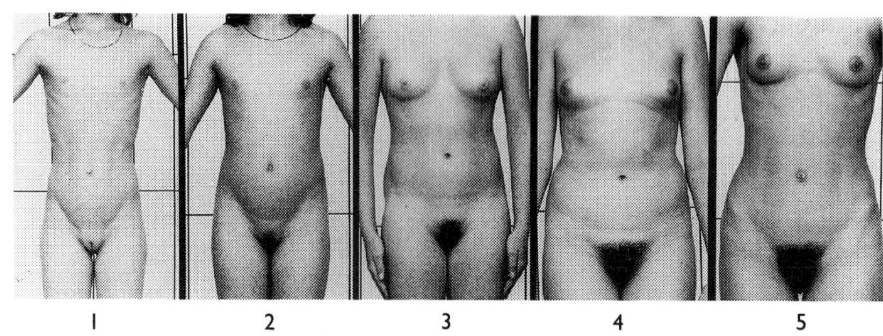

Fig. 14.3 Stages of female pubic hair development, according to Marshall & Tanner [8], Reynolds & Wines [9] and Dupertuis *et al.* [11]. Stage 1: preadolescent; the vellus over the pubes is not further developed than that over the anterior abdominal wall, i.e. no pubic hair. Stage 2: sparse growth of long, slightly pigmented, downy hair, straight or only slightly curled, appearing chiefly along the labia. This stage is difficult to see on photographs. Stage 3: hair is considerably darker, coarser and curlier. The hair spreads sparsely over the junction of the pubes. Stage 4: hair is now adult in type, but the area covered by it is still considerably smaller than in most adults. There is no spread to the medial surface of the thighs. Stage 5: hair is adult in quantity and type, distributed as an inverse triangle of the classic feminine pattern. The spread is to the medial surface of the thighs but not up the linea alba or elsewhere above the base of the inverse triangle.

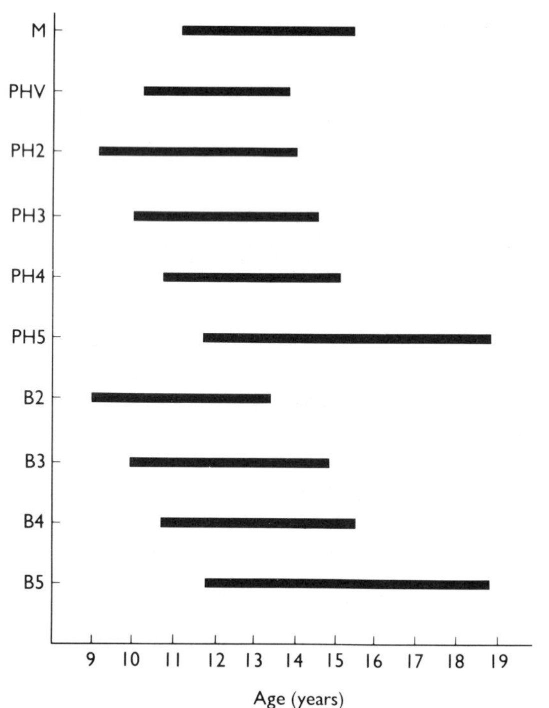

Fig. 14.4 The range of attainment of various stages of puberty in Western European females. M, menarche; PHV, peak height velocity; PH2–5, pubic hair stages; B2–5, breast stages (data from Marshall & Tanner [12] and Van Wieringen *et al.* [13]).

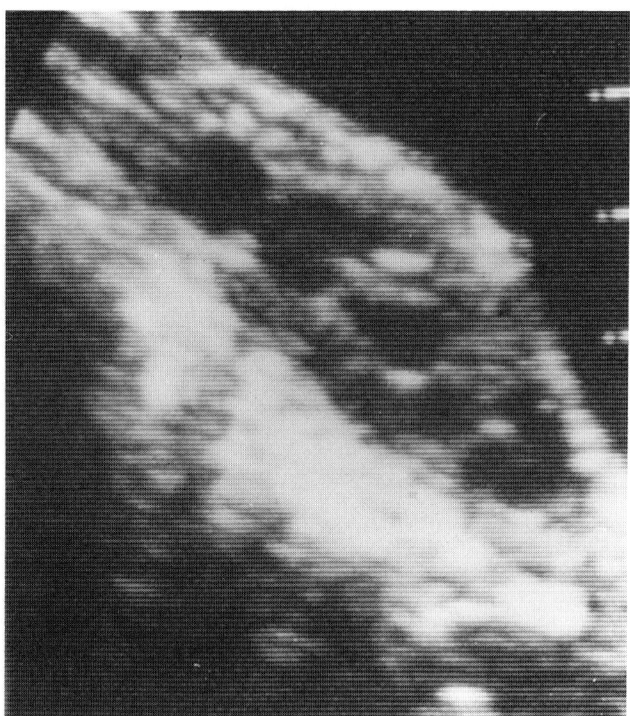

Fig. 14.5 Ovarian ultrasound image from a normal prepubertal 8.8-year-old girl. The ovary has a multi-cystic morphology (more than six cysts of > 4 mm in diameter). The bladder is the dark area above and 1 cm markers are shown (from Stanhope *et al.* [16]).

theca cells. Due to atresia, there are 2–4 million primordial follicles left at birth but only 400 000 remain at menarche.

At the time of the first ovulation the first meiotic metaphase converts the primary oocyte into the secondary oocyte, which is extruded into the fallopian tubes [15]. At the time of sperm penetration the second polar body is eliminated, thereby forming the ovum which contains a haploid set of chromosomes to join with the haploid set of chromosomes of the sperm. While some follicles in the fetus and child progress to the large antral stage, all developing follicles undergo atresia prior to puberty, and few large follicles develop in the child. However, the presence of more than six follicles with a diameter of more than 4 mm indicates the presence of pulsatile gonadotrophin secretion and may be seen in normal prepubertal girls, in pubertal girls prior to menarche and in patients recovering from anorexia nervosa. This 'multicystic appearance' is considered to be characteristic of a phase of pulsatile gonadotrophin secretion prior to positive feedback (see below) (Fig. 14.5) [16]. As will be discussed below, ovulatory periods may develop well before secondary sexual development is complete in the pubertal girl. Immature-appearing girls can be fertile.

OTHER CHANGES IN THE FEMALE

The vagina lengthens early in female puberty, and continues to elongate at least until menarche. The mucosa of the vulva and vagina become softer and thicker, and the hymen thickens with enlargement of the hymenal orifice at puberty [17]. Mucosal changes of the vagina are demonstrable, but the acquisition of a sample of vaginal secretion for clinical diagnosis is rarely indicated, and may be physically or psychologically traumatic to a child. The analysis of a urocytogram is an easier method of collection of a sample of vaginal surface cells but is rarely performed [18]. Before menarche there are about 10% superficial cells in the population and, with oestrogen stimulation, the layer becomes thicker and the cells have an increase in glycogen content. Just before menarche the cells are mostly adult-type cornified cells. Observation of the vaginal secretions in the months prior to menarche reveals a dulling of the mucosa from the reddish tint of prepuberty to a pinkish coloration and an extrusion of whitish disharge. The vaginal fluid becomes acidic with the progression of puberty, while prepubertal secretions are alkaline or neutral. The mons pubis develops more fat and enlarges with puberty. The labia become larger and the surfaces develop fine wrinkles. The clitoris enlarges slightly with normal puberty, but noticeable virilization indicates a process pathological.

The uterus lies in a craniocaudal direction in childhood without the adult flexion. The myometrium enlarges during early puberty, thereby enlarging the corpus leading to the adult corpus to cervix ratio. Although there is a

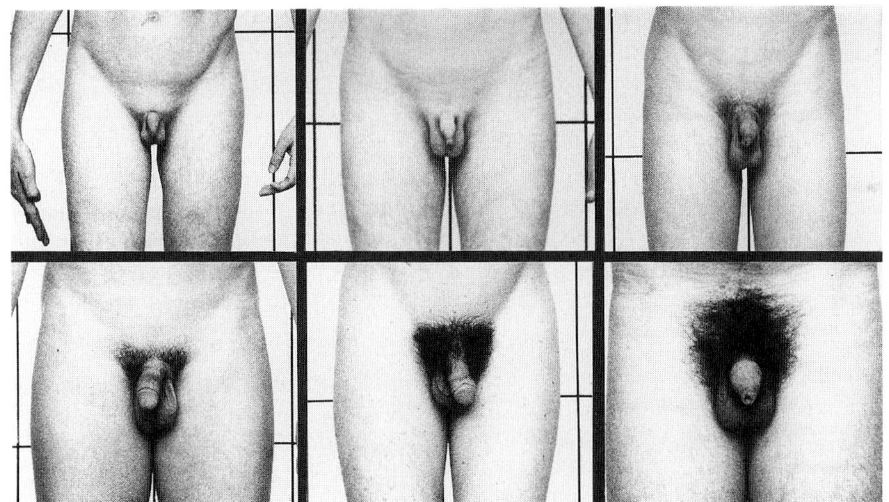

Fig. 14.6 Stages of male genital development and pubic hair development, according to Marshall & Tanner [12], Reynolds & Wines [9] and Dupertuis *et al.* [11]. *Genital.* Stage 1: preadolescent; testes, scrotum and penis are about the same size and proportion as in early childhood. Stage 2: the scrotum and testes have enlarged; there is a change in the texture and also some reddening of the scrotal skin. Stage 3: growth of the penis has occurred, at first mainly in length but with some increase in breadth; there is further growth of the testes and scrotum. Stage 4: the penis is further enlarged in length and breadth with development of the glans. The testes and scrotum are further enlarged. The scrotal skin has further darkened. Stage 5: genitalia are adult in size and shape. No further enlargement takes place after stage 5 is reached. *Pubic hair.* Stage 1: preadolescent; the vellus over the pubes is not further developed than that over the abdominal wall, i.e. no pubic hair. Stage 2: sparse growth of long, slightly pigmented, downy hair, straight or slightly curled, appearing chiefly at the base of the penis. Stage 3: hair is considerably darker, coarser and curlier, and spreads sparsely over the junction of the pubes. Stage 4: hair is now adult in type, but the area it covers is still considerably smaller than in most adults. There is no spread to the medial surface of the thighs. Stage 5: hair is adult in quantity and type, distributed as an inverse triangle. The spread is to the medial surface of the thighs but not up the linea alba or elsewhere above the base of the inverse triangle. Stage 6: most men will have further spread of the pubic hair.

single layer of cuboidal cells lining the uterine cavity in prepuberty, the increase in depth of the endometrium occurs just before menarche [16]. The cervix develops its adult shape and size just before menarche, and the cervical canal enlarges. Due to oestrogen stimulation the epithelial glands begin to produce a clear mucoid secretion which forms threads when dry, similar to the pattern found in the adult female at the middle of the menstrual cycle.

Male

TANNER STAGING

The growth of the penis and genitalia in the male usually correlates with pubic hair development, since both features are under androgen control, but for the most accurate assessment the stages of pubic hair development and genital development should be determined independently (Fig. 14.6) [19]. Growth of the testes is usually the first sign of puberty in the male (Fig. 14.7), and begins at a chronological age approximately 6 months after the average age of initiation of breast development in girls. In general, when the longitudinal measurement of a testis is greater than 2.5 cm, pubertal testicular enlargement has begun: most of the increase is due to enlargement of the Sertoli cells rather than the Leydig cells. A useful method of assessing testicular size utilizes the Prader orchidometer, a string of ellipsoids of known volume which are compared with the size of the testes of the subject (Fig. 14.8 & Table 14.2) [20]. The phallus is best measured in the flaccid state stretched, and the length should be recorded. The length of the erectile tissue (excluding the foreskin) increases from an average of 6.2 cm in the prepubertal state to 13.2 cm in the adult.

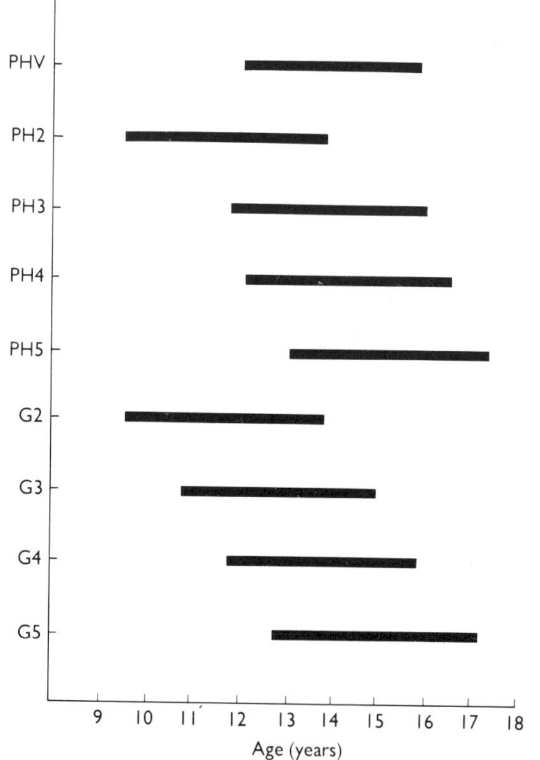

Fig. 14.7 The range of attainment of various stages of puberty in Western European males. PHV, peak height velocity; PH2–5, pubic hair stages; G2–5, genital stages (data from Marshall & Tanner [12] and Van Wieringen *et al.* [13]).

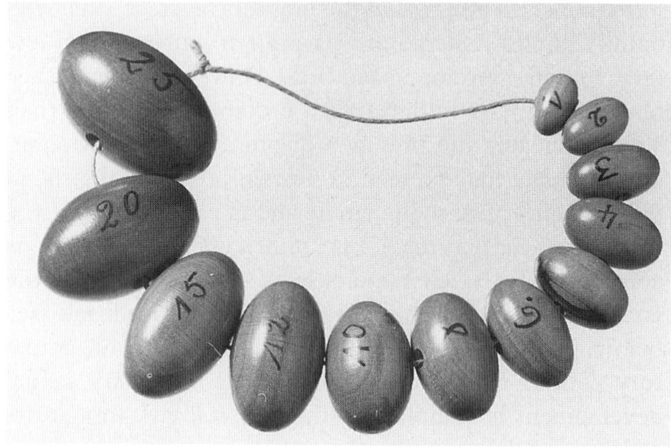

(a)

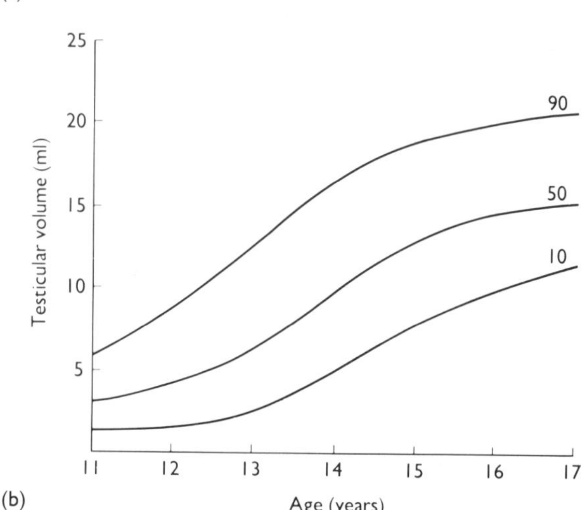

(b)

Fig. 14.8 (a) The Prader orchidometer. The numbers noted on the ellipsoids indicate the volume in millilitres. (b) 10th, 50th and 90th centiles of testicular size in boys at different ages (redrawn from Zachmann *et al.* [20]).

TESTES

The prepubertal testes consist mainly of Sertoli cells but the adult testes are mostly composed of germ cells in the seminiferous tubules. The seminiferous tubules enlarge during puberty and form tight occlusive junctions leading to the development of the blood testicular junction [21].

Table 14.2 Correlation of testicular volume with stage of pubertal development

	Pubertal stage				
	1	2	3	4	5
TVI*	1.8	4.5	8.2	10.5	–
Volume (cm^3)†	2.5	3.4	9.1	11.8	14
Volume (cm^3)‡	1.8	4.2	10.0	11.0	15
Volume (cm^3)§	1.8	5.0	9.5	12.5	17

* Testicular volume index calculated by (length × width of right testis and length × width of left testis)/2 (data from Burr *et al.* [●●] and August *et al.* [55]).
† Volume estimated by comparison with ellipsoid of known volume (orchidometer) that is equal to or smaller than the testes (data from Zachmann *et al.* [20]).
‡ Volume by comparison with orchidometer (data from Waaler *et al.* [85]).
§ Measurement with calipers and average volume of both testes calculated by 0.52 × longitudinal axis × transverse axis (data from Waaler *et al.* [85]).

Leydig cells are present in small numbers in prepuberty, although the interstitial tissue is mainly composed of mesenchymal tissue; however, it is at puberty that the Leydig cells become more apparent.

Spermatogenesis can be detected histologically between 11 and 15 years of age [22]. Ejaculation occurs by a mean of 13.5 years [23]. Thus boys are fertile before finishing their secondary sexual development. Immature-appearing boys can be fertile.

GYNAECOMASTIA

Gynaecomastia occurs in about 75% of boys to some degree, usually during the first stages of puberty [24,25]. In most cases the tissue regresses within 2 years, but occasionally in normal boys, often obese boys, and frequently in pathological conditions such as Klinefelter syndrome or partial androgen resistance where the effective amount of testosterone is reduced, gynaecomastia remains permanently.

Other changes of puberty

Axillary hair appears at an average of 13 years in American girls and 14 years in American boys; circumanal hair in boys precedes the axillary hair in boys [25]. Acne, comedones and seborrhoea of the scalp appear at about 13 years in girls. Voice change occurs at a mean age of 13 years in boys and the adult voice appears by 15 years, both phenomena occurring as a result of the enlargement of the larynx, cricothyroid cartilage and laryngeal muscles [26]. Periodontal disease rarely occurs in subjects younger than the pubertal age range. In the 6 months or so prior to menarche, girls experience a whitish vaginal discharge due to increasing oestrogen effect.

Facial characteristics change at puberty. Facial hair in boys begins to develop on the corners of the upper lips and the upper cheeks at approximately 15 years, and then spreads to the midline of the lower lip and cheek by 16 years, ultimately to the sides and the lower border of the chin at or after pubic hair and genital stage 5. The jaw becomes more prominent, as does the nose, during pubertal development [27].

Body composition

Percentages of lean body mass, skeletal mass and body fat are equal between prepubertal boys and girls. An increase in lean body mass starts at 6 years in girls and 9.5 years in boys, and is the earliest change in body composition of puberty [28]. By maturity, men have 1.5 times the lean body mass and almost 1.5 times the skeletal mass of women, while women have twice as much body fat as men.

Growth in puberty

The pubertal growth spurt encompasses the most rapid phase of growth after the neonatal period. The pubertal growth spurt begins in girls prior to the onset of secondary sexual characteristics, but only the most careful observation reveals this earliest stage of the phenomenon [29]. Boys' growth spurt starts on average 2 years after the average age of onset in girls. Thus the pubertal growth spurt is an early pubertal event in girls but a late pubertal event in boys. A girl who has experienced menarche usually has no more than 5 cm of growth remaining as menarche closely correlates with a bone age of 13 years [30]. There is no such single event in males to indicate approximate remaining growth, but a boy who has not reached the last stages of puberty is likely to have significant growth remaining. A bone age determination will reveal the amount of remaining growth in a pubertal patient.

The mean difference in adult height between men and women of 12.5 cm is due approximately 50% to the taller stature of boys at the onset of the pubertal growth spurt (on average 2 years later than onset in girls) and approximately 50% to the increased height gained during the pubertal growth spurt in boys compared to girls [31].

The pubertal growth spurt is mediated by several endocrine influences. Sex steroids exert a direct effect upon the growing cartilage and stimulate local production of insulin-like growth factor I (IGF-I) (Fig. 14. 9) [32]. Increasing sex-steroid production stimulates increased amplitude (but not increased frequency) of growth hormone secretion at puberty. The increased growth hormone

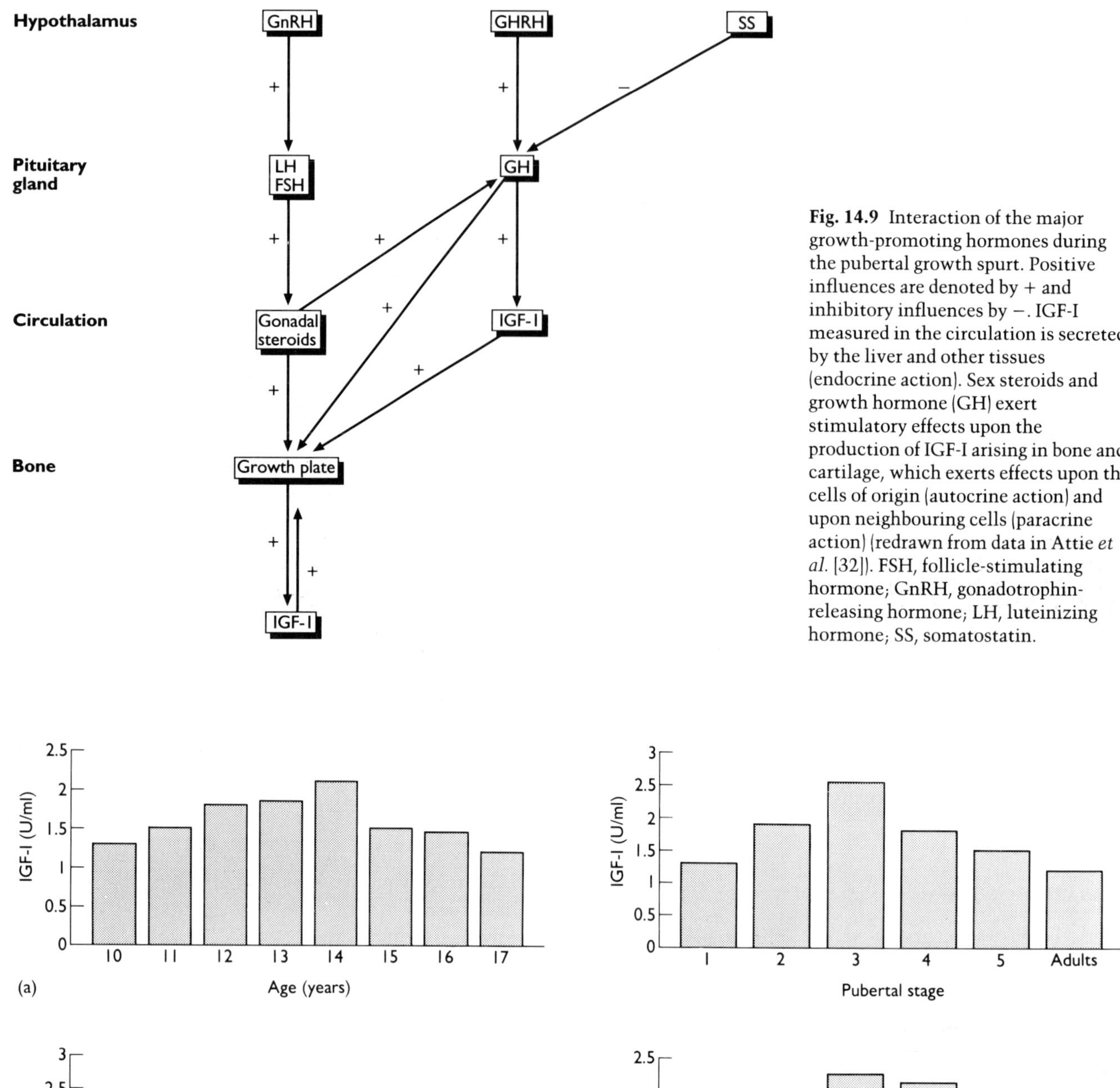

Fig. 14.9 Interaction of the major growth-promoting hormones during the pubertal growth spurt. Positive influences are denoted by + and inhibitory influences by −. IGF-I measured in the circulation is secreted by the liver and other tissues (endocrine action). Sex steroids and growth hormone (GH) exert stimulatory effects upon the production of IGF-I arising in bone and cartilage, which exerts effects upon the cells of origin (autocrine action) and upon neighbouring cells (paracrine action) (redrawn from data in Attie *et al.* [32]). FSH, follicle-stimulating hormone; GnRH, gonadotrophin-releasing hormone; LH, luteinizing hormone; SS, somatostatin.

(b) IGF-I (U/ml) Age (years) Pubertal stage

Fig. 14.10 Serum IGF-I displayed by age and pubertal stage in (a) females, and (b) males. The peak found during puberty is evident (redrawn from data in Grumbach & Styne [33]).

in turn stimulates increased production of IGF-I. Thus pubertal growth is accompanied not only by higher serum sex steroids but by increased episodic secretion of growth hormone and serum IGF-I (Fig. 14.10) [34]. These direct and indirect effects of sex steroids cause the increased growth rate characteristic of the pubertal growth spurt. Thyroid hormone is necessary in sufficient amounts to allow the pubertal growth spurt to proceed. The rapid growth rate is accompanied by an increase in serum alkaline phosphatase and serum Gla protein; thus normal adult values of these proteins are lower than concentrations found in puberty [35].

Limits of normal pubertal development

American boys and girls are similar to British and Swiss children in the age of attainment of most stages of pubertal development, except for menarche (Tables 14.3 & 14.4) [36–39]. There is no difference between black and white boys in the age of attainment of the stages of pubertal development in the USA. Black American girls are advanced in their secondary sexual development compared with white American girls during the first three stages of puberty. Some sign of puberty between 8 and 13 years of age (mean 10.5) is shown by 95% of normal American girls, whereas 95% of boys enter puberty between 9 and 14 years of age (mean 11.5). English girls complete secondary sexual development in a mean of 4.2 years, but the range is 1.5–6 years; the mean for boys is 3.5 years, with a range of 2 to 4.5 years [12].

Table 14.3 Age at stage of puberty in girls

	British girls*		Swiss girls†	
Stage	Mean (years)	SD	Mean (years)	SD
Breast stage 2	11.50	1.10	10.9	1.2
Pubic hair stage 2	11.64	1.21	10.4	1.2
Peak height velocity	12.14	0.88	12.2	1.0
Breast stage 3	12.15	1.09	12.2	1.2
Pubic hair stage 3	12.36	1.10	12.2	1.2
Pubic hair stage 4	12.95	1.06	13.0	1.1
Breast stage 4	13.11	1.15	13.2	0.9
Menarche‡	13.47	1.12	13.4	1.1
Pubic hair stage 5	14.41	1.21	14.0	1.3
Breast stage 5	15.33	1.74	14.0	1.2

* Determined in a prospective study of sequential photographs by Marshall & Tanner [8].
† Determined in a prospective longitudinal study of physical examinations as part of the First Zurich Longitudinal Study of Growth and Development (reported by Largo & Prader [38]).
‡ Mean age of menarche is 12.8 years ± 1.22 (SD) in American girls (from a prospective study from the National Health Survey (DHEW) publication No. (HRA) 74-1615, 1973).

Table 14.4 Age at stage of puberty in boys

	British boys*		Swiss boys†	
Stage	Mean (years)	SD	Mean (years)	SD
Genitalia stage 2	11.64	1.07	11.2	1.5
Genitalia stage 3	12.85	1.04	12.9	1.2
Pubic hair stage 2	13.44	1.09	12.2	1.5
Genitalia stage 4	13.77	1.02	13.8	1.1
Pubic hair stage 3	13.90	1.04	13.5	1.2
Peak height velocity	14.06	0.92	13.9	0.8
Pubic hair stage 4	14.36	1.08	14.2	1.1
Genitalia stage 5	14.92	1.10	14.7	1.1
Pubic hair stage 5	15.18	1.07	14.9	1.0

* Determined in a prospective study of sequential photographs by Marshall & Tanner [12].
† Determined in a prospective longitudinal study of physical examinations as part of the First Zurich Longitudinal Study of Growth and Development (reported by Largo & Prader [39]).

ENDOCRINE CHANGES OF PUBERTY (Figs 14.11 & 14.12)

Hypothalamic control

Gonadotrophin-releasing hormone (GnRH) is a 10 amino acid peptide produced from a larger prohormone precursor; human placental GnRH is cleaved from a 69 amino acid precursor. The gene coding for GnRH is located upon

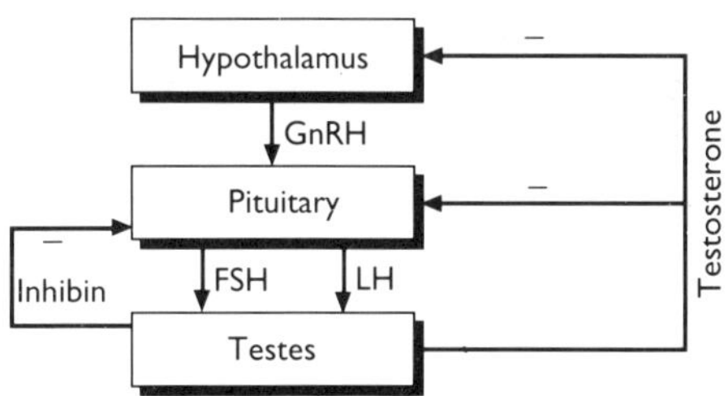

Fig. 14.11 Schematic representation of the hypothalamic–pituitary–testicular axis with stimulatory and inhibitory influences demonstrated.

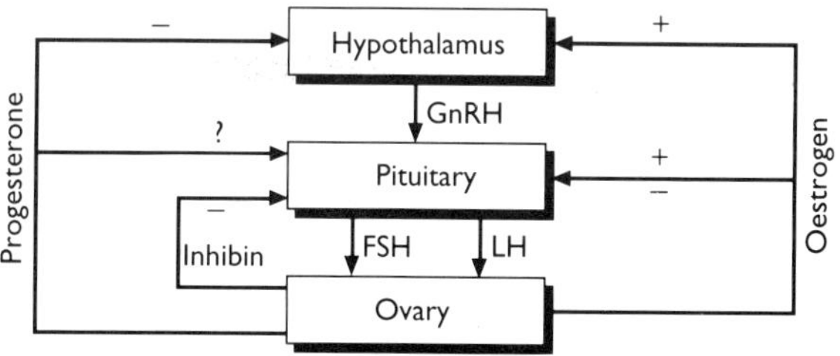

Fig. 14.12 Schematic representation of the hypothalamic–pituitary–ovarian axis with stimulatory and inhibitory influences demonstrated.

chromosome 8 [40]. Neurons producing GnRH originate in the primitive olfactory placode early in development of mammals and then migrate to the medial basal hypothalamus [41]. The control of this migration is related to a gene in the Xp22.3 locus of the X chromosome, the KAL gene. The absence of the KAL gene causes the Kallman syndrome, which consists of a decrease in or lack of gonadotrophin secretion joined with hyposmia due to disordered development of the olfactory bulb [42]. The gene product of KAL is probably an adhesion molecule.

Animal studies demonstrate that GnRH is released in episodic boluses into the hypothalamic–pituitary portal system, whereby it reaches the anterior pituitary gonadotrophs [43]. The half-life of GnRH is only 2–4 min and the daily metabolic clearance is $800\,l/m^2$. The frequency of episodic release varies with development, sex and the stage of the menstrual period. A theory remains that separate factors control luteinizing hormone (LH) and follicle-stimulating hormone (FSH). However, a variation of the frequency of secretion of GnRH will change the amount of LH and FSH released, and the serum levels of each, while sole replacement of GnRH in GnRH-deficient hypogonadal patients will restore the release of both LH and FSH. This supports the theory that this single hypothalamic factor controls both LH and FSH [44].

GnRH is localized mainly in the hypothalamus of the adult, but is also found in the hippocampus, cingulate cortex and the olfactory bulb [45]. GnRH is secreted into milk and is found in the placenta. Although it is not clear that GnRH has any effect upon human behaviour, it will stimulate the sex drive in rodents.

Isolated cultured GnRH neurons exhibit pulsatile release of GnRH, demonstrating an intrinsic rhythm that might be responsible for the coordinated pulsatile release of GnRH from the hypothalamus [46]. The GnRH pulse generator is affected by biogenic amine neurotransmitters, peptidergic neuromodulators, neuroexcitatory amino acids and neural pathways; adrenaline and noradrenaline increase GnRH release while dopamine, serotonin and opioids decrease GnRH release. Testosterone and progesterone inhibit the GnRH pulse frequency. Opioid peptides and corticotrophin-releasing hormone inhibit GnRH release in human beings [45].

Isolation of the arcuate nucleus of the mediobasal hypothalamus from the rest of the brain does not stop menstruation in monkeys, although ablation of the arcuate nucleus does. Pulsatile administration of GnRH to monkeys with ablated arcuate nuclei can restore pulsatile gonadotrophin secretion and varying the frequency of administration will change the ratio of LH to FSH [47]. This suggests that the arcuate nucleus is a locus of control of GnRH secretion.

GnRH affects gonadotrophs by binding to cell surface receptors [48,49]. This attachment to GnRH receptors triggers increased from intracellular calcium concentration and phosphorylation of protein kinase C in a manner similar to other peptide–receptor mechanisms. Continuous infusion of GnRH will decrease LH and FSH secretion and down-regulate the pituitary receptors for GnRH (Fig. 15.13). A decrease in the number of GnRH receptors occurs at first, and a decrease in the action of the occupied receptor upon the gonadotroph follows. Oestrogens increase and androgens decrease GnRH receptors. These alterations in GnRH receptors have an important role in regulating gonadotroph function. There are receptors for GnRH on gonads, but there is no evidence that these receptors are of physiological importance in human beings.

GnRH stimulates the production and secretion of LH and FSH from the gonadotrophs [44]. There appear to be readily releasable pools of LH which lead to a rise in serum

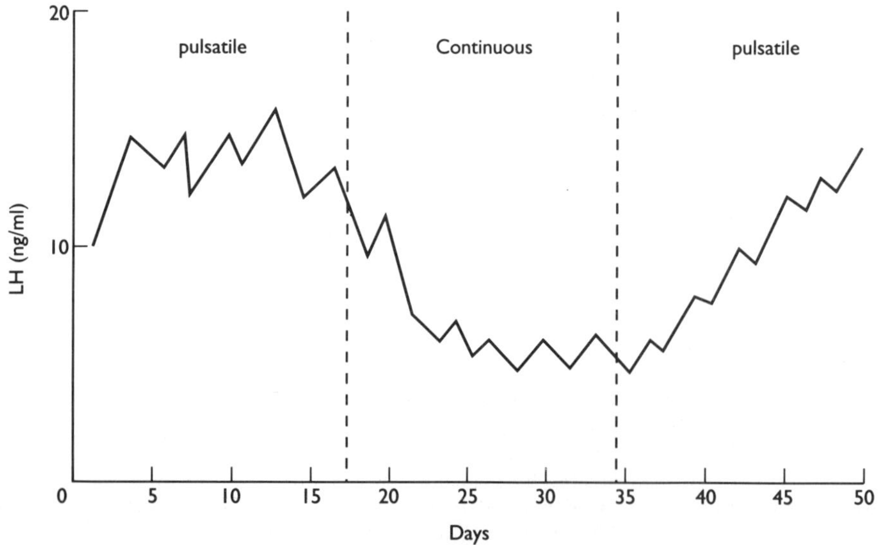

Fig. 14.13 Effect of pulsatile administration of GnRH on LH levels in contrast to continuous infusion of GnRH in adult oophorectomized rhesus monkeys in which gonadotrophin secretion has been abolished by lesions that ablated the medial basal hypothalamic GnRH pulse generator. There is suppression by continuous infusion of the same dose per hour in the same animals and resumption of episodic secretion of LH and FSH with the resumption of pulsatile administration of GnRH (redrawn from data in Belchetz *et al.* [47]).

LH within minutes after a bolus of GnRH, and other pools of LH which take longer to mobilize.

The decrease in gonadotrophin secretion during childhood before the onset of puberty, the juvenile pause, appears to be mediated by the central nervous system (CNS). Damage to the CNS due to increased intracranial pressure or tumour may release the inhibition and bring about premature pubertal development [50].

Gonadotrophins

The two pituitary gonadotrophins, FSH and LH, are glycoproteins composed of two subunits, an α-subunit which is identical for all the pituitary glycoproteins and distinct β-subunits that confer specificity upon each of the pituitary glycoproteins [51]. The β-subunits are 115 amino acids long with two carbohydrate side chains. Human chorionic gonadotrophin (hCG), produced by the placenta, is almost identical in structure to LH (except for an additional 32 amino acids and additional carbohydrate groups), and causes all of the same biological effects as pituitary LH. The LH β-subunit gene is on chromosome 19q13.32, close to the gene for β-hCG, while the FSH gene is at 11p13 [52].

The same gonadotroph cells produces LH and FSH. The gonadotrophs are spread throughout the anterior pituitary gland and abut upon the capillary basement membranes to allow access to the systemic circulation. Gonadotrophins are released into the blood stream in a pulsatile manner due to the pulsatile nature of GnRH secretion. Inactive gonadotroph cells that are not stimulated, e.g. due to disease affecting GnRH secretion, are small in diameter, while the gonadotroph cells of castrated individuals or those with absence of gonads such as in Turner syndrome, which are stimulated by large amounts of GnRH, are large in diameter and demonstrate prominent rough endoplasmic reticulum (RER) [53].

GnRH must stimulate gonadotrophin release before any other factors can affect gonadotrophin secretion. However, in the presence of GnRH stimulation, sex steroids and inhibin can change gonadotrophin secretion.

After injection of LH, a first half-life is 18 min and a second 90 min, while half-lives of FSH are 1.7 h and 8.3 h respectively. Metabolic clearance of LH is 34 ml/min m^{-2} and of FSH is 6–14 ml/min m^{-2}. These metabolic differences are used to explain the differing levels of LH and FSH in response to a single hypothalmic peptide, GnRH.

Serum gonadotrophins change during the progression of pubertal development. Because of the episodic nature of gonadotrophin secretion a single gonadotrophin determination will not reveal the stage of pubertal develop-

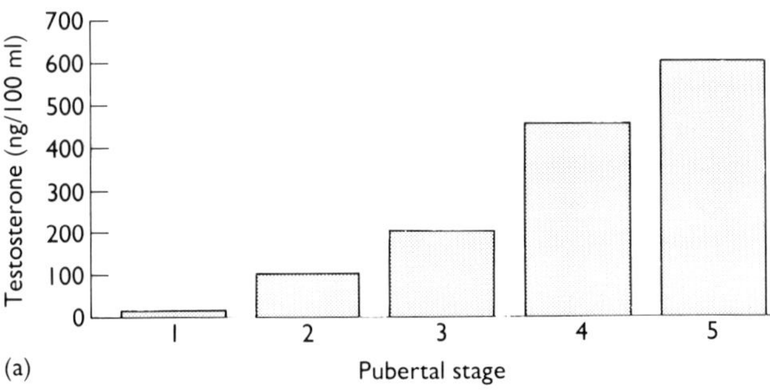

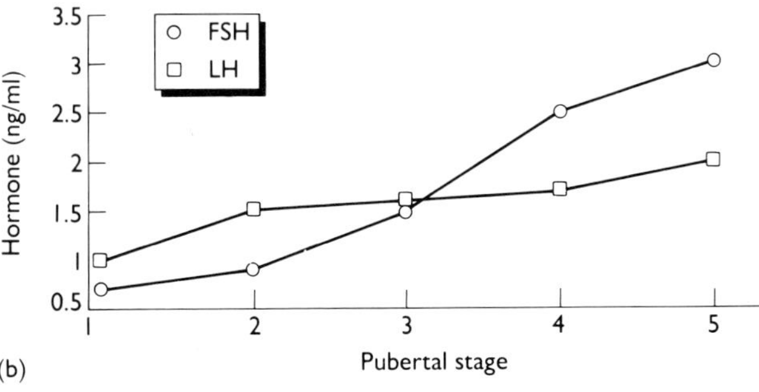

Fig. 14.14 Mean plasma testosterone (a) and gonadotrophins (FSH, LH) (b) in normal boys by stage of maturation (stage 1, prepubertal; stage 5, adolescent male) (redrawn from data in Grumbach [1]).

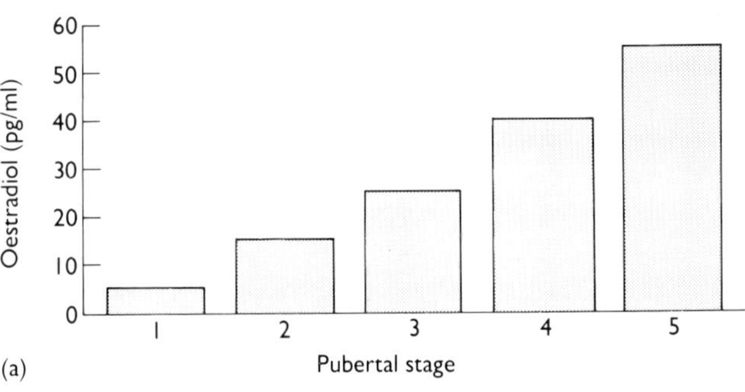

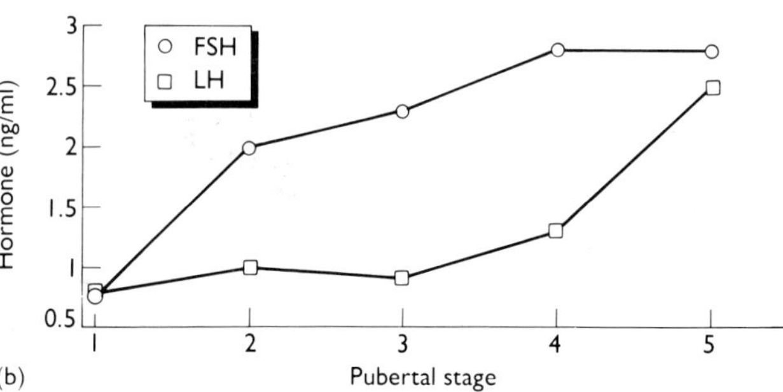

Fig. 14.15 Mean plasma oestradiol (a), FSH and LH concentrations (b) in prepubertal and pubertal females by pubertal stage of maturation (stage 1, prepubertal; stage 5, menstruating adolescents). Single daytime values of gonadotrophins have limited usefulness in the evaluation of individuals due to pulsatility of gonadotrophins during sleep through puberty. The sex steroid values, however, are useful in determination of stage of pubertal development (redrawn from data in Grumbach [1]).

ment. A sequence of nocturnal measurements will demonstrate the nadir and zenith of the pulses, although the method is cumbersome and usually reserved for clinical research. Measurement of LH and FSH after a bolus of GnRH is more convenient, and will determine the stage of development of the hypothalamic–pituitary axis. Nonetheless large surveys of subjects reveal certain patterns of serum gonadotrophins during pubertal development (Figs. 14.14 & 14.15) [54,55].

Leydig cells respond when LH binds to their membrane receptors. The ligand–receptor complex stimulates membrane-bound adenyl cyclase to increase cyclic adenosine monophosphate (cAMP), which then stimulates protein kinase, which in turn causes the stimulation of the conversion of cholesterol to pregnenolone by $P450_{scc}$ (side-chain cleavage enzyme), the first step in the production of testosterone [56]. After exposure to LH, the number of receptors for LH and the postreceptor pathway decrease their responsiveness to LH for at least 24 h. This explains the clinical finding of resistance to LH after daily injections of LH compared to every-other-day injections of LH. When assessing the response of testes to LH, hCG or LH must be administered at 2–3-day intervals to eliminate such down-regulation.

FSH binds to specific receptors on the cell surface of Sertoli cells and causes a sequence of events that culminates in increased protein kinase in a manner similar to the stimulatory effect of LH on Leydig cells [57]. FSH causes an increase in the mass of seminiferous tubules, and in an undefined way supports the development of sperm. A boy with an hCG-secreting tumour will have Leydig cell stimulation without FSH effect and without seminiferous tubule enlargement; the result will be virilization without much testicular enlargement [50].

In the female, LH binds to membrane receptors of ovarian cells and stimulates the activity of adenyl cyclase to produce cAMP, which stimulates the production of the low-density lipoprotein (LDL) receptor to increase binding and uptake of LDL cholesterol and the formation of cholesterol esters. LH stimulates the rate-limiting enzyme $P450_{scc}$ which converts cholesterol to pregnenolone, initiating steroidogenesis. After the onset of ovulation, LH exerts major effects upon the theca of the ovary. FSH binds to its own cell-surface receptors on the glomerulosa cells and stimulates the conversion of testosterone to oestrogen.

Gonadotrophins were previously measured by radioimmunoassays in clinical studies. Biological assays (using cells in culture responsive to the gonadotrophins) reveal different patterns of secretion than when gonadotrophins are measured by immunological assays (Fig. 14.16) [60].

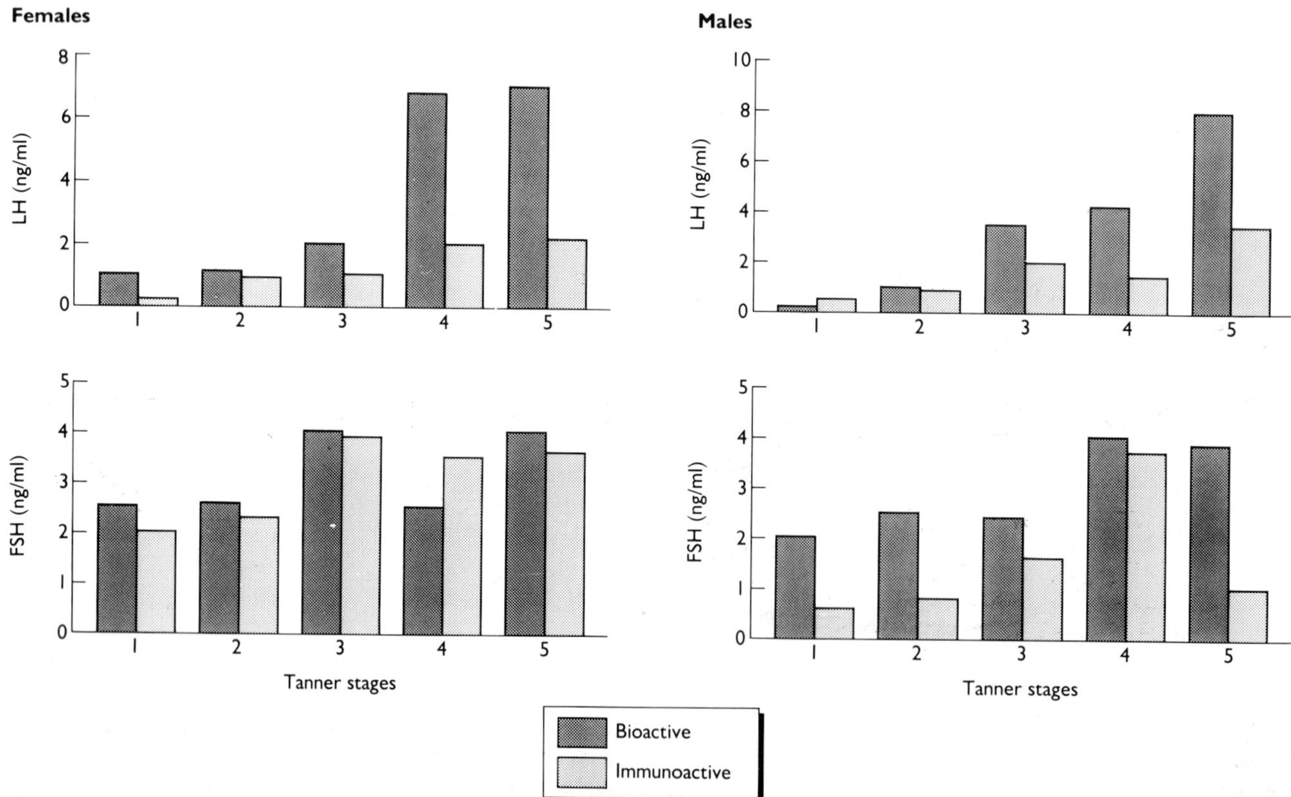

Fig. 14.16 Bioactive and immunoreactive plasma LH and FSH in prepubertal and pubertal girls and boys. Filled bars designate bioactive LH and FSH, and open bars immunoreactive LH and FSH. The concentration of LH is expressed as nanograms per millilitre (LER 960O) and that of FSH as nanograms per millilitre (hFSH-1-3) (redrawn from data in Reiter *et al.* [59] and Beitins *et al.* [60]).

The cause of the difference between these two methods of detection is unclear, but may be related to glycosylation of the molecules. It is postulated that such changes in glycosylation occur in puberty.

Sex steroids

The Leydig cells of the testes produce the major male sex steroid, testosterone, through a series of enzymatic conversions for which cholesterol is the precursor. When testosterone is secreted into the circulation it is bound to sex-hormone-binding globulin [61,63]. The remaining free testosterone is the active moiety. At the target cell, testosterone dissociates from the binding protein, diffuses into the cell and may be converted by 5α-reductase to dihydrotestosterone or converted to oestrogen by aromatase. Testosterone or dihydrotestosterone attaches to androgen receptors which are encoded by a gene on the q arm of the X chromosome [62]. The receptor has a two-fold greater affinity for dihydrotestosterone than for testosterone. Either sex steroid attaches to a nuclear receptor which changes in conformation by the act of binding. The testosterone–receptor complex then attaches to the steroid-responsive region of genomic DNA. Transcription and translation occur by androgen effect, which leads to protein production.

The effects of testosterone are different from those of dihydrotestosterone as a patient without dihydrotestosterone will not virilize fully. Testosterone will suppress LH secretion and will maintain Wolffian ducts while dihydrotestosterone is mostly responsible for the virilization of the external genitalia and for much of the secondary sexual characteristics of puberty. Androgens exert other effects in the body: testosterone causes muscle development, stimulates enzymatic activity in the liver and stimulates haemoglobin synthesis; androgens stimulate bone maturation at the epiphyseal plate.

Oestrogen is produced by the follicle cells of the ovary utilizing the same initial steps as testosterone production with a final aromatization process [15]. The main active oestrogen in human beings is oestradiol. Oestrogen also circulates bound to sex-hormone-binding globulin (SHBG), and follows the same pattern of action as described for testosterone. Oestradiol produces effects upon the breast and uterus and the distribution of adipose tissue and bone.

Sex-hormone-binding globulin

Less than 3% of circulating sex steroid is free and active; the rest is bound to SHBG. SHBG consists of heterogeneous monomers [61,63]. Androgen decreases SHBG and oestrogen stimulates SHBG formation. Thus, with the secretion of testosterone and the resulting decrease in SHBG, and therefore increase in free testosterone, there is a magnification of androgen effect.

Prolactin

Lactotrophs produce prolactin and are suppressed by prolactin-inhibitory factor (dopamine) in the basal state [64]. Thus hypothalamic disease may destroy prolactin inhibitory factor leading to increased prolactin secretion, and pituitary disease may destroy the lactotrophs leading to decreased prolactin secretion.

Inhibin

Inhibin is a heterodimeric glycoprotein produced by the Sertoli cells in the male and by the ovarian granulosa cells and the placenta of the female. Inhibin suppresses FSH secretion from the pituitary gland and provides another explanation for different levels of LH and FSH with only one hypothalamic peptide (GnRH) stimulating secretion of both gonadotrophins. Activin is a subunit of inhibin and has the opposite effect to inhibin, as activin stimulates the secretion of FSH from the pituitary gland. Originally measured decades ago by bioassay, immunoassays are now available to detect inhibin concentrations, and there is considerable interest in determining inhibin physiology [65].

Anti-Müllerian hormone

Anti-Müllerian hormone (AMH) belongs to the same family as inhibin and is produced from the Sertoli cells of the fetal testes and the granulosa cells of the fetal ovary [66,67]. In normal males AMH is high in the fetus and newborn, but decreases thereafter with a further drop at puberty. Girls have low levels of AMH in the newborn period.

Insulin-like growth factors

IGF-I serum concentrations are low at birth but rise throughout childhood until approximately the time of the pubertal growth spurt, when a several-fold increase in serum IGF-I occurs [33]. Serum values of IGF-I then fall to the adult concentration range (see Fig. 14.10).

The rise in serum IGF-I concentrations at puberty appears multifactorial. Increased secretion of GH, which occurs at the time of puberty due to increased sex steroid secretion, stimulates IGF-I production [32]. Thus sex steroids indirectly stimulate IGF-I production. Further, sex steroid secretion appears to cause increased production of IGF-I directly from the cartilage independent of changes in GH (see Fig. 14.9).

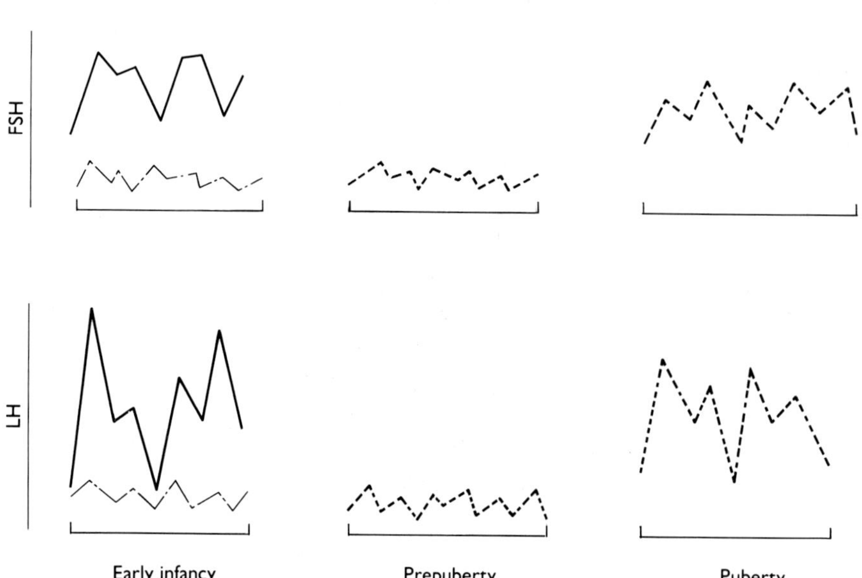

Fig. 14.17 Schematic diagram of the change in the pattern of pulsatile FSH and LH secretion in early infancy, childhood and puberty. There is a pronounced sex difference in amplitude between the male and female infant. After infancy the activity of gonadotrophin secretion diminishes during the juvenile pause which lasts for almost a decade.

Growth hormone

Growth hormone (GH) secretion increases at the time of puberty, apparently due to increased secretion of sex steroids [68]. Children with delayed puberty lack this rise, and may even approximate the concentrations of GH seen in GH deficiency. Thus the diagnosis of GH secretion becomes problematic in delayed puberty.

Control of the hypothalamo – pituitary – gonadal axis

Episodic secretion of gonadotrophins appears to be an intrinsic property of the hypothalamic neurons that produce and secrete GnRH. All gonadotrophin secretion is episodic in normal physiological circumstances [69].

Negative-feedback inhibition is manifest when sex steroids decrease pituitary LH and FSH secretion at the hypothalamic and pituitary levels. Inhibin exerts a potent direct inhibitory effect upon FSH secretion at the pituitary level.

Positive feedback may be demonstrated at midpuberty in female subjects. Rising serum oestrogen secretion primes the gonadotrophs to produce LH until, at a critical stage at the middle of the menstrual period, a large surge of LH is released, causing ovulation [70].

Ontogeny of endocrine pubertal development
(Fig. 14.17)

The fetal hypothalamus contains GnRH-containing neurons by 14 weeks of gestation, and the fetal pituitary contains LH and FSH by 20 weeks [71]. The hypothalamo–pituitary portal system develops by 20 weeks of gestation, allowing hypothalamic GnRH to reach the pituitary gonadotrophs. Gonadotrophin secretion rises to extremely high values at midgestation with a decrease thereafter towards term. Elevated serum testosterone concentrations emanating from the fetal testes demonstrate the bioactivity of the fetal gonadotrophins. At term, gonadotrophin concentrations are lower than midgestation but still relatively high. However, the increased circulating oestrogen concentrations characteristic of gestation exert a restraining effect upon gonadotrophin secretion until after birth. Gonadotrophin values rise once again in an intermittent pattern after birth with episodic peaks noted for the 2–4

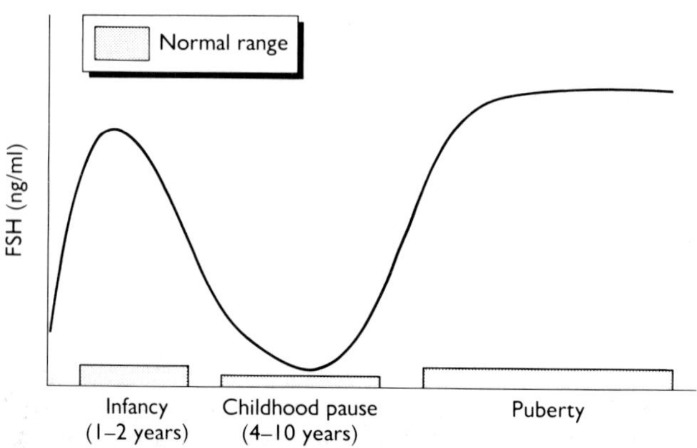

Fig. 14.18 The change in the pattern of the plasma concentration of FSH with age in patients with Turner syndrome (redrawn from data in Conte *et al.* [73]).

years after birth [72]. Oestrogen and testosterone from the infantile gonads also rise episodically during this period; however, mean serum values of gonadotrophins and sex steroids during infancy remain much lower than found in the fetus and the pubertal subject, but higher than found during the juvenile pause of approximately 4–9 years of age. Because sex steroids suppress gonadotrophin secretion to a significant degree during the first years after birth, agonadal patients such as those with Turner syndrome

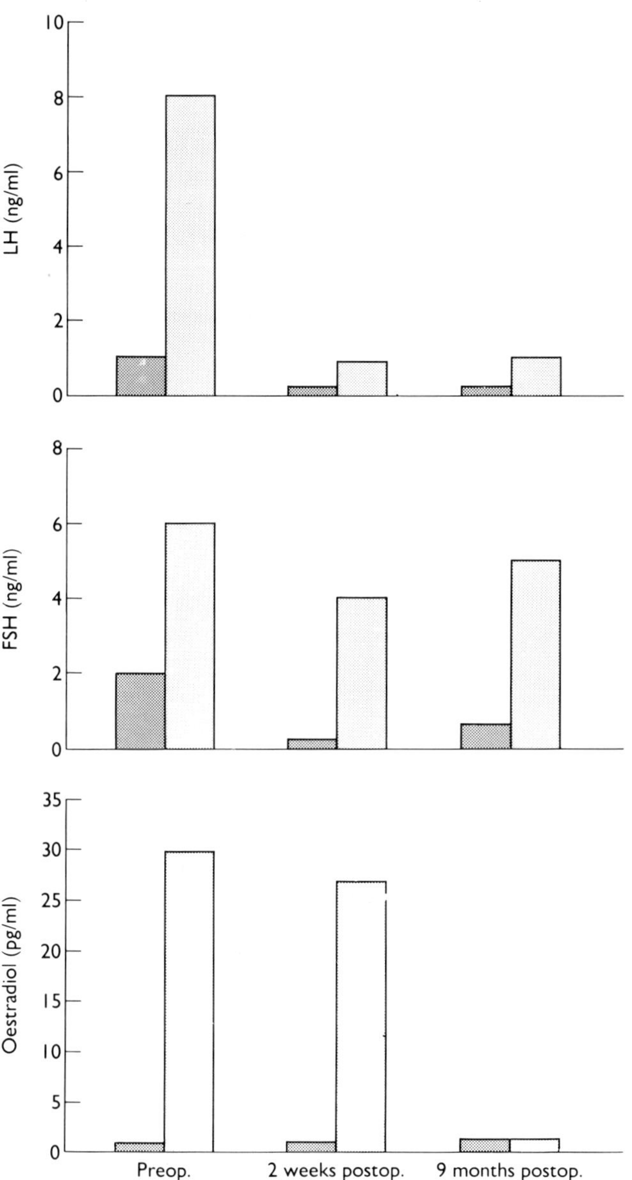

Fig. 14.19 The change in gonadotrophin and oestradiol secretion before and after removal of a subarachnoid cyst in a 3-year-old girl with central precocious puberty. The open bars indicate response to administration of 100 μg GnRH to test secretory activity. The closed bars are basal values (redrawn from data in Grumbach & Styne [33]).

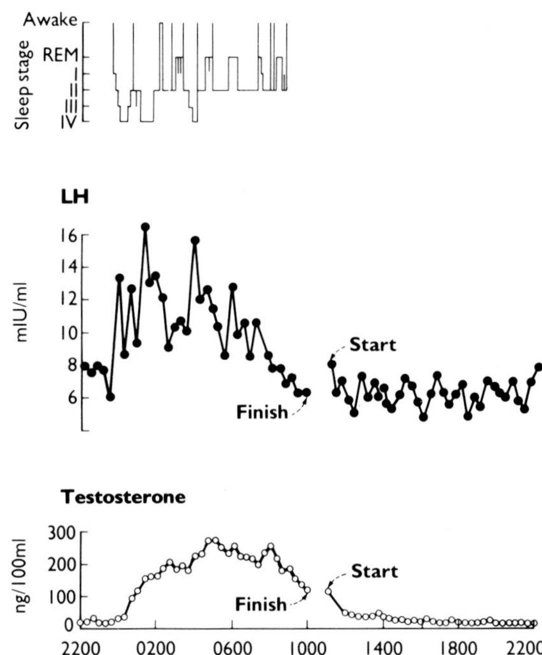

Fig. 14.20 Plasma LH and testosterone levels every 20 min in a 14-year-old boy in pubertal stage 2. The histogram displaying sleep stage sequence is depicted above the period of nocturnal sleep. Sleep stages are REM with stages I–IV shown by depth of line graph. Plasma LH (●) is expressed as mIU/ml. Plasma T (○) is expressed as ng/100 ml (from Boyar *et al.* [86]).

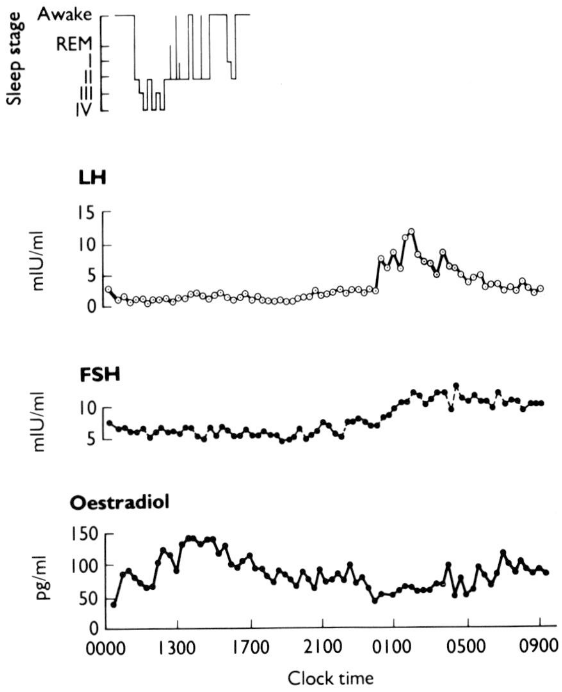

Fig. 14.21 Plasma LH, FSH and oestradiol in a 13.6-year-old girl in breast stage 3 studied as described in Fig. 14.20.

exhibit extremely high (castrate) values of serum gonadotrophins (Fig. 14.18) [73].

During the childhood pause, gonadotrophin concentrations and gonadal activity remain at a low level of activity, restrained by the CNS. Even in children without gonadal function, such as those with Turner syndrome, serum gonadotrophin concentrations are low, demonstrating that the presence of the gonads is not necessary to suppress gonadotrophin secretion during the childhood pause. Nonetheless, testosterone and oestrogen are measurable in the infant circulation, demonstrating low but definite activity of the infantile gonads.

While gonadotrophin secretion is suppressed during the juvenile pause, supersensitive assays now demonstrate pulsatile gonadotrophin secretion at the same frequency as noted during puberty, but at decreased amplitude [74, 75]. Thus the major change of puberty may involve the amount of gonadotrophin secreted, but not the timing of the pulses.

Particular clinical situations indicate the CNS restraint characteristic of the juvenile pause. Hydrocephalus, subarachnoid cysts or posterior hypothalamic tumours may destroy the restraining mechanism and allow central precocious puberty to progress as early as the first postnatal year. When some of these conditions are reversed, such as by the removal of the cyst or shunting of the hydrocephalus, puberty will cease (Fig. 14.19) [69]. Central precocious puberty may also occur due to a hamartoma of the tuber cinereum [76]. This mass of heterotopic hypothalamic tissue contains GnRH neurons and may secrete pulsatile GnRH during childhood due to lack of CNS restraint.

During the peripubertal period, prior to physical changes, gonadotrophin secretion rises first at night [77]. Sequential sampling demonstrates a rise in sex steroid secretion during the night also. Early morning serum testosterone values are higher just prior to the onset of secondary sexual development. As puberty progresses, the

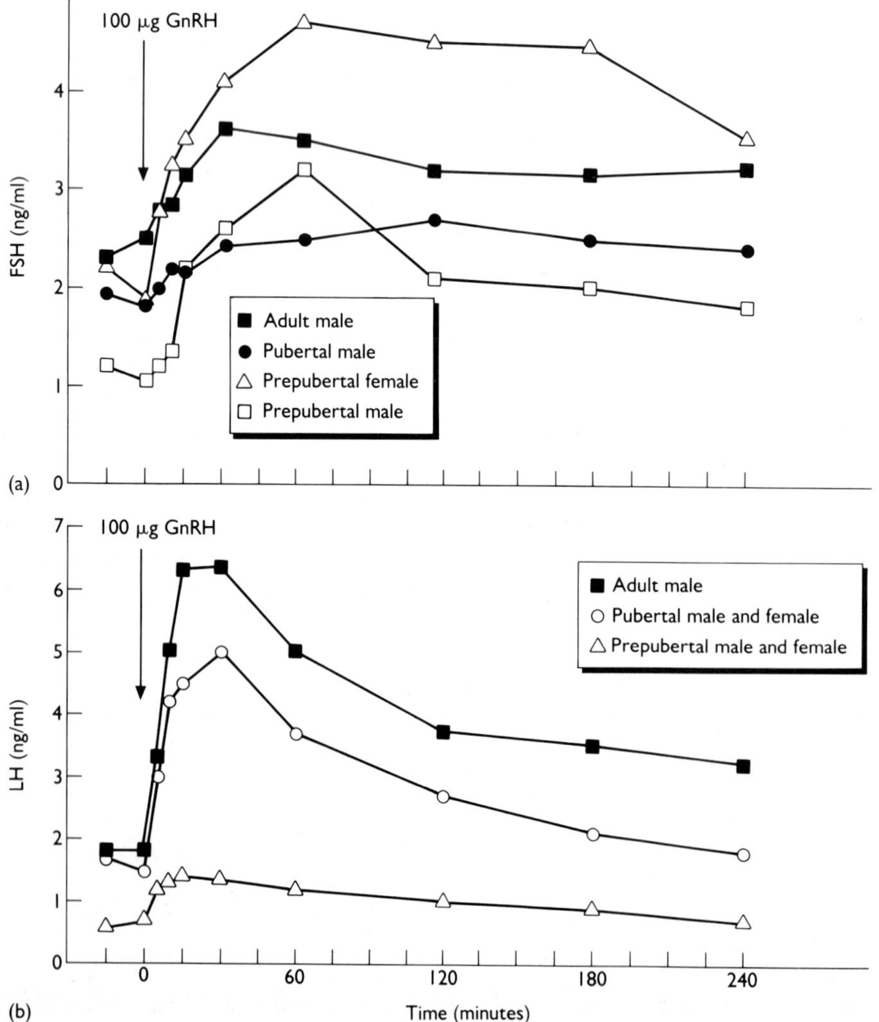

Fig. 14.22 (a) Basal FSH (LER 1364) and the peak and delta increment following intraverous GnRH (100 μg) are compared in normal prepubertal and pubertal females with IPP. (b) Schematic representation of the basal plasma LH (LER 960) and the peak and delta increment following intraverous GnRH (100 μg) are compared in normal prepubertal and pubertal females with the responses of females with IPP. The peak and delta increment of plasma LH is higher in IPP than in normal pubertal females (redrawn from data in Grumbach *et al.* [80]).

secretion of gonadotrophins occurs more during the day until no diurnal rhythm remains.

During the peripubertal period there is also a change in the response of pituitary gonadotrophs to exogenous GnRH administration [79]. The pattern of LH release increases, so that the adult pattern is achieved during puberty. The release of FSH shows no such change with development, although female subjects have more FSH release than male subjects at all developmental stages (Fig. 14.22).

This change in LH secretion after exogenous GnRH administration indicates a change in endogenous GnRH release with pubertal development. If GnRH is administered in low-dose boluses at 60–120-min intervals for 5 days a prepubertal subject will convert the pattern of gonadotrophin release and sex steroid secretion to a pubertal pattern of peaking LH values every 60–120 min [81]. Thus the pituitary response 'matures' with exogenous GnRH administration, suggesting that increasing endogenous GnRH secretion induces puberty in the same way. Patients with gonadotrophin deficiency can be treated with episodic GnRH boluses administered by a miniature programmable pump to induce secondary sexual development, menses and ovulation or spermatogenesis.

Gonadotrophin secretion is episodic, and individual serum samples may not demonstrate a clear pattern of change with puberty. Thus the determination of individual gonadotrophin concentrations is not a useful indication of the stage of puberty. New ultrasensitive assays can differentiate basal gonadotrophin concentrations in a subject in the prepubertal stage from a pubertal subject. Sex steroids, however, are less variable than gonadotrophin concentrations and show a general stepwise increase with each stage of puberty. Thus sex steroid determinations serve a better diagnostic purpose than the measurement of gonadotrophin concentrations in the assessment of puberty.

Positive feedback develops in females at approximately midpuberty [70]. By this process a rising concentration of oestrogen triggers the release of a bolus of LH from the pituitary gonadotrophs which stimulates ovulation. Thus a follicle must be of adequate size to produce appropriate oestrogen to exert the positive feedback effect, the pituitary gland must have sufficient readily releasable LH to affect a surge of LH release and the hypothalamus must be able to secrete adequate GnRH to cause the stimulation for pituitary release. These conditions do not develop until well into the pubertal process.

The first 2 years of menses are anovulatory in 55–90% of cycles. Not until 5 years after menarche are only 20% anovulatory [82,83]. Nonetheless, it is clear that girls may be fertile in many cases at midpuberty before physical sexual maturity.

ADRENARCHE

The adrenal androgens, dehydroepiandrosterone and androstenedione, produced by the zona reticularis, rise 2 or more years before gonadotrophins and sex steroids rise [84]. This process of adrenarche begins by 6–8 years of age in normal subjects, and continues until late puberty (Table 14.5).

The control of the increased activity of the adrenal gland at the time of secondary sexual development remains an enigma. In the absence of adrenocorticotrophin (ACTH) no change in the minimal secretion of these androgens occurs; but there is no change in ACTH secretion at adrenarche to explain the phenomenon, and ACTH appears to be necessary but not sufficient. Adrenarche occurs years before a rise in gonadotrophin secretion occurs, eliminating gonadotrophins as the cause of adrenarche. There may be an internal adrenal mechanism related to increasing size of the adrenal gland which causes adrenarche. Alternatively, there may be another pituitary hormone, as yet undiscovered, that triggers the process of adrenarche.

The presence or absence of adrenarche does not seem to influence the onset of puberty. Addisonian patients experience puberty at an appropriate age and children with premature adrenarche also enter gonadarche at a

Table 14.5 Mean serum concentrations of dehydroepiandrosterone sulphate during childhood

Chronological age (years)	1–6	6–8	8–10	10–12	12–14	14–16	16–20
Boys (μg/dl)	15.4 ± 6.8	18.8 ± 4.1	58.6 ± 10.1	126.4 ± 28.0	133.4 ± 22.2	264.3 ± 19.4	264.1 ± 61.8
Girls (μg/dl)	24.7 ± 11.1	30.4 ± 7.6	117.3 ± 41.7	112.7 ± 16.4	168.9 ± 19.3	253.5 ± 41.3	232.5 ± 49.8
Bone age (years)	**1–6**	**6–8**	**8–10**	**10–12**	**12–14**	**14–16**	**16–20**
Boys (μg/dl)	16.6 ± 6.1	36.3 ± 6.7	57.4 ± 8.5	125.0 ± 22.7	214.9 ± 30.1	403.4 ± 99.4	–
Girls (μg/dl)	2.5 ± 2.5	27.2 ± 9.6	–	112.9 ± 27.6	159.7 ± 26.3	261.0 ± 45.0	145.3 ± 32.2

From Reiter *et al.* [86].

normal age. Thus adrenarche is usually coordinated with gonadarche in the pubertal process, but appears not to play an important role in the progression of gonadarche.

REFERENCES

1 Grumbach MM. Onset of puberty. In: Berenberg SR, Leiden HW, Krose BV, eds. *Puberty, Biologic and Social Components*. Leiden: H.E. Stenfert Krose, 1975:1–21.

2 Tanner JM. Trend toward earlier menarche in London, Oslo, Copenhagen, the Netherlands and Hungary. *Nature* 1973;243: 95–7.

3 MacMahon B. Age at menarche. In: *National Survey DHEW Publication*, No. 133 (HRA), Series 11. Bethesda, MD, 1973:1.

4 Tanner M, Eveleth PB. In: Berenberg SR, ed. *Puberty, Biologic and Psychosocial Components*. Leiden: H.E. Stenfert Krose, 1975:256.

5 Zacharias LM, Rand M, Wurtman R. A prospective study of sexual development in American girls: the statistics of menarche. *Obstet Gynecol Surv* 1976;31:325–37.

6 Hartz AJ, Barboriak PN, Wong A. The association of obesity with infertility and related menstrual abnormalities in women. *Int J Obes* 1979;3:57–73.

7 Warren MP. The effects of exercise in pubertal progression and reproductive function in girls. *J Clin Endocrinol Metab* 1980;51:1150–70.

8 Marshall WA, Tanner JM. Variations in pattern of pubertal changes in girls. *Arch Dis Child* 1969;44:291–303.

9 Reynolds EL, Wines JV. Individualized differences in physical changes associated with adolescence in girls. *Am J Dis Child* 1948;75;329–50.

10 Rohn RD. Papilla (nipple) development during female puberty. *J Adolesc Hlth Care* 1982;2:217–20.

11 Dupertuis CW, Atkinson WB, Elftman H. Sex differences in pubic hair distribution. *Hum Biol* 1945;17:137–42.

12 Marshall WA, Tanner JM. Variations in the pattern of pubertal changes in boys. *Arch Dis Child* 1970;45:13–23.

13 Van Wieringen JD, Wafelbakker F, Verbrugge HP *et al*. *Growth Diagrams* 1965 Netherlands; Second National Survey on 0–24-year-olds. The Netherlands Institute for Preventative Medicine TNO. Groningen: Wolters-Noordhoff, 1971.

14 Peters H, Byskov AG, Grinsted J. Follicular growth in fetal and prepubertal ovaries of humans and other primates. *Clin Endocrinol Metab* 1978;7:469–85.

15 Ross, GT. Follicular development: the life cycle of the follicle and puberty. In: Grumbach MM, Sizonenko PC, Aubert ML, eds. *Control of the Onset of Puberty*. Baltimore: Williams & Wilkins, 1990:376–86.

16 Stanhope R, Adams RJ, Jacobs HS, Brook CG. Ovarian ultrasound assessment in normal children, idiopathic precocious puberty, and during low dose pulsatile gonadotrophin releasing hormone treatment of hypogonadotrophic hypogonadism. *Arch Dis Child* 1985;60:116–19.

17 Wheeler MD. Physical changes of puberty. In: Styne DM, ed. *Endocrinology and Metabolism Clinics of North America*. Philadelphia: W.B. Saunders, 1991;20:1–14.

18 Collett-Solberg PR, Grumbach MM. A simplified procedure for evaluating estrogenic effects and the sex chromatin pattern in exfoliated cells in urine: studies in premature thelarche and gynecomastia of adolescence. *J Pediatr* 1965;66:883–90.

19 Reynolds EL, Wines JV. Physical changes associated with adolescence in boys. *Am J Dis Child* 1951;82:529–47.

20 Zachmann M, Prader A, Kind HP *et al*. Testicular volume during adolescence. *Helv Paediatr Aca* 1974;29:61–72.

21 Gondos B, Kogan SJ. Testicular development during puberty. In: Grumbach MM, Sizonenko PC, Aubert ML, eds. *Control of Onset of Puberty*. Baltimore: Williams & Wilkins, 1990: 387–402.

22 Richardson DW, Short RV. Time of onset of sperm production in boys. *J Biosoc Sci* (Suppl.) 1978:15–25.

23 Nielsen CT, Skakkebaeck NE, Darling JA *et al*. Longitudinal study of testosterone and luteinizing hormone (LH) in relation to spermarche, pubic hair, height and sitting height in normal boys. *Acta Endocrinol* 1986;Suppl.279:98–106.

24 Carlson SE. Gynecomastia. *N Engl J Med* 1980;303:795–9.

25 Nuttall FQ. Gynecomastia as a physical finding in normal men. *J Clin Endocrinol Metab* 1979;48:338–40.

26 Karlberg P, Taranger J. The somatic development of children in a Swedish urban community. *Acta Paediatr Scand* 1976; Suppl.256:1–148.

27 Thompson GW, Popovich F, Anderson DL. Maximum growth changes in mandibular length, stature and weight. *Hum Biol* 1976;48:285.

28 Cheek DB. Body composition, hormones, nutrition and adolescent growth. In: Grumbach MM, Grave GD, Mayer FE, eds. *Control of the Onset of Puberty*. New York: John Wiley & Sons, 1974:424–47.

29 Tanner JM, Whitehouse RH, Marubini E, Resele LF. The adolescent growth spurt of boys and girls of the Harpenden Growth Study. *Ann Hum Biol* 1976;3:109–26.

30 Greulich WS, Pyle SI. *Radiographic Atlas of Skeletal Development of the Hand and Wrist*. Stanford, CA: Stanford University Press, 1959.

31 Largo RH, Gasser TH, Prado A. Analysis of the adolescent growth spurt using smoothing spline funcitions. *Ann Hum Biol* 1978;5:421–34.

32 Attie MK, Ramirez NR, Conte FA, Kaplan SL, Grumbach MM. The pubertal growth spurt in eight patients with true precocious puberty and growth hormone deficiency: evidence for a direct role of sex steroids. *J Clin Endocrinol Metab* 1990;71:975–83.

33 Grumbach MM, Styne DM. Puberty: ontogeny, neuroendocrinology, physiology and disorders. In: Wilson JD, Foster MD, eds. *Williams Textbook of Endocrinology*. Philadelphia: W.B. Saunders, 1992:1139–212.

34 Harris DA, Van Vliet G, Egli CA *et al*. Somatomedin-C in normal puberty and in true precocious puberty before and after treatment with a potent luteinizing hormone-releasing hormone agonist. *J Clin Endocrinol Metab* 1985;61:152–9.

35 Kattwinkel J, Taussig LM, Statland BE, Verter JI. The effects of age on alkaline phosphatase and other serologic liver function tests in normal subjects and patients with cystic fibrosis. *J Pediatr* 1973;82:234.

36 Harlan WR, Grillo GP, Coroni-Huntley J, Leaverton PE. Secondary sex characteristics of boys 12 to 17 years of age: The U.S. Health Examination Survey. *J Pediatr* 1979;95:293–7.

37 Harlan WR, Harlan EA, Grillo GP. Secondary sex characteristics of girls 12 to 17 years of age: The U.S. Health Examination Survey. *J Pediatr* 1980;96:1074–8.

38 Largo RH, Prader A. Pubertal development in Swiss girls. *Helv Paediatr Acta* 1983;38:229–43.

39 Largo RH, Prader A. Pubertal development in Swiss boys. *Helv Paediatr Acta* 1983;38:211–28.

40 Adelman JP, Mason AJ, Hayflick JS, Seeburg PH. Isolation of the gene and hypothalamic cDNA for the common precursor

of gonadotropin-releasing hormone and prolactin release-inhibiting factor in human and rat. *Proc Natl Acad Sci USA* 1986;83:179–83.

41 Schwanzel-Fuduka M, Bick MD, Pfaff DW. Luteinizing hormone-releasing hormone (LHRH)-expressing cells do not migrate normally in an inherited hypogonadal (Kallmann) syndrome. *Mol Brain Rese* 1989;6:11–326.

42 Hardelin JP, Levilliers J, Young J *et al.* Xp22.3 deletions in isolated familial Kallmann's syndrome. *J Clin Endocrinol Metab* 1993;76:827–31.

43 Gorski RA. Maturation of neural mechanisms and the pubertal process. In: Grumbach MM, Sizonenko PC, Aubert ML, eds. *Control of the Onset of Puberty*. Baltimore: Williams & Wilkins, 1990:259–81.

44 Crowley WF, Filicori M, Spratt DI, Santoro NF. The physiology of gonadotropin releasing hormone (GnRH) secretion in men and women. *Rec Prog Horm Res* 1985;41:473–526.

45 Reichlin S. Neuroendocrinology. In: Wilson J, Foster D, eds. *Williams Textbook of Endocrinology*. Philadelphia: W.B. Saunders, 1992:174–5.

46 Mellon PL, Windle JJ, Goldsmith PC, Padula CA, Roberts JL, Weiner RI. Immortalization of hypothalamic GnRH neurons by genetically targeted tumorigenesis. *Neuron* 1990;5:1–10.

47 Belchetz PE, Plant TM, Nakai Y, Keogh EJ, Knobil E. Hypophyseal responses to continuous and intermittent delivery of hypothalamic gonadotropin-releasing hormone. *Science* 1978; 202:631–3.

48 Huckle W, Conn PM. Molecular mechanism of gonadotropin releasing hormone action II. The effector system. *Endocrine Rev* 1988;9:387–95.

49 Hazum E, Conn PM. Molecular mechanism of gonadotropin releasing hormone (GnRH) action. The GnRH receptor. *Endocrine Rev* 1988;9:379–86.

50 Kaplan SL, Grumbach MM. Pathogenesis of sexual precocity. In: Grumbach MM, Sizonenko PC, Aubert ML, eds. *Control of the Onset of Puberty*. Baltimore: Williams & Wilkins, 1990:620–68.

51 Pierce JG, Parsone TF. Glycoprotein hormones: structure and function. *Annu Rev Biochem* 1981;50:465–95.

52 Fiddes JC, Talmadge K. Structure, expression, and evolution of the genes for the human glycoprotein hormones. *Rec Prog Horm Res* 1984;40:43–78.

53 Kovacs K, Horvath E. Gonadotrophs following removal of the ovaries: a fine structural study of human pituitary glands. *Endokrinologie* 1975;66:1–8.

54 Jenner MR, Kelch RP, Kaplan SL, Grumbach MM. Hormonal changes in puberty IV. Plasma estradiol, LH, and FSH in prepubertal children, pubertal females, and in precocious puberty, premature thelarche, hypogonadism, and in a child with a feminizing ovarian tumor. *J Clin Endocrinol Metab* 1972;34:521–30.

55 August GP, Grumbach MM, Kaplan SL. Hormonal changes in puberty. III. Correlation of plasma testosterone, LH, FSH, testicular size and bone age with male pubertal development. *J Clin Endocrinol Metab* 1972;34:319–26.

56 Means AR, Fakunding JL, Huckins C *et al.* Follicle-stimulating hormone, the Sertoli cell, and spermatogenesis. *Rec Prog Horm Res* 1976;32:477–527.

57 Doody KJ, Lorence MC, Mason IJ *et al.* Expression of messenger ribonucleic acid species encoding steroidogenic enzymes in human follicles and corpora lutea throughout the menstrual cycle. *J Clin Endocrinol Metab* 1990;70:1041–5.

58 Carr BR. Disorders of the ovary and female reproductive tract. In: Wilson JD, Foster DW, eds. *Williams textbook of Endocrinology*. Philadelphia: W.B. Saunders, 1992:745.

59 Reiter EO, Beitins IZ, Ostrea TR *et al.* Bioassayable luteinizing hormone during childhood and adolescence and in patients with delayed pubertal development. *J Clin Endocrinol Metab* 1982;54:155–61.

60 Beitins IZ, Padmanabhan V. Bioactivity of gonadotropins. In: Styne DM, ed. *Endocrinology and Metabolism Clinics of North America*. Philadelphia: W.B. Saunders, 1991;20:85–120.

61 Bartsch W, Horst HJ, Derwah KM. Interrelationships between sex hormone-binding globulin and 17 beta-estradiol, testosterone, 5 alpha-dihydrotestosterone, thyroxine, and triiodothyronine in prepubertal and pubertal girls. *J Clin Endocrinol Metab* 1980;50:1053–6.

62 Lubahn DB, Joseph DR, Sullivan PM *et al.* Cloning of the human androgen receptor complementary DNA and localization to the X chromosome. *Science* 1988;240:327–30.

63 Horst HJ, Bartsch W, Dirksen-Thedens I. Plasma testosterone, sex hormone binding globulin capacity and per cent binding of testosterone and 5 alpha-dihydrotestosterone in prepubertal and adult males. *J Clin Endocrinol Metab* 1977;45:522–7.

64 Reichlin, S. Neuroendocrine regulation of prolactin secretion. *Adv Biosci* 1988;69:277–92.

65 De Jong FH. Inhibin. *Physiol Rev* 1988;68:555–607.

66 Hudson PL, Douglas I, Donahoe PK *et al.* An immunoassay to detect human Mullerian inhibiting substance in males and females during normal development. *J Clin Endocrinol Metab* 1990;70:16–22.

67 Josso N, Legeai L, Forest MG, Chaussain J, Brauner R. An enzyme linked immunoassay for anti-Mullerian hormone: a new tool for the evaluation of testicular function in infants and children. *J Clin Endocrinol Metab* 1990;70:23–7.

68 Martha PM Jr, Rogol AD, Veldhuis JD. Alterations in the pulsatile properties of circulating growth hormone concentrations during puberty in boys. *J Clin Endocrinol Metab* 1989; 69:563–70.

69 Grumbach MM, Kaplan SL. The neuroendocrinology of human puberty: an ontogenetic perspective. In: Grumbach MM, Sizonenko PC, Aubert ML, eds. *Control of the Onset of Puberty*. Baltimore: Williams & Wilkins, 1990:1–68.

70 Reiter EO, Kulin HE, Hamwood SM. The absence of positive feedback between estrogen and luteinizing hormone in sexually immature girls. *Pediatr Res* 1974;8:740–5.

71 Gluckman PD, Grumbach MM, Kaplan SL. The neuroendocrine regulation and function of growth hormone and prolactin in the mammalian fetus. *Endocr Rev* 1981;2:363–95.

72 Forest MG. Pituitary gonadotropin and sex steroid secretion during the first two years of life. In: Grumbach MM, Sizonenko PC, Aubert ML, eds. *Control of the Onset of Puberty*. Baltimore: Williams & Wilkins, 1990:451–78.

73 Conte FA, Grumbach MM, Kaplan SL, Reiter EO. Correlation of LRF-induced LH and FSH release from infancy to 19 years with the changing pattern of gonadotropin secretion in agonadal patients: relation to the restraint of puberty. *J Clin Endocrinol Metab* 1980;50:163–8.

74 Goji K, Tanikaze S. Comparison between spontaneous gonadotropin concentration profiles and gonadotropin response to low dose gonadotropin-releasing hormone in prepubertal and early pubertal boys and patients with hypogonadotropic hypogonadism: assessment by using ultrasensitive, time-resolved immunofluorometric assay. *Pediatr Res* 1992; 31(5):535–9.

75 Dunkel L, Alfthan H, Stenman U, Perheentupa J. Gonadal control of pulsatile secretion of luteinizing hormone and follicle-stimulating hormone in prepubertal boys evaluated by ultrasensative time-resolved immunofluorometric assays. *J Clin Endocrinol Metab* 1990;70:107–14.

76 Judge DM, Kulin HE, Santen R, Trapukdi S. Hypothalamic hamartoma: a source of luteinizing-hormone-releasing factor in precocious puberty. *N Engl J Med* 1977;296:7–10.

77 Boyar R, Finkelstein J, Roffwarg H, Kapen S, Weitzman ED, Hellman L. Synchronization of augmented luteinizing hormone secretion with sleep during puberty. *N Engl J Med* 1972;287:582–6.

78 Reiter EO, Beitins IZ, Ostrea T, Gutai JP. Bioassayable luteinizing hormone during childhood and adolescence and in patients with delayed pubertal development. *J Clin Endocrinol Metab* 1982;54:155–61.

79 Roth JC, Grumbach MM, Kaplan SL. Effect of synthetic luteinizing hormone-releasing factor on serum testosterone and gonadotropins in prepubertal, pubertal, and adult males. *J Clin Endocrinol Metab* 1973;37:680–6.

80 Grumbach MM, Roth JC, Kaplan SL *et al.* Hypothalamic-pituitary regulation of puberty in man: Evidence and concepts derived from clinical research. In: Grumbach MM, Grave GD, Mayer FE, eds. *Control of the Onset of Puberty.* New York: John Wiley & Sons, 1974:115–66.

81 Corley KP, Valk TW, Kelch RP, Marshall JC. Estimation of GnRH pulse amplitude during pubertal development. *Pediatr Res* 1981;15:157–62.

82 Apter D, Vihko R. Serum pregnenolone, progesterone, 17-hydroxyprogesterone, testosterone and 5 alpha-dihydrotestosterone during female puberty. *J Clin Endocrinol Metab* 1977;45:1039–48.

83 Lemarchand-Beraud T, Zufferey MM, Reymond M. Maturation of the hypothalamo-pituitary ovarian axis in adolescent girls. *J Clin Endocrinol Metab* 1982;54:241–6.

84 Grumbach MM, Richards GE, Conte FA, Kaplan SL. Clinical disorders of adrenal function and puberty: an assessment of the role of the adrenal cortex in normal and abnormal puberty in man and evidence for an ACTH-like pituitary adrenal androgen stimulating hormone. In: Serio M, ed. *The Endocrine Function of the Human Adrenal Cortex.* Serono Symposium. New York: Academic Press, 1977:583–612.

85 Waaler PE, Thorsen T, Stoa KF *et al.* Studies in normal male puberty. *Acta Paediatr Scand* (Suppl.) 1974:1–36.

86 Boyar RM, Rosenfeld RS, Kapen S *et al.* Simultaneous augmented secretion of luteinizing hormone and testosterone during sleep. *J Clin Invest* 1974;54:609–18.

15: Disorders of Puberty

N.A. BRIDGES and C.G.D. BROOK

INTRODUCTION

The timing and pattern of physical development in males and females at puberty follow a relatively consistent pattern. In girls breast enlargement is usually the first sign of puberty, but pubic hair development follows soon after, and menarche does not occur until the attainment of Tanner breast stage 4 or 5. In boys, genital growth and pubic hair development keep pace with testicular enlargement. Pubertal development is abnormal if this normal consonance of development is lost, or if the events of puberty occur at the wrong time. Clinically, disorders of puberty present with the development of signs of puberty at an abnormally early age, failure to develop at an appropriate age (pubertal delay or pubertal failure), or with problems of development at an age appropriate for puberty.

SEXUAL PRECOCITY

Sexual precocity is defined by the appearance of secondary sexual characteristics before 8 years of age in a girl or before 9 years in a boy. This development may be consonant, with a normal temporal relationship between the development of the various physical features of puberty, the timing of menarche and the pubertal growth spurt. The development may not be consonant, with breast development alone (premature thelarche), pubic and axillary hair development alone (signs of adrenarche) or loss of consonance between the development of the different physical features of puberty (for example, the virilization seen in untreated congenital adrenal hyperplasia results in genital and pubic hair development but no increase in testicular volume). This distinction is important to the differential diagnosis of precocious puberty, which is summarized in Table 15.1. Table 15.2 gives the proportion of individuals in each diagnostic group seen over a 15-year period at the Middlesex Hospital. Less than 10% of those seen were boys.

CENTRAL PRECOCIOUS PUBERTY

In centrally mediated precocious puberty there is premature activation of the hypothalamopituitary–gonadal axis. The pattern of endocrine changes (Fig. 15.1) is the same as that seen in normal puberty and the pubertal development is consonant. The majority of cases are idiopathic and all are girls (over the past 15 years there has been no case of idiopathic central precocious puberty in a boy at the Middlesex Hospital, compared with 85 girls). The sex incidence of central precocious puberty secondary to cerebral lesions is equal. Hydrocephalus, tumours (for example, hamartoma, optic nerve gliomas and pineal tumours) and trauma can all cause central precocious puberty [1–3]. A number of rare congenital syndromes have been described associated with central precocious puberty, for example 'Kabuki make-up syndrome' [4]. The clinical features of sexual precocity in these individuals do not appear to differ from those of individuals with idiopathic central precocious puberty.

Girls who have had cranial radiotherapy (for example those who have had prophylactic radiotherapy for leukaemia), have an increased incidence of precocious puberty [5]. Girls who have been adopted from developing coutries have been documented to have an increased incidence of early puberty, earlier than that seen either in their country of origin or their adoptive country [6]. Sexual abuse has been reported as a precipitating cause of central precocious puberty, and in these cases the development can regress with a change in environment [7].

GONADOTROPHIN-INDEPENDENT PRECOCIOUS PUBERTY

In gonadotrophin-independent precocious puberty there is secretion of sex steroids from the gonads accompanied by low gonadotrophin levels [8]. The pubertal development is not necessarily consonant, because the pattern of endocrine changes seen is not the same as in normal puberty (for example, menstruation may occur at an inappropriately early stage of breast development). Most

Table 15.1 Causes of precocious puberty

Centrally mediated precocious puberty (consonant pubertal development)
Idiopathic – exclusively female
Secondary – equal sex distribution
Tumours
Hydrocephalus
Trauma
Radiotherapy
Sexual abuse
Abnormal patterns of gonadotrophin secretion
Premature thelarche
Thelarche variant
Hypothyroidism
Gonadotrophin-independent precocious puberty
Testotoxicosis
McCune–Albright syndrome
Virilization
Adrenarche
Congenital adrenal hyperplasia
Cushing disease
Adrenal tumours
Others
Gonadotrophin or sex-steroid-secreting tumours
Exogenous steroids

Table 15.2 Diagnosis of 213 children presenting to the Middlesex Hospital with signs of sexual precocity over a 15-year period (numbers of patients in brackets)

Girls 92% (n = 197)	Boys 8% (n = 16)
Idiopathic central precocious puberty 39% (85)	Secondary central precocious puberty 2% (4)
Secondary central precocious puberty 1.5% (3)	Gonadotrophin-independent precocious puberty 1% (2)
Premature thelarche 24.5% (52)	Undertreated congenital adrenal hyperplasia 1% (2)
Thelarche variant 14% (30)	Adrenarche 4% (8)
Hypothyroidism 0.5% (1)	
Adrenarche 9.5% (20)	
Gonadotrophin-independent precocious puberty 3% (6)	

children with this disorder have either testotoxicosis [9], which is familial, or McCune–Albright syndrome, which has an equal sex distribution and is not inherited. Some children appear to have neither disorder, and it is possible that the abnormality described in McCune–Albright syndrome could be expressed only in the gonadal tissue of these individuals.

In McCune–Albright syndrome the sexual precocity is associated with polyostotic fibrous dysplasia of bone and patches of skin pigmentation with a characteristic serrated edge (Fig. 15.2). Girls may have large ovarian cysts at ultrasound [10]. An abnormality of the intracellular messenger of gonadotrophin action, the G protein, has been described in individuals with McCune–Albright syndrome. The G protein activates pyruvate kinase within the cell when gonadotrophin binds to the receptor. In normal individuals this activation occurs for a limited time, but the abnormality of the G protein in McCune–Albright syndrome results in the continued activation of pyruvate kinase and steroid secretion without gonadotrophin stimulation [11,12].

It has been suggested that the mutation which causes the G protein defect occurs during embryonic development, and that individuals with McCune–Albright syndrome are mosaic for the mutation, because the expression of the abnormality in every cell would not be compatible with life [13]. This would explain the variable expression seen in the condition. Hyperfunction of other endocrine glands has been described in McCune–Albright syndrome, presumably due to the manifestation of the G protein abnormality in other cell lines [14]. Less is known about the defect in testotoxicosis. In a study in monkeys, injections of plasma from boys with testotoxicosis resulted in a rise in testosterone, suggesting that the defect is secondary to a circulating stimulatory factor [15].

PREMATURE THELARCHE AND THELARCHE VARIANT

In premature thelarche there is breast development without other signs of puberty. Growth velocity is normal and bone age is not advanced. Sometimes the breast development has been present from infancy and there may be a history of fluctuation in size. Girls with premature thelarche have a characteristic pattern of pulsatile follicle-stimulating hormone (FSH) secretion which is unlike that seen in normal puberty, where luteinizing hormone (LH) predominates (Fig. 15.3) [16]. Pelvic ultrasound may demonstrate ovarian cysts, which are presumably caused by the stimulatory action of FSH (Fig. 15.4) [17]. Geographical clusters of cases of premature thelarche have been reported in which environmental factors such as the use of oestrogens in chicken rearing have been implicated [18].

It is not always easy to classify girls with isolated breast development because not all of them fit the criteria for premature thelarche. Some have an increase in growth velocity and an advanced bone age. We have called this condition thelarche variant because the girls have a variant pattern of pulsatile gonadotrophin secretion with FSH predominant, which does not resemble that seen in normal puberty and appears to be intermediate between premature thelarche and central precocious puberty. Pelvic ultrasound appearances are also intermediate between those seen in premature thelarche and central precocious puberty (Fig. 15.4) [19]. We suspect that this condition is quite common, and it has been described elsewhere as a 'slowly progressive variant of precocious puberty in girls' [20]. Final height is not affected in premature thelarche and thelarche variant.

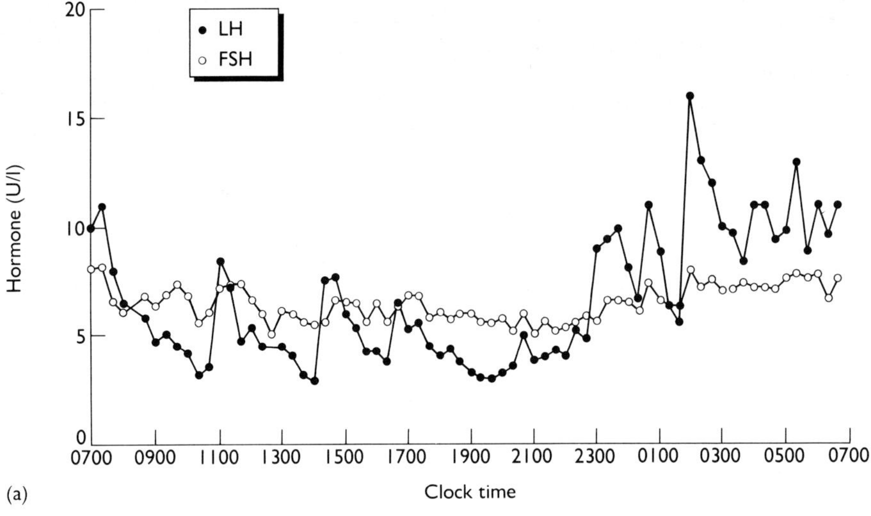

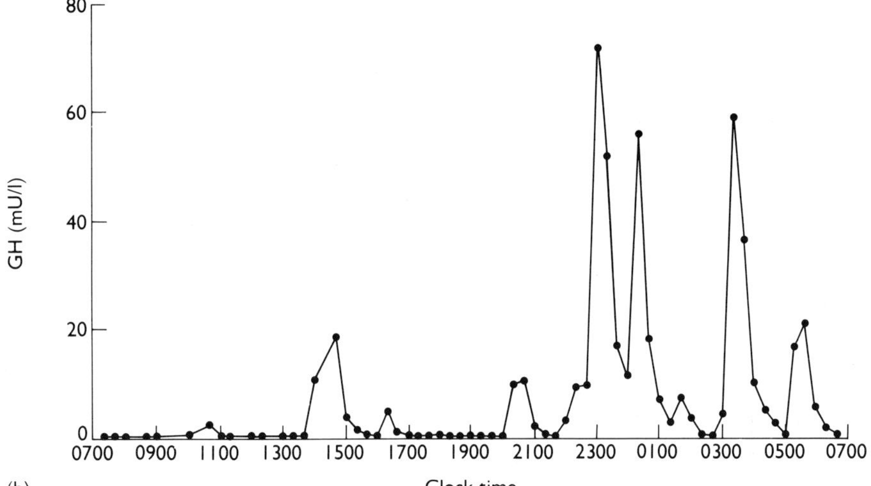

Fig. 15.1 Gonadotrophin and growth hormone (GH) secretion in centrally mediated precocious puberty. 24-h profile (using 20-min sampling) of (a) LH and FSH and (b) GH secretion in a girl of 5 years presenting with consonant pubertal development. The pattern of gonadotrophin and GH secretion is the same as that seen in normally timed puberty.

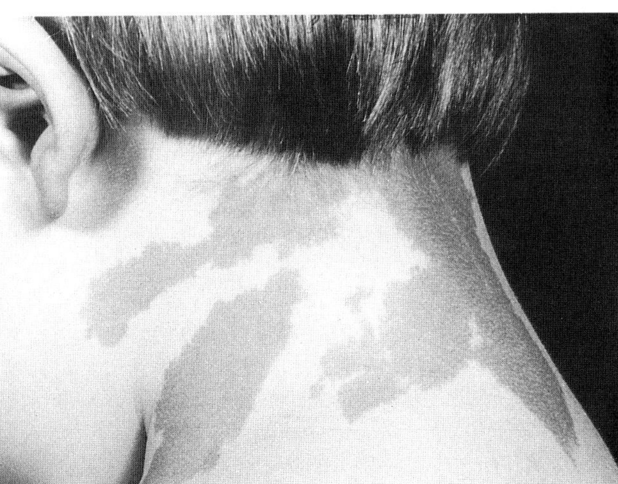

Fig. 15.2 Skin pigmentation in the McCune–Albright syndrome.

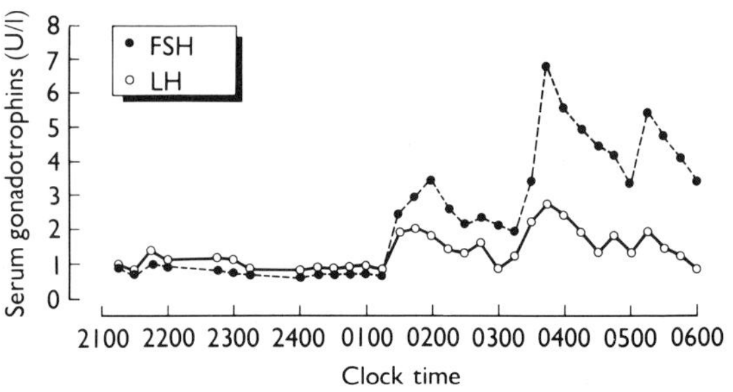

Fig. 15.3 Twenty-four-hour profile of serum gonadotrophin concentrations in premature thelarche.

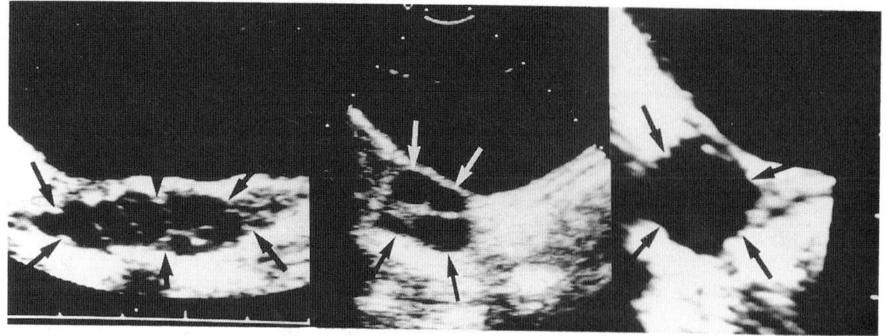

Fig. 15.4 Ovarian ultrasound appearances in premature thelarche (right-hand panel), thelarche variant (centre) and central precocious puberty (left-hand panel).

HYPOTHYROIDISM

Some children with primary hypothyroidism and elevated thyroid-stimulating hormone (TSH) levels also have increased FSH secretion, which may be sufficient to stimulate gonadal steroidogenesis. The development is not consonant; girls typically have breast development without pubic hair development and boys have some genital changes with more testicular enlargement than would be expected, but no pubic hair. FSH concentrations fall with treatment, but the elevated sex steroid levels may 'mature' the hypothalamus and stimulate puberty at an inappropriately early age. This may affect the final height [21,22].

SEXUAL PRECOCITY DUE TO ADRENAL ANDROGENS

At the age of 5–7 years the zona reticularis develops in the adrenal cortex and starts to secrete adrenal androgens. These cause an increase in growth velocity (the midchildhood growth spurt), and often the secretion of apocrine sweat. In a few children there is development of pubic and axillary hair with no other features of puberty. This has been called premature adrenarche or pubarche, but it occurs within the normal age range for adrenarche and the signs are probably a normal variant.

There may be a marked increase in growth velocity and an advance in bone age, but final height is not affected [23]. The reason why some children develop these features at adrenarche is not known: they could be more sensitive to the androgens produced, or they could represent those at the top of the normal range for secretion. There is no evidence that the spontaneous androgen secretion of these children is abnormal, although some investigators using adrenocorticotrophic hormone (ACTH) testing have suggested that there is an increased prevalence of minor defects of adrenal steroidogenesis (such as late-onset 21-hydroxylase deficiency) [24]. Premature adrenarche is more common in children of Mediterranean, Indian and African ancestry. Some of these children present with height over the 97th centile and marked bone age advance (Fig. 15.5). Final height is normal, and this picture probably represents a racial variant of midchildhood growth.

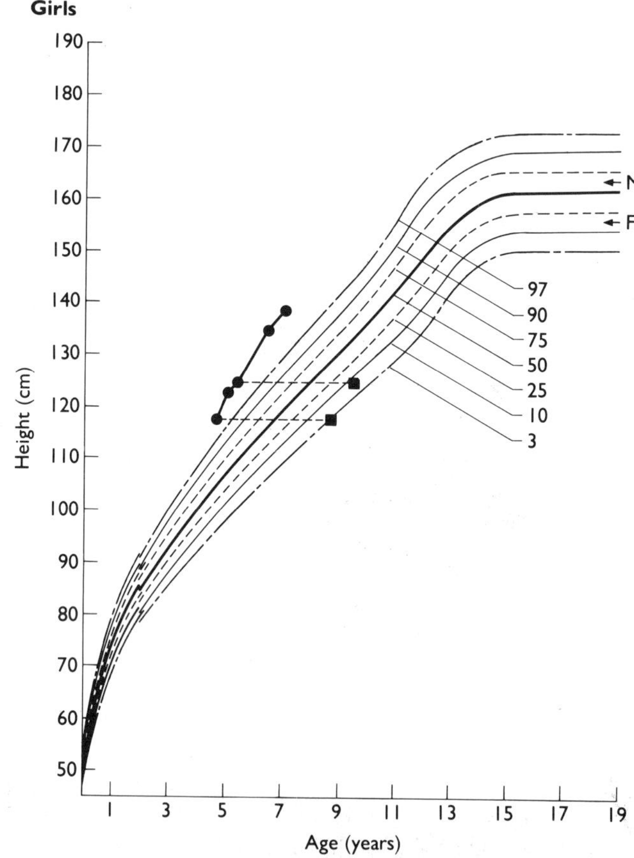

Fig. 15.5 Premature adrenarche. This girl of West Indian origin presented at 4.6 years with pubic and axillary hair. Height is over the 97th centile and bone age is advanced but height velocity is normal. The height prediction remains appropriate for the child's parents. This extreme form of premature adrenarche probably represents a racial variant of midchildhood growth. F, Father's height centile; M, Mother's height centile; ■, bone ages.

Untreated or undertreated congenital adrenal hyperplasia (CAH) may present with virilization. In the severe classical forms of CAH, girls are usually diagnosed at birth because of virilization and boys because of a salt-losing crisis. In less severely expressed enzyme defects, boys may not manifest salt loss and may present with axillary and pubic hair development, penile growth, and pigmentation of the scrotum without testicular enlargement in early childhood. Girls may present with pubic and axillary hair, acne and, sometimes, cliteromegaly. Both boys and girls become tall for their families, and bone age is usually advanced. Centrally mediated precocious puberty is common because of the maturational effect of androgens on the hypothalamus, and this may further compromise final height [25].

The virilization induced by an adrenocortical adenoma or carcinoma normally has a short history, and is characterized by increased growth velocity. The clinical picture may be of virilization alone, but there may be also be hypersecretion of cortisol inducing Cushing syndrome. Feminizing adrenal tumours have also been described, but are extremely rare. The distinction between adrenal tumour, CAH or signs of adrenarche may be very difficult on clinical grounds alone, and children in whom this diagnosis is suspected should be investigated (see below).

Treatment of tumours is by surgical resection, but neither operative findings nor histology are of much help in determining prognosis. An immediate fall in serum or urinary androgen markers of tumour secretion is encouraging and, in these children, adjuvant chemotherapy (mitotane) or radiotherapy has not been demonstrated to improve long-term prognosis [26]. In a group of 156 adults with the disease, 5-year survival after surgery was 34% [27]. Survival was better in younger patients. There are no large series of paediatric patients, but the prognosis should be guarded even where there is apparent complete resection.

OTHER CAUSES OF SEXUAL PRECOCITY

Gonadotrophin- or sex steroid-secreting tumours are an extremely rare cause of sexual precocity. Gonadotrophins are usually secreted in the form of human chorionic gonadotrophin (hCG). Most of these tumours are intracranial, such as pineal germ cell tumours and teratomas, and almost all of the patients are male [28,29]. hCG secretion has also been described in hepatoblastomas and teratomas [30]. Tumour markers such as α-fetoprotein and pregnancy-specific β_1-glycoprotein may be produced by hCG-secreting tumours [29]. Gonadotrophin-secreting adenomas of the pituitary have been described in children. These tumours demonstrate an abnormal increase in the secretion of LH in response to thyrotrophin-releasing hormone (TRH) [31].

Testosterone-secreting Leydig cell tumours of the testis are associated with virilization, but there may also be gynaecomastia with elevated oestradiol concentrations, because of aromatization of testosterone to oestradiol within the tumour. Granulosa cell and germ cell tumours of the ovary have been described which secrete both androgens or oestradiol. Ascites may be a feature, even if the tumour has not metastasized [32].

Problems of sexual precocity

Psychological problems occur in central precocious puberty both because pubertal levels of sex steroids in young children result in disruptive behaviour and because the child looks so much older than its true age. Most children experience some problems at school, which are frequently compounded by the difficulties that teachers and other children have in understanding the problem [33]. The child and his or her family may later have problems dealing with normally timed pubertal development, and are frequently apprehensive about stopping suppressive treatment. In girls, menstruation at an early age presents practical difficulties.

In precocious puberty the pubertal growth spurt occurs in the same manner as in normally timed puberty [34], but it commences when insufficient childhood growth has been completed. The situation is identical to the cause of the differences in adult heights of normal men and women: women are smaller than men because the puberty growth spurt starts early in the sequence of pubertal events at a height about 10 cm less than that of the take-off of the spurt in men. The spurts are of similar magnitude, so this delay (the continuation of childhood growth for a further 2 years) is the main cause of the final height differences. The management of tall predicted stature by inducing puberty at an appropriate height (page 202) is an example of turning this phenomenon to advantage.

Pubertal levels of sex steroids result in rapid bone age advance. This means that the child will initially be tall and have an increased growth velocity. The rapid bone age advance results in diminishing potential for adult height (Fig. 15.6). Children with precocious puberty may present with tall stature, but their height prediction is diminished at presentation, and final height is reduced in both centrally mediated precocious puberty and gonadotrophin-independent precocious puberty [35,36].

Assessment of sexual precocity

Any child with signs of sexual precocity should have his or her height measured, a bone age, and Tanner pubertal stage recorded. If there is any doubt about an apparently benign diagnosis, growth velocity and pubertal progress should be monitored for at least a year. The diagnosis of premature thelarche or of signs of adrenarche requires that a lack of pubertal progress is documented.

The combination of consonant pubertal development with a pattern of LH, FSH and sex steroid secretion ident-

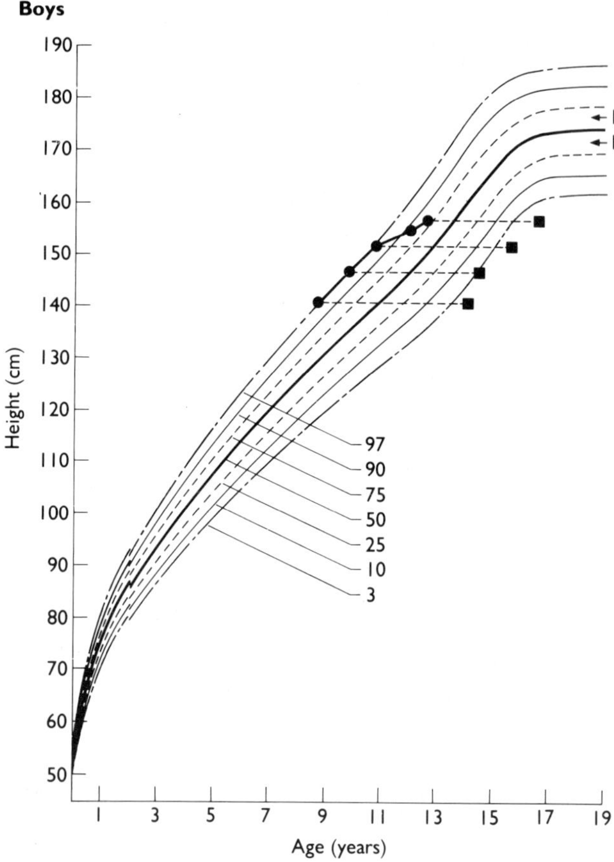

Fig. 15.6 Growth chart for a boy with untreated central precocious puberty. The boy presented at the age of 8 years with centrally mediated precocious puberty secondary to a hypthalamic hamartoma with a testicular volume of 8 ml. Rapid growth accompanied by bone age advance resulted in a diminishing height prediction. F, Father's height centile; M, Mother's height centile; ■, bone ages.

ical to that seen in normal puberty (see Fig. 15.1) confirms the diagnosis of central precocious puberty. Ultrasound findings of multicystic ovaries and an appropriately enlarging uterus support the diagnosis.

Gonadotrophins and sex steroids are secreted in a pulsatile manner, and there is a circadian variation with concentrations of gonadotrophins highest at night and sex steroids highest in the early morning. Spot samples of sex steroid or gonadotrophin concentrations are rarely informative, but the response to gonadotrophin-releasing hormone (GnRH) stimulation may be useful. Normal prepubertal children have an increment of 3–4 IU/l LH and 2–3 IU/l FSH in response to 100 μg given intravenously: regardless of age, the increment will be greater in puberty [37]. The response in premature thelarche and adrenarche will be prepubertal. In gonadotrophin-independent precocious puberty sex steroids are secreted in the absence of gonadotrophins. Spontaneous gonadotrophin secretion is suppressed by the autonomous sex steroid secretion, baseline concentrations are low and a response to GnRH absent.

As idiopathic central precocious puberty in boys has not been seen by us, or reported in any large series, boys should be presumed to have a central lesion and must have a cranial computerized tomography (CT) scan or magnetic resonance image (MRI) undertaken. The sex incidence of intracranial lesions is equal, and girls with precocious puberty outnumber boys 20 times, so most girls have idiopathic central precocious puberty and do not require imaging. CT or MRI should be performed in any girl with signs of increased intracranial pressure or neurological signs, but sexual precocity is rarely the presenting complaint and the diagnosis usually follows the documentation of a neurological lesion.

All girls with sexual precocity should have transabdominal ultrasound examination of the pelvis [38]. If the bladder is full, the uterus and ovaries can be visualized in even the youngest girls, and measurements of the length of the uterus, diameter at fundus and cervix and endometrial thickness should be made. Ovarian volume can be calculated using the formula for an oblate ovoid (the ovary is measured in three directions, and volume = dimension 1 × dimension 2 × dimension 3 × 0.5233) [39]. Prepubertally the fundus of the uterus is narrower than, or the same size as, the cervix and in early puberty the fundus expands and the uterus starts to adopt a pear shape (the diameter of the fundus becomes greater than that of the cervix) (Fig. 15.7). In central precocious puberty the changes are the same as those seen in normal puberty, but in premature thelarche or thelarche variant the uterus remains prepubertal in shape. A few girls apparently presenting with premature thelarche are in fact in the earliest stages of central precocious puberty [40], and ultrasound is helpful in distinguishing them. Endometrial thickening indicates pubertal concentrations of oestrogen, and an endometrium of 5 mm or over suggests that menarche is imminent (Fig. 15.7).

The neonatal ovary may be active with multiple large follicles because of the relatively high levels of gonadotrophins seen at this age. Activity decreases as the gonadotrophin levels fall, but individual follicles more than 4 mm across appear intermittently throughout childhood. Ovaries with multiple larger follicles do not develop until just before puberty (multicystic ovaries, defined as more than six follicles more than 4 mm across [41]) (Fig. 15.8). The ovaries increase in volume throughout childhood, and there is an increase in growth rate before puberty [42]. In central precocious puberty the ovaries are active with multiple follicles with diameters over 4 mm. Larger cysts are sometimes seen in McCune–Albright syndrome and premature thelarche [10,17]. When central precocious puberty is treated the uterus does not return to a prepu-

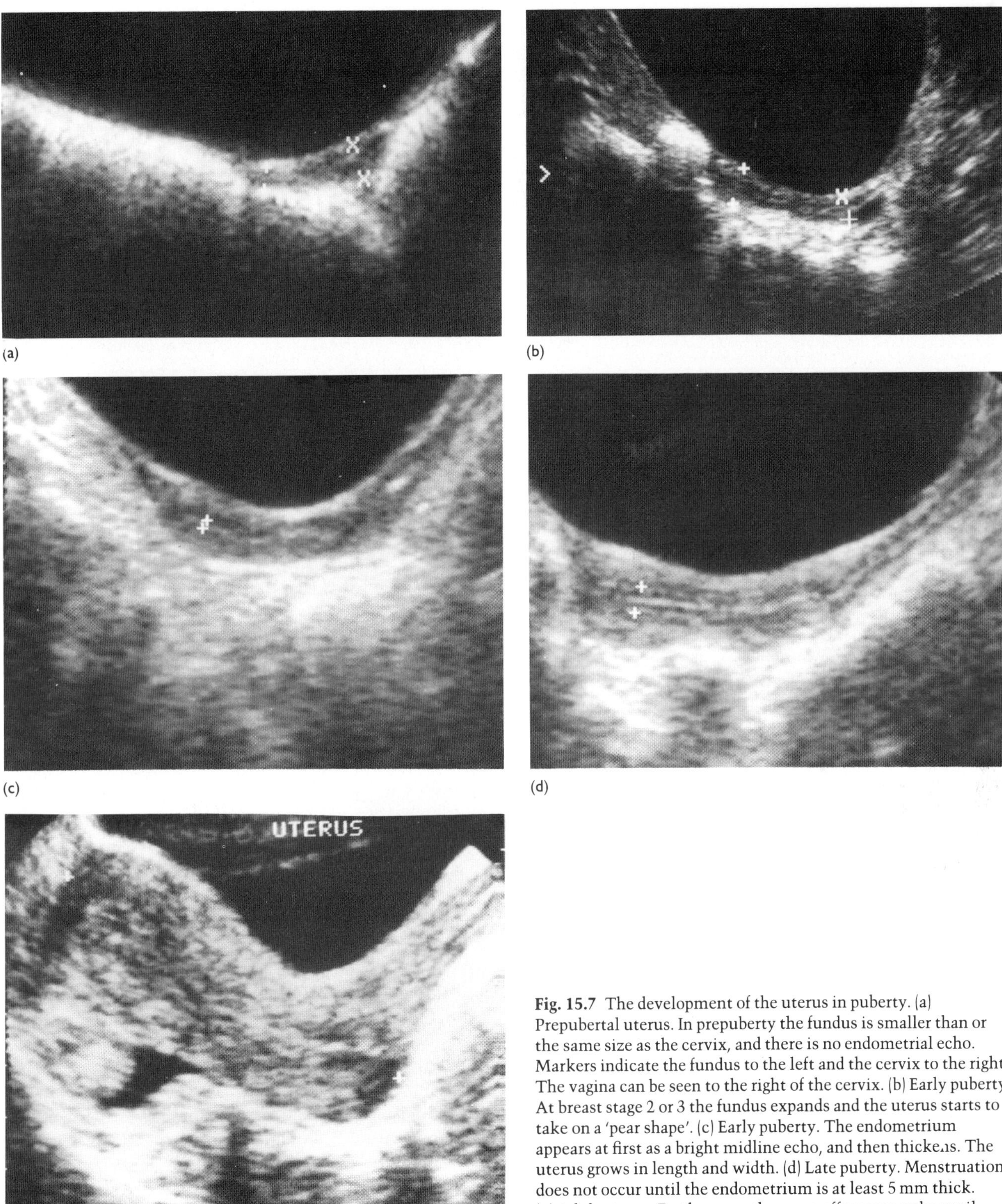

(a) (b) (c) (d) (e)

Fig. 15.7 The development of the uterus in puberty. (a) Prepubertal uterus. In prepuberty the fundus is smaller than or the same size as the cervix, and there is no endometrial echo. Markers indicate the fundus to the left and the cervix to the right. The vagina can be seen to the right of the cervix. (b) Early puberty. At breast stage 2 or 3 the fundus expands and the uterus starts to take on a 'pear shape'. (c) Early puberty. The endometrium appears at first as a bright midline echo, and then thickens. The uterus grows in length and width. (d) Late puberty. Menstruation does not occur until the endometrium is at least 5 mm thick. (e) Adult uterus. Further growth occurs affter menarche until the uterus is of adult dimensions.

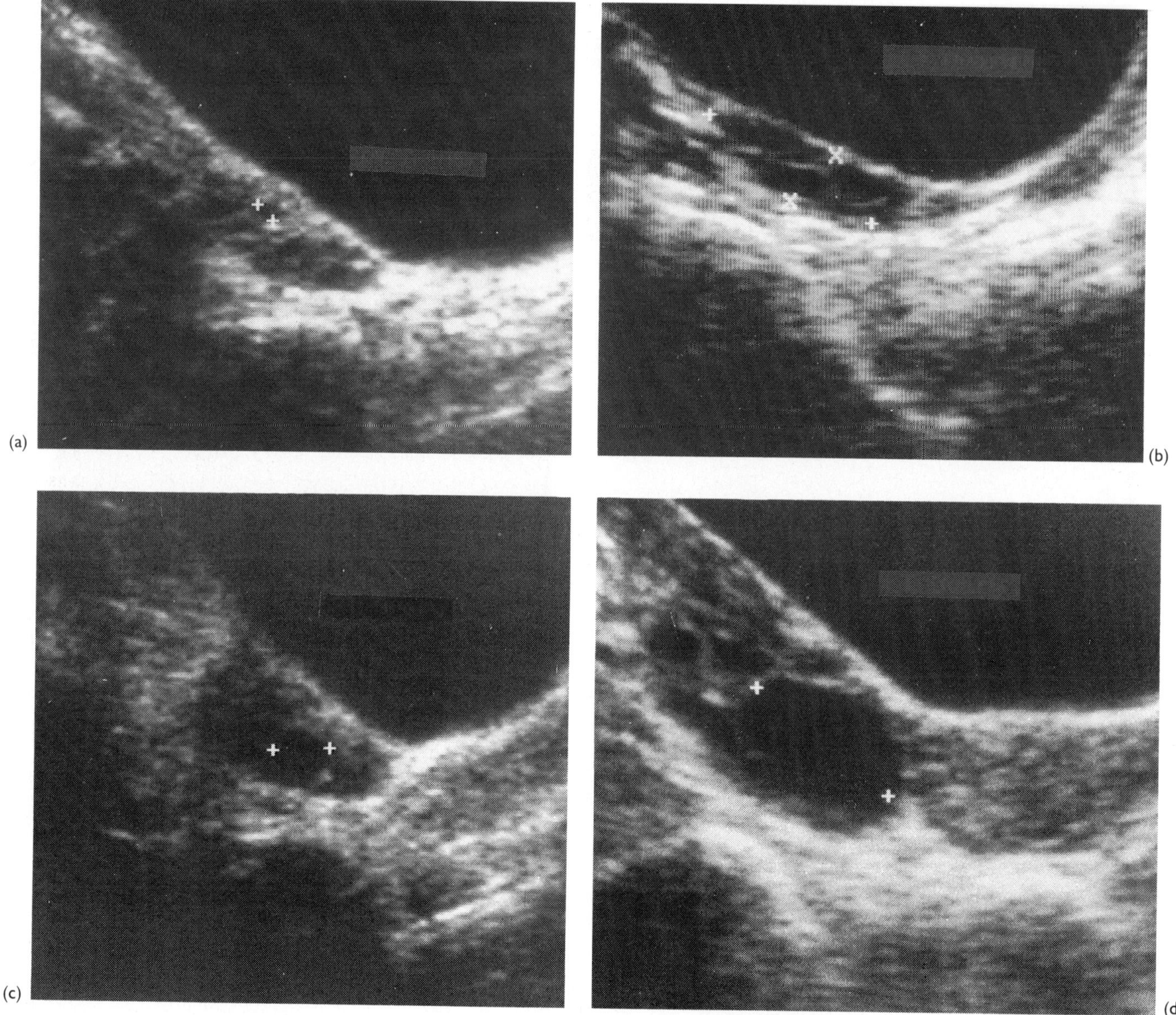

Fig. 15.8 The development of the ovary. (a) Prepubertal ovary. The ovary increases in volume throughout childhood. Small follicles are usually visible; the majority are 4 mm across or less, although the low levels of gonadotrophin secretion at this time can occasionally stimulate larger follicles. (b) A multicystic ovary. In the years before puberty increasing gonadotrophin secretion stimulates an increase in ovarian volume and the growth of multiple larger follicles. (c) Midpuberty. During puberty larger follicles appear in the ovaries, as gonadotrophin and oestrogen concentrations increase. (d) A dominant follicle. Cycles may not be ovulatory for some time after menarche.

bertal shape, but the endometrium should remain thin. The ovaries may remain large for the child's age, but the continuing development of large follicles indicates inadequate suppression.

Rapid growth or virilization, the development of hirsutism (hair other than normal pubic or axillary), deepening of the voice, or clitoromegaly in a girl suggest that the problem is not adrenarche, and the child should be investigated. Serum levels of adrenal androgens may be elevated in an adrenal tumour, and 17-hydroxyprogesterone will be elevated in the commoner forms of CAH. Patterns of urinary steroid excretion are characteristic in adrenal tumours and CAH [43]. If an adrenal tumour is suspected, an abdominal CT or MRI scan should be performed.

Treatment of sexual precocity

Adrenarche, premature thelarche and thelarche variant do not require treatment because final height is not affected.

In both centrally mediated and gonadotrophin-independent precocious puberty the impact on final height and the psychological problems are usually worst in the youngest children and most of these will need treatment. The impact on final height may be less severe in older children, and they are often mature enough to cope with the physical changes. The decision to treat should be based on assessment of growth prognosis and of the child's psychological maturity. Pelvic ultrasound may be helpful in assessing the imminence of menstruation. Treatment will restore a childhood pattern of growth but will not regain lost growth potential. There is no evidence that treatment to suppress puberty will improve final height either in precocious or normally timed puberty.

GONADOTROPHIN-RELEASING HORMONE ANALOGUES

When puberty or fertility is induced using GnRH the pulsatile pattern seen in endogenous GnRH secretion must be mimicked. If a continuous infusion or too high a dose of GnRH is given, there is a brief period of stimulation but the receptors on the gonadotrophs down-regulate and gonadotrophin secretion ceases [44]. The introduction of synthetic analogues of GnRH with enhanced activity and a longer half-life than natural GnRH has meant that this effect can be used in the treatment of central precocious puberty and GnRH analogues have become the first-line treatment for central precocious puberty. A range of different formulations are in use, given as nasal spray, daily injections or as a long-acting subcutaneous depot [45–47]. Monthly depot injections have some practical advantages in children. If the endometrium was thickened, vaginal bleeding may occur at the start of treatment because of the withdrawal of oestrogen.

CYPROTERONE ACETATE AND MEDROXYPROGESTERONE

Cyproterone is an anti-androgen (that is, it has action in blocking androgen receptors) with some progestagenic properties [48]. It suppresses gonadotrophin secretion, but gonadotrophin pulsatility has been detected in girls treated with cyproterone and its effectiveness in halting pubertal progress is probably partly progestational and partly because of its action in blocking androgen receptors [48]. Cyproterone has mineralocorticoid-like actions which suppress adrenal function [49]; many children report feeling tired while on treatment, and severe side-effects secondary to adrenal suppression have been reported. [50].

GnRH analogues are ineffective in gonadotrophin-independent precocious puberty (because pubertal progress in these children is not mediated by gonadotrophins) and cyproterone remains the drug of choice [51]. Cyproterone is useful in suppressing the initial stimulatory effect of GnRH analogue treatment. Our current practice is to give $100\,mg/m^2$ surface area each day for the first 6 weeks. Medroxyprogesterone has similar actions to cyproterone and has been used in the treatment of precocious puberty [52].

KETOCONAZOLE

The antifungal drug ketoconazole is an inhibitor of cytochrome P450 enzymes and has a generalized action in inhibiting steroid biosynthesis [53]. It is effective in halting pubertal progress (in doses much greater than those used for antifungal action) [54]. It has been used in the treatment of Cushing syndrome because it also suppresses ACTH and cortisol secretion, and thus there is a risk of inducing adrenal insufficiency [55]. It occasionally causes severe hepatic dysfunction.

OTHER AGENTS

Testolactone inhibits the aromatization of testosterone to oestradiol and therefore abolishes the actions of testosterone which depend on conversion to oestradiol. Spironolactone has anti-androgen activity. Both have been used in the treatment of gonadotrophin-independent precocious puberty [56,57].

Effect of treatment on growth and final height

Skeletal growth in puberty is mediated both by the action of sex steroids directly and by an increase in growth hormone (GH) secretion which is stimulated by the action of sex steroids on the hypothalamus [58,59]. Treatment of precocious puberty results in a withdrawal of sex steroids and a fall in GH and insulin-like growth factor I (IGF-I) secretion [60]. This means that treatment which suppresses pubertal development also results in a fall in growth rate [61], which is most severe for those with a more advanced bone age [62].

Several studies have documented that treatment with GnRH agonists improves predicted height [63], but improvement with time has also been documented in untreated precocious puberty [64] (Fig. 15.9). Some of the gain in height prediction seen on treatment may be lost in the period of growth between stopping treatment and reaching final height [65]. Data on actual (not predicted) final height following treatment of central precocious puberty with GnRH analogues and with cyproterone acetate demonstrate that these agents are largely ineffective in recovering lost height potential. Children treated with GnRH analogues do not attain their target (parental-based) height [47,65–67]. The small gain seen in final height over height

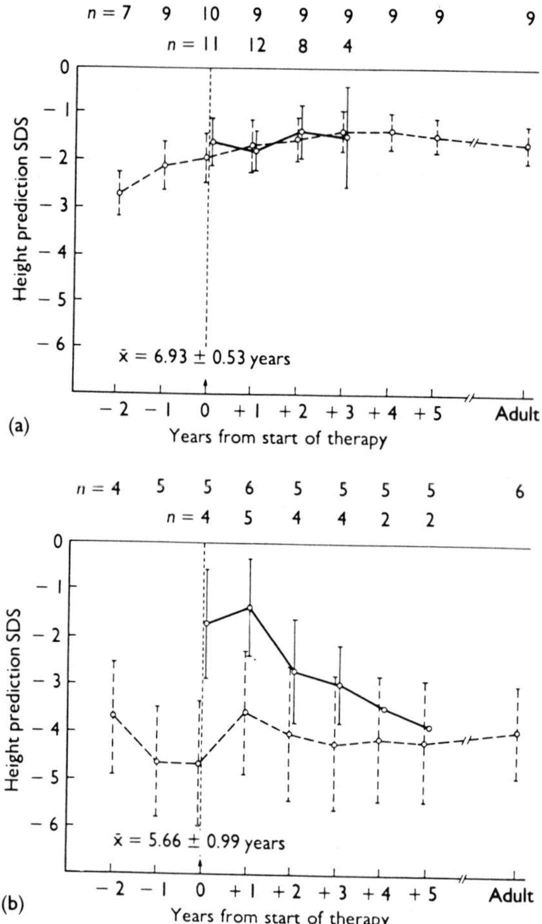

Fig. 15.9 Height prediction SDS (standard deviation score) in (a) girls, and (b) boys with central precocious puberty. The height predictions are identical between those children who were untreated (broken lines) and those treated with cyproterone acetate (solid lines) (redrawn from Werder *et al.* [64]).

prediction in some studies at the start of treatment with GnRH analogues is difficult to assess, because height predictions based on bone ages of normal children are not directly applicable to pathological conditions such as precocious puberty [68].

The observation that the treatment of GH-insufficient children with a combination of GH analogue and GnRH (delaying either a normally times or precocious puberty) resulted in an increase in final height [69,70] has raised the possibility that treatment of central precocious puberty with a combination of GnRH and GH would improve final height, and a number of studies have commenced but there are no data on final heights. Because the combination of GH and GnRH analogue results in polycystic ovarian disease, we recommend caution in adopting this strategy until further data are available.

Stopping treatment and long-term follow-up

For psychological reasons it is best to stop treatment once the child has reached an age acceptable for the onset of puberty. There is no evidence that longer treatment improves final height. Hypothalamic maturity is not affected by treatment, and pubertal growth and development is thus recommenced at an advanced stage. Kauli reported that long-term suppression with depot GnRH analogues persisted for about 4 months before gonadotrophin secretion recovered, but most girls menstruated within a year of stopping treatment [47]. Normal fertility has been documented in children with central precocious puberty, untreated and following treatment with cyproterone and GnRH analogues [35,71,72] Children with gonadotrophin-independent precocious puberty have been reported to experience centrally mediated puberty at an appropriate time [73] but, for girls with McCune–Albright syndrome, there is evidence of abnormal ovarian function continuing into adult life, with development of ovarian cysts and menstrual irregularities.

PUBERTAL DELAY

Ninety-seven per cent of girls have developed the first signs of puberty by 13.2 years, and 97% of boys by 14.2 years. Most of those who have not developed signs of puberty by these ages have delayed activation of the hypothalamopituitary–gonadal axis and will develop signs of puberty eventually. The majority of these cases are idiopathic, and most of those presenting with so-called constitutional delay of puberty are boys. This may reflect the relative insensitivity of the male pituitary to GnRH stimulation (larger doses of GnRH are required to induce puberty in boys than in girls [74]) and contrasts with the preponderance of females with precocious puberty. Chronic disease may delay puberty, for example, in children with inflammatory bowel disease, cystic fibrosis and renal disease [75].

The combination of high levels of exercise and low weight seen in athletes and ballet dancers is a cause of significant delay of puberty. Warren [76], in a study comparing 15 young female ballet dancers with young musicians (who were thought to have the same stress of performance), found that there was a significant delay in the onset of puberty and menarche in the ballet dancers. The ballet dancers were significantly lighter than the musicians, and in 10 of the 15 menarche occurred during a period of reduced exercise due to injury. Similar delays in menarche have been documented in girls who participate in sports, particularly those where an emphasis on thin physique is combined with intensive training, such as gymnastics and distance running [77]. The intensive training of young female athletes may also blunt the pubertal growth spurt and result in impaired final height [78,79], as may anorexia nervosa or bulimia.

Failure to progress in puberty

HYPOGONADOTROPHIC HYPOGONADISM

There are a number of developmental defects of the central nervous system that can be detected at CT or MRI (for example septo-optic dysplasia) which result in failure of GnRH secretion. The hypothalamic secretion of GnRH can be disrupted by a number of tumours (for example, craniopharyngioma). Some children with deficiency of GnRH resulting in failure to progress in puberty have no hypothalamic abnormality detectable on CT or MRI. Haemochromatosis following repeated transfusion with inadequate chelation therapy in thalassaemia can result in hypogonadotrophic hypogonadism [80], although this may not be the whole explanation of the disorder. Defects in the gene encoding for GnRH have not been detected in subjects with hypogonadotrophic hypogonadism [81].

Kallmann syndrome is an X-linked dominant disorder characterized by hypogonadotrophic hypogonadism and loss of the sense of smell. The neurons which secrete GnRH originate outside the central nervous system and migrate through the olfactory placode early in fetal life [82]; failure of this migration has been proposed as the underlying defect in Kallmann syndrome [83]. Xp22.3 deletions have been identified in individuals with Kallmann syndrome [84]. This gene is immediately proximal on the X chromosome to the genes for steroid sulphatase (the cause of X-linked ichthyosis), and individuals with larger deletions at this region may have both conditions. Boys with another X-linked condition, congenital adrenal hypoplasia, have pubertal failure due to hypogonadotrophic hypogonadism in addition to their adrenal problem [85,86].

Pituitary defects, such as developmental abnormalities [87], tumours of the pituitary (such as prolactinoma or germinoma) and damage to the pituitary stalk (such as traumatic transection or infiltration with tumour) may also result in hypogonadotrophic hypogonadism.

At birth, 3% of boys have unilateral, and 1.92% have bilateral, undescended testes, but most these testes descend in the first few months of life [88]. The integrity of the hypothalamopituitary–testicular axis in the fetus is important for testicular descent – pregnant rats treated with the anti-androgen flutamide at a critical stage of gestation deliver male offspring with undescended testes [89], indicating that testosterone is important for initiating testicular descent to the inguinal region: the action of anti-Müllerian hormone (AMH) completes the descent to the scrotum.

Boys with panhypopituitarism have an increased rate of cryptorchidism because of congenital LH deficiency. Both GnRH and hCG have been shown to promote the descent of retractile testes, with hCG more effective (stimulating descent in 23% [90,91]) but, in true hypopituitarism, neither will be effective because the function of the undescended testes may be abnormal. This will persist even when the testis has been brought down to the scrotum [92], since the fetal and neonatal activity of the hypothalamopituitary–testicular axis may be important for subsequent function [93,94]. The higher the undescended testis, the less likely is its structure and function to be normal (which is why it is high); ectopic testes are not affected in this way and need surgical treatment.

GONADAL FAILURE – HYPERGONADOTROPHIC HYPOGONADISM

Gonadal failure results in failure of the normal sex steroid feedback on the hypothalamus and pituitary, and there are elevated FSH and LH concentrations with a rapid pulse frequency [95,96] (Fig. 15.10). The commonest cause of gonadal failure in girls is Turner syndrome. Many girls with Turner syndrome are diagnosed in the neonatal period, or because of poor growth in childhood, but some present with failure to develop at puberty. Twenty per cent of Turner girls have some ovarian function and develop signs of puberty, but many fewer complete puberty. Scanty pubic hair develops spontaneously in a majority of Turner girls, but the administration of oestrogen greatly increases its amount. Fertility has been reported, but this is exceptional [97].

Premature ovarian failure may present as primary or secondary amenorrhoea; it occurs in Turner syndrome (as described above), in women with a 46XO/XX mosaic or XXX karyotype, and is common in those with galactosaemia and mucopolysaccharidosis [98]. In some women, ovarian failure appears to be immune-mediated with lymphocytic infiltration seen on ovarian biopsies, and circulating antibodies to gonadotrophin receptors [99]. Circulating antisteroid cell antibodies have been identified in some women presenting with a combination of autoimmune adrenal failure and ovarian failure. In many women with premature ovarian failure the cause is unknown – the ovaries may be depleted of follicles as in a normal menopause, or there may be multiple primordial follicles which are resistant to gonadotrophin action [98].

Failure of the development of the testes in 46XY individuals results in the development of a female phenotype (so-called pure gonadal dysgenesis). Gonadal dysgenesis has been described in siblings [100]. These individuals usually have a normal appearance, but girls who are 45XO/46XY mosaic may have the phenotype of Turner syndrome. It is important to identify individuals with streak gonads and Y chromosome material because,

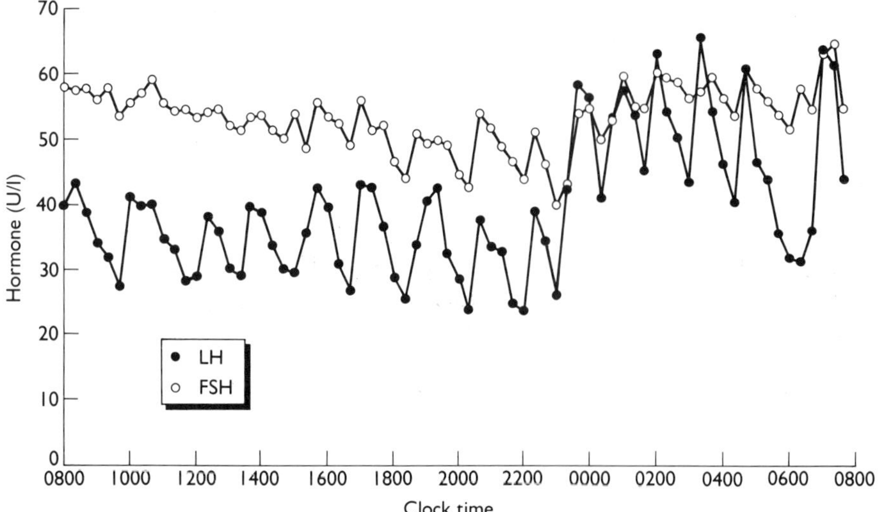

Fig. 15.10 Gonadotrophin secretion in ovarian failure: 24-h LH and FSH profile in a girl who had radiotherapy treatment for a pelvic sarcoma. Without sex steroid feedback, FSH and LH are secreted with a rapid pulse frequency and concentrations are elevated (note the different scale).

unlike girls with 45XO chromosomes, they have an increased risk of gonadal malignancy (gonadoblastoma) [101].

Gonadal failure in either sex may be due to radiotherapy (for example the inclusion of the ovaries in the field for craniospinal or pelvic irradiation and the irradiation of testes in leukaemia) or chemotherapy. In boys, torsion, mumps orchitis and surgical problems associated with orchidopexy may result in gonadal failure.

In anorchia the testes are absent but there are otherwise normal male external genitalia. This suggests there was normal testicular function in early fetal life and normal male differentiation occurred, but the testes regressed for some reason. There may be an entirely normal vas deferens. Mutations in the SRY gene have not been detected in these individuals [102] and torsion in fetal life has been suggested as a cause. Boys may also present with rudimentary, non-functioning testes palpable in the scrotum. Both these groups must be distinguished from bilateral intra-abdominal testes – if there is a testosterone response to hCG there is testicular tissue present, and it should be looked for, because of the increased risk of malignancy in intra-abdominal testes.

Several of the steroid enzymic deficiencies (for example, 3β-hydroxysteroid dehydrogenase, 17α-hydroxylase deficiency, 17,20-lyase and 17β-hydroxysteroid dehydrogenase) can present with gonadal failure in apparent females. Cortisol secretion is reduced in the first three defects, and oestradiol or testosterone production in the gonads is affected in all of them, which means that males with the disorders are inadequately virilized and both sexes suffer pubertal failure [103].

Problems associated with late puberty

Growth velocity gradually diminishes through childhood until the onset of the pubertal growth spurt. Children whose puberty is late will thus grow increasingly slowly, and their peers with normally timed puberty will overtake them. The pubertal growth spurt is diminished in delayed puberty, and late puberty does not increase adult height [104,105]. This pattern of growth means that many children with pubertal delay present with concerns about their height. The lack of secondary sexual characteristics can cause considerable psychological distress, and the fact that these individuals look so young can be a great practical disadvantage in seeking work or higher education.

Pubertal delay results in decreased bone density because of lack of the mineralization induced by sex steroids. Reduced bone mineral density has been documented in young men with a history of delayed puberty [106], and studies in ballet dancers have demonstrated an increased incidence of fractures and scoliosis which correlated with late menarche [107]. This may be a permanent effect – studies of postmenopausal women with osteoporosis have identified late menarche as a risk factor [108].

Investigation of delayed puberty

A plan for the investigation of delayed puberty is given in Fig. 15.11. The differential diagnosis of failure to progress into puberty is given in Table 15.3. Some individuals will have signs of puberty at presentation and require no more than measurement of height, assessment of pubertal stage and a bone age. Children with no signs of puberty should have measurement of height, assessment of pubertal stage and bone age, measurements of gonadotrophin and prolactin concentrations and a test of thyroid function.

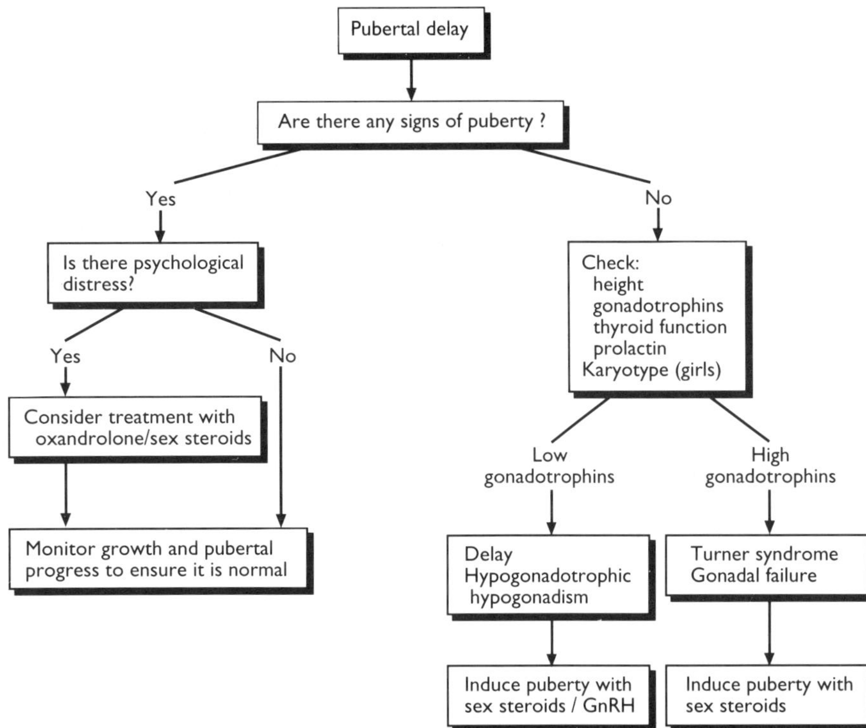

Fig. 15.11 Algorithm for the management of pubertal delay.

Table 15.3 Causes of pubertal delay and pubertal failure

Causes of pubertal delay
Constituitional delay
Chronic disease
Asthma
Gastrointestinal problems
Renal failure
Undernutrition and exercise
Anorexia nervosa
Hypothalamic and pituitary causes of pubertal failure – low gonadotrophins
Congenital defects
Kalmann syndrome
Congenital adrenal hypoplasia
Septoptic dysplasia
Developmental defects of the pituitary
Tumours, direct effects or following radiotherapy or surgery
Haemochromatosis
Gonadal causes of pubertal failure – elevated gonadotroplnins
Radiotherapy or chemotherapy
Females
Turner syndrome
Premature menopause
Males
Anorchia
Bilateral undescended testes
Bilateral orchidectomy
Orchitis

The basal concentrations of gonadotrophins will be expected to be low in children of pubertal age and are measured to exclude gonadal failure [96]. There is no advantage in measuring the response of gonadotrophins to GnRH stimulation, since children with hypogonadotrophic hypogonadism may respond and children with constitutional delay may not do so. A 24-h profile demonstrating very low gonadotrophin secretion does not preclude normal development later on (Figs 15.12 & 15.13). Sex steroid levels are low for much of the day in early puberty, and there is little point in measuring basal concentrations, although early-morning levels of testosterone have been used to distinguish boys about to go into puberty [109].

In girls a pelvic ultrasound examination should be performed to look for signs of ovarian activity or change in the shape of the uterus. Many girls with Turner syndrome (particularly Turner mosaics) do not have a typical phenotypic appearance, and chromosomes should be checked if there is suspicion (for example, if the girl is unusually short for her parents or if gonadotrophin concentrations are unexpectedly raised).

For children growing slowly in late prepuberty there may be a temptation to undertake investigations of GH secretion. This should be resisted, because basal and stimulated levels are low at this time. If it is necessary to predict whether they will rise as spontaneous puberty is

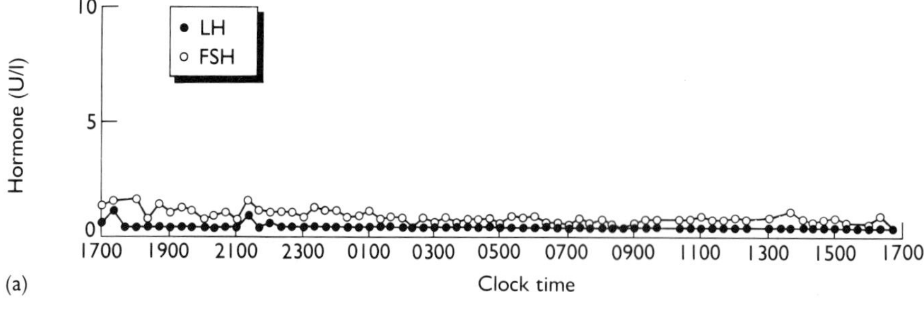

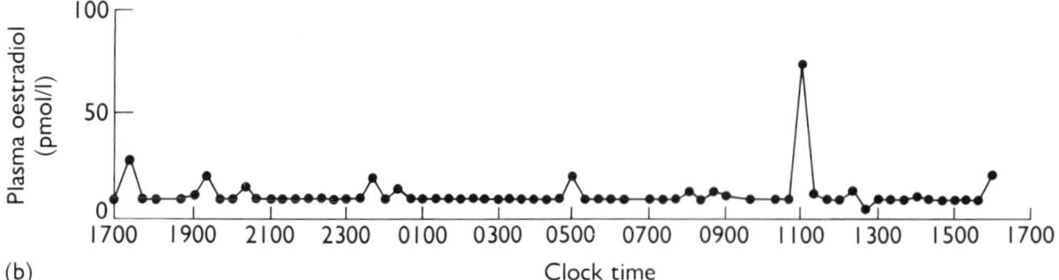

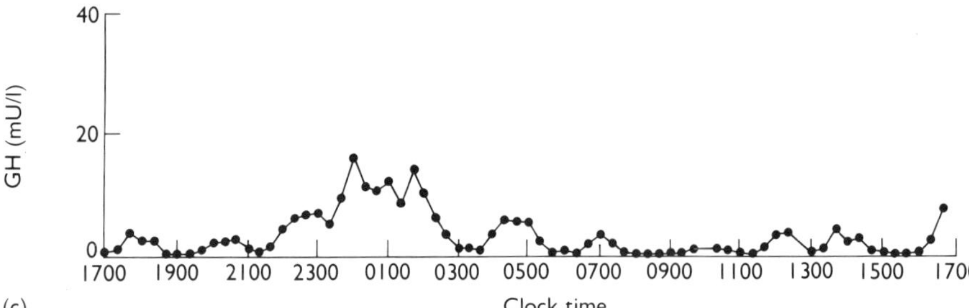

Fig. 15.12 Pubertal delay: 24-h profiles of (a) LH and FSH, (b) oestradiol, and (c) GH in a girl aged 14.0 years with no signs of puberty. The increase in gonadotrophin secretion overnight, which would normally precede pubertal development, is not present. The slow growth seen in pubertal delay is secondary to the low levels of secretion of both GH and sex steroids.

entered, for example, in a patient after cranial irradiation, a test should be done after a dose of sex steroids has been administered (an injection of testosterone esters 100 mg 2 days before the test in a boy, or ethinyloestradiol 20–30 μg daily for 3 days up to the day of the test in a girl). In a patient who has entered puberty but is not growing as expected, a test of GH secretion is required, but should not be primed artificially because the endogenous sex steroids are already present.

Treatment of pubertal delay and pubertal failure

The problems associated with pubertal delay mean that treatment can be of great benefit, even for those who have some signs of puberty or will go into puberty spontaneously at a later stage. For this reason, given that it is difficult, if not impossible, to distinguish hypogonadotrophic hypogonadism from constitutional delay of puberty in adolescent patients, it may be best to treat first and to diagnose later, when time will tell if spontaneous gonadotrophin secretion is effective at maintaining reproductive capability.

If there are no signs of puberty and the gonadotrophin concentrations are low, in other words the patient is suffering either severe constitutional delay or hypogonadotrophic hypogonadism, puberty can be induced with exogenous GnRH or sex steroids. GnRH has to be given by a pulsatile subcutaneous pump, initially overnight (mimicking the pattern seen in normal puberty) (Fig. 15.13) and later changing to treatment throughout the whole 24 h [74]. GnRH treatment is closer to the physiology of normal puberty and induces fertility. This may be of some benefit in the induction of fertility in adult life in individuals with hypogonadotrophic hypogonadism, but the use of subcutaneous infusion pumps presents many more practical difficulties than sex steroid treatment, and is much less widely used.

For boys in early puberty there may, at presentation, may still be over a year to wait before they reach the 10 ml testicular volume at which they will commence a pubertal growth spurt. If lack of stature is the only problem, a short course of oxandrolone (2.5 mg daily for 3 months) will precipitate a growth spurt which will become sustained [110].

If pubertal development is a problem as well as stature, a low dose of testosterone will accelerate pubertal devel-

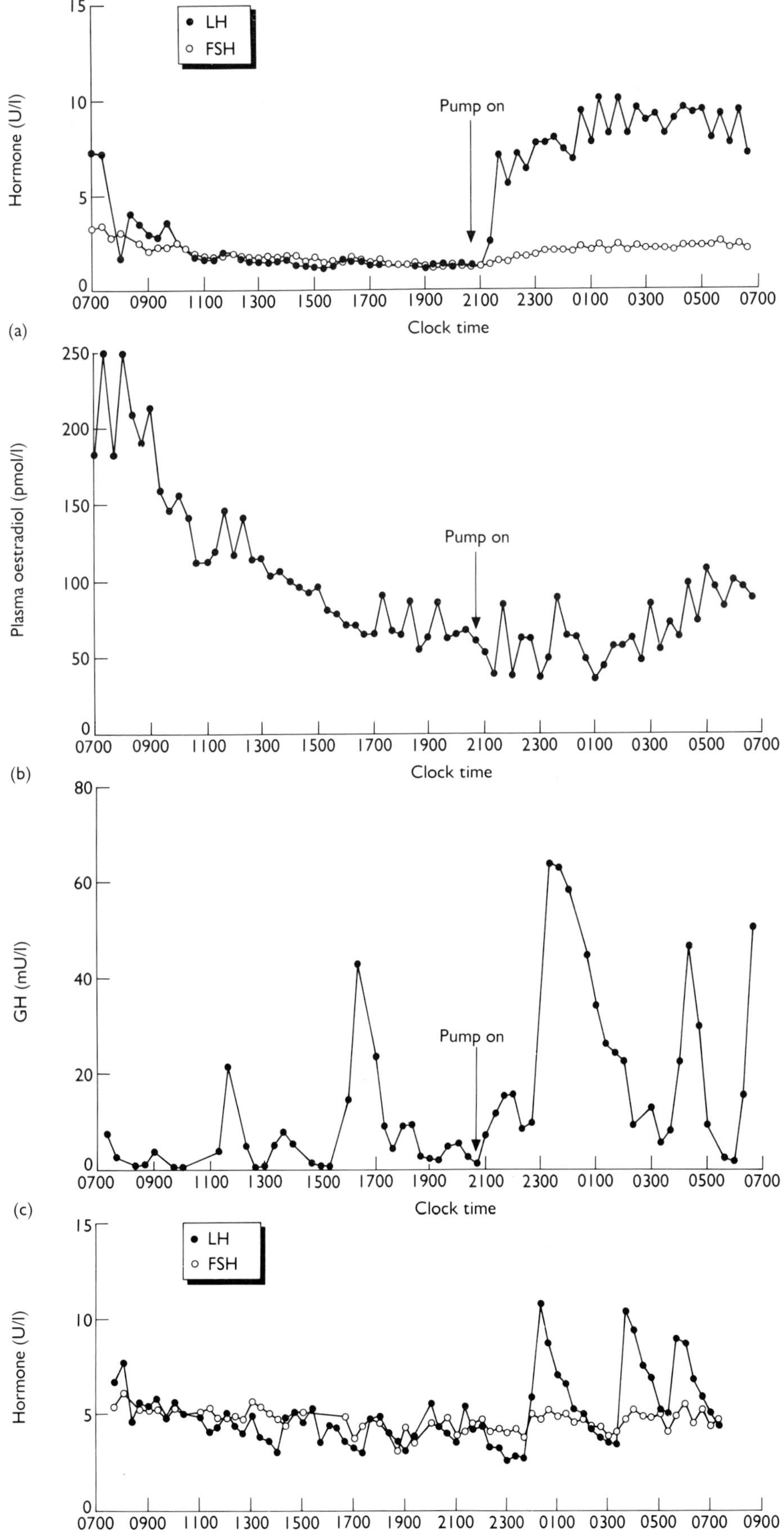

Fig. 15.13 Induction of puberty with GnRH. The girl portrayed in Fig. 15.12 at breast stage 2, following 3 months treatment with subcutaneous GnRH (2 μg every 45 min overnight using a pump). 24-h profiles of (a) LH and FSH, (b) oestradiol, and (c) GH. The rise in oestradiol concentrations has stimulated an increase in GH secretion and the girl has commenced her pubertal growth spurt; she reached breast stage 4 after 16 months on GnRH and stopped treatment; she then progressed spontaneously in puberty. (d) 24-h profile 2 years after the first profile, demonstrating spontaneous gonadotrophin pulsatility with no treatment. She menstruated 3 months after this profile; the diagnosis was therefore constitutional delay.

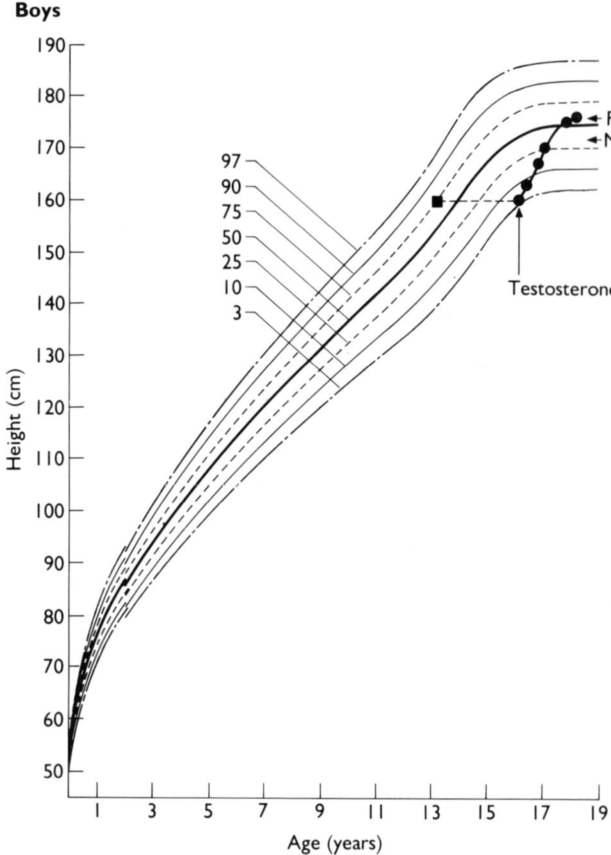

Fig. 15.14 Induction of puberty with testosterone. This boy presented with no signs of puberty at 16 years and was treated with testosterone. Virilization and a normal pubertal growth spurt were induced. His testicular volume did not progress to greater than 6 ml, and testosterone levels fell when the treatment was stopped. The diagnosis was hypogonadotrophic hypogonadism. F, Father's height centile; M, Mother's height centile; ■, bone age.

opment and produce an increase in growth rate (Fig. 15.14). Our current practice is to use 100 mg of testosterone esters intramuscularly every 4–6 weeks, depending upon age and stage of puberty, for 4–6 months. Used at these low doses, neither oxandrolone nor sex steroids will compromise final height [111].

Sex steroid treatment in girls should commence with 5 μg ethinyloestradiol daily orally. This dose is gradually increased to maintain a normal pace of pubertal development; our policy is to increase in 5 μg steps every 6 months to reach a dose of 20–30 μg adult replacement, depending on size and symptomatology. A progestagen should be added when 15 μg of ethinyloestradiol has been reached, or if there is breakthrough bleeding at a lower dose. The thickness of the endometrium should be monitored with ultrasound; if it is over 5 mm there is a likelihood of bleeding and a progestagen should be added.

In the first cycle this should be administered as norethisterone acetate 10 mg for 10 days followed by a break of all therapy for 2 weeks. Subsequent cycles should be of 5 mg norethisterone or 30 μg levonorgestrel for days 21–28 in every 28-day cycle of continuous ethinyloestradiol. The aim is to give regular periods and some girls may need to increase to 30 μg of ethinyloestradiol for this. The oral contraceptive pill is a convenient way of administering higher doses of oestrogen in a cyclical manner, although some young women with gonadal failure find objectionable the idea of taking a contraceptive pill for a disorder that makes them infertile. Increasing the dose of oestrogen too quickly results in poor breast development with prominent nipples. The addition of a progestagen can improve breast development but the normal contour of a female breast may be hard to achieve, and we do not hesitate to seek the advice of a plastic surgeon interested in augmentation mammoplasty.

GH should not be used to treat the short stature of delayed puberty. Not only does it accelerate pubertal development [112] but it is also less effective in promoting final height as compared to small doses of sex steroids [110]. It should be reserved for patients with true insufficiency of growth hormone secretion at puberty.

Individuals with hypergonadotrophic hypogonadism should be treated with sex steroids to induce puberty at the normal time. The pubertal growth spurt induced by oestrogen in girls with Turner syndrome is less than in normal girls because of the skeletal dysplasia which is associated with the syndrome (and is no better when the puberty is spontaneous). Boys with anorchia may wish to have silicone implants at the end of puberty to improve the cosmetic appearance.

Other problems in puberty

A child who commences in puberty and then stops (arrested puberty) requires investigation to exclude a brain tumour (MRI or CT). Some of these individuals have a hypothalamic defect which means that they can produce enough GnRH to start in puberty but not to complete development [113]. The onset of severe illness such as inflammatory bowel disease can halt pubertal development, as can the development of anorexia nervosa [114,115].

Gynaecomastia is extremely common in puberty, but for some boys the problem is severe and causes great embarrassment. Mastectomy can cure the problem in severe cases. Severe gynaecomastia is sometimes associated with Klinefelter syndrome, when testosterone levels are relatively low and the ratio of oestrogen to testosterone is increased.

POLYCYSTIC OVARIES

The endocrine and reproductive consequences of polycystic ovaries were described as the polycystic ovarian (Stein–Leventhal) syndrome before the invention of ultrasound. The introduction of this revolutionary technology has demonstrated that 22–25% of adult women have ovaries with a polycystic appearance [116]. Polycystic ovaries are larger than normal, have increased stroma and a characteristic arrangement of follicles around the periphery of the ovary [117] (Fig. 15.15). Many women with polycystic-appearance ovaries at ultrasound have no problems, but polycystic ovaries account for 87% of menstrual irregularities in women [117].

Some women have severe symptoms referrable to their polycystic ovaries, ranging from mild hirsutism and menstrual irregularity to having classical polycystic ovarian syndrome – obesity, insulin resistance, excessive androgen secretion, ammenorrhoea, hirsutism and acanthosis nigricans [118]. In a study in 190 normal adult women, Clayton *et al.* [116] found 41 with polycystic ovaries at ultrasound (22%); these women had an increased prevalence of hirsutism, but they did not demonstrate an increase in the prevalence of menstrual irregularity or infertility over normal women. The endocrine consequences of polycystic ovaries are a common reason for presentation to gynaecology and infertility clinics, but this study suggests that in the general population polycystic-appearance ovaries at ultrasound are very rarely symptomatic.

The cause of polycystic ovaries is unknown; it has been described in girls with hypogonadotrophic hypogonadism, and thus is probably primarily an ovarian disorder rather than the secondary effect of abnormal pituitary function [119]. Some conditions predispose to the development of polycystic ovaries. The insulin-like growth factor system (IGF-I and the IGF-binding proteins) is an important mediator of follicular growth and maturation in the ovary; IGF-I and its binding proteins are found in follicular fluid, and have an important paracrine action in the ovary [120]. Abnormalities of IGF-I have been detected in women with polycystic ovaries [121,122], and polycystic ovaries are more common in a number of situations where IGF-I or insulin are elevated: those with diabetes, tall girls [42], and those with syndromes of insulin resistance (such as leprechaunism) [123]. The elevated androgen levels seen in polycystic ovarian syndrome may be due either to peripheral androgen production in adipose tissue or to the effect of hyperinsulinaemia on ovarian steroidogenesis [124]. Polycystic-appearance ovaries are also more common in women with high androgen levels: adrenal hyperplasia (where the prevalence is 100% in adult life) and transsexuals [125,126]. There may be an inherited element in polycystic ovaries because familial cases have been described [127].

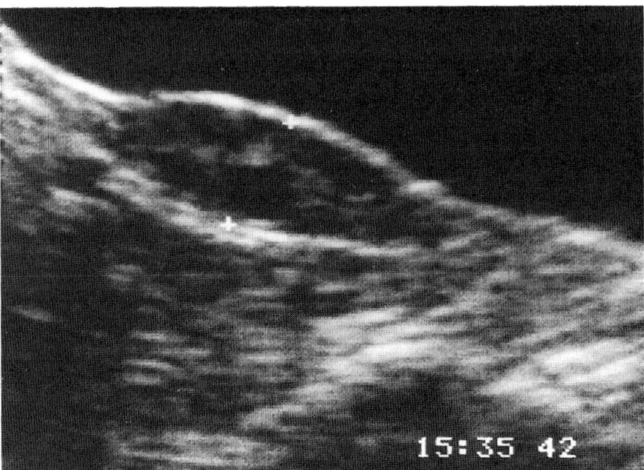

Fig. 15.15 A typical ultrasound appearance of a polycystic ovary in a 12-year-old girl. The ovary is large and has increased stroma (seen as bright echodense areas in the centre). There are multiple follicles arranged around the perimeter of the ovary.

In children the prevalence of polycystic appearance at ultrasound rises from about 6% at 6 years of age until by the end of puberty it is the same as that seen in adult women (22–25%) [42]. It seems likely that polycystic appearance does not disappear once present, and so most women with a polycystic ovarian appearance probably develop it in adolescence. Many of these individuals will never have symptoms referrable to their polycystic ovaries, and for many more the symptoms will be trivial. A few girls with polycystic ovaries develop the features of classical polycystic ovarian syndrome by the end of puberty, with hirsutism, severe acne, obesity and, more rarely, acanthosis nigricans. Polycystic ovaries are the commonest cause of delayed menarche in girls who are otherwise well developed in puberty, and some girls commence immediately on a pattern of irregular menses similar to that seen in some adult women with the condition. Girls with polycystic ovaries may have a long-term problem with impaired fertility which is exacerbated by allowing themselves to become obese.

There is no way to predict which child with polycystic ovaries will become symptomatic. Adolescents with polycystic-appearance ovaries should be encouraged to avoid becoming obese. Obese women with polycystic ovarian syndrome have more severe symptoms [124]. Weight loss can improve both the insulin resistance and the excessive androgen secretion, and result in improved reproductive function [128]. Hirsutism and acne in patients with completed puberty can be greatly improved by the cyclical administration of cyproterone acetate; our current regimen for a 28-day cycle is ethinyloestradiol 30 μg on days 1–21 with cyproterone acetate 50 mg on days 5–15 for 3 months, reducing to 25 mg on days 5–15 for 3 months, then changing to cyclical ethinyloestradiol and levonorgestrol or an oral contraceptive pill, as described above.

LONG-TERM FOLLOW-UP OF CHILDREN WITH PUBERTAL DISORDERS

Individuals who are unable to maintain adult levels of sex steroids must have long-term treatment to maintain normal sexual function and to prevent osteoporosis. In girls this means cyclical oestrogen and progesterone, since unopposed oestrogen increases the risk of endometrial carcinoma. The oestrogen dose should be sufficient to maintain regular normal periods. In boys the dose of testosterone should be sufficient to maintain genital development, sexual function and facial hair growth. The serum testosterone level should remain within the normal adult range.

Individuals with pubertal problems should have their long-term prospects for fertility explained. Those with hypogonadotrophic hypogonadism can attain fertility with gonadotrophin treatment or pulsatile GnRH [129]. Women with ovarian failure, but with a normal-sized uterus, can become pregnant by ovum donation, and this technique has been used to achieve pregnancies in women with Turner syndrome [130]. To grow a normal uterus requires phased introduction of oestrogen and progestagen treatments and concomitant growth hormone secretion. Developments such as ovum donation and the potential for improvements in the administration of sex steroids mean that individuals requiring continuing treatment should maintain contact with a physician with an interest in reproductive endocrinology.

REFERENCES

1 Boyko OB, Curnes JT, Oakes WJ, Burger PC. Hamartomas of the tuber cinereum: CT, MR and pathologic findings. *Am J Neuroradiol* 1991;12:309–14.
2 Junier MP, Wollf A, Hoffman G, Ma YJ, Ojeda SR. Effect of hypothalamic lesions that induce precocious puberty on the morphological and functional maturation of the luteinising hormone releasing hormone neuronal system. *Endocrinology* 1992;131:787–98.
3 Reith KG, Comite F, Dwyer AJ *et al.* CT of cerebral abnormalities in precocious puberty. *Am J Roentgenol* 1987;148:1231–8.
4 Kuroki Y, Katsumata N, Eguchi T, Fukishama Y, Suwa S, Kajii T. Precocious puberty in the Kabuki make up syndrome. *J Pediatr* 1987;110:750–2.
5 Shalet SM, Crowne EC, Didi MA, Ogilvy Stuart AL, Wallace WH. Irradiation induced growth failure. *Ballières Clin Endocrinol Metab* 1992;6:513–26.
6 Proos LA, Hofvander Y, Tuvemo T. Menarcheal age and growth pattern of Indian girls adopted in Sweden. I. Menarcheal age. *Acta Paediatr Scand* 1991;Suppl.80:852–8.
7 Herman ME, Giddens AD, Sandler NE, Freidman NE. Sexual precocity in girls: an association with sexual abuse? *Am J Dis Child* 1988;142:431–3.
8 Holland FJ. Gonadotrophin independent precocious puberty. *Endocrinol Metab Clin N Am* 1991;20:191–210.
9 Laue L, Kenigsberg D, Pescovitz OH *et al.* Treatment of familial male precocious puberty with spironolactone and testolactone. *N Engl J Med* 1989;320:496–502.
10 Mauras N, Blizzard RM. The McCune–Albright syndrome. *Acta Endocrinol Scand* (Suppl.) 1986;279:207–17.
11 Weinstein LS, Shenker A, Gejman PV, Merino MJ, Freidmen E, Speigel AM. Activating mutations of the stimulatory G protein in the McCune–Albright syndrome. *N Engl J Med* 1991;325:1688–95.
12 Levine MA. The McCune–Albright syndrome: the whys and wherefores of abnormal signal transduction. *N Engl J Med* 1991;325:1738–40.
13 Endo M, Yamada Y, Matsua N, Niikawa N. Monozygotic twins discordant for signs of McCune–Albright syndrome. *Am J Med Genet* 1991;41:216–20.
14 Cremonini N, Graziano E, Chiarini V, Sforza A, Zampa GA. Atypical McCune–Albright syndrome associated with growth hormone prolactin pituitary adenoma: natural history, long term follow up and SMS 201-995-bromocriptine combined treatment results. *J Clin Endocrinol Metab* 1992;75:1166–9.
15 Manasco PK, Girton ME, Diggs RL *et al.* A novel testis stimulating factor in familial male precocious puberty. *N Engl J Med* 1991;324:227–31.
16 Stanhope R, Abdulwahid NA, Adams J, Brook CGD. Studies of gonadotrophin pulsatility and pelvic ultrasound examinations distingush between isolated premature thelarche and central precocious puberty. *Eur J Pediatr* 1986;145:190–4.
17 Freedman SM, Krietzer PM, Elkovitz SS, Saberman N, Leonidas JC. Ovarian microcysts in girls with isolated premature thelarche. *Pediatrics* 1993;122:246–9.
18 Freni-Titulaer LW, Cordero JF, Haddock L, Lebron G, Martinez R, Mills JL. Premature thelarche in Puerto Rico. A search for environmental factors. *Am J Dis Child* 1986;140:1263–7.
19 Stanhope R, Brook CGD. Thelarche variant: a new syndrome of precocious sexual development? *Acta Endocrinol* 1990;123:481–6.
20 Fontoura M, Brauner R, Prevot C, Rappaport R. Precocious puberty in girls: early diagnosis of a slowly progressing variant. *Arch Dis Child* 1989;64:1170–6.
21 Pringle PJ, Stanhope R, Hindmarsh PC, Brook CGD. Abnormal pubertal development in primary hypothyroidism. *Clin Endocrinol* 1988;28:479–86.
22 Buchanan C, Stanhope R, Jones J, Grant DB, Preece MA. Gonadotrophin, GH and prolactin secretion in children with primary hypothyroidism. *Clin Endocrinol* 1988;29:427–36.
23 Ibanez L, Virdis R, Potau N *et al.* Natural history of premature pubarche: an auxological study. *J Clin Endocrinol Metab* 1992;74:254–8.
24 Del Balzo P, Borelli P, Cambiaso P, Danielli E, Cappa M. Adrenal steroidogenic defects in children with precocious pubarche. *Horm Res* 1992;37:180–4.
25 Pescovitz OH, Comite F, Cassorla F *et al.* True precocious puberty complicating congenital adrenal hyperplasia: treatment with a LHRH analogue. *J Clin Endocrinol Metab* 1984;58:857–61.
26 Pommier RF, Brennan MF. An eleven-year experience with

adrenocortical carcinoma. *Surgery* 1992;112:963–70.
27 Icard P, Chapuis Y, Andreassian B, Bernard A, Proye C. Adrenocortical carcinoma in surgically treated patients: a retrospective study on 156 cases by the French Association of Endocrine Surgery. *Surgery* 1992;112:972–9.
28 Perilongo G, Rigon F, Murgia A. Oncologic causes of precocious puberty. *Pediatr Hematol Oncol* 1989;6:331–40.
29 Englund AT, Geffner ME, Nagel RA, Lippe BM, Braunstein GD. Pediatric germ cell and human chorionic gonadotropin producing tumors. *Am J Dis Child* 1991;145:1294–7.
30 Root AW, Bongiovanni AM, Eberlein WR. A testicular interstitial cell stimulating gonadotrophin in a child with hepatoblastoma and sexual precocity. *J Clin Endocrinol Metab* 1968;28:1317–22.
31 Ambrosi B, Bassetti M, Ferrario R, Medri G, Giannattasio G, Faglia G. Precocious puberty in a boy with a PRL-, LH- and FSH-secreting pituitary tumour: hormonal and immunocytochemical studies. *Acta Endocrinol* 1990;122:569–76.
32 Lacson AG, Gillis DA, Shawwa A. Malignant mixed germ-cell–sex cord–stromal tumors of the ovary associated with isosexual precocious puberty. *Cancer* 1988;61:2122–33.
33 Souis WA, Comite F, Blue J *et al.* Behaviour problems and social competence in girls with true precocious puberty. *J Pediatr* 1985;106:156–60.
34 Ross JL, Pescovitz OH, Barnes K, Loriaux DL, Cutler GB. Growth hormone secretory dynamics in children with precocious puberty. *J Pediatr* 1987;110:369–72.
35 Murram D, Dewhust J, Grant DG. Precocious puberty: a follow up study. *Arch Dis Child* 1984;59:77–8.
36 Lee PA, Van Dop C, Midgeon CJ. McCune Albright syndrome: long term follow up. *J Am Med Assoc* 1986;256: 2980–4.
37 Hughes IA. *Handbook of Endocrine Investigations in Children*. London: Wright, 1986.
38 Salardi S, Orsini L, Cacciari E *et al.* Pelvic ultrasonography in girls with precocious puberty, congenital adrenal hyperplasia, obesity or hirsutism. *J Pediatr* 1988;112:880–7.
39 Sample WF, Lippe BM, Gyeppes MT. Grey scale ultrasonography of the normal female pelvis. *Radiology* 1977;125: 477–83.
40 Tenore A, Franzese A, Quattrin T *et al.* Prognostic signs in the evaluation of premature thelarche by discriminant analysis. *J Endocrinol Invest* 1991;14:375–81.
41 Stanhope R, Adams J, Jacobs HS, Brook CDG. Ovarian ultrasound assessment in normal children, idiopathic precocious puberty and during low dose pulsatile GnRH treatment of hypogonadotrophic hypogonadism. *Arch Dis Child* 1985;60:116–19.
42 Bridges NA, Cooke A, Healy MJR, Hindmarsh PC, Brook CGD. Standards for ovarian volume in childhood and puberty. *Fertil Steril* 1993;60:456–60.
43 Honour JA, Price DA, Taylor NF, Marsden HB, Grant DB. Steroid biochemistry of virilising adrenal tumours in childhood. *Eur J Pediatr* 1984;142:165–9.
44 Conn PM. The molecular basis of gonadotrophin releasing hormone action. *Endocr Rev* 1986;7:3–10.
45 Stanhope R, Adams J, Brook CGD. The treatment of central precocious puberty using an intranasal LHRH analogue (Buserelin). *Clin Endocrinol* 1985;22:795–806.
46 Parker KL, Lee PA. Depot Leuprolide acetate for treatment of precocious puberty. *J Clin Endocrinol Metab* 1989;69: 689–91.
47 Kauli R, Kornreich L, Laron Z. Pubertal development, growth and final height in girls with sexual precocity treated with the GnRH analogue D-TRP-6-LHRH. *Horm Res* 1990; 33:11–17.
48 Stanhope R, Pringle J, Adams J, Jeffcoate SC, Brook CGD. Spontaneous gonadotrophin pulsatility in girls with central precocious puberty treated with cyproterone acetate. *Clin Endocrinol* 1985;23:547–53.
49 Phan Huu Trung MT, de Smitter N, Bogyo A, Girard F. Effects of cyproterone acetate on adrenal steroidogenesis *in vitro*. *Horm Res* 1984;20:108–15.
50 Savage DCL, Swift PGF. Effect of cyproterone acetate on adrenocortical function in children with precocious puberty. *Arch Dis Child* 1981;56:218–22.
51 Foster CM, Comite F, Pescovitz OH, Ross JL, Loriaux DL, Cutler GB. Variable response to a long acting agonist of LHRH in girls with McCune–Albright syndrome. *J Clin Endocrinol Metab* 1984;59:801–5.
52 Lee PA. Medroxyprogesterone therapy for sexual precocity in girls. *Am J Dis Child* 1981;135:443–5.
53 Sonino N. The use of ketoconazole as an inhibitor of steroid production. *N Engl J Med* 1987;317:812–18.
54 Holland FJ, Fishman L, Bailey JD, Fazekas ATA. Ketoconazole in the treatment of precocious puberty not responsive to LHRH analogue therapy. *N Engl J Med* 1985;312:1023–8.
55 Stalla GK, Stalla J, Huber M *et al.* Ketoconazole inhibits corticotropic cell function *in vitro*. *Endocrinology* 1988: 122:618–23.
56 Laue L, Kenigsberg D, Pescovitz OH *et al.* Treatment of familial male precocious puberty with spironolactone and testolactone. *N Engl J Med* 1989;320:496–502.
57 Feuillan PP, Foster CM, Pescovitz OH *et al.* Treatment of precocious puberty in the McCune–Albright syndrome with the aromatase inhibitor testolactone. *N Engl J Med* 1986; 315:1115–19.
58 Wennink JMB, Delamarre Vandewaal HA, Schoemaker R, Blaaw G, Van den Braken C, Schoemaker J. GH secretion patterns in relation to LH and testosterone secretion throughout normal male puberty. *Acta Endocrinol* 1990; 123:263–70.
59 Moll GW, Rosenfeld RL, Fang VS. Adminsitration of low dose estrogen rapidly and directly stimulates GH production. *Am J Dis Child* 1986;140:124–7.
60 DiMartino Nardi J, Wu R, Fishman K, Saenger P. The effect of long acting analogue of luteinising hormone releasing hormone on growth hormone secretory dynamics in children with precocious puberty. *J Clin Endocrinol Metab* 1991; 73:902–6.
61 Boepple PA, Mansfield MJ, Link K *et al.* Impact of sex steroids and their supression on skeletal growth and maturation. *Am J Physiol* 1988;255:E559–66.
62 Boepple PA, Mansfield MJ, Crawford JD, Crigler JF, Blizzard RM, Crowley WF. Gonadotrophin releasing hormone agonist treatment of central precocious puberty: an analysis of growth data in a developmental context. *Acta Paediatr Scand* 1990;Suppl.367:38–43.
63 Lee PA, Page JG. The Leuprolide study group. Effects of Leuprolide in the treatment of central precocious puberty. *J Pediatr* 1989;114:321–4.
64 Werder EA, Murset G, Zachmann M, Brook CGD, Prader A. Treatment of precocious puberty with cyproterone acetate. *Pediatr Res* 1974;8:248–56.
65 Oerter KE, Manasco P, Barnes KM, Jones J, Hill S, Cutler GB. Adult height after long term treatment with deslorelin. *J Clin Endocrinol Metab* 1991;73:1235–40.
66 Sorgo W, Kiraly E, Homoki J *et al.* The effects of cyproterone

acetate on statural growth in children with precocious puberty. *Acta Endocrinol* 1987;115:44–56.
67 Stanhope R, Hueh KF, Buzi F, Preece MA, Grant DB. The effect of cyproterone acetate on the growth of children with central precocious puberty. *Eur J Pediatr* 1987;146:500–3.
68 Zachmann M, Sobradillo B, Frank M, Frisch H, Prader A. Bayley Pinneau, Roche Wainer Thissen, and Tanner height predictions in normal children and in patients with various pathological conditions. *J Pediatr* 1978;93:749–55.
69 Cara JF, Kreiter ML, Rosenfield RL. Height prognosis of children with true precocious puberty and growth hormone deficency: effect of combination therapy with gonadotropin releasing hormone agonist and growth hormone. *J Pediatr* 1992;120:709–15.
70 Hibi I, Tanaka T, Tanae A *et al.* The influence of gonadal function and the effect of gonadal suppression treatment on final height in growth hormone treated growth hormone deficient children. *J Clin Endocrinol Metab* 1989;69:221–6.
71 Jay N, Mansfield MJ, Blizzard RM *et al.* Ovulation and menstrual function of adolescent girls with central precocious puberty after therapy with gonadotrophin releasing hormone agonists. *J Clin Endocrinol Metab* 1992;75:890–4.
72 Cisternino M, Pasquino A, Bozzola M *et al.* Final height attainment and gonadal function in girls with precocious puberty treated with cyproterone acetate. *Horm Res* 1992; 37:86–90.
73 Boepple PA, Frisch LS, Weirman ME, Hoffman WH, Crowley WF. The natural history of autonomous gonadal function, adrenarche and central puberty in gonadotrophin independent precocious puberty. *J Clin Endocrinol Metab* 1992; 75:1550–5.
74 Stanhope R, Brook CGD, Pringle PJ, Adams J, Jacobs HS. Induction of puberty by pulsatile GnRH. *Lancet* 1987; 2:522–55.
75 Guisti M, Perfumo F, Verrina E *et al.* Delayed puberty in uremia: pituitary gonadal function during short term pulsatile luteinising hormone releasing hormone administration. *J Endocrinol Invest* 1992;15:709–17.
76 Warren MP. The effects of exercise on pubertal progression and reproductive function in girls. *J Clin Endocrinol Metab* 1980;51:1150–7.
77 Warren MP. Amenorrhea in endurance runners. *J Clin Endocrinol Metab* 1992;75:1393–7.
78 Theintz GE, Howald H, Weiss U, Sizononko PC. Evidence for a reduction of growth potential in adolescent female gymnasts. *J Pediatr* 1993;122:306–13.
79 Mansfield MJ, Emans SJ. Growth in female gymnasts: should training decrease during puberty? *J Pediatr* 1993;122:273–4.
80 Oerter KE, Kamp GA, Munson PJ, Nienhaus AW, Cassorla FG, Manasco PK. Multiple hormone deficiencies in children with hemochromatosis. *J Clin Endocrinol Metab* 1993; 76:357–61.
81 Weiss J, Crowley WF, Jamieson JL. Normal structure of GnRH gene in patients with GnRH deficiency and idiopathic hypogonadotrophic hypogonadism. *J Clin Endocrinol Metab* 1989;69:299–309.
82 Schwanzel-Fukuda M, Pfaff DW. Origin of luteinising hormone releasing hormone neurons. *Nature* 1989;338:161–4.
83 Schwanzel-Fukuda M, Bick D, Pfaff DW. Luteinising hormone releasing hormone (LHRH) expressing cells do not migrate normally in an inherited hypogonadal (Kallmann) syndrome. *Mol Brain Res* 1989;6:311–26.
84 Hardelin JP, Levilliers J, Young J *et al.* Xp22.3 deletions in isolated familal Kallmann's syndrome. *J Clin Endocrinol Metab* 1993;76:827–31.
85 Hay ID, Smail PJ, Forsythe CC. Familial cytomegalic adrenocortical hypoplasia – an X linked syndrome of pubertal failure. *Arch Dis Child* 1981;56:715–21.
86 Zachmann M, Fuchs E, Prader A. Progressive high frequency hearing loss – an additional feature in the syndrome of congenital adrenal hypoplasia and gonadotrophin deficiency. *Eur J Pediatr* 1992;151:167–9.
87 Stanhope R, Hindmarsh P, Kendall B, Brook CGD. High resolution CT scanning of the pituitary in growth disorders. *Acta Paediatr Scand* 1986;Suppl.75:779–86.
88 John Radcliffe Hospital Cryptorchidism Study Group. Cryptorchidism: a prospective study of 7500 consecutive male births, 1984–8. *Arch Dis Child* 1992;67:892–9.
89 Husmann DA, McPhaul MJ. Reversal of flutamide induced cryptorchidism by prenatal time specific androgens. *Endocrinology* 1992;131:1711–15.
90 De Muinck Keizer-Schrama SMPF, Hazebroek FJW, Matroos AW, Drop SLS, Molenaar JC, Visser HKA. Double blind placebo controlled study of LHRH nasal spray in treatment of undescended testes. *Lancet* 1986;1:876–79.
91 Bica DT, Hadziselimovic F. Buserelin treatment of cryptorchidism: a randomized, double-blind, placebo-controlled study. *J Urol* 1992;148:617–21.
92 Werder EA, Illig R, Torresani T *et al.* Gonadal function in young adults after surgical treatment of cryptorchidism. *Br Med J* 1976;2:1357–9.
93 Garnelo P, Pinilla L, Gaytan F, Aguilar E. Pituitary testis function in rats treated neonatally with a gonadotrophin relasing hormone agonist: short and long term effects. *J Endocrinol* 1992;134:269–77.
94 Mann DR, Gould KG, Collins DC, Wallen K. Blockade of neonatal activation of the pituitary testicular axis: effect on peripubertal luteinising hormone and testosterone secretion and on testicular development in male monkeys. *J Clin Endocrinol Metab* 1989;68:600–7.
95 Rossmanith WG, Liu CH, Laughlin GA, Mortola JF, Sun BY, Yen SSC. Relative changes in LH pulsatility during the menstrual cycle: using data from hypogonadal women as a reference point. *Clin Endocrinol* 1990;32:647–60.
96 Conte FA, Grumbach MM, Kaplan SL. A diphasic pattern of gonadotrophin secretion in patients with the syndrome of gonadal dysgenesis. *J Clin Endocrinol Metab* 1975;40: 670–4.
97 Kaneko N, Kawagoe S, Hiroi M. Turners syndrome – review of the literature with reference to a successful pregnancy outcome. *Gynecol Obstet Invest* 1990;29:81–7.
98 Fox H. The pathology of premature ovarian failure. *J Pathol* 1992;167:357–63.
99 Aksel S. Immunologic aspects of reproductive diseases. *J Am Med Assoc* 1992;268:2930–4.
100 Popovic V, Micic D, Damjanovic S *et al.* Further evidence for differential regulation of follicle-stimulating hormone (FSH) and luteinizing hormone (LH): increased FSH and decreased LH levels in a patient with familial pure gonadal dysgenesis. *Postgrad Med J* 1992;68:925–7.
101 Savage MO, Lowe DG. Gonadal neoplasia and abnormal sexual differentiation. *Clin Endocrinol* 1990;32:519–33.
102 Lobaccaro JM, Medlej R, Berta P *et al.* PCR analysis and sequencing of the SRY sex determining gene in four patients with bilateral congenital anorchia. *Clin Endocrinol (Oxf)* 1993;38:197–201.
103 D'Armiento M, Reda G, Kater C, Shackleton CH, Biglieri EG. 17α-hydroxlase deficiency: mineralocorticoid hormone profiles in an affected family. *J Clin Exper Metab* 1983;56: 697–701.

104 Crowne EC, Shalet SM, Wallace WHB, Eminson DM, Price DA. Final height in girls with untreated constitutional delay of puberty. *Eur J Pediatr* 1991;150:708–12.

105 Bourguignon J-P and the Belgian Study Group for Paediatric Endocrinology. Variations in duration of pubertal growth: a mechanism compensating for differences in timing of puberty and minimising their effects on final height. *Acta Paediatr Scand* 1988;Suppl.347:16–24.

106 Finkelstein JS, Neer RM, Biller BM, Crawford JD, Klibanski A. Osteopenia in men with a history of delayed puberty. *N Engl J Med* 1992;326:600–4.

107 Warren MP, Brooks Gunn J, Hamilton LH, Fiske Warren L, Hamilton WG. Scoliosis and fractures in young ballet dancers. *N Engl J Med* 1986;314:1348–53.

108 Vico L, Prallet B, Chappard D, Pallot Prades B, Pupier R, Alexandre C. Contributions of chronological age, age at menarche and menopause and of anthropometric parameters to axial and peripheral bone densities. *Osteoporos Int* 1992; 2:153–8.

109 Wu FCW, Brown DC, Butler GE, Stirling HF, Kelnar CJH. Early morning plasma testosterone is an accurate predictor of imminent pubertal development in prepubertal boys. *J Clin Endocrinol Metab* 1993;76:26–31.

110 Buyukgebiz A, Hindmarsh PC, Brook CGD. Treatment of constitutional delay of growth and puberty with oxandrolone compared with growth hormone. *Arch Dis Child* 1990; 65:448–52.

111 Uruena M, Pansiotou S, Preece MA, Stanhope R. Is testosterone therapy for boys with constitutional delay of growth and puberty associated with impaired final height and suppression of the hypothalamo–pituitary–gonadal axis? *Eur J Pediatr* 1992;151:15–18.

112 Darendeliler F, Hindmarsh PC, Preece MA, Cox L, Brook CGD. Growth hormone increases the rate of pubertal maturation. *Acta Endocrinol* 1990;122:414–16.

113 Barkan AL, Reame NE, Kelch RP, Marshall JC. Idiopathic hypogonadotrophic hypogonadism in men: dependence of the hormone responses to GnRH on the magnitude of the endogenous secretory defect. *J Clin Endocrinol Metab* 1985;61:1118–25.

114 Van der Spuy Z. Nutrition and reproduction. *Clin Obstet Gynecol N Am* 1985;12:579–604.

115 Suttie JM, Foster DL, Veenvleit BA, Manley TR, Corson ID. Influence of food in take but independence of body weight on puberty in female sheep. *J Reprod Fertil* 1991;92:33–9.

116 Clayton RN, Ogden V, Hodgkinson J *et al.* How common are polycystic ovaries in normal women and what is their significance for the fertility of the population? *Clin Endocrinol* 1992;37:127–34.

117 Polson DW, Adams JA, Wadsworth J, Franks S. Polycystic ovaries: a common finding in normal women. *Lancet* 1988; 1:870–2.

118 Dunaif A, Hoffman AR, Scully RE *et al.* Clinical biochemical and ovarian morphological features in women with acanthosis nigricans and masculinisation. *Obstet Gynecol* 1985;66:545–52.

119 Stanhope R, Adams J, Pringle PJ, Jacobs HS, Brook CGD. The evolution of polycystic ovaries in a girl with hypogonadotrophic hypogonadism before puberty and during puberty induced with pulsatile GnRH. *Fertil Steril* 1987;47:872–5.

120 Adashi EY, Resnick CE, Hurwitz A *et al.* Insulin like growth factors – the ovarian connection – review. *Hum Reprod* 1991;6:1213–19.

121 Slowinska-Srzednicka J, Zgliczynski W, Makowska A *et al.* An abnormality of the growth hormone/insulin like growth factor 1 axis in women with polycystic ovary syndrome due to coexistent obesity. *J Clin Endocrinol Metab* 1992;74: 1432–5.

122 Nobels F, Dewailly D. Puberty and polycystic ovarian syndrome – the insulin/insulin like growth factor 1 hypothesis. *Fertil Steril* 1992;58:655–66.

123 Geffner ME, Kaplan SA, Bersch N *et al.* Leprechaunism: *in vitro* insulin action despite genetic insulin resistance. *Pediatr Res* 1987;22:286–91.

124 Pasquali R, Casimirri F. The impact of obesity on hyperandrogenism and polycystic ovary syndrome in premenopausal women. *Clin Endocrinol* 1993;39:1–16.

125 Hague WM, Adams J, Rodda C *et al.* The prevalence of polycystic ovaries in patients with congenital adrenal hyperplasia and their close relatives. *Clin Endocrinol* 1990;33:501–10.

126 Spinder T, Spijkstra JJ, Van den Tweel JG *et al.* The effects of long term testosterone administration on pulsatile LH secretion and on ovarian histology in eugonadal female to male transexual subjects. *J Clin Endocrinol Metab* 1989;69: 151–7.

127 Givens JR. Familial polycystic ovarian disease. *Endocrinol Metab Clin N Am* 1988;17:771–83.

128 Kiddy DS, Hamilton Fairley D, Seppala M *et al.* Diet induced changes in sex hormone binding globulin and free testosterone in women with normal or polycystic ovaries: correlation with serum insulin and IGF 1. *Clin Endocrinol* 1989; 31:757–63.

129 Finkel DM, Phillips JL. Stimulation of spermatogenesis by gonadotrophins in men with hypogonadotrophic hypogonadism. *N Engl J Med* 1985;313:651–5.

130 Abdalla HI, Baber RJ, Kirkland A, Leonard T, Studd JWW. Pregnancy in women with premature ovarian failure using tubal and intrauterine transfer of cryopreserved zygotes. *Br J Obstet Gynaecol* 1989;96:1071–5.

16: Gynaecology

J.S. SANFILIPPO

INTRODUCTION

A paediatric patient undergoing gynaecological examination should be handled with particular care. The initial encounter will set the tone for all future gynaecological examinations, and if the examination is painful or uncomfortable or if there is a significant lack of rapport between the patient and the examiner, the patient may well suffer lasting psychological consequences. A gentle, caring attitude on the physician's part will go far in helping the patient relax for the present as well as for future examinations.

HISTORY

It is important to obtain a comprehensive history. This may sometimes be difficult, especially if a paediatric patient in apparent distress is accompanied by distraught parents. The clinician should be well versed with respect to appropriate questions regarding the chief complaint of the paediatric and adolescent patient.

Newborn and infant

Evaluation of the external genitalia of the neonate is of the utmost importance. The procedure conveys to the parents that assessment of the genitalia is an integral part of the general physical examination. Appropriate history should be obtained, especially if there is any abnormality identified at the time of examination. Problems such as congenital adrenal hyperplasia are usually associated with a significant family history. Early diagnosis may well prove to be life-saving. Presence of imperforate hymen also should be diagnosed at this time.

After completion of the inspection of the genitalia and appropriate palpation, consideration should be provided to gentle placement of a paediatric feeding tube into the vagina in an effort to identify any outflow tract obstruction. In the newborn, normal appearance of the external genitalia includes somewhat prominent labia and a thick protuberant hymen, all of which reflect the increase in maternal endogenous oestrogenic milieu. When the infant is several months of age the external genitalia are characterized by more firm, rigid, relatively inflexible vulvar tissue in association with normal anatomy. Presence of clitoromegaly or other abnormality of the genitalia should be diagnosed at this time.

The abdominal examination is important for the identification of organomegaly. Outflow tract obstruction can indicate vaginal agenesis and may present as an abdominal mass when associated with fluid accumulation in the vagina. Other anomalies that should be considered at this time include bladder exstrophy, cloacal defects and vaginal prolapse. Cystic hygroma, lymphoedema and coarctation of the aorta may be early evidence of gonadal dysgenesis, as with Turner syndrome. Ideally, this should be diagnosed in the newborn period.

Toddler or young child

The history should be obtained primarily from the parent(s) or caretaker, but the child, when appropriate, should be involved in the gynaecological experience. The history should include inquiry with respect to developmental milestones, immunizations and past medical problems, as well as duration of the specific complaint. With respect to vaginitis it is important to determine whether or not there has been a change in detergents, bubble bath, type of underwear or play habits (such as sandbox exposure) which can be associated with the introduction of various forms of vulvovaginal irritants.

The physical examination in this age group should include a 'just-looking' approach with appropriate interaction from the child, letting her handle the instruments to build confidence and rapport. This approach has been noted repeatedly to be helpful to the examination process. Use of anatomically correct dolls, in association with communication 'beforehand' on how the examination will proceed, is also helpful.

In this age group the patient is placed in a frog-legged or knee–chest position. The dorsal lithotomy position is reserved for older paediatric patients. The younger patient may choose to sit on her mother's lap, either in a chair or with the mother in the dorsal lithotomy position holding the child. The knee–chest position is helpful for girls aged 2 or older, and allows appropriate access for inspection of the introitus and lower third of the vagina, as well as allowing for cultures or other wet preps as deemed necessary. The use of a calcium alginate (Calgi swab, Spectrum Labs, Houston) is minimally if at all traumatic, making possible a good sampling of vaginal secretions.

The hymen should be inspected carefully. A number of normal hymeneal variants have been reported, including annular, crescent, septate and cribriform types.

The diameter of the hymen continues to be a point of controversy. It is influenced by age, relaxation, type of measurement (that is transverse or anterior–posterior), whether the child tends to masturbate, places foreign objects in the vagina, etc. The hymen appears larger when the patient is in the knee–chest position than in the frog-legged or dorsal lithotomy position. Emans [1] has reported a mean transverse hymeneal diameter of 2.9 ± 1.3 mm with a range of 1–6 mm in 3–6-year-old patients. The mean anterior–posterior diameter is 3.3 ± 1.3 mm with a range of 1–7 mm. A good rule of thumb for determining the appropriateness of hymeneal diameter is 1 mm for each year of age.

The gynaecological examination should also discern the state of perineal hygiene, and a bimanual (recto-abdominal) examination should be performed. Abnormalities more commonly identified include urethral prolapse; labial agglutination; lichen sclerosis; vaginitis, trauma, condyloma, psoriasis; molluscum contagiosum; and evidence for sexual abuse (Plates 16.1–16.5, facing p. 290).

Adolescent girl

A first pelvic examination should be performed only when the patient is sexually active, 18 years of age, or has one or more of the following concerns: abnormal vaginal bleeding, suspected pregnancy or abdominal–pelvic pain.

EXAMINING THE ADOLESCENT

Depending upon the circumstance, the clinician may be called upon to play the role of detective in order to determine why the adolescent seeks gynaecological evaluation. It is imperative that the adolescent be given time (ideally, during the physical examination process) to provide any history which would be germane. Confidentiality must be clearly respected and efforts at establishing a good doctor–patient relationship cannot be overemphasized. Varying degrees of maturity of the adolescent should be taken into account regarding the queries made.

Once the history is completed, the examination process should be explained. This provides an appropriate forum for communication regarding anatomy and physiology. As with all physical examinations, a general examination, complemented by Tanner staging of the breasts and pubic hair followed by a pelvic examination, is indicated. In general the adolescent is placed in the dorsal lithotomy position. Ideally, the patient must remain 'in control'. A mirror to aid in instruction with respect to external genitalia is often helpful. Use of a cotton bud to point out structures easily accomplishes this goal. The hymeneal opening is first inspected. Degree of vaginal epithelialization, pubic hair distribution and clitoral size should be noted. The speculum examination is facilitated by the use of a small Huffman or Pedersen speculum in a virginal female. In general this speculum is no larger than a tampon; information which should be conveyed to the adolescent prior to insertion. Ideally, the speculum is placed first on the patient's thigh with continued communication maintained during the examination process, thus eliminating any 'surprises'. A Papanicolaou (Pap) smear is obtained and, as appropriate, cultures for venereal disease. Any vaginal discharge should be evaluated with use of a wet prep.

After the examination is completed, the findings should be communicated first to the adolescent. As previously mentioned, ground rules should be established with the patient regarding confidentiality, with a clear understanding of the need for establishing a *modus operandi* of dealing with parents, in case a significant clinical problem occurs during the course of therapy. The adolescent should have the option of letting her parent(s) be present during the postexamination discussion. All queries should be answered in a direct and simple manner, and an appropriate plan of management relayed. Ideally, all questions posed by the parent(s) should be thoroughly answered, preferably with active involvement of the adolescent. The patient should have a strong sense of participation in her management.

SPECIFIC MEDICAL PROBLEMS

Throughout life the vulvar skin responds in a different physiological manner from other areas of body skin; for example, in absorption capacity, transepidermal water evaporation, water-holding capacity of the stratum corneum and susceptibility to irritant factors and blood flow. There appears to be an increased bacterial count at the vulva compared with other sites of the body. Table 16.1 illustrates the chief complaints of paediatric patients presenting for gynaecological evaluation.

Table 16.1 Chief complaints of paediatric patients presenting for gynaecological evaluation (from [3])

	Number	Percentage
Vaginal discharge	129	45
Abnormal bleeding	52	18
Contraception	25	9
Abdominal pain	27	9
Suspected anomaly	9	3
Suspected sexual abuse	6	2
Trauma	3	1
All others	37	13
Total	288	100

Vaginal discharge

The paediatric patient with a vaginal discharge can often present a clinical challenge. It is important to note colour, odour, duration and associated pruritus. Several vaginal flora microorganisms commonly believed to be pathogenic may be 'normal' for patients in this age group. Diphtheroids and *Staphylococcus epidermidis* are quite prevalent. Less common forms include streptococci, lactobacilli and coliforms. *Gardnerella vaginalis* has also been isolated from the vagina in asymptomatic younger children.

PHYSIOLOGICAL DISCHARGE

An increase in vaginal discharge normally occurs 6–12 months before menarche. Although there is often a copious discharge, with associated yellow staining of the patient's underpants, it usually has no smell. The discharge is composed of Doderlein's bacilli. Cultures are unnecessary, and reassurance is the best treatment. Spontaneous resolution will occur when the vaginal pH, which is 4.5–5.0 at this age, becomes adjusted for the menstrual cycle from pH 3.8 (follicular phase) to 4.5 (luteal phase).

Non-specific vulvovaginitis

Patients who practise poor perineal hygiene often develop a condition known as non-specific vaginitis. In 68% of reported cases this is associated with coliform bacteria. The discharge is characteristically brown or green with a foetid odour. The vaginal pH is 4.7–6.5. Therapy requires instruction in bowel and bladder habits, with special emphasis on the necessity for wiping faecal material away from the vulvovaginal area. The second most common bacterial organism associated with non-specific vulvovaginitis is β-haemolytic *Streptococcus* or coagulase-positive *Staphylococcus*. These organisms are often contaminants from the nasopharynx which have been transmitted manually to the vulvar area.

On occasion, non-specific vulvovaginitis can result in a state of 'chronic infection', the symptoms of which may cause significant psychological consequences for the child and parent alike. The physician should stress the importance of avoiding 'vaginal fixation', while at the same time giving instruction in good perineal hygiene.

Specific vulvovaginitis

PERIANAL DERMATITIS

In the newborn the skin may be characterized by erythema and an eroded appearance. There may or may not be an associated nappy rash. Treatment consists of careful cleansing, bland lubricants and protective agents (e.g. Vaseline).

MILIARIA

Miliaria is related to obstruction of the eccrine sweat ducts and is common in neonates and infants. The nappy area (nappy dermatitis) is a common site. In general, keeping the affected area clean is all that is usually necessary; however, secondary infection may occur.

INTERTRIGO

Intertrigo in the genitourethral area is common, and develops in relation to friction, obesity and moisture. Miliaria and secondary infection are often associated with intertrigo. Keeping the area dry, and application of a corticosteroid cream, is usually effective.

IMPETIGO

Impetigo is an abnormality primarily found in the newborn. It is associated with *Staphylococcus aureus*, usually phage group II, especially type 71, which may be acquired from the mother, other relatives or hospital personnel. Impetigo tends to affect the vulva and umbilical areas, causing lesions and blisters. Treatment with antibiotics should be instituted to include *Staphylococcus* coverage.

NAPPY DERMATITIS

Irritant dermatitis from friction and wetting, exacerbated by the effects of ammonia, urine of pH >8 and secondary infection with *Candida* or bacteria results in nappy dermatitis. The erythema may become somewhat glazed in its appearance and tends to be marked around the edges. Clearing occurs when the child no longer wears nappies.

SEBORRHOEIC DERMATITIS

This condition of the vulva is often associated with lesions, particularly on the scalp. The nappy area tends to be more diffusely red than in irritant types. There may be associated pruritus. Use of cleansing agents (sulfa and/or salicylic acid) is helpful.

INFANTILE GLUTEAL GRANULOMAS

These lesions are categorized by oval nodules with eroded surfaces on the buttocks, usually but not always associated with a previously existing nappy rash. Fluorinated topical corticosteroids and *Candida* have been suspected aetiologies. Treatment with a mild corticosteroid (0.5–1% hydrocortisone cream) with or without a topical antifungal (for example clotrimazole hydrocortisone ointment) results in regression, but sometimes associated scarring occurs.

MOLLUSCUM CONTAGIOSUM

Molluscum contagiosum presents as an umbilicated dome-shaped papule (Plate 16.1). The central umbilication is usually associated with a pulpy core. It is a fairly common infection of the skin and is associated with the poxvirus group. Vulvar lesions appear to result from autoinoculation or close contact with an affected individual. The incubation period is 2–7 weeks. Diagnosis is confirmed by light microscopic visualization of viral inclusions (molluscum bodies) in the central core. Treatment requires elimination of the lesions. Silver nitrate can be applied following gentle curettage. Other methods of therapy include cryosurgery or electrocautery.

LABIAL ADHESIONS

The labia minora present with a central line of adherence from an area immediately inferior to the clitoris down to the fourchette (Plate 16.2). It is commonly observed in patients under 6 years of age, and is quite often asymptomatic. However, recurrent urinary tract symptoms are seen in 20–40% of patients. The lesions are usually associated with local inflammation in association with the hypo-oestrogenic state of the preadolescent. Pooling of urine in the vagina and recurrent vulvovaginitis appear to provide a continuous nidus of inflammation and infection which results in recurrent urinary tract infections.

If the patient is asymptomatic there is no specific need for treatment; however, in the case of recurrent urinary symptoms, treatment should be offered. Topical oestrogen cream applied each evening is effective in over 90% of cases. Elimination of the lesions may require from 2 to 8 weeks. Daily cleansing, followed by application of a bland ointment such as petrolatum, should be continued for 1–2 months after separation of the adhesions occurs. Manual separation of the adhesions is advisable only if they separate easily and do not cause significant trauma to the child. Labial adhesions are benign and quite common; therapy consists merely of reassurance to the patient and parents. Once the vaginal pH becomes more acid during adolescence, recurrent labial adhesions almost always cease.

PREPUTIAL ADHESIONS

Adhesions of the prepuce to the glans of the clitoris are frquently present in children until they reach the age of 7 or 8. They are not associated with specific symptoms and spontaneous separation occurs around menarche. Nightly application of a cream containing oestrogen for 10 days to 2 weeks is an excellent means of obtaining separation of these adhesions.

LICHEN SCLEROSUS

Lichen sclerosus (LS) is characterized by small, pink-to-ivory flat-topped papules, several millimetres in diameter. The papules appear to coalesce into plaques that become wrinkled and atrophic. The anogenital lesions frequently resemble an hourglass or figure of 8 (Plate 16.3). Vesicles and bullae may occur over the vulva with associated haemorrhage. A biopsy may be required for diagnosis.

LS usually presents before the age of 7, but the youngest person reported was only a few weeks old. Menarche often results in spontaneous improvement.

The cause of LS is unknown, but it is believed to be related to an autoimmune disorder and an associated organ-specific autoimmune disease. Positive immunofluorescence for fibrin, C'3 or immunoglobulin M (IgM) in involved areas has been demonstrated in 75% of patients. Treatment is symptomatic: emollients and topical corticosteroids usually provide relief. Topical oestrogens and/or androgens are also recommended. Any secondary infection should be treated with antibiotics. Some affected individuals demonstrate what is known as the Loebner phenomenon – precipitation of lesions secondary to trauma. They should avoid tight clothing and genital trauma.

LICHEN SIMPLEX CHRONICUS

Lichen simplex chronicus (neurodermatitis) is a chronic, lichenified plaque that causes pruritus. This in turn causes scratching and inflammation, and a vicious scratch–itch cycle is established. The condition is rare in children. Treatment is use of antihistamines and topical or intralesional corticosteroids.

ATOPIC DERMATITIS

Atopic dermatitis affects 3% of all children. Patients

present with hay fever and/or asthma as well as a positive family history of such allergies. The vulvar lesions are characterized by intense pruritus, erythema, papules and vesicles, with oozing and crusting of the involved areas. There may be associated circumscribed, lichenified scaly patches on the vulvar area. Pruritus often causes scratching, which results in excoriation of the lesions. Secondary bacterial or candidal infection is common.

Antihistamines are necessary to control pruritus. Sitz baths with use of mild soap and lubricants are essential. Topical corticosteroids such as 1% hydrocortisone are also effective; secondary bacterial or candidal infections require specific treatment.

CONTACT DERMATITIS

There are two primary types – allergic contact dermatitis, an immunologically mediated phenomenon, and irritant dermatitis which has no immunological association.

The allergic type appears as a result of sensitization to an allergen; the irritant dermatitis may appear instantaneously. In either case the vulva is characterized by oedematous, erythematous, oozing lesions, sometimes accompanied by vesicles or pustules. Chronic contact dermatitis is often associated with thickened and lichenified lesions. The clue for correct diagnosis of this condition is the limitation of the dermatitis to the area of contact with the aetiological agent. There may also be a secondary candidal or bacterial infection. Some common aetiological agents include soaps, powders, bubble baths, feminine hygiene sprays, topical medications, toilet paper, rubber and certain types of clothing. Treatment should include avoiding the offending agent, sitz baths or compresses and use of aluminium acetate topical solution (Burrow's solution) during acute episodes. Mild topical corticosteroids such as 0.5–1% hydrocortisone cream, applied several times daily, may further aid healing and alleviate vulvar irritation. Recurrence can be prevented by removal of the offending aetiological agent.

VULVAR PSORIASIS

Vulvar psoriasis is frequently associated with lesions on other parts of the body and characterized by violaceous papules or plaques with a thick adherent silvery scale (Plate 16.4). The intertriginous areas may manifest inverse psoriasis, a variant associated with sparing of the extremities. Vulvar lesions are usually poorly demarcated and may present as a scaly patch, most commonly on the mons pubis. Therapy is multifaceted. Corticosteroid cream should be used in conjunction with control of secondary infection and pruritus. These lesions are often resistant to therapy, especially if located in the vulvar area. A 1% hydrocortisone cream is beneficial in relieving acute episodes.

PITYRIASIS VERSICOLOR

This lesion is caused by *Pityrosporum orbiculare*, and is manifested by scaly macules of the trunk in postpubertal patients; however, lesions have been reported on the face and the genital area, especially in West Indian infants of African background. The diagnosis is easily established by visualization of hyphae and spores with 10% potassium hydroxide solution. Treatment with topical imidazoles such as clotrimazole, is effective.

PINWORMS

Pinworms (*Enterobius vermicularis*) appear to carry colonic bacteria to the perineum, causing recurrent vulvovaginitis. The female emerges from the anus to deposit eggs. It is believed that 20% of girls infected with *Enterobius vermicularis* develop vulvovaginitis. The 'Scotch tape' test should be used to search for this organism if there is any suspicion for pinworms, or in the case of undiagnosed recurrent vulvovaginitis. Victims typically suffer pruritus and nocturnal episodes of scratching exacerbations. Treatment can be accomplished by administration of mebendazole.

SHIGELLA

Shigella flexneri and *Shigella sonnei* present in various ways in association with vaginitis. About 47% of patients have a bloody vaginal discharge and 2% present with diarrhoea. Systemic antibiotics are the treatment of choice. Bowel colonization with *Shigella* can result in subclinical gastrointestinal symptoms in 10% of household members. Treatment for *Shigella* vaginitis includes ampicillin, amoxicillin, trimethoprim, sulphamethoxazole, nalidixic acid, tetracycline or penicillin.

FOREIGN BODIES

Foreign bodies are sometimes responsible for vaginal bleeding in the paediatric patient. The presence of a foreign body in the vagina is often accompanied by a foul odour and discharge.

Plates 16.5 and 16.6, facing p. 290, attest to the variety of substances that have been found in the vagina and associated symptomatology. Plate 16.5 depicts wadded toilet paper noted with a greater than 1 year history of recurrent vulvovaginal symptoms in a 4-year-old child. Plate 16.6 shows a pen-top identified in the vagina of a 5-year-old. The clinician must suspect the presence of a foreign body any time there is vaginal discharge and bleeding in a young patient.

HERPES SIMPLEX VIRUS

Types 1 and 2 of this virus can be involved in vulvar lesions. Although the types are not site-specific, type 1 is commonly responsible for facial and oral lesions; type 2 for genital lesions. The virus lies latent in the dorsal root ganglia and is periodically reactivated, causing outbreaks on the skin or mucosa. Papules become vesicles, which in turn become eroded and crusted. Primary lesions tend to be more severe than recurrences. Precipitating factors for genital lesions include stress, intercourse and menstruation.

HUMAN PAPILLOMA VIRUS

Human papilloma virus has many serotypes. Types 6, 11, 16 and 18 are more commonly associated with anogenital lesions; 16, 18, 31, 33 and 35 with malignant and premalignant lesions. Lesions may be transmitted by casual domestic contact, including bathing and fomites, as well as vertical transmission, which occurs through maternal infection at the time of delivery. Sexual transmission is the most common means of delivering the organisms in the adolescent and adult populations.

Vulvar neoplasia

Vulvar tumours in children are rare but neurofibromas, granular cell myoblastomas, teratomas, lipomas and lymphangiomas occur in this age group. Neoplasms in children are more commonly malignant than benign and squamous-cell carcinoma, adenocarcinoma, sarcoma botryoides, embryonal carcinoma and endodermal sinus tumours have all been reported.

Vulvar neurofibromas have been noted in association with von Recklinghausen disease. Treatment necessitates operative intervention. Granular cell myoblastoma of the vulva is sometimes seen in the prepubertal girl. This tumour is believed to be of Schwann-cell origin and has the potential for being malignant. Excision must be complete, as recurrence is common. Teratomas of the perineum in newborn infants have been reported and treated with wide excision. Lipoma of the vulva is best treated by excisional biopsy. Haemangiofibrolipomas have been diagnosed in association with distorted vulvar anatomy, and require total excision. Lymphangioma of the vulva may present as a soft, round, symmetrical enlargement of the labia majora and can cause discomfort for the child when she sits down. Lymphangiomas affect pelvic lymphatics rather than acting as a true neoplasm.

Haemangiomas are not true neoplasms but instead represent anomalous development of blood vessels. Capillary haemangiomas are usually asymptomatic and many regress spontaneously (Plate 16.7). Usually no treatment is necessary. Cavernous haemangiomas are composed of larger vessels and may bleed profusely if injured. Surgical treatment should be delayed until toilet training has been completed. Labial papillomas appear as soft, flesh-coloured, pedunculated structures which arise from the labia. They are usually asymptomatic, but torsion of the stalk can result in infarction. Biopsy is necessary for a proper diagnosis.

In the UK, malignant neoplasms of the vulva represent 16% of primary non-ovarian genital tract tumours in children with an incidence of 0.5 cases per million children annually [4]. Clinical presentation of the neoplasm is usually a solid, polypoid, or cystic mass. A chronic ulcer is the more unusual presentation. Sarcomas are the most common of the malignant vaginal tumours in this age group, representing 80% of vulvar neoplasms; carcinomas and germ-cell tumours follow. Radical surgery is often required with postoperative radiation and chemotherapy.

Urethral prolapse

Urethral prolapse, defined as a circular eversion of the urethral mucosa protruding through the meatus, presents as a friable, reddish-blue annular mass (Plate 16.8, facing p. 290). It may be ulcerated, infected or even gangrenous. Careful examination allows identification of the urethral meatus in the centre of the mass and the normal posterior vaginal introitus. Differentiation of a urethral prolapse from neoplasm is essential. Young patients with urethral prolapse are usually premenarcheal. The great majority are an average age of 5 years. The typical presentation is of painless genital bleeding. There may be associated dysuria, urinary frequency or introital pain. There may be a history of genital trauma, increased intra-abdominal pressure from sustained episodes of crying or chronic constipation.

Treatment is by surgical excision and/or ablative procedures resulting in strangulation of the prolapsed tissue. Conservative measures include sitz baths and systemic antibiotics if secondary infection is identified. Topical oestrogens have been the primary mode of therapy. The most common surgical treatment is excision of the prolapsed tissue under general anaesthesia. Strangulation of prolapsed mucosa by suture ligation over a urethral catheter is advocated. Cauterization and cryosurgery are other options to be considered. Hospitalization is minimal in most cases; complications and recurrence rates are low.

Cervical prolapse

Cervical prolapse is rare in children. The usual presentation is a mass protruding from the vagina during the first few days after birth. Most cases are associated with meningomyelocele or other central nervous system anomalies. Repeated digital reduction is usually effective.

Hymenal tags

This problem is seen is 6% of female neonates; the hymenal tag presents as a smooth, firm, pink nodule protruding from the margin of the hymen. The usual location for the tag is the dorsal margin of the hymen near the fourchette. Spontaneous resolution of the tag occurs as the oestrogenic effect decreases during the first few weeks after birth. Persistence of the lesions for more than a few weeks requires biopsy evaluation.

Epidermoid cysts

Epidermoid cysts are benign inclusion cysts. Although rare in children, they present as firm nodular masses which are usually symptomatic. Infection or rupture can cause inflammation and tenderness. Treatment is by simple excision with a histopathological confirmation to rule out a neoplasm.

Chronic vulvar granulomas

Chronic vulvar granulomas are painful, ulcerative, polypoid lesions most often seen in malnourished children. There is usually a long-standing history of vulvovaginitis and vaginal discharge. Treatment includes improvement in nutrition and local eradication of the vulvovaginitis, as well as any ulcerations. The lesions should be cleansed several times a day and kept dry. Topical oestrogens aid healing.

GENITAL TRACT INJURIES IN THE PREPUBERTAL CHILD

Most vulvar injuries in prepubertal children are accidental. However, physical abuse, especially sexual abuse, must be considered. Many vaginal lacerations are superficial and limited to the mucosal and submucosal tissues. Treatment for this type of lesion is expectant. However, continuation of active bleeding may necessitate ligation of the involved vasculature to attain haemostasis. As the vaginal mucosa is distended with blood, intense pain and haematoma formation can result. Usually, the haematoma resolves as the blood clots resorb and the swelling disappears. When a traumatic haematoma extends into the broad ligament or peritoneal cavity, exploratory laparotomy may be necessary. Plane film of the abdomen should be obtained, to rule out a foreign body. Bladder and bowel integrity must be carefully examined and evaluated, and any lacerations surgically corrected.

Vulvar haematomas

The perineum, vulva and vagina are all extremely vascular, with subcutaneous tissue loosely arranged. Blunt injury from a direct blow or fall can cause blood vessels underneath the perineal skin to rupture with resulting haematoma formation (Plate 16.9, facing p. 290). This usually presents as a rounded, tense, tender, purplish-red swelling, the size of which depends upon the amount of blood involved. Tissues spread apart by the bleeding can cause intense pain. In most cases, further haematoma formation can be prevented by the application of pressure on the blood vessels. If secondary infection occurs, there may be sloughing of the involved tissue. If the haematoma is small it can be controlled by applying pressure, perhaps with an ice-pack. Massive swelling of the vulva frequently subsides spontaneously with external pressure from a cold pack. A large haematoma that continues to increase in size may necessitate surgical intervention to remove clots and ligate actively bleeding vessels. Packing around the haematoma may also be helpful. Broad-spectrum antibiotics are used as prophylaxis when the vulvar haematoma is large, especially if operative intervention is required. Sitz baths help remove secretions and contaminants. Treatment for acute symptoms may include use of an air-filled rubber or foam 'doughnut' which can prevent pressure necrosis of the swollen external genitalia. An X-ray of the pelvis is advisable to rule out pelvic bone fracture, especially if the haematoma obstructs the urethra and necessitates insertion of a catheter. When swelling subsides there may be urinary retention, indicating an evulsion of the urethra. In such cases a cystourethrogram is necessary for further evaluation.

BREAST DISORDERS

Mammary glands are derived from the epidermal layer of the foetus. Beginning at approximately 6 weeks of development *in utero*, epidermal cells migrate to the mesenchyme and form the mammary ridges. Breast buds, lactiferous ducts and fully developed mammary glands eventually result. Breast development normally occurs in girls between the ages of 8.5 and 13 years (see Chapter 4). The rate of breast growth is variable and development often asymmetrical. Complete development may not occur until a woman is in her early 20s. The Tanner classification of breast development remains the hallmark for assessment of the mammary glands.

INFANT AND YOUNG CHILD

Examination of the breasts should begin in the delivery room. The presence of normally palpable breast buds is important to differentiate from any congenital anomaly. Polymastia may be detectable in the newborn infant, but usually is not recognized until the child is older (pubertal). Examination of the infant with the parent(s) present, provides an opportunity to educate the family about normal breast anatomy and physiology.

PUBERTAL GIRL

As noted above, examination of the pubertal girl should include Tanner staging of the breasts. Evaluation for asymmetry as well as for masses, congenital anomalies, developmental abnormalities or nipple discharge is appropriate.

ADOLESCENT GIRL

The adolescent should understand that the breast examination is an integral part of the gynaecological evaluation. Tanner staging should be determined, as well as instruction with respect to breast self-examination.

Congenital anomalies

Complete absence of breast tissue is termed amastia. Although quite rare, the condition is frequently unilateral and often associated with other abnormalities such as Poland syndrome (aplasia of the pectoralis musculature, rib deformities, webbed fingers and radial nerve aplasia). Amastia may be iatrogenic, as in the case of inadvertent excision of a breast bud. Athelia is defined as absence of nipple(s). This condition is also rare and may not be associated with absent breast tissue. Both abnormalities require surgical correction. Supernumerary breasts (polymastia) and supernumerary nipples (polythelia) are relatively common (Plate 16.10, facing p. 290); they occur along the 'milk lines' and are usually asymptomatic. There appears to be an association between polythelia and anomalies of the urinary and cardiovascular systems. In general, surgical excision of accessory breasts or nipples is not necessary. However, if this breast tissue or nipple(s) becomes symptomatic, excision may be indicated. Hypoplasia of the breast varies in degree from a nearly total absence to well-formed breasts that are considered by the patient to be 'too small'.

There are three general causes for poor or absent breast development. First, there may be delayed onset and slow breast development which is otherwise normal. Second, there may be a family history of late breast development. Third, there may be failure or suppression of ovarian function. Treatment depends upon the underlying cause. Breast atrophy is occasionally seen in adolescents and is almost uniformly secondary to dietary changes such as anorexia nervosa. Correction of the underlying problem results in re-establishment of breast tissue.

Neonatal breast abnormalities

Bilateral breast hypertrophy secondary to elevated circulating endogenous steroid hormones of late gestation can sometimes occur. It may be associated with discharge from the nipples known as 'witch's milk'. Repeated manipulation of the breasts can exacerbate the condition. On occasion the hypertrophy is associated with mastitis caused by *Staphylococcus* infection. Treatment is administration of antibiotics and manual expression of purulent material.

Premature thelarche

Premature thelarche is isolated breast development that occurs in a child most often under age 4, but can be seen in a child up to 8 years of age. If there are no other signs of pubertal development, no treatment is necessary other than continued close observation for further signs of precocious puberty (see Chapter 15).

The mechanism of premature thelarche is frequently associated with oestrogen production from an ovarian cyst. These transient steroid-producing follicular cysts are usually a self-limiting problem. However, increased oestrogen output can occur from the adrenal gland or ingestion of oestrogens.

Galactorrhoea

Spontaneous flow of milk from the nipples is termed galactorrhoea. Evaluation of this condition is the same for adolescents and adults, and consists of determining the serum prolactin (PRL) level for the possibility of pituitary prolactinoma. One other cause for galactorrhoea is hypothyroidism associated with elevated thyrotrophin-releasing hormone which also stimulates PRL release. Treatment depends upon the underlying aetiology.

Trauma and inflammation

Breast trauma in adolescent females has not been common in the past, but it is now occurring in ever-increasing frequency because of the great rise in the number of young women participating in contact sports. The trauma usually takes the form of contusion or haematoma, and often resolves without incidence. Occasionally fat necrosis occurs, and results in either cystic changes in the breast or fibrosis with retraction of skin or nipple over the injured area. Either of these changes may mimic that associated with malignancy. A biopsy may be the only means of differentiating the two.

Mastitis can occur in a newborn, and presents as erythema, tenderness and sometimes swelling of the affected breast. The problem is usually unilateral, but certainly can be bilateral. Obstruction of a mammary duct appears to be the underlying pathophysiology. Treatment with warm compresses is generally effective. If there is engorgement in the neonate breast, the physician may express milk to relieve pressure, increase comfort and hasten the healing process. Though antibiotics are not usually necessary, these infants must be watched carefully for signs of infection. Mastitis, although uncommon, also occurs in older infants and children. If there is evidence of infection (as noted above), and thus a decision made to proceed with antibiotic therapy, consideration of the appropriate spectrum of coverage should be made. Specifically, *Staphylococcus*, *Streptococcus* and *Escherichia coli* are the most common bacterial organisms. On occasion, *Pseudomonas* may be cultured.

Mammary dysplasia

A breast examination is necessary for a diagnosis of mammary dysplasia. This is a common lesion in the female breast, characterized by changes associated with the menstrual cycle. The aetiology may be related to a hormonal imbalance – possibly a relative excess of oestrogen and deficient corpus luteum activity. This imbalance produces exaggerated responses in the breast tissue, especially in the upper outer quadrants during the premenstrual phase of the cycle. Treatment depends on the degree of symptomatology. Danazol (an isoxazole derivative of testosterone) therapy in daily doses of 200 mg can be beneficial, as well as the avoidance of methylxanthines (coffee, tea, carbonated drinks and the like). In addition, elimination of chocolate in the diet is advisable.

Mastodynia

Breast pain, mastalgia or mastodynia, undoubtedly occurs in the adolescent. The exact aetiology is unknown; however, oestrogen therapy, trauma, hypertrophy, infection and mammary dysplasia appear to play a role.

Treatment includes proper-fitting brassieres and avoidance of caffeine and dairy products. In addition, vitamin E may be useful, although prospective placebo-controlled studies question the efficacy of vitamin E in treatment of mastodynia.

Virginal juvenile hypertrophy

This problem is manifested by pathologically large breasts in the adolescent. It is often familial. Pain, hypovascularization, tissue necrosis and rupture of the skin can be associated with virginal juvenile breast hypertrophy. Some patients have benefited from medical treatment with danazol, but most require surgical intervention in the form of reductive mammoplasty.

Cytosarcoma phylloides

A firm non-tender, well-defined mass, cystosarcoma phylloides, is usually slow-growing and must be differentiated from fibroadenoma. Excision is required, although most are benign, since some have been reported to be malignant with/without metastasis.

Malignancy

Malignant breast tumours are rare in children and adolescents. An incidence of primary breast cancer of 0.2% has been reported, but most of the literature consists of isolated case reports. Two per cent of all breast cancers occur in women under the age of 25. Diagnosis is established by biopsy.

Unilateral breast mass in childhood

A breast mass in a child is a concern for the parent(s) as well as the clinician. A number of masses have been identified in the paediatric-aged patient, including haemangiomas, lipomas, papillomas, lymphangiomas, benign cysts, fibrosis, localized mastitis, haematoma, fat necrosis and benign tumours. The most common of these lesions is the breast haemangioma. This problem is self-limited, and usually surgical excision is not necessary.

Breast cysts are rare in this age group, but do indeed occur. Transillumination of the mass, ultrasonography and needle aspiration are useful from both the diagnostic and therapeutic perspectives. One must be cautioned that asymmetrical breast development is a frequent finding, and biopsy should not be undertaken under such a circumstance. As noted above, malignancy of the breast is extremely rare.

Breast enlargement and masses in the prepubertal child

Breast tumours occur infrequently in the prepubertal girl. Although more common in the adolescent, the probability for malignancy is low. The most common neoplasm in the adolescent breast is the fibroadenoma, which may be variable in size and texture. Most are firm, mobile solitary lesions; but they may be multiple in one-fifth of patients. These tumours are hormone-dependent, as evidenced by the fact that they may change in size during the menstrual cycle. Treatment for a fibroadenoma is by excisional biopsy.

Evaluation of the breast mass in the adolescent female

Complementing the history, physical examination should be directed toward signs of asymmetry, mass effect and overlying skin changes. Dimpling of the skin, prominent venous pattern and ulceration are ominous and raise the suspicion of malignancy. Palpation to distinguish cystic from solid masses may be augmented by transillumination. Examination of lymph nodes should routinely be undertaken when a breast mass is palpable. If a cystic lesion is identified, fine-needle aspiration (FNA) is appropriate. If the FNA is positive, surgical excision is indicated.

Imaging in the adolescent with a breast mass primarily involves use of ultrasound to distinguish cystic from solid masses. Mammography has not proved helpful because of the stromal proliferation in association with normal pubertal mammary development. Computerizd tomography (CT) has also been advocated, as has magnetic resonance imaging (MRI). High-resolution CT scanning appears to be helpful in evaluating bony rib lesions, as well as the overlying soft tissue. Calcifications within the soft tissue may represent previous trauma. Extension of the CT scan through the chest and abdomen may reveal the full extent of an inflammatory process or lesion. Biopsy can be attempted under CT or fluoroscopic guidance. MRI remains an investigational tool in evaluating the adolescent breast mass.

PAEDIATRIC GYNAECOLOGICAL IMAGING

Ultrasonography clearly plays an important and integral role in the clinical evaluation of gynaecological problems in this age group. The opportunity to highlight a number of somewhat unique aspects of imaging in the child with a gynaecological problem should provide particular clinical relevance. Consultation between the clinician and imaging expert is the best means of determining the type of examination best suited for the clinical problem posed. Indications are noted in Table 16.2.

Most examinations in infants and young children can be performed with a 5 or 7.5 MHz transducer. Knowledge of normal dimensions of reproductive organs in the paediatric patient is especially helpful (see Table 16.3 and Chapter 15).

Table 16.2 Indications for ultrasound of the pelvis

Pelvic mass or other pelvic abnormality
Primary amenorrhoea
Gonadal dysgenesis
Precocious puberty
Ambiguous or anomalous genitalia
Anorectal anomalies
Acute or chronic pelvic pain
Suspected congenital Müllerian anomaly
Determination of gestational age in the pregnant adolescent

Table 16.3 Normal dimensions of pelvic organs in the paediatric patient

Ovary
Birth
15 mm long, 3 mm wide, 2.5 mm thick
Volume 0.7 cm^2*
Puberty
Volume 2.5 cm^2
Postpuberty
2.5–5.0 cm long
1.5–3 cm wide
0.6–1.5 cm thick
Volume 1.5–5.7 cm^2
Uterus
Neonate
2.3–4.6 cm long
0.8–2.2 cm AP diameter
Infant to 7 years of age
2.5–3.3 cm long
0.4–1.0 cm AP diameter

* Ovarian volume can be determined by using the formula length × height × width × 0.523.
AP, anteroposterior.
From Sanfillipo & Lavery [5].

In the evaluation of Müllerian anomalies, ultrasound is particularly helpful, as CT scanning in young prepubertal girls may be difficult. However, as puberty approaches with an associated increase in uterine size, both techniques have been used to good effect. With respect to evaluation of a pelvic mass, the imaging techniques of ultrasound, CT or MRI have all been advocated. In the neonate, ovarian cysts, hydrocolpos or hydrometrocolpos account for the majority of pelvic masses. Neonatal ovarian cysts may represent a reflection of exaggerated normal follicular development in association with maternal endogenous hormones. In general, the ovarian cyst is an anechoic thin-walled mass with through transmission. CT may be useful to determine the full extent of the lesion.

With respect to uterine–vaginal anomalies one should consider haematocolpos or haematometrocolpos or the rare malignancy sarcoma botryoides. Haematocolpos and haematometrocolpos are associated with outflow tract obstruction, which results in vaginal and/or uterine distension. Imaging is particularly helpful in facilitating the diagnosis.

Sarcoma botryoides is the most common vaginal and uterine tumour in the paediatric patient, usually presenting with a vaginal discharge and/or mass and associated bleeding. On ultrasound the tumour is of soft-tissue density, and homogeneous unless there is necrosis. Either CT or MRI is required for staging, especially to evaluate haematogenous or lymphatic spread to the liver, lymph nodes or lungs.

Ambiguous genitalia are also, in part, evaluated via imaging. Determining the presence and type of internal reproductive organs is of particular benefit.

In the adolescent with acute onset of pelvic pain, consideration of adnexal torsion and/or ovarian cyst(s) is appropriate. The presence of an ovarian cyst provides increased probability of adnexal torsion. A complex mass may be noted with torsion associated with an intra-ovarian cyst or tumour. Although controversial, CT and MRI appear to be more useful than ultrasound in this particular case.

CHRONIC PELVIC PAIN

The incidence of chronic pelvic pain (CPP) is more frequent in the late adolescent, although it has certainly been reported during early adolescence. The youngest patient known to have endometriosis has been reported to be 10.5 years of age. By definition, CPP requires 6 or more months of persistent lower abdominal pain. The CPP may represent a means of attracting attention, which makes it imperative that the physician assesses interaction between the patient and her parent(s), as well as siblings, who might contribute to a psychological cause of the pelvic pain.

Endometriosis is a chronic process which can begin in young women soon after menarche. Theories of retrograde menstruation [6] and coelomic metaplasia [7] remain in vogue. Endometriosis can cause chronic or acute pelvic pain. CPP in an adolescent can sometimes be an indication of the presence of endometriosis.

Endometriosis is defined as the presence of endometrial tissue in aberrant locations, primarily in the pelvic area. However, phenomena such as cyclic haemoptysis and endometriosis in incisional areas have been reported. In a series by Goldstein *et al.* [8], a 47% incidence of endometriosis was noted in adolescent patients, the youngest of whom was 10.5 years of age. A polygenic/multifactorial mode of inheritance has been proposed for endometriosis. Other studies indicate that between 4% and 17% of all menstruating women have pelvic endometriosis [9]. Thus, the exact incidence of the disease remains to be determined.

Endometriosis may represent an immunological abnormality since endometrial cells normally implant ectopically, whereas this process theoretically could result in implantation in the form of endometriosis if there is an alteration in the immune function. Alteration in humoral immunity is normally manifested by B lymphocytes producing antibodies. Increased T-cell reactivity occurs in women with endometriosis or adenomyosis (endometriosis involving the myometrium). An increase in total immunoglobulin levels occurs as complement is consumed, indicative of the presence of endometriosis. Cell-mediated immunity (T-lymphocyte-related) may also be a factor in the pathophysiology of endometriosis. An increase in the number of T and B cells, as well as T helper cells, has been reported with endometriosis. Interleukins, fibronectin and alteration in natural killer cell activity appear to be integral parts of the mechanism for developing endometriosis.

Initial evaluation of CPP requires a thorough history and physical examination. A gastrointestinal problem such as spastic colon or regional enteritis, genitourinary abnormalities such as recurrent cystitis or other gynaecological disorders must be considered. The latter might involve a müllerian tract anomaly, sequelae of pelvic inflammatory disease, recurrent ovarian cyst formation, etc. Childhood diseases rarely cause pelvic pain; however, infections such as mumps oophoritis must also be ruled out when the history is obtained.

A general physical examination, including pelvic examination, is mandatory. A rectovaginal examination is an integral part of the assessment. The cul-de-sac uterosacral ligaments should be carefully palpated for the presence of nodularity, although it is rare in this age group.

Patients with dysmenorrhoea should be treated initially with non-steroidal anti-inflammatory drugs (NSAIDs). These prostaglandin synthetase inhibitors often produce marked symptomatic improvement. However, if cyclical pain persists, consideration of ovulation suppression with a low-dose (20 or 30 μg) oral contraceptive is indicated. If both of these measures fail, the clinician should proceed to laparoscopy to determine whether the patient is suffering from endometriosis. Intraoperative use of lasers or fulguration of sites of endometriosis have resulted in marked improvement in dysmenorrhoea associated with endometriosis.

Other methods of treatment include the use of Danazol, usually prescribed in 400–800 mg daily dosages (70 kg patient) for 6 months on average, or use of gonadotrophin-releasing hormone agonists. With prompt diagnosis and medical management the adolescent patient can often be given relief from painful menstrual periods.

CONTRACEPTION

The paediatrician is often called upon to counsel adolescent patients on various types of contraception. Various methods are outlined in Table 16.4. By the age of 18, 51% of young women have engaged in sexual activity. Compared with other nations, the UK ranks second (the USA is first) with respect to the incidence of pregnancy and abortion for teenagers aged 15–19 years in industrialized nations (Fig. 16.1). Sex education remains a focal point in

Table 16.4 Contraceptive methods for adolescents

- Combined birth control pill (oestrogen and progestin)
- Mini-pill (progestin-only pill)
- Barrier methods
  - Condom
  - Diaphragm
  - Cervical cap
  - Vaginal contraceptives (creams, foams, jellies, powders, pastes, suppositories, tablets, others)
  - Vaginal sponge
- Intrauterine contraceptive devices
- Postcoital contraceptives
  - Diethylstilboestrol
  - Other oestrogens (ethinyloestradiol or conjugated oestrogens)
  - Mini-pill
  - Oestrogen and progestin combination
  - Intrauterine contraceptive devices
- Injectable contraceptives
  - Medroxyprogesterone acetate
  - Norethindrone acetate
  - Others
- Rhythm methods
  - Basal body temperature
  - Calendar method
  - Fertility awareness of Billing's ovulation method
  - Combinations
  - Others
- Lactation
- Sterilization
- Abortion
- Miscellaneous methods
  - Douche
  - Coitus interruptus ('strategic withdrawal')
  - Masturbation
  - Other non-coital sexual activity (abstinence)

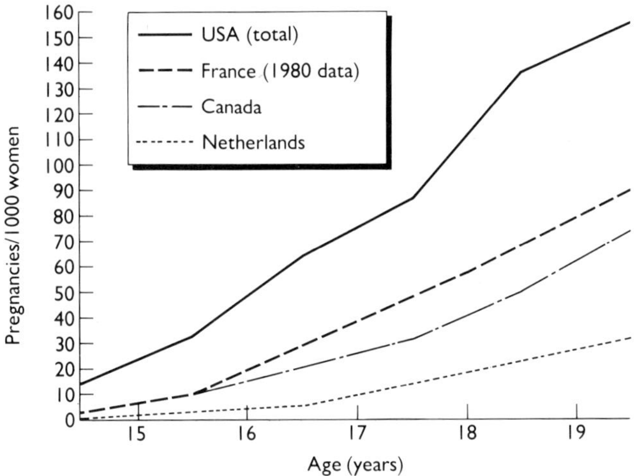

Fig. 16.1 Teenage pregnancy rates – USA versus other industrialized countries. Note that pregnancies are defined here as births plus abortions during 1981; age is age at outcome (from Jones *et al.* [10]).

the hope of decreasing the incidence of adolescent pregnancy. Industrialized nations in which a priority has been established for both the dissemination of contraceptive information via public media and the distribution of contraceptives to adolescents appears to have a significant difference in lowering the incidence of teenage pregnancies. In a number of nations, pharmacies are used as primary educators concerning birth control, and in the Netherlands contraceptives are advertised on television. A number of socioeducational groups provide a safe environment for teenagers to discuss sexuality and learn of the major fallacies regarding pregnancy, parenting, etc. Programmes focusing on adolescent/parent problems and the right to self-determination in contraception seem most effective. The emphasis placed on postponement of intercourse until after secondary school or marriage has repeatedly proved to be beneficial in terms of health-care cost containment.

Oral contraceptives are composed mainly of a synthetic oestrogen, ethinyloestradiol, and one of several progestagens such as norethindrone, norethindrone acetate, ethynodiol diacetate, norgestrel, norgestimate, desogestrel or gestodene. The latter three progestins appear to have beneficial effects on the lipid profile, as well as causing less sebaceous secretion, and are noted to be associated with a lower incidence of breakthrough bleeding. They have also been promoted from the perspective of lower incidence of pregnancy, even if several pills are missed.

The oral contraceptive prevents ovulation by having its effect at a central level, that is by altering luteinizing hormone (LH) secretion. In addition, minimal stimulation of the endometrium and production of hostile cervical mucus results.

Birth control pills have side-effects (Table 16.5). The major problem preventing successful oral contraception is compliance. Oral contraceptives should be prescribed with the lowest possible dose, since the side-effects are related to the dose of oestrogen. Management of a number of oral contraceptive-related problems is outlined in Table 16.6. Contraindications as well as benefits which should be clearly outlined before prescribing oral contraceptives are listed in Table 16.7.

When prescribing oral contraceptives the clinician should keep in mind that simultaneous consumption by

Table 16.5 Side-effects of oral contraceptives

Oestrogen-induced	Progestin-induced
Nausea and/or emesis	Decreased menses
Dysmenorrhoea and/or premenstrual tension (with or without oedema)	Reduced vaginal secretion
	Breast regression
	Weight gain (with increased appetite)
Elevated blood pressure	
Vascular headaches	Fatigue
Cervical erosion and/or polyposis	Depression
	Acne
Increased mucoid vaginal discharge	Hirsutism
	Reduced libido
Tender breasts or fibrocystic breast disease	Leg cramps
	Alopecia
Fluid retention (weight gain)	Others

Table 16.6 Management of oral contraceptive-related problems

Problem	Management
Weight gain or oedema	Use low-dose oestrogen pill
Acne	Usually controlled with anti-acne medications: benzoyl peroxide, tretinoin and antibiotics (topical or systemic). For a youth with acne or hirsutism, try a pill with low androgenic progestagens, such as desogestrel
Acute monilial vaginitis	Usually controlled with antifungal agents given intravaginally: miconazole nitrate 2% for 7 nights: clotrimazole vaginal cream or vaginal tablets for 7 nights; nystatin vaginal tablets b.i.d. for 14 days
Chronic monilial vaginitis	Treat for an entire menstrual cycle; evaluate for other factors (broad-spectrum antibiotic use, endocrinopathies, infected male genital tract); male partner can use a condom; use of oral nystatin to reduce gastrointestinal reservoir
Breakthrough bleeding (intermenstrual spotting)	Usually resolves without treatment after two or three subsequent cycles. Otherwise use a 50 µg pill. Finally, give 10–20 µg ethinyloestradiol for 7–10 days. Be sure patient is taking the pill every day
Possible pregnancy	Stop the pill immediately, since some consider it to be a mild teratogen
Other side-effects	Monitor any side-effects very carefully. Patient must allow frequent evaluation as determined by the physician. Some problems (melasma syn. chloasma) requires cessation of the pill

Table 16.7 Contraindications and benefits of oral contraceptives

Absolute contraindications
Pregnancy
Undiagnosed genital bleeding
Oestrogen-dependent cancer
Active liver disease (acute or chronic)
History of thromboembolic disease
Severe migraine headaches (especially with prolonged auras)
Severe hypertension
Hyperlipidaemia
Cyanotic heart disease
Inability to take the pill each day for a prolonged length of time
Inability to return for follow-up visits to the physician as needed

Relative contraindications
Diabetes mellitus
Epilepsy
Sickle-cell disease
Collagen vascular disease
Uterine leiomyomas
Lactation
Oligomenorrhoea
Depression
Oestrogen-related dermatological disorders (melasma, erythema nodosum)
Gall bladder disease
Inflammatory bowel disease
Hypothalamopituitary dysfunction
Chorea
Porphyria
Coagulation defects
Renal disease
Pulmonary disease
Cardiac disease
Retinal disorders
Severe, chronic monilial vaginitis
Various drug interactions
Severe chest or abdominal pain of unknown aetiology
Others

Benefits of oral contraception
Reversible pregnancy prevention
Menstrual regulation
Improvement in menstrually induced anaemia
Improvement in dysmenorrhoea
Protection from pelvic inflammatory disease
Less benign breast disease
Less ovarian cyst formation
Improved protection from ectopic pregnancy
Cancer protection (lower incidence of endometrial, ovarian and breast cancer)
Improved protection from rheumatoid arthritis
Others

the patient of other medications or drugs may affect the efficacy of the birth control pill medication (Table 16.8). Other methods of contraception include the 'mini-pill' (progestin-only pill). This preparation causes a thickening of the cervical mucus, making it difficult for sperm to penetrate. In addition, the altered endometrium inhibits blastocyst implantation. The effectiveness of the mini-pill is approximately 96%; it has a higher failure rate than the combination birth control pill, which is less than 1%.

The intrauterine contraceptive device is not recommended for adolescents. Barrier methods of contraception such as the diaphragm, foam and condoms are effective

Table 16.8 Drugs interfering with oral contraceptives

Antibiotics	Anticonvulsants	Others
Rifampin	Phenytoin	Chlordiazepoxide
Chloramphenicol	Primidone	Phenylbutazone
Ampicillin	Phenobarbital	Meprobamate
Penicillin	Ethosuximide	Cyclophosphamide
Sulphonamides		Chlorpromazine
Nitrofurantoin		Phenacetin
Neomycin		
Isoniazid		

means of birth control, with 85–96% effectiveness when used routinely.

Intradermal progestin implants are also available. The Norplant system (Wyeth Ayerst, Philadelphia) provides subdermal placement of the synthetic progestin, levonorgestrel: six silastic (siloxane copolymer) cylindrical capsules containing the medication, 36 mg 1-norgestrel, are implanted subdermally through a small incision. The mechanism of action of the exogenous progestin appears to be a decrease in gonadotrophin output (FSH and LH), and thus suppression of ovulation. Failure rates for Norplant have been reported as 4–5/1000 users per year.

Side-effects include irregular menses, although menses can occur at normal intervals. Local reactions, including hyperpigmentation and irritation at the site of placement of the subdermal implants, occur in 5% of patients and infection in 1%; acne has been reported in 15% and persistent headaches in 24%.

Injectable contraceptives are also available, including depo-medroxyprogesterone acetate. This preparation requires injection of the progestin, usually every 3 months. The patient becomes amenorrheic as a rule in association with ovulation suppression.

It has been noted that adolescents are sexually active for an average of 15 months before initiating regular contraceptive use; then, unfortunately, they often use the chosen method inconsistently [11]. A number of young women continue to have psychological barriers to contraceptive use, despite choosing to be sexually active, and the clinician must be 'attuned' in counselling this patient population. The importance of appropriate communication between the patient and the health-care provider will hopefully remove such barriers. Teenagers who are properly counselled and can make intelligent decisions whether to abstain or use contraception will clearly have a positive impact on lowering the current incidence of teenage pregnancy. The paediatrician should be aware of the various methods of contraception and inquire during the gynaecological examination, depending on the patient's age, whether there is a need for contraception. Initial counselling of an adolescent should include laboratory tests to include cervical cultures for gonorrhoea and *Chlamydia*, a serological test for syphilis and, if indicated, human immunodeficiency virus (HIV) as well as a Pap smear. Methods of contraception such as coitus interruptus and postcoital douching are not recommended, because of their low reliability.

REFERENCES

1 Emans SJH, Goldstein DP. *Pediatric and Adolescent Gynecology*, 3rd edn. Boston: Little, Brown, 1990.
2 *The Adolescent Obstetric–Gynecologic Patient.* ACOG Technical Bulletin no. 145, 1990.
3 Talbor CW. The gynecologic examination of the pediatric patient. *Pediatr Ann* 1986;15:501–8.
4 Ridley CM. Vulvar disorders. In: Sanfilippo JS, ed. *Pediatric Adolescent Gynecology*. Philadelphia: W.B. Saunders 1994; pp 203–21.
5 Sanfillipo JS, Lavery JP. The spectrum of ultrasound: antenatal to adolescent years. *Semin Reprod Endocrinol* 1988;6:47.
6 Sampson J. The development of the implantation theory for the origin of peritoneal endometriosis. *Ann J Obstet Gynecol* 1940;40:549–57.
7 Meyer R. Über Endometrium in der Tube sowie über die Hieraus intstehenden wirkiehen und rermeintlichen tolgen. *Zentralbl Gynaekol* 1927;51:1482–91.
8 Goldstein D, DeCholnoky C, Emans SJ. Adolescent endometriosis. *J Adol Health Care* 1980;1:37–41.
9 Ranney B. Etiology, prevention and inhibition of endometriosis. *Clin Obstet Gynecol* 1980;23:875.
10 Jones EF, Forrest JD, Goldman N *et al.* Teen pregnancy in developed countries: determinants and policy implications. *Fam Plann Perspect* 1985;17:53–63.
11 White J, Kellinger K. Teenagers perceptions of unplanned adolescent pregnancies and oral contraceptive use. *J Am Acad Nurse Pract* 1989;21(2):55–62.

FURTHER READING

Lavery JP, Sanfilippo JS, eds. *Pediatric and Adolescent Obstetrics and Gynecology*. New York: Springer Verlag, 1985.
Sanfilippo J. Adolescent girls with vaginal discharge. *Pediatr Ann* 1986;15:509–19.
Sanfilippo J, Wakim N, Schikler K *et al.* Endometriosis in association with a uterine anomaly. *Am J Obstet Gynecol* 1986; 154:39–43.
Simmons P. Breast disorders. In: Sanfilippo JS, ed. *Pediatric Adolescent Gynecology*. Philadelphia: W.B. Saunders 1994: pp 583–63.
Spence J, Dewhurst J. The vulva and its anomalies in the newborn. *Pediatr Adoles Gynecol* 1984;2:83–106.

17: Reproductive Endocrinology – The Ovary

D.F. WOOD and S. FRANKS

INTRODUCTION

Ovarian activity involves the production of gametes and synthesis of the hormones which determine female sexual development and reproductive function. The two functions are closely related and both are controlled by the hypothalamopituitary axis. In addition, the complex changes of cellular differentiation which occur within the ovary are dependent upon a series of locally produced growth-regulating factors which also modulate gonadotrophin action and which therefore function as a 'fine-tuning' system at the level of the target organ. While clinical disorders of ovarian function are uncommon in childhood, normal ovaries are not quiescent during these years. Throughout prepubertal life there is an increase in ovarian size with active follicular growth and attendant atresia, culminating in puberty, menarche and, subsequently, ovulatory menses.

In this chapter normal ovarian development is described, together with the physiology of the mature ovary and the events of the menstrual cycle. The diagnosis and management of disorders of ovarian development and function which may present in childhood and adolescence are described.

DEVELOPMENT OF THE NORMAL OVARY

The fetal ovary

Genetic sex is determined at the time of conception, and gonadal differentiation occurs in early fetal life. The ovary develops from the bipotential gonad; it contains germ cells, which are derived from the yolk sac, and somatic cells originating from coelomic epithelium, mesenchyme and the mesonephros. From the third week of fetal life, germ cells migrate from the yolk sac to the gonadal ridge. Germ-cell replication begins during migration and continues in the fetal ovary up to the fifth month of gestation when a maximum of six to seven million oogonia is reached [1]. During early fetal development the ovary lies close to the mesonephros. Mesonephric cells invade the ovary to form the medulla, causing the germ cells to lie peripherally in the developing cortex.

This association of the ovary and the mesonephros is essential for two important events in ovarian development: the onset of meiosis and the formation of follicles [2]. Primary oocytes continue replication but are arrested in the diplotene phase, not completing the first meiosis until many years later at the onset of ovulation. Meiosis-arrested oocytes become surrounded by a layer of primitive mesonephros-derived granulosa cells to form primordial follicles, a process which continues until the sixth month of postnatal life. Those oocytes which are not incorporated into follicles undergo atresia. Follicular growth and atresia continue throughout life, accounting for the fact that the number of germ cells has fallen to about one million by birth and less than 50% that number at menarche [1].

Development of primordial follicles can be seen from the fourth month of gestation and, by 6 months, many preantral follicles are observed at the interface between the cortex and medulla. Antral follicles develop during the last 2 months of fetal life and are present in large numbers at birth, although many of these early follicles have an abnormal appearance [3]. Human fetal ovaries do not contain detectable binding sites for luteinizing hormone (LH) or human chorionic gonadotrophin (hCG), although follicle-stimulating hormone (FSH) receptors appear towards the end of intrauterine life [4]. The impaired ovarian follicular development observed in anencephalic human fetuses indicates that full follicular maturation is dependent upon gonadotrophin action [5]. Fetal ovaries possess some of the enzymes necessary for steroid hormone production from cholesterol, but they do not appear to secrete significant amounts of these hormones [6].

The development of the Müllerian duct system is not dependent upon gonadal hormone secretion.

The ovary in childhood

Mean ovarian weight increases in childhood, and histological studies of postmortem ovaries show that this is

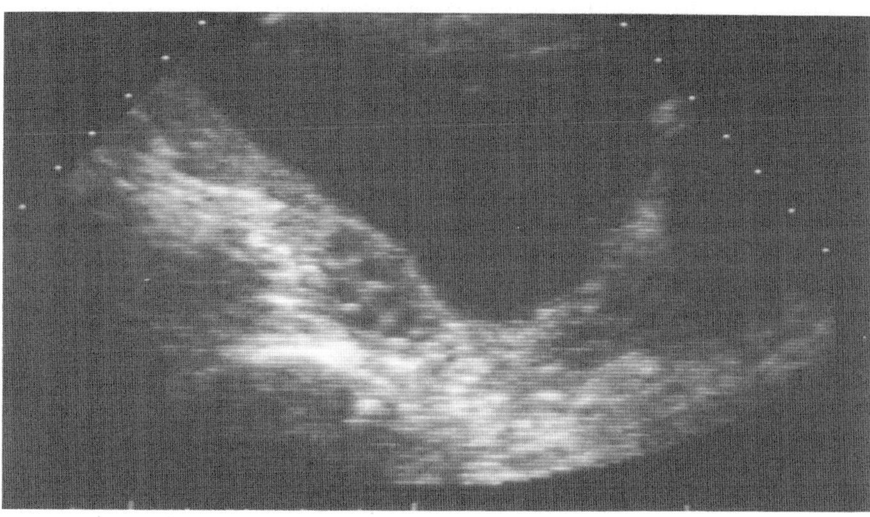

Fig. 17.1 Ultrasound scan to show a prepubertal ovary demonstrating a multifollicular appearance.

due both to increasing amounts of stroma and to increased size and number of follicles [7]. The size of these follicles varies and they may become atretic at any stage in their development.

Although the gonadotrophin levels are low in the latter half of intrauterine life, as a result of the effects of high levels of oestrogen and progesterone secreted by the placenta the hypothalamopituitary axis is potentially functional. The high levels of gonadotrophins seen in the first few months of postnatal life are thought to be due to removal of this steroid-negative feedback [8]. Gonadotrophins fall to low levels by 1–3 years and remain so throughout childhood; the mechanism of this reduction in hypothalamopituitary activity in infancy remains unclear. However, despite overall low levels of gonadotrophins, detectable pulses of secretion are observed and mean concentrations start to rise at about the age of 6 years. This is associated with an increase in the number of antral follicles and a subsequent rise in oestrogen levels [3,9].

By the age of 8 years multifollicular ovaries can be observed by ultrasound scanning in all normal girls but they can be seen in many long before this age. The presence of multifollicular ovaries heralds puberty [10] (Fig. 17.1). At the time of puberty there is a characteristic increase in pulsatile gonadotrophin secretion at night which appears to be controlled, primarily, by the central nervous system (reviewed in [11]). This pattern of gonadotroph in secretion continues until late puberty when the amplitude of LH pulses reaches adult levels throughout the day. Puberty ends in girls with the establishment of regular ovulatory menses associated with adult ovarian morphology and characteristic cyclical changes in hypothalamopituitary–gonadal function.

The mature ovary

In the mature ovary, the functions of gametogenesis and steroid hormone production are regulated by a wide range of hormones and peptides acting in an endocrine, paracrine or autocrine fashion. Gametogenesis occurs in granulosa cells which lie within the follicle in close proximity to the theca interna cells. The two cell types are interdependent for hormone production such that androgens synthesized by theca cells diffuse into the granulosa layer where they are metabolized to oestrogens by the action of aromatase.

The principal regulators of ovarian function are the anterior pituitary hormones LH and FSH. In the mature ovary, receptors for LH are present on theca cells and develop on granulosa cells during the preovulatory phase of follicular growth under the influence of FSH. FSH receptors are localized exclusively to granulosa cells (reviewed in [12]). The ovary also produces a large number of peptide hormones and growth factors which have a potential role in the paracrine and autocrine regulation of follicular growth and steroidogenesis. These include insulin-like growth factors (IGFs), transforming growth factors α and β (TGF-α, TGF-β), epidermal growth factor (EGF), angiogenic factors, prostaglandins, eicosanoids, gonadotrophin-releasing hormone (GnRH)-like peptides, angiotensin II, inhibin, activin, follistatin, growth hormone-releasing hormone (GHRH), catecholamines and interleukins.

While the exact nature of their action *in vivo* remains to be established, it is clear that these factors are involved in diverse intraovarian regulatory functions (reviewed in [13]). For example, in addition to growth promotion, IGF-I promotes follicular development by enhancing the actions of LH and FSH (Fig. 17.2). EGF and TGF-α inhibit basal and gonadotrophin-stimulated granulosa cell function, actions which may reflect stimulation of mitosis with concurrent inhibition of differentiation in these cells [15]. The

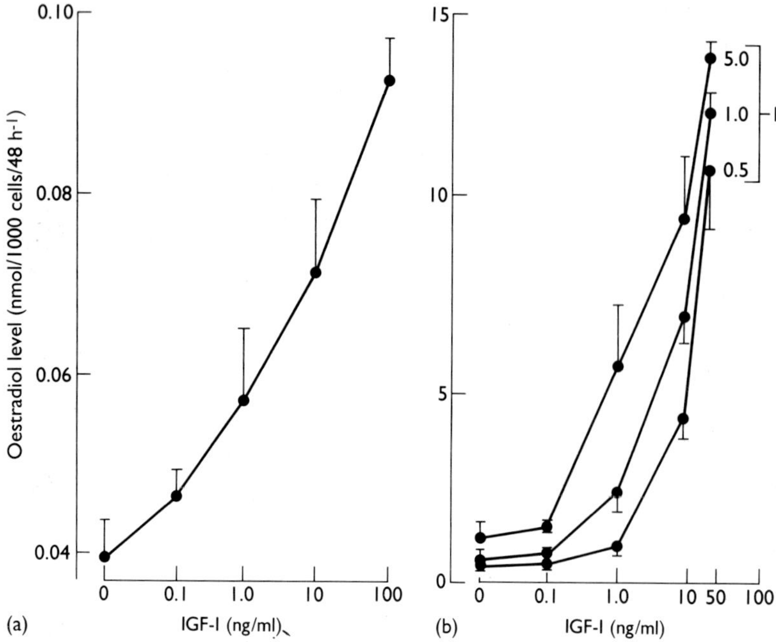

Fig. 17.2 Effects of IGF-I and FSH on oestradiol production by cultured granulosa cells. Oestradiol response to increasing doses of IGF-I in granulosa cells from a normal ovary in the presence of 1 ng/ml FSH (a) and from a polycystic ovary in the presence of three doses of FSH (b) (from Mason *et al.* [14]).

opposing actions of TGF-β and EGF/TGF-α on granulosa cells [16] suggest a mechanism whereby the interaction of local growth factors may subserve gonadotrophin-dependent regulation of cyclical changes in growth and differentiation of follicular cells.

A number of these peptide hormones also have an endocrine effect: inhibin, activin, follistatin, TGF-β and GnRH-like peptides are involved in the regulation of gonadotrophin secretion whereas relaxin, secreted by the corpus luteum in pregnancy, controls the remodelling of the reproductive tract prior to parturition.

The menstrual cycle

The menstrual cycle represents a process of ovarian follicular maturation, ovulation of a dominant follicle and formation of a corpus luteum, with consequent hormonally mediated changes in the reproductive tract. The establishment of regular ovulatory menses is the final stage of ovarian development and reflects maturation of the entire hypothalamopituitary–gonadal axis. The median length of the menstrual cycle is 28 days (25–31) but this varies widely at the two extremes of reproductive life. In the first 1–2 years after menarche, cycle length is often prolonged and bleeding erratic due to inadequate follicular development and the higher rate of anovulatory cycles [17,18].

The menstrual cycle is traditionally divided into two components: the follicular phase, during which the selection, maturation and ovulation of a dominant follicle occurs, and the luteal phase, characterized by high progesterone levels and associated endometrial changes. The endocrine and morphological changes occurring in each phase are shown schematically in Fig. 17.3 and are reviewed in [19].

Initiation of follicular growth occurs during the final few days of the preceding menstrual cycle under the influence of the rising FSH concentrations which follow the decline in oestradiol and progesterone levels. Follicular recruitment occurs during the first 4 days of the cycle, following which one follicle is selected to become dominant. As oestradiol concentrations rise in the midfollicular phase, FSH levels fall and maturation of the other follicles is suppressed as the dominant follicle grows. These events culminate in ovulation of a single follicle at days 13–15. During the follicular phase, under the influence of FSH, oestrogen levels rise in proportion to follicular growth and the increasing number of granulosa cells. FSH also induces aromatase activity and the development of LH receptors on granulosa cells. LH stimulates theca interna cells to secrete androgens, which are aromatized to oestrogens in the granulosa cells. In the latter part of the follicular phase, LH contributes to the production of oestradiol and the small amount of progesterone which is secreted by the preovulatory granulosa layer. The locally produced peptides and growth factors discussed above are intimately involved in controlling ovarian steroidogenesis.

Follicular growth is associated with increasing oestrogen concentrations in the follicular phase. Just before ovulation there is a dramatic rise in oestrogen secretion by the preovulatory follicle which triggers the LH surge. In addition to inducing ovulation this massive rise in LH

Plate 8.1 Model of hGH binding to the hGH receptor. Crystallographic studies of the complex between hGH and the extracellular domains of the GH receptors have shown that one molecule of hormone (red) is bound to two receptor molecules (blue and green). Different surfaces of the hGH molecule interact with the same surface in each receptor, and there is extensive contact between the two receptor molecules close to the cell membrane (yellow pebbled surface). Other evidence suggests that this dimerization is crucial for signal transduction (from De Vos *et al.* [1992]).

8.1

16.1

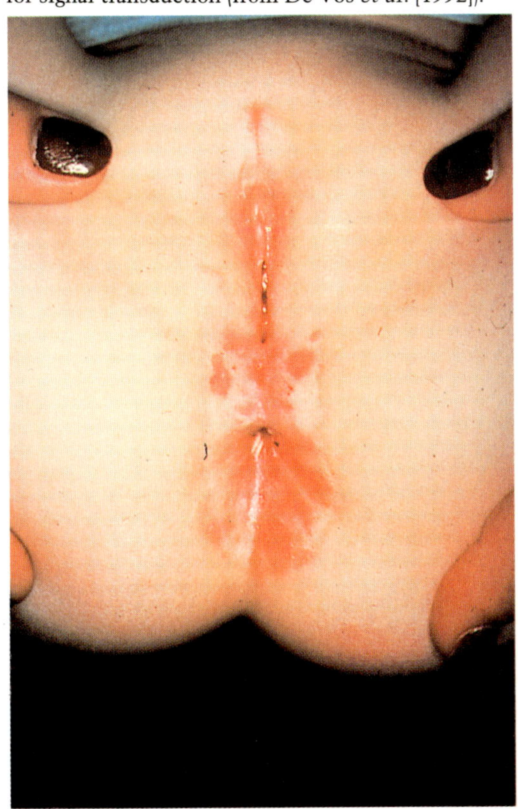

16.2

Plate 16.1 (*above left*) Molluscum contagiosum and evidence of sexual abuse.

Plate 16.2 (*above right*) Labial agglutination.

16.3

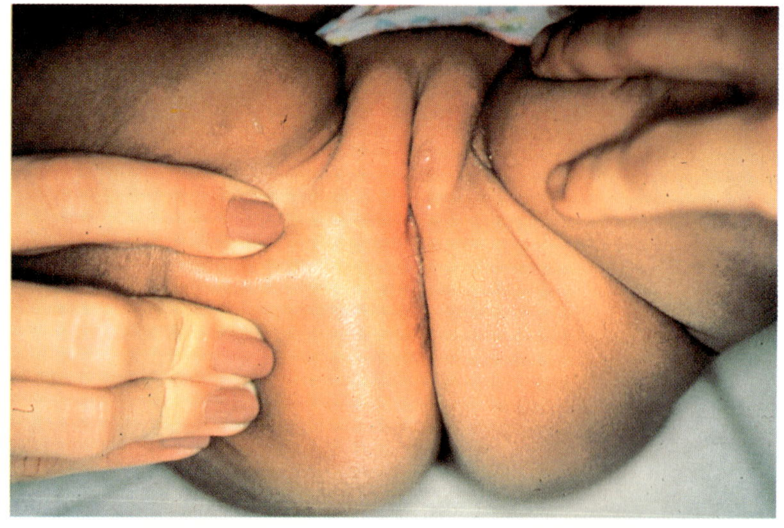

16.4

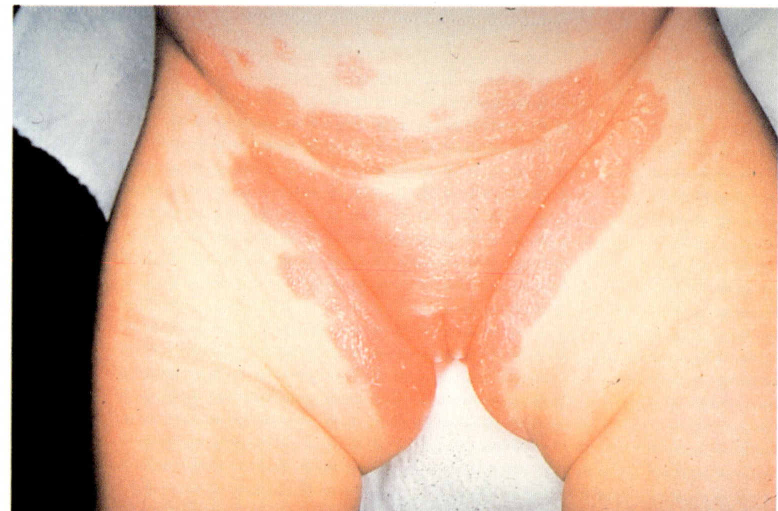

16.5

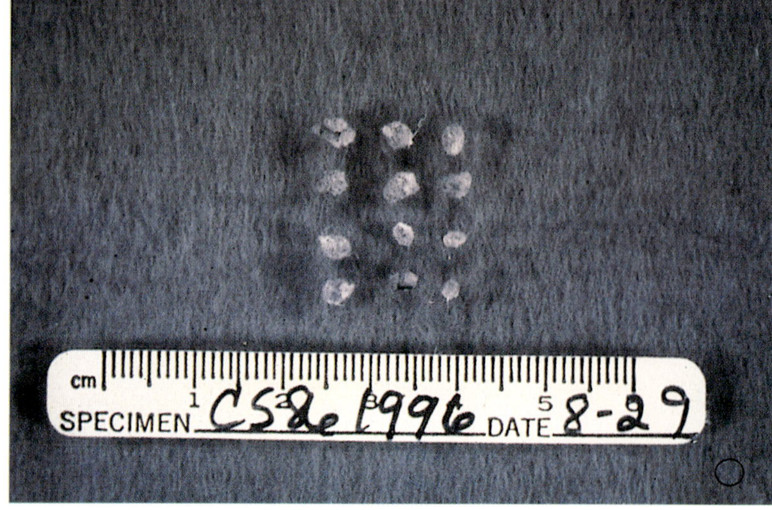

Plate 16.3 (*top left*) Lichen sclerosus.

Plate 16.4 (*centre*) Vulvar psoriasis.

Plate 16.5 (*bottom left*) Rolled toilet paper in the vagina caused chronic vaginitis.

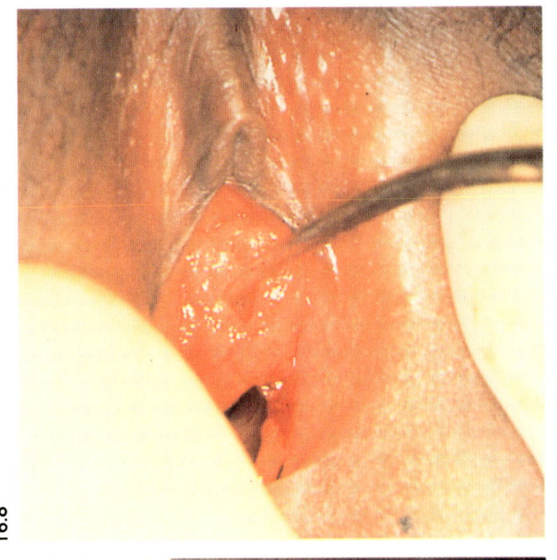

16.8

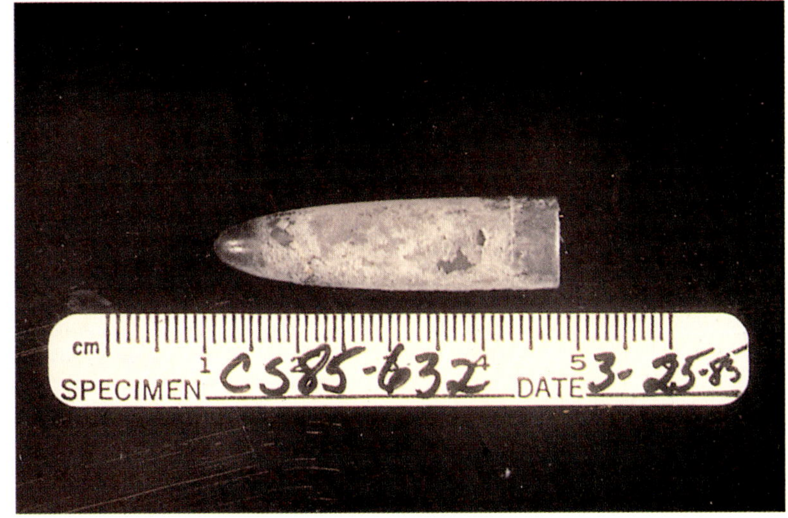

16.6

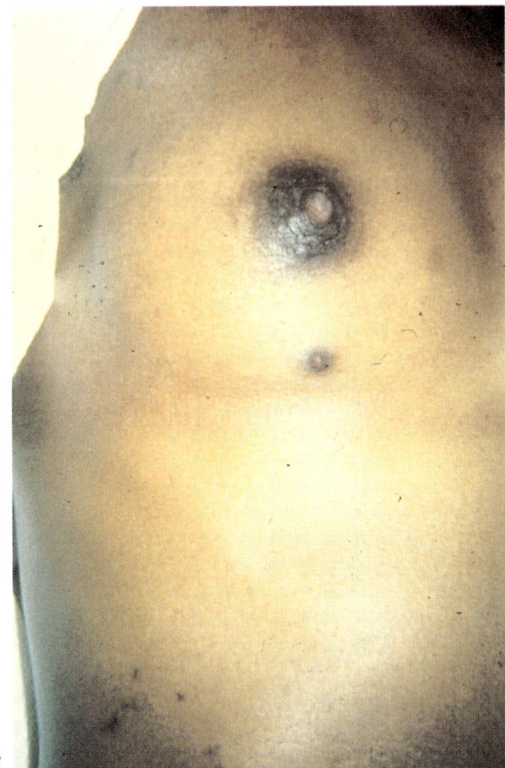

16.10

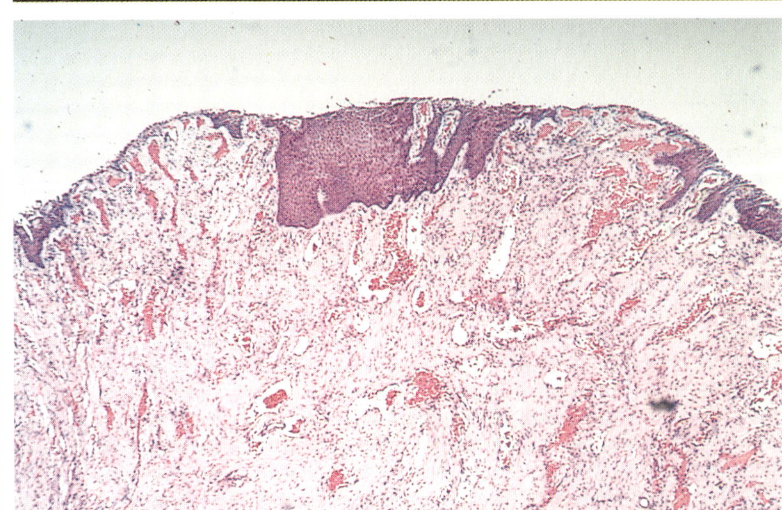

16.7

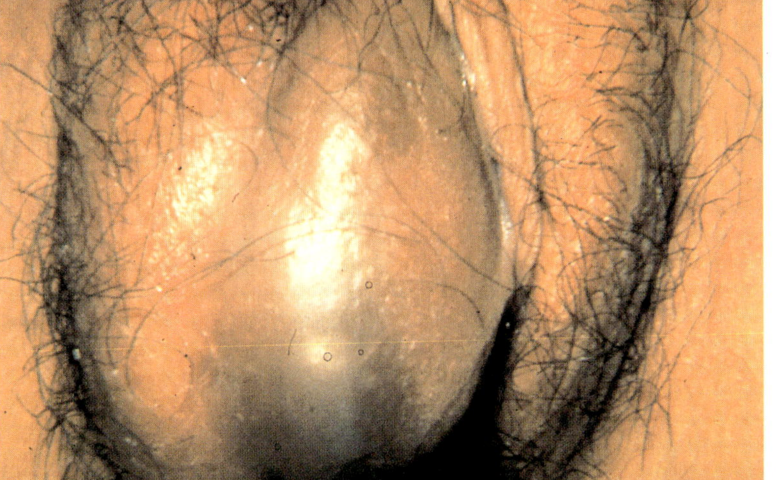

16.9

Plate 16.6 (*top right*) Pen top lodged in the vagina caused vaginal bleeding and vaginitis.

Plate 16.7 (*centre right*) Capillary haemangioma of the vulva in a 5-year-old child.

Plate 16.8 (*above left*) Urethral prolapse.

Plate 16.9 (*bottom right*) Vulvar haematoma.

Plate 16.10 (*above*) Polythelia.

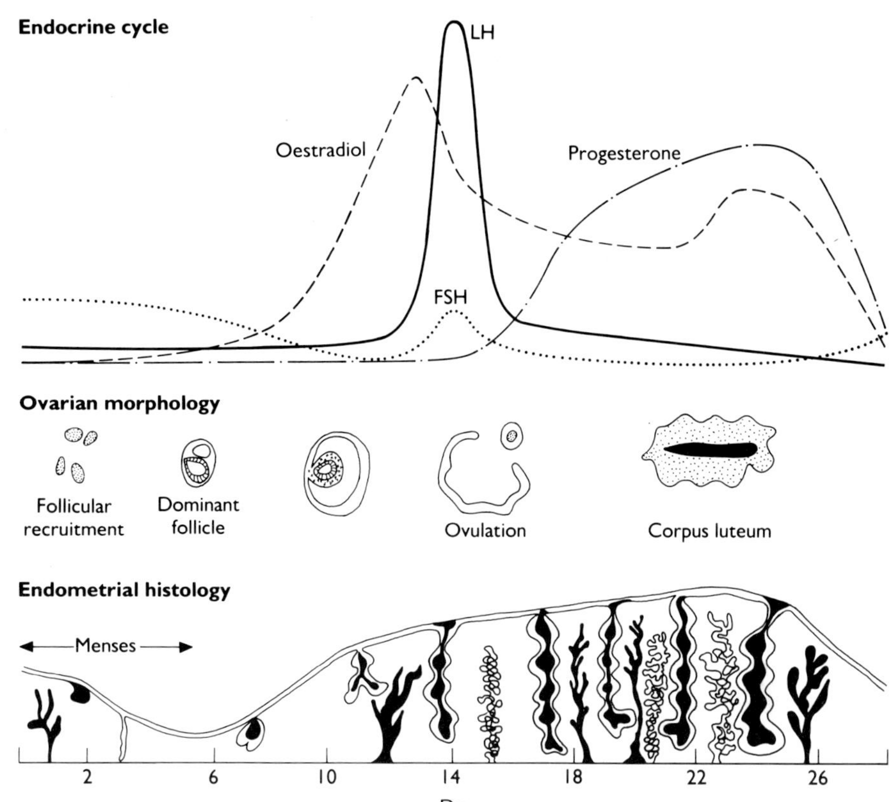

Fig. 17.3 The menstrual cycle. Hormonal, ovarian morphological and endometrial histological changes during the menstrual cycle.

stimulates the resumption of oocyte meiosis, and initiates the process of luteinization of the granulosa cells, producing the rise in progesterone secretion characteristic of the luteal phase.

After ovulation the follicle undergoes morphological change to produce the corpus luteum. Granulosa–lutein cells enlarge, become surrounded by cells of thecal origin and undergo vascularization in response to locally produced angiogenic factors. The primary function of the corpus luteum is to secrete progesterone, allowing development of the oestrogen-primed endometrium prior to implantation of a fertilized ovum. Control of steroid secretion by the corpus luteum is complex. LH concentrations are low but LH is nevertheless essential to maintain the steroidogenic capacity of the corpus luteum. Locally produced peptides may also be important in this role. In the absence of pregnancy, corpus luteum function declines by 9–11 days after ovulation when it starts to undergo luteolysis.

The changes in the reproductive tract associated with the menstrual cycle are well recognized. In the follicular phase the endometrium thickens and narrow tubular glands develop. After ovulation, under the influence of changing steroid concentrations, the glands become more tortuous and dilated, producing intraluminal secretions by day 19. The endometrial stroma subsequently becomes oedematous and the stromal cells around the spiral arteries become enlarged and transformed into the predecidua. By the end of the luteal phase a sheet of well-developed decidual-like cells is present. In the absence of conception the decline in corpus luteum function produces changes in the vascular supply of the endometrium, resulting in cell death and shedding of the superficial layers during menstruation.

DISORDERS OF OVARIAN FUNCTION PRESENTING IN CHILDHOOD AND ADOLESCENCE

Abnormal ovarian function in postpubertal females presents clinically with oligomenorrhoea, amenorrhoea or irregular menstrual cycles. Oligomenorrhoea is defined as an intermenstrual interval of more than 6 weeks, whereas amenorrhoea indicates the absence of menses for more than 6 months. Amenorrhoea may be either primary or secondary. Patients complaining of primary amenorrhoea have never menstruated, whereas those with secondary amenorrhoea have lost previously existing menstrual function. In adolescent girls it is clearly essential to assess these symptoms in the context of pubertal development. It is also important to note that the distinction between primary and secondary amenorrhoea is largely artificial, so

Table 17.1 Causes of primary amenorrhoea

Ovarian disorders	
Gonadal dysgenesis	Turner syndrome, mixed gonadal dysgenesis, pure gonadal dysgenesis
Ovarian insensitivity	17α-hydroxylase deficiency, ovarian resistance syndromes
Gonadal irradiation	
Chemotherapy	
Polycystic ovary syndrome	
Genital tract disorders	Müllerian dysgenesis, disorders of genital differentiation
Hypothalamopituitary disease	Hypogonadotrophic hypogonadism, pituitary/hypothalamic tumours, radiotherapy/chemotherapy
Delayed puberty	Constitutional delay, chronic illness, psychogenic

that many of the causes of secondary amenorrhoea may present in adolescence with primary amenorrhoea and rarely some girls with congenital lesions may menstruate [20].

Primary amenorrhoea

Primary amenorrhoea is uncommon. The majority of cases are due to developmental abnormalities of the ovaries, genital tracts or external genitalia, with syndromes of gonadal dysgenesis accounting for about 50% of these. The causes of primary amenorrhoea are shown in Table 17.1. Many patients will have delayed puberty, and it is important to identify those causes not directly related to the hypothalamopituitary–gonadal axis.

CLINICAL ASSESSMENT OF THE PATIENT WITH PRIMARY AMENORRHOEA

The history should include detailed questions about the age of onset, synchrony and progression of pubertal development (Chapter 15). Features which are of particular importance in identifying those girls with an underlying primary ovarian disorder should be sought. These include coexistent growth failure, musculoskeletal abnormalities, cutaneous lesions, congenital heart disease, recurrent ear infections or deafness and structural renal anomalies. Examination should begin with height and weight and accurate assessment of pubertal stage. Particular attention should be paid to dysmorphic body features, ambiguous genitalia, inguinal herniae, palpable masses in the labia or a blind-ending vaginal canal.

The investigation of girls with primary amenorrhoea is largely dictated by the clinical findings. Thyroid function tests and bone age should be performed in all cases of delayed puberty. Measurement of basal gonadotrophin concentrations will distinguish primary from secondary ovarian failure. Ovarian ultrasound scanning is helpful to identify ovarian tissue and examine its morphology. The presence of multifollicular ovaries in a girl with delayed puberty suggests that the hypothalamopituitary–gonadal axis is functioning, and puberty will eventually progress. Polycystic ovary syndrome (PCOS) occasionally presents with primary amenorrhoea [21] and this also will be demonstrated on ultrasound scanning. Chromosome analysis should be performed if dysmorphic features are observed and in all cases of short stature and delayed puberty as Turner mosaics may be phenotypically normal (see below).

The treatment of primary amenorrhoea is varied, being dictated by the clinical findings.

Ovarian causes of primary amenorrhoea

SYNDROMES OF GONADAL DYSGENESIS

The clinical presentation of patients with gonadal dysgenesis is variable, depending upon the underlying chromosomal abnormality. The complete absence of a second sex chromosome is associated with features of Turner syndrome, sexual immaturity, short stature and a variety of somatic abnormalities [22]. These may be modified by the pattern of sex chromosome deficiency. The usual classification depends on the X-chromatin material present in addition to the monosomic X. In general those patients with additional X chromatin fall in the range of sexually infantile to normal females whereas those who are X-chromatin-negative range between sexually infantile females and hypogonadal males.

TURNER SYNDROME

The typical features of 45XO Turner syndrome are well recognized (reviewed in [23]) and are shown in Table 17.2. The two constant features of this syndrome are short stature and sexual infantilism with normal external genitalia. The mechanism of growth failure in Turner syndrome remains unclear (reviewed in [24]). No typical abnormality of growth hormone (GH) pulsatility has been established, nor is there any obvious abnormality of IGF-I secretion [25]. The contribution played by end-organ resistance associated with skeletal dysplasia remains to be clarified.

Sexual infantilism is associated with 'streak gonads', the term used to describe the streaks of connective tissue located in the mesosalpinges. These are composed of fibrous stroma arranged in whorls, similar to the pattern in normal ovaries but lacking in primordial follicles. Occasionally ovarian function is preserved and there are

Table 17.2 Features of Turner syndrome

Short stature	In 100%
Sexual infantilism	In 100%
Dysmorphic body features	All common
Examples: short webbed neck, micrognathia, epicanthal folds, ptosis, 'shield'-shaped chest, widely spaced nipples, cutaneous lesions	
ENT abnormalities	Common
Examples: recurrent otitis media, sensineural deafness	
Musculoskeletal abnormalities	In 50%
Examples: cubitus valgus, short fourth metacarpals, high arched palate, vertebral hypoplasia (less commonly)	
Renal anomalies	In 30%
Examples: horseshoe kidney, other structural abnormalities	
Congenital lymphoedema	In 30%
Cardiovascular abnormalities	In 10–20%
Examples: dissection of aorta, coarctation of aorta, aortic stenosis	

ENT, ear, nose and throat.

reports of fertility [26]. Ultrasound studies have shown 'non-streak' ovaries in up to one-third of girls with Turner syndrome, a finding which correlated with spontaneous breast development and preservation of the long arm of the second X chromosome [27]. This karyotype has been observed to be associated with a high prevalence of puberty and menstruation in these patients [28]. Ovarian ultrasonography is therefore useful in predicting puberty in girls with Turner syndrome, although statements about future fertility remain doubtful.

A wide range of somatic disorders is associated with Turner syndrome, as shown in Table 17.2. The most common are musculoskeletal, renal, cardiovascular and otological abnormalities. Congenital lymphoedema occurs in about one-third of cases (Bonnevie–Ullrich syndrome). An increased incidence of autoimmune conditions has been reported, namely rheumatoid arthritis, thyroid disease, inflammatory bowel disease and insulin-dependent diabetes. The incidence of mental retardation is not increased in Turner syndrome.

Treatment of Turner syndrome involves the achievement of maximal height, induction of secondary sexual characteristics and the correction of somatic abnormalities where possible. GH therapy allows increased growth velocity to occur in advance of bone maturation [29,30] and certainly has a part to play in management. The optimal dose of human GH and the age when its effect is most beneficial remains unknown. Once-daily injection is certainly as satisfactory as twice-daily dosage [31]. The anabolic steroid oxandrolone may be of value in combination with GH therapy [25]; its growth-promoting effects are not dose-related, whereas its side effects, such as virilization and insulin resistance are. Low-dose ethinyloestradiol accelerates growth velocity in conjunction with GH [30] and with oxandrolone. Large doses (> 2 μg daily) promote early epiphyseal fusion and therefore offer little benefit for final height.

Secondary sexual characteristics should be induced in girls with Turner syndrome by sex hormone therapy. Low-dose ethinyloestradiol (2 μg daily) should be commenced at the age of 12–13 years, being replaced by a low-dose combined oestrogen–progestagen preparation once growth has ceased and breast development has reached Tanner stage 4–5.

VARIANT FORMS OF GONADAL DYSGENESIS

The features associated with Turner syndrome may be modified by sex chromosome mosaicism or partial sex chromosome monosomy. The genetics of the condition has been reviewed recently [24]. In mosaic patients the ratio of 45XO to 45XX primordial germ cells determines the degree of ovarian abnormality, and the relationship between 45XO and 45XX cells in the periphery may be important in the development of somatic disorders. Patients with the most common chromatin-positive mosaicism, 45XO/45XX, are often of normal height, may menstruate and are occasionally fertile. More often these patients have short stature and streak gonads, but few other features of Turner syndrome.

Patients with chromatin-negative mosaicism, structural abnormalities of a Y chromosome or occult Y chromosome material [32] have a modified Turner phenotype with varying degrees of masculinization of the external genitalia. Patients with 'mixed gonadal dysgenesis' usually have the karyotype 45XO/46XY and possess a streak gonad and fallopian tube in association with a contralateral testis. The phenotype depends upon the degree of testicular development and, as gonadal tumours are more common in these patients, removal of the testis is advised in phenotypic females. Patients with 'pure gonadal dysgenesis' have a 45XX or 45XY karyotype and have streak gonads, sexual infantilism and primary amenorrhoea. Varying degrees of genital ambiguity occur in these patients, and the gender of rearing should be determined carefully. In all cases of gonadal dysgenesis removal of dysgenetic gonads, appropriate plastic surgery to the external genitalia and detailed counselling should be undertaken.

OVARIAN RESISTANCE SYNDROMES

This term is used to describe situations where the ovary is unable to respond to gonadotrophin stimulation. Patients with 17α-hydroxylase deficiency have impaired synthesis of 17-hydroxyprogesterone and 17-hydroxypregnenolone, and hence of oestradiol, testosterone and cortisol. Hypergonadotrophic hypogonadism and primary amenorrhoea are associated with elevated adrenocorticotrophin levels and hypertension with hypokalaemic alkalosis secondary to elevated deoxycorticosterone and 18-hydroxycorticosterone concentrations. Recent studies have shown that a number of different mutations in the cytochrome P450 17α gene may be responsible for this enzyme defect [33,34]. Treatment is with replacement doses of glucocorticoids and sex steroids.

The term 'resistant ovary syndrome' is used to describe part of the spectrum of primary ovarian failure, and may present with primary amenorrhoea. More commonly it develops later in life, presenting as secondary amenorrhoea.

GONADAL IRRADIATION AND CHEMOTHERAPY

The importance of gonadal irradiation and chemotherapy for malignant disease in childhood on reproductive function is becoming increasingly recognized. When such therapy has been given early in childhood, girls may present with primary amenorrhoea, although secondary amenorrhoea is a more common outcome.

POLYCYSTIC OVARY SYNDROME

PCOS usually presents with secondary amenorrhoea, and is discussed further below. Rarely, young women with PCOS present with primary amenorrhoea [21].

Other causes of primary amenorrhoea

A number of other mechanisms for primary amenorrhoea exist which are not directly caused by ovarian dysfunction, although that is the ultimate presenting feature. Thus, developmental abnormalities of the genital tract (Müllerian dysgenesis) are common, with congenital absence of the vagina being reported in 1 in 5000 live births [35]. The intersex disorders of genital differentiation are well recognized. Finally, any of the hypothalamopituitary disorders which generally present with secondary amenorrhoea may occur in childhood, causing primary amenorrhoea, usually with features of delayed puberty and other anterior pituitary hormone deficiencies. Primary amenorrhoea of hypothalamic origin may also be caused by childhood chemotherapy or irradiation.

Secondary amenorrhoea

The symptom of secondary amenorrhoea reflects a wide range of underlying pathology, as shown in Table 17.3.

Table 17.3 Causes of secondary amenorrhoea

Primary ovarian failure	'Resistant ovary syndrome'; irradiation/chemotherapy; gonadal dysgenesis; postoperative
Secondary ovarian failure	
Hypothalamopituitary dysfunction	Hyperprolactinaemia, hypothalamopituitary tumours, irradiation/chemotherapy, empty sella syndrome, postoperative
Functional disorders	Weight loss/anorexia nervosa, exercise, psychogenic, chronic illness
Polycystic ovary syndrome	
Genital tract disorders	
Functional ovarian tumours	

The majority of these disorders occur in older women, although all of them may occasionally present in postpubertal adolescent girls. As discussed above, the distinction between primary and secondary amenorrhoea is not absolute, so that occasionally patients with syndromes of gonadal dysgenesis present with secondary amenorrhoea and those girls who have received treatment for malignant disease in childhood may present with either. The most common cause of secondary amenorrhoea in the adolescent population is functional amenorrhoea related to weight loss and exercise.

CLINICAL ASSESSMENT OF THE PATIENT WITH SECONDARY AMENORRHOEA

A detailed menstrual history should be taken from all patients. A history of irregular cycles dating back to the menarche is suggestive of PCOS. Symptoms of oestrogen deficiency may be present, and headaches and visual disturbance should be enquired after. The question of weight loss should be dealt with carefully, and a detailed dietary history obtained. A patient with weight-loss-related amenorrhoea may not necessarily be underweight at the time of presentation. The amount of physical exercise should be established. A history suggestive of other endocrine disorders or of previous chemotherapy or radiotherapy should be sought. Sexual history is important and may not be proffered by younger patients unless specifically asked. A history of pelvic inflammatory disease is important. The examination should begin with measurement of height and weight and the body mass index calculated (BMI = weight (kg)/height^2 (m^2); normal range 20–25 kg/m^2). Signs of hyperandrogenism such as hirsutism, acne or virilization should be noted, and the breasts examined for galactorrhoea. Features of other endocrine disorders may be present, and the visual fields should be assessed.

Investigations are aimed initially at establishing the site of a lesion. Thus, basal FSH measurement will determine those patients with primary ovarian dysfunction. LH is also raised but this is non-specific as LH levels are also elevated in 60–70% of patients with PCOS [36]. Serum prolactin and thyroid function tests should be measured, although unsuspected thyroid disease is a rare cause of secondary amenorrhoea. The use of the GnRH test is of little or no value in the investigation of secondary amenorrhoea as it provides poor discrimination between patients with hypothalamic amenorrhoea and normal women [37]. Oestrogen activity is best assessed by the response to a progestagen challenge, as measurements of plasma oestradiol overlap between hypogonadal patients and normal subjects in the early follicular phase of the menstrual cycle. Vaginal bleeding after a short course of a progestagen (for example medroxyprogesterone acetate, 5 mg daily by mouth for 5 days) indicates adequate tissue oestrogen activity [38]. Pelvic ultrasound scanning, in skilled hands, will distinguish between polycystic and multifollicular ovaries [10].

Causes of secondary amenorrhoea

WEIGHT-LOSS-RELATED AMENORRHOEA

Weight-loss-related amenorrhoea is the commonest cause of secondary amenorrhoea in young women, and may be associated with anorexia nervosa or other defined eating disorders in adolescent girls. A BMI of less than 16 kg/m^2 is associated with severely impaired GnRH activity, resulting in a prepubertal pattern of gonadotrophin secretion [39]. Less severe weight loss is also important, and in these patients the endocrine and ovarian morphological pattern exactly replicates that seen during normal puberty [10,40]. Treatment of weight-loss-related amenorrhoea is weight gain – this is specific therapy and requires the assistance of dieticians, with psychiatric or psychological input in more severe cases. Patients who remain amenorrhoeic should be treated with hormone replacement therapy in the form of a low-dose combined oestrogen/progestagen preparation.

EXERCISE-RELATED AMENORRHOEA

This form of amenorrhoea, related to strenuous physical exercise, is also common in young women. The endocrine and ovarian changes are similar to those seen in girls with weight-related amenorrhoea. While psychological factors may be important in both these groups, the contribution of body weight or body composition itself appears to play a role, as the same changes are observed in patients with chronic illness [41]. Young women with exercise-related amenorrhoea, such as athletes or ballet dancers, may be unable or unwilling to reduce their exercise level, which is the treatment of choice. It is advisable to check oestrogen status, and replacement therapy should be offered to those who do not respond to a progestagen challenge [42].

POLYCYSTIC OVARY SYNDROME

Polycystic ovaries can be observed in 23% of 'normal' women on ultrasound examination, making this the most common structural abnormality of the ovary [43]. Women with the full PCOS have disorders of menstrual function which may present as oligomenorrhoea or secondary amenorrhoea in association with hirsutism and obesity. Patients with PCOS may present in adolescence, usually complaining of hirsutism and oligomenorrhoea/amenorrhoea. The pathology and clinical management of this condition are extensively dealt with in the adult literature (for reviews see [36,44]). Hirsutism in adolescence may cause severe psychological distress, and attention should be given to a clear explanation of the various options for treatment.

POLYCYSTIC OVARY SYNDROME AND PUBERTY

It is well recognized that women who present with PCOS have a history which dates back to puberty. Irregular menstrual cycles are common in adolescent girls, and endocrinological evaluation shows a high proportion of them to have hyperandrogenaemia and polycystic ovaries, features which resolve with time in the majority of girls [45]. Much recent evidence exists to suggest that the features of hyperinsulinaemia, insulin resistance and elevated IGF-I levels characteristic of puberty are also found in PCOS (reviewed in [46]). At the onset of puberty, fasting insulin levels rise, associated with peripheral insulin resistance thought to be related to the pubertal rise in GH secretion [47,48]. Insulin and IGF-I are important regulators of ovarian function, and insulin also regulates sex-hormone-binding globulin (SHBG) concentrations, thus modulating free sex steroid levels. Hyperinsulinaemia is also a feature of PCOS (reviewed in [36]) and has been reported in 30–63% of subjects.

A number of other associated metabolic changes, such as suppression of IGF-binding protein 1 (IGFBP-1, an important regulator of IGF-I activity) and SHBG concentrations are common to both puberty and PCOS. These observations have led to the hypothesis that the transient hyperinsulinaemia and elevated IGF-I levels seen in puberty produce a temporary polycystic ovary-like state in a significant number of adolescent girls, with those bearing a genetic predisposition to ovarian hyperandrogenism have persistent endocrinological and ovarian morphological change, i.e. the polycystic ovary *syndrome*.

This is supported by a follow-up study which showed that girls with the highest serum androgen concentrations in puberty went on to have the lowest fertility rates in the third decade of life, suggesting that anovulation and hyperandrogenism evolve from puberty through to adulthood [49]. Further evidence for a link between PCOS and puberty comes from recent studies which showed an increased incidence of hyperandrogenaemia and PCOS in postpubertal girls previously diagnosed as having precocious pubarche in childhood [50].

CONCLUSION

The mature ovary is a complex organ regulated by a large number of endocrine, paracrine and autocrine factors. Ovarian development begins in early fetal life when oocyte replication and folliculogenesis commence. The changing activity of the hypothalamopituitary–ovarian axis observed throughout childhood culminates in the menarche with the establishment of regular ovulatory menstrual cycles.

Clinical disorders of ovarian function in childhood and adolescence are uncommon. However, due to their profound effects on pubertal development, and their implications for adult life, their early diagnosis and treatment are of great significance.

REFERENCES

1 Baker TG. A quantitative and cytological study of germ cells in human ovaries. *Proc R Soc Lond (Biol)* 1963;158:417–33.

2 Byskov AG. The role of the rete ovarii in meiosis and follicle formation in different mammalian species. *J Reprod Fertil* 1975;45:201–9.

3 Peters H, Byskov AG, Grinsted J. Follicular growth in fetal and prepubertal ovaries of humans and other primates. *Clin Endocrinol Metab* 1978;7:469–85.

4 Huhtaniemi IL, Yamamoto M, Ranta T, Jalkanen J, Jaffe RB. Follicle-stimulating hormone receptors appear earlier in the primate fetal testis than in the ovary. *J Clin Endocrinol Metab* 1987;65:1210–14.

5 Baker T, Scrimgeour J. Development of the gonad in normal and anencephalic human fetuses. *J Reprod Fertil* 1980;60:193–9.

6 Miller W. Molecular biology of steroid hormone synthesis. *Endocr Rev* 1988;9:295–311.

7 Peters H, Himmelstein-Braw R, Faber M. The normal development of the ovary in childhood. *Acta Endocrinol* 1976;82:617–30.

8 Winter JSD, Hughes IA, Reyes FI. Pituitary-gonadal steroid concentrations in man from birth to two years of age. *J Clin Endocrinol Metab* 1976;42:679–86.

9 Brook CGD, Jacobs HS, Stanhope R, Adams J, Hindmarsh P. Pulsatility of reproductive hormones: applications to the understanding of puberty and to the treatment of infertility. *Ballières Clin Endocrinol Metab* 1987;1:23–41.

10 Adams J, Franks S, Polson D *et al.* Multifollicular ovaries: clinical and endocrine features and response to pulsatile gonadotrophin-releasing hormone. *Lancet* 1985;2:1375–9.

11 Wood DF, Franks S. Delayed puberty. *Br J Hosp Med* 1989;4:223–30.

12 Leung PK, Steele GL. Intracellular signaling in the gonads. *Endocr Rev* 1992;13:476–98.

13 Findlay JK. Growth factors in endocrinology – the ovary. *Ballières Clin Endocrinol Metab* 1991;5:755–69.

14 Mason HD, Margara R, Winston RML, Seppala M, Koistinen R, Franks S. Insulin-like growth factor-1 (IGF-1) inhibits production of IGF-binding protein-1 while stimulating oestradiol secretion in granulosa cells from normal and polycystic human ovaries. *J Clin Endocrinol Metab* 1993;76:1275–9.

15 Carson RS, Zhang Z, Hutchinson LA, Herington AC, Findlay JK. Growth factors in ovarian function. *J Reprod Fertil* 1989;85:735–46.

16 Adashi E, Resnick CE. Antagonistic interactions of transforming growth factors in the regulation of granulosa cell differentiation. *Endocrinology* 1986;119:1879–81.

17 Apter D, Raisanen I, Ylostalo P. Follicular growth in relation to serum hormonal patterns in adolescence compared with adult menstrual cycles. *Fertil Steril* 1987;47:82–8.

18 Fraser IS, Michie EA, Wide L. Pituitary gonadotrophin and ovarian function in adolescent dysfunctional uterine bleeding. *J Clin Endocrinol Metab* 1973;37:407–14.

19 Carr BR. Disorders of the ovary and female reproductive tract. In: Wilson JD, Foster DW, eds. *Williams Textbook of Endocrinology*. Philadelphia: W.B. Saunders, 1992:733–98.

20 Franks S. Primary and secondary amenorrhoea. In: *Gynaecology Clinical Algorithms*. London: British Medical Journal, 1989:41–5.

21 Canales ES, Zarate A, Castelazo Ayala L. Primary amenorrhoea associated with polycystic ovaries. Endocrine, cytogenetic and therapeutic considerations. *Obstet Gynecol* 1971;37:205–10.

22 Turner HH. A syndrome of infantilism, congenital webbed neck and cubitus valgus. *Endocrinology* 1938;23:566–74.

23 Wood DF, Franks S. Hypogonadism in women. In: Grossman A, ed. *Clinical Endocrinology*. Oxford: Blackwell Scientific Publications, 1992:669–84.

24 Saenger P. The current status of diagnosis and therapeutic intervention in Turner's syndrome. *J Clin Endocrinol Metab* 1993;77:297–301.

25 Massarano AA, Brook CGD, Hindmarsh PC. Growth hormone secretion in Turner's syndrome and the influence of oxandrolone and ethinyl oestradiol. *Arch Dis Child* 1989;64:587–92.

26 Muram D, Jolly EE. Pregnancy and gonadal dysgenesis. *J Obstet Gynecol* 1982;3:87–8.

27 Massarano AA, Adams J, Preece MA, Brook CGD. Ovarian ultrasound appearances in Turner syndrome. *J Pediatr* 1989;114:568–73.

28 Park E, Bailey JD, Cowell CA. Growth and maturation of patients with Turner's syndrome. *Pediatr Res* 1983;17:1–7.

29 Rongen Westerlaken C, Wit JM, Drop SLS. Methionyl human growth hormone in Turner's syndrome. *Arch Dis Child* 1988;63:1211–17.

30 Vanderschueren Lodeweyckx M, Massa G, Maes M. Growth-promoting effect of growth hormone and low dose ethinyl oestradiol in girls with Turner's syndrome. *J Clin Endocrinol Metab* 1990;70:122–6.

31 Van Teunenbroek A, De Muinck Keizer-Schrama SMPF, Stijnen T *et al.* Dutch Working Group on Growth Hormone. Effect of growth hormone administration frequency on 24-hour growth hormone profiles and levels of other growth related parameters in girls with Turner's syndrome. *Clin Endocrinol* 1993;39:77–84.

32 Medlej R, Lobacarro JM, Berta P. Screening for Y-derived sex determining gene SRY in 40 patients with Turner syndrome. *J Clin Endocrinol Metab* 1992;75:1289–92.

33 Yanase T, Kagimoto M, Matsui N, Simpson ER, Waterman MR. Combined 17α-hydroxylase/17,20 lyase deficiency due to a stop codon in the N-terminal region of 17α-hydroxylase cytochrome P450. *Mol Cell Endocrinol* 1988;59:249–53.

34 Yanase T, Sanders D, Shibata A, Matsui N, Simpson ER, Waterman MR. Combined 17α-hydroxylase/17,20-lyase deficiency due to a 7 base pair duplication in the N-terminal region of the cytochrome P450 (CYP 17) gene. *J Clin Endocrinol Metab* 1990;70:1325–9.

35 Griffin JE, Edwards C, Madden JD, Harrod MJ, Wilson JD. Congenital absence of the vagina. The Mayer–Rokitansky–Kuster–Hauser syndrome. *Ann Intern Med* 1976;85:224–36.

36 Franks S. Polycystic ovary syndrome: a changing perspective. *Clin Endocrinol* 1989;31:87–120.

37 Franks S. Diagnostic uses of LHRH. In: Shaw RW, Marshall JC, eds. *LHRH and its Analogues*. London: Wright, 1989: 80–91.

38 Hull MGR, Knuth UA, Murray MAF, Jacobs HS. The practical value of the progestagen challenge test, serum oestradiol estimation or clinical examination in assessment of the oestrogen state and response to clomiphene in amenorrhoea. *Br J Obstet Gynaecol* 1979;86:799–805.

39 Nillius SJ, Wide L. The pituitary responsiveness to acute and chronic administration of gonadotrophin releasing hormone in acute and recovery stages of anorexia nervosa. In: Vigersky RA, ed. *Anorexia Nervosa*. New York: Raven Press, 1977: 225–41.

40 Stanhope R, Adams J, Jacobs HS, Brooks CGD. Ovarian ultrasound assessment in normal children, idiopathic precocious puberty and during low dose pulsatile gonadotrophin releasing hormone treatment of hypogonadotrophic hypogonadism. *Arch Dis Child* 1985;60:116–19.

41 Stead RJ, Hodson ME, Batten JC, Adams J, Jacobs HS. Amenorrhoea in cystic fibrosis. *Clin Endocrinol* 1987;26: 187–95.

42 Davies MC, Hall ML, Jacobs HS. Bone mineral loss in young women with amenorrhoea. *Br Med J* 1990;301:790–3.

43 Polson DW, Adams J, Wadsworth J, Franks S. Polycystic ovaries—a common finding in normal women. *Lancet* 1988; 1:870–2.

44 McKenna TJ. Hirsutism and polycystic ovary syndrome. In: Grossman A, ed. *Clinical Endocrinology*. Oxford: Blackwell Scientific Publications, 1992:691–712.

45 Venturoli S, Porcu E, Fabbri R *et al.* Menstrual irregularities in adolescents: hormonal pattern and ovarian morphology. *Horm Res* 1986;24:269–79.

46 Nobels F, Dewailly D. Puberty and polycystic ovary syndrome: the insulin/insulin-like growth factor 1 hypothesis. *Fertil Steril* 1992;58:655–66.

47 Amiel SA, Caprio S, Sherwin RS, Plewe G, Haymond MW, Tamborlane WV. Insulin resistance of puberty: a defect restricted to peripheral glucose metabolism. *J Clin Endocrinol Metab* 1991;72:277–82.

48 Hindmarsh P, Di Silvio L, Pringle PJ, Kurtz AB, Brook CGD. Changes in serum insulin concentration during puberty and their relationship to growth hormone. *Clin Endocrinol* 1988; 28:381–8.

49 Apter D, Vikho R. Endocrine determinants of fertility: serum androgen concentrations during follow up of adolescents into the third decade of life. *J Clin Endocrinol Metab* 1990;71: 970–4.

50 Ibanez I, Potau N, Virdis R *et al.* Postpubertal outcome in girls diagnosed as premature pubarche during childhood: increased frequency of functional ovarian hyperandrogenism. *J Clin Endocrinol Metab* 1993;76:1599–603.

18: Reproductive Endocrinology – The Testis

E.M. RITZÉN

INTRODUCTION

The endocrine function of the testis is responsible for both sex differentiation and pubertal signs in the male. However, there are reasons to believe that a normal milieu for the testis during childhood is of vital importance for spermatogenesis in adult life. Therefore, both the endocrine and spermatogenic functions of the testis should be considered in the management of testicular problems in childhood.

Being the prerequisite for propagation of the species, all reproductive organs are supplied with a variety of safeguards to make sure that functions are maintained under almost all circumstances. This may be the reason for the numerous regulatory mechanisms of testicular function that are being gradually unravelled: endocrine, paracrine and autocrine. These signals together direct the two major tasks of the testis, which are the secretion of testosterone by Leydig cells and the production of spermatozoa by seminiferous tubules.

DEVELOPMENT OF THE NORMAL TESTIS

Testicular differentiation

The earliest morphological characteristic that distinguishes the fetal testis from the primitive undifferentiated gonad is the formation of cords of epithelioid cells in the gonadal stroma during the sixth week of gestation. These cells, which will form the future Sertoli cells, are probably derived from the mesonephros, a primitive kidney anlage which otherwise disappears completely. The primordial germ cells, the stem cells of the spermatogonia, can first be identified at the base of the yolk sac. Later, they migrate to the gonadal anlage to be embedded in the seminiferous cords.

At an early stage the fetal testes acquire the ability to produce testosterone from the Leydig cells, which are probably of mesenchymal origin. Testosterone secretion is supported by placental gonadotrophins (human chorionic gonadotrophin, hCG) until the ninth to tenth gestational week. When the hCG concentration in blood drops after 12 weeks, fetal pituitary luteinizing hormone (LH) and follicle-stimulating hormone (FSH) are essential for the further stimulation of both testosterone production and growth of the seminiferous tubules. The prenatal development of the testis is described in more detail by Müller & Skakkebaek [1].

Testicular descent

The mechanisms behind testicular descent have been a matter of argument among researchers. In early fetal development the testis is located in the retroperitoneal space. A mesenchymal structure, the gubernaculum, anchors the cauda epididymides to the abdominal wall at the site where the scrotum will develop as a pouch, containing the different layers of the wall (Fig. 18.1). After the scrotal sac has been formed, the gubernaculum increases in volume within the scrotum, thereby creating a space for the testis, after it has been reduced in size again.

Hormonal factors may influence descent; administration of large doses of oestrogens to pregnant mice will produce cryptorchidism; in androgen insensitivity the testes, which are often of normal size in neonatal and prepubertal ages, mostly stay in the abdomen or the inguinal canals. In anencephalic fetuses and in congenital hypogonadotrophic hypogonadism, testicular descent is impaired. Furthermore, during the first year of life the LH response to an acute challenge with gonadotrophin-releasing hormone (GnRH) has been found to be lower in boys with cryptorchidism than in controls. Finally, in about 50% of boys with cryptorchidism, descent can be induced by hCG treatment. All of this indicates that gonadotrophins (mediated through testosterone) are essential for testicular descent. Special factors that induce growth of the gubernaculum have also been sought, and a possible role for anti-Müllerian hormone is as a growth factor for the gubernaculum.

The process of testicular descent is not completed at birth in some boys; in 3% of full-term boys, and more in premature infants, one or both testes cannot be found in

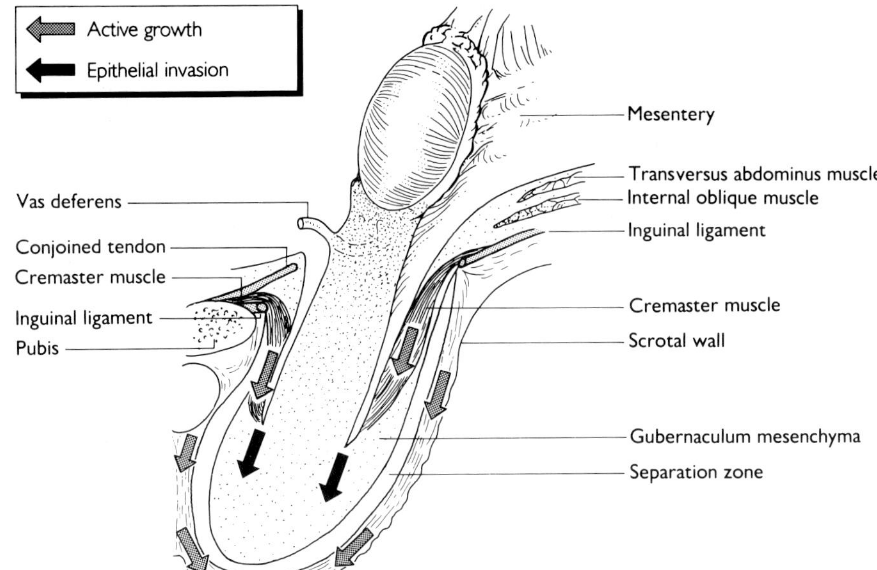

Fig. 18.1 The mechanism of descent of the testis through the inguinal canal to the scrotum. After the abdominal wall has bulged out to form the beginning of the scrotal sac (with the gubernaculum attached to its bottom), the gubernaculum increases in volume and clears the way for the testis through the canal. Later, the gubernaculum is again reduced in size, to become an inconspicuous structure between the cauda epididymides and the bottom of the scrotum (from Backhouse [2]).

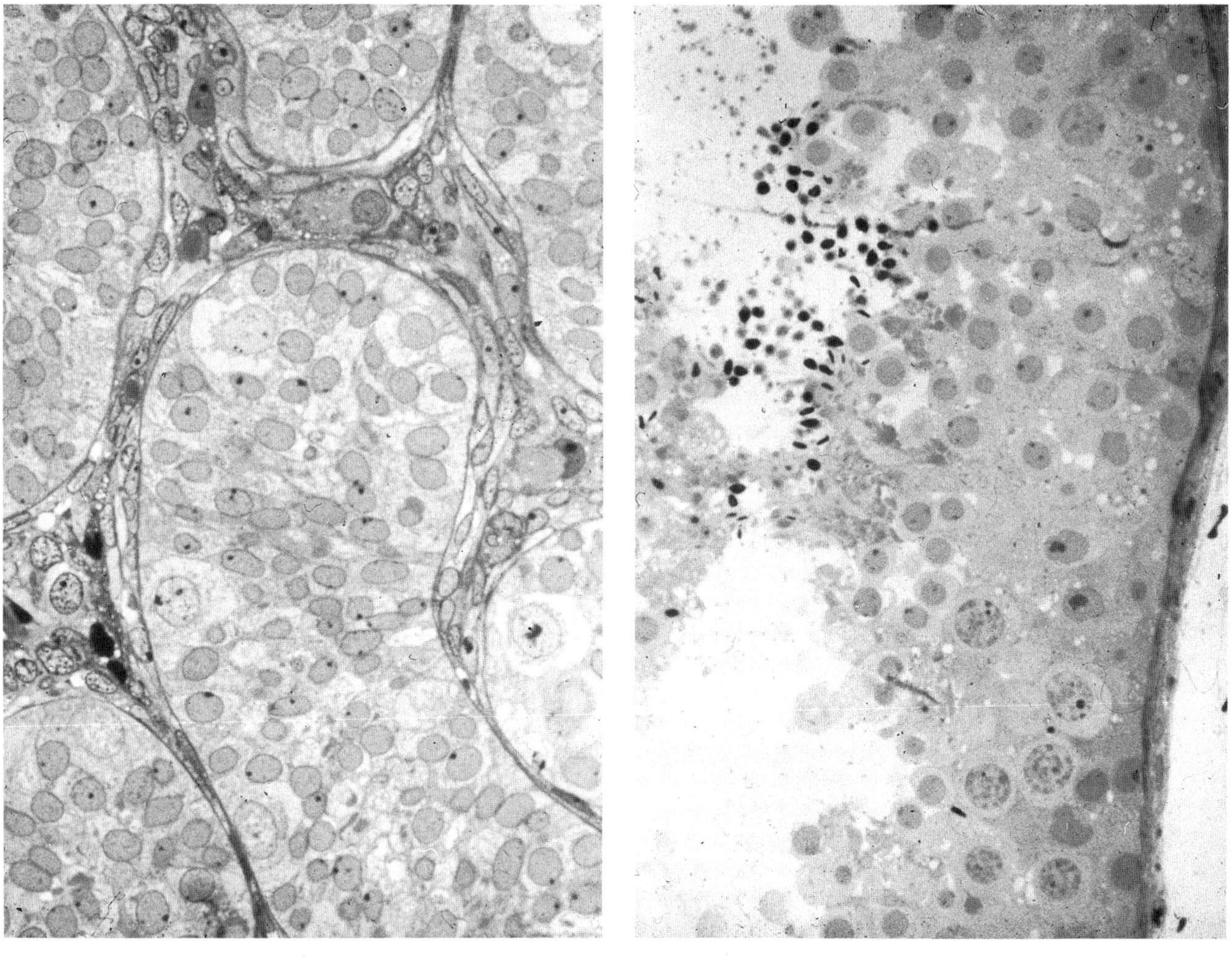

Fig. 18.2 Section through a prepubertal (left) and an adult testis (right) at the same magnification. The seminiferous tubule is increased in size through the germ-cell proliferation in the adult tubule. In the prepubertal tubule only Sertoli cells, spermatogonia and spermatocytes are seen, while the adult tubule shows all stages of germ-cell maturation.

the scrotum. However, by 1 year of age about 50% of these have descended.

The incidence of cryptorchidism at 1 year of age has increased from 0.8 to 1.5% over recent decades. This has parallelled an increase in the incidence of hypospadias, a worsening of sperm quality in adults and an increased incidence of testicular tumours. The rather rapid changes suggest that an environmental factor is harming testicular development. Although not proven, chemicals with some oestrogenic effects have been incriminated.

Testicular morphology

The fetal testis shows maximal production of testosterone at about 12 weeks of gestational age. This is manifested as an abundance of Leydig cells in the interstitial compartment. The germ cells progress in maturation from primitive spermatogonia to reach premeiotic spermatocytes at the time of birth. At this stage the germ-cell maturation comes to a halt, which lasts until puberty begins.

The early prepubertal testis is characterized by small seminiferous tubules and abundant interstitial tissue. Within the tubules, Sertoli cells and spermatogonia dominate, with a few spermatocytes. There is no lumen visible until tubular fluid production begins in puberty (Fig. 18.2). The interstitial Leydig cells cannot be seen in ordinary histological staining, but may still be active in secreting steroids at a very low level.

There is little growth of the testis from 1 to 10 years of age. This reflects the standstill of spermatogenesis. In

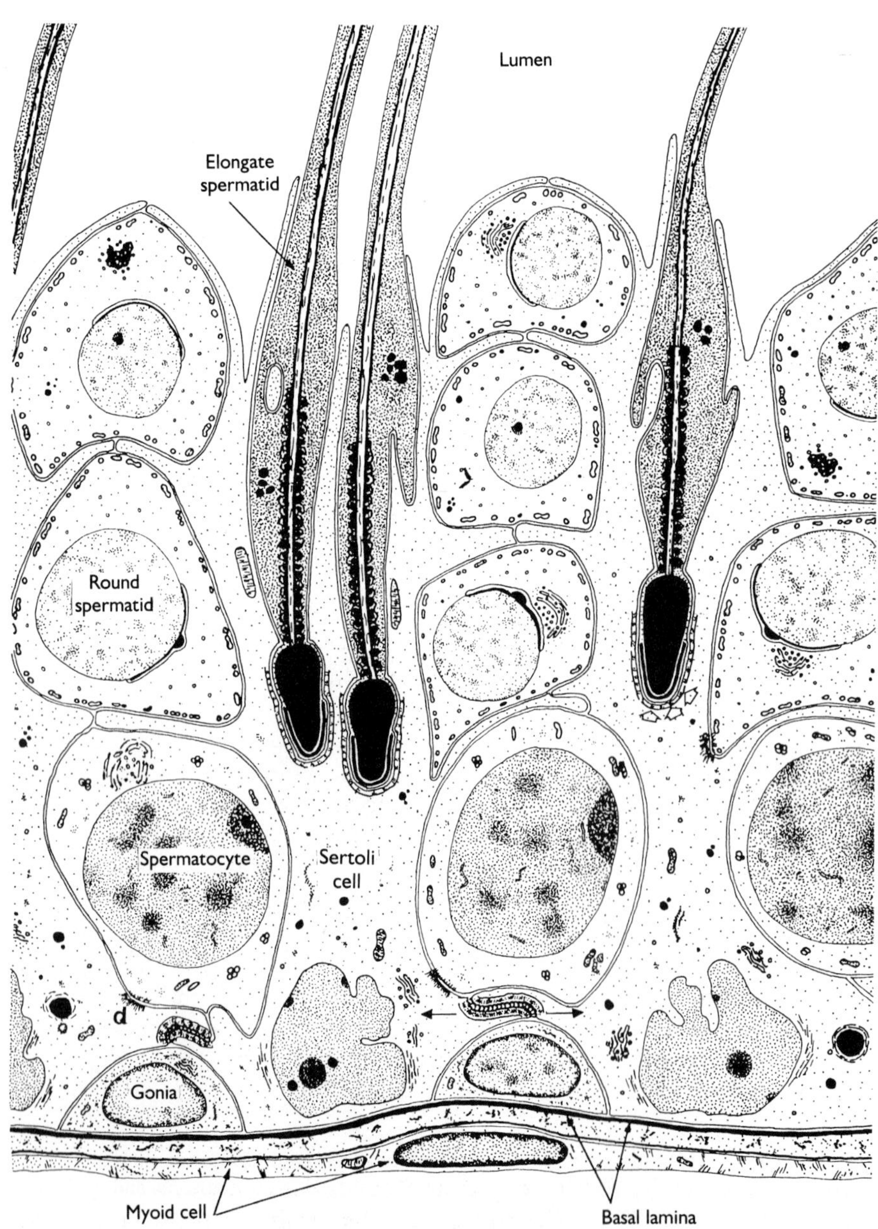

Fig. 18.3 The seminiferous tubule. The tight junctions between the adjacent Sertoli cells form the most important part of the 'blood–testis barrier'. All cells adluminal to the barrier reside in a microenvironment that is very different from that outside the tubule (see text) (from Russel [3]).

the adult testis more than 90% of the testis volume is made up of the seminiferous tubules, while the hormone-producing Leydig cells may constitute a small percentage. The tubules are surrounded by a basement membrane and a single layer of contractile peritubular myoid cells. The germ cells are proliferating at a remarkable rate; a daily production of 200 million spermatozoa makes the testes the most active organ of the body when it comes to cell proliferation.

An important functional aspect of the seminiferous tubule is the so-called blood–testis barrier (Fig. 18.3). This is partly made up of the peritubular cells and the basement membrane, but the tight intercellular junctions between adjacent Sertoli cells form the most important part. It prohibits passage of any macromolecules from the basal compartment into the lumen of the tubule. It also forms a barrier to simple ions; for example, the potassium concentration within the adluminal compartment averages 40 mmol/l. Since this barrier is so tight, the Sertoli cells have to function as 'nurses' for the proliferating germ cells; all nutrients and other regulatory substances must pass through Sertoli cell cytoplasm before reaching the postmeiotic germ cells. It also shields the adluminal compartment from the immune system of the rest of the body. Several cell surface molecules of the spermatids and spermatozoa are therefore regarded as 'foreign' to the immune system and will evoke an immunological response if the blood–testis barrier 'leaks' antigens. In all, the interior of the seminiferous tubule constitutes a very particular secluded 'milieu interieur' of the human body.

Further information on the morphology of the testis can be found in the excellently illustrated publication by Russell [3].

Regulation of testicular function

The regulation of the fetal testis has been described briefly above. Since the fetus is shielded from the maternal peptide hormones it must provide its own regulatory mechanisms. Although the major part of placental peptides are secreted towards the mother, sufficient hCG reaches the fetal circulation to permit adequate stimulation of the fetal Leydig cells. However, there are few data available on the variability of hCG concentrations in fetal blood during the first weeks of fetal life. Therefore, the possibility remains that some instances of deficient masculinization of the male external genital organs may be due to insufficient secretion of hCG to the fetus. If this is followed by a normal fetal pituitary LH and FSH secretion, after the organogenetic phase has passed, the result will be some degree of hypospadias in an otherwise normally masculinized boy. In fact, most cases of hypospadias remain unexplained even after the most careful study of endocrine function. Conversely, a normal hCG-stimulated Leydig

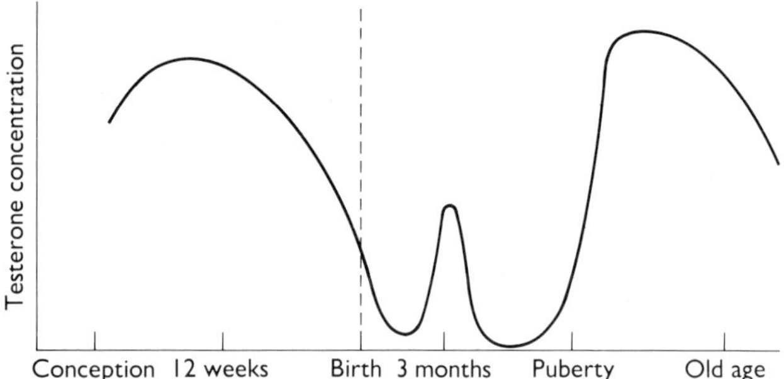

Fig. 18.4 Blood levels of testosterone in fetal, neonatal, prepubertal and adult life. This largely mirrors the testicular activity at the different stages of maturation – high in prenatal and postpubertal life, low in childhood, except for the transient increase at 2–3 months of age.

cell testosterone secretion during the first trimester of pregnancy will succeed in forming a normally shaped but very small penis and scrotum, even if fetal pituitary gonadotrophins are subnormal. This may be the case in anencephaly, panhypopituitarism or in hypogonadotrophic hypogonadism (Kallmann syndrome), where micropenis is a common finding along with small testes.

During the first 1–2 months of postnatal life there is a temporary fall in testosterone blood levels, followed by a major but short-lived peak at 2–4 months of age (Fig. 18.4). At these ages, gonadotrophin levels are still high enough to stimulate testicular activities. Thus, significant testicular testosterone secretion can be measured in blood during the first few days of life, and again at 2–4 months, without exogenous stimulation tests. The ensuing suppression of the hypothalamopituitary–gonadal axis, which lasts until puberty, lays the ground for the long childhood period, unique to humans among other mammals. It has been suggested that this is one of the major reasons for the remarkable degree of sophistication of humankind; the long, almost asexual prepubertal period of the human race gives an extended undisturbed period of learning, before the struggle for sexual dominance starts.

Although the prepubertal testis is developing very slowly compared to both the fetal and the pubertal periods, it has been shown to be active at a low level. The concentration of testosterone around the testis and in the spermatic vein is higher than in peripheral blood throughout childhood. Since the prepubertal ovary has also been shown to develop small follicles on and off during childhood, it is not surprising to see that there is a gradual shaping of the bodies of boys and girls in a male and female pattern, even before puberty.

REGULATION OF LEYDIG CELLS

LH is the principal and major stimulus for Leydig cell steroidogenesis, except for the first trimester of pregnancy

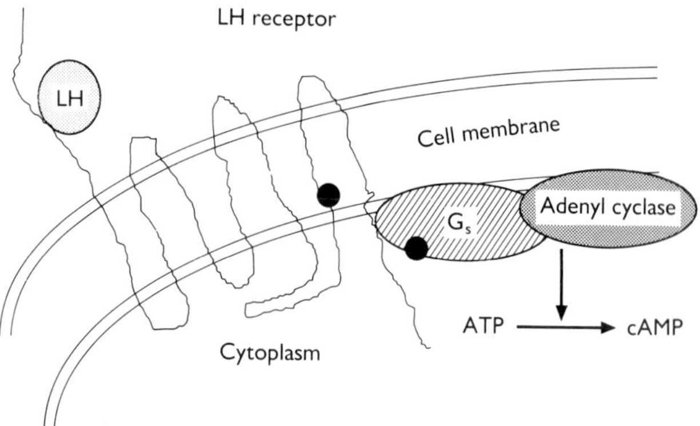

Fig. 18.5 Binding of LH to the extracellular domain of its receptor in the membrane of a Leydig cell, which in its turn causes dissociation of the subunits of the stimulatory G protein (G_s). This increases the activity of adenylate cyclase, to elevate intracellular levels of cAMP. The small black dots symbolize mutations of the LH receptor and G_s protein that have been associated with autonomous activation of andenylate cyclase. ATP, adenosine triphosphate.

when placental hCG dominates (see above). In the male, LH receptors are found only on Leydig cells. LH receptors also bind hCG at a high affinity, actually somewhat higher than LH. The fetal Leydig cells have been shown to be less sensitive to down-regulation by hCG than adult Leydig cells. The ligand-activated receptor then induces a dissociation of the stimulatory G protein into its subunits, which activate adenylate cyclase to produce its second messenger, cyclic adenosine monophosphate (cAMP) (Fig. 18.5). This series of events is amply demonstrated in human disease, in the rare experiments of nature which cause precocious puberty in boys without gonadotrophin stimulation: testotoxicosis and McCune–Albright syndrome.

Testotoxicosis was initially named when it was realized that one form of hereditary precocious puberty was independent of pituitary gonadotrophins. It was proposed that a mechanism similar to thyrotoxicosis would be responsible. However, it has been shown that the disease

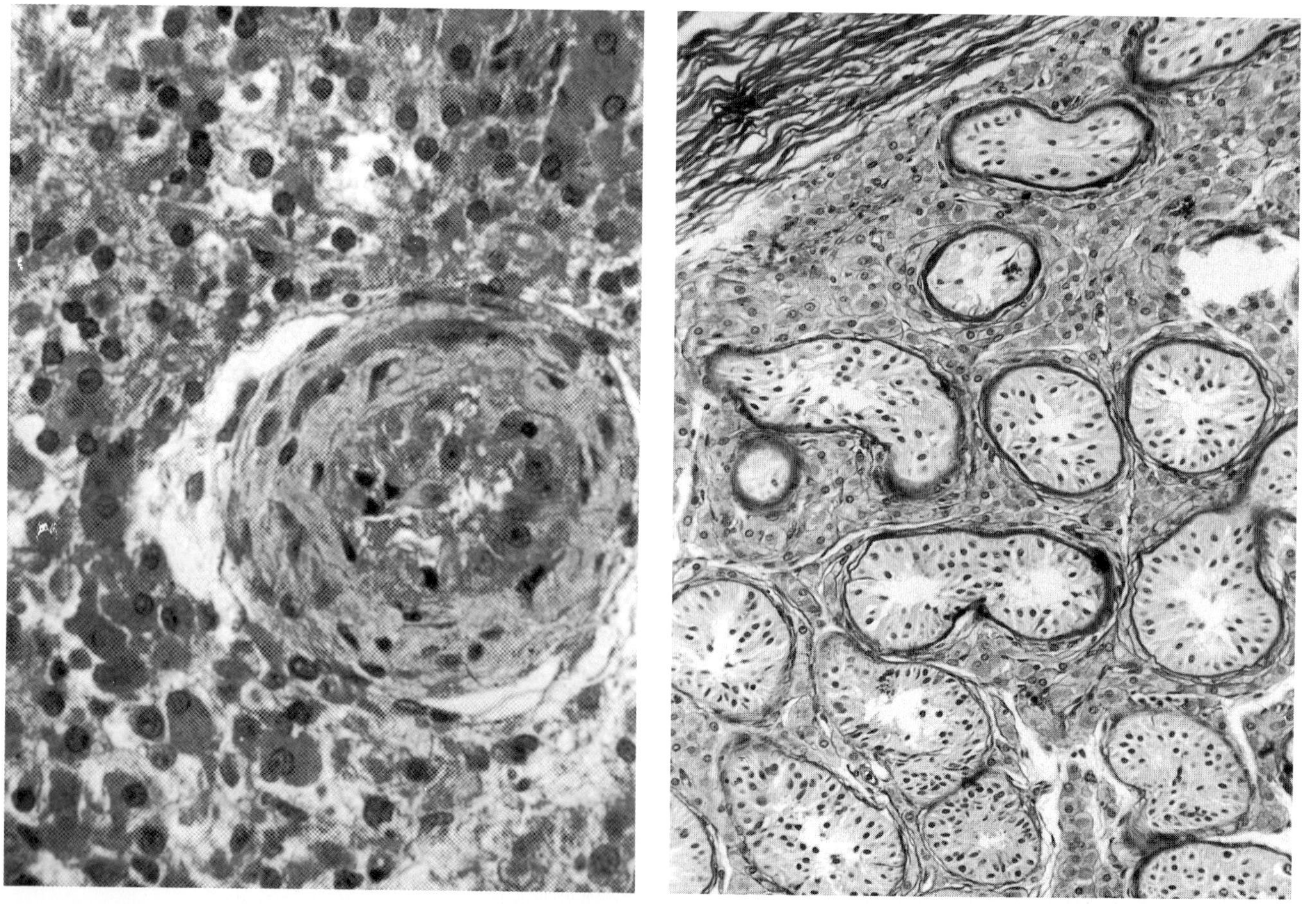

Fig. 18.6 Section of the testis from an adult man with Klinefelter syndrome (left) and from a woman with androgen insensitivity syndrome (AIS) (right). The seminiferous tubules of the Klinefelter testis are sclerotic; in AIS they show no spermatogenesis beyond primary spermatocytes. Both display an enormous hyperplasia of Leydig cells. In spite of this hyperplasia, testosterone levels in both subjects were subnormal for adult men.

depends on a mutation of the LH receptor gene, which causes a constant activation of the G protein even in the absence of ligand [4]. In the McCune–Albright syndrome the G protein itself is mutated in the cells affected [5]. The baseline production of cAMP is elevated to cause overfunction of Leydig cells, adrenal, thyroid and other cells which use cAMP as the second messenger. This does not, however, affect all cells in the body. The mutation probably occurred in a somatic cell early in the embryogenesis, and only the tissues that derive from this particular cell will show an abnormal function – the body will thus be a mosaic of areas of normal and abnormal tissues. The abnormality would otherwise be incompatible with life.

In addition to LH, a large number of endocrine and paracrine factors have been shown to modify Leydig cell function. Testosterone secretion is lowered by oestrogens, not only through suppression of gonadotrophins, but also by direct effects. Glucocorticoids have been suggested to have a similar inhibitory effect on Leydig cells. Early indirect evidence pointed at FSH as a factor potentiating LH action on Leydig cells. For a long time this was a puzzle, since FSH receptors could be found only on Sertoli cells. The probable solution came through the discovery that FSH stimulates production of insulin-like growth factor I (IGF-I) by Sertoli cells, and also potentiates LH action on Leydig cells. However, at least in the rat, seminiferous tubules also produce factors which inhibit testosterone secretion by Leydig cells. The intimate relations between seminiferous tubules and Leydig cells are also exemplified in human disease; marked Leydig cell hyperplasia but poor steroidogenesis is found in cases of tubular damage, such as Klinefelter syndrome, cryptorchidism and androgen insensitivity (Fig. 18.6).

REGULATION OF SPERMATOGENESIS

Hormonal regulation of spermatogenesis is to a large extent the story of the regulation of the Sertoli cell function. The previous role given to the Sertoli cells as a mechanical framework for germ cells has been completely revised over the past two decades. As described above, the tight 'blood–testis barrier' puts the postmeiotic germ cells at the mercy of Sertoli cells; the latter cells thus have an important role of supplying germ cells with nutrients, growth factors and any other specific or non-specific factors. Germ cells are particular in their requirement for energy; they cannot use glucose, but are instead effectively supplied with lactate and pyruvate by the Sertoli cells.

The primary stimuli for Sertoli cell activity are FSH and testosterone (Fig. 18.7). The adjacent Leydig cells provide the Sertoli cells with testosterone concentrations that are

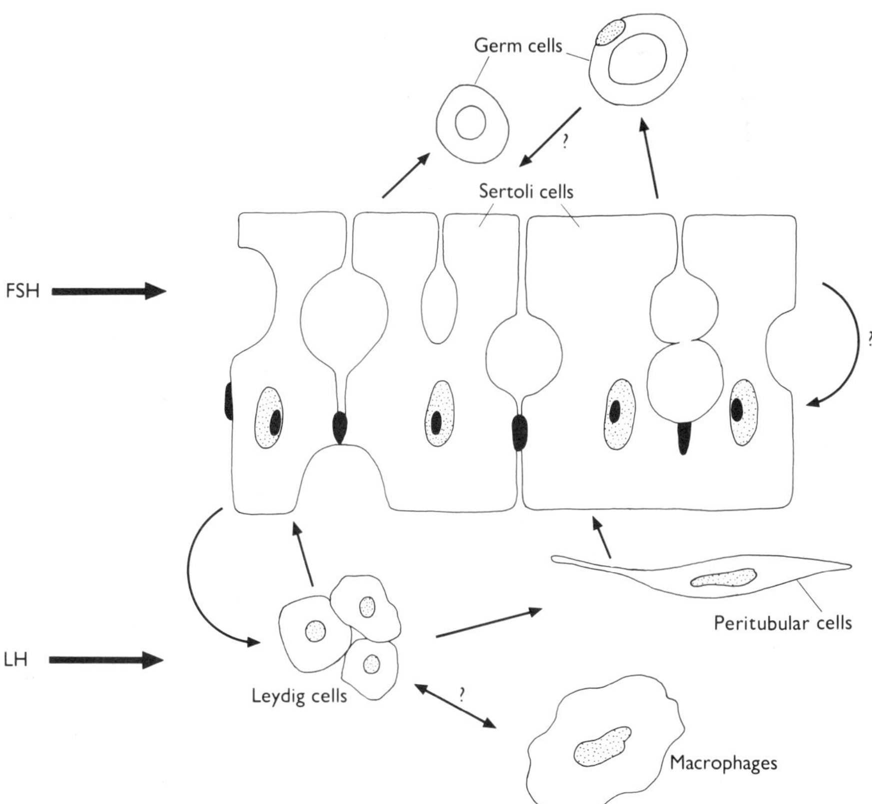

Fig. 18.7 Different cell types of the testis known to be active in endocrine (thick arrows) or paracrine (thin arrows) regulation of its neighbouring cells. Each arrow shows an effect that has been demonstrated *in vitro*.

20–50 times higher than those in peripheral blood. These levels are virtually impossible to reach by systemic administration of testosterone in cases of impaired Leydig cell function. On the contrary, testosterone medication might reduce testicular levels of testosterone due to negative feedback on the pituitary.

Testosterone freely diffuses into the seminiferous tubule to stimulate many different aspects of Sertoli cell function, directly through androgen receptors and indirectly through an androgen-dependent peptide (PMOD-S) produced by peritubular cells. In most species the tubular content of testosterone is augmented by androgen-binding protein (ABP), a specific Sertoli cell product. Germ cells have not been shown to express androgen receptors. On the contrary, in animal experiments, even spermatozoa, which carry the mutated androgen receptor gene and must thus be regarded as androgen-insensitive, can fertilize an egg if they derive from a seminiferous tubule of a chimaeric animal where at least some of the Sertoli cells have a normal androgen sensitivity.

Sertoli cells have been shown to produce numerous regulatory peptides: IGF-I, inhibin, activin, transforming growth factor β (TGF-β), anti-Müllerian hormone, interleukin 1α (IL-1α), IL-6 and TGF-α, among others. The target cells are not always known; most of the growth factors increase germ-cell proliferation *in vitro*, some of them have also been shown to do so *in vivo* [6]. The multitude of factors may secure the rapid cell divisions during spermatogenesis. However, they are also secreted towards the interstitium, where they may influence Leydig cell function (see above). The interleukins and TGF-β may be involved in creating the special immunological milieu in the testis; in several species homografts can survive much longer in the testis than in other tissues. The testis is, for example, the most frequent site of recurrence of acute lymphoblastic leukaemia [7].

The relation between Sertoli and germ cells are not a one-way street. Spermatocytes and spermatids have been shown to produce several active signal peptides, some of which seem to exert their actions on Sertoli cells. Surprisingly, the testes and the brain are often the most active sites of expression of such peptides: nerve growth factor (NGF), glutamic acid decarboxylase (GAD, involved in the synthesis of γ-aminobutyric acid), choline acetyltransferase (the key enzyme for acetylcholine synthesis) and pro-opiomelanocorticoid peptides are some examples. The NGF receptors that have been shown to be located on Sertoli cells are *negatively* regulated by testosterone, opposite to most other Sertoli cell products. This provides a possible local feedback system for maintaining Sertoli cell function even when testosterone supplies are scarce. Another mode of regulation of Sertoli cells is exerted by the excess cytoplasm that is pinched off from the late spermatids; the phagocytosis of these residual bodies by Sertoli cells is a potent stimulus for their interleukin production.

The regulation of cell function in the testis is a good example of the complex endocrine, paracrine and autocrine mechanisms that are involved in cell regulation. It is obvious from this that studies of isolated cells *in vitro* may provide interesting information, but they cannot be accepted to be of physiological importance until the *in vitro* findings have been shown to be of importance in the 'cloud' of regulatory factors present *in vivo*. Reviews in this area can be found in [8–10].

CLINICAL EXAMINATION OF THE TESTIS

In normal development, the activity of the hypothalamo-pituitary–gonadal axis in the male can readily be determined by simple physical examination. Testicular growth indicates the start of the surge of gonadotrophin secretion in early puberty. The testicular growth curve mirrors the low activity during the prepubertal childhood years and the rapid acceleration of sexual maturation at puberty (Fig. 18.8). On the other hand, early signs of androgen action on genitals, growth, skin and muscle without a prior growth of the testes point to the adrenals as the source of androgenic hormones. The Prader orchidometer for measuring testicular volume can be a useful instrument for health

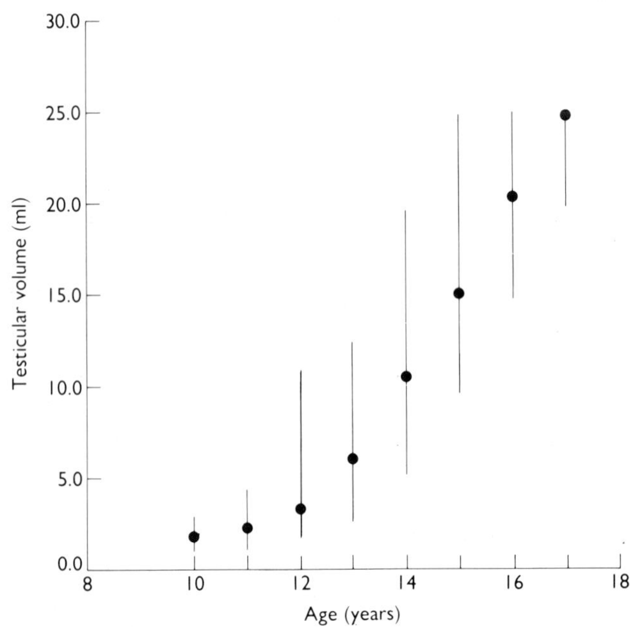

Fig. 18.8 Testicular growth curve constructed from longitudinal measurements of 122 healthy Swedish boys from birth until 20 years of age. From 1 to 10 years of age there is a very slow growth of the testes. Medians and 10th–90th percentiles are indicated. Note the very large variation within this normal population (redrawn from data in Taranger *et al.* [11]).

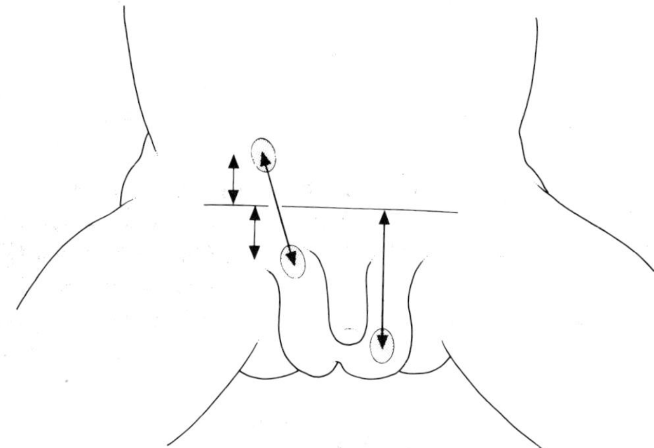

Fig. 18.9 Illustration of the various positions that a testis may have at examination. In a boy with cryptorchidism or with retractile testes, the position of the testis in centimetres from the transverse plane through the pubic tubercles can be exactly recorded before and after treatment. Both the spontaneous position and that during maximal (gentle!) traction downwards, as well as that attained after the traction have been released. The traction should last at least 30 s in order to exhaust the cremasteric reflex (from Karpe *et al.* [12]).

personnel as well as patients in illustrating the progress of puberty.

Cryptorchidism is defined as a permanent location of the testis above the scrotal entrance. Repeated examinations in a warm and unstressed environment may be necessary to separate this condition from so-called retractile testes, when the testes sometimes can be found in the scrotum and sometimes in the inguinal canal. If a testis cannot be palpated when the patient is lying down, the examination should be repeated when standing up, to increase the abdominal pressure. Asking the boy to sit 'like a tailor' while pulling his own feet towards his buttocks during the examination might bring down to the scrotum a testis that previously was not palpable.

The position of the testis should be recorded in a reproducible way, for example in relation to the transverse plane of the pubic tubercles, as shown in Fig. 18.9. This method makes it possible to describe the results of treatment in a quantitative way, rather than as 'success' or 'failure' – terms that are ill-defined and preclude quantitative statistical analysis.

While a permanent position of the testes in the warmer milieu of the abdomen or the inguinal canal definitely prevents normal spermatogenesis, it has not been shown whether retractile testes have a completely normal spermatogenesis later in life. Thus, there is a lot of confusion about the definition of the situation that calls for treatment. Since the seminiferous tubules form the bulk of the testicular volume, the size of the testis is an overall good measure of spermatogenic activity. When the testis reaches a volume of 8–10 ml, the average boy produces his first spermatozoa in morning urine specimens. This is quite early in puberty; the growth spurt has just gained speed and pubic hair may be at stage 2 or 3. Indeed, occasional boys have been described to produce spermatozoa in urine samples already at a testicular volume of 2 ml and 3 ml without other signs of androgen actions. Generally, 4 ml (or 3 cm in testis length) is accepted as the size that gives a clear indication of beginning puberty.

The texture of the testis is important. The prepubertal testis has a quite firm texture, and becomes more fluctuant in puberty and adulthood. The identification of a hydrocele of the testis is easily made by transillumination. A soft testis should always raise suspicion of pathology, irrespective of age; primary dysgenesis, sequelae to treated cryptorchidism, secondary hypogonadotrophic hypogonadism, damage by toxic or ionizing radiation are examples of such abnormalities. Naturally, the presence of a firm nodule within the testis must be suspected of malignancy until otherwise proven.

The epididymis can readily be identified as an elongated mass along the dorsal aspect of the testis. It may be malformed, but is otherwise rarely a site of disease in children. A rounded nodule at the caput epididymidis of an adolescent boy may be found to be a translucent spermatocele.

Varicocele is a common finding in adolescents. It can be observed and palpated if the patient is standing up during the examination, but not if lying down. Varicocele in adult men has been associated with infertility but since the incidence is so high in normal men, it does not call for treatment in most cases.

THE ABNORMAL TESTIS

Cryptorchidism

Retention of one or both testes in the abdomen or in the inguinal canal is known to be associated with impaired fertility in adulthood. The underlying mechanisms behind this fertility problem are probably several: increased temperature of the retained testis, primary dysgenesis of the testis, or both. In almost all mammals (the elephant is one exception) spermatogenesis demands a lower temperature than that of the abdominal cavity. In humans, the temperature gradient between abdomen and scrotum is 2°C.

No incidence of fertility has been reported in truly bilateral cryptorchidism. In animal experiments the derangement (or lack of development) of spermatogenesis upon elevation of the testicular temperature to 'body temperature' can be readily demonstrated. However, after 'therapeutic success' in terms of bringing the testis down into the scrotum by surgical or endocrine therapy, fertility is also compromised. This has raised questions whether in some cases of cryptorchidism the primary defect lies in the testis itself – a dysgenetic testis would not show normal descent. A third explanation of the poor fertility also seen in unilateral cryptorchidism has been put forward: like the example of sympathetic ophthalmopathy, where the originally undamaged eye may be attacked by an autoimmune reaction following laceration of the contralateral eye, the scrotal testis might be damaged if the cryptorchid testis is leaking antigens. However, this hypothesis has not found experimental support, and in the case of primary unilateral cryptorchidism in humans, the postmeiotic germ cell antigens will never appear, due to arrested spermatogenesis already at the spermatogonial or spermatocyte level.

Leydig cell function is only partially compromised in boys with treated cryptorchidism. The rise in testosterone concentrations in puberty is somewhat delayed, but eventually they reach normal levels.

Since elevated temperature does cause damage to spermatogenesis, most researchers agree that retained testes should be brought down to the scrotum; at least one cause of poor spermatogenesis will be eliminated. It is here where the consensus starts and ends; the most suitable age and the most efficient mode of treatment have been the subject of intense discussions. Histological studies of retained testes agree that the slow progress of spermatogenesis seen in a normal scrotal testis from 1 to 2 years of age does not occur in the abdominal or inguinal testis. At first glance it therefore seems logical to place it in the scrotum at 1–2 years of age. There are drawbacks to this approach: the younger the patient, the greater is the risk of damaging the vas deferens and the vasculature to the testis during surgery. Therefore, in the past, most surgeons have elected to wait until after 2 years of age or later. With increasing skill and better instrumentation this tradition now seems to be changing towards younger and younger ages of the patients.

There are so far no convincing studies showing that treatment at an early age actually ends up with a better adult testis than later treatment. The follow-up study with a second biopsy has, for ethical reasons, not been performed, and non-randomized studies of fertility after surgery at different ages can always be criticized for a bias in selection of patients for surgery – in infancy it is even more difficult to exclude patients with retractile testes from those with truly retained testes.

An alternative to surgery is hormonal treatment. In most studies, hCG treatment after age 4 is successful in about 50% of the cases, if the testis is palpable in the inguinal canal. The treatment protocols vary; traditionally 500–1000 IU has been given as an intramuscular injection twice weekly for 5 weeks. However, the results with hCG are not so good before 4 years of age.

Synthetic GnRH has been used as an alternative to hCG, with variable success. Most placebo-controlled studies have failed to show a significant effect. However, a 4-week course of nasal GnRH (1.2 mg/day divided into three doses) does cause a relaxation of the cremasteric muscle, and will help in identifying testes that are retractile rather than truly cryptorchid, thereby avoiding unnecessary surgery. Lately, in an uncontrolled study, a first course of GnRH (doses as above) for 4 weeks immediately followed by hCG (500 IU three times a week for 3 weeks) for the non-responders has been found to lead to descent in about 30% of the retained testes even when treated before 2 years of age. Also in this case the best results were found when the testis was in a 'prescrotal' position – if it was not palpable at all, there was a very poor effect of treatment [13].

Damage to the testis may be a complication of surgery. This would indicate a trial with hormonal therapy before surgery is chosen. However, lately a possible side-effect of hCG treatment has also been pointed out: in experimental animals, hCG and large doses of LH have been shown to produce increased intratesticular pressure and accumulation of inflammatory cells in the interstitium. The latter is also seen in testicular biopsies taken from boys within a few days and as long as 1 year after the last dose of hCG, in cases where descent did not occur. Whether this will cause any harm to the testis is still unknown.

With the above discussion in mind, the strategy for treatment of cryptorchidism will depend on the facilities available. In borderline cases (so-called prescrotal testes, where the distinction between retractile and cryptorchid states is difficult) GnRH therapy provides a gentle and probably safe way to improve the diagnosis – the retractile testes will 'descend' due to relaxation of the cremasteric muscle. Hormonal therapy is most (maybe only?) effective in boys who had scrotal testes at birth, which later ascended. Otherwise, an experienced surgeon should be consulted for boys younger than 4 years. After this age, hCG treatment will bring down the retained testis in about 50% of the cases – the other 50% goes directly to surgery after the (unsuccessful) trial.

A comprehensive summary of various aspects of cryptorchidism can be found in [14].

The absent testis

If the scrotum of a prepubertal boy is found to be empty, and no testes are palpable in the inguinal canals, it is not possible to say whether the testes have vanished completely after fulfilling male sex differentiation (testicular atrophy) or whether one or both testes can be found in the abdomen. The distinction between the two can be made by an hCG stimulation test; 4 days after an intramuscular injection of 3000 IU hCG, the plasma testosterone concentration should be significantly higher than before if an intra-abdominal testis is present. If not, there is little chance that surgery will localize an intra-abdominal testis. Determination of anti-Müllerian hormone in blood has been shown to be of value for the same clinical problem; a measurable level of this hormone in blood proves the existence of at least one testis.

In unilateral absence of a testis, ultrasound examination may sometimes be of help to localize the missing testis before surgery.

Risk of tumours in cryptorchid testes

There is general agreement on the increased risk of testicular cancer in patients with a history of cryptorchidism. In large reviews of patients with testicular tumours, about 10% have a history of previous cryptorchidism. This has been the rationale for recommending testicular biopsy of cryptorchid testes, especially since it has been shown that 2% of these testes carry carcinoma-*in-situ* (CIS) cells. However, in order to arrive at a correct risk assessment, a population-based calculation has to be performed. This has been published by Pinczowski *et al.* [15], who found four cases of testicular cancer among 2918 adult patients operated for cryptochidism 1–18 years earlier, giving a risk ratio of 7.4 (confidence interval 2.0–19) compared to the whole population. In 30 199 patients operated for inguinal hernia and 22 915 men undergoing appendicectomy during the same time period, the risk ratio was the same as that of the general population (1.1 versus 1.0).

Although this study confirmed the increased risk for testicular cancer in formerly cryptorchid men, a larger series of formerly cryptorchid men would be needed to get a more precise estimate of the increased risk. The authors concluded that the low overall risk (four cases in 25 360 human years) did not justify special surveillance after an operation for undescended testes. However, since dysplastic, small and soft testes constitute a special risk factor, it seems not inappropriate to advise a biopsy of such testes after completion of pubertal development to look for CIS.

The testis in sex chromosome abnormalities

47,XXY (KLINEFELTER SYNDROME)

This syndrome occurs with a much higher frequency than is generally recognized in clinical practice. Through the mass screening of neonates for chromosomal abnormalities, the true incidence and the natural history of patients with sex chromosome aberrations have become known, and changed our opinions on what a typical case is like [16,17]. The incidence at birth is about 1:600 boys. Few of them are diagnosed during childhood and adolescence: many are never diagnosed. The testes seem to function normally during fetal and prepubertal life but show progressive tubular degeneration during puberty. There is only one man with 47,XXY reported who has proven to be fertile.

From puberty onwards, testosterone levels in blood are in the low-normal or subnormal range. Histologically, the seminiferous tubules show thickening of the basement membranes and progressive loss of both germ cells and eventually Sertoli cells. The end-result is sclerotic, hyalinized tubules. In spite of the poor testosterone production, Leydig cell hyperplasia can sometimes be conspicuous (see Fig. 18.6). This may be interpreted as a loss of factors from the tubules that are essential for normal Leydig cell steroidogenesis. On physical examination, the degeneration of the tubules is manifested by small (less than 5 ml), firm testes in adult men with Klinefelter syndrome, while they may have had a volume of 6–8 ml in adolescence.

In rare cases, boys may be born with more than one extra X chromosome (48,XXXY, 49,XXXXY). From the sparse information available on these men, testicular function seems to be more affected than in men with 47,XXY. Micropenis and very small testes are reported, and there is little or no testosterone production at any time after birth.

XX MALES

Although sexual differentiation and masculinization in puberty is normal, spermatogenesis is severely impaired and the testes are smaller than normal.

MIXED GONADAL DYSGENESIS (46,XY/45,X)

These patients with a mosaic of normal XY cells and cells devoid of a Y chromosome show a large spectrum of phenotypes – from completely female over various degrees of hypospadias to completely male. In the former case, the gonads are both degenerated into fibrous streaks; in the latter case, one might find gonads that show a good testicular differentiation on one or both sides, with a streak gonad or tumour on the other side. The phenotype can be very variable. Patients with mixed gonadal dysgenesis may occasionally be diagnosed *in utero*, when amniocentesis is performed to detect fetuses with Down syndrome. Some of these patients may show a normal masculinization at birth, others may have hypospadias, some show normal female external genitalia. Thus, the phenotype cannot be predicted by the karyotype alone. The most important aspect of this condition is the very high incidence of testicular tumours in and after puberty.

The enlarged testis

Unilateral enlargement of a testis is dangerous; malignancy should be excluded. The most obvious causes of a swollen scrotum, hydrocele and spermatocele, are easily identified by transillumination. In adolescents and adults, but not in prepubertal boys, epididymitis and orchitis can be found. A tender, swollen scrotum in a prepubertal boy is a medical emergency – it may be a torsion of the testis or the testis appendix that needs immediate surgery. Varicocele has been dealt with above. A previously unilaterally cryptorchid testis is often smaller and has a softer texture than the contralateral one that is of normal size. Compensatory hypertrophy of the scrotal testis may be found in unilateral fetal atrophy of the testis, but not in unilateral cryptorchidism or in postnatal destruction of the other testis.

Malignant testicular tumours may arise from smooth muscle cells (rhabdomyosarcoma) or from germ cells (seminoma, embryonic carcinoma, dysgerminoma, teratoma). Some disorders of sex differentiation are especially prone to develop testicular malignancies (mixed gonadal dysgenesis, androgen insensitivity). Therefore, prophylactic removal of the gonads at puberty is often practised for these patients. However, germ-cell carcinomas have in some cases been shown to be preceded for several years by CIS, which are characterized by large, clear periodic acid Schiff-staining cells within the seminiferous tubules that mostly are devoid of other germ cells. Thus, one might elect to follow the possible appearance of such CIS cells by repeated biopsies of patients at risk. If the lesion is bilateral, low-dose irradiation has been shown to be an effective way to eliminate the CIS cells. Such testes are generally infertile even before irradiation so this side-effect of ionizing radiation is not a problem. Leydig cells do not seem to be damaged by such doses; therefore, future replacement therapy is not necessary. For many boys, avoiding castration is a major psychological advantage of irradiation treatment compared to surgical removal of the testes.

The testis is a frequent site of malignant lymphoid cell infiltration in the course of acute lymphoblastic leukaemia and lymphoma. Other kinds of metastasis are rare, which points to the special environment in the testis that favours growth of lymphoid cells.

In adolescent boys with poorly controlled congenital adrenal hyperplasia due to 21- or 11β-hydroxylase deficiency, multiple hard tumours may occasionally be found in testes which are otherwise small for the stage of pubertal development. Such tumours, which decrease dramatically in size when glucocorticoid therapy is (re)instituted, are believed to be formed by hypertrophy of small islets of adrenocortical cells that may normally reside in the testis.

Bilaterally enlarged testes without other signs of puberty can be found in occasional patients who have been treated for brain tumours. The mechanism behind this and the testicular histology in this condition are unknown. The sometimes extreme enlargement of the testes in the fragile X syndrome (elongation of the seminiferous tubules without obvious pathology) is not marked during the prepubertal period. The term 'fertile eunuch' syndrome is sometimes used for clinical situations when some spermatogenesis can be noticed in sections from testicular biopsies, but few and inconspicuous Leydig cells are seen, and poor masculinization is present. These patients are rarely fertile – the term is based solely on histology.

Iatrogenic damage to testes by irradiation or chemotherapy

In rats all future germ cells can be depleted from the testes of the offspring if the pregnant dam is irradiated by 100 rad a few days before delivery. So-called 'Sertoli cell only' seminiferous tubules are found when these rats reach adulthood. Although similar data are missing for humans, this shows that the immature testis may be even more sensitive to irradiation than the adult. Leydig and Sertoli cell function is much more resistant to irradiation than germ cells. However, even if spermatogenesis is severely damaged by irradiation, a few surviving spermatogonia may eventually repopulate the tubules with germ cells. Alkylating agents used in the treatment of malignancy or autoimmunity may also cause similar damage to spermatogenesis.

REFERENCES

1 Müller J, Skakkebaek NE. The prenatal and postnatal development of the testis. In: de Kretser DM, ed. *Baillière's Clinical Endocrinology and Metabolism*. London: Baillière Tindall, 1992:251–71.

2 Backhouse KM. Embryology of the normal and cryptochid testis. In: Fonkalsrud EW, Mengel W, eds. *The Undescended Testis*. Chicago: Year Book Medical, 1981:5–29.

3 Russel LD. Normal testicular structure and methods of evaluation under experimental and disruptive conditions. In: Clarkson TW, Nordberg GF, Sager PR, eds. *Reproductive and Developmental Toxicity of Metals*. New York: Plenum, 1983: 227–52.

4 Shenker A, Laue L, Kosugi S, Merendino JJ Jr, Minegishi T, Cutler GB. A constitutively activating mutation of the luteinizing hormone receptor in familial male precocious puberty. *Nature* 1993;365:652–4.

5 Weinstein LS, Shenker A, Gejman PV, Merino MJ, Friedman E, Spiegel AM. Activating mutations of the stimulatory G protein in the McCune–Albright syndrome. *N Engl J Med* 1991;325:1688–95.

6 Söder O, Parvinen M, Bang P, Persson H, Ritzén EM. Regulation of germ cell proliferation by growth factors. In: Spera G, Fabbrini A, Gnessi L, Bardin CW, eds. *Molecular and*

Cellular Biology of Reproduction. Serono Symposia Publications, Vol. 90. New York: Raven Press, 1992:109–13.
7 Ritzén EM. Testicular relapse of acute lymphoblastic leukemia (ALL). *J Reprod Immunol* 1990;18:117–21.
8 Burger H, de Kretzer D, eds. *The Testis*, 2nd edn. New York: Raven Press, 1989.
9 de Kretser DM, ed. *Ballière's Clinical Endocrinology and Metabolism. International Practice and Research – The Testes*, Vol. 6, No. 2. London: Baillière Tindall, 1992.
10 Ritzén EM, Hansson V, French FS. The Sertoli cell. In: Burger H, de Kretser D, eds. *The Testis*, 2nd edn. New York: Raven Press, 1989:269–302.
11 Taranger J, Engström I, Lichtenstein H, Svennberg-Redegren I. Somatic pubertal development. *Acta Paediatr Scand* 1976; Suppl.258:121–35.
12 Karpe B, Eneroth P, Ritzén EM. LHRH treatment in unilateral cryptorchidism: effect on testicular descent and hormonal response. *J Pediatr* 1983;103:892–7.
13 Lala R, Matarazzo P, Chiabotto P, de Sanctis C, Canavese F, Hadziselimovic F. Combined therapy with LHRH and HCG in cryptorchid infants. *Eur J Pediatr* 1993;152:S31–3.
14 Sharpe RM, Müller J, Skakkebaek NE. Proceedings of an ESPE Symposium on Cryptorchidism. *Horm Res* 1988;30:212–31.
15 Pinczowski D, McLaughlin JK, Läckgren G, Adami H-O, Persson I. Occurrence of testicular cancer in patients operated on for cryptorchidism and inguinal hernia. *J Urol* 1991;1146: 1291–4.
16 Nielsen J, Wohlert M. Sex chromosome abnormalities found among 34 910 newborn children: results from a 13-year incidence study in Arhus, Denmark. *Birth Defects* 1990;26: 209–23.
17 Ratcliffe SG, Butler GE, Jones M. Edinburgh study of growth and development of children with sex chromosome abnormalities. IV. *Birth Defects* 1990;26:1–44.

19: Anatomy and Physiology of the Hypothalamopituitary Axis

S.L. CHEW and A.B. GROSSMAN

INTRODUCTION

The anatomical relationship of the hypothalamus and pituitary has been known since Galen's time. However, it was Geoffrey Harris's elegant work in the 1940s that provided evidence for the function of the hypothalamus and pituitary as a physiological unit [1]. The hypothalamic releasing and inhibiting hormones involved were progressively isolated, identified and synthesized from the late 1970s, largely by the fiercely competing groups of Schally and Guillemin [2]. In recent years research has increasingly concentrated on the molecular mechanisms of the hypothalamopituitary interaction, and on the influence of other signalling systems (for example immunological) on neuroendocrine function.

EMBRYOLOGY

The human pituitary develops as the combined product of the outgrowth of ectodermal tissue from the buccal cavity, Rathke's pouch, and the down-growth of neural tissue referred to as the infundibulum [3]. The infundibulum is not thought to grow down as such, but to be left as a pocket of tissue when the rest of the brain undergoes its various foldings and conformational changes. The front of Rathke's pouch forms the anterior pituitary or pars distalis, while the back of the pouch forms the intermediate lobe or pars intermedia. The infundibulum borders onto the pars intermedia to form the posterior lobe. It is now clear that there is no distinct structural or functional pars intermedia in the human beyond fetal life. The stalk of the pituitary is composed of neural tissue, but becomes partially ensheathed by migratory buds from Rathke pouch, the pars tuberalis. The portal vasculature develops in the fetus as a complex network of vessels that comes to dominate the function of the pituitary during the second trimester.

While Rathke's pouch is already visible at 4 weeks gestation, only by 18–20 weeks is the pituitary well vascularized and capable of function. At the same time the hypothalamus has been differentiating into discrete nuclei, although these are much less evident in humans than in the rat. Axonal processes extend downwards from these nuclei to the external layer of the median eminence, where regulatory hormones are secreted into the portal blood. By 15 weeks the adult form of the hypothalamus has appeared, with evidence of an exogenous input of neuroamines and an endogenous supply of neuropeptides. There appears initially to be intimate contact between the hypothalamus and pituitary, with possible direct modulation of pituitary hormone secretion by hypothalamic neurons, but as maturation progresses beyond 20 weeks the development of the portal system ensures that the adult type of hypothalamopituitary interaction can occur.

Hypothalamic control of pituitary function is evident in the late-gestation fetus; levels of circulating prolactin (PRL) and growth hormone (GH) vary during fetal life, and are higher than in the neonate. There is a progressive rise in serum thyroid-stimulating hormone (TSH) towards the end of the second trimester, concomitant with a rise in thyroid hormones, while follicle-stimulating hormone (FSH) and luteinizing hormone (LH) are maximal during midgestation, thereafter falling towards term as sensitivity to gonadal steroid feedback increases (Fig. 19.1). The hypothalamopituitary axis is also functional prenatally, at least in terms of changes in peripheral hormone levels, but the effects of these variations are uncertain. The rise in TSH is necessary for full development of the thyroid, although partial growth of the gland is possible in its absence. Similarly, the pituitary–gonadal axis is required for maximum growth of the external genitalia, at least in the male, while adrenocorticotrophic hormone (ACTH) and related peptides (particularly from the fetal pars intermedia) almost certainly play a role in the growth of the fetal adrenal and possibly the initiation of parturition.

The fetal hypothalamus and pituitary develop independently of maternal influences at their own rate. Maldevelopment is uncommon, but when it occurs it mostly involves the formation of 'rests' of embryonal tissue which may become autonomous. Thus, remnants of Rathke's pouch may produce simple intrasellar cysts lined by stratified squamous epithelium or epidermoid cysts, or

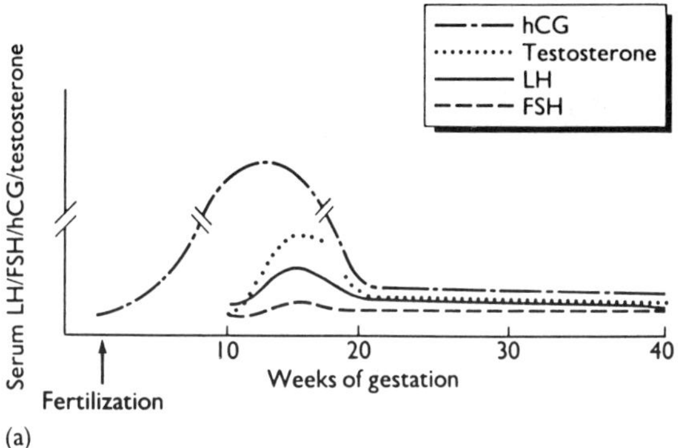

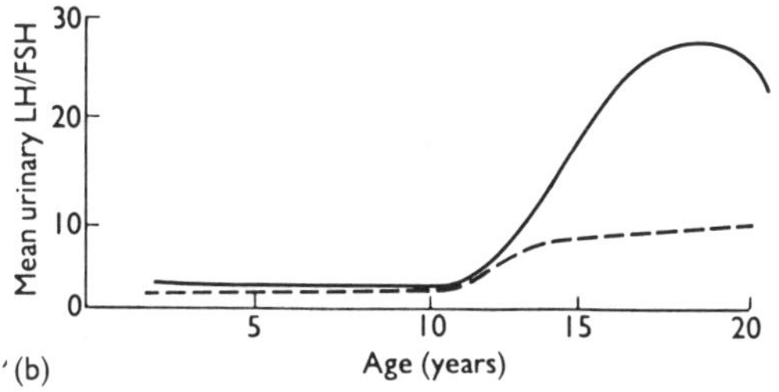

Fig. 19.1 Changes in hormone levels in the human male fetus (a) and during childhood (b) (redrawn from Forsling & Grossman [3]).

may form a matrix of epithelial and connective tissue with variable numbers of cysts, the craniopharyngioma. A simple cyst lined by ciliated columnar epithelium is referred to as 'Rathke's pouch cyst'. Residual tissue from the primitive notochord can also go on to produce chordomas, unpleasant suprasellar tumours usually originating in the region of the clivus.

There are several rare syndromes of congenital midline neuroanatomical anomalies associated with neuroendocrine deficiencies, including agenesis of the corpus callosum and septo-optic dysplasia (de Morsier syndrome). In the latter, unilateral or bilateral hypoplasia of the optic nerves is often (but not invariably) associated with an absent septum pellucidum and a spectrum of endocrine defects, especially GH deficiency [4]. The defect is characteristically hypothalamic, such that GH responsiveness to growth-hormone-releasing hormone (GHRH – see below) is preserved [5]. Other neurological abnormalities may be present, including 'see-saw nystagmus' and agenesis of the cerebellar vermis. The precise locus of the endocrine abnormalities associated with agenesis of the corpus callosum has not been established.

Hamartomas of this region may interfere with stalk function, giving rise to anterior pituitary hormone deficiencies and/or diabetes insipidus, or may consist of secretory neuroendocrine tissue and thus induce, for example, precocious puberty by abnormal production of gonadotrophin-releasing hormone (GnRH). Secretory gangliocytomas or ganglioneuromas of the hypothalamus may also arise as a developmental defect, and have been reported to cause acromegaly and Cushing syndrome later in life.

In 1989 it was shown that GnRH-secreting neurons were derived from epithelial cells of the olfactory apparatus, situated outside the central nervous system [6]. During development these cells migrate through, and populate, the olfactory bulb and tract to reach the hypothalamus. Examination of an aborted fetus with a deletion of the X chromosome confirmed that migration of GnRH-secreting cells was abnormal, reaching only as far as the cribriform plate. Since then deletions of the X chromosome involving a gene (the KALIG gene) coding a protein of the fibronectin family have been identified in Kallmann syndrome [7]. These findings provide an elegant molecular and embryological basis to Kallmann syndrome.

VASCULAR SUPPLY

The superior and inferior hypophyseal arteries arise as branches of the internal carotid, and run respectively to the median eminence and pituitary stalk, and to the posterior lobe (Fig. 19.2). From a capillary plexus in the median eminence, blood then runs down the portal system of long and short veins into a second capillary plexus around the anterior pituitary [8]. It seems probable that the long portal veins arise from the superior hypophyseal artery and the short veins from the inferior hypophyseal artery. The anterior pituitary drains laterally and indirectly into the cavernous sinus, while the inferior hypophyseal veins drain the posterior lobe, and possibly also part of the anterior lobe. Although this unidirectional flow

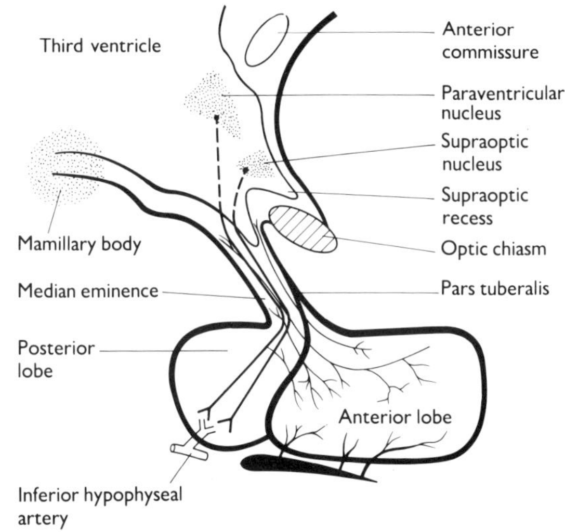

Fig. 19.2 Gross anatomy of the pituitary gland: sagittal section.

of blood corresponds to the original concept of Wislocki and King [7a], there is also some (disputed) evidence in favour of a reversed flow, particularly from the neurohypophysis to the median eminence. Similarly, the short portal veins may serve to interconnect the anterior and posterior lobes.

The portal vessels themselves are tightly coiled into helical structures, and may preserve a topographical distribution between the median eminence and pituitary. As both these latter structures may also be spatially organized, there may be compartmentalization of the releasing factors and their transportal routing. Taken together with studies on the bidirectionality of portal blood, it would seem that the hypothalamopituitary axis is structurally and functionally more complex than the simple mass transfer of hormones from one site to another.

ANATOMY AND PHYSIOLOGY

The human pituitary is situated inferiorly to the hypothalamus within the pituitary fossa, above the sphenoid sinus, which is usually (but not always) aerated [3,8]. The commonest surgical approach to pituitary tumours is trans-sphenoidal (avoiding the necessity of craniotomy), with postoperative cerebrospinal fluid (CSF) rhinorrhoea, meningitis, and sinusitis as potential complications.

The lateral relations of the pituitary are the cavernous sinuses, which are honeycombed by septa and contain the internal carotid arteries, as well as the third, fourth and sixth cranial nerves (Fig. 19.3). Rarely, lateral extensions of pituitary tumours may cause disorders of eye movements, and may eventually invade the temporal lobe.

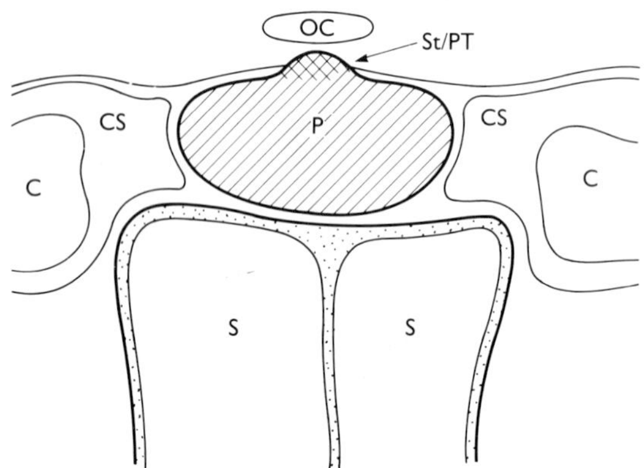

Fig. 19.3 Coronal section of the pituitary gland. Figure drawn from a standard histological section of human autopsy material with permission from Professor I. Doniach. Note that as the pituitary stalk curves sharply backwards it appears to merge with the pituitary (P). C, carotid artery; CS, cavernous sinus; OC, optic chasm; S, sphenoid sinus; St/PT, stalk/pars tuberalis.

Complete surgical resection of some tumours is prevented by venous bleeding from the cavernous sinus, and the important structures often encased by the tumours.

The pituitary itself is encompassed by a split in the dura and relates superiorly to the arachnoid and subarachnoid space which contains CSF. The stalk passes through the small foramen of Lillequist, although occasionally this may be enlarged sufficiently to allow CSF to herniate into the fossa; this is one putative cause of the 'empty sella syndrome'. Arachnoid cysts may form within or above the fossa, which may require surgical drainage and marsupialization. The optic chiasma is directly above the subarachnoid space; as this may vary in position, being very anterior (prefixed), or posterior (postfixed), field defects due to suprasellar tumours may also vary from the classical bitemporal hemianopia.

The hypothalamus extends from the preoptic area and fornix anteriorly to the mamillary bodies posteriorly, and includes the slit-like third ventricle. Its anatomical boundaries are arbitrary. It has reciprocal connections with the frontal cortex and thalamus, but particularly with the limbic circuits (amygdala, hippocampus, subiculum) and the brainstem nuclei involved in autonomic regulation (Fig. 19.4). It is thus ideally placed to integrate neuroendocrine and autonomic responses to motivational and emotional processes. It also appears to be involved in appetite and sexual behaviour, so that large or infiltrative lesions of the hypothalamus may be associated with marked behavioural changes.

The hypothalamus has various nuclei with complex internal pathways, as well as a vital efferent channel of neurosecretory terminals bordering on the portal vessels. In the rat this area of release is seen as a bulge on the floor of the brain – the median eminence – but this is less apparent in humans. Hypothalamic regulatory hormones are secreted, possibly topographically, into the portal vessels for transport to the pituitary, where the signal is amplified and transduced to release the anterior pituitary hormones. It should be noted that most of our knowledge on hypothalamic nuclei and neuropeptides is derived from

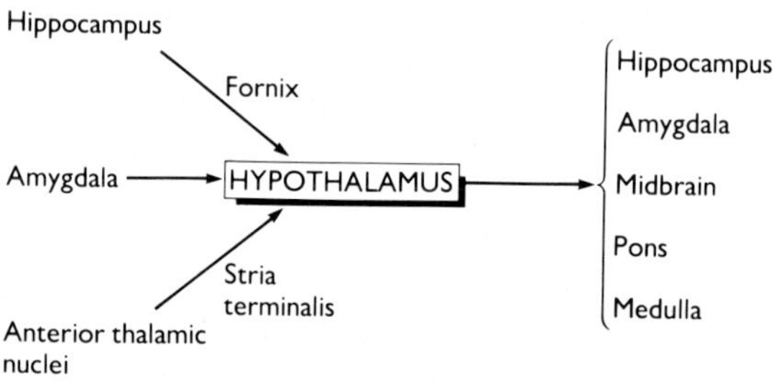

Fig. 19.4 Main afferent and efferent pathways of the hypothalamus.

the rat; there may not be direct correspondence between hypothalamic hormones and similarly named nuclei in humans.

The secretory cells of the anterior pituitary are arranged in irregular cords separated by vascular channels. Conventional staining techniques demonstrate the presence of a predominance of acidophils, basophils and occasional chromophobe cells. Immunohistochemistry has shown that acidophils situated in the posterolateral wings secrete GH, while those distributed throughout the pituitary are PRL-containing lactotrophs. Basophils, situated medially and anteriorly, secrete the glycoproteins FSH, LH, TSH and ACTH-related peptides. Chromophobe cells probably represent a non-secretory stage of the cell cycle. Folliculostellate cells are also present; they were formerly considered to play a nutritive/supportive role, but recent studies have suggested that they may also have a direct neuromodulatory function. The posterior pituitary consists of non-myelinated nerve fibres terminating around vascular sinusoids and pituicytes, which may be a type of glial cell.

ANTERIOR PITUITARY HORMONES

Prolactin

Prolactin was shown to be distinct from GH in the early 1970s. Its sequence similarity to GH suggests that both are descended from a common precursor. In addition, the prolactin receptor is part of a superfamily of transmembrane receptors, which includes the GH and erythropoietin receptors. In the rat, PRL is luteotrophic; it is involved in a variety of functions in other species, including osmoregulation in fish and in the laying down of calcium in eggshell in birds. However, in humans, the principal, if not the only, physiological role of PRL is the induction of lactation and the cessation of menses during the puerperium [9].

Serum PRL rises gradually during pregnancy, but lactation is inhibited at this time by the direct effect of fetoplacental oestrogen production on the breast. At parturition the fall in oestrogens leads to the onset of lactation, which is maintained as long as breast-feeding continues. Serum PRL gradually falls over the next few months, but will still respond with burst release to suckling stimulation.

In non-pregnant women and in men, PRL remains at a level usually less than 400 mU/l or 20 ng/ml throughout the day, although there is a slight increase in the early morning hours. PRL also rises in response to certain forms of stress, particularly hypotension (as in syncopal attacks), hypoglycaemia and surgery. In the neonate, serum PRL may be very high secondary to fetoplacental oestrogens. Thereafter the level is constant during childhood, rising slightly during puberty. There is no good evidence that PRL is important in the endocrine changes associated with puberty.

The principal hypothalamic regulator of PRL release is dopamine, which is secreted into the portal vessels in quantities sufficient to inhibit lactotroph PRL secretion. As PRL is predominantly under inhibitory dopaminergic control, any process or lesion which disturbs or disrupts the neuroendocrine axis will give rise to hyperprolactinaemia.

The dopamine neurons are thought to originate in the arcuate nuclear area at the base of the third ventricle, forming the 'tuberoinfundibular dopamine system'. Drugs that interfere with dopamine storage (such as methyldopa or reserpine) or block dopamine receptors (for example the major tranquillizers, such as chlorpromazine and haloperidol, or the antiemetics, such as metoclopramide and domperidone) will induce hyperprolactinaemia. γ-aminobutyric acid (GABA) may also be a PRL inhibitory factor, but is much less potent than dopamine. Two other hypothalamic peptides, TRH (thyrotrophin-releasing hormone) and VIP (vasoactive intestinal peptide), are PRL secretagogues, and may be physiological stimulators of PRL release under certain circumstances.

Hyperprolactinaemia may be seen in patients with primary hypothyroidism or chronic renal failure, but is most commonly seen in young women with PRL-secreting pituitary microadenomas. In men, prolactinomas usually present late as macroadenomas (more than 10 mm in diameter), with symptoms and signs of local compression. Serum PRL may be normalized in almost all patients following treatment with dopamine agonist drugs such as bromocriptine and the majority of prolactinomas undergo shrinkage. Newer dopamine agonist drugs (based on the ergot structure), such as pergolide, lisuride, cabergoline and terguride, as well as the non-ergot quinagolide, are currently under investigation in some centres, but, except for cabergoline, firm evidence of different spectra of side-effects and duration of action is still lacking.

In childhood, microprolactinomas have been reported but are rare. More commonly, persistent hyperprolactinaemia is indicative of a suprasellar lesion either in the hypothalamus or compressing the portal vasculature, and thus reducing dopamine delivery to the lactotrophs. Possible causes include craniopharyngiomas, Langerhans cell histiocytosis, germinomas, or radiation-induced damage. Hyperprolactinaemia in these patients is generally moderate, usually less than 1000 mU/l, but levels up to 8000 mU/l may be seen.

Hyperprolactinaemia may delay the onset of puberty or arrest its development. Galactorrhoea is rare prepubertally and hyperprolactinaemia is rarely a cause of gynaecomastia. PRL deficiency is seen in patients with pituitary aplasia or Sheehan syndrome and occasionally in postoperative hypopituitarism but is not associated with clinical symptoms or signs.

Growth hormone

Growth hormone is a 191 amino-acid residue peptide secreted by anterior pituitary somatotrophs which causes bone and soft-tissue growth. The hormone circulates in blood both unbound and attached to binding proteins of several sizes which are portions of the extracellular domain of the GH receptor. Insulin-like growth factor I (IGF-I) mediates the growth-promoting effects of GH. Although hepatectomy experiments in animal models suggest that most circulating IGF-I is produced in the liver, other tissues (for example kidney and muscle) also bear high concentrations. Serum IGF-I levels do not always correlate with the degree of anabolism or growth, and a paracrine mode of action of IGF-I is probably important. A variety of binding proteins have been identified for IGF-I: IGFBP-3 appears to be the main carrier protein in the blood, while the physiological and pathological roles of the other binding proteins remain uncertain [10].

GH is secreted in occasional bursts during the day and thus may be undetectable by conventional assays (<1 mU/l) in random samples. There is a sleep-entrained release of GH, with increase in GH pulse amplitude at night, particularly during the first one or two sleep cycles. It is generally considered that the nocturnal release of GH is closely linked with non-dreaming or 'slow-wave' sleep, especially stages III and IV. There is a gradual increase in the 24-h (that is both diurnal and nocturnal) integrated GH secretion during childhood, but this is greatly increased once puberty is established (see Chapter 14). This is probably secondary to the effect of gonadal steroids on GHRH [11], but a direct interaction between the somatotrophs and the gonadotrophs has also been suggested. Pubertal changes in GH release involve an increase in the amplitude of pre-existing pulses rather than a change in pulse frequency. Postpubertally there is a decrease in GH release, followed by a further fall in later life. In the adult GH may be relevant to the maintenance of skeletal muscle and connective tissue function. Some groups have identified a higher prevalence of cardiovascular disease and its surrogate markers in GH-deficient adults; the results of definitive trials of GH treatment in adults will be of considerable interest.

GH release is regulated by two hypothalamic peptides, GHRH, which is stimulatory, and somatostatin, which is inhibitory. GHRH was originally isolated from separate pancreatic tumours in two patients with acromegaly; in one patient from Charlottesville all the GH-releasing activity was contained in a single 40-residue peptide, while the second tumour, from Lyon, France, contained both a truncated 37-residue and an extended (and amidated) 44-residue peptide (Fig. 19.5) [12,13]. Neurons containing GHRH messenger (m)RNA have been identified in the arcuate nucleus of the human hypothalamus. The C-terminal of GHRH does not appear to be critical for its activity, and the C-terminal-abbreviated peptides, down to GHRH (1–29) NH_2, have been shown to be highly active in humans.

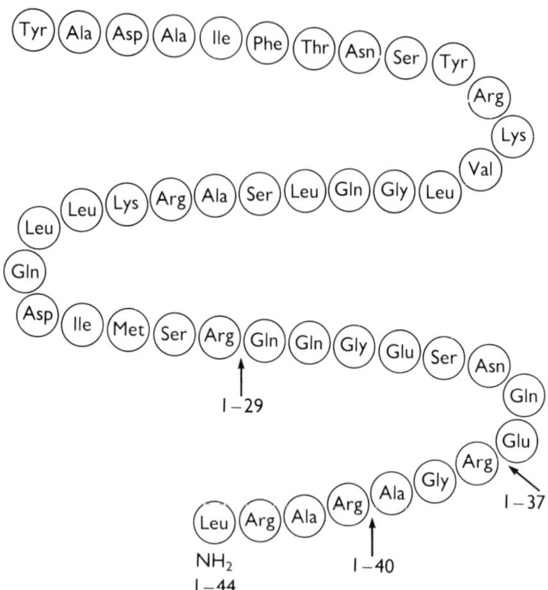

Fig. 19.5 The structures of the family of growth hormone-releasing hormones.

Somatostatin is a 14-residue cyclic peptide (Fig. 19.6) which directly inhibits somatotroph synthesis and release of GH; it was originally isolated after work on a quarter of a million ovine hypothalami [2].

GH pulses are the result of a release of GHRH into the portal blood, although there may also be transient inhibition of somatostatin release. These two peptides are in turn influenced by an array of neurotransmitters, which may be why various drugs cause changes in serum GH. Thus, clonidine and diazepam may stimulate the release of GHRH at α_2-adrenoreceptors and GABA receptors respectively, while bromocriptine, propranolol and cholinergic agonists probably inhibit the release of somatostatin. Dopamine agonists may also inhibit pituitary GH release directly. There is a tight feedback control

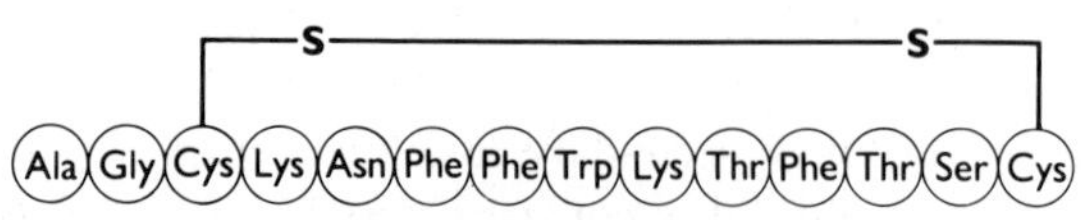

Fig. 19.6 The structure of the cyclic peptide, somatostatin 14.

of GH release, involving GH and IGF-I regulation of somatostatin and probably of GHRH.

At the molecular level both GHRH and somatostatin act on transmembrane receptors, which are linked to the G protein second messenger system. GHRH increases intracellular levels of stimulatory G protein subunits ($G_s\alpha$), while somatostatin increases inhibitory subunits (G_i). $G_s\alpha$-subunit activity increases cyclic adenosine monophosphate (cAMP) levels, while G_i does the converse. The GHRH receptor gene has been found to carry a mutation in its intrinsic guanine triphosphata (GTP)ase region (leading to constitutive activation of adenylate cyclase) in some 30% of GH-secreting pituitary adenomas. According to one group, tumours bearing this mutation appear to be smaller, have higher GH levels, and are more sensitive to somatostatin, than those without the mutation. [14].

Luteinizing hormone and follicle-stimulating hormone

The gonadotrophins, LH and FSH, are glycoproteins secreted by a common cell, the gonadotroph; they may even be stored within the same granule. Their release is stimulated by a single hormone, the decapeptide GnRH. GnRH is released in a pulsatile fashion into the portal capillary plexus from neurons in the preoptic area in the rat, but in humans probably principally from the infundibular or arcuate nucleus at the base of the third ventricle [15]. The synthesis and secretion of both peptides is stimulated by GnRH.

FSH expression and secretion are inhibited by inhibin, a glycoprotein of gonadal origin, which is a heterodimer of an α-subunit and one of two β-subunits (β_A or β_B) [16]. Inhibin has no effect on LH secretion. Dimers of the β-subunits, β_A/β_A and β_A/β_B (activin), release FSH more potently than GnRH, but less rapidly. The full physiological roles of these glycoproteins are still poorly understood, but they may also possess paracrine and tumour-supressing properties.

Knobil and colleagues in Pittsburgh [16a] have shown that GnRH must be released in a pulsatile mode in the primate, in order to produce a consistent release of the pituitary gonadotrophins, especially LH. In animals with hypothalamic ablation the administration of exogenous GnRH every 90 min gives rise to the pulsatile release of LH and FSH; in female animals this gives rise to a normal menstrual cycle, while prepubertal animals can be induced to develop in an accelerated but otherwise normal progression through puberty. Thus, the changes in LH and FSH responsiveness to GnRH seen during puberty can be explained by alteration in the steroidal and peptide milieu without postulating the need for changes in central regulation. In practice it seems likely that the hypothalamic generator can amplify or attenuate these changes and is responsible for the fine-tuning of the system.

In the adult human male the pulse generator appears to discharge at approximately 2-hourly intervals, while in the female the pulse interval of 60–90 min in the follicular phase slows drastically in the luteal phase. This inhibition of pulsatility may be a consequence of progesterone-induced activation of hypothalamic β-endorphin, which is a recognized inhibitory modulator of GnRH release. Little else is known of neurotransmitters affecting GnRH in humans, although changes in dopaminergic tone have been postulated in certain pathological states.

High levels of gonadotrophin (Gn) and gonadal steroids are seen in the neonate and these decline progressively over the years of life, initially very rapidly and then more slowly. Serum Gn starts to increase, initially only nocturnally, at the onset of puberty (see Fig. 19.1). This process involves an amplification of pre-existing low-amplitude pulses of GnRH, which can be detected as isolated increases in LH in all children from time to time at night, although an increase in GnRH frequency has also been suggested.

Thyroid-stimulating hormone

Pituitary TSH is a glycoprotein consisting of the α-subunit common to LH and FSH and a specific β-subunit (Fig. 19.7); it is secreted under the control of TRH. TRH stimu-

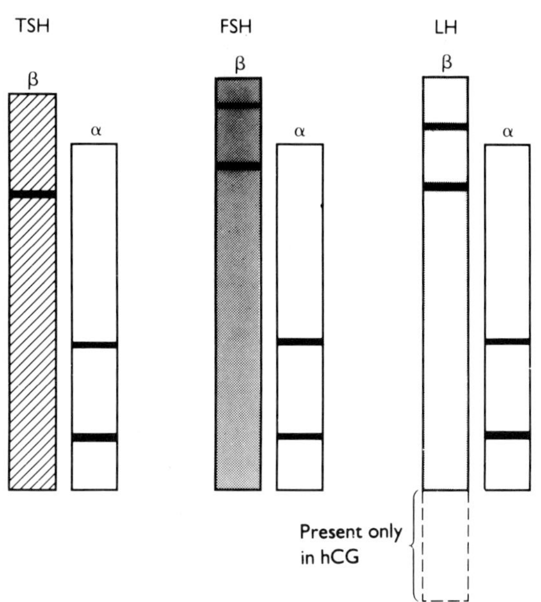

Fig. 19.7 Structures of TSH, FSH and LH. The β-subunits are unique to each hormone, and vary between 110 and 115 residues; they are non-covalently bound to a common α-subunit. Bars denote approximate attachment points of principal carbohydrate moieties.

lates both the synthesis and the release of serum TSH, which increases thyroidal iodine uptake, organification, synthesis and release of thyroxine (T_4). Feedback occurs principally via the binding of triiodothyronine (T_3) to pituitary nuclear receptors, although there may be indirect feedback by T_4 which is deiodinated to T_3 within the pituitary.

Neurotransmitter control of TRH and TSH release has been extensively studied in species other than humans, in which there appear to be excitatory α-adrenoreceptors and inhibitory dopaminergic pathways to TSH release. In humans the only generally agreed evidence is in favour of dopaminergic inhibition of serum TSH directly at the level of the thyrotroph.

There is a circadian rhythm of serum TSH concentration, with peak values being seen around 23.00 h; there is also a circadian rhythm in the dopaminergic control of TSH, this inhibitory tone being proportionally greater at high levels of TSH. Somatostatin also potently inhibits TSH under basal and stimulated conditions.

Following parturition there is a surge of TSH release in the neonate followed by a slower rise then fall in thyroid hormone; this may be a response to the fall in ambient temperature. Serum TSH returns to normal within 3–7 days, and thereafter principally reflects circulating thyroid hormone levels.

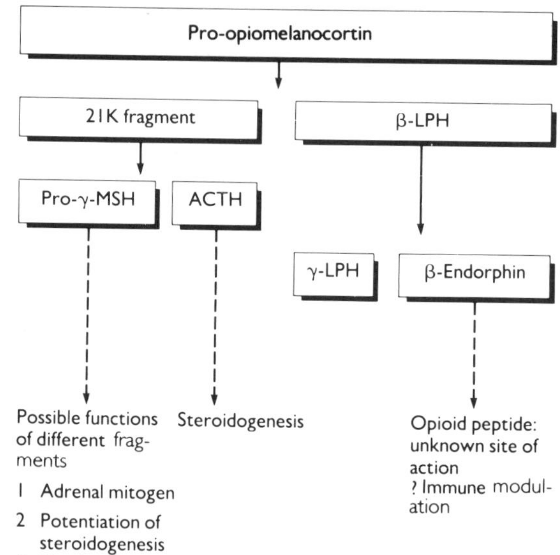

Fig. 19.8 The processing of the ACTH precursor, pro-opiomelanocortin, in the human pituitary, and possible functions of the peptide fragments produced.

Adrenocorticotrophin

ACTH is a 39-amino acid residue peptide secreted by the corticotrophs, which are usually basophilic using conventional staining. This staining was thought to be paradoxical, as ACTH contains no sugar moiety, until it was discovered that ACTH is cleaved from a large glycosylated precursor, pro-opiomelanocortin, of molecular weight 31 kD. This precursor is cleaved to a variety of peptides in addition to ACTH, including β-lipotrophin (β-LPH), β-endorphin and γ-melanocyte-stimulating hormone (γ-MSH) (Fig. 19.8). None of these ACTH-related peptides have been ascribed definitive functions. In species with a distinct pars intermedia, the processing of these peptides proceeds further, with the generation of α-MSH, corticotrophin-like intermediate peptide (CLIP), and greater amounts of β-endorphin. This does not occur in postfetal life in humans, but may well occur *in utero*.

ACTH stimulates adrenocortical activity, especially the synthesis and release of cortisol. It has been speculated that γ-MSH-related peptides may be involved in adrenal growth and/or mineralocorticoid steroidogenesis. A non-ACTH-related adrenal growth factor, gastric inhibitory polypeptide (GIP) has been implicated in rare cases of Cushing syndrome [17].

The principal ACTH-releasing peptide, corticotrophin-releasing hormone (CRH), was identified in 1981, and is a large peptide with strong cross-species structural homology. CRH stimulates ACTH release through an increase in intracellular cAMP levels. Vasopressin also stimulates ACTH release and potentiates the release of ACTH in response to CRH [18]. Current evidence strongly suggests that there is a macromolecular complex concerned with ACTH release, including CRH, vasopressin and possibly further factors. This is in turn modulated by central neurotransmitters. In humans these include an excitatory α-adrenoreceptor pathway, probably serotoninergic and histaminergic excitatory inputs, and an inhibitory GABA synapse. These modulate the release of ACTH in response to circadian rhythmicity (with peak levels at 07.00–08.00 h and a nadir at midnight–02.00 h) as well as stress. There are also data in favour of fast and slow cortisol feedback loops at hypothalamic and pituitary levels. Thus, the levels of ACTH and cortisol at any given time are the result of an interplay of many influences, which complicates the interpretation of single random levels.

POSTERIOR PITUITARY HORMONES

Vasopressin and oxytocin are small peptides consisting of nine amino acids, and differing from each other at two sites. They are synthesized and secreted from magnocellular neurons in the supraoptic and paraventricular nuclei, whence they are transported axonally along the supraoptic–hypophyseal tract to terminate beside capillaries in the posterior pituitary. Both are secreted together with much higher molecular weight peptides, neurophysins I and II, which have no known function.

Vasopressin is secreted in response to small changes in plasma osmolality, an osmolality change as little as 1% being associated with a change in circulating level. Vasopressin also responds to other stimuli, although with less sensitivity. In general terms, plasma vasopressin reflects plasma osmolality, and regulates osmolality to keep it in the range 275–290 mosmol/kg throughout life. It is a difficult hormone to measure, and in most centres information about its level is ascertained indirectly by measurement of plasma and urine osmolality, and calculation of free water clearance.

Oxytocin causes an increase in uterine contractility, and is responsible for the milk let-down reflex in response to suckling. The most interesting aspect of its control is that its release (in non-human species) is inhibited by endogenous opioids, which appear to be responsible for the spacing of births within a litter. Stress-induced inhibition of oxytocin release during suckling is also opioid-mediated. There are no known clinical syndromes associated with oxytocin excess or deficiency.

PEPTIDE HORMONE ASSAYS

Peptide hormones were originally measured by means of relatively sensitive but extremely tedious bioassays which relied on the biological characteristics of the hormone. Standards were derived from highly purified tissue extracts, a process still used for some peptide hormones. In the past decade, using peptide-sequencing techniques cDNA cloning and expression, synthetic peptide hormones have been prepared. These may then be used as standards for the more rigorous biochemical assay of these hormones.

The technique most commonly applied has been 'saturation analysis', in which the peptide to be assayed partitions itself between two phases. The two phases are then separated and the relative partitioning measured by means of a marker. The most popular use of this technique has been as radioimmunoassay (RIA), in which the peptide is partially bound to a specific antibody and exists, in part, as free peptide. The marker is a radioactive tracer attached to a known amount of peptide which will also bind to the antibody in a competitive manner. Thus, the higher the signal the lower the concentration of peptide present. An alternative method is the immunoradiometric assay (IRMA) where two antibodies (one radioactively labelled), raised to different epitopes on the hormone molecule, are used. This method, in which the signal increases with increasing amounts of peptide, is now in common use for many pituitary peptides.

The label may be a fluorescent dye (immunofluorescence and chemiluminescence assays) or an enzyme (ELISA). Separation of the two phases can be by centrifugation, magnetically, by solid-phase adherence or colorimetrically. However, there can be problems in the interpretation of results. The antibody may bind to an antigenic epitope which may not be biologically relevant. Fragments or variants of hormone of different or no biological activity, but which contain the epitope recognized by the detecting antibody, may give spuriously elevated results. Conversely, the presence of binding proteins in the serum of the patient may mask the relevant epitope from the detecting antibodies. Chromatographic separation of molecular moieties, particularly high-performance liquid chromotography (HPLC), can be useful, but are too time-consuming and expensive for routine use.

In interpreting the results of different assays it is important to understand the errors to which assays are prone. RIAs are usually very precise, as assessed by the coefficient of variation, which is a measure of the degree of variability expected if the same sample is assayed several times. For most RIAs, coefficients of variation of 5–10% are to be expected, which implies that reported small changes in hormone levels may be statistical artefacts and of no biological significance. The lowest level of detection of an assay is not zero, and the precision of the assay decreases as the limit of detection is approached. In addition, assays which require an extraction step, that is, those in which the hormone is removed from the plasma and then redissolved (usually necessary to concentrate the hormone and/or remove interfering substances), have a further source of error added. However, in clinical practice all that is often required is to know whether the peptide is undetectable, within the normal range or grossly elevated, and good precision, whilst desirable, may not be essential.

It should be emphasized that RIAs, and other chemical assays, detect physicochemical rather than biological properties, and the two do not always correlate closely. Differences between immunological and biological activities may also vary according to the antibody or binding protein used in the assay system. Many routine laboratories now have access to commercial solid-phase assays, often using enzyme-linked chemical detection methods. Although rapid and generally reliable, they are expensive. Some of this expense can be offset by automation, but it remains important that the clinician understands the usefulness and limitations of any hormone estimation he or she may wish to order.

MOLECULAR PHYSIOLOGY OF THE HYPOTHALAMOPITUITARY AXIS

Although every cell has the full complement of genes, the type and quantity of genes transcribed are limited. The transcription products dictate the specificity and function of cells. The past decade has seen an exponential growth in our understanding of the molecular controls of the hypothalamopituitary axis. Three broad areas have been explored: the regulation of transcription of hormone genes, the detection of mRNA for various hormones in the hypothalamus and pituitary and mechanisms of hormone–receptor action.

Growth of lactotrophs, somatotrophs and thyrotrophs is dependent on a pituitary-specific transcription factor, Pit-1 [19]. Pit-1 appears to be stimulated by activation of the GHRH receptor. GHRH causes a rise in intracellular cAMP levels through $G_s\alpha$ subunit activity of the GHRH receptor; cAMP in turn activates protein kinase A, which then phosphorylates a protein (cAMP response element-binding protein, CREBP) capable of binding DNA. The region of DNA bound by CREBP is known as the cAMP response element (CRE), and is found close to the promotor region of the Pit-1 gene. Transcription of the Pit-1 gene occurs after CREBP binds to this promotor region.

CREs, as well as binding sites for the c-fos/c-jun (AP-1) transcription factor and the glucocorticoid receptor (GRE), have been found close to the promoter regions of the CRH and TRH genes. Elements responsive to steroid receptors are found in the human GnRH gene promoter region. An upstream CRE appears to be critical for somatostatin (and probably GHRH) gene transcription.

In situ hybridization techniques have localized mRNA for many hormones and their receptors (for example GHRH in the cells of the arcuate nucleus, CRH in the paraventricular nucleus). In addition, a number of other mRNAs have been found (such as vasoactive intestinal polypeptide (VIP)) in the hypothalamus and pituitary, and the levels can vary depending on physiological conditions. These findings suggest that numerous factors and hormones interact, probably in a paracrine fashion, to regulate pituitary function. *In situ* hybridization has shown that cells may have high levels of hormone mRNA even when little or no hormone itself is detectable by immunocytochemistry. This may occur under certain conditions when rapid release of the hormone depletes the cellular peptide pool.

The cloning of the complementary (c)DNA for many of the hypothalamopituitary hormone receptors has revealed that the receptors are usually members of a superfamily of G protein-coupled membrane-bound peptides. The prototype for this receptor is the β-adrenoceptor, which is a single chain that crosses the cell membrane seven times (hence often referred to as a seven-transmembrane domain receptor). The intracellular signalling pathway involves G proteins and often adenylate cyclase. The hypothalamic hormone receptors (TRH, dopamine, GnRH) and vasopressin tend to have smaller extracellular domains, while the glycoprotein hormone receptors (FSH, LH/chorionic gonadotrophin and TSH) have large N-terminal extracellular domains. Prolactin and GH receptors are single transmembrane domain peptides which interact with intracellular protein kinases.

The interaction between hormone and receptor may be influenced by binding proteins. The best example of this is the role of IGF-binding proteins in regulating the access of free IGF to its receptor. Although pituitary and hypothalamic hormones are associated with binding proteins (CRH with CRH-binding protein; GH with circulating fragments of the extracellular domain of the GH receptor), the physiology of these binding proteins is currently not well understood.

INTERACTIONS BETWEEN THE HYPOTHALAMOPITUITARY AXIS AND IMMUNE SYSTEMS

The identification and synthesis of cytokines as mediators of inflammation has led to extensive studies on the influence of cytokines on hypothalamopituitary function. Interleukin-1 (notably the β form, IL-1β) releases CRH, and the administration of endotoxin results in expression of IL-1β mRNA in the rat hypothalamus. IL-2, IL-6 and tumour necrosis factor (TNF) also activate the hypothalamopituitary–adrenal axis, while IL-1 and TNF inhibit the thyroid and gonadal axes [20]. These results demonstrate the close interplay between the immune system and the neuroendocrine axis, and further emphasize the sensitivity of the hypothalamopituitary unit to circulating influences.

REFERENCES

1 Harris GW. Neural control of the pituitary gland. *Physiol Rev* 1948;28:139.

2 Wade N. A race spurred by rivalry. *New Sci* 1978:358–60.

3 Forsling M, Grossman A. *Neuroendocrinology: a Clinical Text*. London: Croom Helm, 1986:1–206.

4 Stanhope R, Preece MA, Brook CGD. Hypoplastic optic nerves and pituitary dysfunction. *Arch Dis Child* 1984;59:111–14.

5 Lam KSL, Wang C, Ma JTC, Leung SP, Yeung RTT. Hypothalamic defects in two adult patients with septo-optic dysplasia. *Acta Endocrinol* 1986;112:305–9.

6 Schwanzel-Fukuda M, Pfaff DW. Origin of luteinizing hormone-releasing hormone neurons. *Nature* 1989;338:161–4.

7 Crowley WF Jr, Jameson JL. Clinical counterpoint: gonadotrophin-releasing hormone deficiency: perspectives from clinical investigation. *Endocr Rev* 1992;13:635–40.

7a Wislocki GB, King LS. Permeability of the hypophysis and hypothalamus to vital dyes, with study of the hypophyseal blood supply. *Am J Anat* 1936;58:421–72.

8 Daniel PM, Prichard MML. Studies of the hypothalamus and the pituitary gland. *Acta Endocrinol* (Suppl.) 1975;201:1–63.

9 Franks S, Jacobs HS. Hyperprolactinaemia. *Clin Endocrinol Metab* 1983;12:641–68.

10 Holly JMP, Wass JAH. Insulin-like growth factors; autocrine, paracrine or endocrine? New perspectives of the somatomedin hypothesis in the light of recent developments. *J Endocrinol* 1989;122:611–18.

11 Ross RJM, Grossman A, Davies PSW, Savage MO, Besser GM. Stilboestrol pre-treatment of children with short stature does not affect the GH response to growth-hormone releasing hormone. *Clin Endocrinol* 1987;27:155–61.

12 Grossman A, Savage MO, Besser GM. Growth hormone releasing hormone. *Clin Endocrinol Metab* 1986;15:607–28.

13 Thorner MO, Cronin MJ. Growth-hormone-releasing factor: clinical and basic studies. *Neuroendocr Perspect* 1985;4:95–144.

14 Spada A, Arosio M, Bochicchio D *et al.* Clinical, biochemical, and morphological correlates in patients bearing growth hormone-secreting pituitary tumors with or without constitutively active adenylyl cyclase. *J Clin Endocrinol Metab* 1990;71:1421–6.

15 Marshall JC, Kelch RP. Gonadotropin-releasing hormone: role of pulsatile secretion in the regulation of reproduction. *N Engl J Med* 1986;315:1459–67.

16 Robertson DM, Risbridger GP, de Kretser DM. The physiology of testicular inhibin and related proteins. *Clin Endocrinol Metab* 1992;6:355–72.

16a Belchetz PE, Plant TM, Nakai Y *et al.* Hypophyseal responses to continuous and intermittent delivery of hypothalamic gonadotrophin-releasing hormone. *Science* 1978;202:631–3.

17 Bertagna X. New causes of Cushing's syndrome. *N Engl J Med* 1992;327:1024–5.

18 Al-Damluji S, Thomas R, White A, Besser GM. Vasopressin mediates alpha-1 adrenergic stimulation of ACTH secretion. *Endocrinology* 1990;126:1989–95.

19 Ruvkun G. A molecular growth industry. *Nature* 1992;360: 711–12.

20 Imura H, Fukata J, Mori T. Cytokines and endocrine function: an interaction between the immune and neuroendocrine systems. *Clin Endocrinol* 1991;35:107–15.

20: Neuroradiology

B.E. KENDALL

INTRODUCTION

Neuroradiological studies may be useful in the elucidation of paediatric endocrine disturbances which could be related to congenital abnormalities or lesions affecting directly or indirectly the hypothalamopituitary region or, less commonly, the pineal gland.

THE PITUITARY AND HYPOTHALAMIC REGIONS

Development and structure

The pituitary gland consists of two lobes formed by the juxtaposition of tissues of different origins, the anterior part from the stomodaeum and the posterior part from the diencephalon.

The anterior pituitary commences development in the third week of intrauterine life from an ectodermal placode at least partly of neural crest origin in the roof of the stomodaeum as a diverticulum, Rathke's pouch, lying just proximal to the foregut, rostral to the notochord and below the forebrain. The pouch becomes surrounded by mesoderm, forming the craniopharyngeal canal. The pharyngeal connection is occluded during normal intrauterine development, although it may occasionally persist *in toto* or, more commonly, as vestiges in the body of the sphenoid. The proximal end of the craniopharygeal canal constitutes the pituitary fossa. Rathke's pouch is lined by cuboidal mucus-secreting epithelium; the lumen persists as an ill-defined cleft in the newborn but it is soon largely obliterated, leaving behind tiny scattered cavities, a few millimetres in diameter, which are the basis of colloid or pars intermedia cysts commonly demonstrated in the posterior part of the adenohypophysis.

The ectodermal cells of the cleft mostly develop into the glandular epithelium of the adenohypophysis, but they also form nests of squamous cells which may be found in both the pars distalis and the pars tuberalis of the adenohypophysis, extending along the pituitary stalk even as far as the hypothalamus. A few adenohypophyseal cells persist in the roof of the nasal cavity. These usually remain non-functional, but they may hypertrophy to form a 'pharyngeal pituitary', and may secrete if the pituitary is totally ablated and the level of trophic hormones is particularly high. The cells of the adenohypophysis are arranged in irregular cords surrounded by a highly vascular network of sinusoids, which is particularly well developed as the so-called capillary tuft in the superior part of the anterior lobe.

The neurohypophysis is formed from a diverticulum which extends ventrally from the diencephalon, just posterior to the optic commissure, before the 35th day of gestation. This site becomes the tuber cinereum, a low elevation on the floor of the third ventricle, between the optic chiasm and mamillary bodies and the infundibulum, continuing inferiorly into the pituitary stalk, which descends from its central part. The neurohypophysis forms about 25% by volume of the whole pituitary gland. It becomes enveloped on its anterior and lateral aspects by Rathke's pouch and, hence, by the pars tuberalis and distalis of the adenohypophysis. The pituitary gland is fully formed by the 14th week of gestation [1]. The neurohypophysis contains non-myelinated axons extending from the hypothalamus. These are supported in specialized glia-containing pituicytes within a rich network of sinusoids continuous with those in the pituitary stalk.

There are two major pathways between the hypothalamus and pituitary.

1 The hypothalamic–hypophyseal tract of unmyelinated nerve fibres carrying oxytocin and antidiuretic hormone from the large cells of the supraoptic and paraventricular nuclei into the sinusoidal bed of the posterior pituitary.

2 The tuberoinfundibular pathway, mediating the release of anterior pituitary hormones. This is controlled by parvicellular nuclei lying in the ventromedial regions of the hypothalamus and infundibulum. These manufacture releasing and inhibiting hormones which are transferred through myelinated nerve fibres into the capillary bed of the median eminence of the tuber cinereum. This capillary bed, together with the hypothalamus, is supplied directly from the superior hypophyseal arterial branches of the circle of Willis, and the rich capillary network extends down the pituitary stalk and continues into the capillary bed of the neurohypophysis. The anterior lobe of the pituitary gland receives most of its blood from long and short portal veins draining from the capillary bed of the median eminence and pituitary stalk. These veins open into the sinusoids of the adenohypophysis: they transport the neurotransmitter hormones released into the capillaries of the tuber cinereum to their site of action on the appropriate cells of the anterior pituitary.

The venous drainage of each lobe of the pituitary gland is to the ipsilateral cavernous sinus and to the interconnecting veins and, hence, predominantly towards the ipsilateral inferior petrosal sinus.

THE SELLA TURCICA

The pituitary fossa or sella turcica is a depression in the body of the sphenoid bone containing the pituitary gland. The sella is lined by a thin shell of cortical bone called the lamina dura. The superior margin of the anterior wall projects above the superior margin of the gland to form the tuberculum sellae. There are two major ossification centres for the body of sphenoid, and the synchondrosis between these in the floor of the sella may be visible well after birth. The craniopharyngeal canal or remnants of it may also be visible as a corticated tubular band behind the plane of the synchondrosis. The pneumatized sphenoid sinus relates to the anterior wall of the sella and extends a variable distance beneath the floor, and even into the plate of bone forming the posterior wall or dorsum sellae.

The lateral walls of the sella are lined by the dura constituting the medial walls of the cavernous sinuses and the roof by the dura of the diaphagma sellae, which is supported by the tuberculum, dorsum sellae and clinoid processes. The diaphragma is penetrated by the pituitary stalk, which traverses a hole of variable size. When the hole is large, it is common for the chiasmatic cistern to extend into and occupy a variable proportion of the sella, which is correspondingly increased in volume to accommodate the cerebrospinal fluid (CSF). The pituitary gland is then confined towards the lower part of the sella and sometimes forms a thin rim along the floor and posterior wall; this constitutes a physiological variety of empty sella.

Differences between individuals in the volume of intrasellar CSF constitute the main factor responsible for the large normal variation in sellar size and configuration. Intrasellar extension of the chiasmatic cistern has been shown to be present in 54% of individuals in an autopsy series [2], and correlation has been made between sellar shape and depth. Central concavity of the sellar floor can reach up to 6 mm in normal cases, and sloping of more than 2 mm to either side is not infrequent. Focal depression of the floor of the sella is also a normal variant, being particularly frequent opposite the site of the intersphenoid septum; it may be associated with slight thinning of the lamina dura. Although, in another series [3], erosion of the sellar floor was related to adjacent microadenomas, it is evident that factors other than the volume of the pituitary influence the size and shape of the fossa and measurements are not generally useful in the assessment of equivocal appearances.

Radiographs usually reveal sellar expansion and erosion with macroadenomas, local erosion with large supra- and parasellar tumours, sclerosis with meningioma arising from bone and calcification in the majority of craniopharyngiomas. The anatomy of the paranasal sinuses necessary for surgical planning is also shown. However, conventional radiographs of the sella are of no value in excluding small intrasellar lesions, and can give a misleading impression of the presence of a small mass. Conventional tomography is obsolete, and any clinical or radiological suspicion of pituitary disease, even if the latter is based on incidental discovery of a large sella, is best elucidated by magnetic resonance imaging (MRI) supplemented by, or replaced by, computerized tomography (CT) if the former is not easily available.

In front of the tuberculum sellae there is a flat or slightly concave surface of sphenoid bone of variable length, the sulcus chiasmaticus, limited anteriorly by the posterior margin or limbus of the planum sphenoidale. This region is incompletely ossified in early childhood and the sulcus chiasmaticus appears long and deep, contributing to an appearance sometimes termed an omega sella. The lateral margins of the sulcus are bounded by the optic canals, which are enclosed by the body of the sphenoid and the roots of its lesser wings. The junction of the intracanalicular and intracranial segments of the optic nerves are thus closely related to the sella, but the intracranial segments of the optic nerves and the sagittal diameter of the optic chiasm vary considerably in length between individuals. A chiasm lying above and posterior to the plane of the dorsum sellae is termed postfixed. Variations in anatomy are reflected in the differing degrees of vulnerability of the chiasm to compression by suprasellar extensions of pituitary tumours.

The cavernous segments of the internal carotid arteries run close to the lateral margins of the sella and the pituitary gland. They may occasionally approximate so closely to the midline, towards the anterior aspect of the sella, that they cause a significant hazard during transsphenoidal hypophysectomy. The carotid arteries produce a groove of varying prominence, the carotid sulcus, along the lateral border of the sphenoid bone, adjacent to the floor of the sella.

THE CHIASMATIC CISTERN

The subarachnoid space above the sella turcica is the chiasmatic cistern. It continues anterosuperiorly into the cistern of the lamina terminalis, anterolaterally into the Sylvian fissures, and posteriorly into the interpeduncular and ambient cisterns. The cistern and related structures are well shown on T_1-weighted MRI*. They are usually seen satisfactorily in the axial and coronal planes on CT. The anterior margins of the cistern are demarcated by the posterior borders of the gyri recti and the lateral boundaries by the medially convex borders of the temporal lobes. The shape of the posterior boundary on axial images varies with the angle of section; if the section passes through the basis pedunculi and interpeduncular cistern the suprasellar subarachnoid space is shown as a hexagon, but if it passes more obliquely, so as to section the anterior surface of the upper pons, it appears pentagonal. The vessels of the circle of Willis are shown with variable clarity around the margins of the cistern, particularly after intravenous contrast enhancement.

The optic nerves and chiasm are visible ascending obliquely from the optic canals to the chiasmatic recess of the third ventricle. The long axis of the chiasm is transverse, continuing posteriorly into the optic tracts which are, in most normal cases, only recognizable as such as far as the point where they cross the cerebral peduncle. Optic nerve gliomas often grow along and maintain the characteristic cruciate form of the optic apparatus: tumours may differ in signal and/or density from normal brain substance sufficiently to demarcate the tracts as far as the geniculate bodies. The pituitary stalk descends as a tubular structure from the infundibular recess, through the central part of the cistern, to enter the pituitary fossa posterior to the midpoint of the roof of the sella.

* The strength of a magnetic resonance signal and of the images produced from it depend on the density of hydrogen nuclei and on two exponential magnetic relaxation times. Relaxation in this context refers to the time taken for individual tissues in the strong magnetic field to lose energy that has been added by radiofrequency stimulation delivered at the natural resonant frequency of the system. These times for each individual tissue depend on its physical state, which in turn is determined by the pre-existing fields within it. The energy is lost in two ways.

1 By thermal interactions or molecular collisions. The time taken by tissue to magnetize in the strong magnetic field, or to remagnetize following radiofrequency stimulation, is a measure of this function and is referred to as T_1 relaxation time.

2 Interactions with other protons. Following appropriate radiofrequency stimulation, the protons resonate in phase, producing a measurable signal. This signal reduces in magnitude, due to exchange of energy between the protons causing dephasing, in an exponential manner at a rate referred to as the T_2 relaxation time.

THE NORMAL PITUITARY GLAND, STALK AND SURROUNDING STRUCTURES

These are best imaged by MRI, but are also shown by high-resolution CT [4]. The precise technique to be adopted depends upon the clinical features to be elucidated. If these indicate a large mass, thicker sections may be appropriate, whereas a small lesion demands a slice thickness of 1.5–2.0 mm and a pixel size in the region of 0.6 mm. MRI is also generally superior to CT for imaging of the sellar and perisellar structures.

Using CT, normal cases are best elucidated by direct coronal imaging of the sellar region, performed with the neck extended using a scanning plane which avoids any artefact producing dental amalgam as determined from the scout view image. If an appropriate position cannot be achieved, 1.5 mm thick axial slices are obtained at 1.0 mm intervals with the head extended about 10° so as to place the petrous bones, and the low-density artefacts generated from them, below the plane of the sella. The images produced are reformatted in multiple planes for elucidation of supra- and parasellar extension of masses when indicated. These thin-section images are made after bolus injection of intravenous contrast medium. However, it is good policy to obtain a plain CT through the pituitary and suprasellar region using thicker sections (5 mm) as a preliminary measure. This will elucidate any unexpectedly large masses and also show any abnormal precontrast density.

The pituitary is surrounded by bone and the beam-attenuating effects of the surrounding bony structures may cause linear low-density artefacts. Their nature is evident on the original sections, but when reproduced on reformatted images they form rounded low densities which may simulate small tumours (Fig. 20.1). Even with modern CT machines producing good-quality images using relatively high radiation doses, a noise range of approximately 4–10 Hounsfield units is to be expected in the region of the pituitary gland [5]. This statistical electronic noise will produce regions of high and low density which may simulate small tumours. Unless corroborative evidence is present, the constancy of such appearances can be confirmed only by repeating the study in an additional plane: in the same plane it can be overcome by routine use of dynamic scanning.

Pituitary tissue has a density similar to that of normal brain; it lacks a blood–brain barrier and enhances to reach a density similar to that of the adjacent blood vessels after a bolus of intravenous contrast medium. Using dynamic CT the posterior pituitary and the stalk enhance rapidly because of their direct arterial blood supply; the anterior pituitary, which is supplied by the portal venous system, enhances more slowly and is of lower density on early sections [6]. Over the subsequent minute the intensity of

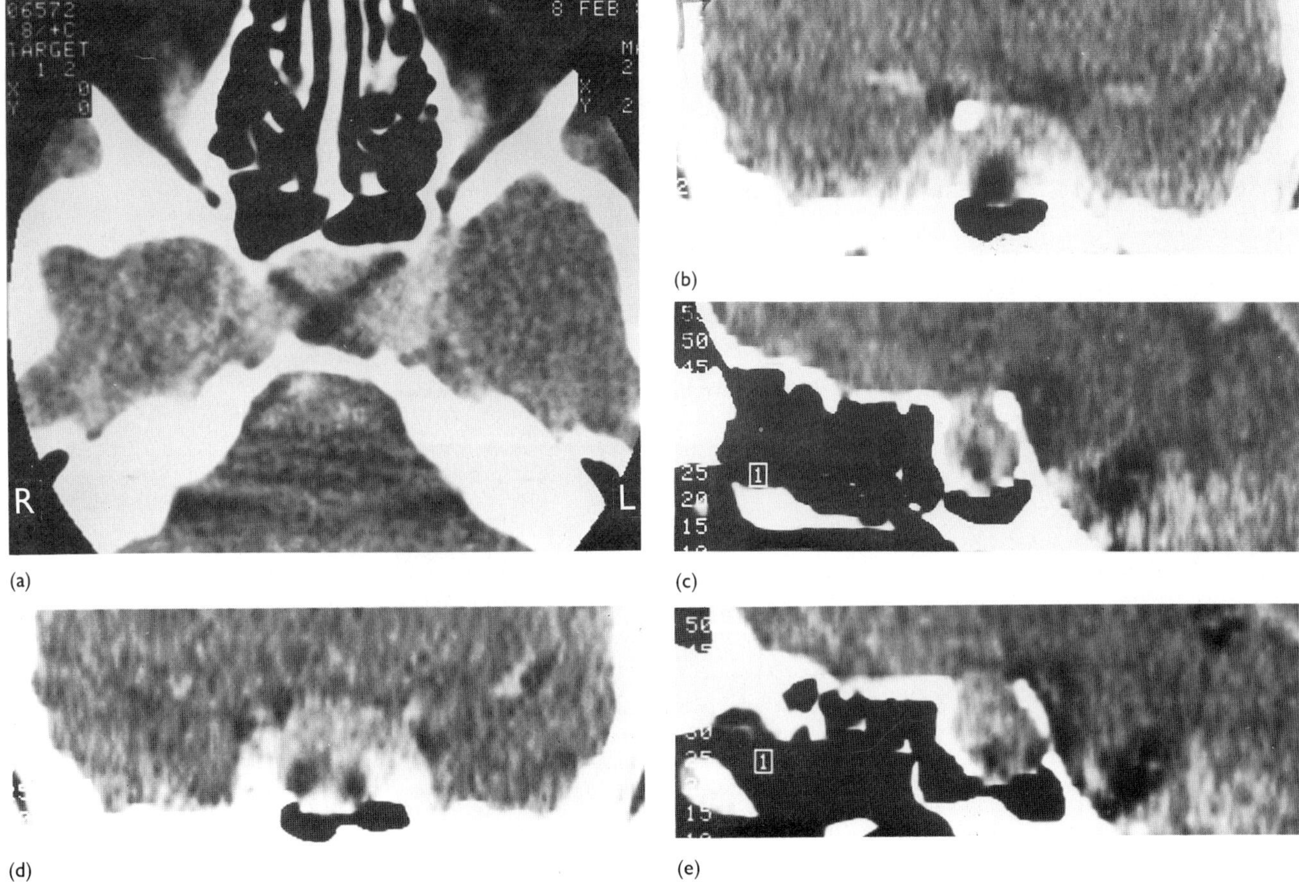

Fig. 20.1 Pituitary tumour with superimposed bone-induced artefacts. CT scan: (a) axial section through enlarged pituitary fossa. Note cruciate low-density artefacts caused by attenuation of the X-ray beam traversing the long axes of the petrous bones and lateral walls of the orbits; (b, c) coronal and sagittal reformatted images at the centre of the cross, showing a single low-density artefact which could be mistaken for a pituitary adenoma in the enlarged gland; (d, e) further reformants through the separated limbs of the cruciate artefact, which are shown as two regions of low density.

the anterior pituitary increases as the portal blood supply opacifies, and eventually it becomes considerably denser than the posterior pituitary due to extravasation through the absent blood–brain barrier. The convex anterior border of the less dense posterior pituitary is shown at this stage impressing the posterior margin of the densely enhancing anterior part. Colloid cysts remain unopacified and less dense than the normal tissue.

Since MRI does not require ionizing radiation it is particularly desirable when imaging children, or when repeated studies are likely to be indicated. MRI has two other major advantages.

1 The capacity, with no patient discomfort, to make thin-section, high-resolution images in any plane, three-dimensional data sets which can be used to produce sectional images in multiple planes and for volume measurements. The planes selected for imaging can be conventional or specifically oriented to a particular therapeutic approach.

2 The type of contrast discrimination within MRI images can vary with the mode of acquisition, so that the method is capable of giving more basic information than CT, which relies entirely on attenuation of the X-ray beam in the tissues traversed.

There are, however, some disadvantages of MRI.

1 It cannot be used in the presence of cardiac pacemakers or ferromagnetic implanted materials, including aneurysm clips, stapes prostheses and orbital metallic foreign bodies.

2 Calcification, which may be significant in the diagnosis of certain conditions, particularly craniopharyngioma, gives a relatively non-specific signal.

On MRI the anterior pituitary gland gives a homogeneous signal generally similar to that from white matter.

Neurosecretory granules, normally present in the cells of the posterior pituitary gland, give rise to a bright T_1 signal associated with a very short T_1 relaxation time (Fig. 20.2). Physiological variation in the bright signal

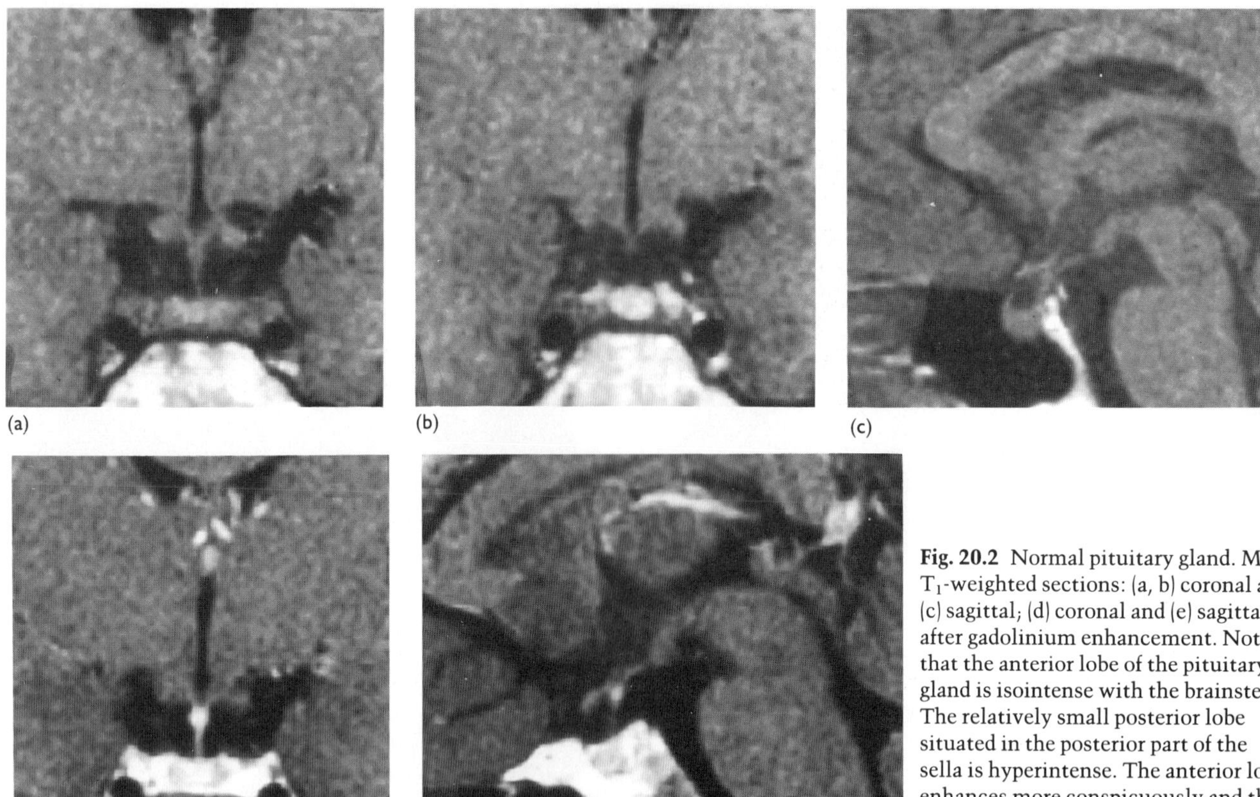

Fig. 20.2 Normal pituitary gland. MRI T_1-weighted sections: (a, b) coronal and (c) sagittal; (d) coronal and (e) sagittal after gadolinium enhancement. Note that the anterior lobe of the pituitary gland is isointense with the brainstem. The relatively small posterior lobe situated in the posterior part of the sella is hyperintense. The anterior lobe enhances more conspicuously and the differential intensity is less marked.

reflects the response of the hypothalamohypophyseal axis to the level of hydration. Bright signal is absent in central diabetes insipidus and occasionally in nephrogenic diabetis insipidus, but not in primary polydipsia.

Occasionally a little fat is visible anterior to the pituitary gland [7]. The carotid arteries and cavernous sinuses are outlined by flow effects in the parapituitary regions and the intracavernous veins are also usually visible. Seconds after gadolinium injection, the infundibulum and posterior pituitary enhance. This is followed by centrifugal enhancement of the anterior pituitary from the infundibular attachment. The pituitary usually becomes brightly and homogeneously enhanced after about 90 s. However, in about 20% of patients, varying compactness of the tissue, small cysts and sometimes gliotic changes may cause signal irregularity. This is followed by washout of contrast medium, which is slightly quicker from the posterior than the anterior pituitary lobes. The cavernous sinuses enhance early and the non-enhancing cranial nerves within them are frequently outlined, particularly in the coronal plane.

Various measurements have been stated for the size of the normal pituitary gland on CT and MRI. The most useful of these concern the height of the gland, which may be taken as lying between 2.5 and 9.0 mm on CT, being larger in females (mean 6.2 mm) than in males (mean 5.1 mm) [8]; the range of these measurements is a little larger than those produced by Syvertsen *et al.* [9] and by Mark *et al.* [7] for MRI, where the height of the gland varied between 4.0 and 8.0 mm, with a mean of 5.7 mm. In preadolescent children the height of the gland increases slightly in a linear fashion from birth, but remains less than the height of the adult gland, not exceeding 6 mm until adolescence, when the mean increases. Elster *et al.* [10] recorded maximum heights of 10 mm in teenage girls and 7 mm in teenage boys. The gland height then decreases by about 20 years to adult levels, then slowly decreases in size over the subsequent decades.

The upper surface of the gland may be concave (43%) or flat (5%) [11] or convex superiorly, particularly during puberty and in young women [5] in whom the gland may become rounded.

In the neonate the signal from the pituitary gland on T_1-weighted images is relatively bright, being higher than that returned from the brainstem. In two-thirds of neonates the upper border of the gland is convex. After about 2 months the T_1 signal becomes isointense with that of the brainstem, and the upper border of the gland tends to become flat. In the first year of life bright signal from the posterior pituitary is visible in only about two-thirds of children [12].

The pituitary stalk, consistently shown extending through the central part of the chasmatic cistern on axial sections on CT; this was shown on about 70% of MRI

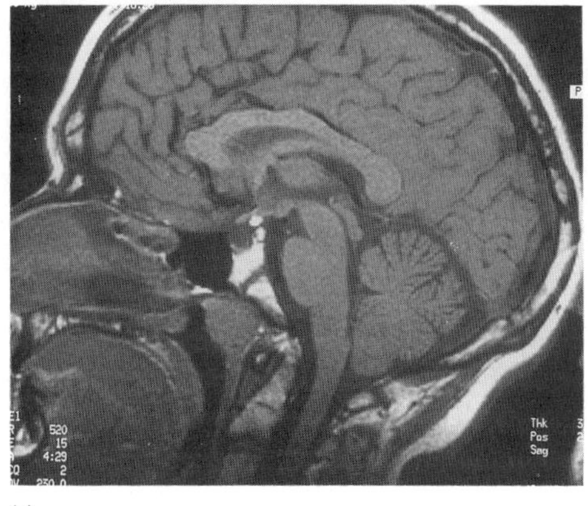

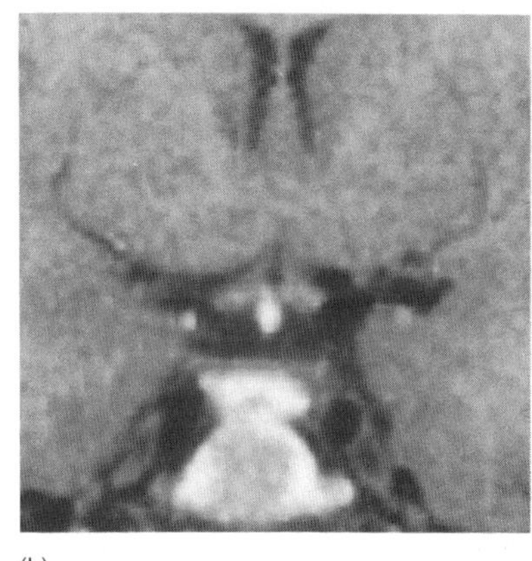

(a) (b)

Fig. 20.3 Child with growth hormone deficiency and a history of breech delivery. MRI: (a) T_1-weighted midsagittal section; (b) T_1-weighted coronal section. The pituitary fossa is small and no anterior pituitary substance is visible. There is a high-intensity nodule just below the tuber cinereum due to the presence of posterior pituitary substance.

scans in one early series [13], but is almost always visible on high-resolution studies. In about 50% of cases the stalk is slightly asymmetrically attached to the gland [11]. Its lower two-thirds has no blood–brain barrier and normally enhances densely, to a similar extent as the adjacent arteries, and it varies in size from very small up to slightly over 2 mm diameter. In young children it becomes more prominent with age and is larger in girls than in boys [14].

THE ABNORMAL PITUITARY GLAND

Congenital abnormalities

The pituitary gland may be aplastic [15], hypoplastic [16] or ectopic.

Disruption of the infundibulum, possibly due to trauma or ischaemia, most likely to occur in the perinatal period, may interrupt the hypophyseal portal system, which impairs anterior pituitary growth and function with severe growth hormone (GH) deficiency and variable degrees of other anterior pituitary hormone deficits due to lack of the hypothalamic releasing factors [16]. The anterior pituitary gland and the pituitary fossa are small and the bright T_1 signal of the neurohypophysis is absent from its usual site [14,17–20]. Axonal transmission of posterior pituitary hormone continues, and stimulates development of the pituicytes at the base of the infundibulum. It may be evident as a small enhancing nodule of T_1 high signal on MRI and brain density on CT (Fig. 20.3).

Hypoplasia of the pituitary [21] is also associated with a small fossa, though the converse does not apply [4]; the infundibulum and pituitary stalk are normal. The chiasmatic cistern often extends into the small sella, which may appear empty, with the stalk outlined by CSF (Fig. 20.3). The patients have isolated and less severe GH deficiency.

The term 'empty sella' is inaccurate, since there is usually a small amount of pituitary substance adjacent to the floor of the fossa: a more correct description is intrasellar arachnoid herniation. This may develop as a secondary effect of congenital underdevelopment of the diaphragma sellae, leaving a wide communication between the chiasmatic cistern and the intrasellar cistern.

The developmental type of empty sella is usually an insignificant anatomical variant. However, it may be associated with CSF rhinorrhoea, particularly in the presence of benign intracranial hypertension. The presence of CSF within the sella, outlining the pituitary stalk and the relationships of the structures within the chiasmatic cistern to the arachnoid herniation, are best elucidated by MRI.

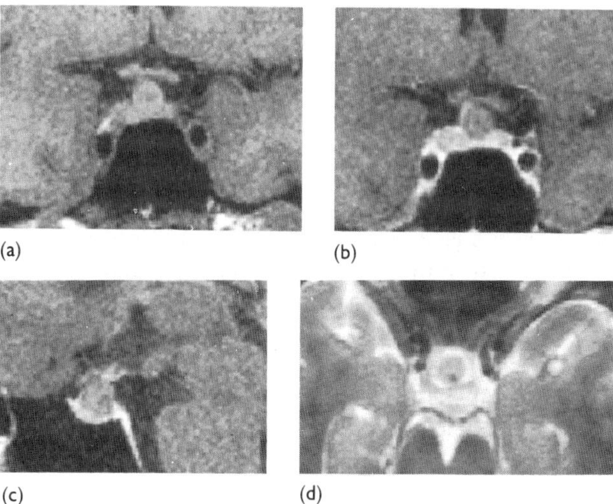

Fig. 20.4 Rathke cyst. MRI: (a, b) coronal T_1-weighted section before (a) and after (b) gadolinium; (c) sagittal T_1-weighted section after gadolinium; (d) axial T_2-weighted section. This cyst is similar in intensity to white matter on T_1- and T_2-weighted sequences and does not enhance. On enhanced images it is a well-demarcated mass distinct from pituitary tissue lying partly within the upper part of the sella, but mainly suprasellar to the left of the pituitary stalk, which is displaced to the right, and reaching up to, but not displacing, the optic chiasm. At surgery the cyst contained clear fluid, and tissue from the wall revealed typical cuboidal epithelium.

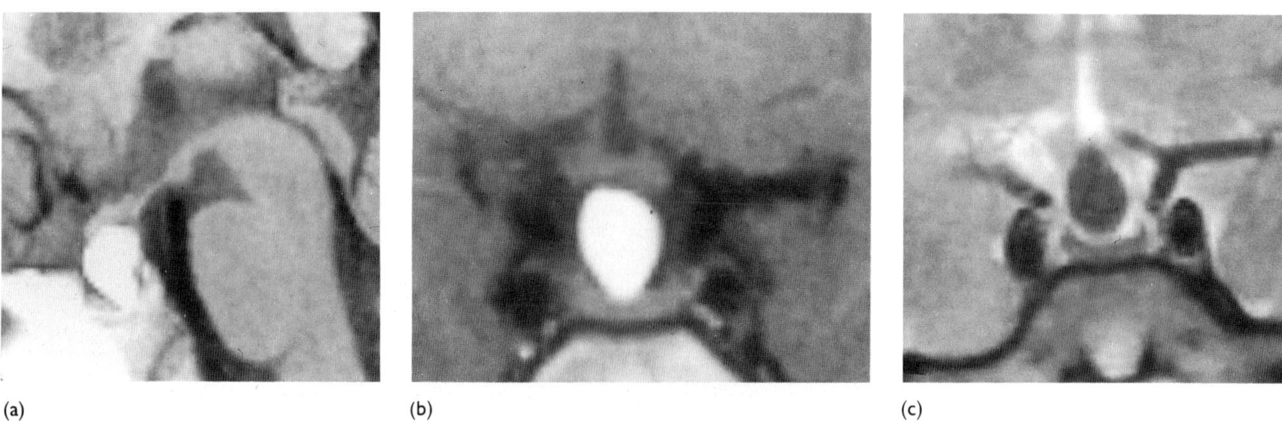

(a) (b) (c)

Fig. 20.5 Rathke's pouch cyst. MRI: (a) midsagittal; (b) coronal T_1-weighted sections; (c) coronal T_2-weighted section. The cyst is partly intra- and partly suprasellar, extending through the chiasmatic cistern to slightly elevate the optic chiasm. It contains fluid returning high signal on the T_1-weighted sequences, presumed to be due to the presence of methaemoglobin, and markedly low signal on the T_2 sequence, presumed to be due to the haemosiderin. The cyst contained altered blood.

Empty sella may also be acquired following pituitary surgery or regression of a tumour as the result of radiation therapy, hormone suppression or spontaneous infarction of tumour or of normal gland.

Hyperplasia of the pituitary gland occurs during puberty, including precocious puberty, and pregnancy. In the first 6 months the gland enlarges to a height of 10 mm and over the last 3 months and first postpartum week reaches 12 mm before returning to normal size. Hyperplasia also occurs in response to thyroid failure: the enlarged gland responds to thyroid replacement therapy.

Ectopic pituitary tissue may develop anywhere along the route of the craniopharyngeal canal: it is usually accessory but rarely constitutes the majority of the anterior hypophyseal cells in association with a hypoplastic, normally placed gland [22].

Rathke's cleft cysts may form from remnants of the pharyngeal pouch. They are usually small and asymptomatic, but they may be over 2 cm in diameter and cause compression of the hypothalamus, infundibulum or pituitary gland, producing hypopituitarism or diabetes insipidus, and/or compress the optic chiasm with visual symptoms. Rarely the contents may leak into the subarachnoid space, causing a septic meningitis or hypocephalus. The majority are intrasellar, though there may be a suprasellar component (Fig. 20.4), and some are entirely suprasellar.

The cyst wall is composed of a single layer of epithelium and the contained fluid varies in composition. It may be serous with signal characteristics similar to CSF, or it may be mucoid, producing a hyperintense signal on T_1-weighted sections and iso- or hyperintense on T_2-weighted sections. The cyst may also contain desquamated debris and give a heterogeneous signal, which may lead to confusion with craniopharyngioma, though enhancement does not occur. Finally, haemorrhage may occur into the cyst, producing methaemoglobin giving hyperintensity on both T_1- and T_2-weighted images and eventually susceptibility effects as haemosiderin is formed (Fig. 20.5). Rathke cleft cysts may be associated with persistence of the craniopharyngeal canal, and rarely they may form a small mass within the nasopharynx [23–26].

Tumours

Tumours of the pituitary and suprasellar region constitute 15–20% of intracranial tumours of childhood and over 30% of supratentorial masses. Prognosis of these neoplasms is related to early diagnosis, which is facilitated by the high sensitivity and multiplanar capability of MRI, supplemented if necessary by CT to show calcification and bone changes, and considered in the clinical context. Overlap of radiological features requires histology to be used for confirmation of differential diagnosis in most cases.

The relative incidence of the mass lesions differs considerably from that found in the adult population, the latter being approached after puberty. Overall, gliomas constitute over 50% (average age 6–7 years), craniopharyngiomas over 20% (average age 9–10 years), pituitary adenomas and germ-cell tumours (average age 15 years) each account for about 5%, and other developmental masses combined for a similar number, the rest being of inflammatory or uncertain aetiology.

Pituitary adenomas

An active pituitary adenoma is diagnosed clinically and confirmed biochemically. The function of imaging is to detect, localize and delineate the extent of the tumour

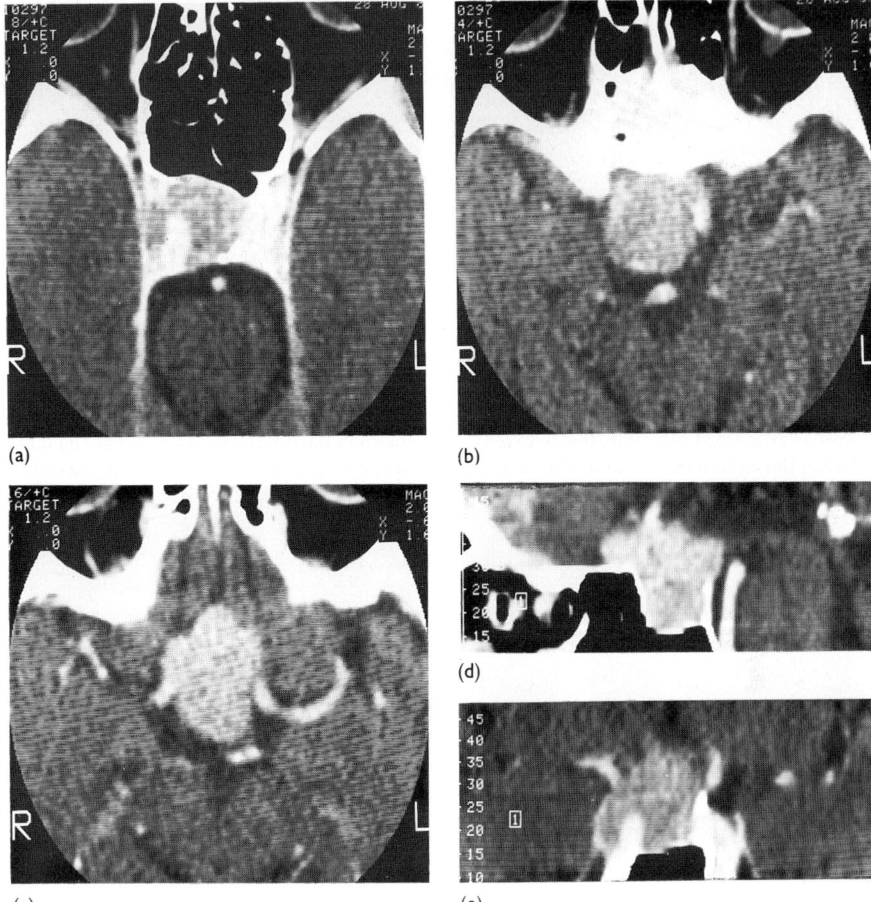

Fig. 20.6 Pituitary macroadenoma. CT scan after intravenous contrast medium: (a–c) axial sections through pituitary fossa and chiasmatic cistern; (d) reformatted axial section; (e) reformatted coronal sections. The enhanced adenoma is denser than brain tissue but less dense than the blood vessels. It forms a mass enlarging the pituitary fossa more on the right side and the floor is deeper on this side. There is a lobulated extension through the chiasmatic cistern, elevating the anterior recesses of the third ventricle. The tumour has invaded and enlarged the right cavernous sinus and surrounded the internal carotid artery.

prior to surgery or radiation therapy, and to document response to treatment. Hormonally inactive tumours usually present with mass effect, usually hemianopia or headache, and imaging should also suggest the differential diagnosis.

Pituitary adenomas are conveniently subdivided into macroadenomas larger than 1.0 cm in diameter, and microadenomas. With CT, using either axial or coronal sections, there is no difficulty in identifying macroadenomas. They may cause local or generalized erosion of the sella, which tends to recorticate but remain thinned with slow-growing lesions. Adenomas may erode through the bone of the sella and form a mass within the sphenoid sinus or clivus; they may extend laterally to encroach on the cavernous sinuses and displace the internal carotid arteries, or superiorly through the chiasmatic cistern to elevate the optic chiasm, third ventricle and/or anterior cerebral arteries. A very large lesion may extend further in any direction, but most frequently into the middle cranial fossae to displace the temporal lobe(s) and middle cerebral artery(s).

The cardinal feature of pituitary adenomas is that they are continuous with, and inseparable from, the pituitary tissue within the sella turcica. On CT the tumour tends to be approximately isodense with brain substance and to enhance considerably (Fig. 20.6). It may contain non-enhancing low-density regions, due to necrotic or cystic change. High-density regions may be due to haemorrhagic components or frank haematoma within the tumour. Calcification is relatively uncommon: it tends to occur in the periphery of the tumour, but may form a more central nodule.

MRI reveals the adenoma and its relationships to suprasellar structures to best advantage using sagittal and coronal T_1-weighted section (Fig. 20.7). Assessment of cavernous sinus invasion is less satisfactory, since the medial wall of the sinus is often not shown as a separate structure. However, enlargement of the superior or inferior compartment of a sinus and, in particular, narrowing of the cavernous segment of a carotid artery indicating tumour encasement, allow positive prediction of invasion in over 60% and negative prediction in over 80% of surgically proven cases [27]. The tumour is usually of lower intensity on long T_1-weighted sequences, isointense

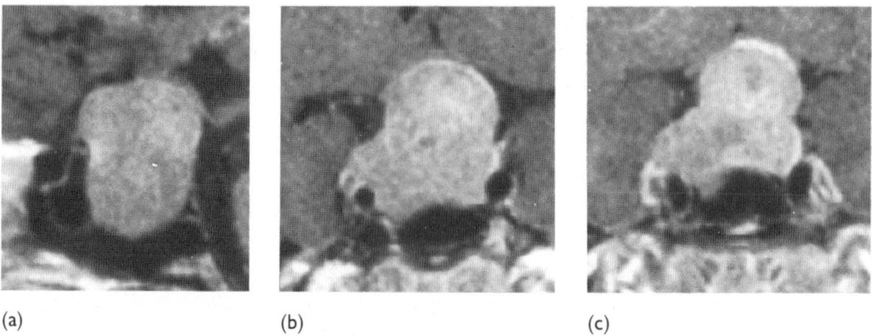

(a) (b) (c)

Fig. 20.7 Pituitary macroadenoma. (a) Midline sagittal T_1-weighted section (b, c) contiguous T_1-weighted coronal sections after intravenous gadolinium enhancement. The tumour causes asymmetrical enlargement of the pituitary fossa, the floor being more depressed and eroded on the right side. The tumour extends superiorly through the chiasmatic cistern to elevate the chiasm and anterior recesses of the third ventricle. It also extends into the right cavernous sinus, as far as the lateral wall, which is shown as a dark band between the enhancing tumour and the temporal lobe. The carotid artery is also displaced laterally and the limbs of the carotid syphon are stretched apart by the tumour extending between them. The left cavernous sinus is also displaced laterally, but does not appear to be invaded by the tumour.

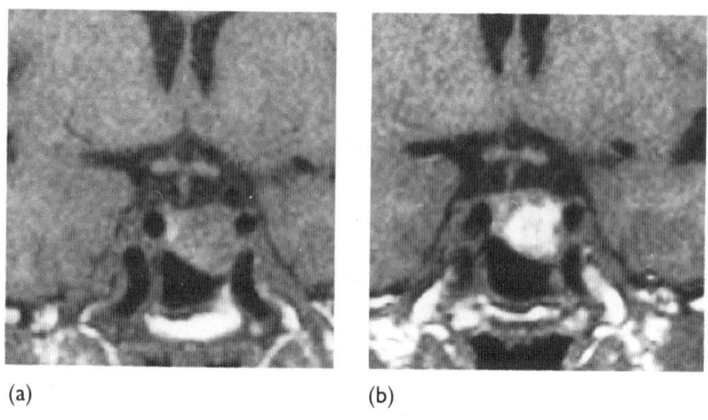

(a) (b)

Fig. 20.8 Pituitary macroadenoma. (a) Coronal section through the pituitary gland. The pituitary adenoma expands the left side of the sella turcica and displaces laterally the cavernous segment of the left internal carotid artery. (b) Similar section 4 months later during bromocriptine therapy. There is a large area of high signal in the left lobe of the pituitary gland due to haemorrhage.

on moderately T_2-weighted sequences and of higher intensity on heavily T_2-weighted sequences. About 85% of tumours are homogeneous.

Regions of high intensity on T_1-weighted sequences suggest haemorrhage (Fig. 20.8); these regions are generally abnormal on CT also, but only 25% have high CT density and 25% have acute deterioration of vision, oculomotor palsy or meningism suggesting pituitary apoplexy [28]. Well-defined, non-enhancing regions of T_1 low, T_2 high signal, but differing in intensity from CSF on bone sequences, are indicative of cystic or necrotic foci.

After treatment with bromocriptine, sensitive tumours may decrease in size, sometimes within a week, usually by 3 weeks, and this may continue for 2 years. Intensity increases on T_1-weighted sequences, often associated with haemorrhagic changes, and also on T_2-weighted sequences. Follow-up MRI is necessary for early detection of regrowth of the tumour.

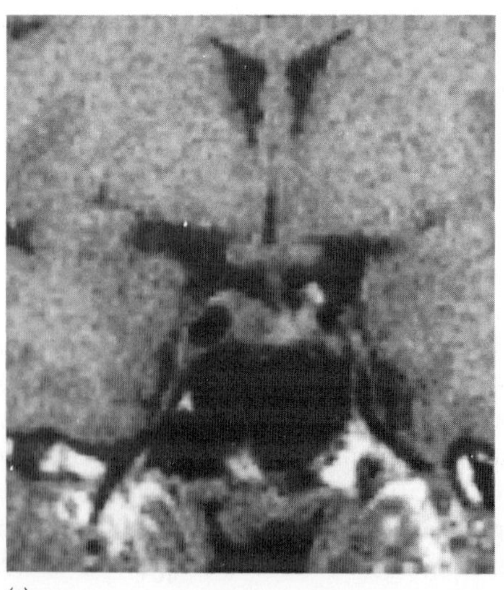

(a)

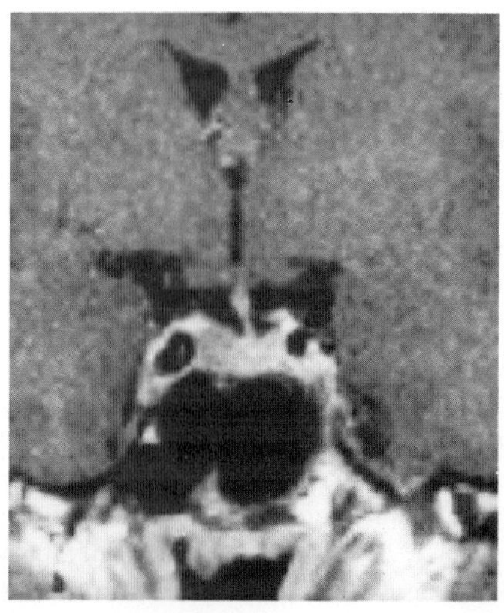

(b)

Fig. 20.9 Pituitary microadenoma. Coronal T_1-weighted sections through pituitary gland: (a) before, (b) after intravenous gadolinium. There is a small low-density, non-enhancing mass enlarging the right lobe of the pituitary gland. Its lateral margin is adjacent to the cavernous sinus. The pituitary stalk is deviated to the left.

Microadenomas, can be more difficult to recognize. Typical microadenomas are CT low-density lesions which enhance less than normal pituitary tissue or not at all, and show as low-attenuation regions on contrast-enhanced CT scans [21]. These appearances are not specific: small low-density regions may occasionally be due to colloid cysts, epidermoids, Rathke pouch cysts, and even metastases, infarcts, abscesses or granulomas [30]. It should also be noted that autopsy series have shown pituitary microadenomas to be present in 10–20% of the general population; these are in the main very small and asymptomatic [19,31]. Also, particularly in the puerperium [32], foci of hyperplasia may be almost impossible to distinguish from adenomas even histologically [33]. Occasional microadenomas have been isodense with normal pituitary tissue, and remain so after contrast enhancement or even become hyperdense [34].

On MRI the majority of microadenomas (Fig. 20.9) are well-defined hypointense foci within the pituitary gland substance on T_1-weighted images [35]. About 10% are hyperintense or isointense, usually due to small areas of haemorrhage within the tumour, and this is more frequent after bromocriptine therapy. Tumours may produce local mass, the effect of which varies with the position of the tumour in the gland – it may cause a convex upper border to one lobe, displacement of the pituitary stalk, or impinge against one side of the sellar floor with focal depression or a cavernous sinus. Microadenomas enhance more slowly than normal anterior pituitary tissue. Relative hypointensity of the adenoma is maximal immediately after gadolinium injection, and decreases progressively over the following 4 min [36]. Between 5 and 10 min after injection the tumour may become iso- or hyperintense.

In practice it can be difficult directly to visualize a small microadenoma because of the heterogeneous appearance of normal pituitary substance, caused by the noise range of the imaging system and by the normal variation in height and shape of the pituitary gland substance. Corroborative evidence of the presence of an adenoma includes a gland exceeding 9.0 mm in height, an eccentric upper convexity of the gland with asymmetrical increase in thickness of one lobe, focal erosion of the sella, displacement of the pituitary stalk from the side of greater thickness, contralateral displacement of the capillary tuft (shown on dynamic scanning) or an impression on the normally convex anterior border of the less enhancing posterior pituitary. However, such indirect signs can be misleading and should be interpreted conservatively [29]. In appropriate clinical circumstances it is reasonable to suggest that a solitary, well-demarcated low-density area larger than 3 mm diameter within the pituitary gland, thickening a lobe and causing focal displacement, is likely to be an adenoma [13].

If imaging fails to reveal a hormone-secreting adenoma [37], venous sampling may be diagnostic. This is best performed by simultaneous catheterization of both cavernous sinuses from the femoral route and taking samples before and during stimulation by appropriate releasing hormones. Adrenocorticotrophin hormone (ACTH)-secreting adenomas tend to present for diagnosis when they average 5 mm in diameter, but may be as small as 2 mm. Currently up to one-third cannot be visualized on imaging and can be localized only by venous sampling, although in children this can be difficult because of blood mixing.

MUCOCOELE OF THE SPHENOID SINUS

This is a rare condition in childhood, but may complicate fibrous dysplasia of the skull base. It may simulate a pituitary tumour on CT. Sagittal MRI shows a high signal mass separate from and below the pituitary gland, and there is often rim enhancement on T_1-weighted sections with gadolinium in infected mucocoeles.

SUPRASELLAR TUMOURS DEVELOPING FROM EMBRYONIC REMNANTS

Craniopharyngiomas

These tumours originate from squamous-cell remnants of the Rathke's pouch and usually form non-invasive, slowly expanding, well-defined masses. They are by far the commonest tumour type affecting the hypothalamopituitary region in childhood, and account for 8–13% of all intracranial tumours under 14 years of age. Craniopharyngiomas are, in the majority of cases, suprasellar tumours which, as they enlarge, impinge upon the sella from above, tending to flatten and erode the dorsum or to extend into the sella, causing it to enlarge. The tumours frequently extend posterosuperiorly, displacing the hypothalamus and midbrain. Large tumours may extend inferiorly behind the clivus, even as far as the foramen magnum, and asymmetrically beneath the frontal or, less frequently, temporal lobes. Hydrocephalus is common with large tumours. Occasionally craniopharyngiomas arise within the sella and rarely within the third ventricle.

Almost all craniopharyngiomas in children contain calcium and many are heavily calcified: the calcification may be curvilinear in the capsule or nodular within the tumour substance. The tumours may be solid, but the majority have cystic components. The cysts often contain cholesterol crystals, causing well-defined low CT attenuation regions (Fig. 25.10). Cysts may also contain cellular debris and, occasionally, altered blood, and may then be similar in density to brain or even hyperdense on CT. Cystic and calcified parts of craniophyaryngiomas do not enhance: solid components show great variation

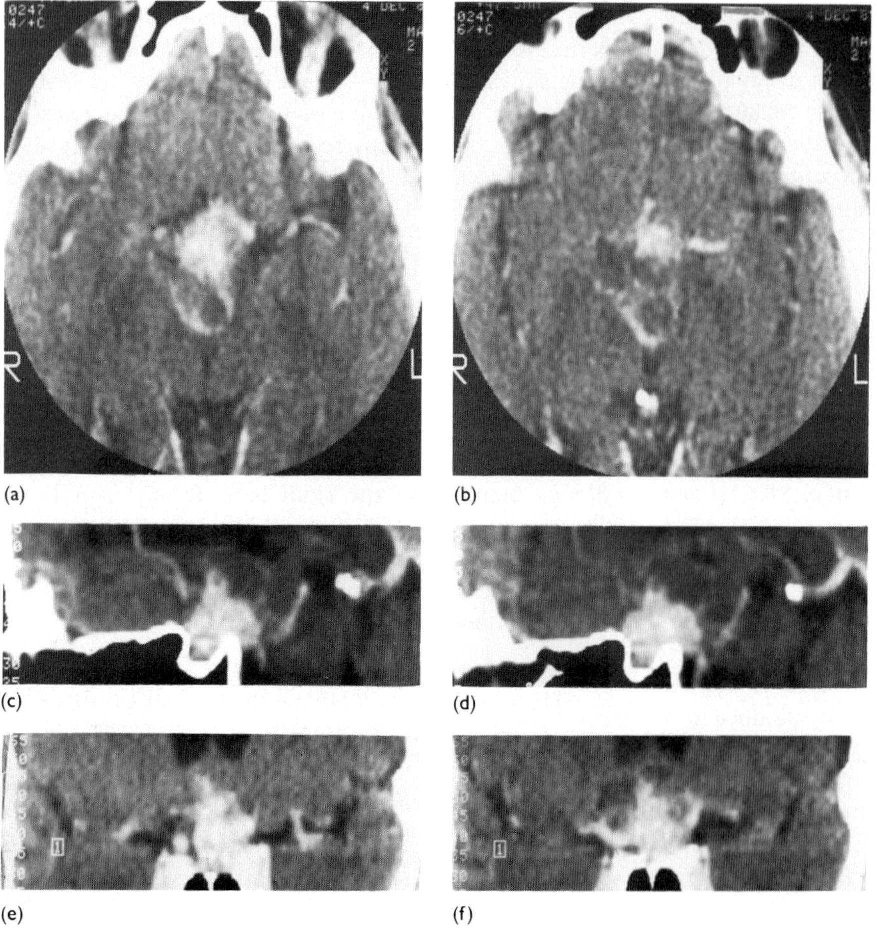

Fig. 20.10 Craniopharyngioma. CT scan after intravenous contrast medium: (a, b) axial sections through the suprasellar cistern; (c, d) sagittal and parasagittal reformats; (e, f) coronal reformats. There is a large mass expanding the chiasmatic and interpeduncular cisterns and extending posteriorly and superiorly to elevate and almost obliterate the third ventricle. It also extends into the upper half of the sella turcica. The lower and anterior half of the mass is of high density and the upper posterior part of mixed, mainly low density, with a partly enhancing rim containing a little curvilinear calcification posteriorly. The lower part of the tumour was solid, but the upper lower-density part contained fluid heavily laden with cholesterol crystals.

in the degree of contrast enhancement which may be moderate, slight or absent.

On MRI the solid parts of the tumour usually return low signal on T_1-weighted sequences and markedly high signal on T_2-weighted sequences and enhance with gadolinium. About two-thirds of tumours are heterogeneous (Fig. 20.11): there may be low signal on all sequences from calcified parts, and fatty fluid in cystic craniopharyngiomas commonly and charactistically returns high signal on both T_1-weighted and T_2-weighted sequences. The latter may simulate the rarer lipomas, teratomas and dermoids, which are also found as congenital tumours in the suprasellar region. Small, mainly calcified tumours, which are obvious on CT, may be almost impossible to detect on MRI.

Uncommonly, craniopharyngiomas behave as invasive tumours infiltrating brain substance and causing reactive oedema, which may spread along the optic tracts and even into the radiations, simulating an optic glioma.

Epidermoids

On CT these most frequently form masses of approximately CSF density, similar to arachnoid cysts but generally more irregular in shape. They may extend into and dilate a temporal horn, causing a virtually pathognomonic appearance. Epidermoids may also be of density similar to brain, or even higher, and occasionally there may be calcification and/or enhancement peripherally in the capsule. Intrathecal non-ionic contrast media may be required for CT diagnosis: the tumour is outlined as a lobulated cauliflower-like filing defect in the opacified cistern.

On T_2-weighted MRI sequences the epidermoid gives a high signal often similar to but sometimes greater than CSF. On T_1-weighted sequences a high signal may also be obtained if the tumour contains a high proportion of fat; more commonly the signal is low, tending to approximate that of the CSF. On proton-density-weighted sequences the tumour intensity may differ sufficiently to be distinguished from CSF (Fig. 20.12).

Dermoids and teratomas

Intracranial dermoids (Fig. 20.13) and teratomas are rare tumours, but the suprasellar region is second in incidence

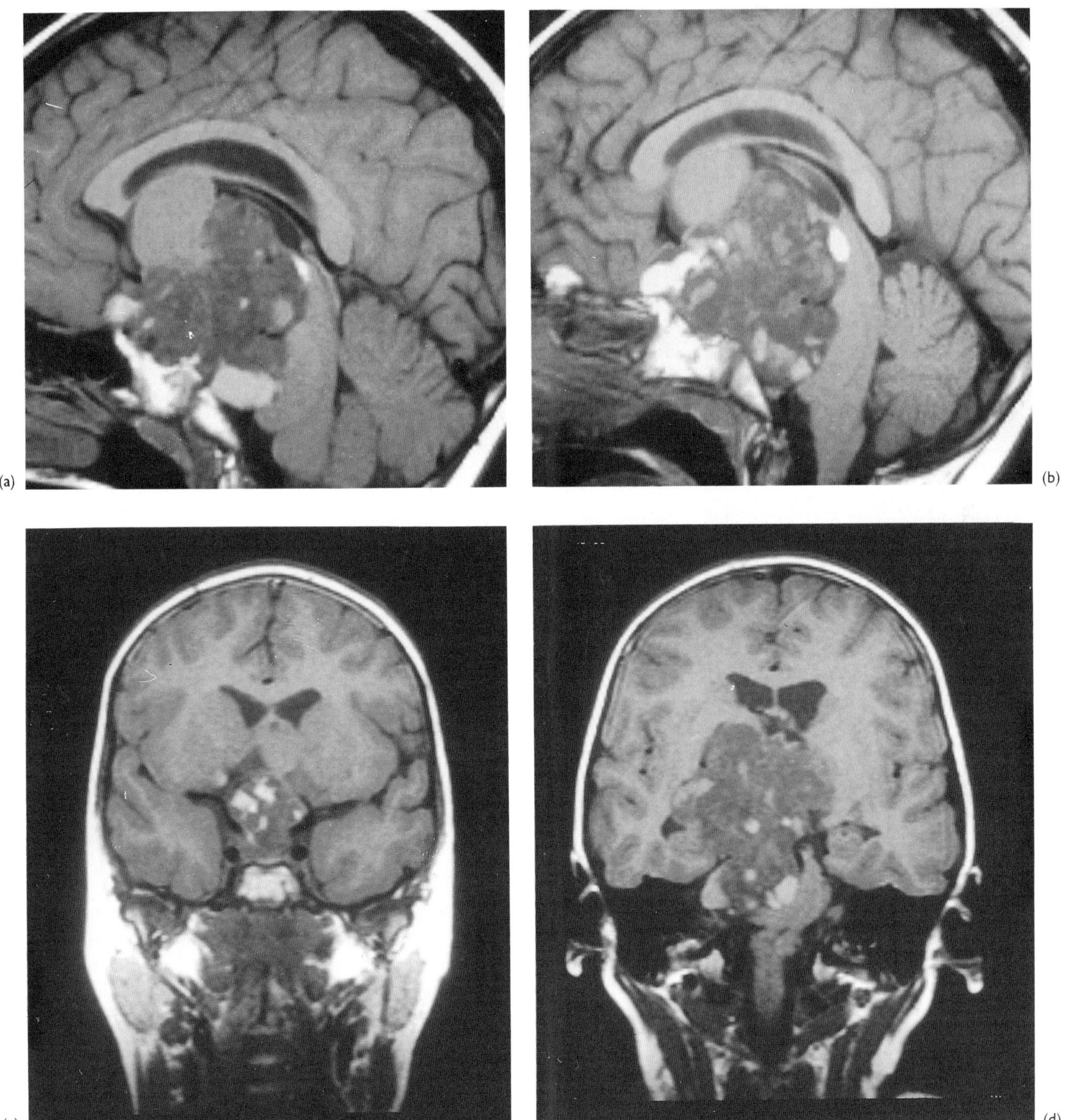

Fig. 20.11 Craniopharyngioma. (a, b) Contiguous sagittal, (c, d) contiguous coronal T_1-weighted sections. There is a mixed intensity mass which has eroded the sella turcica and extended above and behind the sphenoid bone. It fills the chiasmatic cistern and elevates the floor of the third ventricle. It fills the interpeduncular and pontine cisterns and displaces and compresses the midbrain and the pons posteriorly. The tumour contains regions which are of similar intensity to brain substance, and others which are of higher signal due to fluid containing cholesterol, and others which are of lower signal caused by small cysts containing watery fluid.

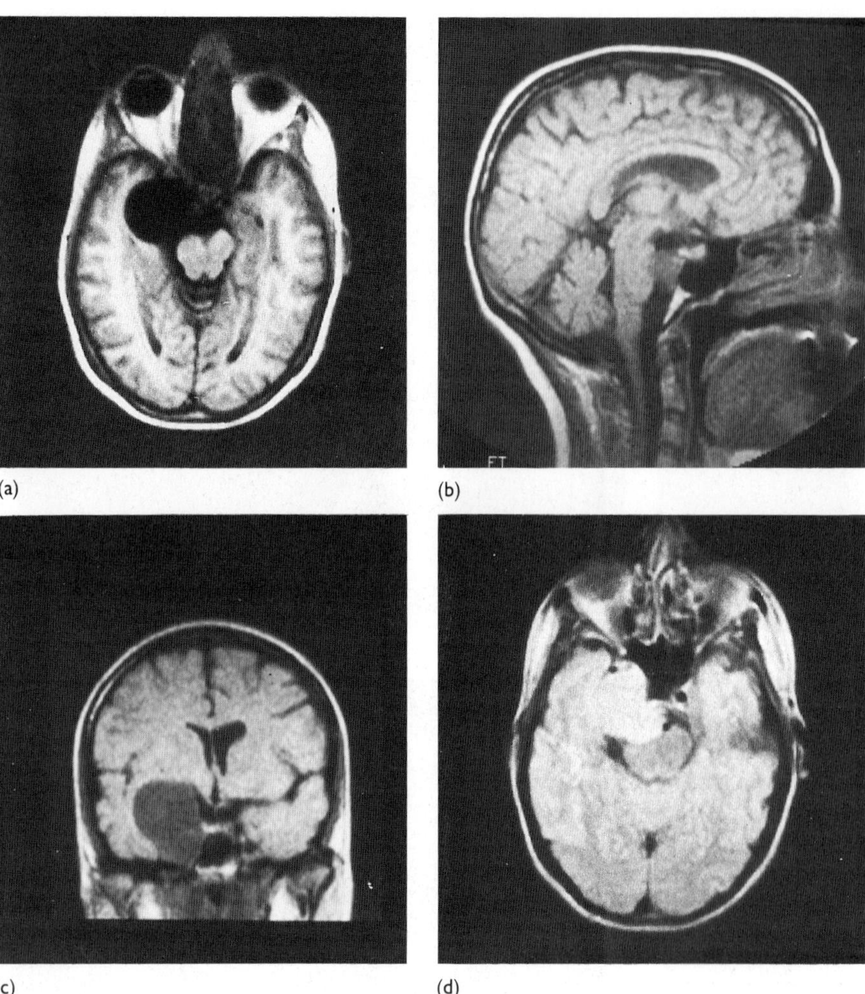

Fig. 20.12 Epidermoid. (a) Axial inversion recovery sequence; (b, c) sagittal and coronal short TR, short TE, SE sequences with T_1-weighting; (d) axial T_2-weighted SE sequence. The epidermoid forms a lobulated mass in the right parasellar region and within the right side of the crural cistern and Sylvian fissure. Its intensity on (a) is similar to CSF, on (b) it is slightly higher and on (d) markedly higher than CSF and brain substance. The lobulated mass displaces laterally the temporal lobe, and elevates the basal ganglia. The crural and ambiens cisterns are widened and the right crus cerebri is displaced and compressed.

only to the pineal as the site of origin. They may present at any age from birth to adult life with chiasmal compression or endocrine disturbances, including delayed growth or precocious puberty. They are recognized on both CT and MRI from the presence of fat in association with one or more other tissues, including bone or calcification, muscle, brain or fluid-containing cysts; enhancement may be patchy or absent.

Lipomas

Lipomas also occur in this region. They present as a homogeneous mass of fat, having negative CT attenuation reaching as low as 50 Hounsfield units, and the typical high signal associated with a very short T_1 on appropriate magnetic resonance sequences. Lipomas are malformations of the meninx primitiva: fat occupies the malformed subarachnoid space and encloses any structures such as nerves and vessels traversing the malformed region.

Arachnoid cysts

Most arachnoid cysts are formed by abnormal splitting of the arachnoid during development. Some are acquired due to meningeal adhesions following an inflammatory process. Most cysts are in the middle fossae, but these may extend into the parasellar region. About 15% of cysts are confined to the parasellar or intrasellar regions [38]. Suprasellar arachnoid cysts usually present with hydrocephalus in infancy, or with symptoms of chiasmatic compression in early life, but they may cause precocious puberty. They form well-defined masses, with tissue characteristics on CT and MRI similar to those of CSF (Fig. 20.14), and they do not enhance. The surrounding brain is displaced by larger cysts; there is no surrounding oedema and the signal intensity remains normal. The skull base may be eroded and remodelled by the cyst.

Large cysts tend to be rounded and wider than the third ventricle, which generally retains its anatomical contours even when hydrocephalic. These characteristics serve to

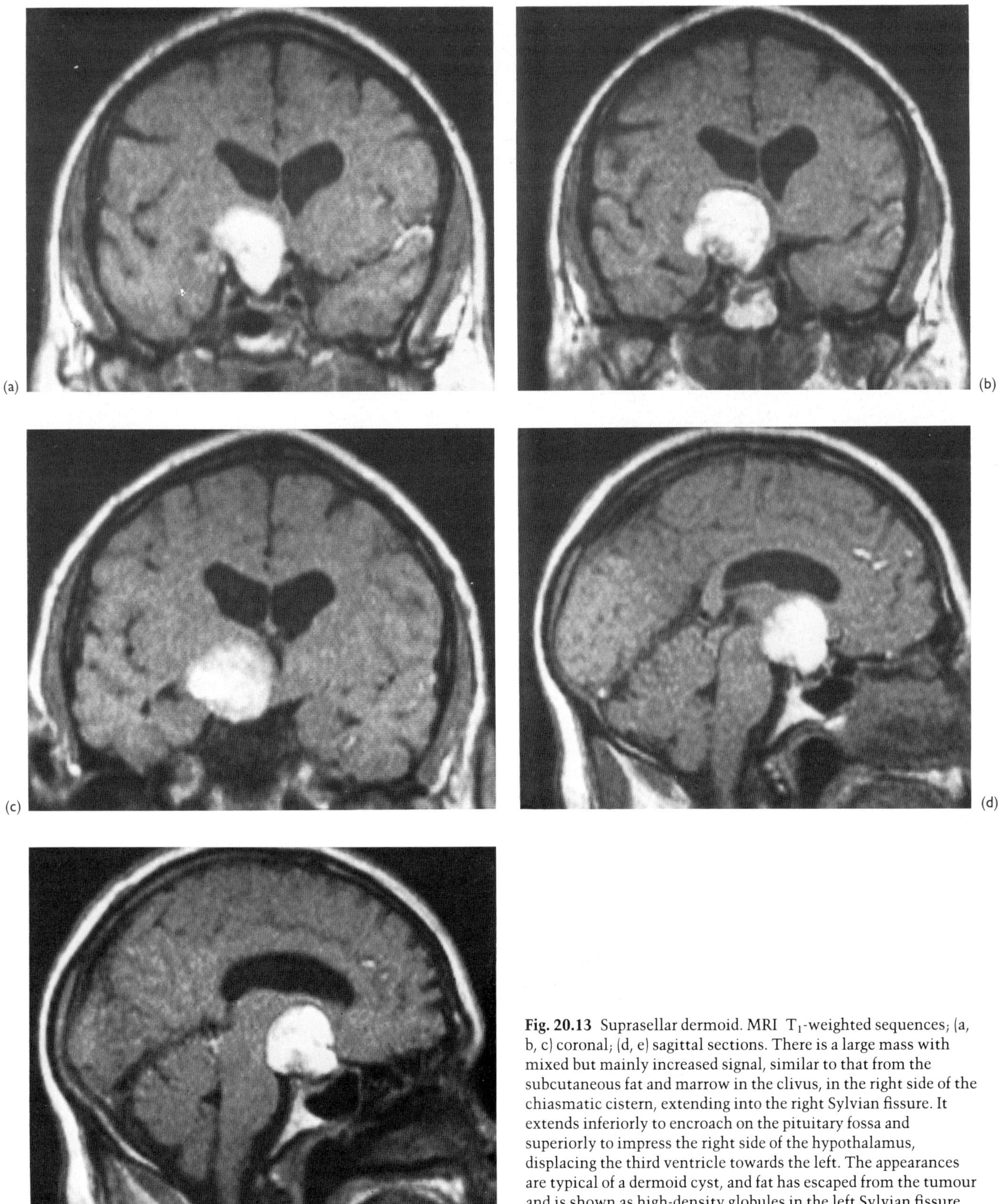

Fig. 20.13 Suprasellar dermoid. MRI T_1-weighted sequences; (a, b, c) coronal; (d, e) sagittal sections. There is a large mass with mixed but mainly increased signal, similar to that from the subcutaneous fat and marrow in the clivus, in the right side of the chiasmatic cistern, extending into the right Sylvian fissure. It extends inferiorly to encroach on the pituitary fossa and superiorly to impress the right side of the hypothalamus, displacing the third ventricle towards the left. The appearances are typical of a dermoid cyst, and fat has escaped from the tumour and is shown as high-density globules in the left Sylvian fissure and medial hemispheric sulci.

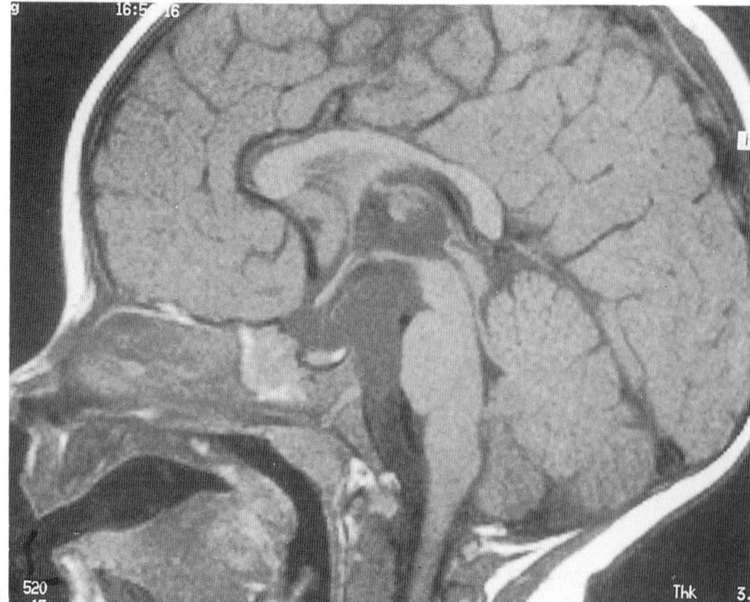

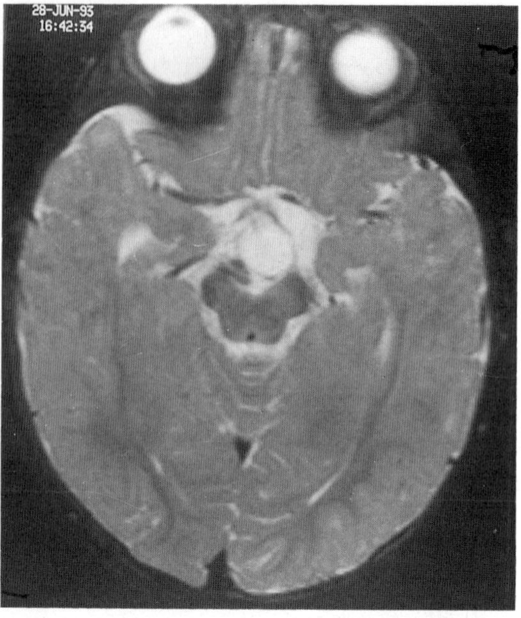

(a) (b)

Fig. 20.14 Arachnoid cyst. (a) Midsagittal T_1-weighted section; (b) axial T_2-weighted section. There is a smooth, well-demarcated mass in the chiasmatic, interpeduncular and pontine cisterns. It returns signal similar to the CSF. The mass elevates the floor of the third ventricle, displaces the midbrain and pons posteriorly and stretches the pituitary stalk. Note the flat superior border of the pituitary gland and the normal high signal return from the posterior pituitary on the T_1-weighted section.

distinguish cysts which have obstructed the foramen of Monro from other causes of hydrocephalus.

INTRINSIC LESIONS OF THE FLOOR OF THE THIRD VENTRICLE, TUBER CINEREUM AND HYPOTHALAMUS

Optic chiasm gliomas

These are usually low-grade astrocytomas, but some are more malignant; they form about 5% of intracranial tumours presenting before the age of 10 years. They may remain confined to the chiasm, but tend to spread along and expand the optic tracts and/or nerves, maintaining their characteristic shape on CT and MRI (Fig. 20.15). They may, however, invade the hypothalamus or cerebral hemispheres and may then be indistinguishable from a glioma arising in any part of the involved region. The usual presenting symptom is visual loss, but endocrine disturbances, including precocious puberty, may be present.

The mass is usually homogeneous with similar CT density and MRI signal characteristics as those of brain substance, but large tumours may be of low CT attenuation (Fig. 20.15). Calcification is unusual but, when present, may lead to difficulty in distinction from craniopharyngioma, and cystic or necrotic regions are present in about 40% of tumours. These are usually but not invariably small, and cause non-enhancing regions of T_1 low, T_2 high signal. Although many optic gliomas are adequately shown by CT, MRI, particularly in the sagittal plane, can more exactly define the smaller tumours deforming the anterior recesses of the third ventricle. Axial MRI demonstrates particularly well the degree of extension into or through the optic canals and along the optic tracts (Fig. 20.16). Superior extension with involvement of the foramina of Munro causing hydrocephalus is present in about one-third of tumours. Extension may also occur beneath the frontal lobes, towards the middle fossae, displacing the temporal lobes, or inferiorly to displace the basilar artery and brainstem. Encasement of arteries of the circle of Willis occurs in a minority of the larger tumours.

Gliomas and hamartomas of the hypothalamus

Gliomas, when small, may present with precocious puberty in males or, if larger, with symptoms of hypothalamic disturbance, diabetes insipidus or pituitary insufficiency. The glioma is usually of low grade, of close to brain MRI intensity and CT density, and with minor to moderate enhancement, though a minority, and particularly the more extensive tumours, have prolonged T_1 and T_2 values, and prominent enhancement. Larger tumours may extend in any direction, and about 40% undergo cystic or necrotic degeneration. They are undistinguishable from gliomas arising in any part of the involved region.

The hamartoma in this region usually presents with precocious puberty or seizures which may be gelastic [39].

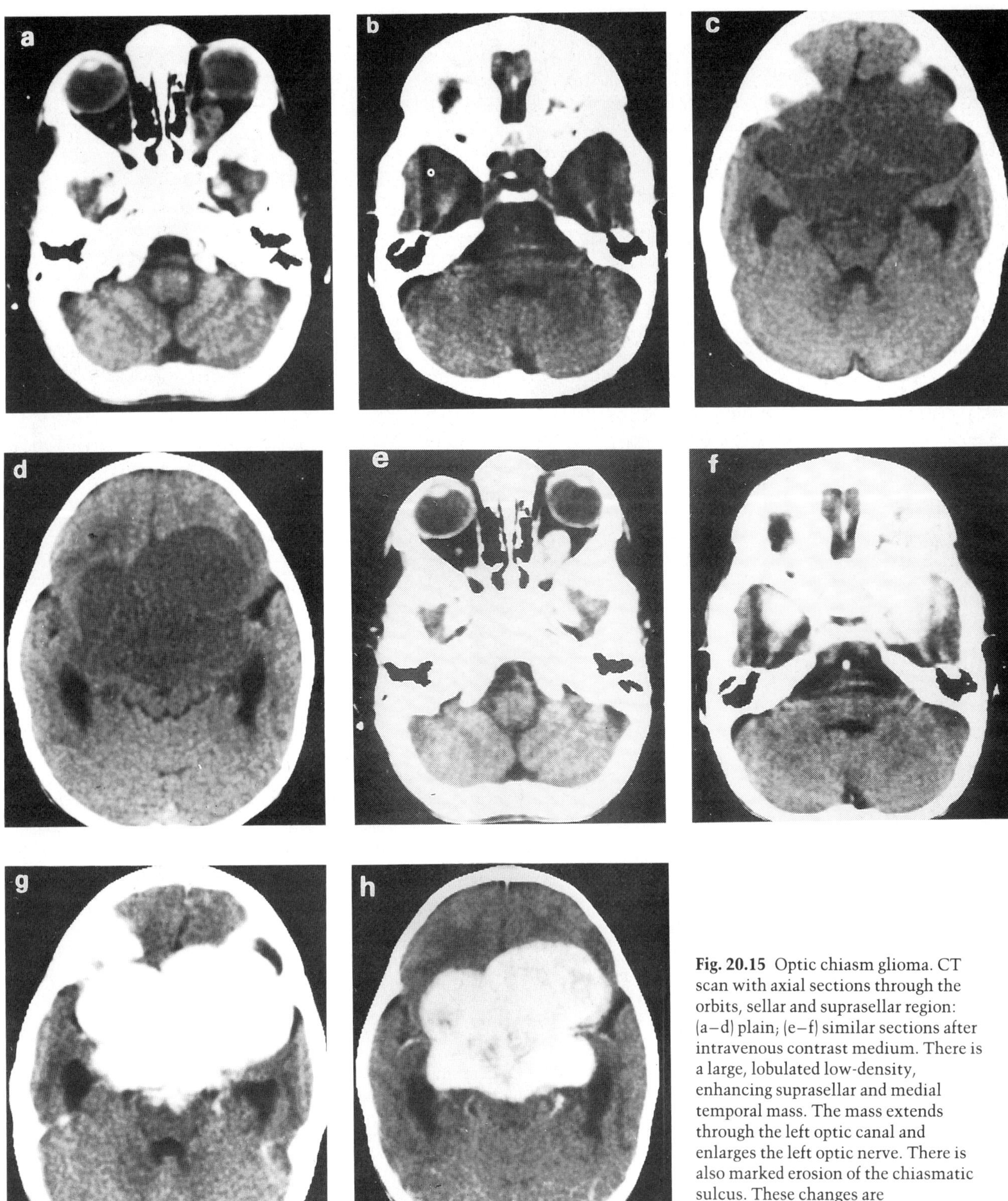

Fig. 20.15 Optic chiasm glioma. CT scan with axial sections through the orbits, sellar and suprasellar region: (a–d) plain; (e–f) similar sections after intravenous contrast medium. There is a large, lobulated low-density, enhancing suprasellar and medial temporal mass. The mass extends through the left optic canal and enlarges the left optic nerve. There is also marked erosion of the chiasmatic sulcus. These changes are characteristic of an optic glioma.

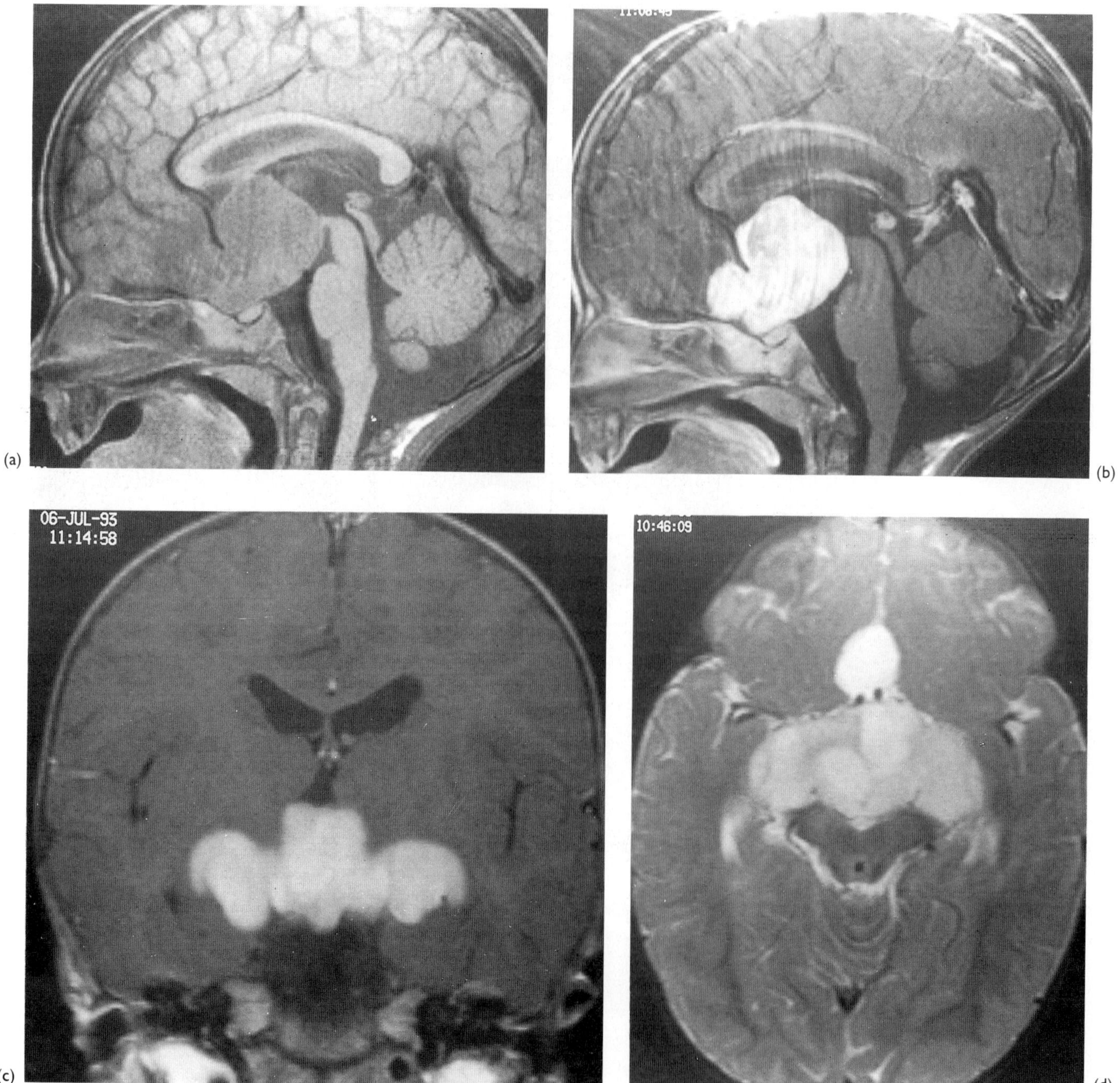

Fig. 20.16 Optic glioma. (a) T_1-weighted sagittal before and (b) after gadolinium; (c) T_1-weighted coronal section after gadolinium; (d) T_2-weighted axial section. There is a lobulated enhancing mass in the chiasmatic cistern extending into the interpeduncular cistern and both crural cisterns. It preserves the shape of the optic chiasm and extends into the proximal parts of both optic tracts. The anterior communicating and anterior cerebral arteries are elevated and displaced anteriorly by the tumour, which returns lower signal than white matter on the T_1-weighted sections and mixed high signal on the T_2-weighted section. Note that the pituitary gland, compressed inferiorly by the mass on the sagittal section, returns higher signal than the tumour substance and is thereby distinguished from it. Note also the elongation of the chiasmatic sulcus due to erosion by the tumour.

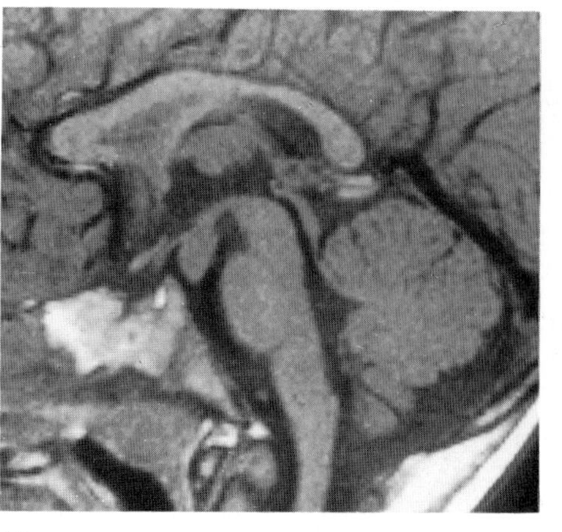

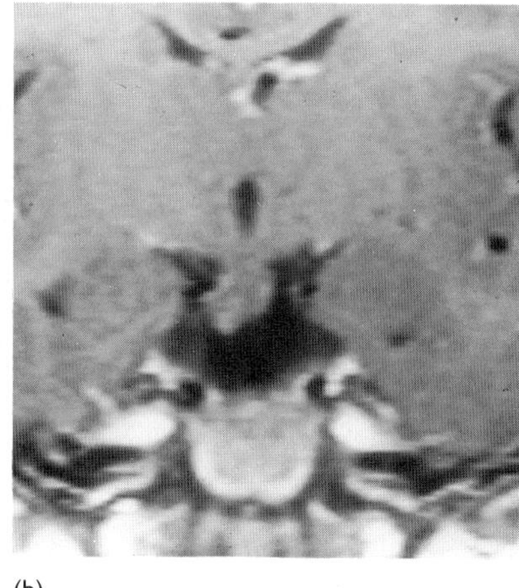

(a) (b)

Fig. 20.17 Hypothalamic hamartoma. (a) Plain midsagittal T_1-weighted section; (b) coronal T_1-weighted section after intravenous gadolinium. There is a pedunculated mass extending from the region of the tuber cinereum into the junction of the chiasmatic and interpeduncular cisterns. It returns signal similar to brain substance and shows no enhancement. Note the normal high signal return from the posterior pituitary substance. The appearances are typical of a hypothalamic hamartoma.

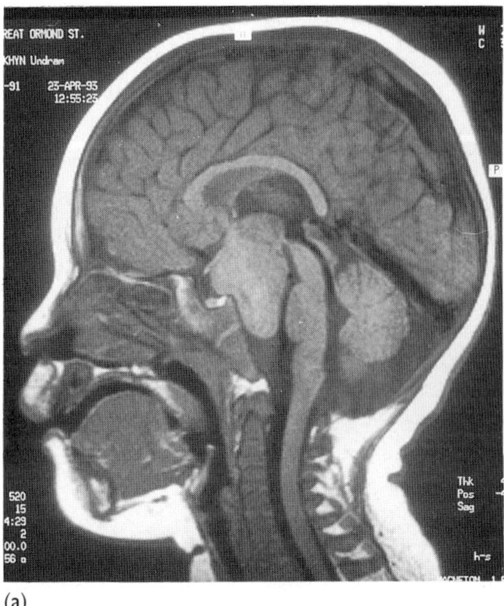

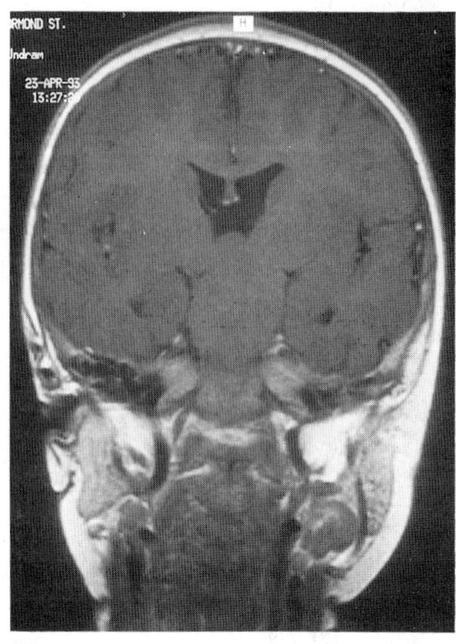

(a) (b)

Fig. 20.18 Hamartoma. (a) Plain midsagittal T_1-weighted section; (b) coronal T_1-weighted section after intravenous gadolinium. The tumour is considerably larger than that shown in Fig. 20.17. It forms a lobulated mass in the chiasmatic interpeduncular and pontine cisterns, elevating the floor of the hypothalamus, displacing the optic chiasm superiorly, and the midbrain and pons posteriorly. Note that the normal high signal from the posterior pituitary is preserved. The appearances are typical of a hypothalamic hamartoma.

Vision is usually normal, and other focal signs are generally absent. The lesion is usually a small, clearly defined, rounded or pedunculated mass involving the region of the tuber cinereum and/or mamillary bodies and lying in the interpeduncular region (Fig. 20.17); large hamartomas also occur as exophytic masses isointense to grey matter on T_1-weighted sections and iso- or hyperintense on T_2-weighted sections (Fig. 20.18). The high T_1 signal from the posterior pituitary is preserved. On CT the tumour is typically isodense with grey matter without calcification, and there is no enhancement on either CT or MRI. However, cystic changes, fat formation, calcification and enhancement have all been recorded in unusual cases [12,40]. Glioma and hamartoma are best distinguished and the relationships to adjacent structures elucidated by sagittal and coronal MRI sections [41].

Germ-cell tumours

Germ-cell tumours constitute about 1% of intracranial tumours and they mostly involve the pineal, though about 20% of them occur in the suprasellar region or pituitary fossa. The suprasellar tumours may be primary or due to transventricular spread from the pineal region. They are tumours of children or young adults and the diagnosis is usually suggested by the clinical combination of visual disturbance, diabetes insipidus and anterior pituitary dysfunction. The more malignant subgroup of germ-cell tumours, the non-germinomatous types, produce a high level of α-fetoprotein and/or human chorionic gonadotrophin in the CSF, which are useful indicators of the nature of the tumour (Fig. 20.19).

The tumour is usually centred behind the infundibulum and has ill-defined edges which may extend along the walls of the third ventricle. It is usually homogeneous

(a)

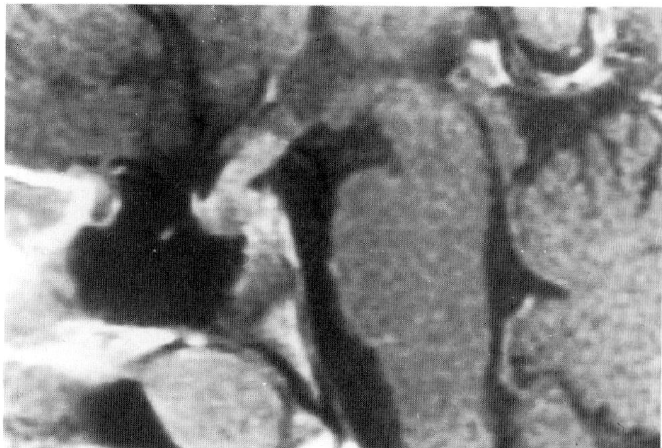

(b)

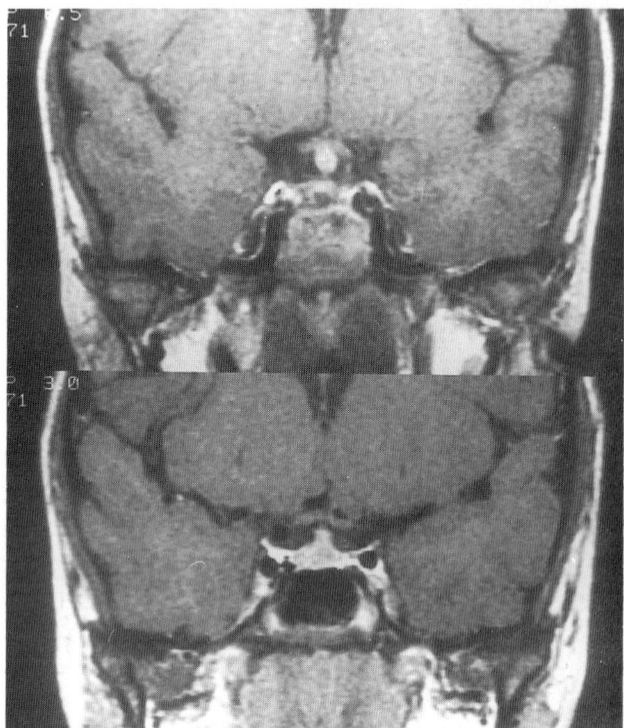

Fig. 20.19 Non-germinomatous germ-cell tumour. T_1-weighted MRI after gadolinium enhancement: (a) sagittal, and (b) contiguous coronal sections. A girl aged 6 presented with failure of growth and diabetes insipidus. High levels of α-fetoprotein were present in the CSF. The enhancing pituitary stalk is abnormally thick. There was a good response to chemotherapy.

without cystic or calcified components, though small cysts may be present. On MRI it returns T_1 isointense or slightly lower, and T_2 higher signal than brain. On plain CT it is of brain or slightly greater attenuation and it enhances homogeneously on both modalities. It should be noted that hypothalamic lesions have been demonstrated many years after onset of symptoms in cases with previously negative studies. Particularly with diabetes insipidus, follow-up studies with pre- and post-gadolinium MRI are indicated.

Metastases, particularly from medulloblastoma and retinoblastoma, may occur in this region and cause indistinguishable masses. These rarely give rise to endocrine upset and the primary tumour is usually already evident. MRI tends to show more exactly the extent of pathology, and is particularly useful for distinguishing between a primary tumour and metastatic spread.

Granulomas and inflammatory lesions

The hypothalamus and the pituitary stalk are regions of predilection for Langerhans cell histiocytosis and sarcoidosis; they may also be involved in tuberculosis. Diabetes insipidus may result without detectable abnormality on CT, or there may be visible thickening of the pituitary stalk and considerable abnormal enhancement. The thickening and detailed anatomy is shown to best advantage in the sagittal plane by thin-section MRI. The abnormal tissue is hyperintense on T_2-weighted sections (Fig. 20.20).

In histiocytosis, lytic bone defects are present in about 25% of cases, and exophthalmos secondary to involvement of the orbital walls is not uncommon. In Langerhans cell histiocytosis, changes in brain substance may occur. These tend to be symmetrical in the white matter, most commonly in the cerebellar hemispheres but occasionally in the occipital and posterior temporal lobes. Enhancement and a minor degree of mass effect may be present in the early phase with progression to resolution or to non-enhancing regions with atrophy.

Symptoms of pituitary and hypothalamic dysfunction are uncommon in tuberculosis. They may occur due to spread of infection from basal meningitis, in which enhancing high-signal granulation tissue within the basal cisterns will be revealed by MRI or CT. Intracerebral oedema or infarcts, particularly in the basal ganglia, may become evident during healing with fibrosis, and calcification may be shown on CT.

Meningeal reaction in sarcoidosis is less florid, and tends to be more localized, but it may be sufficient to cause communicating hydrocephalus. Though enhancing granulomas have a predilection for the suprasellar structures, other juxta-arachnoid and/or ependymal regions may be involved [42].

Syphilis, cysticerosis and pyogenic infections may rarely involve the pituitary and hypothalamic regions. They are recognized by associated intracranial or systemic involvement. Pyogenic infections, usually by Gram-positive cocci, may complicate a pre-existing disease such as a pituitary adenoma, craniopharyngioma or Rathke cleft cyst [43]. Intense ring enhancement around a fluid collection may suggest the diagnosis in an appropriate clinical setting.

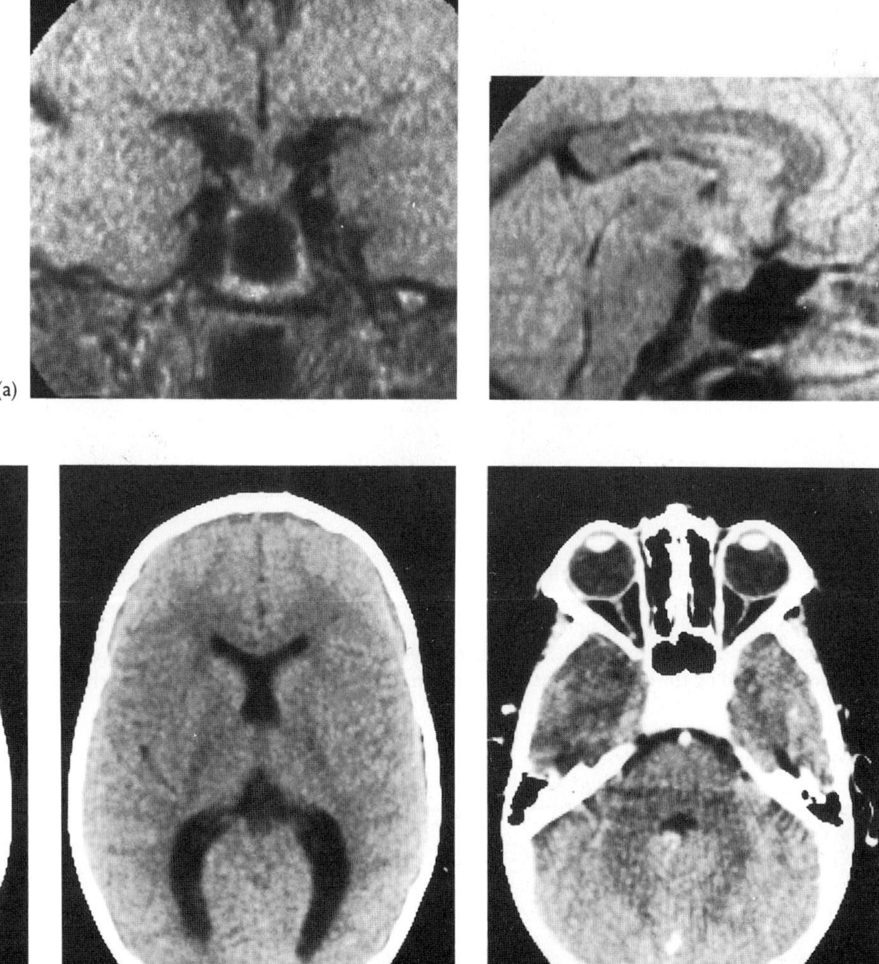

Fig. 20.20 Histiocytosis X. The child had skeletal histiocytosis X and presented with diabetes insipidus. MRI: (a) T_1-weighted coronal section through pituitary gland and stalk; (b) more T_2-weighted midline sagittal section. There is thickening of the pituitary stalk, isointense with brain on the coronal section, and of higher intensity on the sagittal section.

Fig. 20.21 Septo-optic dysplasia. CT scan, axial sections. The septum pellucidum is absent and there is lack of the central deviation of the corpus callosum, which occurs towards a normal septum. The optic nerves are hypoplastic.

CONGENITAL ABNORMALITIES ASSOCIATED WITH ENDOCRINE DISTURBANCES

Disturbance of hypothalamic function presenting as recurrent episodes of hypothermia or secondary effects on pituitary function, resulting in deficiency of gonadotrophins, somatotrophin and antidiuretic hormones, have been described in dysgenesis of the corpus callosum [44], septo-optic dysplasia [45] and sphenoidal encephalocoele. In Kallmann syndrome hypogonadotrophic hypogonadism is associated with anosmia or hyposmia.

Septo-optic dysplasia

In this condition there is a varying degree of hypoplasia of the optic nerves, chiasm and infundibular region of the hypothalamus. The septum pellucidum may be absent, and this is associated with lack of deviation of the central part of the corpus callosum towards the septal insertion (Fig. 20.21). All these features may be shown on thin-section, high-resolution CT or MRI.

The chiasmatic cistern is large and the anterior extremity of the third ventricle is bulbous, with a single dilated anterior recess. These changes are difficult to recognize on CT, but are revealed by sagittal MRI. There is a rare association of glioma of the optic chiasm with septo-optic dysplasia, and this should be suspected if a prominent chiasm or suprasellar mass is present in an otherwise typical case.

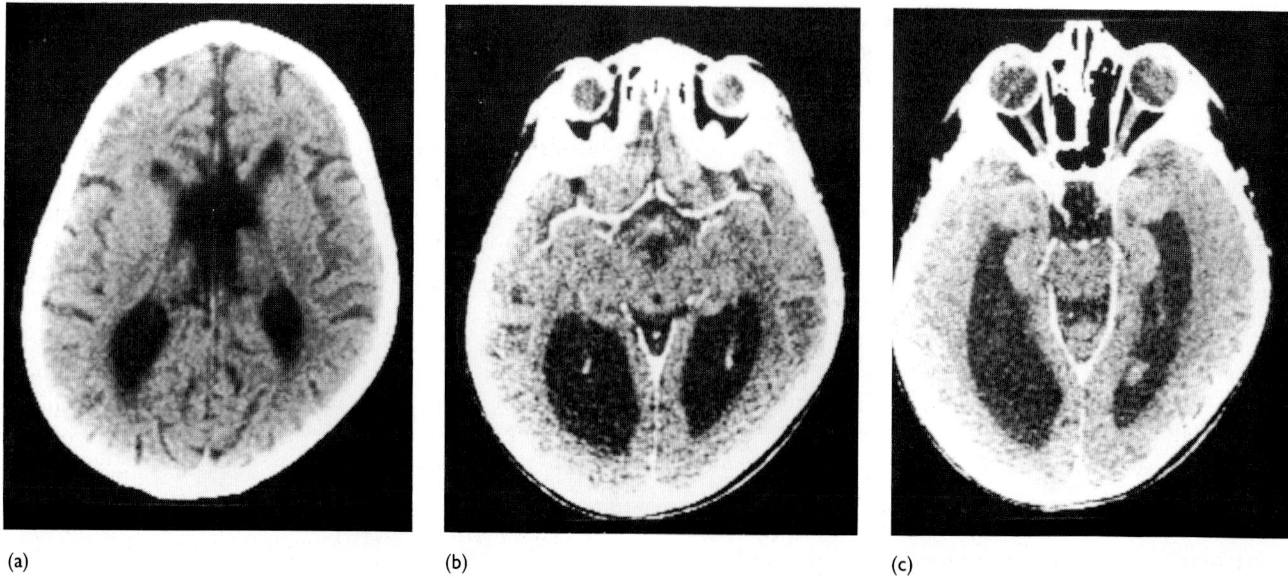

Fig. 20.22 Agenesis of the corpus callosum. Clinically there was hypertelorism, with hypoplasia of the optic nerves and delayed puberty with testicular atrophy. CT scan, axial sections: (a) at the level of the lateral and third ventricles; (b) through the chiasmatic cistern; (c) through the optic nerve and the upper border of the sella turcica. The third ventricle extends superiorly between the widely separated lateral ventricles. The interhemispheric fissure extends back to the level of the third ventricle, transgressing the region which normally would be occupied by the corpus callosum. The optic nerves and chiasm are smaller than usual.

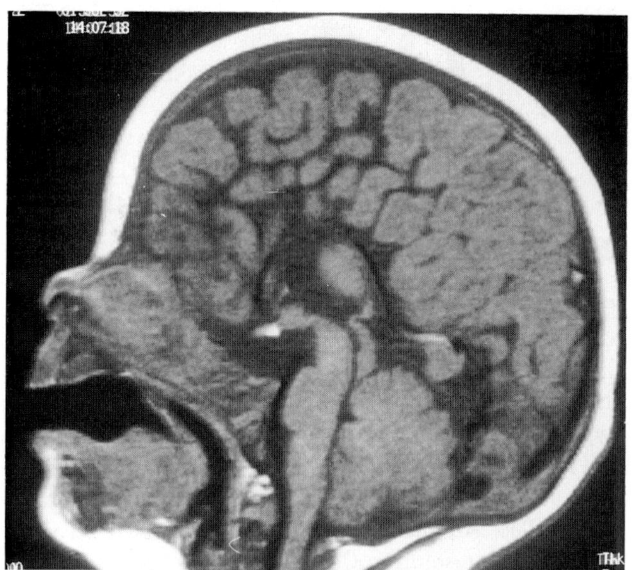

Fig. 20.23 Agenesis of the corpus callosum. Midsagittal T_1-weighted section. The corpus callosum is completely absent. The cerebral gyri on the medial surface of the hemisphere radiate down to the third ventricle. The optic chiasm, pituitary stalk, sella turcica and anterior pituitary gland are not evident. Posterior pituitary substance, reflecting high signal, is present in the region of the tuber cinereum.

Dysgenesis of the corpus callosum

Endocrine deficits are uncommon, but occur with the complete form, the anatomy of which is usually well shown on axial CT (Fig. 20.22) or MRI (Fig. 20.23). The loss of the supporting structure of the corpus callosum leads to separation of the lateral ventricles, widening of the third ventricle and superior extension of the roof of the ventricle between the hemispheres. The foramina of Monro are wide, and the deep cerebral white matter is generally underdeveloped, particularly in the region of the forceps major, resulting in dilatation of the trigones, occipital horns and posterior parts of the temporal horns, sometimes referred to as colpocephaly. The axons which have failed to cross in the corpus callosum form longitudinal bundles of myelinated fibres, which lie ventral to the cingula and are inverted on the medial surface of the hemispheres to form straight or medially concave medial walls of the laterally displaced ventricles.

The sulci and gyri on the medial surface of the hemispheres have an abnormal pattern, which is well shown on MRI. The predominant features include dysplasia of the central part of the cingulate gyri, with poor demarcation of the cingulate sulci. The parieto-occipital and calcarine sulci may fail to converge, so that the medial gyri and sulci radiate from the narrow inferior margin of the hemisphere.

Defects in neuronal migration are frequently associated with dysgenesis of the corpus callosum. This may result in focal cortical thickening intracerebral nodules or subependymal heterotopias forming non-calcified nodules of CT density and magnetic resonance intensity similar to grey matter, which may cause irregular protrusions into the lumen of the lateral ventricles.

Sphenoidal encephalocoele

The precise aetiology of this condition is uncertain. The cranial defect passes through the basisphenoid at the site of the craniopharyngeal canal which normally closes at 50 days of gestation. The typical clinical presentation is with obstruction of the nasopharynx, causing breathing difficulties or alteration of voice. Hypertelorism is constant, and there may be labial, palatine or median nasal fissures. Optic malformations are commonly associated and include unilateral coloboma or hypoplasia of the eye and orbit, optic nerve or chiasm hypoplasia and retinal defects. These craniofacial deformities should alert the clinican to the probability of a trans-sphenoidal encephalocoele when such patients present with endocrine defects.

Sphenoidal encephalocoeles are best demonstrated by coronal and sagittal MRI [46]. The bone defect involves the centre of the sellar floor and typically extends anteriorly to include the anterior wall of the sella, and may extend between the anterior clinoids or even into the ethmoid region; the dorsum sellae is always normal. The encephalocoele contains the inferior part of third ventricle, together with the infundibulum and the hypophysis. It is often difficult to precisely locate the optic chiasm, but it is likely to be within the encephalocoele in the majority of cases. The first segments of the anterior cerebral arteries are usually deviated inferiorly towards the encephalocoele.

Kallmann syndrome

Kallmann syndrome is a rare disorder with a frequency of 1 in 10 000 males and 1 in 50 000 females. It is most frequently transmitted by a specific gene on the X chromosome, and this form may be associated with renal abnormalities and ichthyosis due to deletion of a contiguous gene. The condition may also be inherited in an autosomal recessive manner, and it may then be associated with cleft lip and palate. In addition, an autosomal dominant form also occurs.

The association of anosmia and hypogonadism has been elegantly explained by recent immunohistochemical studies. At approximately 41 days of fetal life the olfactory placode situated high in the nasal fossa produces fibres and cells that migrate towards the telencephalic vesicle to form the olfactory nerves. The nerve fibres grow into the brain, and the olfactory bulbs are induced to develop as diverticuli from the telencephalic ventricles. These diverticuli are pinched off to form the olfactory ventricles; later the ventricles are obliterated to leave solid olfactory bulbs. Finally, the cartilaginous cribriform plate forms below the bulb around the bundles of the olfactory nerves. Cellular migration also occurs from the medial part of the olfactory placode to the region of the hypothalamus, and to the septum pellucidum to form the medial septal nuclei. These contain the cells which control gonadotrophin-releasing hormones (GnRH).

In Kallmann syndrome the olfactory axons fail to reach the brain, or to induce neuronal migration, resulting in olfactory hypogenesis or agenesis and absence of the GnRH cells. Using high-resolution MRI in the coronal plane, hypoplasia of the olfactory sulci and olfactory bulbs can be demonstrated. In some cases abnormally prominent soft tissue is shown in the region of the olfactory bulbs, which is consistent with arrest in an abnormal position of the migrating neurons [47].

THE PINEAL GLAND

The precise role of the pineal gland in the inhibitory control of gonadotrophin secretion, and in the timing of human puberty, is uncertain, but almost one-third of young male patients with pineal tumours develop precocious puberty [20].

The pineal gland is a cone-shaped structure, 5–9 mm in length and 3–6 mm in diameter, attached by a pedicle to the posterior border of the third ventricle, just above the entry of the cerebral aqueduct. A small diverticulum of the ventricle, the pineal recess, extends into the base of the gland, with the habenular commissure in its upper margin and the posterior commissure in its lower margin. The gland nestles in the quadrigeminal cistern in the groove between the superior colliculi, covered by the splenium of the corpus callosum. Thin neural strands of postganglionic sympathetic fibres from the superior cervical ganglia pass to the pineal along the tentorium in the region of the straight sinus.

The specific cells of the gland, pineocytes, are arranged in cords and follicles around fenestrated capillaries which do not have a blood–brain-type barrier. Between these cells there are astrocytes, and within the stroma of the gland there are many laminated calcareous structures, corpora aranacea. Ganglion cells in the habenular nuclei and base of the pineal gland transmit autonomic impulses from the anterior nuclei of the thalamus, hypothalamus, superior colliculi, tegmentum and the reticular formation. Sympathetic fibres project, via the thalamus and red nucleus, through the interpenduncular nucleus to the reticular formation.

In addition to precocious puberty in males, pineal tumours may present with diabetes insipidus without evidence of direct involvement of the hypothalamus. Involvement of the superior colliculi and accessory ocular motor nuclei may cause Parinaud syndrome, and blockage of the posterior part of the third ventricle or aqueduct may result in hydrocephalus.

Radiological features of the normal pineal gland

The incidence of calcification visible on routine skull radiographs varies between races, being evident in approximately 10% of adult Japanese, 20% of Indians and Africans, and 44% of Caucasians. It also varies with age; it is rare before 6 years, occurs in 2% up to the age of 8 years and 10% by the age of 15 years. Below the age of 6 years calcification in the pineal gland suggests the presence of a neoplasm; between 6 and 10 years it is suspicious and may be an indication for further elucidation by CT or MRI, as may any calcified gland with a diameter greater than 1.0 cm.

The solid pineal gland is similar to brain in CT density and MRI signal, and enhances with intravenous contrast media. CT reveals calcification in up to 30% of pineal glands at the age of 15 years. Asymptomatic pineal cysts are shown not infrequently on MRI as well-defined non-enhancing masses returning signals similar to CSF on T_1-weighted sequences, and sometimes of slightly higher intensity on moderately T_2-weighted sequences. Even when a little larger than 1.0 cm diameter and causing slight impression of adjacent structures, cysts are not usually considered significant.

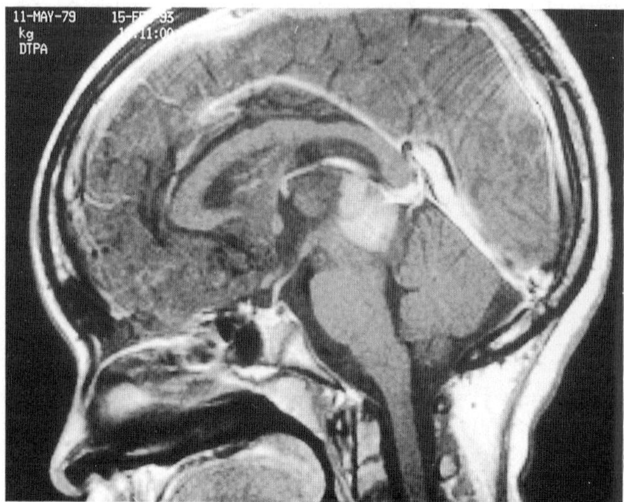

Fig. 20.24 Non-germinomatous germ-cell tumour. Sagittal T_1-weighted section made after gadolinium enhancement. An enhancing mass arising from the pineal gland encroaches into the posterior third of the third ventricle and extends into the upper half of the aqueduct, displacing posteriorly the superior corpora quadrigemina away from the tegmentum. The terminal part of the internal cerebral vein is elevated.

TUMOURS OF THE PINEAL REGION

These constitute 0.4–1.0% of all intracranial tumours. Those arising in the pineal gland itself may originate from germ cells, pineal cells or glial cells. Tumours may also originate in the adjacent brain substance, choroid plexus or in the meninges, and involve the pineal gland secondarily, but these tumours are not associated with endocrine disturbance.

All masses in this region tend to impress the posterior border of the third ventricle, to depress and compress the aqueduct, causing hydrocephalus, and to extend through the tentorium to impress the upper surface of the cerebellum. Extrinsic tumours compress the quadrigeminal plate and flatten the midbrain. Conversely, intrinsic tumours tend to enlarge the midbrain and expand the tectum. The multiplanar imaging facility of MRI demonstrates these anatomical changes to best advantage [48] (Fig. 20.24) and may also give an indication of the degree of vascularity of the mass, and the size of the blood vessels supplying it. Only when the exact disposition of the blood vessels is required for surgical planning is angiography generally indicated.

Tumours of germ-cell origin

Though rare, only 10–20 occurring in the UK per year, these are the commonest tumours of pineal origin. They are subdivided into germinomatous germ-cell tumours (GCTs) (65%), which rarely produce tumour markers, and non-germinomatous germ-cell tumours (NGCTs) in which the presence of high levels of α-fetoprotein and/or human chorionic gonadotrophin in the CSF is common and the level may give some indication of the histological composition of the tumour. They occur in childhood and have a marked male preponderence. GCTs are well-defined masses of homogeneous T_1 low and T_2 high signal on MRI, and of slightly greater than brain density on CT without calcification in the tumour matrix, though it may occur prematurely in the pineal gland substance. These tumours show intense uniform enhancement. They are well demarcated from the adjacent structures in the early stages, but tend to infiltrate and extend along the walls of the third ventricle in more advanced cases (Fig. 20.25). Haemorrhage into the tumour is not uncommon. Metastatic spread within the ventricles and subarachnoid space is common.

Non-germinomatous germ-cell tumours (Fig. 20.24) may show calcification within the tumour matrix and tend to undergo cystic haemorrhagic and necrotic changes resulting in non-enhancing regions on examinations made after intravenous contrast medium.

Differentiated teratomas which form a small proportion of NGCT constitute heterogeneous masses. In addition

Fig. 20.25 Germinoma (proven by biopsy). CT scan, axial sections at the level of the pineal gland: (a) plain; (b) enhanced. There is a mass of slightly higher than brain density, which enhances considerably, surrounding the calcified pineal gland and extending into the quadrigeminal cistern. There is enhancing tissue of slightly lower density around the left frontal horn, with a small hyperdense, possibly partly calcified nodule adjacent to the tip of the horn.

(a) (b)

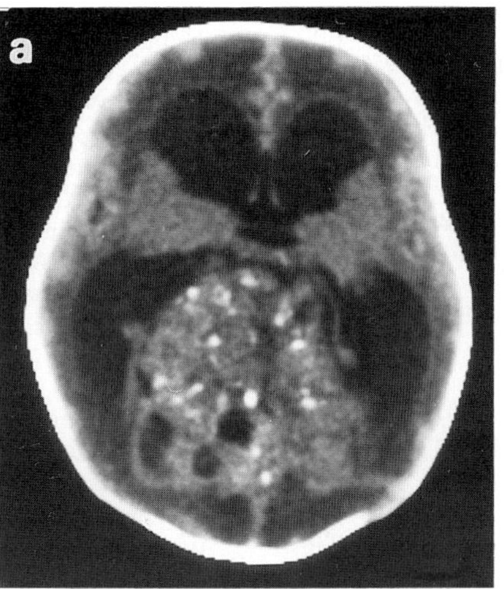

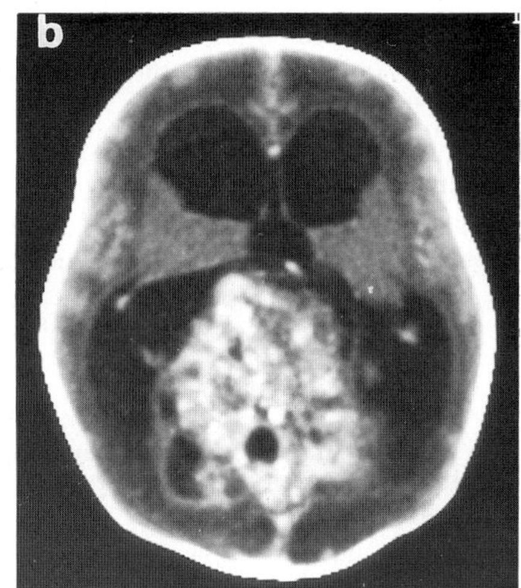

Fig. 20.26 Pineal region teratoma. CT scan, axial sections at level of pineal gland: (a) plain; (b) after intravenous contrast medium. The large tumour impresses the posterior margin of the third ventricle and separates the trigones. It has caused three ventricular hydrocephalus and low density in the hemispheric white matter due to retrograde passage of CSF through the ependyma. Most of the tumour is of higher than brain density and enhancing, but there are calcified and low-density, non-enhancing components, some of which are less dense than the CSF due to the presence of fat. These appearances are typical of a teratoma, which was confirmed at surgery.

to calcified areas and soft-tissue components with similar CT density and MRI signal to brain substance, but enhancing after intravenous contrast medium, the presence of fat is characteristic (Fig. 20.26), and ossification or tooth formation occasionally occurs. Haemorrhage into these tumours is common, and contributes to the heterogeneous appearance. The tumour may rupture with leakage of fat globules, which may remain free within the ventricular system but tend to become fixed, and may cause a chemical reaction associated with adhesion formation and hydrocephalus.

GCTs are curable by radiation; indeed the complete and rapid response to radiotherapy confirms a putative (radiological) diagnosis because biopsy can be very damaging. Other germ-cell tumours are also sensitive, but generally recur after a period of regression, and are most successfully treated with chemotherapy controlled by serial estimates of tumour markers.

Tumours of pineal cell origin

Pineoblastomas occur in children and pineocytomas in adults, and are distributed equally between the sexes. The matrix of the tumour is often calcified. The uncalcified tumour is usually of grey matter intensity on MRI and brain density on CT, and enhances after intravenous contrast medium. Though not specific, calcification throughout a pineal region tumour in a female patient suggests that it is of pineal cell origin.

Astrocytomas arising in the mesencephalic tectum and posterior part of the hypothalamus may invade the pineal region. They are usually of T_1 low and T_2 high signal, and of lower than brain density on CT. They may contain calcification and tend to enhance irregularly.

CONCLUSION

Taken together with the clinicobiochemical context, analysis of magnetic resonance images, supplemented when necessary by other neuroradiological studies, allows a confident diagnosis of most intracranial conditions presenting as a disturbance of endocrine function in the paediatric age group.

REFERENCES

1 Gluckman PD, Grumbach MM, Kaplan SL. The human foetal hypothalamus and pituitary gland. In: Tulchinsky D, Ryan KH, eds. *Maternal–Foetal Endocrinology*. Philadephia: WB Saunders, 1980.

2 Sage MR, Blumberg PC, Fowler GW. The diaphragma sellae: its relationship to normal sellar variations in frontal radiographic projections. *Radiology* 1982;145:699–701.

3 Turski PA, Neuton TH, Horlen BH. Sellar contour: anatomic polytomographic correlation. *Am J Roentgenol* 1981;137: 213–16.

4 Matsui T, Ueno I, Miki Y, Funchinoue T, Kobayashi N. Flattened sella turcica and CT appearance of normal pituitary gland. *Neuroradiology* 1984;26:75–7.

5 Wolpert SM, Molitch ME, Goldman JA, Wood JB. Size, shape and appearance of the normal pituitary gland. *Am J Roentgenol* 1984;143:377–81.

6 Bonneville JF, Cattin F, Moussa-Bacha K, Portha C. Dynamic computed tomography of the pituitary gland: the 'tuft sign'. *Radiology* 1983;149:145–8.

7 Mark L, Pech P, Daniels D, Charles C, Williams A, Haughton V. The pituitary fossa: a correlative anatomic and NMR study. *Radiology* 1984;153:453–7.

8 Sipponen P, Similä S, Collan Y, Autere T, Herva R. Familial syndrome with panhypopituitarism, hypoplasia of the hypophysis, and poorly developed sella turcica. *Arch Dis Child* 1978;53:644–7.

9 Syversen A, Haughton VM, Williams AL, Cusick JF. Computed tomographic appearance of the normal pituitary gland and pituitary microadenomas. *Radiology* 1979;133:385–91.

10 Elster AD, Chen MYM, Williams DW, Key LL. Pituitary gland: MR imaging of physiologic hypertrophy in adolescence. *Radiology* 1990;174:681–5.

11 Roppolo HMN, Latchaw RE. Normal pituitary gland: II. Microscopic anatomy – CT correlation. *Am J Neuroradiol* 1983;4:938–44.

12 Cox TD, Elster TD. Normal pituitary gland changes in shape, size and signal intensity during the first year of life on MR imaging. *Radiology* 1991;179:721–4.

13 Davis PC, Hoffman JC, Tindall GT, Braun IF. Prolactin-secreting pituitary microadenomas: inaccuracy of high resolution CT imaging. *Am J Roentgenol* 1985;144:151–6.

14 Seidel FG, Towbin R, Kaufman RA. Normal pituitary stalk size in children; a CT study. *Am J Roentgenol* 1985;145: 1297–302.

15 Brewer DB. Congenital absence of the pituitary gland and its consequences. *J Pathol Bacteriol* 1957;73:59–67.

16 Johnson JD, Hansen RC, Albritton WL, Wertemann U, Christiansen RO. Hypoplasia of the anterior pituitary and neonatal hypoglycemia. *J Pediatr* 1973;82:634–71.

17 Kelly WM, Kucharczyk W, Kucharcyzk J *et al.* Posterior pituitary ectopia: an MR feature of pituitary dwarfism. *Am J Neuroradiol* 1988;9:453–60.

18 Reid JD. Congenital absence of the pituitary gland. *J Pediatr* 1950;56:658–64.

19 Burrow GN, Wortzman G, Rewcastle NB, Holgate RC, Kovacs K. Microadenomas of the pituitary and abnormal sellar tomograms in an unselected autopsy series. *N Engl J Med* 1981;304:156–8.

20 Kitay TI. Pineal lesions and precocious puberty: a review. *J Clin Endocrinol Metab* 1954;14:622–5.

21 Mosier HD. Hypoplasia of the pituitary and adrenal cortex: report of occurrence in two siblings and autopsy findings. *J Pediatr* 1956;48:633–9.

22 Ehrlich RM. Ectopic and hypoplastic pituitary with adrenal hypoplasia. *J Pediatr* 1957;51:377–84.

23 Mize Y, Ball WS, Towbin RB, Han BK. Atypical CT and MR appearances of a Rathke cleft cyst. *Am J Neuroradiol* 1989; 10:S83–4.

24 Asari S, Ito T, Tsuchida S, Tsutsui T. MR appearances and cyst content of Rathke's cleft cysts. *J Comput Assist Tomogr* 1990;14:532–5.

25 Nemoto Y, Inouue Y, Fukuda T *et al.* MR appearance of Rathke's cleft cysts. *Neuroradiology* 1988;30:155–9.

26 Maggio WW, Cail WS, Brookeman JR, Persing JA, Jane JA. Rathke's cleft cyst: computed tomographic and magnetic resonance imaging appearances. *Neurosurgery* 1987;21:60–2.

27 Scotti, G, Chin-Yin Y, Dillon WP *et al.* MR imaging of cavernous sinus involvement by pituitary adenomas. *Am J Neuroradiol* 1988;9:657–64.

28 Ostrov SG, Quencer RM, Hoffman JC, Davis PC, Hasso AN, David NJ. Haemorrhage with pituitary adenomas. *Am J Neuroradiol* 1989;10:503–10.

29 Teasdale E, Teasdale G, Mohsen F, Macpherson P. High resolution computed tomography in pituitary microadenomas. *Clin Radiol* 1986;37:227–32.

30 Chambers EF, Turski PA, LaMasters D, Newton TH. Regions of low density in the contrast-enhanced pituitary gland: normal and pathologic processes. *Radiology* 1982;144: 109–13.

31 Parent AD, Bebin J, Smith RR. Incidental pituitary adenomas. *J Neurosurg* 1981;54:228–31.

32 Hinshaw DB, Hasso AN, Thompson AN, Thompson JR, Davidson BJ. High resolution computerised tomography of the post-partum pituitary gland. *Neuroradiology* 1984;26: 299–301.

33 Collins WF. Adenomas of the pituitary gland – an epidemic? *Surg Clin N Am* 1980;61:1201–6.

34 Carr D, Sandler LM, Joplin GG. Computed tomography of sellar and parasellar lesions. *Clin Radiol* 1984;35:281–6.

35 Posjunas KW, Daniels DL, Williams AL, Haughton VM. MR imaging of prolactin-secreting microadenomas. *Am J Neuroradiol* 1986;7:209–13.

36 Miki Y, Nishizawa S, Maksuo M *et al.* Pituitary adenomas and normal pituitary tissue: enhancement patterns on gadopentate enhanced MR imaging. *Radiology* 1990;177:35–8.

37 Hill SA, Falko JM, Wilson CB, Hunt WE. Thyrotrophin-producing pituitary adenomas. *J Neurosurg* 1982;57:515–19.

38 Wiener SN, Pearistein AE, Eiber A. MR imaging of intracranial arachnoid cysts. *J Comput Assis Tomogr* 1987;11: 236–41.

39 Boyko OB, Curnes JT, Oakes WJ, Burger PC. Hamartomas of

the tuber cinereum: CT, MR and pathological findings. *Am J Roentgenol* 1991;156:1053–8.

40 Burton EM, Ball WS Jr, Crane K *et al.* Hamartomas of the tuber cinereum: comparison of CT and MR findings in 4 cases. *Am J Neuroradiol* 1989;10:497–502.

41 Hubbard AM, Egelhoff JC. MR imaging of large hypothalamic hamartomas in two infants. *Am J Neuroradiol* 1989;10:1277.

42 Weisberg LA, Jacobs L. Clinical and computed tomography findings in intracranial sarcoidosis involving the juxtasellar region. *Comput Radiol* 1984;8:107–11.

43 Daningue JM, Wilson CB. Pituitary abcesses: report of 7 cases and review of the literature. *J Neurosurg* 1977;46:601–8.

44 Noel P, Hubert HP, Ectors M, Frankel L, Flaminent-Durand J. Agenesis of the corpus callosum associated with relapsing hypothermia. A clinico-pathological report. *Brain* 1983;96: 359–68.

45 Hoyt WF, Kaplan SL, Grumbach MM, Glaser JS. Septo-optic dysplasia and pituitary dwarfism. *Lancet* 1970;1:893–4.

46 Diebler C, Dulac O. Cephalocoeles: clinical and neuroradiological appearances. *Neuroradiology* 1983;25:199–216.

47 Truwit CL, Barkovich AJ, Grumbach MM, Martini JJ. MR imaging of Kallmann syndrome, a genetic disorder of neuronal migration affecting the olfactory and geneital systems. *Am J Neuroradiol* 1993;14:827–43.

48 Kilgore DP, Strother RJ, Haughton VM. Pineal germinoma MR imaging. *Radiology* 1986;158:435–8.

21: The Neurosurgical Approach to Hypothalamohypophyseal Tumours

M. POWELL and D. THOMPSON

INTRODUCTION

The hypothalamopituitary axis is vulnerable to compression or invasion by any mass lesion in the parasellar area. In childhood, craniopharyngioma is not only the most common parasellar lesion but also one of the commonest intracranial tumours, in contrast to adulthood where it is comparatively rare. Pituitary adenomas are less common in children, although they are by far the most common parasellar lesion (95% of all in the area) in adults. This chapter will concentrate on the presentation, diagnosis and surgical management of the two main tumours, and give an outline of the principles on management of the less common lesions. The possible lesions in the parasellar area are listed in Table 21.1.

CRANIOPHARYNGIOMA

Proximity to vital structures, relentless tendency for recurrence and resistance to surgical and medical therapies are combined in the craniopharyngioma to pose a formidable challenge to neurosurgical management. These features have been responsible for the controversies which continue to surround a tumour whose benign histological appearance belies its 'malignant' natural history.

Craniopharyngiomas comprise about 9% of intracranial childhood neoplasms [1] and show a peak incidence between 5 and 15 years of age. There is no consistent preponderance in either sex.

Embryology and pathology

Before the closure of the anterior neuropore, a diverticulum of the stomatodeum appears at the level of the buccopharyngeal membrane which is inclined dorsally towards an outpouching of the floor of the primitive diencephalon with which it comes into contact. This infundibulum from the neural plate retains its neural connection both anatomically and functionally in the form of the stalk and pars nervosa of the pituitary gland. The foregut diverticulum (hypophyseal recess or Rathke's pouch) meanwhile gives rise to the pars anterior, pars intermedia and pars tuberalis of the pituitary. The original connection with the stomatodeum gradually involutes. It is from squamous cell rests along the path of an incompletely involuted Rathke's pouch that the craniopharyngioma is believed to arise. This is invariably the case in childhood but about half of adult craniopharyngiomas show histological differences which have been cited in support of an origin from metaplasia of squamous cells within the pituitary gland itself [2], this form of the tumour having a more favourable prognosis.

The tumour is characterized by the presence of solid and cystic components. The solid component comprises trabeculae of (mainly) squamous cells in a stroma of connective tissue (Fig. 21.1). Degeneration of the stromal component may give rise to the cyst formation. Cysts are lined with an epithelium of variable thickness which may keratinize and desquamate. The cyst fluid contains cellular debris and large amounts of cholesterol crystals which can be clearly seen by their reflections of ambient light at the time of surgery. Although calcification is sometimes absent in the adult, it is seen in almost all childhood craniopharyngiomas and may vary from a grainy consistency to large and extremely hard concretions.

Craniophryngiomas have a tendency to excite an intense gliotic reaction in the adjacent brain parenchyma. The ease with which this can be used as a plane of tumour resection, however, varies markedly both between individuals and even within a particular tumour. Distinguishing between brain and tumour can be extremely difficult in the region of the hypothalamus and the integrity of the infundibulum and the pituitary stalk are at particular risk in such situations. Damage to these structures at the time of surgery can seriously compromise postoperative recovery and long-term functional outcome.

Anatomical relations and classification

Craniopharyngiomas arise in the pituitary stalk in remnants of the hypophyseal recess between the tuber cinereum and the pituitary gland. Rare reports of pharyngeal

Table 21.1 Intracranial pathology involving the hypothalamo-pituitary axis

Parasellar tumours
Glial origin
Hypothalamic and thalamic gliomas
Optic nerve gliomas
Colloid cysts
Other parasellar tissue origin
Pituitary adenomas
Germinomas
Meningiomas
Developmental cysts
Craniopharyngiomas
Rathke pouch cysts
Dermoids
Epidermoids
Hydocephalus
Inflammatory lesions
Granulomas
Postirradiation changes

craniopharyngioma attest the original full extent and origin of the hypophyseal recess. The occasional finding of posterior fossa and even intraventricular craniopharyngiomas is, however, less easy to reconcile with a purely embryological mechanism.

The growth of the tumour in relation to the adjacent anatomical structures (Fig. 21.2) significantly influences both the mode of presentation and the options for surgical treatment, and has been used as a basis of classification [3].

INTRASELLAR CRANIOPHARYNGIOMAS

These are confined below the diaphragma sellae. Local expansive growth may lead to erosion of the bony confines of the sella turcica with thinning of the clinoid process and the sella floor, through which the tumour may erode into the sphenoidal sinus. Lateral growth of an intrasellar craniopharyngioma can compress the cavernous sinus and the neural structures therein, sometimes presenting with cranial nerve signs.

The infundibular stalk lies immediately behind the optic chiasm and upward growth of the tumour brings it into direct relationship to the hypothalamus and chiasm. The relationship of the tumour to the chiasm is both of surgical and prognostic significance.

PRECHIASMATIC CRANIOPHARYNGIOMAS

These extend toward the planum sphenoidale, obliterating the prechiasmatic cerebrospinal fluid cistern. The tumour insinuates itself between the two optic nerves which become stretched and more vertically disposed, lifting both the chiasm and the anterior cerebral arteries in the process. This direction of growth brings the tumour in front of the lamina terminalis, so third ventricular involvement with risk of obstructive hydrocephalus is less likely.

RETROCHIASMATIC EXTENSION

Retrochiasmatic extension of craniopharyngiomas is seen most commonly [4]. The optic tracts are splayed and stretched in the process, and hypothalamic compression and obstruction of the third ventricle are most commonly seen in association with this type of craniopharyngioma. One-third of all retrochiasmatic cranipharyngiomas oc-

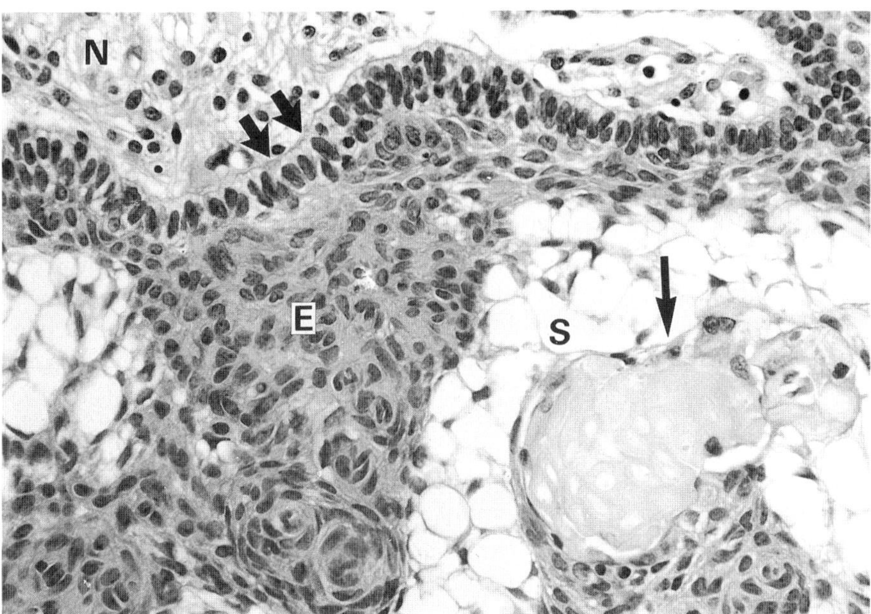

Fig. 21.1 Photomicrograph showing craniopharyngioma with: E, compact squamous epithelium; S, stellate reticulum; double arrow, peripheral palisading epithelial cells; arrow, keratinized nodule. Gliotic neural tissue can be seen at the periphery of the tumour. (Haematoxylin and eosin × 300.)

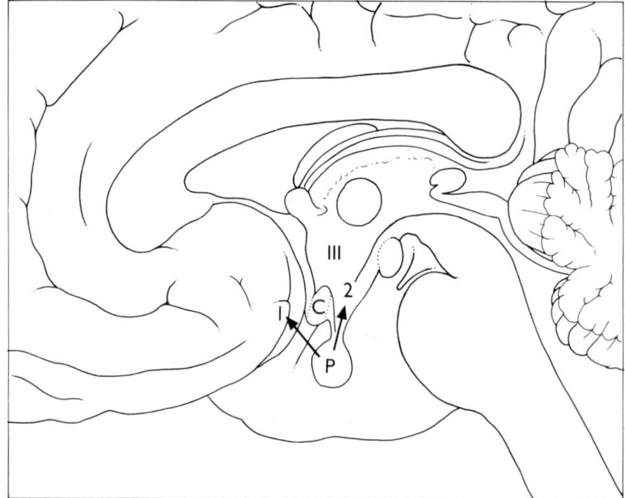

Fig. 21.2 Sagittal view of the brain illustrating directions of craniopharyngioma growth in relation to local anatomical structures: (1) prechiasmatic, (2) retrochiasmatic, (P) pituitary gland, (C) optic chiasm, (III) third ventricle.

cur in the under-10-years age group. Small perforating branches of the circle of Willis destined for the diencephalic structures are particularly vulnerable in these tumours, and severely compromise their safe surgical excision. Few are amenable to radical surgery and attempts to do so are associated with significant morbidity and mortality.

GIANT CRANIOPHARYNGIOMAS

On occasion, particularly in the paediatric age group, these tumours may reach large dimensions extending into all cranial fossae. They frequently comprise a number of loculated cysts, the walls of which may show heavy calcification.

ATYPICAL CRANIOPHARYNGIOMAS

This term encompasses a heterogeneous population of rarely encountered craniopharyngiomas, which are unusual in their anatomical localization in the pharynx, posterior fossa, within the ventricular system or in the region of the pineal gland, sites difficult to reconcile with the embryological aetiology proposed.

Clinical presentation

Raised intracranial pressure, ophthalmological impairment and endocrine disturbance are the principal modes of presentation. Headache and endocrine upset are more commonly seen in childhood, in contrast to visual impairment which is more likely to herald the diagnosis in adults (Table 21.2). Headache will accompany raised intracranial pressure and hydrocephalus in a number of instances, but may occur because of local meningeal distortion due to tumour growth.

Table 21.2 Presenting features (percentages) of craniopharyngiomas in adults and children

Complaint	Children	Adults
Headache	80	30
Nausea/vomiting	60	20
Visual loss	40	80
Short stature	30	15
Mentation defects	5	15
Diplopia	10	20

From Carmel [5].

Table 21.3 Endocrine anomalies at presentation in 45 cases of childhood craniopharyngioma

Endocrine abnormality	Frequency (%)
Hypopituitarism	91
Multiple hormone deficiency	83
Isolated hormone deficiency	9
Pituitary dwarfism	24
Hyperprolactinaemia	36
Galactorrhoea	4
Diabetes insipidus	41
Precocious puberty	0
Syndrome of inappropriate antidiuretic hormone secretion	0
Obesity	42
Emaciation	7

Adapted from Imura *et al.* [6].

Hypopituitarism of variable degree is the usual endocrine disturbance. The presenting endocrinological abnormalities were reviewed by Imura *et al.* [6] in 46 cases, and are summarized in Table 21.3. Isolated hormonal loss is usually of growth hormone but growth retardation is not common as a primary presenting feature, although height, height velocity and bone age are impaired in up to 90% of childhood cases at presentation [7]. Thomsett *et al.* [8] identified clinical evidence of growth retardation in 53% of a childhood series and established growth hormone deficiency in 72%. Diabetes insipidus, failure to develop secondary sexual characteristics and mild obesity are occasional associated findings. Pituitary dwarfism may be seen in those children whose disease began before puberty.

Visual impairment can relate to loss of acuity or fields, and may be secondary to direct pressure on the optic nerves, chiasm or tracts, or a consequence of papilloedema related to sustained elevated intracranial pressure. Visual field reductions are rather more common than defects of visual acuity. A bitemporal hemianopia associated with chiasmal compression is the classical deficit, but since the major compression may occur in the optic nerve, monocular visual loss or a homonymous hemianopia due to compression of the optic tract is also common. Visual loss can occur to an advanced degree in children before it becomes evident to observers, and may thus delay diagnosis.

Investigation

Endocrinological evaluation may be performed preoperatively to establish a baseline, but it is needed mainly after surgical intervention with or without radiotherapy to enable planning of long-term maintenance therapy. The preoperative identification of fluid balance and electrolyte disturbance secondary to diabetes insipidus, which can adversely affect neurological evaluation and put the child at risk during anaesthesia, is of particular surgical importance. Fluid replacement, combined with vasopressin therapy where indicated, should be instituted and closely monitored. Steriod treatment should be commenced preoperatively, its role being two-fold: firstly the correction of any hypophyseal–adrenal impairment produced by the tumour and secondly as a means of reducing local oedema in the vicinity of the tumour.

Good-quality imaging is essential to diagnosis and the planning of surgical intervention. Plain radiology of the skull may reveal calcification in the suprasellar region, enlargement of the sellar turcica or erosion of its walls. Computerized tomography (CT) and magnetic resonance imaging (MRI), however, are the mainstays of imaging modalities. The role of CT scanning in craniopharyngiomas and anatomically allied lesions is established [9]. CT scanning is able to delineate tumour extent and the solid/cystic composition (Fig. 21.3), although craniopharyngioma cyst fluid appearances may vary markedly on CT. The consequences of mass effect, such as hydrocephalus, are also revealed. Calcification is also particularly well demonstrated by CT.

MRI has been a further advance in the management of these tumours; although poor in the detection of calcification compared with CT, diagnostic sensitivity is improved, and the soft-tissue definition obtainable on MRI allows accurate preoperative determination of the position of the tumour in relation to the optic pathways, the circle of Willis and the sella (Fig. 21.4) [10].

Ophthalmological assessment should be routinely performed preoperatively. This will encompass assessment of visual acuity, visual fields and fundoscopy. Even in the very young child, electrophysiological tests using visual evoked potentials can identify these deficits. Repeated ophthalmological assessment will be performed regularly during follow-up, and can be a useful early indicator of recurrence.

Treatment

Patient survival statistics are an insufficient measure of therapeutic outcome in the management of craniopharyngioma. Reports of prolonged disease-free intervals following radical surgical extirpation of tumours may obscure the more perinent question of functional recovery. Profound psychosocial disability, behavioural lability, memory impairment and sleep disturbance in addition to the physical handicap of visual loss are the frequently recognized, although sometimes understated, long-term sequelae of craniopharyngioma surgery [10a,11,12]. The relative merits of surgery and radiotherapy in the primary treatment of craniopharyngioma have been the source of long-standing and continued debate.

Although total removal of the tumour remains the aim

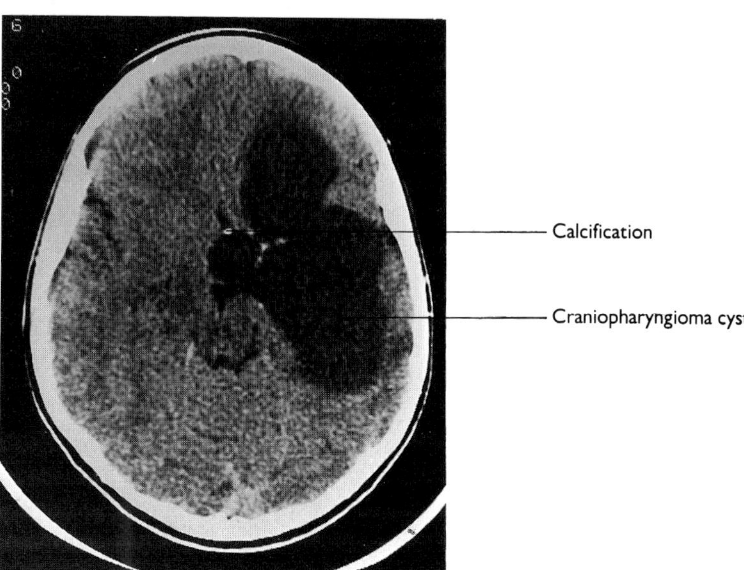

Fig. 21.3 Axial CT scan of a predominantly cystic craniopharyngioma. There is mural calcification and giant cyst formation which extends into the frontal, temporal and parietal lobes.

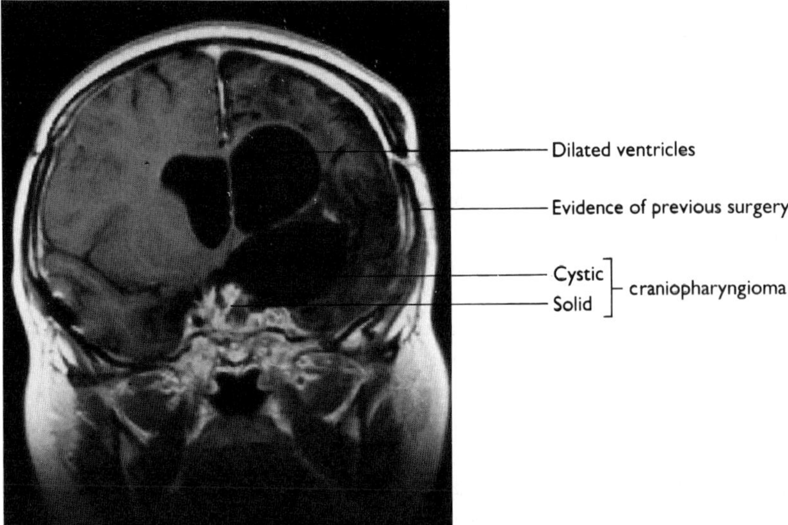

Fig. 21.4 Coronal MRI scan of a recurrent craniopharyngioma with solid and cystic components. The third ventricle has been obstructed producing hydrocephalus.

of neurosurgical management, this is clearly not possible in a significant proportion of cases. There are clinical and radiological features which may help to identify this poor prognostic group before surgery, and guide the surgeon toward adopting a more conservative approach in the resection or at least heighten his or her awareness to the potential hazards of attempting radical surgery. Hypothalamic dysfunction at the time of presentation manifested by weight increase, appetite disturbance, etc. indicates involvement of the extremely sensitive diencephalic structures. Attempts at radical removal in this instance carry risk of severe additional functional damage. Similarly, radiological characteristics such as hydrocephalus, large solid component (particulary if the hypothalamus is involved), thick cyst walls and tumour extending into adjacent cranial fossae suggest advanced tumour growth and should alert the surgeon to the potential dangers of embarking upon aggressive surgery. In these situations subtotal surgical resection with subsequent close clinical and radiological surveillance may help avert iatrogenic functional disability. Additional surgical procedures such as cyst drainage or repeat conservative surgery can then be carried out as necessary and radiotherapy delayed until the child is older (Fig. 21.5).

Surgery

The surgery of craniopharyngioma has been considerably advanced by the routine use of microsurgical techniques, which allow the sugeon much greater confidence in assessing the limits of safety in the extent of resection. The anatomical approach is largely dictated by tumour localization. In craniopharyngiomas that are entirely or mainly infradiaphragmatic, the trans-sphenoidal approach, more commonly used in pituitary adenoma surgery, can be employed either as a definitive treatment [13,14] or as part of a staged procedure [15]. The trans-sphenoidal approach is associated with lower operative morbidity than craniotomy in first-time surgery, and useful preliminary tumour decompression can be achieved by this route. The approach has been said to be associated with greater risk of postoperative pituitary failure in patients who had some preservation of pituitary function preoperatively. Despite the expected anatomical limitations in the paediatric patient, the trans-sphenoidal route is not precluded in this group assuming the sphenoidal air sinus is pneumatized.

Tumours with suprasellar extension require a craniotomy for definitive surgical treatment. Large sellar and prechiasmatic tumours are well visualized using a subfrontal approach. Following frontal craniotomy the frontal lobe is gently elevated, ideally on the non-dominant side, and the arachnoid of the chiasmatic cistern is opened between the elevated optic nerves to display the underlying tumour. In situations of predominantly retrochiasmatic extension, a pterional approach is advocated: elevation of the frontal lobe and posterior retraction of the temporal lobe provides a view of the tumour lying in the enlarged interval between the optic nerve and the internal carotid artery through which the resection can be performed.

It may sometimes be necessary to enter the third ventricle through the lamina terminalis or the corpus callosum in order to gain access to a tumour that has expanded into the ventricle and cannot be seen adequately by the extra-axial route. This manoeuvre must be performed with

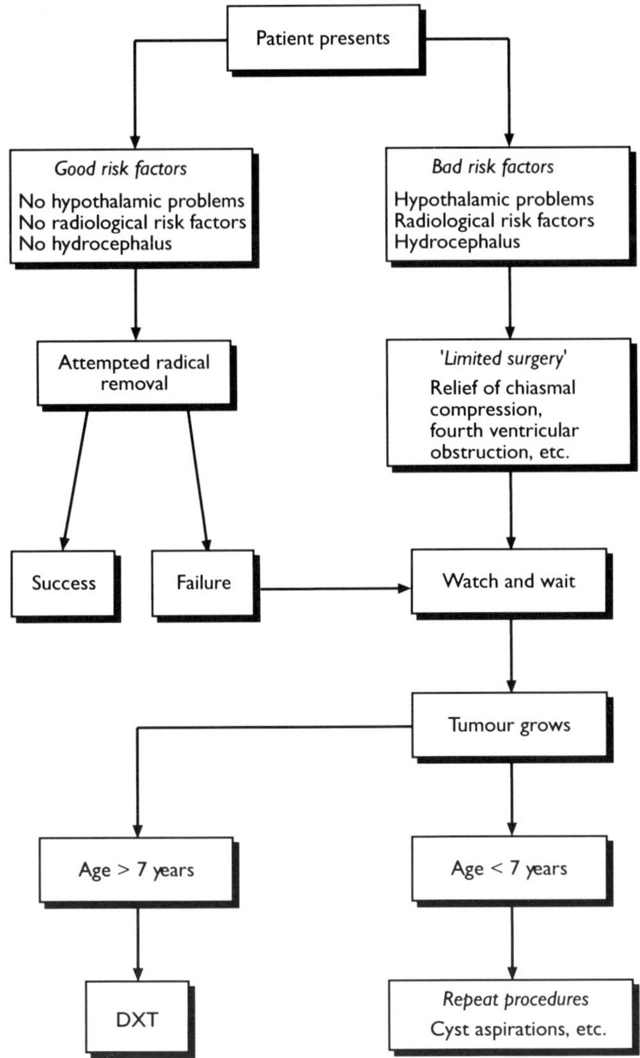

Fig. 21.5 Suggested management plan for childhood craniopharyngioma. DXT, radiotherapy (from Hayward RD, personal communication).

caution, since it has an increased risk of hypothalamic damage.

Once the tumour has been identified, thermocoagulation and incision of the cyst wall is usually possible. Microsuction and ultrasonic aspiration can be used to drain the cyst contents, thus decompressing the tumour internally and greatly facilitating the subsequent resection of the mural component which is gently teased from adjacent structures. The wall thickness varies markedly, and in places it may not be possible to identify a plane of cleavage between tumour and brain parenchyma: in such instances attempts at total resection are to be avoided.

Using these techniques total removal of craniopharyngioma is possible in a large proportion of cases [16,17]. Concern about the long-term consequences of irradiation of the nervous system in children, and the particular biological features of childhood craniopharyngioma with faster growth rates and greater propensity for recurrence [2,18], are used as arguments in favour of the radical approach. Yet despite radical surgery, tumour recurrence remains a significant problem. Seventeen of 45 childhood craniopharyngiomas treated by radical surgery recurred after a mean period of 2.5 years in a recent series [17]. Furthermore, the functional morbidity associated with radical surgical excision is great [19]. Level of employment and educational achievement may be more adversely affected by radical surgery than by more conservative surgery and radiotherapy [20].

Other surgical techniques which have a place in the management of craniopharyngiomas include cyst drainage and the insertion of silastic drainage catheters which can be attached to subcutaneous reservoirs; these allow repeated percutaneous aspiration, either for relief of symptoms attributable to cyst growth or the placement of radioactive sources for treatment. Stereotactic localization using computer-generated target measurements has allowed surgical access to relatively small symptomatic tumour cysts, enabling the surgeon to aspirate the cyst through a single burr-hole.

Radiotherapy

Radiotherapy has an effect on the tumour epithelium which can reduce the secretory potential and result in a reduced incidence of recurrence. When surgery is combined with radiotherapy the long-term outcome in terms of disease-free interval appears to be independent of whether the surgery was radical or subtotal [21]. Furthermore, the combination of conservative surgery and irradiation is better in terms of both reduced recurrence and functional outcome [7,19–22]. Baskin & Wilson [7] report a 91% remission rate in their series, and Fischer [20] observed only a 14% recurrence rate over a 10-year period.

The use of radiation for a benign pathology is of particular concern in a paediatric population. Delayed hypopituitarism, neuronal necrosis, optic neuritis, brain mineralization and induction of new neoplasms are all recognized sequelae of radiotherapy and, in childhood, there is the added concern of long-term intellectual development. It has not been established at what age radiotherapy can be used without this risk. An increasing body of neurosurgical opinion takes the view that, even following subtotal surgery, a policy of close clinical radiological follow-up should be pursued in children where possible.

Intracyst radiotherapy

The tendency towards cyst formation has been used to therapeutic advantage in craniopharyngioma management with the placement of localized radioactive sources via cyst reservoirs, so-called brachytherapy. The ideal properties for such an isotope are a β-emitter of high energy and short half-life [23]. Yttrium, gold and phosphorus have been used with good effect on cyst appearances when followed radiologically. The techniques is, however, limited to tumours with single or bilocular cysts of sufficient volume. There is no consensus on the most appropriate isotope or its dosage calculation. Furthermore, local neuronal toxicity is a problem, and worsening of already compromised visual function has been reported [24]. The precise role of brachytherapy in the management of craniopharyngioma is not established; at present its use is likely to be restricted to selected cases presenting particular problems.

The problem of recurrence

Despite the therapeutic armamentarium available, or the skill of the surgeon, recurrence remains an ever-present threat long after the initial treatment of craniopharyngioma. There are unfortunately no clearly identifiable histological features which serve to identify those tumours more likely to recur. The child who develops symptoms after treatment should be thoroughly investigated to exclude other causes for deterioration. The long-term effects of radiotherapy, endocrine imbalance, electrolyte disturbance secondary to diabetes insipidus and disordered cerebrospinal fluid circulation are some of the more commonly seen causes for late deterioration [25].

In the event of established recurrent tumour the therapeutic options are limited. Further surgery should be considered; this may involve a relatively straightforward procedure, such as the placement of a reservoir for cyst drainage. Repeat tumour resection is more difficult and more hazardous by any route other than the initial operation. Adherence to local blood vessels, loss of arachnoid planes and the possible tissue effects of previous radiotherapy are but some of the difficulties.

Additional radiotherapy can be of benefit, though it may result in optic nerve damage, compromising existing visual impairment, local brain damage and vascular changes. Stereotactically directed radiation can at best limit these effects.

Chemotherapy has been employed with some success [26]. Bleomycin injected into tumour cysts led to shrinkage and symptomatic improvement, though the treatment appeared to be more effective for cystic than for solid tumours, and the results have not been shared by others [19]. Other regimes of chemotherapeutic agents have been employed, but long-term results in adequate numbers of patients are awaited.

In summary, the goal of management of craniopharyngiomas must be tumour eradication with functional preservation, but this goal remains elusive in a large proportion of patients. The relative roles of surgery and radiotherapy in striving to achieve this aim continue to be a source of debate. The biological behaviour of craniopharyngiomas, their clinical presentation, the therapeutic options and longterm prognosis impose particular considerations with regard to the childhood form of the disease. Advances in neuroimaging and microsurgical techniques have had a considerable impact on operative management, but no single strategy of management or surgical approach can be considered appropriate for this capricious neoplasm. The surgeon requires a repertoire of approaches and techniques which can be adapted to the prevailing circumstances. Foremost in the mind of the neurosurgeon must remain the potential lifelong functional consequences of radical procedures. The doctrine of *primum non nocere* (first, do no harm) is paramount in this condition.

PITUITARY ADENOMAS

Although pituitary adenomas constitute 12–14% of adult intracranial tumours, in childhood they make up only 1–2%. Not only are they less common, but there are considerable differences in both frequency of tumour type and mode of presentation between childhood (Table 21.4) and adult adenomas. In adulthood, prolactinomas are the most common, usually presenting as a disturbance of menstrual cycle in women of reproductive age. 'Acromegalic' growth hormone-secreting tumours and non-secreting tumours make up the second and third most common types, and 'Cushing' tumours secreting adrenocorticotrophic hormone (ACTH) are relatively infrequent.

Prolactinomas seldom present in childhood, although they can cause delayed pubenty. The characteristic dis-

Table 21.4 Paediatric pituitary adenoma series (percentages)

	ACTH	Prolactin	Non-secreting tumours	GH	TSH
Laws *et al.* [27]*	28.9 (7–19)	57.0 (12–19)	1.3 (18)	11.8 (15–19)	1.3 (18)
Ludeke *et al.* [28]	42.3	30.7	–	–	26.9
Wilson [29]*	39.6	39.6 (12–19)	–	13.5	–

* American series include children to the age of 19. Age ranges where available are given in parentheses.
ACTH, adrenocorticotrophic hormone; GH, growth hormone; TSH, thyroid-stimulating hormone.

turbance of the menstrual cycle may come to notice in the final years of paediatric care. The few existing series of paediatric pituitary adenomas (Table 21.4) cite this type infrequently, except in American series which include the later teenage years. Gigantism in children is also uncommon, although many acromegalic adults are very tall and the condition must have originated in childhood. Cushing disease is more common in paediatric practice. If the androgenic features are prominent, a failure of growth may not be very obvious. The diagnosis is easy when the child is small and has the other features of Cushing disease. Large non-secreting tumours, although rare, are most likely to present with growth problems, for children seldom report visual symptoms until they are virtually blind.

Embryology and pathology

Pituitary adenomas derive from the anterior part of the pituitary gland and are probably monoclonal, that is, deriving from a single cell undergoing loss of replication control. Most adenomas in children are microadenomas, technically under 1 cm but in practice often far smaller, often in the range of 3–5 mm. On the rare occasions that paediatric pituitary tumours extend outside the pituitary fossa, as in adulthood, they usually grow upwards into the suprasellar recess, compressing the optic chiasm, although lateral extension through the cavernous sinus also occurs.

The pituitary gland is bounded laterally by the cavernous sinuses. This complex venous structure containing the carotid siphon and the third, fourth and sixth cranial nerves poses little barrier to lateral extension of the larger tumours. Once invasion into the sinus occurs, tumour removal becomes a very difficult technical problem. Fortunately this is relatively rare in paediatric practice. Small tumours, however, lying alongside the medial wall of the cavernous sinus are easy to overlook at surgery. In the majority of normal-sized fossae, there is a fold of arachnoid, which dips down in front of the anterior lobe of the gland and becomes the source of cerebrospinal fluid leaks if torn during a trans-sphenoidal surgical exploration.

The pituitary fossa lies within the sphenoid air sinus. Pneumatization of this sinus is complete by 4 years and thus before the age of presentation of the majority of these tumours, however, a non or partially pneumatized fossa is not a bar to surgical exploration, as access can be obtained using the high-speed air drill to remove the obstructing bone.

Clinical presentation

CUSHING DISEASE

ACTH-secreting adenomas, causing Cushing syndrome, make up half of most paediatric series of pituitary adenomas, except those including a majority of adolescent prolactinoma patients. The management of Cushing disease has undergone significant improvement since the introduction of MRI and inferior petrosal sinus sampling with corticotrophin-releasing factor (CRF) stimulation. The new imaging technology identifies 70–80% of all intracellular microadenomas—a significant improvement over the best of CT scanning. Venous sinus sampling differentiates, absolutely, Cushing disease from peripheral ectopic ACTH production, such as from a carcinoid tumour or bronchial carcinoma, although it is less accurate in terms of lateralizing the tumour nodule within the fossa, especially in children in whom venous mixing from the two sides complicates the issue.

In paediatric practice the incidence of ectopic ACTH production is so low as not to warrant consideration in the majority of cases. Furthermore the identification of a lesion on MRI makes surgical exploration mandatory, thus avoiding the need for an unpleasant radiological examination.

Although, in adult practice, conclusive evidence and localization of a Cushing tumour is now very much more efficient, in paediatric practice radiological demonstration of the lesion is not as successful. Professor Wilson states that only approximately 45% of paediatric Cushing tumours are localized on modern high-quality MRI (personal communication).

PROLACTINOMAS

Prolactinomas make up the bulk of adult pituitary practice. Presentation in the child is unusual, occurring almost exclusively in adolescent girls in whom the failure of menarche leads to the investigation of sex hormone and thus prolactin levels. Prolactinomas in teenage or younger boys are exceedingly rare but, as in adult practice, the presentation is usually with visual disturbance rather than failure of secondary sexual characteristics.

GROWTH HORMONE-SECRETING TUMOURS

Acromegaly presents in children as gigantism. Reports exist of children of toddler age presenting with the classic feature of acromegaly. Endocrinological diagnosis in adults is made on the demonstration of both raised resting growth hormone (GH) and the failure of suppression of GH to below 2 ng/ml following a glucose load. In the child GH levels may already be raised as part of the consequences of normal growth, and the decision that growth rate is abnormally high may be difficult.

MRI should show the lesion, usually a microadenoma. Wilson reports that half his personal series of children with gigantism from GH-secreting tumours had large aggressive semi-malignant tumours (C.B. Wilson, personal communication).

OTHER PITUITARY TUMOURS

Both non-secreting and thyroid-stimulating hormone (TSH)-secreting tumours in childhood have been reported, but are extremely rare. The former, although relatively common in adulthood, has not been seen by this author in a child. In adulthood, presentation is with a combination of optic chiasmal compression, headaches and panhypopituitarism in one-third of cases. Non-secreting tumours may often contain active granules on immunocytochemical staining, such as follicle-stimulating hormone (FSH), luteinizing hormone (LH) or precursor hormones. Nevertheless their expression as hormone syndromes is unknown. TSH-secreting tumours constitute the rarest of all pituitary adenomas. This author has the experience of only one such tumour in adulthood, and none in paediatric practice, although anecdotal reports of such tumours do exist in which the child presents with mild thyrotoxicosis.

Investigation

Investigation of the patient with a pituitary adenoma has two parts: endocrine and radiological.

Endocrine investigations are dealt with in detail elsewhere in this book. All children referred to this author have had an extensive endocrine workup covering every aspect of pituitary function.

Radiology of the pituitary has undergone great improvement since the introduction of CT techniques. Since the first reconstructed sella pictures from early CT, which seldom gave much information with regard to sella pathology except in the most gross of cases, there have been impressive advances. Dynamic coronal CT scanning using fourth-generation CT scanners (such as the Somaton DRG and GE9800) can, in expert hands, identify tumours of 3–4 mm in size (Fig. 21.6).

Over the past 5 years, high magnet strength MRI (1.5 Te) with gadolinium enhancement has given the best information to date, and virtually replaced CT.

Both CT and MRI techniques require considerable skill, particularly in children. In coronal dynamic CT, positioning is all-important, so that the slightest movement can ruin the images obtained, and is also uncomfortable with the head tipped far back. As the scan is 'dynamic', depending on the changes between sequential images after a bolus dose of contrast, a failure cannot be repeated for approximately 24 h, until the contrast has been excreted completely. The technique, quite apart from the long-term dangers of radiation, is not suitable for restless and uncooperative children. It is also less accurate than the best MRI.

MRI with gadolinium enhancement, paticularly if dynamic enhancement sequences can be used, gives the best chance of showing a microadenoma down to a size of 3–5 mm. The technique is not foolproof and is accurate only in a maximum of 80% of cases. Small cystic areas within the gland need not necessarily be tumour, although they are usually identified as such until surgery. MRI scanning is a noisy and claustrophobic experience, and movement significantly degrades the images, so that there are practical limitations on scanning small children, which cannot as easily be overcome by anaesthetizing the child as with CT.

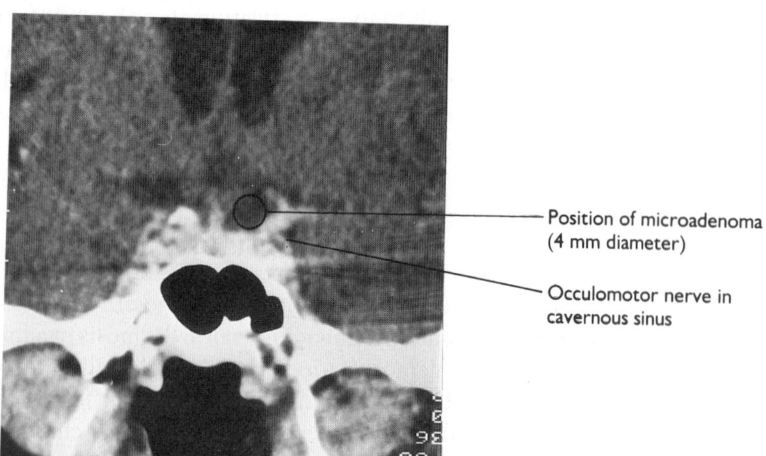

Fig. 21.6 Coronal CT image (postcontrast) of a microadenoma in Cushing disease. The occulomotor nerve can be seen.

Surgery

SURGICAL STRATEGY

All paediatric pituitary tumours requiring surgery should be operated via the trans-sphenoidal route. There is no justification for 'first-approach' transcranial surgery in the child. Virtually all tumours are small, and good endocrine results cannot be obtained through a subfrontal or pterional craniotomy. Even large tumours can usually be decompressed satisfactorily using the trans-sphenoidal route. This approach is very little different from that used in the adult, although the scale is smaller and the surgeon's touch is therefore required to be rather more delicate.

The child should have a confirmed endocrine diagnosis, and where possible a radiological localization of the tumour, which if present can allow the surgery to proceed to selective adenomectomy, plus removal of a thin rim of adjoining normal gland, which will often contain tumour cell nests. If the tumour is not localized, the surgeon must use radiological pointers. These include pituitary stalk deviation away from the tumour, unilateral thinning or slight ballooning of the sella floor or unilateral upward bulging of the fossa diaphragm.

In the event of these pointers being present a careful search is made on the side suggested by the pointers, and if a microadenoma is found, selective adenomectomy is performed with a thin rim of the normal tissue as before. If there are no pointers and no tumour is found, the surgeon must take a chance and resect according to clinical suspicion. It is important to discuss the failure rate of surgery with parents before the procedure and to discuss strategies if a cure is not obtained the first time. A second or even a third exploration is always possible and parents usually agree to this if a careful plan is put forward.

If the tumour is large, even if it is invasive or multilobular, there is little to be lost by attempting a trans-sphenoidal approach first. The tumours are usually soft and suckable, and various safe manoeuvres are available for bringing the tumour into the fossa. If trans-sphenoidal surgery fails the child can be given a craniotomy.

SURGICAL TECHNIQUE

Trans-sphenoidal approach (Fig. 21.7)

The child is anaesthetized and a throat pack placed. The nose is prepared with otrovine drops to constrict the nasal mucosa and thus minimize blood loss. The child is positioned supine with slight head uptilt and the neck extended. The thigh is prepared for a fascia lata graft in case of a peroperative cerebrospinal fluid leak, caused by perforation of the arachnoid layer over the dome of the gland.

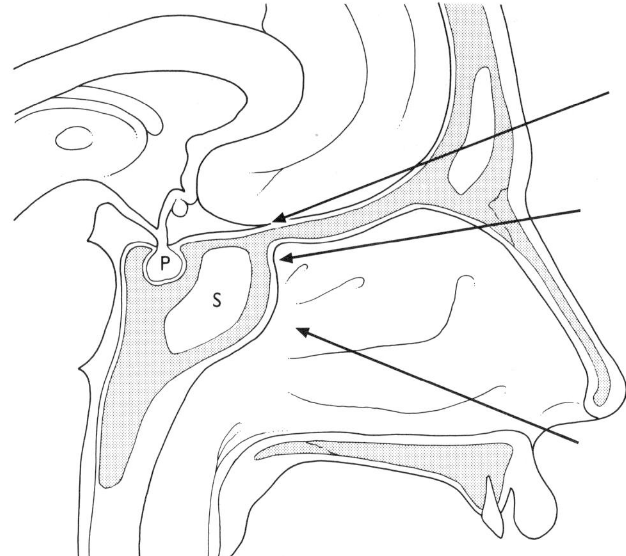

Fig. 21.7 Diagram illustrating the surgical approaches to the pituitary gland. Transcranial (upper arrow), transethmoidal (middle arrow) and trans-sphenoidal (lower arrow). P, pituitary; S, sphenoid bone.

The 'C' arm of the image intensifier is placed laterally to allow a true lateral view of the skull. This device is not always needed, but it is difficult to bring into position if wanted after the procedure has started. The operating microscope is prepared with a 300 mm or longer focal-length lens.

There are a variety of approaches to the sphenoid air sinus, this author preferring the 'endonasal' approach of Landolt, which offers the easiest route with the least trauma to the nose, as well as the least scar tissue should repeat surgery be neccessary (see Fig. 21.4). A submucosal pocket along the nasal septum is created using a small incision along the columella inside the right nostril, and the cartilage mobilized to the left. The bony septum is removed and the sinus entered in the midline at the vomer (the base of the bony septum) at the sphenoid ostia. The sinus mucosa is stripped and the septum, which is usually in the midline, removed. The floor of the pituitary fossa is then opened with a diamond burr, and the opening extended with 1 and 2 mm upcut bone punches to the cavernous sinus laterally and the floor of the anterior fossa superiorly. The intercavernous sinuses are identified and the dura of the fossa opened between these venous lakes to expose the anterior surface of the pituitary gland.

The tumour may be obvious on the surface of the gland as a white creamy soft tumour, in which case it may be possible to dissect it out as one or, failing that, piecemeal; an adjacent 'normal' fringe of gland is removed along with it. If no tumour is seen a grid pattern of exploratory incisions into the gland is made until the tumour is identified, when it is removed as above. If no tumour is seen, a previously agreed plan for removal of half the gland is usually performed. It is important to inspect the lateral border of the gland where it abuts the cavernous sinus, as tumour may lie alongside this part.

Haemostasis is seldom a major problem, and CSF leaks are infrequent. If all is well, the nose can be closed without a permanent repair to the fossa floor, which will reconstitute itself within a few months. If a leak has occurred, a fascial graft will incorporate as a watertight seal within 2 days, although this incorporation is considerably aided by a lumbar drain during this period. The nose is gently packed with soft sponges, which are removed the next day.

The child can be up and about the following day, if a cerebrospinal fluid leak is not present, and usually leaves hospital at about 5–7 days, the endocrine management usually being the determining factor in hospital stay beyond the fourth postoperative day.

Transcranial approach

The child is anaesthetized and a bicoronal skin flap made with either a limited or minimal head shave. This incision gives the best cosmetic result. A small bone flap is made, based on the right pterion, the outer point of the wing of the sphenoid. Most UK neurosurgeons use a myoplastic flap leaving the muscle attached to supply blood to the bone, although this is not strictly necessary in a child. The dura is opened and the posterior frontal lobe gently elevated along the sphenoid ridge to the right optic nerve, and the carotid behind. The tumour is usually found in the space between and in front of the two optic nerves. The tumour is gently separated from the pia of the adjacent brain, entered and gutted from within. The capsule of the tumour is then peeled from the surrounding structures and the remnants of the capsule carefully coagulated to control any bleeding points. Both the optic chiasm and the pituitary stalk are usually easily seperated. Identification of the normal gland is often more difficult in this approach, but it is usually a flattened structure above the tumour attached to the stalk. Once tumour removal is achieved, the skull and scalp are reconstructed. The child may often be up and about the following day, and the same restrictions on time in hospital apply as with the trans-sphenoidal approach.

Postoperative management

IMMEDIATE MANAGEMENT

While the child is still in hospital, the most imporant part of early management is to assess the residual posterior lobe pituitary function.

The child has cortisol cover during the procedure, and needs this reduced to replacement levels in the days following. In children, as in adults, with Cushing disease the cortisol replacement is usually left at a level above normal for a period, until the residual normal corticotrophs resume ACTH output. This may be several months later. The choice of replacement is between hydrocortisone (15 mg/m^2 a day in two divided doses) and prednisolone (4 mg/m^2 a day). The other anterior pituitary hormone levels are less critical in the early period but thyroxine levels may sometimes fall precipitately. Posterior lobe function is usually intact after pituitary surgery and the passing of large volumes of dilute urine cannot be taken as evidence of diabetes insipidus without demonstrating a low urine osmolality in the presence of a high plasma value. In the first 24 h there is often a mild diuresis, which is physiological and can be ignored, and thirst related to mouth breathing through a temporarily blocked nose. Desamino-D-arginine vasopressin (DDAVP) (1 μg intramuscularly) is given to control diabetes insipidus until the nasal mucosa recovers when DDAVP is given as a spray. Ultimately, the majority of postoperative diabetes insipidus disappears in the ensuing months.

LONG-TERM MANAGEMENT

The aim of surgery is to remove the tumour while retaining normal function. Endocrine cure is established by repeating the diagnostic tests that established the condition. Cure rates for the different tumour types are well known, and depend on the size and position of the tumour in the fossa, its relationship to the normal gland and, most of all, the absence of presence of cavernous sinus invasion. Small central tumours have a better than 80% cure rate with surgery. Laterally placed tumours have a slightly lower cure rate, and if sinus invasion has occurred the cure rate falls dramatically. The larger tumours, especially with suprasellar extension, also have a lower cure rate, falling to 35–40% for the largest. Conversely, if no tumour is found, the chances for cure also fall.

If surgery fails it may be repeated, as radiotherapy is not particularly successful in controlling Cushing disease and, although successful with acromegaly, controls the disease slowly, taking a number of years. There are now well-recognized long-term dangers of radiotherapy in pituitary failure and second tumour induction, quite apart from the effect on intellect and general brain growth.

OTHER PARASELLAR LESIONS

Glial origin

The common tumours of childhood in this category are optic nerve gliomas (ONGs) (3.6% [1]) and thalamic low-grade astrocytomas (TLGAs) (9% [29]). MRI diagnosis is extremely accurate, and it is questionable whether surgery should be involved, except to control hydrocephalus, since ONGs are likely only to have effects on the hypothalamopituitary axis if within the optic chiasm and tract. In these axis they are irresectable, and the only use for surgery would be to confirm diagnosis by biopsy in aggressive progressive tumours. Similarly, the only effective use for surgery in TLGAs is in biopsy, in which case CT-guided systems would be used.

Other parasellar tumours

Pituitary tumours, the commonest lesions in the area, have been covered in detail above. Meningiomas from the planum sphenoidale and cavernous sinus are extremely uncommon in childhood (<0.4% [1]). In adulthood, these tumours seldom affect the hypothalamopituitary axis, except by mild 'stalk effect' causing mildly raised prolactin levels and consequent disturbance of the menstrual cycle. Surgical removal is the only cure, and is carried out through a pterional or subfrontal craniotomy. Germinomas and teratomas (1.2% and 0.9% [29]) may be found in the parasellar area causing disturbance of growth or puberty. Both should be approached by craniotomy, altough complete resection may be impossible. Teratomas in the pineal region in boys may also lead to growth disorder through the development of precocious puberty.

Developmental cysts

The management of dermoids, epidermoids and other non-inflammatory cysts of the parasellar area, such as that of Rathke's cleft origin, is surgical. Their rarity, even in adults, makes generalization difficult. All may cause compression of the hypothalamopituitary axis. When symptoms arise from expansion which threatens vision, and, if it is possible through an expanded fossa, it is reasonable to approach these lesions via the trans-sphenoidal route; if not, a craniotomy may be necessary.

Inflammatory parasellar lesions

Pituitary abscess is the only inflammatory lesion that may directly affect the sella itself, although tuberculous and mycotic granulomas may be found in the parasellar area. Both types of lesion are very rare and should be managed by craniotomy and the appropriate antibiotic or antimycotic therapy.

Hydrocephalus

Many intracranial lesions may cause hydrocephalus by blockage of cerebrospinal fluid pathways, either within the brain or the basal cerebrospinal fluid cisterns, either at the time of presentation or through their subsequent treatment. Enlargement of the third ventricle may, through downward pressure on the hypothalamus, cause disorders of the hypothalamopituitary axis. The pressure may lead to precocious puberty. Treatment of hydrocephalus is a complex subject, but in principle, if the primary cause is irreversible, the child will need some form of cerebrospinal fluid diversion. At present the most reliable form of this is the ventriculoperitoneal shunt.

REFERENCES

1 Matson DD. *Neurosurgery of Infancy and Childhood*, 2nd edn. Springfield: Thomas, 1969.

2 Khan E, Gosch H, Seeger J *et al.* Forty-five years experience with craniopharyngiomas. *Surg Neurol* 1973;1:5–12.

3 Rougerie J. What can be expected from the surgical treatment of craniopharyngiomas in children. *Childs Brain* 1979;5: 443–9.

4 Hoffman H. Craniopharyngiomas. *Prog Exp Tumor Res* 1987; 30:325–34.

5 Carmel P. Craniopharyngiomas. In: Wilkins RH, Rengacharry SS, eds. *Neurosurgery*. New York: McGraw Hill, 1985:905–16.

6 Imura H, Kato Y, Nakai Y. Endocrine aspects of tumours arising from suprasellar, third ventricular regions. *Prog Exp Tumor Res* 1987;30:313–24.

7 Baskin D, Wilson C. Surgical management of craniopharyngiomas. A review of 74 cases. *J Neurosurg* 1986;65:22–7.

8 Thomsett M, Conte F, Kaplan S, Grumbach M. Endocrine and neurological outcome in childhood craniopharyngiomas. Review of the effects of treatment in 42 patients. *J Paediatr* 1980;97:728–35.

9 Nadich T, Pinto R, Kushner M *et al.* Evaluation of sellar and parasellar masses by CT. *Radiology* 1976;120:91–9.

10 Karnaze M, Sartor K, Winthrop J, Gado M, Hodges F. Suprasellar lesions: evaluation with MR imaging. *Radiology* 1986;161(1):77–82.

10a Palm L, Nordin V, Elmqvist D, Blennow G, Persson E, Westgren U. Sleep and Wakefulness after treatment for craniopharyngioma in childhood; influence on the quality and maturation of sleep. *Neuropaediatrics* 1992;23(1):39–45.

11 Galatzer A, Nofar E, Beit-Halachmi N *et al.* Intellectual and psychosocial functions of children, adolescents and young adults before and after operation for craniopharyngioma. *Child Care Health Dev* 1981;7:307–16.

12 Cavazzuti V, Fisher EG, Welch K, Bell JA, Winston KR. Neurological and psychophysiological sequelae following different treatments of craniopharyngioma in children. *J Neurosurg* 1983;59:409–17.

13 Landholt A, Zachmann M. Results of transphenoidal extirpation of craniopharyngiomas and Rathke's cysts. *Neurosurgery* 1991;28:410–15.

14 Honnegger J, Buchfelder M, Fahlbusch R, Dauble B, Dorr H. Transphenoidal microsurgery for craniopharyngioma. *Surg Neurol* 1992;37:189–96.

15 Kobayashi T, Nakane T, Kageyama N. Combined transphenoidal and intracranial approach for craniopharyngioma surgery. *Prog Exp Tumor Res* 1987;30:341–9.

16 Yasergill M, Curcic M, Kis M, Siegenthaler G, Teddy P, Roth P. Total removal of craniopharyngiomas. *J Neurosurg* 1990; 75:3–11.

17 Hoffman H, De Silva M, Humphreys R, Drake J, Smith M, Blaser S. Aggressive surgical management of craniopharyngioma in children. *J Neurosurg* 1992;76:47–52.

18 Hoff JT, Patterson RH. Craniopharyngiomas in children and adults. *J Neurosurg* 1972;36:299–302.
19 Fischer E, Welch K, Schillito J, Winston K, Tarbell N. Craniopharyngiomas in children. Long-term effects of conservative surgical procedures combined with radiation therapy. *J Neurosurg* 1990;73:534–40.
20 Graham P, Gattmaneni H, Birch J. Paediatric craniopharyngiomas: a regional review. *Br J Neurosurg* 1992;6(3):187–93.
21 Rajan B, Ashley S, Gorman C *et al.* Craniopharyngioma – long term results following limited surgery and radiotherapy. *Radiother Oncol* 1993;26(1):1–10.
22 Wen D, Seljeskog E, Haines S. Microsurgical management of craniopharyngiomas. *Br J Neurosurg* 1992;6(5):467–74.
23 Kobayashi T, Kagemyama N, Ohara K. Internal irradiation for cystic craniopharyngioma. *J Neurosurg* 1981;55:896.
24 Van der Berge J, Blaauw G, Breeman W, Rahmy A, Wijngaarde R. Intracavity brachytherapy of cystic craniopharyngiomas. *J Neurosurg* 1992;77(4):545–50.
25 Sweet WH. Recurrent craniopharyngiomas: therapeutic alternatives. *Clin Neurosurg* 1980;27:206–29.
26 Takahashi H, Nakazawa S, Shimura T. Evaluation of postoperative intratumoural injection of bleomycin for craniopharyngioma in children. *J Neurosurg* 1985;62:120–7.
27 Laws ER. Sheithauer BW, Groover RV. Pituitary adenomas in children and adolescence. *Prog Exp Tumor Res* 1987;30:359–61.
28 Ludecke DK, Herrman H-D, Schulte FJ. Special problems with neurosurgical treatment of hormone secreting pituitary adenomas in children. *Prog Exp Tumor Res* 1987;30:362–70.
29 Hoffman HJ. Supratentorial brain tumors in children. In: Youman JR, ed. *Neurological Surgery*. Philadelphia: WB Saunders, 1982:2702–32.

22: Thyroid, Adrenal and Pancreatic Surgery

R.C.G. RUSSELL

INTRODUCTION

Endocrine conditions requiring surgical intervention are uncommon in the paediatric age group. When diagnosed, such problems are a source of great interest and, often, considerable debate. This is understandable since few centres (and even fewer individual surgeons) can draw on a wealth of experience. A great divergence of opinion regarding management is understandable in that paediatric endocrine lesions often differ from their adult counterparts in histology, natural history and response to treatment [1]. Paediatric endocrine tumours are also less frequently malignant. In addition to the great strides made in surgical and anaesthetic technique and operative monitoring, progress in three areas has substantially advanced the surgical management of endocrine disorders in the past decade: imaging, pathology and pharmacology.

The new imaging tools of ultrasonography, computerized tomography (CT) (particularly the recent introduction of spiral CT) and magnetic resonance imaging (MRI) have provided the surgeon with an anatomical map on which he or she can design the operation. The need for the explorative laparotomy has largely been displaced.

Developments in the field of tagged antibodies and radiopharmaceuticals create opportunities for accurate localization of aberrant structures so that a blind procedure is outdated.

The combination of accurate imaging with fine-needle aspiration biopsy enables a core of tissue to be so characterized with immunocytochemical markers, special stains and enhanced experience that an exact pathological diagnosis can be provided before management decisions have to be made, enabling refinement of surgical technique.

Newer pharmaceutical agents enable the effects of the endocrine syndrome to be well controlled before the operation, thus presenting the patient to the surgeon in a fitter condition, to be more stable during the operation and thus able to make a more rapid recovery.

The principle of management in paediatric surgical endocrinology is that the surgeon must work in conjunction with a specialist paediatric endocrinologist who has the full support of a large adult endocrine unit and an imaging department with state-of-the-art ultrasound, CT scanning and MRI so that the correct imaging modality can be used to achieve the most precise picture. Unfortunately, the surgeon will not find in the current literature a vast experience of endocrine surgical series: present experience in these conditions is limited and many patients are still treated on a one-off basis without adequate follow-up to assess long-term outcome.

It is assumed in this chapter that the diagnosis has been made by a paediatric endocrinologist or, as often occurs with a thyroid swelling, discussed by the surgeon with an endocrinologist before embarking upon treatment. The surgeon needs from his or her colleagues an exact diagnosis, an assessment of the possibilities of associated syndromes, and how these can affect the outcome. He or she needs to know the site of the lesion with the appropriate imaging being discussed with the radiologist and whether a preoperative needle biopsy would be helpful or would merely contaminate the surgical field. Before surgery, the effects of the endocrine condition should have been controlled by the physician and the timing of operation planned according to preoperative therapy. Once these criteria have been met a paediatric anaesthetist should be involved, and a plan of action followed during the immediate pre-, per- and postoperative period such that the endocrine condition and its consequences are stable throughout. To achieve this stability, both vital signs and biochemical monitoring may be required on a continuous basis. Such an approach is not an excuse for surgical ignorance, for an informed discussion on management requires a sound knowledge of the underlying condition by both anaesthetist and surgeon.

THYROID DISEASE

Surgical treatment for thyroid disease in infancy and childhood varies according to geographic and genetic background. Surgical treatment is indicated in the following situations [2]:

1 juvenile goitre of extraordinary size and sufficient regression is not expected;
2 tracheal or oesophageal compression;
3 goitre is retrosternal;
4 conservative treatment is unsuccessful over a 2-year period;
5 autonomous adenoma;
6 thyroid cancer is suspected.

BENIGN THYROID DISEASE

This presents with simple features such as a lump or symptoms due to compression of the trachea, oesophagus or veins. Investigations commonly show a nodular colloid goitre, which is a common finding in parts of the world where iodine deficiency remains common [3]. Surgical treatment is indicated only if the symptoms fail to resolve with appropriate supplementation.

THYROTOXICOSIS

Thyrotoxicosis presents as a result of Graves disease or an autonomous nodule. The latter is extremely rare in childhood, but is a definite indication for surgical management. The indications for surgery in Graves disease are:

1 unsuccessful medical therapy (that is failure of spontaneous remission within a reasonable timescale).
2 a large goitre;
3 insufficient patient compliance;
4 poor control despite compliance;
5 recurrence after successful therapy.

CANCER OF THE THYROID

This is rare in children [4]. It frequently presents with an enlarged cervical lymph node or other metastases, such as in the lung, but the most usual presentation is that of a solitary lump in the neck [5]. Imaging in association with a fine-needle aspiration biopsy will define the diagnosis.

The operation

Preoperative preparation consists of ascertaining that the patient is euthyroid, ensuring with the anaesthetist that the airway is satisfactory and will not present difficulty on intubation, ascertaining that the vocal cords are mobile and assessing that the child is fit for surgery. The major operative decision is the extent of the operation. For a benign lesion affecting both lobes of the thyroid a subtotal thyroidectomy is appropriate, while if the nodule affects only one lobe a simple enucleation is appropriate. For thyrotoxicosis a radical subtotal thyroidectomy is appropriate, leaving very small remnants, such as less than 3 g of tissue. For a cancer, a lobectomy with removal of any affected lymph nodes is probably adequate, although some advocate a total thyroidectomy routinely.

No patient whose thyroid status is not normal should be submitted to surgical treatment.

Results

For benign thyroid disease the results are good with a rapid recovery following surgery, leaving hospital on the second or third postoperative day and returning to full activity by day 14. Complications are few, with a low incidence of recurrent laryngeal nerve damage (less than 5%), hypoparathyroidism or airway impairment. Mortality is nil.

For a nodular colloid goitre and solitary nodules there are no long-term sequelae, but if there is diffuse involvement of the gland by a colloid nodular process, recurrence is likely often in association with hypothyroidism so replacement therapy with thyroxine is mandatory.

In thyrotoxicosis the outcome is less certain with some 20–60% of patients becoming hypothyroid [6–8]. This is influenced by the amount of remaining thyroid tissue and the accompanying lymphocytic thyroiditis. The more thyroid tissue that remains, however, the greater is the likelihood of recurrence of hyperthyroidism. In 12.7% of 558 operations for hyperthyroidism in the literature, hyperfunction of the thyroid gland recurred [9]. To ensure prevention of recurrent hyperthyroidism, Perzik [10] recommends total thyroidectomy; however, this view is unusual. Nevertheless, a near-total thyroidectomy with immediate treatment with thyroxine replacement has much to commend it.

Recent experience with thyroid cancer suggests that the disease can be controlled in 95% of patients who are well treated with the aid of adequate surgery, radioactive iodine and replacement therapy [11].

In conclusion, surgery has a limited but defined role in paediatric thyroidology. Careful selection after an adequate trial of conservative therapy will ensure good results, but postoperative follow-up is essential with replacement therapy being prescribed appropriately.

HYPERPARATHYROIDISM

This is a very rare condition in children [12]. All reported infants with hyperparathyroidism have had parathyroid hyperplasia, while children invariably present with a single adenoma. In infants, once the diagnosis of hyperparathyroidism has been made, surgery appears the only way forward. Similarly in children, surgical treatment is indicated. Careful ultrasound of the parathyroid glands will usually reveal a discrete adenoma. An experienced ultrasonographer interested in parathyroid imaging is required to achieve accuracy.

The surgical treatment for diffuse hyperplasia is removal of all four glands. The glands are now transplanted to a superficial position in the forearm and there marked carefully. Should hyperparathyroidism recur, removal is comparatively simple. Prolonged follow-up is necessary in such instances, as the survival of these grafts in the longer term is unknown [13].

For a solitary adenoma it is probably sufficient to excise that adenoma and avoid biopsy of the other glands to prevent hypoparathyroidism postoperatively. Recurrence is extremely unlikely, and multiple adenoma almost unknown. The results of surgery are excellent.

THE ADRENAL GLAND

Adrenal medulla

Tumours arising from the adrenal medulla include: phaeochromocytoma, neuroblastoma (the commonest malignancy in children), and ganglioneuroma. The latter two have no endocrine effects and will not therefore be discussed further.

PHAEOCHROMOCYTOMA

This is an unusual childhood tumour and one that differs from the adult tumour in that more than 10% are bilateral; however, malignancy remains uncommon. Over 50% are at extra-adrenal sites but 95% are within the abdomen. Familial disease is common [14].

Once the diagnosis has been made, localization of the tumour is essential. A CT scan of the abdomen should be performed with particular emphasis on a sequence through the adrenal glands. A magnetic resonance image may be useful, particularly for identifying unusual sites. The preferred technique at present for diagnosing the site of these tumours, particularly if extra-adrenal, is using the radiopharmarceutical ^{131}I MIBG. A whole-body scan should be done to exclude thoracic or other-sited extra-abdominal disease. The surgeon should not proceed with the operation until the site of the disease has been accurately localized.

Preoperative preparation

It is essential to have the effects of the secretion of the phaeochromocytoma completely controlled in the immediate preoperative period. It is ideal to have both α- and β-adrenergic blockade prior to proceeding or even investigating the child, in order to prevent the potentially fatal complications of acute hypertensive crises and cardiac dysrhythmias. Even with blockade it is essential to dissuade the interventional radiologist from undertaking a biopsy of the adrenal or other mass, as this can cause profound and long-lasting hypertension.

As a result of the ability to control the hypertension rapidly, prolonged preoperative preparation is unnecessary and conservative management of this condition is inappropriate since these tumours can be malignant. The patient should be commenced on an α-blocking agent such as phenoxybenzamine as soon as the diagnosis is made. Propanolol may be used as the β-adrenergic blockade in the immediate preoperative period in order to control the tachycardia and the arrhythmias which may result from α-adrenergic blockade. Patients with phaeochromocytoma tend to be hypovolaemic, experiencing an average 15% reduction of normal plasma volume. Thus, the patient should arrive in theatre normotensive and well hydrated.

Children with phaeochromocytomas who have a high basal metabolic rate and a high plasma level of catecholamines are recognized as a poor anaesthetic risk. The anaesthetic must be approached with care to reduce the blood pressure during the immediate preoperative phase, during induction of anaesthesia and during mobilization of the tumour. Great care is also required to maintain a normal blood pressure after removal of the tumour. In order to titrate the pharmacological agents accurate monitoring of both the arterial blood pressure and the central venous pressure is necessary. Continuous monitoring of these parameters electronically is now essential. A urinary catheter is necessary to monitor the urine output, which may well be poor initially, due to the low plasma volume and the high catecholamine levels.

The operation

With the child normotensive and adequately monitored, the surgeon locates the incision adjacent to the tumour. With the imaging facilities available, a full laparotomy and rough mobilization of the tumour is unnecessary and contraindicated. The tumour is carefully isolated and, using minimally invasive techniques, mobilized with ligation at an early stage of the feeding blood vessels. If sited in the adrenal, ligation of the adrenal arteries should be followed by ligation of the vein. The anaesthetist needs to be acquainted with the stage of the operation so that he or she can assess the titration of blocking agents appropriately. Once the tumour is removed, blood pressure support may be required with adrenergic agents. In order to prevent oliguria, infusion of plasma or colloid substitute may be wise, to ensure an adequate circulating volume for the expanding peripheral circulation due to the release from prolonged pressor stimulation.

Results

In the Mayo Clinic series [13], 18 patients had no intraoperative complication, provided adequate blocking agents were used. Thirteen of the 18 patients became normotensive postoperatively. Three patients had a malignant tumour and all such tumours were at an extra-adrenal site. These children require careful follow-up in order to assess whether the tumours are multiple because second or subsequent tumours may have been suppressed by the high levels of tumour secretion, and thus only become manifest some months later. Such a course of action is better than a careful laparotomy, which usually fails to diagnose second tumours.

Adrenal cortex

Neoplasms of the adrenal cortex, both benign and malignant, are very rare in children. In a recent review from the Mayo Clinic [13], of 27 children with adrenal cortical neoplasms, virilization was the most common clinical finding (55%). Cushing syndrome occurred in 22% and two children had aldosteronism. Whether the tumour was benign or malignant depended on the size of the tumour; the larger the tumour, the more likely was a malignancy to be present. The frequency of virilization was the same in children with adenomas and carcinomas, as was Cushing syndrome.

Once the diagnosis of an adrenocortical endocrine lesion has been made, it is essential to determine the site of the lesion by imaging. Extra-adrenal sites are exceptionally rare. The endocrine effects of these tumours rarely produce the dramatic cardiovascular changes of the medullary tumour; nevertheless it is essential that the patient's condition is controlled and ideal prior to surgery.

At operation, an incision is made on the side of the lesion, and the lesion is removed with minimal trauma. Some of these tumours may be large, particularly those associated with virilization. Such tumours require careful manipulation and handling so as not to breach the capsule. Enucleation from the adrenal is inappropriate, and a complete adrenalectomy should be performed. Removal of the kidney, without evidence of tumour involvement, is contraindicated.

Postoperatively, care is required to maintain the electrolyte balance and, in particular, patients with Cushing syndrome may well require steroid supplementation in the immediate postoperative period to maintain blood pressure and well-being. Very careful follow-up of these patients is frequently required, with slow withdrawal of steroid support, assessing that the contralateral adrenal gland is functioning satisfactorily.

For benign tumours the outlook is excellent and, even in patients with malignant disease, prolonged survival is usual provided the surgical treatment was performed early before the capsule of the gland was breached. Late tumours, however, have a sombre prognosis and those patients with local invasion of surrounding structures usually succumb to their tumour.

HYPERINSULINISM

The most common cause (55%) of persistent hypoglycaemia in infants has been reported to be hyperinsulinism. These infants and children present a clinical appearance of symptomatic hypoglycaemia that responds poorly to medical treatment [15]. The greatest danger is irreversible brain damage if definitive therapy is withheld. All patients subjected to surgery have failed medical management with unstable blood sugar levels. Such patients should be submitted to surgery after a trial of conservative therapy, before frequent hypoglycaemic episodes have taken place.

The preferred procedure is a 95% pancreatectomy [16]. The earlier and more conservative procedure of an 85% removal of the pancreas, leaving much of the head of the pancreas *in situ*, proved less efficacious with a frequent recurrence of hypoglycaemia in the region of 40%. Now, a spleen-preserving distal pancreatectomy is performed, in which the body and tail of the pancreas are mobilized from the left side across to the portal vein. The procedure is then extended to the head of the gland and, in children, there is a good plane of cleavage between the superior mesenteric and portal vein and the uncinate process of the pancreas. The head of the pancreas can thus be lifted out of the C loop of the duodenum and away from the duodenal wall, leaving only a small amount of pancreas between the duodenum and the bile duct, which must be identified and carefully preserved.

Throughout this procedure the blood sugar level is liable to fluctuate wildly. Thus, constant monitoring of the blood sugar level with a reliable glucose meter is essential, in combination with the ability to infuse into a large vessel either glucose, during the mobilization, or insulin following the excision of the gland. During the postoperative period, careful control of the blood sugars is essential, as they may rise or fall and require appropriate management.

The long-term effects of this procedure are good. There should be no operative mortality, and morbidity should be minimal provided the patient suffered no side-effects before the operation. Approximately 10% of patients will require diazoxide for continued low blood sugars. Between 10% and 20% may require insulin in the short term but rarely (less than 10%) in the medium term. Decompensation may occur during the pubertal growth spurt. Interestingly, few patients develop steatorrhoea, although this may be encountered in the early postoperative phase. Appropriate enzyme replacement is indicated.

CONCLUSION

Paediatric endocrine surgery is a cooperative venture between paediatrician, radiologist, anaesthetist and surgeon. This surgery requires accurate endocrine diagnosis, accurate localization of the disease, accurate pathology either before or after the operation and careful monitoring throughout the procedure to counteract the endocrine effects of the disease process. With good teamwork the outcome is excellent. Long-term monitoring is essential to ensure that recurrence or deficiency disease does not occur, and that any replacement therapy that is required is correctly controlled.

REFERENCES

1 Gauderer MWL. Surgery for endocrinological diseases and malformations in childhood. In: Gauderer MWL, Angerpointner TA, eds. *Progress in Pediatric Surgery*, Vol. 26. Berlin: Springer Verlag, 1991:1–2.

2 Röher H-D. *Endokrine Chirurgie*. Stuttgart: Thieme, 1987.

3 Lindinger A, Sitzmann C. Die juvenile struma. *Kinderarzt* 1978; 9:277–81.

4 Joppich S, Röher HD, Hecker WCh, Knorr D, Daum R. Thyroid carcinoma in childhood. *Prog Pediatr Surg* 1983;16:23–7.

5 Hung W, Anderson KD, Chandra RS *et al.* Solitary thyroid nodules in 71 children and adolescents. *J Pediatr Surg* 1992; 27:1407–9.

6 Buckingham BA, Costin G, Roe TF, Weitzman JJ, Kogut MD. Hyperthyroidism in children. *Am J Dis Child* 1981;135:112–17.

7 Farnell MB, van Heerden JA, McConahey WM, Carpenter HA, Wolff LH. Hypothyroidism after thyroidectomy for Grave's disease. *Am J Surg* 1981;142:535–9.

8 Thompson NW, Dunn EL, Freitas JE, Sisson JC, Coran AG, Nishiyama RH. Surgical treatment of thyrotoxicosis in children and adolescents. *J Pediatr Surg* 1977;12:1009–17.

9 Mühlendahl KE, Helge H. Hyperthyreose im kindesalter. 2. Klinik und Therapie. *Padiatr Prax* 1978;20:601–16.

10 Perzik SL. The place of total thyroidectomy in the management of 909 patients with thyroid disease. *Am J Surg* 1976; 132:480–3.

11 Balázs G, Lukács G, Csáky G, Boros P, Ilyés I. Late prognosis of childhood and juvenile thyroid carcinoma. *Prog Pediatr Surg* 1991;26:41–7.

12 Ross AJ III. Parathyroid surgery in children. *Prog Pediatr Surg* 1991;26:48–59.

13 Telander RL, Zimmerman D, Kaufman BH, Van Heerden JA. Pediatric endocrine surgery. *Surg Clin N Am* 1985;65:1551–87.

14 Kaufman BH, Telander RL, van Heerden JA, Zimmerman D, Sheps SG, Dawson B. Phaeochromocytoma in the pediatric age group: current status. *J Pediatr Surg* 1983;18:879–84.

15 Filler RM, Weinberg MJ, Curtz E, Wesson DE, Ehrlich RM. Current status of pancreatectomy for persistent idiopathic neonatal hypoglycaemia due to islet cell dysplasia. *Prog Pediatr Surg* 1991;26:60–75.

16 Martin LW, Ryckman FC, Sheldon CA. Experience with 95% pancreatectomy and splenic salvage for neonatal nesidioblastosis. *Ann Surg* 1984;200:355–62.

23: Gynaecological Endocrine Surgery

S.J. STEELE

INTRODUCTION

The following are some basic principles for paediatric gynaecological surgery.

1 Psychological support. This is required for the parents of infants and young children who may need to be supported through the stress of doubt about the sex of their child, of concern about abnormalities (which may include other parts of the body as well as the reproductive tract), of corrective surgery and of the prospects for sex, marriage and childbearing. It is equally important for older children as they become aware that they are different from their peers, and ongoing support is often required to help them to adjust to these problems as they pass through adolescence and early adult life. With older children the whole family may need support, and this is particularly important where there is confusion over gender, as in androgen insensitivity.

2 Continuity of care. While some conditions are easily corrected, others may involve observation, review and surgery over some years. There are immense advantages if the same gynaecologist can undertake the necessary care for the infant, child, adolescent and adult. It is much easier for adolescents and women to return to a doctor who may have known them over the years, and who is familiar with their condition, than for them to establish a relationship with a gynaecologist they have not met before. This facilitates questions and discussion of problems in relation to fertility, sex, menstruation and the other concerns which are likely to arise as the years pass.

3 No corrective surgery should be undertaken until the exact nature of any abnormality has been defined and the sex of rearing decided.

4 Vaginal examination of children and young adolescents in the outpatient clinic is inappropriate. Where this is necessary it should be done as an examination under anaesthetic.

5 Pressure to operate. In some cases of notably ambiguous genitalia, there is sometimes great pressure on the surgeon to operate as early as possible. Operations on small babies are difficult, and carry an increased risk of both mortality and morbidity. Furthermore total blood volume is small so that minimal blood loss may be significant, and these operations should be delayed until an appropriate time judged by the fitness of the child, minimal risk of surgery and optimal conditions for a good outcome.

6 Vaginal surgery causes scarring, which may be very difficult to overcome, and it is particularly important that the first attempt at corrective surgery in this region is successful. Subsequent attempts will be increasingly difficult and less likely to succeed.

7 Time and privacy. Time is required to assess these cases and even more to explain either to the parents, the patient or all of them what is wrong, what requires to be done and the likely outcome. Small babies and young children should always be seen with their parent or parents. I always offer older children the choice of whether their parent actually observes the examination or not; some prefer them to wait outside. I always see adolescents on their own initially, and then talk to them and the parent or parents afterwards. It should be remembered that adults whose abnormalities have either been diagnosed late, or who have not had the treatment they should have had, may present with problems which cause them immense distress and considerable confusion. This is sometimes exacerbated by previous inadequate communication. Much time and care may be required to explain the situation and the treatment options.

ADHERENT OR FUSED LABIA

This condition is relatively common but causes great anxiety. Rarely it is the result of trauma. It is usually diagnosed in the neonate or infant, but is occasionally not identified until a child is older. The abnormality once identified causes concern to the parents, and may be associated with urinary infection and discharge due to the pooling of urine beneath the labia. The application of oestrogen cream daily, and gentle distraction by the parent in the bath, normally result in resolution of the problem. If this is not successful the labia may be separated under an anaesthetic, and it is not usually necessary to use instruments for this purpose. It is wise to advise the parent to separate the labia in the bath at night and to apply oestrogen cream for 7–10 days subsequently, otherwise the labia will occasionally re-adhere.

URETHRAL PROLAPSE

This condition is seen rarely in babies or young children. The whole urethra prolapses below the external meatus; it may strangulate and become infected or ulcerated. If there is infection, a swab should be taken for culture and appropriate antibiotic treatment given. The prolapsed tissue should be excised, the external urethral meatus tightened so that the prolapse cannot recur and the urethral mucosa sutured to skin. The use of a small amount of 0.5% bupivacaine hydrochloride will minimize the discomfort to the child on waking, and in most cases will avoid the need for a catheter. Unless there is infection, the child should be able to go home the following day.

VAGINAL DISCHARGE AND/OR BLEEDING

Infection with *Candida* can be diagnosed by external examination, and a swab taken from the vulva or introitus. If the discharge is persisent or bloodstained, and cannot be otherwise explained, further investigation is required. Ultrasound may be helpful in revealing the presence of a foreign body or rarely a tumour. In any event an examination under anaesthesia will be required, and this will include inspection of the vagina using a small endoscope to exclude the presence of a foreign body and tumours of the vagina and cervix. Foreign bodies are normally easily removed. Tumours are rare and include the mixed mesodermal or Müllerian tumour known as sarcoma botryoides. Clear-cell adenocarcinoma is seen rarely in girls whose mothers received treatment with diethyl stilboestrol [1]. If there is any question of the bleeding coming from the urinary tract then a cystoscopy should be carried out at the same time. The possibility of abuse should be considered in any case where there is evidence of trauma in the region of the vulva or perineum.

LONGITUDINAL VAGINAL SEPTA

These septa which run in the midline longitudinally may be partial or complete. In the latter case there is a double vagina which may be associated with a double cervix and uterus. These are detected during an examination, or when there is difficulty in inserting a tampon after menarche. They should be divided because of the problems which they cause with tampons, coitus and delivery. Occasionally the septum will be eccentric and fused laterally so that the vagina on that side ends blindly (Fig. 23.1). In this situation blood may accumulate (cryptomenorrhoea) and this will require drainage which can be achieved by dividing the septum.

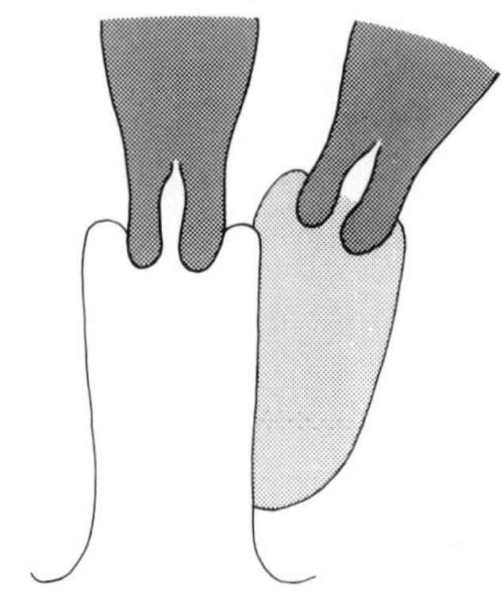

Fig. 23.1 Double vagina and uterus with vaginal septum and cryptomenorrhoea.

TRANSVERSE VAGINAL SEPTA

The commonest form is low in the vagina and may be confused with vaginal atresia. These forms are occasionally detected before menarche, in which case they should be treated before that event occurs. If the periods start before diagnosis, as is usually the case, menstrual blood will accumulate in the vagina. These girls may present with primary amenorrhoea, an abdominal mass, pain or acute retention of urine. There is often a history of reasonably regular episodes of dysmenorrhoea-type pain, and inspection of the abdomen and perineum makes the diagnosis relatively simple. Ultrasound will show the fluid-filled vagina, which may be very large. If the condition continues until the vagina is fully distended, the blood will pass upwards through the tubes into the peritoneal cavity, where endometriosis may occur. Treatment is by incision of the septum and drainage..No further measures should be undertaken at that time because of the risk of ascending infection. The normal acid pH of the vagina is re-established after drainage and the stay in hospital need not be more than 2 or 3 days. There is an association with congenital abnormalities of the urinary tract, and ultrasound scans and an intravenous pyelogram will show whether these are present or not. Septa higher in the vagina should be managed as for absence or partial absence of the vagina (see page 368).

AMBIGUOUS GENITALIA

Virilizing congenital adrenal hyperplasia

This abnormality is normally detected at birth, and its cause should be investigated promptly, particularly when there is salt loss. A karyotype is required to confirm

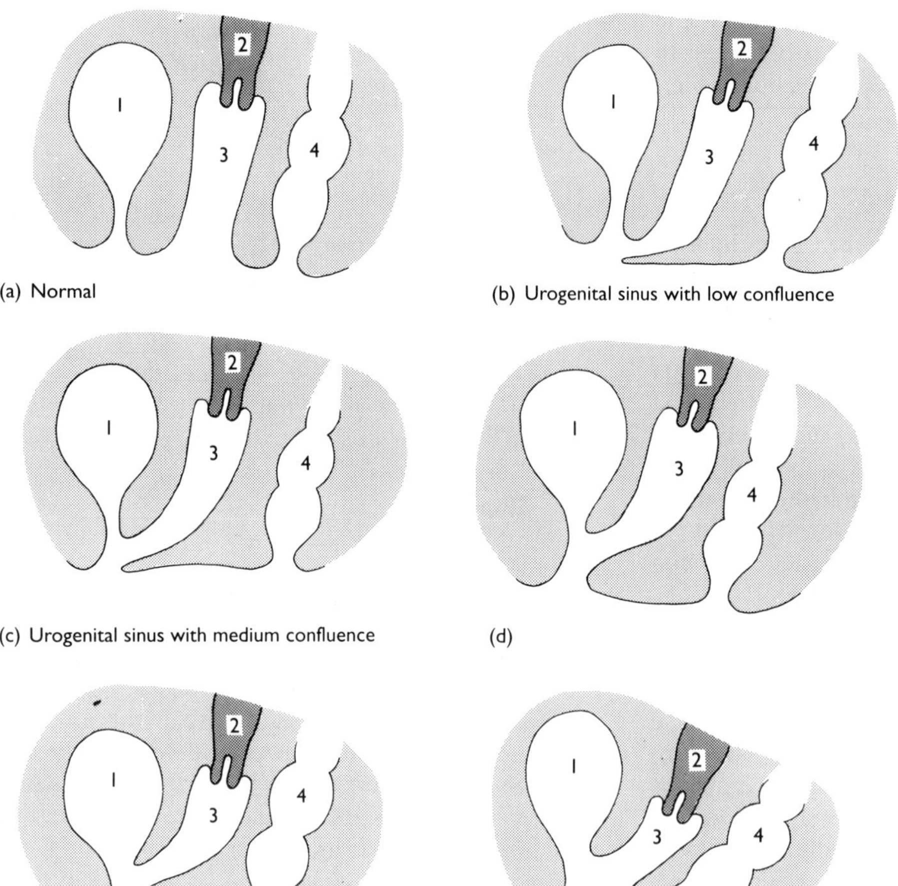

Fig. 23.2 Anomalies of the confluence of the urethra, vagina and rectum. 1, bladder; 2, uterus; 3, vagina; 4, rectum.

gender, and ultrasound may be helpful in identifying the uterus, ovaries and vagina.

The principles of correcting anatomical abnormalities of the genital tract are the same, subject to the diagnosis and treatment of any underlying endocrine abnormality and the decision to raise a child as a female. The degree of abnormality with congenital adrenal hyperplasia varies. The size and appearance of the clitoris are variable, and the skin of the labia may be rugose and similar to scrotal skin in some cases. The labial folds are fused in virilized females so that there is one external orifice for the urethra and vagina (urogenital sinus). The site of this must be identified – it is most often at the base of the clitoris but may be on the clitoris itself. The lower vagina may be considerably narrowed, and the vagina and urethra join as a urogenital sinus at variable levels up to the bladder neck (Fig. 23.2a–e). Assessment of the abnormality can be made either by X-ray taken with introduction of radiopaque medium into the vagina or by endoscopy.

Reduction of the enlarged clitoris

Clitoromegaly is the most obvious manifestation of ambiguous genitalia and causes immense distress to the parents. There is therefore always pressure to perform corrective surgery at an early date, and surgeons differ both in the procedures they undertake and in their timing. The first few weeks of life are often far from straightforward for these children, and I believe the best time to operate is between 3 and 6 months. Surgery in very small children is inevitably more difficult, and the risks decrease with increasing age and maturity. The operation can be combined with an assessment of the rest of the genital tract as indicated above, and should be carried out before the age of 2 years.

Of the techniques described, flexion and burial of the enlarged clitoris is not acceptable because the bent phallus may cause great discomfort and embarrassment to the adolescent or woman when it becomes engorged on sexual arousal. The best approach is to remove an appropriate portion of the clitoris so that what remains is of the right size for a female. A good technique is to raise a ventral flap of the skin from the clitoris with the glans attached, and to dissect out the clitoris, removing an appropriate portion distal to the bifurcation of the corpora cavernosa. Some surgeons preserve the dorsal neurovascular bundle, and the glans can be sutured onto the base of the clitoris. Blood loss is reduced by local infiltration with adrenaline 1:200000 and 0.5% bupivacaine hydrochloride. Babies seem to tolerate this procedure well and can normally leave hospital in 2–4 days, provided that their endocrine control is satisfactory. Some of the skin from the clitoris can be used to create labia minora, and the labia majora may be reduced if the appearance is grossly scrotal or advanced towards the perineum if this improves the appearance. The clitoris is sensitive and responsive in adults who have had this operation. Where I have had to reduce the clitoris in a young woman, sensation and function have returned within 6 months.

Some gynaecologists and urologists advocate opening up the vaginal introitus at the same time, but this is usually unnecessary and unwise [2]. The anatomy is more difficult to define in the young child, the procedure appreciably increases the duration of the operation and blood loss and, most important of all, if the lower vagina is narrowed, any scarring which occurs as a result of this initial procedure will make it more difficult to obtain a satisfactory lower vagina later. The situation should be reassessed in puberty before menarche. At this stage it is much easier to open up the vagina and do any necessary corrective surgery.

If the fused tissue is relatively thin, a straight incision through the fused labia is all that is required, followed by suturing of the skin to the vagina on each side. If the tissue is thicker, or if there is narrowing, either a posterior-based skin flap may be reflected and the underlying tissue incised in the midlines so that the flap can then be used to form the posterior wall of the vagina or, alternatively, two flaps may be raised from each side of the introitus which can then be rotated and laid into the vagina. If there is major concern about creating a vagina of adequate calibre, it may be better to do the minimum necessary procedure in puberty, and defer other surgery until the patient is ready to start sexual activity, because of the problems which may arise from scarring. Dilatation will then prevent this from occurring.

If the vagina enters the urethra high up, the opening of the urethra may be adjusted posteriorly and a lower urethra fashioned separate from the vagina, which can then be enlarged posteriorly as described above. If the union occurs in the region of the sphincter (Fig. 23.2e), it is essential that a urologist is involved. Abnormalities of the urogenital sinus are found in other conditions, and the level and degree of confluence vary. In some cases the urethra, vagina and rectum join as a persistent cloaca, and a sigmoid colostomy is required before reconstructing the component parts.

DYSGENETIC GONADS

If streak gonads are discovered in a 46,XX female, no surgical treatment is necessary. If the karyotype is 46,XY, or there is a mosaic with XY, the dysgenetic gonads should be removed because of the risk of neoplasia, for example gonadoblastoma. As streak gonads are not functional, and do not contribute to development, they should be removed as soon as is convenient after diagnosis. In some cases it may be possible to do this laparoscopically, although great care is required because of the close proximity of the streaks to large vessels and the ureters. The tumours may be very small and not visible on a macroscopic examination of a 'streak'. Gonadoblastoma and dysgerminoma are the commonest tumours.

ANDROGEN INSENSITIVITY

These patients usually present in adolescence with primary amenorrhoea. Some advocate removal of the testes before puberty, but we believe the testis should not be removed until the secondary sexual characteristics have developed; others recommend gonadectomy in the young child. Breast development is very satisfactory in these individuals, although there will no pubic or axillary hair if insensitivity is complete. There is a significant risk of tumours in the testis including hamartomas, gonadoblastomas and seminomas [7]. If the gonad is intra-abdominal it may be removed by laparotomy, or in some cases by laparoscopic surgery. If it is in the groin or labia, removal is relatively simple. Identification of intra-abdominal testes by ultrasound is not wholly reliable because they may be sited away from the normal position of the ovary.

The vagina is short in this condition and inadequate for intercourse. It can usually be stretched fairly easily, and if this is done regularly, either digitally or using dilators, it is possible to create a vagina 8 cm long [3]. The anatomy and procedure need to be explained very carefully to the patient, and many gynaecologists do the initial stretch under a general anaesthetic. Thereafter, regular dilatation is necessary over a period of 3–4 months. Some of these patients will have attempted to have sexual intercourse unsuccessfully and, once the vagina has reached a reasonable length, coitus itself provides a very effective method of stretching. The best results are obtained in those who are motivated to have intercourse, or who have already tried to do so, and the involvement of the sexual partner is often helpful. Where a woman has difficulty, regular visits to see a nurse who is trained to teach the technique of dilatation will often overcome the problems.

This technique may be tried in patients other than those with androgen insensitivity. As it does not involve any invasive procedure it has a great deal to commend it, and is well worth a trial. It is least likely to succeed in those who are unable or unwilling to do anything active to improve their situation, and in some slim patients in whom the tissues cannot be dilated to a sufficient extent.

True hermaphrodites

These are very rare, and it is crucial that there is full investigation, assessment and discussion before surgery is contemplated. The abnormal external genitalia are usually the first indication of the problem, and the findings in some cases are similar to those associated with 21-hydroxylase deficiency in the female. The gonad may be palpable in the labioscrotal region or the groin, or may be within the abdomen. Van Niekirk reported 26% of ovotestes in the labioscrotal fold, 24% in the inguinal canal and 46% within the abdomen [4]. The karyotype is important, but may be 46,XX even when there is a testis present.

The commonest finding is of an ovotestis with the two types of tissue arranged end to end. In one-third of those who have an ovotestis the condition is bilateral. When a testis is present it is commoner to find this on the right, and an ovary is commoner on the left. An ovotestis may have either a fallopian tube or a vas, but not both. If there is a fallopian tube it is usually not patent. The gonad must be inspected if necessary by laparotomy (46% will be intra-abdominal). Careful examination and a long biopsy is necessary to establish the precise picture. Frozen-section histology enables appropriate action to be taken immediately. If there is a normal ovary on one side and it has been agreed that the child is to be reared as a female, the testis or ovotestis can be removed. If there are bilateral ovotestes it may be possible to preserve the ovarian part of the gonad while removing the testicular portion. The external genitalia will require correction with reduction of the clitoris and correction of the urogenital sinus if this exists.

ABSENCE OF THE VAGINA

There are a number of techniques available for construction of a vagina in those who are born with vaginal agenesis. Most of the surgical procedures are complex, with a significant risk of major complications, such as vesicovaginal fistula formation. A successful outcome implies the ability to have satisfactory sexual intercourse. Due to the problems which arise with specific methods and their limitations, together with the marked tendency of a newly created vagina to stenose, many of these operations have an unsuccessful outcome. Great care is required in selecting the time and operation for an individual patient. The adolescent or woman needs to be well prepared psychologically for the procedure and the follow-up treatment, and adequately informed to make a decision to go ahead with the operation. Discussion with someone else who has been through the same procedure may be helpful.

Absence of a vagina is usually associated with the absence of a uterus, and there is therefore no reason to embark on corrective surgery until the patient is fully grown, able to understand all the implications of what is to be done and ready to start sexual activity. Some young women are particularly keen to have the abnormality corrected, but their expectations are often unrealistic. The best results are obtained in those who are ready for sexual activity, or have already tried it, and have good relationships with supportive partners.

If the uterus is present a vagina must be created, otherwise retrograde menstruation will occur with the risk of dysmenorrhoea and endometriosis. The situation may not be diagnosed until menarche, and therefore will require to be treated relatively expeditiously. The state of the uterus can be assessed by ultrasound and laparoscopy. In some cases the uterine cervix is also abnormal. Hysterectomy would, of course, avoid the complications of this situation, but every attempt should be made to preserve the uterus.

It is, however, unwise to assure a girl or young woman with confidence that she will be able to carry a pregnancy. The uterus in some of these patients with extensive abnormalities is capable of menstruation, but is not normal and does not respond fully and normally to oestrogen and progesterone.

Vaginoplasty

A number of techniques have been used for the creation of a vagina, but with one exception all involve major surgery and have a very significant complication rate, while success, as judged by normal sexual activity, is limited.

1 McIndoe vaginoplasty – this involves opening up the space between the urethra and the rectum and then inserting a split-thickness skin graft on a mould into the space created [5]. The dissection may be difficult. The mould has to be changed after 7–10 days and it is essential to keep a mould in the vagina and continue dilating for some 3 months. Fistula formation, haematomas, infection, expulsion of the mould and stenosis are the major complications of this procedure. Unless the artificial vagina is kept dilated it will naturally stenose, and the need to have repeated dilatation is discouraging and depressing for the woman. The original technique has been modified and meshed grafts are now used on perforated moulds.

2 A similar technique using amnion has been described which was reasonably successful [6], but problems arose with this because of the need to check the HIV status of the donor of the amnion.

3 Peritoneal flaps may be used anteriorly and posteriorly with labial skin flaps or vulval skin laterally.

4 Caecovaginoplasty – the caecum may be used to create a vagina. This adds the potential complications of bowel surgery and anastomosis to the problems of creating the vagina. Caecal or colon vaginoplasty are appropriate methods in cases where the uterus is present, because stenosis is less of a problem than with the skin graft vaginoplasty. A 2-week hospital stay is required for the procedure, and close follow-up and initial dilatation afterwards are essential. Discharge of mucus is troublesome to patients, and some find it necessary to douche in order to reduce this to a minimum.

5 A segment of colon may be used instead of caecum. This is narrower than the caecum and can provide a very satisfactory result, though again there is a possibility of stenosis and there will be mucus secretion. In these procedures the omentum may be used to reinforce suture lines and enhance healing.

When the upper third of the vagina is atretic, and the uterus is present, it may be necessary to open the uterine cavity and identify the cervical canal. If the cervical canal is atretic it can be split and the canal closed over a T-drain placed in the uterus and stitched to the vaginal introitus. The ability of the cervix to stenose, however, is considerable.

Vulvovaginoplasty

This is a relatively simple procedure designed by Williams [8], in which a pouch on the perineum is created using the skin of the labia and perineum. It does not carry the risk of major complication, and the vagina does not tend to stenose unless there is infection. This method has much to commend it for its simplicity, and it is certainly compatible with satisfactory intercourse, although the direction and depth do not quite match up to the normal vagina, or even perhaps to the successful but much more complicated vaginoplasties. The complication and failure rates of the latter procedures, however, must be taken into account.

In selecting the appropriate procedure for a particular patient the experience of the surgeon with particular procedures and the wishes and motivation of the woman determine the best approach. With most vaginoplasties, if there is not regular and frequent intercourse, there will be a natural tendency for stenosis to occur.

OVARIAN DISORDERS

Functional cysts

These cysts, which may be up to 5 cm in diameter, are detected by ultrasound examination or found at laparotomy. They may be either follicular cysts or corpus luteum cysts and haemorrhage in the latter group will occasionally cause presentation with acute abdominal pain. If they are detected by ultrasound, they should be observed and will normally resolve within 3–4 weeks. Physiological cysts are normally recognizable to the gynaecologist. If there is any doubt they may be aspirated, but ovarian surgery should not be undertaken.

Endometriosis

Adolescents may present with dysmenorrhoea and persistent cysts on ultrasound scanning and laparoscopy will result in the diagnosis of endometriosis. Conservative surgery with resection of endometriotic cysts, laser or diathermy destruction of cysts, endometriotic deposits or small endometriomas is the rule.

Ovarian tumours

The commonest tumours are sex-cord tumours and germ-cell tumours. Ultrasound is helpful in distinguishing between solid and cystic tumours, and determining whether both ovaries are involved.

The benign teratomas are often identified by ultrasound, and are easily recognizable at laparotomy or laparoscopy. The cyst can usually be removed with conservation of the rest of the ovary, but it is important to check the contralateral ovary as these tumours are bilateral in 10–20%.

Solid tumours have a one in three chance of being malignant. Ascitic fluid and peritoneal washing should be taken for cytology, careful assessment of the extent of the disease within the abdomen carried out and the affected ovary and tube removed. Provided that the remaining ovary appears healthy it should be conserved. Frozen-section histology enables the diagnosis to be made at the time of laparotomy, but is unlikely to affect the surgery performed unless there is a macroscopic lesion in the remaining ovary. The granulosa tumour, which is usually unilateral and must be regarded as of low malignancy, may produce oestrogen and therefore present with precocious puberty. The thecoma, which is a benign tumour but more frequently bilateral, may present in the same way. These tumours should be removed by unilateral salpingo-oophorectomy. If there is doubt about the remaining ovary it may be bisected and a biopsy taken, but particular care should be taken in repairing it afterwards, to avoid the formation of adhesions and reduction of fertility subsequently.

COMPLICATIONS OF OVARIAN TUMOURS

Solid tumours particularly, and the heavy benign cystic teratomas, may present with torsion. Unless surgery is carried out promptly the ovary will be infarcted and have to be removed. It is particularly important in each case to check there is no tumour in the remaining ovary. If there is, this should be removed by an ovarian cystectomy to avoid the risk of the same complication.

Rupture of the tumour may occur. The patient presents with an acute abdomen. Malignant tumours such as the endodermal sinus tumour may present in this way, and the ovary should be removed and appropriate assessment of the peritoneal cavity made in every case so that appropriate treatment, if it is indicated, can be planned once the histology is available.

REFERENCES

1 Herbst AL. Clear cell adenocarcinoma and the current status of DES-exposed females. *Cancer* 1981;48:484.

2 Edmonds DK. *Practical Paediatric and Adolescent Gynaecology.* London: Butterworths, 1989.

3 Frank RT. The formation of an artificial vagina without operation. *Am J Obstet Gynecol* 1938;35:1053.

4 Nickirk WA Van. True hermaphrodism. In: Josso N, ed. *Paediatric and Adolescent Endocrinology (The Intersex Child),* Basel: Karger, 1981:80–99.

5 McIndoe AH, Bannister JB. An operation for the cure of congenital absence of the vagina. *Br J Plast Surg* 1938;45:490.

6 Morton KE, Dewhurst CJ. Human amnion in the treatment of vaginal malformations. *Br J Obstet Gynaecol* 1986;93:50.

7 Snyder HMcL. In: King LR, ed. *Urologic Surgery in Neonates and Young Infants.* Philadelphia: W.B. Saunders, 1988:360.

8 Williams EA. Congenital absence of the vagina: a simple operation for its relief. *J Obstet Gynaecol Br Commonw* 1964; 71:511.

24: Endocrine-related Urological Surgery

J.M. HUTSON

AMBIGUOUS GENITALIA

Surgical considerations

The management of ambiguous genitalia is complex and best achieved with a team including an endocrinologist, social worker and urologist in the neonatal period, followed by the assistance of a psychiatrist, psychologist, gynaecologist and endocrinologist in adult life. The gender of rearing is dependent on the basic underlying anomaly, as well as the degree of masculinization of the external and internal genitalia.

Genital anomaly presents with one of three patterns (Fig. 24.1). In congenital adrenal hyperplasia, and in most patients with androgen insensitivity syndrome, the gender of rearing will be female. In adrenal hyperplasia this is because of the ultimate prospect of normal female fertility, while in androgen insensitivity it is because the genital tissues cannot respond to exogenous androgens. For patients with gonadal dysgenesis, or for the rare patient with true hermaphroditism, the gender of rearing is determined on the size of the phallus.

Since androgen exposure *in utero* is directly responsible for masculinization of the external genitalia (Fig. 24.2), the size of the phallus is directly correlated with: (i) the degree of fusion of the inner genital folds to form a masculine urethra; (ii) the degree of fusion, pigmentation and wrinkling of the outer genital folds to form the scrotum; and (iii) the degree of regression of the urogenital sinus part of the vagina. The correlation between the phallic size and the urethral fusion on the one hand, and size of the vaginal remnant on the other hand, is important, since if the urethral fusion is only moderate and the phallus small, a moderate-sized vagina will be present opening low near the exterior. Masculine gender assignment would be considered only if the length of the phallus was greater than 2.5 cm in stretched length.

A key feature in the assessment of the genitalia is the presence and position of the gonads: if they are palpable in the labioscrotal folds or inguinal region one can assume that they are testes, and that the child is a genetic male. This is because ovaries presenting in an inguinal hernia are always associated with normal female genitalia and there is no suggestion of ambiguity. Although the cause of transabdominal descent of the testis to the inguinal region is highly controversial, the author has proposed that this is caused by Müllerian-inhibiting substance (MIS) [1]. Certainly, there is a very strong correlation between the degree of Müllerian duct regression and the transabdominal descent of the testis:

Transabdominal testicular descent	$\propto$	Müllerian duct regression
∴ Palpable gonads at or below groin	$\equiv$	Normal MIS secretion; absent uterus and tubes

This suggests that both features may be under common hormonal control [2]. In the clinical situation, this association can be put to advantage: the presence of testes in the groin or labioscrotal folds correlates with complete Müllerian duct regression, so that one can predict the absence of a uterus.

Asymmetry of the labioscrotal folds with one descended gonad is the common presentation of mixed gonadal dysgenesis and true hermaphroditism, as one gonad may be a non-functional streak or contain ovarian tissue. If only one testis is palpable in the groin, and the other one is impalpable, Müllerian duct regression is commonly asymmetrical also. The clinical assessment of the genital development is supplemented by a retrograde urogenital sinugram to demonstrate the size of the vagina and its site of connection with the urethra (Fig. 24.3). A pelvic ultrasound will confirm the presence of ovaries and the uterus in a child with adrenal hyperplasia, and may show a vaginal cavity. If the gonads are absent from the groin, a rectal examination will determine the presence of a uterus by palpation of the cervix.

Female reconstruction

Female reconstruction of the genitalia is performed in more than 50% of the patients with ambiguous genitalia because patients with adrenal hyperplasia and androgen

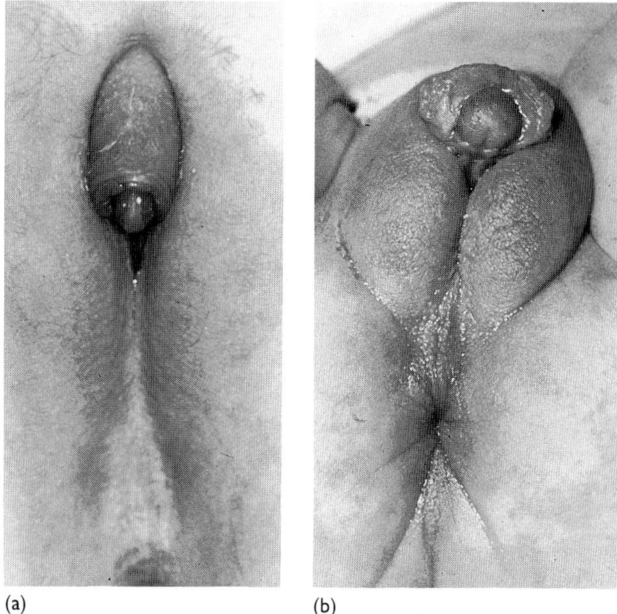

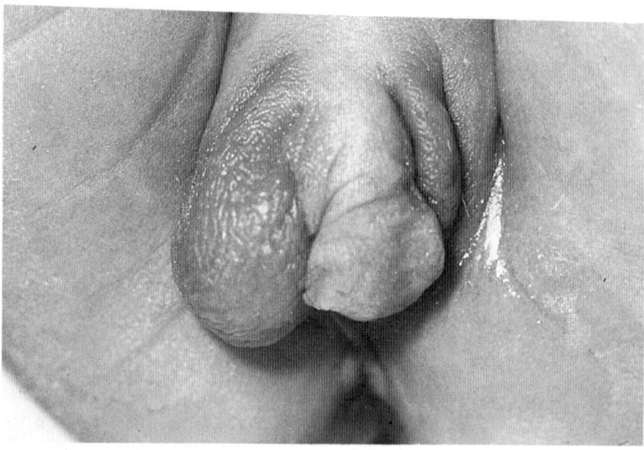

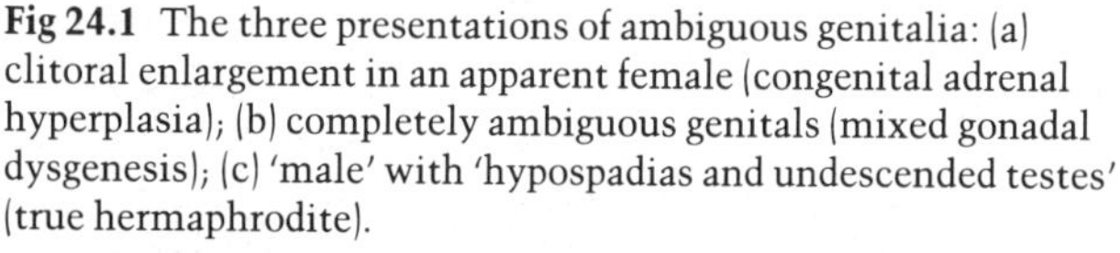

Fig 24.1 The three presentations of ambiguous genitalia: (a) clitoral enlargement in an apparent female (congenital adrenal hyperplasia); (b) completely ambiguous genitals (mixed gonadal dysgenesis); (c) 'male' with 'hypospadias and undescended testes' (true hermaphrodite).

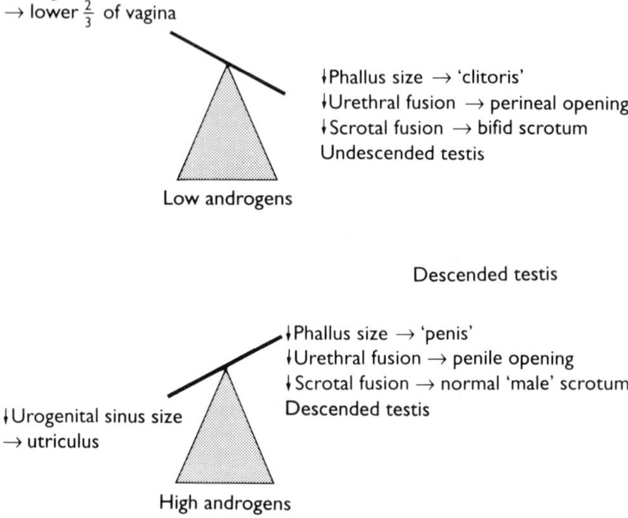

Fig 24.2 The effect of androgens on the external genitalia and its correlation with regression of the urogenital sinus.

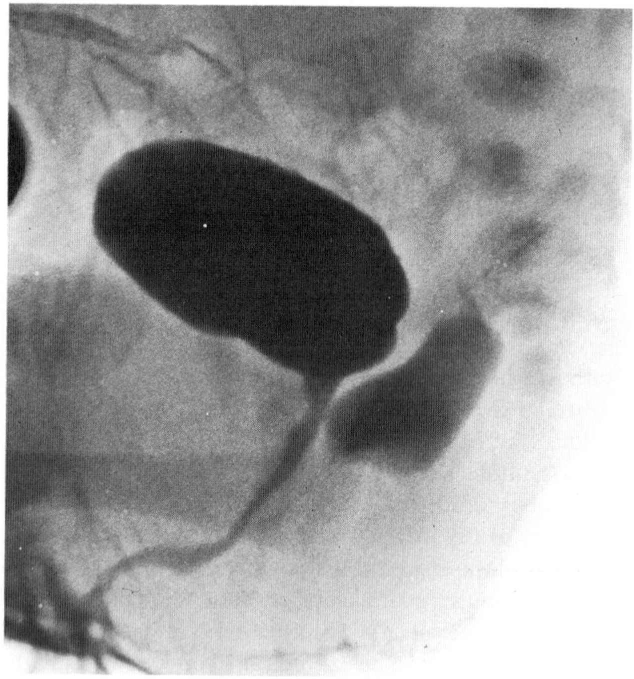

Fig 24.3 A urogenital sinugram showing a long vagina (with the indentation of a cervix) in congenital adrenal hyperplasia.

insensitivity will be raised as females. In babies with gonadal dysgenesis containing some testicular tissue, the gonads themselves should be removed at the time of reconstruction, which ideally should be before 2 months of age. This avoids any unnecessary postnatal exposure to circulating androgens, which commonly are elevated between 2 and 4 months after birth. The author prefers to correct the genital anomaly at 4–6 weeks, combining reconstruction of the external genitalia with removal of the gonads, if required.

There are four main features of genital reconstruction: (i) a vaginoplasty (usually a V–Y flap repair, since a pull-through vaginoplasty is usually unnecessary); (ii) clitoral reduction aiming to preserve blood supply and sensation; (iii) creation of the labia minora from the foreskin and shaft of the enlarged phallus; and (iv) removal of the masculinized labia majora by excision of the pigmented and wrinkled skin. The normal labia majora of a female infant are smooth and non-pigmented. Removal of this pigmented skin in children with ambiguous genitalia greatly improves the cosmetic appearance.

The operative procedure is relatively standard, apart from the fact that the clitoris is reduced in length and size by a method that is different from many other centres [3]. After isolation of the corpora cavernosa with tourniquets, the ventral surface of the glans and shaft of the phallus are removed completely and the phallus folded over and sutured to itself, recreating the hairpin bend in the female clitoris. This preserves the dorsal neurovascular supply to the clitoris but enables the bulk and length of the clitoris to be reduced, as well as enabling the glans clitoris to be 'pruned' to a feminine size.

No postoperative dressings are applied apart from Betadine ointment, and a catheter may be used to drain the bladder for 24–48 h. Regular dilatations of the neovagina are not performed. However, where the vaginal reconstruction has been performed in adolescence (because of late diagnosis or deliberate delay), postoperative dilatations are useful. In some children after neonatal flap vaginoplasty, a further introitoplasty may be necessary in adolescence to enlarge the opening of the vagina to enable insertion of a tampon.

Male reconstruction

Following the less common decision to raise the child as a boy, reconstructive surgery, which is more complicated than in a female, is usually begun at about 6 months. Release of the very severe penoscrotal chordee is accompanied by ventral rotation of the dorsal hood of the foreskin to enable the ventral surface of the straightened phallus to be covered by skin. If there has been significant inhibition of masculinization, the suspensory ligament of the penis may be lax and need tightening to enable the penis to point forward, rather than downwards. It may need to be accompanied by tucks in the Buck fascia posteriorly to straighten any curvature in the corpus cavernosum. Testicular biopsy, or even excision, may be required if the child has mixed gonadal dysgenesis. Finally, at this first operation penoscrotal transposition can be performed to place the scrotum caudal to the phallus. Six months after release of the chordee, the urethra is reconstructed along standard lines for hypospadias repair.

Simultaneously with one of the operations for external genital reconstruction, the urogenital sinus anlagen of the vagina can be removed. This is most easily performed via the transvesical method [4]. As the proximal vas deferens usually drains into the cranial end of the Müllerian duct and/or urogenital diverticulum, its excision is inevitably associated with disconnection of the ejaculatory apparatus.

Rare genital anomalies

Persistence of the primitive cloaca is a rare, severe anomaly which may masquerade as ambiguous genitalia (Fig. 24.4) [5]. However, this is a morphological abnormality of the urogenital system and hindgut, rather than a hormonally mediated abnormality, as in the usual cases of ambiguous genitalia. It is associated with an imperforate anus and often there is apparent phallic enlargement and labioscrotal fusion. The enlarged phallus is mostly illusory, since the erectile tissue is of normal size for a female but may be associated with an enlarged foreskin and stenosis of the external opening of the cloaca. Obstruction of the urinary outflow or vaginal secretions may produce hydrometrocolpos or obstructed ureters. If the cloacal channel is narrow, urine may drain into the vagina or colon, where mixing of the urine with meconium causes precipitation of ammonium magnesium phosphate [6]. This produces speckled intramural calcification along the line of the colon on a plain abdominal X-ray.

Children with cloacal abnormalities commonly have other major anomalies which may preclude active treatment. They should be investigated by sinugram and endoscopy, as well as careful X-rays of the spine, since sacral agenesis is a common accompaniment and may indicate

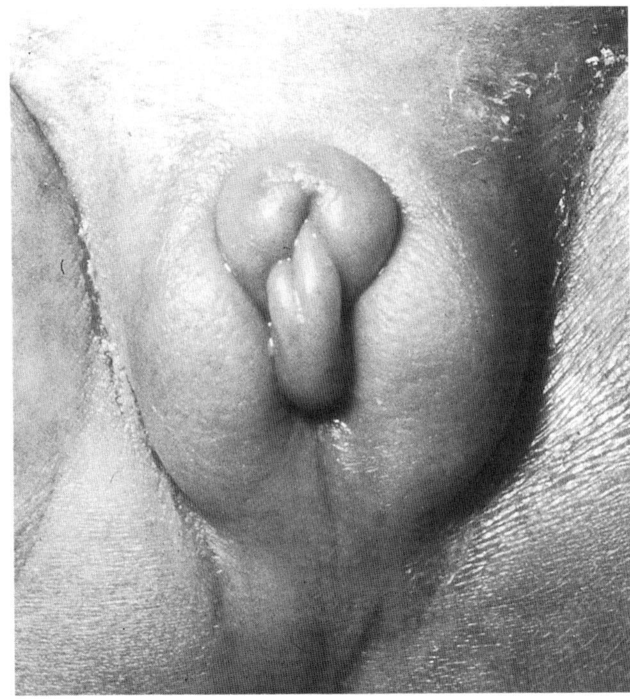

Fig 24.4 Cloacal abnormality in a female with an imperforate anus, a small external opening and enlarged skin folds around the clitoris. The lack of scrotalization of the labia and absence of excess erectile tissue suggest a complex morphological anomaly, rather than excess androgens.

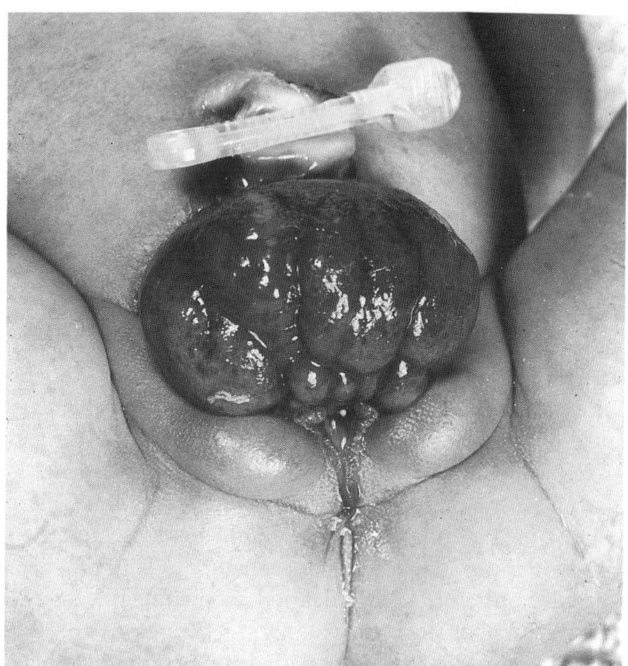

Fig 24.5 Exstrophy of the bladder (ectopia vesicae) is a complex lower abdominal wall defect with separation of the pubic skeleton and the genitalia.

a very poor outlook for urinary and faecal continence. Should surgery be undertaken, a preliminary colostomy with or without bladder or vaginal decompression in the neonatal period is followed by a definitive posterior sagittal procedure to bring the vagina and the bowel to the perineum, as described by Hendren [7] and Pena [8].

Exstrophy of the bladder is another major lower abdominal wall and perineal malformation which may be mistaken for a complex case of ambiguous genitalia. Failure of the lower abdomen to close leaves the bladder mucosa exposed on the surface, with accompanying separation of the pubic bones and, in severe cases, complete separation of the external genitalia (Fig. 24.5). Reconstruction of this complex and rare deformity is beyond the scope of this chapter, but includes reconstruction of the bladder, the urethral sphincter, the urethra itself and the genitalia.

FEMALE GENITALIA

Development of the female external genitalia is less complex than in the male, and is more likely to be normal. Consequently, congenital anomalies are rare in girls. Imperforate hymen is a rare condition which presents either at birth or at puberty. In the perinatal period, mucus produced by the vagina in response to maternal hormones may cause bulging of the introitus (a mucocolpos). At puberty, an imperforate hymen presents with primary amenorrhoea caused by failure of evacuation of the menstrual flow, leading to haematocolpos, or even haematometrocolpos. Clinical presentation is a phenotypic female with primary amenorrhoea and cyclical abdominal pain. Between the neonatal period and puberty, imperforate hymen or other variants of vaginal atresia almost never present because there is no vaginal mucus to cause obstruction.

Abnormalities of Müllerian duct fusion or development may come to the attention of the urologist because of unilateral renal agenesis [9]. This is often associated with Müllerian duct agenesis when the ureter is absent. Complete Wolffian duct agenesis, or failure of the Wolffian duct to reach the cloaca, will prevent normal development of the Müllerian duct as well as the ureteric bud, leading to the combined abnormality of vaginal or uterine atresia

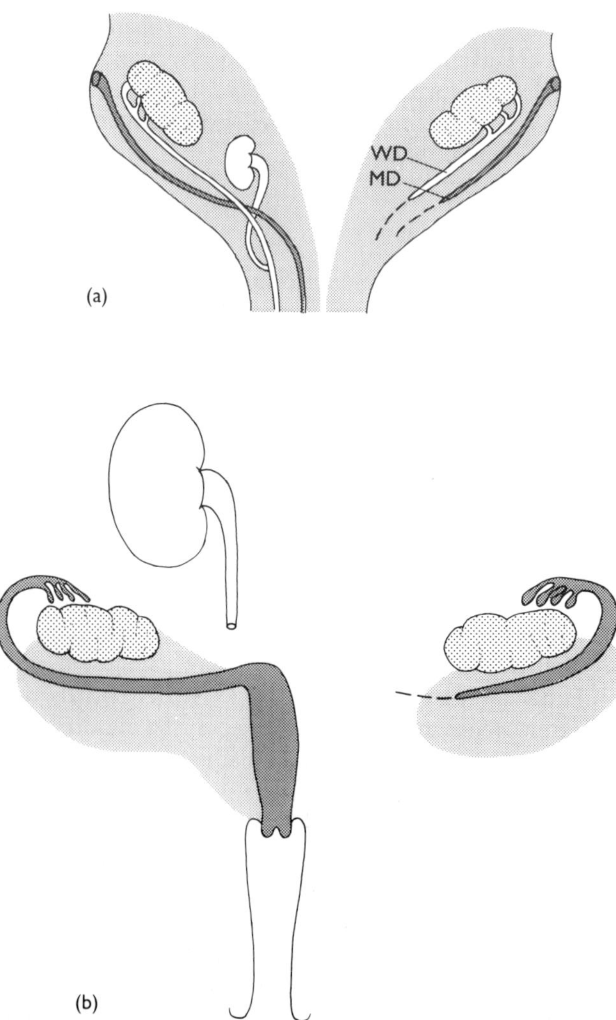

Fig 24.6 The Rokitansky–Mayer syndrome is caused by an abnormality of the Wolffian duct (WD) (a), which leads to secondary Müllerian duct (MD) agenesis associated with ipsilateral ureteric and renal agenesis (b).

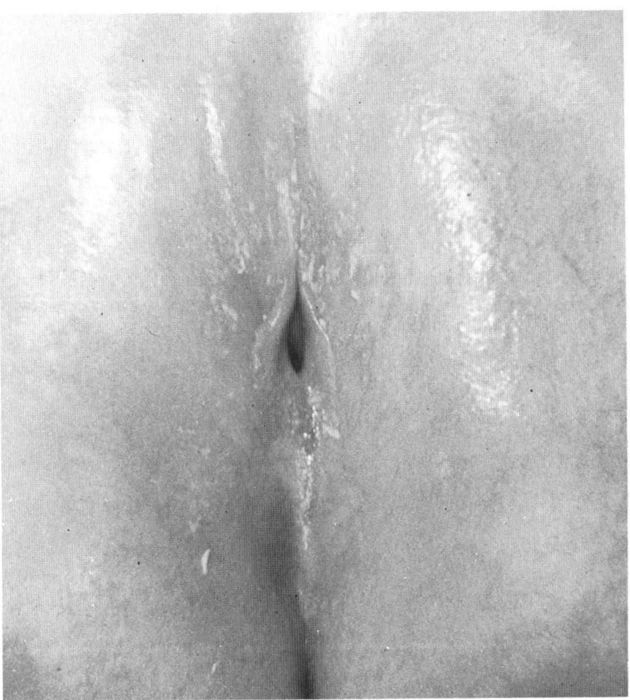

Fig 24.7 Labial adhesion is an acquired condition caused by ammoniacal dermatitis and labial ulceration with secondary adhesion during healing.

and fusion deficiency and unilateral renal agenesis. This syndrome is known as Rokitansky–Mayer syndrome (Fig. 24.6).

A common acquired anomaly of the female genitalia is labial adhesion (Fig. 24.7), which is often misdiagnosed by the inexperienced attendant as vaginal atresia [10]. Characteristically, the parents notice in a 1–3-year-old girl following a bath that the vaginal opening is not visible. In fact, the introitus is covered over by the adherent inner edges of the labia minora following ulceration from ammoniacal dermatitis and re-epithialization. The anomaly can be distinguished from true vaginal atresia by the fact that the introitus is hidden by the labia minora. Simple separation of the labia by pressure with the fingers or a Vaseline-coated thermometer resolves the parental anxiety immediately. Vaseline is applied afterwards for 1–2 weeks to prevent re-adhesion of the labia minora. Oestrogen cream can be applied topically to separate the labia without any minor trauma, but this has the disadvantage that it takes 1–2 weeks to cause desquamation with separation. Simple separation of the labia by digital retraction during the physical examination is preferable, despite the small amount of pain induced, because it reveals the normal vagina in the introitus immediately, thereby reassuring the family that all is well.

MALE GENITALIA

The penis

THE FORESKIN

The genital tubercle enlarges during embryogenesis in response to androgenic stimulation, to form the penis. The inner genital folds are fused together to form the urethra on the ventral surface, and the prepuce develops around the glans as an invagination of the epithelium. Initially, this epithelial invagination is solid, but in the first few years after birth it begins to separate, forming a separate foreskin. The timing of spontaneous separation of the foreskin is quite variable, and may take 5 or even 10 years to become completely separate from the glans.

During infancy, partial separation of the glans allows accumulation of epithelial debris (smegma). This presents as a deposit of white cheesy material building up under the foreskin, and is commonly mistaken for a tumour. It has no special significance, apart from the fact that it indicates that the foreskin and glans are undergoing normal separation. Once they are completely separated, the deposits of smegma wash out in the bath.

Routine circumcision of boys seems unnecessary in most circumstances. Occasionally, the child with complicated urinary tract malformation may benefit from prophylactic circumcision to reduce the incidence of urinary infection. The only common indication for circumcision is phimosis with secondary urinary obstruction. Less common indications would be recurrent balanitis or paraphimosis. In children who have associated hypospadias with ventral deficiency of the foreskin, circumcision should be actively discouraged, as the skin is required for surgical repair of the hypospadias.

HYPOSPADIAS

Hypospadias occurs when the fusion of the inner genital folds to form the urethra along the shaft of the penis is deficient, so that the urethral meatus is proximal to its normal site. This common anomaly of the male genitalia occurs in 1 : 300 male births, and is related to a deficiency of androgen stimulation in some patients. In many children, however, no hormonal defect can be identified, suggesting that it is a primary morphological defect of penile development.

Because hypospadias is a form of inadequate virilization of the penis, its presentation may overlap with that of true ambiguous genitalia. It is important, therefore, to be able to differentiate between hypospadias in a male and the rare child with ambiguous genitalia of more serious import. Clinically, the presence of 'intersex' can be suspected when there is an associated abnormality of fusion of the scrotum or descent of the testis. Significant genital anomalies with associated hypospadias have a bifid scrotum and/or maldescent of one or both gonads. Conversely, normal boys with hypospadias should have a fused scrotum containing two fully descended testes. Any baby who has apparent hypospadias at birth should be immediately investigated for ambiguous genitalia if one or other testis is impalpable or the scrotum is bifid. Although hypospadias can be associated with an undescended testis in otherwise normal boys, this is also the presentation for mixed gonadal dysgenesis and, occasionally, for true hermaphroditism.

The degree of hypospadias can be quite variable with the ventral opening of the urethra anywhere between the glans distally and the perineum proximally. Commonly, the urethra opens near the coronal groove of the glans. When urethral fusion is deficient, the periurethral tissues on the ventral surface of the penis also fail to grow to the normal length. This causes the common associated abnormality of chordee, which is ventral curvature of the penile shaft. The corpora cavernosa on the dorsal side of the shaft are the normal length, while the ventral periurethral tissues are shorter. With erection, the shaft bends because the ventral surface is shorter than the dorsal surface. The final defect in hypospadias is ventral deficiency of the foreskin to produce a dorsal hood. Associated abnormalities occur commonly in the urinary tract in association with severe hypospadias, where the proximal opening is on the scrotum or perineum. By contrast, distal hypospadias is rarely related to urinary tract anomaly.

Clinical examination reveals a shallow groove in the glans where the urethra should have formed, often associated with some blind-ending pits. The ventral skin raphe on the shaft is usually deviated to one or other side, related to the inadequate fusion of foreskin and shaft skin. Occasionally, chordee can be present without an abnormal urethra, a condition called by the French 'hypospadie sans hypospadie'. The cause of this variant is unknown, but may be related to pressure necrosis on the ventral surface of the penis from compression by the heel of the fetus [11]. Certainly, this variant of hypospadias has been associated with urethral fistula and other evidence of superficial skin ischaemia and necrosis.

Hypospadias is an important condition because the urinary stream is deflected downwards, forcing a small boy to sit on the toilet. During primary school years this leads to discrimination against the child because he cannot manifest outwardly normal masculine behaviour. In many cases it leads to psychological trauma during development of the personality, as well as to physical abuse. Because of this we would aim to correct the urinary stream prior to primary school years. Later in life the chordee is the more serious abnormality because of painful erections and difficulty with intercourse.

The aim of treatment is to correct the chordee to allow normal adult sexual function and to correct the urethral opening to allow normal micturition, which is an expression of male sexuality during the paediatric years. Surgery can be performed at any time prior to school age, with a recent preference for surgery between 6 and 18 months. In the common forms of hypospadias, with a distal opening and minimal chordee, the surgery can be accomplished in a simple one-stage procedure [12]. However, where the chordee is severe and the hole proximal on the shaft or in the perineum, two-stage procedures are available [13]. In the first procedure the chordee is corrected, followed by construction of the urethra from residual skin of the foreskin at the second operation.

EPISPADIAS

This is a rare condition of the phallus related to exstrophy of the bladder, where the lower abdomen fails to close in the pubic region (Fig. 24.8). The posterior urethra opens between the pubic bones on the dorsal surface of the phallus, and the penile urethra is usually completely absent. The phallus has a ventral hood and reversed chordee with a bend upwards, producing an unusual button-shaped appearance. Fortunately, this abnormality is rare (1:30000 livebirths) for the outlook is uncertain, as many children remain incontinent of urine, despite

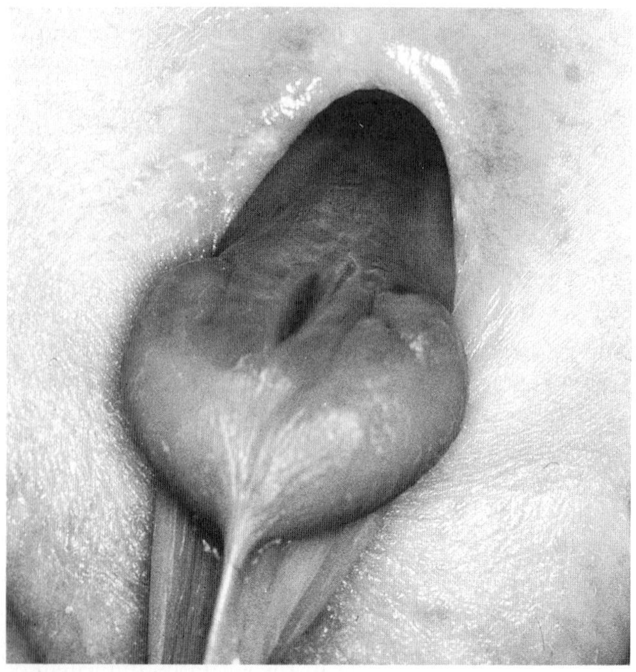

Fig 24.8 The bladder neck and urethra are deficient in epispadias, where the urinary meatus is dorsal to the abnormally short and curved phallus.

attempts to reconstruct the bladder neck. As the pubic rami are separated as part of the fusion defect, the penis is shortened as the corpora cavernosa are not fused normally.

The testis

UNDESCENDED TESTIS

Migration of the testis from the urogenital region of the abdominal cavity to the extra-abdominal scrotum is a precarious journey, and deficiency of this phase of migration is one of the commonest abnormalities in paediatric surgery. Undescended testis is present in 4–5% of males at birth, with delayed descent in the first 12 weeks occuring in about 50% of these. This leaves approximately 2% of boys with congenital undescended testis at 3–6 months. At one time these children had surgery between 5 and 10 years of age, but nowadays elective surgery is being performed in infancy in the belief that earlier treatment will improve the long-term results [14].

Some children appear to develop undescended testis later in childhood, despite having had no evidence of an abnormality in infancy. These apparently acquired variants of undescended testis are known as retractile testes or ascending testes.

Retraction of the testis by the cremaster muscle in response to low temperature or trauma is a normal reflex, but during childhood is enhanced when the circulating testosterone levels in the serum are low. This occurs between 2 and 10 years, when the level of androgen in the serum is low. In many children the degree of retraction during this time is greater than at other times of life, but in some children the degree of retraction appears to be actually pathological, with the testis not residing normally in the scrotum [15].

Another apparently acquired variant of undescended testis is now called the ascending testis [16]. These testes descend postnatally into the scrotum by 12 weeks. Subsequently, they appear to ascend back out of the scrotum as the child grows, often leading to an operation later in childhood. This phenomenon could well account for the fact that, although only 2% of boys have true congenital undescended testis, approximately 4–5% of males end up undergoing orchidopexy, consistent with the possibility that many retractile or ascending testes are treated surgically. The cause of ascending testes is unknown, but appears to be related to failure of the spermatic cord to elongate in proportion to growth of the boy.

Undescended testis is a major clinical problem because of the cosmetic defect, the loss of fertility, and the increased risk of developing a testicular tumour. There is still great controversy about whether the testis is primarily or secondarily abnormal in undescended testis. Many authors [14] have suggested that an abnormally formed testis will not descend, and also will have abnormal fertility and increased cancer risk. Alternatively, it has been recently proposed that most testes which are undescended are morphologically and probably physiologically normal prenatally, but develop secondary abnormality and subsequent dysplasia postnatally, caused by the abnormally high temperature of the non-scrotal environment. The scrotum is a specialized low-temperature environment that maintains the testis at 33°C, compared with 37°C for the core temperature of the body [17]. Where the testis does not reside spontaneously in the scrotum, it is likely to suffer secondary abnormality if the abnormal position is long-standing.

Most children with an undescended testis have no obvious hormonal abnormality at birth, or any indication of having had one prenatally since the genital development is normal. After birth, when the testis normally would begin functioning at 33°C, physiological derangements are first observed in the hormone levels of testosterone [18] and MIS [19], followed by microscopic, and eventually macroscopic, evidence of dysplasia (Fig. 24.9). It is this progressive secondary degeneration which causes the death

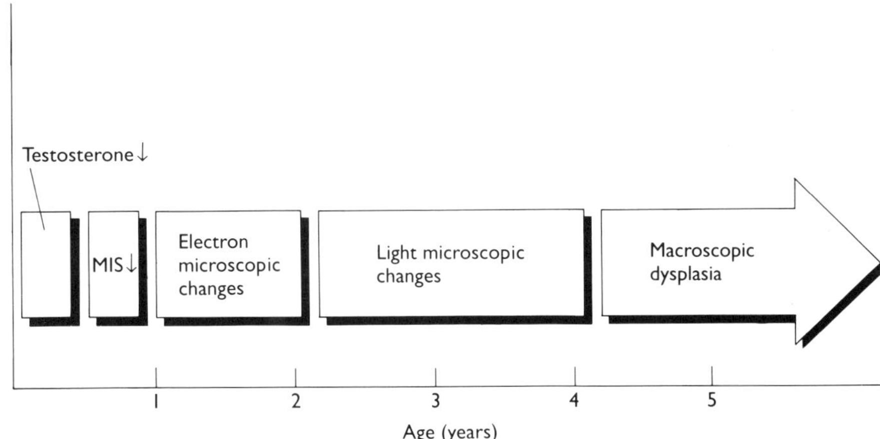

Fig 24.9 Schema showing how abnormalities of testicular function and morphology are related to age in boys with cryptorchidism.

of the germ cells and the increased risk of malignancy [20]. At present it is not possible to predict accurately how significant is the risk of infertility and malignancy, since the age for surgery in children has been falling dramatically in the last 20–30 years. As the lag time between treatment and assessment of fertility or malignancy risk is between 20 and 40 years, there has not been adequate time for feedback to allow clinicians to determine whether intervention in infancy is really better than treatment in the 10-year-old boy. Despite this dilemma, there is a significant body of experimental evidence which would suggest that early surgery should produce a significantly improved result in outcomes of poor fertility and cancer risk [21–23].

Aetiology

The aetiology of undescended testes depends on understanding the normal process of testicular descent. This begins at approximately 10 weeks of gestation, shortly after the onset of sexual differentiation at 8 weeks. There are two morphological steps. Initially, the testis moves from the urogenital ridge to the inguinal region at between 10 and 15 weeks. This has been called transabdominal descent. Secondly, the testis then migrates from the inguinal canal to the scrotum between 28 and 35 weeks [24] (Fig. 24.10).

The descent of the testis is controlled by a mesenchymal column or ligament, known as the gubernaculum, which connects the testis in the urogenital ridge to the inguinal region at the site of the future inguinal canal. Under the action of male hormones, the gubernaculum in the male enlarges to form a solid mesenchymal cord with an enlarged caudal end known as the bulb [25]. The thickened gubernaculum in the male anchors the testis near the inguinal region as the fetus enlarges. By contrast, in the female the gubernaculum remains thin and fails to hold the ovary near the inguinal region with fetal growth.

The inguinoscrotal phase of descent requires the gubernaculum to move from the inguinal region to the scrotum. This second phase is dependent on androgen secretion, and recent evidence suggests that it also requires a normal genitofemoral nerve [26]. The genitofemoral nerve may release a neurotransmitter (calcitonin gene-related peptide) which may be important for controlling this migration phase. As the gubernaculum elongates towards the scrotum, it is hollowed out by a diverticulum of the peritoneal cavity, the processus vaginalis. The effect of these combined mechanisms is that the gubernaculum is somewhat like an elongating windsock as it moves towards the scrotum, with the testis inside the processus vaginalis.

These ideas help explain some variants of undescended testis. Children with primary defects of testicular develop-

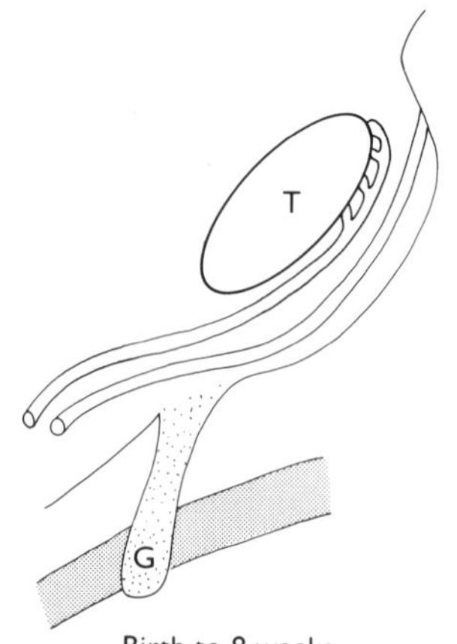

Birth to 8 weeks

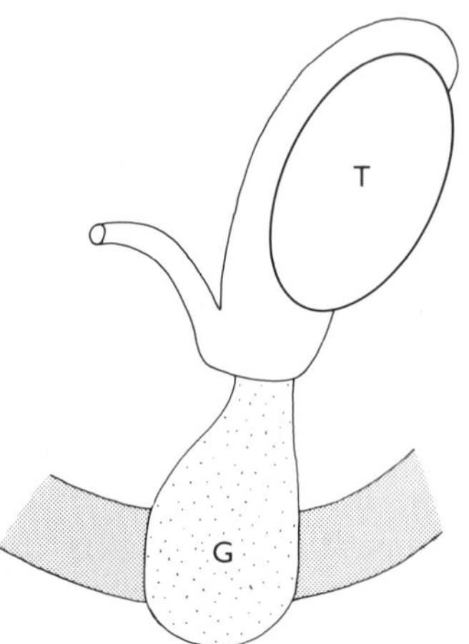

8–15 weeks: MIS (?) → gubernacular enlargement

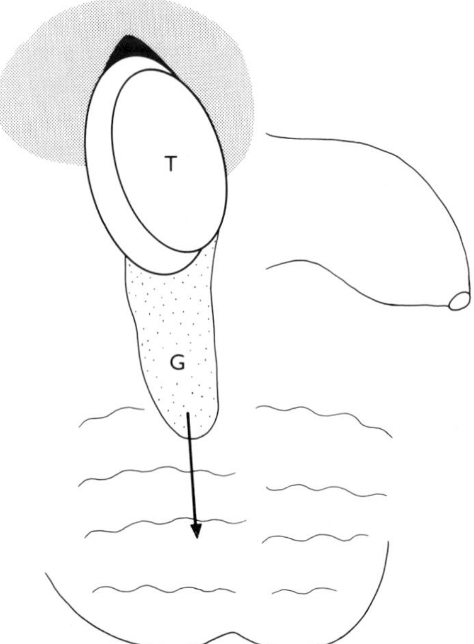

28–35 weeks: testosterone → gubernacular migration

Fig 24.10 Schema of the two-stage hypothesis for testicular descent. G, gubernaculum; T, testis.

ment or hormone production may have undescended testis, such as those children with proven MIS [27] or androgen deficiency [28]. Such hormonal abnormalities are rare, and most children have no obvious hormonal deficiency. The first phase of descent is rarely abnormal, and nearly all undescended testes have an abnormality of the migration phase of the gubernaculum. Consequently, the testis is usually palpable in the groin. Testes that have migrated to ectopic positions, such as the perineum, may be caused by an abnormal location of the genitofemoral nerve.

Diagnosis

Diagnosis of an undescended testis depends on localizing the testis and finding the lowest position towards the scrotum that it can occupy. Where the testis resides within the scrotum at least some of the time, no treatment is indicated. Even when the testis has not reached the scrotum during development, it is still within the processus vaginalis inside the gubernaculum. Therefore, it has significant mobility, which may make diagnosis difficult. Unless the inguinal region is palpated carefully, the mobility of the testis may cause it to elude the examiner's fingers. The essential points in the clinical examination are shown in Figs 24.11 & 24.12 [30].

In approximately 5–10% of children the testis is impalpable. This occurs if it is cranial to the external inguinal ring, as even the testis within the canal is usually impalpable. Where the testis cannot be felt, approximately one-third will be in the canal, another one-third will lie in the abdomen (usually just near the internal inguinal ring), and one-third will be absent. Investigations that have been suggested to locate the impalpable testis include ultrasound, computerized tomography and magnetic resonance imaging. Operative laparoscopy would now appear to be the best method of finding an impalpable testis. Where the child has bilateral impalpable testes a human chorionic gonadotrophin (hCG) stimulation test will indicate whether or not there is testicular tissue present prior to any further intervention.

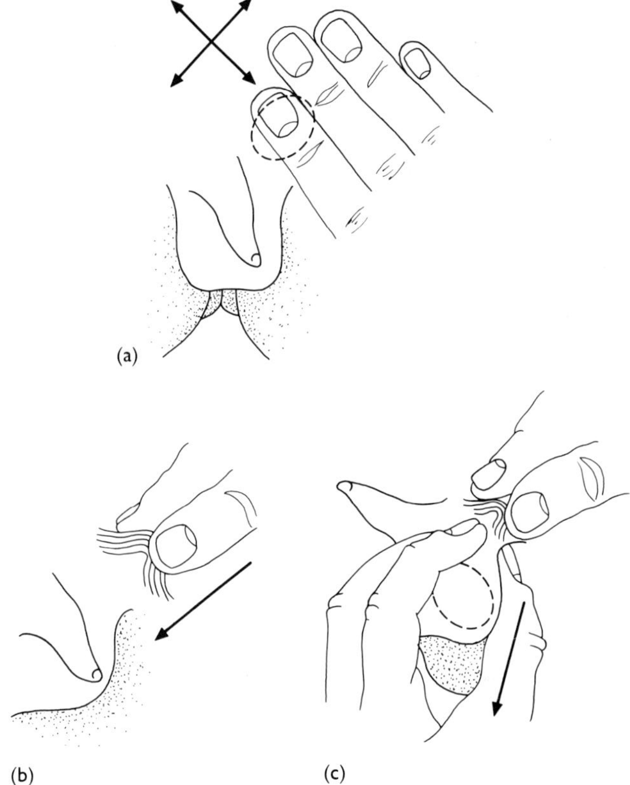

Fig 24.12 The technique of locating and delivering an undescended tesits to the top of the scrotum. (a) Palpating the inguinal testis by using its natural mobility. (b) Pushing the testis towards the scrotal neck. (c) Determining the lowest position that the testis can reach should distinguish between cryptorchid and normally retractile testes (redrawn from Hutson & Beasley [30]).

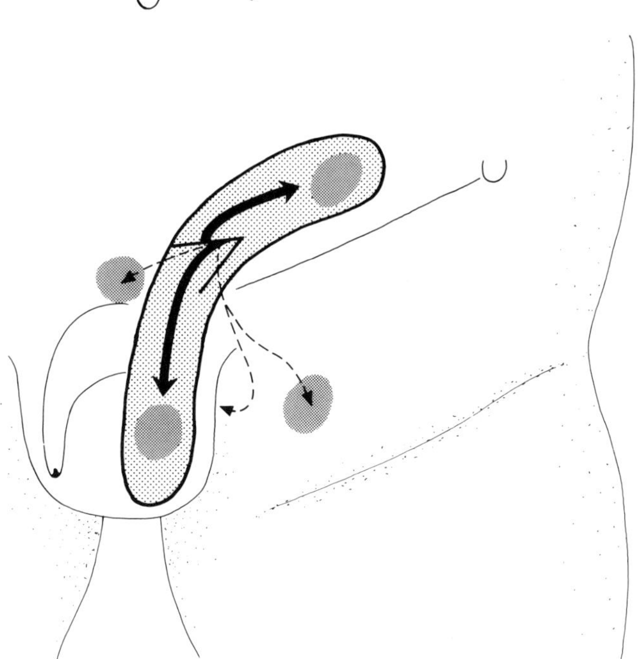

Fig 24.11 The surface anatomy of the inguinal region and the arc along which the testis normally is located. The ectopic positions shown are all rare (redrawn from Hutson & Beasley [30]).

Treatment

The aim of treatment of an undescended testis is to place the testis within the scrotum early in childhood to prevent secondary germ-cell degeneration and dysplasia. It is believed that this can be achieved by surgery between 6 months and 2 years. Operation in infancy requires skill and experience to avoid damage to the testicular vessels and the vas deferens. Occasionally, a concomitant hernia necessitates neonatal herniotomy when the orchidopexy would be done simultaneously. Surgery is performed under general anaesthesia in a day surgical unit, with discharge a few hours postoperatively. The testis is located through an inguinal skin crease incision and the spermatic cord mobilized inside the canal with dissection and ligation of any residual processus vaginalis. The vas and the vessels are dissected free of surrounding tissues until they can be stretched so that the testis will reach the scrotum. The testis is placed in the subcutaneous pouch which is made in the scrotum, and is held there either by 'buttonholing' the testis through the deep fascia or by a stitch to the scrotal septum.

Hormonal treatment with hCG or luteinizing-hormone-releasing hormone (LHRH) have both been tried, but have proved to be relatively ineffective for true undescended testis [29,31]. By contrast, those children with abnormally retractile or ascending testis may respond to hCG or LHRH. In an older child, therefore, where ascending or retractile testes are statistically more likely, a trial of hCG therapy may be appropriate [32]. In the infant with true congenital undescended testis, however, early surgery is probably a better alternative, given current knowledge.

The long-term outcome for undescended testes remains uncertain because of the changing treatment and the long lag time between therapy and results. At present the role of surgery in avoiding infertility or malignancy is uncertain, but there is every reason to anticipate improved results when the children who are currently being treated reach adult life.

ANORCHIA

Complete absence of the testis may be caused by primary agenesis or secondary ischaemic necrosis during development [33]. Where there is complete agenesis of the urogenital ridge there may be deficiency of the ipsilateral kidney. Ischaemic necrosis during descent of the testis is a more common cause for anorchia. This occurs during testicular migration, when the testis is mobile and vulnerable to torsion. The vas deferens and the testicular vessels end at the internal inguinal ring where there is a small nubbin of fibrous tissue containing haemosiderin. Testicular prostheses are required occasionally to overcome psychological problems related to anorchia, particularly in adolescence. There are prostheses suitable for prepubertal children, but these are not commonly required.

ACUTE SCROTUM

The 'acute scrotum' includes a group of conditions where there is acute inflammation of the scrotal contents [34]. There are four main diagnoses: epididymo-orchitis, torsion of the testis, torsion of the testicular appendages and acute idiopathic scrotal oedema. Acute local allergic reactions cause superficial scrotal oedema, but the other three causes are related to inflammatory or mechanical problems in the testis and epididymis. Their aetiology is related to hormonal stimulation, and they tend to present at characteristic times at childhood in relation to the serum hormone levels (Fig. 24.13).

The most common abnormality is torsion of a testicular appendage, which can occur throughout childhood but is most common between 11 and 12 years. The appendage, or hydatid of Morgagni, is at the cranial pole of the testis adjacent to the head of the epididymis, and is believed to be the cranial remnant of the Müllerian duct. It is a small pedunculated cyst which enlarges between 11 and 13 years of age, when there is often a low level of circulating oestrogen in the serum of prepubertal boys (which also may cause transient gynaecomastia). The Müllerian duct remnant responds to oestrogen by enlargement, thereby predisposing to torsion around the narrow stalk. This produces acute pain and secondary inflammation in the scrotum, which may be so profound that it is impossible to differentiate the small twisted appendage from torsion of the testis itself. Treatment is by immediate scrotal exploration, to exclude torsion of the testis and to excise the twisted appendage, which is immediately curative.

Torsion of the testis is the next most common abnormality seen in childhood, and has two peaks of incidence, one in the first year of life and another at about 13–14

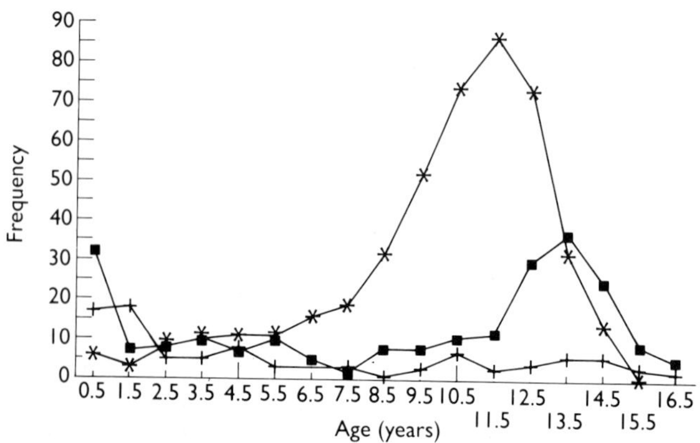

Fig 24.13 The relationship between age and frequency of different causes of acute scrotum. ■, Torsion of testis; *, torsion of testicular appendage; +, epididymitis (redrawn from Clift & Hutson [34]).

years. The first peak is related to perinatal torsion during descent, and here the entire gubernacular apparatus, including the testis, is twisted. Frequently, testicular torsion has occurred prenatally, and by the time of delivery the testis is infarcted and atrophies postnatally. Rarely, the torsion might occur immediately after birth and may be salvaged by immediate scrotal exploration.

In adolescent boys, torsion of the testis occurs most commonly at 13–14 years and is caused by twisting of the testis within the tunica vaginalis. It is predisposed to by a long mesorchium, a minor anatomical variant whereby the mesentery of the testis and the epididymis is elongated so that the testis hangs loosely inside the tunica vaginalis. This predisposes to torsion, which can occur any time, but is most common when the testis enlarges rapidly in response to pubertal androgens. Treatment is by immediate exploration, untwisting, and fixation of the testis if it is still viable, or excision if it is necrotic. Fixation of the contralateral testis is important to prevent torsion, since the long mesorchium is bilateral.

Epididymitis, or epididymo-orchitis, is relatively uncommon in childhood. After puberty, a common cause is viral infection by mumps, or bacterial infection related to sexual activity. Prior to puberty, epididymitis is caused by retrograde spread of organisms from the urinary tract along the vas deferens, and is therefore only common in children with urinary malformations and secondary urinary infection. Postnatal testosterone secretion may predispose to epididymitis at this time by transient stimulation of the vas deferens and adjacent glandular structures. Beyond 2 years of age, epididymitis is a very rare condition until after puberty, when the vas again becomes a patent structure containing secretions which predispose to organisms being transmitted retrogradely.

VARICOCELE

Varicocele is a dilatation of the veins in the pampiniform plexus of the spermatic cord. It develops with the onset of puberty and is more common on the left side. It is caused by a defect of the valves in the testicular veins, allowing back-pressure and varicose dilatation of the veins in the scrotum. When the boy is supine, the varicocele may be hard to feel or see, with just a vague, soft swelling in the upper scrotum. However, on standing, the varicosities are filled and characteristically feel like a 'bag of worms'. Varicocele causes no symptoms until it becomes of moderate size, when it may cause an aching sensation in the groin. The primary concern and reason for intervention is that it is associated with decreased fertility, presumed to be caused by the increased temperature of the testis when surrounded by varicose veins.

The management of varicocele is controversial, because no single operation has demonstrated superior efficacy over alternatives, and because of the high risk of complications such as recurrence of the varicocele or secondary hydrocele in the scrotum [35,36]. Surgical alternatives include exploration of the inguinal spermatic cord with ligation of the varicosities, with or without a microscope, retroperitoneal ligation of the varicose testicular veins via a small supra-inguinal incision or more recently laparoscopic ligation of the testicular veins. It has been demonstrated in varicoceles that ligation of the testicular artery, as well as the vein, rarely causes testicular atrophy, and may in fact be a useful adjunct to treatment. If all the veins are ligated, the arterial blood will have no convenient exit to leave the testis, which may predispose to recurrence of the varicocele. By contrast, when the testicular vessels, including the artery, are ligated, the total flow through the testis should be reduced, thereby reducing the risk of recurrence. In this condition there seem to be good secondary collaterals already formed along the artery to the vas deferens, which is probably why ligation of the testicular artery does not cause testicular necrosis.

Where the varicocele occurs before the onset of puberty, the physical examination should include careful assessment of the kidneys to exclude a retroperitoneal tumour, such as a neuroblastoma or Wilms tumour, which may cause compression of the proximal end of the testicular vein leading to a secondary varicocele.

TESTICULAR TUMOURS

In childhood, testicular tumours are quite rare. In early infancy, teratomas or embryonal carcinomas are seen, along with rhabdomyosarcomas in the spermatic cord later in childhood. After puberty, hormone-secreting tumours are seen occasionally. Secondary leukaemic infiltration has been a common cause of testicular tumours, but is now less common with changing practice in oncology.

REFERENCES

1 Hutson JM, Donahoe PK. The hormonal control of testicular descent. *Endocr Rev* 1986;7:270–83.
2 Scott JES. The Hutson hypothesis. *Br J Urol* 1987;60:74–6.
3 Hutson JM, Voigt RW, Kelly H, Luthra M, Fowler R. Girth-reduction clitoroplasty: a new technique with 15 years' experience in 38 patients. *Pediatr Surg Int* 1991;6:336–40.
4 Johnston JH. The surgery of upper tract duplication. In: Frank JD, Johnston JH, eds. *Operative Paediatric Urology.* Edinburgh: Churchill Livingstone, 1990:12–18.
5 McMullin ND, Hutson JM. Female psuedohermaphroditism in children with cloacal anomalies. *Pediatr Surg Int* 1991;6: 56–9.
6 Goh DW, Middlesworth W, Stephens FD, Kelly JH, Hutson JM. Intracolonic lithiasis: a result of prenatal admixture of urine and meconium? *Pediatr Surg Int* 1993;8:222–5.
7 Hendren WH. Repair of cloacal anomalies: current techniques. *J Pediatr Surg* 1986;21:1159–76.

8 Pena A. The surgical management of persistent cloaca: results in 54 patients treated with a posterior sagittal approach. *J Pediatr Surg* 1989;24:590–8.
9 Tarry W, Duckett J, Stephens FD. The Mayer–Rokitansky syndrome: pathogenesis, classification and management. *J Urol* 1986;136:648–52.
10 Leung AKC, Robson WLM, Tay-Uyboco J. The incidence of labial fusion in children. *J Paediatr Child Health* 1993;29: 235–6.
11 Stephens FD. Embryology and pathoembryology of the urinary tract. In: Webster G, Kirby R, King L, Goldwasser B, eds. *Reconstructive Urology*. Oxford: Blackwell Scientific Publications, 1993:93–104.
12 Duckett JW. Hypospadias repair. In: Frank JD, Johnston JH, eds. *Operative Paediatric Urology*. Edinburgh: Churchill Livingstone, 1990:197–208.
13 Belman AB. Hypospadias. In: Welch KJ, Randolph JG, Ravitch MM, O'Neill JA, Power MI, eds. *Pediatric Surgery*, 4th edn. Chicago: Year Book Medical, 1986:1286–302.
14 Hutson JM, Beasley SW. *Descent of the Testis*. London: Edward Arnold, 1992.
15 Farrington GH. The position and retractability of the normal testis in childhood with reference to the diagnosis and treatment of cryptorchidism. *J Pediatr Surg* 1968;3:53–9.
16 John Radcliffe Hospital Cryptorchidism Study Group. Boys with late descending testes: the source of patients with 'retractile' testes undergoing orchidopexy. *Br Med J* 1986;293: 289–90.
17 Zorgniotti AW, ed. Temperature and environmental effects on the tesits. In: Zorgniotti AW, ed. *Advances in Experimental Medicine and Biology*, Vol. 286. New York: Plenum Press, 1991.
18 Gendrel D, Roger M, Job J-C. Plasma gonadotropin and testosterone values in infants with cryptorchidism. *J Pediatr* 1980;97:217–20.
19 Yamanaka J, Baker M, Metcalfe S, Hutson JM. Serum levels of Müllerian inhibiting substance in boys with cryptorchidism. *J Pediatr Surg* 1991;26:621–3.
20 Giwercman A, Bruun E, Frimodt-Moller CAI, Skakkebaek NS. Prevalence of carcinoma-*in-situ* and other histopathological abnormalities in testes of men with a history of cryptorchidism. *J Urol* 1989;142:998–1002.
21 Hadziselimovic F, Herzog B, Seguchi H. Surgical correction of cryptorchidism at 2 years: electron microsopic and morphometric investigations. *J Pediatr Surg* 1975;10:19–26.
22 Mengel W, Heinz HA, Sippe WG, Hecker WC. Studies on cryptorchidism: a comparison of histological findings in the germinative epithelium before and after the second year of life. *J Pediatr Surg* 1974;9:445–50.
23 Stewart RJ, Brown S. Fertility in experimental unilateral cryptorchidism. *J Pediatr Surg* 1990;25:672–4.
24 Hutson JM. A biphasic model for the hormonal control of testicular descent. *Lancet* 1985;2:419–21.
25 Wensing CJG, Colenbrander B. Normal and abnormal testicular descent. In: Clarke JR, ed. *Oxford Review of Reproductive Biology*, Vol. 8. Oxford: Clarendon Press, 1986: 125–30.
26 Hutson JM, Baker ML, Griffiths AL *et al.* Endocrine and morphological perspectives in testicular descent. *Reprod Med Rev* 1992;1:165–77.
27 Hutson JM, Chow CW, Ng WD. Persistent Mullerian duct syndrome with transverse testicular ectopia. An experiment of nature with clues for understanding testicular descent. *Pediatr Surg Int* 1987;2:191–4.
28 Mason AJ, Pitts SL, Nikolics K *et al.* The hypogonadal mouse: reproductive functions restored by gene therapy. *Science* 1986;234:1372–8.
29 Rajfer J, Handelsman DJ, Swerdloff RS. Hormonal therapy of cryptorchidism. A randomised double-blind study comparing human chorionic gonadotropin and gonadotropin-releasing hormone. *N Engl J Med* 1986;314:466–70.
30 Hutson JM, Beasley SW. *The Surgical Examination of Children*. Oxford: Heinemann Medical, 1988.
31 De Muinck Keizer-Schrama SMPF. Hormonal treatment of cryptorchidism. *Horm Res* 1988;30:178–86.
32 Karpe B. Prognosis of hormonal treatment of undescended testis related to testicular position at birth. *Pediatr Surg Int* 1991;6:221–2.
33 Oesch I, Ransley PG. Unilaterally impalpable testis. *Eur Urol* 1987;13:324–6.
34 Clift VL, Hutson JM. The acute scrotum in childhood. *Pediatr Surg Int* 1989;4:185–8.
35 Beck EM, Schlegel PN, Goldstein M. Intraoperative varicocele anatomy: a macroscopic and microscopic study. *J Urol* 1992; 148:1190–4.
36 Goldstein M, Gilbert BR, Dicker AP, Duroth J, Gnecco C. Microsurgical inguinal varicocelectomy with delivery of the testis: an artery and lymphatic sparing technique. *J Urol* 1992;148:1808–11.

25: Growth and Endocrine Sequelae Following the Treatment of Childhood Cancer

S.M. SHALET

INTRODUCTION

The overall cure rate for childhood cancer is now over 60% and is over 90% for some tumours. It has been estimated that at least 1 : 1000 young adults will have been cured of childhood cancer by the year 2000. This improved survival has stimulated great interest in the adverse late effects of radiotherapy and cytotoxic chemotherapy on growth and the endocrine system.

Radiation therapy may directly impair hypothalamic, pituitary, thyroid and gonadal function or, alternatively, it may induce the development of thyroid adenomas or carcinomas. Cytotoxic chemotherapy may damage the gonads. Both irradiation and cytotoxic chemotherapy may interfere with the normal growth of bone.

A variety of clinical presentations, which require endocrine expertise in management, may result from these complications of treatment (Table 25.1).

GROWTH IMPAIRMENT

There are a number of factors which may adversely affect growth in children treated for the common malignant diseases. These include direct radiation damage to the hypothalamopituitary axis, the long bones and the spine. Other important factors include malnutrition, steroid therapy and the presence of residual tumour. Cytotoxic chemotherapy may be a potent influence on growth, and studies indicate that growth is more adversely affected in children treated for brain tumours with a combination of chemotherapy and central nervous system (CNS) irradiation than with CNS irradiation alone [1]. The most studied of these adverse factors, however, are radiation-induced growth hormone (GH) deficiency, impaired spinal growth and precocious or early puberty.

GH deficiency

RADIATION SCHEDULE

The radiobiological impact of an irradiation schedule is dependent on the total dose, the number of fractions and duration. The same total given in fewer fractions over a shorter time period is likely to cause a greater incidence of GH deficiency than if the schedule were spread over a longer time interval with a greater number of fractions [2].

The radiation schedule for total-body irradiation (TBI) consists of approximately 750–1300 cGy administered either as a single dose or as multiple fractions over several days. Either schedule may induce GH deficiency [3–6], but it is unclear if the single-dose schedule does so more frequently.

The degree of pituitary hormonal deficit is related to the radiation dose received by the hypothalamopituitary axis. Thus, after lower radiation doses, isolated GH deficiency ensues, whilst higher doses may produce panhypopituitarism. In the vast majority of children the GH deficiency is isolated; however, in certain centres, children with brain tumours or nasopharyngeal carcinomas may receive a higher dose of irradiation to the hypothalamopituitary axis leading to other pituitary hormone deficits [7].

The greater the radiation dose, the earlier GH deficiency will occur after treatment. Between 2 and 5 years after irradiation 100% of children receiving $\geq$ 3000 cGy (over 3 weeks) to the hypothalamopituitary axis showed subnormal GH responses to an insulin tolerance test (ITT), while 35% of those receiving $<$ 3000 cGy (over 3 weeks) still showed a normal GH response [8]. The prospective studies, however, have concentrated on GH responses to provocative tests; the speed of onset of GH deficiency detected by measurement of spontaneous GH secretion following radiation-induced damage, and the natural history of GH deficiency after TBI, remain unknown. Furthermore, while there is no dispute about the capacity of radiotherapy to render a child GH-deficient, recent prospective studies have suggested that the GH response to an ITT may already be perturbed before radiotherapy [9], contrary to the findings of earlier studies [10].

AGE AND PUBERTAL STATUS

Investigations of GH secretion after cranial irradiation in

Table 25.1 Clinical endocrine problems following childhood cancer treatment

Short stature
Lack of pubertal development
Precocious puberty
Hypothyroidism
Thyroid tumours
Gynaecomastia
Infertility
Hypopituitarism

humans support experimental animal data, which show the CNS of young animals to be more radiosensitive than those of older animals. After a mean time of 2.8 years following TBI (1000–1320 cGy in five or six fractions over 3 days), 18 of 18 adults still showed a normal GH response to an ITT [11], while 15 out of 29 children showed subnormal GH responses to an ITT after a mean time of 2.4 years and a similar TBI schedule (1100–1520 cGy in three to eight fractions over 2–5 days) [5]. Admittedly, three of the 15 children had received cranial irradiation previously, which might have explained the GH deficiency, but no other irradiation had been administered to the remaining 12.

Thus the CNS of children appears more radiosensitive than those of adults and there is evidence that the younger the child receiving prophylactic cranial irradiation for acute lymphoblastic leukaemia (ALL), the greater the susceptibility to radiation-induced GH deficiency [12].

GROWTH HORMONE TESTS

A factor influencing the prevalence of radiation-induced GH deficiency is the type of investigation used to assess GH secretion. Chrousos *et al.* [13] showed that physiological GH secretion could be severely reduced in quantity in an irradiated primate which still showed a normal GH response to arginine or L-dopa stimulation. Similarly Blatt *et al.* [14] reported normal GH responses to an ITT but subnormal spontaneous GH secretion in three children who received prophylactic cranial irradiation for ALL. This phenomenon has been described as radiation-induced GH neurosecretory dysfunction. In complete contrast Ryalls *et al.* [15] have observed essentially normal spontaneous GH secretion but blunted GH responses to an ITT in children treated for ALL, who had never received any radiotherapy. Some of the apparent contradiction may be explained by the gradual evolution over time of damage to different centres concerned with the control of GH secretion.

It is likely that the higher irradiation doses (≥2700 cGy) received by children with brain tumours affect both spontaneous GH secretion and stimulated GH responses with time fairly completely and therefore, ultimately, equally. Radiation-induced GH neurosecretory dysfunction may only be a real clinical problem in the children treated for ALL who have received a radiation dose in the range of 1800–2400 cGy. The exact prevalence of this problem is unknown.

Reduced spontaneous GH secretion during 24-h profiles has been described in both prepubertal and pubertal girls following cranial irradiation for ALL (2400 cGy) with a failure of the expected increase in GH secretion at puberty [16] associated with attenuated pubertal growth [17]. After 1980 the dose of irradiation employed in prophylactic cranial irradiation for ALL was reduced to 1800 cGy in an attempt to minimize neuropsychological disturbance and abnormalities of GH secretion.

Results of recently completed studies of GH secretion [18] differ from those obtained by Moell *et al.* [16] in that spontaneous GH secretion was normal in the prepubertal children following low-dose cranial irradiation (1800 cGy). The pubertal children, however, showed abnormalities of spontaneous GH secretion, despite the fact that each underwent puberty spontaneously and showed normal pubertal progression. Apart from a reduction in the total amount of GH secreted, there was also a significant disturbance in the periodicity of GH secretion in the irradiated (1800 cGy) pubertal children [18] (Fig. 25.1); a finding which has also been observed in the first year after TBI for childhood leukaemia [15]. Furthermore, preliminary data suggest that low-dose cranial irradiation administered below the age of 7 years is associated with suboptimal pubertal growth subsequently [19].

Impaired spinal growth

Skeletal disproportion due to impaired spinal growth has been described in children following craniospinal irradiation for brain tumours [20], TBI for leukaemia [4] and abdominal irradiation for Wilms tumour [21]. The younger the child at treatment, the more severe is the restriction on spinal growth and the shorter and more disproportionate such children become as adults [20,21]. There is no evidence that the spine is more radiosensitive at any particular phase of childhood [22] but the effect is, of course, particularly evident during puberty when spinal growth is so important.

GH replacement therapy after craniospinal irradiation does not alter the growth of an irradiated spine [23]; thus the effect of GH is to exaggerate disproportion, albeit to a limited extent, in a situation where marked disproportion already exists (Fig. 25.2). Currently studies are under way to determine if an increase in GH dosage can improve the height prognosis for this form of radiation-induced skeletal dysplasia [24].

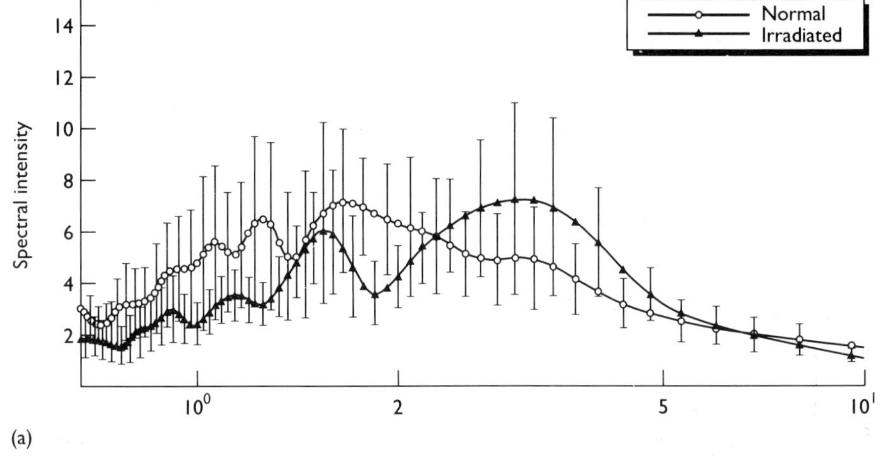

(a)

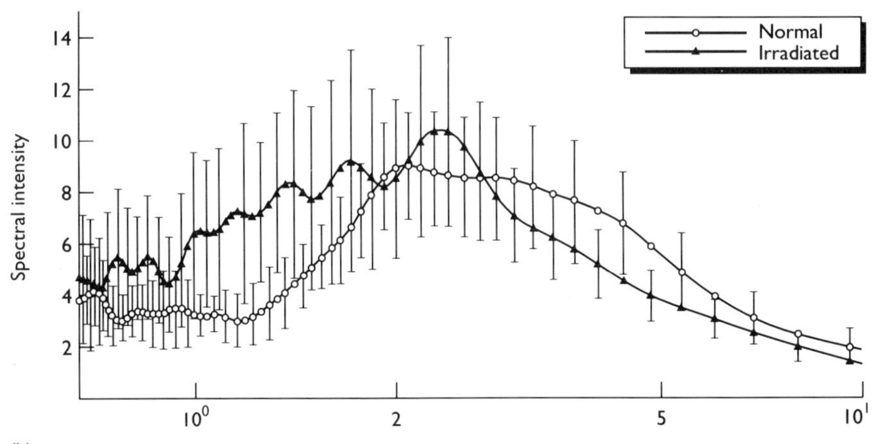

(b)

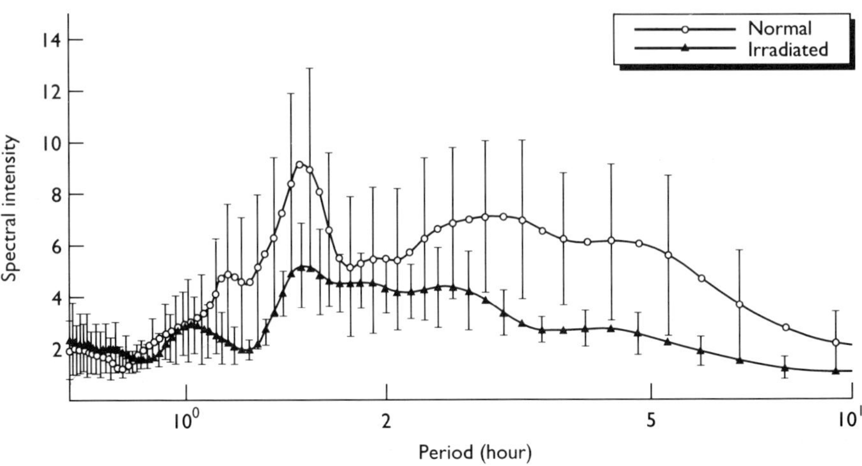

(c)

Fig. 25.1 Pooled estimated power spectra for the GH profiles of (a) prepubertal, (b) pubertal and (c) postpubertal groups. Results for both normal children and those treated with low-dose cranial irradiation (1800 cGy) are depicted. Note the spectral flattening for both pubertal and postpubertal irradiated groups. In particular, the pubertal irradiated group exhibits increased spectral intensities for all short periods, indicating a randomization of GH pulsing.

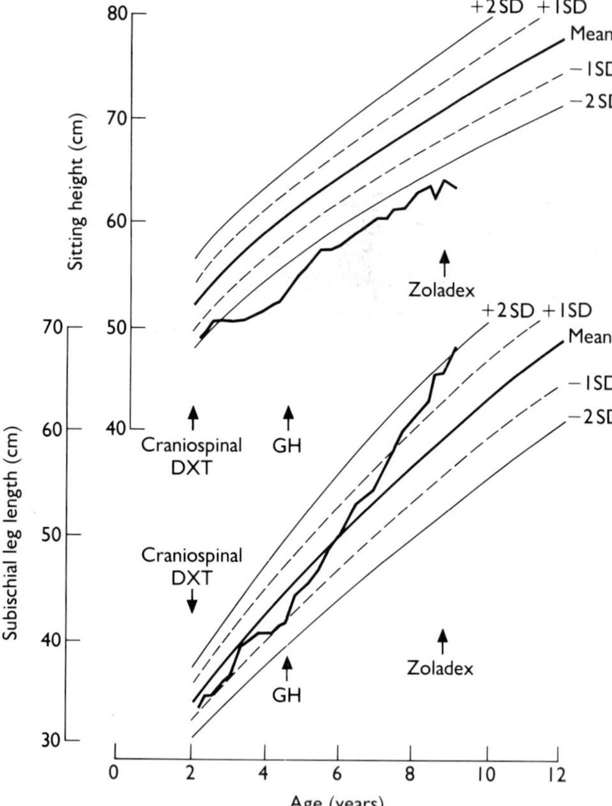

Fig. 25.2 Response in leg length and sitting height to GH therapy in a boy who received craniospinal irradiation (DXT) for a medulloblastoma at the age of 2 years. GH therapy was initiated between the ages of 4 and 5 years. Note the contrast between the excellent increment in growth in the legs and the lack of any change in sitting height.

Early or precocious puberty

The low doses of cranial irradiation (1800–2400 cGy) employed in the management of ALL may cause early or precocious puberty in girls but not in boys [17,25]. To determine if this sexual dichotomy existed at higher irradiation doses (2500–4700 cGy) the onset of puberty was identified in 46 children (30 male), previously irradiated for a brain tumour not involving the hypothalamo-pituitary axis, and compared with the normal pubertal standards of Marshall & Tanner [26].

In the patients, the onset of puberty occurred at an early age in both sexes (mean 8.5 years in girls and 9.2 years in boys). In the context of GH deficiency, which is usually associated with a delay in the onset of puberty, this is abnormal. There was a significant linear association between age at irradiation and age at onset of puberty in both sexes. At each age of irradiation the estimated age at the onset of puberty was approximately 0.7 years earlier in girls than in boys. A similar trend was seen for bone age, which was abnormally early at the time of pubertal onset. Thus, radiation-induced early puberty is not restricted to females at the doses of irradiation employed in the treatment of brain tumours.

The impact of early puberty in a child with radiation-induced growth failure is to foreshorten the time available for GH therapy. Consequently a number of these children are now treated with a combination of a gonadotrophin-releasing hormone (GnRH) analogue and GH therapy. It is relatively easy to halt the progression in pubertal development, but it is too early to analyse the impact of this approach on final height.

Indications for GH therapy

To determine if GH has had a significant impact on growth in children with radiation-induced GH deficiency, the growth velocity during the first year of GH therapy has been compared with the pretreatment growth velocity. This will indicate if there has been a significant short-term improvement in growth rate, but not if there will be a substantial gain in final height. Thus long-term studies are the most critical, and ideally these should include an analysis of the final height and gain or loss in stature (standard deviation score) from initiation of GH therapy until the end of growth in children with radiation-induced GH deficiency, contrasted with the growth pattern in those who did not receive GH therapy.

Our own final height studies [23,27] indicated that GH therapy was of significant benefit in children with radiation-induced GH deficiency but the height gained, or rather the 'height loss' that had been prevented, was disappointingly small, and much less than that seen in GH-treated children with idiopathic GH deficiency. Similarly disappointing results were reported by Sulmont *et al.* [28].

A number of factors contributed to the suboptimal growth response, including spinal irradiation, precocious or early puberty, the excessively long time interval (mean 5.5–6.7 years) between irradiation and the initiation of GH therapy and the inadequacy of the GH schedule used in the early studies.

Since the first children with radiation-induced GH deficiency treated with GH therapy reached their final height, our clinical criteria for whom to treat and when to initiate GH therapy have continued to evolve, in order to improve the final height prognosis.

The chances of recurrence of a brain tumour are greatest within 2 years of the primary treatment of the tumour. If GH treatment was offered within the first 2 years it would be associated with a number of tumour recurrences and deaths. Therefore, despite a lack of proof of a causal relationship, many families and doctors would associate GH therapy with tumour recurrence. On the other hand there is no evidence that treatment with GH increases the risk of late recurrence of a brain tumour (≥2 years from primary treatment) in children with radiation-induced GH deficiency [29].

A reasonable approach, therefore, would be to consider GH therapy for all children with brain tumours treated by standard radiation schedules, including a dose to the hypothalamopituitary axis in excess of 3000 cGy at 2 years after the completion of the primary treatment. By this time they would no longer be receiving cytotoxic chemotherapy, the chance of recurrence of a tumour would be low and it is established that most, if not all, will be GH-deficient. In certain centres, GH therapy might be offered routinely at 2 years without recourse to GH tests or evidence of impaired growth. Others would insist on biochemical evidence of GH deficiency and a subnormal growth rate. In our own centre we establish GH deficiency biochemically but would consider GH therapy independent of the growth rate, nor least because a number of children who are GH-deficient after radiotherapy grow apparently normally because of either an excessive calorie intake, early puberty or both.

Where the natural history of radiation-induced GH deficiency is less predictable or less well-known, for example after a radiation dose of 2000–3000 cGy, standard provocative tests of GH release are performed at 2 years, and if the results are abnormal the children receive GH therapy. If GH secretion appears normal, and the growth rate is appropriate for pubertal status, then growth is observed and the GH-stimulation tests repeated annually. However, if the growth rate is subnormal in the presence of normal GH responses to pharmacological stimuli, a combination which is very unusual in our centre, then GH neurosecretory dysfunction may be a possible explanation. Alternative approaches would be either an appraisal of physiological GH secretion, such as a 24-h profile, or an empirical trial of GH therapy. In practice, 24-h GH profiles are reserved for research studies and not clinical management.

These guidelines assume that growth is assessed in craniospinal irradiated children by leg length velocity, and that other causes of poor growth such as radiation-induced hypothyroidism, recurrent tumour and malnutrition have been excluded.

The timing of the introduction of GH therapy is matched with the special circumstances, age, pubertal status and needs of an individual child. Early treatment is particularly suitable for the craniospinally treated young child of short parents.

Acute lymphoblastic leukaemia

Much confusion and controversy have been generated over the growth patterns and growth hormone requirements of the child with ALL treated with prophylactic cranial irradiation and combination cytotoxic chemotherapy for several years. The dispute arose because some groups found no adverse effects on final height, while others noted a modest adverse effect on growth [30]. As final height was unknown in most of the children, the possibility of impaired pubertal growth may have meant that final height loss was substantial in a minority of children. Finally, there was a third group [31] which studied children with ALL and found a much greater retardation of growth. Analysis of the radiation schedules and chemotherapy protocols used in the different centres has led to some understanding of the explanation for the differences in height loss observed between groups.

There is *in vitro* evidence that cytotoxic chemotherapy may affect growth mechanisms and *in vivo* evidence of an effect on growth [30,31]. In the child with ALL, the duration and nature of the combination cytotoxic chemotherapy will influence the growth prognosis. After treatment with regimes used in the UK, the effects of cytotoxic chemotherapy are likely to be minor, but more intense cytotoxic chemotherapy regimes have had a profound impact on growth [31]. Children irradiated prophylactically for ALL rather than for a brain tumour tend to receive a lower radiation dose to the hypothalamo-pituitary axis. Most of the growth studies have been carried out in children who received a total cranial radiation dose of 2400–2500 cGy. As discussed earlier, the incidence of GH deficiency in such children will depend on the number of fractions, fraction size and duration of the radiation schedule [2].

For a number of reasons the demand for treatment with GH is more difficult to predict after treatment for ALL than after a brain tumour. Some of the reasons for the dissimilar growth patterns in children with ALL studied by different groups [32,33] have already been discussed. In children with severe growth retardation, even though cytotoxic chemotherapy is a serious adverse factor, radiation-induced GH deficiency is common [31]. It is appropriate, therefore, that most of these children be offered treatment with GH, whereas only a minority of the children with ALL in the UK, in whom chemotherapy appears to be only a minor adverse factor, have been treated with GH. The clinical dilemma is how to identify the few who should receive treatment.

Final height data from a number of studies are now available, and the vast majority indicate that final height is significantly compromised following 1800 cGy as well as 2400 cGy cranial irradiation for ALL [19,32–35]. Interpretation of these data is complicated by the recent observation that 23% of irradiated leukaemic children show significant skeletal disproportion at final height (Fig. 25.3) whereas GH deficiency *per se* is associated with proportionate short stature. We have suggested that in the

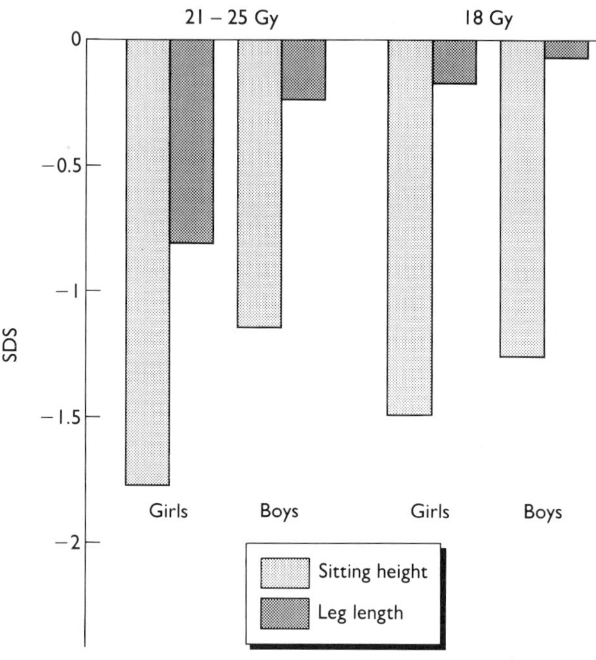

Fig. 25.3 Mean sitting height standard deviation score (SDS) and leg length SDS at final height in 101 children previously treated for ALL with combination chemotherapy and cranial irradiation but no spinal irradiation. In 60% the cranial irradiation dose was 21–25 Gy and in 40% it was 18 Gy.

presence of biochemical evidence of GH deficiency those children who are below the 10th centile, or whose growth rate is persistently poor after completion of cytotoxic chemotherapy, should be considered for a therapeutic trial of GH [30]. It should be understood, however, that this is an arbitrary definition of GH requirement.

Total-body irradiation

Marrow transplantation has become lifesaving for an increasing number of children and young adults with haematological disorders, particularly leukaemia. Follow-up studies evaluating growth and development have shown that the delayed effects are related to the regime used for preparation for marrow transplantation. Few endocrine abnormalities have been observed after regimes containing only high doses of cyclophosphamide, but growth disturbance and multiple endocrine abnormalities have been seen after regimes that include TBI [4–6].

Following TBI, severe growth disturbance is common, and may be caused by various aetiological factors including GH deficiency, thyroid dysfunction, radiation-induced impairment of skeletal growth or graft-versus-host disease and its treatment. GH deficiency may occur, even if the child has not received prophylactic cranial irradiation previously, irrespective of the TBI schedule being single-dose [3] or fractionated [5], although this is not a universal finding [36].

Preliminary data suggest a modest benefit from GH therapy in children with growth failure following TBI. Papadimitriou *et al.* [37] concluded that such children respond to treatment with GH in either of the two dose regimes with an increase in height velocity that is adequate to restore a normal growth rate but not catch-up. The heterogeneous nature of the 13 patients studied by Papadimitriou *et al.* [37], however, makes firm conclusions difficult. In their study several children were pubertal, others were receiving additional endocrine therapy and two had graft-versus-host disease. Furthermore the mean age at which GH therapy was introduced was 12.2 years.

There is a desperate need for more information on the impact of single and fractionated courses of 1000–1300 cGy TBI on the incidence of GH deficiency, frequency of GH neurosecretory dysfunction, speed of onset of GH deficiency and the natural history of radiation-induced skeletal dysplasia. Without such information the growth problems of this group of patients remain among the most difficult encountered in clinical practice. Once graft-versus-host disease and hypothyroidism have been excluded, standard provocative tests of GH secretion are required in a child growing poorly after TBI. If the GH responses are subnormal, GH therapy should be offered. If GH responses are normal, a number of questions remain. Is the child growing slowly because of radiation-induced skeletal dysplasia or GH neurosecretory dysfunction? Should the child receive an empirical trial of GH therapy? If GH therapy is instituted, what is the optimal schedule in the likely presence of GH deficiency and radiation-induced skeletal dysplasia?

THYROID DISEASE

The most important complications of radiation to the thyroid gland are hypothyroidism and thyroid tumours [38]. An association between X-ray exposure and thyroid cancer was suggested by Duffy & Fitzgerald [39]. More recently Ron *et al.* [38] studied 10 834 children who received X-ray therapy for tinea capitis between 1948 and 1960. These were compared with 10 834 non-irradiated controls and 5392 non-irradiated siblings. Ninety-eight thyroid tumours (1 : 100) were identified among the exposed and 57 (1 : 280) among the non-irradiated. An estimated dose of 9 cGy was linked to a four-fold increase of malignant tumours and a two-fold increase of benign tumours. The risk of thyroid cancer rises with increasing dose, but this is derived almost entirely from the increase from less than 200 cGy to greater than 200 cGy [40]. The risk of thyroid cancer did not decrease, however, at radiation doses as high as 6000 cGy [40].

THYROID DYSFUNCTION

Thyroid dysfunction after irradiation and cytotoxic chemotherapy in adults with Hodgkin disease ranges from frank hypothyroidism (with increased thyroid-stimulating hormone (TSH) and low thyroxine (T_4) concentrations) to compensated thyroid dysfunction (with raised TSH, but normal T_4 levels) [41]. It is not clear whether thyroid dysfunction is more common after the same dose of irradiation in children compared to adults but most large studies with prolonged follow-up have been carried out in adults [41]. After a radiation dose to the neck of 4000–5000 cGy was administered to adult patients with Hodgkin disease [33], approximately 25% of patients showed elevated TSH and low T_4 concentrations while a further 41% had raised TSH levels in the presence of normal T_4 levels. The time interval between thyroid irradiation and the peak incidence of thyroid dysfunction is unknown. However, the low incidence of thyroid dysfunction (14%) after 1 year rose to a cumulative incidence of 66% at 6 years postirradiation [42].

Children whose thyroid glands are irradiated during craniospinal irradiation for brain tumours, or during TBI before bone marrow transplantation, are vulnerable to thyroid dysfunction. Of significant importance is the finding that the incidence of thyroid dysfunction (16%) following fractionated TBI [5] is much lower than that reported after single fraction TBI (39–59%) [6]. The incidence may vary with time, as recovery of thyroid function has been observed in patients with documented thyroid dysfunction following TBI.

Thirty per cent of children treated for brain tumours with cranial or craniospinal irradiation, with or without adjuvant cytotoxic chemotherapy, will develop thyroid dysfunction at some time after treatment. The most frequent abnormality is compensated thyroid dysfunction and thyroid function reverts to normal with time in a significant minority. It appears that the combined effect of direct irradiation to the thyroid gland during craniospinal irradiation plus cytotoxic chemotherapy is the most deleterious to the thyroid gland, and is associated with the highest incidence of thyroid dysfunction and fastest time to onset of thyroid dysfunction [43,44].

In children with obvious biochemical hypothyroidism, T_4 replacement is indicated. In patients with compensated thyroid dysfunction who have been irradiated, treatment with T_4 is indicated for several reasons. First, there is strong circumstantial evidence that an increased concentration of TSH may increase the risk of thyroid tumour developing in an irradiated thyroid gland. Secondly, in a child in whom growth may be compromised for a number of reasons, it is important to maximize the remaining growth potential by ensuring that the child is euthyroid. In those children who are at risk of developing radiation-induced thyroid disease, annual palpation of the neck and measurement of the basal TSH and T_4 concentrations are recommended.

GONADAL DYSFUNCTION

The impact of combination cytotoxic chemotherapy on gonadal function is dependent on the nature and dosage of the drugs received by the child. Drugs that have been shown to cause gonadal damage include the alkylating agents, such as cyclophosphamide, chlorambucil and the nitrosoureas, in addition to procarbazine, vinblastine, cytosine arabinoside and cisplatinum.

It is known that the normal adult testis is extremely sensitive to the effects of external irradiation. However, neither the threshold dose of irradiation required to damage the germinal epithelium in childhood nor the dose above which irreversible damage occurs are known. In irradiated women the response of the ovary involves a fixed pool of oocytes which once destroyed cannot be replaced. The LD_{50} for the human oocyte has recently been estimated not to exceed 400 cGy [45].

ACUTE LYMPHOBLASTIC LEUKAEMIA

Combination chemotherapy and the testis

Lendon *et al.* [46] studied testicular histology in 44 boys treated with combination chemotherapy for ALL. At the time of testicular biopsy, 21 boys were still receiving cytotoxic drugs and 23 had completed their chemotherapy some time earlier. Based on a count of at least 100 cross-sections of tubules per biopsy, the tubular fertility index (TFI) was calculated as the percentage of seminiferous tubules containing identifiable spermatogonia. The mean TFI in the 44 biopsies was 50% of that in age-matched controls, and 18 of the biopsies showed a severely depressed TFI of 40% or less. Previous chemotherapy with cyclophosphamide or cytosine arabinoside (total dose $> 1\,g/m^2$) depressed the TFI; TFI improved with increasing time after completion of chemotherapy. These conclusions were supported by the findings of Uderzo *et al.* [47].

Shalet *et al.* [48] studied testicular function in the 44 boys whose testicular biopsies were reported by Lendon *et al.* [46]. They reported normal Leydig cell function as assessed by the testosterone response to human chorionic gonadotrophin (hCG) but described abnormalities of FSH secretion consistent with germ-cell damage in the pubertal boys. In this study all the boys subsequently achieved normal adult secondary sex characteristics and had a serum testosterone concentration within the normal adult range consistent with normal Leydig cell function.

In a recent study of testicular function in 25 boys treated with a modified LSA_2L_2 protocol [49], that consisted of 10 cytotoxic agents including cyclophosphamide and cytosine arabinoside for 3 or 4 years, severe testicular damage was reported. In 24 testicular biopsies assessed at the time of completion of chemotherapy there was an absence of germ cells in 13 and the germ cells were markedly depleted in the remaining 11. Raised basal FSH levels and an exaggerated FSH response to an acute bolus of GnRH were reported in the majority of boys who were pubertal at assessment.

To assess the reversibility of documented germ-cell damage after chemotherapy for ALL in childhood, our group [50] has studied testicular function in 37 male long-term survivors. This study was conducted at two separate time points; initially a wedge testicular biopsy was performed at or near completion of chemotherapy to assess the incidence of occult testicular relapse. The TFI was calculated as described earlier [46]. Subsequently, at a median time of 10.7 years after stopping chemotherapy, the patients were reassessed by clinical examination, measurement of gonadotrophins and testosterone levels and by semen analysis in 19. The median TFI for all 37 biopsies was 74% and six men had evidence of severe damage to the germinal epithelium at reassessment. Five of these men had azoospermia and one, who did not provide semen for analysis, had a reduced mean testicular volume and a raised basal FSH consistent with severe germ-cell damage.

Of 11 males who had a TFI $< 50\%$ at testicular biopsy, five recovered normal germ-cell function at a median of 10.1 years after completing chemotherapy. Twenty-three of the 26 males who had a TFI $> 50\%$ showed completely normal testicular function when reassessed subsequently, and in the remaining three men the results were inconclusive. Clearly, with increasing time after completion of treatment, germ-cell function can improve so that normal fertility may be a possibility for some patients who have sustained damage to the germinal epithelium. Nonetheless, the long-term prognosis for fertility may remain poor for at least 10 years in those most severely affected.

Combination chemotherapy and the ovary

Ovarian damage following combination chemotherapy for ALL has been reported rarely [51]. By contrast, morphological studies have shown that the ovaries from girls treated for ALL between 1 and 12 years of age, and studied 1 week to 4 years after diagnosis, demonstrated inhibition of follicular development [52]. The girls who had received chemotherapy for a short period of time had normal ovaries with ample follicular growth and many small non-growing follicles. This implied that cytotoxic drugs, rather than the disease itself, had disrupted ovarian morphology.

To evaluate ovarian function and pregnancy outcome after treatment of ALL, Green *et al.* [53] reported 27 pregnancies in 12 of 39 women who had been treated for ALL during childhood or adolescence. There were four spontaneous abortions, one stillbirth and 22 liveborn infants. Two of the liveborn infants had congenital anomalies (one heart murmur, one epidermal naevus) and none of the children (aged 1 month to 10 years) had developed cancer.

Two recent studies emphasize that the prevalence of ovarian dysfunction partly reflects the length of follow-up. Quigley *et al.* [49] described a high incidence of ovarian damage in 20 girls treated with a modified LSA_2L_2 protocol. Basal and peak FSH levels after administration of GnRH were significantly higher in both the prepubertal and pubertal girls than in the comparable contral groups. Further evidence of ovarian damage was an undetectable concentration of serum inhibin, a granulosa cell product, in a high proportion of the girls. Despite clear evidence of primary ovarian damage, none of the girls had a delay in reaching puberty and oestradiol levels were normal.

By contrast, Wallace *et al.* [54] studied ovarian function in 40 women who had remained in first remission following combination chemotherapy for childhood leukaemia over 10 years earlier. All achieved adult sexual development and 37 had regular menses. Ten patients produced 14 livebirths and evidence of ovulation was obtained in a further 11. Four showed biochemical evidence of ovarian damage, three of whom received craniospinal irradiation and one cyclophosphamide. Thus, the long-term outlook for ovarian function is good for the majority of childhood ALL survivors. A premature menopause, however, remains a possibility if significant follicular depletion has occurred at the time of cytotoxic treatment.

Testicular irradiation

Brauner *et al.* [55] studied 12 boys with ALL who had received direct testicular irradiation (2400 cGy in 12 fractions over 18 days) between 10 months and 8.5 years earlier for a testicular relapse (in nine) and as testicular prophylaxis (in three). Leydig cell dysfunction, manifested by a low or absent testosterone response to hCG or an increased basal level of plasma luteinizing hormone (LH) or both was present in 10 of the 12 boys. Similar findings were reported by Leiper *et al.* [56] who studied 11 prepubertal boys who had received 2400 cGy in 10–12 fractions over 14–16 days.

It has been shown subsequently that severe Leydig cell damage was present fairly soon after irradiation, often within the first year, and that there was no evidence of Leydig cell recovery up to 5 years after irradiation [57].

Castillo *et al.* [58] have examined the effect of 'intermediate' doses of testicular irradiation on Leydig cell function in boys treated for ALL. Fifteen boys were studied, 12 receiving 1200 cGy 'prophylactic' testicular irradiation in six 200 cGy fractions over 8 days; three patients were treated for overt testicular relapse, two with 2400 cGy and one with 1500 cGy. The seven patients old enough to provide semen were azoospermic. Eleven of the 12 patients who received 1200 cGy, as well as the patients who received 1500 cGy, had normal pubertal development for their age, with an appropriate basal testosterone level and response to hCG. Elevated basal, or post-GnRH stimulation LH levels in the pubertal boys suggest that subclinical Leydig cell damage is common after this dose of testicular irradiation.

All boys who have received direct testicular irradiation for ALL require biochemical assessment of testicular function. In the presence of results that indicate Leydig cell failure, if there are no signs of puberty by 13 years of age or if there is failure to progress through puberty, androgen replacement therapy should be initiated.

Brain tumours

Both the adjuvant cytotoxic chemotherapy and the spinal fields of irradiation may damage the gonads in children treated for brain tumours. Ahmed *et al.* [59] studied gonadal function in children treated previously for medulloblastoma with surgery and postoperative craniospinal irradiation. The nine children in the group receiving adjuvant chemotherapy with nitrosoureas (carmustine (BCNU) or lomustine (CCNU)) plus procarbazine (in three patients) showed clinical and biochemical evidence of gonadal damage, with elevated FSH concentrations and, in the boys, small testes for their stage of pubertal development. There was no evidence of gonadal damage in the group of eight children who did not receive chemotherapy, all completing puberty normally. Ahmed *et al.* [59] concluded that nitrosoureas were responsible for the gonadal damage, with procarbazine contributing to the damage in the three children who received this drug.

Subsequently, long-term follow-up in 21 girls and 29 boys who had received nitrosoureas (carmustine or lomustine) with or without procarbazine has shown that there is a high prevalence of primary gonadal dysfunction [60,61]. Both sexes progressed normally through puberty but with consistently raised basal concentrations of FSH and, occasionally, increased concentrations of LH. The girls achieved menarche at an appropriate age. As adults, most of the boys had inappropriately small testicular volumes, which are likely to be associated with severe oligospermia or azoospermia, and infertility. A sex difference in the reversibility of damage was observed. The boys showed no evidence of recovery of germinal epithelial function and no deterioration in Leydig cell function in a follow-up extended to 11 years. By contrast, several girls, who had been shown previously to have ovarian damage, have continued with regular menses and normal FSH and oestradiol concentrations. Although it was not known whether these cycles were ovulatory, it is likely that these girls had recovered from the ovarian damage. The prospects of fertility among such girls are good in the early childbearing years but a premature menopause remains possible.

Many of these children also received spinal irradiation, which results in a scattered irradiation dose to the gonads. In the boys this results in a small dose to the testes estimated at 46–120 cGy (following a fractionated course of radiotherapy delivering a total dose of 3500 cGy to the whole spine in the Manchester centre). This small radiation dose is likely to contribute to the observed testicular damage. At other centres individual boys who were treated with craniospinal irradiation but no chemotherapy have developed testicular dysfunction, but the scattered testicular irradiation dose is unknown.

In girls the dose of irradiation received by the ovary may show greater variation. In the Manchester centre a total dose in the range 90–1000 cGy has been estimated to reach the ovaries. The position of the ovaries in relation to the spinal field, and therefore the radiation dose received, can be difficult to estimate, as the ovaries are mobile and their position may vary throughout the course of treatment. Nonetheless, the radiation dose received may contribute appreciably to ovarian dysfunction, and this may be irreversible.

The scattered dose to the ovary will vary depending on the radiotherapy technique used at different centres. In a large study of gonadal dysfunction following treatment of intracranial tumours [62], 18 of 42 girls (43%) showed evidence of primary ovarian dysfunction. Seven of 11 girls who received craniospinal irradiation but no chemotherapy and nine of 14 who had both craniospinal radiotherapy and adjuvant chemotherapy had ovarian dysfunction. The authors concluded that spinal irradiation was the dominant gonadotoxic treatment. Hence the individual contributions of spinal irradiation and cytotoxic chemotherapy to ovarian damage following the treatment of intracranial tumours will vary depending on the radiotherapy techniques used as well as the nature of the adjuvant chemotherapy.

ABDOMINAL TUMOURS

Radiation damage to the ovary

There have been few studies of ovarian function following ovarian irradiation uncomplicated by the effects of other cytotoxic agents in humans. Ovarian morphology following whole abdominal radiation (2000–3000 cGy) has been studied by Himmelstein-Braw *et al.* [63] in seven girls who died from malignant disease. They found that follicle growth was inhibited and the number of oocytes was markedly reduced in the majority.

The natural history of radiation-induced ovarian failure [64] was studied in 53 children treated for an abdominal malignancy by surgery and radiotherapy. Of 38 who received whole abdominal irradiation (2000–3000 cGy), 27 failed to undergo or complete pubertal development (pubertal failure) and a premature menopause (median age 23.5 years) occurred in a further 10. Of 15 girls who received flank irradiation (2000–3000 cGy), ovarian function was normal in all but one, in whom pubertal failure occurred. The median age at last assessment of this latter group is only 15 years. In only one patient, who developed pubertal failure after whole abdominal irradiation and required sex steroid replacement therapy to achieve normal secondary sex characteristics, has there been evidence of reversibility of ovarian function with a documented conception at the age of 22.7 years. Five patients who developed pubertal failure required bilateral augmentation mammoplasties despite sex steroid replacement therapy.

It is clear that outlook for normal ovarian function following whole abdominal irradiation is poor. Flank irradiation, which was introduced intermittently from 1972, has resulted in less pubertal failure, but the possibility of a premature menopause still exists. By further study of the 18 of these girls who received megavoltage whole abdominal radiotherapy (3000 cGy), and developed pubertal failure [45], the LD_{50} for the human oocyte has been estimated not to exceed 400 cGy. Knowledge of the radiosensitivity of the human oocyte provides a more factual basis on which to provide fertility counselling for such patients. The dose of irradiation received by an ovary is dependent on the position in relation to the radiation field; this can be determined by pelvic ultrasound examination. If the dose received by the ovary furthest from the radiation field is calculated, then the surviving fraction of oocytes can be estimated, and the predicted age at ovarian failure determined assuming an average complement of oocytes for age at the time of irradiation. With knowledge of the relationship between radiation dose and ovarian function, oophoropexy can be performed in carefully selected individuals with Hodgkin disease or other pelvic tumours, thereby reducing the subsequent incidence of ovarian failure [65,75].

Radiation damage to the uterus

In women in whom ovarian function is preserved, but in whom the uterus has been involved in the radiation field, there is evidence that radiation to the uterus often results in failure to carry a pregnancy. In 38 women who received whole abdominal irradiation (2000–3000 cGy) during childhood, there were six conceptions in four patients, all ending in second-trimester miscarriages [64]. The majority of these 38 developed radiation-induced ovarian failure following whole abdominal irradiation. The uterine physical characteristics and blood flow were evaluated in 10 women, as was the functional uterine response to exogenous sex steroid replacement [66]. Those who received whole abdominal irradiation in childhood had significantly shorter uteri than women with premature ovarian failure not attributable to irradiation (Fig. 25.4). This implies that prepubertal exposure to irradiation may have an irreversible effect on uterine development and vasculature. In addition, the endometrium was unresponsive to physiological serum levels of oestradiol and progesterone, which were given by exogenous administration. Doppler signals from the uterine arteries were absent in most. It is unclear whether there is damage to the vasculature of the uterus, although this is possible as appropriate vascularization and subsequent growth of the endometrium are essential for implantation and successful continuation of pregnancy. In summary, it is unlikely that women receiving a significant dose of abdominal irradiation in childhood will be able to sustain a pregnancy to term.

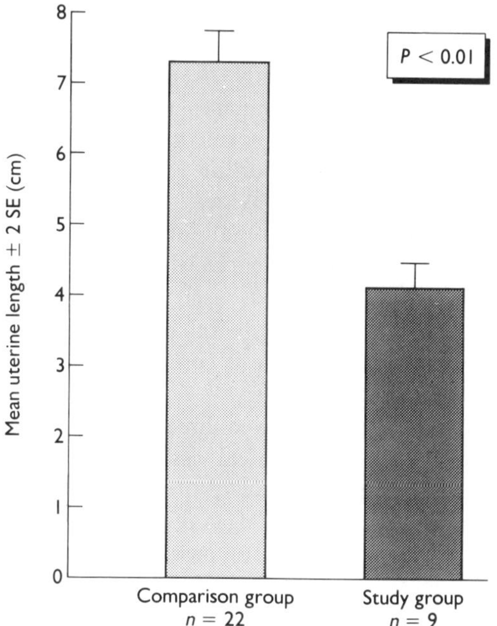

Fig. 25.4 Mean uterine length in nine women exposed to whole abdominal irradiation in childhood compared with a control group of 22 women with premature ovarian failure who had not received whole abdominal irradiation (mean 4.0 versus 7.3 cm; $P < 0.01$).

Radiation damage to the testis

There are very few studies of testicular function following low-dose irradiation to the testes in childhood. Shalet *et al.* [67] studied testicular function in 10 men aged between 17 and 36 years who had received irradiation for a Wilms tumour in childhood. The dose of scattered irradiation to the testes ranged from 270 to 980 cGy (20 fractions over 4 weeks). Eight men had either oligospermia or azoospermia (sperm count 0–5.6 million/ml), and seven of these had an elevated FSH level. All patients progressed through puberty spontaneously.

The impact of larger doses of testicular irradiation has been described on pages 390–1. Additional comparative studies examining the age dependency of radiation-induced Leydig cell damage have shown a much greater vulnerability to Leydig cell failure following the same dose of testicular irradiation in the prepubertal boy compared with the adult male [68].

BONE MARROW TRANSPLANTATION

The testis

Sklar *et al.* [69] examined eight males aged between 10 and 17 years at the time of transplant, who were followed up for 13–77 months after bone marrow transplant. Therapy before bone marrow transplant consisted of high-dose cyclophosphamide alone (two patients); high-dose cyclophosphamide plus total lymphoid irradiation (one patient); the remaining five patients received TBI and either high-dose cyclophosphamide or a combination of BCNU, cyclophosphamide and cytosine arabinoside. Total lymphoid irradiation was given as a single dose of 750 cGy; the calculated dose of irradiation to the testis was 35–99 cGy. TBI was delivered as a single dose of 750 cGy.

Basal serum FSH was elevated in six patients and small testes were noted in four. Of the six with abnormal FSH levels, four who were followed serially showed a return of the basal FSH level to the normal range. Semen analysis, performed in one patient, revealed oligospermia despite normal basal gonadotrophins. Leydig cell function was less impaired in that seven of the eight patients had normal adult male levels of testosterone and all eight progressed through puberty normally.

The largest study to date of growth and development following bone marrow transplantation in childhood is from the Seattle group [70]. They studied 142 patients, aged 1–17 years at the time of transplant, who have survived disease-free for more than 1 year after marrow transplantation for haematological malignancies. Before transplant all children received multi-agent chemotherapy and 55 also received central nervous system irradiation given as a single dose of 920–1000 cGy (79 patients) or as fractionated doses of 200–225 cGy/day for 6–7 days (63 patients).

Sixty-three boys between 1 and 13 years of age were prepubertal at transplant. At study, 31 of these were aged 13–22 years and 21 showed delayed development of secondary sexual characteristics. Biochemical investigations in 25 of the 31 boys who had entered puberty revealed isolated elevation of FSH concentration in seven boys and both FSH and LH levels raised in 10 of the remainder, four of whom had an undetectable testosterone level. All 10 showed delayed development.

Biochemical investigations in 25 of 27 boys who were postpubertal at the time of transplant revealed raised FSH levels in 23, raised LH in 10 and a normal testosterone level in all. Semen analysis in four boys revealed azoospermia, thereby confirming the severe damage to the testicular germinal epithelium.

These results are in agreement with earlier conclusions on radiation-induced testicular damage. The Leydig cells of the prepubertal testis appear more vulnerable than those of the postpubertal testis to damage induced by TBI. Severe damage to the germinal epithelium after TBI is inevitable, and the chances of reversibility remain to be quantified.

The ovary

In view of the radiosensitivity of the human oocyte (LD_{50} < 400 cGy) [45] it is not surprising that a high prevalence of primary ovarian failure is found after TBI. In the large study by Sanders *et al.* [70], 35 girls were prepubertal at transplant (age 2–12 years), and 16 of the 35 were progressing through puberty at the time of the study. Six girls achieved menarche at an appropriate age (four of these six had received fractionated TBI) but the remaining 10 girls showed delayed development of secondary sexual characteristics. Gonadotrophin and oestradiol levels in 11 of the 16 girls over the age of 12 years showed very high FSH and LH levels, and an oestradiol level in the prepubertal range in seven, with transiently abnormal results in two of the remaining four girls.

Of the 17 girls who were postpubertal at the time of transplant, all had amenorrhoea with elevated FSH and LH levels and low oestradiol levels for the first 2 years post-transplant. Among 14 girls followed up between 3 and 14 years after transplant, four have shown recovery of ovarian function between 3 and 5 years after transplant.

The majority of girls who have received high-dose chemotherapy and TBI before bone marrow transplantation are likely to develop irreversible ovarian failure. Appropriate sex steroid replacement therapy may be necessary to induce secondary sexual characteristics, alleviate symptoms of oestrogen deficiency, prevent osteoporosis, and decrease the risk of ischaemic heart disease in these patients.

HODGKIN DISEASE

Combination chemotherapy has greatly improved the prognosis for patients treated for Hodgkin disease. This has resulted in the survival of an increasing number of young patients, cured of this cancer, but at risk from the late effects of the treatment.

Combination chemotherapy and the testis

Sherins *et al.* [71] were the first to report chemotherapy-induced testicular damage in patients treated for Hodgkin disease in childhood. They studied 19 Ugandan boys who had been treated for Hodgkin disease with nitrogen mustard (Mustine), vincristine (Oncovin), procarbazine and prednisolone (MOPP) and were at least 2 years from treatment. Eight of nine pubertal boys had a raised basal FSH level and, in all six boys biopsied, testicular histology revealed germinal aplasia. Whitehead *et al.* [72] also found evidence of severe damage to the germinal epithelium in patients who received MOPP in childhood. Six patients, two of whom had also received a small dose of testicular irradiation, provided semen analysis between 2.4 and 8 years after completion of chemotherapy and were found to be azoospermic. Four boys studied while still prepubertal had normal basal gonadotrophin levels and normal gonadotrophin responses to GnRH. However, several subjects treated when prepubertal showed normal serum gonadotrophin levels in prepubertal life but an evolving pattern of abnormally elevated gonadotrophin levels in early puberty, despite the increasing length of time since completion of chemotherapy. Despite the gloomy prognosis over the first 10 years after completion of chemotherapy, recovery of spermatogenesis has been described in one young man 12 years after six cycles of MOPP for childhood Hodgkin disease [65].

There is no doubt that the cytotoxic drugs which damage the testis predominantly affect the germinal epithelium. However, subtle impairment of Leydig cell function has also been suggested in adult men and boys treated with MVPP (Mustine, vinblastine, procarbazine and prednisolone) for Hodgkin disease. While the circulating testosterone concentration and response to hCG are normal, the basal LH concentration is frequently elevated and the LH response to a GnRH test exaggerated. The bioactive to immunoactive LH ratio is normal and there is no disturbance of LH pulse frequency but the amplitude of the LH pulses is significantly elevated. Because of this compensatory process, androgen replacement therapy is rarely indicated following chemotherapy-induced testicular damage [73] in adult life, while all boys treated with MVPP for Hodgkin disease progress through puberty unaided.

Combination chemotherapy and the ovary

There are few reports about ovarian function in girls treated for Hodgkin disease with combination chemotherapy alone, but the prognosis appears reasonable for the majority [74].

In adulthood, the age of a woman is an important factor in determining if ovarian failure is likely to follow MOPP or MVPP for Hodgkin disease. As the number of oocytes decreases steadily with increasing age, it is likely that ovarian function in prepubertal and pubertal girls may be less susceptible to cytotoxic-induced damage than in adult life.

CONCLUSION

There are a number of reasons why an endocrinologist might be interested in the growth and endocrine sequelae following the treatment of childhood cancer. First the increasing success of the oncologist and radiotherapist leads to a growing number of survivors who require endocrine expertise on an individual basis. Secondly accurate documentation of the prevalence of these endocrine sequelae will lead to modification of the cancer schedules, providing survival rates are not compromised. Finally, analysis of the impact of cytotoxic drugs and radiotherapy provides the potential for further understanding of certain endocrine systems in the human.

REFERENCES

1 Olshan JS, Gubernick J, Packer RJ *et al.* The effects of adjuvant chemotherapy on growth in children with medulloblastoma. *Cancer* 1992;70:2013–17.
2 Shalet SM, Price DA, Beardwell CG, Jones PH, Pearson D. Normal growth despite abnormalities of growth hormone secretion in children treated for acute leukaemia. *J Pediatr* 1979;94:719–22.
3 Borgstrom B, Bolme P. Growth and growth hormone in children after bone marrow transplantation. *Horm Res* 1988; 30:98–100.
4 Leiper AD, Stanhope R, Lau T *et al.* The effect of total body irradiation and bone marrow transplantation during childhood and adolescence on growth and endocrine function. *Br J Haematol* 1987;67:419–26.
5 Ogilvy-Stuart AL, Clark DJ, Wallace WHB *et al.* Endocrine deficit following fractionated total body irradiation. *Arch Dis Child* 1992;67:1107–10.
6 Sanders JE, Buckner CD, Sullivan KM *et al.* Growth and development in children after bone marrow transplantation. *Horm Res* 1988;30:92–7.
7 Constine LS, Woolf PD, Cann D *et al.* Hypothalamic–pituitary dysfunction after radiation for brain tumours. *N Eng J Med* 1993;328:87–94.

8 Clayton PE, Shalet SM. Dose dependency of time of onset of radiation-induced growth hormone deficiency. *J Pediatr* 1991; 118:226–8.

9 Spoudeas HA, Hindmarsh PC, Matthews DR, Brook CGD. Discrepancies between physiological and pharmacological tests of growth hormone secretion in children with brain tumours. *Pediatr Res* 1993;33(Suppl. 5):abstract 141.

10 Shalet SM, Beardwell CG, Aarons BM, Pearson D, Morris Jones PH. Growth impairment in children treated for brain tumours. *Arch Dis Child* 1978;53:491–4.

11 Littley MD, Shalet SM, Morgenstern GR, Deakin DP. Endocrine and reproductive dysfunction following fractionated total body irradiation in adults. *Q J Med* 1991;78:265–74.

12 Brauner R, Czernichow P, Rappaport R. Greater susceptibility to hypothalamopituitary irradiation in younger children with acute lymphoblastic leukaemia. *J Pediatr* 1986;108:332.

13 Chrousos GO, Poplack D, Brown T, O'Neill D, Schwade J, Bercu BB. Effects of cranial radiation on hypothalamic–adenohypophyseal function: abnormal growth hormone secretory dynamics. *J Clin Endocrinol Metab* 1982;54:1135–9.

14 Blatt J, Bercu BB, Gillin JC, Mendelson WB, Poplack DG. Reduced pulsatile growth hormone secretion in children after therapy for acute lymphoblastic leukaemia. *J Pediatr* 1984; 104:182–6.

15 Ryalls M, Spoudeas HA, Hindmarsh PC *et al.* Short-term endocrine consequences of total body irradiation and bone marrow transplantation in children treated for leukaemia. *J Endocrinol* 1993;136:331–8.

16 Moell C, Garwicz S, Westgren U, Wiebe T, Albertsson-Wikland K. Suppressed spontaneous secretion of growth hormone in girls after treatment for acute lymphoblastic leukaemia. *Arch Dis Child* 1989;64:252–8.

17 Moell C, Garwicz S, Westgren U, Wiebe T. Disturbed pubertal growth in girls treated for acute lymphoblastic leukaemia. *Pediatr Haematol Oncol* 1987;4:1–5.

18 Crowne EC, Moore C, Wallace WHB *et al.* A novel variant of growth hormone (GH) insufficiency following low dose cranial irradiation. *Clin Endocrinol* 1992:36:59–68.

19 Uruena M, Stanhope R, Chessells JM, Leiper AD. Impaired pubertal growth in acute lymphoblastic leukaemia. *Arch Dis Child* 1990;66:1403–7.

20 Shalet SM, Gibson B, Swindell R, Pearson D. Effect of spinal irradiation on growth. *Arch Dis Child* 1987;62:461–4.

21 Wallace WHB, Shalet SM, Morris-Jones PH, Swindell R, Gattamaneni HR. Effect of abdominal irradiation on growth in boys treated for a Wilms' tumor. *Med Pediatr Oncol* 1990;18:441–6.

22 Clayton PE, Shalet SM. The evolution of spinal growth after irradiation. *Clin Oncol* 1991;3:220–2.

23 Clayton PE, Shalet SM, Price DA. Growth response to growth hormone therapy following craniospinal irradiation. *Eur J Pediatr* 1988;147:597–601.

24 Sauvion S, Brauner R, Sulmont V *et al.* The effect on growth of increased GH dosage following cranial or craniospinal irradiation. *Horm Res* 1991;35(Suppl. 2):Abstract 117.

25 Leiper AD, Stanhope R, Kitching P, Chessells JM. Precocious and premature puberty associated with the treatment of acute lymphoblastic leukaemia. *Arch Dis Child* 1987;62:1107–12.

26 Ogilvy-Stuart AL, Clayton PE, Shalet SM. Cranial irradiation and early puberty. *J Clin Endocrinol Metab* 1994;78:1282–6.

27 Clayton PE, Shalet SM, Price DA. Growth response to growth hormone therapy following cranial irradiation. *Eur J Pediatr* 1988;147:593–6.

28 Sulmont V, Brauner R, Fontoura M, Rappaport R. Response to growth hormone treatment and final height after cranial or craniospinal irradiation. *Acta Paed Scand* 1990;79:542–9.

29 Ogilvy-Stuart AL, Ryder WDJ, Gattamaneni HR, Clayton PE, Shalet SM. Growth hormone and tumour recurrence. *Br Med J* 1992;304:1601–5.

30 Clayton PE, Shalet SM, Morris Jones PH, Price DA. Growth in children treated for acute lymphoblastic leukaemia. *Lancet* 1988;1:460–2.

31 Kirk JA, Raghupathy P, Stevens MM *et al.* Growth failure and growth hormone deficiency after treatment for acute lymphoblastic leukaemia. *Lancet* 1987;1:190–3.

32 Bramswig JH, Zielinski G, Schellong G. Adult height, target height and siblings' adult height in 107 patients treated for acute lymphoblastic leukaemia (ALL). Comparison of the effects of 4 different chemotherapeutic regimens and different doses of cranial irradiation. *Horm Res* 1990;33(Suppl. 3): abstract 123.

33 Schriock EA, Schell MJ, Carter M, Hustu O, Ochs JJ. Abnormal growth patterns and adult short stature in 115 long-term survivors of childhood leukaemia. *J Clin Oncol* 1991;9:400–5.

34 Davies HA, Didi M, Didcock E *et al.* Final height and disproportion after cranial radiotherapy for leukaemia. *Arch Dis Child* 1994;70:472–5.

35 Sklar C, Mertens A, Walter A *et al.* Final height after treatment for childhood acute lymphoblastic leukemia: comparison of no cranial irradiation, 1800 cGy and 2400 cGy cranial irradiation. *J Pediatr* 1993;123:59–64.

36 Brauner R, Fontoura M, Zucker JM *et al.* Growth and growth homone secretion after bone marrow transplantation. *Arch Dis Child* 1993;68:458–63.

37 Papadimitriou A, Urena M, Hamill G, Stanhope R, Leiper AD. Growth hormone treatment of growth failure secondary to total body irradiation and bone marrow transplantation. *Arch Dis Child* 1991;66:689–92.

38 Ron E, Modan B, Preston D, Alfandlary E, Stovall M, Boice JD Jr. Thyroid neoplasia following low-dose radiation in childhood. *Radiat Res* 1989;120:516–31.

39 Duffy BJ, Fitzgerald PJ. Thyroid cancer in childhood and adolescence. *Cancer* 1950;3:1018–32.

40 Tucker MA, Morris Jones PH, Boice JD *et al.* Therapeutic radiation at a young age is linked to secondary thyroid cancer. *Cancer Res* 1991;51:2885–8.

41 Hancock SL, Cox RS, McDougall IR. Thyroid diseases after treatment of Hodgkin's disease. *N Engl J Med* 1991;325: 599–605.

42 Schimpff SC, Diggs CH, Wiswell JG *et al.* Radiation-related thyroid dysfunction: implications for the treatment of Hodgkin's disease. *Ann Intern Med* 1980;92:91–8.

43 Livesey EA, Brook CGD. Thyroid dysfunction after radiotherapy and chemotherapy of brain tumours. *Arch Dis Child* 1989; 64:593–5.

44 Ogilvy-Stuart AL, Shalet SM, Gattamaneni HR. Thyroid function after treatment of brain tumors in children. *J Pediatr* 1991;119:733–7.

45 Wallace WHB, Shalet SM, Hendry JH, Morris-Jones PH, Gattamaneni HR. Ovarian failure following abdominal irradiation in childhood: the radiosensitivity of the human oocyte. *Br J Radiol* 1989;62:995–8.

46 Lendon M, Hann IM, Palmer MK, Shalet SM, Morris-Jones PH. Testicular histology after combination chemotherapy in childhood for acute lymphoblastic leukaemia. *Lancet* 1978; 2:439–41.

47 Uderzo C, Locasciulli A, Marzorati R *et al.* Correlation of gonadal function with histology of testicular biopsies at treatment discontinuation in childhood acute leukaemia. *Med Pediatr Oncol* 1984;12:97–100.

48 Shalet SM, Hann IM, Lendon M, Morris-Jones PH, Beardwell CG. Testicular function after combination chemotherapy in childhood for acute lymphoblastic leukaemia. *Arch Dis Child* 1981;56:275–8.

49 Quigley C, Cowell C, Jimenez M *et al.* Normal or early development of puberty despite gonadal damage in children treated for acute lymphoblastic leukaemia. *N Engl J Med* 1989;321:143–51.

50 Wallace WHB, Shalet SM, Lendon M, Morris-Jones PH. Male fertility in long-term survivors of childhood acute lymphoblastic leukaemia. *Int J Androl* 1991;14:312–19.

51 Siris ES, Leventhal BG, Vaitukaitis JL. Effects of childhood leukaemia and chemotherapy on puberty and reproductive function in girls. *N Engl J Med* 1976;294:1143–6.

52 Himmelstein-Braw R, Peters H, Faber M. Morphological study of the ovaries of leukaemic children. *Br J Cancer* 1978;38:82–7.

53 Green DM, Hall B, Zevon A. Pregnancy outcome after treatment for acute lymphoblastic leukaemia during childhood or adolescence. *Cancer* 1989;64:2335–9.

54 Wallace WHB, Shalet SM, Tetlow LJ, Morris-Jones PH. Ovarian function following the treatment of childhood acute lymphoblastic leukaemia. *Med Pediatr Oncol* 1993;21:333–9.

55 Brauner R, Czernichow P, Cramer P, Schaison G, Rappaport R. Leydig cell function in children after direct testicular irradiation for acute lymphoblastic leukaemia. *N Engl J Med* 1983;309:25–8.

56 Leiper AD, Grant DB, Chessells JM. The effect of testicular irradiation on Leydig cell function in prepubertal boys with acute lymphoblastic leukaemia. *Arch Dis Child* 1983;58: 906–10.

57 Shalet SM, Horner A, Ahmed SR, Morris-Jones PH. Leydig cell damage after testicular irradiation for lymphoblastic leukaemia. *Med Pediatr Oncol* 1985;13:65–8.

58 Castillo LA, Craft AW, Kernahan J, Evans RG, Aynsley-Green A. Gonadal function after 12-Gy testicular irradiation in childhood acute lymphoblastic leukaemia. *Med Pediatr Oncol* 1990;18:185–9.

59 Ahmed SR, Shalet SM, Campbell RHA, Deakin RHA. Primary gonadal damage following treatment of brain tumours in childhood. *J Pediatr* 1983;103:562–5.

60 Clayton PE, Shalet SM, Price DA, Morris-Jones PH. Ovarian function following chemotherapy for childhood brain tumours. *Med Pediatr Oncol* 1989;17:92–6.

61 Clayton P, Shalet SM, Price DA, Campbell RHA. Testicular damage after chemotherapy for childhood brain tumors. *J Pediatr* 1988;112:922–6.

62 Livesey EA, Brook CGD. Gonadal dysfunction after treatment of intracranial tumours. *Arch Dis Child* 1988;63:495–500.

63 Himmelstein-Braw R, Peters H, Faber M. Influence of irradiation and chemotherapy on the ovaries of children with abdominal tumours. *Br J Cancer* 1977;36:269–75.

64 Wallace WHB, Shalet SM, Crowne EC, Morris-Jones PH, Gattamaneni HR. Ovarian function following abdominal irradiation in childhood: natural history and prognosis. *Clin Oncol* 1989;1:75–9.

65 Ortin TTS, Shostak CA, Donaldson SA. Gonadal status and reproductive function following treatment for Hodgkin's disease in childhood: the Stanford experience. *Int J Radiat Oncol Biol Phys* 1990;19:873–80.

66 Critchley MOD, Wallace WHB, Shalet SM, Mamtora H, Higginson J, Anderson DC. Abdominal irradiation in childhood; the potential for pregnancy. *Br J Obstet Gynaecol* 1992;99:392–4.

67 Shalet SM, Beardwell CG, Jacobs HS, Pearson D. Testicular function following irradiation of the human prepubertal testis. *Clin Endocrinol* 1978;9:483–90.

68 Shalet SM, Tsatsoulis A, Whitehead E, Read G. Vulnerability of the human Leydig cell to radiation damage is dependent upon age. *J Endocrinol* 1989;120:161–5.

69 Sklar CA, Kim TH, Ramsay KC. Testicular function following bone marrow transplantation performed during or after puberty. *Cancer* 1984;53:1498–501.

70 Sanders JE, Pritchard S, Mahoney P *et al.* Growth and development following marrow transplantation for leukaemia. *Blood* 1986;68:1129–35.

71 Sherins RJ, Olweny CLM, Ziegler JL. Gynacomastia and gonadal dysfunction in adolescent boys treated with combination chemotherapy for Hodgkin's disease. *N Engl J Med* 1978:299:12–16.

72 Whitehead E, Shalet SM, Morris-Jones PH, Beardwell CG, Deakin DP. Gonadal function after combination chemotherapy for Hodgkin's disease in childhood. *Arch Dis Child* 1982;57:287–91.

73 Talbot JA, Shalet SM, Tsatsoulis A, Grabinski M, Robertson WR. Luteinizing hormone pulsatility in men with damage to the germinal epithelium. *Int J Androl* 1990;13:223–31.

74 Bramswig JH, Heiermann E, Heimes U, Schlegel W, Hanker JP, Schellong G. Ovarian function in 63 girls treated for Hodgkin's disease (HD) according to the West German DAL-HD-78 and DAL-HD-82 therapy study. *Med Ped Oncol* 1989;17:344.

75 Thibaud E, Ramirez M, Brauner R *et al.* Preservation of ovarian function by ovarian transposition performed before pelvic irradiation during childhood. *J Pediatr* 1992;121: 880–4.

26: The Thyroid Gland

F. DELANGE and D.A. FISHER

INTRODUCTION

The function of the thyroid gland is to concentrate iodide from the blood and to return it to the peripheral tissues in the form of thyroid hormones (TH). The effects of TH on energy metabolism and on the metabolism of nutrients and inorganic ions are well known, and these actions are qualitatively similar in children and in adults. TH also exert important effects on growth and development and, in contrast to the metabolic effects, these developmental actions are uniquely manifested during the first two decades of life [1–5]. In particular, TH play a determining role in growth and differentiation of the brain which takes place from prenatal life up to the end of the third postnatal year [6]. Consequently, a deficit in thyroid hormones and/or in iodine during early life will result not only in general hypometabolism but also in brain damage, expressed clinically by irreversible mental retardation [7–9]. An excess of thyroid hormones during the critical period of brain development can also result in alterations in brain growth [10] and mental development [11]. In this chapter the processes of TH synthesis and metabolism, and the congenital and acquired disorders of thyroid function in the paediatric age groups, are reviewed. Embryological and genetic abnormalities involving TH production or action are prominent in the differential diagnosis of thyroid disorders during childhood.

THYROID PHYSIOLOGY AND BIOCHEMISTRY

General aspects

FUNCTIONAL ANATOMY [12]

The functional unit of the thyroid is the follicle, a spheroidal mass made of colloid surrounded by the follicular cells and a basal membrane. Thyroid hormones are synthesized at the cellular level and stored in thyroglobulin (Tg), a glycoprotein which is the main constituent of the colloid. The follicles are in close contact with blood and lymphatic vessels, and adrenergic nerve terminals. The size and shape of the follicles and epithelial cells are variable and depend principally on the degree of stimulation of the thyroid by thyrotrophin or thyroid-stimulating hormone (TSH) and other stimulating factors: under normal resting conditions the epithelial cells are flat and the colloid abundant. Under conditions of stimulation the epithelial cells are hyperplastic and columnal and the colloid is rare. Between the follicle cells are the parafollicular cells or C cells of neurogenic origin, which secrete calcitonin.

METABOLISM OF IODINE [13]

The major thyroid hormone, tetraiodothyronine or thyroxine (T_4) is approximately 60% iodine by weight. Consequently, the quantity of iodine available in the environment is a determining factor in the yield of the synthesis of thyroid hormones. Although adaptative mechanisms to an unphysiological supply of iodine to the thyroid allow the maintenance of thyroid hormone synthesis within the limits of normal, both severe iodine deficiency and excess can result in thyroid failure and hypothyroidism.

Dietary iodine (I_2) is transformed in the gastrointestinal tract into iodide, which is rapidly absorbed in the blood. Iodide is distributed within the extrathyroidal iodide pool, which represents 30–40% of body weight. The concentration of iodide in the serum (plasma inorganic iodide (PII) varies from 0.1 to 0.5 μg/dl, depending on iodine intake. Its half-life in the serum is only 8 h because the pool of extrathyroidal iodide is constantly cleared of iodide by two competing mechanisms, active transport into the thyroid cells and excretion by the kidney. The mechanism of concentrating iodide by the thyroid cells, often called the iodide pump, confers on the thyroid the ability to concentrate iodide to 20–40 times its levels in plasma under normal conditions. Under such conditions the thyroid clearance of iodide is 10–35 ml/min. It varies markedly with the dietary intake of iodine. The renal clearance of iodide is about 35 ml/min in normal adults

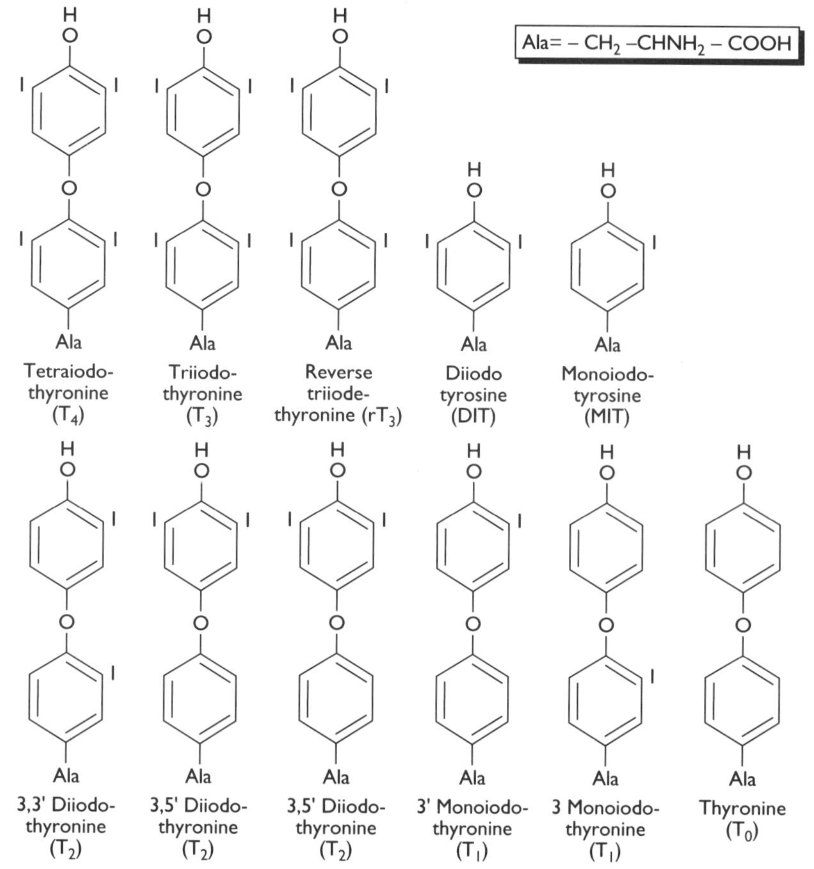

Ala= – CH_2 –$CHNH_2$ – COOH

Tetraiodothyronine (T_4)	Triiodothyronine (T_3)	Reverse triiodethyronine (rT_3)	Diiodo tyrosine (DIT)	Monoiodotyrosine (MIT)	
3,3' Diiodothyronine (T_2)	3,5' Diiodothyronine (T_2)	3,5' Diiodothyronine (T_2)	3' Monoiodothyronine (T_1)	3 Monoiodothyronine (T_1)	Thyronine (T_0)

Fig. 26.1 Structure of thyroid hormones and analogues. Ala represents the alanine side-chain, the structure of which is shown in the box. Positions of the iodine molecules are shown.

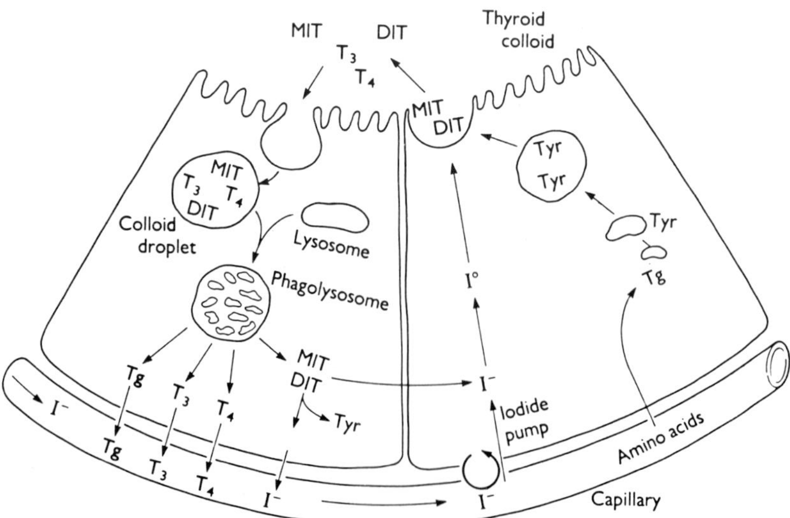

Fig. 26.2 Diagram showing the pattern and events of TH synthesis and secretion by thyroid follicular cells. These processes proceed simultaneously in the same cell. Synthesis and secretion are shown in separate cells for clarity. Thyroglobulin (Tg) with its tyrosine residues is synthesized and transported to the luminal membrane where it interacts with reactive iodine species to form iodotyrosines which couple to form triiodothyronine (T_3) and thyroxine (T_4). These products are stored in extracellular colloid. Secretion involves invagination and formation of intracellular colloid droplets which fuse with enzyme-laden lysosomes to form phagolysosomes in which thyroglobulin is hydrolysed to release iodotyrosines T_3 and T_4. The iodotyrosines are deiodinated and the iodide reutilized; T_3 and T_4 are released into the circulation. DIT, diiodotyrosine; I^-, iodide; I^0, oxidized iodide species; MIT, monoiodotyrosine.

and is not influenced by the dietary intake of iodine. There is no substantial faecal excretion of iodine under normal conditions. Consequently, in conditions of dietary equilibrium, the excretion of iodide in the urine is equal to the level of intake of iodine, so intake can be evaluated by the measurement of the daily urinary excretion of iodine. A small fraction of plasma inorganic iodide (1–2%) may be excreted in sweat under basal conditions, and as much as 10% with severe sweating. Iodide secreted by the salivary glands is reabsorbed in the gut.

SYNTHESIS OF THYROID HORMONES [14–17]

Thyroid hormones and analogues are tyrosine derivatives. Their structures are shown in Fig. 26.1. The steps in the synthesis and release of thyroid hormones are summarized in Fig. 26.2. They include:

1 iodide trapping by the thyroid gland;
2 synthesis of thyroglobulin;
3 organification of trapped iodide as iodotyrosines (monoiodotyrosine (MIT) and diiodotyrosine (DIT));
4 coupling of the iodotyrosines to form the iodothyronines (T_4 and triiodothyronine (T_3)) and storage in follicular colloid;
5 endocytosis of colloid droplets and hydrolysis of thyroglobulin to release MIT, DIT, T_4 and T_3;
6 deiodination of MIT and DIT with intrathyroidal recycling of the iodine.

Iodide-concentrating mechanism

The transport of iodide across the thyroid cell membrane is the first and rate-limiting step in TH biosynthesis [18]. This transport is an energy-requiring process but the exact mechanism remains unclear. Normally the thyroid follicular cell generates a thyroid/serum (T/S ratio) concentration gradient of 30–40. This gradient increases markedly when stimulated by a low-iodine diet, by TSH, by thyroid-stimulating immunoglobulins (TSI), or by drugs that impair the efficiency of hormone synthesis. The salivary glands, gastric mucosa, uterus, mammary glands, small intestine and placenta are also able to concentrate iodide, but they are not capable of iodothyronine synthesis. Several anions are capable of competitively inhibiting iodide transport. These include bromide (Br^-), nitrite (NO_2), thiocyanate (SCN^-), perchlorate (ClO_4), and technetium (TcO_4).

Synthesis of thyroglobulin

The thyroid cell synthesizes Tg, which is secreted by exocytosis into the follicular lumen of the thyroid follicle where it becomes the substrate of a complex series of reactions catalysed by thyroperoxidase and requiring iodide and hydrogen peroxide. Thyroglobulin is a thyroid hormone precursor that permits storage of iodine and storage of iodinated tyrosyl residues covalently bound within the protein structure. Tg is an iodinated glycoprotein with a molecular weight of approximately 660 000 and a sedimentation rate of 19.4 (19S). It is composed of two 12S subunits, each of which is composed of two to four peptide chains. The thyroid gland normally contains 50–100 mg Tg for every 1 g of gland. The abundance and degree of iodination of Tg vary greatly depending on the activity of the gland. The tyrosyl residues, which are the iodine acceptors of Tg, comprise about 3% of the weight of the protein, and about two-thirds of these are spatially oriented to be susceptible to iodination. Dimers (27S) and trimers (37S) of 19S Tg are formed in varying amounts during the oxidative iodination of the molecule by thyroperoxidase.

Organification of trapped iodide: coupling of iodotyrosines

The oxidation of iodide to an active intermediate is followed by iodination of thyroglobulin-bound tyrosyl residues to form MIT and DIT. Both iodide oxidation and organification are catalysed by thyroid peroxidase. Iodination also requires generation of hydrogen peroxide (H_2O_2). These processes are very rapid; the half-life of incorporation of iodide into protein is approximately 2 min. In addition to catalysing the iodination of tyrosines, thyroid peroxidase catalyses the coupling of iodotyrosines within the Tg molecule to form T_3 and T_4. DIT and MIT couple to form T_3; DIT and DIT couple to form T_4. The relative proportions of T_3 and T_4 formed depend on the amount of available iodide and the extent of Tg iodination. In the absence of iodine deficiency, about 30% of the iodoproteins are iodotyronine with a T_4/T_3 ratio of 10/1–20/1. Low-iodine diet increases the MIT/DIT ratio, T_3 synthesis, and the Tg T_3/T_4 ratio. High-iodine diets decrease the MIT/DIT ratio and favour T_4 synthesis. Coupling efficiency is also dependent on TSH.

Digestion of thyroglobulin and secretion of thyroid hormones

Thyroglobulin is stored in the colloid after iodination and coupling have occurred at or near the cell colloid–apical membrane interface. Before thyroid hormones are released, the colloid droplets must first be incorporated into the follicular cells by endocytosis, which is under the control of TSH. Within minutes after administration of TSH or other thyroid stimulators, large pseudopods can be observed at the apical surface of the thyroid follicular cell. The ingested colloid droplets fuse with apically streaming proteolytic enzyme-containing lysosomes to form phagolysosomes, wherein thyroglobulin hydrolysis occurs. The free MIT, DIT, T_3 and T_4 within the phagolysosomes are then released into the follicular cells.

Deiodination of iodotyrosines and intrathyroidal recycling of iodine

After the enzymatic digestion of Tg, T_3 and T_4 are released and diffuse from the thyroid follicular cell into the thyroid capillary blood. The MIT and DIT released are largely deiodinated under the influence of a deiodinase. The released iodide enters the intracellular iodide pool and is reutilized through the organification process for new hormone synthesis.

METABOLISM OF THYROGLOBULIN

Until recently, Tg was believed to be present only in thyroid tissue. It is now clear that some Tg escapes degradation in thyroid phagolysosomes and appears in serum in association with secreted iodothyronines [17]. The serum concentration of Tg in adults varies from 1 to 30 ng/ml with a mean of approximately 5 ng/ml. In normal children, serum Tg varies from undetectable values to 80 ng/ml. The values are high in premature infants during the first weeks of life, and values decrease with age throughout infancy and childhood [19] (Table 26.1). The secretion of Tg by the thyroid is at least partly under TSH control: Tg values increase after TSH administration and decrease during thyroid hormone administration. Circulating Tg levels may be elevated in patients with a variety of thyroid disorders reflecting thyroidal hyperactivity, including endemic goitre, subacute thyroiditis, Graves disease and toxic multinodular goitre [17]. In Hashimoto thyroiditis, serum antithyroglobulin antibody precludes reliable measurement of Tg. Serum Tg concentrations are also increased, often markedly, in patients with thyroid adenoma and papillary follicular carcinoma, although not in those with anaplastic or medullary carcinoma. In iodine deficiency, elevated serum Tg levels in adults [25,26] and newborns [27] are not entirely due to increased serum TSH. They are correlated with the serum T_3/T_4 ratio, suggesting that iodine availability, which affects the degree of thyrogobulin iodination, may be more responsible for elevated Tg secretion than TSH hyperstimulation [25]. The average half-life of circulating 19S Tg varies from 4.3 days to 13.8 days. Clearance presumably occurs within the liver. There is good evidence that Tg reaches the general circulation via thyroidal lymphatics. However, the mechanism of Tg secretion or release remains obscure and its role in serum or plasma is not known.

REGULATION OF THYROID FUNCTION [28–32]

Thyroid follicular cell function is largely regulated by circulating TSH and iodide levels. TSH acutely stimulates the binding of iodide to proteins, iodotyrosine oxidative coupling, thyroid hormone release, and many pathways of intermediary metabolism, such as the oxidation of glucose by the pentose phosphate pathway. With a delay of several hours, TSH enhances the trapping of iodide and the synthesis of thyroglobulin RNA and proteins. When it is administered over a long period it induces cell growth and multiplication, i.e. cell hypertrophy and thyroid hyperplasia. TSH interacts with the thyroid follicular cell at the level of plasma membrane by binding to specific receptors coupled to effectors or catalytic units.

TSH activates adenylate cyclase and stimulates the production and accumulation of cyclic adenosine mono-

Table 26.1 Changes with age in serum concentrations of thyroid hormones, TSH, thyroxine-binding globulin (TBG) and thyroglobulin (Tg)

Age	TSH* (μU/ml)		T_4† (μg/dl)		T_3‡ (ng/dl)		Reverse T_3‡ (ng/dl)		TBG† (mg/dl)		Tg† (ng/ml)	
Cord blood	10.0	(1–20)	10.8	(6.6–15.0)	50	(14–86)	224	(100–501)	3.0	(0.8–5.2)	24	(2–54)
1–3 days	12.0	(1–20)	16.5	(11.0–21.5)	420	(100–740)			3.0	(0.8–5.2)	45	(1–110)
4–7 days												
Fullterms	5.6	(1–10)§	14.1	(8.1–20.1)	186	(36–316)	146	(34–258)	2.8	(0.6–5.0)	42	(2–106)
Preterms, 26–33 weeks	10.2	(1–20)§	7.3	(1.0–13.4)§	95	(10–178)§	137	(60–210)	2.1	(1.1–3.1)	106	(6–230)
1–4 weeks	2.3	(0.5–6.5)	12.7	(8.2–17.2)	225	(105–345)§	90	(26–290)	2.8	(0.6–5.0)		
1–12 months	2.3	(0.5–6.5)	11.1	(5.9–16.3)	175	(105–245)	40	(11–129)	2.6	(1.6–3.6)		
1–5 years	2.0	(0.6–6.3)	10.5	(7.3–15.0)	168	(105–269)	33	(15–71)	2.1	(1.4–2.8)	35	(2–65)
6–10 years	1.9	(0.6–6.3)	9.3	(6.4–13.3)	150	(94–241)	36	(17–79)	2.1	(1.4–2.8)	35	(2–65)
11–15 years	1.9	(0.6–6.3)	8.1	(5.5–11.7)	133	(83–213)	41	(19–88)	2.1	(1.4–2.8)	18	(2–36)
16–20 years	1.5	(0.5–6.0)	8.0	(4.2–11.8)	130	(80–210)	41	(25–80)	2.1	(1.4–2.8)	18	(2–36)
21–50 years	1.5	(0.5–6.0)	7.3	(4.3–12.5)	123	(70–204)	42	(30–80)	1.9	(1.2–2.6)	4	(2–25)

* Mean and 95% range; † mean and 2 SD range; ‡ geometric mean and range; § in Brussels, in moderately iodine-deficient infants. From Fisher [2], Fisher & Vanderschueren-Lodeweyckx [20], Walfish & Tseng [21], Delange *et al.* [22], Pezzino *et al.* [23] and Delange [24].

phosphate (cAMP) in thyroid homonogenates and slices. cAMP appears to mediate most of the effects of TSH on thyroid metabolism (iodide trapping, iodotyronine synthesis, Tg synthesis, glucose oxidation, pinocytosis, hormone release and thyroid growth). The thyroid receptor antibodies (TRAbs) found in the serum of patients with Graves disease produce the effects of TSH and bind to the same receptors. TSH receptor-blocking antibodies, on the other hand, cause hypothyroidism. Noradrenaline and other adrenergic agents have also been shown to bind to thyroid follicular cell membranes and to stimulate cAMP production in humans. Other extracellular stimulatory signals have also been implicated in thyroid regulation, including serotonin, histamine and the prostaglandins. However, these agents are much less effective than TSH, and their significance in the control of thyroid function and growth in humans is not clear.

The average level of plasma iodide is also an important factor in the control of thyroid function. Variations in iodine intake in the physiological range modulates thyroid membrane iodide trapping and, in pharmacological doses, iodide has been shown to block organification (the Wolff–Chaikoff effect) [33–35], Tg synthesis, hormone release and thyroid growth. At least one important mechanism for these effects is the inhibitory action of iodide on the stimulation of cAMP by TSH.

Hypothalamic control of pituitary TSH secretion is summarized in Fig. 26.3. TSH functions as a trophic hormone, and removal of the pituitary reduces thyroid cell function to a basal level. TSH secretion is modulated by thyrotrophin-releasing hormone (TRH), a peptide synthesized in the hypothalamus and secreted into the pituitary portal vascular system for transport to the anterior pituitary thyrotroph cell. TRH production is modulated by environmental temperature via both peripheral and central (hypothalamic) thermal receptors. These receptors modulate neuronal output to the hypothalamic centres regulating TRH secretion. Decreasing environmental and body temperatures increase TRH and increase the tonic level of TSH release. Somatostatin and dopamine can inhibit TSH release, and these transmitters probably contribute to central nervous system modulation of TSH release. Noradrenaline and serotonin may inhibit TSH release but their significance is not clear. Glucocorticoids inhibit TSH release at hypothalamic level.

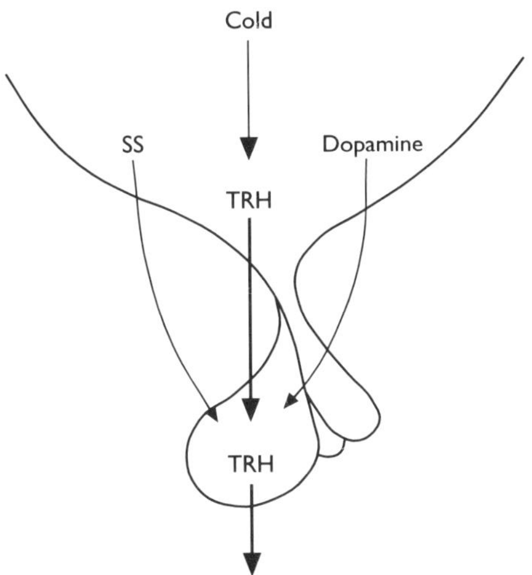

Fig. 26.3 Regulation of TSH release. The synthesis and release of TSH are directly modulated by hypothalamic thyrotrophin-releasing hormone (TRH) by way of TRH receptors on thyrotroph cells of the anterior pituitary gland. TRH secretion is modulated via central anterior hypothalamic as well as peripheral thermal receptors. Body cooling stimulates TRH release. Somatostatin (SS) and dopamine probably can inhibit TSH release at the pituitary thyrotroph level. T_3 negative feedback at the pituitary thyrotroph level modulates the TRH effect such that TRH stimulates and T_3 inhibits TSH release.

THYROID HORMONE TRANSPORT, METABOLISM AND ACTION [36–42]

Thyroid hormones are present in the blood in noncovalent linkage with the carrier proteins: thyroxine-binding globulin (TBG), prealbumin or transthyretin and albumin. The bound form is in equilibrium with free hormones. The peripheral metabolism of the main secretory product of the thyroid, T_4, generates iodothyronines that are more potent (T_3) or less potent (reverse (r)T_3) than the parent compound.

Thyroid hormone-binding proteins

When T_4 and T_3 are released into the circulation they readily and almost completely bind to specific transport proteins, principally to TBG, a globulin with an electrophoretic mobility between the α_1- and α_2-globulins. TBG is the most important carrier protein for T_4; TBG and albumin seem equally important for T_3. The binding reactions are nearly complete so that the euthyroid steady-state concentration of free T_4 and T_3 approximate 0.03% and 0.30% respectively of the total hormone concentrations. Absolute mean free T_4 and T_3 concentrations approximate 10 and 4 pg/ml respectively. In adolescents and adults the plasma concentrations of the several binding proteins are 1.0–3.0 mg/dl for TBG, 20–30 mg/dl for thyroxine binding prealbumin (TBPA) and 2–5 g/dl for albumin. TBG levels are higher in children than in adults and decrease progressively to adult levels during adolescence (see Table 26.1).

In adults, the production rate of T_4, 90 µg/day, is almost three times higher than that of T_3. Most (80%) of circulating T_3 and almost all (94%) of circulating rT_3 result from extrathyroidal monodeiodination of T_4. Monodeiodination of the β or outer (hydroxyl) ring produces T_3, which has three to four times the metabolic potency of T_4. Monodeiodination of the α or inner ring produces rT_3 which is metabolically inactive. About 70–90% of circulating T_3 is derived from peripheral conversion and 10–25% from the thyroid gland; values for rT_3 are probably 96–98% and 2–4% respectively. Progressive tissue monodeiodination reactions degrade T_3 and rT_3 to deiodo-monoiodo- and non-iodinated thyronine (see Fig. 26.1).

Deiodination occurs in several tissues and especially in the liver, kidney, cerebral cortex and pituitary. A particularly important finding is that the intracellular deiodination of T_4 to T_3 varies from one tissue to another and that, consequently, the relative amounts of T_4 and T_3 in the serum do not necessarily correspond to the intracellular proportions of the hormones and thus to the biological effects of the hormones. For example, in the pituitary and in the cerebral cortex, >50% of the intracellular T_3 is derived from the intracellular deiodination of T_4, which therefore acts as a prohormone for T_3; while in the liver only 25% of the intracellular T_3 is generated from T_4 and virtually all the specifically bound nuclear T_3 derives from plasma [43]. This concept explains the state of clinical euthyroidism and normal serum concentrations of TSH in patients with the low T_3 syndrome [44] as observed during fetal life [20], in malnutrition [45], and in chronic illness [46]. It also explains persistently elevated serum TSH in spite of elevated T_3 in conditions such as congenital hypothyroidism due to ectopic thyroid gland [47] and iodine deficiency [48–50] in which the production rate of T_4 is decreased. The existence of an adaptative mechanism to anomalies of thyroid function at a cellular level, especially in the cerebral cortex, has been described. In hypothyroid rats the nuclear contribution of T_3 derived from T_4 decreases in the liver and kidney, whereas it increases in the pituitary [3,51], resulting in a partial protection against the effects of hypothyroxinaemia. Conversely, in hyperthyroidism, the conversion of T_4 to T_3 is increased in the liver but decreased in the pituitary.

Thyroid hormone effects

Thyroid hormone penetrates the cell membrane and binds to a specific nuclear, chromosomal, non-histone receptor protein. T_3 binds to a nuclear receptor with 10 times the affinity of T_4. T_3 also binds to plasma membrane and mitochondrial and cytosolic sites; but the major effects of TH are probably mediated via the nuclear T_3 receptors. Nuclear T_3 receptor binding modulates gene transcription and synthesis of messenger (m)RNA and cytoplasmic proteins. The significance of the plasma membrane, mitochondrial and cytosolic binding sites is not clear.

TH influences nearly all cells by stimulating synthesis of mitochondrial enzymes and structural elements and increasing mitochondrial activity. T_3 binding to mitochondrial receptors may play a role. Various tissues and cell functions are modified through varying patterns of genome activation and protein and receptor synthesis, to account for the multiple physiological actions of TH. In addition to thermogenesis these include stimulation of water and ion transport, acceleration of substrate turnover (including cholesterol) and amino acid and lipid metabolism, and stimulation of growth and development of various tissues at critical periods, including the central nervous system and skeleton. There is increasing evidence that the effects on growth and development may be mediated by TH modulation of growth factor production and action.

TH also potentiate the action of catecholamines; increased catecholamine effects are prominent manifestations of the hyperthyroid state. These effects are mediated via increased β-adrenergic receptor binding as well as postreceptor responsiveness, and occur in spite of normal or lowered circulating catecholamine concentrations. The β-adrenergic effects, such as tachycardia, tremor and lid lag, can be blocked in hyperthyroid subjects by propranolol, a β-receptor blocking agent; but propranolol does not alter thyroid function or the basal level of cellular activity.

Paediatric aspects of the physiology of thyroid function and regulation

ONTOGENESIS OF THYROID FUNCTION AND REGULATION IN HUMANS [52–54]

The thyroid gland forms as a midline outpouching of the endoderm of the primitive buccal cavity. It is first visible at 16–17 days gestation. Lateral contributions are derived from the ultimobranchial portion of the fourth pharyngeal pouch. The thyroid migrates caudally and has reached its final shape and position by the seventh week of fetal life. Active trapping of iodide by the thyroid is detectable by the 12th week of gestational age. TRH is detected in the human hypothalamus by the eighth week of gestation and the concentration increases progressively thereafter (Fig. 26.4). TSH is present in the pituitary by 10–12 weeks. Between 18 and 24 weeks there is a progressive increase in pituitary TSH content and concentration, and a progressive increase in fetal serum TSH concentration with a parallel increase in fetal thyroid radioiodine uptake. This stimulation of TSH synthesis and secretion at midgestation probably correlates with maturation of the hypothalamopituitary portal blood supply and/or maturation of hypothalamic TRH production. Between midgestation and term, fetal serum TSH concentration remains relatively high, and there is a progressive increase in fetal serum T_4 and free T_4 concentrations. These data suggest

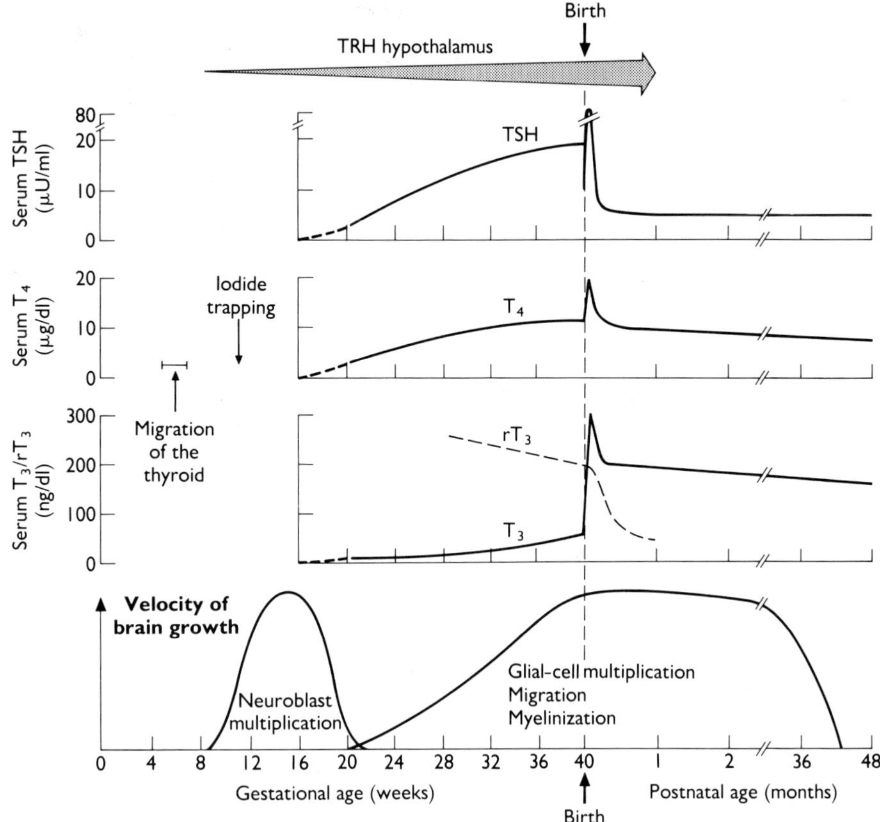

Fig. 26.4 Ontogenesis of thyroid function and regulation in humans during fetal and early postnatal life in relation to the velocity of brain growth (from Fisher [52] and Dobbing & Sands [6]).

the progressive increase in fetal T_4 secretion during the last trimester of pregnancy.

Fetal serum T_3 concentrations are low throughout gestation. Studies in fetal sheep have shown a low T_3 production rate and high T_4/T_3 and rT_3/T_3 production ratios. The low fetal T_3 production rate is associated with low levels of outer ring iodothyronine deiodinase activity in fetal liver. Fetal blood rT_3 levels are high by 20–24 weeks due to predominant rT_3 production in fetal tissues. T_4 to rT_3 conversion is quite active in the liver, and probably accounts for most of the fetal rT_3 production. However, placental conversion of T_4 to rT_3 may contribute [55]. Fetal pituitary, brain and brown adipose tissues contain active outer ring iodothyronine deiodinase and appear to be capable of local T_3 production from T_4 [2]. The significance of these tissues to fetal T_3 production is unclear.

Near-term fetal serum T_3 levels increase modestly from 20 to about 52 ng/dl. Data in sheep suggest that this near-term increase in fetal serum T_3 levels is mediated by an increasing fetal cortisol secretion; cortisol increases fetal serum T_3 levels by increasing the capacity of fetal liver to convert T_4 to T_3. Immediately after delivery there is a sharp (2–8-h) increase in T_3 levels in newborn serum due to a further increase in T_4 to T_3 conversion. In addition, there is a marked postnatal TSH surge; newborn TSH levels peak at 30 min in the range of 70–100 μU/ml, probably stimulated by cooling of the neonate in the extra-uterine environment. In response, both T_4 and T_3 secretion from the thyroid gland are stimulated, and serum T_4 and T_3 concentrations increase briskly [54,56]. Serum TBG concentrations, in contrast, remain unchanged at levels approximating 2 mg/dl, so that the serum free T_4 and free T_3 levels abruptly increase. The high levels of serum rT_3 only gradually decrease to adult values during the first 2–3 weeks. The physiological significance of the neonatal hyperthyroid state remains speculative, but it has been shown that the increased TH levels stimulated catecholamine-mediated brown adipose tissue thermogenesis and mobilization of fatty acids from body fat stores, as well as catacholamine-mediated non-shivering thermogenesis [57]. Other catecholamine-mediated as well as non-catecholamine effects of TH may also be stimulated.

TRANSFER ACROSS THE PLACENTA OF SUBSTANCES AFFECTING FETAL AND NEONATAL THYROID FUNCTION

Among the substances which are easily or actively transferred are iodide, TRH, somatostatin, dopamine agonists and antagonists, antithyroid drugs and thyroid autoantibodies, including antithyroglobulin antibody (ATA),

Table 26.2 Changes with age and iodine supply of thyroid weight, iodine content and estimated turnover rate of thyroidal iodine (based on a daily requirement of 150 µg in adults and 50 µg in neonates)

Age	Median urinary iodine of newborn populations (µg/dl)	Thyroid Weight (mg)	Thyroid Iodine content (µg)	Thyroid Estimated turnover rate (% /day)
Fetus (days)				
95–100		90	1.09	
105–120		131	3.93	
122–130		139	1.80	
145–165		261	7.15	
166–230		728	21.93	
Term				
Toronto	14.8	1 000	292.0	17
Brussels	4.8	760	80.8	62
Leipzig	1.6	3 270	42.7	125
Northern Italy		1 430	49.0	
1 year		2 500		
5 years		6 100		
10 years		8 700		
15 years		15 800	16 300	
Adults		20 000	15 800	1

Adapted from Delange [24] and Delange & Ermans [177].

antimicrosomal (AMA), thyroid stimulating immunoglobulin (TSI), growth-blocking antibody (TGI) and TSH-binding inhibitor immunoglobulins (TBII) [58,59].

The transfer of iodide is particularly important because maternal serum iodide is the only source for the build-up of the iodine stores of the fetal thyroid. This is illustrated by Table 26.2 which shows the changes in thyroid weight and iodine content with age and iodine supply: the iodine stores of the thyroid progressively increase during fetal life. They reach about 300 µg in fullterm newborns when the iodine intake in the general population is above 500 µg/day (Toronto) but are only 80 µg when the intake is about 50–70 µg/day (Brussels) and are as low as 40 µg/day when the intake is severely deficient, as in Leipzig (20 µg/day). The differences in iodine intake in the adult populations in Toronto, Brussels and Leipzig are accompanied by parallel changes in the urinary iodine in healthy newborn infants. These data indicate that the iodine stores of the thyroid in newborn infants are clearly related to the iodine intake of the general population [60]. This is not the case later in life during adolescence and adulthood, probably because chronic stimulation of the iodide pump over years in iodine-deficient individuals allows the maintenance of the iodine absolute uptake within the limits of normal. Biochemical studies of human fetal thyroids have evidenced organification defects, inefficiently iodinated thyroglobulin and reduced lysosomal function [61]. Low iodine stores, elevated T_4 requirements and consequently elevated turnover rate of intrathyroidal iodine stores (see Table 26.2), minor biochemical anomalies in hormone synthesis and release, and the lack of maturation of the autoregulatory process of iodide uptake in the case of acute iodine overload evidenced in preterm infants [54,61] may explain why newborn infants, and especially preterms, are more sensitive than adults to the antithyroid effects of both iodine deficiency and iodine excess.

Before 1950 it was assumed that the placenta was permeable to thyroid hormones because maternal and cord blood protein-bound iodine (PBI) levels were similar [58]. Investigations during the next 25 years indicated that maternal to fetal transfer of thyroxine is limited, and that there are marked maternal to fetal gradients of T_4 and T_3 in all mammals studied: studies in the early 1960s showed that loading of pregnant women at term with large amounts of T_4, varying from 4 to 8 mg/day, resulted in a transfer of not more than 1–3% of this dose, and that the administration of T_3 to pregnant women at a dose of 300 µg/day for several weeks produced only a modest and barely significant reduction in mean cord serum T_4 concentration. In addition, chronic administration of 500 µg of T_4 a day to pregnant woman treated with propylthiouracil during pregnancy did not necessarily prevent the development of fetal goitre [53,62]. Vulsma and coworkers [63] have shown that serum T_4 levels in athyroid newborns or those with complete organification defect are about 30% of normal values. The authors concluded that, in infants with severe congenital hypothyroidism, substantial amounts of T_4 are transferred from mother to fetus during late gestation. Another possible explanation is that a small ectopic thyroid rapidly loses its functional capacity after birth [64].

Studies in rats indicate that the limited placental transfer of thyroid hormones is significant. This maternal hormone may be important to the developing fetus before the onset of significant fetal thyroid function at midgestation [65–71]. The concentrations of thyroid hormones in rat fetuses born to thyroidectomized mothers were much lower than in control rat fetuses from day 9 onwards; that is, before the onset of fetal thyroid function. This indicates transfer of thyroid hormones from mother to fetus before the onset of fetal thyroid function. The difference between the two groups of rat fetuses disappeared in late gestation with increased secretion of thyroid hormones by the intact fetal thyroid. This adaptative mechanism, however, could not function if fetal thyroid was also impaired, for example, as a consequence of severe iodine deficiency. In this case the concentration of T_4 and T_3 in the plasma, carcass, liver and also in the brain of 21-day-old rat fetuses (that is at term) were lower in those fetuses born to severely iodine-deficient mothers than in the controls. In addition, there is a significant transfer of T_4 from mother to fetus even during late gestation: as much as 17% of the T_4 in term rat fetus tissues is of maternal origin [71].

Finally, activity of the unique (type II) enzyme in fetal brain tissue for converting T_4 to T_3 increases in the hypothyroid state, and can preferentially normalize fetal brain T_3 levels in the face of low circulating T_4 concentrations [51].

Table 26.3 Changes with age in serum concentrations of free T_4 and free T_3 (mean ± SD)

Age	No. of cases	Free T_4 (pg/ml)	Free T_3 (pg/ml)
Cord blood	7	13.8 ± 3.5	1.9 ± 1.1
5–10 days	7	22.3 ± 3.9	3.7 ± 1.2
1–10 years	90	11.4 ± 2.0	4.9 ± 1.0
10–12 years	10	11.9 ± 1.1	4.8 ± 0.8
12–14 years	10	10.3 ± 0.7	4.4 ± 0.9
14–16 years	10	10.3 ± 1.1	3.8 ± 0.8
20–60 years	57	10.3 ± 3.1	3.7 ± 0.6

Adapted from Lucas *et al.* [72] and Delange [24].

THYROID FUNCTION IN INFANCY, CHILDHOOD AND ADOLESCENCE [2,20,24,72]

After the period of physiological neonatal hyperthyroidism, the serum T_4 and T_3 concentrations both decrease significantly with age (see Table 26.1). This results in part from a decrease in serum TBG which is accompanied by an increase in serum TBPA. The mechanism involved in the changes of binding protein is unclear. Oestrogens of maternal origin partly explain elevated TBG in early life, and gonadal sex steroids partly explain low levels of TBG at puberty. But binding protein changes begin to manifest themselves before the pubertal secretion of gonadal steroids is evident. The serum concentration of rT_3 remains unchanged, or increases slightly, during childhood and adolescence. Because circulating rT_3 is probably derived almost entirely from peripheral monodeiodination of T_4, these observations suggest that the relative rate of T_4 conversion to rT_3 increases with age. Concurrently, with the progressive decrease in total T_4 and T_3, there is also a trend toward decreasing free T_4 and especially free T_3 with age (Table 26.3).

Peripheral turnover of T_4 is relatively high in young infants and progressively decreases with age (Table 26.4). The thyroxine turnover rate per unit weight decreases and thus the thyroxine requirements are higher in young infants than in adolescents and adults. The extrathyroidal organic iodine pool increases with age, as does the intrathyroidal organic iodine pool.

Thus, thyroid hormone metabolism during infancy, childhood and adolescence is characterized by progressively decreasing serum T_4 and T_3 with stable rT_3. The decreasing total T_4 and T_3 are attributable both to a decrease in mean serum TBG concentration with age and to decreasing T_4, and especially T_3, production with age. The relative rate of rT_3 production from T_4 probably increases with age, suggesting that the decreasing T_3 production rate is attributable both to decreased thyroid secre-

Table 26.4 Changes with age in peripheral thyroxine metabolism (mean ± SEM)

Age	Half-life (days)	Plasma disappearance rate (%/day)	Distribution volume (l/kg)	Extrathyroidal organic iodine pool (μg)	Thyroxine turnover (μg/kg day^{-1})
Children (3–9 years)	5.0 ± 0.1	13.9 ± 0.5	0.16 ± 0.008	145 ± 8	1.0 ± 0.9
Adolescents (10–15 years)	5.6 ± 0.4	12.5 ± 0.7	0.16 ± 0.014	418 ± 63	1.5 ± 0.07
Adults (23–26 years)	6.7 ± 0.3	10.5 ± 0.4	0.12 ± 0.005	548 ± 38	1.1 ± 0.06
Elderly adults (80–90 years)	9.3 ± 0.9	7.6 ± 0.8	0.12		0.7

From Delange [24].

tion and to decreased peripheral conversion from T_4. The mechanism for the relative decrease in thyroid function with age is not clear. Data on variations in serum TSH with age are conflicting: after the physiological stage of neonatal hyperthyrotropinaemia, both stable TSH concentrations with age and a decrease in concentration with age were reported. Decreasing TSH stimulation and thyroid function at least partly explain the decreasing serum Tg levels.

The concept of decreasing thyroid activity with age could account for two observations made in young infants with permanent primary congenital hypothyroidism: (i) the quantity of T_4 per unit weight required for the substitutive therapy is much higher in young infants than in children and adults; (ii) in order to achieve normal growth, bone maturation and intellectual development, and to revert serum TSH and TSH responses to TRH to normal values, serum free T_4 has to be maintained at the extreme upper limit of normal for adults.

HYPOTHYROIDISM

The main causes of hypothyroidism are listed in Table 26.5.

The aetiological distinction between congenital hypothyroidism, that is hypothyroidism present at birth or even during fetal life, and acquired hypothyroidism, correspond fairly well from a clinical point of view to neonatal and juvenile hypothyroidism respectively. However, when congenital anomalies of thyroid development or function are minor, as observed for example in large ectopic thyroid glands, minor congenital defects in thyroid hormonogenesis or in some cases of resistance to thyroid hormones, the development of hypothyroidism can be delayed until adolescence or even adulthood, and it appears clinically as acquired hypothyroidism. Conversely, severe hypothyroidism can occasionally be acquired during early postnatal life, for example as a consequence of pre- and postnatal iodine overload, and be expressed clinically as neonatal hypothyroidism, indistinguishable from permanent primary hypothyroidism, with the same potential harmful consequences on brain development. Therefore, from an operational point of view it appears reasonable, independently of the aetiology, to consider as congenital hypothyroidism thyroid failure detected by neonatal thyroid screening, and as acquired hypothyroidism a state of thyroid failure not detected by screening.

Table 26.5 Aetiology of sporadic hypothyroidism

Congenital hypothyroidism
Permanent hypothyroidism
Due to thyroidal abnormalities (primary hypothroidism)
Developmental defects (thyroid dysgenesis)
Thyroid agenesis (athyreosis)
Thyroid hypoplasia
Ectopic thyroid
Inborn errors of thyroid hormone biosynthesis
Due to extrathyroidal abnormalities
Hypothalamopituitary defects (tertiary–secondary hypothyroidism)
Peripheral resistance to thyroid hormones
General tissue resistance
Extrapituitary resistance
Isolated pituitary resistance
Transient neonatal disorders of thyroid function and regulation
Transient hypothyroxinaemia
Transient primary hypothyroidism
Transient hyperthyrotropinaemia
Low T_3 syndrome
Acquired hypothyroidism
Autoimmune thyroiditis
Post-thyroidectomy or cervical irradiation
Action of antithyroid drugs and goitrogenic agents
In systemic disorders (cystinosis, renal failure)
Endemic iodine deficiency
Iodine overload
Low T_3 syndrome
Hypothalamopituitary acquired defects

Congenital hypothyroidism [9,73,74]

BEFORE THE ERA OF SYSTEMATIC NEONATAL THYROID SCREENING

The prevalence of permanent congenital hypothyroidism (CH) detected on the basis of clinical findings before the era of systematic screening varied from 1/5000 to 1/10 000 [75–78].

The full clinical picture of severe congenital hypothyroidism (Fig. 26.5) included growth retardation; puffy features with myxoedema; flat nose and sunken immature nasal bridge; macroglossia; micrognathia; delayed closure of the fontanelles, especially the posterior fontanelle; abundant hair; abdominal distension with umbilical hernia; dry, cold and scaly skin; mottling; persistent neonatal icterus; lethargy; feeding problems; constipation; a hoarse cry; and hypothermia [79,80]. Muscle impairment could occur with hypertrophy of muscles and slowness of contraction and movement, a syndrome entitled Kocher–Debré–Semelaigne syndrome [81,82]. Bone maturation was retarded, with delayed epiphyseal ossification and epiphyseal dysgenesis. The stippled appearance of the epiphysis is due to abnormal calcification and ossification. The finding of dysgenesis indicated the time of life when thyroid deficiency began. For example, dysgenesis of the epiphysis of the knee indicated hypothyroidism of prenatal onset [79].

Hypothyroid infants could exhibit a variety of metabolic abnormalities. Insensible water loss is greatly diminished and the glomerular filtration rate is impaired.

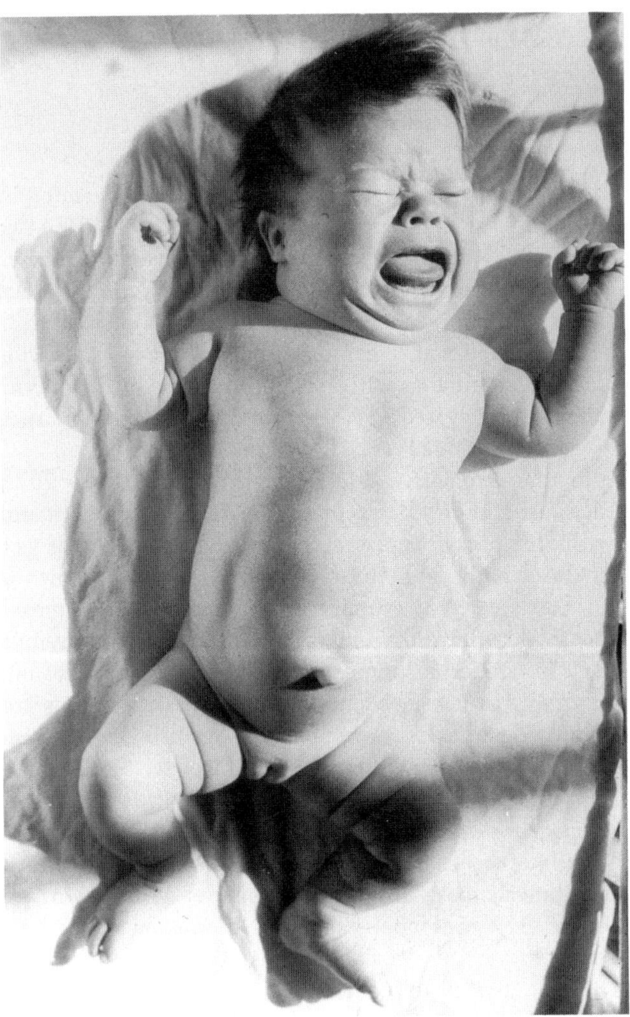

Fig. 26.5 Clinical aspects of severe congenital hypothyroidism before the era of screening. Diagnosis was established on the basis of clinical findings at the age of 4 months. There was no thyroidal uptake of radioiodine, almost undetectable serum protein-bound iodine and a prenatal bone age.

Inappropriate secretion of antidiuretic hormone (ADH) has been described, and administration of forced feedings or intravenous fluid may lead to water intoxication and hyponatraemia. The conjugation and excretion of drugs and bilirubin are impaired, accounting for prolonged neonatal jaundice. Most affected infants were moderately anaemic and failed to respond to iron.

Because of the rarity and lack of specificity of the clinical signs and symptoms of CH in the young infant (Table 26.6), the diagnosis was usually delayed: only 10% of the affected infants were diagnosed within the first months of life; 35% within 3 months; 70% within the first year and 100% only within 3–4 years [75,77]. As a consequence of late diagnosis and therapy the neuro-intellectual prognosis of CH was poor. In a series of 651 CH infants collected from the literature, the mean IQ was

Table 26.6 Prevalence of signs and symptoms of congenital hypothyroidism in infancy (values recorded as percentage of patients)

	Age			
	1–7 days	1–3 months	4–6 months	7–24 months
Symptoms				
Constipation		65	48	59
Feeding problems		60	61	35
Lethargy		55	48	31
Respiratory (signs and/or symptoms)		30	13	1
Signs				
Umbilical hernia	10	68	65	44
Enlarged protruding tongue	22	65	91	100
Facial puffiness	19	25	91	100
Neonatal jaundice	57	28	17	15
Hoarse cry		23	30	21

Adapted from Raiti & Newns [83] and Virtanen [84].

76% with only a handful of children in the 110–120 range and none above [85]. The percentage of infants with an IQ above 85% was 78% when the diagnosis was established before the age of 3 months, 19% when it was established between 3 and 6 months and 0% after the age of 7 months [85]. The mentally retarded hypothyroid infants frequently exhibited additional neurological signs [80] including spasticity, shifting gate, incoordination, awkwardness, jerky movements, coarse tremor and increased deep-tendon reflexes, cerebellar ataxia [86,87], strabismus [88], nystagmus [89] and sensorineural hearing loss [80]. Due to screening, these anomalies are no longer seen in sporadic CH. However, they are still observed in the myxoedematous type of endemic cretinism [90,91], as seen in areas of severe iodine deficiency, and for which other explanations than CH have also been proposed [90].

Even when early therapy prevented severe mental retardation, infants with congenital hypothyroidism, especially of prenatal onset, frequently had neurointellectual sequelae including fine motor and learning disabilities, especially with mathematics [92]. These findings partly explain why these infants occasionally had poorer scholastic achievement and social integration than would be expected from infants with their IQ. The data suggested that, in order to improve the prognosis of CH, therapy has to be initiated in early life, optimally during the first days of life, before the appearance of clinical symptoms. This is the reason why systematic screening for CH during the neonatal period was introduced in 1974 when the techniques became available [93–95]. As a consequence of this screening, the full clinical picture of congenital myxoedema should no longer be seen.

CONGENITAL HYPOTHYROIDISM DETECTED BY SYSTEMATIC SCREENING [2,73,76,96–106]

Organization

Serum concentrations of TSH or/and T_4 are measured from an eluate of whole blood collected on filter paper by a heel-prick on days 4–6 of life. Sampling for thyroid screening between 1 and 3 days of life is not done because of the physiologically elevated serum TSH and T_4 at that age. Screening data confirm that serum T_4 values are low and TSH concentrations high in most newborns with primary hypothyroidism. However, 10–20% of infants with congenital hypothyroidism have T_4 values in the low normal range and the screening programmes using primary T_4 followed by TSH maintain the T_4 cut-off for TSH testing at the 10th or even 20th centile levels with a substantial recall rate of infants. Therefore, primary TSH screening can be considered as the method of choice in the early detection of overt and subclinical primary congenital hypothyroidism, and is recommend by the European Society for Paediatric Endocrinology [106].

Sensitive TSH assays can also be used to identify the effects of moderate to mild iodine deficiency at a population level, and to monitor the effects of iodine supplementation [107]. This is an important issue in many European countries which are still iodine-deficient [108]. However, of infants with congenital hypothyroidism, 8–10% will have a screening TSH value less than 50 μU/ml blood (100 μU/ml serum) and 1/10–1/30 hypothyroid infants will have a screening TSH level less than 20 μU/ml blood with a delayed postnatal rise to hypothyroid levels. Therefore, the cut-off point for recall should be 20–30 μU/ml blood (40–60 μU/ml serum) [2,98,105,109,110].

Primary TSH screening is presently used in all European countries [111,112] except the Netherlands [113], and in Japan, Australia and parts of North America [97,104,114]. Finland has developed a national programme based on the determination of cord blood TSH [115]. Whatever the method used, the number of false-positives has to be maintained as low as possible, particularly in view of the persistent emotional disturbances created in parents by the recall [116].

The cost–benefit ratio of thyroid screening is highly favourable for society [117] and has the invaluable advantage to families of preventing the burden of raising a mentally handicaped child. However, because of the potentially persisting minor pitfalls in the system, it is important for the clinician to remember that an occasional infant with CH will escape detection in newborn screening programmes, and that these infants must be diagnosed on clinical grounds.

Results

The incidence of congenital hypothyroidism detected by screening varies from 1/3500 to 1/4500 [97,104]—two times higher than the prevalence of the disorder detected on a clinical basis. The discrepancy results from the fact that a number of affected infants are missed by clinical detection, and that screening based on TSH determination also detects infants with no clinical signs of hypothyroidism with elevated TSH levels and normal or subnormal T_4 concentrations [111].

In a large majority of CH infants (approximately 90%), the cause is thyroid dysgenesis. The term describes infants with ectopic or hypoplastic thyroid glands (or both) as well as those with total thyroid agenesis. In large series of infants detected by primary TSH screening [109], approximately 30% have thyroid agenesis, 60% ectopic thyroids and 10% eutopic glands (glands in normal location). Thyroid dysgenesis occurs approximately twice as frequently in females as in males. The disorder has been reported to be less common in black (1/32 000) than in white infants, and may be more frequent (1/2000) in Hispanic infants [118,119]. Although the disorder is usually sporadic, rare familial cases have been described. The prevalence is increased in infants with Down syndrome [120]. Seasonal variations in the incidence have been observed in Japan and Australia [121]. In rare instances, thyroid dysgenesis has occurred in association with maternal autoimmune thyroiditis. However, there usually is no correlation between thyroid dysgenesis and the presence of maternal circulating thyroid antimicrosomal or antithyroglobulin antibodies [9,73]. Immunoglobulins blocking TSH-stimulated thyroid cell growth in tissue culture have been found in the blood of both mothers and infants in approximately 50% of sporadic CH by some authors [122,123]. These findings have not been confirmed by others [124], and the role of such growth-blocking immunoglobulins in the pathogenesis of CH has not been established [76].

Infants recalled because of high TSH or low T_4 serum levels should be investigated without delay by clinical examination and with determinations of blood TSH and thyroid hormones, possibly also with thyroid echography and thyroid scintigraphy. T_4 substitutive therapy should be initiated immediately after withdrawal of blood for confirmation tests in infants with serum TSH above 100 μU/ml at the time of screening because of the very high (98%) probability of CH in such instances. The diagnosis should be considered in any infant exhibiting prolonged jaundice, transient hypothermia and enlarged (> 1 cm) posterior fontanelle, failure to nurse properly or respiratory distress

Table 26.7 Inborn errors of thyroid hormones biosynthesis

Anomalies	Important diagnostic features
Iodide trapping defect	Very low thyroidal uptake of radioactive iodine (^{123}I). ^{123}I salivary/serum ratio below 10 (normal: above 20). Response to iodine medication
Iodine oxidation and tyrosil iodination defects (organification – peroxidases defects)	Rapid uptake of ^{123}I. Discharge of thyroidal ^{123}I above 50% of the 2-h value by perchlorate (500 mg) or thiocyanate (1000 mg). Occasional sensorineural hearing loss (Pendred's syndrome)
Iodotyrosine coupling defect	Rapid uptake of ^{123}I. No discharge by perchlorate. Thyroid biopsy: elevated MIT/DIT and T_3/T_4 ratios
Thyroglobulin (Tg) defects	Rapid uptake of ^{123}I. No discharge by perchlorate. Abnormal serum iodoproteins: increased protein-bound thyroxine/iodine ratio. Low serum Tg
Iodotyrosines deiodinase defect	Rapid uptake of ^{123}I. Elevated serum and urinary iodotyrosines MIT and DIT. Inability to deiodinate injected radioactive DIT. Response to iodine medication

Adapted from Foley [127] and Dumont *et al.* [14].

with feeding (see Table 26.6) [84,125,126]. Goitre is a rare finding which suggests an inborn error in thyroid hormone synthesis (Table 26.7) [14,127]. Length at birth of affected infants is normal, but a significant decrease in the growth rate has been shown during the first weeks of life [128].

Athyreotic patients have significantly higher TSH and lower T_4 and T_3 levels than patients with other types of defects. However, there is a substantial overlap between individual values (Table 26.8). Measurements of thyroglobulin may contribute to the classification of congenital hypothyroidism [64,129,130]. It is usually but not always undetectable in athyreosis and in some inborn errors of thyroid hormone synthesis.

Thyroid scintigraphy with [^{123}I] Na or [^{99m}]Tc provides information concerning the location of the thyroid gland and consequently on the prognosis of the disease [131]; it also helps to make, without any delay, a decision regarding the need for lifelong therapy. It can still be performed 2–5 days after the initiation of therapy since serum TSH levels still remain elevated. Ultrasonography of the thyroid gland may detect the presence of a thyroid gland in the normal position in the hands of experienced paediatric radiologists, but is presently of very limited help in localizing an ectopic thyroid gland. In all cases of thyroid dysgenesis, meticulous thyroid echography identifies small hyperechogenic masses in the thyroid area which probably represent remnants of ultimobranchial bodies, and which have to be distinguished from thyroid lobes [132].

TREATMENT [2,133–137]

The treatment of hypothyroidism is accomplished with exogenous thyroid hormone. Sodium-l-thyroxine (NaT_4) is the drug of choice, because of its uniform potency and reliable absorption; appropriate doses of synthetic T_4 also produce normal serum levels of T_3 via peripheral conversion. The doses of thyroxine recommended in therapy decrease progressively with age (Table 26.9) but are stable for surface area at 100 μg/m^2 a day. The best guide to adequacy of therapy is periodic measurement of circulating levels of T_4 and TSH; during the initial stage of treatment a T_3 determination also may be of value. The history and physical examination are important in follow-up, but mild hypothyroidism or hyperthyroidism cannot always be excluded on clinical grounds. Using NaT_4 for treatment, the serum T_4 should be adjusted to the upper normal range (10–14 μg/dl), at which time serum T_3 should be normal (70–220 ng/dl), together with a serum

Table 26.8 Serum concentrations of T_4 at screening and of T_4, T_3, Tg and bone age at diagnosis (mean ± SEM) in the first 85 infants with congenital hypothyroidism detected by screening in Brussels. Serum TSH was above 50 μU/ml at screening in all infants and above 100 μU/ml in all except two infants with large ectopic thyroids who had a serum TSH at diagnosis of 77 and 80 μU/ml respectively

		Levels at diagnosis			
Final diagnosis	Screening T_4 (μg/dl)	T_4 (μg/dl)	T_3 (ng/dl)	Tg (ng/dl)	Bone age (weeks)
Athyreosis (n = 17)	1.7 ± 0.2	1.2 ± 0.2	56 ± 12	4 ± 2	35 ± 1
Ectopic gland (n = 59)	4.1 ± 0.3	4.3 ± 0.5	139 ± 10	62 ± 12	38 ± 1
Eutopic gland (n = 9)	2.3 ± 0.7	2.0 ± 0.8	55 ± 11	222 ± 218	36 ± 2

Table 26.9 Recommended dose of NaT_4 in the therapy of congenital hypothyroidism

	Daily dose of NaT_4	
Age	μg	μg/kg
0–6 months	25–50	8–10
6–12 months	50–75	6–8
1–5 years	75–100	5–6
6–12 years	100–150	4–5
> 12 years	100–200	2–3

From Guyda [136] and Foley [74].

TSH below 5 μU/ml, although still detectable. Persistently elevated TSH levels in spite of normal T_4 and T_3, especially if accompanied by retardation in bone maturation, should be considered to indicate insufficient dosage or insufficient compliance with therapy [73] rather than abnormality in the pituitary–thyroid axis [138,139].

Overtreatment can induce tachycardia, excessive nervousness, disturbed sleep patterns and other findings suggesting thyrotoxicosis. Excessive NaT_4 over a long period (3–12 months) can produce premature synostosis of cranial sutures and undue advancement of bone age [133]. For these reasons TSH concentrations should be measured and maintained within the normal range. Rapid shedding of lanugo, and in older infants devitalized scalp hair, are normal consequences of treatment and do not indicate a need to reduce the dosage.

Follow-up of infants and children is routine. Clinical examination, evaluation of growth and growth maturation, determination of serum total and free T_4 and T_3 and of TSH and an evaluation of the psychomotor and intellectual development will be performed at regular intervals. With a follow-up period of 10–14 years, infants with congenital hypothyroidism who were adequately treated in an appropriate psychosocial environment will reach normal IQ values [76,140–146]. However, infants with evidence of hypothyroidism of prenatal onset and/or with severe clinical signs, particularly those with a low T_4 and delayed bone maturation at diagnosis, have slightly poorer mental prognosis than controls, even if their intellectual or developmental quotients remain within the normal limits for age [146,147]. Infants with congenital hypothyroidism, in spite of normal IQ and normal neurological scores resulting from early and appropriate therapy, may exhibit subtle but significant impairment in specific neurological areas involving coordination and fine manipulative skills. The severity of these anomalies correlates with development quotient, serum T_4 levels and delayed bone maturation at the time of diagnosis [148,149]. These defects can impair social and school performances and require appropriate psychomotor rehabilitation.

CONGENITAL HYPOTHYROIDISM DUE TO EXTRATHYROIDAL ABNORMALITIES

Hypothalamopituitary defects [150,151]

Congenital hypothyroidism due to decreased effective TSH stimulation of TH production can result from a variety of abnormalities in TSH synthesis and metabolism. These include anomalous hypothalamic or pituitary development, isolated, sporadic or familial deficiency in TRH or TSH secretions, or TSH deficiency in association with other pituitary hormone deficiencies. Several syndromes have been described: hypothalamic hypopituitarism with TRH deficiency or insensitivity, or both; isolated TSH deficiency; familial panhypopituitarism; congenital absence of the pituitary; and panhypopituitarism with absence of the sella turcica. The combined prevalence of these abnormalities associated with CH approximates 1/60 000–1/140 000 births. The clinical signs of hypothyroidism are usually modest except for retardation in growth and bone maturation. The mental prognosis is good. Basal serum TSH as serum T_4, free T_4 and T_3 are low. The distinction between hypothyroidism from hypothalamic or pituitary origin is based on the results of TRH stimulation tests. In hypothalamic hypopituitarism TRH induces a delayed and sustained elevation of serum TSH. In pituitary hypothyroidism there is no TSH response to TRH [152].

Resistance to thyroid hormones [14,153]

Thyroid hormone resistance syndromes are rare. The defect is located at the level of the target tissues, with decreased affinity or capacity of T_3 nuclear binding sites. In the most common form, high serum levels of free thyroid hormones are found in the absence of clinical manifestations of hyperthyroidism. TSH levels are elevated early, but are normal as thyroid hyperplasia occurs, and the defect is compensated. The first cases were described as a familial syndrome combining deaf-mutism, delayed bone maturation with stippled epiphysis, goitre and elevated serum levels of protein-bound iodine [154]. The patients also had a peculiar body habitus consisting of bird-like facies, pigeon breast and winged scapulae. Such patients have been shown to have a general tissue resistance to thyroid hormones. Both the pituitary and extrapituitary tissues are involved. The defect is congenital and is predominantly familial. Basal TSH and TSH responses to TRH are normal or elevated. The usual clinical presentation includes a small goitre and absence of hypermetabolism despite elevated serum free hormone levels. No therapy is required unless peripheral indexes of thyroid hormone action indicate cellular hypometabolism. In such cases therapy with relatively large doses of thyroid hormone is initiated, and occasionally results in a marked improvement.

Other types of thyroid hormone resistance have been described. Isolated extrapituitary resistance to thyroid hormones is a very rare form combining clinical hypothyroidism, normal or elevated serum levels of thyroid hormones and normal basal TSH and TRH stimulation test response. Isolated pituitary resistance to thyroid hormones is manifested by inappropriate TSH secretion. This gradually leads to increased T_4 secretion and elevated levels of TSH in patients who are clinically hyperthyroid. These patients can be distinguished from those with Graves disease by their increased TSH levels.

TRANSIENT NEONATAL DISORDERS OF THYROID FUNCTION [54,61]

These disorders are detected at screening, are still present at the time of the control examinations but disappear subsequently in a few days or weeks. They are mainly observed in premature babies (Table 26.10).

Transient hypothyroxinaemia

Serum T_4 concentrations increase progressively with gestational age, and all premature infants have some degree of hypothyroxinaemia [54,155,156]. About 98% of term infants have serum T_4 concentrations $>6.6\,\mu g/dl$, but serum T_4 values $<6.6\,\mu g/dl$ are found in approximately 50% of infants delivered before 30 weeks gestation. The prevalence of such levels in all premature infants approximates 25%. Infants with hypothyroxinaemia also have low levels of free T_4, although these levels are not in the low range of neonates with congenital primary hypothyroidism. The relatively low free T_4 levels in premature infants are associated with normal or low basal serum TSH values and normal TSH and T_4 responses to TRH, the latter indicating responsive pituitary and thyroid glands. The hypothyroxinaemia is transient, correcting spontaneously (over 4–8 weeks) with progressive maturation [22,155]. Postnatal growth and development of these infants is normal, so that they do not require treatment, although treatment does not increase growth rate [155, 157]. Thus, such infants appear to manifest a state of hypothalamic (or tertiary) hypothyroidism or immaturity which represents a normal stage of thyroid system development which does not require substitutive therapy with T_4.

Table 26.10 Mean features of the transient disorders of thyroid function and regulation reported in early infancy, mainly in preterm infants, as diagnosed through neonatal screening

Disorders	Serum levels of T_4	Serum levels of TSH	Aetiology
Transient hypothyroxinaemia	↓	N	Immaturity of the hypothalamopituitary–thyroid axis
Transient primary hypothyroidism	↓	↑	Antithyroid therapy in the mother. Iodine deficiency. Iodine excess. Immunological factors. Idiopathic
Transient hyperthyrotropinaemia	N	↑	Pitfalls in TSH assays. Iodine deficiency. Iodine excess. Idiopathic
Low T_3 syndrome in preterm infants	N	N	Prematurity, infections or surgical stress, malnutrition

N, normal.
From Delange *et al.* [61].

Transient primary hypothyroidism [22,158,159]

Transient hypothyroidism in the neonate, characterized by low serum T_4 and high TSH concentrations, is more common in Europe than in the USA, and the prevalence varies geographically relative to iodine intake. The prevalence of transient hypothyroidism in Belgium approximated 20% of premature infants with the incidence increasing with decreasing gestational age. These infants manifest a reduction in free T_4 levels in to the range observed in infants with congenital hypothyroidism, and serum TSH concentrations increased in to the primary hypothyroid range. Cord blood T_4 and TSH values in these infants are usually in the normal range for premature infants. The primary hypothyroid state develops during the first 1–2 weeks of extrauterine life and is often superimposed on the transient hypothyroxinaemia characteristic of prematurity. Urinary iodine excretion and thyroid iodine content are relatively reduced in these infants, suggesting that the acquired primary hypothyroidism is the result of limited iodine availability for the mother during pregnancy [160] and for the infant [22]. Correction of both iodine deficiency (systematic supplementation with potassium iodide, 40 µg daily) and prevention of iodine overload (iodinated skin disinfectants in mother and child) prevented entirely transient primary hypothyroidism in preterm infants in Belgium.

The hypothyroidism is transient but may persist for 2–3 months, so that treatment is recommended. The average time to recovery of function and discontinuation of treatment in Belgium was 50 days.

Premature infants also are particularly susceptible to

transient, iodine-induced hypothyroidism [61]. Either *in utero* or in the postnatal period, administration of iodine-containing drugs to the mother, or amniotic injection of radiographic contrast agents for amniofetography, has induced hypothyroidism. The hypothyroidism, with or without goitre, is characterized by low serum T_4 and free T_4 concentrations and high levels of TSH. Transient hypothyroidism has also been reported in term infants exposed to iodine *in utero*. Treatment of these infants at birth is indicated. T_4 is the treatment of choice.

Transient hyperthyrotropinaemia

Idiopathic hyperthyrotropinaemia is a rare disorder. In Japan the prevalence is 1 in 16 000–19 000 newborns; the prevalence in Europe and the USA is not precisely known, but is much lower [54,159,161]. Thyroid function tests in these infants are normal except for the serum TSH concentration, which remains elevated for 3–9 months before reducing spontaneously. Affected infants do not require treatment, but prolonged follow-up is necessary to exclude the possibility of a permanent disorder, such as an ectopic thyroid or an inborn defect in thyroid hormonogenesis. The mechanism of transient idiopathic hyperthyrotropinaemia is not clear. Delayed maturation of thyroid responsiveness to TSH and/or of iodothyronine feedback control of pituitary TSH secretion have been suggested. Transient hyperthyrotropinaemia without hypothyroxinaemia in the newborn may also occur in response to intrauterine antithyroid drug exposure, intrauterine iodine excess or deficiency, and has been recorded as a TSH assay artefact.

Low T_3 syndrome in preterm infants

In the preterm infant the changes in thyroid function tests during neonatal adaptation are qualitatively similar to those in term infants, but quantitatively lesser in degree [54]. The early TSH surge and the neonatal T_4 peak decrease in amplitude with decreasing gestational age. The neonatal T_3 peak is less, and in small premature infants serum T_3 levels reach values comparable to term infants only after several weeks. This transient low T_3 state is the result of a variety of factors. There is a likelihood of a transient period of relative undernutrition in the neonatal period. Premature infants also have an increased susceptibility to neonatal morbidity, including respiratory distress, an increased risk of birth trauma, vascular accidents, hypoxia, hypoglycaemia, hypocalcaemia and infection [54,61]. All of these factors tend to inhibit T_4 to T_3 conversion in the neonatal period and aggravate the low T_3 state characteristic of prematurity. Serum T_3 values may remain low in these infants for 1–2 months.

Features of the low T_3 syndrome in premature infants include a low serum T_3 concentration (due to a decreased rate of conversion of T_4 to T_3 in non-thyroidal tissues), variable serum rT_3 levels and normal or low total serum T_4 concentrations [54,61]. Free T_4 levels are usually in the range of values for healthy premature infants of matched gestational age and weight. In some infants serum TBG levels are low and there may be an inhibitor of T_4 binding to TBG, as described in adults with the low T_3 syndrome. Serum TSH concentrations are normal.

Acquired hypothyroidism

Growth retardation and goitre are the most common presenting symptoms of hypothyroidism in childhood. Other signs are a mild to moderate excess in weight, fatigue, dry skin, myxoedema and cold intolerance. Mental retardation does not occur in acquired hypothyroidism, although mental sluggishness might be present. Muscular hypertrophy has been described (Kocher–Debré–Semelaigne syndrome) [81]. Most of the time, delayed puberty is seen at adolescence but early breast development and testicular enlargement are common in girls and boys as a result of follicle-stimulating hormone (FSH) stimulation. Serum TSH is elevated and serum T_4 and T_3 are low or occasionally normal (subclinical hypothyroidism).

AUTOIMMUNE (HASHIMOTO) THYROIDITIS

Autoimmune thyroiditis (chronic thyroiditis, lymphadenoid goitre, autoimmune thyroiditis) was described by Hashimoto in 1912 in four patients with goitre. The thyroid glands were infiltrated with plasma cells and lymphocytes and demonstrated fibrosis, parenchymal atrophy and eosinophilic degeneration in some of the acini. It is the most common cause of acquired hypothyroidism in non-endemic goitre areas [162–165]. The disease occurs in a genetically predisposed population and there is a family history of thyroid disease in 30–40% of patients; females are much more commonly affected than males. The onset of the disorder is usually insidious and most children present with a euthyroid goitre and mild hypothyrodism [163,164,166,167]. The thyroid gland is usually irregularly enlarged and firm, with accentuation of the normal lobular architecture (bosselated). On occasion the goitre gives rise to the sensation of local pressure and difficulty in swallowing. Some 5–10% of patients, particularly those in adolescence, may present with tachycardia, nervousness and other signs suggesting thyrotoxicosis. The course of autoimmune thyroiditis is variable. Usually the gland undergoes progressive atrophy, and the patient presents with acquired hypothyroidism. In adult populations the yearly incidence of hypothyroidism among patients with subclinical autoimmune thyroiditis is 5–7% [168,169]. Spontaneous remission has been reported to occur in some 30% of adolescent patients [164].

The spectrum of the disease in children includes

Table 26.11 The clinical spectrum of autoimmune thyroiditis

Euthyroid goitre
Hypothyroid goitre
Idiopathic hypothyroidism
Painless thyroiditis*
Thyrotoxicosis
Nodular goitre
Reidel's (fibrous) thyroiditis*
Congenital hypothyroidism
Thyroid antigen–antibody complex nephritis
Thrombocytopenia
Multiple endocrine deficiency syndromes

* Predominantly adult syndromes

euthyroid goitre, hypothyroid goitre, thyrotoxicosis, nodular goitre, thyroid antigen–antibody nephritis and multiple endocrine deficiency disease [162,170–174]. The latter includes diabetes mellitus, adrenal insufficiency, hypoparathyroidism, moniliasis and, less commonly, pernicious anaemia and thrombocytopenia [170,172]. The commonest clinical association with autoimmune thyroiditis is diabetes mellitus with or without adrenal cortical insufficiency (Schmidt syndrome). Recent studies have shown a prevalence of thyroid autoantibodies of 30% in children with type I diabetes mellitus and a prevalence of elevated serum TSH levels approximating 10% [171, 172]. All children with diabetes mellitus should be screened for autoimmune thyroid disease. The clinical spectrum of autoimmune thyroiditis is summarized in Table 26.11.

In patients with autoimmune thyroiditis the histological picture of the thyroid gland suggests an autoimmune reaction of the delayed hypersensitivity type [162,165]. There is prominent lymphoid and plasma cell infiltration with varying degrees of thyroid cell atrophy and fibrosis. In addition, most patients have detectable circulating antithyroid antibodies. Several types of antibodies have been described including antithyroglobulin, antimicrosomal, antiperoxidase, TSH-receptor blocking, TSH-receptor stimulating, thyroid growth-inhibiting, thyroid growth-stimulating, and non-thyroglobulin antibodies [165,175,176]. Antithyroglobulin and antimicrosomal antibodies are the most useful in diagnosis. The prevalence of such antibodies measured by sensitive methods such as radioimmunoassay in patients with autoimmune thyroiditis approaches 95%; the presence of these antibodies, however, is not pathognomonic. In 15–20% of patients without thyroiditis significant antibody titres occur. At least some of these subjects represent genetically predisposed individuals who have not yet developed thyroiditis. Antithyroid antibodies also are present in patients with untreated Graves disease. The familial prevalence of antiperoxidase, antimicrosomal or antithyroglobulin antibodies serves to identify the familial predisposition to autoimmune thyroid disease.

A genetically determined defect in the immune surveillance system has been postulated as the basic defect in patients with autoimmune thyroid disease [162,165]. Clones of T lymphocytes sensitized against thyroidal components explain the cell-mediated immune response as well as the presence of humoral antibodies directed at various thyroid and other tissue components. The humoral antibodies are produced by T lymphocytes and it is known that the interaction of T and B lymphocytes plays a crucial role in the elaboration of immunoglobulins by the latter cells.

EXPOSURE TO GOITROGENIC AGENTS [177–179]

Any food or drug that interferes with TH synthesis is a potential cause of goitre and hypothyroidism. These include selected anions, such as iodide, perchlorate and thiocyanate; cations, such as cobalt, arsenic and lithium; antithyroid drugs, including the thionamides; aminosalicylic acid, aminoglutethimide and phenylbutazone; and a variety of naturally occurring goitrogens, such as cabbage, soya beans, cassava and water pollutants.

HYPOTHALAMOPITUITARY ACQUIRED DEFECTS

Hypothalamic or pituitary disorders may be acquired secondary to head trauma, tumours, granulomatous disease, meningitis, head irradiation or rare vascular accidents, including Sheehan syndrome. Growth failure due to growth hormone (GH) and/or to TSH deficiency is usually the first manifestation of pituitary hypofunction, but other signs and symptoms related to the primary disease, neurological disorder and/or hypothalamic dysfunction may occur. Secondary (TSH deficiency) or tertiary (TRH deficiency) hypothyroidism also may be precipitated by treatment of GH-deficient children with exogenous GH if they have a progressive multiple pituitary hormone endocrinopathy [180]. An inhibitory effect of GH on the pituitary–thyroid axis has also been postulated [181].

MISCELLANEOUS CAUSES

Hypothyroidism appears to occur with increasing frequency in association with several syndromes associated with abnormal chromosome karyotypes, including Turner syndrome, Down syndrome, Klinefelter syndrome and Noonan syndrome [15,120,182]. In Down syndrome there is an increased prevalence of thyroid dysgenesis. Autoimmune thyroiditis has been said to be more prevalent in all of the disorders. Compensated hypothyroidism occurs frequently and early in children with nephropathic cystinosis, and some children with the disorder manifest overt hypothyroidism [183]. The thyroid glands show extensive destruction and infiltration of the epithelium with cystine crystals.

DIAGNOSIS

The most important sign of acquired hypothyroidism in childhood is growth failure. The possibility of thyroid deficiency should be considered in any child who is not growing normally. Usually a number of years elapse between the onset of hypothyroidism and the emergence of classic signs of myxoedema. However, if growth records are available, the onset of hypothyroidism can be documented as the beginning of a progressive downward deviation from a previously normal growth channel. Weight tends to increase modestly, and in most instances weight is proportionately greater than height. The retardation of bone age in hypothyroidism usually equals, but can sometimes greatly exceed, the retardation in linear growth; bone age retardation is common in problems of growth and a mild delay does not assist diagnosis. However, if bone age is extremely delayed, hypothyroidism should be considered in the absence of other signs.

Other signs of hypothyroidism and varying clinical manifestations of myxoedema related to organ hypofunction (cardiac, gut, skin, renal, etc.) usually occur, and are helpful in differential diagnosis. However, in some children the predominant manifestation is growth retardation, which may be difficult to distinguish from primary hypopituitarism [184]. Muscle weakness is observed in 30–40% of children with hypothyroidism. Muscle bulk is usually normal or increased, but atrophy may occur [185].

Muscular hypertrophy may be marked in hypothyroid children, and this phenomenon has been referred to as the Kocher–Debré–Semelaigne syndrome [81]. Creatinine phosphokinase levels may be elevated [145]. The proximal musculature of the pelvic and shoulder girdles is primarily affected, but hypertrophy may involve the calves, thigh, hands, neck, tongue and facial muscles [81,185]. As in adults, the prolongation of muscle contraction produces the characteristic slow relaxation phase of the tendon reflex reaction. Muscle dysfunction resembling dermatomyositis or polymyositis has also been described [185].

Sexual development of most hypothyroid children is delayed approximately in proportion to the retardation of skeletal age. However, some children with hypothyroidism present with manifestations of sexual precocity [186–188]. Females present with breast development in association with large ovarian follicles. Males show excessive enlargement of the testes and sometimes of the penis. Most patients lack sexual hair; galactorrhoea may occur in patients of both sexes. Bone age is retarded, in keeping with the duration of the hypothyroid state. The sella turcica may be enlarged. Serum gonadotrophin (Gn) and prolactin (PRL) levels are elevated [189,190]. The increased serum PRL may be explained by the fact that TRH directly stimulates both TSH and PRL release from the pituitary. Other non-TSH pituitary hormone secretion may be due to paracrine effects of TSH-stimulated second messenger in pituitary tissue. With treatment the manifestations of sexual precocity regress, and normal puberty ensues at the appropriate time relative to maturity.

Table 26.12 Characteristics of autoimmune (Hashimoto) thyroiditis*

Characteristics	Percentage
Thyroid gland moderately enlarged, firm, bosselated	80–90
Abnormal thyroid scan with spotty pattern of radioiodine uptake	60–70
Circulating antithyroid autoantibodies	90–95
Positive perchlorate discharge test	60–70
Increased serum TSH or increased TSH response to TRH	30–40

* Percentage of patients with each characteristic is shown.

The diagnosis of autoimmune thyroiditis in euthyroid patients is based on a series of five characteristic findings, as outlined in Table 26.12 [191]. The presence of two of these five markers provides a presumptive diagnosis; three of five positive criteria support the diagnosis with 85–90% reliability. A presumptive diagnosis of autoimmune thyroiditis is warranted in an overtly hypothyroid patient with elevated antithyroid antibody titres.

The diagnosis should be supported by objective test criteria before treatment is instituted. Minimal documentation should include measurement of serum T_4 and TSH levels. If a goitre exists, antithyroid antibodies should be measured. If not, a thyroid scan is useful to exclude thyroid dysgenesis. An elevated blood TSH level establishes that the disease originates in the thyroid rather than the pituitary gland. A low T_4 (and free T_4) with a low serum TSH level indicates hypothalamic or pituitary hypothyroidism. A TRH stimulation test helps differentiate hypothalamic and pituitary defects. A normal (or prolonged) TSH response to TRH implies hypothalamic TRH deficiency; a low or absent TSH response indicates pituitary TSH deficiency. Whenever TSH deficiency is suspected, other pituitary hormone deficiencies should be identified by pituitary function studies. Appropriate neurological and specialized studies should be carried out to exclude a pituitary tumour in patients with acquired TSH deficiency.

TREATMENT

The treatment of children with hypothyroidism should be accomplished with NaT_4 as in infants with congenital hypothyroidism. Most children respond well to a dose of NaT_4 equivalent to about 100 μg/m^2 body surface daily [192–194]. Treated children resume growth at a rate greater than normal; the period of transient catch-up growth. Excessive dosage is marked by disproportionate advancement in skeletal age. This should be avoided, since it will hasten the closure of epiphyses and may shorten adult stature. In patients with pituitary TSH deficiency with deficiency of other anterior pituitary hormones, treatment should be provided as necessary. Treatment of patients with compensated hypothyroidism due to autoimmune thyroiditis is indicated. Treatment of such patients during the euthyroid phase of the disease is controversial. TH therapy prevents the development of mild and subtle hypothyroidism and may suppress autoantibody titres. However, there is no evidence that the natural progression of the disease is altered [164].

NON-THYROIDAL ILLNESS (THE LOW T_3 SYNDROME)

Sullivan *et al.* first described in 1973 a selective deficiency of serum and tissue T_3 in patients dying with severe prolonged illness [195–197]. They referred to these patients as the 'euthyroid sick'. More recently other terms, including low T_3 syndrome and non-thyroidial illness (NTI), have been applied. This syndrome of low total and free serum T_3, normal, low or high total serum T_4, normal to high free T_4 and normal serum TSH concentrations has now been reported in a variety of situations. These include the premature neonate, patients with protein–calorie malnutrition or anorexia nervosa, fasting subjects, postoperative patients and patients with a variety of severe acute and chronic illnesses. The latter have included patients with diabetic ketoacidosis, severe trauma, burns, febrile states, cirrhosis and renal failure. In addition, a number of drugs have been observed to produce a similar syndrome of selective T_3 deficiency; these drugs include dexamethasone, selected radiographic contrast agents, propylthiouracil, propranolol and amiodarone.

Three patterns of change in TH levels have been described (Table 26.13); low T_4, normal T_4 and high T_4 NTI syndromes. The low serum T_3 levels in these syndromes occur as a result of inhibition of iodothyronine β-ring monodeiodinase activity and a decreased rate of T_3 production from T_4 in non-thyroidal tissues [195,197]. α-Ring monodeiodination is not impaired so that rT_3 production is not reduced. Moreover, rT_3 degradation is decreased because the conversion of rT_3 to diiodothyronine appears to be mediated by the same deiodinase that mediates T_4 to T_3 conversion. Thus, serum T_3 levels fall and rT_3 levels tend to remain normal or increase. In some patients serum T_4 levels also fall (the low T_4 syndrome). TBG levels may be reduced in such patients, and an inhibitor of T_4 binding to TBG has been described in the serum and derived from the tissues of such patients [198]. The high T_4 NTI syndrome probably involves one or more induced abnormalities in the disposal pathways of T_4.

There is no convincing evidence that treatment with TH, either T_4 or T_3, is indicated in NTI [157,195]. Treatment is directed to the primary systemic illness. The T_3 deficiency has been interpreted as a compensatory mechanism to reduce metabolic rate and tissue catabolism in sick patients with reduced substrate intake. Treatment would increase tissue metabolism.

Table 26.13 Patterns of thyroid function abnormalities in non-thyroidal illness

	Serum hormone levels			
Syndrome	T_3	T_4	rT_3	TSH
Low T_3 syndrome	D	N	N or I	N
Low T_4 syndrome	D	D	N or I	N
High T_4 syndrome	D	I	N or I	N

D, decreased; I, increased; N, normal.

IODINE DEFICIENCY

Iodine is a trace element present in the human body in minute amounts (15–20 mg; that is 0.02×10^{-3}% of body weight). Iodine is an essential substrate for synthesis of thyroid hormones. The recommended dietary allowance of iodine is 100 μg/day for adolescents and adults (150 μg/day for pregnant and lactating women). It is 60–100 μg/day for children aged 1–10 years; 40 μg/day for infants aged 6–12 months and 30 μg/day for infants 6 months of age or younger, which represents about 8 μg/kg a day, 7 μg/100 kcal and 5 μg/dl milk [199]. A re-evaluation of the iodine requirements in young infants based on iodine balance studies showed that, at least in conditions of marginally low iodine intake as observed in Europe, the recommended dietary allowance should be increased to 90 μg for infants aged less than 1 year [200].

When the physiological requirements of iodine are not met in a given population, a series of functional and developmental abnormalities occur, including thyroid function abnormalities and, when iodine deficiency is severe, endemic goitre and cretinism, decreased fertility rate, increased perinatal death and increased infant mortality. These complications, which constitute a hindrance to the development of the affected populations, are grouped under the general heading of iodine-deficiency disorders, IDD [201].

Currently available data indicate that *at least 800 million people,* living largely in developing countries, are at risk of IDD [177]. Recent figures from Europe increase this number by another 100–120 million [108,202,203]. These disorders therefore constitute a major public health issue. Although theoretically entirely preventable, the disorders still prevail because of various socioeconomic, cultural and political limitations to adequate programmes of iodine supplementation [204].

Physiopathology

The fundamental mechanism by which the thyroid gland adapts to an insufficient iodine supply is to increase the trapping of iodide. This results in the accumulation within the gland of a larger percentage of the ingested exogenous iodide [13,205–207]. The increase in iodide trapping is the result of both TSH-independent augmentation of membrane iodide trapping (thyroid autonomy) and TSH stimulation of the iodide pump [14,208]. In addition, chronic TSH stimulation leads to an increased mass of thyroid tissue, resulting in the development of goitre. Increased TSH stimulation also provokes a marked acceleration of all steps of intrathyroidal iodine metabolism with a fast turnover rate of this compartment. The reduced iodine content of the thyroid results in a low iodination level of thyroglobulin with a reduced efficiency of iodothyronine synthesis due to an abnormal tertiary structure of the protein. The major modification is an increase of the poorly iodinated thyroid compounds MIT and T_3, with an increased T_3/T_4 ratio within the gland [177,205,207, 209,210].

The pattern of circulating thyroid hormones in clinically euthyroid adults in conditions of severe iodine deficiency [47–49,211–213] is characterized by low serum T_4, elevated TSH but normal or supranormal T_3 levels (Table 26.14). The mechanisms responsible for this pattern are unclear, but include thyroidal secretion of T_4 and T_3 in the proportion in which they exist within the gland, preferential secretion of T_3, and an increased level of peripheral conversion of T_4 to T_3. The shift to increased T_3 to T_4 secretion and serum ratios may play an important role in the adaptation to iodine deficiency since T_3 possesses approximately four times the metabolic potency of T_4 while requiring only 75% as much iodine for synthesis.

Paediatric aspects of adaptation to iodine deficiency

CONDITIONS OF SEVERE IODINE DEFICIENCY

The metabolic pattern observed in adults in severe endemic goitre represents the final stage of an adjustment process which is critically influenced by growth. The acceleration of the main steps of iodine kinetics is much more marked in childhood and adolescence than in adulthood, and progressively decreases with age. Goitre does not constitute the optimal mechanism of adaptation to

Table 26.14 Comparison of epidemiological and biochemical findings in Brussels, Belgium and in the Ubangi endemic goitre area (Zaire). The number of patients is shown in parentheses. The differences for each variable between Brussels and Ubangi are highly significant ($P < 0.0001$) except for T_4 ($P < 0.01$) and T_3 (n.s.) in infants

Population	Daily urinary excretion of iodine (μg)	Prevalence of goitre (%)	Serum concentration (mean ± SEM) T_4 (μg/dl)	T_3 (ng/dl)	TSH (μU/ml)	Thyroidal uptake of ^{131}I/24 h (% dose)
Brussels						
Adults	51.2 ± 5.8 (38)	3	8.1 ± 0.1 (125)	144 ± 3 (124)	1.7 ± 1.1 (255)	46.4 ± 1.1 (255)
Mothers at delivery			12.7 ± 0.3 (112)	182 ± 5 (109)	3.6 ± 0.2 (111)	
Newborns (cord)			11.4 ± 0.2 (204)	50 ± 1 (202)	8.2 ± 0.4 (201)	
Infants 1–30 months			8.7 ± 0.3 (53)	181 ± 9 (55)	3.5 ± 0.2 (56)	
Ubangi						
Adults	15.5 ± 1.3 (243)	76.8	4.9 ± 0.2 (358)	166 ± 3 (299)	18.6 ± 2.1 (365)	65.2 ± 0.9 (167)
Mothers at delivery			8.0 ± 0.5 (117)	196 ± 6 (118)	14.0 ± 2.4 (120)	
Newborns (cord)			7.4 ± 0.4 (83)	96 ± 7 (84)	70.7 ± 13.1 (83)	
Infants 1–30 months			6.9 ± 0.7 (54)	185 ± 7 (56)	53.6 ± 11.6 (56)	

Data from Delange *et al.* [214] and Lagasse *et al.* [215].

iodine deficiency. Rather, it constitutes an unfavourable side-effect of the process [216].

By studying the time-course (as a function of age) of the serum concentrations of TSH, T_4 and T_3 in clinically euthyroid patients in severe endemic goitre areas [217], it was shown that the highest values of serum TSH were observed in the youngest infants in spite of the fact that they also had the highest serum T_4 values. These variations of the TSH/T_4 ratio as a function of age are poorly understood. They could reflect the increase in iodine stores within the thyroid as a function of age. They also could be explained by modifications with age of the turnover rate of T_4 [24], and/or by modifications in thyroid gland sensitivity to TSH, including progressive development of thyroid tissue autonomy [218].

One of the major achievements of recent years in the field of paediatric thyroidology in severe endemic goitre areas has been the concept of hypersensitivity of the neonate to the antithyroid effect of iodine deficiency. Newborns in severe endemic goitre regions have much more elevated serum concentrations of TSH than pregnant and non-pregnant adults (see Table 26.14). Eleven per cent of these infants have both a cord serum TSH above 100 μU/ml and a cord serum T_4 below 3 μg/dl, indicating congenital hypothyroidism [177,219,220]. The picture of CH was only transient in some infants, but remained unchanged in others. The abnormalities of neonatal thyroid function were prevented by correcting iodine deficiency in mothers before or during pregnancy [220,221]. Permanent CH in severe endemic goitre starting during the perinatal period is responsible for the development of myxoedematous endemic cretinism. Transient hypothyroidism occurring during the critical period of brain development is responsible for the endemic mental retardation frequently observed in clinically euthyroid children in areas of severe iodine deficiency [222].

CONDITIONS OF MODERATE IODINE DEFICIENCY

Impairment of neonatal thyroid function due to iodine deficiency is not limited to severely iodine-deficient areas in developing countries, but is also a public health issue in some parts of Europe today. In many European regions or countries, the iodine intake is far below the value of

Finland
>300
Sweden
150–330
Norway
150–250
North Sea
Ireland
60–180
Denmark
40–90
Baltic
Sea
UK
70–130
Netherlands
100–160
Germany
20–70
Poland
40–70
Belgium
50–60
Czech Republic
and Slovakia
30–80
Former USSR
70–90
Atlantic Ocean
France
60–70
Austria
150
Hungary
30–120
Romania
40–130
Switzerland
130–160
Italy
10–130
Croatia 90
Portugal
10–130
Black Sea
Spain
30–110
Bulgaria
20–60
Greece
40–180
Mediterranean Sea

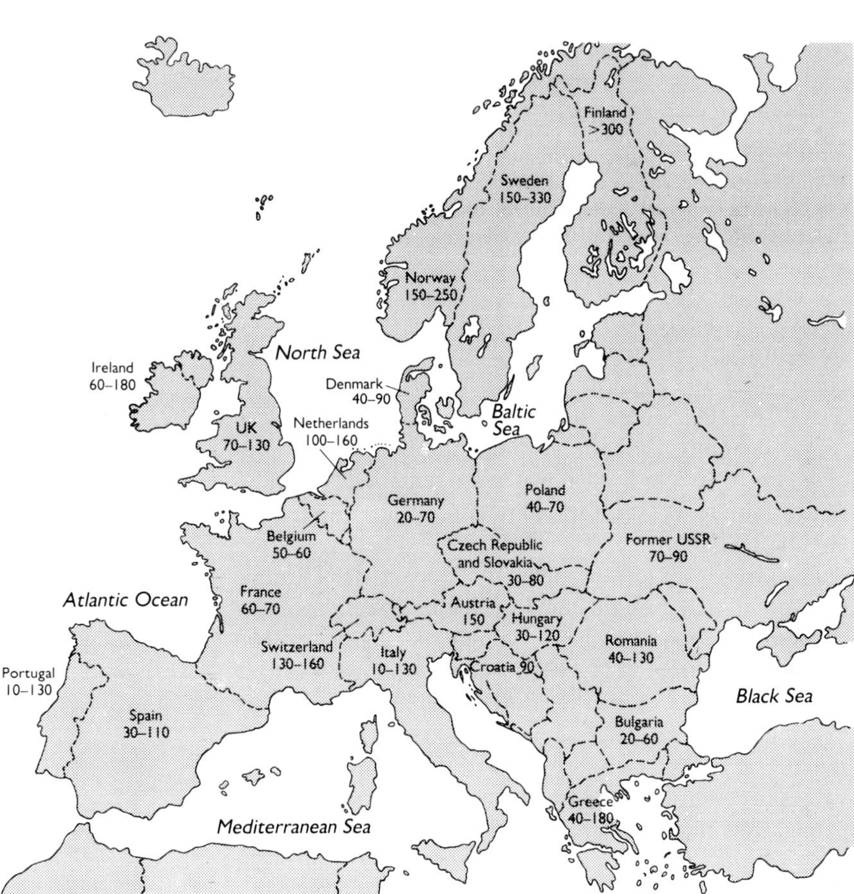

Fig. 26.6 Iodine intake in Europe (μg/day). Range of the values obtained during regional or national surveys for the daily urinary excretion of iodine (redrawn from data in Delange *et al.* [108].)

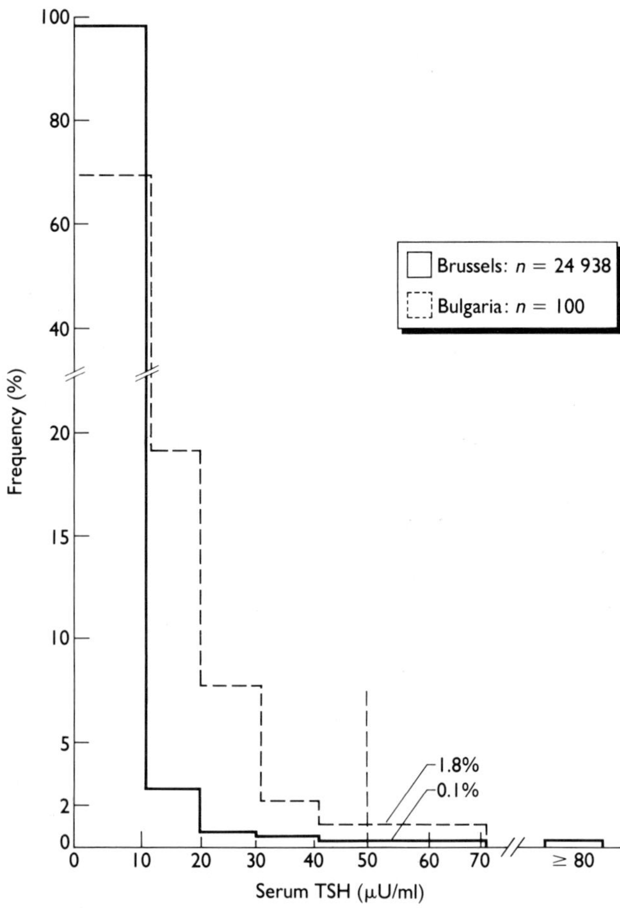

Fig. 26.7 Comparison of the frequency distribution of serum TSH on day 5 in healthy fullterm neonates in Brussels (neonatal thyroid screening) and in an endemic goitre area in Bulgaria. The cut-off point for recall under suspicion of congenital hypothyroidism is 50 μU/ml (from Delange *et al.* [60]).

Table 26.15 Comparison of the results obtained in different European cities in infants at day 5 for urinary iodine concentrations, for the recall rate at systematic screening for congenital hypothyroidism (CH) under suspicion of CH and for the incidence of confirmed permanent primary hypothyroidism

City	Median urinary iodine concentration, day 5 (μg/dl)	Recall rate at screening for CH (%)	Incidence of CH
Stockholm	11.0	0.07	1/2200
Catania	7.1	0.16	1/3700
Brussels	4.8	0.21	1/3200
Freiburg	1.2	0.89	1/3000
Iena	0.8	⩾0.74	1/3500

Adapted from Delange & Gürgi [202].

100 μg/day classically recommended, and is accompanied by significant problems of goitre, especially in the southern, central and eastern parts of the European continent (Fig. 26.6) [108]. There are also marked differences in the iodine content of breast milk and the iodine supply to newborn infants in Europe which are remarkably parallel to the differences in the iodine intake in the general population [159].

The changes in iodine intake in various parts of Europe have no influence on the incidence of permanent sporadic congenital hypothyroidism, which is about 1/3500 throughout Europe [111,112]. In contrast, these changes are accompanied by marked differences in the frequency distribution of neonatal serum TSH at the time of systematic thyroid screening with a shift towards elevated values in conditions of iodine deficiency (Fig. 26.7) accompanied by a marked increase in the recall rate of infants with results suspicious of CH (Table 26.15). The recall examinations were normal in all recalled infants except in the very few with confirmed sporadic CH. This indicates that the frequency of very transiently elevated TSH at screening, the so-called 'false-positives', using primary TSH screening, is inversely related to the iodine intake of newborn populations and represents a very transient alteration of thyroid function [107,177]. In contrast, in spite of the changes in the iodine supply, thyroid function in adults is unmodified, except in areas with overt endemic goitre. Consequently, these data clearly confirm that newborn infants are more sensitive than adults to the antithyroid effects of iodine deficiency.

It has been suggested that the hypersensitivity of newborn infants to iodine deficiency is related to the fact that the iodine stores of the thyroid are particularly low in newborn infants and that, consequently, the turnover rate of intrathyroidal iodine is particularly accelerated in young infants (see Table 26.1) [60]. The same mechanisms were proposed in Belgium for explaining why preterm infants are more susceptible to developing transient hypothyroidism during early postnatal life than are fullterm infants [22,158]. The validity of the proposal was shown by the fact that systematic supplementation of all preterm infants with 40 μg of iodide a day prevented any further occurrence of transient hypothyroidism in preterm infants. Another important recent contribution in the field of iodine nutrition of young infants in Europe is the demonstration that, even in Europe today, as reported earlier in developing countries [222], moderate iodine deficiency results in impaired mental development in euthyroid schoolchildren [223–225].

DIFFUSE NON-TOXIC GOITRE (SIMPLE COLLOID GOITRE, ADOLESCENT GOITRE)

A syndrome of euthyroid diffuse goitre has been described during adolescence in non-endemic goitre areas. Many such patients have autoimmune thyroiditis but some have no evidence of thyroid lymphocytic infiltration. A common finding in such patients is a family history of goitre, but detailed tests of thyroid function fail to reveal identifiable defects [167,226]. The genetic pattern in such families is suggestive of an autosomal dominant mode of transmission with greater expression in the female [226]. The goitrous adolescent may manifest circulating non-thyroxine iodine (a PBI–T_4 difference which exceeds 2 μg/dl), but other thyroid function tests are normal and thyroid biopsy reveals only 'colloid goitre'. The thyroid enlargement usually regresses spontaneously without therapy, but many patients who develop nodular goitres in the third, fourth and fifth decades of life have a history of mild diffuse thyroid enlargement during childhood or adolescence [226,227]. There is increasing evidence for the presence of modest levels of thyroid autoantibodies in the serum of such patients, so that simple goitre of adolescence may represent a mild form of autoimmune thyroid disease [122,228–231].

SUBACUTE THYROIDITIS

Subacute thyroiditis is a self-limited inflammation of the thyroid that usually follows or is associated with an upper respiratory illness [230,231]. Patients have been identified with evidence of associated mumps virus infection and others with cat-scratch fever. It is likely that a variety of viral agents may be responsible for this condition. The incidence is similar in males and females. The onset is accompanied by fever and pain that may be local or referred to the angles of the jaws. The thyroid gland may be exquisitely sensitive to palpation or only mildly tender.

Characteristically there is an increase in serum T_4 and T_3 levels due to release of stored hormone, and signs and symptoms of hyperthyroidism develop. Thyroidal radioiodine uptake at this time is low or absent, indicating thyroid cell damage. Signs and symptoms of hyperthyroidism usually persist for 1–4 weeks. After this time there is a period of transient hypothyroidism as the thyroid gland recovers. The total course runs 2–9 months [232, 233]. A syndrome of painless (subacute) thyroiditis has also been described with a similar pattern of transient hyperthyroidism associated with a low thyroid radioiodine uptake. The 'painless thyroiditis' syndrome, however, resembles autoimmune thyroiditis histologically, and often occurs in the postpartum period in women with a history of autoimmune thyroid disease [165]. This syndrome has not yet been described in children.

Treatment of subacute painful (viral) thyroiditis includes large doses of acetylsalicylic acid or other antiflammatory drugs; in severe cases corticosteroid medication may be helpful. Most patients do not develop antithyroid antibodies, and recover without residual defect in thyroid function. Subacute thyroiditis may be difficult to distinguish from acute purulent thyroiditis, but the latter condition is now rare.

HYPERTHYROIDISM

Graves disease

PATHOGENESIS

Thyrotoxicosis in childhood and adolescence is usually caused by Graves disease, a multisystem disorder involving hyperthyroidism, eye manifestations and dermopathy [234–236] (Table 26.16). The disease occurs in preschool children and rarely may begin in infancy, but there is a sharp increase in incidence as children approach adolescence. Girls are afflicted six to eight times more often than boys. A high proportion of patients have a family history positive for goitre, hyperthyroidism or hypothyroidism. Graves disease is an autoimmune disorder and, like autoimmune thyroiditis, occurs in a genetically predisposed population.

Among the thyroid system-directed autoimmune antibodies in patients with Graves disease are immunoglobulins with thyroid-stimulating properties (TSI). The first TSI described was referred to as the long-acting thyroid stimulator (LATS) because it had a much more prolonged action than normal TSH when injected into mice. More recently, other immunoglobulins with human thyroid-stimulating activity have been identified by bioassay and receptor assay techniques [176]. TSI stimulate adenylate cyclase in thyroid cell membranes in a manner similar to TSH. TSI also displace radiolabelled TSH from thyroid membrane TSH receptors; TSI measured in this way is referred to as TSH binding–inhibiting immunoglobulin (TBII). The prevailing hypothesis is that TSI represents antibody directed at the TSH receptor molecule.

CLINICAL FEATURES

The onset of thyrotoxicosis may be abrupt or insidious. Patients present with nervousness, palpitations, increased

Table 26.16 Causes of hyperthyroidism

Diffuse toxic goitre (Graves disease)
Nodular toxic goitre (Plummer disease)
Thyroiditis with hyperthyroidism
Subacute thyroiditis
Chronic lymphocytic thyroiditis
TSH-induced hyperthyroidism
TSH-producing pituitary tumour
Inappropriate secretion of TSH
Factitious hyperthyroidism

From Malvaux [237].

Table 26.17 Frequency of symptoms in Graves disease

Symptoms	Percentage of patients		
	Saxena [235] (n = 100)	Maenpaa [240] (n = 39)	Barnes [238] (n = 100)
Goitre	100	100	97
Nervousness	80	66	92
Tachycardia	91	38	88
Systolic hypertension	84	53	80
Exophthalmos	77 }	69	78
Staring eyes	100 }		
Tremor	76	51	68
Increased appetite	71		67
Weight loss	67	58	50
Hyperhydrosis	70	64	50
Cardiac murmur	36		48
Thyroid bruit	71		48
School problems	43		40
Hyperkinesis	63		38
Palpitation	41	23	30
Heat intolerance	40		25
Weight gain	4		15
Sleep disturbance	17	25	15
Fatigue	71	41	13
Diarrhoea	16	35	13
Polyuria			7

From Malvaux [237].

appetite and muscle weakness (Table 26.17). Marked weight loss may occur. Except for the eye signs the symptoms of thyrotoxicosis are non-specific. Behaviour abnormalities and declining school performance may dominate the clinical picture. In other patients cardiovascular signs are more prominent. Tiredness and objective muscle weakness occur in 60–70% of patients. As in adult Graves disease, the juvenile disorder may occur in association with myasthenia gravis or periodic paralysis. Many of the signs and symptoms of Graves disease are due to hyperactivity of the sympathetic nervous system. Tachycardia, a widened pulse pressure and an overactive praecordium are common signs which include tremor, excessive perspiration, rapid tendon reflex relaxation time and emotional instability.

The size of the thyroid gland is highly variable, and the goitre may escape notice in a patient whose gland is only slightly enlarged. Careful thyroid examination is essential. The eye signs of Graves disease are variable, but severe Graves ophthalmopathy is much less common in children than in adults, and malignant exophthalmos is virtually unknown. Some of the eye findings are secondary to the sympathetic hyperactivity. There is a stare owing to retraction of the upper lid and wide palpebral aperture and a lag in the descent of the upper lid on looking downward (lid lag). These latter findings parallel the severity of the disease, improve with propranolol treatment and disappear as the patient is rendered euthyroid.

In addition, there is infiltration of the orbit with mucopolysaccharides, lymphocytes and oedema fluid involving the ocular muscles, lachrymal glands and retro-orbital fat. These changes lead to exophthalmos, ophthalmoplegia, chemosis of the conjunctiva, pain, swelling and irritation. Although such inflammatory changes usually improve with treatment of the hyperthyroid state, the course of the thyroid and eye manifestations may differ, and exophthalmos may remain after recovery from the thyrotoxicosis.

The accumulation of mucopolysaccharides in skin and subcutaneous tissues (Graves dermopathy) is rare in children. Graves disease and autoimmune thyroiditis are occasionally encountered in the same patient. Such children have clinical and laboratory features of autoimmune thyroiditis, and in addition exhibit thyrotoxicosis. In these patients a thyroid-stimulating antibody develops among the spectrum of autoimmune antibodies and, if the titre is high enough, clinical thyrotoxicosis develops. The term 'hashitoxicosis' has been applied to these patients, but they may be indistinguishable from the routine patient with Graves disease, except by history.

LABORATORY DIAGNOSIS

Initial laboratory tests should include serum T_4 (with T_3 resin uptake) and T_3 determinations and a sensitive serum TSH measurement to rule out TSH-dependent hyperthyroidism. In patients with borderline results, measurement of free T_4 and/or a TRH response test will be helpful. Patients with thyrotoxicosis have absent or depressed TSH response to TRH. Thyroid radioactive iodine uptake assessment is not usually necessary. Measurements of serum levels of TSH and/or thyroid-stimulating antibodies may be very helpful in confirming the diagnosis in selected patients.

TREATMENT

Treatment of thyrotoxicosis is directed to reducing the secretory rate of TH and blunting their effects. Three principal methods are available for reducing TH secretion: antithyroid drug treatment, subtotal thyroidectomy and radioactive iodine. Antithyroid drug treatment is most commonly employed [234–236,238–240]. Close supervision by the physician is necessary for a period of several years. A permanent remission is achieved in 60–70% of patients. A small percentage of patients are hypersensitive to propylthiouracil or methimazole, but these reactions are usually mild and disappear when the drug is withdrawn.

With proper surgical management most patients achieve satisfactory remission, and requirements for intensive medical follow-up are less rigorous than in those patients treated exclusively with drugs [236,239]. The availability of an experienced thyroid surgeon is an important criterion for successful surgical treatment. With proper preparation of the patient for surgical thyroidectomy the immediate operative mortality approximates that for other major surgical procedures. The incidence of permanent hypoparathyroidism and recurrent laryngeal nerve damage following subtotal thyroidectomy are still appreciable, and these serious complications will persist and may require lifelong treatment.

In terms of ease, cost, efficacy and short-term safety, treatment with radioactive iodine is superior [241]. However, this approach has not been extensively used in childhood and adolescence because of the high prevalence of post-treatment hypothyroidism, and concern about radiation oncogenesis and genetic damage. Late development of primary hypothyroidism after radioactive iodine therapy has occurred in every series of patients studied, regardless of the dosage or radioiodine employed. Approximately 10–20% of patients treated with radioiodine are hypothyroid within 1 year, and the incidence of hypothyroidism is 3–5% a year thereafter. The fear of inducing leukaemia and thyroid carcinoma in adult patients with radioiodine treatment has been largely alleviated [241]. However, the thyroid glands of young animals are much more susceptible to induction of thyroid carcinoma by ionizing radiation than those of older animals, and radiation has been incriminated as an important cause of thyroid cancer in children [241].

Thus, it has been the practice in most clinics to reserve the use of radioiodine for treatment of thyrotoxicosis in older adolescents who fail to follow a medical regime and who cannot be adequately prepared for surgical thyroidectomy. However, the recent report by Hamburger of the successful treatment of 191 children and adolescents with radioiodine over a 23-year period suggests that this approach may be safe enough to consider as initial treatment in some patients [241]. In Hamburger's series, one dose of radioiodine provided effective treatment in 85% of cases.

The choice of therapy in thyrotoxicosis must be individualized, taking into consideration any illness, the quality of surgery available and the socioeconomic factors which condition the success of a prolonged medical regime. In most instances treatment is begun with an antithyroid drug and a decision regarding continuing drug therapy, surgery or radioiodine is made when the patient becomes euthyroid.

β-Adrenergic-blocking drugs are useful to control the sympathetic hyperactivity. These drugs have also proved life-saving in critically ill patients in thyroid storm, but cannot be relied upon as the only therapy in such patients. β-Receptor blockade is potentially dangerous in patients with cardiac failure or arrhythmias.

The drugs derived from thiourea inhibit oxidation of iodide and thereby block synthesis of TH [242]. Neither the release of TH nor the effect of TSH on the iodide pump is affected. Of the commonly used drugs, carbimazole and methimazole have a longer half-life of degradation than propylthiouracil, and maintenance therapy with these drugs can sometimes be accomplished with a single daily dose (Table 26.18). There always is a time lag between institution of drug treatment and achievement of a euthyroid state, since the biosynthetic block is not complete and the stores of preformed hormone must first be discharged. The rapidity of response to therapy correlates best with the initial size of the thyroid gland. Those patients with a small gland usually exhibit improvement in a few weeks, whereas those with very large glands may not respond for 2–3 months.

Table 26.18 Characteristics of common antithyroid drugs

Drug	Initial daily dose (mg/kg)	Maintenance daily dose (mg/kg)	Incidence of major toxic reactions (%)
Methimazole	0.4–0.6	0.1–0.3	1.4
Carbimazole	0.4–0.6	0.1–0.3	0.5
Propylthiouracil	4–6	1–3	0.9

From Marchant *et al.* [242].

The initial dosage of propylthiouracil varies from 300 to 600 mg daily (175 mg/m^2 or 4–6 mg/kg) in dosages spaced at 6- or 8-h intervals (Table 26.18). Skin rashes occur in about 2% of patients treated with propylthiouracil or carbimazole and in 5% of patients treated with methimazole early in the course of therapy; they disappear when the drug is withheld. Often these rashes are mild and can be controlled with antihistamines. Severe reactions are rare, 0.5–1.4%. Granulocytopenia, when it occurs, is usually delayed (4–8 weeks of therapy). Protective isolation and antibiotic treatment usually allow recovery.

Usually it is necessary to continue drug therapy for 1–2 years. In many instances treatment has been continued for 3–6 years before the gland has lost its hyperplastic character. The best clinical prognostic guide is the size of the thyroid gland. Most patients with continued thyroid enlargement will relapse if antithyroid drugs are discontinued. It is also possible to monitor the levels of circulating TSI. When circulating TSI disappear in a patient in clinical remission on drug treatment, a permanent remission of treatment is likely. Antithyroid drugs probably have no influence on the fundamental disease process. However, drug treatment does permit the patient to remain euthyroid and in good health until such time as the disease has spontaneously run its course.

Iodide in large doses will block TH synthesis, inhibit the release of preformed TH and render the gland less vascular. Iodine blockade can be maintained for only a limited period of time (4–16 weeks) before escape occurs, and a fully euthyroid state may not be achieved. The use of inorganic iodine is reserved for severely toxic patients with impending thyroid storm, and for the immediate preoperative preparation of patients who are about to undergo subtotal thyroidectomy.

Iodinated radiographic contrast agents (ipodate or iopanoic acid) have been employed in drug treatment of Graves hyperthyroidism [243,244]. Doses of 0.01 μg/mg day^{-1} or 0.04–0.05 μg/kg every 3 days have been utilized successfully, and have maintained remission for 6–8 months. There is only limited experience with their use in children.

NEONATAL THYROTOXICOSIS

Neonatal Graves disease is rare, probably due to the low incidence of thyrotoxicosis in pregnancy (one or two cases in a 1000 pregnancies) and the fact that the neonatal disease ocurs only in about one in 70 thyrotoxic pregnancies [245]. In most cases the disease is due to transplacental passage of TSI from a mother with active or inactive Graves disease or autoimmune thyroiditis [246–251]. Thus, prediction of neonatal Graves disease from the maternal clinical status is not always possible. However, it is possible to predict neonatal disease in the offspring of women wih high TSI titres. In a recent report all women with TSI titres (measured by stimulation of cAMP in human thyroid slices) exceeding 500% of control values delivered thyrotoxic infants, whereas those with lower titres delivered euthyroid infants [252]. Some infants acquire multiple TSH-receptor antibodies from the mother, and the presence of TBII has been reported to block the effect of TSI transiently and to delay the onset of neonatal thyrotoxicosis by several weeks [251].

Graves disease in the newborn is manifested by irritability, flushing, tachycardia, hypertension, poor weight gain, thyroid enlargement and exophthalmos. Thrombocytopenia, hepatosplenomegaly, jaundice and hypoprothrombinaemia have also been observed. Arrhythmias, cardiac failure and death may occur if the thyrotoxicity is severe and the treatment is inadequate. Mortality approaches 25% in disease severe enough to be diagnosed.

Although neonatal Graves disease may be manifested at birth, in some infants the onset of symptoms and signs in the newborn may be delayed as long as 8–9 days. This is due to the postnatal depletion of transplacentally acquired blocking doses of antithyroid drugs, and to the fact that there is an abrupt increase in conversion of T_4 to T_3 shortly after birth [246]. The diagnosis is confirmed by measuring high levels of T_4, free T_4 and T_3 in postnatal blood [249]. Cord blood values may be normal or near-normal, while levels at 2–5 days may be markedly increased; the serum TSH is low. Neonatal Graves disease resolves spontaneously as maternal TSI in the newborn is degraded; the half-life approximates 12 days. The usual clinical course of neonatal Graves disease extends for 3–12 weeks [251].

The treatment of hyperthyroidism in the newborn includes sedatives and digitalization as necessary. Iodide or antithyroid drugs are administered to decrease TH secretion [246,249]. These drugs have additive effects with regard to inhibition of hormone synthesis; in addition, iodide will rapidly inhibit hormone release. Lugol solution (5% iodine and 10% potassium iodide; 126 mg of iodine/ml) is given in doses of one drop (about 8 mg) three times daily. Methimazole, carbimazole or propylthiouracil is administered in doses of 0.5–1 mg, 0.5–1 mg or 5–10 mg, respectively, per kilogram daily in divided doses at 8-h intervals. A therapeutic response should be observed within 24–36 h. If a satisfactory response is not observed, the dose of antithyroid drug and iodide can be increased by 50%. Adrenal corticosteroids in anti-inflammatory dosage and propranolol (1–2 mg/kg a day) may also be helpful. Radiographic contrast agents may be useful in treatment (100 mg/day or 0.5 g every 3 days) either alone or in conjuction with antithyroid drug treatment [253].

Thyrotrophin-dependent hyperthyroidism

Rarely, hyperthyroidism may be associated with hypersecretion of TSH. Two syndromes have been described: TSH-dependent hyperthyroidism due to a pituitary TSH-secreting tumour and non-neoplastic hypersecretion of TSH associated with a defect in feedback inhibition of TSH secretion by thyroid hormones [254,255]. The latter represents a rare syndrome of isolated pituitary resistance to thyroid hormone. Both disorders are associated with goitre and clinical hyperthyroidism, and these disorders should be suspected in any child who presents with goitrous hyperthyroidism and hyperthyroxinaemia in whom the serum TSH concentration is not suppressed.

PITUITARY TUMOURS

TSH-secreting pituitary tumours associated with clinical hyperthyroidism are quite rare, but have been reported in children as well as adults [254]. Most have been chromophobe or basophilic adenomas. Local manifestations of the tumour are prominent, including visual changes, optic atrophy, hydrocephalus and amaurosis. Children with hyperthyroidism should be examined for evidence of neurological dysfunction and visual abnormalities; skull X-rays for evaluation of the sella turcica are indicated if clinical evaluation arouses suspicion, or if the serum TSH concentration is elevated. A lesion in the pituitary can usually be demonstrated and the circulating level of free α-subunits of TSH is elevated. The serum TSH level falls to respond to exogenous TRH.

SELECTED PITUITARY T_3 RESISTANCE

Hyperthyroidism with diffuse goitre and elevated serum TSH levels has been reported in several patients without pituitary enlargement [255,256]. These patients manifest resistance to the feedback effect of T_3 on TSH release. The TSH response to TRH has been variable. These patients seem to represent selective pituitary resistance to TH. Features of thyroid autoimmune disease are absent and the serum TSH level is inappropriately elevated in relation to the serum T_4 and T_3 concentrations. In contrast to patients with pituitary TSH-secreting tumours, the TSH α-subunit level is not elevated and the TSH response to TRH is increased. Treatment of the disorder is difficult. Thyroid ablation controls the hyperthyroidism but aggravates the TSH hypersecretion and increases the risk of development of a pituitary adenoma. Suppression of TSH by exogenous TH may aggravate the hyperthyroidism. However, this approach has been successful [257] and treatment with 2,5,3′-triiodothyroacetic acid (TRIAC) has been proposed [258].

Autonomous (nodular) hyperthyroidism

Autonomous functioning thyroid nodules are uncommon in childhood and adolescence. Thyroid function in patients with thyroid nodules is variable; most patients are euthyroid. Rarely, single or multiple autonomously functioning nodules may be associated with clinical hyperthyroidism [259,260]. Such nodules are true follicular adenomas and nearly always benign; the incidence of thyroid carcinoma in functioning nodules is less than 1%. It is generally felt that function in a thyroid nodule essentially excludes a diagnosis of thyroid carcinoma, but the possibility must be considered. Small functional nodules usually do not produce clinical thyrotoxicosis; large nodules (in excess of 3 cm diameter) are more likely to do so.

Nodular autonomy is usually discerned by thyroid radioiodine scan. A nodule is autonomous if it is the only thyroid tissue showing uptake. If the nodule shows increased radioiodine uptake but the remaining thyroid tissue is still visible on scan, autonomy is likely. Autonomy is confirmed if the serum TSH concentration measured by a highly sensitive method is suppressed and/or is unresponsive to TRH stimulation [259,260]. The absence of clinical thyrotoxicosis and the presence of normal range serum T_4 and T_3 concentrations is compatible with a blunted TSH response to TRH. T_4 or T_3 suppression testing has been used to confirm autonomy; radioiodine uptake in autonomous nodules is not suppressible by exogenous TH.

The natural history of functioning thyroid nodules in individual patients is variable. Most likely, if euthyroid, such patients will remain euthyroid, but there may be a gradual increase in autonomous TH production with development of clinical evidence of hyperthyroidism. Nodule enlargement or thyrotoxic symptoms may create the need for ablative therapy. Functioning nodules producing clinical and chemical thyrotoxicosis require surgical removal. Radioiodine treatment now tends to be reserved for older patients (those over 40 years of age). Antithyroid drug therapy is considered only for short-term management. Complete lobectomy with removal of pericapsular lymph nodes and preservation of the recurrent laryngeal nerve is the most desirable procedure.

THYROID NEOPLASIA

Classification

A solitary thyroid mass with a consistency differing from that of the rest of the thyroid gland suggests neoplasia [261,262]. The prevalence of malignancy in adult thyroid nodules approximates 4% [262]. In children with thyroid nodules the current prevalence has been estimated to be 30–40% [263]. Nodular enlargement in the male is somewhat more likely to be cancerous than in the female. The ratio of females to males among children with thyroid cancer is only 2:1, in contrast to the much higher predominance of females with thyroid enlargement from other causes. External radiation therapy to the head and neck area during infancy and childhood has been shown to predispose to thyroid cancer. In a series of children reported in the 1950s with thyroid cancer, 80% had a history of prior head and neck radiotherapy [264–266]. The average time between irradiation and the recognition of the tumour was 10 years. However, in the 1980s the aetiology of most childhood thyroid carcinoma has been obscure since head and neck irradiation is no longer administered for benign disease in children.

A classification of thyroid neoplasms is shown in Table 26.19. Of solitary thyroid nodules presented during childhood, 50% or more prove to be cystic lesions or benign adenomas. Hyperfunctioning adenomas are rare in the

Table 26.19 Types of thyroid neoplasia in childhood

Tumours of the follicular epithelium
Follicular adenoma
Papillary carcinoma
Follicular carcinoma
Anaplastic carcinoma
Tumours of non-follicular origin
Medullary carcinoma
Metastatic tumours
Teratoma
Lymphoma
Other

first two decades of life. Well-differentiated thyroid follicular carcinomas account for over 90% of the malignant lesions in this age group. Well-differentiated carcinomas are further classified into papillary and follicular adenocarcinoma. If sufficient tissue sections are examined, most well-differentiated carcinomas will contain both cell patterns, and management and prognosis are similar for both tumour types. Other malignant tumours of the thyroid gland during childhood include medullary carcinomas, undifferentiated carcinomas and tumours such as lymphomas and metastatic tumours arising in other tissues. The prognosis in these cases is much worse than in well-differentiated follicular cell adenocarcinomas; hence it is important to establish a tissue diagnosis as early as possible and design the treatment accordingly.

HORMONAL MANIFESTATIONS OF MEDULLARY CARCINOMAS

Medullary thyroid carcinomas (MTC) arising from the parafollicular of C cells of the thyroid gland, comprise 4–10% of thyroid carcinomas [267,268]. The histological picture includes large deposits of amyloid situated among sheets of pleomorphic epithelial cells. Both sporadic and familial cases of MTC have been described. The familial cases seem to be transmitted as an autosomal dominant trait and may be associated with multiple endocrine neoplasia (MEN). Thus MTC is part of a syndrome, referred to as MEN II, that can be distinguished from MEN I (with parathyroid, pituitary and pancreatic tumours). MEN IIA includes MTC, phaeochromocytomas and hyperparathyroidism; MEN IIB includes MTC, phaeochromocytomas and multiple mucosal neuromas. The common feature of all the tumours is a neuroectodermal origin. Patients with mucosal neuromas usually have a distinctive appearance with protruding, thick, often bumpy lips, occasional prognathism and a marfanoid habitus.

MTC is associated with excessive secretion of calcitonin [268]. Other substances, including adrenocorticotrophin, melanocyte-stimulating hormone, histaminase, serotonin, prostaglandins, somatostatin and β-endorphin, may also be produced. Although calcitonin levels are invariably elevated in patients with palpable tumours, small tumours can be detected in children before development of a palpable mass by serum calcitonin measurement before and/or after stimulation tests with intravenous calcium of pentagastrin. Using such stimulation tests it is possible to identify MTC in prepubertal children of affected parents and remove the thyroid at a time when the tumour is only a few millimetres in size. The tests can easily be done as an office procedure, and can thus be carried out at regular intervals (1–2 years) on all children of affected families.

Diagnosis and management

A scan of the neck following administration of radioiodine or technetium is important in the diagnosis of thyroid nodules during childhood. If the nodule concentrates iodide, carcinoma is unlikely. If there is associated autoimmune thyroiditis, carcinoma is unlikely; 10–15% of such patients present with thyroid nodules which are lymphoid in type, or represent areas of thyroid hyperplasia [191]. Scanning the neck with ultrasound is of value in distinguishing cystic lesions, and this is useful since cystic lesions are likely to be benign. However, the most useful approach to diagnosis is small-needle biopsy of the nodule. If the nodule is large enough and accessible, small-needle aspiration allows diagnosis of cystic nodules and is helpful in differentiating malignant and benign lesions. An experienced cytologist should be involved in interpretation [262,269]. The presence of colloid and benign follicular cells in the needle aspirate indicates a pseudonodule or adenoma. The absence of colloid and the presence of cellular malignancy criteria suggest a papillary–follicular carcinoma or medullary carcinoma.

Surgery is recommended for a cold nodule in an otherwise normal thyroid gland if malignancy criteria are present. These include a history of radiation to the head or neck, rapid growth of a nodule that is very firm or hard, satellite lymph nodes, hoarseness or dysphagia or evidence of distant metastases. When there are no malignancy criteria, and the nodule is large enough, management is based on results of needle biopsy. Surgery is necessary if the biopsy is positive or suspicious. A negative biopsy allows thyroid suppression treatment with observation. The initial approach to surgery is simple removal of the affected lobe. No further surgery is necessary if the mass proves to be a cystic lesion or benign adenoma. If frozen section reveals carcinoma, total thyroidectomy should be carried out with preservation of the parathyroid glands and recurrent laryngeal nerves.

Although accessible regional nodes should be removed, a mutilating neck dissection is not warranted [262]. Routine radioiodine treatment following surgery is of questionable benefit in children with well-differentiated thyroid carcinoma and no evidence of metastases. In patients with lymph-node involvement or distant metastases, postoperative radioiodine should be given to ablate any residual functioning thyroid tissue and identifiable metastatic loci. Patients are then followed after surgery and radioiodine treatment by measurement of serum Tg concentrations as a reliable tumour marker. Serum Tg levels of < 1 ng/ml on thyroxine suppression treatment or < 10 ng/ml off thyroxine suppression indicate remission; higher values suggest the presence of metastases. Metastatic disease is usually treated with high-dose radioiodine. It is important following surgery or surgery and radioiodine that the patient be maintained on full substitution dosages of exogenous TH to avoid stimulation of tumour growth by endogenous TSH [262].

The prognosis in children with metastatic well-differentiated thyroid follicular cell carcinomas is good. The course is usually an indolent one, with long periods in which there is little progression. In most instances spread is confined to regional lymph nodes with little tendency to metastasize by the blood. Life expectancy in such patients is normal. Most recurrences are local in patients without initial metastatic disease, and repeated surgery and radioiodine treatments may be necessary. TH suppression cannot be overemphasized and should be prescribed in doses adequate to suppress serum TSH as assessed by a high-sensitivity TSH assay while avoiding toxicity. Mortality in thyroid carcinoma during childhood and adolescence is primarily accounted for by the relatively uncommon instances of medullary carcinoma and undifferentiated carcinoma. In these cases more radical surgery combined with radiation or cancer chemotherapy is fully justified.

DISORDERS OF THE CARRIER PROTEINS

The serum proteins represent an extremely heterogeneous group of protein molecules produced in large part by the liver. The major groups include prealbumin, albumin and globulins, and genetic heterogeneity is marked within each group. Abnormalities of the levels or patterns of serum albumin concentration have been described. The major categories are bisalbuminaemia and analbuminaemia. Since albumin usually binds only about 10% of the circulating T_4 and 30–50% of T_3, and the concentrations of TBG and prealbumin are normal or increased in these disorders, the levels of TH in these patients are usually in the normal range [15,270,271]. No confirmed disorder of prealbumin involving abnormalities of TH levels has been described to date. Thus the plasma protein disorders associated with abnormal serum T_4 levels include only the variations in TBG and the recently described hyperthyroxinaemic state 'familial dysalbuminaemic hyperthyroxinaemia.'

Abnormalities of thyroxine-binding globulin

THYROXINE-BINDING GLOBULIN DEFICIENCY

Thyroxine-binding globulin deficiency was first described in 1959 in a euthyroid male. Since that time many reports of a familial TBG deficiency syndrome have appeared [15,272]. The prevalence of the disorder varies from 1 in 5000 to 1 in 10 000 newborns. The disorder is transmitted as an X-linked trait; serum TBG levels measured either by immunoassay or T_4 binding capacity are very low in affected males and approximately half-normal in carrier females. Serum T_4 levels vary similarly. Male-to-male transmission has not been observed, but there is invariable transmission of the trait from affected males to female offspring. An abnormality in hepatic TBG synthesis has been postulated. Affected subjects are euthyroid with normal serum TSH responses to exogenous TRH. Treatment is not indicated.

LOW THYROXINE-BINDING GLOBULIN

A second disorder is characterized by diminished but not absent TBG. A number of families have been reported [38,39,42]. In these families, as in those with very low serum TBG levels, serum free T_4 and TSH levels are normal. The TBG levels were diminished in affected males and there was a tendency to decreased concentrations in carrier females. This abnormality also seems to be transmitted as an X-linked trait. Kinetic studies using purified TBG in these patients have shown that the total daily degradation rate of TBG is proportional to the serum concentration of the protein, indicating that the abnormality, like the absent TBG abnormality, is due to an altered rate of hepatic TBG production. Another disorder associated with decreased TBG levels and decreased TBG affinity for T_4 has been reported in Australian Aborigines [270].

HIGH THYROXINE-BINDING GLOBULIN

Subjects with increased levels of TBG have increased total serum T_4 concentrations with normal free T_4 and normal TSH levels; thus they are euthyroid [15]. Studies in these subjects, as in those with low TBG concentrations, have shown a correlation between TBG production rates and serum levels, suggesting that the mechanism for the high TBG concentrations is increased production, presumably by the liver. TBG levels are increased up to 4.5 times normal levels in affected individuals, and carrier females have serum concentrations intermediate between normal values and the high levels in affected males. Early reports suggested a dominant mode of inheritance, but subsequent studies are compatible with an X-linked mode of inheritance. This disorder, too, is probably heterogeneous.

Familial dysalbuminaemic hyperthyroxinaemia

Several groups of investigators have reported euthyroid subjects with increased serum T_4 concentrations not corrected by the use of the free T_4 index correction and with normal free T_4, total serum T_3 and TSH levels [272–274]. There is increased binding of T_4 to albumin, and the albumin in these patients has an affinity for T_4 binding intermediate between TBG and TBPA. T_3 is less avidly bound, accounting for the preferential increase in serum

T_4 concentration. Patients with the disorder are euthyroid with normal thyroid hormone production rates. The abnormal albumin seems to be transmitted as an autosomal dominant trait. There is male-to-male transmission and an affected to unaffected ratio of one or greater in first-degree relatives.

REFERENCES

1 Fisher DA. Thyroid hormone effects on growth and development. In: Delange F, Fisher DA, Malvaux P, eds. *Pediatric Thyroidology*. Basel: Karger, 1985:75–89.

2 Fisher DA. Thyroid development and thyroid disorders in infancy. In: Van Middlesworth L, ed. *The Thyroid Gland, a Practical Clinical Treatise*. Chicago, IL: Year Book, 1986: 111–29.

3 Larsen PR. Regulation of thyroid hormone metabolism in the brain. In: De Long GR, Robbins J, Condliffe PG, eds. *Iodine and the Brain*. New York: Plenum Press, 1989:5–18.

4 Porterfield SP, Hendrich CE. The role of thyroid hormones in prenatal and neonatal neurological development. Current perspectives. *Endocr Rev* 1993;14:94–106.

5 Walker P. Developmental action of thyroid hormones. In: Dussault JH, Walker P, eds. *Congenital Hypothyroidism*. New York: Dekker, 1983:63–84.

6 Dobbing J, Sands J. Quantitative growth and development of human brain. *Arch Dis Child* 1973;48:757–67.

7 Delange F. Relation of thyroid hormones to human brain development. In: Hetzel BS, Smith RM, eds. *Fetal Brain Disorders. Recent Approaches to the Problem of Mental Deficiency*. Amsterdam: Elsevier/North-Holland, 1981: 285–96.

8 De Long G, Robbins J, Condliffe PG. *Iodine and the Brain*. New York: Plenum Press, 1989.

9 Dussault JH, Walker P. *Congenital Hypothyroidism*. New York: Dekker, 1983.

10 Weichsel ME. Thyroid hormone replacement therapy in the perinatal period: neurologic considerations. *Pediatrics* 1978;92:1035–8.

11 Hollingsworth DR, Mabry CC. Congenital Graves' disease. Four familial cases with long-term follow-up and perspective. *Am J Dis Child* 1976;130:148–55.

12 Capen CC. Anatomy, comparative anatomy, and histology of the thyroid. In: Braverman LE, Utiger RU eds. *The Thyroid. A Fundamental and Clinical Text*. Philadelphia, PA: JB Lippincott, 1991:22–40.

13 Wayne EJ, Koutras DA, Alexander WD. *Clinical Aspects of Iodine Metabolism*. Oxford: Blackwell Scientific Publications, 1964.

14 Dumont JE, Vassart G, Refetoff S. Thyroid disorders. In: Scriver CR, Beaudet AL, Fly WS, Valle D, eds. *The Metabolic Basis of Inherited Diseases*, 6th edn, Vol. 2. New York: McGraw-Hill, 1989:1843–79.

15 Fisher DA. Thyroid disorders. In: Emery AEH, Rimoin PL, eds. *The Principles and Practice of Medical Genetics*. Edinburgh: Churchill Livingstone, 1983:1152–63.

16 Taurog A. Hormone synthesis: thyroid iodine metabolism. In: Braverman LE, Utiger RD, eds. *The Thyroid. A Fundamental and Clinical Text*. Philadephia, PA: Lippincott, 1981:51–97.

17 Van Herle AJ, Vassart G, Dumont JE. Control of thyroglobulin synthesis and secretion. *N Engl J Med* 1979;301: 239–49; 307–17.

18 Wolff J. Congenital goiter with defective iodine transport. *Endocr Rev* 1983;4:240–54.

19 De Nayer P, Cornette C, Vanderschueren M *et al*. Serum thyroglobulin levels in preterm neonates. *Clin Endocrinol* 1984;21:149–53.

20 Fisher DA, Vanderschueren-Lodeweyckx M. Laboratory tests for thyroid diagnosis in infants and children. In: Delange F, Fisher DA, Malvaux P, eds. *Pediatric Thyroidology*. Basel: Karger, 1985:127–42.

21 Walfish PG, Tseng KH. Thyroid physiology and pathology. In: Collu R, Ducharme JR, Guyda HJ, eds. *Pediatric Endocrinology*. New York: Raven Press, 1989:367–448.

22 Delange F, Dalhem A, Bourdoux P *et al*. Increased risk of primary hypothyroidism in preterm infants. *J Pediatr* 1984; 105:462–9.

23 Pezzino V, Filetti S, Belfiore A, Proto S, Donzelli G, Vigneri R. Serum thyroglobulin levels in the newborn. *J Clin Endocrinol Metab* 1981;52:364–6.

24 Delange F. Thyroid hormones. Biochemistry and physiology. In: Bertrand J, Rappaport R, Sizonenko, eds. *Pediatric Endocrinology*. Baltimore, MD: Williams & Wilkins, 1993:242–51.

25 Pezzino V, Vigneri R, Squatrito S, Filetti S, Camus M, Polosa P. Increased serum thyroglobulin levels in patients with nontoxic goiter. *J Clin Endocrinol Metab* 1978;46:653–7.

26 Van Herle AJ, Chopra IJ, Hershman JM, Hornabrook RW. Serum thyroglobulin in inhabitants of an endemic region of New Guinea. *J Clin Endocrinol Metab* 1976;43:512–16.

27 Sava L, Tomaselli L, Runello F, Belfiore A, Vigneri R. Serum thyroglobulin levels are elevated in newborns from iodine-deficient areas. *J Clin Endocrinol Metab* 1986;62:429–32.

28 Dumont JE, Lamy F. The regulation of thyroid cell metabolism, function, growth, and differentiation. In: de Visscher M, ed. *The Thyroid Gland*. New York: Raven Press, 1980: 153–68.

29 Larsen PR. Thyroid–pituitary interaction. Feedback regulation of thyrotropin secretion by thyroid hormones. *N Engl J Med* 1982;306:23–32.

30 Morley JE. Neuroendocrine control of thyrotropin secretion. *Endocr Rev* 1981;2:326.

31 Scanlon MF. Neuroendocrine control of thyrotropin secretion. In: Braverman LE, Utiger RD, eds. *The Thyroid. A Fundamental and Clinical Text*. Philadelphia, PA: Lippincott, 1991:230–56.

32 Yamada T. Control of thyroid hormone secretion. In: Hershman J, Bray GA, eds. *The Thyroid. Physiology and Treatment of Disease*. Oxford: Pergamon Press, 1979:83–98.

33 Nagataki S. Effect of excess quantities of iodide. In: Greer MA, Solomon DS, eds. *Handbook of Physiology*, Section 7: *Endocrinology*, Vol. III: *Thyroid*. Washington, DC: American Physiology Society, 1974:329–44.

34 Roti E, Vagenakis AG. Effect of excess iodide: clinical aspects. In: Braverman LE, Utiger RD, eds. *The Thyroid. A Fundamental and Clinical Text*. Philadelphia, PA: Lippincott, 1991:390–402.

35 Wolff J, Chaikoff IL. The inhibitory action of excessive iodine upon the synthesis of diiodotyrosine and of thyroxine in the thyroid gland of the normal rat. *Endocrinology* 1948; 43:174–9.

36 Bernal J, De Groot LJ. Mode of action of thyroid hormones. In: de Visscher M, ed. *The Thyroid Gland*. New York: Raven Press, 1980:123–43.

37 Davis PJ. Cellular actions of thyroid hormones. In: Braverman LE, Utiger RD, eds. *The Thyroid. A Fundamental*

and Clinical Text. Philadelphia, PA: Lippincott, 1991: 190–203.

38 De Nayer P, Glinoer D. Thyroid hormone transport and action. In: Delange F, Fisher DA, Malvaux P, eds. *Pediatric Thyroidology*. Basel: Karger, 1985:57–74.

39 Gershengorn MC, Glinoer D, Robbins J. Transport and metabolism of thyroid hormones. In: de Visscher M, ed. *The Thyroid Gland*. New York: Raven Press, 1980:81–121.

40 Köhrle J, Hesch D, Leonard JL. Intracellular pathways of iodothyronine metabolism. In: Braverman LE, Utiger RD, eds. *The Thyroid. A Fundamental and Clinical Text*. New York: Lippincott, 1991:144–89.

41 Larsen PR, Silva JE, Kaplan MM. Relationship between circulating and intracellular thyoid hormones: physiological and clinical implications. *Endocr Rev* 1981;2:87–102.

42 Robbins J. Thyroid hormone transport proteins and the physiology of hormone binding. In: Braverman LE, Utiger RD, eds. *The Thyroid. A Fundamental and Clinical Text*. Philadelphia, PA: Lippincott, 1991:111–25.

43 Silva JE, Dick TE, Larsen PR. The contribution of local tissue thyroxine monodeiodination to the nuclear 3,5,3'-triiodothyronine in pituitary, liver and kidney of euthyroid rats. *Endocrinology* 1978;103:1196–207.

44 Hesch RD. *The 'Low T3 Syndrome'*. London: Academic Press, 1981.

45 Ingenbleek Y. Thyroid function in nutritional disorders. In: Delange F, Fisher DA, Malvaux P, eds. *Pediatric Thyroidology*. Basel: Karger, 1985:345–68.

46 Chopra IJ. Nature, sources, and relative biologic significance of circulating thyroid hormones. In: Braverman LE, Utiger RD, eds. *The Thyroid. A Fundamental and Clinical Text*. Philadelphia, PA: Lippincott, 1991:126–43.

47 Verelst J, Delange F, Bourdoux P, Vu Q, Ermans AM. Circulating thyroid hormones in thyroid dysgenesis. In: Naruse H, Irie M, eds. *Neonatal Screening*. Amsterdam: Excerpta Medica, 1983:138–9.

48 Chopra IJ, Hershman JM, Hornabrook RW. Serum thyroid hormone and thyrotropin levels in subjects from endemic goiter regions of New Guinea. *J Clin Endocrinol Metab* 1975;40:326–33.

49 Delange F, Hershman JM, Ermans AM. Relationship between the serum thyrotropin level, the prevalence of goiter and the pattern of iodine metabolism in Idjwi Island. *J Clin Endocrinol Metab* 1971;33:261–8.

50 Delange F, Camus M, Ermans AM. Circulating thyroid hormones in endemic goiter. *J Clin Endocrinol Metab* 1972; 34:891–5.

51 Obregon MJ, Ruiz de Ona C, Escobar del Rey F, Morreale de Escobar G. Regulation of intracellular thyroid hormones concentrations in the fetus. In: Delange F, Fisher DA, Glinoer D, eds. *Research in Congenital Hypothyroidism*. New York: Plenum Press, 1989:79–94.

52 Fisher DA. Ontogenesis of hypothalamic–pituitary–thyroid function in the human fetus. In: Delange F, Fisher DA, Malvaux P, eds. *Pediatric Thyroidology*. Basel: Karger, 1985:19–32.

53 Fisher DA, Dussault JH, Sack J, Chopra IJ. Ontogenesis of hypothalamic–pituitary–thyroid function and metabolism in man, sheep and rat. *Rec Prog Horm Res* 1977;35:59–116.

54 Fisher DA, Klein AH. Thyroid development and disorders of thyroid function in the newborn. *N Engl J Med* 1981;304: 702–12.

55 Roti E, Gnudi A, Braverman LE. The placental transport, synthesis and metabolism of hormones and drugs which affect thyroid function. *Endocr Rev* 1983;4:121–49.

56 Polk DH, Wu SY, Fisher DA. Serum thyroid hormone and tissues 5' monodeiodinase activity in acutely thyroidectomized newborn lambs. *Am J Physiol Endocrinol Metab* 1986;14:E151–5.

57 Polk DH, Padbury JE, Callegari C *et al*. Effect of fetal thyroidectomy and newborn thermogenesis in lambs. *Pediatr Res* 1987;21:435–57.

58 Bachrach L, Burrow GN. Thyroid function in pregnancy. Fetal–maternal relationships. In: Delange F, Fisher DA, Malvaux P, eds. *Pediatric Thyroidology*. Basel: Karger, 1985: 1–18.

59 Braverman LE. Placental transfer of substances from mother to fetus affecting fetal pituitary–thyroid function. In: Delange F, Fisher DA, Glinoer D, eds. *Research in Congenital Hypothyroidism*. New York: Plenum Press, 1989:3–17.

60 Delange F, Bourdoux P, Laurence M, Peneva L, Walfish P, Willgerodt H. Neonatal thyroid function in iodine deficiency. In: Delange F, Dunn JT, Glinoer D, eds. *Iodine Deficiency in Europe. A Continuing Concern*. New York: Plenum Press, 1993:199–209.

61 Delange F, Bourdoux P, Ermans AM. Transient disorders of thyroid function and regulation in preterm infants. In: Delange F, Fisher D, Malvaux P, eds. *Pediatric Thyroidology*. Basel: Karger, 1985:369–93.

62 Dussault JH. The developing fetal thyroid gland and the maternal fetal placental unit. In: Dussault JH, Walker P, eds. *Congenital Hypothyroidism*. New York: Dekker, 1983:3–9.

63 Vulsma T, Gons MH, De Vijlder JJM. Maternal–fetal transfer of thyroxine in congenital hypothyroidism due to a total organification defect or thyroid agenesis. *N Engl J Med* 1989; 321:13–16.

64 Delange F, de Vijlder J, Morreale de Escobar G, Rochiccioli P, Varrone S. Significance of early diagnostic data in congenital hypothyroidism: report of the Subcommittee on neonatal hypothyroidism of the European Thyroid Association. In: Delange F, Fisher DA, Glinoer D, eds. *Research in Congenital Hypothyroidism*. New York: Plenum Press, 1989:225–34.

65 Ekins R, Sinha A, Ballabio M *et al*. Role of maternal carrier proteins in the supply of thyroid hormones to the feto-placental unit: evidence of a feto-placental requirement for thyroxine. In: Delange F, Fisher DA, Glinoer D, eds. *Research in Congenital Hypothyroidism*. New York: Plenum Press, 1989:42–60.

66 Emerson CH. Role of the placenta in fetal thyroid homeostasis. In: Delange F, Fisher DA, Glinoer D, eds. *Research in Congenital Hypothyroidism*. New York: Plenum Press, 1989:31–41.

67 Escobar del Rey F, Pastor R, Mallol J, Morreale de Escobar G. Effects of maternal iodine deficiency on T4 and T3 contents of rat concepta, both before and after onset of fetal thyroid function. In: Medeiros-Neto GA, Gaitan E, eds. *Frontiers of Thyroidology*. New York: Plenum Press, 1986:1033–8.

68 Morreale de Escobar G, Pastor R, Obregon MJ, Escobar del Rey F. Effect of maternal hypothyroidism on the weight and thyroid hormone content of rat embryonic tissues, before and after onset of fetal thyroid function. *Endocrinology* 1985;117:1890–900.

69 Morreale de Escobar G, Obregon MJ, De Ona CR, Escobar del Rey F. Transfer of thyroxine from the mother to the rat fetus near term: effects on brain 3,5,3'-triiodothyronine deficiency. *Endocrinology* 1988;122:1521–31.

70 Morreale de Escobar G, Obregon MJ, De Ona CR, Escobar del

Rey F. Comparison of maternal to fetal transfer of 3,5,3′-triiodothyronine versus thyroxine in rats, as assessed from 3,5,3′-triiodothyronine level in fetal tissues. *Acta Endocrinol* 1989;120:20–30.

71 Morreale de Escobar G, Calvo R, Obregon MJ, Escobar del Rey F. Contribution of maternal thyroxine to fetal thyroxine pools in normal rats near term. *Endocrinology* 1990;126: 2765–7.

72 Lucas C, Carayon P, Bellilchi J, Giraud F. Evolution du taux d'hormones thyroïdiennes libres chez l'enfant de 1 à 16 ans. *Pédiatrie* 1980;35:197–204.

73 Delange F, Fisher DA, Glinoer D. *Research in Congenital Hypothyroidism*. New York: Plenum Press, 1989.

74 Foley TP Jr. Sporadic congenital hypothyroidism. In: Dussault JH, Walker P, eds. *Congenital Hypothyroidism*. New York: Dekker, 1983:231–59.

75 Alm J, Larsson A, Zetterström R. Congenital hypothyroidism in Sweden. Incidence and age at diagnosis. *Acta Paed Scand* 1978;67:1–3.

76 Delange F. Neonatal hypothyroidism: recent developments. *Baillières Clin Endocrinol Metab* 1988;2:637–52.

77 Jacobsen BB, Brandt NJ. Congenital hypothyroidism in Denmark. Incidence, types of thyroid disorders and age at onset of therapy in children 1970–1975. *Arch Dis Child* 1981;56:134–6.

78 Klein AH, Meltzer S, Kenny FM. Improved prognosis in congenital hypothyroidism treated before age three months. *J Pediatr* 1972;81:912–15.

79 Andersen HJ. Studies of hypothyroidism in children. *Acta Paediatr (Copenh)* 1961;50(Suppl. 125):1–150.

80 Smith DW, Blizzard RM, Wilkins L. The mental prognosis in hypothyroidism of infancy and childhood. A review of 128 cases. *Pediatrics* 1957;19:1011–22.

81 Najjar SS. Muscular hypertrophy in hypothyroid children; the Kocher–Debre–Semelaigne syndrome. *J Pediatr* 1974; 85:236–9.

82 Rosman P. Neurological and muscular aspects of thyroid dysfunction in childhood. *Pediatr Clin N Am* 1976;23: 575–94.

83 Raiti S, Newns GH. Cretinism: early diagnosis and its relation to mental prognosis. *Arch Dis Child* 1971;46: 692–4.

84 Virtanen M. Manifestations of congenital hypothyroidism during the 1st week of life. *Eur J Pediatr* 1988;147:270–4.

85 Klein R. History of congenital hypothyroidism. In: Burrow GN, Dussault JH, eds. *Neonatal Thyroid Screening*. New York: Raven Press, 1980:51–9.

86 Hagberg B, Westphal O. Ataxic syndrome in congenital hypothyroidism. *Acta Paed Scand* 1970;59:323–7.

87 Wiebel J. Cerebellar–ataxic syndrome in children and adolescents with hypothyroidism under treatment. *Acta Paed Scand* 1976;65:201–5.

88 Kirkland RT, Kirkland JL, Roberson MC, Librik L, Clayton GW. Strabismus and congenital hypothyroidism. *J Pediatr* 1972;80:648–50.

89 Schulman JD, Crawford JD. Congenital nystagmus and hypothyroidism. *N Engl J Med* 1969;280:708–10.

90 Boyages SC, Halpern JP, Maberly GF *et al.* A comparative study of neurological and myxedematous endemic cretinism in Western China. *J Clin Endocrinol Metab* 1988;67:1262–71.

91 Delange F, Ermans AM, Vis HL, Stanbury JB. Endemic cretinism in Idjwi Island (Kivu Lake, Republic of the Congo). *J Clin Endocrinol Metab* 1972;34:1059–66.

92 Wolter R, Noel P, Craen M *et al.* Neuropsychological study in treated thyroid dysgenesis. *Acta Paed Scand* 1979; Suppl. 227:41–6.

93 Delange F, Camus M, Winkler M, Dodion J, Ermans AM. Serum thyrotropin determination on the fifth day of life as screening procedure for congenital hypthyroidism. *Arch Dis Child* 1977;52:89–96.

94 Dussault JH, Laberge C. Dosage de la thyroxine (T4) par méthode radioimmunologique dans l'éluat de sang séché: nouvelle méthode de dépistage de l'hypothyroïdie néonatale? *Union Med Can* 1973;102:2062–4.

95 Rochiccioli P, Dutau G, Bayard F, Augier D. Neonatal detection of hypothyroidism by radioimmunoassay of the thyroxin in the eluate of dried blood. *Pediatr Res* 1975;9:685.

96 American Academy of Pediatrics. Newborn screening for congenital hypothyroidism: recommended guidelines. *Pediatrics* 1993;91:1203–9.

97 Burrow GN, Dussault JH. *Neonatal Thyroid Screening*. New York: Raven Press, 1980.

98 Fisher DA. Background, strategies and problems of newborn screening for congenital hypothyroidism. In: Carter TP, Willey AM, eds. *Genetic Disease Screening and Management*. New York: Liss, 1986:233–51.

99 Fisher DA. Effectiveness of newborn screening programs for congenital hypothyroidism: prevalence of missed cases. *Pediatr Clin N Am* 1987;34:881–90.

100 Grant GA, Carsson DJ, McReid M, Hutchinson JM. Congenital hypothyroidism missed on screening. *Arch Dis Child* 1986;61:189–90.

101 Illig R. Primary TSH screening. In: Dussault JH, Walker P, eds. *Congenital Hypothyroidism*. New York: Dekker, 1983: 169–78.

102 La Franchi SH, Hanna CE, Krainz PL, Skeels MR, Miyahara RS, Sesser DE. Screening for congenital hypothyroidism with specimen collection at two time periods: results of the northwest regional screening program. *Pediatrics* 1985;76: 734–40.

103 Mitchell ML, Larsen PR. Screening for congenital hypothyroidism: the T4-TSH approach. In: Dussault JH, Walker P, eds. *Congenital Hypothyroidism*. New York: Dekker, 1983:169–78.

104 Naruse H, Irie M. *Neonatal Screening*. Amsterdam: Excerpta Medica, 1983.

105 New England Regional Screening Program and the New England Congenital Hypothyroidism Collaborative. Pitfalls in screening for congenital hypothyroidism. *Pediatrics* 1982; 70:165–200.

106 Working Group on Congential Hypothyroidism of the European Society for Paediatric Endocrinology. Guidelines for neonatal screening programmes for congenital hypothyroidism. *Eur J Pediatr* 1993;152:974–5.

107 Delange F, Bourdoux P, Ermans AM. Neonatal thyroid screening used as an index of an extra physiological supply of iodine. In: Hall R, Köbberling J, eds. *Thyroid Disorders Associated with Iodine Deficiency and Excess*. New York: Raven Press, 1985:273–82.

108 Delange F, Dunn JT, Glinoer D. *Iodine Deficiency in Europe. A Continuing Concern*. New York: Plenum Press, 1993.

109 Czernichow P. Analyse critique de la méthode de dépistage de l'hypothyroïdie congénitale en France. *Arch Fr Pediatr* 1987;44:681–6.

110 Pomarede R, Czernichow P, Farriaux JP. Analyse des échecs du dépistage de l'hypothyroïdie congénitale par dosage de la TSH sur sang capillaire. *Arch Fr Pediatr* 1986;43:15–18.

111 Delange F, Beckers C, Höfer R, König MP, Monaco F, Varrone S. Progress report on neonatal screening for congenital hypothyroidism in Europe. In: Burrow GN, Dussault JH, eds. *Neonatal Thyroid Screening*. New York: Raven Press, 1980:107–31.

112 Toublanc JE. Comparison of epidemiological data on congenital hypothyroidism in Europe with those of other parts in the world. *Horm Res* 1992;38:230–5.

113 Verkerk PH, Buitendijk SE, Verloove-Vanhorick SP. Congenital hypothyroidism screening and the cutoff for thyrotropin measurement: recommendations from the Netherlands. *Am J Publ Health* 1993;83:868–71.

114 Therell BL. *Advances in Neonatal Screening*. Amsterdam: Excerpta Medica, 1987.

115 Virtanen M, Perheentupa J, Mäenpäa J, Pitkanen L, Pikkarainen J. Finnish national screening for hypothyroidism. Few false positives, early therapy. *Eur J Pediatr* 1984;143:2–5.

116 Bodegard G, Fryo K, Larsson A. Psychological reactions in 102 families with a newborn who has a falsely positive screening test for congenital hypothyroidism. *Acta Paed Scand* 1983;Suppl. 304:1–21.

117 Laberge C. Cost benefit evaluation of neonatal thyroid screening: the Quebec experience 1973–1982. In: Dussault JH, Walker P, eds. *Congenital Hypothyroidism*. New York: Dekker, 1983:209–16.

118 Brown AL, Fernhoff PM, Milner J, McEwen C, Elsas LS. Racial differences in the incidence of congenital hypothyroidism. *J Pediatr* 1981;99:934–6.

119 Frasier SD, Penny R, Snyder R. Primary congenital hypothyroidism in Spanish surnamed infants in Southern California. *J Pediatr* 1982;101:315.

120 Fort P, Lifshitz F, Bellissario R *et al.* Abnormalities of thyroid function in infants with Down's syndrome. *J Pediatr* 1984;104:545–9.

121 Miyai K, Connelly JF, Foley TP Jr *et al.* An analysis of the variation of incidence of congenital dysgenetic hypothyroidism in various countries. *Endocrinol Jpn* 1984;31:77–81.

122 Drexhage HA, Bottazzo GF. The thyroid and autoimmunity. In: Delange F, Fisher DA, Malvaux P, eds. *Pediatric Thyroidology*. Basel: Karger, 1985:90–105.

123 Van Der Gaag RD, Drexhage HA, Dussault JH. Role of maternal immunoglobulins blocking TSH-induced thyroid growth in sporadic forms of congenital hypothyroidism. *Lancet* 1985;1:246–50.

124 Chiovato L, Vitti P, Marcocci C *et al.* TSH-blocking antibodies and congenital hypothyroidism. In: Delange F, Fisher DA, Glinoer D, eds. *Research in Congenital Hypothyroidism*. New York: Plenum Press, 1989:141–50.

125 Grant DB, Smith I, Fuggle PW, Tokar S, Chapple J. Congenital hypothyroidism detected by neonatal screening: relationship between biochemical severity and early clinical features. *Arch Dis Child* 1992;67:87–90.

126 Letartre J, Guyda H, Dussault JH. Clinical, biochemical and radiological features of neonatal hypothyroid infants. In: Burrow GN, Dussault JH, eds. *Neonatal Thyroid Screening*. New York: Raven Press, 1989:225–35.

127 Foley TP Jr. Familial thyroid dyshormonogenesis. In: Delange F, Fisher DA, Malvaux P, eds. *Pediatric Thyroidology*. Basel: Karger, 1985:174–88.

128 Leger J, Czernichow P. Congenital hypothyroidism: decreased growth velocity in the first weeks of life. *Biol Neonate* 1989;55:218–23.

129 Czernichow P, Schlumberger M, Pomarede R, Fragu P. Plasma thyroglobulin measurements help determine the type of thyroid defect in congenital hypothyroidism. *J Clin Endocrinol Metab* 1983;56:242–5.

130 Muir A, Daneman D, Daneman A, Ehrlich R. Thyroid scanning, ultrasound, and serum thyroglobulin in determining the origin of congenital hypothyroidism. *Am J Dis Child* 1988;142:214–16.

131 Ermans AM, Verelst J, Chanoine JP, Delange F. Scintigraphy in congenital hypothyroidism. In: Delange F, Fisher DA, Glinoer D, eds. *Research in Congenital Hypothyroidism*. New York: Plenum Press, 1989:187–92.

132 Chanoine JP, Toppet V, Body JJ *et al.* Contribution of thyroid ultrasound and serum calcitonine to the diagnosis of congenital hypothyroidism. *J Endocrinol Invest* 1990;13:103–9.

133 Fisher DA. Management of congenital hypothyroidism. *J Clin Endocrinol Metab* 1991;72:523–9.

134 Fisher DA, Foley BL. Early treatment of congenital hypothyroidism. *Pediatrics* 1989;83:785–9.

135 Frost GJ, Parkin JM. Management of patients with congenital hypothyroidism. *Br Med J* 1985;290:1485–9.

136 Guyda HJ. Treatment of congenital hypothyroidism. In: Dussault JH, Walker P, eds. *Congenital Hypothyroidism*. New York: Dekker, 1983:385–96.

137 Van Vliet G, Barboni Th, Klees M, Cantraine F, Wolter R. Treatment strategy and long term follow-up of congenital hypothyroidism. In: Delange F, Fisher DA, Glinoer D, eds. *Research in Congenital Hypothyroidism*. New York: Plenum Press, 1989:245–52.

138 McCrossin RB, Sheffield LJ, Robertson EF. Persisting abnormality in the pituitary–thyroid axis in congenital hypothyroidism. In: Nagataki S, Stockigt JHR, eds. *Thyroid Research VIII*. Canberra: Australian Academy of Science Publishers, 1980:37–40.

139 Sato T, Suzuki Y, Taketani T, Ishiguro K, Nakajima H. Age-related change in pituitary threshold for TSH release during thyroxine replacement therapy for cretinism. *J Clin Endocrinol* 1977;44:553–9.

140 Barnes ND. Screening for congenital hypothyroidism: the first decade. *Arch Dis Child* 1985;60:587–92.

141 Farriaux JP, Dhondt JL, Lebecq MP. Intellectual outcome in hypothyroid children screened at birth. In: Delange F, Fisher DA, Glinoer D, eds. *Research in Congenital Hypothyroidism*. New York: Plenum Press, 1989:253–64.

142 Glorieux J, Dussault JH, Morissette J, Desjardins M, Letarte J, Guyda H. Follow-up at ages 5 and 7 years on mental development in children with hypothyroidism detected by Quebec screening program. *J Pediatr* 1985;107:913–15.

143 Hulse JA, Grant DB, Jackson D, Clayton BE. Growth development, and reassessment of hypothyroid infants diagnosed by screening. *Br Med J* 1982;284:1435–7.

144 Illig R, Largo RH, Qin Q, Torresani T, Rochiccioli P, Larsson A. Mental development in congenital hypothyroidism after neonatal screening. *Arch Dis Child* 1987;62:1050–5.

145 New England Congenital Hypothyroidism Collaborative. Neonatal hypothyroidism screening: status of patients at 6 years of age. *J Pediatr* 1985;107:915–19.

146 Rovet J, Ehrlich R, Sorbara D. Intellectual outcome in children with fetal hypothyroidism. *J Pediatr* 1987;5:700–4.

147 Glorieux J, Dussault JH, Van Vliet G. Intellectual development at age 12 years of children with congenital hypothyroidism diagnosed by neonatal screening. *J Pediatr* 1992;121:581–4.

148 Rochiccioli P, Alexandre F, Roge B. Neurological devel-

opment in congenital hypothyroidism. In: Delange F, Fisher DA, Glinoer D, eds. *Research in Congenital Hypothyroidism*. New York: Plenum Press, 1989:301–10.
149 Rochiccioli P, Roge B, Alexandre T, Tauber MT. School achievement in children with hypothyroidism detected at birth and search for predictive factors. *Horm Res* 1992;38:236–40.
150 Foley TP Jr. Congenital hypopituitarism. In: Dussault JH, Walker P, eds. *Congenital Hypothyroidism*. New York: Dekker, 1983:331–48.
151 Miyai K. Defect in hypothalamic–pituitary function. In: Delange F, Fisher DA, Malvaux P, eds. *Pediatric Thyroidology*. Basel: Karger, 1985:143–53.
152 Suter SN, Kaplan SL, Aubert ML, Grumbach MM. Plasma prolactin and thyrotropin and the response to thyrotropin-releasing factor in children with primary and hypothalamic hypothyroidism. *J Clin Endocrinol Metab* 1978;47:1015–20.
153 Refetoff S, Weiss RE, Usala SJ. The syndromes of resistance to thyroid hormones. *Endocr Rev* 1993;14:348–99.
154 Refetoff S, Dewind LT, De Groot LJ. Familial syndrome combining deafmutism, stippled epiphyses, goiter and abnormally high PBI: possible target organ refractoriness to thyroid hormone. *J Clin Endocrinol Metab* 1967;27:279–94.
155 Hadeed AJ, Asay LD, Klein AH, Fisher DA. Significance of transient postnatal hypothyroxinemia in premature infants with and without respiratory distress syndrome. *Pediatrics* 1981;68:494–8.
156 Klein AH, Oddie TH, Parslow M, Foley TP Jr, Fisher DA. Developmental changes in pituitary–thyroid function in the human fetus and newborn. *Early Human Dev* 1982; 6:321–30.
157 Chowdhry P, Scanlon JW, Auerbach R, Abbassi V. Results of controlled double blind study of thyroid replacement in very low birth weight premature infants with hypothyroxinemia. *Pediatrics* 1984;73:301.
158 Delange F, Dodion J, Wolter R *et al.* Transient hypothyroidism in the newborn infant. *J Pediatr* 1978;92:974–6.
159 Delange F, Heidemann P, Bourdoux P *et al.* Regional variations of iodine nutrition and thyroid function during the neonatal period in Europe. *Biol Neonate* 1986;49:322–30.
160 Glinoer D, De Nayer P, Bourdoux P *et al.* Regulation of maternal thyroid during pregnancy. *J Clin Endocrinol Metab* 1990;71:276–87.
161 Miyai K, Karada T, Nose O, Mizuta H, Amino N, Yabuuchi H. Hyperthyrotropinemia with normal thyroid hormone concentrations in newborn babies. In: Naruse H, Irie M, eds. *Neonatal Screening*. Amsterdam: Excerpta Medica, 1983: 44–9.
162 Fisher DA, Beall GN. Hashimoto's thyroiditis. *Pharmacol Ther* 1976;1:445–58.
163 Inoue M, Taketani N, Sato T, Nakajima H. High incidence of chronic lymphocytic thyroiditis in apparently healthy school children: epidemiological and clinical study. *Endocrinol Jpn* 1975;22:483–8.
164 Rallison M, Dobyns BM, Keating FR, Rall JE, Tyler FH. Chronic lymphyocytic thyroiditis in children. *J Pediatr* 1975;86:675–82.
165 Volpé R. *Auto-immunity in the Endocrine System*. Berlin: Springer Verlag, 1981.
166 Greenberg AH, Czernichow P, Hung W, Shelley W, Winship T, Blizzard RW. Juvenile chronic lymphocytic thyroiditis: clinical laboratory, and histological correlations. *J Clin Endocrinol Metab* 1970;30:293–301.
167 Ling SM, Kaplan SA, Weitzman JJ, Reed GB, Costin G, Landing BH. Euthyroid goiters in children: correlation of needle biopsy with other clinical and laboratory findings in chronic lymphocytic thyroiditis and simple goiter. *Pediatrics* 1969;44:695–708.
168 Gordin A, Lamberg BA. Spontaneous hypothyroidism in symptomless autoimmune thyroiditis. A long term follow-up study. *Clin Endocrinol* 1981;15:537–43.
169 Hayashi Y, Tamai H, Fukata S *et al.* A long term clinical, immunological and histological follow-up of patients with goitrous chronic lymphocytic thyroiditis. *J Clin Endocrinol Metab* 1985;62:1172–8.
170 Bright GM, Blizzard RM, Kaiser DL, Clarke WL. Organ specific autoantibodies in children with common endocrine diseases. *J Pediatr* 1982;100:8–14.
171 Gilani BB, MacGillivray MH, Voorhess ML, Mills BJ, Riley RJ, MacLaren NK. Thyroid hormone abnormalities at diagnosis of insulin-dependent diabetes mellitus in children. *J Pediatr* 1984;105:218–22.
172 Gray RS, Borsey DQ, Seth J, Herd R, Brown NS, Clarke BF. Prevalence of subclinical thyroid failure in insulin-dependent diabetes. *J Clin Endocrinol Metab* 1980;50:1034–7.
173 Hymes K, Blum M, Lackner H, Karpatkin S. Easy bruising, thrombocytopenia, and elevated platelet immunoglobulin G in Graves' disease and Hashimoto's thyroiditis. *Ann Intern Med* 1981;94:27–30.
174 Jordan SG, Buckingham B, Sakai R, Olson D. Studies of immune complex glomerulonephritis mediated by human thyroglobulin. *N Engl J Med* 1981;304:1212–15.
175 Portmann L, Hamada N, Heinrich G, Degroot LJ. Anti-thyroid peroxidase antibody in patients with autoimmune thyroid disease. Possible identity with antimicrosomal antibody. *J Clin Endocrinol Metab* 1985;61:1001–3.
176 Rees Smith B, Mc Lachlan SM, Furmaniak J. Autoantibodies to the thyrotropin receptor. *Endocr Rev* 1988;9:106–21.
177 Delange F, Ermans AM. Iodine deficiency. In: Braverman LE, Utiger RD, eds. *The Thyroid. A Fundamental and Clinical Text*. Philadelphia, PA: Lippincott, 1991:368–90.
178 Gaitan E. *Environmental Goitrogenesis*. Boca Raton, CA: CRC Press, 1989.
179 Vagenakis AG, Braverman LE. Drug-induced hypothyroidism. In: Hershman JM, Bray GA, eds. *The Thyroid: Physiology and Treatment of Disease*. Oxford: Pergamon Press, 1979:389–99.
180 Lippe BM, Van Herle AJ, La Franchi SH, Uller RP, Lavin N, Kaplan SA. Reversible hypothyroidism on growth hormone deficient children treated with human growth hormone. *J Clin Endocrinol Metab* 1975;40:612–18.
181 Rodriguez Arnao J, Miell JP, Ross RJM. Influence of thyroid hormones on the GH-IGF axis. *Trends Endocrinol Metab* 1993;4:169–73.
182 Pai GS, Leach DC, Weiss L, Wolf C, Van Dyke DL. Thyroid anormalities in 20 children with Turner syndrome. *J Pediatr* 1977;91:267–9.
183 Lucky AW, Howley PM, Megylesi K, Spielberg SB, Schulman JD. Endocrine studies in cystinosis: compensated primary hypothyroidism. *J Pediatr* 1977;91:204–10.
184 Raiti S, Trias E, Maclaren NK. Primary hypothyroidism: differentiation from primary hypopituitarism. *Am J Dis Child* 1975;129:1397–9.
185 Newman AJ, Lee C. Hypothyroidism simulating dermatomyositis. *J Pediatr* 1980;97:772–4.
186 Barnes ND, Hayles AB, Ryan RJ. Sexual maturation in juvenile hypothyroidism. *Mayo Clin Proc* 1973;48:849–56.

187 Hemady ZS, Siler-Khodr TM, Najjar S. Precocious puberty in juvenile hypothyroidism. *Pediatrics* 1978;92:55–9.
188 Van Wyk JJ, Grumbach MM. Syndrome of precocious menstruation and galactorrhea in juvenile hypothyroidism: an example of hormonal overlap in pituitary feedback. *J Pediatr* 1960;57:416–35.
189 Costin G, Kershnar AK, Kogut MD, Turkington RW. Prolactin activity in juvenile hypothyroidism and precocious puberty. *Pediatrics* 1972;50:881–9.
190 Lee PA, Blizzard RM. Serum gonadotropins in hypothyroid girls with and without sexual precocity. *Johns Hopkins Med J* 1974;135:55–60.
191 Fisher DA, Oddie TH, Johnson DE, Nelson TC. The diagnosis of Hashimoto's thyroiditis. *J Clin Endocrinol Metab* 1975;40:795–801.
192 Abbassi V, Aldige C. Evaluation of sodium L-thyroxine (T4) requirement in replacement therapy of hypothyrodism. *J Pediatr* 1977;90:298–301.
193 Niimi H, Sasaki N, Inomota H, Nakajima H. Evaluation of l-thyroxine requirement in treatment of congenital hypothyroidism. *Endocrinol Jpn* 1980;27:733–8.
194 Rezvani IR, Digeorge AM. Reassessment of the daily dose of oral thyroxine for replacement therapy in hypothyroid children. *J Pediatr* 1977;90:291–7.
195 Brent GA, Hershman JM. Thyroxine therapy in patients with severe nonthyroidal illness and low serum thyroxine concentration. *J Clin Endocrinol Metab* 1986;63:1–8.
196 Chopra IJ, Hershman JM, Pardridge WM, Nicoloff JT. Thyroid function in nonthyroidal illness. *Ann Intern Med* 1983;98: 946–57.
197 Engler D, Burger AG. The deiodination of iodothyronines and of their derivatives in man. *Endocr Rev* 1984;5:131–84.
198 Chopra IJ, Solomon DH, Chua Teco GN, Eisenberg JB. An inhibitor of the binding of thyroid hormones to serum proteins is present in extrathyroidal tissues. *Science* 1982;215: 407–9.
199 Food and Nutrition Board, US National Research Council. Iodine. In: *Recommended Dietary Allowances*, 10th edn. Washington: National Academy Press, 1989:213–17.
200 Delange F. Requirements of iodine in humans. In: Delange F, Dunn TJ, Glinoer D, eds. *Iodine Deficiency in Europe. A Continuing Concern.* New York: Plenum Press, 1993:5–16.
201 Hetzel BS. Iodine deficiency disorders (IDD) and their eradication. *Lancet* 1983;2:1126–9.
202 Delange F, Bürgi H. Iodine deficiency disorders in Europe. *Bull WHO* 1989;67:317–26.
203 Gutekunst R, Scriba PC. Goiter and iodine deficiency in Europe. The European Thyroid Association report as updated in 1988. *J Endocrinol Invest* 1989;12:209–20.
204 Thilly CH, Hetzel BS. An assessment of prophylactic programs: social, political, cultural and economic issues. In: Stanbury JB, Hetzel BS, eds. *Endemic Goiter and Endemic Cretinism.* New York: Wiley, 1980:475–90.
205 Ermans AM. Etiopathogenesis of endemic goiter. In: Stanbury JB, Hetzel BS, eds. *Endemic Goiter and Endemic Cretinism.* New York: Wiley, 1980:287–301.
206 Stanbury JB, Brownell GL, Riggs DS, Perinetti H, Itoiz J, Del Castillo EB. *Endemic Goiter. The Adaptation of Man to Iodine Deficiency.* Cambridge, MA: Harvard University Press, 1954.
207 Studer H, Kohler H, Bürgi H. Iodine deficiency. In: Greer MA, Solomon DH, eds. *Handbook of Physiology.* Section 7, *Endocrinology*, Vol. III: *Thyroid.* Washington, DC: American Physiological Society, 1974:303–28.
208 Brabant G, Bergmann P, Kirsch CM, Köhrle J, Hesch RD, von zur Mühlen A. Early adaptation of thyrotropin and thyroglobulin secretion to experimentally decreased iodine supply in man. *Metabolism* 1992;41:1093–6.
209 Abrams GM, Larsen PR. Triiodothyronine and thyroxine in the serum and thyroid glands of iodine-deficient rats. *J Clin Invest* 1973;52:2522–31.
210 Lamas L, Morreale de Escobar G. Iodoaminoacid distribution in the thyroid of rats on different iodine intakes and with normal plasma protein bound iodine. *Acta Endocrinol (Copenh)* 1972;69:473–87.
211 Hershman JM, Due DT, Sharp B *et al.* Endemic goiter in Vietnam. *J Clin Endocrinol Metab* 1983;57:243–9.
212 Patel YC, Pharoah POD, Hornabrook PW, Hetzel BS. Serum triiodothyronine, thyroxine and thyroid-stimulating hormone in endemic goiter: a comparison of goitrous and nongoitrous subjects in New Guinea. *J Clin Endocrinol Metab* 1973;37:783–9.
213 Pharoah POD, Lawton NF, Ellis SM, Wiliams ES, Ekins RP. The role of triiodothyronine (T3) in the maintenance of euthyroidism in endemic goitre. *Clin Endocrinol* 1973;2: 193–9.
214 Delange F, Bourdoux P, Lagasse R *et al.* Effects of thiocyanate during pregnancy and lactation on thyroid function in infants. In: Ermans AM, Mbulamoko NM, Delange F, Ahluwalia R, eds. *Role of Cassava in the Etiology of Endemic Goitre and Cretinism.* Ottawa: International Development Research Centre, Publication No. 135e, 1980:121–6.
215 Lagasse R, Bourdoux P, Courtois P *et al.* Influence of the dietary balance of iodine/thiocyanate and protein on thyroid function in adults and young infants. In: Delange F, Iteke FB, Ermans AM, eds. *Nutritional Factors Involved in the Goitrogenic Action of Cassava.* Ottawa: International Development Research Centre, 1982:34–9.
216 Delange F. *Endemic Goitre and Thyroid Function in Central Africa.* Monographs in Pediatrics, Vol. 2. Basel: Karger, 1974.
217 Delange F. Adaptation to iodine deficiency during growth: etiopathogenesis of endemic goiter and cretinism. In: Delange F, Fisher DA, Malvaux P, eds. *Pediatric Thyroidology.* Basel: Karger, 1985:295–326.
218 Bachtarzi H, Benmiloud M. TSH-regulation and goitrogenesis in severe iodine deficiency. *Acta Endocrinol (Copenh)* 1983;103:21–7.
219 Delange F, Thilly C, Camus M, *et al.* Evidence for fetal hypothyroidism in severe endemic goiter. In: Robbins J, Braverman LE, eds. *Thyroid Research.* Amsterdam: Excerpta Medica, 1976:493–6.
220 Thilly CH, Delange F, Lagasse R *et al.* Fetal hypothyroidism and maternal thyroid status in severe endemic goiter. *J Clin Endocrinol Metab* 1978;47:354–60.
221 Thilly CH, Vanderpas J, Bourdoux P *et al.* Prevention of myxedematous cretinism with iodized oil during pregnancy. In: Ui N, Torizuka K, Nagataki S, Miyai K, eds. *Current Problems in Thyroid Research.* Amsterdam: Excerpta Medica, 1983:386–9.
222 Delange F. Endemic cretinism. In: Braverman LE, Utiger RD, eds. *The Thyroid. A Fundamental and Clinical Text.* Philadelphia, PA: JB Lippincott, 1991:942–55.
223 Bleichrodt N, Escobar del Rey F, Morreale de Escobar G, Garcia I, Rubio C. Iodine deficiency. Implications for mental and psychomotor development in children. In: De Long GR, Robbins J, Condliffe PG, eds. *Iodine and the Brain.* New York: Plenum Press, 1989:269–87.
224 Fenzi GF, Giusti LF, Aghini-Lombardi F *et al.* Neuropsy-

chological assessment in schoolchildren from an area of moderate iodine deficiency. *J Endocrinol Invest* 1990;13: 427–31.
225 Vermiglio F, Sidoti M, Finocchiaro MD *et al.* Defective neuromotor and cognitive ability in iodine-deficient schoolchildren of an endemic goiter region in Sicily. *J Clin Endocrinol Metab* 1990;70:379–84.
226 Nilsson LR, Persson PS. Cytological aspiration biopsy in adolescent goitre. *Acta Paediatr* 1964;53:333–8.
227 Studer H, Rameli F. Simple goiter and its variants: euthyroid and hyperthyroid multinodular goiters. *Endocr Rev* 1982;3: 40–61.
228 Drexhage HA, Botazzo GF, Doniach D, Bitensky L, Chayen J. Evidence for thyroid growth stimulating immunoglobulins in some goitrous thyroid diseases. *Lancet* 1980;2:287–92.
229 Fisher DA, Pandian MR, Carlton E. Autoimmune thyroid disease, an expanding spectrum. *Pediatr Clin N Am* 1987;34: 907–18.
230 Smyth PPA, McMullan NM, Grubek Loebenstein B, O'Donovan DK. Thyroid growth stimulating immunoglobulins in goitrous disease: relationship to thyroid stimulating immunoglobulins. *Acta Endocrinol* 1986;111:321–30.
231 Wadeleux PA, Winand RJ. Thyroid growth modulating factors in the sera of patients with simple non-toxic goiter. *Acta Endocrinol* 1986;112:502–8.
232 Cassidy CE. Subacute painful thyroiditis. In: Van Middlesworth L, Givens JR, eds. *The Thyroid Gland, a Practical Clinical Treatise.* Chicago: Year Book, 1986:363–70.
233 Volpé R. Subacute thyroiditis. In: Delange F, Fisher DA, Malvaux P, eds. *Pediatric Thyroidology.* Basel: Karger, 1985: 252–64.
234 Fisher DA. Thyrotoxicosis in childhood. In: Braverman LE, Utiger RD, eds. *The Thyroid. A Fundamental and Clinical Text.* Philadelphia, PA: Lippincott, 1991:1238–46.
235 Saxena KM, Crawford JD, Talbot NB. Childhood thyrotoxicosis, a long term perspective. *Br Med J* 1964;2:1153–8.
236 Zimmerman D, Hayles AB. Hyperthyroidism in children. In: Delange F, Fisher DA, Malvaux P, eds. *Pediatric Thyroidology.* Basel: Karger, 1985:223–39.
237 Malvaux P. Hyperthyroidism. In: Bertrand J, Rappaport R, Sizonenko P, eds. *Pediatric Endocrinology.* Baltimore, MD: Williams & Wilkins, 1993:264–9.
238 Barnes V, Blizzard RM. Antithyroid drug therapy for toxic diffuse goiter (Graves' disease): thirty years experience in children and adolescents. *J Pediatr* 1977;91:313–20.
239 Howard CP, Hayles AB. Hyperthyroidism in childhood. *J Clin Endocrinol Metab* 1978;7:127–43.
240 Maenpaa J, Kuusi A. Children hyperthyroidism. *Acta Paed Scand* 1980;69:137–42.
241 Hamburger JL. Management of hyperthyroidism in children and adolescents. *J Clin Endocrinol Metab* 1985;60:1019–24.
242 Marchant B, Lees JFH, Alexander WD. Antithyroid drugs. In: Hershman JM, Bray GA, eds. *The Thyroid: Physiology and Treatment of Disease.* Oxford: Pergamon Press, 1979: 209–52.
243 Shen DC, Wu SY, Chopra IJ *et al.* Long-term treatment of Graves' hyperthyroidism with sodium ipodate. *J Clin Endocrinol Metab* 1985;61:723–7.
244 Wu SY, Shyh TP, Chopra IJ *et al.* Comparison of sodium ipodate (Oragrafin) and propylthiouracil in early treatment of hyperthyroidism. *J Clin Endocrinol Metab* 1982;54:630–4.
245 Harve P, Francis HH. Pregnancy and thyrotoxicosis. *Br Med J* 1962;2:817–22.
246 Fisher DA. Neonatal thyroid disease in the offspring of women with autoimmune thyroid disease. In: Oppenheimer JH, ed. *Thyroid Today*, Vol. 9, No. 4. Flint Laboratories, 1986:1–7.
247 Maisey MN, Stimmler L. The role of long acting thyroid stimulator in neonatal thyrotoxicosis. *Clin Endocrinol* 1972;1:81–90.
248 McKenzie JM, Zakarija M. Pathogenesis of neonatal Graves' disease. *J Endocrinol Invest* 1978;2:183–9.
249 Smallridge RC, Wartofsky L, Chopra IJ *et al.* Neonatal thyrotoxicosis: alterations in serum concentrations of LATS protector, T4, T3, reverse T3 and 3,3'T2. *J Pediatr* 1978;93:118–20.
250 Sunshine P, Kusumoto H, Kriss JP. Survival time of circulating long-acting thyroid stimulator in neonatal thyrotoxicosis: implications for diagnosis and therapy of the disorder. *Pediatrics* 1965;36:869–76.
251 Zakarija M, McKenzie JM, Munro DS. Immunoglobulin G inhibitor of thyroid-stimulating antibody is a cause of delay in the onset of neonatal Graves's disease. *J Clin Invest* 1983;72:1352–6.
252 Zakarija M, McKenzie JM, Hoffman WH. Prediction and therapy of intrauterine and late onset neonatal hyperthyroidism. *J Clin Endocrinol Metab* 1986;62:368–71.
253 Karpman BA, Rapoport B, Filetti S, Fisher DA. Treatment of neonatal hyperthyroidism due to Grave's disease with sodium ipodate. *J Clin Endocrinol Metab* 1987;64:119–23.
254 Tolis G, Bird C, Bertrand G, McKenzie JM, Ezrin C. Pituitary hyperthyroidism: case report and review of the literature. *Am J Med* 1978;64:177–81.
255 Weintraub BD, Gershengorn MC, Kourides IA, Fein H. Inappropriate secretion of thyroid stimulating hormone. *Ann Intern Med* 1981;95:339–51.
256 Gershengorn MC, Weintraub BD. Thyrotropin induced hyperthyroidism caused by selective pituitary resistance to thyroid hormone: a new syndrome of inappropriate secretion of TSH. *J Clin Invest* 1975;56:633–42.
257 Rosler A, Litvin Y, Hoge C, Gross J, Cerasi E. Familial hyperthyroidism due to inappropriate thyrotropin secretion successfully treated with triiodothyronine. *J Clin Endocrinol Metab* 1982;54:76–82.
258 Beck Peccoz P, Piscitelli G, Cattaneo MG *et al.* Successful treatment of hyperthyroidism due to non-neoplastic pituitary TSH secretion with 2,5,3'-triiodothyroacetic acid (TRIAC). *J Endocrinol Invest* 1983;6:217–23.
259 Abe K, Konno M, Sato T, Matsuura N. Hyperfunctioning thyroid nodules in children. *Am J Dis Child* 1980;134: 961–3.
260 Osburne RC, Goren EN, Bybee DE, Johnsonbaugh RE. Autonomous thyroid nodules in adolescents: clinical characteristics and results of TRH testing. *J Pediatr* 1982;100:383–6.
261 Hung W. Thyroid nodules and cancer. In: Delange F, Fisher DA, Malvaux P, eds. *Pediatric Thyroidology.* Basel: Karger, 1985:271–94.
262 Robbins J. Thyroid cancer. In: Van Middlesworth L, Givens JR, eds. *The Thyroid Gland, a Practical Clinical Treatise.* Chicago, IL: Year Book, 1986:405–28.
263 Scott MD, Crawford JD. Solitary thyroid nodules in childhood: is the incidence of thyroid carcinoma declining? *Pediatrics* 1976;58:521–5.
264 Refetoff S, Harrison J, Karanfilski BT, Kaplan EL, De Groot LJ, Bekerman C. Continuing occurrence of thyroid carcinoma after irradiation to the neck in infancy and childhood. *N Engl J Med* 1975;292:171–206.

265 Shore RE, Hildreth N, Dvoretsky P, Andresen E, Moseson M, Pasternack B. Thyroid cancer among persons given X-ray treatment in infancy for an enlarged thymus gland. *Am J Epidemiol* 1993;137:1068–80.
266 Winship T, Rasvoll RV. Thyroid carcinoma in children. Final report and 20 year study. *Clin Proc Child Hosp Washington, DC* 1970;26:327–48.
267 Cobin RH. Medullary carcinoma of the thyroid. In: Cobin RH, Sirota DK, eds. *Malignant Tumors of the Thyroid.* New York: Springer Verlag, 1992:112–41.
268 Melvin KEW. Familial medullary carcinoma of the thyroid. In: Van Middlesworth L, Givens JR, eds. *The Thyroid Gland, a Practical Clinical Treatise.* Chicago, IL: Year Book, 1986: 429–47.
269 Miller JM, Kini SR, Hamburger JL. *Needle Biopsy of the Thyroid.* New York: Traeger, 1983.
270 Glinoer D, De Nayer P. Anomalies in thyroid hormone transport proteins. In: Delange F, Fisher DA, Malvaux P, eds. *Pediatric Thyroidology.* Basel: Karger, 1985:394–406.
271 Hollander CS, Bernstein G, Oppenheimer JH. Abnormalities of thyroxine binding in analbuminemia. *J Clin Endocrinol Metab* 1968;28:1064–9.
272 Lee WNP, Golden MP, Van Herle AJ, Lippe BM, Kaplan SA. Inherited abnormal thyroid hormone binding protein causing selective increase in total serum thyroxine. *J Clin Endocrinol Metab* 1979;49:292–9.
273 Ruiz M, Rajatanavin R, Young RA *et al.* Familial dysalbuminemic hyperthyroxinemia. *N Engl J Med* 1982;306: 635–9.
274 Stockigt JR, Topliss DJ, Barlow JW, White EL, Hurley DM, Taft P. Familial euthyroid thyroxine excess: an appropriate response to abnormal thyroxine binding associated with albumin. *J Clin Endocrinol Metab* 1981;53:353–9.

27: The Adrenal Cortex

J.W. HONOUR

INTRODUCTION

The adrenal cortex undergoes a number of changes of structure and function during childhood which need to be understood when evaluating the role of the gland in normal and pathological circumstances. The purpose of the fetal adrenal cortex remains enigmatic, but the presence of steroids from this zone during the neonatal period causes a number of analytical problems for other steroid hormones. The execution and interpretation of laboratory tests need special considerations throughout childhood, particularly with regard to reference ranges for age, development and body size.

Radioimmunoassay is the major technique for measuring the concentrations of steroid hormones in biological fluids, although production rates can now be determined using stable (as opposed to radioactive) isotopes. The analysis of urinary steroids by gas chromatography with mass spectrometry has an important place in assessing adrenal function in childhood.

EMBRYOLOGY

The adrenal cortex originates from the mesoderm at the cranial end of the mesonephros. During the fifth week of fetal development, mesothelial cells proliferate and invade the underlying stroma. A compact mass, the adrenal blastema, is penetrated on the medial aspect by cells from the neural crest to form the basis for the adrenal medulla. During fetal life, these chromaffin cells secrete noradrenaline but some cells begin to synthesize adrenaline just after birth. The first mesothelial cells form the fetal adrenal cortex, which has a different steroid synthetic capacity to a second outer layer of differentiated mesothelial cells which become the adult or definitive zones of the cortex. Around the 10th week of fetal development, mesenchymal cells surround the adrenal to provide the collagenous capsule. The blood and nerve supplies also develop during this time. The differentiation of cells in the cortex, and the development of function in the fetus, appear to be under the control of the fetal pituitary gland. The adrenals are small in anencephaly.

ANATOMY

The adrenal glands are triangular and positioned at superior poles of the kidneys usually embedded in fat. Changes in structure and size of the adrenal cortex during childhood affect the weight and function of the glands. At the end of fetal life, the adrenal glands are almost as large as the kidneys. Adrenal glands weight then decreases rapidly, by 30% during the first weeks after birth. Following a period of further, slower shrinkage, the adrenals grow throughout childhood to achieve the adrenal weight at birth in late puberty. The combined adrenals weigh 8–12 g by the end of puberty.

At birth the fetal adrenal zone occupies 80% of the enlarged adrenal gland volume (Fig. 27.1). This is unique to higher primates. The adult or definitive zones are incomplete at this time, being scattered in groups around the periphery of the gland. The adrenal medulla is relatively small. After birth, the fetal cortex decreases in size by involution [1] so that, by 4 weeks of postnatal age, the fetal adrenal zone comprises a mere 20% of the total cortex. Some remnants of the fetal cortex can persist, but most have disappeared by the sixth month, except perhaps in the case of infants delivered prematurely [2,3]. The evidence for these changes in adrenal structure comes mainly from adrenals taken at autopsy, although there are biochemical data that support it *in vivo* [4–7]. Data from the monkey, *Mucaca mulatta*, suggest that the fetal zone disappears after birth without necrosis [8].

Each adrenal gland is supplied by three arteries, the superior suprarenal from the inferior phrenic artery, the medial suprarenal from the aorta and the inferior suprarenal from the renal artery. Arteries pierce the capsule and form a capillary plexus. Straight capillaries run through the adrenal cortex and anastomose to form a plexus outside the medulla. The capillaries fuse with medullary capillaries to form venules that run into a large central vein. Blood from the left adrenal drains into the left renal

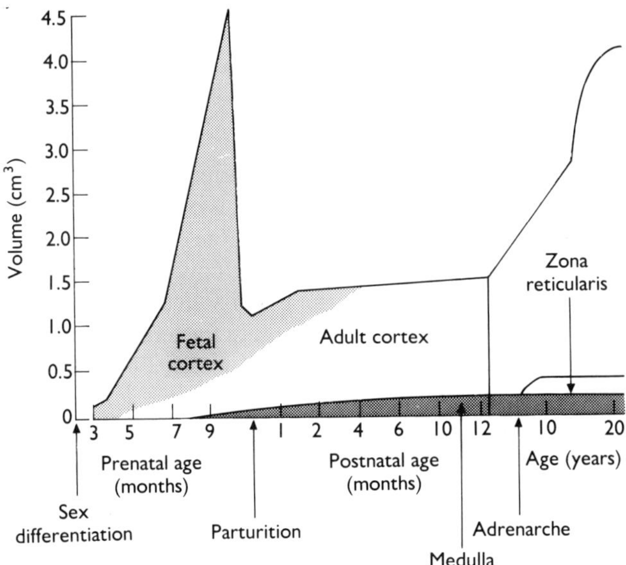

Fig. 27.1 Adrenal size during childhood.

vein and the right adrenal directly to the inferior vena cava [9]. Blood flow through the adrenals may contribute to the regulation of adrenal function [10].

CYTOLOGY

All the cells of the adrenal cortex possess the general characteristics of steroid-producing cells. They have relatively little rough endoplasmic reticulum but abundant smooth endoplasmic reticulum. Many lipid droplets are present and the mitochondria are usually round or elongated and possess laminal cristae.

The outer zona glomerulosa under the capsule is recognizable as small ill-defined clumps. The fasciculata cells are larger than those in the zona glomerulosa and form long cords arranged radially with respect to the medulla. Cholesterol esters in the fasciculata cells contribute to the yellow colour of the adrenal cortex; the medulla is reddish-brown. The zona glomerulosa comprises 5–10% of the cortex and the fasciculata 75–85% of the volume of the adrenal cortex in the young child. The adrenal glands of children from 2 years of age show new reticularis cells appearing at the boundary with the medulla, and these cells form a network of short cords with interdigitating capillaries. The reticularis cells have less smooth endoplasmic reticulum and lipid droplets than are seen in the fasciculata, but there are more lysozymes and lipofuscin granules, which increase in number with age. The mitochondria tend to be more elongated and have both short and long cristae. The zona reticularis becomes a continuous zone usually after the age of 6 years. By age 13–15 years the histological pattern ceases to change.

FUNCTIONS OF THE ADRENAL CORTEX

Cortisol and aldosterone are the most active hormones secreted by the adrenal cortex and they affect respectively carbohydrate metabolism and electrolyte balance (glucocorticoid and mineralocorticoid effects). Cortisol has a number of effects on carbohydrate metabolism which lead to elevation in plasma glucose concentration. An increase in gluconeogenesis occurs through a number of mechanisms including an increase in protein catabolism, hepatic glycogenolysis and ketogenesis. Cortisol is necessary for the action of noradrenaline and adrenaline, glucagon and catecholamines, as well as for the normal functions of blood vessels, cardiac and skeletal muscle, the nervous system and gastrointestinal tract (permissive effects). Glucocorticoids also inhibit the inflammatory response to tissue injury. Adrenal insufficiency is characterized by a failure to excrete a water load. Aldosterone and other steroids with mineralocorticoid activity (deoxycorticosterone, corticosterone) increase sodium reabsorption from the urine, sweat, saliva and gastric juice. Sodium ions are retained by exchange for potassium and hydrogen ions.

The steroid hormones act by stimulating DNA-dependent synthesis of certain messenger (m)RNAs in the nuclei of target cells. This leads in turn to formation of proteins that alter cell function. Each of the steroid groups acts generally through specific receptors [11] which become transcription factors, although there may be some exceptions to this rule [12].

Many steroids have trivial names and can be named systematically, although at the time of their discovery they were given alphabetical characters in order of their characterization (Table 27.1). Along with the histological distinction of the zones of the adrenal cortex, each layer produces a spectrum of steroids. Aldosterone is produced only in the zona glomerulosa. The zona fasciculata produces mainly cortisol. Other steroids from this zone include deoxycorticosterone (DOC), 11-deoxycortisol, corticosterone and some adrenal androgens, of which 11-hydroxyandrostenedione is a specific adrenal androgen. Most of the adrenal androgen is secreted by the zona reticularis as dehydroepiandrosterone sulphate (DHEAS). There is an excellent correlation between plasma DHEAS concentrations and the development of the zona reticularis [13].

The fetal adrenal zone produces increasing amounts of adrenal androgens, predominantly DHEAS, from 8 weeks of gestation. In the placenta, DHEAS is converted to oestrogens by the action of sulphatase and aromatase. The fetoplacental unit acts as an integrated endocrine organ [14,15]. Oestrogen production used to be monitored as an index of fetal viability, but this has been largely superseded by ultrasound. Glucocorticoid and mineralocor-

Table 27.1 Trivial, alphabetical and systematic names of steroids

Trivial name	Alphabetical abbreviation	Systematic name
11-Dehydrocorticosterone	A	21-Hydroxy-4-pregnene-3,11,20-trione
Corticosterone	B	11β,21-Dihydroxy-4-pregnene-3,20-dione
Cortisone	E	17α,21-Dihydroxy-4-pregnene-3,11,20-trione
Cortisol (hydrocortisone)	F	11β,17α,21-Trihydroxy-4-pregnene-3,20-dione
11-Deoxycortisol	S	17α,21-Dihydroxy-4-pregnene-3,20-dione
11-Deoxycorticosterone (DOC)		21-Hydroxy-4-pregnene-3,20-dione
Aldosterone		11β,21-Dihydroxy-4-pregnene-3,20-dione-18-al
Pregnenolone		3β-Hydroxy-5-pregnen-20-one
17-Hydroyxpregnenolone		3β,17α-Dihydroxy-5-pregnen-20-one
Progesterone		4-Pregnene-3,20-dione
17-Hydroxyprogesterone (17-OHP)		17α-Hydroxy-4-pregnene-3,20-dione
Dehydroepiandrosterone (DHEA)		3β-Hydroxy-5-androsten-17-one
Androstenedione		4-Androstene-3,17-dione
Testosterone		17β-Hydroxy-4-androsten-3-one

ticoid production by the fetal adrenal is largely dependent on placental progesterone as substrate. A key enzyme in the production of active steroid hormone (with 3-keto-4-ene structure) is 3β-hydroxysteroid dehydrogenase with 5/4 isomerase, which seems to be inactivated in the fetal adrenal zone throughout pregnancy [16–18]. The fetal adrenal gland secretes DOC, corticosterone, 17-hydroxyprogesterone and 11-deoxycortisol rather than cortisol and aldosterone, and many of the products are sulphated [19]. Glucocorticoids secreted by the fetal adrenal gland affect maturation of a number of enzyme systems in the liver, pancreas and gastrointestinal tract [20,21]. Glucocorticoids induce the development of surfactant in the lung. The fetus is protected from exposure to high cortisol concentrations by the action of 11β-hydroxysteroid dehydrogenase, which oxidizes cortisol to inactive cortisone [22].

PATHWAYS OF STEROID BIOSYNTHESIS

Steroid hormones of the adrenal cortex are derived from cholesterol. The *de novo* biosynthesis of cholesterol from acetate provides only a small part of the cholesterol necessary for steroid production [23,24]. Low-density lipoprotein (LDL)–cholesterol is the major source of cholesterol for adrenal steroidogenesis, except in the fetus. Proteolytic and lipolytic enzymes act on LDL to release cholesterol esters for storage in lipid droplets in the adrenal cells [25–28]. In order for the adrenal cortex to synthesize active steroid hormones, a number of changes are required in the structure of cholesterol. Several of these enzyme-catalysed reactions involve cytochrome P450 (CYP) enzymes. Adrenal steroidogenesis (Fig. 27.2) follows three distinct routes which reflect the zonal differences in function and regulation, and help to interpret the consequences of metabolic diseases affecting any of the enzymes. Substrates which cannot then be metabolized through the usual pathways can themselves be active, or be subject to the action of side-chain cleavage to give androgens.

Cortisol is produced from cholesterol in the zona fasciculata by the sequential action of five enzyme systems under the control of adrenocorticotrophic hormone (ACTH). The carbon content is first reduced from 27 to 21 in a reaction which leaves an oxygen group at C-20 (pregnenolone). The 3β-hydroxysteroid-5-ene structure is changed to 3-keto-4-ene (progesterone) before hydroxylation reactions at positions 17, 21 and 11.

Aldosterone is produced in the zona glomerulosa under the drive of renin/angiotensin. The 17-hydroxylase is not expressed in the zona glomerulosa, but progesterone can be hydroxylated at C-21 and at C-11 before insertion of an aldehyde at C-18.

The adrenal gland makes androgens from cholesterol by the action of three enzymes to dehydroepiandrosterone (DHEA) and four to androstenedione. The carbon content of 17-hydroxypregnenolone is reduced in number to 19 in a reaction leaving an oxygen at C-19 (DHEA) before 3-keto-4-ene conversion (androstenedione). Testosterone is not an important product of the adrenal cortex but is formed in the periphery through conversion of DHEA and androstenedione.

Several of the reactions in steroid biosynthesis are catalysed by CYP-type enzymes and these resemble other P450s. The cellular locations of the enzymes involved in steroid biosynthesis can be on the endoplasmic reticulum (ER) (microsomal) or attached to membranes within mitochondria (Table 27.2). Twenty to 30 amino acids of the N termini of the microsomal P450s serve to anchor these enzymes to the lipid bilayer of the ER. Mitochondrial

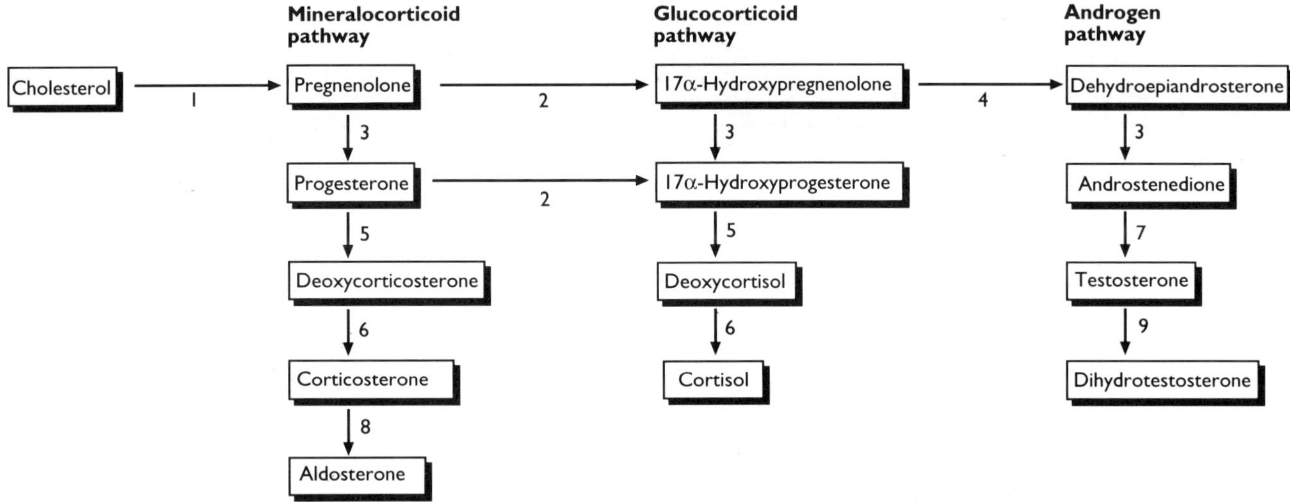

Fig. 27.2 Pathways of adrenal steroid biosynthesis, divided according to function. 1: side-chain cleavage; 2: 17-hydroxylase; 3: 3β-hydroxysteroid dehydrogenase; 4: 17,20-lyase; 5: 21-hydroxylase; 6: 11-hydroxylase; 7: 17-reductase; 8: 18-hydroxylase and 18-oxydase; 9: 5α-reductase.

Table 27.2 Cell location of adrenal steroidogenic enzymes

Endoplasmic reticulum (microsomes)
3β-Hydroxysteroid dehydrogenase
17α-Hydroxylase
21-Hydroxylase
Mitochondria
Side-chain cleavage ($P450_{scc}$)
11β-Hydroxylase

Table 27.3 Electron transport proteins for steroid biosynthesis

Side-chain cleavage	Adrenodoxin reductase
	Adrenodoxin
$P450_{c17}$	Flavoprotein P450 reductase
$P450_{c21}$	Cytochrome b5

P450s are synthesized through the normal channels for protein and then imported into the mitochondria. The membrane-binding regions of these P450s to the inner mitochondrial membrane are not known.

All steroidogenic cytochrome P450s are b-type cytochromes within which haem forms the active site of the enzyme that binds the substrate and molecular oxygen. Carbon monoxide (CO) competes with oxygen for binding to this site, and this can inhibit enzyme activity. The name P450 derives from the distinct ultraviolet absorption maximum at 450 nm of the reduced and CO-bound forms of the enzyme [29]. The reactions catalysed by steroidogenic P450s are either a single hydroxylation at a specific position on the steroid molecule or a series of consecutive mono-oxygenations which precede a C–C bond cleavage or aromatization of the steroid A ring. Each catalysed hydroxylation has the following equation:

$$\text{Steroid–H} + \text{NADPH} + \text{H}^+ + \text{O}_2 \rightarrow \text{Steroid–OH} + \text{NADP} + \text{H}_2\text{O}$$

The single oxygen atom incorporated into the steroid (mono-oxygenation) derives from molecular oxygen. Electrons are transferred from NADPH to cytochrome P450 by specific carrier proteins (Table 27.3).

The microsomal steroidogenic P450s share low (< 40%) sequence homology with each other and poor homology with P450 systems (such as many xenobiotic liver enzymes). The three mitochondrial P450s share high sequence homology with each other. The microsomal and mitochondrial P450s show sequence homology only around limited haem-binding segments close to the carboxy termini.

ENZYMES IN STEROID BIOSYNTHESIS

Side-chain cleavage

In the synthesis of active steroids, cholesterol with 27 carbons is converted first to pregnenolone with 21 carbon atoms. This reaction is catalysed by side-chain cleavage (SCC) or desmolase in three cycles of cytochrome $P450_{scc}$ in rapid succession (Fig. 27.3). Hydroxylations of cholesterol at C-20 and C-22 precede C–C bond cleavage.

17-Hydroxylase and 17,20-lyase (CYP17)

Pregnenolone is used for cortisol synthesis in the zona fasciculata or androgen synthesis in the zona reticularis. 17α-Hydroxylase acting on pregnenolone is the first

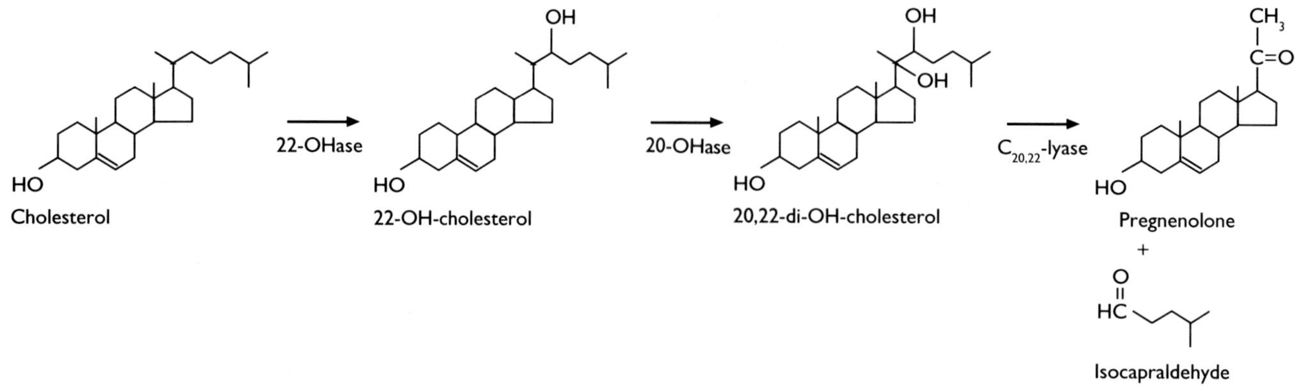

Cholesterol → 22-OHase → 22-OH-cholesterol → 20-OHase → 20,22-di-OH-cholesterol → $C_{20,22}$-lyase → Pregnenolone + Isocapraldehyde

Fig. 27.3 The side-chain cleavage of cortisol.

step in cortisol synthesis. In the zona reticularis the conversion of 17-hydroxypregnenolone to dehydroepiandrosterone (DHEA–C-19 steroid) is catalysed by 17, 20-lyase (coded CYP17). The two enzyme activities (17-hydroxylase and lyase at C-17 to C-20) are functions of the same gene product [30]. How each of the activities is controlled to maintain a physiological balance between glucocorticoid and C-19 steroid production remains to be elucidated. 17-Hydroxylase activity is not expressed in the zona glomerulosa [31].

3β-Hydroxysteroid dehydrogenase and 5/4 isomerase

17-Hydroxypregnenolone is the substrate for 3β-hydroxysteroid dehydrogenase (3β-OHS-DH), which liberates 17-hydroxyprogesterone. Pregnenolone can be utilized in the zona glomerulosa for mineralocorticoid synthesis, in which case pregnenolone is a substrate for 3β-OHS-DH/5,4-isomerase. This conversion gives rise to progesterone with a 3-keto-4-ene structure.

21-Hydroxylase (CYP21)

Further hydroxylation of 17-hydroxyprogesterone and progesterone at C-21 gives 11-deoxycortisol and 11-deoxycorticosterone respectively.

11-Hydroxylase (CYP11)

11-Deoxycortisol is acted on by 11β-hydroxylase (CYP11B1) and converted to cortisol. Deoxycorticosterone is converted by 11β-hydroxylation to corticosterone. This 11-hydroxylase gene product (CYP11B2, aldosterone synthase) will also induce the aldehyde group at C-18 characteristic of aldosterone. The latter is a two-step reaction of 18-hydroxylation before aldehyde formation [32–35].

GENETIC BASIS FOR STEROIDOGENIC ENZYMES

The human $P450_{scc}$ is coded by a single gene on chromosome 15 [36]. A large precursor protein is synthesized which must be processed by proteolysis before or on insertion into mitochondria [37].

Two genes have been found within chromosome 1p11–p13 for 3β-OHS-DH sharing 93% sequence homology. Type II mRNA is the almost exclusive form in the adrenal cortex (ovaries and testes), whereas type I mRNA is prominent in skin (placenta and mammary tissue). The 3β-OHS-DH genes have little sequence homology with other steroid dehydrogenases [38].

The human P450c17 gene is a single copy with eight exons mapped to 10q24–q25 [39]. The full-length complementary (c)DNA have been isolated from the testes [30] and adrenal gland [40] independently; their structures are identical.

21-Hydroxylase has a molecular weight of 52 000 and is the product of a gene in 10 exons on the short arm of chromosome 6 within a 1000 kb region coding for class III cell surface antigens, including complement C4 (A and B genes), complement cascade factors B and C2, as well as tumour necrosis factor (α and β) and heat-shock protein (HSP70) [41,42]. Gene duplications are particularly common in the region of chromosome 6p21 coding for the human leukocyte antigen (HLA) compatibility locus, and about 6 kb away from CYP21B there is a homologous gene (CYP21A) the sequence of which has several mutations which render it a non-functional pseudogene [43]. The two C4 human genes encode functional C4 protein. Two genes coded XA and XB are encoded by the opposite strand of DNA [44] and overlap the CYP21 genes – the XA gene fits between C4A and CYP21B. The product of XA may be a small extracellular matrix protein [45].

Two genes coding for 11-hydroxylase are about 45 kb apart on the human chromosome 8q21–q22 [46,47]. The two genes are approximately 11 kb long and contain nine exons. The genes are 95% identical in coding regions and 90% identical in introns. The enzymes are predicted to be 93% identical in amino-acid sequence [35]. CYP11B2 has 11-hydroxylase activity and will 18-hydroxylate corticosterone and further oxidize this to aldosterone. CYP11B1 has only 11-hydroxylase activity and is expressed in the zona fasciculata at levels significantly higher than CYP11B2 in the zona glomerulosa [48].

CONTROL OF STEROID SECRETION

Cortisol secretion by the adrenal cortex is regulated by ACTH, a single polypeptide of 39 amino acids. ACTH is cleaved from a single precursor protein (pro-opiomelanocortin (POMC)) with a molecular weight of 30 000 and from the sequences of melanocyte-stimulating hormones (MSH), lipotrophin (LPH), endorphin and enkephalin. Some of these peptides are neurotransmitters in the central nervous system (CNS) and are not usually found in the peripheral circulation, although certain tumours may secrete them along with ACTH. A 1–24 synthetic peptide (Synacthen) has biological activity similar to the natural hormone, except that the half-life is shorter.

ACTH is secreted in regular pulses of variable amplitude over 24 h with most activity during the night (0200–0900 h), which is the basis of the circadian rhythm of plasma cortisol concentrations [49] (Fig. 27.4). High concentrations of cortisol inhibit ACTH secretion (negative feedback) (Fig. 27.5). Trauma, emotional stress and some drugs initiate secretion of corticotrophin-releasing hormone (CRH) by nerve endings in the posterior hypothalamus and median eminence. CRH is a 41 amino acid peptide transmitted by the hypophyseal portal vessels to the adenohypophysis evoking release of ACTH [50]. Low circulating cortisol concentrations lead to an increase in CRH–ACTH secretion. The pituitary inhibitory activity of steroids parallels their glucocorticoid potency, although the effect varies and steroid medication at night seems to be more effective in suppressing ACTH than at other times. ACTH may itself exert a negative feedback on its own release by a pituitary short-loop feedback [51,52].

The acute action of ACTH is to increase the flux of cholesterol through the steroidogenic pathway, resulting in rapid production of steroids [53–55]. ACTH binds to receptors on the adrenal cell membranes prior to activation of adenylate cyclase. In turn the cyclic adenosine monophosphate (cAMP) generated activates phosphoprotein kinase and several enzymes likewise by phosphorylation. The newly activated enzymes stimulate several processes, the most important of which is the hydrolysis of cholesterol esters.

In the newborn infant, cortisol is readily converted to the inactive, oxidized product cortisone, which can be at concentrations up to 2000 nmol/l, whereas cortisol can be

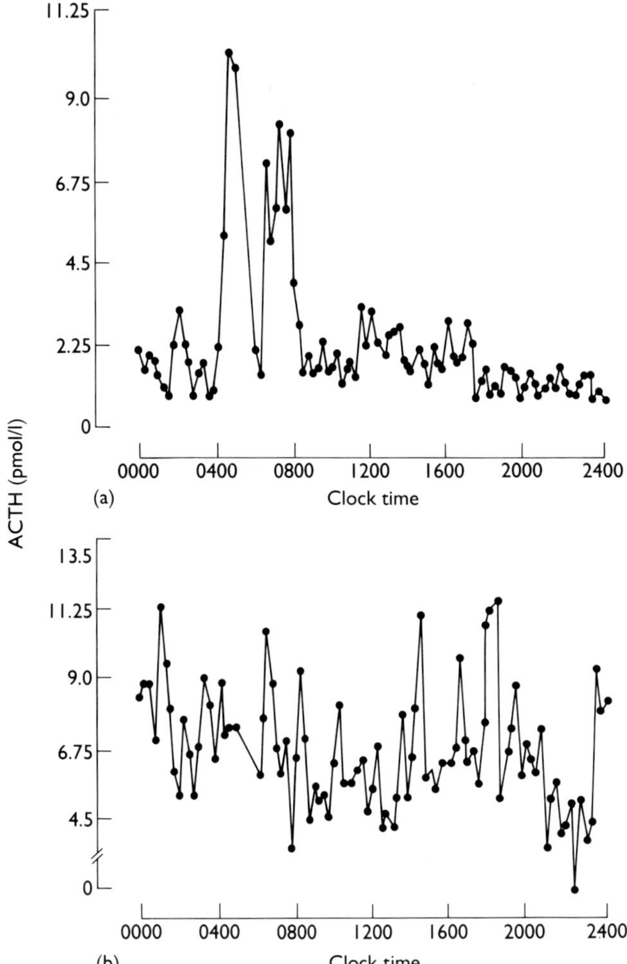

Fig. 27.4 Plasma ACTH concentrations at intervals over a 24-h period in two patients: (a) normal subject; (b) patient with Cushing disease.

less than 400 nmol/l. After 6 months of age there are noticeable changes in the pattern of cortisol levels. First the ratio of cortisol : cortisone is about 5 : 10, as is found throughout the remainder of life. The circadian rhythm is also established around that time [56]. Care should be taken in the selection of assay methods for cortisol measurement in paediatric samples in the first 6 months of life. A low cross-reaction of cortisone in the assay is important.

Adrenal androgen secretion varies with age [57,58] and the response of androgens to ACTH stimulation of the adrenals (during the circadian rhythm and in response to exogenous ACTH) does not always parallel the response of cortisol. DHEAS concentrations are high in the newborn and decline over the first 6 months. There is a rise in concentration in childhood (adrenarche), which may lead to pubic and axillary hair growth. The plasma concentrations of DHEA and DHEAS during sexual development are

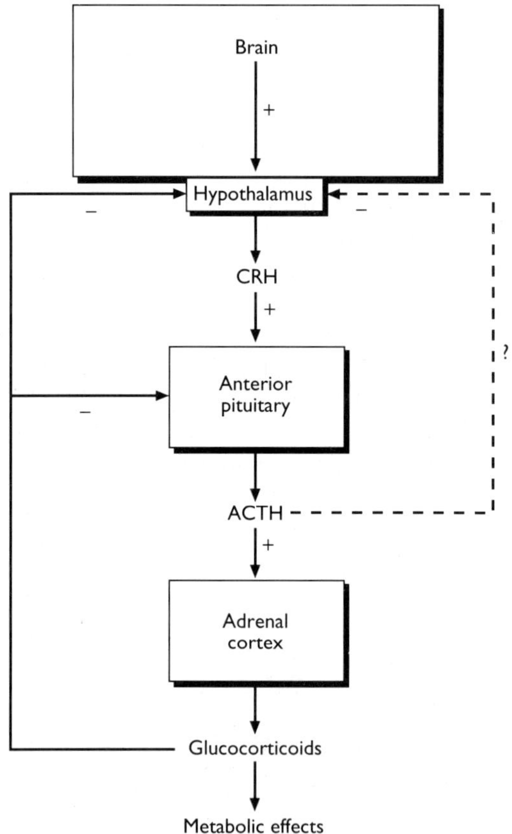

Fig. 27.5 Feedback inhibition for cortisol on corticotrophin-releasing hormone (CRH) secretion by the hypothalamus and ACTH release from the pituitary.

normally suppressed by dexamethasone and stimulated by ACTH [57], but this is not the case before adrenarche [59]. DHEA and 11-hydroxyandrostenedione are secreted episodically and concurrently with cortisol [60,61]. Although the secretion of androgens is under ACTH control, a number of other hormones, both pituitary and extra-pituitary, may have a role [62–67].

The changes in adrenal function before puberty are attributed to remodelling of the adrenal cortex as the gland grows to adult size [68,69]. Adrenocortical cells arise from stem cells under the capsule and migrate inward towards the medulla. As cells move inward they change from glomerulosa to fasciculata cells, and at a critical adrenal size the cells adjacent to the medulla differentiate into reticularis cells [70]. The mechanism for the development of an additional population of zona reticularis cells has been controversial [71–73]. A POMC fragment was isolated as the androgen-stimulating hormone but this action was not confirmed [74,75].

The developmental changes in adrenal androgen secretion reflect changes in relative enzyme activity induced by the necessity to maintain cortisol secretion in the face of adrenal growth [76]. During fetal life, in spite of high ACTH stimulation, adrenal 3β-OHS-DH activity is markedly reduced by the combined inhibitory effects of placental and fetal adrenal steroids [77]. After birth, when placental steroids have been removed and the metabolic clearance of cortisol reduced, there is a decline of ACTH so that adrenal size regresses and the V_{max} for 3β-OHS-DH decreases [78]. Growth factors may participate in intra-adrenal mechanisms which mediate the steroidogenic changes that characterize the adrenarche. Steroids may also act within the gland as pseudosubstrates [79]. The concentrations of androstenedione in the inner region of the cortex have been shown to increase with age as the adrenal reaches maximum size [80]. Similar information can be inferred from the ratios of urine metabolites [81]. The androstenedione levels can be within the range that cause reduction in 21-hydroxylase activity in cultured cells [79].

Aldosterone production is regulated principally by the renin–angiotensin system, which is responsive to the electrolyte balance and to plasma volume. ACTH can induce a temporary rise in aldosterone synthesis [82], but this is not sustained. Hyponatraemia can itself lead to an increase in aldosterone secretion [83]; hyperkalaemia also stimulates aldosterone biosynthesis.

Renin is a glycoprotein (molecular weight 42 000) synthesized in the juxtaglomerular apparatus. An inactive proenzyme is stored in cells of the macula densa of the convoluted distal tubules. Renin release is stimulated by reduced renal perfusion, by hyperkalaemia and by reduced sodium concentration in the macula densa. Renin is a proteolytic enzyme which hydrolyses a decapeptide (angiotensin I) from renin substrate (angiotensinogen – an α_2-globulin synthesized in the liver) (Fig. 27.6). Angiotensin I has very little intrinsic biological activity but is hydrolysed to angiotensin II, an octapeptide, by the action of angiotensin-converting enzyme (ACE). The converting enzyme is present in high concentrations in the lung, although widely distributed in the vasculature and other tissues so that local production of angiotensin II may be important under some circumstances. Angiotensin II only has a short plasma half-life of 1–2 min, being rapidly destroyed by angiotensinase.

The synthesis of aldosterone is regulated at two steps.

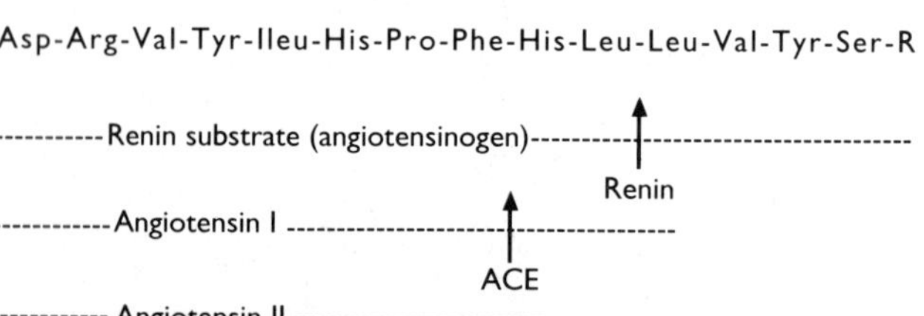

Fig. 27.6 The generation of angiotensins from renin substrate. Cleavage points for the enzymes are shown by arrows.

The first is the conversion of cholesterol to pregnenolone. This early step is stimulated by angiotensin II, ACTH and potassium ions. The second (or late) step in the conversion of corticosterone to aldosterone is stimulated by potassium and high concentrations of angiotensin II [84,85]. Sodium depletion enhances aldosterone biosynthesis through activation of both early and late steps [86,87].

Prostaglandins stimulate aldosterone release from the adrenal glomerulosa cells. The site of action is unknown. Inhibitors of prostaglandin synthesis have been reported by many (but not all) investigators to reduce aldosterone release stimulated by angiotensin.

The CNS acts on the adrenal cortex through the regulation of renin release [88,89]. Serotonin (at least *in vitro*) is a potent stimulator of aldosterone synthesis [90]. The evidence that dopaminergic mechanisms inhibit aldosterone secretion derives from *in vitro* studies employing the dopamine antagonist, metoclopramide [83,91,92]. Administration of this drug to humans increases aldosterone concentrations in blood and urine with no change in the clearance rate. In children the significance of the modulatory effect of dopamine needs clarification.

An aldosterone-stimulating factor (ASF) has been purified to homogeneity and shown to be a glycoprotein with a molecular weight of 26000 [83]. ASF stimulates aldosterone secretion by a cAMP-independent mechanism, and the response is not blocked by specific competitive antagonists of ACTH or angiotensin II. ASF concentrations in blood increase with dietary sodium restriction and are not suppressed when dexamethasone is given. ASF does not respond to upright posture in normal subjects, but increases in patients with idiopathic hyperaldosteronism. A prepubertal boy with bilateral adrenal hyperplasia had hyperaldosteronism with normal circadian variation of cortisol, growth hormone, prolactin and low renin. An elevation of ASF appeared to explain the hyperaldosteronism [93].

Plasma aldosterone concentrations and urinary aldosterone excretion rates are high in term infants during the newborn period. There are age-related differences in these parameters which reflect the plasma renin activity, which is very much higher in newborn infants than older children and adults [94–97] (Fig. 27.7). A significant age-related decrease in angiotensin II is also observed, but not for ACE, which is comparable to values in adults [95]. Inactive forms of renin in plasma are known which are activated by acid, cold or proteolytic treatment [98]. In contrast to adults, trypsin exposure appears to degrade renin in plasma from children. Inactive renin is not detectable in blood taken from children in the supine position, but active renin is high (8–30 ng/ml h^{-1}). Inactive renin represents 80–90% of the total renin in adults.

Fullterm, breast-fed infants are usually in positive sodium balance. Very preterm infants receiving formula feeds may develop a negative sodium balance with hyponatraemia [99–102]. High concentrations of atrial natriuretic peptide and poor renal tubule development may contribute to the poor aldosterone response to angiotensin seen in the newborn infant [103,104].

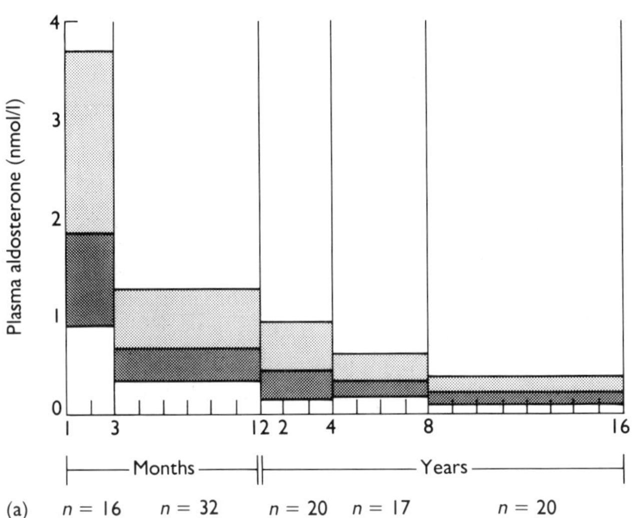

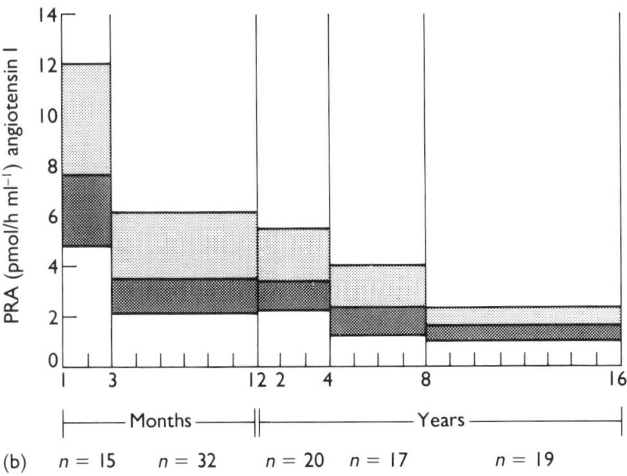

Fig. 27.7 Plasma renin activity (PRA) (b) and aldosterone (a) concentrations during childhood.

TRANSPORT OF ADRENAL STEROIDS

Cortisol is largely bound (70%) in the circulation to an α_2-macroglobulin called transcortin or corticosteroid-binding globulin (CBG). This protein (molecular weight 52000) has a single binding site for cortisol per molecule. CBG is synthesized in the liver and the production is increased by oestrogens. CBG concentrations are lowered in cirrhosis, nephrosis and multiple myeloma. A rare benign condition of CBG deficiency has been described [105]. Cortisol is also bound to albumin to a lesser degree (20%) than to CBG. At normal cortisol concentrations there is very little free cortisol in the plasma. At cortisol concentrations above 600 nmol/l, CBG is saturated and the plasma-free cortisol increases dramatically. Corticosterone, 11-deoxycortisol, 17-hydroxyprogesterone, DOC, progesterone, cortisone and aldosterone are bound to CBG, but to a lesser extent than cortisol. The synthetic steroids dexamethasone and 9α-fluorocortisol are only weakly bound to CBG. The half-life of cortisol is 60–90 min. Aldosterone is bound to albumin more than to CBG, but the binding of aldosterone to protein is weak and the half-life is about 20 min.

STEROIDS IN PLASMA

Immunoassay is the technique most widely used for the measurement of adrenal steroid concentrations in biological fluids. High-performance liquid chromatography (HPLC), coupled to a ultraviolet detection, can be useful in a few situations (to measure cortisol or intermediates in steroid biosynthesis when a patient has a genetic defect of one of the steroidogenic enzymes) [106,107], but in general terms HPLC is insufficiently sensitive. A method has been described for androgen sulphates in plasma based on HPLC of chemically derivatized steroids (dansyl derivatives) and electrochemical detection [108].

There has been a growing tendency to use direct immunological methods in which specific antisera and radiolabel are added directly to plasma samples. Ideally steroids should first be extracted from the plasma into an organic solvent. This step is essential if interference with steroid measurements in blood from newborn infants is to be reduced [109]. The extraction step leaves the steroid sulphates secreted from the large fetal adrenal gland in the aqueous phase. In many clinical circumstances direct assays are functional, but antisera are rarely specific so chromatography may be necessary to purify steroids in an organic extract. This approach has the additional advantage in paediatric studies that several steroids can be measured from a single plasma extract, although it may then be necessary to perform column chromatography or HPLC to separate individual steroids prior to quantitative analysis by radioimmunoassay (RIA) [110–113].

Throughout most of childhood the concentrations of cortisol in plasma are minimal around midnight (less than 150 nmol/l) and rise in a series of peaks to reach maxima (200–800 nmol/l) between 0600 and 0900 h, thereafter falling slowly throughout the day. This circadian rhythm is found in all normal children except newborn infants up to 6 months of age [56]. In the neonate cortisol circulates at very much lower concentrations than cortisone, and the choice of assay to measure cortisol concentrations should consider the cross-reaction with cortisone. Care must also be taken with samples from children being treated with prednisolone and where plasma 11-deoxycortisol concentrations are high (substrate for 11-hydroxylase, which may be inactivated by drugs or increased by a genetic defect). Prednisolone and 11-deoxycortisol are the steroids most likely to cross-react with the antisera, but may be distinguished by HPLC analysis. Cortisol is normally the major form after 6 months of age.

17α-Hydroxyprogesterone (17-OHP) concentrations in plasma are above 40 nmol/l during the first 48 hours of life. Normal levels in children after that time are less than 10 nmol/l. In very ill children, particularly preterm infants, persistently raised concentrations can be found [114,115]. This may reflect partly the quality of the assays, since assays performed directly without extraction of steroid into an organic solvent give abnormally high results [114]. Steroids from the fetal adrenal cortex must be tested for cross-reactivity in any assay used to measure 17-OHP in newborn infants. 17-hydroxypregnenolone sulphate has been shown to be at high concentrations in newborn plasma and to bind to certain 17-OHP antisera [116].

DHEAS has a long half-life of 10–20 h and consequently there are only small fluctuations in the concentration in plasma, as opposed to the episodic secretion of androstenedione and DHEA. In neonates high levels of DHEAS reflect the low activity of 3β-OHS-DH in the fetal adrenal cortex. Plasma DHEAS concentrations are higher in preterm infants compared with fullterm babies [117,118]. DHEAS concentrations are low from 6 months to 6–8 years but the levels are increasing by 8–10 years (Table 27.4) as the zona reticularis develops. Children with premature adrenarche have increased plasma concentrations of DHEA and DHEAS for age [57]. DHEAS concentrations are grossly elevated in children with adrenal tumours and somewhat raised in congenital adrenal hyperplasia (CAH) due to 3β-OHS-DH deficiency. Testosterone and androstenedione production and plasma concentrations (Table 27.5) are lower during childhood than in

Table 27.4 Plasma concentrations of dehydroepiandrosterone sulphate in the neonate and throughout childhood (μmol/l)

Age	Female	Male
Cord blood	0.4–7.6	0.6–6.9
1 day	0.5–10.7	1.0–13.5
1 month	0.1–1.2	0.2–2.6
1–6 months	0–0.3	0–0.8
5–12 months	0–0.3	0–0.3
1–5 years	0–0.3	0–0.3
6–8 years	0.1–0.6	0.1–0.6
8–10 years	0.3–1.6	0.2–2.8
10–12 years	0.8–3.2	0.9–3.8
12–14 years	1.0–5.0	1.3–4.0

Table 27.5 Plasma concentrations of testosterone and androstenedione (nmol/l) during childhood

Age	Androstenedione	Testosterone	
		Male	Female
Cord blood		4–14	0.5–2
7 days		0.5–1.5	<0.5
14 days to 3 months		4–10	<0.5
4 months to start of puberty	0.3–1.8	0.1–0.5	<0.5
Tanner stage 2		0.5–5*	<1
Tanner stage 3		3.5–11*	<1
Tanner stage 4	2–8‡	7–20†	<1.5

* Nocturnal peak levels, must take blood before 1000 h.
† Levels sustained throughout the day.
‡ Circadian rhythm 0800 h peak values.

the first year and at puberty. Androgen production during childhood is largely from the adrenal cortex [119].

11-Deoxycortisol (compound S) is usually determined by RIA and the plasma concentrations are normally 5–20 nmol/l [120]. HPLC has been useful in displaying excess 11-deoxycortisol in patients with CAH due to 11-hydroxylase defects, and in patients receiving metyrapone medically to suppress cortisol production by blocking 11-hydroxylase [121,122].

Aldosterone shows a circadian rhythm due to the transient influence of ACTH on aldosterone production. Plasma aldosterone concentrations are affected by posture, but this is less easy to control in children than adults. In childhood it is important to judge aldosterone levels in relation to the plasma renin activity. High plasma concentrations of aldosterone and plasma renin activity are seen in the newborn infant (see Fig. 26.7). Both decline over the first 3 years of life and adult values are reached at 3–5 years of age.

CATABOLISM AND EXCRETION OF STEROIDS

Steroids are inactivated before clearance from the body. Most of the steroid is excreted in the urine but some is lost through the intestinal tract. In general, steroid catabolism is reductive and occurs mainly in the liver. Enzymes act principally on the A ring and side-chain (Table 27.6). The 4-ene-3-keto configuration is reduced by the addition of four hydrogen atoms so that many steroid hormone metabolites are tetrahydro products (Table 27.7) of the systemic or trivially named hormones. Positional (α and β) isomers in combinations are possible. The 5β-reductases are microsomal while the 5α-reductases are soluble enzymes, but both use NADPH as a cofactor. 3α- and 3β-hydroxysteroid dehydrogenases are mainly liver enzymes with different substrate and cofactor requirements.

Table 27.6 Enzymes in steroid catabolism

Reduction of 4-ene-3-keto structure
5α-Reductase
5β-Reductase
3-Ketosteroid reductase
Reduction of 20-ketone
20α-Reductase
20β-Reductase
Oxidative formation of androgens
Side-chain cleavage
17-Ketosteroid reductase

Table 27.7 Principal metabolites of adrenal steroids

Circulating hormone	Principal conjugates of steroids in urine
Cortisol (F)	Tetrahydrocortisol (THF) 5α-THF (allo-THF) Cortol 11β-Hydroxyandrosterone 11β-Hydroxyaetiocholanolone
Cortisone (E)	Tetrahydrocortisone (THE) Cortolone
Corticosterone (B)	Tetrahydrocorticosterone (THB) 5α-THB
17-Hydroxyprogesterone	Pregnanetriol
11-Deoxycorticosterone (DOC)	Tetrahydrodeoxycorticosterone (THDOC)
11-Deoxycortisol (S)	Tetrahydrodeoxycortisol (THS)
Testosterone	Aetiocholanolone
Androsterone	Androsterone

Reductions at the 20-oxo group in the side-chain of cortisol are catalysed by 20β-OHS-DH and 20α-OHS-DH producing isomeric hydroxyls at C-20, of which the 20α predominates in humans. A tetrahydro-reduced steroid becomes a hexahydro-reduced steroid once further reduced at the C-20 position. Some of these steroids have trivial names (cortols and cortolones). Cortisol and cortisone are converted by side-chain cleavage to androgens.

The majority of steroid metabolites are excreted in the urine as sulphate and glucuronide conjugates formed mainly in the liver through transferase enzyme systems (phosphoadenosine phosphosulphate and uridine diphosphoglucuronic acid).

In newborn children a number of steroid hydroxylases (1β, 6α and 6β, 15β, 16α and 16β, 18) act on steroids, possibly to increase the polarity of the steroid for excretion [123,124]. The metabolites are extremely polar and difficult to extract from aqueous phase. These enzymes

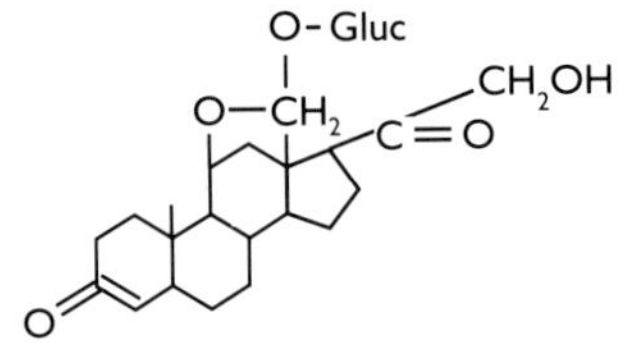

Fig. 27.8 Structure of 18-glucuronide conjugate of aldosterone (hemiacetal form).

become less active over the first year of life and, apart from the induction of some of the enzymes by drugs (notably the 6-hydroxylase by anticonvulsants), do not influence the metabolism of steroids outside the newborn period.

Aldosterone is catabolized in a fashion similar to cortisol with the formation of 3α,5β-tetrahydroaldosterone. A unique conjugate of aldosterone in urine occurs as a highly polar conjugate from which aldosterone can be liberated by hydrolysis at pH 1. The structure of the conjugate has been confirmed as the 18-glucuronide of aldosterone (Fig. 27.8) [125]. This metabolite is produced primarily by the kidney.

ADRENAL STEROIDS IN URINE

The measurements of steroid excretion rates in urine collected over 24 h are important integers of daily adrenal activity. The major problem with children is the reliable collection of the sample. Urine collection bags for babies are notoriously difficult to retain on an active newborn, although some paediatric departments have special cots, in which the baby lies on a porous nylon sheet which allows urine to pass through, with flow directed to a collection vessel (preferably cooled). In young children 24-h collections are possible under close supervision.

STEROID METABOLITES IN URINE

Free cortisol in the blood is filtered by the kidney and excreted in the urine. Once plasma-binding proteins have become saturated, the free cortisol excretion will increase in proportion to the increased production of the hormone. Free cortisol excretion is therefore a useful measure of excess cortisol production (Cushing syndrome) but not for adrenal insufficiency. There are a number of drugs which interfere with the determination [126]. The free cortisol in urine is usually measured by RIA, preferably after a solvent extraction which will not take up the many steroid conjugates from the urine. Antisera should be tested for their binding of metabolites since the latter are present in urine at much higher concentrations than cortisol itself.

Cortisol secretion rates need no longer be measured in children using radioactive tracer techniques. The use of stable isotopes for the purpose has proved more accurate, and the experiments can be conducted more physiologically [127]. Secretion rates are estimated to be around 6 mg/m^2, which are lower than previously reported from radioactive experiments. These new figures are closer to the combined excretion rates of all of the cortisol and cortisone metabolites, so that these excretion rates approximate the production rate of cortisol [128]. Assessment of cortisol metabolite excretion has been effectively used to assess the degree of cortisol excess in obese children and the extent of adrenal suppression in children with asthma taking inhaled steroids [129].

Pregnanetriol is the main urinary metabolite of 17α-hydroxyprogesterone in children and adults. This steroid is a poor marker for CAH due to 21-hydroxylase deficiency in a newborn infant. Using capillary column gas chromatography and mass spectrometry 17-hydroxypregnanolone and 15β,17-dihydroxypregnanolone are better neonatal markers for the disease [130–132].

The acid-labile conjugate of aldosterone (18-glucuronide) is a convenient index of aldosterone production. This conjugate is cleaved by acid at pH 1, whereas other glucuronides at C-3 and C-21 are not affected by this degree of acid exposure. After extraction of free steroids from urine and acid hydrolysis, a dichloromethane extract will contain only aldosterone liberated by the acid hydrolysis, and this can be measured by RIA. The excretion rate of aldosterone 18-glucuronide correlates with the sodium excretion rate (Fig. 27.9) [133]. Measurements of 3α,5β-tetrahydroaldosterone excretion have proved useful in paediatric studies, but require the specialized facilities of a research laboratory [134]. Free aldosterone and 18-hydroxycorticosterone can be determined using HPLC [135].

PROFILES OF URINE STEROIDS BY GAS CHROMATOGRAPHY AND MASS SPECTROMETRY

The term 'profile' is often used when examining temporal changes of hormone concentrations in a fluid under basal conditions or in response to stimuli. A profile of urinary steroids gives information about the mix of all steroid metabolites in urine. Capillary column gas chromatography is used for the separation of individual steroids. The column outlet can be either a non-specific flame ionization detector or a mass spectrometer, in which case the steroid in each peak can be identified by the resulting fingerprint of molecular weight and fragmentation pattern.

Steroid excretion rates in a 24-h urine collection give indices of daily hormone production. In addition to the excretion rates it is also useful to examine ratios of various groups of metabolites (for example α to β reduced met-

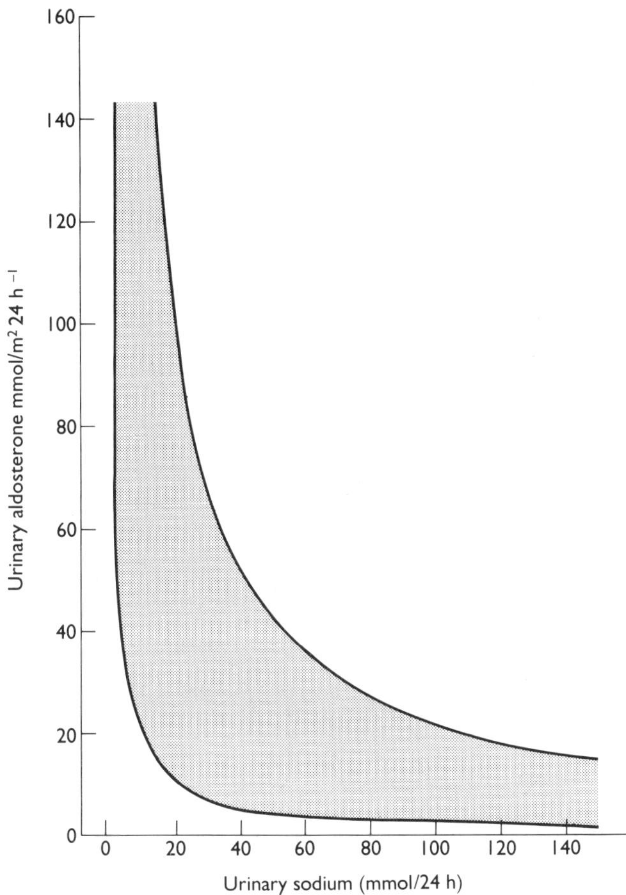

Fig. 27.9 Ranges for urine excretion rates of aldosterone 18-glucuronide in relation to sodium excretion.

abolites, and cortisol to cortisone). In general the urine steroid profile is an assessment of adrenal cortical function. Few drugs interfere with the assay (for example carbamazepine). Prednisone and prednisolone metabolites can be recognized from the mass spectra (two mass units less than the equivalent endogenous cortisone and cortisol metabolites). Cyproterone acetate and megesterol are two of the few steroid drugs used in clinical practice which give peaks in the analysis. Despite the range of steroids in use, few interfere with the analysis but synthetic steroids, such as beclomethasone used for the treatment of asthma, can lower steroid production and hence excretion rates [129]. The drawback of urine profile analysis is that several metabolites arise from each hormone.

The most important metabolites in a normal child are from cortisol and cortisone but only cortisone metabolites are seen up until about 4–6 months of age [136]. For the sum of excretion rates of cortisol and cortisone metabolites there is a close agreement of absolute steroid excretion (μg/day) with the body surface area. Steroid excretion when corrected for body size is constant throughout childhood from 2 to 16 years [128] and close to the value for steroid production calculated by stable isotopic techniques. These parameters have been useful when judging adrenal excess in an obese child, and in evaluating the effect of synthetic steroids in suppressing the hypothalamopituitary–adrenal axis [129] which may otherwise only be revealed by blood sampling throughout the night to demonstrate suppression of nocturnal cortisol pulses [137].

Androgen excretion rates are low for the first 7 years then rise 10–12-fold over the next 7 years to achieve adult excretion rates (Fig. 27.10). The increased androgen metabolites which appear in the urine reflect the increased production of DHEAS. 'Premature' adrenarche (recognized by early appearance of pubic hair) is a benign condition resulting from advanced adrenal growth with precocious differentiation of the zone reticularis. Androgen and cortisol metabolite excretion rates are marginally elevated for age and, to a lesser extent, for body size. The timing of this condition is often not premature; it is the appearance of the signs of androgen action which give rise to concern, chiefly because they may have a more sinister origin (e.g. adrenal carcinoma).

Congenital adrenal hyperplasia due to 21-hydroxylase deficiency is generally diagnosed reliably by measurements of 17-OHP in serum or blood spots. Assays for 17-OHP concentrations in the blood of newborn infants may not distinguish results from normal levels in the first 36 h but thereafter there are very much higher concentrations in affected cases. The assay should include a solvent extraction step, as discussed earlier. The urine steroid profile of a child with 21-hydroxylase deficiency is characteristic after the third day of life, although pregnanetriol is not a major metabolite. The diagnosis is made from the appearance of high concentrations of 17-hydroxypregnanolone and 15,17-dihydroxypregnanolone [130–132] and 16-hydroxypregnenolone [132]. Cortisol production may be normal, but at the expense of excess production of intermediates.

In the case of 11-hydroxylase deficiency there is an obvious excess of tetrahydo-11-deoxycortisol (THS) and 6-hydroxy-THS in a newborn. The 6-hydroxy steroid is not seen later on, and there are also hexahydro-S peaks seen [138]. Cortisol is not produced in 11-hydroxylase deficiency. Hypertension is frequently said to be a complication of CAH due to 11-hydroxylase deficiency, but this is not usually the case before puberty. The diagnosis may sometimes be confused with 21-hydroxylase deficiency due to the apparently high 17-hydroxyprogesterone concentrations. A steroid profile with mass spectrometric proof of the nature of all steroids detected is a definitive test [139].

The steroid products of virilizing adrenal tumours are sometimes from unusual steroids for which hormone assays are not widely available (11-hydroxyandrostenedione, pregnenolone) [140–142]. The commonest

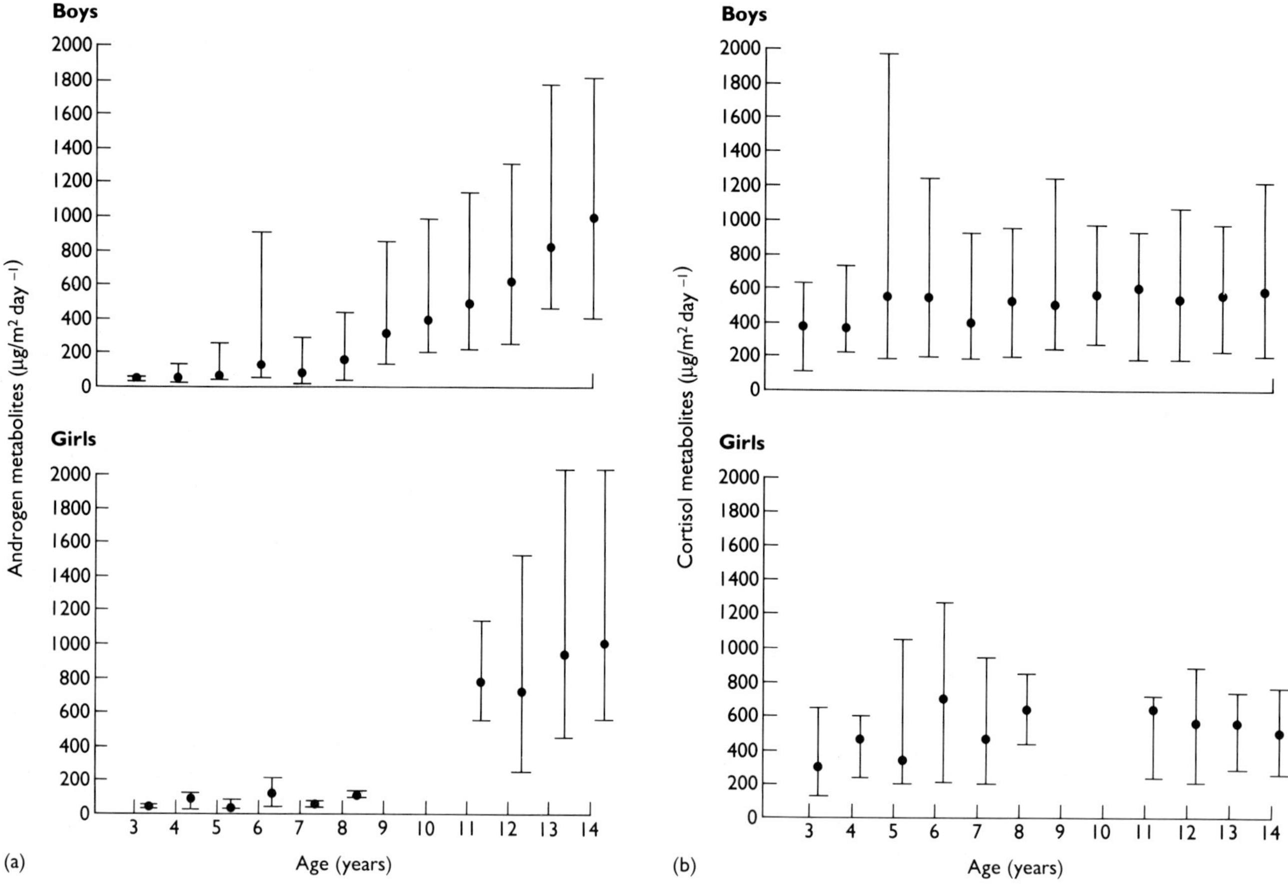

Fig. 27.10 Excretion rates for (a) androgen metabolites and (b) cortisol metabolites during childhood.

adrenal tumour encountered in children secretes DHEA(S), but since this is a weak androgen the tumours may get quite large before there are clinical signs from the high androgen production. Tumours secreting more potent androgens may present with a rapid clinical history, and scanning techniques may be necessary to detect small tumours.

In salt-losing states of infancy, urinary steroid profiles will reveal excess excretion of metabolites from corticosterone, 18-hydroxycorticosterone and aldosterone metabolites. The relative amounts of each can reveal information about the site of a metabolic block in aldosterone production. This is difficult when the child is treated, but when salt loss leads to high plasma renin activity, the urinary steroid profiles display the excess mineralocorticoid metabolites [143].

Severe hypertension in children is usually the result of renal disease. A rare defect in cortisol metabolism (a defect of 11-hydroxysteroid dehydrogenase which is involved in the oxidation of cortisol to cortisone) may prevent equilibrium of cortisol [144]. It is thought that this enzyme normally protects the kidney against the action of cortisol by the oxidation of the steroid [145]. If the enzyme is ineffective, cortisol acts at the mineralocorticoid receptor and aldosterone and renin will be low, which is a picture of apparent mineralocorticoid excess (hence the acronym AME). The hypertension may be severe, but the benefit of early diagnosis is that the response to spironolactone is rapid and impressive. The urinary steroid profile shows a low excretion of cortisone relative to cortisol metabolites (Fig. 27.11) [144,146].

Urinary steroid analysis is helpful if a female infant (46,XX) is born with ambiguous genitalia (congenital adrenal hyperplasia). If a 46,XY infant has an ambiguous phenotype, the urinary steroid profile is not usually helpful. 17-Hydroxylase deficiency may be detected [147]. Defects of androgen production, such as 5α-reductase deficiency, can be revealed from the ratio of reduced metabolites of cortisol when there are no adrenal or gonadal androgens in the urine. In the newborn period only cortisone metabolites are seen, and there is no suitable pair of α- and β-reduced products to look at. The analysis is, however, useful in older patients with 5α-reductase deficiency [148,149]. Cortisol metabolites can

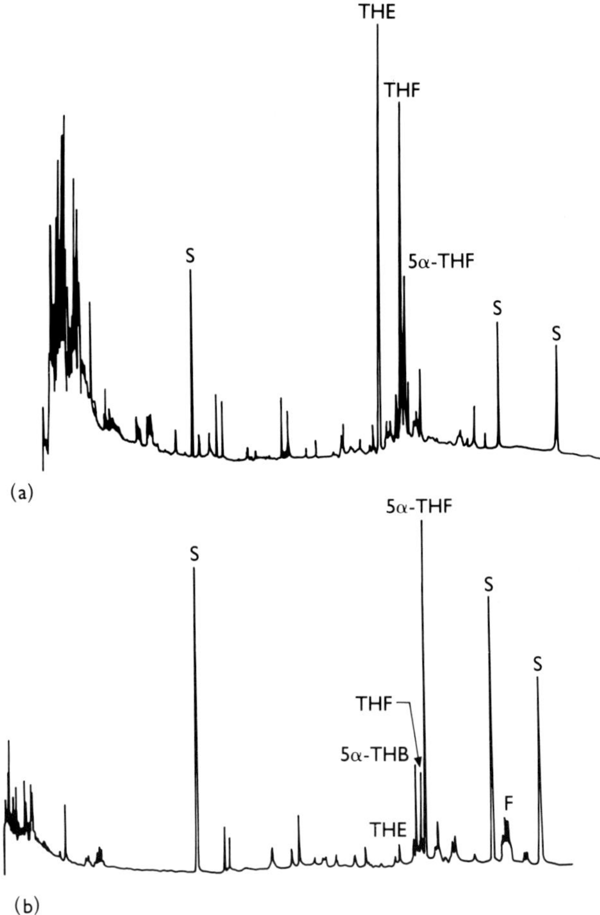

Fig. 27.11 Steroid profile analysis from GC separation of urine steroids: (a) normal child, and (b) child with defect on conversion of cortisol to cortisone – 11β-hydroxysteroid dehydrogenase defect or AME syndrome of apparent mineralocorticoid excess. For abbreviations, see Table 27.7.

be examined from 6 months of age. 5α-Reductase deficiency is often suspected only at puberty when testosterone production affects the clitoris as well as muscle and hair growth in a more masculine manner. Androgen and cortisol metabolites then show low ratios of 5α to 5β products.

STIMULATION AND SUPPRESSION TESTS

The ACTH test has frequently been used to diagnose abnormalities of steroid biosynthesis which are not necessarily apparent under basal conditions. Data for the response of several steroids to ACTH in childhood have been produced, and are a good reference point to which any new assay could be compared for performance [112,113]. When measuring low levels of steroids in samples from children, it is not always possible to use an assay used in the laboratory for adults. Particularly when using radioactive-iodine labels, there can be a positive bias to results at low level if the assay does not reach equilibrium [109]. There are also differences in the concentrations of binding proteins in the blood of children from the levels seen in adults, which must be considered.

The ACTH test is usually conducted with an injection of 250 μg of ACTH 1–24 (Syacthen), but 500 ng/m^2 of body surface area is a maximal stimulus [150]. In the future, lower-dose tests may be more helpful in resolving endocrine problems than the response to a huge and unphysiological dose.

Hypothalamopituitary function is sometimes tested by insulin-induced hypoglycaemia. This should be undertaken only with medical supervision. Glucose (10% solution) and hydrocortisone should be ready in the event of an emergency, but must be used with care since hyperglycaemia can be an additional problem [151]. Insulin injected at 0.15 U/kg body weight is sufficient to produce hypoglycaemia in normal children. If the patient is suspected to have adrenal insufficiency, the dose should be reduced to 0.1 U/kg. A number of disturbing symptoms are experienced by the patient (sweating, tremor, disorientation and occasionally coma). Blood glucose should be tested with stick tests at regular intervals during the procedure and the blood glucose should be brought back to normal after 30 min. Less than 5 g of glucose is usually all that is necessary to achieve this aim in a child, so that a sweet drink will usually be sufficient. Glucose (10%) can be given at 0.7 ml/kg min^{-1} over 3 min, then at 0.1 ml/kg min^{-1} until blood glucose is kept at 5–8 mmol/l.

Dexamethasone suppression tests may be useful in children with possible Cushing syndrome and autonomous steroid-secreting tumour. The overnight low dose test can be 0.3 mg/m^2 [152].

ROLES OF BIOCHEMISTRY AND MOLECULAR BIOLOGY

The sequence of all the genes in steroid biosynthesis has been elucidated by molecular biology, although the regulation of the genes is still not clear. Using linkage analysis [153] and gene amplification techniques, a prenatal diagnosis of congenital adrenal hyperplasia can be offered to families with an affected child [154]. Virilization of the female genitalia can be prevented in subsequently affected infants if the fetal adrenal function is suppressed from as early in gestation as possible [155]. Biochemical techniques are still essential for the first diagnosis of the index case.

REFERENCES

1 Benner MC. Studies on the involution of the fetal cortex of the adrenal glands. *Am J Pathol* 1940;16:787–98.
2 Lanman JT. The fetal zone of the adrenal gland. Its devel-

opmental course, comparative anatomy, and possible physiologic functions. *Medicine* 1953;32:389–430.
3 Johannisson E. Aspects of the ultrastructure and function of the human fetal adrenal cortex. *Contr Gynecol Obstet* 1979;5:109–30.
4 De Peretti E, Forest MG. Patterns of plasma dehydroepiandrosterone sulfate levels in humans from birth to adulthood: evidence for testicular production. *J Clin Endocrinol Metab* 1978;47:572–7.
5 Wallace AM, Beesley J, Thomson M, Giles CA, Ross AM, Taylor NF. Adrenal status during the first month of life in mature and immature infants. *J Endocrinol* 1987;112: 473–80.
6 Midgley P, Oates N, Shaw JCL, Honour JW. Virilisation of preterm infants. *Arch Dis Child* 1990;27:338–44.
7 Honour JW, Wickramaratne K, Valman HB. Adrenal function in preterm infants. *Biol Neonate* 1992;61:214–21.
8 McNulty WP, Novy MJ, Walsh SW. Fetal and postnatal development of adrenal glands in *Macaca mulatta*. *Biol Reprod* 1981;25:1079–89.
9 Dobbie JW, Symington T. The human adrenal gland with special reference to the vasculature. *J Endocrinol* 1966;34: 479–89.
10 Hinson JP, Vinson GP, Whitehouse BJ. The relationship between perfusion medium flow rate and steroid secretion in the isolated perfused rat adrenal gland *in situ*. *J Endocrinol* 1986;111:391–6.
11 Edelman IS. Mechanism of action of steroid hormones. *J Steroid Biochem* 1975;6:147–59.
12 Duval D, Durant S, Homo-Delarche F. Non-genomic effects of steroids. Interactions of steroid molecules with membrane structures and functions. *Biochim Biophys Acta* 1983; 737:409–42.
13 Reiter EO, Fuldauer VG, Root AW. Secretion of the adrenal androgen, dehydroepiandrosterone sulfate during normal infancy, childhood and adolescence, in sick infants and in children with endocrinologic abnormalities. *J Pediatr* 1977; 90:766–70.
14 Diczfalusy E. Steroid metabolism in the human foetoplacental unit. *Acta Endocrinol (Copenh)* 1969;61:649–64.
15 Jaffe RB, Seron-Ferre M, Crickard K, Koritnik D, Mitchell BF, Huhtaniemi IT. Regulation and function of the primate fetal adrenal gland and gonad. *Rec Prog Horm Res* 1981; 37:41–103.
16 Fujeida K, Faiman C, Reyes FI, Winter JSD. The control of steroidogenesis by human fetal adrenal cells in tissue culture. I. Responses to adrenocorticotropin. *J Clin Endocrinol Metab* 1981;53:34–8.
17 Hirato K, Yanaihara T, Nakayama T. A study of Δ^5-3-hydroxysteroid dehydrogenase in human foetal adrenal glands. *Acta Endocrinol* 1982;99:122–8.
18 Voutilainen R, Miller WL. Developmental expression of genes for the steroidogenic enzymes P450scc (20,22-desmolase), P450c17 (17α-hydroxylase/17,20-lyase), and P450c21 (21-hydroxylase) in the human fetus. *J Clin Endocrinol Metab* 1986;63:1145–50.
19 Hall CStG, Branchaud C, Klein GP *et al.* Secretion rate and metabolism of the sulfates of cortisol and corticosterone in newborn infants. *J Clin Endocrinol* 1971;33:98–104.
20 Liggins GC. Adrenocortical-related maturational events in the fetus. *Am J Obstet Gynecol* 1976;126:931–41.
21 Pasqualini JR, Sumida C. Receptors and mechanism of action of steroid hormones in the foetal compartment. In: Pal SB, ed. *Hormones in Normal and Abnormal Human Tissues*. Berlin: Walter de Gruyter, 1981:251–80.
22 Murphy BEP. Ontogeny of cortisol–cortisone interconversion in human tissues: a role for cortisone in human fetal development. *J Steroid Biochem* 1981;14:811–17.
23 Borkowski A, Delcroix C, Levin S. Metabolism of adrenal cholesterol in man. I. *In vitro* studies. *J Clin Invest* 1972; 51:1664–79.
24 Borkowski A, Delcroix C, Levin S. Metabolism of adrenal cholesterol in man. II. *In vitro* studies. *J Clin Invest* 1972; 51:1679–87.
25 Brown MS, Kovanen PT, Goldstein JL. Receptor-mediated uptake of lipoprotein in cholesterol and its utilisation for steroid synthesis in the adrenal cortex. *Rec Prog Horm Res* 1979;35:215–57.
26 Carr BR, Simpson ER. Cholesterol synthesis by human fetal hepatocytes: effect of lipoproteins. *Am J Obstet Gynecol* 1984;150:551–7.
27 Boggaram V, Funkenstein B, Waterman NR, Simpson ER. Lipoproteins and the regulation of adrenal steroidogenesis. *Endocr Res* 1985;10:387–409.
28 Simpson ER, Boggaram V, Funkenstein B, Waterman MR. Lipids in the regulation of hormone-responsive cells. *Biochem Soc Trans* 1985;13:55–7.
29 Hall PF. Cellular organization for steroidogenesis. *Int Rev Cytol* 1983;86:53–95.
30 Chung B-C, Picado-Leonard J, Haniu M *et al.* Cytochrome P450c17 (steroid 17α-hydroxylase/17,20 lyase): cloning of human adrenal and testis cDNAs indicates the same gene is expressed in both tissues. *Proc Natl Acad Sci USA* 1987; 84:407–11.
31 Zuber MX, John ME, Okamura T, Simpson ER, Waterman MR. Bovine adrenocortical cytochrome P-$450_{17\alpha}$. Regulation of gene expression by ACTH and elucidation of primary sequence. *J Biol Chem* 1986;261:2475–82.
32 Aupetit B, Accarie C, Emeric N, Vonarx V, Legrand J-C. The final step of aldosterone biosynthesis requires reducing power, it is not a dehydrogenation. *Biochim Biophys Acta* 1983;752:73–8.
33 Ulick S. Diagnosis and nomenclature of the disorders of the terminal portion of the aldosterone biosynthetic pathway. *J Clin Endocrinol Metab* 1976;43:92–6.
34 Marusic ET, White A, Aedo AR. Oxidative reactions in the formation of an aldehyde group in the biosynthesis of aldosterone. *Arch Biochem Biophys* 1973;157:320–1.
35 Mornet E, Dupont J, Vitek A, White PC. Characterisation of two genes encoding human steroid 11β-hydroxylase (P$450_{11\beta}$). *J Biol Chem* 1989;264:20961–7.
36 Chung B-C, Matteson KJ, Voutilainen R, Mohandas TK, Miller WL. Human cholesterol side-chain cleavage enzyme, P450scc: cDNA cloning, assignment of the gene to chromosome 15, and expression in the placenta. *Proc Natl Acad Sci USA* 1986;83:8962–6.
37 Morohashi K-I, Sogaya K, Omura T, Fujii-Kuriyama Y. Gene structure of human cytochrome P-450 (SCC) cholesterol desmolase. *Biochem J* 1987;101:879–87.
38 Lachance Y, Luu-The V, Verreault H *et al.* Structure of the human type II 3β-hydroxysteroid dehydrogenase/5-4 isomerase (3β-HSD) gene: adrenal and gonadal specificity. *DNA Cell Biol* 1991;10:701–11.
39 Sparkes RS, Klisak I, Miller WL. Regional mapping of genes encoding human steroidogenic enzymes: P450scc to 15q23–q24; adrenodoxin to 11q22; adrenodoxin reductase to 17q24–q25; and P450c17 to 10q24–q25. *DNA Cell Biol* 1991;10:359–65.

40 Bradshaw KD, Waterman MR, Couch RT, Simpson ER, Zuber MX. Characterisation of complementary deoxyribonucleic acid for human adrencortical 17α-hydroxylase: a probe for analysis of 17α-hydroxylase deiciency. *Mol Endocrinol* 1987;1:348–53.

41 Levine LS, Zachmann M, New MI *et al.* Genetic mapping of the 21-hydroxylase-deficiency gene within the HLA linkage group. *N Engl J Med* 1978;299:911–15.

42 Higashi Y, Yoshioka H, Yamane M, Gotoh O, Fujii-Kuriyama Y. Complete nucleotide sequence of two steroid 21-hydroxylase genes tandomly arranged in human chromosome: a pseudogene and a genuine gene. *Proc Natl Acad Sci USA* 1986;81:2841–5.

43 White PC, New MI, Dupont B. Structure of human steroid 21-hydroxylase genes. *Proc Natl Acad Sci USA* 1986;83: 5111–15.

44 Morel Y, Bristow J, Gitelman SE, Miller WL. Transcript encoded on the opposite strand of the human steroid 21-hydroxylase/complement component C4 gene locus. *Proc Natl Acad Sci USA* 1989;86:6582–6.

45 Miller WL, Gitelman SE, Bristow J, Morel Y. Analysis of the duplicated human C4/P450c21/X gene cluster. *J Steroid Biochem* 1992;8:961–71.

46 Lifton RP, Dluhy RG, Powers M *et al.* Hereditary hypertension caused by chimaeric gene duplications and ectopic expression of aldosterone synthase. *Nature Genet* 1992; 2:66–74.

47 Kawamoto T, Mitsuuchi Y, Toda K *et al.* Role of steroid 11β-hydroxylase and steroid 18-hydroxylase in the biosynthesis of glucocorticoids and mineralocorticoids in humans. *Proc Natl Acad Sci USA* 1992;89:1458–92.

48 Curnow KM, Tusie-Luna M-T, Pascoe L *et al.* The product of the CYP11B2 gene is required for aldosterone biosynthesis in the human adrenal cortex. *Mol Endocrinol* 1991;5:1513–22.

49 Wallace WHB, Crowne EC, Shalet SM *et al.* Episodic ACTH and cortisol secretion in normal children. *Clin Endocrinol* 1991;34:215–21.

50 Vale W, Spiess J, Rivier C, Rivier J. Characterization of a 41-residue ovine hypothalamic peptide that stimulates secretion of corticotropin and β-endorphin. *Science* 1981;213: 1394–7.

51 Beckford U, Holmes MC, Gillham B, Jones MT. Biphasic inhibition of bioactive hypothalamic corticotrophin releasing factor secretion in vitro by corticosterone and prevention of the second phase by various steroids. *J Endocrinol* 1983;97:339–46.

52 Mahmoud SN, Scaccianoce S, Scraggs PR, Nicholson SA, Gillham B, Jones MT. Characteristics of corticosteroid inhibition of adrenocorticotrophin release from the anterior pituitary of the rat. *J Endocrinol* 1984;102:33–42.

53 Hall PF. Trophic stimulation of steroidogenesis: in search of the elusive trigger. *Rec Prog Horm Res* 1985;41:1–39.

54 John ME, Simpson ER, Boggaram V, Waterman MR. Molecular cloning of steroid hydroxylases. *Endocr Res* 1985;10: 319–33.

55 Zuber MX, Simpson ER, Hall PF, Waterman MR. Effects of adrenocorticotropin on 17α-hydroxylase activity and cytochrome P-$450_{17\alpha}$ synthesis in bovine adrenocortical cells. *J Biol Chem* 1985;260:1842–8.

56 Onishi S, Miyazawa G, Nishimura Y *et al.* Postnatal development of circadian rhythm in serum cortisol levels in children. *Pediatrics* 1983;72:399–404.

57 Korth-Schutz S, Levine LS, New MI. Dehydroepiandrosterone sulfate (DS) levels – a rapid test of abnormal adrenal androgen secretion. *J Clin Endocrinol Metab* 1976;42: 1005–13.

58 Nieschlag E, Loriaux DL, Ruder HJ, Zucker IR, Kirschner MA, Lipsett MB. The secretion of dehydroepiandrosterone and dehydroepiandrosterone sulphate in man. *J Endocrinol* 1973;57:123–34.

59 Kreitzer PM, Blethen SL, Festa RS, Chasalow FI. Dehydroepiandrosterone sulfate levels are not suppressible by glucocorticoids before adrenarche. *J Clin Endocrinol Metab* 1989;69:1309–11.

60 James VHT, Tunbridge D, Wilson GA *et al.* Central control of steroid hormone secretion. *J Steroid Biochem* 1978; 9:429–36.

61 Rosenfeld RS, Hellman L, Roffwarg H, Weitzman ED, Fukushima DK, Gallagher TF. Dehydroisoandrosterone is secreted episodically and synchronously with cortisol by normal man. *J Clin Endocrinol* 1971;33:87–92.

62 Albright F, Smith PH, Fraser R. A syndrome characterised by primary ovarian insufficiency and decreased stature. Report of 11 cases with a digression on hormonal control of axillary and pubic hair. *Am J Med Sci* 1942;204:625–48.

63 Carter JN, Tyson JE, Warne GL, McNeilly AS, Faiman C, Eriesen HG. Adrenocortical function in hyperprolactinemic women. *J Clin Endocrinol Metab* 1977;45:973–80.

64 Vermeulen A, Suy E, Rubens R. Effects of prolactin on plasma DHEA(S) levels. *J Clin Endocrinol Metab* 1977; 44:1222–7.

65 Parker LN, Odell WD. Evidence for existence of cortical-androgen stimulating hormone. *Am J Physiol* 1979;236: 616–20.

66 Warne GL, Carter JN, Faiman C, Ryes FI, Winter JSD. Hormonal changes in girls with precocious adrenarche; a possible role for estradiol or prolactin. *J Pediatr* 1978;92: 743–7.

67 Sklar CA, Kaplan SL, Grumbach MM. Evidence for dissociation between adrenarche and gonadarche: studies in patients with idiopathic precocious puberty, gonadal dysgenesis, isolated gonadotrophin. *J Clin Endocrinol Metab* 1980;51: 548–56.

68 Chester Jones I. Variation in the mouse adrenal cortex with special reference to the zona reticularis and to brown degeneration, together with a discussion of the 'cell migration' theory. *Q J Microsc Sci* 1948;89:53–74.

69 Crowder RE. The development of the adrenal gland in man, with special reference to origin and ultimate location of cell types and evidence in favor of the 'cell migration' theory. *Carnegie Contrib Embryol* 1957;251:195–210.

70 Zajicek G, Ariel I, Arber N. The streaming adrenal cortex: direct evidence of centripetal migration of adrenocytes by estimation of cell turnover rate. *J Endocrinol* 1986;111: 477–82.

71 Cutler GB Jr, Davis SE, Johnsonbaugh RE, Loriaux DL. Dissociation of cortisol and adrenal androgen secretion in patients with secondary adrenal insufficiency. *J Clin Endocrinol Metab* 1979;49:604–9.

72 Anderson DC. The adrenal androgen-stimulating hormone does not exist. *Lancet* 1980;2:454–6.

73 Wierman ME, Beardsworth DE, Crawford JD *et al.* Adrenarche and skeletal maturation during luteinizing hormone releasing hormone analogue suppression of gonadarche. *J Clin Invest* 1986;77:121–6.

74 Mellon SH, Shiveley JE, Miller WL. Human pro-opiiomelanocortin-(79–96), a proposed androgen stimulatory hormone, does not affect steroidogenesis in cultured human

fetal adrenal cells. *J Clin Endocrinol Metab* 1991;72:19–22.

75 Penhoat A, Sanchez P, Jaillard C, Langlois D, Begeot M, Saez JM. Human proopiomelanocortin-(79–96), a proposed cortical androgen-stimulating hormone, does not affect steroidogenesis in cultured human adult adrenal cells. *J Clin Endocrinol Metab* 1991;72:23–26.

76 Byrne GC, Perry YS, Winter JSD. Steroid inhibitory effects upon human adrenal 3β-hydroxysteroid dehydrogenase activity. *J Clin Endocrinol Metab* 1986;62:413–18.

77 Byrne GC, Perry YS, Winter JSD. Kinetic analysis of adrenal 3β-hydroxysteroid dehydrogenase activity during human development. *J Clin Endocrinol Metab* 1985;60:934–9.

78 Couch RM, Muller J, Winter JSD. Regulation of the activities of 17-hydroxylase and 17,20-desmolase in the human adrenal cortex: kinetic analysis and inhibition by endogenous steroids. *J Clin Endocrinol Metab* 1986;63:613–18.

79 Hornsby PJ. Regulation of 21-hydroxylase activity by steroids in cultured bovine adrenocortical cells: possible significance for adrenocortical androgen synthesis. *Endocrinology* 1982;111:1092–101.

80 Dickerman Z, Grant DR, Faiman C, Winter JSD. Intra-adrenal steroid concentrations in man: zonal differences and developmental changes. *J Clin Endocrinol Metab* 1984; 59:1031–6.

81 Kelnar CJH, Brook CGD. A mixed longitudinal study of adrenal steroid excretion in childhood and the mechanism of adrenarche. *Clin Endocrinol* 1983;19:117–29.

82 McKenna TJ, Island DP, Nicholsen WE *et al.* ACTH stimulates late steps in aldosterone biosynthesis. *Acta Endocrinol (Copenh)* 1979;90:122–32.

83 Carey RM, Sen S. Recent progress in the control of aldosterone secretion. *Rec Prog Horm Res* 1986;42:251–96.

84 McKenna TJ, Island DP, Nicholsen WE *et al.* The effects of potassium on early and late steps in aldosterone biosynthesis in cells of the zona glomerulosa. *Endocrinology* 1978;103: 1411–16.

85 Müller J, Hofstetter L, Schwendener-Canlas P, Brunner DB, Lund E-G. Role of the renin–angiotensin system in the regulation of late steps in aldosterone biosynthesis by sodium intake of potassium-deficient rats. *Endocrinology* 1984; 115:350–6

86 Kramer RE, Gallant S, Brownie AC. The role of cytochrome P-450 in the action of sodium depletion on aldosterone biosynthesis in rats. *J Biol Chem* 1979;254:3953–8.

87 Kramer RK, Gallant S, Brownie AC. Actions of angiotensin II on aldosterone biosynthesis on the rat adrenal cortex; effects of cytochrome P-450 enzymes on the early and late pathway. *J Biol Chem* 1980;255:3442–7.

88 Johnson JA, Davis JO, Witty RT. Effects of catecholamines and renal nerve stimulation on renin release in the non-filtering kidney. *Circul Res* 1971;29:646–53.

89 McKenna TJ, Island DP, Nicholsen *et al.* Dopamine inhibits angiotensin stimulated aldosterone biosynthesis in bovine adrenal cells. *J Clin Invest* 1979;64:287–91.

90 Racz K, Wolf I, Kiss R *et al.* Corticosteroidogenesis by isolated human adrenal cells. Effects of serotonin and serotonin antagonists. *Experientia* 1979;35:1532–4.

91 Sowers JR, Berg G, Tuck ML, Martin VI, Chandler DW, Mayes DM. Dopaminergic modulation of 18-hydroxycorticosterone secretion in man. *J Clin Endocrinol Metab* 1982; 54:523–7.

92 Sulyok E, Ertl T, Varga L, Bodis J, Csaba IF. The effect of metoclopramide administration on electrolyte status and activity of renin-angiotensin-aldosterone system in premature infants. *Paediatr Res* 1985;19:912–15.

93 Oberfield SE, Levine LS, Firpo A *et al.* Primary hyperaldosteronism in childhood due to unilateral macronodular hyperplasia. Case report. *Hypertension* 1984;6:75–84.

94 Dillon MJ, Gillin MEA, Ryness JM, de Swiet M. Plasma renin activity and aldosterone concentration in the human newborn. *Arch Dis Child* 1976;51:537–40.

95 Fiselier T, Lijnen P, Monnens L, Van Munster P, Jansen M, Peer P. Levels of renin, angiotensin I and II, angiotensin converting enzyme and aldosterone in infancy and childhood. *Eur J Pediatr* 1983;141:3–7.

96 Hayduk K, Krause DK, Huenges R, Unbehaun V. Plasma renin concentration at delivery and during the newborn period in humans. *Experientia* 1972;28:1489–90.

97 Sassard J, Sann L, Vincent M, Francois R, Cier JF. Plasma renin activity in normal subjects from infancy to puberty. *J Clin Endocrinol Metab* 1975;40:524–5.

98 Blazy I, Dechaux M, Guillot F *et al.* Inactive renin in infants and children: evidence for its physiological response to orthostasis in children. *J Clin Endocrinol Metab* 1984; 59:321–7.

99 Al-Dahhan J, Haycock GB, Chantler C, Stimmler L. Sodium homeostasis in term and preterm neonates. I. Renal aspects. *Arch Dis Child* 1983;58:335–42.

100 Honour JW, Valman HB, Shackleton CHL. Aldosterone and sodium homeostasis in preterm infants. *Acta Paed Scand* 1977;66:103–9.

101 Rees L, Brook CGD, Shaw JCL, Forsling ML. Hyponatraemia in the first week of life in preterm infants. Part I. Arginine vasopressin secretion. *Arch Dis Child* 1984;59:414–22.

102 Rees L, Shaw JCL, Brook CGD, Forsling ML. Hyponatraemia in the first week of life in preterm infants. Part II. Sodium and water balance. *Arch Dis Child* 1984;59:423–9.

103 Atlas SA, Laragh JH. Atrial natriuretic peptide: a new factor in hormonal control of blood pressure and electrolyte homeostasis. *Ann Rev Med* 1986;37:397–414.

104 Anderson JV, Struthers AD, Payne NN, Slater JDH, Bloom SR. Atrial natriuretic peptide inhibits the aldosterone response to angiotensin II in man. *Clin Sci* 1986;70:507–12.

105 Roitman A, Bruchis S, Bauman B, Kaufman H, Laron Z. Total deficiency of corticosteroid-binding globulin. *Clin Endocrinol* 1984;21:541–8.

106 Hofreiter BT, Mizera AC, Allen JP, Masi AM, Hicok WC. Solid-state extraction of cortisol from plasma or serum for liquid chromatography. *Clin Chem* 1983;29:1808–9.

107 Wei J-Q, Wei J-L, Zhou X-T, Cheng J-P. Isocratic reversed phase high performance liquid chromatography determination of twelve natural corticosteroids in serum with on-line ultraviolet and fluorescence detection. *Biomed Chromatogr* 1990;4:161–4.

108 Shimada K, Tanaka M, Nambara T. Studies on steroids. CC. Determination of 17-ketosteroid sulphates in serum by high-performance liquid chromatography with electrochemical detection using pre-column derivatization. *J Chromatogr* 1984;307:23–8.

109 Honour JW, Rumsby G. Problems in diagnosis and management of congenital adrenal hyperplasia. *J Steroid Biochem Mol Biol* 1993;45:69–74.

110 Sippell WG, Becker H, Versmold HT, Bidlingmaier F, Knorr D. Longitudinal studies of plasma aldosterone, corticosterone, deoxycorticosterone, progesterone, 17-hydroxyprogesterone, cortisol, and cortisone determined simultaneously in mother and child at birth and during the early neonatal period. I. Spontaneous delivery. *J Clin Endocrinol*

Metab 1978;46:971–84.
111 Schöneshöfer M, Fenner A, Bulce HJ. Assessment of eleven adrenal steroids from a single serum sample by combination of automatic high-performance liquid chromatography and radioimmunoassay (HPLC-RIA). *J Steroid Biochem* 1981; 14:377–86.
112 Lashansky G, Saenger P, Fishman K *et al.* Normative data for adrenal steroidogenesis in a healthy pediatric population: age- and sex-related changes after adrenocorticotropic stimulation. *J Clin Endocrinol Metab* 1991;73:674–86.
113 Lashansky G, Saenger P, DiMartino-Nardi J *et al.* Normative data for the steroidogenic response of mineralocorticoids and their precursors to adrenocorticotropin in a healthy pediatric population. *J Clin Endocrinol Metab* 1992;75:1491–6.
114 Wallace AM, Beastall GH, Cook B *et al.* Neonatal screening for congenital adrenal hyperplasia: a programme based on a novel direct radioimmunoassay for 17-hydroxyprogesterone in blood spots. *J Endocrinol* 1986;108:299–308.
115 Walker RF, Read GF, Hughes IA *et al.* Radioimmunoassay of 17α-hydroxyprogesterone in saliva, parotid fluid and plasma of congenital adrenal hyperplasia patients. *Clin Chem* 1979; 25:542–5.
116 Wong T, Shackleton CHL, Covey TR, Ellis G. Identification of the steroids in neonatal plasma that interfere with 17α-hydroxyprogesterone radioimmunoassays. *Clin Chem* 1992;38:1830–7.
117 Turnipseed MR, Bentley K, Reynolds JW. Serum dehydroepiandrosterone sulfate in premature infants and infants with intrauterine growth retardation. *J Clin Endocrinol Metab* 1976;43:1219–25.
118 Grueters A, Korth-Schutz S. Longitudinal study of plasma dehydroepiandrosterone sulfate in preterm and fullterm infants. *J Clin Endocrinol Metab* 1982;55:314–20.
119 Bidlingmaier F, Dörr HG, Eisenmenger W, Kuhnle U, Knorr D. Contribution of the adrenal gland to the production of androstenedione and testosterone during the first two years of life. *J Clin Endocrinol Metab* 1986;62:331–4.
120 Perry LA, Al-Dujaili EAS, Edwards CRW. A direct radioimmunoassay for 11-deoxycortisol. *Steroids* 1982;39:115–28.
121 Reardon GE, Caldarella AM, Canalis E. Determination of serum cortisol and 11-deoxycortisol by liquid chromatography. *Clin Chem* 1979;25:122–6.
122 Canalis E, Caldarella AM, Reardon GE. Serum cortisol and 11-deoxycortisol by liquid chromatography. Clinical studies and comparison with radioimmunoassay. *Clin Chem* 1979; 25:1700–3.
123 Derks HJG, Drayer NM. The identification and quantification of three new 6-hydroxylated corticosteroids in human neonatal urine. *Steroids* 1978;31:289–305.
124 Taylor NF, Curnow DE, Shackleton CHL. Analysis of glucocorticoid metabolites in the neonatal period: catabolism of cortisone acetate by an infant with 21-hydroxylase deficiency. *Clin Chim Acta* 1978;85:219–29.
125 Carpenter PC, Mattox VR. Isolation determination of structure and synthesis of the acid-labile conjugate of aldosterone. *Biochem J* 1976;157:1–14.
126 Schöneshöfer M, Fenner A, Dulce HJ. Interferences in the radioimmunological determination of urinary free cortisol. *Clin Chim Acta* 1980;101:125–34.
127 Estaban NV, Loughlin T, Yergey AL *et al.* Daily cortisol production rate in man determined by stable isotope dilution/mass spectrometry. *J Clin Endocrinol Metab* 1991;71:39–45.
128 Honour JW, Kelnar CJH, Brook CGD. Urine steroid excretion in childhood reflect growth and activity of the adrenal cortex. *Acta Endocrinol (Copenh)* 1991;124:219–24.
129 Priftis K, Milner AD, Conway E, Honour JW. Adrenal function in asthma. *Arch Dis Child* 1990;65:838–40.
130 Joannou GE. Identification of 15β-hydroxylated C_{21} steroids in the neo-natal period: the role of 3α,15β,17α-trihydroxy-5β-pregnan-20-one in the perinatal diagnosis of congenital adrenal hyperplasia (CAH) due to a 21-hydroxylase deficiency. *J Steroid Biochem* 1981;14:901–12.
131 Honour J. Biochemical aspects of congenital adrenal hyperplasia. *J Inher Metab Dis* 1986;9(Suppl. 1):124–34.
132 Homoki J, Teller WM. Increased urinary excretion of total 16α-hydroxypregnenolone in newborn infants with congenital adrenal hyperplasia due to 21-hydroxylase deficiency. *Klin Wochenschr* 1982;60:407–10.
133 New MI, Baum CJ, Levine LS. Nomograms relating aldosterone excretion to urinary sodium and potassium in a pediatric population and their application to the study of childhood hypertension. *Am J Cardiol* 1976;37:658–66.
134 Honour JW, Shackleton CHL. Mass spectrometric method for tetrahydroaldosterone. *J Steroid Biochem* 1977;8:299–305.
135 Schöneshöfer M, Weber B, Dulce HJ, Belkien L. Estimation of free urinary aldosterone and 18-hydroxycorticosterone by a combination of automatic high-performance liquid chromatography and radioimmunoassay. *J Chromatogr* 1982; 227:492–6.
136 Shackleton CHL, Gustafsson J-A, Mitchell FL. Steroids in newborns and infants. The changing pattern of urinary steroid excretion during infancy. *Acta Endocrinol* 1973;74:157–67.
137 Law CM, Marchant JL, Honour JW, Preece MA, Warner JO. Nocturnal adrenal suppression in asthmatic children taking inhaled beclomethasone dipropionate. *Lancet* 1986;1:942–4.
138 Hughes IA, Arisaka O, Perry LA, Honour JW. Early diagnosis of 11β-hydroxylase deficiency in two siblings confirmed by analysis of a novel steroid metabolite in newborn urine. *Acta Endocrinol* 1986;111:349–54.
139 Ratcliffe WA, McClure JP, Auld WH, Honour JW, Fraser R, Ratcliffe JG. Precocious pseudopuberty due to a rare form of congenital adrenal hyperplasia. *Ann Clin Biochem* 1982; 19:145–50.
140 Lisboa BP, Strassner M, Nocke-Finck L, Brener H, Bayer JM. Metabolism of steroid hormones in a virilising adenoma of adrenal cortex. *Acta Endocrinol* (Suppl.) 1975;199:395.
141 Lee PDK, Winter RJ, Green OC. Virilizing adrenocortical tumors in childhood: eight cases and a review of the literature. *Pediatrics* 1985;76:437–44.
142 Honour JW, Price DA, Taylor NF, Marsden HB, Grant DB. Steroid biochemistry of virilising adrenal tumours in childhood. *Eur J Pediatr* 1984;142:165–9.
143 Honour JW, Dillon MJ, Shackleton CHL. Analysis of steroids in urine for differentiation of pseudohypoaldosteronism and aldosterone biosynthetic defect. *J Clin Endocrinol Metab* 1982;54:325–31.
144 Shackleton CHL, Honour JW, Dillon MJ, Chantler C, Jones RWA. Hypertension in a four-year-old child: gas chromatographic and mass spectrometric evidence for deficient hepatic metabolism of steroids. *J Clin Endocrinol Metab* 1980;50: 786–92.
145 Stewart PM, Corrie JET, Shackleton CHL, Edwards CRW. Syndrome of mineralocorticoid excess – a defect in the cortisol–cortisone shuttle. *J Clin Invest* 1988;82:340–9.
146 Honour JW, Dillon MJ, Levin M, Shah V. Fatal, low renin hypertension associated with a disturbance of cortisol metabolism. *Arch Dis Child* 1983;58:1018–20.
147 Dean HJ, Shackleton CHL, Winter JSD. Diagnosis and natural

history of 17-hydroxylase deficiency in a newborn male. *J Clin Endocrinol Metab* 1984;59:513–20.

148 Imperato-McGinley J, Gautier T, Pichardo M, Shackleton C. The diagnosis of 5α-reductase deficiency in infancy. *J Clin Endocrinol Metab* 1986;63:1313–18.

149 Corrall RJM, Wakelin K, O'Hare JP, O'Brien IAD, Ishmail AAA, Honour J. 5α-reductase deficiency: diagnosis via abnormal plasma levels of reduced testosterone derivatives. *Acta Endocrinol* 1984;107:538–43.

150 Crowley S, Holownia P, Hindmarsh P, Brook CGD, Honour JW. The acute adrenal response to physiological ACTH. *J. Endocrinol* 1991;130:475–9.

151 Shah A, Stanhope R, Matthew D. Hazards of pharmacological tests of growth hormone secretion in childhood. *Br Med J* 1992;304:173–4.

152 Hindmarsh PC, Brook CGD. Single dose dexamethasone suppression test: dose relationship to body size. *Clin Endocrinol* 1985;23:67–70.

153 Rumsby G, Honour JW. *In vitro* gene amplification for prenatal diagnosis of congenital adrenal hyperplasia. *J Med Genet* 1990;27:676–8.

154 Rumsby G, Honour JW, Rodeck C. Prenatal diagnosis of congenital adrenal hyperplasia by direct detection of mutations in the steroid 21-hydroxylase gene. *Clin Endocrinol* 1993;38:421–5.

155 Rumsby G, Skinner C, Honour JW. Genetic analysis of the steroid 21-hydroxylase gene following *in vitro* amplification of the genomic DNA. *J Steroid Biochem Mol Biol* 1992;41:827–9.

28: Adrenal Steroid Deficiency States

M.G. FOREST

INTRODUCTION

Disorders of the adrenal gland are related to hypo- or hyperfunction of either the adrenal cortex or medulla. Function in a broad sense defines the normality of hormonal secretions and/or metabolism. As detailed in the present chapter, and summarized in Fig. 28.1, hormonal secretions of the adrenal cortex are dependent upon central regulation in a cybernetic fashion (feedback control). Mineralocorticoid secretions, although corticotrophin (ACTH)-dependent are controlled by the renin–angiotensin system [1–3].

Disorders of the adrenal gland can result from abnormal adrenal secretion, primary disorders, or from altered hypothalamohypophyseal control, secondary disorders. They occur in both hypo- and hyperfunction of the adrenal.

Increased or decreased function of the adrenal cortex may be complete or dissociated, that is resulting in inadequate production of glucocorticoids, mineralocorticoids, androgens or oestrogens. In some instances the unbalanced hormonal status may result in disruption of the normal feedback controls and lead to syndromes in which selective adrenal hypofunction and hyperfunction are mixed: typical examples are the multiple forms of congenital adrenal hyperplasia and adrenal tumours. Thus classification of adrenal disorders is sometimes arbitrary, being made on the prominent clinical or biochemical disorders.

Understanding of the pathophysiological conditions is based on our knowledge of the physiology and development of the hypothalamohypophyseal–adrenal axis which have greatly improved in the past two decades. However, complete pathophysiological bases are still lacking in some adrenal disorders.

Diagnosis of any dysfunction of the adrenal glands is directed by clinical findings, but it is fully established by hormonal measurements, dynamic testing and morphological studies which require technical abilities and are best performed in specialist centres.

ADRENOCORTICAL HYPOFUNCTION

The term 'adrenocortical hypofunction' includes all conditions in which the production of one or several adrenal hormones is impaired, whether this results from destruction of the organ or a congenital defect of the enzymes implicated in steroidogenesis (primary disorder) or from a functional disorder of the hypothalamohypophyseal complex (secondary and tertiary adrenal hypofunction) (Fig. 28.2). In secondary adrenal insufficiency the adrenal cortex is atrophic but intact, and the disease is due to inadequate stimulation by the pituitary gland. In tertiary adrenal insufficiency the defect is a lack of normal secretion of corticotrophin-releasing hormone (CRH), and the pituitary is intrinsically normal. Primary disorders can be either congenital or acquired and are chronic in the sense that there is no possible healing of the adrenal defect. Several of them are revealed by acute adrenal insufficiency, particularly those which are congenital or hereditary, but acute adrenal insufficiency ('Addisonian crisis') may occur in primary as well as in secondary chronic adrenal insufficiency, and in treated as well as untreated patients exhibiting the same clinical and biochemical findings. The adrenal crisis might thus be considered in itself a special illness.

Transient hypofunction of the adrenal cortex is also observed, either due to a delay in maturational processes (delay in the timing of the normal production for age of a given hormone, or delay in the maturation of the target cell response) or due to partial atrophy, damage or surgical resection of the adrenal glands. The term 'Addisonism', which has long been used to define a vague entity of clinical signs including weakness, pallor, hypotension and so on not due to hypoadrenalism, does not correspond to any precise aetiology or pathophysiological definition and should be abandoned since it is misleading, and since these patients do not require treatment with adrenocortical hormones.

The various aetiologies of adrenocortical hypofunction are listed in Table 28.1. From this list it is obvious that primary adrenocortical insufficiency in infancy and

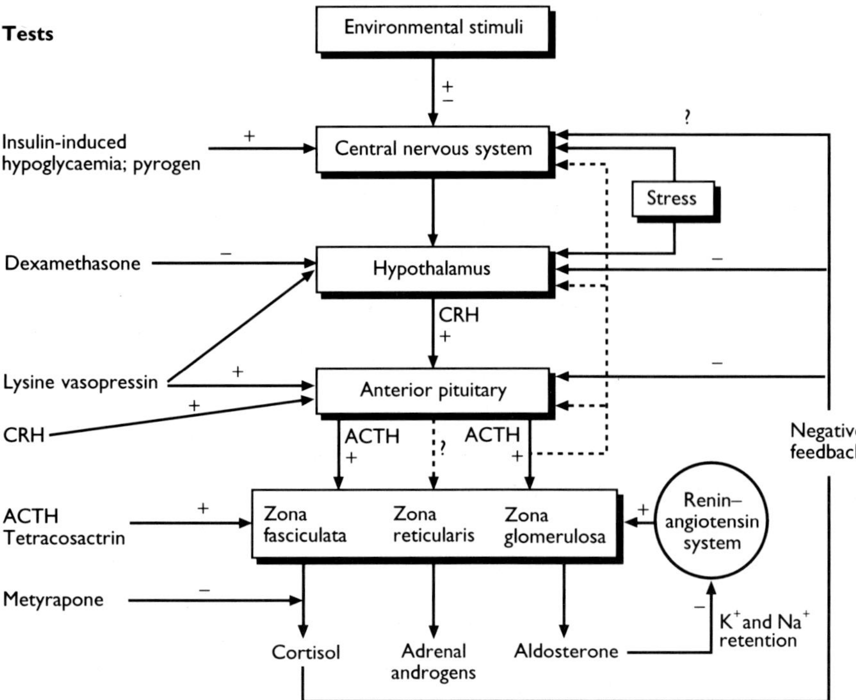

Fig. 28.1 Schematic representation of the regulation of adrenal function. Each level of the hypothalamo-hypophyseal–adrenal axis may be explored by specific dynamic function tests (on the left).

childhood is heterogeneous. However, the conditions have in common many clinical signs and biological findings, and the same replacement treatment. Selective deficiency in adrenal oestrogen secretion has not been described.

The timing of presentation can also vary and can be used arbitrarily for classification (Tables 28.2 & 28.3). Early manifestations are frequently seen in congenital adrenal hypoplasia or in various forms of congenital adrenal hyperplasia, or after bilateral neonatal adrenal haemorrhage, but they can also become symptomatic rather later in childhood. Secondary adrenal failure, very rare in early life, might well be manifest in the neonatal period. On the other hand chronic adrenal insufficiency ('Addison disease') is usually seen in children but not infants.

Congenital adrenal hypoplasia

DEFINITION AND INCIDENCE

This diagnosis attaches to newborns presenting with primary adrenocortical failure due to hypoplasia or atrophy of the adrenal glands. It includes functional defects which are similar, but several different anatomical abnormalities. According to Favara *et al.* [4], diagnostic criteria of hypoplasia of the adrenals are when the combined adrenal glands weigh < 1 g or $< 0.1\%$ of the total body weight.

The term 'congenital adrenal hypoplasia' has been used for years to describe hypoadrenalism and/or anatomical findings in newborns dying from adrenal failure. Idiopathic congenital adrenal hypoplasia is rare but not all that uncommon. Its incidence has been estimated to be 1 in 12 500 births and 0.19% [5] or 0.26% [4,6] of perinatal autopsies. In the series of 5687 autopsies studied, there were 11 cases of adrenal hypoplasia in children aged over 13 years and 112 cases (2%) of adrenal hypoplasia associated with brain deformity, all but four of whom were anencephalic. One other infant had a mother who had received long-term glucocorticoid therapy but none had adrenal haemorrhage. Of the 11 infants with congenital adrenal hypoplasia, maternal pre-eclamptic toxaemia was a feature in nine.

HISTORY

In 1948, Sikl [7] first reported a 1-month-old male infant who was pigmented, presented with diarrhoea and died suddenly. At necropsy the adrenals were markedly atrophied (< 1 g) while the pituitary was normal. Approximately half of the subsequently reported cases unassociated with anencephaly have presented in early infancy with a salt-losing syndrome which became apparent during the first month of life, and rarely at a later age (2–4 months). Other children presenting with respiratory symptoms, cyanosis, vomiting or diarrhoea have died suddenly within 48 h of birth. Although a few infants survived, most of them died within a few months, even during recent years [8,9].

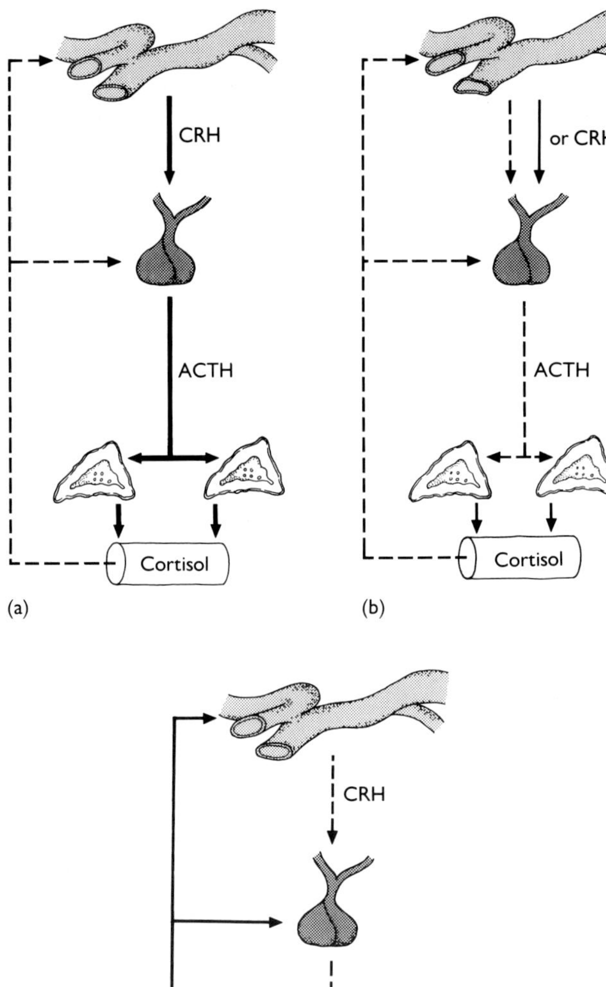

Fig. 28.2 Schematic representation of the changes in the hypothalamohypophyseal–adrenal relationships in adrenal hypofunction: (a) primary form; (b) secondary form; (c) iatrogenic form.

Congenital hypoplasia may be sporadic [4,5,10–18] or familial [8,9,19–32]. It has been described in uniovular female twins by Mosier *et al.* [24], in male twins and their sister by Cathro [33] and affecting only one of dizygotic male twins by Seeliger [34].

Adrenal hypoplasia has also been described in infants dying from various congenital malformations: polydactyly, hemihypertrophy, omphalocele, multiple kidneys or com-

Table 28.1 Aetiologies of adrenal hypofunction

PRIMARY ADRENAL HYPOFUNCTION

Complete adrenocortical insufficiency (decreased production of glucocorticoids, mineralocorticoids and androgens)

Idiopathic congenital adrenal hypoplasia or aplasia
Congenital adrenal hyperplasia due to defect in cholesterol 20,22-Desmolase (lipoid adrenal hyperplasia)
Adrenal haemorrhage, cyst
Wolman syndrome
Adrenal apoplexy: Waterhouse–Friedrichsen syndrome in fulminating infections
Adrenal necrosis following adrenal vein thrombosis or anticoagulant treatment
Addison disease (tuberculosis, syphilis)
Chronic adrenal insufficiency following adrenocortical retraction (autoimmune adrenalitis)
Multiple endocrinopathies: Schmidt syndrome, Whitaker syndrome, diabetes mellitus, hyperthyroidism or other associations (vitiligo, pernicious anaemia)
Mycosis (blastomycosis, histoplasmosis, coccidiomycosis) or parasitoses
Addison – Schilder syndrome
Iatrogenic: *Chemical, metabolic or toxic effect*: antibiotics, antimitotics, synthetic inhibitors of cortisol biosynthesis. *Surgical*: bilateral adrenalectomy or ablation of an adrenal tumour

Selective adrenocortical insufficiency

Glucocorticoids
Isolated glucocorticoid deficiency (or ACTH unresponsiveness)
Congenital adrenal hyperplasia: so-called mild form of 21-hydroxylase deficiency, 17α-hydroxylase deficiency, 11β-hydroxylase deficiency
Respiratory distress syndrome?
Iatrogenic

Mineralocorticoids
Isolated hypoaldosteronism (defect in 18-hydroxylase or 18-dehydrogenase, aldosterone synthase)
Pseudohypoaldosteronism
Hypokalaemic alkalosis with low aldosterone
Transient hypoaldosteronism
Iatrogenic

Gluco- and mineralocorticoids
Congenital adrenal hyperplasia due to defect in cholesterol desmolase, Δ^4-3β-hydroxysteroid dehydrogenase-isomerase, 21-hydroxylase

Androgens
17,20-Desmolase, or lyase, deficiency
Delayed adrenarche

Adrenal medullary insufficiency

SECONDARY ADRENAL HYPOFUNCTION
Anencephaly
Congenital adrenal hypoplasia associated with pituitary hypoplasia
Isolated ACTH insufficiency
Panhypopituitarism
Hypothalamohypophyseal tumours (craniopharyngioma, etc.)
Hypothalamic defect
Iatrogenic: glucocorticoid therapy

Table 28.2 Main causes of adrenal hypofunction in the newborn in decreasing frequency

Inborn defects of steroidogenic enzymes (congenital adrenal hyperplasia)
Congenital adrenal hypoplasia – cytomegalic, anencephalic, miniature
Destruction of the adrenal by haemorrhage, cyst, haemorrhagic diathesis, Waterhouse–Friedrichsen syndrome in fulminating infections
Congenital isolated hypoaldosteronism, isolated glucocorticoid deficiency
Maternal Cushing syndrome or steroid therapy during pregnancy
Congenital panhypopituitarism

Table 28.3 Main causes of adrenal hypofunction in infants and children in decreasing frequency

Iatrogenic: pituitary and/or adrenal hypofunction secondary to glucocorticoid therapy
Inborn errors in steroidogenesis (congenital adrenal hyperplasia) whether the onset is early in life (surviving treated patients) or manifests later
Secondary adrenal insufficiency: ACTH deficiency isolated or associated with deficiency of other pituitary hormones (hypopituitarism)
Chronic Addison disease as the consequence of adrenal atrophy due to autoimmune disease
Surviving infants with any of the aetiologies of adrenal hypofunction seen in neonates (Table 28.2)
Adrenal destruction due to tuberculosis, mycosis or parasitoses

plex cardiac malformations [35]. It is not clear whether adrenal insufficiency has been the cause of death in all these cases. Precise biochemical data are still very few in these conditions, and those available have not been correlated with adrenal hypophyseal or cerebral lesions [8,10]. Although the earlier reports lack hormonal data they have provided numerous post-mortem anatomical studies.

PATHOLOGICAL ANATOMY

Reviews of about 40 cases [5,29,36] indicated heterogeneity of pathological findings. While the degree of hypoplasia of the adrenal glands may vary between absence of adrenal tissue and considerable hypoplasia or rudimentary aspect, histological appearances differ markedly: the adrenal medulla is either normal or reduced to a few cellular aggregates. The three cortical zones may be hypoplastic but normally differentiated [7,18,24,37,38]; selective absence of a cortical zone has been reported [12,35,38]; the cortex may be reduced to small aggregates of undifferentiated cells [37,39].

In some instances the adrenal structure is disordered; the zones are not differentiated and the cortex contains large cells, not arranged in any particular form but clumped together with abundant eosinophilic cytoplasm and nuclei with large nucleoli. Mitoses are not found [7,23,35]. These cells have been described as 'giant' by Kampmeier [40], 'anaplastic' by Craig & Landing [41] and 'cytomegalic' by Beatty & Hawes [42], and are thought to derive from the cells of the fetal zone. In other reports the adrenal tissue was totally replaced by fibrous tissue [14], contained deposits of haemosiderin [18] or was reduced to large bilateral cysts [15].

In half of the 30 cases where both pituitary and adrenal glands have been examined at autopsy they were both abnormal. The pituitary might be absent [37,43,44], ectopic [38] or hypoplastic with a decreased number of acidophilic cells [24,33,45].

The confusion in anatomical findings has been clarified by recent studies, and it now appears that three distinct histological patterns are found in so-called idiopathic adrenal hypoplasia (Fig. 28.3). In all three patterns the medulla is usually normal.

1 The 'cytomegalic' or 'primary' pattern. The atrophic adrenal glands show abnormal architecture; the cortex is poorly differentiated with no distinct granulosa or fasciculata zones. The cells are abnormally large, show pleiomorphism and cytomegaly and resemble the giant cells occasionally found in the normal fetal zone [40,48]. Only 20 cases documented at autopsy have been reported [49], and only in males.

2 The 'anencephalic' pattern or 'secondary' pattern. In the small adrenals the fetal zone is markedly reduced or absent, while the permanent cortical zone is well differentiated [17,46]. It would appear to be the commonest pattern found [5,6] either in sporadic or familial cases [25,47] and resembles that seen in the adrenals in anencephaly [46].

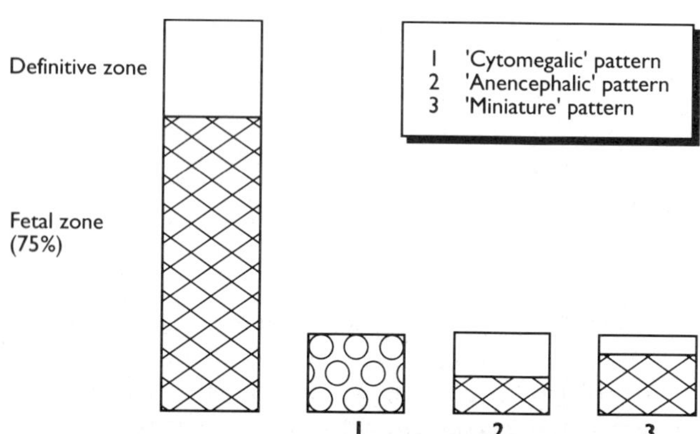

Fig. 28.3 Different histological patterns of the adrenal gland observed in congenital adrenal hypoplasia as compared with normal full-term adrenal glands (on the left) (redrawn from Laverty *et al.* [5]).

3 The 'miniature' pattern [4]. The adrenal glands are simply very small, 'miniature' with a normal ratio between fetal and adult cortex. This pattern occurs in between 30% [5] and 90% [4] of cases.

CLINICAL AND LABORATORY FINDINGS

Whatever the morphological type of congenital adrenal hypoplasia, clinical signs are those of complete adrenal insufficiency which manifests very early in life [50,51] or even at birth (convulsions, cyanosis, apnoeic spells). The clinical features of those who survive the first 2 days of life are those of dehydration, poor feeding, failure to thrive, intermittent fever and vomiting or diarrhoea. These infants have on more than one occasion been misdiagnosed as cases of upper alimentary tract obstruction and submitted to dramatic surgery [19,32,52,53]. Hyperpigmentation has been noted once at birth [54], but several times before the third week of life [14,15,18,25]. Hyperpigmentation when present or developing after the initiation of treatment [30,39] is a good indicator of pituitary activity. Prolonged neonatal jaundice has been reported [18] and it is clear that cortisol deficiency for any reason causes conjugated hyperbilirubinaemia.

Association of congenital adrenal hypoplasia with isolated gonadotrophin deficiency first reported in one adult [55], and is increasingly reported in adolescents [22,56–64]. Whether isolated gonadotrophin deficiency is invariable or not in congenital adrenal insufficiency is not yet established, but failure of gonadotrophin secretion, whether complete or partial, is a constant feature of X-linked congenital adrenal hypoplasia. A patient presenting with this form of the disease, initially reported by Zachmann *et al.* [64], was subsequently shown to have progressive high-frequency hearing loss [65]. This appears to be to an additional feature of X-linked congenital adrenal hypoplasia, suggesting that any patient with this syndrome should be examined for hearing loss.

The earliest biochemical abnormality is hyperkalaemia, hyponatraemia and metabolic acidosis. Severe hypoglycaemia is often associated. Plasma cortisol and aldosterone levels are low. Plasma renin activity is extremely high. Determination of basal ACTH levels is important to differentiate primary and secondary adrenal deficiency. When elevated, and they are usually extremely elevated, they prove normal pituitary function and are the best parameter to document primary adrenal failure.

Dynamic studies are difficult in these fragile infants. An ACTH test will show no rise in steroid hormones but must be performed only after correction of salt loss and preferably under mineralocorticoid treatment. Any other tests, even manipulation for electrocardiagraphy (ECG), electroencephalography (EEG) or X-ray, should be delayed in these very fragile infants as rapid treatment is mandatory. Later, after recovering good health with replacement therapy, determination of thyroid hormonal status, of growth hormone and gonadotrophin reserve is recommended. Antibodies to the adrenals or other tissues have never been found in congenital adrenal hypoplasia.

PATHOGENESIS AND GENETICS

The causes of the condition are several, and their pathogenesis is not well understood. Congenital adrenal hypoplasia has been viewed as an arrest in the development of the adrenal glands [29,42], as a failure of the cortex to develop [66], as the result of non-involution of the fetal zone [47] which usually occurs soon after birth [67] or as an isolated defect of organogenesis [9]. It has also been suggested that hypoplasia of the adrenal glands may not be primary but may occur secondary to pituitary atrophy [24,56], as it does in anencephalic patients [68,69].

Hereditary forms of congenital adrenal hypoplasia

From conclusions based on adrenal morphology, histology and familial studies, it has become clear that primary or idiopathic congenital adrenal hypoplasia may be hereditary [27,70] and that there are two forms.

1 *X-linked inheritance.* The condition was first recognized by Sikl in 1948 [7], and the first reported description of two affected siblings was by Mitchell & Rhaney [23]. It affects only boys, and the X-linked inheritance demonstrated in 1968 [59] has been largely confirmed [5,27,30,49,66,71,72]. This condition is apparently associated with the 'cytomegalic' histological pattern [73] but the 'miniature' pattern has also been reported as occurring exclusively in males [5] and gonadotrophin deficiency with [64] or without cryptorchidism, is a prominent association [60,63,64,74,75].

The pathogenesis of the condition is unknown. The cause of adrenal atrophy has been attributed to 'an organogenetic injury' of the adrenal gland in early fetal life [76], or to the failure of an 'inducer substance' normally responsible for the formation of the adult cortex [66]. The cause (and site) of the gonadotrophin deficiency is unclear. Some endocrinologists believe it to be secondary to a hypothalamic defect [74,77,78] but this view is not supported by a poor acute response to gonadotrophin-releasing hormone (GnRH) [56] nor by a lack of luteinizing hormone (LH) response to the pulsed administration of GnRH for 3 months [61]. This opinion is reinforced by several other reports suggesting that pituitary gland dysfunction is the primary defect based on the lack of response to prolonged pulsatile GnRH stimulation (see review in [79]). To add to the confusion, sexual precocity has been reported in this disease [31].

This form of congenital adrenal hypoplasia is associated

with other X-linked metabolic defects, such as glycerol kinase deficiency (GKD) [80–83] and Duchenne muscular dystrophy (DMD) [84]. The genes for X-linked congenital adrenal hypoplasia, GKD and DMD have been mapped using patients' breakpoints in Xp21.2 [85]. The X-linked congenital adrenal hypoplasia locus has been mapped to region Xp21.3–p21.2. Interstitial deletions of the X chromosome overlapping this region have been observed to cause complex clinical problems, with congenital adrenal hypoplasia as a prominent component. The various clinical syndromes resulting from different overlapping deletions have been referred to as contiguous deletion syndromes (see [79]). Patients present with a variety of clinical problems depending on which contiguous genes have been disrupted. A molecular Xp deletion has been suggested as a locus for hypogonadotrophic hypogonadism distal to the GKD and congenital adrenal hypoplasia loci. The locus for the progressive deafness may be in the same area [65].

2 *Autosomal recessive inheritance.* Adrenal hypoplasia occurs in both sexes and the histological pattern is usually the 'miniature' one, although there are reports of its association with the 'anencephalic' pattern. The autosomal recessive form of cytomegalic type has been described in two sisters in association with a chronic nephropathy due to focal hyalinosis [86].

The intriguing association of unexplained isolated LH deficiency has recently been reported in a family with autosomal recessive congenital adrenal hypoplasia, in whom an X-linked inheritance was ruled out [87].

Sporadic congenital adrenal hypoplasia

All three histological patterns have been described as sporadic. In such instances it is possible that the family history has been incomplete, and that the patients have one of the two hereditary forms [49].

Secondary congenital adrenal hypoplasia

Infants dying from acute adrenal crisis and found to have abnormal development of the pituitary gland have secondary adrenal deficiency. Atrophy or incomplete development of the adrenal cortex follows lack of trophic stimulation, whether due to ACTH or an ACTH-like pituitary factor [88] or to a mechanism of direct stimulation of steroidogenic enzymes [8] of the fetal zone. Predominantly, these infants have been females, whether or not the occurrence was familial. In the author's opinion such disorders, even if they encompass adrenal insufficiency, should not be called congenital adrenal hypoplasia but variants of either congenital deficiency of corticotrophin, congenital panhypopituitarism or anencephaly. There may be several causes of atrophy of the adrenal gland in subjects in whom no abnormality of the pituitary gland is found at autopsy.

Local damage of the adrenal glands, such as cysts or haemorrhage, may be secondary to an underlying problem. The high incidence (82%) of pre-eclampsia in one report [5] has suggested a possible role for extreme overactivity of the maternal gland, as seen in adrenal hypoplasia secondary to maternal Cushing syndrome [89,90] or steroid therapy during pregnancy [91]. However, in the latter conditions the adrenal glands are of the anencephalic type, while the three patterns of idiopathic congenital adrenal hypoplasia have been found in the fetuses of mothers presenting with pre-eclamptic toxaemia.

It has been suggested that viruses could be responsible for the 'anaplastic' transformation of the fetal cells into cytomegalic cells [92]. This is unlikely. Beatty & Hawes, when describing cytoplasmic inclusions in the giant fetal cells, probably observed the rare congenital variety of cytomegalovirus disease or cytomegalic inclusion disease [42], which is not to be confused with the cytomegalic form of idiopathic congenital adrenal hypoplasia.

AETIOLOGICAL DIAGNOSIS

The 'anencephalic' form is suspected by the association with pituitary disorders, the frequency of other malformations, lack of pigmentation, extremely precocious onset and low ACTH levels. In this form there should be some response to ACTH stimulation [30,93].

The 'cytomegalic' type can be suspected by the absence of other endocrine abnormality, male sex and family history [49]. In a male infant from an affected kindred, the finding of normal results of adrenal function does not rule out the possibility of X-linked adrenal hypoplasia, as onset of symptoms may be delayed in some patients [58–60,79]. Indeed, early onset is not an indication of the disorder, since it may occur from birth to adult age [94]. A peculiar adrenal secretion (20α-hydroxyprogesterone) has been described only in this adult case.

ANTENATAL DIAGNOSIS

As the diagnosis of congenital adrenal hypoplasia is difficult to ascertain, and the clinical disorder may develop in the first few hours of life, its antenatal diagnosis is of potential interest. In many countries oestriol determination is routinely made in pregnant women. By such systematic studies, or by search in a mother who has previously lost a child from adrenal insufficiency, the antenatal diagnosis of congenital adrenal hypoplasia has been made by several authors [5,33].

The diagnosis of congenital adrenal hypoplasia in the fetus should be considered when the fetus is alive and low oestriol secretion is found in the mother. In a male fetus the finding does not differentiate placental sulphatase deficiency [95,96], since this is sex-linked and apparently more frequent than congenital adrenal hypoplasia [5]. The infants with placental sulphatase deficiency are normal and do not require therapy. Recent studies [97] suggest that the ratio of urinary levels of oestriol over those of oestrone plus 17β-oestradiol might distinguish sulphatase deficiency (low ratio) and fetal adrenal hypoplasia (subnormal ratio), but it has not yet been proved that such studies would lead to unambiguous diagnosis.

Low oestriol levels are also found in eclamptic toxaemia. Diagnosis of this condition in the mother does not exclude the possible occurrence of congenital adrenal hypoplasia as its coincidence has been very high (nine of 11 sporadic cases) in the study by Laverty *et al.* [5]. Although it was suspected in one case, the delay in treatment was the cause of fatal adrenal crisis.

DIFFERENTIAL DIAGNOSIS

Differential diagnosis is essentially that of the various types of congenital adrenal hyperplasia. Buccal smear or karyotype should be performed in females presenting with either normal or ambiguous genitalia and in cryptorchid males to confirm diagnosis of either virilized genetic females or exclude the diagnosis of genital male with congenital lipoid adrenal hyperplasia [98–101]. In true females it is not currently possible to distinguish this disease from congenital adrenal hypoplasia. Clinical and biological findings are exactly the same. In both diseases plasma steroid concentrations and excretion are extremely low and do not rise after ACTH stimulation. Plasma renin activity is high and electrolyte disturbances are identical. Severe hypoglycaemia is frequent. Plasma ACTH is elevated and hyperpigmentation is also found in both. Differential diagnosis with other steroid enzyme defects, on the other hand, is easy by finding abnormal steroids.

PROGNOSIS

Prognosis of congenital adrenal hypoplasia was classically very poor [49]. Most of the reported patients have died early in infancy. With the use of improving diagnostic means, including antenatal diagnosis, appropriate treatment is now given more rapidly than in the past, and longer survival results [102].

Adrenal haemorrhage, adrenal cysts and adrenal calcifications

Adrenal haemorrhage in the newborn is not uncommon. Its incidence has been estimated to be 0.05% in 3657 autopsies by Snelling & Erb [103], and birth trauma the pathogenic factor. The adrenal gland at birth is nearly as large as the kidney. The normal involution of the fetal zone of the adrenal cortex is preceded by a hyperaemia of the gland which renders it particularly fragile at this stage. Haemorrhagic diathesis of the newborn (hypoprothrombinaemia) [104], treatment by anticoagulant [105,106], and anoxia [107] are other major factors responsible. The incidence of adrenal haemorrhage is higher in premature babies and in difficult or prolonged labour, particularly in breech or forceps deliveries. Adrenal haemorrhage may also result from anoxia, shock or infections. The reasons why adrenal haemorrhage may occur *in utero* [103,108] in the absence of the above conditions are less evident. The congenital forms of syphilis or tuberculous infection of the adrenals may cause extensive haemorrhage and acute adrenal failure [109]. In older children (or adults) bilateral adrenal infarction associated with adrenal haemorrhage may result in embolus, sepsis or, very rarely, adrenal vein thrombosis after a back injury [110].

Adrenal haemorrhage may be unilateral [104,111] or bilateral [112–114]; it can be variable in intensity [115, 116] and of considerable size, giving abdominal distension and it may be palpable as an abdominal mass. Intra-adrenal haematomas may rupture into the peritoneum [117]. In other instances a large haemorrhage remains encapsulated in the adrenal glands and, when unilateral, can be mistaken for a Wilms tumour [36]. Haemorrhage into a large cyst causing intestinal obstruction is occasionally seen [118,119].

CLINICAL SIGNS

These are hypotension or acute shock, pallor, cyanosis, tachycardia and pain in the abdomen, flank or back. Lower chest pain, hyperpyrexia and dyspnoea may be present. These symptoms are often mistaken for acute pneumonia, but X-rays of the chest are normal. Other symptoms include anorexia, nausea or vomiting, abdominal rigidity or rebound [110], and neuropsychiatric manifestations. Hypotension is observed in about half the cases before shock develops. On the other hand, hypertension, due to compression of the kidney or the renal artery, has been reported [120]. Collapse and death are frequent as a result of massive bleeding, even if emergency resuscitation including intravenous corticoid therapy has been commenced rapidly.

DIAGNOSIS

Diagnosis is usually made between 2 and 7 days of life [115] and is difficult: clinical symptoms are non-specific in the severe form described above, as well as in the other forms. Attention might be alerted when a palpable mass is discovered. Ultrasonography is helpful to visualize the mass as a large pseudocystic suprarenal zone and hence to recognize its origin. This non-invasive imaging technique is very helpful for the diagnosis in the asymptomatic forms [121]. Until the development of the computerized tomography (CT) scan the diagnosis was often made at autopsy. Unexplained prolonged jaundice [122] or symptoms of renal failure [123,124] are seldom observed. Discovery of suprarenal calcification as early as the fifth day of life [125] is helpful, but calcifications may be manifest only several months later [126,127], or never occur. On the other hand, adrenal haemorrhage may be totally unrecognized and suprarenal calcification discovered fortuitously. Adrenal haemorrhage may be associated with intracranial haemorrhage and renal atrophy secondary to thrombosis of the renal vein (Orsini, cited in [128]).

In infants recovering from the acute phase, as well as in those in whom signs of adrenal hypofunction are the first manifestations later in life, differential diagnosis from other causes of adrenal failure is often not possible unless the haemorrhage has been clearly diagnosed at birth. Suprarenal calcification, shown best if the X-rays are taken standing, is very suspicious. Adrenal calcification may, however, be seen in association with simple adrenal cysts, adrenocortical carcinoma, neuroblastoma, ganglioneuroma, phaechromocytoma, adrenal tuberculosis, Nieman–Pick disease, Wolman syndrome and xanthomatosis [129,130]. Exact diagnosis may be extremely difficult and made only at laparotomy.

The incidence of the association of adrenal haemorrhage with adrenal insufficiency is difficult to estimate accurately. Histological examination of the adrenal glands of the neonates who have died from massive adrenal haemorrhage shows complete destruction of the adrenal tissue, including the medulla. This suggests that acute adrenal failure was responsible for death [131]. On the other hand there is no relation with the apparent intensity of the bleeding and the severity or the chronicity of adrenal hypofunction. Bilateral adrenal haemorrhage associated with neonatal tuberculosis is not necessarily fatal [109,132].

RESULTS

When associated with adrenal haemorrhage, adrenal insufficiency is usually transient [120]. The adrenal gland has a great capacity for regeneration [133]. Thus adrenal hypofunction manifesting soon after the critical period has elapsed might recover later on. The writer has observed two such cases in whom severe neonatal adrenal insufficiency had completely recovered by 12 and 18 months of age (as proved by subsequent ACTH testing) and a third child in whom clinical signs of adrenal insufficiency developed around 12 years of age and in whom adrenal calcification was clearly seen retrospectively on a chest radiograph taken in the neonatal period.

Thus at whatever age adrenal calcification is found, a complete check of adrenal function (basal levels of gluco- and mineralocorticoid hormones but also plasma ACTH and renin activity levels) and reserve (ACTH test) should be performed. The latter testing is necessary whether normal or subnormal basal levels are found, since adrenal remnants functioning at a maximal level are unable to increase their hormonal production in the face of stress. On the other hand, in subjects in whom adrenal insufficiency follows adrenal haemorrhage, dynamic testing of adrenal function should be repeated at intervals in order to discontinue an unnecessary treatment in case of full recovery.

ADRENAL CYSTS

Adrenal cysts result from tubulocystic dilation of the superficial cortical sinusoids [134]. With the exception of one observation in which the massive bleeding inside the cyst *in utero*, rather than the cyst itself, was considered responsible for the destruction of the adrenal gland [119], there seems to be no relation between cyst formation and risk of adrenal failure. Cysts, commonly seen in otherwise normal adrenal glands of infants before 34 weeks of gestation, are interpreted as a degenerative process due to intrauterine stress [135]. They should be distinguished from adrenal haematoma or neuroblastoma [120], since they do not regress spontaneously, and have to be surgically removed.

Acute adrenal insufficiency (adrenal crisis)

Acute forms of adrenal insufficiency with salt loss, circulatory collapse and hypoglycaemia are due to inadequate secretion of glucocorticoids and/or mineralocorticoids. Adrenal crisis may be the first symptom in any of the aetiological forms of adrenal insufficiency listed in Table 28.1, except in isolated androgen deficiency. Adrenal crisis is common. More frequent in newborns or infants, it may be seen at all ages in untreated as well as in treated patients. Acute illness, surgery, trauma, emotional shock, exposure to excessive heat (salt loss by excessive sweating), or excessive diuretic treatment may precipitate a patient into adrenal crisis. Hypoglycaemic episodes may occur independently of the symptoms caused by salt and water loss, and can be precipitated by fasting and acute infections.

An acute episode may be preceded by unusual fatigue, irritability or nausea and abdominal pain, but usually its onset is very abrupt. The child becomes suddenly very ill with signs of circulatory failure. Signs and symptoms include vomiting, diarrhoea, dehydration and fever, which may be followed by hypothermia, vascular collapse, confusion and coma. Hyponatraemia, hyperkalaemia and metabolic acidosis are found.

TREATMENT

This consists of replacement of fluids and adrenal hormones, and treatment of hypotension and of the underlying disease [136]. Cortisol hemisuccinate (or phosphate) (1–2 mg/kg) should be given intravenously at once. If the intravenous infusion is not possible because of vascular venous collapse the intramuscular route is used, but dosages are doubled. Glucocorticoid therapy is continued as an infusion of cortisol hemisuccinate (20–150 mg in small children, 150–200 mg in older children) during the first 24 h. Cortisone acetate (1–2 mg/kg) may also be injected i.m. immediately, and repeated daily to ensure slow release over 24 h and allow reduction of i.v. doses. Aldosterone may be given i.v. and/or i.m. in a dose of 25 mg and injections repeated as indicated clinically. However, the half-life of injected aldosterone is short so an i.m. injection of 1–3 mg of deoxycorticosterone acetate (DOCA) (if available) is usually given at once. The daily dose of DOCA will be reduced to 1–2 mg in the following days.

Dehydration must be rapidly corrected, with i.v. saline in 5% or 10% glucose started. Fluid requirements for the first 24 h are 100–120 ml/kg when body weight is less than 20 kg; and 75 ml/kg over this weight. In cases of severe shock, replacement of part of this volume by blood (5 ml/kg of body weight) or plasma is recommended. The fluid should be given rapidly at first, 20–25% of the total volume in the first 2 h. Fluid replacement after the second day will be calculated according to losses and laboratory findings. The child may need additional salt for a short period (1 g/10 kg of body weight).

PREVENTION

In cases of minor stress, such as a fever less than 38°C, tooth extraction without anaesthesia, or intense physical effort, a two- to three-fold increase in the oral maintenance dose is recommended on that day. When there is excessive sweating, ingestion of sodium chloride pills (1–3 g) is advisable.

In cases of high fever, intramuscular injection of cortisol (25–50 mg) should be given. Mineralocorticoid treatment is increased only in cases of vomiting, and is then preferably given intramuscularly.

In cases of major stress, such as anaesthesia, surgery or serious illness, the patients must be given a stress dose of cortisone. Preparation for surgery must begin the day before. Just before surgery, cortisol hemisuccinate (1–2 mg/kg i.v.) and DOCA (1–3 mg i.m.) are injected. After the operation, return to maintenance therapy is achieved over a week.

Waterhouse–Friderichsen syndrome

The earliest records of overwhelming sepsis and fulminating purpura associated with sudden onset of adrenal failure due to adrenal apoplexia, were made in the UK [137,138]. Waterhouse in 1911 [139] reviewed the 15 cases of the literature and favoured the theory that the cause of the syndrome was a bacterial infection. Later on Friderichsen [140,141] made comprehensive reviews on the subject. Since then the name of Waterhouse–Friderichsen has been given to the clinical syndrome associating overwhelming sepsis, extensive purpura or petechiae, and circulatory collapse. In this syndrome the toxaemic invasion is constant but adrenal insufficiency is not [142], and the issue is not always fatal [143,144]. It has thus been proposed to restrict the term Waterhouse–Friderichsen syndrome to those cases in which bilateral adrenal haemorrhage is found at autopsy, and to call 'fulminant infectious diseases' those cases in which acute sepsis, petechiae, purpura and vascular collapse are not associated with significant adrenal pathology [36,145].

AETIOLOGY

Waterhouse–Friderichsen syndrome is more severe and more constantly observed in invasive meningococcaemia [146] or diphtheria than in other sepsis. Adrenal destruction may also be due to influenza, pneumococcus, haemolytic streptococcus of group A, acute pemphigus and, more exceptionally, to a number of other causes including leukaemia, purpura and early accidents (6–10 days) of anticoagulant therapy or abdominal operations [106,147,148].

CLINICAL FEATURES

First symptoms may be irritability, headache, abdominal pain or gastrointestinal disturbances; but usually the onset of the syndrome is extremely abrupt and the evolution seldom lasts more than 1–2 days. A perfectly healthy child may suddenly develop high fever, overwhelming sepsis, extensive purpura and cutaneous petechiae. There is a fall in blood pressure and signs of severe shock such as pallor or general cyanosis, rapid shallow breathing and eventually peripheral vascular collapse. Symptoms such as stiff neck, convulsions or coma are concomitantly observed. Severe dehydration or disturbance in electrolytic balance (as hyponatraemia, hyperkalaemia or hypoglycaemia) might not have time to develop before death occurs. In other instances adrenal apoplexy is fatal before there is any clinical or biological evidence of meningitis or sepsis. The cortisol levels in plasma or cortisol secretion rate, being elevated in most cases, are severely impaired only in those subjects who die [142].

PATHOLOGY

Morphological and histological changes found at autopsy are often the same as those found in subjects who have died of any type of stress [149–151]. Adrenal glands are barely enlarged but show signs of lipid deletion and cellular necrosis. Sinusoids are filled with clotted blood. The medulla is always necrotic even if damage to the cortex is not very extensive. Thrombi are frequently seen in small vessels but only rarely in large ones. It is generally thought that thrombosis of the adrenal gland is a secondary phenomenon. Macroscopic adrenal haemorrhage, which is a frequent finding (74%), may be only one manifestation of multiple system organ failure caused by septic shock [152].

PATHOGENESIS

In the Waterhouse–Friderichsen syndrome, circulatory collapse is probably the result of severe toxaemia rather than being primarily due to acute adrenal failure. According to present concepts the adrenal haemorrhage would be the consequence of a generalized Schwartzmann reaction [150,153,154]. Bacterial toxins sensitize the endothelium of vessels which react to repeated exposure by intravascular clotting. Hypofibrinogenaemia and haemorrhagic diathesis occur secondarily. Infarction of the adrenal may occur, and is only one extension of the disease. Thrombosis leads to haemorrhage in many organs.

DIFFERENTIAL DIAGNOSIS

Attempts to make a differential diagnosis between peripheral vascular collapse due to bacterial endotoxin and shock due to acute adrenal failure are not completely theoretical. Indeed, the use of adrenal steroids and noradrenaline in the prophylaxis or treatment of fulminant infections is probably not justified, but they should be used in the presence of adrenal insufficiency.

However, diagnosis is difficult. Due to the life-threatening situation in both conditions, prompt therapeutic decisions are to be taken, since laboratory help is often too slow. The history and a knowledge of any bacterial epidemic may help; onset of adrenal failure seems to be less rapid than that of overwhelming sepsis, and is rapidly responsive to glucose in saline solution and to glucocorticoid therapy.

TREATMENT AND PROGNOSIS

Complete agreement on the best therapeutic approach is still lacking. The use of large doses of cortisol was of no benefit in a study of over 300 extremely ill patients [155,156]. Adrenal steroids have no beneficial effect on the course of Waterhouse–Friderichsen syndrome itself.

The harmfulness of cortisol in this syndrome has been claimed as altering body resistance to infection, inhibiting formation of antibodies and increasing the risks of a Schwartzmann reaction [150,157]. The biological half-life of exogenous cortisol is increased in patients having fatal shock, probably as the result of impairment of hepatocellular metabolism, hepatic blood flow or renal function [158]. This reduction in metabolic disposal of cortisol might be responsible for additional undesired pharmacological effects [159] and for blocking the pituitary–adrenal axis [160]. However, there is not yet enough evidence for not using short-course therapy of glucocorticoids to prevent circulatory collapse. It should be kept in mind that cortisol potentiates the effects of noradrenaline [161]; thus the maintenance of normal blood pressure depends upon the presence of cortisol. In the absence of cortisol, response to adrenaline is progressively lost, the collapse might become irreversible and adrenal insufficiency grow worse [162]. In addition, on finding low plasma levels of cortisol shortly before death in patients with severe meningococcal meningitis [142], it has been felt that a high dose of cortisol should be given [33,36,136,163].

Adequate antibiotic therapy or other supportive treatment of the underlying disease should be given immediately. Heparin treatment has been advised to prevent the formation of fibrin [150]. Blood transfusion or exchange transfusion should be considered. Shock should be treated by epinephrine, angiotensin II or noradrenaline. If the pressor agents are not rapidly effective, stress doses of cortisol should be administered for 2 days and decreasing doses are given thereafter. Morphine or barbiturates should not be given until cortisol has been administered in case of adrenal insufficiency [164]. Treatment is otherwise the same as in the other aetiologies of adrenal insufficiency, and is detailed above.

Prognosis of acute bacterial sepsis has considerably improved with the use of antibiotics, but that of unequivocal cases of Waterhouse–Friderichsen syndrome is still very poor.

Primary chronic adrenocortical insufficiency: Addison disease

Addison disease is caused by damage to the adrenal glands which leads to both glucocorticoid and mineralocorticoid deficiency. The adrenal failure as described originally by Addison [165] is typically a chronic illness; however, acute adrenal crisis may occur at any time and may lead to the diagnosis [166].

Addison disease is rare. Its incidence has been differently estimated, and is difficult to assess accurately as some cases are unrecognized and many others unpublished. Its general incidence is estimated as 0.04% of the death rate in the USA [145] and UK [167] and 1.4% in autopsy studies in Switzerland [168]. It is observed mostly in adults between 20 and 50 years of age. In children the disease is rare but not exceptional [169], and 2 years after the description by Addison, the disease was described in children. An early review of 62 proven cases [170] showed that 95% of the subjects were 10–15 years old and the others younger. From successive reviews of nearly 2000 cases [21,171–174] it now appears that the disease is more often diagnosed in young children or infants. Addison disease has been found in 0.014% of paediatric patients in both the USA and Switzerland, in 1% of children with endocrine disorders in the former USSR [175] or ≤0.5% in the author's experience. All races are affected, and the apparent higher incidence in some is probably related to the higher incidence of tuberculosis or other infections in those populations [176].

AETIOLOGY, PATHOGENESIS AND GENETICS

Until about 1950 the main cause of Addison disease was tuberculosis [177], accounting for 68%, 76% or 95% of all cases recorded by Guttman [172], Conybeare & Millis [178] and de Gennes [179] in the USA, UK and France respectively. This cause has markedly decreased in the past three decades [180], although it presents as the cause in 21% of cases in UK [181], and 45% in France [182].

Tuberculosis causes a progressive destruction of the adrenal glands which are extensively caseated. The caseation extends to the medulla, which is totally destroyed, and occasionally to the surrounding adipose tissue. The destructive process is very slow; it may take 7–27 years [25]. Adrenal failure manifests only when over 90% of both glands are destroyed.

Infections such as mycosis, histoplasmosis [183], North or South American blastomycosis [184–186], coccidiomycosis, tolurolis or parasitoses (*Echinococcus alveolaris*) may cause extensive destruction of the adrenals. Their incidence is anyway minor in children, but may become significant in adults in some areas where those infections are frequently encountered. Amyloidosis may also be a cause of adrenal insufficiency.

Whatever the aetiology, primary adrenal insufficiency results from a process that destroys the adrenal cortex. The relative causes vary according to ethnic origin, age and/or living conditions: disseminated tuberculosis, and fungal infections are still major causes of adrenal insufficiency in populations which have a high prevalence of these diseases, while bilateral metastatic disease is one of the most common causes in oncology services [187,188], though rarely in children.

The main cause of chronic Addison disease in children, as in adults, is autoimmune destruction of the adrenal glands, a condition termed 'autoimmune adrenalitis'. The histological aspect of adrenal retraction or contraction has been known for many years [189] and was noted by Addison. At pathological examination, adrenal glands are atrophic but never calcified. The outstanding aspect is that of extensive lymphocytic infiltration [190].

Patients with isolated autoimmune adrenalitis are predominantly male in the first two decades of life, equally male and female in the third decade, and predominantly female thereafter [191,192]. These age- and sex-related differences are unexplained. On the other hand, patients with polyglandular autoimmune syndromes are at all ages predominantly female [191].

Humoral immunity

Following reports that patients with Addison disease have circulating adrenal antibodies [193–197], the autoimmune basis for primary adrenal atrophy has been suspected [198,199]. These antibodies, reacting with all three zones of the cortex, are immunoglobulins (Ig) (class IgG) that have been identified by immunofluorescence, complement fixation, gel diffusion or tanned red cell agglutination [200,201]. There are antibodies both to adrenal microsomes and mitochondria. Their titre is usually low (<1/64) and decreases either with age or in the course of treatment [190,195,200]. They are more common in women, particularly those with polyglandular autoimmune syndrome. Their presence seems to precede the development of adrenal insufficiency by several years [202,203]. They may also be found in first-degree relatives of Addison patients, or even in normal subjects [181,202, 204,205]. Not all subjects who have antiadrenal antibodies have adrenal insufficiency, but as a group they develop the disease at a rate of up to 19% per year. The earliest symptom is increased plasma renin activity (PRA) with normal to low aldosterone levels, suggesting that the zona glomerulosa is first affected [203]. Several months to years later the dysfunction of the zona fasciculata becomes progressively apparent, first by decreased ACTH-stimulated plasma cortisol levels, later by increased plasma ACTH levels, finally by decreased basal cortisol levels and overt clinical symptoms [202,203].

The antigen(s) are located in adrenal microsomes and/or plasma membranes, in all cortical cells, but are more abundant in the zona fasciculata [206]. They disappear from adrenal cells following steroid treatment. Their nature is still a matter of controversy. They have been described as carbohydrate-containing lipoproteins with no species specificity [200]. Some antibodies were found to react with an adrenal-specific 55 kD microsomal protein [207]. Most adrenal autoantibodies block the stimulatory effect of ACTH on cortisol secretion and DNA synthesis *in vitro* [208]. This finding was the basis of a belief that autoantibodies interfere with the binding of ACTH to its receptor.

Another interesting hypothesis is that steroid enzymes are the autoantigens in immune adrenalitis. Indeed, it was recently shown that the 55 kD adrenal-specific protein which reacts with adrenal autoantibodies, has the biochemical characteristics of 21-hydroxylase and reacts on Western blots with rabbit antibodies to recombinant 21-hydroxylase [209–211]. In another study, steroid 17α-hydroxylase and 21-hydroxylase were both recognized as being adrenal autoantigens in patients with autoimmune adrenocortical insufficiency [212]. This led to the suggestion that adrenal-specific steroid enzymes are major autoantigens involved in adult-onset autoimmune Addison disease. However, the pathological nature of these antigens is not yet proven.

An alternative possibility is that production of autoantibody against enzymes is a secondary phenomenon, the initiating event being T-cell-mediated cytotoxicity directed against endogenous, enzyme-derived peptides coexpressed with class I (or II) major histocompatibility complex on target cells.

Cell-mediated immunity

Cell-mediated immunity may be important in the development of adrenal insufficiency. It is evidenced either by positive intradermal reaction towards adrenal homogenates [213] or by the test of migration of leukocytes or migration-inhibiting factor (MIF) test [214]. The antigen responsible for the secretion of MIF is localized in the mitochondrial preparation from adrenal homogenates. Decreased suppressor T lymphocyte function and increased levels of circulating Ia-positive T lymphocytes have also been described [215]. Evidence of positive cellular or humoral immune reactions is found in nearly 90% of patients with idiopathic primary hypoadrenalism. The former is more frequently found (80%) than the latter (50–60%). Although autoimmune adrenalitis and humoral immunity is preponderant in females, the cellular immunity is more frequent in males with this disease [200,202].

Associated endocrine autoimmunity

In about 70% of patients with idiopathic Addison disease, circulating antibodies to adrenal tissue can be detected. Antibodies to other endocrine tissues, including thyroid, ovary, testis, parathyroid and islet cells, have also been demontrated in these patients with or without clinical evidence for other organ failure [194,195,200,202,216–221]. These various organ-specific antibodies found in nearly 70% of adult patients are less frequent in children (43%) but, when they do occur, they do so predominantly in females (82%). Circulating antibodies described in the polyglandular deficiency syndromes are of various types – simple binding (with various tissue or protein components, for example adrenal cortex cell, thyroglobulin), cytotoxic (for example to pancreatic β cells), receptor stimulating (such as thyroid-stimulating immunoglobulins) and receptor blocking (for example ACTH receptor blockers). It is possible that an autoimmune reaction directed to the proteins of either hair-root follicles or skin may occur in alopecia totalis and vitiligo. However, in most instances it is not certain whether the antibodies are the cause of the problem or only a sign. There are also experimental data, mainly *in vitro*, suggesting cell-mediated autoimmunity, perhaps related to T cell dysfunction.

Polyglandular autoimmune syndromes

Addison disease can occur in association with other conditions believed to be 'autoimmune' in nature. The condition was described as 'insuffisance pluriglandulaire' by Claude & Gougerot [222] and as 'multiple endocrine sclerosis' by Falta [223]. Despite the clear description of primary multiple endocrine failures, the syndrome has often been mistaken for hypopituitarism.

The list of associated endocrine and other diseases includes: acquired primary hypogonadism, alopecia, chronic active hepatitis, chronic lymphocytic thyroiditis, chronic mucocutaneous moniliasis, exophthalmos, Graves disease, hypophysitis, insulin-requiring diabetes, keratoconjunctivitis and Sjögren syndrome, malabsorption syndrome, myasthenia gravis, pernicious anaemia/atrophic gastritis, primary anaemia/atrophic gastritis, primary biliary cirrhosis, quantitative immunoglobulin abnormalities, spontaneous acquired hypoparathyroidism and vitiligo. When a combination of the above conditions occurs in the same patient (usually in association with the demonstration of circulating antibodies), this constitutes the polyglandular deficiency syndrome [224] or the polyglandular autoimmune syndrome [225]. A number of associations or syndromes have been described [204,226–228].

Thyroid disease is frequently hyperthyroidism in adults [229] but, in children, is more often hypothyroidism. Its association with Addison disease is known as Schmidt syndrome [230–233]. Diabetes mellitus may be associated with Addison disease [234,235] or with Schmidt syndrome [230,236].

The association of hypothyroidism and superficial

moniliasis with Addison disease was described by Whitaker *et al.* [237] and by Di George & Paschkis [238]. Hashimoto disease [239] or pernicious anaemia [199] are also encountered. Due to the frequency of hypoparathyroidism (35%) in these diverse associations, careful examination of calcium balance should be made in all cases of autoimmune adrenalitis to detect, as early as possible, the possible development of hypoparathyroidism. Conversely, testing of adrenal function must be performed in all cases of hypoparathyroidism.

Ovarian failure is frequent in older patients [240] and may also complicate the syndrome of Whitaker [241]. There is no correlation between the titre of respective tissue antibodies and/or the severity of the endocrine failure or their clinical manifestations.

The polyglandular deficiency syndromes have been classified into three types [225,242,243]. Type I, also called autoimmune polyendocrinopathy–candidiasis–ectodermal dystrophy (APECED) [244], associates chronic mucocutaneous moniliasis, hypoparathyroidism and Addison disease. At least two of the three conditions must be present. When all three are present they have usually occurred in the order listed above. Other immune disorders may be present, with a high incidence of alopecia [245] and malabsorption (about 25%) and a disturbing incidence of chronic active hepatitis (about 10%) [244]. The syndrome has a broad clinical spectrum; the majority of patients have three to five manifestations, some of which may not appear until the fifth decade [244].

Type II associates Addison disease with autoimmune thyroid disease and insulin-requiring diabetes. Addison disease plus one of the other two must be present. Other immune disorders may be present, especially gonadal failure and vitiligo.

In type III there is autoimmune thyroid disease without Addison disease, but with one the following: insulin-requiring diabetes, pernicious anaemia, vitiligo and/or alopecia. A patient may progress from type III to type II if Addison disease develops subsequently. Characteristics of type I and type II polyglandular deficiency syndromes are summarized in Table 28.4.

Diagnosis of the polyglandular deficiency syndromes must be based on a high index of suspicion, that is simple screening in any patient with evidence for one primary endocrine gland failure (or hyperthyroidism). For example, if Addison disease is primary, screening should consist of menstrual history or testosterone measurement, free thyroxine levels, 2-h postprandial blood glucose, calcium, blood count with red cell indices and serum glutamic oxaloacetic transaminase (SGOT). Studies should be repeated at 1–2-year intervals. Remember that multiple organ failures may be confused with primary pituitary dysfunction, but trophic hormone measurements should enable differentiation. Measurement of circulating antibodies against other endocrine tissues is of questionable predictive value, but measurable levels are most likely to precede the onset of clinical disease when islet cells or adrenal antibodies are present. In addition, the occurrence of the disease in families should be systematically screened every 2 years by ACTH testing of siblings of an Addisonian patient.

Table 28.4 Characteristics of type I and type II polyglandular deficiency syndromes [242,243]

	Type I	Type II
Inheritance, autosomal	Recessive	Dominant
Age at onset	Childhood (< 12 years)	Adulthood (peak at 30 years)
Female : male ratio	1.5 : 1	1.8 : 1
HLA association	Not found	With -B6, -Dw3, -DR3
Disease components		
Addison disease	65%	100%
Hypoparathyroidism	80%	None
Mucocutaneous moniliasis	75%	None
Alopecia	25%	< 1%
Malabsorption syndrome	22%	None
Gonadal failure	20%	20%
Pernicious anaemia	13%	< 1%
Autoimmune thyroid disease	10%	70%
Chronic active hepatitis	10%	None
Vitiligo	8%	5%
Diabetes mellitus	4%	50%

HLA, human leukocyte antigen.

The adrenal glands in acquired immune deficiency syndrome

The adrenal gland is the most commonly involved endocrine organ in acquired immune deficiency syndrome (AIDS) [246–250]. Histopathological evidence of adrenal disease is common in AIDS, but most lesions (due to opportunistic infections, most commonly cytomegalovirus (CMV), followed by mycobacterial and fungal infection) are not sufficiently extensive to result in clinical adrenal insufficiency. In contrast to previous reports stressing the importance of CMV adrenalitis as a possible cause of adrenal insufficiency [250–252], tuberculosis is the most likely cause of total cortical destruction [253]. An intriguing observation was that some AIDS patients with clinical symptoms of adrenal insufficiency have unexpectedly high cortisol values. This finding has been interpreted as a stress pattern of response to illness [249], or a result of ectopic production by lymphocytes or monocytes of factors which stimulate the adrenal cortex [254]. More recent studies have shown such AIDS patients to have abnormal glucocorticoid receptors on lymphocytes [255]. This acquired cortisol resistance syndrome implies complex changes in immune-endocrine function, which may in turn influence the course of the disease.

Pathogenesis of the disease

Typical adrenal lesions of human autoimmune adrenalitis in human and circulating antiadrenal antibodies may be produced experimentally by the injection of adrenal homogenates [193]. However, it is unlikely that, in the human disease, the liberation of adrenal antigens is a sufficient factor for activating the immunological system. Indeed antibodies are not found in Addison disease due to tuberculosis or other infections [204].

There is no correlation between the presence of antibodies in the sera and the severity or even the occurrence of the disease [200,216]. It is thus probable that antibodies reflect the disturbance in the immunological system rather than that they mediate the destruction of adrenal cortical tissue. It is currently believed that cell-mediated immunity plays an important part in producing adrenocortical destruction [256]. Serum of patients with polyendocrinopathies has a cytotoxic effect *in vivo* [257] and adrenal lesions are reproduced in animals by transfer of lymphocytes [258]. The mechanism by which T lymphocytes mediate the adrenal lesions is unknown.

Familial occurrence is frequent in immune adrenalitis [166,191,192,220,227,243,259–262] and results from inherited abnormalities of the immune response mechanism. The inheritance is probably autosomal recessive [192,220,263]. In autoimmune polyendocrinopathies, type I may be an autosomal recessive condition and type II an autosomal dominant condition [243,265].

Finally there is a significant association of histocompatibility antigens (HLA-A1, -B8, -A3, -DR4) but not of chromosome 6 with idiopathic Addison disease [262,264, 266]. There are several reports regarding HLA (human leukocyte antigen) typing in patients with the polyglandular deficiency syndromes [231,262,265]. Most of the type IIs are associated with an increased prevalence of HLA-B8, -Dw3, -DR3. HLA associations with type I are not clear-cut.

CLINICAL FEATURES

These are related to the deficits in gluco- and mineralocorticoid hormones either directly or indirectly by the fact of unrestrained pituitary secretions. Their dependence and pathogenesis are listed in Table 28.5. From the classical description by Addison and the review by Thorn [270], the major clinical symptoms in adult patients with Addison disease are weakness and fatigue (100%), weight loss (97–100%), hyperpigmentation of the skin (94–98%) or mucosae (82%), anorexia (90%), vomiting (84%) or nausea (81%), and hypotension (87%). Other symptoms are less frequent: abdominal pain (32–34%), constipation (28%), diarrhoea (21%), salt craving (19%), syncope (16%), muscular pain (16%) and vitiligo (9%). All symptoms become progressively manifest and increase with time. In children, the outstanding features are hyperpigmentation, hypoglycaemia, gastrointestinal disturbance and progressive general weakness [261,271,272].

Pigmentation

Pigmentation is caused by increased production of melanin and its catabolite, melanoid. The hyperpigmentation affects the whole body but especially areas exposed to light, areas physiologically pigmented, such as nipples, the perianal region or genitalia, areas submitted to friction, skin folds or creases and operative scars. Skin is otherwise dry and brittle.

In children, the skin pigmentation seldom reaches the degree observed in adults. It is often unnoticed and found only on direct questioning. Typical histories are that parents are proud of the quality and lasting suntan in their child, or that the mother complains that the child is apparently more negligent in washing. The mother may try excessively to wash apparently dirty knees, ankles, elbows or finger knuckles and damage the skin. Skin hyperpigmentation may be absent, so-called white Addison disease [273] or limited to freckles or hyperpigmented naevi in blond or red-haired subjects. Spotty, bluish-brown pigmentation of the gums, inner face of the cheeks or other mucosae are less common in children with Addison disease than in adult patients.

Thus changes in complexion rather than degree of pigmentation should call for attention. Only scars acquired after the onset of the disease are pigmented. Coexistence of uncoloured and pigmented scars might exceptionally give very precise dating of the adrenal destructive process. Indeed, pigmentation may precede the other clinical symptoms by up to 10 years, particularly in patients with latent Addison disease (that stage at which adrenal remnants maximally stimulated are still able to maintain normal basal adrenal function).

Hypoglycaemia

Hypoglycaemia occurs in Addison disease [274,275]. In children it is a very frequent symptom ($\geqslant 90\%$). Easy to recognize when it is accompanied by sudden weakness, cold sweating, hunger and pallor in the morning or before meals, it is often misdiagnosed because it may occur 1 or 2 h after meals rich in carbohydrate, because clinical symptoms of hypoglycaemia appear at higher levels of glycaemia (60–80 mg%) than in normal subjects (< 50 mg%) and because, when complicated by gastro-

Table 28.5 Clinical and biological consequences of hormonal deficits in primary chronic adrenal insufficiency

Glucocorticoid deficit

Energy metabolism
Decreased gluconeogenesis and lipolysis and decreased glycogen mobilization; decreased carbohydrate turnover; increased sensitivity to insulin
Anorexia
Hypoglycaemia → decreased resistance to fasting, coma, mental retardation
Muscular weakness

Water balance
Reduced glomerular filtration, possible increase in antidiuretic hormone (ADH) secretion or delayed breakdown of ADH; increased facultative water reabsorption in distal renal tubules
Opsiuria, nocturia, danger of water intoxication

Calcium homeostasis
Increased calcium absorption, decreased active calcium excretion
Normal or elevated serum phosphate levels
Hypercalcaemia (increased protein-bound calcium), hypercalciuria
Thirst, hyposthenuria, polyuria

Lipid metabolism
Insufficient fat resorption, fat intolerance, steatorrhoea, periodic diarrhoea, lipid depletion in the organs

Cardiovascular system
Reduced sensitivity to catecholamines, hence reduced tonic action of adrenaline upon arterioles and capillaries
Orthostatic hypotension

Gastrointestinal tract
Increased secretion of sodium chloride into the intestinal lumen, reduced production of hydrochloric acid and pepsin by the gastric mucosa and sometimes histamine-refractory achlorhydria
Irritation of gastrointestinal mucosa
Anorexia, gastric or abdominal pains, nausea, vomiting
Some hypochloraemia

Haematopoietic system
Normocytic, normochromic anaemia, increased osmotic resistance of the erythrocytes by unknown mechanism
Increased lymphocytosis (> 35%), eosinophils (8–10%) probably by increasing their efflux from organs where they are formed, stored or degraded or redistribution to other body compartments [164]
Decreased neutrophil leukocytes, particularly evident during infections by lack of stimulation of bone marrow

Olfactory threshold
Lowered gustatory threshold for salt, lowered olfactory and acoustic threshold
Increased sensory acuities

Hypersensitivity to drugs
These include narcotics, morphine, codeine, or sedatives such as barbiturates and bromides; possibly linked to increased endorphin synthesis [267,268]
Possible accidents of such treatments

Mineralocorticoid deficit (disturbed electrolyte balance)

Increased renal excretion of sodium and water
Results in hypovolaemia, extracellular dehydration
Hyponatraemia, masked or not by haemoconcentration; increased excretion of sodium in urine, saliva and sweat
Incapacity to cope with salt restriction
Weight loss, extremely restricted drinking, salt craving, hypotension
In case of severe salt loss, decrease in renal circulation, severe renal insufficiency and increased blood urea nitrogen and shock

Decreased renal excretion of potassium
Hyperkalaemia which stimulates ACTH release [269], muscular weakness and cramps; EEG changes

Shift of H^+ ions from intracellular to extracellular space
Deficient ammonium formation and deficient renal tubular excretion of H^+ ion
Metabolic acidosis

Androgen deficit
Delay or decreased development of sexual hair
Negative influence on women's psychosexuality with reduced sexual drive and appetite

Loss of feedback controls
Increased pituitary secretion of ACTH, ACTH-related peptides including β-melanocyte-stimulating hormone, β-lipotrophin
Hyperpigmentation of skin and mucosae; increased pigmentation of the hair
Increased plasma renin activity, primarily due to hypovolaemia and unbalanced sodium homeostasis [1]

intestinal disorders, hypoglycaemia can be masked by severe dehydration and hypovolaemia. Testing of adrenal function (see below) must be undertaken in all children with clinical or biological symptoms of hypoglycaemia, recurrent convulsions or unexplained coma with apparently isolated metabolic acidosis.

Hypotension

Hypotension is often not evident in young children, except in acute adrenal crisis. Decreased intravascular volume is responsible for small heart size and, together with a reduced cardiac output, leads to a small and retarded pulse. Exceptionally, cardiovascular changes may mimic heart disease [276]. Electrocardiogram disturbances are either non-specific or typical of hypokalaemia: high, pointed, symmetrical, T waves with normal QT intervals [261].

Renal function

The capacity to secrete dilute urine is always impaired,

while renal-concentrating ability is usually preserved [277]. Severe renal insufficiency is seen only during acute renal crisis.

Sensory thresholds

Changes in sensory thresholds are related to cortisol deficiency. Taste [278,279], olfactory [280] and auditory [281] thresholds are decreased in Addison disease. These are less evident in children, probably because they have not been sought.

PUBERTAL DEVELOPMENT AND FERTILITY

Development of sexual hair and beard is classically said to be poor in adults, but this is not our experience. We have observed patients with an onset of the disease before 2 years of age, who became particularly hairy in adulthood. Macrogenitosomy [282], and excessive hair in the first months of life and advanced pubertal development in two girls [173,283] have been reported in association with adrenal insufficiency in children. True isosexual precocity and regression following cortisol treatment has been described in a 3.5-year-old boy with Addison disease [284]. A younger brother of this patient developed the same clinical features, but diagnosis was made 18 months earlier, on growth acceleration, slight pigmentation and increased ACTH, LH and follicle-stimulating hormone (FSH) levels, and lack of rise of cortisol after an ACTH test (unpublished observation by the same group of authors). Pathogenesis in this apparently exceptional association is not fully explained [284,285].

In most children on treatment, linear growth and pubertal development is normal [166,286,287]. There does not seem to be general agreement on whether or not onset of puberty is delayed in Addison disease. Given adequate steroid treatment, patients are fertile, pregnancy is uneventful and babies are normal, even though they may have transient circulating adrenal antibodies.

LABORATORY FINDINGS

Electrolyte abnormalities are the rule. Hyperkalaemia is due to aldosterone deficiency. Hyponatraemia, occurring with glucocorticoid deficiency, is caused by elevated arginine vasopressin (AVP) levels and the resulting increased free water retention, descreased sodium pump activity and consequent shift of extracellular sodium into cells [288]. Other common findings are low fasting blood glucose and anaemia, a direct effect of glucocorticoid deficiency [261]. Hypercalcaemia is not uncommon [191, 289], due in part to increased calcium-binding proteins resulting from haemoconcentration. However, volume repletion does not normalize calcium concentrations, which occurs after the institution of glucocorticoid therapy.

The classical water load test [290,291] and its correction by glucocorticoid treatment is now obsolete and may be dangerous due to water intoxication [145].

Measurement of basal levels of plasma cortisol and aldosterone or of urinary 17-oxogenic steroids is commonly of no help in the diagnosis of Addison disease [261,292]. Basal hormone levels are decreased only in advanced Addison disease. The diagnosis of glucocorticoid deficiency is easily and unambiguously made on the findings of elevated plasma ACTH levels, generally well above 300 pg/ml [293,294], with persistent diurnal rhythm [295–297] and biological activity [298].

The same pattern (high levels but persistence of diurnal rhythms) is found for β-lipoprotein and β-endorphin [299]. These is a lack of rise of plasma cortisol to ACTH or CRH stimulation. Stimulation tests of carbohydrate metabolism (insulin-induced hypoglycaemia), pyrogen stimulation tests or metyrapone tests are risky and should be avoided.

The natural evolution of Addison disease is towards total destruction of the adrenal glands with complete failure of cortical adrenal function, although spontaneous recovery may exceptionally be seen [300].

Mineralocorticoid deficiency is evident when characteristic electrolyte disturbances are found. These are, however, often subclinical and only demonstrated by salt restriction (10 mmol of sodium a day for 5 days). This test may precipitate acute salt loss and should be performed with great caution. Dynamic tests of aldosterone secretion [301] may also be risky and are no more informative than combined measurements of plasma or urinary levels of aldosterone and plasma renin activity.

Assessment of adrenal medullary function is not easy. Adrenaline is the catecholamine produced in the adrenal medulla. Evidence of a decreased excretion of adrenaline in basal conditions is difficult to obtain due to the large range of normal values [302,303]. Stimulation tests by 2-deoxyglucose [304], or by insulin (1.7 IU/m^2) once the glucocorticoid deficit is corrected [305], have proved reliable in a number of cases. However, interpretation is difficult and these tests are not commonly used. In autoimmune adrenalitis, adrenomedullary function is normal.

The presence of antibodies to the adrenal cortex may precede the clinical onset of adrenal insufficiency. Their discovery may allow the early diagnosis of subclinical adrenocortical failure, even in the absence of specific clinical symptoms [191,200]. In such patients, repeated testing of adrenal function is necessary to detect subclinical Addison disease and the need for therapy, in order to avoid subsequent adrenal crisis. Also, because of the familial character of the autoimmune adrenalitis, siblings of affected patients should have their adrenal function evaluated.

IMAGING OF THE ADRENAL GLANDS

During the past decade, radiological evaluation of the adrenal glands has been revolutionized by tomographic techniques, particularly CT, that have permitted a direct 'visualization' of the adrenal glands [306]. CT can be very useful in the evaluation of Addison disease, by distinguishing idiopathic atrophy from other aetiologies such as granulomatous infection, neoplasm and haemorrhage. More recently magnetic resonance imaging (MRI) has provided a new imaging tool. Although MRI appears inferior to CT in evaluating adrenal hypofunction, it might be useful in the differential diagnosis between adrenal haemorrhage and other masses [306].

DIFFERENTIAL DIAGNOSIS

The diagnosis of chronic adrenal insufficiency is difficult [307] because symptomatology is often incomplete and because none of the clinical symptoms is specific *per se*, and all can be found in a great variety of other conditions.

Hyperpigmentation

Hyperpigmentation may be racial, due to excessive exposure to sun or ultraviolet light, to chronic skin irritation, to nutritional deficiencies of vitamins (pellagra) or iron, or to ingestion of toxic substances such as arsenic, bismuth, lead and silver or of medicaments, such as hydantoin. A number of gastrointestinal diseases are associated with skin pigmentation: regional enteritis, ulcerative colitis, cirrhosis, polyposis of the small intestine associated with melanosis in the Peutz–Jegher syndrome.

Other syndromes associated with increased melanin pigmentation can be differentiated by different skin manifestations and associated symptoms: von Recklinghausen disease (neurofibromatosis), Albright syndrome (polyostotic dysplasia) and acanthosis nigricans.

Melanosarcoma, dermatomyositis, scleroderma pernicious anaemia, thyrotoxicosis or chronic tuberculosis

Without adrenal insufficiency these may all be accompanied by hyperpigmentation. Sprue can mimic Addison disease, but pigmentation is dirty grey and localized to the face, anaemia is more severe, osteomalacia and tetany are present and the bulky nature of the stools is characteristic. Melanin deposition in haemochromatosis commonly mimics that seen in Addisonian patients and the two diseases may coexist. Brown pigmentation of the skin and buccal mucosa is often seen in end-stage chronic renal failure. Increased melanin concentration here is likely to be due to decreased clearance of β-lipotrophin [308]. Severe salt-loss is seen but, unlike Addison disease, renal concentration is lost.

General weakness or weight loss

These are features of myasthenia gravis. Extreme fatigue and irritability are typical symptoms of hyperparathyroidism. Anorexia, vomiting, hypotension and weight loss are more severe in anorexia nervosa than in Addison disease. However, anorexia nervosa is more commonly seen in young girls and its progressive onset may sometimes be misleading, since deficiency of thyroid-stimulating hormone occurs and, later, deficiency of ACTH.

Hypoglycaemia

Hypoglycaemia, one of the cardinal symptoms for which differential diagnosis is most important in young children, may be due to glycogen storage disease, spontaneous hypoglycaemia, McQuarrie–Zetterström syndrome (idiopathic hypoglycaemia), adenomas and hyperplasia of the islet cells. Low plasma cortisol levels are found in cases of familial cortisol-binding globulin deficiency [309]. In this condition, however, there are no clinical signs of Addison disease since only the bound fraction of cortisol is decreased and plasma cortisol levels rise sharply after ACTH.

TREATMENT

Because of unresolved immunological problems, adrenal transplantation [310] has not yet been successful. Replacement therapy must thus be given for life.

Under normal conditions, glucocorticoid and mineralocorticoid replacement is required but no special diet is recommended. Treatment of Addison disease requires replacement [311] of normal cortisol production, that is 12–15 mg/m^2 of body surface area a day. Cortisol rather than cortisone acetate is currently used. The oral route is the method of choice [312]. When fast action is desired, i.m. or i.v. cortisol hemisuccinate should be used, not i.m. cortisone acetate because it is too slowly absorbed (>4 h). If cortisol hemisuccinate is not available, parenteral administration of prednisolone hemisuccinate or phthalate or another synthetic compound at a dose adjusted for glucocorticoid potency (Table 28.6) can be given twice a day [313]. The use of synthetic steroids is otherwise pointless. Since they have no salt-retaining activity, higher doses of mineralocorticoid are required.

Table 28.6 Approximate values comparing the activities of natural and synthetic steroids

Natural or synthetic corticoids	Dose (mg)* physiological range	Potency		
		Glucocorticoid	Mineralo-corticoid	Anti-inflammatory
Glucocorticoids				
Cortisol (cp F; hydrocortisone; 11β,17α,21-trihydroxy-pregn-4-ene-3, 20-dione)†	20–30	1	1	1
Cortisone (cp E; 17α,21-dihydroxy-pregn-4-ene-3,11,20-trione)	25–37	0.8	0.3	1
Prednisone (1-2-dehydrocortisol)	7.5	3.5	0.06	4
Prednisolone (1-2-dehydrocortisone)	5–7	4	0.05	4
Triamcinolone (9α-fluoro-16α-hydroxyprednisolone)	4–6	5.5	0	6
Methylprednisolone (9α-fluoro-6α-methylprednisolone)	4–6	5	0	6
Betamethasone (9α-fluoro-16β-methylprednisolone)	0.75	25	0	20
Dexamethasone (9α-fluoro-16α-methylprednisolone)	0.5–1	30	0	30
Paramethasone (6α-fluoro-16α-methylprednisolone)	2–3	10	0	5
Mineralocorticoids				
Aldosterone (11β,21-dihydroxy-18-oxo-pregn-4-ene-3,20-dione)	0.04–1.5	0.3	160	9
11-Deoxy corticosterone (DOC; pregn-4-ene-21-ol-3,20-dione)	0.05–0.16	0	4.5	0
Corticosterone (cp B; pregn-4-ene-11β,21-diol-3,20-dione)	1–3	0.5	0.45	0.3
Fludrocortisone (9α-fluorohydrocortisone)	0.05–0.2	80	125	10

* Doses for adults. They must be recalculated on body surface area basis in children.
† Physiological needs are 12 mg/m^2; oral doses are about twice i.m. doses. Cortisol hemisuccinate contains 75% of active compound F.

Synthetic 9α-fluorocortisone (fludrocortisone) is the sole mineralocorticoid used orally. In combination with cortisone (cortisol) therapy, daily fludrocortisone requirement is 150 μg/m^2, regardless of age.

In the course of replacement therapy all clinical symptoms of hypoadrenalism must be corrected. Indication of adequate cortisone dosage is given by general well-being, normal appetite and activity, weight gain and normal growth. Measurement of cortisol levels is of little help, but measurements of ACTH levels are useful, particularly at the onset of treatment. Adequate doses of cortisol theoretically reduce serum ACTH levels to normal values. However, recent studies have shown that peak ACTH levels in well-controlled patients are three to ten times higher than normal in the morning but fell to within the normal range between 1200 and 1400 h, although plasma levels peaked twice a day [314]. This study indicates that timing in sampling is most important in interpreting ACTH levels [294,315].

Control of mineralocorticoid therapy is less precise and is often determined empirically. Its adequate dosage is nevertheless of considerable importance. Even when asymptomatic, insufficient replacement leads to minor degrees of hypovolaemia, leaving the child vulnerable to circulatory insufficiency. Measurement of plasma renin activity is not always easy to interpret because of diet or postural factors [316]. Although useful to detect insufficient mineralocorticoid replacement, it cannot distinguish between adequate and excessive dosage, even in the absence of hypertension [317]. The much simpler determination of serum potassium is as good. Adrenal androgen insufficiency does not warrant therapy in children but it may be required (as testosterone undecanoate by mouth) in older patients.

When tuberculosis is suspected, appropriate treatment is recommended. Rifampicin, widely used for this purpose, increases hepatic 6-hydroxylase activity and increases cortisol breakdown [318]. Thus the daily requirement of cortisol increases.

When hypothyroidism is associated with chronic adrenal insufficiency, adequate glucocorticoid therapy should be given before starting the treatment with thyroid hormones. By increasing the clearance of adrenal hormones, thyroid therapy given alone may precipitate an adrenal crisis. This is the only instance of adrenal insufficiency where the use of cortisol and not cortisone is required, since inactivity of 11β-hydroxysteroid dehydrogenase in hypothyroid patients results in a slow conversion of cortisone to cortisol.

Intercurrent illness or stress

Any intercurrent illness, stress or physical effort (such as sports) will increase the requirement for cortisone. Stress effect of psychological problems or psychological trauma or fear should not be overlooked. In such conditions, increase of the dosage of oral cortisone by 50–100% is mandatory and is sufficient in most instances. Parents and physicians should, however, remain attentive if vomiting or high fever occur, in the event i.m. injection of 25–50 mg of cortisone and 1–3 mg of DOCA should be given immediately. Immediate hospitalization is recommended in cases of severe illness because of the risk of acute adrenal crisis. For surgery or anaesthesia, stress doses should be given. The basis for giving high doses of cortisol before stress occurs is the knowledge that cortisol production rate in acute stress may reach 100–300 mg/day.

Education of the parents and child is of great importance. Parenteral preparations should always be kept at home. The child should carry cortisone tablets and a tag explaining the nature of the disease and what should be done in case of accident.

PROGNOSIS

The course of Addison disease may be complicated at any time by acute adrenal crisis. Salt loss is usually more rapidly diagnosed and related to adrenal disease than severe hypoglycaemia. Both may be life-threatening and the parents must be taught to recognize the symptoms and to give prompt treatment (glucose and high doses of cortisol i.v.) at home before transfer to hospital. Even if the diagnosis is uncertain, there is no harm in treating the patient: the only risks are delay in treatment and stressful diagnostic procedures. Given correct treatment and parental support, patients with Addison disease have a normal life and normal lifespan. However, whether the patients are well treated or not, the development of pituitary adenoma (Nelson syndrome) may complicate the course of the disease [319] and necessitate trans-sphenoidal surgery [320].

Hypoadrenalism and central nervous system: adrenal insufficiency related to peroxisomal disorders

Adrenoleukodystrophy (ALD), adrenomyeloneuropathy (AMN) and Zellweger syndrome are inherited disorders, characterized by progressive neurological dysfunction associated with primary adrenal insufficiency. An uncommon form of familial adrenal insufficiency associated with progressive diffuse cerebral sclerosis [321] or spastic paraplegia [322] was first described by Siemerling & Creutzfeld in 1923 [323] and is also referred to as Addison–Schilder disease or ALD [324,325]. Cases without evident adrenal insufficiency have been previously classified as Schilder syndrome or sudanophilic leukodystrophy. Until the past two decades, a score of cases had been reported [326–336] but it appears that the diseases are more common than had been realized [337,338] and that they show a wide range of phenotypic variation.

PATHOLOGICAL FINDINGS

Pathological changes are similar in all forms of ALD [331,333,339]. There is atrophy of the cortex with few remaining cortical cells and no signs of inflammation. There is severe, diffuse or patchy, extensive demyelinization of the cerebellum and cerebrum, particularly in the occipital and posterior parietal areas, with destruction spreading in a caudal–rostral direction. The demyelinization of the central nervous system is progressive and does not appear to be secondary to the adrenal insufficiency [333]. The adrenal glands are atrophic, and show ballooned cortical cells in the zona reticularis and fasciculata. Apart from demyelinization of the mammillary bodies, and decreased number of basophilic cells reflecting long-term glucocorticoid administration, the hypothalamus and the pituitary gland are usually normal at histopathological examination. Schaumburg *et al.* [333] and Powell *et al.* [339] made the important observation that adrenal and cortical cells contain characteristic cytoplasmic inclusions. An abnormal accumulation of cytoplasmic striated inclusions is found in brain macrophages, cells of the central nervous system, adrenocortical cells, Schwann cells, and occasionally in testicular interstitial cells [333]. At the ultrastructural level, the inclusions appear as electron-lucent spicules bounded by 25 Å wide membranes [339].

CLINICAL FORMS

ALD classically refers to the association of Addison disease and progressive demyelinization of the cerebrum. As true for other disorders, the demonstration of a specific biochemical abnormality has let to a reappraisal of the clinical manifestations of the disorder. Two types of ALD are currently recognized, and Zellweger syndrome is considered as a related disorder.

X-linked ALD

This is the juvenile or childhood form [333], representing the most common form (about 60%) of ALD [337,338]. In this disorder, the biochemical abnormalities would be confined to very long chain fatty acids (VLCFA), and peroxisomal structure is normal. The disorder involves primarily the cerebral white matter and adrenal cortex. The subcortical white matter is atrophic, which can be observed by CT and MRI imaging of the brain [340]. The clinical presentation is more varied than has been originally thought [341]. ALD begins in childhood and progresses rapidly to dementia, blindness, and quadriparesis. In many cases the first symptoms of a psychiatric or neurological disorder and signs of primary adrenal failure usually occur at 4–8 years of age. Behavioural changes associated with cognitive impairment are frequently the first symptoms [333] such as school failure, emotional outbursts, memory loss or dementia. Visual disturbances are common and present as homonymous hemianopia, visual agnosia, loss of visual acuity and, later, motor impairment. A clinical variant, the so-called adult ALD, has been ascribed to patients in whom the first symptoms occur later in life. In both, adrenal insufficiency is mild to severe, and may precede or follow the onset of neurological disturbances. In general adrenal insufficiency becomes evident in younger patients before neurological symptoms, while in older patients initial symptoms tend to be neurological [338,342].

Adrenomyeloneuropathy is currently considered a variant of ALD, since it shows the same structural and biochemical abnormalities as ALD [334]. It represents 17–28% of ALD [337,338]. AMN may begin in adolescence and early childhood with weakness, spasticity and distal polyneuropathy as the initial complaints. It is milder and more progressive [338,343]. AMN occurs mainly in adults and, in addition to the adrenal cortex, involves mainly the white matter of the spinal cord and peripheral nerves. It presents in the third decade of life with progressive spastic paraparesis combined with evidence of peripheral polyneuropathy, bowel and bladder disturbances, sensory changes, severe adrenal insufficiency and hypogonadism, but intact intellect [334]. AMN may be misdiagnosed as multiple sclerosis [343].

The association of spastic paralysis or polyneuritis with adrenal insufficiency and sometimes hypogonadism may be observed [342]. The clinical appearance of this syndrome may occur in families affected by ALD. Indeed, unlike most other storage diseases, in X-linked ALD there is a striking variability in phenotype among members of the same kindred. In both childhood ALD and AMN, the liver is normal, there is no retinopathy, no dysmorphic features, a normal number and appearance of peroxisomes and normal pipecolic acid levels [338]. ALD and AMN have been observed in the same kindred [343], and even in siblings [344], and are thus viewed as different expressions of the same disease.

It was long thought that the neurological symptoms developed before adrenal insufficiency, but five of eight boys with idiopathic adrenal insufficiency have been described to have adrenomyeloneuropathy [345]. Thus AMN should be considered in any boy presenting with adrenal insufficiency.

Symptomatic heterozygotes. Progressive paraparesis which resembles that seen in AMN has been observed in women who are heterozygous carries of ALD [346]. The discovery of a biochemical marker of the disease has permitted extensive study of affected families. It was found that a number of obligate heterozygote carriers were symptomatic [347] or presymptomatic as judged on brainstem auditory evoked potentials (BAER) [348].

Neonatal ALD

Neonatal ALD has been recognized as a distinct form of ALD [349–351]. It resembles other peroxisomal disorders (Zellweger syndrome or infantile Refsum disease) in that the number and size of the peroxisomes are diminished and the function of at least six peroxisomal enzymes is impaired [337]. Reported cases have been sporadic [351] or familial with either two affected brothers [350] or occurring in a sister and a brother [349]. Neonatal ALD has never been described in the same family or kindred as childhood ALD or AMN.

In neonatal ALD the typical ultrastructural and biochemical changes characteristic of X-linked ALD are present. However, in one case the demyelinization relatively spared the occipital and parietal lobes [351] and the leukodystrophy was moderate with severe involvement of the thymus in another [349]. Since then, about 35 other case have been reported (7% of the ALD cases reviewed in [338]). Unlike the appearance in childhood ALD, abnormal neuronal migration and polymicrogyria is frequently found. In addition, in the neonatal form there may be enlargement of the liver (50%), retinopathy (41%), dysmorphic features (36%), diminished or absent liver peroxisomes [352] and increased pipecolic acid levels [338].

Neonatal ALD has the same degree of accumulation of VLCFA as childhood ALD or AMN, but differs from them in that it involves a wider range of tissues and involves girls as frequently and as severely as it does boys. Clinical onset is very early in life in the first few days. Clinical symptoms may be hypotonia and poor feeding followed by either severe seizures and hypsarrhythmia on EEG [351] or severe psychomotor retardation, blindness and deafness [350], opisthotonos and mental retardation.

Although most patients have biological evidence of adrenocortical dysfunction, none develops isolated adrenal insufficiency before the onset of neurological deterioration; they usually die before 5 years of age.

Related disorders

These refer to diseases associated, more or less frequently, with some degree of adrenal insufficiency. They occur in many metabolic diseases, and are probably more common than is usually thought in lipid storage diseases [70].

Zellweger syndrome or cerebrohepatorenal syndrome has many features in common with the neonatal form of ALD (see review in [338]). It affects both sexes. Neurological symptoms are hypotonia, severe retardation and seizures. Cytoplasmic inclusions are found in the adrenals. There is abnormal neuronal migration and polymicrogyria. Enlarged liver, retinopathy, dysmorphic features, increased levels of plasma pipecolic acid and absence of liver peroxisomes are constantly found [353]. There may be renal cortical cysts or chondrodysplasia calcificans.

However, in Zellweger syndrome plasmalogen and bile acid syntheses are impaired, whereas they are normal in neonatal ALD.

Among the other diseases of the peroxisomal group (infantile Refsum disease, and punctuata rhizomelic chondrodysplasia), adrenal insufficiency is almost symptom-free, but can be suspected on the basis of the results of laboratory explorations of the hypothalamopituitary axis [354].

Exceptionally, other metabolic diseases may be accompanied by adrenal insufficiency. This is the case in Gaucher disease or xanthomatosis. The latter, also named Wolman disease, is a rare disorder with autosomal recessive inheritance, characterized by intracellular triglyceride and cholesteryl ester storage caused by the absence of lysosomal acid lipase activity [70,354].

GENETICS

Childhood ALD and AMN are transmitted in an X-linked fashion. Study of a large kindred with patients heterozygous for both ALD and an electrophoretic variant of glucose-6-phosphatase dehydrogenase (G6PD) deficiency has made it possible to locate the ALD gene at Xq28, in close proximity to the G6PD locus, along with colour blindness and haemophilia [355,356]. The origin and genetic transmission are the same in ALD and AMN, implicating the Xq28 region of the X chromosome [356].

The study of fibroblast clones from heterozygotes demonstrated an unusual phenomenon: the great majority of clones were of the ALD type. Thus, in contrast to what has been observed at other X-linked loci, selection in ALD appears to favour the mutant population in the heterozygous state. This observation may explain the relatively frequent occurrence of symptoms in women who are heterozygous for ALD.

The neonatal form of ALD, as well as Zellweger syndrome, have an autosomal recessive inheritance [338]. This further emphasizes that there is a fundamental distinction between these disorders and childhood ALD–AMN.

DIAGNOSIS

Moser *et al.* [338] have extended earlier observations [333,357] to develop diagnostic assays for the ALD homozygote, carrier detection and prenatal diagnosis [358]. In patients with ALD, elevated levels of VLCFA are found in virtually all tissues [358–361]. Diagnosis of the disease is done most conveniently by measuring hexacosanoate (C26:0) levels in red blood cell phospholipids or total plasma lipids [338], although reliable results have been obtained on cultured skin fibroblasts [346] or white blood cells [359]. Normal plasma levels of C26:0 are 0.33 ± 0.15 μg/ml. Values are unambiguously elevated in childhood ALD–AMN (1.6 ± 0.84 μg/ml), or in neonatal ALD (2.4 ± 0.73 μg/ml) [338].

According to Moser *et al.* [338], a reliable diagnostic procedure should include the determination of the plasma levels of C24:0, which are elevated, and of docosanoic acid (C22:0), a saturated unbranched fatty acid, which is normal in ALD. The increase in VLCFA can be expressed most readily by calculating the ratio of C26:0/C22:0 and C24:0/C22:0 in a total lipid extract of plasma and then in cultured skin fibroblasts if there is any doubt. With this precaution no false-positive tests have been observed. Strikingly elevated levels of C26:0 are found in Zellweger syndrome (2.5 ± 0.85 μg/ml), or in a related disorder, hyperpipecolic acidaemia [338]. ALD differs from these two disorders in its pattern of VLCFA accumulation: in the former the increase is confined to saturated VLCFA, while there is an increase in both monounsaturated and saturated VLCFA in the latter.

Carrier detection

Plasma levels of C26:0 are intermediate in heterozygotes (0.81 ± 0.33 μg/ml) [338]. Several approaches used in sequence (plasma assay, followed by fibroblast assay and study of BAER, and possibly an oral C26:0 loading test with peanut butter) permit the identification of 95% or more of women heterozygous for ALD. Systematic biochemical studies have enabled the disease to be recognized in young adults with cerebral dysfunction and misdiagnosed as having a brain tumour or psychosis, and in patients with adrenal insufficiency with a familial history of ALD. Abnormalities characteristic of ALD have also been found in the asymptomatic male relatives of ALD patients [338,346].

Carrier detection is of particular importance in view of the progressive neurological involvement that heterozygous carrier females may develop with age. This is possible by conventional biochemical analysis of VLCFA levels, but the test may lead to false-negative results and/or be difficult to interpret [341]. The use of multiple polymorphic DNA probes linked to the ALD gene is a second novel approach [362]. The combination of biochemical and molecular genetic analysis now allows extremely high accuracy in carrier detection [363].

Prenatal diagnosis

Prenatal diagnosis has been successfully made in both ALD [358] and Zellweger syndrome [338] on the elevation of the C26:0/C22:0 ratio in cultured amniocytes. Prenatal diagnosis of the disease has first been made by assay of VLCFA on amniocytes [341,364] and later on trophoblastic tissue [365]. More recently, molecular genetic studies, using multiple DNA probles from Wq28, allow a more accurate analysis of the genotypes in ALD families. Thus, linkage analysis at the Xq28 locus is now proposed in informative families for a more accurate prenatal diagnosis [366].

PATHOGENESIS

ALD belongs to the group of inherited lipid storage diseases. They are caused by abnormal fatty acid metabolism that leads to the accumulation of VLCFA as cholesterol esters and gangliosides in the brain, adrenal cortex and other organs [338]. The early observations of Schaumburg *et al.* [333] and Igarashi *et al.* [357] have pointed to the biochemical abnormalities in ALD–AMN, namely to the accumulation of saturated unbranched or monosaturated fatty acids with a carbon chain length of 24–30, particularly hexacosanoic acid (C26:0). These VLCFA may account for up to 40% of the total fatty acids of the cholesterol esters and gangliosides of the cerebral white matter and the adrenal cortex [346,357]. Accumulation of VLCFA is also found in sphingomyelin and other lipid fractions of plasma, red blood cells, white blood cells, cultured skin fibroblasts, cultured muscle cells and cultured amniocytes [338,361]. It is believed that normal catabolism of VLCFA involves a metabolic pathway which is distinct from that of other fatty acids, and that this pathway is genetically deficient in ALD patients [361]. Detailed studies have shown that oxidation of palmitate (C16:0) or stearate (C18:0) in ALD is normal, while that of lignolcerate (C24:0) or C26:0 is impaired [338]. Moser *et al.* suggest that ALD patients have a defect in the oxidation of VLCFA (C24:0 and longer), but not for the degradation of fatty acids with a chain length of 18 carbons or less. Such a defect probably accounts for the accumulation of VLCFA in virtually all tissues and lipid fractions. The enzymatic basis for the accumulation of VLCFA is still unknown. There are no abnormalities in the cholesterol esterase activity [361], but cholesterol synthesis capacity is impaired in cultured skin fibroblats [367].

Based on the observations that the oxidation of C24:0 is localized to the peroxisomes [360], that patients with Zellweger syndrome lack hepatic and renal peroxisomes and have striking elevation of VLCFA, Goldfisher [368] has proposed that ALD and Zellweger syndrome both represent peroxisomal disorders. These derive their name from the fact that enzymes involved in lipid metabolism are localized in peroxisomes [354,367]. The name of these intracellular organelles originates from the fact that enzymes which produce and degrade hydrogen peroxide are localized within this compartment. Peroxisomes also contain all or part of a number of different biochemical pathways. There is now considerable evidence that peroxisomes have a role not only in cholesterol oxidation but also in cholesterol biosynthesis [367]. However, a problem in assigning a single predominant function to the peroxisomes is that the complement of peroxisomal enzymes varies among organisms and cell types.

It has been shown that the activation of the VLCFA to their coenzyme A (CoA) derivatives is defective in the peroxisomal β-oxidation (review in [354]). Attempts to purify the VLCF–CoA synthetase have so far been unsuccessful. The gene coding for VLCFA–CoA synthetase, considered as a candidate gene for ALD, failed to detect homologous sequences on the X chromosome [356]. The putative ALD gene has recently been identified in the distal part of Xq28 which has deletions in one or several exons in six of 85 independent patients [369]. Surprisingly, this putative ALD gene not only does not code for VLCFA–CoA synthetase but has a very significant sequence identity with a 70 kD human and rat peroxisomal membrane protein (PMP 70) involved in peroxisome biogenesis belonging to the adenosine triphosphate (ATP)-binding cassette (ABC) superfamily [369]. Further studies are necessary to determine the role of this transport protein in the pathogeneis of ALD.

The adrenal insufficiency appears secondary to a destruction of the adrenal cortex, since there is substantial evidence that the accumulation of abnormal cholesterol esters is detrimental to adrenal cortical cells [338]. A contributing factor is that the abnormal fatty acid content of cholesterol esters transforms them into an abnormal substrate for cholesterol ester hydroxylase which may impair the availability of cholesterol for normal steroidogenesis. The pathogenesis of the ALD brain, spinal cord and peripheral nerve lesions is not understood. Furthermore, there is no correlation between levels of VLCFA in plasma and fibroblasts and the severity of the neurological disturbances [338].

Clinical heterogeneity and lack of correlation between plasma VLCFA and severity of the neurological manifestations has led to the conclusion that the lipid abnormalities are necessary but not sufficient for the pathogenesis of the neuropathology, and that additional pathogenetic mechanisms must play a role. Moser [370] hypothesized that immunological mechanisms are involved, and this is one of the bases for modern treatment (see below).

TREATMENT AND PROGNOSIS

Treatment of the adrenal insufficiency in ALD is replacement with gluco- and mineralocorticoids as in other cases of adrenal failure. There is no specific therapy for the neurological disorder and, except in isolated cases [338, 371], glucocorticoid therapy does not appear to improve the neurological status. Demonstration that the C26:0 acid which accumulates in the brain is of dietary origin [338] had led to the hope that dietary restriction might improve the course of the disease, but unfortunately this has not been the case [338]. Other therapeutic trials such as dietary oleic acid [372], association of plasmaphaeresis and diet, or immunosuppression have been disappointing [370].

Currently, two therapeutic approaches are used in an attempt to modify the neurological evolution of the disorders [337]. One consists of a lipid diet and the other is bone-marrow transplantation. The diet is both restricted in VLCFA and enriched in glycerol trioleate and trierucate. It is used in AMN, neurologically asymptomatic ALD patients with or without Addison disease, and in symptomatic heterozygotes. The diet is associated with immunological treatment in advanced cerebral forms.

First trials with bone-marrow transplant have normalized fatty acids, but did not influence the evolution of the neurological disease [370,372]. More recent experience suggests that bone-marrow transplantation can still be an approach aimed at reversing early cerebral lesions if made early enough [337]. At the moment the indication is in children with very early signs of the cerebral form [337]. It is too early to answer the important question whether the diet given to asymptomatic patients can prevent neurological deterioration.

The prognosis of the condition is that of the neurological disorder, which progresses inexorably. The average survival after clinical onset is 1–6 years in neonatal ALD, 1–9 years in childhood ALD, two decades or more in AMN and more than two decades in symptomatic heterozygotes [338] and in Zellweger syndrome.

Selective glucocorticoid deficiency

ISOLATED GLUCOCORTICOID INSUFFICIENCY

Isolated glucocorticoid insufficiency is a rare syndrome first reported by Shepard *et al.* [373] and also described by Migeon *et al.* [374] in six patients as 'congenital adrenal unresponsiveness to ACTH'. It is defined as isolated glucocorticoid deficiency unassociated with hypoaldosteronism. About 45 cases have been reported [375–390].

Genetics

Familial occurrence has been observed in all cases but one. The incidence is higher in males, but girls are also affected [377]. This disease is hereditary and is probably transmitted by autosomal recessive genes [385,387].

Pathological findings

The adrenal glands show a thick capsule, decreased thickness of the cortex and a normal medulla [374,387]. The morphological changes in the cortex differ markedly from those observed in congenital adrenal hypoplasia (see Fig. 28.3). The zona fasciculata and zona reticularis are almost absent, reduced to a narrow band of fibrous tissue hardly wider than the remnant of the involuted fetal zone which is seen normally between cortex and medulla in the first 2 years of life. In contrast, the zona glomerulosa is rather broad, has a normal structure but may be lipid-depleted. There is usually no lymphocytic infiltration as seen in autoimmune adrenalitis.

Clinical manifestation

First symptoms usually appear in early childhood (1–2 years) with convulsions, muscle weakness, severe hypoglycaemia or coma. Hyperpigmentation is characteristic. Tall stature has been reported in four children [379,381, 384]. The clinical features are those of primary adrenocortical insufficiency in general, without problems of salt loss. An uncommon association of the syndrome of ACTH insensitivity with achalasia and alacrima is described as the triple-A syndrome [377,385].

Familial isolated glucocorticoid deficiency associated with achalasia of the cardia and deficient tear production was first described by Allgrove *et al.* [391]. Since then a number of similar cases have been reported [377,392–395]. Recent studies indicate that there may be a loss of parasympathetic function in the disorder [377], and motor and sensory neuropathy have also been described [393,396]. Some patients develop more widespread neurological abnormalities (polyneuropathy with sensory, motor and autonomic components, Parkinsonism, signs of dorsal and pyramidal tract damage, and mental retardation) [389,397].

Laboratory findings

These confirm a selective defect in glucocorticoid production: low plasma cortisol, low 17-oxo and 17-oxogenic steroids which do not rise or rise only very little after ACTH stimulation. In contrast, the response of plasma aldosterone to ACTH is usually large [375], but it is variable, and may be absent [398]. Plasma ACTH levels are high. Mineralocorticoid function is usually normal or partially deficient [389] and aldosterone secretion rate before and after salt depletion and aldosterone plasma levels are normal [381,384,387]. Plasma renin activity is also normal and responds normally to orthostasis, salt restriction or to frusemide-induced diuresis [382]. Hypoglycaemia is frequent and associated with ketosis and hypoalaninaemia. Recently, adrenomedullary hyporesponsiveness has been described in this disease [382]. Whether this is a common feature is not yet established, since most patients have not been tested for adrenomedullary function. In one patient presenting with a multisystem involvement but no achalasia, alteration of plasma medium-chain fatty acid levels was found, suggesting a genetic disease of lipid metabolism [399]. The findings of low red-cell folate concentrations, and neurotransmitter amine metabolism disturbance in another case remain unexplained [397].

Pathogenesis

The pathogenesis of the disease is not fully understood. Migeon *et al.* [374] have observed that the *in vitro* cortisol production of a surgically removed adrenal gland was stimulated neither by ACTH nor by cyclic adenosine monophosphate (cAMP). However, cAMP increased corticosterone production. Hence, the pathogenesis of the adrenal disorder has long been thought to be due to an inherited defect within the adrenal gland causing primary unresponsiveness to ACTH [374]. The absence of steroidogenic response to ACTH has suggested a possible defect of the ACTH receptor. However, *in vitro* studies of ACTH binding showed no difference from normal, but the physiological significance of this binding is doubtful [385]. The ACTH receptor, belonging to the family of receptors coupled to guanine nucleotide-binding proteins, has recently been cloned [400]. Molecular genetic studies have been undertaken, but do not as yet explain the pathogenesis of the associated disorders. In one patient a point mutation was found in the sequence coding for the second transmembrane domain of the ACTH receptor [401], but no genetic lesion was found in five other families [402].

On the other hand, it is difficult to define a single genetic defect which could cause the characteristic triad of the triple-A syndrome. Moreover the occurrence of achalasia without adrenal insufficiency has been reported in several families [403]. It thus appears that the various manifestations observed in the triple-A syndrome, as well as in related syndromes [70], may well represent diseases due to mutations at distinct but adjacent gene loci, and the combination of the symptoms due to the extent of gene loss, as seen in X-linked congenital adrenal hypoplasia. Alternatively, the abnormalities may be, at least in some cases, secondary to an inherited progressive degenerative process of both the adrenal gland and the nervous system [377].

In favour of this view is the rather late onset of clinical signs (after 1 year of life) for a congenital defect and the deterioration of the response of the 17-oxogenic steroids to ACTH before the appearance of the clinical manifestations of mineralocorticoid deficiency, or before their increase in severity [384,390]. On the other hand, because of the association with achalasia and alacrima in some patients, it has been suggested, but not demonstrated experimentally, that the glucocorticoid failure may be the consequence of the loss of parasympathetic input to the adrenal gland [404].

Differential diagnosis

The differential diagnosis is that of primary adrenal hypofunction in general, other causes of severe hypoglycaemia, the various forms of secondary adrenal insufficiency such as hypopituitarism, and withdrawal of glucocorticoid therapy.

Differentiation from chronic Addison disease may be difficult since, in isolated glucocorticoid insufficiency, the mineralocorticoid function which is normal under basal conditions may show a slightly decreased functional capacity [387]. In another instance there was a lack of rise in urinary aldosterone in a 10-year-old patient, while the response was normal in the 5-year-old sister [390]. There may be dissociation in timing of the onset of gluco- and mineralocorticoid failure in Addison disease [405]. Definitive diagnosis can be made only after prolonged follow-up and repeated testing to provide evidence of no mineralocorticoid dysfunction.

Treatment

Replacement of glucocorticoids is the only therapy needed. Management is as in chronic adrenal insufficiency, and adequate preventive treatment should also be provided in cases of intercurrent infection, stress or surgery.

GLUCOCORTICOID RECEPTOR RESISTANCE

This rare disorder, also called primary cortisol resistance, is due to a functional abnormality of the glucocorticoid receptor. It is characterized by an increased activity of the hypothalamopituitary–adrenal axis, resulting in high ACTH and cortisol levels in order to overcome the peripheral decreased efficacy of cortisol at the target cell level. This hypercortisolism is not associated with other clinical or biochemical features of Cushing syndrome.

The disorder was first described in a patient presenting with hypertension and hypokalaemia [406], and was subsequently shown to be a familial disease [407] with an autosomal dominant inheritance pattern with variable penetrance, although a sporadic case has been reported [408]. Clinical manifestations are variable among patients, and partial cortisol resistance has been suggested in some [409]. Clinical symptoms are seldom observed and, when present, result from ACTH-dependent overproduction of nonglucocorticoid adrenal steroids. Elevated mineralocorticoid production causes hypertension in adults of both sexes. Elevated adrenal androgen production is asymptomatic in adult males, but in females it is responsible for acne, hirsutism and irregular menses [409,410].

Overproduction of adrenal androgens may cause inappropriate and early virilization in children presenting with primary cortisol resistance [411]. In a 6.5-year-old boy, isosexual precocity was the first symptom of the disease: despite high cortisol levels and moderately elevated ACTH levels the child had no clinical symptom of hypercortisolism but accelerated linear growth, advanced bone age, pubic hair stage 3, and elevated adrenal androgen levels, contrasting with prepubertal size testes and normal LH and FSH levels. Androgens were suppressed to the normal range for age only by high doses of dexamethasone, demonstrating both the ACTH dependence of the abnormal androgen secretion and the pituitary resistance to cortisol feedback. Thus, the diagnosis should be considered in boys with unexplained isosexual precocity and in girls with unexplained androgen excess.

Functional studies of the glucocorticoid receptor (GR) on peripheral mononuclear leukocytes or fibroblasts showed changes either in the apparent dissociation constant (reduced affinity) and/or in the number of receptors in most patients [410], but also qualitative abnormalities such as thermolability [409,410]. Direct analysis of messenger RNA (mRNA) and genomic DNA from two patients showed decreased levels of GR-mRNA, and an altered restriction enzyme pattern, suggesting a defect in the steroid-binding domain of the human GR gene [412]. Molecular studies of the GR in two other cases showed that the genetic defect involved only a single amino-acid substitution within the glucocorticoid-binding domain of the receptor [413,414].

Selective mineralocorticoid deficiency

CONGENITAL HYPOALDOSTERONISM

This term is restricted to cases of inborn errors of the last step of aldosterone biosynthesis [415,416]. The biosynthesis of aldosterone from corticosterone involves two enzymes successively: first a 18-hydroxylase (or corticosterone methyloxidase type I (CMO-I)) between corticosterone and 18-hydroxycorticosterone, and a last step between 18-hydroxycorticosterone and aldosterone catalysed by a 18-hydroxysteroid dehydrogenase (called isomerase, 18-oxidase or corticosterone methyloxidase type II, CMO-II) [416]. The corresponding inborn errors were identified by Ulick in 1976, and termed CMO-I and CMO-II deficiencies. These are rare inherited disorders transmitted as an autosomal recessive trait.

The clinical onset may occur as salt loss in infancy [417–420] with failure to thrive, vomiting, progressive dehydration, hyponatraemia, hyperkalaemia and normal renal function. However, clinical presentation is highly variable, from severe salt-losing crisis in infancy, failure to thrive or apparently isolated growth disturbance in young infants or children to asymptomatic forms in adults [417,421–424]. Associations with juvenile-onset diabetes mellitus or idiopathic hyperparathyroidism have been reported [425,426] but are probably coincidental. The pathogenesis of salt loss is still not fully understood, since it occurs in spite of high deoxycorticosterone (DOC) levels which are not suppressed by dexamethasone [424,427].

Diagnosis of the enzyme deficiency relies on the findings of decreased aldosterone production, elevated PRA or prorenin [428], but normal ACTH levels and normal glucocorticoid and androgen production [429] (Table 28.7).

Table 28.7 Main characteristics of the various causes of mineralocorticoid deficiency

	Aetiology	Inheritance	PRA	Aldosterone	Kalaemia	Treatment	Reference
Deficiency of aldosterone biosynthesis	Deficit in						
Type I	CMO-I	Autosomal recessive	↗	↘ $\frac{\text{18-OHB}}{\text{aldo}} < 5$	↗ or *n*	9α-Fluorocortisol	[416]
Type II	Deficit in CMO-II	Autosomal recessive	↗	↘ $\frac{\text{18-OHB}}{\text{aldo}} > 10$	↗ or *n*	9α-Fluorocortisol	[430]
Pseudohypoaldosteronism	Target cell insensitivity	Autosomal dominant	↗	↗↗	↗ or *n*	Sodium	[431,432]
Hyporeninaemic hypoaldosteronism	Primary renin deficiency	Sporadic or familial	↘	↘	↗	9α-Fluorocortisol	[433,434]
Syndrome hypokalaemia, normal blood pressure, and hyperreninaemia with hypoaldosteronism	Unknown	Sporadic	↗	↘	↘	Potassium	[435]

Determination of the ratio of 18-hydroxycorticosterone (18-OHB) to aldosterone (normal levels are 2 regardless of age) or that of their urinary metabolites (normal levels >6), have classically been used to recognize the site of the enzyme block [417,436]. The ratios are elevated in type II but normal in type I CMO deficiency [420]. These ratios are also useful in detecting mild or late-onset forms [433] or asymptomatic forms [436].

It is classically said that an increased corticosterone/18-OHB ratio is the more reliable index for the diagnosis of the CMO deficiency type I [430], and that the persistence of subnormal levels of 18-OHB did not rule out its diagnosis [419,430]. In fact, most reports of CMO deficiency have been of type II, whether in a large series of Iranian Jews [424] or in isolated families in Europe or North America [416,419]. In addition, reanalysis of original reports of CMO-I deficiency [420,437] indicate that the subjects actually had CMO-II deficiency [429,430]. However, a North American kindred was recently reclassified as being CMO type I [438].

Understanding of the molecular basis of primary aldosterone deficiency is rapidly progressing. It was first shown that a single cytochrome ($P450_{c11}$) catalysed the last two steps of aldosterone biosynthesis as well as the 11β-hydroxylation of DOC to corticosterone [439]. More recent studies indicate that in humans there are two distinct cytochrome P450 isoenzymes: the first (termed $P450_{c11}$ or P450X1BI) catalyses hydroxylation at position 11β in the zona fasciculata, while the second (termed $P450_{aldo}$, $P450_{c18}$, $P450_{cmo}$, P450X1B2 or aldosterone synthase P450) catalyses all three reactions (that is the conversion of DOC to aldosterone) in the zona glomerulosa [440]. These isoenzymes are encoded by two highly homologous structural genes, named respectively CYP11B1 and CYP11B2, which are both located on chromosome 8q22 [441]. The CYP11B2 gene was initially postulated to be a pseudogene or a closely related less active gene for $P450_{11\beta}$ [442]. It is in fact transcribed, but only in the zona glomerulosa [443]. The gene is regulated by angiotensin II, and mutations are found in persons who are unable to synthesize aldosterone, because of CMO-II deficiency [444–446]. Although not yet proven, it is believed that the biochemical phenotype seen in CMO-I deficiency results from different mutations in the CYP11B2 gene [438].

Differential diagnosis includes the syndrome hyperreninaemic hypoaldosteronism seen in critically ill children [447] which often has a bad prognosis independently of plasma potassium and 18-OHB levels, pseudohypoaldosteronism and other rare syndromes associated with hypoaldosteronism (see below and Table 28.7).

Treatment is mineralocorticoid replacement therapy (oral 9α-fluorocortisol, that is fludrocortisone) at a mean dosage of 150 μg/m^2 of body surface area per day. In infants the daily dose of about 20–30 μg is divided into two portions and a sodium chloride supplement of 2–3 g (34–51 mmol) is added to the daily diet and equally divided in feeds. In case of febrile acute illness supplements of both water and salt are indicated, especially during the night. If vomiting or symptoms of dehydration appear, i.v. infusion of sodium chloride may be necessary. The condition has a good prognosis, especially as symptoms of salt-wasting decrease with age [424]. This coincides with the maturation of the kidney for sodium reabsorption by a mechanism independent of aldosterone. Whether treatment should be maintained in adult life is controversial [430]. Although older subjects may remain asymptomatic after discontinuing therapy, the biochemical abnormalities persist. Evidence of chronic natriuresis and intravascular volume depletion suggest the need for lifelong therapy.

PSEUDOHYPOALDOSTERONISM

This disorder was first described in 1958 by Cheek & Perry [448] in a male infant in whom renal salt-wasting was associated with normal renal and adrenal function. Because the condition improved with sodium chloride supplementation, but was refractory to exogenous mineralocorticoid administration without added salt, these authors postulated that the disease was due to a defective renal tubular response to mineralocorticoids. Since then, more than 100 cases have been reported in the literature [449–454]. Familial occurrence has been recorded in most instances [455–458] but sporadic cases have been observed. In spite of a slight male predominance (58%), this disease appears to be inherited as an autosomal trait, but the data in the literature so far conflict with evidence of autosomal-dominant [452,457,458] as well as autosomal-recessive inheritance [456,459].

It is believed that the disorder is due to an end-organ defect, but the underlying mechanism is not yet fully established, although abnormal or absent mineralocorticoid receptors [431,460] or a postreceptor defect [461] have been demonstrated. Both modes of inheritance agree with the mapping of the mineralocorticoid receptor gene to chromosome 4 [462]. Two recent studies [450,452] provide further evidence for two autosomal modes of inheritance, and demonstrate the frequency of hormonal and receptor abnormalities in asymptomatic members of affected families. Thus the frequency of the disease may be underestimated.

The natural history and clinical presentation are variable [455,463], from fulminant presentation in a premature infant [464] to asymptomatic forms in adults [424]. It may even manifest *in utero*, causing fetal polyuria and hydramnios [465]. In the severe forms the constant feature is early onset (before the seventh month of life) of progressive or severe salt-wasting. In other infants the symptoms are chronic failure to thrive, lethargy, vomiting and poor feeding [456,457]. In older children the history may be limited to growth failure and ultimate short stature [456]. Diagnosis may be made incidentally later in life, at the occasion of family studies of a patient with pseudohypoaldosteronism (PHA) [463].

Diagnosis is made on the findings of high levels of plasma aldosterone (up to 3000–15 000 pg/ml, or about 8000–45 000 pmol/l) or urinary aldosterone metabolites, high PRA and normal renal histology and function [446]. In older children or adults with asymptomatic forms the diagnosis can easily be made on the concomitant elevation in plasma aldosterone levels and plasma renin activity (or active renin) [405,428]. Unresponsiveness to the administration of mineralocorticoids is typical, not only in distal or proximal tubules but also in other salt-retaining organs such as the colon, sweat and salivary glands [467]. In order to estimate the action of aldosterone at the level of late distal and cortical collecting tubules, a new non-invasive test has been designed [468,469] and validated [470]. The calculation of transtubular potassium concentration gradient (TTKG) is made by dividing the ratio of urinary potassium concentration : (urine/plasma) osmolality by the potassium concentration in venous blood. TTKG is >5 when aldosterone is present, and <3 in the absence of mineralocorticoid activity [470, 471].

Pseudohypoaldosteronism is a complex syndrome which includes several mechanisms and aetiologies, since salt loss may be of renal and/or salivary and sweat gland origin. Several clinical entities may be recognized: (a) the classical form of primary PHA, due to renal tubular insensitivity as described above; (b) a general target cell insensitivity to aldosterone with kidney, intestine, and sweat and salivary gland dysfunction [467,472]; (c) PHA due to sweat gland dysfunction, without urinary salt loss and without cystic fibrosis [473]; (d) PHA due to salivary gland dysfunction [474].

Distinction is now made between PHA type I and type II. Type I PHA is the primary form of PHA, with two clinically and genetically distinct entities, that is with either renal or multiple target organ defect [451]. Type II HPA is the 'chloride-shunt syndrome'. This was described in a patient with mineralocorticoid-resistant renal hyperkalaemia in whom renal potassium excretion increased normally when the distal delivery of sodium was increased with non-chloride anions, such as sulphate and bicarbonate [475]. The proposal was that the primary defect was an abnormal increase in the reabsorption of chloride by the renal tubule (chloride shunting). This hypothesis was confirmed in other patients presenting the same tubular defect with a presumably autosomal-dominant inheritance [476].

Differential diagnosis is also with secondary forms of PHA, which are rarely observed in children. Partial tubular insensitivity to aldosterone may account for hyperkalaemia observed after unilateral renal vein thrombosis or neonatal medullary necrosis [477]. A syndrome of transient renal tubular resistance has been observed in infants with obstructive uropathy and urinary tract infection, the diagnosis of which should always be ruled out before the diagnosis of primary PHA is accepted. The last differential diagnosis is with a variant of PHA described as the syndrome of 'early-childhood hyperkalaemia' in infants and young children with failure to thrive or growth retardation in whom the only biochemical abnormalities were hyperkalaemia and metabolic acidosis [478]. This syndrome is probably due to a maturation disorder in the function of aldosterone receptors. This is transient and, at about 5 years of age, therapy is no longer needed [478, 479].

Treatment is still symptomatic with high-sodium diet. Therapeutic trials with high doses of mineralocorticoids [432], or indomethacin [449] remain isolated experiences. Daily doses of salt supplementation vary according to the severity of salt wastage. In infants the dose is 10–25 mmol/kg a day (0.6–1.5 g/kg) in four or five divided doses. Sodium balance is monitored by measuring sodium and other electrolytes. It is more hazardous to adjust sodium needs to plasma renin levels because of the marked (daily, individual and age) variations in this parameter. Spontaneous clinical improvement occurs with advancing age, despite the persistence of elevated aldosterone production and other biochemical features. This is unexplained, but enables a patient eventually to discontinue therapy. However, it appears advisable to maintain salt supplementation for several years in order to avoid growth retardation [424]. With this precaution, growth and development are otherwise normal.

SYNDROMES ASSOCIATED WITH HYPOALDOSTERONISM (see Table 28.7)

Hyporeninaemic hypoaldosteronism

This syndrome is characterized by an inappropriately low aldosterone secretion without an associated impairment in cortisol synthesis. It was first described in 1957 [480], as a syndrome of aldosterone deficiency, and the hyporeninaemia recognized in 1972 [481]. It is the most common form of isolated hypoaldosteronism in adulthood and is attributed to impaired renin release from the kidney. The typical clinical presentation is unexplained asymptomatic hyperkalaemia and mild to moderate renal insufficiency (creatinine clearance >15 ml/min) in 50–70-year-old subjects. Muscle weakness or cardiac arrhythmia is seldom seen, but diabetes mellitus is present in about half the cases, often associated with either pyelonephritis, nephrolithiasis, polycystic disease, nephrosclerosis or drug abuse [433]. Other associated diseases include systemic lupus erythematosus, multiple myeloma, renal amyloidosis, cirrhosis, sickle-cell anaemia and AIDS [247,482].

This syndrome has rarely been reported in infancy [483] but its frequency may be higher than usually recognized in children with moderate renal insufficiency [471]. The condition has been observed in a 5-month-old boy, co-existing with severe lactic acidosis, mental retardation and deafness [434], and in a 3-month-old boy presenting with growth failure and severe psychomotor retardation [483]. A familial occurrence has been reported [433] where the clinical onset was congenital in the two affected brothers who presented with salt loss, growth retardation, low basal levels of PRA and aldosterone, but a normal aldosterone rise in response to ACTH, and normal to subnormal angiotensinogen levels. Systematic studies revealed normal PRA but low angiotensinogen levels in the father, and normal biological parameters in the mother. An interesting feature of all these cases was the presence of salt-wasting, a condition rarely observed in cases of hyporeninaemic hypoaldosteronism associated with chronic renal insufficency.

The pathogenesis of this syndrome is not clear [484]. The anomalies may result from damage to the juxtaglomerular apparatus, impaired conversion of precursors of renin to the active hormone, insufficient sympathetic stimulation of renin-producing cells, inhibition of renin release by hyperkalaemia, physiological suppression of renin release by volume expansion and altered synthesis of renal prostaglandins. The most recent hypothesis supports the view that prostacyclin deficiency is a key factor in the development of the syndrome [485]. These proposed mechanisms do not not explain why the disease is an acquired secondary aldosterone deficiency in adults, but a congenital, and possibly hereditary, disorder in the paediatric age group. Treatment must take into consideration the age of the patient and the other associated disorders. Mineralocorticoid replacement is usually necessary in children, but is reserved in adult patients for those who have severe hyperkalaemia and no hypertension or congestive heart failure.

Hyperreninaemic hypoaldosteronism

A syndrome associating hypokalaemia, normal blood pressure, hyperreninaemia and hypoaldosteronism has been described in rare sporadic cases (see Table 28.7). A similar condition is exceptionally seen in patients with metastatic cancer to the adrenal gland [486]. Persistent hypotensive, critically ill patients also have inappropriately low plasma aldosterone concentrations contrasting with an active renin–angiotensin system [447]. In this subgroup of patients the defect is probably in zona glomerulosa function, because it is not associated with any particular state of the underlying disease or therapy [487]. For some authors this selective hypoaldosteronism results from an impairment in angiotensin production [487] or a combination of insensitivity to angiotensin II and tubular unresponsiveness to mineralocorticoid [488].

The hereditary syndrome of low production of aldosterone, severe hypertension and hypokalaemic alkalosis [489] was in the past believed to represent a secondary form of hypoaldosteronism, due to the renal tubular wastage of potassium. This syndrome is rather a form of apparent mineralocorticoid excess, recently identified as being specifically associated with a defect in 3β-hydroxysteroid dehydrogenase (see Chapter 29).

TRANSIENT HYPOALDOSTERONISM IN INFANCY

It has been proposed that delay in the normal process of maturation of the zona glomerulosa which normally follows birth, and/or immaturity of the renal distal tubular response to aldosterone, could explain some transient hypoaldosteronism states in which no enzymatic defect and normal renal function are found.

ACQUIRED AND IATROGENIC HYPOALDOSTERONISM

The impairment of aldosterone production may be acquired [490]. It has also been shown that autoimmune disorders [491] or amyloidosis [492] induce some clinical manifestations of aldosterone deficiency in adults. These are exceptional in paediatric patients. Hypoaldosteronism is observed with some brain tumours and in orthostatic hypotension, in which aldosterone secretion is not stimulated by salt restriction, ACTH or angiotensin II [493]. The condition results from chronic hypostimulation due to impaired renin secretion rather than from a primary disturbance in adrenal biosynthesis. In chronic treatment by indomethacin [494] or chronic lead poisoning [495], hypoaldosteronism is secondary to decreased renin activity and renal insufficiency. Specific inhibition of aldosterone secretion may occur by an unknown mechanism in long-term heparin treatment [496]. Orthostatic hypotension, the common feature of these various conditions, is improved by mineralocorticoid therapy.

Selective androgen deficiency

Production of adrenal androgen, as reflected by decreased urinary excretion of Δ^5-3β-hydroxysteroids, is relatively more impaired than that of glucocorticoids in certain forms of congenital adrenal hyperplasia or in anencephalic babies (see below). In the premature neonate with intrauterine growth retardation the urinary excretion of Δ^5-3β-hydroxysteroids may also be selectively decreased, while urinary excretion of cortisol metabolites and the response of plasma cortisol to ACTH are normal [497].

The prepubertal rise in the secretion of adrenal androgens (adrenarche) may be delayed in patients with constitutional delay of gonadal puberty (gonadarche) but is not in hypogonadotrophic, hypogonadal patients [498]. In the author's experience delayed adrenarche is found in patients with severe constitutional short stature, whether or not gonadarche is delayed. Absence or delay in adrenarche is also observed in subjects presenting with isolated growth hormone deficiency, but normal ACTH reserve [499].

All these apparently unrelated situations have some common features: the functional impairment is selectively related to one of the morphological zones of the adrenal cortex, deficient fetal zone in the premature infant or neonate, and deficient activation of the reticular zone in older children. The non-ACTH dependence and apparent lack of specific stimulation of either zone has been discussed in all these conditions. Growth problems are associated in all situations. The evidence for a pituitary hormone controlling adrenal androgen secretions, either in the fetal cortex or the adult reticulosa [8,88,500,501] is not yet convincing [502].

This putative hormone has been named AASH (adrenal androgen-stimulating hormone [503]) or cortical androgen-stimulating hormone (CASH) [504]. Recently it has been proposed that CASH was the proximal 18 amino-acid hinge region of the joint peptide of pro-opiomelanocortin (POMC) [505]. However, the identity of POMC-(79-86) as a physiologically important CASH remains uncertain, since this peptide was unable to affect steroidogenesis in primary cultures of either fetal [506] or adult [507] human adrenal cells.

Secondary hypoadrenocorticism

DEFINITION, PATHOGENESIS AND AETIOLOGY

Adrenal hypofunction secondary to a decreased secretion of ACTH can be caused by a variety of pituitary and hypothalamic abnormalities, either congenital or acquired. In all brain malformations such as anencephaly, rhinencephaly, cobocephaly or porencephaly [69,70,508, 509], pituitary atrophy is usually secondary to the hypothalamic defect. Congenital aplasia of the pituitary gland may be associated, however [43]. Isolated aplasia of the anterior pituitary [510,511] or an empty sella [512,513] have also been described.

Isolated corticotrophin deficiency may occur but is rare [513–517], and may be congenital [518]. It is classically reported that isolated ACTH deficiency is not associated with other endocrine abnormalities. However, it becomes apparent that the association with primary thyroid insufficiency is not uncommon. Several cases have been described [512], in whom adrenal insufficiency has been precipitated during thyroxine replacement therapy. Whether the association is coincidental is not established. Finally, isolated ACTH deficiency has been seen as one of the autoimmune polyendocrine syndromes [264,519].

The defect is probably at the pituitary level because the ACTH response to corticotrophin-releasing hormone (CRH) is usually blunted [520]. The disorder has many causes, but is due to an autoimmune process in most instances. This belief is based on the frequent association with other autoimmune disorders [521], the finding of antipituitary antibodies in half the cases in one series [522], or of anticorticotroph antibodies in another case [523].

Most frequently, ACTH deficiency occurs as part of hypopituitarism either idiopathic, following irradiation of the head, or due to tumours such as craniopharyngioma in children or chromophobe adenoma after adolescence. In the two latter conditions, complete panhypopituitarism usually follows surgical treatment. Congenital forms of hypopituitarism have been reported [524,525].

CLINICAL AND BIOLOGICAL FEATURES

Glucocorticoid and androgen deficiencies are typical of secondary hypoadrenalism. Aldosterone production is normal and responds normally to salt deprivation. With the exception of the congenital form of hypopituitarism, which is associated with severe neonatal hypoglycaemia and micropenis [525], adrenal hypofunction is less severe in isolated ACTH deficiency or in hypopituitarism than in primary adrenal insufficiency. However, acute adrenal crisis including salt loss and vascular collapse can also be precipitated by an intercurrent stress. Neonatal chlolestasis, often associated with hypoglycaemia, may be a consequence of cortisol deficiency [526]. Associated growth hormone deficiency accentuates the tendency to hypoglycaemia, whereas associated hypothyroidism somewhat compensates for the low secretion of cortisol by decreasing its metabolic clearance. On the other hand, an impaired growth hormone response to stimuli may be the consequence of the hypocortisolism, and thus be reversible during glucocorticoid replacement therapy [527].

Plasma levels of ACTH are low. Levels of plasma cortisol or urinary 17-oxogenic steroids are usually at the lower limit of normal. The association of low dehydroepiandrosterone sulphate (DHEAS) levels [528,529] reflects the deficient secretion of ACTH and may be of the putative pituitary factor involved in adrenal androgen secretions (see above). A positive diagnosis is made by dynamic tests of ACTH reserve. Fetal ACTH deficiency is one of the specific causes of low maternal oestriol levels throughout pregnancy [530]. Therefore, a prenatal diagnosis based on longitudinal study of maternal oestriol levels, can be made in families with a clinical history of the disease.

DIFFERENTIAL DIAGNOSIS BETWEEN PRIMARY AND SECONDARY HYPOADRENALISM

Absence of hyperpigmentation and low plasma levels of ACTH are strong indicators of pituitary defect [531]. One should bear in mind that these findings do not totally exclude secondary hypoadrenalism, since low ACTH levels and skin hyperpigmentation are found in exceptional cases of hypothalamic deficiency of CRH [532]. Lipotrophin deficiency may be associated with that of ACTH [533].

Metyrapone tests

The standard test involves giving 750 mg of metyrapone orally every 4 h, or 24 h starting at 0800 h. Dosages are adapted for body size in small children. Urine is collected the day before, the day of and the day after administration of metyrapone, and 17-oxogenic steroids measured. Specific measurement of 11-deoxycortisol in plasma or urine, and daily determination of the plasma levels of ACTH, are preferable. Normal response is characterized by the doubling of urinary steroids and ACTH levels. Even during the test the diurnal variation of ACTH is conserved [534].

Shorter oral or intravenous metyrapone tests have been proposed [535,536]. The oral test consists of giving 40 mg/kg of metyrapone with milk at about midnight and collecting blood 8 h later, prior to food ingestion. Response is considered as normal when the concentration of 11-deoxycortisol in plasma is greater than 7 μg/gl. In this protocol, because of the vomiting effect of the drug, plasma cortisol should be measured specifically to ensure that blockade in cortisol biosynthesis has occurred [537].

The intravenous test is widely used nowadays. Metyrapone (30 mg/kg in normal saline) is infused over a 4-h period and blood collected 4 h after ending the perfusion. In both protocols, response is considered as normal when the concentration of 11-deoxycortisol in plasma is > 7 μg/dl at the end of the tests.

ACTH-stimulation tests

These tests are performed using tetracosactrin (1–24 ACTH, Cortrosyn, Synacthen). The compound is short-lived but when adsorbed onto zinc phosphate its effect is prolonged.

Short ACTH tests are easy to perform in ambulatory conditions [538]. There is no need for fasting and the test can be done at any time of the day. A basal blood sample is taken. Tetracosactrin (250 μg) is administered either i.m. or i.v. Blood samples are taken 30 and 60 min later. Normal response is when cortisol levels rise at either time by more than 7 μg/dl (190 nmol/l) or to above 20 μg/dl (600 nmol/l) [538–540]. Lower doses may have a greater sensitivity in detecting mild adrenal insufficiency.

Long ACTH tests use depot tetracosactrin. After a single i.m. injection of 1 mg, maximal cortisol response (30–50 μg/dl) is seen at 8 h, whereas after six 12-hourly i.m. injections of 0.5 μg/m^2 of the drug, plasma cortisol levels normally reach 50–80 μg/dl at all ages except in the first 6 months of life, where the rise in cortisol is much greater [541].

ACTH testing is necessary to differentiate primary and secondary adrenal failure when the metyrapone test is abnormal. A lack of rise of cortisol is typical of Addison disease, but in patients with secondary adrenal insufficiency there may be a small rise in cortisol after short ACTH stimulation. These two groups can be further differentiated by the 3-day stimulation test.

Other dynamic tests

Pyrogen test, lysin vasopressin test or insulin-induced hypoglycaemia stimulate the release of CRF and thus of ACTH. The first two have been abandoned because of unpleasant side-effects and the third should be performed with caution. It has, however, the advantage that it can be used to assess growth hormone as well as ACTH release. Normal response is when plasma corticosteroids rise by at least 6 μg/dl (165 nmol/l) to a maximum over 20 μg/dl (550 nmol/l). More recently, the use of CRH stimulation has been advocated as quite useful in the differential diagnosis between primary and secondary adrenal insufficiency [542,543].

TREATMENT AND PROGNOSIS

Secondary adrenal insufficiency requires glucocorticoid replacement. Treatment is the same as in Addison disease, but smaller doses are required.

Tertiary hypoadrenalism

Any process that involves the hypothalamus and interferes with the secretion of CRH can cause tertiary adrenal insufficiency. Such processes involve tumours, cranial irradiation or infiltrative disease such as sarcoidosis. Tertiary adrenal insufficiency also occurs in patients who are cured of Cushing syndrome by removal of a pituitary or non-pituitary ACTH-secreting or adrenal cortisol-secreting tumour. However, the most frequent cause of tertiary hypoadrenalism is chronic pharmacological administration of glucocorticoids. Such treatment decreases CRH synthesis and secretion by the hypothalamus, blocking its tropic and secretagogue actions on the pituitary corticotrophs, which decrease in size and in amount of ACTH synthesized and stored. This represents one form of iatrogenic adrenal insufficiency.

The differentiation between secondary and tertiary adrenal insufficiency can be made with a CRH test. There is little or no ACTH response in patients with secondary adrenal insufficiency, whereas patients with tertiary adrenal insufficiency usually have an exaggerated and prolonged ACTH release [543–545]. However, making this distinction is rarely important from a therapeutic standpoint.

Iatrogenic hypoadrenalism

GLUCOCORTICOID THERAPY

Adrenal atrophy resulting from exogenous administration of glucocorticoids is by far the commonest cause of hypoadrenalism in paediatric patients, but it is also the only reversible one. Primary and tertiary adrenal hypofunctions and combined adrenal atrophy are secondary to the suppression of CRH and ACTH by the glucocorticoid treatment via the negative-feedback mechanism (see Fig. 28.2). However, adrenal atrophy often persists after the pituitary has recovered. Natural or synthetic glucocorticoids (see Table 28.6) are used at physiological or pharmacological doses in a wide variety of diseases. Whether the underlying disease is well controlled, there is eventually an attempt to withdraw glucocorticoid therapy.

During the course of such treatment, except for the risk of developing severe osteopenia [546], the patient may remain healthy but, when treatment is interrupted or when there is intercurrent illness or stress, the demand for cortisol cannot be met by the atrophic adrenal glands, and an Addisonian crisis may be observed, even during a course of high-dose glucocorticoid therapy [547]. The same situation occurs in a neonate whose mother has been treated over a long period with glucocorticoids [91,548,549] or who has developed Cushing syndrome during pregnancy [89,90]. The extent of adrenal insufficiency relates both to dosage and duration of treatment, and also to the timing and mode of administration. The parenteral route causes more suppression than the oral route. Topical administration has the least suppressive effect. However, adrenal suppression may occur after long-term treatment at subnormal levels, or after steroid administration for as little as 3 days, depending on the dose and time of the day [163,164,550–552]. Unexpected side-effects can even be observed in asthmatic children treated with normal-dose long-term inhaled steroids, such as growth failure [553], and acute adrenal insufficiency may occur after discontinuation of therapy [554].

In the management of the condition four types of problems must be considered: prevention and recovery of adrenal atrophy, withdrawal from glucocorticoid therapy and assessment of the return to normal functioning of the hypothalamopituitary–adrenal axis (HPA).

Prevention

Prevention of iatrogenic hypoadrenalism has been attempted by giving the total 48-h dose as a single dose every other day rather than in daily doses. The well-known diurnal variations of the HPA activity governed by the sleep–wake pattern are the basis for the alternate-day steroid therapy which has been widely employed for over 20 years. It would appear that, with this protocol, inhibition of HPA and side-effects are less severe; in particular, growth is less inhibited [555].

Recovery

The sequence of recovery, at least after a short treatment period of 1–2 weeks, is characterized first by a return to normal of ACTH secretion, followed by sequential returns to normal of CRH and adrenal steroid secretion [556]. The inhibitory effect of chronic glucotherapy is more persistent on adrenal androgen secretions (dehydroepiandrosterone (DHEA), DHEAS) than it is on cortisol secretion [528]. Long-term and high-dose treatment would require a longer period of recovery. CRH testing appears to be most useful for the detection of the disturbed HPA function upon the discontinuation of steroid therapy [543,557].

As long as recovery of the HPA is incomplete, patients should be treated as Addisonian in case of intercurrent stress, illness or surgery. The best policy is to maintain this preventive attitude for the whole year following cessation of steroid therapy.

Withdrawal of steroid therapy

Several protocols have been proposed [163,551,558,559]. It is generally considered that acute steroid treatment with short-acting drugs administered for <3 days can be discontinued at once. When duration of steroid treatment is 3–10 days the daily dose must either be tapered, changed to a single morning dose, then to an alternate-day regime, or be weaned by reducing the daily dose by 30%, before discontinuation. Treatment is stopped when the therapeutic dosage reaches the equivalent of half the physiological secretion rate of cortisol.

In cases of chronic high-dose therapy, gradual tapering of the dosage must be accomplished over several weeks or months, but the proposed protocols differ: one can consider whether to reduce the dose by 25% each week [163] or to taper the high dosage as quickly as possible to 40 mg of cortisol or its equivalent, then to reduce the dosage by 10% every month to the stopping point defined above. A more detailed protocol has been advised by Byyny [551]. It starts with rapid decrements (2–5 mg of prednisone or equivalent every 3–7 days) to physiological doses. At that point, whatever the drug used before, the patient is switched to a single oral morning dose of short-acting cortisol, as the evening dose must be withdrawn first. Between 2 and 4 weeks later the morning dose of cortisol is reduced by 2.5 mg every week to 10 mg or the lower limits of physiological secretion, according to body size, to enhance pituitary recovery. This maintenance dose is stopped when circulating cortisol levels are > 10 μg/dl in the morning before taking the daily medication. Supplement or 'coverage' therapy is continued until complete recovery of HPA function. This may take 9 months.

Assessment of HPA function

The major problem in steroid withdrawal is the difficulty of determining when complete recovery from steroid suppression has occurred. Intermittent stimulation by ACTH has been proposed to stimulate adrenal secretion; the metyrapone test or insulin-induced hypoglycaemic tolerance test should theoretically be preferred, but these tests are not easy to perform. The short i.m. or i.v. ACTH test (250 μg of tetracosactrin) can easily be performed monthly until the response is normal (see above). At this point it is assumed that HPA recovery is complete, since the adrenal cortex usually lags behind the pituitary in recovering normal function. One should, however, bear in mind that the steroid withdrawal syndrome (consisting of anorexia, nausea, vomiting, fever, headache, weight loss, postural hypotension and lethargy) may develop even when a normal adrenal response to ACTH is observed. Although it is not clear if, in these conditions, the syndrome is related to adrenal deficiency or to the underlying disease, complete testing of the HPA must be performed before considering that adrenal function has definitely recovered. Finally, it must be kept in mind that primary adrenal insufficiency may be masked by intercurrent glucocorticoid therapy [560].

OTHER IATROGENIC CAUSES OF ADRENAL INSUFFICIENCY

These include surgical and medical treatment of adrenal tumours. During surgery, treatment should be that explained above. Bilaterally adrenalectomized patients must be treated for life as Addisonian patients. After removal of an adrenocortical adenoma, maintenance therapy and coverage should be maintained as long as the contralateral adrenal has not recovered from atrophy.

Medical treatment by inhibitors of steroid biosynthesis such as *o,p*′DDD or aminoglutethimide lead to clinical and biochemical adrenocortical insufficiency [561]. Aminoglutethimide may also have indirect virilizing effects, as in the case of pseudohermaphroditism reported in a female child whose mother was treated up to the eighth month of pregnancy [537].

A number of drugs may be an iatrogenic cause of primary adrenal sufficiency. The first group are drugs interfering with steroid biosynthesis [562], such as the antiepileptic aminoglutethimide [563,564], the antimycotic ketoconazole [565], the antiparasitic suramin [566], or the anaesthetic etomidate [567], also danazol [568] or metyrapone [569]. Drugs inducing hepatic mixed-function oxygenase enzymes, thus accelerating the metabolism of cortisol and of most synthetic steroids, include barbiturates [562], phenytoin [570], or rifampicin [562,571]. In neither case do these drugs usually lead to hypocortisolism in subjects with a normal HPA, because they are able to increase their ACTH secretion, which in turn overrides the blockade and the incipient fall in cortisol. The drugs produce clinical adrenal insufficiency in patients with limited adrenal or pituitary reserve or in those with adrenal insufficiency who are receiving replacement steroids. This is the case for AIDS patients in whom ketoconazole or rifampicin used to treat opportunistic infections may precipitate adrenal crisis in those with unsuspected partial adrenal insufficiency [572]. Therapy with cortisol in physiological doses is recommended in any case of drug-induced adrenal insufficiency.

ADRENAL MEDULLA HYPOFUNCTION

Production of adrenaline by the chromatin cells of the adrenal medulla is impaired after severe stress such as extensive burns, after adrenalectomy (when a destruction process of the adrenal cortex extends to the medulla) and in other forms of adrenocortical hypofunction. It also results from reduced phenylethanol amine-*N*-methyl transferase activity, which is cortisol-dependent. However, the clinical consequences are few.

Diseases such as idiopathic orthostatic hypotension, McQuarrie–Zetterström syndrome or idiopathic hypoglycaemia affecting young infants up to about the sixth year of life do not appear to be due to defective synthesis of epinephrine by the medulla. Hypothalamic defect or functional disorder of the sympathetic nervous system is responsible.

Familial dysautonomia, Riley–Day syndrome, is a recessive disease associated with disturbance in the liberation of catecholamines (inadequate release of norepinephrine on orthostatism) and is characterized by defective lacrimation in all cases. This disease affects only Jewish families; onset is very early in life. Dysphagia, recurrent bronchopneumonia, hypotension or hypertensive crisis, relative indifference to pain, motor incoordination, hyporeflexia, hyperhydrosis and absence of taste buds on the tongue are the clinical features. Typical biological findings are a decrease in vanilmandelic acid and an increase in homovanillic acid excretions [573]. The basic disorder is an inborn defect in dopamine-β-hydroxylase enzyme [574]. Treatment is only symptomatic.

REFERENCES

1 Oparil S, Haber E. The renin–angiotensin system. *N Engl J Med* 1974;291:389–401;446–57.

2 Peart WS. The functions for renin and angiotensin. *Rec Prog Horm Res* 1965;21:73–118.

3 Quinn SJ, Williams GH. Regulation of aldosterone secretion. *Ann Rev Physiol* 1988;50:409–26.

4 Favara BE, Franciosi RA, Miles V. Idiopathic adrenal hypoplasia in children. *Am J Clin Pathol* 1972;57:287–96.

5 Laverty CR, Fortune DW, Beischer NA. Congenital idiopathic adrenal hypoplasia. *Obstet Gynecol* 1973;41:655–64.

6 Daamen CBF. Adrenal hypoplasia during the perinatal period. *Arch Dis Child* 1970;45:148.

7 Sikl R. Addison's disease due to congenital hypoplasia of the adrenals in an infant aged 33 days. *J Pathol Bacteriol* 1948; 60:323–9.

8 Shackleton CHL, Swift PGF, Savage DCL *et al.* Deficient 3β-hydroxy-5-ene steroid secretion by newborn infants. *J Clin Endocrinol Metab* 1974;49:247–51.

9 Sperling MA, Wolfsen AR, Fisher DA. Congenital adrenal hyperplasia: an isolated defect of organogenesis. *J Pediatr* 1973;82:444–9.

10 Carlström FG, Björk G, Eneroth P *et al.* Perinatal adrenal anomaly associated with total absence of 3β-hydroxy-5-ene steroids in the infant's urine. *J Steroid Biochem* 1975;6: xxxiii–iv (Abstr. 75).

11 Crabbé J, Vandeput Y, Blizzard RM. Diminution de l'excrétion urinaire d'adrènaline dans l'insuffisance corticosurrénale primaire. *Ann Endocrinol* 1972;33:544–7.

12 Denys P, Corbeel L, Malbrain H. Hypocorticisme simple congénital. *Acta Paediatr Belgica* 1955;9:169–82.

13 Dunn JM. Anterior pituitary and adrenal absence of a liveborn normocephalic infant. *Am J Obstet Gynecol* 1966;96: 893–4.

14 Geppert LJ, Spencer WA, Richmond AM. Adrenal insufficiency in infancy. *J Pediatr* 1950;37:1.

15 Moore FP, Cermak E. Adrenal cysts and adrenal insufficiency in an infant with fatal termination. *J Pediatr* 1950; 36:91–5.

16 Provenzano RW. Adrenocortical hypoplasia in the newborn infant. *N Engl J Med* 1950;242:87.

17 Welsh JB, Mehlin GB. Congenital adrenal aplasia. *Am J Dis Child* 1954;87:319–20.

18 Williams A, Robinson MJ. Addison's disease in infancy. *Arch Dis Child* 1956;31:265–9.

19 Boyd JF, MacDonald AM. Adrenal cortical hypoplasia in siblings. *Arch Dis Child* 1960;35:561–8.

20 Brook CGD, Bambach M, Zachmann M *et al.* Familial congenital adrenal hypoplasia. *Helv Paediatr Acta* 1973;28:277–82.

21 Fournier A, Pauli A, Cousin J *et al.* L'insuffisance surrénale du nourrisson. *Pédiatrie* 1972;27:243–56.

22 Hay JD. Pubertal failure in congenital adrenocortical hypoplasia. *Lancet* 1977;2:1035.

23 Mitchell RG, Rhaney K. Congenital adrenal hypoplasia in siblings. *Lancet* 1959;1:488–92.

24 Mosier HD. Hypoplasia of the pituitary and adrenal cortex. Report of occurrence in twin siblings and autopsy findings. *J Pediatr* 1956;48:633–9.

25 O'Donohoe NV, Holland PDJ. Familial congenital adrenal hypoplasia. *Arch Dis Child* 1968;43:717–23.

26 Pakravan P, Kenny FM, Depp R *et al.* Familial congenital absence of adrenal glands: evaluation of glucocorticoids, mineralocorticoid and estrogen metabolism in the perinatal period. *J Pediatr* 1974;84:74–8.

27 Petersen KE, Bille T, Jacobsen BB, Versen T. X-linked congenital adrenal hypoplasia. A study of five generations of a Greenlandic family. *Acta Paed Scand* 1982;71:947–51.

28 Polonovski C, Zittoun R, Mary F. Hypocorticisme global, hypoaldostéronisme du nourrisson (trois observations). *Arch Fr Pédiatr* 1965;22:1061–86.

29 Rosseli A, Barbosa LT. Congenital hypoplasia of the adrenal glands. Report of two cases in sisters with necropsy. *Pediatrics* 1965;35:70–5.

30 Uttley WS. Familial congenital adrenal hypoplasia. *Arch Dis Child* 1968;43:724–30.

31 Wittenberg DF. Familial X-linked adrenocortical hypoplasia. Association with androgenic precocity. *Arch Dis Child* 1981;56:633–6.

32 Zondek LH, Zondek T. Congenital adrenal hypoplasia in two infants. *Acta Paed Scand* 1968;57:250–4.

33 Cathro DM. Adrenal cortex and medulla. In: Hubble D, ed. *Pediatric Endocrinology*. Oxford: Blackwell Scientific Publications, 1969;187–327.

34 Seeliger H. Nebennierenrindeninsuffizienz bei angeborener Nebenierenhypoplasie. *Dtsch Med Wochenschr* 1969;94: 169–75.

35 McMahon H, Wagner R, Weiner D. Acute adrenal insufficiency due to congenital defect. *Am J Dis Child* 1957;94: 282–6.

36 Visser HKA. The adrenal cortex in childhood. Part 1. Physiological aspects; Part 2: Pathological aspects. *Arch Dis Child* 1966;41:2–16;113–36.

37 Blizzard RM, Alberts M. Hypopituitarism, hypoadrenalism and hypogonadism in the newborn infant. *J Pediatr* 1956;48: 782–92.

38 Ehrlich RM. Ectopic and hypoplastic pituitary with adrenal hypoplasia. *J Pediatr* 1957;51:377–84.

39 Deamer WC, Silver HK. Abnormalities in the secretion of the adrenal cortex during early life. *J Pediatr* 1950;37:490.

40 Kampmeier OF. Giant epithelial cells of the human fetal adrenal. *Anat Rec* 1927;37:95–102.

41 Craig JM, Landing BH. Anaplastic cells of fetal adrenal cortex. *Am J Clin Pathol* 1951;21:940–9.

42 Beatty EC, Hawes CR. Cytomegaly of the adrenal gland. *Am J Dis Child* 1955;89:463–71.

43 Brewer DD. Congenital absence of the pituitary gland and its consequences. *J Pathol Bacteriol* 1957;73:59–67.

44 Moncrieff MW, Hill DS, Archer J *et al.* Congenital absence of pituitary gland and adrenal hypoplasia. *Arch Dis Child* 1972; 47:136–7.

45 Reid JD. Congenital absence of the pituitary gland. *J Pediatr* 1969;56:658–64.

46 Kerenyi N. Congenital adrenal hypoplasia: report of a case with extreme adrenal hypoplasia and neurohypophyseal aplasia, drawing attention to certain aspects of etiology and classification. *Arch Pathol* 1961;71:336–43.

47 Winquist PG. Adrenal hypoplasia. *Arch Pathol* 1961;71: 324–9.
48 Aterman K, Kerenyi N, Lee M. Adrenal cytomegaly. *Virchows Arch* 1972;355:105–22.
49 Mamelle JC, David M, Riou D *et al.* Hypoplasie surrénalienne congénitale de type cytomégalique, forme récessive liée au sexe. A propos de trois observations. *Arch Fr Pédiatr* 1975; 32:139–59.
50 Bertoye A, Carron R, Bertrand J *et al.* Un cas d'insuffisance surrénale chronique évolutive à manifestation néonatale. *Pédiatrie* 1964;19:353–8.
51 McMahon H, Wagner R. Acute adrenal insufficiency due to congenital defect of the gland: case report. *Am J Dis Child* 1956;92:517.
52 Cox PJN. Congenital adrenal hypoplasia. *Proc R Soc Med* 1962;55:981–2.
53 Weens HS, Golden A. Adrenocortical insufficiency in infants simulating intestinal obstruction. *Am J Roentgenol* 1955;74: 213.
54 Sparrow GR. Neonatal Addison's disease. *Proc R Soc Med* 1957;20:719.
55 Perlmutter M, Numeroff M, Manulkin T. Primary adrenocortical insufficiency and hypogonadotrophic eunuchoidism. *Metabolism* 1961;10:647–53.
56 Black S, Brook CGD, Cox PJN. Congenital adrenal hypoplasia and gonadotrophin deficiency. *Br Med J* 1977;2:996.
57 Brook CGD. Pubertal failure in congenital adrenal hypoplasia. *Lancet* 1977;2:1360.
58 Golden MP, Lippe BM, Kaplan SA. Congenital adrenal hypoplasia and hypogonadotropic hypogonadism. *Am J Dis Child* 1977;131:1117–18.
59 Hay ID, Smail PJ, Forsyth CC. Familial cytomegalic adrenocortical hypoplasia: an X-linked syndrome of pubertal failure. *Arch Dis Child* 1981;56:715–21.
60 Kelly WF, Joplin GF, Pearson GW. Gonadotropin deficiency and adrenocortical insufficiency in children: a new syndrome. *Br Med J* 1977;2:98.
61 Kikuchi K, Kaji M, Momoi T *et al.* Failure to induce puberty in a man with X-linked congenital adrenal hypoplasia and hypogonadotropic hypogonadism by pulsatile administration of low-dose gonadotropin-releasing hormone. *Acta Endocrinol* 1987;114:153–60.
62 Lippe MB, Golden M. Pubertal failure in congenital adrenal hypoplasia. *Lancet* 1978;1:392–3.
63 Prader A, Zachmann M, Illig R. Luteinizing hormone deficiency in hereditary congenital adrenal hypoplasia. *J Pediatr* 1975;86:421–2.
64 Zachmann M, Tassinari D, Prader A. Gonadotropin deficiency and cryptorchidism in three prepubertal brothers with congenital adrenal hypoplasia. *J Pediatr* 1980;97: 255–7.
65 Zachmann M, Fuchs E, Prader A. Progressive high frequency hearing loss: an additional feature in the syndrome of congenital adrenal hypoplasia and gonadotrophin deficiency. *Eur J Pediatr* 1992;151:167–9.
66 Weiss L, Mellinger RC. Congenital adrenal hypoplasia. An X-linked disease. *J Med Genet* 1970;7:27–32.
67 Lanman JT. The adrenal gland in the human fetus. An interpretation of its physiology and unusual developmental pattern. *Pediatrics* 1961;27:140–58.
68 Angevine DM. Pathologic anatomy of hypophysis and adrenals in anencephaly. *Arch Pathol* 1938;26:507–18.
69 Ch'in KY. Endocrine glands of anencephalic foetuses. Quantitative and morphologic study of 15 cases. *Chinese Med J* 1938;2(Suppl.):63–90.
70 McKusick VA. *Mendelian Inheritance in Man*, 3rd edn. Baltimore, MD: Johns Hopkins Press, 1971.
71 Virdis R, Levine LS, Pang S *et al.* Congenital adrenal hypoplasia: two new cases. *J Endocrinol Invest* 1983;6:51–4.
72 Hammond J, Howard NJ, Brookwell R *et al.* Proposed assignment of loci for X-linked adrenal hypoplasia and glycerol kinase genes. *Lancet* 1985;4:54.
73 Mardsen HB, Zakhour HD. Cytomegalic adrenal hypoplasia with pituitary cytomegaly. *Virchows Arch (Pathol Anat)* 1978;378:105–10.
74 Kruse K, Sippell WG, Schnakenburg KV. Hypogonadism in congenital adrenal hypoplasia: evidence for a hypothalamic origin. *J Clin Endocrinol Metab* 1984;58:12–17.
75 Martin MM, Martin LA. The syndrome of congenital hereditary adrenal hypoplasia and hypogonadotropic hypogonadism. *Int J Adol Med Health* 1985;1:119–37.
76 Harlem OK, Myhre E. Congenital adrenal hypoplasia: report of a case with the characteristic clinical features of dysadrenocorticism and autopsy findings of extreme hypoplasia of the adrenal glands. *Am J Dis Child* 1957;94:696–701.
77 Richards GE, Conte FA, Kaplan SL, Grumbach MM. Congenital adrenal hypoplasia and isolated gonadotropin deficiency: ability of gonadotrophs to respond to LRF. *Clin Res* 1978;26:171A.
78 Kruse K, Sippel WG, Schnakenburg KV. Hypogonadism in congenital adrenal hypoplasia: evidence for a hypothalamic origin. *J Clin Endrocrinol Metab* 1984;58:12–17.
79 Kletter GB, Gorski JL, Kelch RP. Congenital adrenal hypoplasia and isolated gonadotropin deficiency. *Trends Endocrinol Metab* 1991;2:123–8.
80 Bartly JA, Miller DK, Hayford JT. Concordance of X-linked glycerol kinase deficiency with X-linked congenital adrenal hypoplasia. *Lancet* 1982;2:733–6.
81 Matsumoto T, Kondoh T, Yoshimoto *et al.* Complex glycerol kinase deficiency: molecular-genetic, cytogenetic, and clinical studies of five Japanese patients. *Am J Med Genet* 1988;32:603–16.
82 Oleesky DA, Hakeem V. Congenital adrenal hypoplasia and glycerol kinase deficiency. *Acta Paed Scand* 1989;78: 893–5.
83 Wise JE, Matalon R, Morgan AM *et al.* Phenotypic features of patients with congenital adrenal hypoplasia and glycerol kinase deficiency. *Am J Dis Child* 1987;141:744–7.
84 Chelly J, Marlhens F, Dutrillaux G *et al.* Deletion proximal to DXS 68 locus (L1 probe site) in a boy with Duchenne muscular dystrophy, glycerolkinase deficiency, and adrenal hypoplasia. *Hum Genet* 1988;78:222–7.
85 Worley KC, Ellison KA, Zhang YH *et al.* Yeast artificial chromosome cloning in the glycerol kinase and adrenal hypoplasia congenita region of Xp21. *Genomics* 1993;16: 407–16.
86 Ohlbaum P, Hehunstre PP, Bouchet JL, Deminiere C. Insuffisance surrénale chronique et hyalinose segmentaire et focale familiale. Une nouvelle association. *Pédiatrie* 1986; 41:86.
87 Burke BA, Wick MR, King R *et al.* Congenital adrenal hypoplasia and selective absence of pituitary hormone: a new autosomal recessive syndrome. *Am J Med Genet* 1988; 31:75–97.
88 Grumbach MM, Richards GE, Conte FA *et al.* Clinical disorders of adrenal function and puberty: an assessment of the role of the adrenal cortex in normal and abnormal

puberty in man and evidence for an ACTH-like pituitary adrenal androgen stimulating hormone. In: James VHT, Serio M, Giusti G, Martini L, eds. *The Endocrine Function of the Adrenal Cortex*. London: Academic Press, 1978: 583–612.

89 Kreines K, DeVaux WD. Neonatal adrenal insufficiency associated with maternal Cushing's syndrome. *Pediatrics* 1971;47:516–19.

90 Kreines K, Perin E, Salzer R. Pregnancy in Cushing's syndrome. *J Clin Endocrinol Metab* 1964;24:75–9.

91 Bongiovanni AM, McPadden AJ. Steroids during pregnancy and possible fetal consequences. *Fertil Steril* 1960;11:181–6.

92 Birdwell TR, Dimmette RM. Cytomegaly of the adrenal gland. *Am J Clin Pathol* 1967;47:585.

93 Roberts G, Cawdery JE. Congenital adrenal hypoplasia. *J Obstet Gynaecol Br Commonw* 1970;77:654–6.

94 Ehrlich EN, Strauss FH II, Hunter RL *et al.* Cytomegalic adrenocortical hypoplasia and increased plasma 20α-hydroxy-pregnen-4-en-3-one in a man exhibiting the features of selective mineralocorticoid deficiency. *J Clin Endocrinol Metab* 1969;29:523–38.

95 France JT, Liggins GC. Placental sulfatase deficiency. *J Clin Endocrinol Metab* 1969;29:138–41.

96 Oakey RE. Placental sulphatase deficiency: antepartum differential diagnosis from foetal adrenal hypoplasia. *Clin Endocrinol* 1978;9:81–8.

97 Mujaji BW, Toumba KJ, Oakey RE. Urinary excretion of oestrone, oestradiol-17β and oestriol in pregnancies complicated by steroid sulphatase deficiency. *J Endocrinol* 1979; 83:95–100.

98 O'Doherty NJ. Lipoid adrenal hyperplasia. *Guy's Hosp Rep* 1964;113:368–79.

99 Prader A, Anders GJPA. Zur genetik der Kongenitalen lipoid hyperplasie der Nebennieren. *Helv Paediatr Acta* 1962;17: 285–9.

100 Prader A, Gurtner HP. Das syndrom des pseudohermaphroditismus masculinus bei kongenitaler nebenniereuredenhyperplasie oline androgenberproduktion. *Helv Pediatr Acta* 1955;10:397–412.

101 Prader A, Siebenmann RE. Nebenniereninsuffizienz bei konigenitaler lipoid hyperplasie der Nebennieren. *Helv Paediatr Acta* 1957;12:569–95.

102 Sills IN, Voorrhess ML, MacGillivray MH, Peterson RE. Prolonged survival without therapy in congenital adrenal hypoplasia. *Am J Dis Child* 1983;137:1186–8.

103 Snelling CE, Erb EH. Haemorrhage and subsequent calcification of the suprarenal. *J Pediatr* 1935;6:22–41.

104 Kaplan M, Straus P, Grumbach R *et al.* Hématomes surrénaliens unilatéraux chez le nouveau-né à terme. A propos de deux observations. *Ann Pédiatr* 1964;11:405.

105 Harper JR, Ginn WM Jr, Taylor WJ. Bilateral adrenal hemorrhage. A complication of anticoagulant therapy. *Am J Med* 1962;32:984.

106 Tönz O, Aufdermauer F. Erfolgreiche Behandlung eines Waterhouse–Friderichsen Syndroms mit Heparin. *Schweiz Med Wochenschr* 1967;97:1611.

107 Gruenwald P. Asphyxia, trauma and shock at birth. *Arch Fr Pediatr* 1950;67:103–15.

108 Gardner LI. Newer knowledge of adrenocortical disturbances: hypoadrenocorticism in infants. *Pediatr Clin N Am* 1957;4:895.

109 Coleman R, Eric W, Arneil GC. Acute tuberculosis adrenocortical failure with clinical recovery. *Lancet* 1962;1:885.

110 Rao RH, Vagnucci AH, Amico JA. Bilateral massive adrenal hemorrhage: early recognition and treatment. *Ann Intern Med* 1989;110:227–35.

111 Castello MA, Rezza E, Iannaccone G. Hemorragia suprarenal unilateral en el recien nacido. *Rev Esp Pediatr* 1967;23: 273–92.

112 Arneil GC. Acute bilateral suprarenal haemorrhage. *Arch Dis Child* 1946;21:171.

113 Lotti A. Emorragie surrenaliche nel neonato: considerazioni etiopatogenetiche, anatomopatologiche e cliniche su 15 case osservati. *Aggiornamento Pediatrico* 1965;XVI:371–92.

114 Peluffo E, Delgado B, Correa JC *et al.* A proposito de quatro casos de hemorragia suprarrenal en recien nacidos. *Arch Pediatr Uruguay* 1950;21:128–38.

115 Black J, Williams DI. Natural history of adrenal haemorrhage in the newborn. *Arch Dis Child* 1973;48:183–90.

116 Kuhn J, Jewett T, Munschauer R. The clinical and radiographic features of massive neonatal adrenal hemorrhage. *Radiology* 1971;99:647–52.

117 Hill EE, Williams JA. Massive adrenal haemorrhage in the newborn. *Arch Dis Child* 1959;34:178–82.

118 Babin SP, Allain D, Demarquez JL *et al.* Kyste angiomateux et pseudokyste hématique de la surrénale chez le nouveau-né. *Pédiatrie* 1976;31:81–2.

119 Corcoran WJ, Strauss AA. Suprarenal hemorrhage in the newborn. *J Am Med Assoc* 1924;82:626–8.

120 Vasmant D, Safran C, Raux-Eurin MC. Hématome de la surrénale chez le nouveau-né: conduite à tenir et complications. In: *Rapports des Journées Parisiennes de Pédiatrie*. Paris: Flammarion Médecine-Sciences, 1983:161–73.

121 Lawson EE, Teele RL. Diagnosis of adrenal hemorrhage by ultrasound. *J Pediatr* 1978;92:423–6.

122 Rose J, Berdon WE, Sullivan T *et al.* Prolonged jaundice as presenting sign of massive adrenal hemorrhage in newborn. *Radiology* 1971;98:263–72.

123 Guibaud P, Racle P, Guerrier M *et al.* Hématome surrénal bilatéral du nouveau-né à manifestations rénales primitives. *Pédiatrie* 1966;21:844–5.

124 See G, Chavannes L, Jurkovitz P *et al.* Hématome surrénal du nouveau-né associé à des troubles rénaux. *Arch Fr Pédiatr* 1967;22:1093–106.

125 Schaffer AJ. *Disease of the Newborn*, 2nd edn. Philadelphia, PA: W.B. Saunders, 1966.

126 Jarvis JL, Seaman WB. Idiopathic adrenal calcification in infants and children. *Am J Roentgenol* 1959;82:510–19.

127 Stevenson J, MacGregor AM, Connelly P. Calcification of the adrenal glands in young children: a report of three cases with a review of the literature. *Arch Dis Child* 1961;36: 316–20.

128 Codaccioni JL, Boyer J, Oliver C *et al.* Calcifications surrénales idiopathiques. Étude d'un cas et revue de la littérature. *Ann d'Endocrinol* 1970;31:879–94.

129 Crocker AC, Vawter GF, Neuhauser EBD *et al.* Wolman's disease: three new patients with a recently described lipidosis. *Pediatrics* 1965;35:627–40.

130 Wolman M, Sterk UU, Gatt S *et al.* Primary familial xanthomatosis with involvement and calcification of the adrenals. Report of two more cases in siblings of a previously described infant. *Pediatrics* 1961;28:742–57.

131 Goldzieher MA, Gordon MB. Syndrome of adrenal hemorrhage in the newborn. *Endocrinology* 1932;16:165–81.

132 Lorber J. Massive bilateral adrenal haemorrhage in the newborn with recovery. *Proc R Soc Med* 1965;58:125.

133 Selye H, Dosne C. Physiological significance of compensatory adrenal hypertrophy. *Endocrinology* 1942;30:581.

134 Babin SP, Allain D, Demarquez JL *et al.* Les kystes de la surrénale chez le nouveau-né. A propos de deux observations. *Arch Fr Pédiatr* 1977;34:130–42.

135 Oppenheimer EH. Cyst formation in the outer adrenal cortex. Studies in the human fetus and newborn. *Arch Pathol* 1969;87:653–9.

136 Smith CA. *The Critically Ill child: Diagnosis and Management*, 2nd edn. Philadelphia, PA; W.B. Saunders, 1977.

137 Little EG. Purpura, ending fatally with haemorrhage into suprarenal capsules. *Br J Dermatol* 1901;13:445.

138 Voelcker AF. Pathological report. *Middlesex Hospital Report.* 1984.

139 Waterhouse R. Suprarenal apoplexy. *Lancet* 1991;1:576–8.

140 Friderichsen C. Nebennierenapoplexie bein Kleinen Kindern. *Jahr Kinderheilk Phys Erziehung* 1918;87:109–25.

141 Friderichsen C. Waterhouse–Friderichsen syndrome. *Acta Endocrinol* 1955;18:482.

142 Migeon CJ, Kenny FM, Hung W *et al.* Study of adrenal function in children with meningitis. *Pediatrics* 1967;40: 163–83.

143 Calafell R, Gilbert P, Perez-Vitoria C. A case of Marchand–Waterhouse–Friderichsen syndrome with recovery. *Med Clin* 1949;13:191–5.

144 Hoffman K, Mamelok SH. Two cases of Waterhouse–Friedrichsen syndrome in the same family, one with recovery under penicillin therapy. *Arch Pediatr 63. Excerpta Medica* 1947;1:114.

145 Forsham PH. The adrenal cortex: diseases of adrenocortical hypofunction. In: Williams RH, ed. *Textbook of Endocrinology.* Philadelphia, PA: W.B. Saunders, 1968:315–19.

146 Bamatter F. Fulminante Meningokokkensepsis. Zur Ätiologie des syndroms von Waterhouse–Friderichsen. *Jahr Kinderheilk* 1934;142:127.

147 Fox B. Adrenal haemorrhage and necrosis resulting from abdominal operations. *Lancet* 1969;1:600.

148 Van der Horst RL. Purpura fulminans in a newborn baby. *Arch Dis Child* 1962;37:436–41.

149 Rich AR. A peculiar type of adrenal cortical damage associated with acute infections, and its possible relation to circulatory collapse. *Bull Johns Hopkins Hosp* 1944;74:1.

150 Stuber HW, Hitzig WH. Zur Pathogenese und therapie des Waterhouse–Friderichsen–syndroms. Beziehungen zum Sanarelli–Schwartzman–phänomen. *Schweiz Med Wochenschr* 1961;91:1612.

151 Thomison JB, Shapiro JL. Adrenal lesions in acute meningococcemia. *Arch Pathol* 1957;63:527.

152 Leclerc F, Delepouille F, Martinot A *et al.* Fréquence des hémorrhagies surrénaliennees au cours des formes fatales de *purpura fulminans* de l'enfant. Considérations étiopathogéniques et thérapeutiques. *Pédiatrie* 1988;43:545–50.

153 Levin J, Cluff LE. Endotoxemia and adrenal hemorrhage. A mechanism for the Waterhouse–Friderichsen syndrome. *J Exp Med* 1965;121:247.

154 Schwartz K, Dieterle P, Hochheuser W *et al.* Zur Klinik der Nebennierenrinden insuffizienz. *Med Klin* 1967;62:551.

155 Bennett IL Jr, Finland H, Hamburger M *et al.* A double-blind study of the effectiveness of cortisol in the management of severe infection. *Trans Assoc Am Phys* 1962;75:198–20.

156 Kass EH. The effectiveness of hydrocortisone in the management of severe infections. A double-blind study. Cooperative study group. *J Am Med Assoc* 1963;183:166.

157 May CD. Circulatory failure (shock) in fulminant meningococcal infection. *Pediatrics* 1960;25:316–28.

158 Melby JC, Spink WW. Comparative studies of adrenal cortisol function and cortisol metabolism in healthy adults and in patients with shock due to infection. *J Clin Invest* 1958;37:1791–8.

159 Justin-Beasançon L, Klotz HP, Sikorow H. Insuffisance surrénale aiguë à forme comateuse. Manie aiguë au 3ème jour d'un traitement par la cortisone. *Sem Hôp Paris* 1951; 27:578–84.

160 Eberlein WR, Bongiovanni AM, Rodriguez CS. Diagnosis and treatment: the complications of steroid treatment. *Pediatrics* 1967;40:279–82.

161 Harisson TS, Chawla RC, Wojtalik RS. Steroidal influences on catecholamines. *N Engl J Med* 1968;279:136–42.

162 Ramey ER, Goldstein MS. The adrenal cortex and the sympthetic nervous system. *Physiol Rev* 1957;37:155.

163 Cope CL. Adrenal inhibition. In: *Adrenal Steroids and Disease.* London: Pitman Medical, 1972:313–44.

164 Fauci AS, Dale DC, Balow JE. Glucocorticoid therapy: mechanism of action and clinical considerations. *Ann Intern Med* 1976;84:304–15.

165 Addison T. *On the Constitutional and Local Effects of Disease of the Suprarenal Capsules.* London: D. Highley, 1855.

166 Grant DB, Barnes ND, Moncrieff MW, Savage MO. Clinical presentation, growth, and pubertal development in Addison's disease. *Arch Dis Child* 1985;60:925–8.

167 Mason AS, Meade TW, Lee JAH *et al.* Epidemiological and clinical picture of Addison's disease. *Lancet* 1968;2:744–7.

168 Labhart A. Adrenal cortex. In: *Clinical Endocrinology.* Berlin: Springer Verlag, 1974:312–32.

169 Pearson GW. Addison's disease in a 6 year-old-boy. *Br Med J* 1962;1:1057.

170 Jaudon JC. Addison's disease in children. *J Pediatr* 1946;28: 737–55.

171 Aceto T, Blizzard RM, Migeon CJ. Adrenocortical insufficiency in infants and children. *Pediatr Clin N Am* 1962;9: 177.

172 Guttman PH. Addison's disease. A statistical analysis of 566 cases and a study of the pathology. *Arch Pathol* 1930;10: 742–85;895–935.

173 Turpin R, Lafourcade J, Gorin R *et al.* L'atrophie corticosurrénale de l'enfant. *Ann Pédiatr* 1961;37:303–14.

174 Welch RG. Addison's disease in a nine year old girl. *Br Med J* 1957;1:980.

175 Zhukovsky M. Characteristics of the adrenal cortex functioning in children in health and disease. In: Ghai OP, Tanega PN, eds. *Current Topics in Pediatrics.* Indian Academy of Science, 1977:100.

176 White FP, Sutton LE. Addison's disease in a negro child. *J Pediatr* 1950;37:778.

177 Gsell O, Uehlinger E. Tuberkulöser Morbus Addison. Stellung der Nebennieren-tuberkulose im Ablauf der tuberkulösen Infektion. *Beitr Klin Tuberkulose spez Tuberkulose-forsch* 1933;83:121.

178 Conybeare JJ, Millis GC. Observations on twenty-nine cases of Addison's disease treated at Guy's Hospital between 1904 and 1923. *Guy's Hosp Rep* 1924;4:369–75.

179 De Gennes JL. *Maladies des Glandes Endocrines.* Paris: Flammarion, 1952.

180 O'Donnell WM. Changing pathogenesis of Addison's disease. *Arch Intern Med* 1965;36:266.

181 Irvine WJ, Barnes EW. Adrenocortical insufficiency. In: *Clin Endocrinol Metab* 1972;1:549–94.

182 Tourniaire J, Darsy P, Chalendar D *et al.* Le diagnostic étiologique de la maladie d'Addison. 58 observations per-

sonnelles. *Lyon Médical* 1977;238:83–7.

183 Crispell KR, Parson W, Hamlin J *et al.* Addison's disease associated with histoplasmosis. *Am J Med* 1956;20:23–9.

184 Del Negro G, Wajchenberg BL, Pereira VG *et al.* Addison's disease associated with South American blastomycosis. *Ann Intern Med* 1961;54:189.

185 Fish RG, Takaro T, Lovell M. Coexistent Addison's disease and North American blastomycosis. *Am J Med* 1960;28:152.

186 Murray HLU, Littman ML, Roberts RB. Disseminated paracoccidioidomycosis (South American blastomycosis) in the United States. *Am J Med* 1974;56:209–20.

187 Cedermark BJ, Blumenson LE, Pickren JW *et al.* The significance of metastases to the adrenal glands in adrenocarcinoma of the colon and rectum. *Surg Gynecol Obstet* 1977;144: 537–46.

188 Girelli ME, Casara D, Rubello D *et al.* Metastatic thyroid carcinoma of the adrenal gland. *J Endocrinol Invest* 1992;15: 139–41.

189 Friedman NB. The pathology of the adrenal gland in Addison's disease with special reference to adrenocortical contraction. *Endocrinology* 1948;42:181.

190 Irvine WJ, Barnes EW. Addison's disease, ovarian failure and hypoparathyroidism. In: Irvine WJ, ed. *Autoimmunity in Endocrine Disease. Clinical Endocrinology and Metabolism*, Vol. 4. Philadelphia, PA: W.B. Saunders, 1975:379–434.

191 Nerup J. Addison's disease – clinical studies. A report of 108 cases. *Acta Endocrinol* 1974;76:127–41.

192 Spinner MW, Blizzard RM, Childs B. Clinical and genetic heterogeneity in idiopathic Addison's disease and hypoparathyroidism. *J Clin Endocrinol Metab* 1968;28:795–804.

193 Anderson JR, Buchanan WW, Goudie RB. *Autoimmunity Clinical and Experimental.* Springfield, IL: Thomas, 1967.

194 Blizzard RM, Kyle M. Studies of the adrenal antigens and antibodies in Addison's disease. *J Clin Invest* 1963;42: 1653–60.

195 Irvine WJ, Chan MMW, Scarth L. The further characterization of auto-antibodies reactive with extra-adrenal steroid-producing cells in patients with adrenal disorders. *Clin Exp Immunol* 1969;4:489–503.

196 Pousset G, Monier JL, Thivolet J. Anticorps anti-surrénaliens et maladie d'Addison. *Ann Endocrinol* 1970;31:995–1002.

197 Pousset G, Tourniaire J, Monier JC *et al.* Les autoanticorps anti-surrénaliens dans l'insuffisance surrénale chronique. *Rev Fr Endocrinol Clin* 1968;9:305–19.

198 Blizzard RM, Kyle MA, Chandler RW *et al.* Adrenal antibodies in Addison's disease. *Lancet* 1962;2:901–3.

199 Hung W, Migeon CJ, Parrott RH. A possible autoimmune basis for Addison's disease in three siblings, one with idiopathic hypoparathyroidism, pernicious anemia and superficial moniliase. *N Engl J Med* 1963;269:658–63.

200 Nerup J. Addison's disease – serological studies. *Acta Endocrinol* 1974;76:142–58.

201 Scherbaum WA, Berg PA. Development of adrenocortical failure in non-addisonian patients with antibodies to adrenal cortex. *Clin Endocrinol* 1982;16:345–52.

202 Ahonen P, Miettinen A, Perheentupa J. Adrenal and steroidal cell antibodies in patients with autoimmune polyglandular disease type I and risk of adrenocortical and ovarian failure. *J Clin Endocrinol Metab* 1987;64:494–500.

203 Betterle C, Scalci C, Presotto F *et al.* The natural history of adrenal function in autoimmune patients with adrenal antibodies. *J Endocrinol* 1988;117:467–75.

204 Blizzard RM, Chee D, Davis W. The incidence of adrenal and other antibodies in the sera of patients with idiopathic adrenal insufficiency (Addison's disease). *Clin Exp Immunol* 1967;2:19–30.

205 Irvine WJ, Stewart AG, Scarth L. A clinical and immunological study of adrenocortical insufficiency (Addison's disease). *Clin Exp Immunol* 1967;2:31–69.

206 Bright GM, Singh I. Adrenal autoantibodies bind to adrenal subcellular fractions enriched in cytochrome-*c* reductase and 5′-nucleotidase. *J Clin Endocrinol Metab* 1990;70:95–9.

207 Furmaniak J, Talbot D, Reinwein D *et al.* Immunoprecipitation of human adrenal microsomal antigen. *FEBS Lett* 1988;231:25–8.

208 Wulffraat NM, Drexhage HA, Bottazzo GF *et al.* Immunoglobulins of patients with idiopathic Addison's disease block the in vitro action of adrenocorticotropin. *J Clin Endocrinol Metab* 1989;69:231–8.

209 Baumann-Antczak A, Wedlock N, Bednarek J *et al.* Autoimmune Addison's disease and 21-hydroxylase. *Lancet* 1992;340:429–30.

210 Bednarek J, Furmaniak J, Wedlock N *et al.* Steroid 21-hydroxylase is a major autoantigen involved in adult onset autoimmune Addison's disease. *FEBS Lett* 1992;309:51–5.

211 Winqvist O, Karlsson FA, Kämpe O. 21-Hydroxylase, a major autoantigen in idiopathic Addison's disease. *Lancet* 1992; 339:1559–62.

212 Krohn K, Uibo R, Aavik E, Peterson P, Savilahti S. Identification by molecular cloning of an autoantigen associated with Addison's disease as steroid 17α-hydroxylase. *Lancet* 1992;239:770–3.

213 Nerup J, Andersen V, Bendixen G. Anti-adrenal cellular hypersensitivity in Addison's disease. IV. *In vivo* and *in vitro* investigation of the mitochondrial fraction. *Clin Exp Immunol* 1969;4:355–63.

214 Moulias R, Goust JM, Deville G *et al.* Le test de migration des leucocytes du sang périphérique. Un nouveau test d'hypersensibilité retardée *in vitro* chez l'homme. II. Utilisation dans les affections auto-immunes humaines. Résultats préliminaires et interprétation. *Presse Méd* 1970;73: 2315–18.

215 Rabinove SL, Jakson RA, Dluhy RG, Williams G. Ia-positive T lymphocytes in recently diagnosed idiopathic Addison's disease. *Am J Med* 1984;7:597–601.

216 Evans AWH, Woodrow JC, McDougall CDM *et al.* Antibodies in the families of thyrotoxic patients. *Lancet* 1967;1:636.

217 Moore JM, Neilson JMcE. Antibodies to gastric mucosa and thyroid in diabetes mellitus. *Lancet* 1963;2:645–7.

218 Murthy GG, Peress NS, Khan SA. Demonstration of antibodies to testicular basement membrane by immunofluorescence in a patient with multiple primary endocrine deficiencies. *J Clin Endocrinol Metab* 1976;42:637–41.

219 Riley WJ, Maclaren NK, Neufeld M. Adrenal autoantibodies and Addison disease in insulin-dependent diabetes mellitus. *J Pediatr* 1980;97:191–5.

220 Spinner MW, Blizzard RM, Gibbs J *et al.* Familial distribution of organ-specific antibodies in the blood of patients with Addison's disease and hypoparathyroidism and their relatives. *Clin Exp Immunol* 1969;5:461–8.

221 Valloton MB, Forbes A. Autoimmunity in gonadal dysgenesis and Klinefelter's syndrome. *Lancet* 1967;1:648–51.

222 Claude H, Gougerot H. Sur l'insuffisance simultanée de plusieurs glandes à sécrétion interne (insuffisance pluriglandulaire). *J Physiol Pathol Gén* 1908;10:468–505.

223 Falta W. Späteunuchoidismus und multiple Blutdrüsensklerose. II. Multiple Blutdrüsensklerose. *Berliner Klin Wochenschr* 1912;49:1477.

224 Loriaux DL. The polyendocrine deficiency syndromes. *N Engl J Med* 1985;312:1568–9.
225 Neufeld M, Maclaren N, Blizzard R. Autoimmune polyglandular syndromes. *Pediatr Ann* 1980;9:43–53.
226 Drury MI, Keelan DM, Timoney FJ *et al.* Juvenile familial endocrinopathy. *Clin Exp Immunol* 1972;7:125–32.
227 Frey HMM, Vogt JM, Nerup J. Familial poly-endocrinopathy. *Acta Endocrinol* 1973;72:401–16.
228 Mershon JC, Dietrich JG. Hereditary Addison's disease and multiple endocrine adenomatosis in a kindred. *Ann Intern Med* 1966;65:252.
229 Edmonds M, Lamki L, Killinger DW *et al.* Autoimmune thyroiditis, adrenalitis and oophoritis. *Am J Med* 1973;54:782–7.
230 Carpenter CCJ, Solomon N, Silverberg SG *et al.* Schmidt's syndrome (thyroid and adrenal insufficiency). A review of the literature and a report of fifteen new cases including ten instances of co-existent diabetes mellitus. *Medicine* 1964;43:153–80.
231 Epstein D, Dale R, Breckenridge WC *et al.* Autoimmune thyroid and adrenal insufficiency (Schmidts syndrome) and familial LCAT deficiency in the same kindred. In: *61st Annual Meeting of the Endocrine Society, Anaheim*, 13–15 June. 1979:190 (Abstr. 471).
232 Genant HK, Hoagland HC, Randall RU. Addison's disease and hypothyroidism (Schmidt's syndrome). *Metabolism* 1967;16:189–94.
233 Schmidt MB. Eine Biglanduläre Erkrankung (Nebennieren und Schilddrüse) bei Morbus Addisonii. *Verhandlung Dtsch Ges Pathol* 1926;21:212–21.
234 Kogut MD, Brinegar CH. Addison's disease and diabetes mellitus. *J Pediatr* 1972;81:307–11.
235 McNicol GP, McNicol MW. Addison's disease complicated by diabetes mellitus. Report of a case. *Scottish Med J* 1957;5:30.
236 Solomon N, Carpenter CCJ, Bennett IL *et al.* Schmidt's syndrome (thyroid and adrenal insufficiency) and coexistent diabetes mellitus. *Diabetes* 1965;14:300.
237 Whitaker J, Landing BH, Esselborn VM *et al.* The syndrome of familial juvenile hypoadrenocorticism, hypoparathyroidism and superficial moniliasis. *J Clin Endocrinol Metab* 1956;16:1374–87.
238 Di George AM, Paschkis K. The syndrome of Addison's disease hypoparathyroidism and superficial moniliasis. *Am J Dis Child* 1957;94:476–8.
239 Kenny FM, Holliday MA. Hypoparathyroidism, moniliasis, Addison's and Hashimoto's diseases. *N Engl J Med* 1964;271:708.
240 H de M Ruehsen, Blizzard RM, Garcia-Bunuel R *et al.* Autoimmunity and ovarian failure. *Am J Obstet Gynecol* 1972;112:693–703.
241 Cortet P, Brun JM, Rifle C *et al.* Candidose, hypoparathyroidie chronique, insuffisance surrénale, insuffisance ovarienne primitive et maladie de Biermer. Extension de la triade de Whitaker. *Ann Méd Interne* 1978;129:449–53.
242 Leor J, Levortowsky D, Sharon C. Polyglandular autoimmune syndrome, type 2. *South Med J* 1989;82:374–6.
243 Neufeld M, Maclaren N, Blizzard R. Two types of autoimmune Addison's disease associated with different polyglandular autoimmune (PGA) syndromes. *Medicine* 1981;60:355–62.
244 Ahonen P, Myllärniemi S, Sipila, Perheentupa J. Clinical variations of autoimmune polyendocrinopathy-candidiasis-ectodermal dystrophy (APECED) in a series of 68 patients. *N Engl J Med* 1990;322:1829–36.
245 Iman K, Mohamed A, Felicetta JV. Alopecia universalis as a feature of polyglandular autoimmunity type I. *West J Med* 1988;149:338–41.
246 Aron DC. Endocrine complications of the acquired immunodeficiency syndrome. *Arch Intern Med* 1989;149:330–3.
247 Dluhy RG, The growing spectrum of HIV-related endocrine abnormalities. *J Clin Endocrinol Metab* 1990;70:563–5.
248 Groll A, Schneider M, Althoff PH *et al.* The morphology and clinical significance of pathologic changes of the adrenal glands and hypophysis in AIDS. *Dtsch Med Wochenschr* 1990;115:483–8.
249 Membreno L, Irony I, Dere W, Klein R, Biglieri EG, Cobb E. Adrenocortical function in acquired immunodeficiency syndrome. *J Clin Endocrinol Metab* 1987;65:482–7.
250 Schlienger JL. Conséquences endocriniennes de l'infection par le virus de l'immunodéficience humaine (VIH). *Pathol Biol* 1989;37:921–6.
251 Pulakhandam U, Dincsoy HP. Cytomegalovirus adrenalitis and adrenal insufficiency in AIDS. *Am J Clin Pathol* 1990;93:651–6.
252 Tapper MI, Rotterdam HZ, Lerner CW *et al.* Adrenal necrosis in the acquired immunodeficiency syndrome. *Ann Intern Med* 1984;100:239–41.
253 Rotterdam H, Dembitzer F. The adrenal glands in AIDS. *Endocrinol Pathol* 1992;4:4–14.
254 Whitcomb RW, Marston Linehan W, Whal LM, Kuazeh RA. Monocytes stimulate cortisol production by cultured human adrenocortical cells. *J Clin Endocrinol Metab* 1988;66:33–8.
255 Norbiato G, Bevilacqua M, Vago T *et al.* Cortisol resistance in acquired immunodeficiency syndrome. *J Clin Endocrinol Metab* 1992;74:608–13.
256 Silverberg J, Volpé R. Autoimmunity in endocrine disease. In: Ingbar SH, ed. *The Year in Endocrinology*. New York: Plenum Press, 1978:345–86.
257 McNatty KP, Short RV, Barnes EW *et al.* The cytotoxic effect of serum from patients with Addison's disease and autoimmune ovarian failure on human granulosa cells in culture. *Clin Exp Immunol* 1975;22:378–84.
258 Levine S, Wenk EJ. The production and passive transfer of allergic adrenalitis. *Am J Pathol* 1968;52:41–53.
259 Bamatter F, Koegel R, Haller J De *et al.* Maladie d'Addison familiale. Insuffisance corticosurrénale chez quatre frères et plusiers cas probables dans deux générations de la même famille. *Helv Paediatr Acta* 1966;21:109–52.
260 Fairchild RS, Schimke RN, Abdou NI. Immunoregulation abnormalities in familial Addison's disease. *J Clin Endocrinol Metab* 1980;51:1074–7.
261 Burke CW. Adrenocortical insufficiency. *Clin Endocrinol Metab* 1985;14:947–76.
262 Valenta LJ, Bull RW, Hackel E, Bottazzo GF. Correlation of the HLA-A1, B8 haplotypes with the circulating autoantibodies in a family with increased incidence of autoimmune disease. *Acta Endocrinol* 1982;100:143–9.
263 Perheentupa J, Tiilikainen A, Lokki ML. Autoimmune polyendocrinopathy–candidosis syndrome (APECS): clinical variation, inheritance and HLA association in 40 Finnish patients. *Pediatr Res* 1978;12:1087 (Abstr. 28).
264 Farid NR, Bear JC. The human major histocompatibility complex and endocrine disease. *Endocr Rev* 1981;2:250–86.
265 Ahonen P, Koskimies S, Likki ML, Tillikainen A, Perheentupa J. The expression of autoimmune polyglandular disease type 1 appears associated with several HLA-A antigens but not with HLA-DR. *J Clin Endocrinol Metab* 1988;66:1151–7.

266 Platz P, Ryder L, Nielsen LS *et al.* HLA and idiopathic Addison's disease. *Lancet* 1974;2:289.
267 Ling N, Burgus R, Guillemin R. Isolation, primary structure, and synthesis of α-endorphin and β-endorphin, two peptides of hypothalamic hypophysial origin with morphinomimetic activity. *Proc Natl Acad Sci USA* 1976;73:3942–6.
268 Simantov R. Glucocorticoids inhibit endorphin synthesis by pituitary cells. *Nature* 1979;280:684–5.
269 Kracier J, Milligan JV, Gosbee JL *et al.* *In vitro* release of ACTH: effects of potassium, calcium and corticosterone. *Endocrinology* 1969;85:1144–53.
270 Thorn GW. *The Diagnosis and Treatment of Adrenal Insufficiency*, 2nd edn. Springfield, IL: CC Thomas, 1951.
271 Artavia-Loria E, Chaussain JL, Bougnères PF *et al.* Frequency of hypoglycemia in children with adrenal insufficiency. *Acta Endocrinol* 1986;276:275–8.
272 Tobin MV, Aldridge SA, Morris AL *et al.* Gastrointestinal manifestations of Addison's disease. *Am J Gastroenterol* 1989;84:1302–5.
273 Fellows RE, Buchanan JR, Peterson RE *et al.* Chronic primary adrenal insufficiency without hyperpigmentation. *N Engl J Med* 1962;267:215.
274 Rochiccioli P, Ribot C, Dutau G *et al.* Hypoglycémie par déficit cortico- et/ou medullo-surrénalien. *Arch Fr Pédiatr* 1973;30:977–88.
275 Rushton JB, Gragg RW, Stalker LK. Spontaneous hypoglycemia due to atrophy of adrenal glands, report of a case. *Arch Intern Med* 1940;66:531–40.
276 Somerville RJ, Nora JJ, Clayton GW *et al.* Adrenal insufficiency mimicking heart disease in infancy. *Pediatrics* 1968;42:691–4.
277 Ackerman GL, Lindley Miller C. Role of hypovolemia in the impaired water diuresis of adrenal insufficiency. *J Clin Endocrinol Metab* 1970;30:252–8.
278 Henkin RI, Gill JR Jr, Barter FS. Studies on taste thresholds in normal man and in patients with adrenal cortical insufficiency: the role of adrenal cortical steroids and of serum sodium concentration. *J Clin Invest* 1963;42:727–35.
279 Kosowicz I, Proszewicz A. The taste test in adrenal insufficiency. *J Clin Endocrinol Metab* 1967;27:214–18.
280 Henkin RI, Bartter FC. Studies on olfactory thresholds in normal man and in patients with adrenal cortical insufficiency: the role of adrenal cortical steroids and of serum sodium concentrations. *J Clin Invest* 1966;45:1631–9.
281 Henkin RI, McGlone RE, Daly R *et al.* Studies of auditory thresholds in normal man and in patients with adrenal cortical insufficiency. The role of adrenal cortical steroids. *J Clin Invest* 1967;46:429–35.
282 Wilkins L, Fleisshmann W, Howard JE. Macrogenitosomia precox with hyperplasia of the androgenic tissue and death from corticoadrenal insufficiency. *Endocrinology* 1940;26:385–95.
283 Ehrengut W. Addison's disease and growth. *Helv Pediatr Acta* 1956;11:63–77.
284 Bertrand J, Loras B, Saez J *et al.* Puberté précoce au cours d'une insuffisance surrénale chronique. Nouvel example d'endocrinopathie complexe par entrainement? *(Semaine des Hôpitaux de Paris) Ann Pédiatr* 1965;41:2892–7.
285 Van Gelderen HH. Precocious menstruation in hypothyroidism. *Arch Dis Child* 1962;37:337–9.
286 Lucky AW, Rebar RW, Blizzard RM *et al.* Pubertal progression in the presence of elevated serum gonadotropins in girls with multiple endocrine deficiencies. *J Clin Endocrinol Metab* 1977;45:673–8.
287 Urban MD, Lee PA, Gutai JP, Migeon CJ. Androgens in pubertal males with Addison's disease. *J Clin Endocrinol Metab* 1980;51:925–9.
288 Ng LL, Evans DJ, Burke CW. The human leucocyte sodium pump in adrenocortical insufficiency. *Clin Endocrinol* 1987;27:235–43.
289 Garnier PE, Luton JP, Leprat J *et al.* L'hypercalcémie au cours de l'insuffisance surrénale primaire. *Rev Fr Endocrinol Clin* 1972;13:391–400.
290 Moses AM, Gabrilove JL, Soffer LJ. Simplified water loading test in hypoadrenocorticism and hypothyroidism. *J Clin Endocrinol Metab* 1958;18:1413–17.
291 Robinson FJ, Power MH, Kepler EJ. Two new procedures to assist in the recognition and exclusion of Addison's disease: a preliminary report. *Proc Staff Meetings Mayo Clinic* 1941;16:577–83.
292 Haydar NA, Marc JR St, Reddy WJ *et al.* Adrenocortical insufficiency with normal basal levels of urinary 17-hydroxycorticosteroids; diagnostic implications. *J Clin Endocrinol Metab* 1958;18:121–9.
293 Besser GM, Cullen DR, Irvine WJ *et al.* Immunoreactive corticotrophin levels in adrenocortical insufficiency. *Br Med J* 1971;1:374–6.
294 Ney RL, Shimizu N, Nicholson WE *et al.* Correlation of plasma ACTH concentration with adrenocortical response in normal human subjects, surgical patients and patients with Cushing's disease. *J Clin Invest* 1963;42:1669–77.
295 Bethune JE, Nelson DH, Thorn GW. Plasma adrenocorticotrophic hormone in Addison's disease and its modification by administration of adrenal steroids. *J Clin Invest* 1957;36:1701–7.
296 Graber A, Givens JR, Nicholson WE *et al.* Persistence of diurnal rhythmicitv in plasma ACTH concentrations in cortisol deficient patients. *J Clin Endocrinol Metab* 1965;25:804–7.
297 Krieger DT, Gewirtz GP. The nature of the circadian periodicity and suppressibility of immunoreactive ACTH levels in Addison's disease. *J Clin Endocrinol Metab* 1974;39:46–52.
298 Oyama K, Shimizu M, Nogawa T *et al.* Plasma bioactive ACTH levels in normal children and the patients with adrenocortical hypofunction. In: Ghia OP, Tanega PN, eds. *Current Topics in Pediatrics.* Indian Academy of Science, 1977:18.
299 Sekiya K, Nawata H, Hato KI *et al.* Diurnal rhythms of proopiomelanocortin-derived N-terminal peptide, β-lipoprotein, β-endorphin and adrenocorticotropin in normal subjects and in patients with Addison's disease and Cushing's disease. *Endocrinol Jpn* 1986;33:713–9.
300 Washburn RG, Bennett JE. Reversal of adrenal glucocorticoid dysfunction in a patient with disseminated histoplasmosis. *Ann Intern Med* 1989;110:86–7.
301 Gaillard RC, Riondel A, Merkelbach O *et al.* Changes in plasma aldosterone following the administration of various combinations of stimuli. *Acta Endocrinol (Copenh)* 1979;92:309–18.
302 Jéquier E. Measure biochimique de la fonction de la médullosurrénale et du système sympathique en clinique. *Schweiz Med Wochenschr* 1970;100:532–6.
303 Woorhess ML. Urinary catecholamine excretion by healthy children. *Pediatrics* 1967;39:252–7.
304 Wegienka LC, Grasso SG, Forsham PH. Estimation of adrenomedullary reserve by infusion of 2-deoxy-D-glucose. *J Clin Endocrinol Metab* 1966;26:37–45.

305 Goldfien A, Moore R, Zileli S *et al.* Plasma epinephrine and norepinephrine levels during insulin-induced hypoglycemia in man. *J Clin Endocrinol Metab* 1961;21:296–304.

306 Glazer GM, Francis IR, Quint LE. Imaging of the adrenal glands. *Invest Radiol* 1988;23:3–11.

307 Paterson JR, Neithercut WD, Spooner RJ. Delayed diagnosis of Addison's disease. *Ann Clin Biochem* 1990;27:378–81.

308 Smith AG, Shuster S, Comaish JS *et al.* Plasma immunoreactive β-melanocyte stimulating hormone and skin pigmentation in chronic renal failure. *Br Med J* 1975;1:658–9.

309 Doe RP, Lohrenz FN, Seal US. Familial decrease in corticosteroid-binding globulin. *Metabolism* 1965;14:940.

310 Kohlenbrener RM, Sheridan JT, Steiner MM *et al.* Fetal adrenal transplantation attempt in juvenile Addison's disease. *Pediatrics* 1963;31:936–45.

311 Khalid BAK, Burke CW, Hurley DM *et al.* Steroid replacement in Addison's disease and in subjects adrenalectomized for Cushing's disease: comparison of various glucocorticoids. *J Clin Endocrinol Metab* 1982;55:551–9.

312 Fariss BL, Hane S, Shinsako J *et al.* Comparison of adsorption of cortisone acetate and hydrocortisone hemisuccinate. *J Clin Endocrinol Metab* 1979;47:1137–40.

313 Goodman LS, Gilman A. *The Pharmacological Basis of Therapeutics*, 5th edn. London: Macmillan, 1975.

314 Scott RS, Donald RA, Espiner EA. Plasma ACTH and cortisol profiles in Addisonian patients receiving conventional substitution therapy. *Clin Endocrinol* 1978;9:571–6.

315 Feek CM, Ratcliffe JG, Seth J *et al.* Patterns of plasma cortisol and ACTH concentrations in patients with Addison's disease treated with conventional corticosteroid replacement. *Clin Endocrinol (Oxf)* 1981;14:451–8.

316 Oparil S. Theoretical approaches to estimation of plasma renin activity: a review and some original observations. *Clin Chem* 1976;22:583–93.

317 Thompson DG, Stuart Mason A, Goodwin FJ. Mineralocorticoid replacement in Addison's disease. *Clin Endocrinol* 1979;10:499–506.

318 Edwards OM. Changes in cortisol metabolism following rifampicin therapy. *Lancet* 1974;2:549–51.

319 Himsworth RL, Lewis JG, Rees LH. A possible ACTH secreting tumour of the pituitary developing in a conventionally treated case of Addison's disease. *Clin Endocrinol* 1978;9:131–9.

320 Krautli B, Müller J, Landotlt AM, Schulthess F von. ACTH-producing pituitary adenomas in Addison's disease: two cases treated by transsphenoidal microsurgery. *Acta Endocrinol* 1982;99:357–83.

321 Hoefnagel D, Noort S, van den Ingbar SH. Diffuse cerebral sclerosis with endocrine abnormalities in young males. *Brain* 1962;85:553–68.

322 Harris-Jones JN, Nixon PGF. Familial Addison's disease with spastic paraplegia. *J Clin Endocrinol Metab* 1955;15:739–44.

323 Siemerling E, Creutzfeld HD. Bronzenkrankenheit und Sklerosierende Encephalomyelitis. *Arch Psychiatr Nervenkr* 1923;68:217–44.

324 Blaw ME. Melanodermic type leucodystrophy (adrenoleucodystrophy). In: Vinkers PJ, Bruyn CW, eds. *Handbook of Clinical Neurology*, Vol. 10. Amsterdam: North Holland, 1970:128–33.

325 Duprey J, Lubertzki J, Lemaignen H. Un cas probable d'adrénoleucodystrophie (maladie de Schilder–Addison) chez un adulte. *Ann d'Endocrinol* 1979;40:77–8.

326 Cohandon F, Vital C, Loiseau P *et al.* Leucodystrophie avec insuffisance surrénalienne (adréno-leucodystrophie). Étude de trois cas familiaux, avec ultrastructure d'un cas biopsié. *Rev Neurol* 1975;131:407–18.

327 Fanconi A, Prader A, Isler W *et al.* Morbus Addison mit Hirnskerose im Kindesalter. *Helv Paediatr Acta* 1963;18:480–501.

328 Forsyth GC, Forbes M, Cumings JN. Adrenocortical atrophy and diffuse cerebral sclerosis. *Arch Dis Child* 1971;46:273–84.

329 Livet MO, Chaussain JL, Lyon G. La maladie de Schilder avec insuffisance surrénale (adrenoleucodystrophie). *Arch Fr Pédiatr* 1977;34:232–47.

330 Malpuech G, Raynaud EJ, Menut G *et al.* Insuffisance surrénale et leucodystrophie. *Pédiatrie* 1973;28:859–966.

331 Powers JM, Schaumburg HH. The adrenal cortex in adrenoleukodystrophy. *Arch Pathol* 1973;96:305–10.

332 Sanchez JE, Lopez VF. Sex-linked sudenophilic leukodystrophy with adrenocortical atrophy (so-called Schilder's disease). *Neurology* 1976;26:261–9.

333 Schaumburg HH, Powers J, Raine CS *et al.* Adrenoleukodystrophy. A clinical and pathological study of 17 cases. *Arch Neurol* 1975;32:577–91.

334 Schaumburg HH, Powers JM, Raine CS *et al.* Adrenomyeloneuropathy: a probable variant of adrenoleukodystrophy. II. General pathologic, neuropathologic and biochemical aspects. *Neurology* 1977;27:1114–19.

335 See G, Dayras JC, Czernichow P *et al.* Association d'une maladie d'Addison et d'une leucodystrophie. *Arch Fr Pédiatr* 1971;28:847–64.

336 Turkington RW, Stempfel RS. Adrenocortical atrophy and diffuse cerebral sclerosis (Addison–Schilder's disease). *J Pediatr* 1966;69:406–12.

337 Aubourg P, Chaussain JL. Adrenoleukodystrophy presenting as Addison's disease in children and adults. *Trends Endocrinol Metab* 1991;2:49–52.

338 Moser HW, Moser AE, Singh I, O'Neil BP. Adrenoleucodystrophy: survey of 303 cases: biochemistry, diagnosis, and therapy. *Ann Neurol* 1984;16:628–41.

339 Powell H, Tindall R, Schultz P *et al.* Adrenoleukodystrophy. Electron microscopic findings. *Arch Neurol* 1975;32:250–60.

340 Aubourg P, Adamsbaum C, Lavallard-Rousseau MC *et al.* Brain MRI and electrophysiologic abnormalities in preclinical and clinical adrenomyeloneuropathy. *Neurology* 1992;42:45–91.

341 Moser HW, Bergin A, Naidu S, Ladenson RW. Adrenoleukodystrophy. *Endocrinol Clin N Am* 1991;20:297–318.

342 Holmberg BH, Hagg E, Hagenfeldt L. Adrenomyeloneuropathy. Report on a family. *J Intern Med* 1991;230:535–8.

343 Griffin JW, Goren E, Schaumburg H *et al.* Adrenomyeloneuropathy: a probable variant of adrenoleucodystrophy. 1. Clinical and endocrinological aspects. *Neurology* 1977;27:1107–13.

344 Davis LE, Snyder RD, Orth DN *et al.* Adrenoleucodystrophy and adrenomyeloneuropathy associated with partial adrenal insufficiency in three generations of a kindred. *Am J Med* 1979;66:342–6.

345 Sadeghi-Nejad A, Senior B. Adrenomyeloneuropathy presenting as Addison's disease in childhood. *N Engl J Med* 1990;322:13–16.

346 Moser HW, Moser AB, Kawamura N *et al.* Adrenoleucodystrophy: studies of the phenotype, genetics and biochemistry. *Johns Hopkins Med* 1980;147:217–24.

347 O'Neil BP, Moser HW, Saxena KM, Marmion LC. Adrenoleucodystrophy: clinical and biochemical manifestations in carriers. *Neurology* 1984;34:798–801.

348 Garg BP, Markand ON, Demeyer WE, Warren C Jr. Evoked response studies in patients with adrenoleucodystrophy and heterozygous relatives. *Arch Neurol* 1983;40:356–9.

349 Jaffe R, Crumrine P, Hashida Y, Moser HW. Neonatal adrenoleucodystrophy: clinical, pathological and biochemical delineation of a syndrome affecting both males and females. *Am J Pathol* 1982;108:100–11.

350 Mantz HJ, Schuelein M, McCullough DC *et al.* New phenotypic variant of adrenoleucodystrophy. Pathologic, ultrastructural, and biochemical study in two brothers. *J Neurol Sci* 1980;45:245–60.

351 Ulrich J, Herschkowitz N, Heitz P *et al.* Adrenoleucodystrophy: preliminary report of a connatal case. *Acta Neuropathol* 1978;43:77–83.

352 Partin JS, McAdams JA. Absence of hepatic peroxisomes in neonatal onset adrenoleucodystrophy. *Pediatr Res* 1983;17: 294A.

353 Singh I, Moser AE, Goldfischer S, Moser HW. Lignoceric acid is oxidized in the peroxisome: implications for the Zellweger cerebro-hepato-renal syndrome and adrenoleucodystrophy. *Proc Natl Acad Sci USA* 1984;84:4203–7.

354 Moser HW, Bergin A, Cornblath D. Peroxisomal disorders. *Biochem Cell Biol* 1991;6:463–74.

355 Migeon BA, Moser HW, Moser AB *et al.* Adrenoleucodystrophy: evidence for X-linkage, inactivation and selection favoring the mutant allele in heterozygous cells. *Proc Natl Acad Sci USA* 1981;78:5066–70.

356 Feil R, Aubourg P, Mosser J *et al.* Adrenoleucodystrophy: a complex chromosomal rearrangement in the Xq 28 red–green-color-pigment gene region indicates two possible gene localizations. *Am J Hum Genet* 1991;4:1361–71.

357 Igarashi M, Shaunmburg HH, Powers J *et al.* Fatty acid abnormality in adrenoleucodystrophy. *J Neurochem* 1976; 26:851–60.

358 Moser HW, Moser AB, Powers JM *et al.* The prenatal diagnosis of adrenoleucodystrophy. Demonstration of increased hexacosanoic acid levels in cultured amniocytes and fetal adrenal gland. *Pediatr Res* 1982;19:172–5.

359 Molzer B, Berheimer H, Heller R *et al.* Detection of adrenoleucodystrophy by increased $C_{26:0}$ fatty acid levels in leucocytes. *Clin Chim Acta* 1982;125:299–305.

360 Singh I, Moser HW, Moser AB, Kishimoto Y. Adrenoleucodystrophy: impaired oxidation of long chain fatty acids in cultured skin fibroblasts and adrenal cortex. *Biochem Biophys Res Commun* 1981;102:1223–9.

361 Singh I, Moser AE, Moser HW, Kishimoto Y. Adrenoleucodystrophy: impaired oxidation of very long chain fatty acids in white blood cells, cultured skin fibroblasts, and amniocytes. *Pediatr Res* 1984;18:286–90.

362 van Oost BA, van Zandvoort PM, Tünte W *et al.* Linkage analysis in X-linked adrenoleukodystrophy and application in post- and prenatal diagnosis. *Hum Genet* 1991;86:404–7.

363 Notarangelo LD, Parolini O, Baiguini G *et al.* Carrier detection in X-linked adrenoleucodystrophy by determination of very long chain fatty acid levels and by linkage analysis. *Eur J Pediatr* 1992;151:761–3.

364 Aubourg P, Bougnères PF, Rochiccioli F. Capillary gas liquid chromatographic mass spectrometric measurement of very long chain (C22 to C26) fatty acid in microliter sample of plasma. *J Lipid Res* 1985;2:263–7.

365 Parent P, Le Meur F, Alix D, Le Fur JM, Toudic L, Castel Y. A propos d'une observation familiale d'adrénoleucodystrophie liée à l'X avec réalisation d'un diagnostic anténatal. *Pédiatrie* 1987;42:297–301.

366 Del Mastro RG, Bundey S, Kilpatrick MW. Adrenoleucodystrophy: a molecular genetic study in five families. *J Med Genet* 1990;27:670–5.

367 Krisans SK. The role of peroxisomes in cholesterol metabolism. *Am J Respir Cell Mol Biol* 1992;7:358–64.

368 Goldfisher S. Peroxisomes and human metabolic diseases: the cerebro-hepato-renal syndrome (CHRS), cerebrotendinous xanthomatosis, and Schilder's disease (adrenoleucodystrophy). *Ann NY Acad Sci* 1982;386:526–9.

369 Mosser J, Douar AM, Sarde O *et al.* Putative X-linked adrenoleucodystrophy gene shares unexpected homology with ABC transporters. *Nature* 1993;361:726–30.

370 Moser HW. X-linked adrenoloeucodystrophy: pathogenesis and treatment. *J Clin Chem Clin Biochem* 1989;27:306–8.

371 Peckham RS, Marshall MC, Rosman PM *et al.* A variant of adrenomyeloneuropathy with hypothalamic–pituitary dysfunction and neurological remission after glucocorticoid replacement therapy. *Am J Med* 1982;72:173–6.

372 Moser AE, Borel J, Odone A *et al.* A new dietary therapy for adrenoleukodystrophy: biochemical and clinical preliminary results in 36 patients. *Ann Neurol* 1987;21:240–9.

373 Shepard TH, Landing BH, Mason DG. Familial Addison's disease. Case reports of two sisters with corticoid deficiency unassociated with hypoaldosteronism. *Am J Dis Child* 1959; 97:154–62.

374 Migeon CJ, Kenny FM, Kowarski A *et al.* The syndrome of congenital adrenocortical unresponsiveness to ACTH. Report of six cases. *Pediatr Res* 1968;2:501–13.

375 Davidai G, Kahana L, Hochberg Z. Glomerulosa failure in congenital adrenocortical unresponsiveness to ACTH. *Clin Endocrinol* 1984;20:515–20.

376 Franks RC, Nance WE. Hereditary adrenocortical unresponsiveness. *Pediatrics* 1970;45:43–8.

377 Geffner ME, Lippe BM, Kaplan SA *et al.* Selective ACTH insensitivity, achalasia, and alacrima: a multisystem disorder presenting in childhood. *Pediatr Res* 1983;17:532–6.

378 Kelch RP, Kaplan SL, Biglieri EG *et al.* Hereditary adrenocortical unresponsiveness to adrenocorticotropic hormone. *J Pediatr* 1972;81:726–36.

379 Kershnar AK, Roe TF, Kogut MD. Adrenocorticotropic hormone unresponsiveness: report of a girl with excessive growth and review of 16 reported cases. *J Pediatr* 1972;80: 610–19.

380 Mozziconacci P, L'Hirondel J, Girard F *et al.* Maladie d'Addison familiale avec insuffisance surrénale dissociée. *Ann Pédiatr* 1960;36:265–74.

381 Petrykowski WV, Burmeister P, Bohm N. Familiäre glucocorticoid-insuffizienz. *Klin Pädiatr* 1975;187:198–215.

382 Soltesz G, Dillon MJ, Jenkins PA *et al.* Isolated glucocorticoid deficiency: metabolic and endocrine studies in a 5-year-old boy. *Eur J Pediatr* 1985;143:297–300.

383 Stempfel RS, Engel FI. A congenital familial syndrome or adrenocortical insufficiency without hypoaldosteronism. *J Pediatr* 1960;57:443–51.

384 Thistlethwaite D, Darling JAB, Fraser R *et al.* Familial glucocorticoid deficiency. *Arch Dis Child* 1975;50:291–7.

385 Moore PSJ, Couch RM, Perry YS, Schuckett EP, Winter JSD. Allgrove syndrome: an autosomal recessive syndrome of ACTH insensitivity, achalasia and alacrima. *Clin Endocrinol* 1991;19:107–14.

386 Völlmin JA. Gas chromatographic separation of steroids on glass capillary columns. *Chromatographia* 1970;3:233.

387 Werder EA, Haller R, Wetter W *et al.* Isolated glucocorticoid insufficiency. *Helv Paediatr Acta* 1975;30:175–83.

388 Williams HE, Freeman M. Primary familial Addison's disease. *Austr Paediatr J* 1965;1:93–7.
389 Lanes R, Plotnick LP, Bynum TE *et al.* Glucocorticoid and partial mineralocorticoid deficiency associated with achalasia. *J Clin Endocrinol Metab* 1980;50:268–70.
390 Moshang T, Rosenfield ML, Bongiovanni AM *et al.* Familial glucocorticoid insufficiency. *J Pediatr* 1973;82:821–6.
391 Allgrove J, Clayden GS, Grant DB, McCauley JC. Familial glucocorticoid deficiency with achalasia of the cardia and deficient tear production. *Lancet* 1978;1:1284–6.
392 Ambrosiano MM, Geneiser NB, Bangaru BS *et al.* The syndrome of achalasia of the esophagus, ACTH insensitivity and alacrima. *Pediatr Radiol* 1986;16:328–9.
393 Dumic M, Radica A, Jusic A *et al.* Selective insensitivity associated with autonomic nervous system disorders and sensory polyneuropathy. *Eur J Pediatr* 1987;146:592–4.
394 Ehrich E, Aranoff G, Johnson WG. Familial achalasia associated with adrenocortical insufficiency, alacrima, and neurological abnormalities. *Am J Med Genet* 1987;26: 637–44.
395 Stukey BG, Mestaglia FL, Reed WD, Pullan PT. Glucocorticoid insufficiency, achalasia, alacrima, with autonomic and motor neuropathy. *Ann Intern Med* 1987;106:62–4.
396 Dumic M, Radica A, Sabol Z *et al.* Adrenocorticotropic hormone insensitivity associated with autonomic nervous system disorders. *Eur J Pediatr* 1991;150:696–9.
397 Grant, DB, Dunger DB, Smith I, Hyland K. Familial glucocorticoid deficiency with achalasia of the cardia associated with mixed neuropathy, long-tract degeneration and mild dementia. *Eur J Pediatr* 1992;151:85–9.
398 Spark RF, Etzkorn JR. Absent aldosterone response to ACTH in familial glucocorticoid deficiency. *N Engl J Med* 1977;297: 917–20.
399 Federico A, Baracchini G, Dotti MT *et al.* Infanto-juvenile encephaloneuropathy and pigmentary retinopathy in a girl associated with congenital insufficiency and altered plasma medium-chain fatty acid levels. *J Inher Metab Dis* 1989; 11(Suppl. 2):178–82.
400 Mountjoy KG, Robbins LS, Mortrud MT, Cone RD. The cloning of a family of genes that encode the melanocortin receptors. *Science* 1992;257:1248–51.
401 Clark AJL, McLoughlin L, Grossman A. Familial glucocorticoid deficiency associated with point mutation in the adrenocorticotropin receptor. *Lancet* 1993;341:461–2.
402 Naville D, Chatelain P, Brunelli V, Bégeot M. A study of the ACTH receptor gene in five different families with ACTH insensitivity. *Proceedings of the 75th Meeting Endocrinology Society, Las Vegas* 1993:237 (Abstr. 747).
403 Haverkamp F, Zerres K, Rosskamp R. Three sibs with achalasia and alacrima: a separate entity different from triple-A syndrome. *Am J Med Genet* 1989;34:289–91.
404 Pombo M, Devesa J, Taborda A *et al.* Glucocorticoid deficiency with achalasia of the cardia and lack of lacrimation. *Clin Endocrinol* 1985;23:237–43.
405 Raux MC, Pham-Huu-Trung MT, Marrec D, Girard F. Plasma aldosterone concentration during neonatal period. *Pediatr Res* 1977;11:1982–5.
406 Vingerhoeds ACM, Thijssen JHH, Scwarts FJ. Spontaneous hypercortisolism without Cushing's syndrome. *J Clin Endocrinol Metab* 1976;43:1128–33.
407 Chrousos GP, Renquist O, Brandon D *et al.* Primary cortisol resistance in man. A glucocorticoid receptor-mediated disease. *J Clin Invest* 1982;69:1261–9.
408 Nawata H, Sekiya K, Higuchi K *et al.* Decreased deoxyribonucleic acid binding of glucocorticoid–receptor complex in cultured skin fibroblasts from a patient with the glucocorticoid resistance syndrome. *J Clin Endocrinol Metab* 1987; 65:219–26.
409 Lamberts SWJ, Koper JW, Biemond P *et al.* Cortisol receptor resistance. The variability of its clinical presentation and response to treatment. *J Clin Endocrinol Metab* 1992;74: 313–21.
410 Lipsett MB, Chrousos GP, Tomita M *et al.* The defective glucocorticoid receptor in man and nonhuman primates. *Rec Prog Horm Res* 1985;41:199–247.
411 Malchoff CD, Javier EC, Malchoff DM *et al.* Primary cortisol resistance presenting as isosexual precocity. *J Clin Endocrinol Metab* 1990;70:503–7.
412 Linder MJ, Thompson EB. Abnormal glucocorticoid receptor gene and mRNA in primary cortisol resistance. *J Steroid Biochem* 1989;32:243–9.
413 Brufsky AM, Malcholl DM, Javier EC *et al.* Glucocorticoid receptor mutation in a subject with primary cortisol resistance. *Trans Assoc Am Phys* 1990;CIII:53–62.
414 Hurley DM, Accili D, Stratakis CA *et al.* Point mutation causing a single amino acid substitution in the hormone binding domain of the glucocorticoid receptor in familial glucocorticoid resistance. *J Clin Invest* 1991;87:680–6.
415 Biglieri E. A perspective on aldosterone abnormalities. *Clin Endocrinol* 1976;5:399–410.
416 Ulick S. Diagnosis and nomenclature of the terminal portion of the aldosterone biosynthetic pathway. *J Clin Endocrinol Metab* 1976;43:92–6.
417 Hauffa BP, Solyom J, Glaz E *et al.* Severe hypoaldosteronism due to corticosterone methyl oxidase type II deficiency in two boys; metabolic and gas chromatography–mass spectrometry studies. *Eur J Pediatr* 1991;150:149–53.
418 Royer H, Lestrader H, de Menibus CH *et al.* Hypoaldostéronisme familial chronique à début néonatal. *Ann Pédiatr* 1961;37:901–6.
419 Veldhuis JD, Kulin HE, Santen RJ *et al.* Inborn error in the terminal step of aldosterone biosynthesis. Corticosterone methyl oxidase type II deficiency in a North American pedigree. *N Engl J Med* 1980;303:117–21.
420 Visser HKA, Cost WS. A new hereditary defect in the biosynthesis of aldosterone: urinary C21-corticosteroid pattern in three related patients with a salt-losing syndrome suggesting an 18-oxidation defect. *Acta Endocrinol (Copenh)* 1964;47: 589–612.
421 Klaus D, Lederle RM, Vecsei P. Primary hypoaldosteronism and secondary pseudohypoaldosteronism. *Klin Wochenschr* 1984;62:753–8.
422 Lebel M, Grose JH. Angiotensin II effect on plasma steroid in selective hypoaldosteronism. *Horm Metab Res* 1982;14: 432–6.
423 Picco P, Garibaldi L, Cotellessa M *et al.* Corticosterone methyl oxidase type II deficiency; a cause of failure to thrive and recurrent dehydration in early infancy. *Eur J Pediatr* 1992;151:170–3.
424 Rösler A. The natural history of saltwasting disorders of adrenal origin. *J Clin Endocrinol Metab* 1984;59:689–700.
425 Lieva de A, Christlieb AR, Melby JC *et al.* Big renin and biosynthetic defect of aldosterone in diabetes mellitus. *N Engl J Med* 1976;295:639–43.
426 Marieb NJ, Melby JL, Lyall SS. Isolated hypoaldosteronism associated with idiopathic hypoparathyroidism. *Arch Intern Med* 1974;134:424–9.
427 Kater CE, Biglieri EG, Brust N *et al.* Stimulation and sup-

pression of the mineralocorticoid hormones in normal subjects and in adrenocortical disorders. *Endocr Rev* 1989;10: 149–64.

428 Blazy I, Guillot F, Laborde K, Dechaux M. Comparison of plasma renin and prorenin in healthy infants and children as determined with an enzymatic method and a new direct immunoradiometric assay. *Scand J Clin Lab Invest* 1989;49: 413–18.

429 Lee PDK, Patterson BD, Hintz RL *et al.* Biochemical diagnosis and management of corticosterone methyl oxidase type II deficiency. *J Clin Endocrinol Metab* 1986;62:225–9.

430 Veldhuis JD, Melby JC. Isolated aldosterone deficiency in man: acquired and inborn errors in the biosynthetic action of aldosterone. *Endocr Rev* 1981;2:495–517.

431 Armanini D, Kunle U, Strasser T *et al.* Aldosterone-receptor deficiency in pseudohypoaldosteronism. *N Engl J Med* 1985; 313:1178–81.

432 Tieder M, Vure E, Gilboa Y *et al.* Syndrome de perte de sel du nourrisson avec hyperaldostéronisme présentant une sensibilité aux hormones minéralocorticoïdes: pseudo-hypoaldostéronisme? *Arch Fr Pédiatr* 1976;33:485–6.

433 Landier F, Guyene TT, Boutignon H *et al.* Hyporeninemic hypoaldosteronism in infancy: a familial disease. *J Clin Endocrinol Metab* 1984;58:143–8.

434 Shuper A, Eisenstein B, Stark H, Varsano I. Hyporeninemic hypoaldosteronism in a child with lactic acidosis, deafness and mental retardation. *J Pediatr* 1982;100:769–72.

435 Bergstein JM, Weinberger MH. Hypokaliemia, normal blood pressure and hyperreninemia with hypoaldosteronism. *J Pediatr* 1981;99:561–4.

436 Kater CE, Biglieri EG, Rost CR *et al.* The constant plasma hydrocorticosterone to aldosterone ratio: an expression of the efficacy of corticosterone methyl oxidase type II activity in disorders with variable aldosterone production. *J Clin Endocrinol Metab* 1985;60:225–8.

437 Degenhart HJ, Frankena L, Visser HKA *et al.* Further investigations of a new hereditary defect in the biosynthesis of aldosterone: evidence for a defect in 18-hydroxylation of corticosterone. *Acta Physiol Pharmacol Neerl* 1966;14: 88–93.

438 Ulick S, Wang JZ, Morton DH. The biochemical phenotypes of two inborn errors in the biosynthesis of aldosterone. *J Clin Endocrinol Metab* 1992;74:1415–20.

439 Yanagibashi K, Hanin H, Shively JE *et al.* The synthesis of aldosterone by the adrenal cortex: two zones (fasciculata and glomerulosa) possess one enzyme for 11β- 18-hydroxylase, and aldehyde synthesis. *J Biochem Chem* 1986;261:3356–62.

440 Curnow KM, Tusie-Luna MT, Pascoe L *et al.* The product of the CYP11B2 gene is required for aldosterone biosynthesis in the human adrenal cortex. *Mol Endocrinol* 1991;5:1513–22.

441 Chua SC, Szabo P, Vitek A *et al.* Cloning of cDNA encoding steroid 11β-hydroxylase (P-450c11). *Proc Natl Acad Sci USA* 1987;84:7193–7.

442 Mornet E, Dupont J, Vitek A, White PC. Characterization of the two genes encoding human steroid 11β-hydroxylase (P45011β). *J Biol Chem* 1985;264:20961–7.

443 Kawamoto T, Mitsuuchi Y, Toda K *et al.* Role of steroid 11β-hydroxylase and steroid 18-hydroxylase in the biosynthesis of glucocorticoids and mineralocorticoids in humans. *Proc Natl Acad Sci USA* 1992;89:1458–62.

444 Globerman H, Rösler A, Theodor R *et al.* An inherited defect in aldosterone biosynthesis caused by mutation in or near the gene for 11-hydroxylase. *N Engl J Med* 1988;319:1193–7.

445 Mitsuuchi Y, Kawamoto T, Rösler A *et al.* Congenitally defective aldosterone biosynthesis in humans: the involvement of point mutations of the P-450c18 gene (CYP11B2) in CMO II deficient patients. *Biochem Biophys Res Commun* 1992;182:974–9.

446 Pascoe L, Curnow KM, Slutsker L, Rösler A, White PC. Mutations in the human CYP11B2 (aldosterone synthase) gene causing cortiscosterone methyloxidase II deficiency. *Proc Natl Acad Sci USA* 1992;89:4996–5000.

447 Zipser RM, Davenport MW, Martin KL *et al.* Hyperreninemic hypoaldosteronism in the critically ill: a new entity. *J Clin Endocrinol Metab* 1981;53:867–72.

448 Cheek DB, Perry JW. A salt wasting syndrome in infancy. *Arch Dis Child* 1958;33:252–6.

449 Bommen M, Brook CGD. Pseudohypoaldosteronism. Response to long-term treatment with indomethacin. *Arch Dis Child* 1982;57:718–20.

450 Cessans C, Berthier M, Labrie C *et al.* Le pseudoaldostéronisme congénital: à propos de 6 observations. *Pédiatrie* 1989;44:649–54.

451 Hanukoglu A. Type I pseudohypoaldosteronism includes two clinically and genetically distinct entities with either renal or multiple target organ defects. *J Clin Endocrinol Metab* 1991;73:936–44.

452 Kuhnle U, Nielsen MD, Tietze HU *et al.* Pseudohypoaldosteronism in eight families; different forms of inheritance are evidence for various genetic defects. *J Clin Endocrinol Metab* 1990;70:638–41.

453 Rampini S, Furrer J, Keller HP *et al.* Congenital pseudohypoaldosteronism: case report and review. *Helv Paediatr Acta* 1978;33:153–67.

454 Speiser PW, Stoner E, New MI. Pseudohypoaldosteronism; a review and report of two new cases. *Adv Exp Med Biol* 1986;196:173–95.

455 Chitayat D, Spirer Z, Ayalon D, Gollander A. Pseudohypoaldosteronism in a female infant and her family: diversity of clinical expression and mode of inheritance. *Acta Paed Scand* 1985;74:916–22.

456 Hanukoglu A, Fried D, Gotlieb A. Inheritance of pseudohypoaldosteronism. *Lancet* 1978;1:1359.

457 Limal JM, Rappaport R, Dechaux M *et al.* Familial dominant pseudohypoaldosteronism. *Lancet* 1978;1:51.

458 Roy C. Pseudohypoaldosteronisme familial. *Arch Fr Pédiatr* 1976;34:37–54.

459 Bonnici F. Pseudohypoaldosteronisme familial à transmission autosomique récessive. *Arch Fr Pediatr* 1977;34: 915–16.

460 Kuhnle U, Dörr H, Strasser T *et al.* Demonstration of mineralocorticoid receptor deficiency in two siblings with pseudohypoaldosteronism (PH). *Pediatr Res* 1985;19:617.

461 Bierich JR, Schmidt U. Tubular Na, K-ATPase deficiency, the cause of the congenital renal salt-losing syndrome. *Eur J Pediatr* 1976;121:81–8.

462 Arriza JL, Weinberger C, Cerelli G *et al.* Cloning of the human mineralocorticoid receptor complementary DNA: structural and functional kinship with the glucocorticoid receptor. *Science* 1987;237:238–75.

463 Shigetomi S, Ojima M, Ueno S *et al.* Two adult familial cases of selective hypoaldosteronism due to insufficiency of conversion of corticosterone to aldosterone. *Endocrinology* 1985;33:787–94.

464 Keszler M, Sivasubramanian KM. Pseudohypoaldosteronism: fulminant presentation in a premature infant. *Am J Dis Child* 1983;137:738–40.

465 Abramson O, Zmora E, Mazor M, Shinwell ES. Pseudohypo-

aldosteronism in a preterm infant: intrauterine presentation as hydramnios. *J Pediatr* 1992;120:129–32.
466 Schindler AM, Bergman GE. Prospective diagnosis of pseudohypoaldosteronism. *Pediatrics* 1986;78:516–18.
467 Oberfield SE, Levine SL, Carey RM *et al.* Pseudohypoaldosteronism: multiple target organ unresponsiveness to mineralocortocoid hormones. *J Clin Endocrinol Metab* 1979; 48:228–34.
468 West ML, Benddz O, Chen CB *et al.* Development of a test to evaluate the transtubular potassium gradient in the cortical collecting duct *in vivo. Miner Electrolyte Metab* 1986;12: 226–33.
469 West ML, Mardsen PA, Richardson RMA *et al.* New clinical approach to evaluate disorders of potassium excretion. *Miner Electrolyte Metab* 1986;12:234–8.
470 Rodriguez-Soriano J, Ubetagoyena M, Vallo A. Transtubular potassium concentration gradient: a useful test to estimate renal aldosterone bio-activity in infants and children. *Pediatr Nephrol* 1990;4:105–10.
471 Rodriguez-Soriano J, Vallo A. Renal tubular hyperkaliemia in childhood. *Pediatr Nephrol* 1988;2:498–509.
472 Popow C, Pollak A, Herkner K *et al.* Familial pseudohypoaldosteronism. *Acta Paed Scand* 1988;77:136–41.
473 Anand SK, Froberg L, Northway JD *et al.* Pseudohypoaldosteronism due to sweat gland dysfunction. *Pediatr Res* 1976; 10:677–82.
474 Sanderson IR, Carter EP, Dillon MJ *et al.* Familial salivary gland insensitivity to aldosterone: a variant of pseudoaldosteronism. *Horm Res* 1989;32:145–7.
475 Schamberlan M, Sebastian A, Rector FC Jr. Mineralocorticoid-resistant renal hyperkalaemia without salt wasting (type II pseudohypoaldosteronism): role of increased renal chloride reabsorption. *Kidney Int* 1981;19:716–27.
476 Take C, Ikeda K, Kurasawa T, Kurkawa K. Increased chloride reabsorption as an inherited renal tubular defect in familial type II pseudoaldosteronism. *N Engl J Med* 1991;324:472–6.
477 Rodriguez-Soriano J, Vallo A, Oliveros R, Castillo G. Transient pseudohypoaldosteronism secondary to obstructive uropathy in infancy. *J Pediatr* 1983;103:375–80.
478 McSherry E. Renal tubular acidosis in childhood. *Kidney Int* 1981;20:859–78.
479 Appiani AC, Marra G, Tirelli SA *et al.* Early childhood hyperkalaemia: variety of pseudohypoaldosteronism. *Acta Paed Scand* 1986;75:970–4.
480 Hudson JB, Chobianian AV, Relman AS. Hypoaldosteronism. A clinical study of a patient with isolated mineralocorticoid deficiency, resulting in hypokalemia and Stokes-Adams attacks. *N Engl J Med* 1957;257:529–36.
481 Schamberlan M, Stockigt JR, Biglieri EG. Isolated hypoaldosteronism in adults. A renin-deficiency syndrome. *N Engl J Med* 1972;287:573–8.
482 Kalin MF, Poretsky L, Seres DS *et al.* Hyporeninemic hypoaldosteronism associated with acquired immune deficiency syndrome. *Am J Med* 1987;82:1035–8.
483 Monnens L, Fiselier T, Bos B, Van Munster P. Hyporeninemic hypoaldosteronism in infancy. *Nephron* 1983;35:140–2.
484 Phelps HR, Lieberman RL, Oh MS, Carroll HJ. Pathophysiology of the syndrome of hyporeninemic hypoaldosteronism. *Metabolism* 1980;29:186–99.
485 Nadler JL, Lee FO, Hsueh W *et al.* Evidence of prostacyclin deficiency in the syndrome of hyporeninemic hypoaldosteronism. *N Engl J Med* 1986;314:1015–20.
486 Otabe S, Moto S, Asano Y *et al.* Hyperreninemic hypoaldosteronism due to hepatocellular carcinoma metastatic to the adrenal gland. *Clin Nephrol* 1991;35:66–71.
487 Findling JW, Adams AH, Raff H. Selective hypoaldosteronism due to endogenous impairment in angiotensin II production. *N Engl J Med* 1987;316:1632–5.
488 Muto S, Fujisawa G, Natsume T *et al.* Hyponatremia and hyperreninemic hypoaldosteronism in a critically ill patient: combination of insensitivity to angiotensin II and tubular unresponsiveness to mineralocorticoid. *Clin Nephrol* 1990; 34:208–13.
489 Liddle GW, Bledsoe T, Coppage WS Jr. A familial renal disorder simulating primary aldosteronism but with negligible aldosterone secretion. In: Baulieu EE, Robel E, eds. *Aldosterone.* Oxford: Blackwell Scientific Publications, 1964:353.
490 Williams FA, Shambelan M, Biglieri E, Carey RM. Acquired primary hypoaldosteronism due to zona glomerular defect. *N Engl J Med* 1983;309:1623–7.
491 Mizuno K, Matsui S, Shigetomi S *et al.* Selective hypoaldosteronism associated with chronic thyroiditis and other endocrine abnormalities. *Jpn J Med* 1981;20:16–25.
492 Agmon D, Green E, Plateau E, Better O. Isolated mineralocorticoid deficiency due to amyloidosis associated with familial Mediterranean fever. *Am J Med Soc* 1984;288:40–3.
493 Slaton PE, Biglieri EG. Reduced aldosterone excretion in patients with autonomic insufficiency. *J Clin Endocrinol Metab* 1967;27:37–45.
494 Kutyrina IM, Androsova SO, Tareyeva IE. Indomethacin-induced hyporeninaemic hypoaldosteronism. *Lancet* 1979; 1:785.
495 McAllister RG Jr, Michelakis AM, Sandstead HH. Plasma renin activity in chronic plumbism. *Arch Intern Med* 1971; 127:919–23.
496 Wilson D, Goetz C. Selective hypoaldosteronism after prolonged heparin administration. *Am J Med* 1964;36:635–40.
497 Reynolds JW, Turnipseed MR, Mirkin BL. Adrenal cortical function in abnormal newborn infants. *J Steroid Biochem* 1975;6:669–72.
498 Sizonenko PC. Preadolescent and adolescent endocrinology. Physiology and physiopathology. 2. Hormonal changes during abnormal development. *Am J Dis Child* 1978;132: 797–805.
499 de Peretti E, Forest MG, David L *et al.* Dehydroepiandrosterone (DHA), its sulfate (DHAS) 17α-hydroxyprogestrone (OHP) and cortisol (F) levels in pànhypopituitarism (group I) and isolated GH deficiency (group II): evidence for a pituitary hormone controlling adrenal androgen biosynthesis. *Pediatr Res* 1978;12:151.
500 Forest MG, de Peretti E, Bertrand J. Developmental patterns of the plasma levels of testosterone, Δ^4-androstenedione, 17α-hydroxyprogesterone, dehydroepiandrosterone and its sulfate in normal infants and prepubertal children. In: James VHT, Serio M, Guisti G, Martini L, eds. *The Endocrine Function of the Human Adrenal Cortex.* 1978:561–82.
501 Parker LN, Odell WD. Control of adrenal androgen secretion. *Endocr Rev* 1980;1:392–410.
502 Adams JB. Control of secretion and the function of C_{19}-Δ^5-steroids of the human adrenal gland. *Mol Cell Endocrinol* 1985;41:1–17.
503 Forest MG, de Peretti E, Bertrand J. Age-related shifts in the response of plasma Δ^4- and Δ^5-androgens, their C21 precursors and cortisol to ACTH from infancy to puberty. In: Cacciari E, Prader A, eds. *Pathophysiology of Puberty.* London: Academic Press, 1980:137–55.
504 Sklar CA, Kaplan S, Grumbach MM. Evidence for dissocia-

tion between adrenarche and gonadarche: studies in patients with idiopathic precocious pubery, gonadal dysgenesis, isolated gonadotropin deficiency, and constitutionally delayed growth and adolescence. *J Clin Endocrinol Metab* 1981;51: 548–56.

505 Parker L, Lifrak E, Shively J *et al.* Human adrenal gland cortical androgen-stimulating hormone (CASH) is identical with a portion of the joining peptide of pituitary proopiomelanocortin (POMC). In: *71th Annual Meeting of the Endocrine Society* 1989:97 (Abstr. 299).

506 Mellon SH, Shively JE, Miller WL. Human proopiomelanocortin-(79-86), a proposed cortical androgen-stimulating hormone, does not affect steroidogenesis in cultured human fetal adrenal cells. *J Clin Endocrinol Metab* 1991;72:19–22.

507 Penhoat A, Sanchez P, Jaillard C *et al.* Human proopiomelanocortin-(79-86), a proposed cortical androgen-stimulating hormone, does not affect steroidogenesis in cultured human adult adrenal cells. *J Clin Endocrinol Metab* 1991;72:23–6.

508 Covell WP. A quantitative study of the hypophysis and adrenals of the human anencephalic monster. *Am J Pathol* 1927;3:1.

509 Haworth JC, Medovy H, Lewis AJ. Cebocephaly with endocrine dysgenesis. Report of 3 cases. *J Pediatr* 1961;59:726.

510 Willard D, Sacrez R, Messer J *et al.* La dysgénésie antehypophysaire primitive. *Nouv Presse Méd* 1972;1:2237–42.

511 Sadeghi-Nejad A, Senior B. A familial syndrome of isolated 'aplasia' of the anterior pituitary. *J Pediatr* 1974;84:79–84.

512 Nakagawa H, Nagasaka A, Koie K *et al.* Isolated adrenocorticotropin deficiency associated with an empty sella. *J Clin Endocrinol Metab* 1982;55:795–7.

513 Stephens WP, Goddard KJ, Laing I, Adams JE. Isolated adrenocorticotrophin deficiency and empty sella associated with hypothyroidism. *Clin Endocrinol* 1985;22:771–6.

514 Aynsley-Green A, Moncrieff MW, Ratter S *et al.* Isolated ACTH deficiency. Metabolic and endocrine studies in a 7-year old boy. *Arch Dis Child* 1978;53:499–502.

515 Cleveland WW, Green OL, Migeon CJ. A case of proved adrenocorticotropin deficiency. *J Pediatr* 1960;57:376–81.

516 Hung W, Migeon CJ. Hypoglycemia in a two-year-old boy with adrenocorticotropic hormone (ACTH) deficiency (probably isolated) and adrenal medullary unresponsiveness to insulin-induced hypoglycemia. *J Clin Endocrinol Metab* 1968;28:146–52.

517 Odell WD, Green GM, Williams RH. Hypoadrenotropism: the isolated deficiency of adrenotropic hormone. *J Clin Endocrinol Metab* 1960;20:1017–28.

518 Stacpoole PW, Interlandi JW, Nicholson WE, Rabin D. Isolated ACTH deficiency: a heterogenous disorder. Critical review and report of four new cases. *Medicine* 1982;61: 13–24.

519 Tovo PA, Lala R, Martino S *et al.* Isolated adrenocorticotropic hormone deficiency associated with common variable immunodeficiency. *Eur J Pediatr* 1991;150:400–2.

520 Koide Y, Kimura S, Inoue S *et al.* Responsiveness of hypophyseal-adrenocortical axis to repetitive administration of synthetic ovine corticotropin-releasing hormone in patients with isolated adrenocorticotropin deficiency. *J Clin Endocrinol Metab* 1986;63:329–35.

521 Shigemasa C, Kouchi T, Ueta Y, Mitani Y, Yoshida A, Mashiba H. Evaluation of thyroid function in patients with isolated adrenocorticotropin deficiency. *Am J Med Sci* 1992; 304:279–84.

522 Sugiura M, Hashimoto A, Shizawa M *et al.* Heterogeneity of anterior pituitary cell antibodies in insulin-dependent diabetes mellitus and adrenocorticotropic hormone deficiency. *Ann Intern Med* 1986;105:200–3.

523 Sauter NP, Toni R, McLaughlin CD *et al.* Isolated adrenocorticotropin deficiency associated with an autoantibody to a corticotroph antigen that is not adrenocorticotropin or other proopiomelanocortin-derived peptides. *J Clin Endocrinol Metab* 1990;70:1391–7.

524 Cacciari E, Cicognani A, Pirazzoli P *et al.* Congenital hypopituitarism associated with neonatal hypoglycaemia and microphallus: effect of GH therapy. *Helv Paediatr Acta* 1977;31:481–5.

525 Lovinger RD, Kaplan SL, Grumbach MM. Congenital hypopituitarism associated with neonatal hypoglycemia and microphallus. 4 cases secondary to hypothalamic hormone deficiencies. *J Pediatr* 1975;87:1171–81.

526 Leblanc A, Odievre M, Hadchouel M *et al.* Neonatal cholestasis and hypoglycemia. Possible role of cortisol deficiency. *J. Pediatr* 1981;99:577–80.

527 Giustina A, Romanelli G, Candrina R, Giustina G. Growth hormone deficiency in patients with idiopathic adrenocorticotropin deficiency resolves during glucocorticoid replacement. *J Clin Endocrinol Metab* 1989;68:120–4.

528 Cutler GP Jr, Davis SE, Johansonbaugh RE, Loriaux DL. Dissociation of cortisol and adrenal androgen secretion in patients with secondary adrenal insufficiency. *J Clin Endocrinol Metab* 1979;49:604–9.

529 Yamaji T, Ishibashi M, Takaku F, Itabashi A, Katayama S, Ishii J. Serum dehydroepiandrosterone sulfate concentrations in secondary adrenal insufficiency. *J Clin Endocrinol Metab* 1987;65:448–51.

530 Zachmann M, Girard J, Duc G *et al.* Low urinary estriol during pregnancy caused by isolated fetal ACTH-deficiency. *Acta Paed Scand* 1979;Suppl. 227:26–31.

531 Holdaway IM, Rees LH, Landon J. Circulating corticotrophin levels in severe hypopituitarism and in the neonate. *Lancet* 1973;2:1170–1.

532 Fehm HL, Voigt KH, Lang R *et al.* Adrenal insufficiency secondary to hypothalamic corticotropin releasing factor (CRF) insufficiency with hyperpigmentation: a case report. *Horm Metab Res* 1976;8:470–4.

533 Nichols ML, Brown RD, Granville GE *et al.* Isolated deficiency of adrenocorticotropin (ACTH) and lipotropins (LPHs). *J Clin Endocrinol Metab* 1978;47:84–90.

534 Donald RA, Espiner EA, Beaven DW. The effect of metyrapone on corticotrophin secretion. *J Endocrinol* 1972;52: 517–24.

535 Gold EM, Kent JR, Forsham PH. Clinical use of a new diagnostic agent, methopyrapone (Su-4885) in pituitary and adrenocortical disorders. *Ann Intern Med* 1961;54:175.

536 Limal JM, Basmaciogullari A, Rappaport R. Evaluation of single oral dose metyrapone tests in children with hypopituitarism. *Acta Paed Scand* 1976;65:177–83.

537 Gower DB. Modifiers of steroid-hormone metabolism: a review of their chemistry, biochemistry and clinical applications. *J Steroid Biochem* 1974;5:501–23.

538 Patel SR, Selby C, Jeffcoate WJ. The short Synacthen test in acute hospital admissions. *Clin Endocrinol* 1991;35:259–61.

539 Musa BU, Dowling JT. Rapid intravenous administration of corticotrophin as a test of adrenocortical insufficiency. *J Am Med Assoc* 1967;201:633.

540 Wood JB, Frankland AW, James VHT *et al.* A rapid test of adrenocortical function. *Lancet* 1965;1:243–5.

541 Forest MG. Age-related response of plasma testosterone, Δ^4-androstenedione and cortisol to ACTH in infants, children

and adults. *J Clin Endocrinol Metab* 1978;47:931–7.

542 Hermus ARMM, Pieters GFFM, Pesman GJ, Smams AGH, Benraad TJ, Kloppenborg PWC. ACTH and cortisol responses to ovine corticotrophin-releasing factor in patients with primary and secondary adrenal failure. *Clin Endocrinol* 1985;22:761–9.

543 Taylor AL, Fishman LM. Corticotropin releasing hormone. *N Engl J Med* 1988;319:213–22.

544 Fukata J, Nakai Y, Imura H *et al.* Human cortocotropin-releasing hormone test in normal subjects and patients with hypothalamic pituitary or adrenocortical disorders. *Endocrinol Jpn* 1988;35:491–502.

545 Schulte HM, Chrousos GP, Avgerinos P *et al.* The corticotropin-releasing hormone stimulation test: a possible aid in the evaluation of patients with adrenal insufficiency. *J Clin Endocrinol Metab* 1984;58:1064–7.

546 Prummel MF, Wiersinga WM, Lips P, Sanders GTB, Sauerwein HP. The course of biochemical parameters of bone turnover during treatment with corticoids. *J Clin Endocrinol Metab* 1991;72:382–6.

547 Jacobs TP, Whitlock RT, Edsall J *et al.* Addisonian crisis while taking high-dose glucocorticoids. *J Am Med Assoc* 1988;260:2082–4.

548 Ballard PL, Ballard RA. Corticosteroids and respiratory distress syndrome: status 1979. *Pediatrics* 1979;63:163–5.

549 Hottinger A. Insuffisance cortico-surrénale chez le nouveau-né de mère traitée par la cortisone. *Ann Pédiatr Paris* 1961;37:357–9.

550 Axelrod L. Glucocorticoid therapy. *Medicine* 1976;55:39–66.

551 Byyny RL. Withdrawal from glucocorticoid therapy. *N Engl J Med* 1976;295:30–2.

552 Graber AL, Ney RL, Nicholson WE *et al.* Natural history of pituitary – adrenal recovery after long-term suppression with corticosteroids. *J Clin Endocrinol Metab* 1965;25:11–16.

553 Priftis K, Everard ML, Milner AD. Unexpected side-effects of inhaled steroids: a case report. *Eur J Pediatr* 1991;150:448–9.

554 Zwaan CM, Odink RJH, Delemarre-van de Waal HA *et al.* Acute adrenal insufficiency after discontinuation of inhaled corticosteroid therapy. *Lancet* 1992;340:1289–90.

555 McGregor RR, Sheagren JN, Lipsett MB *et al.* Alternate-day prednisone therapy. *N Engl J Med* 1969;280:1427–31.

556 Watson AC, Rosenfield RL, Fang VS. Recovery from glucocorticoid inhibition of the responses to corticotrophin-releasing hormone. *Clin Endocrinol* 1988;28:471–7.

557 Streeten DHP, Anderson GH Jr, Dalakos TG *et al.* Normal and abnormal function of the hypothalamic-pituitary-adrenocortical system in man. *Endocr Rev* 1984;5:371–94.

558 Melby JC. Systemic corticosteroid therapy: pharmacology and endocrinologic considerations. *Ann Intern Med* 1974;81:505–12.

559 Thorn GW. *Steroid Therapy*. Kalamazoo: Upjohn, 1971.

560 Marston RA. Primary adrenocortical failure masked by exogenous steroid administration. *Clin Endocrinol* 1992;36:519–20.

561 Santen RJ, Wells SA, Runic S *et al.* Adrenal suppression with aminoglutethimide. I. Differential effects of aminoglutethimide on glucocorticoid metabolism as a rational for use of hydrocortisone. *J Clin Endocrinol Metab* 1977;45:469–79.

562 Elias AN, Gwinup G. Effects of some clinically encountered drugs on steroid synthesis and degradation. *Metabolism* 1980;29:582–94.

563 Fishman LM, Liddle GW, Island DP *et al.* Effects of aminoglutethimide on adrenal function in man. *J Clin Endocrinol Metab* 1967;27:481–90.

564 Vermeulen A, Paridaens R, Heuson JC. Effects of aminoglutethimide on adrenal steroid secretion. *Clin Endocrinol* 1983;19:673–82.

565 Sonino N. The use of ketoconazole as inhibitor of steroid production. *N Engl J Med* 1987;317:812–18.

566 Ashby H, DiMattina M, LineHan WM *et al.* The inhibition of human adrenal steroidogenic enzyme activities by suramin. *J Clin Endocrinol Metab* 1989;68:505–8.

567 Wagner RL, White PF, Kan PB *et al.* Inhibition of adrenal steroidogenesis by the anesthetic etomidate. *N Engl J Med* 1984;310:1415–21.

568 Barbieri RL, Osathanondh R, Canick JA *et al.* Danazol inhibits human adrenal 21- and 11β-hydroxylation *in vitro*. *Steroids* 1980;35:251–63.

569 Liddle GW, Island D, Lance EM *et al.* Alterations of adrenal steroid pattern in man resulting from treatment with a chemical inhibitor of 11β-hydroxylation. *J Clin Endocrinol Metab* 1958;18:906–12.

570 Keilholtz U, Guthrie GP Jr. Adverse effect of phenytoin on mineralocorticoid replacement with fludrocortisone in adrenal insufficiency. *Am J Med Sci* 1986;291:280–3.

571 Kyriazopoulou V, Parparousi O, Vagenakis AG. Rifampicin-induced adrenal crisis in addisonian patients receiving corticosteroid replacement therapy. *J Clin Endocrinol Metab* 1984;59:1204–6.

572 Ediger SK, Isley WL. Rifampicin-induced adrenal insufficiency in the acquired immunodeficiency syndrome: difficulties in diagnosis and treatment. *Postgrad Med J* 1988;64:405–6.

573 Gitlow S, Mendlowitz M, Wilk EK *et al.* Excretion of catecholamine metabolites by normal children and those with familial dysautonomia. *J Clin Invest* 1965;44:1049–50.

574 Goodall MC, Gitlow SE, Alton H. Decreased noradrenaline (norepinephrine) synthesis in familial dysautonomia. *J Clin Invest* 1971;50:27–34.

29: Adrenal Steroid Excess

M.G. FOREST

INTRODUCTION

The term hyperadrenalism encompasses all situations in which the adrenal glands produce excessive amounts of hormones. This may result either from excessive stimulation by trophic hormones, when the adrenal glands become hyperplastic and hypersecreting (secondary forms), or from autonomous adrenal tumours, when the contralateral adrenal gland is usually atrophic (primary form). All forms of hyperadrenalism are rare in childhood but all have serious consequences.

Iatrogenic hyperadrenalism produces similar clinical and biochemical disturbances and may follow either the administration of excessive doses of steroid hormones or steroid-like compounds or the ingestion of drugs which alter the normal metabolism of steroid hormones. The various causes of hyperadrenalism are listed in Table 29.1. This classification is based upon the predominant group of steroid hormones abnormally produced.

Although adrenal hyperfunction is usually confined to one of the four groups of adrenocortical hormones, an increase in glucocorticoid hormones may be accompanied by a lesser increase in androgenic secretions and vice versa.

In congenital adrenal hyperplasia, glucocorticoid hypofunction may be associated with excessive production of either mineralocorticoid or androgens. There is no situation in which adrenocortical and medullary hormones are both produced in excess, but both have hypertension in common.

CUSHING SYNDROME

Definition, aetiologies, incidence and genetics

Cushing syndrome encompasses all pathological conditions secondary to a chronic excessive production of glucocorticoids. Clinical and metabolic abnormalities result primarily from hypercortisolism, whether or not other endocrine abnormalities are associated. Hyperproduction of glucocorticoids usually originates from the adrenal glands but, exceptionally, it can also result from the hyperfunction of ectopic adrenocortical remnants in ovarian or testicular tissue or near the abdominal aorta [1]. Descriptions of typical hypercortisolism in children appeared in the literature [2–5] long before the classical report of Cushing [6].

The term Cushing syndrome [7] comprises four main aetiologies.

1 Primary hypercortisolism, the result of an adrenal tumour, benign or malignant [8], which is adrenal Cushing syndrome.

2 Excessive stimulation of a normal adrenal cortex secondary to excessive pituitary secretion of adrenocorticotrophin (ACTH), which is Cushing disease or pituitary Cushing syndrome [9].

3 ACTH [10,11], corticotrophin-releasing hormone (CRH) [12,13], or both [14,15], produced by malignant extra-pituitary tumours, ectopic ACTH syndrome.

4 Iatrogenic, either primary following glucocorticoid treatment, whether the route is parenteral, oral or topical [16,17], or secondary to excessive and prolonged ACTH administration.

Spontaneous Cushing syndrome is usually more simply divided into two main groups defined by dependency or otherwise on ACTH (Table 29.1). In the first category are Cushing disease, the ectopic ACTH syndrome and the very rare ectopic CRH syndrome; in the second are unilateral adrenocortical adenomas and carcinomas producing cortisol. On some occasions there is evidence that an autonomous, ACTH-independent overproduction of cortisol is associated with bilateral adrenocortical involvement: the enlarged glands being multinodular with an atrophic, normal or hyperplastic intervening non-nodular cortex. This ill-defined disorder has received much attention, but little explanation, and is probably a pot-pourri of disease among which two new aetiologies have recently been characterized.

1 *The Carney complex* [18] is a rare familial Cushing syndrome due to primary pigmented nodular adrenocortical dysplasia which can be part of a large multisystem tumour syndrome, in which the tumours are multicentric

Table 29.1 Aetiology of hyperadrenalism

Adrenocortical hyperfunction

Glucocorticoids

Spontaneous Cushing syndrome, ACTH-dependent*
- Cushing disease and its variants (bilateral nodular adrenocortical hyperplasia, Carney complex, McCune–Albright)
- Ectopic ACTH syndrome
- Ectopic CRH syndrome

Spontaneous Cushing syndrome, ACTH-independent
- Cortisol-producing unilateral adrenocortical tumour (adenoma or carcinoma)
- Bilateral nodular adrenocortical hyperplasia
- Food-dependent (GIP-dependent) cortisol hypersecretion

Iatrogenic Cushing syndrome (glucocorticoid therapy)

Mineralocorticoids

Autonomous primary hyperaldosteronism
- Conn syndrome, adrenal adenoma
- Adrenocortical hyperplasia

Glucocorticoid-remediable aldosteronism

Syndrome of apparent mineralocorticoid excess (AME)
- AME type I (11β-HSD deficiency)
- AME type II

Pseudohyperaldosteronism*
- Liddle syndrome
- Iatrogenic (liquorice intoxication)

Secondary aldosteronism
- Oedematous states, salt-wasting nephropathies, renal artery stenosis, renal malformations
- Renin-secreting tumours
- Bartter syndrome
- Iatrogenic (treatment by diuretics)

Primary hypermineralocorticoidism
- Congenital adrenal hyperplasia due to 17α-hydroxylase or 11β-hydroxylase deficiency
- Adrenal tumours secreting DOC or 18-hydroxylated compounds

Androgen

Virilizing adrenal tumours (carcinoma, adenoma)

Congenital adrenal hyperplasia due to 21-hydroxylase or 11β-hydroxylase deficiency

Premature adrenarche

Oestrogens

Feminizing adrenal tumours

Adrenal medulla hyperfunction

Phaechromocytoma† isolated or associated with multiple endocrine adenomatoses type II (Sipple syndrome) with neurocutaneous syndromes: multiple fibromatoses, von Hippel–Lindau disease, Sturge–Weber syndrome and tuberous sclerosis

* Hypokalaemic hypertension without hypermineralocorticoidism.
† Hypertension without hypokalaemia or hyperaldosteronism.
CRH, corticotrophin-releasing hormone; DOC, deoxycorticosterone; GIP, gastric inhibitory polypeptide; HSD, hydroxyosteroid dehydrogenase.

in affected organs and bilateral in paired organs. It associates myxomas, pigmented skin lesions, peripheral nerve tumours and various endocrine tumours [19]. The disorder is inherited as a Mendelian autosomal dominant, occurring primarily in children and young adults [20].

2 *Food-dependent Cushing syndrome.* This recently discovered disorder has been reported by two groups [21,22]. It may explain rare cases of bilateral nodular adrenocortical hyperplasia that are truly ACTH-independent. In such patients, ACTH levels are normally suppressed, and morning levels of plasma cortisol are subnormal. However, the diurnal rhythm of plasma cortisol is inverted [23]. This led Lacroix *et al.* [21] to hypothesize that a factor other than ACTH, and possibly of gastrointestinal origin, was involved. Both groups brought evidence that nodular hyperplasia and Cushing syndrome may be food-dependent as a result of abnormal responsiveness of adrenal cells to physiological secretion of gastric inhibitory polypeptide (GIP). 'Illicit' ectopic expression of GIP receptors on adrenal cells presumably underlies the disorder (Fig. 29.1).

Cushing syndrome is relatively rare but over 600 cases have been reviewed [24–29]. The general incidence in children is difficult to estimate because aetiological classifications do not use uniform criteria, because it is difficult to identify patients who have been included in several reports at different ages and because cases are often no longer reported. Children comprise 5–10% of reported cases [30]. De Gennes [31], reviewing the literature in 1967, found 110 children, and over 130 other cases have been reported since [30,32–46]. Cushing syndrome has been described in children of all ages. Fetal onset of Cushing disease has been discussed [47] and Cushing syndrome may occur in newborn infants [48–51], the earliest reports being at 4 and 6 weeks [52]. It is very rare between 1 and 8 years of age, and 15 years ago only 32 cases under the age of 16 years had been recorded in a survey of 113 institutions in the USA [53].

The relative frequency of the causes of hypercortisolism is better known. The iatrogenic forms are most frequent but their exact incidence has not been clearly recorded. In adults about 70% of cases of hypercortisolism are secondary to pituitary disorders, with a female:male ratio of 3–4:1, while the 30% remaining are equally distributed between Cushing syndrome and ectopic tumours. This is not the case in children: de Gennes [31] recorded 52% of Cushing disease, 45% of adrenal carcinomas and 11% of adrenal adenomas.

From more recents reviews of the literature, it appears

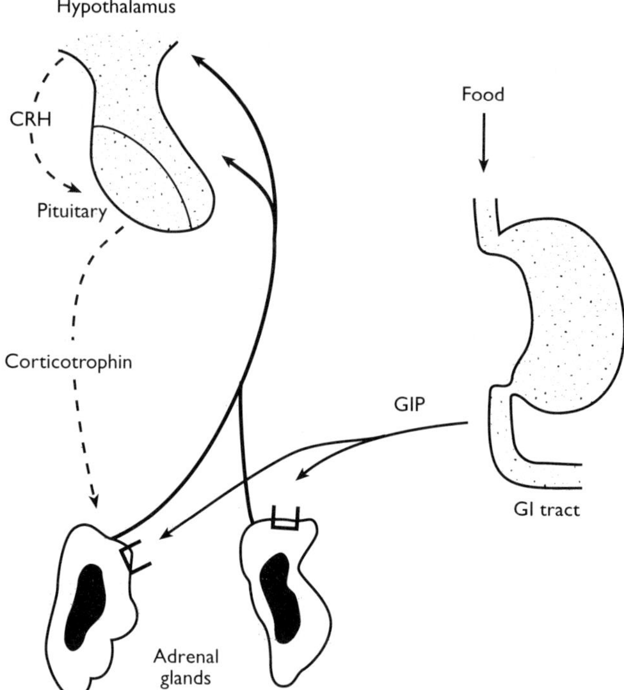

Fig. 29.1 Pathogenesis of food-dependent Cushing syndrome: meal-induced production of gastrointestinal (GI) GIP stimulates cortisol secretion, which in turn suppresses the hypothalamopituitary axis (redrawn from Reznik *et al.* [22]).

that Cushing disease is rare in infancy but represents about two-thirds of cases of adrenal hyperfunction in children between 11 and 15 years of age [54]. In some instances it remains uncertain whether Cushing disease originates from a hypothalamic or a pituitary disorder [55,56], but the evidence of monoclonal corticotroph adenoma in Cushing disease favours the latter hypothesis [57], even though a pituitary macroadenoma is rarely found in children [9].

The distribution between adrenal tumours and Cushing disease varies with age and sex. Adrenal tumours are frequent (82%) and predominate in female infants (76%) under 2 years of age [54]. Frequency and sex differences decrease with age. Adrenal tumours lead to autonomous, non-ACTH-dependent Cushing syndrome, and carcinoma accounts for almost two-thirds of them [58]. In some cases of adrenal carcinoma, other unrelated primary tumours may develop [59]. The high frequency of the association of adrenal tumours with the hemihypertrophic or Wiedemann–Beckwith syndromes [60–63], brain tumours or other congenital anomalies is striking [64–66].

The apparently increasing frequency of ectopic ACTH syndrome probably reflects improvement in diagnosis [67]. Since the first report of a child with ectopic ACTH syndrome by Leyton *et al.* in 1931 [68], 11 cases have been collected by Omenn [11] and only four reports have subsequently appeared in the literature ([37,69] and Pombo *et al.* and Styne *et al.* quoted in [40]). In fact, ectopic ACTH production is extremely rare in children [70,71], and although it has been claimed that in some cases CRF may be the primary cause of the disease [72], these tumours often co-secrete ACTH [73]. Ectopic CRF secretion has not yet been found or proven in children.

Primary adrenal nodular hyperplasia is rare in children and young adults, with possible familial incidence [74]. The pigmented nodular hyperplasia must be differentiated from macronodular hyperplasia, developing in patients presenting with pituitary-dependent Cushing disease [75]. The frequency of bilateral adrenal hyperplasia is 18% under 2 years of age, 32% between age 2 and 10 and 81% after 10 [31]. Female predominance is not found until after adolescence; the sex ratio is about 1 : 1 in patients under 16 years of age [31,40,76].

The rarest cause of Cushing syndrome is adrenal hyperplasia associated with non-endocrine tumours. Over 100 cases were recorded in adults a decade ago. Non-endocrine tumours associated with Cushing syndrome are carcinoma of the lung (50%) [15], particularly those of the oat-cell type and (with a decreasing frequency of 10–5%) epithelial tumours of the thymus [77], pancreatic islet cell carcinoid or adenocarcinoma [78], bronchial carcinoids [79], and medullary carcinoma of the thyroid, all of which are exceptional in children or infants. Rarer associations include liver tumours [11] or neoplasms from the natural crest tissue, ganglioneuroblastomas [1,37,80], Wilms tumours [60,69,81] and phaeochromocytoma [82–84]. Finally, a few cases of cortisol-producing teratoma have been observed in infants.

Cushing syndrome or disease is usually sporadic but adrenal carcinomas may occur in siblings [58,65] and rare forms of familial hypercortisolism have been described, inherited as a dominant autosomal trait with variable penetration [48]: these are part of the Carney complex.

Cushing syndrome is not constantly part of the multiple endocrine neoplasia type 2 (MEN-2) which is believed to be inherited as an autosomal dominant trait [84]. However, other familial causes of adrenal hyperfunction are described. These are secondary to pituitary adenomas which result from the syndromes of glandular hyperfunction involving cells responding to extracellular signals through the activation of hormone-sensitive adenylate systems. These catalyse the formation of cyclic adenosine monophosphate (cAMP) and are not accompanied by elevated plasma concentrations of the relevant trophic hormone [85,86].

The McCune–Albright syndrome (MAS) is characterized by polyostotic fibrous dysplasia, café-au-lait pigmentation of the skin, and autonomous hyperfunction of various endocrine tissues, including pituitary adenoma causing adrenal hyperplasia [85,86]. The disease is caused by mutations in the α-subunit ($G_s\alpha$) of the stimulatory guanine-nucleotide-binding protein (G protein) of adenylate cyclase, which is necessary for the action of hormones such as ACTH which use cAMP as an intracellular second messenger [87]. Single base mutations in $G_s\alpha$ resulting in constitutive activation of adenylate cyclase in affected tissues [88] occur during early embryogenesis, and thus patients with McCune–Albright syndrome are mosaic.

Multiple endocrine neoplasia (MEN) type 1 is an inherited disorder which affects the endocrine glands and is transmitted as an autosomal dominant trait. It is characterized by the formation of pituitary adenomas, pancreatic endocrine tumours and hyperparathyroidism [89]. The mechanism of disease in MEN type 1 is not yet understood, but is believed to be due to the deletion of a recessive oncogene on chromosome 11q13 [89,90]. A recent report of a family pedigree exhibiting features of both MEN-1 and McCune–Albright syndromes [91] supports the concept that they are part of the same complex with a common molecular and biochemical aetiology [92,93].

History, pathogenesis and pathological findings

Cushing [6] clearly delineated the clinical features of the syndrome which bears his name, and proposed the theory of a pituitary-centred disease, although he found basophilic adenomas in only six of his 12 patients. The syndrome was thereafter correctly attributed to a chronic excess of cortisol and the causes of primary and secondary hypercortisolism were delineated (Fig. 29.2).

CUSHING DISEASE

The term Cushing disease is currently restricted to instances in which bilateral adrenocortical hyperplasia is secondary to excessive secretion of ACTH by the pituitary gland. The adrenal glands may be slightly (combined weight > 10 g) or greatly enlarged, reaching the size of the kidney. Their shape and structure are conserved. However, the cortex is thickened with changes in the absolute and relative widths of individual zones. The zona fasciculata is often the most hyperplastic, but this simple form of bilateral adrenal hyperplasia is not invariable. In the nodular form, zones of increased proliferation of cortical tissue develop in the cortex contained within the capsule [94]. The size of nodules is extremely variable between nodular dysplasia and adrenal adenoma.

The pathophysiology of Cushing disease is still not entirely elucidated [95,96] but an understanding of normal regulation of the hypothalamocorticotrophic–adrenal axis is important [97]. ACTH secretion is stimulated by the hypothalamic corticotrophin-releasing hormone (CRH). Bioamines are involved in the control of CRH secretion, although the details of the system are controversial [98].

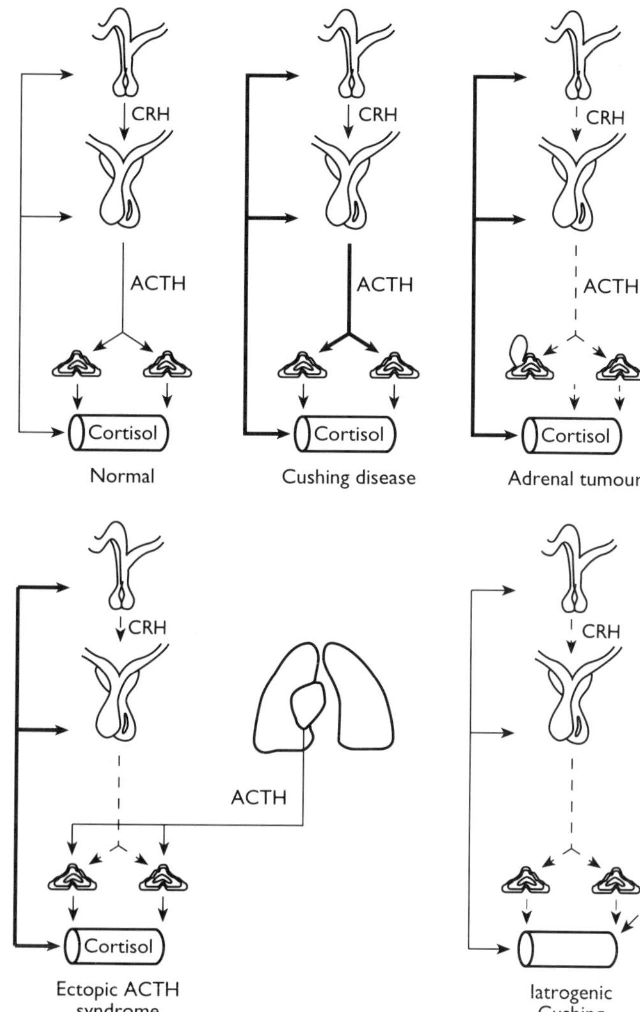

Fig. 29.2 Schematic representation of the hormonal dysregulation in the various causes of Cushing syndrome.

Serotonin may function either as a stimulator or an inhibitor of ACTH release. Cholinergic pathways interact with serotoninergic and noradrenergic systems stimulating ACTH secretion. α-Adrenergic stimuli increase ACTH secretion, while β-neuron stimulation has an inhibitory effect on the release of ACTH. Glucocorticoids act by decreasing ACTH pulse amplitude.

There are at least two pathways of negative feedback control of ACTH, one regulated by the concentration of circulating cortisol, the other by the concentration of ACTH itself [98]. The integration of these regulatory systems is responsible for pulsatile ACTH release superimposed on the well-known circadian variation.

Various aetiologies have been postulated to explain Cushing disease [99]. The first, 'pituitary theory', was based on the description of pituitary tumours, either basophilic, chromophobic or mixed [100–102]. Their common feature is the presence of 'Crooke cells', with increased cytoplasm and nucleus and perinuclear hyaline change in the cytoplasm replacing the basophil granules [26]. Immunohistochemical studies may demonstrate ACTH in granular cells [101]. Pituitary adenomas may metastasize. Absence of detectable pituitary tumours in some patients with lack of suppressibility of pituitary activity by low doses of dexamethasone [56] were the basis for the theory of a hypothalamic disorder, i.e. that the regulatory negative feedback was set to a higher cortisol level (higher threshold of inhibition) (see Fig. 29.2).

Subsequently, the finding that basal ACTH levels are often only slightly elevated [103] and maintain a circadian rhythm [104], and that small tumours of the pituitary gland [105] are frequently detectable at microsurgical exploration or electron microscopic examination of the pituitary gland, has strengthened the 'pituitary' theory. However, other findings have made the theory of a primary autonomous pituitary adenoma questionable, because of alterations in basal circadian, stress-induced and feedback regulation of ACTH release [106]. Other abnormalities of hypothalamic function, such as loss of diurnal variation of growth hormone (GH) and prolactin (PRL) release [107], blunted GH responsiveness to insulin-induced hypoglycaemia and decreased amount of slow-wave sleep [7], persisting after adrenalectomy or pituitary irradiation, and abnormal rise in ACTH induced by thyrotropin-releasing hormone (TRH) [108] were suggestive of abnormal hypothalamic regulation in Cushing disease [109].

The next hypothesis was that Cushing disease is primarily due to an abnormal regulation of the hypothalamic secretion of CRF which leads to ACTH release by the pituitary, and possibly to the development of pituitary tumours which may become autonomous [110].

This concept was based on the fact that although Crooke cells have seldom been observed in iatrogenic hypercortisolism, pituitary tumours are frequently found in adrenalectomized Cushing patients on replacement therapy [111], but not after adrenalectomy for other causes. On the other hand, the return of normal hypothalamo-pituitary function after surgical resection of a pituitary adenoma [112] suggests a pituitary cause [113].

The suggestion that Cushing disease has a central nervous system cause is the most recent hypothesis [96]. Dopaminergic depletion or increased serotonin content of the hypothalamus would stimulate release of CRH. Some of the evidence for these concepts is experimental and indirect. In animals submitted to stressful manipulations there is an increase in hypothalamic serotonin content [96]. Stressful conditions of life appear to have been overlooked in the development of Cushing disease [114]. An antiserotonin agent, cyproheptadine, may produce a remission of Cushing disease in some patients [115] but not in others [107]. The effect of dopamine is even more controversial. However, the underlying mechanisms for possible disturbances of central neurotransmitter regulation of ACTH release in Cushing disease are unknown [98].

Recent studies of 24-h profiles of plasma cortisol (and/or ACTH) have shown that cortisol may be secreted episodically in true Cushing disease, and that the concept of a defect of the neural clock generating the 24-h periodicity in ACTH secretion should be reviewed [27,116]. Circadian periodicity may be maintained at a higher level. Some studies have shown plasma levels of ACTH are sustained by increased ACTH pulse amplitude without significant alterations in pulse frequency in patients with Cushing disease [117]. However, in another study, two patterns of ACTH secretion were found: in one pituitary oversecretion of ACTH was relatively independent of CRH, but in a second there was increased hypothalamic release of CRH or pituitary sensitivity to it. Other abnormalities in the secretion and processing of pro-opiomelanocortin (POMC), the precursor molecule of ACTH, have been reported [96,118]. Thus it becomes more evident that Cushing disease is not a single entity [119], and may result from either pituitary or hypothalamic disturbances.

ECTOPIC ACTH SYNDROME

Although the coexistence of Cushing syndrome with tumour formation was noted by Gabcke at the turn of the century, it was not until 1952 that Thorn first hypothesized that non-pituitary tumours may secrete ACTH-like substances. Later Meador *et al.* [94] supplied the first clinical and biochemical evidence, and Liddle *et al.* [120] named it 'ectopic ACTH syndrome'. Its pathogenesis was demonstrated by the measurement and isolation of polypeptides with ACTH activity in primary tumours, metastases and blood, together with a decreased pituitary content of ACTH (see Fig. 29.2). Ectopic tumours produce a prohormone form of ACTH, so-called 'big-ACTH' [121] and other ACTH-related fragments [122], such as β-melanotrophin-stimulating hormone (β-MSH) and α-MSH and corticotrophin-like intermediate lobe peptide (CLIP), which have little or no ACTH-like activity. γ-Lipotrophin and β-lipotrophin are also secreted by ectopic tumours [123], the latter in a ratio to ACTH twice normal [124]. It is now believed that ectopic ACTH tumours have a disturbance in peptide packaging and release but also possess enzymatic activities degrading the precursor or parent molecule into small peptides characteristic of the pars intermedia lobe, processes which do not normally occur in the human anterior pituitary gland [125].

It is currently thought that 'ectopic' ACTH-secreting cells regain the potential for elaborating ACTH present in their genome before their differentiation. This derepression does not occur at random. Pearse was the first to show that groups of peptide-secreting cells scattered throughout the body and sharing morphological characteristics and the histochemical property of amine precursor uptake and decarboxylation (APU) were all of neural crest origin. Pearse and Polack [80] named cells undergoing neoplastic changes and developing the ability to secrete ACTH and related peptides apudomas. There is increasing evidence that all 'ectopic' ACTH tumours derive from APUD cells [125].

Non-endocrine tumours may also secrete a CRH-like factor [12,13,126,127]. Its presence in some tumours may explain observations made in patients whose plasma ACTH levels rise in response to metyrapone and argininvasopressin tests and are suppressed by dexamethasone. Ectopic secretion of cortisol itself is found exceptionally in tumours such as phaeochromocytomas [128]. Also, corticotrophinoma-like responses to glucocorticoids observed in some ACTH-secreting bronchial carcinoids would result from expression of glucocorticoid receptors and are not necessarily related to the production of CRH [129].

PATHOGENESIS OF CUSHING SYNDROME

In patients with adrenal tumours, pathogenesis is clear. Adrenocortical tumours are the source of excessive and autonomous production of cortisol, which in turn suppresses the pituitary gland (see Fig. 29.2). Isolated hypercortisolism occurs in less than 20% of cases and most tumours also produce androgens [33]. Atrophy of the contralateral gland is frequent (70%) but is less (30%) with predominantly androgen-producing tumours.

Two types of tumour are described: adenomas and carcinomas. Adenomas are benign, well-encapsulated tumours composed of nests of large cells containing lipid and glycogen. These cells are similar to normal fascicular or reticular cells. The surrounding tissue is often compressed and contains haemorrhage or cysts. Tumour size is variable (< 1–20 cm) and palpable tumours (100 g–1 kg) are not uncommon (20%). Adenomas are bilateral in only 1–2% of cases and can develop in ectopic tissue (2%). The incidence of hormone-inactive tumours with the same histological appearance at autopsy is surprisingly high (16%). Differentiation between nodular hyperplasia and adenomas may be very difficult.

Carcinomas are often large, necrotic, haemorrhagic and sometimes calcified tumours. Typical signs of malignancy include invasion of the capsule and adjacent organs, and tumour emboli. Extensions of the tumour may reach the vena cava. The cells are poorly differentiated, but histological examination is often of little help in differentiating adenoma and carcinoma; only the appearance of metastases establishes the true diagnosis.

A peculiar form of adrenal Cushing syndrome has been identified as primary nodular diffuse hyperplasia and has been described in adults as well as in children [43,51,54, 130–133]. Its pathogenesis is not well understood, although it has been suggested that in familial forms [133], often affecting newborn infants [48], microadenomatosis has developed from fetal remnants [48]. Macro- or micronodular adrenal hyperplasia may also be associated with Cushing disease in 15–20% of adult patients [8,130,132, 134] or in infants [135,136]. The condition may be due to increased sensitivity to usually low endogenous ACTH levels [137].

Clinical features and laboratory findings

These are due to cortisol excess which leads to excessive protein catabolism due to transamination of amino groups from amino acids in the liver, increased production of carbohydrates, fat deposition, potassium loss, and enhanced vascular responsiveness to pressor agents. The clinical symptoms are related to both the degree and duration of excessive cortisol secretion. The cardinal features encountered in adults, by decreasing frequency, are:

1 hypertension, obesity predominant on the trunk and the neck, moon-like face (90–95%);
2 disturbance of glucose metabolism, purple striae, hirsutism, osteoporosis, hypogonadism (70–75%);
3 muscular weakness (60%) and susceptibility to ecchymoses and infections.

In children the relative importance and the appearance of these clinical symptoms may differ. The effect of hypercortisolism on growth, bone maturation, pubertal development and protein depletion is often masked or partially compensated by the association of hyperandrogenism which may sometimes dominate the clinical picture (Fig. 29.3).

Progressive obesity is typically the first symptom. Fat deposition over the upper thoracic vertebrae gives the typical 'buffalo hump' and on the cheeks (often obscuring the ears) gives the typical moon face and fish mouth. Increased pectoral, abdominal or pelvic fat deposits appear later on. By contrast, limbs are rather thin. Obesity may progress extremely rapidly in young infants, who in a few months may look like a Buddha.

GROWTH RETARDATION

This is the most frequent symptom in infants or children with Cushing disease [30,44,138–141]. Deceleration of growth velocity and even complete growth arrest may be the only clinical feature of Cushing syndrome [142]. The cause of the growth failure is uncertain [138]. Sleep-associated elevation of plasma GH levels may be absent and the response of GH to insulin-induced hypoglycaemia is often blunted [7]: it may not recover after adrenalectomy

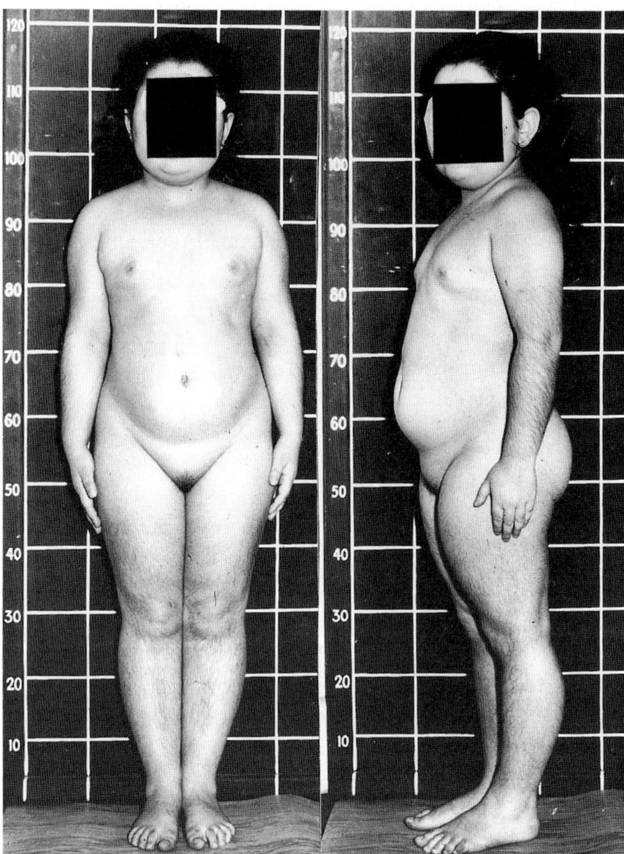

Fig. 29.3 Cushing disease in a 9-year-old girl presenting with the most frequent triad seen in children: growth failure, obesity and hirsutism; there was moderate hypertension, but no evidence of protein depletion.

[143,144]. Somatomedin activity may be decreased [145]. In contrast, steroid-treated children may have a normal GH response to hypoglycaemia but an impaired metabolic response to acute administration of GH. Disturbances in GH secretion [7] are not due solely to cortisol excess and do not entirely account for growth retardation. It is likely that both relative GH deficiency and peripheral inhibition of GH effect at tissue level are involved.

Delay in bone maturation and osteoporosis are frequent (50%) [30,132,140], but less marked than growth retardation. Bony matrices are progressively degraded. Calcium balance is negative, due to diminished intestinal absorption, decreased tubular reabsorption and increased calcium excretion. Serum calcium and inorganic phosphorus levels are normal. Renal calculi may be found, but rarely in children. Alkaline phosphatases are normal. Dorsal pain, severe dorsal kyphosis or spontaneous fractures may reveal the osteoporosis [146]. Deformation of the vertebral bodies with infraction is typical [147].

Osteoporosis is a well-known side-effect of treatment with glucocorticoids [146], but the exact mechanism by which they induce osteopenia is not completely understood [148]. It would appear that glucocorticoid-induced osteopenia is caused by a depressed bone formation in the presence of an unaltered but ongoing bone resorption. Secondary hyperparathyroidism and change in vitamin D metabolism are apparently not involved [149].

MUSCULAR ATROPHY

This results from the catabolic and anti-anabolic effect of cortisol. When associated with severe hypokalaemia it leads to muscular weakness, myopathy and apathy [150, 151], which are rare in children [30]. Hypertrophic cardiomyopathy is exceptional, severe, but reversible [152].

STRIAE

Changes in the skin, which becomes thin and shiny, and stretching due to fat deposition are responsible for skin fractures and striae, but the latter may also occur in simple obesity, particularly in pubertal girls whose breasts are rapidly growing. In those instances striae diverge from the nipples but are thin and pale. Striae are not pathognomonic of Cushing syndrome unless they are very broad and violaceous and are located on the flanks, lower part of the abdomen, thighs and axilla parallel to the lines of tension. The dark colour seems associated with extravasation or capillary injury. Flushing of the skin, a plethoric face and ecchymoses are due to increased capillary fragility; poor wound healing may be observed.

HYPERTENSION

This is a common finding [30,153] but blood pressure is usually only slightly elevated in children. Headaches are uncommon. Multiple factors contribute to the pathogenesis of hypertension [119,154]. Aldosterone levels are usually normal, plasma renin activity is suppressed but plasma renin substrate may be elevated. Hypertension may be due to an ectopic secretion of renin [78], but may also exist in the presence of normal mineralocorticoid production and normal plasma renin concentrations. Hypertension is thought to result from cortisol-induced enhanced responsiveness to pressor agents coupled with increased angiotensin formation [155]. The marked increase in production of glucocorticoids with moderate mineralocorticoid activity, such as 11-deoxycortisol, corticosterone, or 19-nordeoxycorticosterone [156], may play a role. On the other hand overload of the mechanism of cortisol inactivation is sufficient to explain the occurrence of hypertension in the ectopic ACTH syndrome [157]. In this condition, cortisol produced in large excess becomes a significant mineralocorticoid as seen in the syndrome of apparent mineralocorticoid excess (see below).

CARBOHYDRATE METABOLISM

Moderate hyperglycaemia without glycosuria and impaired carbohydrate tolerance are common. Frank diabetes mellitus is rare in children and seen only in patients with a family history of diabetes, hypercortisolism unmasking a latent disease. When present, diabetes mellitus is benign, although insulin-resistant, but vascular complications of diabetes may occur.

THYROID FUNCTION

This may be impaired. Low thyroxin levels result from glucocorticoid suppression of plasma thyroxine-binding globulin and thyroid-stimulating hormone (TSH) [158]. Decreased function of the thyroid gland is secondary. There is usually no rise of TSH after TRH injection. Association of Cushing syndrome with autoimmune thyroiditis would appear fortuitous [159,160].

HIRSUTISM

This is the third cardinal clinical symptom in children. Signs of virilization are more frequent in children than in adults: premature appearance of pubic or axillary hair, penile enlargement, scrotal pigmentation or clitoral hypertrophy. The latter signs are usually found when adrenal tumours produce excessive amounts of androgens. Downgrowth of frontal hairline, seborrhoea and acne vulgaris are commonly seen at all ages, including young infants.

Amenorrhoea is common in adolescent girls [51]. Diminished immune defence against bacterial or fungal infections is classical [161]. Abdominal pain and mass are frequent in adrenal tumours. The tumour is palpable in practically all reported cases of carcinoma, but is less frequently in adenomas [40]. Pain and abdominal mass, and fever, are the only symptoms in non-secreting tumours [68,162,163].

PSYCHOLOGICAL DISTURBANCES

Psychological disturbances and emotional lability are not as conspicuous as in adults. School performance may be poor, but may remain unchanged, despite long-standing disease [28]. In some situations, mental disturbances seem to be related to increased secretion of β-endorphin, which together with ACTH and β-lipoprotein, is part of the common glycoprotein precursor molecule, POMC [108, 164].

OTHER LABORATORY FINDINGS

Increased haematocrit, neutrophilia, eosinopenia and lymphopenia are often observed but are of little diagnostic value. Polycythaemia is rarer. Hypercortisolism promotes urinary excretion of potassium to extracellular spaces. Potassium losses are compensated by uptake of sodium and hydrogen ions from the extracellular space. Hypokalaemic metabolic alkalosis is thus the typical electrolyte pattern found in 15–20% of cases in children. Serum bicarbonate is high and chloride is low. Serum sodium and urinary excretion of sodium are usually normal. Urine pH is acidic.

Positive and differential diagnosis

Any of the four cardinal symptoms of Cushing syndrome in children–growth failure, obesity, hirsutism and hypertension–is highly suggestive of adrenal hyperfunction (see Fig. 29.3).

All clinical features of Cushing syndrome may develop after the administration of pharmacological dosages of ACTH (the common treatment of hypsarrhythmia in infancy) or glucocorticoids for treatment of various diseases. Differential diagnosis of iatrogenic from naturally occurring Cushing syndrome is usually easily made by direct interrogation, but a careful search for intermittent or topical administration of glucocorticoid should be made in all cases.

Iatrogenic Cushing syndrome is always accompanied by a complete suppression of the hypothalamopituitary–adrenal axis. Thus plasma cortisol or urinary 17-oxogenic steroid levels, as well as plasma ACTH levels, are very low. All clinical signs of hypercortisolism disappear when treatment is stopped. In particular, normal physical growth and bone maturation resume. The real danger for the patient at the time of glucocorticoid withdrawal is underlying secondary adrenal insufficiency. Management of this problem is discussed in Chapter 28.

In the presence of obesity, whether or not other clinical features are associated, the first problem is to establish whether adrenal function is normal. This is easy when Cushing syndrome is florid, whatever parameter of cortisol secretion is determined. Basal levels of cortisol over 30–40 μg/dl (800–1100 nmol/l), urinary excretion of free cortisol greater than 200 μg/day (~5000 nmol/day) and marked elevation of 17-oxogenic steroids are typical.

Growth rate is increased in children obese from infancy, while children with Cushing syndrome gain weight in spite of a low-calorie diet, and growth failure is constant. There are, however, less typical situations in which distinction between minor abnormalities in obesity and early stages in Cushing syndrome may be difficult.

Moderate adrenal hyperactivity is found in obese pa-

Table 29.2 Tests of hypothalamopituitary – adrenal function

Basal function tests	Dynamic function tests
Plasma cortisol	*Tests of the control mechanisms*
Plasma ACTH	Nycthemeral control – determination of diurnal variations in plasma cortisol and ACTH levels
Urinary 17-hydroxysteroids (17-OHCS)	Negative-feedback control:
Urinary 17-oxogenic steroids (KGS)	Dexamethasone suppression tests
Urinary 'free' cortisol	Metyrapone test
Cortisol production rate	Stress control:
	Insulin tolerance test
	Lysine-vasopressin
	Pyrogen
	Tests of functional capacity (reserve)
	ACTH tests
	Metyrapone test
	CRH test

tients. Cortisol secretion rate is a function of body cell mass, except when significant losses of cell mass have taken place in adult life. Apparently elevated cortisol secretion rate or elevated 24-h excretion of cortisol metabolites in obese children is normal when corrected for body weight and not for surface area [165]. The observation that urinary excretion and cortisol secretion rate return to normal during fasting in obese adolescents may be helpful to the diagnosis.

Establishment of hypercortisolism can be made on a variety of rather simple screening tests (Table 29.2), none of which is infallible [166,167]. These tests include the determination of basal plasma cortisol levels, basal urinary excretions of free cortisol and 17-oxosteroids, the study of their day-to-day circadian variations and of their suppressibility be dexamethasone.

Several careful studies have demonstrated that most of the screening methods are not 100% reliable for the detection of early or mild hypercortisolism and for the differentiation of obesity from Cushing syndrome. Several of the tests listed in Table 29.2 must be performed.

PLASMA LEVELS OF CORTISOL

The plasma level of cortisol is 7–20 μg/dl (190–550 nmol/l) in the early morning (0800–0900 h) and it decreases by more than 75% after 1800 h to less than 5 μg/dl (138 nmol/l) by midnight. These levels may appear normal on a single measurement in obese patients, as well as in those with Cushing syndrome, primarily because of the large range in physiological value and biological rhythmicity [169]. Measurements should be repeated both in the morning and at 2000 h.

High cortisol levels may be found in normal subjects because of stress due to anxiety or apprehension, but also because of unrelated situations. Cortisol levels are elevated following oestrogen therapy because of a rise in corticosteroid-binding globulin (CBG) and also in the syndrome of glucocorticoid insensitivity [169,170]. The first situation is easily recognized by careful questioning, but the second is exceptionally rare [171]. In both situations there are no clinical signs of hypercortisolism. Abnormality in the functional binding capacity of CBG (increased free fraction of cortisol) might exceptionally be a cause of Cushing syndrome [172].

DIURNAL VARIATION

The determination of isolated plasma cortisol levels is not very helpful for the diagnosis of Cushing syndrome except when a loss of normal circadian variation is clearly demonstrated [104,173]. Cortisol may, however, be secreted episodically in authentic Cushing syndrome [174], but most investigators indicate that elevated cortisol levels at night with or without significant day–night variation should be a constant feature of Cushing syndrome [166]. This may become evident only in the evolution of the disease [116]. Nycthemeral rhythm is abolished in stressed patients, and these studies should not be performed during the first 48 h of hospital admission. They are useless in infants under the age of 2 years. Determination of the mean of four to eight evenly spaced plasma cortisol levels has been advocated as a highly reliable method for positive diagnosis: a mean over 20 μg/dl (~550 nmol/l) is suggestive of hypercortisolism [175]. Study of the pattern of ACTH/cortisol secretion by frequent blood sampling over 24 h and analysis of pulse frequency and amplitude is more useful to establish the level of the abnormality in hypothalamic or pituitary Cushing disease [117,167]. Loss of the postprandial surge in cortisol seems to be a valuable biological marker of the disease [117].

URINARY 'FREE' CORTISOL

An excess of 85–90 μg (200–250 nmol) a day or > 60 μg/m^2 (180 nmol/m^2) a day is very suggestive of Cushing syndrome [169], but about one-third of patients are not discriminated by the test [176]. Measurement of salivary cortisol also allows detection of elevated free cortisol levels [177].

17-HYDROXYSTEROIDS AND 17-OXOGENIC STEROIDS

Determination of the daily excretion of 17-hydroxysteroids (17-OHCS) or that of 17-oxogenic steroids (KGS) has been constantly included in the studies screening for Cushing syndrome. It is a widely available routine test which gives a reasonably good index of the daily secretion in cortisol when related to body surface area or urinary creatinine [40,168]. Urinary excretion of 6β-hydroxycortisol also appears to correlate with cortisol secretion [40]. Urinary 17-ketosteroids (17-KS) are not a reliable indicator of adrenal hyperfunction and are of little interest [56]. Normal urinary excretions are $3.1 \pm 1.1\,\text{mg/m}^2 \cdot 24\,\text{h}^{-1}$ or 2–6.9 mg/g creatinine for 17-OHCS, 0.5–3 mg/24 h in prepubertal children for 17-KS, $<60\,\mu\text{g/m}^2 \cdot 24\,\text{h}^{-1}$ for free cortisol, and $0.23 \pm 0.3\,\text{mg/m}^2 \cdot 24\,\text{h}^{-1}$ for 6β-hydroxycortisol.

SUPPRESSION TESTS

Low-dose dexamethasone suppression tests may be performed in obese children with elevated 17-oxosteroid value (see Fig. 29.3). Two tests are currently used: the first, *a single-dose test*, is easy, rapid and will discriminate a number of obese patients with normal feedback response [178,179]. Following the ingestion of $1\,\text{mg}/1.73\,\text{m}^2$ of dexamethasone at 2300 or 2400 h plasma cortisol levels should be suppressed below 5 μg/dl (135 nmol/l) 8 h later [56]. This short suppression test can be adapted to children, by relating the dose to body size as $0.3\,\text{mg/m}^2$ [180].

The second type of *low-dose dexamethasone* suppression is performed over 2–3 days. The inability of a low-dose ($0.5\,\text{mg}/1.73\,\text{m}^2$ every 6 h for 48 h) to suppress urinary KGS or free cortisol levels is accepted as establishing the diagnosis of Cushing syndrome in adults [166]. Lack of relation of the doses to body size may cause the diagnosis of hypercortisolism in children to be missed or delayed. A dose of 5 μg/kg every 6 h for 2 days and correction for creatinine of the urinary steroid levels measured on the second day of the test would appear to validate the test. Normal suppression is when 17-oxogenic steroids fall to < 1 mg/g creatinine per day [168].

A dose of 10 μg/kg (or $0.3\,\text{mg/m}^2$) every 6 h for 2–3 days should decrease plasma cortisol to less than 5 μg/dl at 6 h after the last dose, urinary 17-OHCS to less that 2 mg/g creatinine, and urinary cortisol to less than half of baseline [169].

The high-dose dexamethasone test consists of ingestion of 40 μg/kg (or $2.2\,\text{mg/m}^2$) every 6 h for 2–3 days. Serum cortisol should be unmeasurable 6 h after the last dose, urinary 17-OHCS less than 1 mg/g creatinine, and androgens significantly suppressed. It is usually used sequentially, after a 2–3-day low-dose test. In both tests, concurrent treatment with diphenylhydantoin therapy, which accelerates steroid metabolism, may lead to false-positive results.

An intravenous dexamethasone suppression test has also been proposed [181,182]. Dexamethasone phosphate is infused i.v. at a dose of 1 mg/h for 4 h starting at 1100 h. Plasma levels of cortisol are estimated every 20 min between 0900 and 1600 h, then every 2 h until midnight and at 0900 h the next day. This test, which investigated ACTH feedback response, can distinguish normal or obese subjects from patients with Cushing syndrome and help the aetiological diagnosis in the latter: a 50% suppression with an escape the next day occurs in Cushing disease, but there is no significant variation in ectopic ACTH syndrome [181].

INSULIN TOLERANCE TEST

Insulin-induced hypoglycaemia stimulates the release of CRH and thus ACTH. Insulin is injected i.v. at a dose of 0.1–0.5 i.u./kg and blood taken 30, 60 and 90 min later. In normal subjects, plasma corticosteroids should rise by at least 8 μg/dl (220 nmol/l) to maximum over 20 μg/dl (550 nmol/l). The response of cortisol is normal in simple obesity and in stressed or severely depressed patients, but not in Cushing syndrome. There are exceptions, however. This test is of no help in distinguishing the cause of hypercortisolism, and should be used only when all other tests are inconclusive [166].

Aetiological diagnosis

Once a positive diagnosis of Cushing syndrome has been made there may be even more problems in delineating the causes of the disease. Aetiological diagnosis can be helped by clinical findings such as the age of the patient, the rapidity of evolution, the presence or not of skin pigmentation, the electrolyte pattern, and also by relative frequency of causes.

In young infants, adrenal tumours are a frequent cause of Cushing syndrome. In only a third of the 234 cases reviewed by Hayles *et al.* [183] were clinical signs of hypercortisolism predominant. Cushing syndrome is due to adrenocarcinoma in half of the cases in infancy and in two-thirds before the age of 2. Rapidly evolving clinical symptoms, discovery of a palpable mass and signs of virilization are highly suggestive of adrenal carcinoma. Absence of obesity, even loss of weight, marked skin hyperpigmentation, severe hypokalaemia and alkalosis are typical of ectopic ACTH syndrome. Cushing disease may be characterized by its slow onset and evolution, a pure hypercortisolism with signs of marked protein catabolism. In cases of pituitary tumours, evolution is more rapid, hyperpigmentation may be present and neurological symptoms may be associated, such as headaches, vomiting, decreased visual acuity and optic atrophy. In most instances the aetiological diagnosis is made not only on further hormonal testing but also in morphological tests (Fig. 29.4).

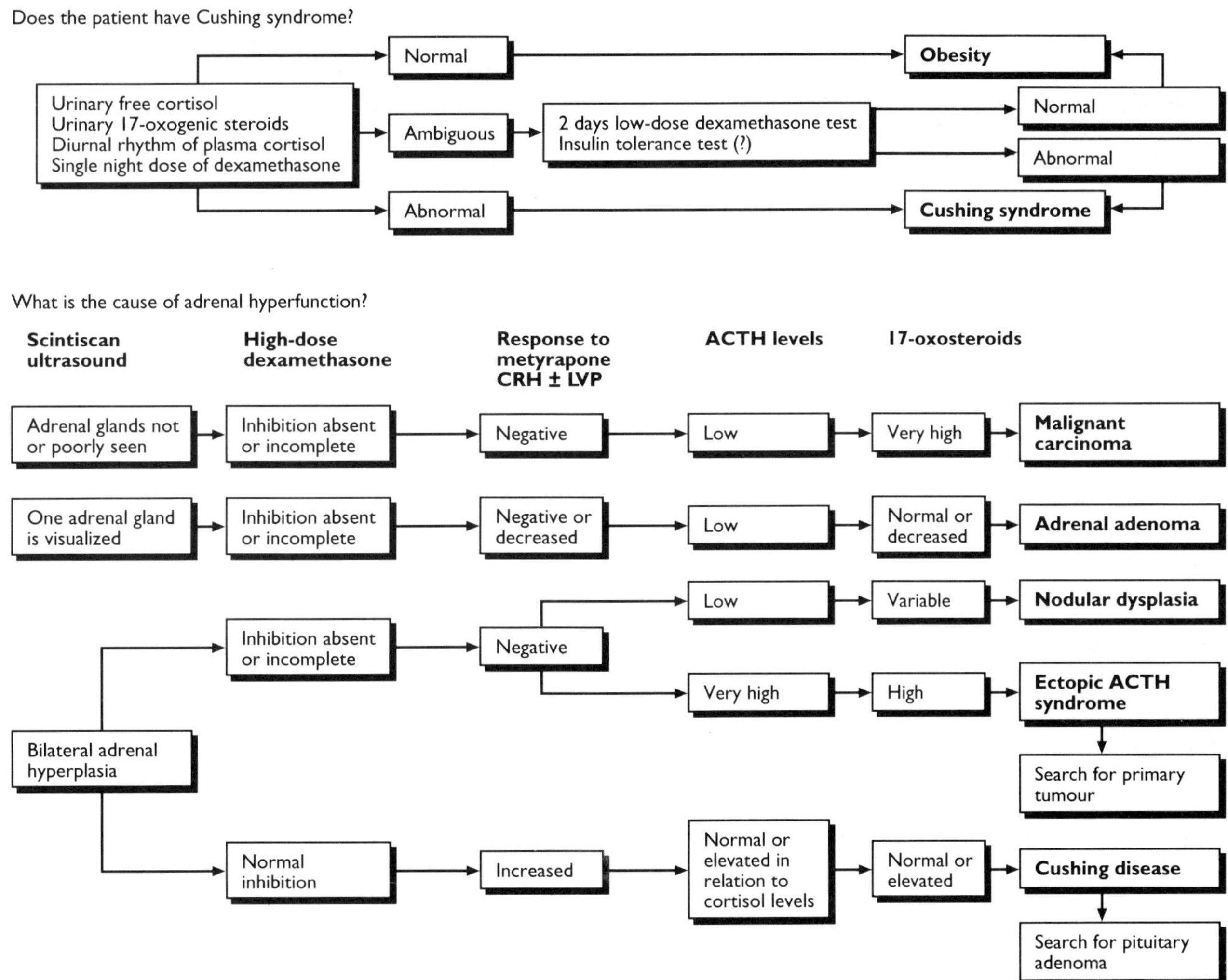

Fig. 29.4 Chronological sequences to use in screening for diagnosis of Cushing disease. LVP, lysine-8-vasopressin.

BASAL ADRENAL FUNCTION TESTS

Determination of plasma ACTH levels and urinary excretion of 17-ketosteroids in basal conditions are useful. Most bioassays are not sensitive enough to measure plasma ACTH levels. Recently developed cytochemical assay or isolated adrenal cell assay are still tedious research tools and not available to the clinician. Radioimmunoassay is the method of choice for measuring plasma ACTH. This should be a routine procedure, since reliable assays are currently available in most countries. An assay using N-terminal antibodies shuld be used to assess biological activity. Normal values are 10–80 pg/ml at 0900 h and < 10 pg/ml at midnight. Determination of plasma ACTH levels will theoretically differentiate non-ACTH-dependent hypercortisolism, i.e. adrenal tumours, from the ACTH-dependent causes of Cushing syndrome [184]. ACTH levels are invariably low or undetectable in adrenal tumours and in autonomous nodular dysplasia [184,185]. They are normal or moderately increased in Cushing disease and markedly increased (> 300 to over 2000 pg/ml) in ectopic ACTH syndromes or in some cases of pituitary adenoma [27,184]. However, circulating ACTH levels may be detectable in some cases of adrenal tumours. In both Cushing disease and adrenal tumours, plasma levels of lipotrophic hormone (β-LPH) parallel that of ACTH and β-LPH/ACTH ratios (0.9–4) and are identical to those observed in normal subjects. In contrast, ACTH levels and the β-LPH/ACTH ratio (ranging from 3 to 19) are both elevated in patients with ectopic ACTH-secreting tumours [124]. ACTH and β-LPH have also been found elevated in tumoral tissue of patients with 'ectopic ACTH tumours' [15,67,184,187]. Diagnosis of such tumours has been confirmed by selective venous sampling showing no gradient concentration between the jugular and peripheral veins, but a positive gradient in other veins of the body, in adults

[188,189] as well as in children [69]. However, measurement of ACTH in lavage fluid obtained during bronchoscopy is not helpful [190].

The finding of extremely elevated urinary excretion of 17-ketosteroids is suggestive of either adrenal carcinoma [191] or ectopic ACTH syndrome. Variable levels are observed in all other aetiologies (see Fig. 29.4). This measurement is often of little help in differentiating adenoma from carcinoma [188,192].

The determination of serum or urinary androgens, oestrogens or aldosterone is useful when virilization, feminization or salt-retention are dominant clinical features, and suggest the possibility of an adrenal tumour, [40,185,193–195]. However, the usefulness of measuring plasma 17α-hydroxypregnenolone, dehydroepiandrosterone sulphate (DHEAS) [12,196] or other steroids [62,197–199] to differentiate adrenal carcinoma from adenoma has not been fully assessed in adults, and not at all in children.

DYNAMIC TESTS OF ADRENAL FUNCTION

The metyrapone test has long been considered useful in differentiating pituitary-dependent hypercortisolism from autonomous adrenal function or ectopic ACTH syndromes in adults [99]. Failure to respond to the test with an increase in either urinary 11-OHCS or 17-oxogenic steroids or plasma 11-deoxycortisol (compound S) indicates a lack of pituitary reserve (pituitary inhibition) or a failure of the adrenal to respond to ACTH, whereas hyperresponsiveness is typical of bilateral adrenal hyperplasia. However, a normal response or lack of response has been reported in Cushing disease [166,167] and a high response in adenoma [200], so this test has limited reliability. The same applies to ACTH stimulation. A failure to respond is indicative of adrenal tumours or of maximally stimulated adrenal glands (ectopic ACTH syndrome). An increased response to ACTH is usually seen in adrenal hyperplasia, but variable responses are also seen in cases of adrenal tumours of all histological types. A lack of response to ACTH has been correlated with selective biochemical defects of adrenal tumour cells [201].

Current protocols for a metyrapone test utilize the ingestion of a single dose of 30 mg/kg at 2200–2300 h, rather than the 'classical' 1-day test. Serum 11-deoxycorticosterone normally rises to 7–20 μg/dl at 0800 h the next morning. The ACTH test which has been most commonly used in the diagnostic approach of Cushing syndrome consist of an i.v. infusion of 25–40 i.u. (0.25–0.40 mg) of cortrosyn over 6–8 h. A normal response is when serum cortisol and/or urinary 17-OHCS increase two- to threefold.

The classical high-dose dexamethasone suppression test (2 mg 6-hourly for 2 or 3 days) is not reliable; suppression should occur in hypothalamic Cushing disease [202] but not in other aetiologies. Anything can be seen, even a paradoxical rise in adrenal steroids, which Fehm *et al.* [106] demonstrated to be due to disturbance of the dual corticosteroid feedback mechanism in stress-induced activation of ACTH secretion.

In some patients with Cushing disease, the rate-sensitive negative-feedback mechanism is converted to a positive one, whereas the level-sensitive mechanism is undisturbed, indicating again that the site of disturbance is at or above the hypothalamus in Cushing disease. Decreased clearance of dexamethasone may account for the normal suppression seen in some patients with Cushing disease. For others [116], resistance to dexamethasone suppression is seen in all stages of Cushing disease, and is evidence of disturbed negative feedback (pituitary Cushing disease). The nocturnal high-dose [203] or the i.v. infusion [181] dexamethasone suppression tests are said to be discriminating in a number of these patients. Limited suppressibility of cortisol secretion with loss of the diurnal rhythm during high-dosage dexamethasone treatment may be the best indicator of macronodular diffuse adrenal hyperplasia [204,205].

The lysine-8-vasopressin (LVP) test (i.v. injection of 6–10 i.u. LVP with the measurement of ACTH 15 and 60 min later) [206], together with the increasing availability of ACTH and β-LPH assays has been used for aetiological diagnosis [27]. In adrenal tumour or nodular dysplasias, low ACTH levels are not stimulated by LVP, whereas the response may be positive in Cushing disease. LVP stimulates the secretion of ACTH and related peptides directly. The principal interest of the test is to differentiate patients with pituitary adenoma, who have an explosive response, from those with ectopic ACTH syndrome, who usually fail to respond. ACTH secretion is greater than that of β-LPH in Cushing disease [103], and the reverse may be seen in ectopic ACTH syndrome or pituitary adenoma [124].

Determination of the pattern of response of ACTH to CRH has in the past been judged not to be useful in the aetiological diagnosis of Cushing disease [126] and is less effective than expected in differentiating patients with primary adrenal hyperfunction or central Cushing disease from those with ectopic ACTH hypersecretion. The CRH-induced response of ACTH is variable in Cushing disease [207,208]. For some authors the low pituitary sensitivity to CRH found in some patients is due to abnormalities in CRH receptors [209]. For others the responsivity to CRH and lack of suppressibility are related phenomena in Cushing disease and are inversely proportional to basal cortisol levels [210]. Recent re-evaluation of the results of the CRH stimulation test (100 μg of ovine CRH) [55,211–213], sometimes augmented by a low dose of LVP (1 unit, i.v. per 1.73 m^2 body surface area) [214], have revealed the interest of the test. CRH or CRH plus LVP-stimulated ACTH levels are particularly elevated in Cushing disease, while there is no significant ACTH response in a case of an adrenal tumour.

CRH stimulation performed 7–10 days after surgery may be helpful in the prediction of remission after transsphenoidal resection of a microadenoma [126]. While patients with the ectopic ACTH syndrome do not usually have ACTH responses to CRH, others have tumours which contain CRH and respond both *in vivo* and *in vitro* to CRH [126].

The long-acting synthetic enkephalin analogue (D-ala; MePhe^4,met-(*O*)enkephalin-ol, FK 33-824) has been used for aetiological diagnosis in Cushing syndrome. The drug blocks the CRH-induced secretion of ACTH, β-endorphin and cortisol in normal subjects, but not in patients with Cushing disease [215].

Morphological tests of the adrenal glands

The development of techniques for visualizing adrenal glands has modified the diagnostic approach in Cushing syndrome. Together with the measurement of plasma ACTH levels, morphological tests should be considered as the most useful in establishing aetiological diagnosis.

On rare occasions an adrenal tumour may be suspected on straight abdominal X-ray or intravenous pyelography [216,217], but a unilateral calcified mass displacing the kidney down and laterally is seldom seen [218,219]. Retroperitoneal air insufflation is obsolete [217].

IODOCHOLESTEROL SCINTIGRAPHY

A tracer dose of cholesterol is injected i.v. and abdominal regions are scanned daily from the fourth to the seventh day [220]. The adrenal uptake of the injected radioactivity is low (0.2–0.4%) and slow. The best images are usually seen on the seventh day.

The following three situations are encountered.

1 Two adrenal glands are clearly visualized similar to normal adrenals. Differentiation between bilateral adrenal hyperplasia and ectopic ACTH syndrome is made by hormonal testing (see above and Fig. 29.4). Asymmetry in the image is suggestive of nodular hyperplasia.

2 The diagnosis of adrenal adenoma is clear when only one adrenal gland is visualized.

3 When no adrenal tissue is seen, or is poorly seen several days later, this is typical of carcinomas which have a low uptake of cholesterol.

This test seems to be reliable and appears first choice for detecting metastatic tissues (lung, liver), ectopic adrenal remnants and non-adrenal tumours secreting ACTH [221].

Adrenal iodocholesterol scans [222] have improved considerably with the recent use of more stable tracers [223, 224]. The major inconvenience of this test is its length. However, it may be useful to identify and localize adrenal tumours, not only preoperatively [221,225,226] but also postoperatively in order to demonstrate recurrence or metastases [227]. Because of *in vivo* deiodination of the ^{131}I-19-iodocholesterol, the thyroid gland should be protected by prior administration of potassium perchlorate. Risks for other tissues are negligible [228].

IMAGING TECHNIQUES [229]

Ultrasound imaging of the adrenal glands [230] is technically difficult, because of their deep location. Although this technique is rapid, simple and non-invasive, its reliability is highly dependent on operator expertise. It has been effective in detecting adrenal tumours as small as 3–5 cm [230,231], and appears useful in investigating extensions of adrenal tumours and for localizing primary tumours in a case of ectopic ACTH syndrome [216].

Computerized tomography (CT) is easier to perform [232], but is an expensive technique. It allows better detection of smaller adrenal tumours or ectopic tumours [233] than conventional methods [216,232,234] and provides indices of malignancy [235].

Receptor imaging is the latest technique used for visualizing small neuroendocrine tumours containing high numbers of somatostatin receptors since the latter are functional. Somatostatin receptor scintigraphy with radiolabelled somatostatin analogue (octreotide) is nowadays widely used for this purpose [236]. It is helpful for the *in vivo* localization of lung tumours, carcinoids [237] and other apudomas, but the differential diagnostic value of octreotide scintigraphy in pituitary tumours is limited [236].

OTHER PROCEDURES

Renal arteriography is a useful preoperative step in cases of adrenal carcinomas because it detects abnormal vasculature and connections to the vena cava. It may also help to discover hepatic metastases.

Invasive techniques such as selective venous catheterization are rarely necessary for the diagnosis. Multiple venous sampling is aimed at demonstrating either a gradient in cortisol and androgen concentrations between the adrenal veins (and thus localizing the side of an adrenal tumour), or a gradient between adrenal and peripheral veins. The technique is difficult but efficient [234,238,239].

Morphological tests of the pituitary

Skull films and tomograms may reveal an enlarged sella turcica. CT of the brain and carotid arteriography may localize a pituitary adenoma over 6–7 mm in size [229]. This cause is exceptional in infants [9] or children.

The aim of CT is to demonstrate the corticotrophin-cell adenoma. In the past, CT has given results difficult to interpret, or negative [240]. The availability of systems with higher resolution [241] and a lateral digital localizer ('scoutview') [242], and above all the introduction of dynamic pituitary CT scans [242], have been of major benefit for the diagnosis of small pituitary adenomas. For pituitary scanning to be successful there must be a well-trained team and a good psychological preparation of the patient. There is also no substitute for experience. When all optimal conditions are met [242], 70% of abnormal pituitary glands are found in patients with presumptive Cushing disease (presumption being based on clinical and biological signs of hypercortisolism, a >40% suppression of adrenal secretions after a high-dose dexamethasone test, an explosive response to the metyrapone test, and normal or moderately elevated ACTH levels), but a clearly defined adenoma is found in only 55% of the cases. ACTH-secreting pituitary adenomas do not present suprasellar extension [242].

Magnetic resonance imaging (MRI) gives more information than CT on hypothalamopituituary anatomy and has the advantages of multiplanar capability, superior soft-tissue discrimination, absence of bone-induced artefacts, and lack of invasiveness and radiation hazards [192, 242–246].

A normal CT scan or MRI of the pituitary gland does not contraindicate surgical exploration if there is a formal diagnosis of Cushing disease, since there are still chances of finding a microadenoma [247].

Selective venous catheterization of the inferior petrosal sinus, demonstrating a gradient in ACTH levels between the inferior petrosal and peripheral veins through simultaneous sampling [248–250], is also successful in differentiating pituitary or ectopic ACTH secretion [188], or localizing pituitary adenomas [189,238–240]. It may give improved diagnostic information if combined with CRH stimulation [189,251–253]. Combination of the procedure with CRH stimulation (with a correction method based on the peak intersinus TSH and/or prolactin ratio obtained after simultaneous TRH stimulation) would improve the diagnostic accuracy in less experienced hands [254].

Treatment, evolution and prognosis

Whatever the cause of Cushing syndrome, early diagnosis and treatment are mandatory because the natural course is severe. In untreated patients, osteoporosis, weakness, diabetes and hypertension may lead to death within a few months from cardiac failure, cerebral haemorrhage or intercurrent infection. The observation of spontaneous remission, possibly due to haemorrhage into an adrenal tumour or pituitary adenoma [256–259], does not justify postponing the treatment. Apparent spontaneous remission might be due to alternative active and inactive phases of secretion in Cushing disease [100]. Treatment may be surgical, physical or medical (Table 29.3). Therapeutic choice is theoretically clearly dictated by the aetiology of the disease, but, in practice the choices may be difficult when the cause of Cushing disease is not clearly established [260].

Table 29.3 Therapeutic means proposed for the treatment of Cushing syndrome

Surgical treatment

Removal of adrenal tumours or ectopic tumours secreting ACTH
Total adrenalectomy followed by adrenal autograft
Trans-sphenoidal resection of pituitary adenoma
Pituitary ablation

Physical treatment

External radiotherapy of the hypothalamopituitary region or of the adrenal region
- Conventional megavoltage (200 kV) irradiation (total of 4000–6000 rad)
- High-energy radiation such as cobalt therapy, cyclobaltotherapy, caesium radiation, betatron or heavy particle (proton beam) radiation (8000–11 000 rad of α-particle radiation)

Intrasellar implantation of radioactive isotopes such as ^{90}yttrium, ^{192}iridium or ^{198}gold

Medical treatment

Control of cortisol secretion: steroid biosynthesis blocking agents (chemical adrenalectomy)
- *o,p'*DDD
- Aminoglutethmide
- Metyrapone
- WIN-24,450
- Ketoconazole

Control of ACTH secretion
- Serotonin antagonists: cyproheptadine or metergoline
- Dopaminergic agents: bromocriptine (CB-154) or L-dopa
- Others: reserpine, morphine, barbiturates

Control of glucocorticoid biological activity
- Glucocorticoid antagonist RU 486

IATROGENIC CUSHING DISEASE

Treatment is discontinuing glucocorticotherapy according to the scheme detailed in Chapter 28.

ADRENAL TUMOURS

The only logical treatment is to remove the tumour and to perform a unilateral adrenalectomy. Because of atrophy of the contralateral gland and complete inhibition of hypothalamohypophyseal function (see Fig. 29.1) patients have no capacity to cope with stress, and present complete adrenal insufficiency as soon as the tumour is removed. It is thus essential to prepare patients for surgery as if for total adrenalectomy or for surgery in an Addisonian patient (see Chapter 28). Except in an emergency (evident malignant carcinoma), surgery is best performed after reducing hypercortisolism by preoperative medical treatment with *o,p'*DDD (see below). This reduces, although it does not eliminate, postoperative morbidity due to the risk of thromboembolic complications [261], frequent respiratory complications due to muscular weakness of the chest and obesity, and poor healing of the frail tissues. Unilateral adrenalectomy usually cures the patient presenting with an adrenal adenoma [262]. Bilateral adenomas may be found at surgery, which should explore both adrenals. However, the dilemma of a possible tumour in the contralateral adrenal is now solved by imaging techniques. Recovery of the contralateral adrenal function, which occurs earlier for cortisol than for androgen biosynthesis [196], and normal feedback control must be followed, as it is for patients with glucocorticoid withdrawal.

Recovery of corticotrophic function may take an extremely long time, as demonstrated by persistent decreased response of ACTH and cortisol to stimulation tests [263]. If complete excision is uncertain, or not possible, a postsurgical treatment with either mitotane [264] or conventional radiotherapy is indicated, because a poor prognosis is not invariable.

Adrenal tumours may be malignant (carcinoma) [33,37, 39,47,163,164,239,266]. Histological examination is often difficult [264]. Necrosis, haemorrhage and capsular and vascular invasion are indicative of malignancy. Histological examination shows an increased number of mitotic figures and cellular pleomorphism in both types of tumours. Staging of the tumour has not been used in children. Results of retrospective staging and treatment may be found in the literature [40].

While adenocarcinomas are monoclonal tumours, about half of adrenal tumours presenting typical features of adenoma also have features of monoclonal tumours [267] and/or overexpression of IGF-II [268,269] and various mutations [268,270,271].

The size of the tumour is important for prognosis [271]. Small tumours (< 5 cm) without local or distant metastases or lymph node infiltration (stage I) have a prognosis as good as adenomas. Larger tumours with (stage III – IV) or without (stage II) infiltration or metastases are usually of poor prognosis, despite adjuvant therapy. The latter includes irradiation, mono- or multiple chemotherapy (5α-fluorouracil, cyclophosphamide, vincristine, adriamycin), *o,p'*DDD alone or in combination [40,59,163,272] and treatment of metastases by cisplatin has been proposed [273].

MULTINODULAR ADRENAL HYPERPLASIA

Bilateral adrenalectomy appears to be the optimal treatment for the condition [30,134,274], followed by replacement therapy for life. Macronodular hyperplasia associated with Cushing syndrome does not require primary adrenal surgery, since it may be cured by successful transsphenoidal surgery [275]. In all patients who undergo bilateral adrenalectomy, postoperative follow-up of skin pigmentation, plasma ACTH [111,207], POMC-related peptides or PRL [276] levels, visual fields, and brain CT scans [243] are necessary for the early detection of the occurrence of Nelson tumours. An increased and prolonged ACTH response to CRH stimulation is also indicative of the syndrome [253]. An incidence of 25–60% has been reported in children [40,53,111,277]. The reasons why the incidence of Nelson syndrome is much lower (10–15%) in adults [278] are unknown. Treatment of Nelson tumours is as in pituitary Cushing disease (see below) but is not as effective. In adults the rates of stabilization or cure are 40% and 10%, after either pituitary surgery, heavy particle irradiation or cyproheptadine treatment [115,275,279–281]. Expansive tumour growth may necessitate total hypophysectomy [282].

For patients with the Carney complex the only alternative is medical treatment, usually with *o,p'*DDD (see below). In the McCune–Albright syndrome treatment must be tailored to the bone disease and endocrinopathies of each individual patient. In those with Cushing syndrome, bilateral adrenalectomy is often required [283]. Finally, in patients with food-dependent Cushing syndrome, treatment with octreotide appears to have transient efficiency in decreasing cortisol secretion, and thus ameliorates clinical symptoms, but long-term results are not available [22].

ECTOPIC ACTH SYNDROME

Elective treatment is the removal of the primary tumour responsible for ACTH hypersecretion. Complete remission may, exceptionally, be observed. Eradication of the tumour is not always possible. Although the final outcome depends on the course of the primary malignant disorder, and is often fatal, medical treatment with *o,p'*DDD is recommended to reduce hypercortisolism and improve the patient's comfort.

CUSHING DISEASE

Treatment aims to control cortisol overproduction, to avoid permanent endocrine deficiency, to eradicate the source of ACTH hypersecretion and to avoid permanent dependence on hormonal medication. None of the therapeutic approaches used completely fulfils these objectives.

Adrenal surgery

The least logical treatment of Cushing disease in children is to remove the source of hypercortisolism by adrenal surgery. Three techniques have been proposed. Subtotal bilateral adrenalectomy should be abandoned because of the high incidence (>50%) of recurrence [30]. The fascinating, but isolated, reports of successful treatment of Cushing disease by adrenal autotransplantation [32] warrant further evaluation. In the past, total bilateral adrenalectomy has been considered the most effective therapeutic approach in children.

It is particularly important to a child to ensure not only normal linear growth but also normal development of secondary sexual characteristics and reproductive capacity. Total bilateral adrenalectomy meets the first two objectives given above, but not the last two. Hypercortisolism is rapidly controlled. Normal catch-up growth usually follows [138,142], with rare exceptions [143]. As long as epiphyses are not fused, osteoporosis is completely reversible in children, in contrast to adults in whom it may remain a difficult problem. Other symptoms and signs usually regress. Normal pituitary function is conserved. Disadvantages of this form of therapy are the need for lifelong steroid replacement therapy by both gluco- and mineralocorticoids and, above all, the risk of development of pituitary adenoma or Nelson syndrome [111]. Replacement treatment should be adapted to patient needs [284], and daily dosages given in fractional doses [285]. Overtreatment may lead to factitious recurrence [286]. Nelson syndrome can be suspected on the appearance of skin pigmentation, sellar enlargement [287] and by a progressive rise in plasma ACTH levels [27]. Pituitary irradiation within 2 months of adrenalectomy may prevent the development of Nelson syndrome, but not always [278]. For these reasons alternative therapies which act on the primary hypothalamopituitary disorder are currently considered [260,288].

Pituitary irradiation and surgery

Treatment of Cushing disease aimed at suppressing corticotroph function by pituitary irradiation or hypophysectomy should not be the first approach [35,76] because of the risks to other pituitary functions. Reports of hypopituitarism after irradiation in children [285,289] have limited the use of this logical form of therapy even though conventional pituitary irradiation may be effective in reducing hypercortisolism and preventing pituitary enlargement without affecting other pituitary functions [25,76]. Safety and efficacy appear, however, to be dose- and age-related [285]. Total dose should be no more than 4000–5000 rad (40–45 Gy) and the rate should be 200 rad (2 Gy), five times a week [76]. Children respond better than adults to this treatment. The full reliability of pituitary irradiation is not yet established since failure of catch-up growth, recurrence of Cushing disease or Nelson syndrome may yet follow [278]. The apparent main disadvantage of this treatment is its slow effectiveness. Several months (2–18) are required to control cortisol overproduction [25,76].

Other forms of pituitary particle beam irradiation (heavy particle or proton beam irradiation) give faster and better results than conventional photons [290,291] and may be useful in the prevention or treatment of Nelson syndrome. The rate of success and of complication is not established, since their use in children has been limited.

A new mode of pituitary irradiation has been reported, according to which conventional γ-rays are focused on the pituitary fossa and are administered through multiple entries. Although recovery has been reported in four children after such treatment, long-term follow-up is not available. Similar or even better results have been reported after interstitial irradiation [35,292]. The limiting factor is the expertise of the neurosurgeon who implants the radioactive gold or yttrium seeds. Since this is an intracranial manipulation, removal of the microadenoma might as well be attempted.

According to Korth-Schutz [40], who reviewed the literature [33,37,39,59,115,151,162,266] and analysed the results of a questionnaire sent to European paediatric endocrinologists, varying forms of pituitary irradiation may prove to be successful in the hands of expert neurosurgeons in specialized centres. However, it now appears that the dose of irradiation used may have deleterious effects on the brain or other pituitary functions, in particular growth hormone secretion [293] and thus normal growth and/or intellectual development are impaired.

Resection of pituitary microadenomas is the method of choice in the treatment of both Cushing disease and Nelson syndrome [105,247,275,282,294] in the hands of surgeons experienced in micropituitary dissection. In adults the cure rate is 65–85% [105,112,113,126,137,207, 247,280,281], and is better in small than in large adenomas. However, if the primary lesion is hypothalamic, pituitary adenomas are likely to recur [137].

Pituitary trans-sphenoidal microadenomectomy gives immediate success in about 90% of children [45] undergoing such treatment. After surgery there is transient ACTH deficiency followed by a progressive return to normal pituitary–adrenal function. Preoperative testing fails to predict a recurrence of pituitary adenoma [295] which occurs in about 15% of the cases [126]. Although panhypopituitarism may result from surgery in some instances, the residual function of the pituitary is usually good [112,296].

Drug treatment

According to the theories which proposed that central

nervous system (CNS) dysfunction is the primary disorder in 'hypothalamic' Cushing disease, logical medical treatments would be those using dopaminergic agents or serotonin antagonists.

Following the report [115] of the remission of Cushing disease by the antiserotonergic agent cyproheptadine, this drug has been used in adults [7,207] and children [139,297]. Sustained remission is observed in up to 60% of cases [7,298]. However, relapse occurs immediately after discontinuing therapy [107], which must therefore be indefinite. A significant side-effect of the drug is polyphagia which leads to excessive weight gain, particularly in children. Comparable results are observed with a similar drug, metergoline, which has no side-effects [40]. Treatments with other CNS drugs, such as bromocriptine, L-dopa, reserpine, opiate agonist or somatostatin [275,299–303] have been variably successful, unless used in association with adrenolytic agents [304]. Other drugs listed in Table 29.3 have been abandoned.

MEDICAL TREATMENT OF CUSHING SYNDROME

Medical treatment has a special place in the control of hypercortisolism in all aetiologies of Cushing syndrome. It has particular value in the preoperative management of patients or in inoperable patients with tumours and as useful adjuncts to therapy in Cushing disease.

Two types of compounds have been used in oral treatments.

Drugs blocking cortisol synthesis [305]

Aminoglutethimide (α-ethyl-α′-*p*-aminophenylglutarimide) inhibits the conversion of cholesterol to pregnenolone. Usual dosages are 1–2 g, four times daily. Larger doses may be used in malignant tumours. Side-effects are rashes, drowsiness, respiratory depression and ataxia. The action of the drug is rapid, and total adrenal insufficiency may occur in the first days of treatment. Replacement therapy by gluco- and mineralocorticoids in physiological doses is mandatory. Remission has been reported [304], although the action of the drug may only be temporary [306].

Metyrapone (SU 4885, 2-methyl-1,2,-bis(3-pyridyl)-1-propanone) inhibits 11β-hydroxylation but also 17-, 18- and 19-hydroxylations; it increases the 21-hydroxylation of progesterone and stimulates ACTH [307]. Biosynthesis of aldosterone is usually maintained. Daily doses may vary between 1 and 2 g. Gastrointestinal side-effects are better tolerated when the drug is given with meals or milk. Metyrapone also increases adrenal androgen production and may produce hirsutism.

Aminoglutethimide and metyrapone seem to be more effective when given in association [308]. This combination enables the dosage of each drug to be lower, thus reducing side-effects to tolerable limits in a long-term regime. Both compounds have a rapid action in decreasing plasma cortisol levels, but they do not overcome ACTH release in Cushing disease. They must be considered only as useful adjuncts to more definitive forms of therapy in Cushing disease, such as waiting for the beneficial effect of pituitary irradiation [224]. They may be useful in obtaining a clinical remission before removal of an adrenal adenoma or bilateral adrenalectomy [306]. Neither drug has an effect on tumours when their use is palliative, as it is in ectopic ACTH syndrome.

Trilostane (*Win*-24,540) (4α-,5-epoxy-17β-hydroxy-3-oxo-5α-androstane-2α-carbonitrile) inhibits 3β-hydroxysteroid dehydrogenase isomerase and has been used with apparent benefit in Cushing syndrome [309]. It acts faster than the two former drugs, but whether it will prove superior has not been established.

o,p′DDD (lysodren; mitotane) (1,1-dichloro-2(*o*-chlorophenyl)-2-(*p*-chlorophenyl) ethane). This drug affects both adrenal secretion and extra-adrenal metabolism of cortisol (inhibition of conversion of Δ5-3β-hydroxy-C21-steroids to their 3α-hydroxy pregnane analogues). In addition, the drug causes severe cytotoxic adrenal atrophy of the fasciculata and reticularis zones. The zona glomerulosa is less affected. The effect is dose-dependent. Normal aldosterone secretion may be maintained at low doses [310] but not at high ones [41]. The drug takes 2–4 weeks to act. At that time, gluco- and mineralocorticoid replacement therapy is needed. Severe gastrointestinal side-effects are less pronounced when the drug is micronized on cellulose acetyl phthalate [24]. Increased serum cholesterol is reversible at the cessation of treatment. This compound has the same indications as explained above for aminoglutethimide and metyrapone. Its additive cytotoxic action may bring about complete remission in some cases of advanced adrenal carcinoma [311]. Sustained remissions have been obtained with *o,p*′DDD in adults [24,52,272,312–315] as well as in children [34,43], even in inoperable cases [41]. Recommended doses are 4–12 g a day for 3 months, then 6–8 g per day, or 6 g/m^2 a day increased to 10 g/m^2 a day if necessary.

Ketoconazole, an imidazole derivative used in clinical practice for its antifungal activity, was recently found to be a potent inhibitor of steroidogenesis. It is a general inhibitor of cytochrome P450-dependent enzymes such as the cholesterol side-chain cleavage enzymatic complex, 11β-hydroxylase or the C17–20 lyase [316]. A glucocorticoid antagonist activity of the drug has been shown *in vitro*. In addition, in some unknown way it prevents the expected rise in ACTH secretion in patients with Cushing disease [317]. The drug has been successfully used (600–800 mg/day) in 12 adult patients, eight of whom had recurrent severe hypercorticolism after selective trans-sphenoidal surgery [316,317], and in one case of adrenal adenoma [317]. The drug has also been used in a patient with a functioning adrenal tumour of the liver in preparation for surgery [36]. Rapid and subsequently persistent improvement is observed. Although further evaluation is needed, ketoconazole may become a serious contender as the drug of choice for the medical treatment of hypercortisolism [318].

All these drugs are palliative and have to be continued indefinitely. They all have side-effects [260] but, in addition, they do not address the cause of the disease. As adjunctive therapy to pituitary irradiation, trilostane or other drugs [315], may be as important in children as they have been in adults, but since lifelong steroid replacement cannot be prevented in most instances, this form of treatment seems to offer no long-term advantage over bilateral adrenalectomy in Cushing disease, and the incidence of Nelson tumours has not been estimated.

Glucocorticoid antagonists

These are an attractive alternative treatment of hypercortisolism in theory and have been researched extensively. By competing for glucocorticoid-receptor sites, they would decrease cortisol biological activity. RU 486 (17β-hydroxy-11β-(4-dimetylaminophenyl) 17α-(1-propyl) estra-4,9-dien-3-one) meets the requirements and binds to the glucocorticoid receptor with high affinity but with no agonist effect [319]. Short-term administration of the drug (400 mg every 3 days) induces a delayed and prolonged pituitary–adrenal response in Cushing disease, but not in non-pituitary-dependent Cushing syndrome [320]. Successful monitoring of hypercortisolism (5–20 mg/kg for 9 weeks) has subsequently been reported in a patient with an ectopic ACTH tumour [319]. No side-effects were observed. The practical efficiency of the drug is not established, since it remains to be determined whether the enhanced cortisol production will overcome the peripheral effect of RU 486 in long-term treatment.

VIRILIZING ADRENAL TUMOURS

Incidence

Adrenal tumours are rare [321]. Although over 200 cases were recorded in the literature of 1966 [183], these tumours are relatively uncommon in children [33,238, 322–324]. Virilizing tumours represent about two-thirds of all adrenal tumours, while non-secreting adrenal tumours [77] are rare ($\leqslant 5\%$) in children [40]. Virilizing adrenal tumours rarely occur at birth [192] and are more likely to occur in children between 1 and 8 years of age with a female ratio of 2–3 : 1 [33,40]. They may complicate untreated 21-hydroxylase deficiency [325,326] or be associated with congenital abnormalities [63,65] or other nonadrenal tumours [59,60], and a familial history of malignancy is found in some cases [8,33]. Geographical distribution appears uneven, as frequency is high in Brazil and very low in Africa.

Pathological findings

Virilizing adrenocortical tumours are often carcinomas but may be adenomas in over one-third of the cases [33, 192,207,327,328]. Both have the same pathological and histological features as adrenal tumours causing Cushing syndrome. As discussed above, the distinction of malignant from benign tumours is only made unambiguously when metastases develop. The size of the tumour may be indicative. Tumours in excess of 200 g are almost invariably malignant [33]. Adrenal carcinomas do not metastasize early [265]. Metastases are most frequent in liver, lungs and corresponding regional lymph nodes. An exceptional case of a tumour developing from an ectopic adrenal remnant within the liver has been observed [329].

Pathogenesis

The possibility that adrenal tumours derive from fetal adrenal cells undergoing 'anaplastic' change has been advanced [330]. Because these tumours grow very slowly, it may be that many of them exist at birth although they rarely become clinically evident [49], which could explain the high incidence found in infants or young children. The great majority of the tumours are autonomous with regard to steroid secretion. However, steroid secretion may initially be suppressed by dexamethasone and the condition misdiagnosed for congenital adrenal hyperplasia [195]. On the other hand, one girl with salt-losing congenital adrenal hyperplasia subsequently developed an adrenal adenoma [331]. These observations have led to the speculation that adenomas might perhaps be due to excessive ACTH stimulation.

Irrespective of histological type, several biochemical abnormalities may be found in the adrenal tumour cell: loss of receptors to ACTH or to prostaglandin E_1 (PGE_1), abnormal ACTH receptor anomaly of the cAMP-dependent protein kinase, or expression of steroid receptors in the tumoral tissue [201,332]. Loss of ACTH-responsiveness may also occur with the development of β-adrenergic receptor-linked adenylate cyclase. Whether these defects are the consequence or the cause of the tumoral process is unknown.

Clinical and hormonal features

Virilizing adrenal tumours differ from those producing Cushing syndrome only by their secretory patterns and clinical symptoms. In virilizing tumours, clinical symp-

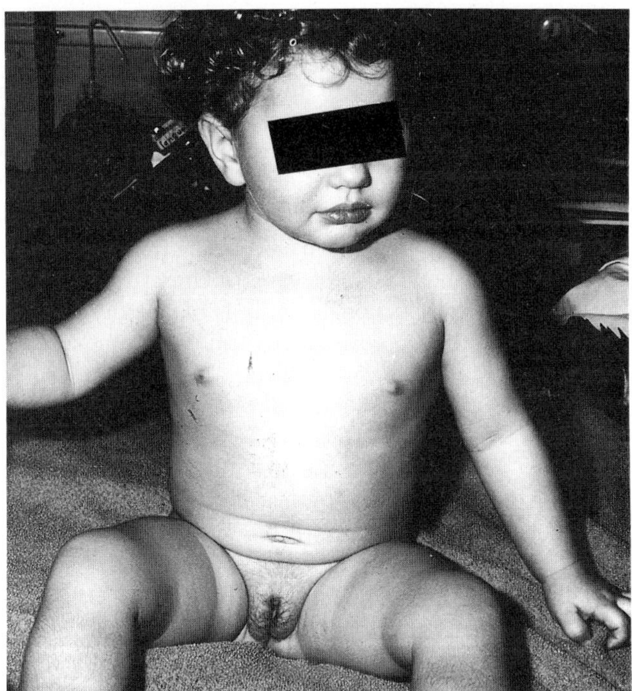

Fig. 29.5 Virilizing adrenal tumour in a 15-month-old female child. Rapid onset of signs of virilization (less than a month prior to this picture) was the only clinical symptom; there was no metastasis. Apparent healing after the total eradication of a 165 g carcinoma, following which the child grew normally and attained perfect health.

toms are those produced by any virilization process which may cause pseudosexual precocity in boys [39,194], and heterosexual development in girls [333,334].

Signs of virilization may be the only symptom. It seems that pure virilizing adenoma [333] are rare, since only 18 cases have been recorded up to 1981 [238]. However, this form of presentation was almost as frequent in adenoma (35%) as in carcinoma (42%) in a series of 55 cases of adrenal tumours in a recent review [40] of the literature [33,37,39,59,60,62,162,163,185,194,195,239,262,265,266, 335,336]. Signs of virilization may appear late in the disease [42]. In rare instances, initial symptoms may be virilization, but feminization occurs and predominates during the course of the disease [8,266,337]. Usually the symptoms of androgen hypersecretion predominate [335] with tall stature, acceleration of growth rate and bone maturation, muscular hypertrophy and early development of pubic and axillary hair. In boys, voice deepening, pigmented scrotum and excessive growth of the phallus contrast with testes of prepubertal size. In girls, enlargement of the labia majora and clitoris is observed (Fig. 29.5) and secondary amenorrhoea may occur.

In a significant proportion of cases, virilizing symptoms are associated with features of hypercortisolism [338] (approximately 20%) such as obesity and hypertension, feminization (approximately 65%) or hyperaldosteronism (approximately 3%) [40]. In addition, rapidly growing tumours may present with non-specific symptoms such as abdominal pain, weight loss or fever. A palpable abdominal mass is found in only one-third of cases [33]. There is usually no particular chemical abnormality, except the rare occurrence of low cholesterol levels associated with large tumours. Spontaneous hypoglycaemia has occasionally been described, probably due to the production of insulin-like substances.

There have been numberous studies of the various steroids produced in adrenal tumours [339]. Various secretory patterns have been described, suggesting that certain enzymes may be more active than in normal adrenal tissue [198]; various enzyme deficiencies may coexist [62,195,197,266,327,339–344]. There is no correlation between the size or the microscopic appearance of the tumour and its endocrine function. A characteristic feature is excessive production of Δ5-pregnene steroids reflecting low 3β-hydroxysteroid dehydrogenase activity in the tumour, as shown by histochemical and *in vitro* studies [185]. Overproduction of dehydroepiandrosterone (DHEA) and DHEAS and of their normal or abnormal metabolites is a frequent finding [62,185,191,195,197,198, 342]. Failure to find excessive DHEA production does not always rule out the possibility of a virilizing adrenal tumour.

Urinary excretion of 17-oxosteroids is often very high [33] but may be subnormal [37] because of the predominant production of androgens such as testosterone [194,333], which contribute little to the measurements. Urinary 17-oxogenic steroids may be normal or moderately increased [195]. Pregnanetriol is usually normal but may be increased when excessive amounts of 17α-hydroxypregnenolone are produced. Urinary oestriol is often elevated. From their detailed hormonal study of 12 infants with virilizing adrenocortical tumours, Honour *et al.* [327] have concluded that in several instances determination of plasma testosterone and DHEAS is not enough for defining the steroidogenic potential of a specific tumour. Measurement of the excretion of 17-KS may be helpful: if greater than 11 mg/day, the tumour primarily produced DHEAS; when it was marginally elevated (2.2–5 mg/day), the major steroid secreted by the tumour was 11β-hydroxyandrostenedione, as in another case [199]. However, some tumours may have low activity of 11β-hydroxylase [194] or 21-hydroxylase [342]. Further evidence of the biochemical heterogeneity is provided by the demonstration that some tumours have enzyme activities which are not normally found, such as the formation of 11β-hydroxy-DHEA [199] or 19-nor-deoxycorticosterone (DOC) [156].

Finally, the hormonal pattern may change, either spontaneously or during therapy [266]. It is not possible to distinguish benign adenoma and malignant carcinoma on the basis of hormonal studies. The detection of a variety of steroid metabolites other than DHEA is, however, suggestive of carcinoma: excessive DOC production, possibly due to a relative 11β-hydroxylation defect [194] and a variety of other enzymatic deficiencies as exist in various forms of congenital adrenal hyperplasia, may be found [343].

Morphological studies

These are important for localization of the adrenal tumours. Straight abdominal X-ray may show calcification in the adrenal region in a quarter of cases [33,192,323]. Intravenous pyelography may reveal the tumour displacing the kidney [33]. Although of significant value, radiological investigations have been superseded by ultrasonography [230] and abdominal CT scans [232,234]. In most cases, arteriography or isotope scanning with ^{131}I or 19-iodocholesterol are no longer essential. In general, the sophistication of the techniques required is inversely related to the size of the tumour.

Adrenal venography with measurement of steroids in the adrenal tumour [234,238,239] is rarely necessary for the diagnosis.

Differential diagnosis

In either sex early development of an adrenal tumour may produce signs not grossly different from precocious pubarche or constitutional sexual precocity (see below). True sexual precocity, either idiopathic or secondary to brain tumours or McCune–Albright syndrome, is distinguished by breast development or pubertal enlargement of the testes and a normal pattern of adrenal androgen secretion. In exceptional cases of interstitial cell tumour of the testis, a unilateral testicular tumour is easily palpable. The major differential diagnosis is with the virilizing forms of congenital adrenal hyperplasia. A very mild enzyme defect in 21-hydroxylase may reproduce the same clinical findings as those given by an adrenal tumour. Differential diagnosis is established by hormonal studies and by dynamic tests. Moderate elevation in cortisol, variable levels of Δ4-androstenedione, normal 17α-hydroxyprogesterone and extremely high levels of DHEA are characteristic of adrenal tumours. Plasma or urinary steroids are not influenced by ACTH stimulation in cases of adrenal tumour, whereas a marked rise in 17α-hydroxyprogesterone with an inadequate rise in cortisol after ACTH is typical of congenital adrenal hyperplasia. Unfortunately adrenal tumours may, however, be responsive to ACTH [201] and be suppressed by dexamethasone [195].

Treatment

This is surgical. Although the contralateral adrenal is often not atrophied in cases of pure virilizing adrenal tumours, the patient should be considered as having potential inhibition of the pituitary–adrenal axis, and be given careful preoperative and postoperative glucocorticoid therapy. There is no harm if the treatment is not necessary. In about 10% of cases bilateral tumours are found, and bilateral adrenalectomy is mandatory. In such cases, in addition to coverage treatment during surgery, substitution therapy should, of course, be given for life.

In cases of inoperable tumour or metastases, medical treatment by *o,p'*DDD may be effective at doses of 2–6 g/m^2 a day [313,314]. Results are variable. The drug has been used extensively in adults [41,77,312–314]. This has resulted in increased life expectancy but rarely eradicated the disease. A complete response to treatment has, however, been found in seven patients [312]. Positive long-term effects of the drug after cessation of treatment are related to storage in adipose tissue and slow release into blood [345]. The few reports of its use in children indicate that it is unlikely to have long-term benefit [40].

Postoperative irradiation of the tumour has been proposed [265], even though adrenocarcinomas are felt to be radioresistant [322]. Maximal dose, safe for neighbouring tissues (35–40 g, 2500–4500 rad/25–45 Gy), is used. Improvement, when noted, has been temporary. Similarly, chemotherapy, used in a number of adults and in a few children, has no real benefit [324]. Cisplatin has been used in a few adult patients with some temporary remission [273].

Prognosis

This is very poor but not always fatal. Prognosis is highly dependent on the surgical problems, since other forms of therapy have been disappointing. Complete remission may be observed in more than 90% of cases of tumours easy to remove and well encapsulated [33]. In contrast, the incidence of recurrence (local or metastatic) is very high when the tumour is adherent or incompletely eradicated. The magnitude of the tumoral secretions and their pattern do not appear to have any prognostic value. Nor does the presence of metastases, since complete remission has been recorded with treatment by *o,p'*DDD in two children with metastases [311]. Prolonged follow-up is necessary, since apparent remission may be complicated by the development of metastases several years later.

FEMINIZING ADRENAL TUMOURS

Feminizing adrenal tumours are the third variant of adrenal tumours [193,346]. Predominant secretion of oestrogens by adrenal carcinoma or adenoma is very rare. A score of cases have been reported in children of both sexes [231,337,341,345,347]. Most feminizing tumours occur in adults between 25 and 45 years of age [346]. In contrast, in the cases reported in children between 21 months and 14 years old, more than half had occurred before 4 years. The sex ratio is about equal.

The first symptoms in girls are the premature appearance of breast development, enlarged labia majora and pubic or axillary hair. Precocious menarche is found in half of the girls. Parents complain of gynaecomastia in boys, but also of tall stature or occurrence of acne in young infants.

In both sexes the differential diagnosis is with precocious puberty, which may be accompanied in boys by gynaecomastia, and pseudoprecocious puberty caused by oestrogen-producing gonadal tumours, such as granulosa cell tumours of the ovary or interstitial testicular tumours.

In boys the clinical features of heterosexual precocity are more suggestive of an endocrine tumour than in girls. However, the practically constant association of clinical signs of virilization, deepening of the voice and marked increase of the phallus, contrasting with the prepubertal size of the testis in boys and clitoromegaly in girls, merely call for attention. Bone maturation is considerably advanced in all cases (bone age of 10–12 years in infants). Symptoms of hypercortisolism are more rarely associated ($\leqslant 20\%$). Hypertension is exceptional. An abdominal mass, often considerable, is palpated in half the cases.

Hormonal studies have been limited but show the association of increased oestrogen and androgen excretion. Relative increases in urinary oestrone, oestradiol or oestriol are variable. The average excess of androgen production is about half that found in virilizing adrenal tumours [33,336]. The predominant androgen is again DHEA. There is an apparent discrepancy between the overproduction of androgens and the relatively modest clinical signs of virilization.

Adenomas are as frequently observed as carcinomas. Their morphological types do not differ from other secreting adrenal tumours. Treatment is surgical. Management of the patients and prognosis are as in the other types of adrenal tumour.

ADRENARCHE

Adrenarche is defined as the selective changes in adrenal secretions, 'adrenal androgen activation', which occur in childhood before puberty. In early childhood, plasma levels of adrenal and gonadal steroids are low in both sexes. Plasma adrenal androgens (DHEA, DHEAS and Δ4-androstenedione) rise by about 6–8 years of skeletal age until 13–15 years of age [348]. Gonadal steroids (testosterone, 17β-oestradiol, 17α-hydroxyprogesterone) and pituitary gonadotrophins increase 2–3 years later (gonadarche).

Premature pubarche

Premature pubarche is defined as the precocious development of sexual hair (pubic and axillary) before 8 years of age in girls or 9 years of age in boys, without the appearance of other signs of sexual maturation [349]. However, other clinical symptoms [350] may include skin changes, acne, adult-type perspiration and a deepening of voice frequency. Accelerated growth is often observed, and may be the only symptom of early adrenarche without pubarche. Skeletal maturation is slightly advanced.

Premature pubarche is attributed to the premature and/or excessive activation of adrenal androgen secretion (premature adrenarche). Plasma levels of DHEA, DHEAS and Δ4-androstenedione and urinary 17-ketosteroids are elevated for age in the range normally seen in older pubertal children [351,352]. The response to ACTH stimulation is also greater than in age-matched controls [350]. The adrenal origin of the increased androgens has clearly been established by dexamethasone suppression [351].

The mechanisms responsible for the normal adrenarche, as well as for premature adrenarche, are unclear. The incidence of premature pubarche is not well documented. It occurs more commonly in girls than in boys, between 3 and 8 years of age [352], and may be associated with CNS abnormalities or brain damage [350,352]. Familial occurrence has been reported, and it has been postulated that predisposition to premature pubarche is transmitted as a dominant non-human leukocyte antigen (HLA) linked trait [350,353].

Isolated premature pubarche is considered as a constitutional variant [349], but must be differentiated from other causes of premature pubarche, such as a first sign of true precocious puberty. A differential diagnosis is made on clinical and biological signs of gonadal activation (increased testicular volume in boys, increased ovarian and uterine size at ultrasonographic examination in girls, and increased levels of gonadal steroids and gonadotrophins in both sexes). In recent years it has progressively emerged that mild forms or late-onset forms of 21-hydroxylase deficiency can mimic premature pubarche [354,355], as DHEA and DHEAS levels are elevated for age in both, although the ratio of DHEA–Δ4-androstenedione is lower in the latter [352]. Dexamethasone suppression tests do not differentiate the two conditions, since adrenal androgens are suppressed in both [351,355]. Differential diagnosis is made on the elevation of basal plasma 17α-hydroxyprogesterone levels or after ACTH stimulation [355–357].

Premature pubarche may also be due to mild forms of

11β-hydroxylase or 3β-hydroxysteroid dehydrogenase (3β-HSD) deficiency [355,358]. However, considerable controversy surrounds the distinction of premature adrenarche (and/or polycystic ovarian syndrome) from non-classical forms of congenital hyperplasia, due to a mild deficiency in either 21-hydroxylase, 11β-hydroxylase or 3β-HSD [359,360]. Diagnostic criteria must be more stringent than in the past, and final diagnosis should now be achieved by molecular genetic studies [358,361–363].

In androgen-producing neoplasms, premature pubarche is accompanied by other symptoms of virilization, skeletal maturation is usually more and dexamethasone does not suppress the markedly elevated androgen levels (see above). Thus a diagnosis of isolated premature pubarche is made only when all other causes of hyperandrogenism have been ruled out.

True puberty usually develops normally at a normal or slightly advanced age in patients with the manifestation of adrenarche defined as premature pubarche. A long-term study of a large group of girls presenting with premature pubarche, in whom steroid enzyme deficiency was ruled out, showed that premature pubarche is associated with a transient acceleration in growth and bone maturation, without significant effect on the onset and progression of puberty and final height [364]. On the other hand, in a longitudinal study we observed that plasma levels of both DHEA/DHEAS and Δ4-androstenedione continued to rise throughout puberty and remained above the normal range for age, even in adulthood in many cases (Fig. 29.6).

These patients frequently develop peripubertal hirsutism and/or polycystic ovarian disease [350,366]. This could result from adrenarche being not only precocious but also exaggerated, with a dysregulation of the 17α-hydroxylase/17,30-lyase enzyme activities in both the adrenal and the ovary [367]. Thus, although isolated premature pubarche is considered as a benign disorder, for which there is no need for treatment, a rational attitude is to follow growth and sexual development, and to repeat annual measurements of plasma androgens and gonadotrophins until the patient has achieved puberty.

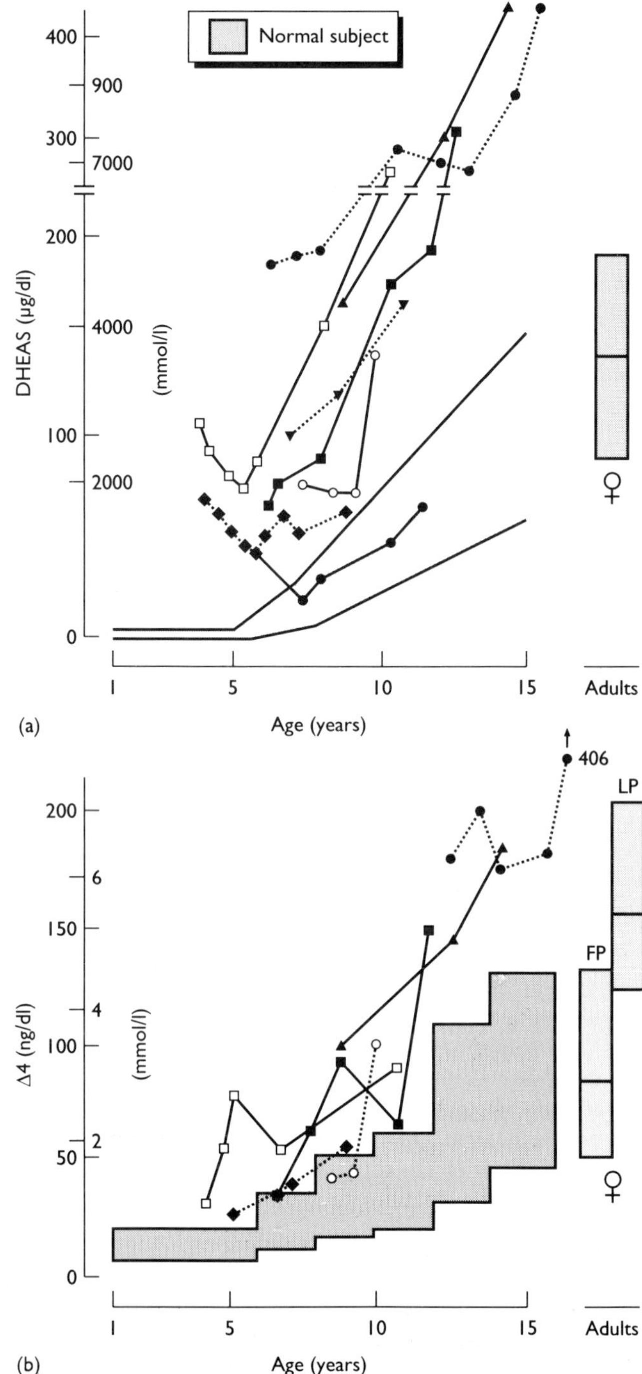

Fig. 29.6 Longitudinal study of plasma DHEAS and Δ4-androstenedione (Δ4) in girls with premature pubarche (MG Forest and F de Peretti, unpublished observations). Mean + SD for DHEAS (redrawn from de Peretti and Forest [365] and 95% confidence limits for Δ4 (MG Forest, unpublished observations). FP, follicular phase; LP, luteal phase.

HYPERALDOSTERONISM AND HYPERMINERALOCORTICISM

Primary hyperaldosteronism or Conn syndrome

Inappropriate hypersecretion of aldosterone is an uncommon (≤1%) cause of hypertension. The first reported patient [368] had asymptomatic hypertension, hypokalaemia and an adrenal adenoma. The condition is very rare in the paediatric age group, in which about 25 cases have been reported, the youngest patient being 3 years of age. Adrenal adenoma classically represents the predominant cause of primary aldosteronism in adults, but is rare in children. The tumours giving rise to primary hyperaldosteronism usually develop from the zona glomerulosa. The second cause of hyperaldosteronism is bilateral adrenal hyperplasia, which may be micronodular [369] and may not be as uncommon as generally believed [370]. Adrenal carcinoma is a rare cause of hyperaldosteronism, and unilateral adrenal hyperplasia is even rarer [371]. Aldosterone synthase cytochrome P450, distinct from cytochrome $P450_{11\beta}$ hydroxylase, is responsible for the biosynthesis of aldosterone in patients presenting with primary aldosteronism [372].

The main clinical symptom is hypertension without oedema. Although the hallmark of hyperaldosteronism is hypokalaemia with inappropriate renal wasting of potassium [373], symptoms are mild in the early course of the disease, and the child may present only with hypertension without hypokalaemia. As the disease progresses, hypokalaemia becomes the predominant cause of symptoms and may be the only sign. Affected children present later with muscular weakness, paraesthesias, tetany, polyuria, nocturia and often enuresis or poor growth [239,374].

Characteristic biochemical disturbances are hypokalaemia, sustained hyperkaluria and alkalosis. However, a normal potassium level has been found in a child with hypertensive hyperaldosteronism [375]. Thus, if hypokalaemia is not present, it can be precipitated by a high-sodium diet for 4 days: this may be dangerous in children. Plasma and urinary levels of aldosterone and its metabolites are variably elevated. As in primary hyperaldosteronism, aldosterone secretion is autonomous, plasma renin is suppressed and is unresponsive to manoeuvres that deplete intravascular volume (see Fig. 29.4). Adrenal calcification and hypomagnesaemia can be observed [375]. Plasma levels of atrial natriuretic peptide (ANP) are elevated, probably due to volume expansion and/or to increased synthesis in the adrenal medulla [376], whereas they are normal in uncomplicated essential hypertension [377]. The loss of physiological inhibition of aldosteronogenesis by ANP in adenoma cells is presumed to be due to the absence of ANP-specific receptors in these tumours [378,379].

A diagnosis is made by typical response to dynamic tests. Aldosterone is not suppressed by dexamethasone [380] or sodium chloride. Plasma renin [381] is not stimulated by ambulation. Salt restriction fails to stimulate either aldosterone or renin. Differential diagnosis is mainly with the syndrome of glucocorticoid-suppressible aldosteronism [131]. It should also exclude 'idiopathic primary aldosteronism', a hyperplasia of the zona glomerulosa or bilateral macronodular hyperplasia thought to be due to the inappropriate secretion of a putative aldosterone-stimulating factor [382]. Response to the ingestion of a single dose of captopril, an inhibitor of the angiotensin-converting enzyme [383], has been proposed as a useful test to discriminate Conn syndrome from idiopathic aldosteronism [384] or other causes of essential hypertension [385]. In patients in whom aldosterone production is autonomous, captopril has little effect on either aldosterone or renin levels. The urinary pattern of 18-oxocortisol provides a basis for the biochemical classification of primary aldosteronism and the differentiation between typical aldosterone-producing adenomas (high levels) from idiopathic hyperaldosteronism associated with bilateral adrenal hyperplasia (low levels) [386].

The next diagnostic step is to identify the exact cause of autonomous aldosterone secretion. Modern imaging of the adrenal gland [229] identifies adenomas, but MRI will perhaps carry more precise information on tumours less than 1 or 2 cm in diameter, which are not detected accurately by abdominal CT. Scintigraphic localization has been useful but in some instances confirmation of the diagnosis and localization of the adenoma has been made only by catheterization and selective sampling in the vena cava, renal and adrenal veins [239,374].

Treatment is surgical. Unilateral adrenalectomy is performed in cases of solitary adenomas [373,387] or unilateral adrenal hyperplasia [371]. Temporary salt supplementation is advisable because of the possible suppression of the contralateral adrenal. In case of bilateral adrenal hyperplasia, bilateral adrenalectomy often does not cure the hypertension, and thus medical treatment is more suitable. Potassium balance can be restored by spironolactone 200–400 mg/day, a competitive antagonist of aldosterone. Amiloride, another diuretic, has recently been proposed as the drug of choice [370]. Acting independently of aldosterone, this compound is an inhibitor of distal tubular sodium transport, but does not always control blood pressure.

Syndrome of apparent mineralocorticoid excess

AN HEREDITARY FORM OF 11β-HYDROXYSTEROID DEHYDROGENASE DEFICIENCY?

The syndrome of apparent mineralocorticoid excess (AME) is a rare cause of juvenile hypertension with an apparent genetic autosomal inheritance, characterized by severe hypokalaemic alkalosis despite low plasma renin activity and subnormal levels of aldosterone and other mineralocorticoids [388]. AME was described in 1979 [389] and about 25 cases have been reported in children [390,391]. It was first speculated that an unknown steroid with gluco- and mineralocorticoid activity was responsible for the disorder [392]. However, it was subsequently shown that the unexplained hypermineralocorticoid clinical state was associated with defective peripheral metabolism of cortisol, the primary defect being a decreased rate of peripheral 11β-hydroxydehydrogenation of cortisol to cortisone [389]. The link between hypertension, hyperkalaemia and the inability to convert cortisol to cortisone remained unexplained until it was understood that the type I renal receptor has the same affinity for cortisol and for aldosterone [393]; thus the dehydrogenase activity of 11β-HSD is necessary to protect the renal type I receptor from normally higher plasma circulating levels of cortisol, allowing aldosterone to regulate homeostasis [100,154,393–395]. This is a unique mechanism for achieving receptor specificity [396] and the present pathogenetic concept is that in AME patients cortisol functions as a mineralocorticoid [397].

Two different types of AME have been described. Type I is believed to represent a deficiency of 11β-HSD by which there is impaired conversion of cortisol to cortisone, and also of 5β-reductase [398]. Plasma cortisol is normal, although its production rate is decreased. In urine there is an increase in the ratio of tetrahydrocortisol (THF) plus alloTHF to tetrahydrocortisone (THE) plus alloTHE. The half-life of cortisol is increased. Since the ability to convert orally administered cortisone to cortisol is intact, it is believed that the defect is only in cortisone reductase ability.

In type II variant of AME, all clinical and biochemical features of AME are present: there is a decrease in the rate of cortisol metabolic clearance, cortisol turnover and decreased ring-A reduction but the urinary THF/THE ratio is normal [399]. It has been suggested that the situation could result from a simultaneous defect in both oxidation and reduction but this has not been demonstrated. Moreover, the term of 11β-HSD deficiency is not an adequate term to define the spectrum of AME, not only because it does not embrace the type 2 variant, but also because no mutation has been found in the HSD11 gene in AME patients believed to have 11β-HSD deficiency [400]. Also, in both types, the major metabolic error is defective ring-A reduction of cortisol [401]. It is likely that more complex abnormalities in the enzymes involved in cortisol metabolism constitute the basis of both type I and type II AME, but the genetic basis of the disorder is still unknown.

Differential diagnosis should exclude the 'Liddle syndrome' which presents the same clinical and metabolic features, but is considered to represent deficient membrane sodium transport in the tubule [402]. The administration of the salt-wasting diuretic triamterene corrects the hypokalaemia in this syndrome but not in AME.

Treatment of AME is difficult. The clinical symptoms respond to the aldosterone antagonist, spironolactone, administered alone or in association with a diuretic or a low-sodium diet, but the effects are usually transient. Patients with type II AME respond better to the suppression of cortisol secretion by dexamethasone [399]. Dexamethasone may be effective because it binds to the mineralocorticoid receptor without expressing mineralocorticoid activity [390]. Long-term experience is lacking.

Acquired 11β-hydroxysteroid dehydrogenase deficiency

The chronic excessive ingestion of liquorice induces hypokalaemia and kaliuresis, and suppresses the renin–aldosterone system. The mechanism was unclear until it was shown that glycyrrizic acid (GZA), a glycosylated saponin which is the major constituent of liquorice, and its aglycone, glycyrrhetinic acid (GRA), inhibit microsomal 11β-HSD, the enzyme which converts active 11-hydroxysteroids to inactive 11-ketosteroids [403,404]. This enzyme deficiency allows glucocorticoids to exert effects through the mineralocorticoid receptor, and explains the development of symptoms similar to those of apparent mineralocorticoid excess [403,404].

Glucocorticoid-suppressible hyperaldosteronism

This rare disorder, also termed glucocorticoid-remediable aldosteronism in the literature, was first described by Sutherland *et al.* [405] as a form of hypertension associated with hyperaldosteronism and low renin which was relieved by small doses of dexamethasone [399]. Autosomal dominant transmission of the syndrome was later demonstrated [406]. This peculiar form of primary aldosteronism appears to be regulated by ACTH rather than by renin–angiotensin [407]. Indeed, plasma aldosterone levels, which fall instead of rising in the morning (in the upright position) [408], are unresponsive to angiotensin II, but can be stimulated by continuous ACTH infusion for over 5 days, instead of the usual transient rise followed by suppression.

High levels of 18-oxocortisol and 18-hydroxycortisol are produced [409]. They are positively regulated by ACTH and their structure is consistent with cortisol being used as a substrate for aldosterone synthetase. These 17α-hydroxylated analogues of 18-hydroxycorticosterone and aldosterone cannot normally be synthesized in the zona glomerulosa because this zone lacks 17α-hydroxylase activity.

Two enzymatic activities distinguish the biosynthesis of gluco- and mineralocorticoids. Normally, the 17-hydroxylation necessary for cortisol biosynthesis is catalysed by the cytochrome $P450_{c17}$, an enzyme present only in the adrenal fasciculata, while the final three steps of aldosterone synthesis, 11β- and 18-hydroxylation and 18-oxidation are mediated by a cytochrome P450, aldosterone synthase, encoded by the CYP11B2 gene, in the zona glomerulosa. A related isoenzyme (genetic locus CYP11B1) is expressed at much higher levels than CYP11B2 in the zona fasciculata, which possesses only the 11β-hydroxylase activity necessary for cortisol biosynthesis. CYP11B1 is regulated by ACTH, while CYP11B2 is normally regulated by angiotensin II but not ACTH (see review [279]).

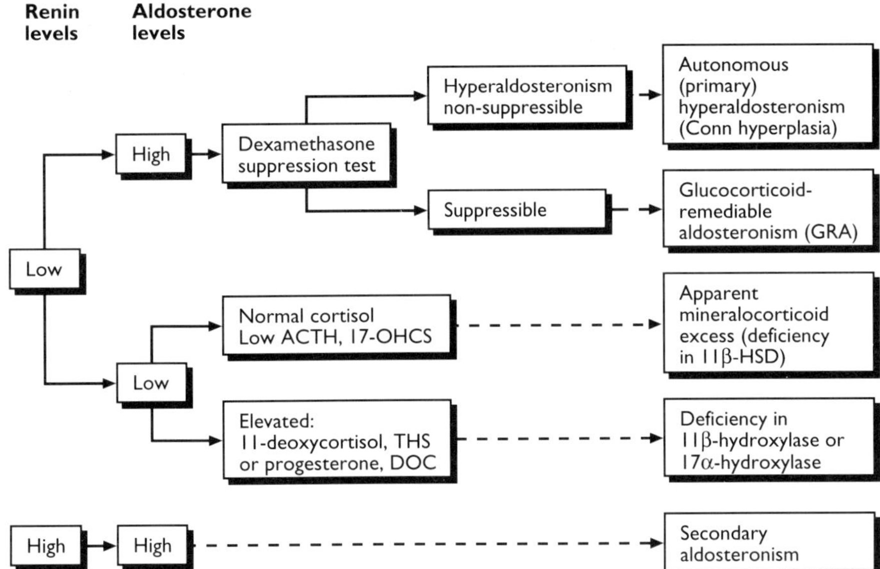

Fig. 29.7 Flow chart of the screening procedure for the aetiological diagnosis of adrenal hypertension. THS, tetrahydro-11-deoxycortisol.

Recent studies have shown that the disorder is caused by fusion of the regulatory sequences of the steroid 11β-hydroxylase gene to coding sequences of the aldosterone synthase gene resulting in an unequal crossing-over between homologous regions of these two closely linked genes on chromosome 8 [410,411]. The mutant allele carries a duplication introducing a novel function, the ectopic expression of aldosterone synthase in the wrong part of the adrenal gland, the zona fasciculata, under the control of ACTH.

The familial occurrence, the abnormal steroids and the ratio of these steroids to urinary tetra-aldosterone and the dexamethasone test are sufficient to suspect the diagnosis and distinguish this disorder from other causes of hypertension (Fig. 29.7). The diagnosis can be confirmed by a simple direct genetic test, since chimaeric gene duplication of 11β-hydroxylase/aldosterone synthase gene, first described in the affected members of a large pedigree [410], is considered a specific marker for glucocorticoid-suppressible hyperaldosteronism (GSH) [279].

Treatment is based on the administration of dexamethasone (0.5 mg/day) [390]. Small doses averaging 0.5 mg/day are often sufficient for prompt relief of symptoms, but there is individual sensitivity to the drug. Treatment of children with GSH poses special problems and, as in 21-hydroxylase deficiency, should be undertaken only by physicians experienced in the management of growth and development and the side-effects of excessive glucocorticoid dosing. The smallest effective dose of hydrocortisone or prednisolone is advised and the addition of a potassium-sparing diuretic may assist the control of blood pressure. In general, the prognosis is better than in AME.

Secondary hyperaldosteronism

Secondary hyperaldosteronism may be due to a variety of conditions in which aldosterone excess is not the primary abnormality, and in which hypertension may or may not be present (see Table 29.4). Plasma aldosterone is increased in a number of diseases, such as congestive heart failure, cirrhosis and nephrotic syndrome, which have in common the formation of peripheral oedema, but are not associated with hypertension. In these situations aldosterone secretion rises in response to a reduced effective circulating blood volume caused by diminished cardiac output or transudation of intravascular fluid into extravascular sites. Also, in these situations there is no potassium wasting because sodium concentration is low in the distal tubule where cation exchange is located, as a result of the increased reabsorption of sodium chloride in

Table 29.4 Causes of secondary hyperaldosteronism

Associated with hypertension	Without hypertension
Primary hyperreninaemia	Oedematous states
Juxtaglomerular cell tumour	Congestive heart failure
Wilms tumour	Hepatic cirrhosis
Secondary reninism	Nephrotic syndrome
Renovascular malformation	Renal tubular disorders
Renal transplantation	Acute (tubular necrosis)
Anephric state	Chronic (Bartter syndrome)
Fibrous encapsulation of the kidneys	Anorexia nervosa
Genitourinary tract obstructions	
Phaeochromocytoma	

the proximal tubule. In all cases the sodium-retaining effect of aldosterone persists because the normal escape mechanism from mineralocorticoid action is not activated. In addition, in a case of liver disease, there is a diminished hepatic metabolism of aldosterone.

In other forms associated with hypertension, hyperaldosteronism is due to increased renin stimulation. Renin is produced in excess either by a tumour (primary hyperreninaemia) or indirectly as the consequence of renal artery stenosis or renovascular malformations (secondary reninism) (see Table 29.4).

RENIN-SECRETING TUMOURS

Renin-secreting tumours are rare; they are usually found near the juxtaglomerular region. A recent review reports six of seven new cases in patients 13–22 years of age [412]. Diagnosis of such tumours is made when hypertension is discovered in a young subject. The prominent features are hypokalaemia, excessively high levels of renin and prorenin and secondary hyperaldosteronism. Renal angiography is necessary to exclude a renovascular cause for the hypertension. The renin-secreting tumours are small (10–15 mm in diameter) and best visualized by CT. Although theoretically the method of choice, selective renin measurement in renal veins is not always successful in localizing the side of the tumour. Treatment is surgical and selective tumorectomy allows complete recovery and restores blood pressure to normal, even after several years of hypertension.

Other tumours, such as nephroblastoma or pancreatic adenocarcinoma [78], may produce renin or other metabolites [10]. Malignant renin-secreting tumours of extrarenal origin have been observed in various organs, including the lung, urogenital tract, liver, pancreas and muscle. The common feature of all these tumours is the association of high levels of both aldosterone and renin. However, these malignant tumours secrete higher levels of prorenin than do juxtaglomerular tumours [413].

In *Wilms tumours*, hypertension is not a common feature. When it occurs it is the result of combined primary and secondary reninism due to both increased renin production by the tumour cells themselves and renal artery obstruction [81,414].

BARTTER SYNDROME

A rare syndrome of hyperreninaemia, hyperaldosteronism, hypokalaemia and alkalosis without hypertension or oedema, was described by Bartter *et al.* in 1962 [186]. The disease may occur in children or adults, and familial cases suggest a recessive autosomal inheritance. Black children are severely affected. The typical patient presents a peculiar facies with bulging forehead and temporal baldness. The disorder usually begins in childhood with vomiting, dehydration, polyuria–polydipsia and failure to thrive [415]. Other symptoms include muscular weakness, cramps or developmental impairment [416]. The findings include severe hypokalaemia (less than 2 mmol/l) with renal wasting of potassium, metabolic alkalosis, hypomagnesaemia and hypercalciuria [417,418]. Sodium concentration is moderately decreased. Aldosterone levels are high for age, but they do not reach values that one would expect for the considerable rise in plasma renin (more than 10 times normal) due to hypokalaemia. Renal juxtaglomerular cell hyperplasia [186] and increased urinary PGE_2 excretion [47] are observed.

A number of primary defects have been proposed to account for the activation of the renin–angiotensin–aldosterone system in this disease, but the cause is still unknown. A chloride reabsorption defect may be present in the thick ascending limb of the loop of Henlé in the renal tubule, but similar defects have been found at other sites of the nephron, and one patient developed the tubular defect after exhibiting other features of the syndrome. The hyperaldosteronism probably is not the primary cause of hypokalaemia because bilateral adrenalectomy does not correct the kaliuresis [419].

Treatment with potassium supplementation and indomethacin (2–3 mg/kg a day), an inhibitor of prostaglandin synthesis, has shown favourable clinical results [416]. Somatostatin has recently been proposed in the treatment of the syndrome for suppressing aldosterone secretion [420] but its long-term efficacy has not yet been ascertained.

REFERENCES

1 Normann T, Havnen J, Mjolnerod O. Cushing's syndrome in an infant associated with neuroblastoma in two ectopic adrenal glands. *J Pediatr Surg* 1971;6:169.

2 Apert E. Dystrophies en rapport avec les lésions des capsules surrénales. Dystrophies variées (hermaphrodisme, puberté précoce, hirsutisme, obésité) en coïncidence avec des lésions des capsules surrénales. *Bull Méd (Paris)* 1910;24:1161.

3 Bauer T, Wassing H. Zur Frage der Adipositas hypophysarea: Basophiles Adenom der Hypophyse. *Berliner Klin Wochenschr* 1913;50:1531.

4 Bullock W, Sequiera JH. On the relation of the suprarenal capsules to the sexual organs. *Trans Pathol Soc Lond* 1905; 56:189–91.

5 Fox TC. Case of primary sarcoma of the left adrenal capsule with extensive thrombosis of the vena cava inferior in a child. *Trans Pathol Soc Lond* 1885;36:460–2.

6 Cushing H. The basophil adenomas of pituitary body and their clinical manifestations (pituitary basophilism). *Bull Johns Hopkins Hosp* 1932;50:137–95.

7 Krieger DT. *Cushing's Syndrome*. Berlin: Springer Verlag, 1982.

8 Lee PDK, Winter RJ, Green OC. Virilizing adrenocortical tumors in childhood: eight cases and a review of the literature. *Pediatrics* 1984;76:437–44.

9 Levy SR, Wynne V Jr, Lorentz WB. Cushing's syndrome in infancy secondary to pituitary adenomas. *Am J Dis Child* 1982;136:605–7.
10 Baylin SB, Mendelsohn G. Ectopic (inappropriate) hormone production by tumours: mechanisms involved and the biological and clinical implications. *Endocr Rev* 1980;1:45–77.
11 Omenn GS. Ectopic syndromes associated with tumors in childhood. *Pediatrics* 1971;47:613–22.
12 Belsky JL, Cuello B, Swanson LW *et al.* Cushing's syndrome due to ectopic production of corticotropin-releasing factor. *J Clin Endocrinol Metab* 1985;60:496–500.
13 Carey RM, Varma SK, Drake CR *et al.* Ectopic secretion of corticotropin-releasing factor as a cause of Cushing's syndrome. A clinical morphologic, and biochemical study. *N Engl J Med* 1984;311:13–20.
14 Schteingart DE, Lloyd RV, Akil H *et al.* Cushing's syndrome secondary to ectopic corticotropin-releasing hormone-adrenocorticotropin secretion. *J Clin Endocrinol Metab* 1986;63:770–5.
15 Suda T, Kondo M, Totani R *et al.* Ectopic adrenocorticotropin syndrome caused by lung cancer that responded to corticotropin-releasing hormone. *J Clin Endocrinol Metab* 1986;63:1047–51.
16 May P, Stein EJ, Ryter RJ *et al.* Cushing syndrome from percutaneous absorption of triamcinolone cream. *Arch Intern Med* 1976;136:612–13.
17 Vaz R, Senior B, Morris M, Binkiewicz A. Adrenal effects of becomethasone inhalation therapy in asthmatic children. *J Pediatr* 1982;100:660–2.
18 Carney JA, Gordon H, Carpenter PC *et al.* The complex of myxomas, spotty pigmentation, and endocrine overactivity. *Medicine (Balt)* 1985;64:270–83.
19 Young FW, Carney JA, Musa BU *et al.* Familial Cushing's syndrome due to primary pigmented nodular adrenocortical disease. *N Engl J Med* 1989;321:1659–64.
20 Ichiba Y, Nishizaki Y, Tanizaki M. Cushing's syndrome due to primary pigmented nodular adrenocortical disease with cardiac myxomas and mucocutaneous lentigines. *Acta Paediatr* 1992;81:91–2.
21 Lacroix A, Bolté E, Tremblay J *et al.* Gastric inhibitory polypeptide-dependent cortisol hypersecretion – a new cause of Cushing's syndrome. *N Engl J Med* 1992;327:974–80.
22 Reznik Y, Allali-Zerah V, Chayvialle JA *et al.* Food-dependent Cushing's syndrome mediated by aberrant adrenal sensitivity to gastric inhibitory polypeptide. *N Engl J Med* 1992:327:981–6.
23 Hamet P, Larochelle P, Franks DJ *et al.* Cushing syndrome with food-dependent periodic hormonogenesis. *Clin Invest Med* 1987;10:530–3.
24 Luton JP, Mahoudeau JA, Bouchard P *et al.* Treatment of Cushing's disease by o,p'DDD, survey of 62 cases. *N Engl J Med* 1979;300:459–64.
25 Orth DN, Liddle GW. Results of treatment in 108 patients with Cushing's syndrome. *N Engl J Med* 1971;285:243–7.
26 Plotz CM, Knowlton AI, Ragan C. The natural history of Cushing's syndrome. *Am J Med* 1952;13:597–614.
27 Raux MC, Binoux M, Luton JP *et al.* Studies of ACTH secretion in 116 cases of Cushing's syndrome. *J Clin Endocrinol Metab* 1975;40:186–97.
28 Soffer LJ, Iannacone A, Gabrilove JL. Cushing's syndrome. A study of fifty patients. *Am J Med* 1961;30:129–46.
29 Thieblot P, Luton JP, Mahoudeau J *et al.* Etude de la fonction gonadotrope dans le syndrome de Cushing chez la femme. *Ann Endocrinol* 1979;40:429–30.
30 McArthur RG, Cloutier MD, Hayles AB *et al.* Cushing's disease in children. *Mayo Clin Proc* 1972;47:318–26.
31 De Gennes JL. Syndrome de Cushing chez l'enfant. In: Soulairac A, ed. *Le Syndrome de Cushing.* Paris: Masson et Doin, 1967:237–82.
32 Barzilai D, Dickstein G, Kanter Y *et al.* Complete remission of Cushing's disease by total bilateral adrenalectomy and adrenal autotransplantation. *J Clin Endocrinol Metab* 1980;50:863–5.
33 Benaily M, Schweisguth O, Job JC. Les tumeurs corticosurrénales de l'enfant. Etude rétrospective de 34 cas observés de 1954–1973. *Arch Fr Pédiat* 1975;32:441–54.
34 Canlorbe P, Vassal J, Job JC. Essai de traitement d'un syndrome de Cushing par l'*o,p'*-DDD chez l'enfant. *Ann Pédiatr* 1971;18:609–16.
35 Casar J, Doyle FH, Mashiter K, Joplin GF. Treatment of Cushing's disease in juveniles with interstitial pituitary irradiation. *Clin Endocrinol* 1979;11:313–21.
36 Contreras P, Altieri E, Liberman C *et al.* Adrenal rest tumor of the liver causing Cushing's syndrome: treatment with ketoconazole preceding an apparent surgical cure. *J Clin Endocrinol Metab* 1985;60:21–8.
37 Dahms WT, Gray G, Vrana M, New M. Adrenocortical adenoma and ganglioneuroblastoma in a child. *Am J Dis Child* 1973;125:608–11.
38 Ernest I, Ekman H. Adrenalectomy in Cushing's disease: a long-term follow-up. *Acta Endocrinol (Copenh)* 1972; 69(Suppl. 160):1–41.
39 Fontaine G, Lacheretz M, Dupont A *et al.* Tumeur de la cortico-surrénale avec puberté précoce et gynécomastie chez un garçon de 3 ans 1/2. *Ann Pédiatr* 1970;17:463–75.
40 Korth-Schutz S. Cushing's syndrome and adrenocortical carcinoma in childhood. In: New MI, Levine LS, eds. *Adrenal Diseases in Childhood. Pediatric and Adolescent Endocrinology,* Vol. 13. Basel: Karger, 1984:185–209.
41 Lubitz JA, Freeman L, Okun R. Mitotane use in inoperable adrenal cortical carcinoma. *J Am Med Assoc* 1973;223: 1109–12.
42 Mardsen HB, Morris Jones B, Lees PD, Hann IM. Late functioning adrenocortical carcinoma in a 5-year old girl. *Arch Dis Child* 1978;53:341–2.
43 Sizonenko PC, Doret AM, Riondel AM, Paunier L. Cushing's syndrome due to bilateral adrenal cortical hyperplasia in a 13-year-old girl: successful treatment with *o,p'*-DDD. *Helv Paediatr Acta* 1974;29:195–202.
44 Solomon IL, Schoen EJ. Juvenile Cushing syndrome manifested primarily by growth failure. *Am J Dis Child* 1976; 130:200–2.
45 Styne DM, Grumbach MM, Kaplan SL *et al.* Treatment of Cushing's disease in childhood and adolescence by transphenoidal microadenomectomy. *N Engl J Med* 1984;310:889–93.
46 Stewart PM, Corrie JET, Shackleton CHL *et al.* Syndrome of apparent mineralocorticoid excess. *J Clin Invest* 1988; 82:340–9.
47 Rocha Artigas JL, D'Avila Niclewicz E, Silva APC, Athayde SL. Congenital adrenal cortical carcinoma. *J Pediatr Surg* 1976;11:247–52.
48 Böhm N, Lippmann-Grob B, von Petroykowski W. Familial Cushing's syndrome due to pigmented multinodular adrenocortical dysplasia. *Acta Endocrinol (Copenh)* 1983;102: 428–35.
49 Gershanik JJ, Elmore M, Levkoff AH. Congenital occurrence of adrenal cortical tumor, ganglioneuroma and toxoplas-

mosis. *Pediatrics* 1973;51:703–8.

50 Goldstein AE, Rubin SW, Askin JA. Carcinoma of adrenal cortex with androgenital syndrome in children: complete review of the literature and report of a case with recovery in a child eight months of age. *Am J Dis Child* 1946;72: 563–603.

51 McArthur RG, Bahn RC, Hayles AB. Primary adrenocortical nodular dysplasia as a cause of Cushing's syndrome in infants and children. *Mayo Clin Proc* 1982;57:58–63.

52 Downing V, Eule J, Huseby RA. Regression of an adrenal cortical carcinoma and its neovascular bed following mitotane therapy. A case report. *Cancer* 1974;34:1882–7.

53 Hopwood NJ, Kenny FM. Incidence of Nelson's syndrome after adrenalectomy for Cushing's disease in children: results of a nationwide survery. *Am J Dis Child* 1977;131:1353–6.

54 Neville AM, Symington T. Bilateral adrenocortical hyperplasia in children with Cushing's syndrome. *J Pathol* 1972; 107:95–106.

55 Gold PW, Loriaux DL, Roy A *et al.* Responses to corticotropin-releasing hormone in the hypercortisolism of depression and Cushing's disease. *N Engl J Med* 1986;314:1329–35.

56 Liddle GW. Tests of pituitary–adrenal suppressibility in the diagnosis of Cushing's syndrome. *J Clin Endocrinol Metab* 1960;20:1539–60.

57 Gicquel C, Le Bouc Y, Luton JP *et al.* Monoclonality of corticotroph macroadenomas in Cushing's disease. *J Clin Endocrinol Metab* 1992;75:472–5.

58 Hartley AL, Birch JM, Mardsen HB *et al.* Adrenal cortical tumours: epidemiological and familial aspects. *Arch Dis Child* 1987;62:683–9.

59 Levine GW. Adrenocortical carcinoma in two children with subsequent primary tumors. *Am J Dis Child* 1978; 132:238–40.

60 Muller S, Gardner H, Weber B *et al.* Wilm's tumor and adrenocortical carcinoma with hemihypertrophy and hamartomas. *Eur J Pediatr* 1978;127:219–26.

61 Pettenatti MJ, Haines JL, Higgins RR *et al.* Wiedemann–Beckwith syndrome: presentation of clinical and cytogenic data on 22 new cases and review of the literature. *Human Genet* 1986;74:143–54.

62 Weinstein RL, Kliman B, Neeman J, Cohen RB. Deficient 17-hydroxylation in a corticosterone producing adrenal tumor from an infant with hemihypertrophy and visceromegaly. *J Clin Endocrinol Metab* 1970;30:457–68.

63 Wiedmann HR. Tumours and hemihypertrophy associated with Wiedemann–Beckwith syndrome. *Eur J Pediatr* 1984;141:129–32.

64 DiGeorge AM. Albright syndrome; is it coming of age? *J Pediatr* 1975;87:1018–20.

65 Fraumeni JF, Miller RW. Adrenocortical neoplasm with hemihypertrophy brain tumors and other disorders. *J Pediatr* 1967;70:129–38.

66 Horrocks PM, Franks S, Hockley AD *et al.* An ACTH-secreting pituitary tumour arising in a patient with congenital adrenal hyperplasia. *Clin Endocrinol* 1982;65: 777–81.

67 Imura H. Ectophic hormone syndromes. *Clin Endocrinol Metab* 1980;9:235–60.

68 Leyton O, Turnbull HM, Bratton AB. Primary cancer of the thymus with pluriglandular disturbance. *J Pathol Bacteriol* 1931;34:635–9.

69 Cummins GE, Cohen D. Cushing's syndrome secondary to ACTH-secreting Wilms' tumor. *J Pediatr Surg* 1974;9:535–9.

70 Pasmore SJ, Berry PJ, Oakhill A. Recurrent pancreatoblastoma with inappropriate adrenocorticotrophic hormone secretion. *Arch Dis Child* 1988;63:1494–5.

71 Ward PS, Mott MG, Smith J *et al.* Cushing's syndrome and bronchial carcinoid tumour. *Arch Dis Child* 1984;59:375–7.

72 Findling JW. The Cushing's syndrome. An enlarging clinical spectrum. *N Engl J Med* 1989;321:1677–8.

73 Raux-Demay MC, Proeschel MF, de Kreser Y *et al.* Characterization of human corticotrophin-releasing hormone and pro-opiomelanocortin-related peptides in a thymic carcinoid tumour responsible for Cushing's syndrome. *Clin Endocrinol* 1988;29:649–57.

74 Larsen JL, Cathey WJ, Odell WD. Primary adrenocortical nodular dysplasia, a distinct subtype of Cushing's syndrome. *Am J Med* 1986;80:976–84.

75 Hermus AR, Pieters GF, Smals AG *et al.* Transition from pituitary-dependent to adrenal-dependent Cushing's syndrome. *N Engl J Med* 1988;318:966–70.

76 Jennings AS, Liddle GW, Orth DN. Results of treating childhood Cushing's disease with pituitary irradiation. *N Engl J Med* 1977;297:957–62.

77 Lewinsky BS, Grogor KM, Symington T *et al.* The clinical pathologic features of 'non-hormonal' adrenocortical tumors: report of twenty new cases and review of the literature. *Cancer* 1974;33:778–90.

78 Ruddy MC, Atlas SA, Salerno FG. Hypertension associated with a renin-secreting adenocarcinoma of the pancreas. *N Engl J Med* 1982;307:993–7.

79 Zarate A, Kovacs K, Flores M *et al.* ACTH and CRF-producing bronchial carcinoid associated with Cushing's syndrome. *Clin Endocrinol* 1986;24:523–9.

80 Pearse AGE, Polak JM. Endocrine tumors of neural crest origin neurolophomas, apudomas and the APUD concept. *Med Biol* 1974;52:3–18.

81 Mitchell JD, Baxter TJ, Blair-West JR *et al.* Renin levels in nephroblastoma (Wilms tumor). Report of a renin secreting tumor. *Arch Dis Child* 1970;45:376–84.

82 Luton JP, Thieblot P, Bricarie H. Association syndrome de Cushing-phéochromocytome. *Nouv Pres Méd* 1977; 6:4053–7.

83 O'Brien T, Young WF, Davilla DG *et al.* Cushing's syndrome associated with ectopic production of corticotrophin-releasing hormone, corticotrophin and vasopressin by a phaeochromocytoma. *Clin Endocrinol* 1992;37:460–7.

84 Steiner AL, Goodman AD, Powers SR. Study of a kindred with pheochromocytoma medullar thyroid carcinoma, hyperparathyroidism and Cushing's disease: multiple endocrine neoplasia type 2. *Medicine* 1968;47:371–409.

85 Levine MA. The MacCune–Albright syndrome. *N Engl J Med* 1991;325:1738–40.

86 Schwindinger WF, Levine MA. McCune–Albright syndrome. *Trends Endocrinol Metab* 1993;4:238–42.

87 Patten JL, Johnes DR, Valle D *et al.* Mutation in the gene encoding the stimulatory G protein of adenylate cyclase in Albright's hereditary osteodystrophy. *N Engl J Med* 1990; 322:1412–19.

88 Weinstein LS, Shenker A, Gejman PV *et al.* Activating mutations of the stimulatory G protein in the McCune–Albright syndrome. *N Engl J Med* 1991;325:1688–95.

89 Thakker RV, Bouloux P, Wooding C *et al.* Association of parathyroid tumours in multiple endocrine neoplasia type 1 with loss of alleles on chromosome 11. *N Engl J Med* 1989; 321:218–24.

90 Nakamura Y, Larsson C, Julier C *et al.* Localization of the genetic defect in multiple endocrine neoplasia type I within

a small region of chromosome 11. *Am J Hum Genet* 1989; 44:751–5.

91 O'Halloran D, Shalet SM. A family pedigree exhibiting features of both multiple endocrine neoplasia type 1 and McCune–Albright syndromes. *J Clin Endocrinol Metab* 1994;78:523–5.

92 Clapham DE. Mutations in G protein-linked receptors: novel insights on disease. *Cell* 1993;75:1237–9.

93 Spiegel AM, Weinstein LS, Shenker A. Abnormalities in G-protein-coupled signal transduction pathways in human disease. *J Clin Invest* 1993;92:1119–25.

94 Meador CK, Bowdoin B, Owen WC *et al.* Primary adrenocortical nodular dysplasia; a rare cause of Cushing's syndrome. *J Endocrinol Metab* 1967;27:1255–63.

95 Grossman A. What is the cause of Cushing's disease? *Clin Endocrinol* 1992;36:451–2.

96 Krieger DT. Physiopathology of Cushing's disease. *Endocr Rev* 1983;4:22–43.

97 Cone RD, Mountjoy KG. Molecular genetics of the ACTH and melanocyte-stimulating hormone receptors. *Trends Endocrinol Metab* 1993;4:242–7.

98 Martin JB, Reichlin S, Brown GM. Clinical neuroendocrinology. *Contemp Neurol* 1977;14:3–394.

99 Liddle GW. Pathogenesis of glucocorticoid disorders. *Am J Med* 1972;53:638–48.

100 Atkinson AB, Chestnutt A, Crothers E *et al.* Cyclical Cushing's disease: two distinct rhythms in a patient with basophil adenoma. *J Clin Endocrinol Metab* 1985;60:328–32.

101 Kruse A, Klinken L, Holck S *et al.* Pituitary histology in Cushing's disease. *Clin Endocrinol* 1992;37:254–9.

102 Teel HM. Basophilic adenoma of the hypophysis with associated pluriglandular syndrome. *Arch Neurol Psychiatry* 1931;26:593–7.

103 Suda T, Liotta A, Krieger DT. Plasma lipotropin (LPH) and ACTH secretion in normal subjects and patients with pituitary–adrenal disorders. In: *60th Meeting of the Endocrine Society*, Miami, 1978:224.

104 Hellman L, Weitzman ED, Roffwarg H *et al.* Cortisol is secreted episodically in Cushing's syndrome. *J Clin Endocrinol Metab* 1970;30:686–9.

105 Tyrrell JB, Brooks RM, Fitzgerald PA *et al.* Cushing's disease. Selective trans-sphenoidal resection of pituitary microadenomas. *N Engl J Med* 1978;298:753–8.

106 Fehm HL, Voigt KH, Kummer G *et al.* Positive rate-sensitive corticosteroid feedback mechanism of ACTH secretion in Cushing's disease. *J Clin Invest* 1979;64:102–8.

107 Allgrove J, Husband P, Brook CGD. Cushing's disease: failure of treatment with cyproheptadine. *Br Med J* 1977; iii:686–7.

108 Krieger DT, Luria M. Plasma ACTH and cortisol responses to TRF, vasopressin or hypoglycemia in Cushing's disease and Nelson's syndrome. *J Clin Endocrinol Metab* 1977; 44:361–8.

109 Stewart PM, Penn R, Gibson R *et al.* Hypothalamic abnormalities in patients with pituitary-dependent Cushing's sydnrome. *Clin Endocrinol* 1992;36:453–8.

110 Boggild MD, Jenkinson S, Pistorello M *et al.* Molecular genetic studies of sporadic pituitary tumors. *J Clin Endocrinol Metab* 1994;78:387–92.

111 Nelson DH, Meaking JW, Thorn GW. ACTH producing pituitary tumors following adrenalectomy for Cushing's syndrome. *Ann Intern Med* 1960;52:560–9.

112 Schnall AM, Brodkey JS, Kaufman B, Pearson OH. Pituitary function after removal of pituitary microadenomas in Cushing's disease. *J Clin Endocrinol Metab* 1978;47:410–17.

113 Lüdecke D, Kautzky R, Saeger W, Schrader D. Selective removal of hypersecreting pituitary adenomas? An analysis of endocrine function, operative and microsurgical findings in 101 cases. *Acta Neurochir* 1976;35:27–42.

114 Gifford S, Gunderson JG. Cushing's disease as a psychosomatic disorder. *Medicine* 1970;49:397–409.

115 Krieger DT, Luria M. Effectiveness of cyproheptadine in decreasing plasma ACTH concentration in Nelson's syndrome. *J Clin Endocrinol Metab* 1976;43:1179–82.

116 Cook DM, Kendall JW, Allen JP, Lagerquist LG. Nyctohemeral variation and suppressibility of plasma ACTH in various stages of Cushing's disease. *Clin Endocrinol* 1976; 5:303–12.

117 Liu JH, Kazer RR, Rasmussen DD. Characterization of the twenty-four hour secretion patterns of adrenocorticotropin and cortisol in normal women and patients with Cushing's disease. *J Clin Endocrinol Metab* 1987;64:1027–35.

118 Bertagna X. Unrestrained production of proopiomelanocortin (POMC) and its peptide fragments by pituitary corticotroph adenomas in Cushing's disease. *J Steroid Biochem Mol Biol* 1992;43:379–84.

119 Saruta T, Suzuki H, Handa M *et al.* Multiple factors contribute to the pathogenesis of hypertension in Cushing's syndrome. *J Clin Endocrinol Metab* 1986;62:275–9.

120 Liddle GW, Givens JR, Nicholson WE *et al.* The ectopic ACTH syndrome. *Cancer Res* 1965;25:1057–61.

121 Yalow RS, Berson SA. Size heterogeneity of immunoreactive human ACTH in plasma and in extracts of pituitary glands and ACTH-producing thymoma. *Biochem Biophys Res Commun* 1971;44:439–45.

122 Stewart PM, Gibson S, Crosby SR *et al.* ACTH precursors characterise the ectopic ACTH syndrome. *Clin Endocrinol (Oxf)* 1994;40:199–204.

123 Crosby SR, Stewart MF, Ratcliffe JG *et al.* Direct measurement of the precursors of adrenocorticotropin in human plasma by two-site immunoradiometric assay. *J Clin Endocrinol Metab* 1988;67:1272–7.

124 Kuhn JM, Proeschel MF, Seurin D *et al.* Comparative assessment of ACTH and lipoprotein plasma levels in the diagnosis and follow-up of patients with Cushing's syndrome: a study of 210 cases. *Am J Med* 1989;86:678–84.

125 White A, Clark AJL. The cellular and molecular basis of the ectopic ACTH syndrome. *Clin Endocrinol* 1993;39: 131–41.

126 Schrell U, Fahlbusch R, Buchfelder M *et al.* Corticotropin-releasing hormone stimulation test before and after trans-sphenoidal selective microadenomectomy in 30 patients with Cushing's disease. *J Clin Endocrinol Metab* 1987; 64:11050–9.

127 Upton GV, Amatruda TT. Tumor peptides with CRF-like activity in the ectopic ACTH syndrome. *N Engl J Med* 1971;285:419–23.

128 Mulrow PJ, Cohn GL, Yesner R. Isolation of cortisol from pheochromocytoma. *Yale J Biol Med* 1959;31:363–5.

129 Florkowski CM, Wittert GA, Lewis JG *et al.* Glucocorticoid responsive ACTH secreting bronchial carcinoid tumours contain high concentrations of glucocorticoid receptors. *Clin Endocrinol (Oxf)* 1994;40:269–74.

130 Mosier HD, Flynn PJ, Will DW, Turner RD. Cushing's syndrome with multinodular adrenal glands. *J Clin Endocrinol Metab* 1960;20:632–40.

131 Oberfield SE, Levine LS, Carey RM *et al.* Adrenal glomerulosa function in patients with dexamethasone suppressible

hyperaldosteronism. *J Clin Endocrinol Metab* 1981;53: 158–64.
132 Ruder HJ, Loriaux DL, Lipsett MB. Severe osteopenia in young adults associated with Cushing's syndrome due to micronodular adrenal disease. *J Clin Endocrinol Metab* 1974;39:1138–47.
133 Schweizer-Cagianut M, Froshch ER, Hedinger C. Familial Cushing's syndrome with primary adrenocortical microadenomatosis (primary adrenocortical nodular dysplasia). *Acta Endocrinol (Copenh)* 1980;94:529–35.
134 Smals AGH, Pieters GFFM, Van Haelst UJG *et al.* Macronodular adrenocortical hyperplasia in long-standing Cushing's disease. *J Clin Endocrinol Metab* 1984;58:25–31.
135 Houven RHJ, Drop SLS, Hazebroek FW, Tenkate FWJ. Pituitary-dependent Cushing disease and primary adrenocortical nodular dysplasia in childhood. Presentation of 4 cases. *Eur J Pediatr* 1983;141:101–8.
136 Klevit HD, Robert MD, Campbell MD *et al.* Cushing's syndrome with nodular adrenal hyperplasia in infancy. *J Pediatr* 1966;68:912–20.
137 Lamberts SWJ, Stefanko SZ, Delange SA *et al.* Failure of clinical remission after transsphenoidal removal of microadenoma in a patient with Cushing's disease: multiple hyperplastic and adenomatous cell nests in surrounding pituitary tissue. *J Clin Endocrinol Metab* 1980;50:793–5.
138 Copinschi G, Nève P, Volter R *et al.* Dwarfism caused by Cushing's syndrome. *Acta Endocrinol (Copenh)* 1969; 60:446–50.
139 Grant DB, Arherden SM. Cushing's disease presenting with growth failure: clinical remission during cyproheptadine therapy. *Arch Dis Child* 1979;54:466–8.
140 Strickland AL, Underwood LE, Voina SJ *et al.* Growth retardation in Cushing's syndrome. *Am J Dis Child* 1972; 123:207–13.
141 Zadik Z, Cooper M, Chen M *et al.* Cushing's disease presenting as pubertal arrest. *J Pediatr Endocrinol* 1993;6:201–4.
142 Lee PA, Veldon VV, Migeon CJ. Short stature as the only clinical sign of Cushing's syndrome. *J Pediatr* 1975;86: 89–91.
143 Mosier HD, Smith FG, Schultz MA. Failure of catch-up growth after Cushing's syndrome in childhood. *Am J Dis Child* 1972;124:251–6.
144 Tyrrell JB, Wiener-Kronish J, Lorenzi M *et al.* Cushing's disease: growth hormone response to hypoglycemia after correction of hypercortisolism. *J Clin Endocrinol Metab* 1977;44:218–21.
145 Elders MJ, Winfield BS, McNatt ML. Glucocorticoid therapy in children: effect on somatomedin secretion. *Am J Dis Child* 1975;129:1393–6.
146 Adinoff AD, Hollister JR. Steroid induced fractures and bone loss in patients with asthma. *N Engl J Med* 1983;309:265–8.
147 Follis RH. The pathology of the osseous changes in Cushing's syndrome in an infant and in adults. *Bull Johns Hopkins Hosp* 1951;88:440–51.
148 Reid IR. Pathogenesis and treatment of osteoporosis. *Clin Endocrinol* 1989;30:83–103.
149 Prummel M, Wiersininga WM, Lips P *et al.* The course of biochemical parameters of bone turnover during treatment with corticosteroids. *J Clin Endocrinol Metab* 1991;72: 382–6.
150 Afifi AK, Bergman RA, Harvey JC. Steroid myopathy. *Bull Johns Hopkins Hosp* 1969;124:158–74.
151 Müller R, Kugelberg E. Myopathy in Cushing's syndrome. *J Neurol Neurosurg Psychiatr* 1959;22:314–19.
152 Lapasset M, De Geeter B, Juif JG *et al.* Myocardiopathie hypertrophique sévère associée à un corticosurrénalome. *Arch Fr Pédiatr* 1986;43:635–6.
153 Oberfield SE, Levine LS, Firpo A *et al.* Primary hypertension in childhood due to unilateral macronodular hyperplasia. Case report. *Hypertension* 1984;6:75–84.
154 Mantero F, Boscaro M. Glucocorticoid-dependent hypertension. *J Steroid Biochem Mol Biol* 1992;43:409–13.
155 Krakoff L, Nicolis G, Amsel B. Pathogenesis of hypertension in Cushing's syndrome. *Am J Med* 1975;36:216–20.
156 Ehlers ME, Griffing GT, Wilson TE, Melby JC. Elevated urinary 19-nor-deoxycorticosterone glucuronide in Cushing's syndrome. *J Clin Endocrinol Metab* 1987;64: 926–30.
157 Ulick S, Wang JZ, Blumfeld JD *et al.* Cortisol inactivation overload: a mechanism of mineralocorticoid hypertension in the ectopic adrenocorticotropin syndrome. *J Clin Endocrinol Metab* 1992;74:963–7.
158 Duick DS, Wahner MW. Thyroid axis in patients with Cushing's syndrome. *Arch Intern Med* 1979;139:767–72.
159 Peillon F, Metzger J, Garnier H *et al.* Syndrome de Cushing par tumeur surrénalienne primitive avec hypothyroïdie d'origine autoimmune. *Ann Méd Int* 1974;125:169–76.
160 Romano A, Blethen SL. Subacute thyroiditis presenting as Cushing's syndrome. *Horm Res* 1991;35:170–2.
161 Britton S, Thorén M, Sjøberg HE. The immunological hazard of Cushing's syndrome. *Br Med J* 1975;xii:678–80.
162 Constantinopoulos A, Karpouzas J, Xypolita A *et al.* Non-hormonal case of adrenal cortical carcinoma. *Arch Dis Child* 1978;53:827–30.
163 Visconti EB, Peters PW, Cangir A *et al.* Unusual case of adrenal cortical carcinoma. *Arch Dis Child* 1978;53:342–4.
164 Orth DN, Guillemin R, Ling N, Nicholson WE. Immunoreactive endorphins, lipotropins and corticotropins in human nonpituitary tumor: evidence for a common precursor. *J Clin Endocrinol Metab* 1978;46:849–52.
165 Savage DCL, Forsyth CC, Cameron J. Excretion of individual adrenocortical steroids in obese children. *Arch Dis Child* 1974;49:946–50.
166 Kaye TB, Crapo L. The Cushing's syndrome: an update on diagnostic tests. *Ann Intern Med* 1990;112:434–44.
167 Rivarola MA, Mendilaharzu H, Dahi V *et al.* Pitfalls of functional tests for the establishment of the etiology of Cushing's syndrome in childhood and adolescence. *J Clin Endocrinol Metab* 1970;31:254–9.
168 Forest MG. Adrenal function tests. In: Ranke MB, ed. *Functional Endocrinological Diagnostics in Children and Adolescents.* Mannheim: J & J Verlag 1992:248–74.
169 Chrousos GP, Vingerhoeds ACM, Loriaux DL, Lipsett MB. Primary cortisol resistance: a family study. *J Clin Endocrinol Metab* 1983;56:1243–5.
170 Vingerhoeds ACM, Thijssen JHH, Schwarz F. Spontaneous hypercortisolism without Cushing's syndrome. *J Clin Endocrinol Metab* 1976;43:1128–33.
171 Malchoff CD, Javier EC, Malchoff DM *et al.* Primary cortisol resistance presenting as isosexual precority. *J Clin Endocrinol Metab* 1990;70:503–7.
172 Rubin LM, Loriaux DL, Slaunwhite WR Jr. Polymorphism of human transcortin and a variant associated with Cushing's syndrome. In: *Proceedings of the International Congress of Endocrinology*, Hamburg 1976:372.
173 Van Cauter E, Refetoff S. Evidence for two subtypes of Cushing's disease based on the analysis of episodic cortisol

secretion. *N Engl J Med* 1985;312:1343–9.

174 Atkinson AB, Kennedy AL, Carson SJ *et al.* Five cases of cyclical Cushing's syndrome. *Br Med J* 1985;291:1453–7.

175 Boscaro M, Sonino N, Mantero F. Diagnosis and treatment of Cushing's syndrome. *J Endocrinol Invest* 1992;15:223–44.

176 Vidal-Trecan G, Laudat MH, Thomopoulos P *et al.* Urinary free corticoids: an evaluation of their usefulness in the diagnosis of Cushing's syndrome. *Acta Endocrinol (Copenh)* 1983;103:110–15.

177 Evans PJ, Peters JR, Dyas J *et al.* Salivary cortisol levels in true and apparent hypercortisolism. *Clin Endocrinol* 1984:20:709–15.

178 Cronin C, Igoe D, Duffy MJ *et al.* The overnight dexamethasone test is a worthwhile screening procedure. *Clin Endocrinol* 1990;33:27–33.

179 Montwill J, Igoe D, McKenna TJ. The overnight dexamethasone test is the procedure of choice in screening for Cushing's syndrome. *Steroids* 1994;59:296–8.

180 Hindmarsh PC, Brook CGD. Single dose dexamethasone suppression test in children: dose relationship to body size. *Clin Endocrinol* 1985;23:67–70.

181 Abou Samra AB, Dechaud H, Estour B *et al.* B-lipotropin and cortisol responses to an intravenous infusion dexamethasone suppression test in Cushing's syndrome and obesity. *J Clin Endocrinol Metab* 1985;61:116–19.

182 Biemond P, de Jong FH, Lamberts F. Continuous dexamethasone infusion for seven hours in patients with the Cushing syndrome. *Ann Intern Med* 1990;112:738–41.

183 Hayles AB, Hahn HB Jr, Sprague RG *et al.* Hormone-secreting tumors of the adrenal cortex in children. *Pediatrics* 1966; 37:19–25.

184 Ratcliffe JG, Knight RA, Besser GM *et al.* Tumor and plasma ACTH concentrations in patients with and without the ectopic ACTH syndrome. *Clin Endocrinol* 1972;1:27–44.

185 Cahen LA, Villee DB, Powers ML *et al.* A virilizing adrenocortical tumour in a female infant: in vivo and in vitro biochemical characteristics. *J Clin Endocrinol Metab* 1978; 47:300–6.

186 Bartter FC, Pronove J, Gill JR *et al.* Hyperplasia of the juxtaglomerular complex with hyperaldosteronism and hypokalaemic alkalosis: a new syndrome. *Am J Med* 1962; 33:811–28.

187 Krieger DT, Liotta AS, Brownstein MJ, Zimmerman EA. ACTH, β-lipoprotein, and related peptides in brain, pituitary and blood. *Rec Prog Horm Res* 1980;36:27–336.

188 Corrigan DF, Schaaf H, Whaley RA *et al.* Selective venous sampling to differentiate ectopic ACTH secretion from pituitary Cushing's syndrome. *N Engl J Med* 1977;296:861–2.

189 Findling JW, Aron DC, Tyrell JB *et al.* Selective venous sampling for ACTH in Cushing's syndrome. Differentiation between Cushing's disease and the ectopic ACTH syndrome. *Ann Intern Med* 1981;94:647–52.

190 Doppman JL, Pass HI, Nieman L *et al.* Failure of bronchial lavage to detect elevated levels of adrenocorticotrophin (ACTH) in patients with ACTH-producing bronchial carcinoids. *J Clin Endocrinol Metab* 1989;69:1302–4.

191 Loras B, Migeon CJ. Metabolism of 7-H^3-dehydroisoandrosterone in patients with virilizing adrenal tumors. *Steroids* 1966;7:459–76.

192 Burrington JD, Stephen CA. Virilizing tumors of the adrenal gland in childhood: report of eight cases. *J Pediatr Surg* 1969;4:291–302.

193 Bhettay E, Bonnici F. Pure estrogen-secreting feminizing adrenocortical adenoma. *Arch Dis Child* 1977;52:241–3.

194 Costin G, Goebelsmann U, Kogut MD. Sexual precocity due to a testosterone-producing adrenal tumor. *J Clin Endocrinol Metab* 1977;45:912–19.

195 Korth-Schutz, S, Levine JA, Saenger P *et al.* Virilizing adrenal tumor in a child suppressed with dexamethasone for three years. Effect of o,p'DDD on serum and urinary androgens. *J Clin Endocrinol Metab* 1977;44:433–9.

196 Yamaji T, Ishibashi M, Sekihara H *et al.* Serum dehydroepiandrosterone sulfate in Cushing's syndrome. *J Clin Endocrinol Metab* 1984;59:1164–8.

197 Gregory T, Gardner LI, Gower DB *et al.* Studies of 16-androstenes in an infant with virilizing adrenal carcinoma. *Am J Dis Child* 1979;133:294–7.

198 Saez JM, Rivarola MA, Migeon CJ. Studies of androgens in patients with adrenocortical tumors. *J Clin Endocrinol Metab* 1967;27:615–23.

199 Weidenfeld J, Shaefer JA, Landau H *et al.* 11β-Hydroxydehydroepiandrosterone in a case of virilizing adrenal adenoma: isolation from urine and mitochondrial conversion from dehydroepiandrosterone. *J Clin Endocrinol Metab* 1978; 47:102–4.

200 Crystal RG, Rose LI, Jagger PI *et al.* Cushing's syndrome caused by a metyrapone responsive adrenocortical adenoma. *J Clin Endocrinol* 1970;31:199–203.

201 Saez JM, Tell GP, Dazord A. Human adrenocortical tumors: alterations in membrane-bound hormone receptors and cAMP protein kinases. In: Sharma RK, Criss WE, eds. *Endocrine Control in Neoplasia.* New York: Raven Press, 1978:53–69.

202 Caro JF, Meikle AW, Check JH, Cohen SN. 'Normal suppression' to dexamethasone in Cushing's disease: an expression of decreased metabolic clearance for dexamethasone. *J Clin Endocrinol* 1978;47:667–71.

203 Bruno OD, Rossi MA, Contreras LN *et al.* Nocturnal high-dose dexamethasone suppression test in the aetiological diagnosis of Cushing's syndrome. *Acta Endocrinol (Copenh)* 1985;109:158–62.

204 Cugini P, Battisti P, Di Palam L *et al.* 'Giant' macronodular adrenal hyperplasia causing Cushing's syndrome: case report and review of the literature on a clinical distinction of adrenocortical nodular pathology associated with hypercortisolism. *Endocrinol Jpn* 1989;36:101–16.

205 Dichek HL, Nieman LK, Oldfield EH *et al.* A comparison of the standard high dose dexamethasone suppression test and the overnight 8-mg dexamethasone suppression test for the differential diagnosis of adrenocorticotropin-dependent Cushing's syndrome. *J Clin Endocrinol Metab* 1994;78: 418–22.

206 Rochiccioli P, Ribot C, Ghisofi J *et al.* Le test à la lysine–vasopressine. Résultats chez 50 enfants normaux. *Pédiatrie* 1971;26:5–13.

207 Mueller OA, Baur X, Fahlbusch R *et al.* Diagnosis and treatment of ACTH-producing tumors. In: Fahlbuch R, Werder V, eds. *Treatment of Pituitary Adenomas.* Stuttgart: Thieme, 1978:343–51.

208 Orth DN, de Bold CR, de Chesney GS *et al.* Pituitary microadenomas causing Cushing's disease respond to corticotropin-releasing factor. *J Clin Endocrinol Metab* 1982;55: 1017–19.

209 Suda T, Tomori N, Tozawa F *et al.* Effect of corticotropin-releasing factor and other materials on adrenocorticotropin secretion from pituitary glands of patients with Cushing's disease *in vitro. J Clin Endocrinol Metab* 1984;55:840–5.

210 Hermus ARMM, Pieters GFFM, Pesman GJ *et al.* Respon-

sivity of adrenocorticotropin to corticotropin-releasing hormone and lack of suppressibility by dexamethasone are related phenomena in Cushing's disease. *J Clin Endocrinol Metab* 1986;62:634–9.

211 Nieman LK, Cutler GB, Oldfield RH *et al.* The ovine corticotrophin-releasing hormone (CRH) stimulation test is superior to the human CRH stimulation test for the diagnosis of Cushing's disease. *J Clin Endocrinol Metab* 1989;69: 165–9.

212 Tabarin A, San Galli F, Leprat F *et al.* The corticotropin releasing factor test in the differential diagnosis of Cushing's syndrome: a comparison with the lysine – vasopressin test. *Acta Endocrinol* 1990;123:331–8.

213 Trainer PT, Grossman A. The diagnosis and differential diagnosis of Cushing syndrome. *Clin Endocrinol* 1991; 34:317–20.

214 Favrod-Coune C, Raux-Demay MC, Proeschel MF *et al.* Potentiation of the classical ovine corticotrophin releasing hormone stimulation test by the combined administration of small doses of lysine vasopressin. *Clin Endocrinol* 1993; 38:405–10.

215 Allolio B, Deuss U, Kaulen *et al.* FK 33-824, a Met-enkephalin analog, blocks corticotropin-releasing hormone-induced adrenocorticotropin secretion in normal subjects but not in patients with Cushing's disease. *J Clin Endocrinol Metab* 1986;63:1427–31.

216 Grossman H. The evaluation of abdominal masses in children with emphasis on non-invasive methods. A roentgenographic approach. *Cancer* 1975;35:884–900.

217 Sutton D. The radiological diagnosis of adrenal tumours. *Br J Radiol* 1975;48:237–58.

218 Bonnin A, Butez J, Tonnelier M. Radiologie des surrénales. *Rev Pract* 1973;23:907–21.

219 Vermees M, Schour L, Jaffe ES. Calcification in a benign nonfunctioning adrenal carcinoma. Report of a case with selective adrenal arteriogram. *Br J Radiol* 1972;45:621–4.

220 Beierwaltes WH, Lieberman LM, Ansart AN *et al.* Visualization of human adrenal glands *in vivo* by scintillation scanning. *J Am Med Assoc* 1971;216:275–7.

221 Gross MD, Shapiro B, Thrall JH *et al.* The scintigraphic imaging of endocrine organs. *Endocr Rev* 1984;5:221–81.

222 Troncone L. Radiocholesterol scintigraphy in adrenal gland tumours. *Eur J Nucl Med* 1980;5:345–56.

223 Forman BH, Antar MA, Touloukian RJ *et al.* Localization of a metastatic adrenal carcinoma by ^{131}I-19-iodocholesterol. *J Nucl Med* 1974;15:332–4.

224 Ortega D, Foz M, Domenech-Torne FM, Tresanchez JM. The diagnosis of Cushing's syndrome using ^{113}I-19-iodocholesterol uptake and adrenal imaging. *Clin Endocrinol* 1980; 13:145–9.

225 Gordon RD, Hamlet SM, Tunny TJ *et al.* Distinguishing aldosterone-producing adenoma from other forms of hyperaldosteronism and lateralizing the tumour preoperatively. *Clin Exp Pharmacol Physiol* 1986;13:325–8.

226 Schteingart DE, Seabold JE, Gross MD, Swanson D. Iodocholesterol adrenal tissue uptake and imaging in adrenal neoplasms. *J Clin Endocrinol Metab* 1981;52:1156–60.

227 Shenker Y, Gross MD, Grekin RJ *et al.* The scintigraphic localization of mineralocorticoid-producing adrenocortical carcinoma. *J Endocrinol Invest* 1986;9:115–20.

228 Barbarino A, Troncone L, Salvo D *et al.* Thyroidal accumulation of ^{131}I during adrenal gland scintigraphy with ^{131}I-19-iodocholesterol: effects of thyroid blocking agents. *J Clin Endocrinol Metab* 1975;41:405–7.

229 Sandler MP, Patton JA, Gross MD *et al.* *Endocrine Imaging.* New York: Appleton & Lange, 1992.

230 Yen HC. Sonography of the adrenal glands: normal glands and small masses. *Am J Roentgenol* 1980;135:1167–77.

231 Itami RM, Amundson GM, Kaplan SA, Lippe BM. Prepubertal gynecomastia caused by an adrenal tumor. Diagnostic value of ultrasonography. *Am J Dis Child* 1982;136:584–6.

232 Dunnick NR, Schaner EG, Doppman JL *et al.* Computed tomography in adrenal tumors. *Am J Roentgenol* 1979;132: 43–6.

233 White FE, White MC, Drury PL *et al.* Value of computed tomography of the abdomen and chest in investigation of Cushing's syndrome. *Br Med J* 1982;284:771–4.

234 Dunnick NR, Doppman JL, Gill JR *et al.* Localization of functional adrenal tumors by computed tomography and venous sampling. *Radiology* 1982;142:429–33.

235 Gussain S, Belldegrun A, Seltzer S *et al.* Differentiation of malignant from benign adrenal masses: predictive indices on computed tomography. *Am J Roentgenol* 1985;144:61–5.

236 Krenning EP, Kwekkeboom DJ, Bakker WH *et al.* Somatostatin receptor scintigraphy with [^{111}In-DTPA-d-Phe^{1}] and [^{123}I-Tyr^{3}]-octeotride: the Rotterdam experience with more than 1000 patients. *Eur J Nucl Med* 1993;20:716–31.

237 Philiponneau M, Nocaudie M, Epelbaum J *et al.* Somatostatin analogs for the localization and preoperative treatment of an adrenocorticotropin-secreting bronchial carcinoid tumor. *J Clin Endocrinol Metab* 1994;78:20–4.

238 Gabrilove JL, Seman AT, Sabet R *et al.* Virilizing adrenal adenoma with studies on the steroid content of the adrenal venous effluent and a review of the literature. *Endocr Rev* 1981;2:462–70.

239 Kafrouni G, Oakes MD, Lurvey AN, De Quatro V. Aldosteronoma in a child with localization by adrenal vein aldosterone: collective review of the literature. *J Pediatr Surg* 1975; 10:917–24.

240 Hemminghytt S, Kalkoff RK, Daniels DL *et al.* Computed tomographic study of hormone-secreting micro-adenomas. *Radiology* 1983;146:65–9.

241 Taylor S. High resolution computed tomography of the sella. *Radiol Clin N Am* 1982;20:207–36.

242 Bonneville JF, Cattin F, Dietemann JL. *Computed Tomography of the Pituitary Gland.* Berlin: Springer Verlag, 1986.

243 Bilaniuk LT, Zimmermann RA, Werhrli FW *et al.* Magnetic resonance imaging of pituitary lesions using 1.0 to 1.5 T field strength. *Radiology* 1984;150:95–8.

244 de Herder WW, Uitterlinden P, Pieterman H *et al.* Pituitary tumour localization in patients with Cushing's disease by magnetic resonance imaging. Is there a place for petrosal sinus sampling? *Clin Endocrinol* 1994;40:87–92.

245 Doppman JL, Frank JA, Dwyer AJ *et al.* Gadolinium DPTA enhanced MR imaging of ACTH-secreting microadenomas of the pituitary gland. *J Comput Assist Tomogr* 1988;12: 728–35.

246 Webb SM, Ruscalleda J, Schwarzstein D *et al.* Computerized tomography versus magnetic resonance imaging: a comparative study in hypothalamic–pituitary and parasellar pathology. *Clin Endocrinol* 1992;36:459–65.

247 Bigos ST, Somma M, Rasio E *et al.* Cushing's disease: management by transphenoidal pituitary microsurgery. *J Clin Endocrinol Metab* 1980;50:348–54.

248 Crook PA, Pestell RG, Calenti AJ *et al.* Multiple pituitary hormone gradients from inferior petrosal sinus sampling in Cushing's disease. *Acta Endocrinol (Copenh)* 1988;119:75–80.

249 Oldfield EH, Chrousos GP, Shuulte HM *et al.* Pre-operative lateralization of ACTH-secreting pituitary microadenomas by bilateral and simultaneous inferior petrosal venous sinus sampling. *N Engl J Med* 1985;312:100–3.
250 Tabarin A, Corcuff JB, Rashedi M *et al.* Multihormonal response to corticotropin-releasing hormone in inferior petrosal sinus blood of one patient with Cushing's disease: comparison with in vitro secretion of the tumoral corticotrophes. *Acta Endocrinol (Copenh)* 1992;127:284–8.
251 Drury PL, Ratter S, Tomlin S *et al.* Experience with selective venous sampling in diagnosis of ACTH-dependent Cushing's syndrome. *Br Med J* 1982;284:9–12.
252 Landolt AM, Schubiger O, Maurer R *et al.* The value of inferior petrosal sinus sampling in diagnosis and treatment of Cushing's disease. *Clin Endocrinol (Oxf)* 1994;40:485–92.
253 Tabarin A, Greselle JF, San-Galli F *et al.* Usefulness of the corticotropin-releasing hormone test during bilateral inferior petrosal sinus sampling for the diagnosis of Cushing's disease. *J Clin Endocrinol Metab* 1991;73:53–60.
254 McNally PG, Bolia A, Absalom SR *et al.* Preliminary observations using endocrine markers of pituitary venous dilution during bilateral simultaneous inferior petrosal sinus catheterization in Cushing's syndrome: is combined CRF and TRH stimulation of value? *Clin Endocrinol* 1993;39:681–6.
255 Extabe J, Vazquez JA. Morbidity and mortality in Cushing's disease: an epidemiological approach. *Clin Endocrinol (Oxf)* 1994;40:479–84.
256 Blau N, Miller WE, Miller ER *et al.* Spontaneous remission of Cushing's syndrome in a patient with an adrenal adenoma. *J Clin Endocrinol Metab* 1975;40:659–63.
257 Ovlisen B, Andersen HJ. Spontaneous remission in a case of Cushing's syndrome presumably due to adrenal tumor. *J Clin Endocrinol Metab* 1966;26:294–300.
258 Pasqualini RW, Gurevich N. Spontaneous remission in a case of Cushing's syndrome. *J Clin Endocrinol Metab* 1956; 16:406–11.
259 Scott RS, Espiner EA, Donald RA. Intermittent Cushing's disease with spontaneous remission. *Clin Endocrinol* 1979; 11:561–6.
260 Atkinson AB. The treatment of Cushing's syndrome. *Clin Endocrinol* 1991;34:507–13.
261 Sjöberg HE, Blomback M, Granberg PO. Thromboembolic complications, heparin treatment and increase in coagulation factors in Cushing's syndrome. *Acta Med Scand* 1976; 199:95–8.
262 Arcadi JA, Cushing's syndrome in a 10-year-old girl associated with a benign adrenal adenoma. *J Urol* 1971;106: 766–9.
263 Gordon D, Semple CG, Beastall GH *et al.* A study of hypothalamic–pituitary–adrenal suppression following curative surgery for Cushing's syndrome due to adrenal adenoma. *Acta Endocrinol (Copenh)* 1987;114:166–70.
264 Freeman DA. Steroid hormone-producing tumors in man. *Endocr Rev* 1986;7:204–20.
265 Stewart DR, Morris-Jones PM, Jolleys A. Carcinoma of the adrenal gland in children. *J Pediatr Surg* 1974;9:59–67.
266 Halmi KA, Lasciari AD. Conversion of virilization to feminization in a young girl with adrenal cortical carcinoma. *Cancer* 1971;27:931–5.
267 Gicquel C, Leblond-Francillard M, Bertagna X *et al.* Clonal analysis of human adrenocortical carcinomas and secreting-adenomas. *Clin Endocrinol* 1994;40:465–79.
268 Gicquel C, Bertagna X, Schneid H *et al.* Rearrangements at the 11p15 locus and overexpression of IGFII gene in sporadic adrenocortical tumors. *J Clin Endocrinol Metab* 1994;78: 1444–53.
269 Ilvesmäki V, Kahri AI, Miettinen PJ *et al.* Insulin-like growth factors and their receptors in adrenal tumors: high IGF-II expression in functional adrenocortical carcinomas. *J Clin Endocrinol Metab* 1993;77:852–8.
270 Lin S-R, Lee Y-J, Tsai J-H. Mutations of the p53 gene in human functional adrenal neoplasms. *J Clin Endocrinol Metab* 1994;78:483–91.
271 Sullivan M, Boileau M, Hodges CV. Adrenal cortical carcinoma. *J Urol* 1978;120:660–5.
272 Helson L, Wollner N, Murphy ML, Schwartz MK. Metastatic adrenal corticol carcinoma: biochemical changes accompanying clinical regression during therapy with *o,p'*-DDD. *Clin Chem* 1973;17:1191–3.
273 Tattersall MH, Lander H, Bain B *et al.* Cis-platinum treatment of metastatic adrenal carcinoma. *Med J Aust* 1980;1: 419–21.
274 Lamberts SWJ, Bons E, Bruining HA. Different sensitivity to adrenocorticotropin of dispersed adrenocortical cells from patients with Cushing's disease with macronodular and diffuse adrenal hyperplasia. *J Clin Endocrinol Metab* 1984;58: 1106–10.
275 Aron DC, Findling JW, Fitzgerald PA *et al.* Cushing's syndrome: problems in management. *Endocr Rev* 1982;3: 229–44.
276 Yamaji T, Ishibashi M, Teramoto A *et al.* Hyperprolactinemia in Cushing's disease and Nelson's syndrome. *J Clin Endocrinol Metab* 1984;58:790–5.
277 McArthur RG, Hayles AB, Salassa RM. Childhood Cushing disease: results of bilateral adrenalectomy. *J Pediatr* 1979; 95:214–19.
278 Moore TJH, Dluhy RG, Williams GH *et al.* Nelson's syndrome: frequency, prognosis and effect of prior pituitary irradiation. *Ann Intern Med* 1976;85:731–4.
279 Lifton RP, Dluhy RG. The molecular basis of a hereditary form of hypertension, glucocorticoid-remediable aldosteronism. *Trends Endocrinol Metab* 1993;4:57–61.
280 Post KD. Transsphenoidal surgery for pituitary tumors. In: Post KD, Jackson I, Reichlin S, eds. *The Pituitary Adenoma.* New York: Plenum Press, 1980:379–400.
281 Wilson CB, Demsey LC. Transphenoidal microsurgical removal of 250 pituitary adenomas. *J Neurosurg* 1978;48: 13–22.
282 Nelson DH. Therapy for acromegaly, Cushing's disease and Nelson's syndrome. *West J Med* 1980;133:244–5.
283 Mauras N, Blizzard RM. The McCune–Albright syndrome. *Acta Endocrinol (Copenh)* (Suppl.) 1986;279:207–17.
284 Khalid BAK, Burke CW, Hurley DM *et al.* Steroid replacement in Addison's disease and in subjects adrenalectomized for Cushing's disease: comparison of various glucocorticoids. *J Clin Endocrinol Metab* 1982;55:551–9.
285 Aristizabal S, Caldwell WC, Avila J. The relationship of time–dose fractionation factors to complications in the treatment of pituitary tumours by irradiation. *Int J Radiat Oncol Biol Phys* 1977;2:667–74.
286 Cook DM, Meikle AW. Factitious Cushing's syndrome. *J Clin Endocrinol Metab* 1985;61:385–7.
287 Young LW, Lim GHK, Forbes GB *et al.* Post-adrenalectomy pituitary adenoma (Nelson's syndrome) in childhood: clinical and roentgenologic detection. *Am J Roentgenol* 1976;126: 550–6.
288 Guilhaume B, Bertagna X, Thomsen M *et al.* Transphenoidal pituitary surgery for the treatment of Cushing's disease:

results in 64 patients and long-term follow-up studies. *J Clin Endocrinol Metab* 1988;66:1056–64.
289 Wara WM, Richards GE, Grumbach MM *et al.* Hypopituitarism after irradiation in children. *Int Radiat Oncol Biol Phys* 1977;2:549–53.
290 Lawrence JH, Tobias CA, Linfoot JA *et al.* Heavy particle therapy in acromegaly and Cushing's disease. *J Am Med Assoc* 1976;235:2307–10.
291 Linfoot JA. Alpha particle pituitary irradiation in the primary and postsurgical management of pituitary microadenomas. In: Faglia G, Giovanilli MA, MacLeod RM, eds. *Pituitary Microadenomas.* New York: Academic Press, 1980:515–29.
292 Casar J, Doyle FH, Lewis PD *et al.* Treatment of Nelson's syndrome by pituitary implantation of yttrium-90 or gold-198. *Br Med J* 1976;ii:269–72.
293 Thoren M, Rahn T, Hallegtren B *et al.* Treatment of Cushing's disease in childhood and adolescence by stereotaxic pituitary irradiation. *Acta Paed Scand* 1986;75: 388–95.
294 Boggoan JE, Tyrrell JB, Wilson CB. Transphenoidal microsurgical management of Cushing's disease. *J Neurosurg* 1983;59:195–200.
295 Buchfelder M, Fahlbusch R, Wentzlaff-Eggebert H *et al.* Does an analysis of the pulsatile secretion pattern of adrenocorticotropin and cortisol predict the result of transphenoidal surgery in Cushing's disease? *J Clin Endocrinol Metab* 1993; 77:720–4.
296 Gomez MT, Magiakou MA, Mastorakos G *et al.* The pituitary corticotroph is not the rate-limiting step in the postoperative recovery of the hypothalamic–pituitary–adrenal axis in patients with Cushing syndrome. *J Clin Endocrinol Metab* 1993;77:173–7.
297 Couch RM, Smail PJ, Dean HJ, Winter JSD. Prolonged remission of Cushing disease after treatment with cyproheptadine. *J Pediatr* 1984;104:906–8.
298 D'Ercole AJ, Morris MA, Underwood LE *et al.* Treatment of Cushing's disease in childhood with cyproheptadine. *J Pediatr* 1977;90:834–6.
299 Ambrosi B, Bochicchio D, Ferrario R *et al.* Effects of the opiate agonist loperamide on pituitary–adrenal function in patients with suspected hypercortisolism. *J Endocrinol Invest* 1989;12:31–5.
300 Benker G, Hackenberg K, Hamburger B *et al.* Effects of growth hormone release-inhibiting hormone and bromocryptine (CB154) in states of abnormal pituitary–adrenal function. *Clin Endocrinol* 1976;5:187–90.
301 Kennedy AL, Sheridan B, Montgomery DAD. ACTH and cortisol response to bromocriptine and results of long-term therapy in Cushing's disease. *Acta Endocrinol (Copenh)* 1978;89:461–9.
302 Miura K, Aida M, Mihara A *et al.* Treatment of Cushing's disease with reserpine and pituitary irradiation. *J Clin Endocrinol Metab* 1975;41:511–26.
303 Hale AC, Coates PJ, Doniach I *et al.* A bromocriptine-responsive adenoma secreting alpha-MSH in a patient with Cushing's disease. *Clin Endocrinol* 1988;28:215–23.
304 Givens JR, Camacho A, Patterson P. Effect of aminoglutethimide and reserpine on the human pituitary–adrenal axis: remission of a case of Cushing's disease. *Metabolism* 1970;19:818–30.
305 Gower DB. Modifiers of steroid-hormone metabolism: a review of their chemistry, biochemistry and clinical applications. *J Steroid Biochem* 1974;5:501–23.
306 Zachmann M, Gitzelmann RP, Zagalak M *et al.* Effect of aminoglutethimide on urinary cortisol and cortisol metabolites in adolescents with Cushing's syndrome. *Clin Endocrinol* 1977;7:63–71.
307 Totani Y, Niinomi M, Takatsuki K *et al.* Effect of metyrapone pretreatment on adrenocorticotropin secretion induced by corticotropin-releasing hormone in normal subjects and patients with Cushing's disease. *J Clin Endocrinol Metab* 1990;70:798–803.
308 Child DF, Burke CW, Burley DM *et al.* Drug control of Cushing's syndrome. Combined aminoglutethimide and metyrapone therapy. *Acta Endocrinol (Copenh)* 1976;82: 330–41.
309 Komanicky P, Spark RF, Melby JC. Treatment of Cushing's syndrome with trilostane (WIN 24,540), an inhibitor of adrenal steroid biosynthesis. *J Clin Endocrinol Metab* 1978; 47:1042–51.
310 Temple TE, Jones DJ, Liddle GW *et al.* Treatment of Cushing's disease. Correction of hypercortisolism by o,p'DDD without induction of aldosterone deficiency. *N Engl J Med* 1969;281:801–5.
311 Rappaport R, Schweisguth O, Cachin O *et al.* Corticosurrénalome malin avec métastases. Exérèse et traitement par o,p'DDD suivi de guérison. *Arch Fr Pédiatr* 1978; 35:551–9.
312 Boven E, Vermorken JB, van Slooten H, Pinedo HM. Complete response of metastasized adrenal cortical carcinoma with o'p'-DDD. *Cancer* 1984;53:26–9.
313 Greig F, Oberfield SE, Levine LS *et al.* Recovery of adrenal function after treatment of adrenocortical carcinoma with o,p'-DD. *Clin Endocrinol* 1984;20:389–99.
314 Hutter AM, Kayhoe DE. Adrenal cortical carcinoma. Results of treatment with o,p'-DDD in 138 patients. *Am J Med* 1966;41:581–92.
315 Schteingart DE, Tsao HS, Taylor CI *et al.* Sustained remission of Cushing's disease with mitotane and pituitary irradiation. *Ann Intern Med* 1980;92:613–19.
316 Sonino N, Boscaro M, Merola G, Mantero F. Prolonged treatment of Cushing's disease by ketoconazole. *J Clin Endocrinol Metab* 1985;61:718–22.
317 Loli P, Berselli E, Tagliaferri M. Use of ketoconazole in the treatment of Cushing's syndrome. *J Clin Endocrinol Metab* 1986;63:1365–71.
318 Tabarin A, Navarranne A, Guérin J *et al.* Use of ketokenazole in the treatment of Cushing's disease and ectopic ACTH syndrome. *Clin Endocrinol* 1991;34:63–9.
319 Nieman LK, Chrousos GP, Kellner C *et al.* Successful treatment of Cushing's syndrome with the glucocorticoid antagonist RU 486. *J Clin Endocrinol Metab* 1985;61:536–40.
320 Bertagna X, Bertagna C, Laudat MH *et al.* Pituitary–adrenal responses to the antiglucocorticoid action of RU 486 in Cushing's syndrome. *J Clin Endocrinol Metab* 1986;63:639–43.
321 Young JL, Miller RW. Incidence of malignant tumors in US children. *J Pediatr* 1975;86:254–8.
322 Didolkar MS, Bescher RA, Elias EG, Moore RH. Natural history of adrenal cortical carcinoma: a clinicopathologic study of 42 patients. *Cancer* 1981;47:2153–61.
323 Gyepes MT, Lindstrom R, Merten D *et al.* Hormonally active adrenal adenomas and carcinomas in children. *Ann Radiol* 1976;20:123–8.
324 Hajjar RA, Hickey RC, Samaan NA. Adrenal cortical carcinoma: a study in 32 patients. *Cancer* 1975;35:549–54.
325 Bhatia V, Shukla R, Mshra SK *et al.* Adrenal tumor com-

plicating untreated 21-hydroxylase deficiency in a 5½-year-old boy. *Am J Dis Child* 1993;147:1321–3.

326 Shimshi M, Ross F, Goodman A *et al.* Virilizing adrenocortical tumor superimposed on congenital adrenocortical hyperplasia. *Am J Med* 1992;93:338–42.

327 Honour JW, Price DA, Taylor NF *et al.* Steroid biochemistry of virilizing adrenal tumours in childhood. *Eur J Paediatr* 1984;142:165–9.

328 Lipsett MB. Benign masculinizing adrenal adnomas. *N Engl J Med* 1973;289:802–3.

329 Wilkins L, Ravitch MM. Adrenocortical tumor arising in the liver of a three year old boy with signs of virilism and Cushing's syndrome. *Pediatrics* 1952;9:671–81.

330 Craig JM, Landing BH. Anaplastic cells of fetal adrenal cortex. *Am J Clin Pathol* 1951;21:940–9.

331 Pang S, Becker D, Cotelingham J *et al.* Adrenocortical tumor in a patient with congenital adrenal hyperplasia due to 21-hydroxylase deficiency. *Pediatrics* 1981;68:242–6.

332 Sanfilipo JS, Wittliff JL. Steroid hormone receptors in adrenal cortical carcinoma. *Am J Obstet Gynecol* 1984;150:326–7.

333 Burr IM, Sullivan J, Graham T *et al.* A testosterone-secreting tumor of the adrenal producing virilization in a female infant. *Lancet* 1973;ii:643–4.

334 Sorgo W, Meyer D, Rodens K *et al.* Testosterone-secreting adrenocortical tumor in a pubertal girl. *Horm Res* 1988;30: 217–23.

335 Bierich JR. Nebennierenrinden-tumoren mit Wirkung auf die Sexualspliäre. *Minerva Pediatr* 1965;17:725–30.

336 Nottelet E, Guillot F, Loiseau C *et al.* Les corticosurrénalomes féminisants de l'enfant. Etude d'une observation et revue de la littérature. *Ann Pédiatr* 1976;23:813–24.

337 Wohltmann H, Mathur RS, Williamson H. Sexual precocity in a female infant due to feminizing adrenal carcinoma. *J Clin Endocrinol Metab* 1980;50:186–9.

338 Guin HG, Gilbert EF. Cushing's syndrome in children associated with adrenal cortical carcinoma. A case report with review of the literature. *Am J Dis Child* 1936;92:297–304.

339 Baulieu EE, Peillon F, Migeon CJ. Adrenogenital syndrome. In: Eisenstein Ab, ed. *The Adrenal Cortex.* Boston: Little Brown, 1967:554–7.

340 Aupetit-Faisant B, Battaglia C, Zenatti M *et al.* Hypoaldosteronism accompanied by normal or elevated mineralocorticosteroid pathway steroid: a marker of adrenal carcinoma. *J Clin Endocrinol Metab* 1993;76:38–43.

341 Howard CP, Takahashi H, Hayles AB. Feminizing adrenal adenoma in a boy. Case report and literature review. *Proc Mayo Clin* 1977;52:354–7.

342 Huhtaniemi I, Kahri AI, Pelkonen R *et al.* Ultrastructural and steroidogenic characteristics of an androgen producing adreno-cortical tumor. *Clin Endocrinol* 1978;8:305–14.

343 Sakai Y, Yanase T, Hara T *et al.* Mechanisms of abnormal production of adrenal androgens in patients with adrenocortical adenomas and carcinomas. *J Clin Endocrinol Metab* 1994;78:36–40.

344 Shibata H, Suzuki H, Ogishima T *et al.* Significance of steroidogenic enzymes in the pathogenesis of adrenal tumour. *Acta Endocrinol (Copenh)* 1993;128:235–42.

345 Moolenaar AJ, Van Seters AP. o.p'DDD values in plasma and tissues during and after chemotherapy of adrenocortical carcinoma. *Acta Endocrinol (Copenh)* 1975;80(Suppl. 199): 226.

346 Gabrilove JE, Sharma DC, Wotiz HH *et al.* Feminizing adrenocortical tumors in the male. A review of 52 cases including a case report. *Medicine* 1965;44:33–56.

347 Millington DS, Golder MP, Conley T *et al. In vitro* biosynthesis of steroids by a feminizing adrenocortical carcinoma: effect of prolactin and other protein hormones. *Acta Endocrinol (Copenh)* 1976;82:561–71.

348 Ducharme JR, Forest MG, de Peretti E *et al.* Plasma adrenal and gonadal sex steroids in human pubertal development. *J Clin Endocrinol Metab* 1976;42:468–76.

349 Silverman SH, Migeon CJ, Rosenberg E *et al.* Precocious growth of sexual hair without other secondary sexual development: 'premature pubarche', a constitutional variation of adolescence. *Pediatrics* 1952;10:426–32.

350 Forest MG, de Péretti E, David M, Sempé M. L'adrénarche joue-t-elle vraiment un rôle déterminant dans le développement pubertaire. Etude des dissociations entre adrénarche et gonadarche. Echec du traitement par la déhydroépiandrostérine sulphate dans les retards d'adrénarche. *Ann Endocrinol (Paris)* 1982;43:465–95.

351 Korth-Schutz A, Levine LS, New MI. Evidence for the adrenal source of androgens in precocious adrenarche. *Acta Endocrinol* 1976;82:342–52.

352 Pang S. Premature adrenarche. In: New MI, Levine LS, eds. *Adrenal Diseases in Childhood. Pediatric Adolescent Endocrinology*, Vol. 13. Basel: Karger, 1984:176–84.

353 Lee PA, Migeon CJ, Bias WB, Jones GS. Familial hypersecretion of adrenal androgen transmitted as a dominant, non-HLA linked trait. *Obstet Gynecol* 1987;69:259–64.

354 Forest MG, de Peretti E, David M. Late onset 21-hydroxylase deficiency (21-OHD) can be misdiagnosed as 'typical' premature pubarche (PP) in childhood. *Pediatr Res* 1985;19: 624.

355 Temeck JW, Pang S, Nelson C, New MI. Genetic defects of steroidogenesis in premature pubarche. *J Clin Endocrinol Metab* 1987;64:609–17.

356 August GP, Hung W, Mayes DM. Plasma androgens in premature pubarche: value of a 17α-hydroxyprogesterone in differentiation from congenital adrenal hyperplasia. *J Pediatr* 1975;87:246–9.

357 Granoff AB, Chasalow FI, Blethen SL. 17-Hydroxyprogesterone responses to adrenocorticotropin in children with premature adrenarche. *J Clin Endocrinol Metab* 1985;60: 409–15.

358 Siegel SF, Finegold DN, Urban MD *et al.* Premature pubarche: etiological heterogeneity. *J Clin Endocrinol Metab* 1992;74:239–47.

359 Azziz R, Dewailly D, Owerbach D. Non-classic adrenal hyperplasia: current concepts. *J Clin Endocrinol Metab* 1994;78:810–15.

360 Cathro DM, Golombeck SG. Non-classic 3β-hydroxysteroid dehydrogenase deficiency in children in Central Iowa. Difficulties in differentiating this entity from cases of precocious adrenarche without an adrenal enzyme defect. *J Pediatr Endocrinol* 1994;7:19–32.

361 Forest MG, Mébarki F, Simard J *et al.* Le déficit en 3β-hydroxystéroïde déshydrogénase: hétérogénéité des formes cliniques et apport de la biologie moléculaire. *Rev Fr Endocrinol Clin* 1994;35:307–19.

362 Morel Y, Bertrand J, Rappaport R. Disorders of hormonosynthesis. In: Bertrand J, Rappaport R, Sizonenko PC, eds. *Pediatric Endocrinology*, 2nd edn. Baltimore: Williams & Wilkins 1993:305–22.

363 Simard J, Rhéaume E, Sanchez R *et al.* Molecular basis of congenital adrenal hyperplasia due to to 3β-hydroxysteroid dehydrogenase deficiency. *Mol Endocrinol* 1993;7:716–28.

364 Ibañez L, Verdis R, Potau N *et al.* Natural history of pre-

mature pubarche: an auxological study. *J Clin Endocrinol Metab* 1992;74:254–7.

365 de Peretti E, Forest MG. Pattern of plasma dehydroepiandrosterone sulfate levels in humans from birth to adulthood: evidence for testicular production. *J Clin Endocrinol Metab* 1978;47:572–7.

366 Ibañez L, Potau N, Virdis R *et al.* Postpubertal outcome in girls diagnosed with premature pubarche during childhood: increased frequency of functional ovarian hyperandrogenism. *J Clin Endocrinol Metab* 1993;76:1599–603.

367 Rosenfield RL, Barnes RB, Cara JF *et al.* Dysregulation of cytochrome P450c17α as the cause of polycystic ovarian syndrome. *Fertil Steril* 1990;53:785–91.

368 Conn JW. Primary aldosteronism, a new clinical entity. *J Lab Clin Med* 1955;45:6–17.

369 Banks WA, Kastin AJ, Biglieri EG *et al.* Primary adrenal hyperplasia: a new subset of primary aldosteronism. *J Clin Endocrinol Metab* 1987;58:783–5.

370 Young WF, Hogan MJ, Klee GC *et al.* Primary aldosteronism: diagnosis and treatment. *Mayo Clin Proc* 1990;65:96–110.

371 Dye NV, Litton NJ, Varma M *et al.* Unilateral adrenal hyperplasia as a cause of primary aldosteronism. *South Med J* 1989;82:82–6.

372 Ogishima T, Shibata H, Shimada H *et al.* Aldosterone synthetase cytochrome P-450 expressed in the adrenals of patients with primary aldosteronism. *J Biol Chem* 1991;266: 10731–4.

373 Melby JC. Diagnosis of hyperaldosteronism. *Endocrinol Metab Clin N Am* 1991;20:247–55.

374 Ganguly A, Bergstein J, Grim CE *et al.* Childhood primary aldosteronism due to an adrenal adenoma: preoperative localization by adrenal vein catheterization. *Pediatrics* 1980; 65:605–9.

375 Kelch RP, Connors MH, Kaplan SL *et al.* A calcified aldosterone producing tumor in hypertensive, normokalaemic, prepubertal girl. *J Pediatr* 1973;83:432–7.

376 Lee Y-J, Lin S-R, Shin S-J *et al.* Increased adrenal medullary atrial natriuretic polypeptide synthesis in patients with primary aldosteronism. *J Clin Endocrinol Metab* 1993;76: 1357–62.

377 Yamaji T, Ishibashi M, Sekihara H *et al.* Plasma levels of atrial natriuretic peptide in primary aldosteronism and essential hypertension. *J Clin Endocrinol Metab* 1986;63: 815–18.

378 Higuchi K, Nawata H, Kato KI *et al.* Lack of inhibitory effect of α-human atrial natriuretic polypeptide on aldosteronogenesis in aldosterone-producing adenoma. *J Clin Endocrinol Metab* 1986;63:192–6.

379 Shionoiri H, Hirawa N, Takasaki I *et al.* Lack of atrial natriuretic peptide receptors in human aldosteronoma. *Biochem Biophys Res Commun* 1988;152:37–43.

380 Imai T, Seo H, Murata Y *et al.* Dexamethasone-nonsuppressible cortisol in two cases with aldosterone-producing adenoma. *J Clin Endocrinol Metab* 1991;72:575–81.

381 Galen FX, Devaux C, Atlas S *et al.* New monoclonal antibodies against human renin. *J Clin Invest* 1984;74: 723–35.

382 Carey RM, Sen SS, Dolan LM *et al.* Idiopathic hyperaldosteronism. A possible role for aldosterone-stimulating factor. *N Engl J Med* 1984;311:94–100.

383 Vidt DG, Bravo EL, Fouad FM. Captopril. *N Engl J Med* 1982;306:214–18.

384 Thibonnier M, Sassano P, Dufloux MA *et al.* Test diagnostique simple de l'hyperaldostéronisme primaire. *Nouv Presse Méd* 1983;12:1461–6.

385 Hambling C, Jung RT, Gunn A *et al.* Re-evaluation of the captopril test for the diagnosis of primary hyperaldosteronism. *Clin Endocrinol* 1992;36:499–503.

386 Ulick S, Blumenfeld JD, Atlas SA *et al.* The unique steroidogenesis of the aldosteronoma in the differential diagnosis of primary aldosteronism. *J Clin Endocrinol Metab* 1933;76: 873–8.

387 Bryer-Ash M, Wilson D, Tune BM *et al.* Hypertension caused by an aldosterone-secreting adenoma. *Am J Dis Child* 1984; 128:673–6.

388 Oberfield SE, Levine LS, Sconer E *et al.* Metabolic and blood pressure responses to hydrocortisone in the syndrome of apparent mineralocorticoid excess. *J Clin Endocrinol Metab* 1983;56:332–9.

389 Ulick S, Levine LS, Gunczler P *et al.* A syndrome of apparent mineralocorticoid excess associated with defects in peripheral metabolism of cortisol. *J Clin Endocrinol Metab* 1979; 49:757–64.

390 Ulick S. Two uncommon causes of mineralocorticoid excess – syndrome of apparent mineralocorticoid excess and glucocorticoid-remediable aldosteronism. *Endocrinol Metab Clin N Am* 1991;20:269–76.

391 Walker BR, Edwards CRW. 11β-Hydroxysteroid dehydrogenase and enzyme-mediated receptor protection: life after liquorice? *Clin Endocrinol* 1991;35:281–9.

392 New MI, Levine LS, Biglieri EG *et al.* Evidence for an unidentified steroid in a child with apparent mineralocorticoid hypertension. *J Clin Endocrinol Metab* 1977;44:924–33.

393 Sheppard KE, Funder JW. Equivalent affinity of aldosterone and corticosterone for type I receptor in kidney and hippocampus direct binding studies. *J Steroid Biochem* 1987;28: 737–42.

394 Funder JW, Perace PT, Smith R *et al.* Mineralocorticoid action: target tissue specificity is enzyme not receptor mediated. *Science* 1988;242:583–5.

395 Edwards CRW, Stewart PM, Burt D *et al.* Localization of 11β-hydroxysteroid dehydrogenase; tissue specific protector of the mineralocorticoid receptor. *Lancet* 1988;ii:986–9.

396 Tannin G, Agarwal AK, Monder C *et al.* The human gene for 11-β-hydroxysteroid dehydrogenase. *J Biol Chem* 1991;266: 16653–8.

397 Edwards CRW. Renal 11-beta-hydroxysteroid dehydrogenase: a mechanism ensuring mineralocorticoid specificity. *Horm Res* 1990;345:114–17.

398 Monder C, Shackleton CHL, Bradlow HL *et al.* The syndrome of apparent mineralocorticoid excess: its association with 11β-dehydrogenase and 5β-reductase deficiency and some consequences for corticosteroid metabolism. *J Clin Endocrinol Metab* 1986;63:550–7.

399 Ulick S, Tedde R, Mantero F. Pathogenesis of the type 2 variant of the syndrome of apparent mineralocorticoid excess. *J Clin Endocrinol Metab* 1990;70:200–6.

400 White PC, Obeid J, Agarval AK *et al.* Genetic analysis of 11β-hydroxysteroid dehydrogenase. *Steroids* 1994;59:111–15.

401 Ulick S, Tedde R, Wang JZ. Defective ring A reduction of cortisol as the major metabolic error in the syndrome of apparent mineralocorticoid excess. *J Clin Endocrinol Metab* 1992;74:593–9.

402 Liddle GW, Bledsoe T, Coppage WS. A familial renal disorder simulating primary aldosteronism but with negligible aldosterone secretion. *Trans Assoc Am Phys* 1963;76: 199.

403 Farese RV, Biglieri EG, Shackleton CHL *et al.* Licorice-

induced hypermineralocorticoidism. *N Engl J Med* 1991;325: 1225–7.

404 Stewart PM, Wallace AM, Valentino R *et al.* Mineralocorticoid activity of liquorice: 11β-hydroxysteroid dehydrogenase deficiency comes of age. *Lancet* 1987;2:821–4.

405 Sutherland DJA, Ruse JL, Laidlaw JC. Hypertension increased aldosterone secretion and low plasma renin activity relieved by dexamethasone. *Can Med Assoc J* 1966;95:1109–19.

406 New MI, Oberfield SE, Levine LS *et al.* Autosomal dominant transmission and absence of HLA linkage in dexamethasone-suppressible hyperaldosteronism. *Lancet* 1980;1:550–1.

407 Ganguly A. Glucocorticoid-suppressible hyperaldosteronism: a paradigm of arrested adrenal zonation. *Clin Sci* 1991; 80:1 – 7.

408 Ganguly A, Grim C, Weinberger MH. Anomalous postural aldosterone response in glucocorticoid-suppressible hyperaldosteronism. *N Engl J Med* 1981;305:991–3.

409 Rich GM, Ulick S, Cook S *et al.* Glucocorticoid-remediable aldosteronism in a large kindred: clinical spectrum and diagnosis using a characteristic biochemical phenotype. *Ann Intern Med* 1992;116:813–20.

410 Lifton RP, Dluhy RG, Powers M *et al.* A chimaeric 11β-hydroxylase/aldosterone synthase gene causes glucocorticoid-remediable aldosteronism and human hypertension. *Nature* 1992;355:262–5.

411 Pascoe L, Curnow KM, Slutsker L *et al.* Glucocorticoid-suppressible hyperaldosteronism results from hybrid genes created by unequal crossovers between CYP11B1 and CYP11B2. *Proc Natl Acad Sci USA* 1992;89:8327–31.

412 Corvol P, Pinet F, Galen FX *et al.* Seven lessons from seven renin secreting tumors. *Kidney Int* 1988;34(Suppl. 25): S38–44.

413 Galen FX, Devaux C, Houot AM *et al.* Renin biosynthesis by human juxtaglomerular cells. Evidence for renin precursor. *J Clin Invest* 1984;73:1144–55.

414 Luciani JC, Baldet P, Dumas RS *et al.* Etude du système rénine-angiotensine dans deux cas de tumeur de Wilms avec hypertension artérielle sévère. *Arch Fr Pédiatr* 1979;36: 240–9.

415 Veldhuis JD, Kulin HE, Santen RJ *et al.* Metabolic mimicry of Bartter's syndrome by covert vomiting. Utility of urinary chloride determinations. *Am J Med* 1979;99:361–3.

416 Proesmans W, Massa G, Vandershueren-Lodeweyckx M. Growth from birth to adulthood in a patient with the neonatal form of Bartter syndrome. *Pediatr Nephrol* 1988; 2:205–9.

417 Restrepo de Rovetto C, Welch TR, Hug G *et al.* Hypercalciuria with Bartter syndrome: evidence for an abnormality of vitamin D metabolism. *J Pediatr* 1989;115:397–404.

418 Stein JH. The pathogenic spectrum of Bartter's syndrome. *Kidney Int* 1985;28:85–93.

419 Trygstad CW, Mangos J, Bloodworth MDJ *et al.* A sibship with Bartter's syndrome: failure of total adrenalectomy to correct the potassium wastage. *Pediatrics* 1969;44:234–42.

420 Shigeta H, Tasaki N, Kitazumi S *et al.* Somatostatin suppresses plasma aldosterone concentration in a case of Bartter's syndrome. *Endocrinol Jpn* 1987;34:309–12.

30: Congenital Adrenal Hyperplasia

Z. HUMA, C. CRAWFORD and M.I. NEW

INTRODUCTION

Congenital adrenal hyperplasia (CAH) is the term applied to a group of genetically determined enzymatic defects in the synthesis of cortisol from cholesterol. The histological finding of hyperplasia is due to the chronic stimulation of the adrenal cortices by adrenocorticotrophin (ACTH), the synthesis and release of which from the anterior pituitary corticotrophs is elevated secondary to the insufficient rate of cortisol production [1].

Severe defects of any of the cortisol-synthesizing enzymes result in the classical forms of CAH, in which sex hormonal imbalances cause some degree of genital ambiguity. Adrenal androgen overproduction causes virilization at birth in females (female pseudohermaphroditism) and precocious development postnatally in both sexes. On the other hand, impairment of androgen synthesis in adrenals and gonads causes insufficient virilization of males at birth (male pseudohermaphroditism) and failure of pubertal development in both sexes. Non-classical forms of adrenal hyperplasia also occur, characterized by signs of postnatal androgen excess. These are more prevalent than the classical forms (Table 30.1).

In well over 90% of cases, classical CAH is due to impaired steroid 21-hydroxylation. The adrenal steroid 21-hydroxylase (21-OH) enzyme is a cytochrome P450 [2]. Another classical form of CAH is due to deficiency of the steroid 11β-hydroxylase (11β-OH) enzyme, also a cytochrome P450 [3]. Cortisol precursors in both of these forms of CAH are channelled into androgen pathways and produce hyperandrogenaemia, which masculinizes the external genitalia of the genetic female fetus. These forms are known as virilizing CAH. No genital abnormalities result at birth in males with 21-OH deficiency or 11β-OH deficiency and although prenatal and perinatal testosterone levels are high, comparable to pubertal levels, this is normal in all male neonates.

The three early steps in the conversion of cholesterol to cortisol (cholesterol side chain-cleavage enzyme (formerly cholesterol desmolase), 3β-hydroxysteroid dehydrogenase (3β-HSD)/$\Delta^{5,4}$-isomerase, and the dual-function steroid 17α-hydroxylase (17-OH)/17,20-lyase enzyme) are common to adrenal and gonadal steroidogenesis and deficiencies of these enzymes cause reduction of all sex steroid synthesis. The result is pseudohermaphroditism in the male and sexual infantilism in the female. The external genitalia and ductal structures of newborn males with these deficiencies are incompletely developed because of insufficient local and systemic amounts of testosterone. Females do not develop in puberty.

Genetic defects at the molecular level have been identified for most forms of CAH. First identified were mutations in the gene encoding the steroid 21-OH enzyme, both because of the frequency of occurrence of this enzyme defect and because of linkage of the disease trait with human leukocyte antigens (HLA), the major histocompatibility complex (MHC) in man. Linkage with HLA, discovered and reported in 1977 [4], had immediate application in predictive diagnosis of 21-OH deficiency CAH in families and gave rise to the definition of non-classical 21-OH deficiency (NC21-OHD) as a distinct disorder by classical genetic criteria. Later and continuing molecular genetic studies have described 21-OH mutant gene sequences.

The 17-OH/17,20-lyase enzyme was the next for which mutations in the structural gene were confirmed to underlie the clinical deficiency. Following this, steroid 11β-OH-encoding gene defects were found, and defects in the gene encoding the adrenal/gonadal isoform of the non-cytochrome P450 enzyme 3β-HSD [5] have now been identified. For the side-chain cleavage enzyme, the gene for which has, like the others, been cloned, no DNA mutation has yet been identified in affected patients; thus the genetic basis of this defect of cortisol synthesis remains to be established.

The frequency of the homozygous affected state for classical 21-OH deficiency CAH ranges from 1/5000 to 1/23 000 in most populations, based on case surveys and neonatal screening [6–8]. International screening reveals the average frequency to be 1 in 15 000 live births [9]. Among the major populations it seems slightly more frequent among Caucasian peoples, and slightly less frequent

Table 30.1 Clinical and laboratory features of various disorders of adrenal steroidogenesis

Newborn with sexual ambiguity		Clinical features				Laboratory findings: Urinary excretion				Laboratory findings: Circulating hormones				
Female	Male	Salt-wasting	Hyper-tension	Postnatal virilization	Enzyme deficiency	17-KS	17-OH	P-triol	Aldo	17-OHP	Δ^4-A	DHEA	Testo-sterone	Renin
+	0	0	0	+	21-hydroxylase: simple-virilizing	↑↑	n or ↓	↑↑	n	↑↑	↑↑	n or ↑	↑	n or ↑
+	0	+	0	+	21-hydroxylase: salt-wasting	↑↑	↓	↑↑	↓	↑↑	↑↑	n or ↑	↑	↑↑
+	0	0	+	+	11β-hydroxylase	↑↑	↑↑ (a)	↑	↓	↑	↑↑	↑	↑	↓↓
+	+	+	0	+	3β-HSD(b)	↑ (c)	↓↓	n or ↓	↓	n or ↑	n or ↑	↑↑	↑ (d)	↑

(a) Mostly tetrahydro-II-deoxycortisol; (b) the values presented apply to the infant and the very young child; (c) mostly Δ^5-17 ketosteroids (17-KS); (d) ↓ or normal in male; ↑ or normal in female.
Δ^4-A, Δ^4-androstenedione; Aldo, aldosterone; DHEA, dehydroepiandrosterone; n, normal; 17-OHP, 17α-hydroxyprogesterone; P-triol, pregnane trial.

in the Japanese. Two isolates carry severe 21-OH defects at very high frequency: Yup'ik Innuits in Alaska and the inhabitants of La Réunion island in the Indian Ocean. The steroid 11β-OH defect has a probable overall frequency of the order of 1/120 000 to 1/200 000, but in Israel and north Africa founder defects account for 20% or more of all CAH cases. There are no frequency estimates for the other defects. NC21-OHD has been suggested to be the most common human autosomal recessive disorder; it occurs with a frequency of 1 in 27 individuals of Ashkenazi Jewish background, and 1 in 100 of heterogeneous New York City Caucasoid population [10]. The frequency has been confirmed by computer reanalysis of data [11], clinical/family study updates [12] and pilot screenings [13].

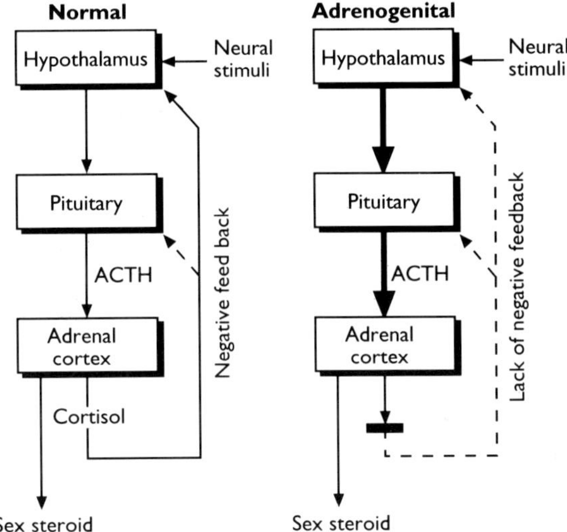

Fig. 30.1 Regulation of cortisol synthesis in normal subjects and in patients with virilizing congenital adrenal hyperplasia.

ADRENAL STEROIDOGENESIS

The adrenal cortex produces cortisol and aldosterone by specific and largely separate regulatory systems. Cortisol is synthesized in cells of the zona fasciculata (ZF) under the trophic control of ACTH; cortisol–ACTH form a negative feedback loop, high serum cortisol centrally inhibiting and low serum cortisol permitting further pituitary release of ACTH. This defines the hypothalamo-pituitary–adrenal axis (Fig. 30.1). Aldosterone is necessary for adequate renal reabsorption of sodium across the tight epithelium of the distal tubule; by determining net retention of this electrolyte it indirectly controls total body fluid volume. Aldosterone synthesis takes place only in cells of the zona glomerulosa (ZG), modulated by the pressor peptide angiotensin II (AII) and by serum potassium. A decrease in renal perfusion results in an increase in plasma renin secretion which stimulates the production of AII and ultimately aldosterone. Serum potassium stimulates aldosterone synthesis independently of volume status; aldosterone increases the exchange of this ion for sodium in the kidney and potassium thus governs its own excretion.

The synthesis of cortisol in the adrenal ZF is under the control of ACTH. The binding of ACTH to receptors on the external membrane of adrenal cortical cells initiates generation of the intracellular second-messenger cyclic adenosine monophosphate (cAMP) which activates one or more cascades of phosphorylation/dephosphorylation leading from protein kinase A (PKA) and producing a biphasic steroidogenic response [14].

Glucocorticoids (17α-hydroxy pathway) (Fig. 30.2)

Cortisol synthesis from pregnenolone in the ZF requires 17α-hydroxylation, 3β-hydroxysteroid dehydrogenation

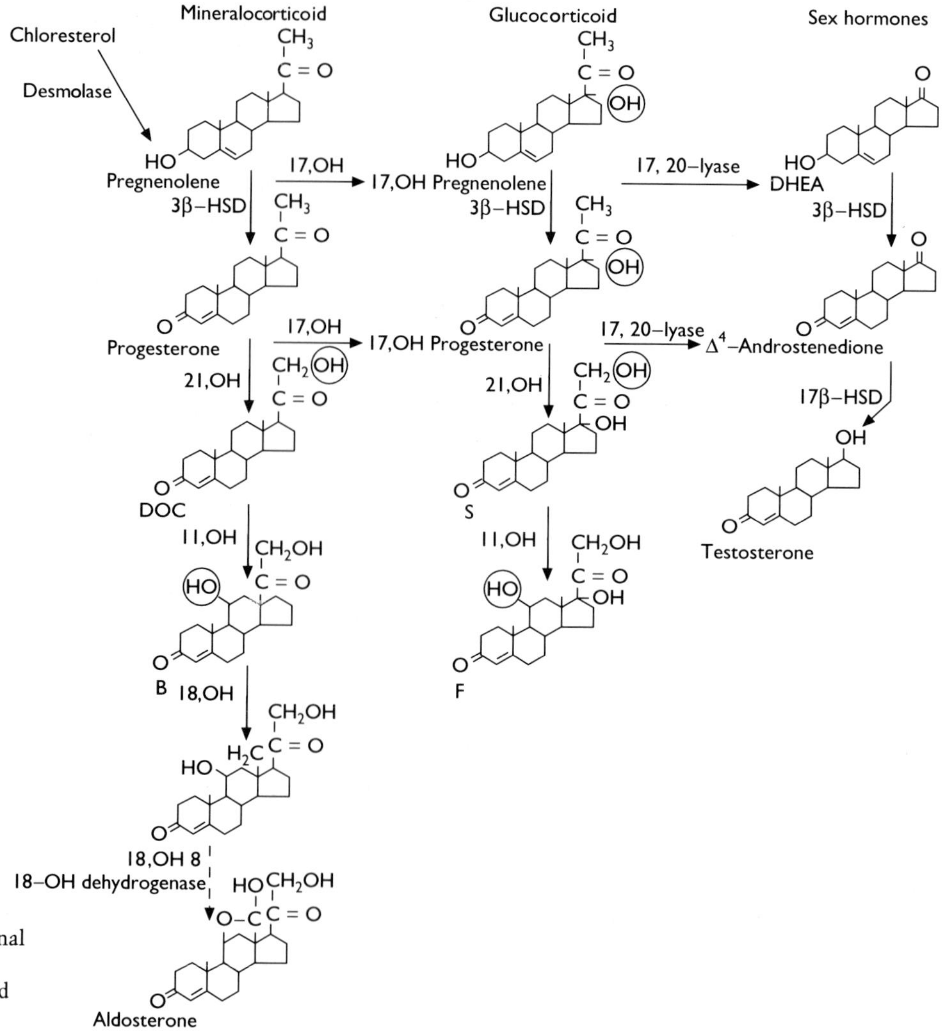

Fig. 30.2 Simplified scheme for adrenal steroidogenesis. Each hydroxylation step is indicated, and the newly added hydroxyl group is circled.

(with concomitant $\Delta^{5,4}$-isomerization) and two further hydroxylations, at the 21- and 11β-positions. An alternative order of conversion is for pregnenolone first to undergo 3β-dehydrogenation, thereby becoming progesterone. Action of the enzyme performing 17α-hydroxylation, 17α-hydroxylase/17,20-lyase, on pregnenolone produces 17α-hydroxypregnenolone (17-Δ^5-P), and on progesterone produces 17α-hydroxyprogesterone (17-OHP). The resultant 17-OHP undergoes 21-hydroxylation to form 11-deoxycortisol (compound S), which is further 11β-hydroxylated in a single step to form cortisol (compound F). Conversion of pregnenolone to 17-OHP in the cortisol pathway is largely via 17-Δ^5-P as intermediate, and in lesser amounts via progesterone.

MINERALOCORTICOIDS

Pregnenolone is converted to aldosterone in the ZG by a series of enzymatic steps, many of which are parallel to the series of conversions leading to cortisol in the ZF. Pregnenolone is first converted to progesterone by 3β-HSD; this is then 21-hydroxylated to deoxycorticosterone (DOC), an active salt-retaining hormone. DOC then undergoes 11β-hydroxylation to produce corticosterone (compound B), a weak mineralocorticoid with some glucocorticoid activity. The final two steps toward aldosterone synthesis in the ZG are 18-hydroxylation to 18-hydroxycorticosterone (18-OHB), and 18-oxidation to aldosterone. These steps are also called corticosterone methyl oxidase (CMO) types I and II. The CMO-I function, 18-hydroxylation, can act before or after the 11β-OH, and thus as well as B, another intermediate in the transformation of DOC to 18-OHB is 18-hydroxy-11-deoxycorticosterone (18-OHDOC). The terminal 18-oxidase – or CMO-II – function which completes aldosterone synthesis takes place only in the ZG. Mineralocorticoid biosynthesis by the ZG is primarily under the control of AII and serum potassium [15], and only secondarily by ACTH.

17-DEOXYSTEROID PATHWAY IN THE ZONA FASCICULATA

The same steroids and conversions that belong to the mineralocorticoid pathway in the ZG comprise what is called the 17-deoxysteroid pathway in the ZF. DOC and B, which are almost exclusively committed to eventual conversion to aldosterone in the ZG, also arise in the ZF by conversion from the minor cortisol intermediate progesterone, and while there is very little secretion of aldosterone precursors from the ZG, progesterone, DOC and B are secreted in measurable amounts from the ZF. These ZF products are called the 17-deoxysteroids and their serum levels represent activity of the cortisol-producing ZF andare thus ACTH-stimulatable and glucocorticoid-suppressible.

The component cells of the adrenal ZG and the ZF differ in certain respects.

1 ZG adrenocortical cells are of a low-output type and ZF cells of a high-output type; the ZG occupies much less than the ZF so the net steroid output of the ZF is 10^2 to 10^3 times greater.

2 The main factors regulating the ZG are AII and serum potassium concentration ([K^+]), whereas the ZF is under the primary control of ACTH. The ZG does respond secondarily to ACTH and exposure to ACTH seems to be involved in conversion of the adrenocortical cell from the ZG to the ZF type.

3 Steroid 17OH/17,20-lyase is expressed only in ZF cells. Production of 17-deoxysteroids in the ZF is at the branch points in the cortisol pathway and arises by enzyme competition for substrates.

4 The aldosterone synthase isozyme of 11β-OH is expressed at levels to dominate the pattern of steroid synthesis only in the ZG, consistent with the production of aldosterone by this zone. Both isozymes appear to have steroid 18-hydroxylating capacity, although to what relative degree has not yet been determined.

As a result of 18-hydroxylation in the ZF (17α-hydroxy substrate affinities are less) minor side-products of steroid synthesis in this zone are 18-hydroxy-11-deoxycortisol (18-OHS), 18-hydroxycortisol (18-OHF) and 18-oxocortisol (18-oxoF) – that is, 17α,18-*di*hydroxysteroids, specific analogues of the ZG 17-deoxysteroids 18-OHDOC, 18-OHB and aldosterone.

Sex steroids

Cleavage of the short (C2) side-chain of 17α-hydroxy-pregnenolone results in a C19 or androgenic steroid, dehydroepiandrosterone (DHEA), which in free and (sulphate-)conjugated form is quantitatively the main steroid secreted by the adrenal cortex. This cleavage conversion is called (C-)17,20-lysis, and is catalysed by 17α-hydroxylase/17,20-lyase, a dual-function enzyme responsible both for forming glucocorticoid precursors and for shunting these same precursors into androgen (sex steroid) pathways [16]. DHEA is readily converted to the much more potent androgen Δ^4-androstenedione (Δ^4-A) by the same 3β-HSD/isomerase enzyme that converts pregnenolone to progesterone and 17α-hydroxy pregnenolone to 17-OHP. With reduction of the oxo group at the C17 position, Δ4-A is converted to testosterone.

Sexual development is covered in another chapter, but underdevelopment of male external genitalia in 17α-hydroxylase deficiency and 3β-HSD deficiency – as well as in other, rarer adrenal/gonadal (cholesterol desmolase) and gonadal (17β-HSD, formerly called also 17-ketosteroid reductase) enzyme defects – is due largely to a lack of secreted testosterone as a substrate for the peripheral enzyme steroid 5α-reductase, which converts testosterone to dihydrotestosterone (DHT). Deficiency of 5α-reductase type II will lead to similar underdevelopment of male external genitalia. The postnatal developmental patterns seen in these enzyme defects have allowed the distinct physiological effects of these two potent end-hormones, testosterone and DHT, to be determined.

Lack of suppression of the breast anlage from low prenatal exposure to sex steroids may be the origin of gynaecomastia observed in some males with 17α-OH deficiency. Conversely, in females with 3β-HSD deficiency, even partial peripheral conversion of the weak Δ^5-steroids, present at impressively high serum concentrations, can result in significant serum levels of more potent androgens and thus in some degree of virilization. The increased androgen environment in this form of CAH, as well as in 21-OH and 11β-OH deficiencies, does not affect the development of the Müllerian ducts in the genetic female into fallopian tubes, uterus and upper vagina: only the Sertoli cells of the fetal testis secreting anti-Müllerian hormone prevents this development in the male.

MAJOR ENZYME DEFECTS

Steroid 21-hydroxylase deficiency

The problems of 21-OH deficiency vary according to chronological age, gender and the type of 21-OH deficiency, that is, classical simple virilizing or salt-wasting, and non-classical.

Classical simple virilizing 21-hydroxylase deficiency

Since adrenocortical function begins in the third month of gestation, the fetus is exposed to increased adrenal androgens at a critical time of sexual differentiation. Thus female infants may be born with genital ambiguity. In extreme cases the masculinization can be so profound that the urethra extends the full length of the phallus, resulting in an appearance indistinguishable from a normal male [17], but usually the genital phenotype is an enlarged clitoris with fusion of the labioscrotal folds. The distal two-thirds of the vagina and urethra are under androgen control and so there may be a urogenital sinus. Internal genital development is normal with the presence of normal ovaries and Müllerian structures.

Males have normal external genitalia, and thus in this form of 21-OH deficiency, diagnosis in the male and the sex-misassigned female is often delayed until progressive virilization becomes apparent. The average time to diagnosis can be long, 19 months in girls and 62 months in boys in one survey [18]. After birth these patients manifest phallic enlargement, precocious development of pubic and axillary hair, acne, deepening of voice, rapid growth and musculoskeletal development, followed by premature epiphyseal fusion. Thus, although statural growth is initially advanced, full height potential is lost and these patients are short in adulthood. Characteristics of the hormonal profile are presented in Table 30.1.

Secondary central precocious puberty is a complication encountered when the diagnosis of 21-OH deficiency has been delayed or when adrenal androgens have been inadequately controlled [19]. The advanced somatic and skeletal maturation in these children is associated with premature activation of the hypothalamopituitary–gonadal axis leading to an onset of puberty that is early for the child's chronological age but appropriate for the skeletal age.

Another complication in boys with insufficient therapy or poor compliance is the development of testicular adrenal rest tissue [20]. Increased secretion of ACTH can cause growth of adrenal rests that can occur unilaterally or bilaterally anywhere along the pathway of testicular descent [20,21]. In the absence of central precocious puberty, adrenal rest tissue is the most likely cause of bilateral testicular enlargement. This can be diagnosed by testicular ultrasound.

Classical salt-wasting

Salt-wasting, stemming from deficient production of aldosterone, which is necessary to support distal renal tubular sodium reabsorption, occurs in up to 75% of all cases of classical 21-OH deficiency. In this form of 21-OH deficiency the same range of physical signs of hyperandrogenism and of excess ACTH secretion is seen in simple virilizing 21-OH deficiency. Salt loss may be aggravated by the natriuretic effects of cortisol precursors. Renal salt-wasting and plasma volume loss with hyperkalaemia can lead to adrenal crisis (azotaemia, vascular collapse, shock and death). Dehydration and shock from salt loss may occur as early as weeks 1–4 of life, when the diagnosis can be made; otherwise a triggering event may be required, such as systemic infection. Male infants with the salt-losing form are at particularly high risk of an adrenal crisis because they do not manifest the genital ambiguity at birth which flags the diagnosis. The prevention of adrenal crisis is a compelling reason for newborn screening programmes and for prenatal diagnosis.

Non-classical

Females with NC21-OHD are born with normal external genitalia. Somatic manifestations of androgen excess are more subtle than in the classical form of the disease. In our experience the earliest presentation of NC21-OHD has been in a 6-month-old girl with premature development of pubic hair [22]; however, clinical manifestations from increased androgen production can occur at any time. Later in childhood or adolescence, symptoms in female patients include hirsutism [23–25], temporal baldness, severe cystic acne [26,27], delayed menarche, menstrual irregularities and infertility [28–30].

Testing of the adrenal axis reveals NC21-OHD in a percentage of women with polycystic ovarian syndrome [6,29]. It is theorized that the usual cyclicity of gonadotrophin release and/or the androgen-synthesizing characteristics of the developing ovarian follicles could be disrupted by altered serum androgen levels issuing from a primary adrenal enzyme defect (the so-called generator stage), and that once this imbalance is established the polyfollicular ovary then continues autonomously to produce excess androgens [31]. The ability to reverse infertility with glucocorticoid treatment in late-onset adrenal hyperplasia has been recognized since the 1950s [32–34]. There have been case reports of subfertility in males with NC21-OHD. There has been a case report of one boy with gynaecomastia [35].

Elevated adrenal androgens promote the early fusion of epiphyseal growth plates, and it is common but not invariable that children with the disorder have advanced bone age, accelerated linear growth velocity and a final height shorter than the height predicted for them based on mid-parental height [36,37]. It is likely that all patients with the biochemical manifestations of NC21-OHD manifest signs of androgen excess at some time [35].

HORMONAL DIAGNOSIS

In classical 21-OH deficiency baseline serum 17-OHP concentrations are diagnostic. Salt-wasting is defined by hyponatraemia and hyperkalaemia, inappropriately high urinary sodium, metabolic acidosis, and low serum and urinary aldosterone with concomitantly high plasma renin

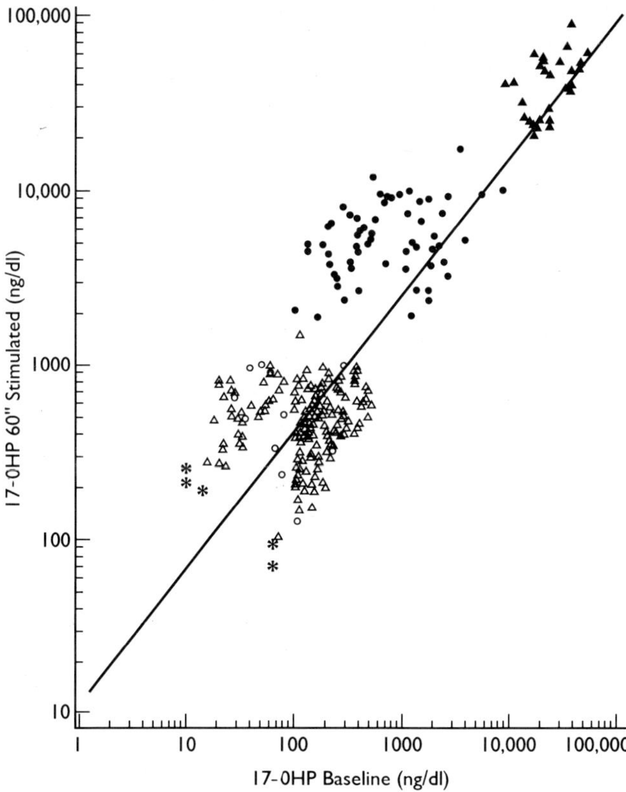

Fig. 30.3 Nomogram relating baseline and 60-min ACTH stimulated serum 17-OHP concentration. *; genetically unaffected. Patients with: ▲, classical congenital adrenal hyperplasia; ●, nonclassical congenital adrenal hyperplasia. Heterozygotes for: △, classical congenital adrenal hyperplasia; ○, nonclassical congenital adrenal hyperplasia. (Redrawn from New [39]).

activity (PRA). In NC21-OHD basal 17-OHP hormonal levels may not differ from normal values when measured randomly, but are elevated during the diurnal peak in cortisol production, so early morning serum values are informative [22,24,25].

The best indicator of any degree of 21-OH deficiency is the excessive rise of serum 17-OHP with ACTH administration. A standard 60-min ACTH test involves serum samples taken at 0 min (baseline) and 60 min (stimulated) after a bolus i.v. injection of 0.25 mg synthetic $ACTH_{1-24}$. The two serum 17-OHP concentrations obtained are mapped on a standard reference nomogram (Fig. 30.3) [39]. The coordinates of the hormonal values segregate into four groups on a regression line in the following descending order: (a) classical 21-OH deficiency patients, (b) NC21-OHD patients, (c) heterozygotes (for either form) and (d) unaffected individuals. The first two groups are easily distinguishable from each other and from the last two groups, which overlap.

Before the advent of radioimmunoassay (RIA) for 17-OHP [40] urinary adrenocorticoid metabolites were diagnostic for 21-OHD: pregnanetriol is selectively elevated in this disorder among all patient classes [41–44]. Siblings are usually concordant for the phenotype of 21-OH deficiency, but important exceptions have been found [45–47].

A screening test for 21-OH deficiency CAH has been developed for newborns, which involves obtaining a small sample of capillary blood (by heel-prick) onto filter paper of a standard gauge. A fixed-sized disc cut from the area wholly impregnated with blood is then assayed for 17-OHP content by RIA [48]. Cost-effectiveness and sensitivity of this test have been proven [49].

A screening protocol for NC21-OHD measures early morning (0800 h) 17-OHP in saliva [13]. Salivary testing has an advantage in being non-invasive, and salivary 17-OHP correlates well with serum values. False-positive results are to be expected from premature infants and infants with unusual stress in the perinatal period, in whom serum 17-OHP may be quite high. On the other hand, while data available on ACTH testing in neonates have been few, anomalous low adrenal steroid (17-OHP and Δ^4-A) response to ACTH has been observed in some newborns with CAH [50].

GENETICS

A genetic basis for CAH was first shown in 1956 by Childs *et al.* [51], who studied 56 kindreds with CAH. Based on these family studies they suspected an autosomal recessive pattern of inheritance for this condition. In 1977 Dupont *et al.* [4] demonstrated by linkage studies that the locus for the 21-OH gene was situated on the short arm of chromosome 6 in the MHC or HLA (human leukocyte antigen A – later 'antigens'). This linkage was subsequently confirmed in other family studies [52] (reviewed in [53]).

The close linkage between the 21-OHD trait locus and the loci for certain of these HLA antigens served for 15 years in the ascertainment of 21-OH genotypes. Certain HLA antigens are known to be associated with particular clinical forms of the disorder, for example, HLA-Bw47; DR7 with the salt-wasting form (especially in Anglo-Saxon populations) and B14;DR1 with the non-classical form. Other interesting haplotype findings included B35 increased in classical patients, and B8 and B14 decreased; conversely, in non-classical patients B14 is increased and B35 is decreased (reviewed in [53]). In the Yugoslav population the HLA associations seen with NC21-OHD in the other ethnic groups are not found, suggesting a different mutation or class of mutations [12,54]. The use of HLA linkage studies to identify affected status in family members may provide erroneous results due to intra-HLA recombination or uninterpretable results due to antigen homozygosity in a parent or antigen sharing between parents.

GENETICS/MOLECULAR BIOLOGY

In 1984 a gene for an adrenal 21-hydroxylating cytochrome P450 was cloned, providing a probe for DNA studies [55]. Southern blots indicated duplication of the 21-OH gene in normal DNA and the absence of one gene band was observed in cases of HLA-linked adrenal hyperplasia [56]. The absence of the other band was noted in some hormonally normal individuals. The two 21-OH genes were found to be arranged in tandem with the two isoforms of serum complement component C4, genes C4A and C4B [57,58]. These genes were sequenced and sequence data confirmed that gene A, or CYP21P, was a pseudogene, and gene B, or CYP21, was the active gene encoding the adrenal 21-OH enzyme [59,60]. These genes both have 10 exons and are 96–98% identical; they are 30 kb apart.

Due to the symmetrical arrangement of the four genes, that is the alternating C4 and CYP21 pairs, there appears to be frequent misalignment and unequal crossing over between chromatids during meiosis. This may result in complete deletion of 30 kb of DNA including CYP21 and one of the complement C4 genes; alternatively perhaps because of the proximity of the CYP21 gene to its pseudogene, there may be the transfer of deleterious mutations from the latter to the active gene by a less understood process (so-called gene conversion) [61–65]. With the exception of rare sporadic mutations [66,67], *de novo* mutations causing classical 21-OH deficiency are expected to be the result of either of the two mechanisms involved in gametogenesis [68,69].

The frequency of gene deletions causing 21-OH deficiency ranges from 11% to 35% (reviewed in [70]) and is highest in northern European populations, which carry HLA-Bw47;DR7 at a high frequency. The single most common mutation may be a point mutation in intron 2 resulting from gene conversion; this accounted for 57% of non-deletional alleles in one study [71]. New mutations continue to be discovered as molecular techniques improve.

Steroid 21-OH deficiency presents in a variety of clinical forms, but results from mutations in a single gene and attempts have been made to link particular mutations to specific clinical presentations. In order to accomplish genotype–phenotype correlations the clinical phenotype must first be clearly defined. In 21-OH deficiency, neither the clinical nor the biochemical distinction between simple virilizing and salt-wasting phenotypes is absolute, and occasional patients have recovered from salt-wasting [72,73]. Most patients can, however, be separated into one of the types of 21-OH deficiency so far described.

Clinical wisdom would suggest that the difference between the phenotypes is essentially a quantitative difference in enzyme activity which should in turn be attributable to the severity of the genetic mutation. Early genotype–phenotype studies have already shown that the correlation between clinical, biochemical and molecular genetic findings in patients with classical 21-OH deficiency is not absolute [73]. As predicted, mutations that completely destroy enzymatic activity (preventing aldosterone synthesis) are caused by deletions and large gene conversions, and result in salt-wasting, whereas most cases of simple-virilizing disease result from single base-pair substitutions. Ile-172 to Asn, a single base-pair change in exon 4, is the only mutation thus far associated exclusively with the simple-virilizing form of the disease [72,74].

Unfortunately, the issue is more complicated than this, since discordance for salt-wasting between siblings with the same mutation has been described, and certain mutations result in salt-wasting in some individuals but not others [47,75,76]. These findings suggest that epigenetic or non-genetic factors can influence the clinical presentation of 21-OH deficiency.

NC21-OHD, the causative mutations of which are allelic with severe defects at the 21-OH gene loci, raises further dilemmas. In the HLA-B14;DR1-associated non-classical disease haplotype, a further duplication has been identified, thus making three C4–21-OH pairs. DNA banding patterns after restriction enzyme digestion and probe labelling showed that the A gene is duplicated [64]. The B gene itself in this haplotype is abnormal, having received a number of point mutations by gene conversion from the pseudogene as reported by Speiser *et al.* [77]. The causative mutation in this mutant B gene is the point mutation causing amino-acid substitution val-281 to leu, which results in an enzyme with about 50% of normal activity [78]. Homozygotes for this mutation have the non-classical form of the disorder with significant hormonal abnormalities and variable symptoms of androgen excess.

Heterozygote carriers of classical 21-OH deficiency would also be expected to have 50% of normal enzymatic activity, but are asymptomatic and have only minor biochemical abnormalities. These findings may be due to the presence of competitive inhibitors for mutant 21-OH enzyme and pseudosubstrate inhibition of other steroidogenic enzymes by accumulation of precursors to the 21-hydroxylating step. The latter may also explain reports of multiple enzyme deficiencies [79–81]. 21-OH deficiency has thus become a paradigm for the correlation between molecular genotype and clinical phenotype.

EPIDEMIOLOGY

The overall frequency of classical 21-OH deficiency has been estimated to be about 1 in 13 500 by case survey and by neonatal screening [7–9] (Table 30.2) Neonatal screening for NC21-OHD has now been instituted in some states in the USA [83]. First estimates of the frequency of NC21-OHD were obtained using ethnic-

Table 30.2 Incidence of CAH by worldwide newborn screening

Population	Number screened	Incidence/live birth
Yupik Innuits	3740	1:288
Native Alaskan	12 131	1:809
LaRéunion, France	82 225	1:4111
Brazil	82 870	1:7533
Switzerland	65 823	1:10 970
Italy	133 198	1:11 100
Sweden	660 000	1:11 786
Germany	12 500	1:12 500
France	270 060	1:12 860
Portugal	100 000	1:14 285
USA	1 806 039	1:15 305
Canada	50 000	1:16 666
Scotland	119 690	1:17 099
Spain	206 875	1:17 239
Japan	2 523 948	1:19 121
New Zealand	404 128	1:21 269

From Pang & Clark [9].

group-specific HLA-B and NC21-OHD associations in conjunction with ACTH testing in obligate heterozygote parents. Disease frequencies are 1 in 27 for Ashkenazi Jews, 1 in 53 for Hispanics, 1 in 63 for Yugoslavs, 1 in 100 in a heterogeneous Caucasian New York City population, and 1 in 333 for Italians (Fig. 30.4).

While these disease frequency estimates refer to the population at large, the occurrence of NC21-OHD is higher in populations preselected for symptoms or signs of hyperandrogenism. Among our clinic population referred for premature pubarche we found a 30% incidence of NC21-OHD [84]. Among female patients referred for hirsutism the incidence of NC21-OHD was 14% [85].

PRENATAL DIAGNOSIS AND THERAPY

Prenatal diagnosis has been used for over 20 years in pregnancies known to be at risk [86,87]. Hormonal diag-

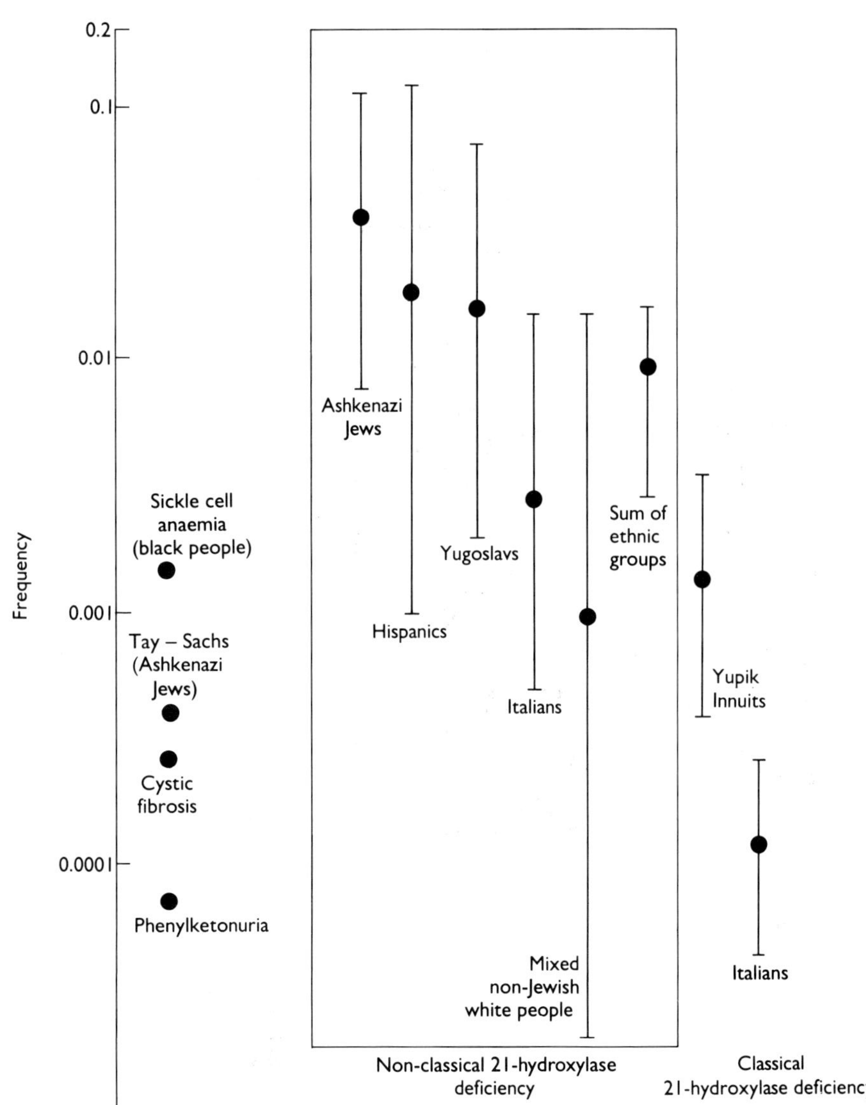

Fig. 30.4 Disease frequencies of NC-21-OHD and classical 21-OH deficiency relative to other common autosomal recessive genetic disorders. Bars represent 95% confidence limits. The lower confidence limit for mixed non-Jewish descent approximates zero.

nosis has been made by the finding of elevated levels of amniotic fluid 17-OHP in the second trimester [88]. Later, genetic diagnosis was performed by HLA serotyping of fetal cells cultured from the amniotic fluid [89]. Although these tests are accurate in most cases, they are performed in the second trimester, when genital ambiguity in the affected female is already established. False-negative 17-OHP levels in non-salt-losing cases and intra-HLA recombination were among the reasons for the imprecision in some prenatal diagnostic studies [90].

With the advent of chorionic villus sampling (CVS), evaluation of the fetus at risk has become possible in the villous tissue by molecular genetic techniques. Since the molecular defect in the index case, and the carrier parents has already been established, a specific molecular diagnosis can be made within 2 weeks [91].

Over the past 10 years prenatal treatment of at-risk pregnancies using dexamethasone has been introduced. When administered to the pregnant woman (at a starting dose of 10–20 μg/kg a day, given three times daily, maximum 1.5 mg a day) at less than 8 weeks gestation it suppresses the abnormal secretion of androgens by the fetal adrenal glands. The adequacy of suppression can be assessed by measuring maternal urinary oestriol excretion. Suppressing the fetal androgen secretion prevents prenatal virilization of affected female infants, resulting in normal female external genitalia, and negates the need for later genital surgery. A suggested algorithm for prenatal diagnosis and treatment is presented in Fig. 30.5.

In order to be effective treatment must be started by 8 weeks, before a hormonal or genetic diagnosis of the fetus is available. Current recommendations include initiation of dexamethasone treatment in all at-risk pregnancies by 8 weeks then subsequent CVS or amniocentesis for karyotype, hormonal and genetic diagnosis. If the fetus is an affected female then treatment is continued through

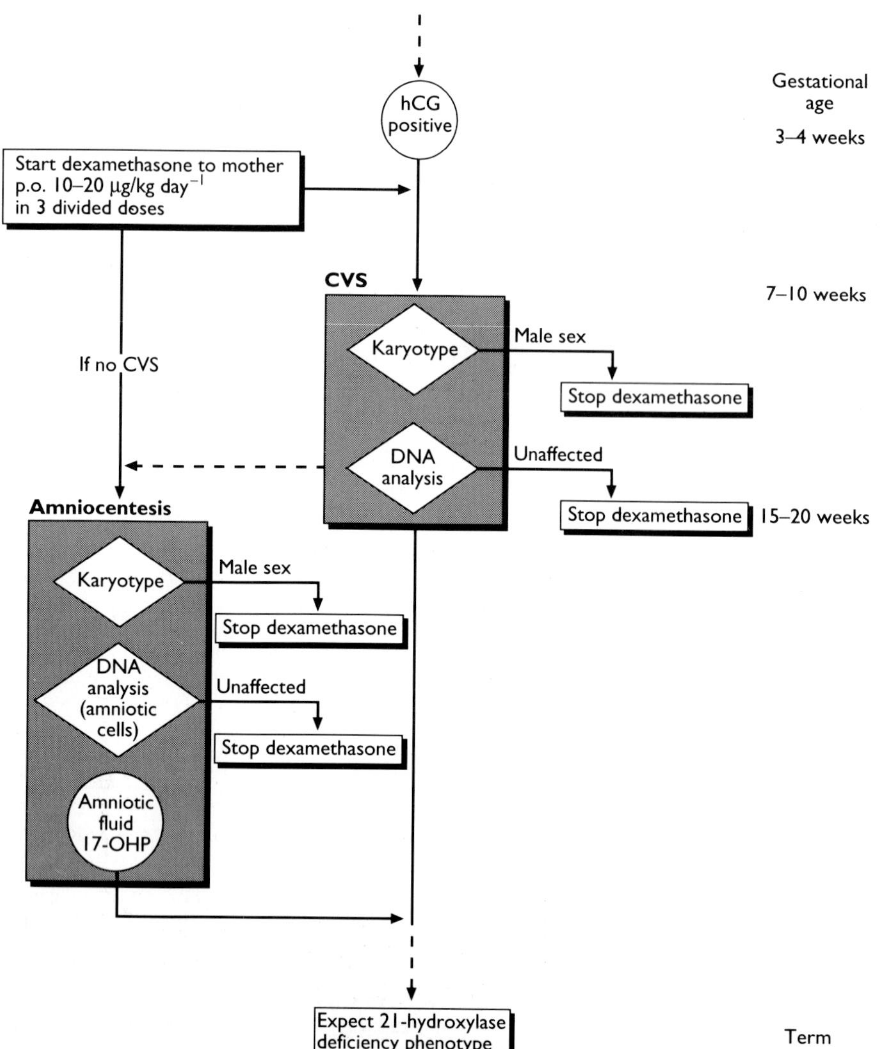

Fig. 30.5 Procedure for management of pregnancies at risk for congenital adrenal hyperplasia due to 21-OH deficiency. hCG, human chorionic gonadotrophin (from Speiser *et al.* [73]).

the pregnancy, and if the fetus is male or an unaffected female then treatment is discontinued.

The safety of prenatal treatment for the fetus with dexamethasone is currently assumed with a substantial degree of confidence. As experience with prenatal treatment grows, information continues to be amassed [92,93]. Low-dose dexamethasone appears to have no teratogenic potential and is judged safe [94]. This is in spite of earlier findings in rodents exposed to dexamethasone in very high dose, which resulted in cleft palate formation *in utero* and placental degeneration with fetal death [95,96]. Infants treated prenatally (both affected and unaffected) have been followed for up to 8 years, and have had normal growth and cognition [92].

Steroid effects on the mother may include mood changes and weight gain, but are mostly well tolerated; even in two cases where side-effects were significant, the mothers indicated they would undergo therapy again if necessary because of the good genital outcome in their affected daughters [97]. The risk–benefit ratio is highly in favour of a prenatal treatment protocol of dexamethasone administration to the mother in pregnancies with a female fetus diagnosed as affected with 21-OH deficiency.

Steroid 11β-hydroxylase deficiency

CLINICAL FEATURES

The second most common classic inborn error of steroid biosynthesis is steroid 11β-OH deficiency. It has an incidence in the order of 1 in 100 000 births in the Caucasian population [98]. Patients with this disorder are unable to convert 11-deoxycortisol (compound S) to cortisol. Elevated levels of ACTH cause S and other non-11β-hydroxylated steroid precursors to be synthesized and secreted in excess, and there is accumulation of precursors proximal to these, such as 17-OHP directly preceding S formation in the cortisol pathway. Shunting of these precursors into the pathway(s) for androgen biosynthesis occurs, as in 21-OH deficiency. Thus, again, females with 11β-OH deficiency have masculinized external genitalia at birth and undergo progressive virilization postnatally; males have normal genitalia and precocious isosexual development, and both sexes undergo precocious adrenarche and rapid somatic growth with premature epiphyseal closure, resulting in short adult stature. This premature virilization of both sexes and genital ambiguity of female newborns is identical to that seen in classical 21-OH deficiency.

In 11β-OH deficiency, as in 21-OH deficiency, the enzymatic defect in the ZF not only increases cortisol precursors, but affects steroid synthesis in the parallel 17-deoxysteroid pathway; in 11β-OH deficiency the 17-deoxysteroid DOC is not able to be converted to corticosterone (compound B), and is oversecreted. This is readily discernible by serum hormonal measurement of high DOC, and this is the index steroid in monitoring treatment of 11β-OH deficiency. The steroid DOC is hormonally active, being a moderately potent mineralocorticoid. Elevated serum levels of DOC and of its metabolites with mineralocorticoid activity induces hypokalaemia with metabolic alkalosis and hypertension. This is in direct contrast to the salt-losing state of the majority of cases with 21-OH deficiency.

The prevalence of hypertension in 11β-OH deficiency has been reported as 61% [99] and 54% [100]. Elevated blood pressure is exceptional in infancy but may develop early and advance to death from cerebrovascular accidents [99]. In other cases hypertension may develop more slowly. There is poor correlation between the degree of virilization and the severity of hypertension and serum levels of DOC or other steroids are not indicative of the degree of hypokalaemia or hypertension.

Mild, late-onset, and even cryptic (detected by hormonal tests only) forms of 11β-OH deficiency have been reported [99,101–103]. As in 21-OH deficiency the clinical variability may represent allelism at the 11β-hydroxylase gene locus.

HORMONAL DIAGNOSIS

The hormonal profile of the untreated patient is characterized by elevated concentrations of DOC and compound S. Both steroids rise disproportionately following ACTH administration, but the relative degrees of elevation of DOC and S (and their metabolites) may differ [100,104]. The 24-h urinary quantities of the principal metabolites THDOC (tetrahydro-11-DOC) and THS (tetrahydro-11-deoxycortisol) are also diagnostic. Renal sodium retention induced by DOC results in volume expansion and suppression of PRA [6]. Thus the ZG is atrophic.

A decade ago it was shown that with glucocorticoid control of ZF activity, the ZG in 11β-OH deficiency could be released from suppression and a basically intact ZG secretory pattern established [6]. In the interim it was observed in human and rat studies [105,106] that a defect in 11β-OH activity is often accompanied by a defect in 18-hydroxylation, and it was proposed that both catalytic functions might reside in a single mitochondrial enzyme. An apparent single protein was purified from porcine and bovine adrenal tissues capable of synthesizing aldosterone from DOC [107,108]. Correlating with the earlier clinical findings [109], however, new molecular studies confirm that aldosterone synthesis is accomplished in the ZG by a B2 form of 11β-OH. The specific isoform of 11β-OH in the ZG is called aldosterone synthase [110]. In the ZF it is the B1 form of 11β-OH that is necessary for the synthesis of corticosterone and cortisol.

As a consequence of high levels of non-11β-hydroxylated precursors, androgens are formed distal to these, preeminent among them Δ^4-androstenedione [109].

Deoxycorticosterone and hypertension

The relationship between DOC and hypertension in 11β-OH deficiency [111] is problematic. Among patients with 11β-OH deficiency there are patients with elevated DOC who are normotensive [42,43] and hypertensive patients with normal to mildly elevated DOC [112–114]. DOC infusion does not necessarily induce hypertension in control subjects [115] and suppression of DOC does not necessarily cause remission of the hypertension [99], although long-standing hypertension of any cause may be refractory to treatments normalizing the hormonal variables. Rösler *et al.* [99] proposed that certain metabolites of DOC, perhaps 18-hydroxy-DOC, may also be factors in the induction and maintenance of hypertension [115].

GENETICS

There are two distinct 11β-OH genes in man: CYP11B1 and CYP11B2 [116] on chromosome 8q21–22 [117] separated by about 30 kb. They encode two isoenzymes, the predicted amino-acid sequences of which are 93% identical. The isozyme encoded by CYP11B1 has 11β-OH activity in *in vitro* expression studies [110,118,119] consistent with a function in cortisol synthesis; it is normally expressed at high levels in the adrenal glands [110,116] and is regulated by ACTH in cultured cells [110]. It is this gene that is mutated in patients with 11β-OH deficiency, in whom cortisol production is affected [120–123].

The product of the CYP11B2 gene has 11β-OH, 18-OH and 18-oxidase activities *in vitro* [110,118,119], is normally expressed at low levels in the adrenal gland, is regulated by AII and is mutated in individuals with a much rarer inherited condition in which there is an isolated inability to synthesize aldosterone, termed CMO type II deficiency [124,125]. This enzyme activity of the B2 isoform of 11β-OH is now termed *aldosterone synthase*. No cases have yet been found of concomitant mutations of this enzyme with the B1 isoform (that is in 11β-OH deficient patients).

3β-Hydroxysteroid dehydrogenase/ $\Delta^{5,4}$-isomerase deficiency

CLINICAL FEATURES

Classical 3β-HSD [126] is characterized by severe impairment of steroid biosynthesis in both the adrenal cortex and the gonads. This enzyme is essential for the biosynthesis of all classes of active steroids from the adrenal or gonads. A complete enzyme defect may have a fatal outcome if not treated early. Affected newborns exhibit signs and symptoms of glucocorticoid and mineralocorticoid deficiencies [127–129]. Non-salt-wasting cases have also been reported [128,130].

Impairment of androgen biosynthesis in the testes results in moderate to severe hypospadias. The testes may be undescended or palpable in the scrotal folds. Pubertal males presenting with classical 3β-HSD deficiency all show some degree of external genital ambiguity [131–134]. Hormonal testing has attempted to assess differing adrenal/gonadal and peripheral contributions to the hormonal profile [135,136].

Affected females may exhibit partial virilization (clitoral hypertrophy), due to the action of potent (Δ^4) androgens which arise from peripheral conversion of DHEA of adrenal origin, which is present in the serum in very high concentrations [130].

Late-onset 3β-HSD deficiency, which may present similarly to NC21-OHD with precocious puberty, menstrual irregularities, acne and hirsutism, has been well documented in females [85,137–139], although still not in males. It was conjectured by Bongiovanni that this disorder like the partial adrenal 21- and 11β-OH defects, would probably be revealed increasingly with improved clinical assessments of mild androgen excess states in adult women [140,141]. Very occasionally there may be clitoromegaly. A feature noted in one series of pubertal patients was that pubarche commenced before thelarche [85]. Late-onset 3β-HSD is a potential underlying basis of polycystic ovarian syndrome.

HORMONAL DIAGNOSIS

A high ratio of Δ^5- to Δ^4-steroids may be seen at or soon after birth, characterized specifically by elevated serum levels of Δ^5-steroids pregnenolone, 17-Δ^5-P and DHEA. Increased urinary excretion of the Δ^5-metabolite pregnanetriol is diagnostic for a severe 3β-HSD defect in an infant. Hepatic and renal steroid-metabolizing systems do not mature until about 6 months of age, thus the steroid profiles in newborn babies with ambiguous genitalia may not permit easy and immediate differentiation of a 3β-HSD enzyme defect from the more likely 21-hydroxylase defect [85,142].

Non-classical (late-onset) 3β-HSD deficiency

Pang *et al.* in 1985 [85] proposed biochemical criteria for establishing the presence of a non-classical (i.e. late-onset) 3β-HSD defect in adult females based on serum steroid concentrations and ratios following a 60-min ACTH stimulation test. The four parameters are:

1 17-Δ^5-P;

2 DHEA;

3 ratio: 17-Δ^5-P to 17α-hydroxyprogesterone (17-Δ^5-P:17-OHP);
4 ratio: 17-Δ^5-P to cortisol (17-Δ^5-P:F).
For confirmation of a 3β-HSD defect, all four values must be more than 2 standard deviations above the post-ACTH stimulation means. Comparable criteria for pubertal children were worked out by Temeck *et al.* [84]. Debate continues whether the criteria of Pang are too strict, since their relaxation has allowed symptomatic androgen excess conditions to be better identified and controlled in some clinical situations [139]. Another question in the non-classical 3β-HSD defect is whether it may be arising, at least in some cases, as a secondary effect from increased systemic levels of androgenic steroids evolving by some other primary endocrine imbalance, since the 3β-HSD system appears to be particularly sensitive to steroid inhibition.

GENETICS/MOLECULAR BIOLOGY

Two isozymes of the 3β-HSD enzyme have been identified by the cloning and sequencing of two genes in humans, a type I and type II gene. Transcripts encoded by the human type II 3β-HSD messenger (m)RNA species are in the adrenal, ovary and testis, while type I is the predominant 3β-HSD gene expressed in the placenta and peripheral tissues such as skin and mammary gland [143]. From comparative studies, this appears to be general in mammals; however, there is a type III isoform in the rat, and it is thought likely that there will be additional isoforms in humans and other species also [144].

The structures of the human genes encoding the type I (placental/peripheral) and type II (adrenal/gonadal) genes have been determined [5,145]. A defect in the type II gene would be expected to lead to disorders of steroidogenesis in the adrenal and gonads. Significant defects in the type I gene would be expected to manifest early as poor placental function and inadequate progesterone synthesis beyond the eighth to 10th week of pregnancy might lead to interruption of pregnancy and fetal loss [146]. If the other putative isoforms exist, mutations in these might be responsible for subtle disturbances such as cause the clinical picture in non-classical 3β-HSD defects.

Clinical genetic studies have identified missense mutations in the gene for type II 3β-HSD in patients with classical 3β-HSD deficiency [145,147–149] consistent with the enzyme activity pattern of deficient glandular and intact peripheral formation of 3-oxo-Δ^4-steroids in this form of CAH. Effects of these mutations on the kinetic properties of the 3β-HSD type II isoenzyme *in vitro* are being investigated [150]. With the exception of a heterozygous missense mutation in the type II gene found in one case (female) [151], the molecular basis of non-classical 3β-HSD deficiency has yet to be defined. The type I 3β-HSD gene has been normal in all patients tested.

Currently, no prenatal hormonal testing is diagnostic for 3β-HSD deficiency because the glandular enzyme activity is very low in the fetus, as a result of which Δ^5-steroids are non-specifically elevated. In pregnancies parented by patients in whom a specific molecular defect has been identified, molecular prenatal diagnosis may be a possibility in the future.

Steroid 17α-hydroxylase/17,20-lyase deficiency

A single protein, cytochrome $P450_{17\alpha}$, supports two enzyme activities in steroidogenesis, 17α-hydroxylation of corticosteroids and 17,20-lyase activity, converting pregnane (C_{21}) steroids to androstane (C_{19}) steroids [152,153]. The single-copy gene CYP17 appears to be transcribed identically in the adrenal cortex and in gonads of both sexes [154]. How the bifunctionality of this enzyme in regulated differently in adrenal cortex and gonadal tissues and modulated is the subject of current basic science investigations. Clinically, there are two main types of defect of this enzyme: (i) 17-OH deficiency: this could theoretically be a primary defect of the hydroxylase function alone or a combined deficiency of the 17α-hydroxylase/17,20-lyase functions; (ii) isolated deficiency of 17,20-lyase. In both cases androgen formation is compromised, and so it would be very difficult to distinguish the two possibilities. It has so far not been possible to identify an isolated deficiency of 17-OH function. The first reports of isolated sex-steroid deficiency supported the notion that 17-OH and 17,20-lyase might be different enzymes before it was conclusively established that these activities are catalysed by the single bifunctional protein, cytochrome P450.

Steroid 17-OH defect has been described in genetic females [83] and genetic males [155]. Between 100 and 120 cases of 17-OH deficiency have been described [156–159]. Cortisol synthesis is affected and this defect is thus a form of CAH. Isolated 17,20-lyase deficiency is much rarer still, having been reported in under 20 cases.

CLINICAL FEATURES

Failure of the adrenal and gonadal steroidogenic tissues to 17α-hydroxylate pregnenolone and progesterone, and subsequently to convert 17α-hydroxypregnenolone and 17-OHP by the 17,20-lyase reaction to DHEA and Δ^4-A leads to deficient production of testosterone and oestrogens [160]. The adrenal block in formation of 17-OHP, precursor to cortisol, leads to an elevation of ACTH with overproduction of 17-deoxysteroids, primarily DOC and 18-OHDOC, whose mineralocorticoid activity in turn results in low renin hypertension, hypokalaemia and metabolic alkalosis. Moderate glucocorticoid activity results in some protection against stress and limited feedback to the pituitary, as a result of which ACTH elevation may be less than in the other forms of CAH [161]. In addition, impaired production of sex hormones causes abnormalities of sexual development in both male and female patients.

Genetic males have an absence of masculinization with female external genitalia when the deficiency is complete. Since anti-Müllerian hormone is produced normally by the testis, Müllerian duct regression still takes place, so these patients have a blind vagina with absent Müllerian structures (fallopian tubes, uterus, upper third of vagina) [156,162–166]. Pubic and axillary hair is absent. Genetic females have normal genitalia at birth but present with primary amenorrhoea, lack of axillary and pubic hair and no pubertal development leading to hypoplastic breasts in adolescence.

Clinical evidence of glucocorticoid insufficiency is unusual, episodes similar to adrenal crises having been reported in only three cases despite impaired cortisol production [167,168]. The reason for this is the glucocorticoid action of corticosterone (B), serum concentrations of which may be elevated 30–60 times or more above normal. Elevation of DOC with its mineralocorticoid action probably accounts for the suppression of PRA and very low aldosterone secretion from the ZG. DOC may be the cause of hypertension, which may be very mild or very severe [165,169]. Hypertension appears at any time from early infancy to the fifth decade [167,170]. Severity of hypertension and degree of hypokalaemia may differ and do not always correlate with gonadal steroid insufficiency. This may reflect different degrees of expression of the mutant $P450_{17\alpha}$ between adrenal cortex and gonad. Other complications include tall stature, bone age retardation and osteoporosis [171]. These are relatively frequent and closely related to the reduced production of sex steroids.

HORMONAL DIAGNOSIS

Patients with 18-OHB deficiency have increased levels of B, DOC, 18-B and 18-OHDOC, subnormal levels of 17-OHP and S and suppressed aldosterone and renin [172]. The C19 steroids (DHEA and Δ^4-A) are markedly reduced, as are testosterone and oestrogen. Administration of ACTH amplifies these findings and administration of human chorionic gonadotrophin (hCG) fails to stimulate testosterone production. In addition the levels of luteinizing hormone (LH) and follicle-stimulating hormone will be elevated (hypergonadotrophic hypogonadism).

Patients with isolated 17,20-lyase deficiency may be separated by the finding of increased urinary pregnanetriolone, a metabolite of 17-OHP, which rises further after the administration of ACTH and hCG, while low levels of T and DHEA do not rise following ACTH or hCG.

Elevated levels of DOC in 17α-OH deficiency suppress plasma renin activity, which causes blood volume expansion, secondarily suppressing levels of aldosterone [173]. There are several paradoxical reports of cases in which the aldosterone is normal while the renin remains suppressed [174,175].

It should be noted that some genetic males with partial 17-OH deficiency have been reported with normal or ambiguous external genitalia [155,171,174,175] suggesting some ability to produce testosterone. Some genetic females have been reported to have normal or irregular menstruation [176], suggesting some degree of oestrogen production.

Hypertension accompanied by hypokalaemic alkalosis may be the presenting clinical picture leading to the diagnosis of this adrenal enzyme defect. The haemodynamic features of 17-OH deficiency are somewhat like those of 11β-OH deficiency in that there is overproduction of DOC and its metabolites, but in this instance 18-OHB is high and 17-OHP and S are low. Mineralocorticoid excess produces low PRA and suppression of the ZG; as a result of slow recovery of this cortical layer, aldosterone may remain low for some months after hormonal therapy begins, even though glucocorticoid administration quite promptly decreases ZF DOC production and normalizes blood volume [170].

A recent study has suggested that ACTH testing in obligate heterozygotes with 17-OH deficiency can be diagnostic [177].

GENETICS

Detection of the heterozygous state has been based on hormonal abnormalities [178]. Pedigree patterns based on DNA findings clearly show an autosomal recessive mode of transmission. Concordance between gonadal and adrenal 17-OH deficiency suggests that a structural gene defect is responsible for this syndrome.

The human $P450_{17\alpha}$ gene (CYP17) is a single-copy gene [179] and has been mapped to chromosome 10 [180]. The complementary DNA inserts of full-length $P450_{17\alpha}$ isolated from the testis and adrenal have been identical. Expression of the gene is predominantly regulated by ACTH in a cAMP-dependent manner in the adrenals [181], and by LH in the Leydig cells of the testis and theca interna of the ovary (reviewed in [182]).

Although we now know that this gene catalyses two distinct reactions required for the synthesis of cortisol and androgens (17-OH and 17,20-lyase), we cannot yet fully explain the dissociation between secretion of androgens and cortisol observed in specific physiological and clinical states, for example the developmental stage of puberty.

Molecular analysis of the gene in affected patients reveals a different mutation in almost every unrelated case. Siblings with presumably the same genetic defect have exhibited different phenotypes [159].

Cholesterol desmolase deficiency

The rate-limiting step of steroidogenesis is oxidative cleavage of a C_6 fragment from the cholesterol side-chain at position C20,22; a single cytochrome P450 responsible for this complex biochemical step, cytochrome $P450_{scc}$, has been cloned [183]. Side-chain cleavage produces pregnenolone, the common precursor essential to the biosynthesis of all mineralocorticoids, glucocorticoids and sex steroids. There are very early reports conforming with apparent inability to generate any steroids whatsoever, and the clinical picture expected from deficiency of the cholesterol desmolase enzyme. The first case reported by Prader, of a male pseudohermaphrodite with severe salt-wasting and impaired production of all adrenal cortical hormones, gave this defect the name Prader syndrome [184]. Histological examination of the adrenals at autopsy would reveal massively hyperplastic adrenals with cholesterol-laden cells, hence the disease was also termed lipoid adrenal hyperplasia [185]. Few patients have been detected [186–189]. Extended survival of some patients has been achieved on hormonal treatment [189].

In vitro assay of adrenal cortical tissue from autopsy confirmed a biochemical block between cholesterol and pregnenolone formation. Recent attempts by molecular genetic analysis to identify a mutation or mutations in the gene encoding the cytochrome $P450_{scc}$ enzyme apoprotein have, however, been unsuccessful.

TREATMENT

Hormonal therapy

The prime object of treatment is to normalize growth and development in the affected child and to maintain a normal hormonal environment in the adult. The mainstay of endocrine therapy is hormonal replacement, which provides essential hormonal functions, and suppresses adrenal overproduction of precursors. Hydrocortisone directly replaces the low or absent cortisol, providing essential glucocorticoid function (averting adrenal crisis) in all forms of CAH, and suppresses pituitary release of ACTH.

STEROID 21-HYDROXYLASE DEFICIENCY

Replacement therapy is with the smallest dose of glucocorticoid that normalizes growth velocity and the rate of physical maturation, at the same time as maintaining hormonal values within acceptable limits. Serum 17-OHP and Δ^4-A levels obtained by RIA provide the most sensitive index of biochemical control in the child and adult, but Δ^4-A values are the most useful single parameter in the adolescent. In the first instance hydrocortisone is used in the dose range of 10–20 mg/m^2 a day [190–192]. The total daily dose of hydrocortisone is usually administered two or three times daily, with the largest portion given in the morning. Although the opinion exists that the dosage schedule may not be critical [192], one recent trial claims more normal rates of growth and skeletal maturation with twice-daily rather than once-daily dosing [193]. Longer-acting forms of glucocorticoids, such as prednisone and dexamethasone, should not generally be used in infants or young children because of the long half-lives and increased incidence of growth suppression. An adult with 21-OH deficiency can, however, be treated with a single daily dose of dexamethasone which simplifies the therapeutic regime and can improve compliance.

Individual responses to therapy differ widely. Inadequate treatment and non-compliance can result in increased adrenal androgen secretion, aggravating symptoms of androgen excess and accelerating growth. This may also lead to secondary central precocious puberty. Overtreatment can result in growth suppression and all the signs and symptoms of hypercortisolism, especially striae, obesity and hypertension. It should be borne in mind that the need for treatment is life-long, not only for the patient with salt-wasting, but also for simple-virilizing patients, in whom continued glucocorticoid replacement will be of benefit in enhancing fertility and, in the adult male, in preventing the formation of adrenal rests.

In instances of salt-wasting, addition of a mineralocorticoid to the regime is necessary. The synthetic mineralocorticoid 9α-fluorocortisol (9α-fluorohydrocortisone acetate, Florinef) in a dose of 0.05–0.2 mg daily orally is suggested (0.15 mg/m^2 a day). Patients should have unlimited access to salt. Salt supplements (0.5–1 g NaCl/10 kg a day) should be added to infant formula to ensure adequate sodium intake. An increase in salt-craving is often the first sign of inadequate mineralocorticoid replacement. Some children have been observed to crave unusual foods (hot chilies, peppers, pickle juice, etc.) and demonstrate increased irritability and mood swings. These salt-cravings and behavioural responses resolve when the mineralocorticoid dose is increased.

Mineralocorticoid steroids may also be given as replacement therapy in the absence of overt salt-wasting. The renin–angiotensin–aldosterone (RAA) system and the hypothalamopituitary–adrenal axis interact, so that PRA is commonly found to be elevated in simple-virilizing patients. In these patients, Florinef is effective in lowering the PRA towards normal, and this is found to bring down ACTH levels further, resulting in better control of androgens without increase in the glucocorticoid dose [194].

Treatment of NC21-OHD (and the non-classical 3β-

HSD deficiency) is usually with low-dose, long-acting glucocorticoids, such as dexamethasone. Treatment may be augmented with the use of progestational and oestrogenic agents, which inhibit gonadotrophin release, thereby suppressing ovarian excess androgen production [195,196]. Other hormonal agents that may help to reduce androgen effects include anti-androgens spironolactone and cyproterone acetate, and the newer, more experimental, androgen receptor blocker flutamide. The aim of treatment in these patients is to minimize symptoms without giving rise to glucocorticoid side-effects. Possible use of glucocorticoids should be remembered in the case of non-classical patients free of androgen-related symptoms in whom the benefits of such treatment would include improved adult height [37] and fertility [197].

STEROID 11β-HYDROXYLASE DEFICIENCY

Treatment of 11β-OH deficiency consists of glucocorticoid therapy, which replaces cortisol, reduces adrenal over-secretion of androgens and controls hypertension by reducing serum DOC levels and normalizing serum biochemistry. The usual choice of glucocorticoid in 11β-OH deficiency is hydrocortisone, or in adults either prednisone or dexamethasone; dosage in this defect is highly variable depending on the clinical presentation. Glucocorticoid administration results in the suppression of ACTH and consequently of DOC secretion with normalization of plasma volume. Renin is released from DOC suppression, resulting in increased AII production and a rise in aldosterone levels to normal [198]. Measurement of PRA is of great use in monitoring treatment of this enzyme defect (in fact, in all forms of CAH). In contrast to the elevated PRA and the tendency to salt loss in 21-OH deficiency, PRA will be suppressed in 11β-OH deficieny because of volume expansion in the untreated state. On treatment the PRA should rise to normal, and this will indicate good control. Inadequacy of hormonal management will be signalled by lowering of the PRA.

Transitional salt-wasting may occur in 11β-OH deficiency cases starting hormonal replacement [199–201]. This reflects the fact that restoration of function of the ZG (as in the case when the entire cortex has been suppressed), involves induction of many cell factors and thus takes some time. Synthesis of aldosterone depends on induction of the intact B2 isoform of the 11β-OH enzyme. In addition to this, different lengths of duration of this transient reponse may represent diversity of other genetic factors, such as stimulatability of renin formation, inducibility of hepatic renin substrate production, and tissue expression of angiotensin-converting enzyme.

STEROID 17α-HYDROXYLASE/17,20-LYASE DEFICIENCY

The hypertension of 17-OH deficiency is similarly controlled by glucocorticoid replacement therapy, with normalization of serum DOC and hypertension. In this form of CAH, therapy is aimed principally at this feature, since the lack of cortisol is not a problem. Sex steroids must be provided to these patients, in the form of testosterone from early infancy to those with a male sex assignment, and in the form of oestrogens, starting at puberty, in patients with a female sex of assignment. In isolated 17,20-lyase deficiency, sex steroid replacement therapy only is required.

3β-HYDROXYSTEROID DEHYDROGENASE DEFICIENCY

Treatment of classical 3β-HSD deficiency in the neonate is by steroid replacement and salt. Continued management is as for salt-wasting 21-OH deficiency; that is with a combined glucocorticoid/mineralocorticoid regime with monitoring of PRA for an index of volume status. Inadequate virilization of the genetic male 3β-HSD deficiency patient requires testosterone replacement from infancy, whereas in females, in whom potent androgens formed by peripheral conversion have caused virilization, administered glucocorticoid suppresses the high adrenal precursor output.

Sex assignment

The most critical aspect of sex assignment is that it be done as soon as the relevant diagnostic information is obtained. Delay in this matter or ambiguity in the minds of the parents or the child's medical staff as to the sex of the child may cause permanent and irreparable damage in child-rearing. Parents are usually very anxious to know the sex of their child so that a name can be given. They should not be encouraged to give an ambiguous name while a sex assignment is being sought.

In cases of 21-OH and 11β-OH in genetic females, female sex assignment is the rule, as these individuals have entirely normal female internal sex organs and a reasonably good chance of successfully bearing children. The experience in one series indicated that 64% of female patients with 21-OHD starting therapy between the ages of 6 and 20 years were fertile [202]. If clitoromegaly is not severe, the relative size of the clitoris may become less prominent with age and, if the family is receptive, surgery may not always be necessary. Vaginal reconstruction may be required at some point.

In cases of 3β-HSD deficiency, 17-OH deficiency and cholesterol desmolase deficiency, any of which results in inadequate masculinization in a genetic male, sex assignment will depend in large part on whether the phallic anatomy after surgical reconstruction will ultimately allow urination in the standing position, and intromission in sexual intercourse. If the decision is made to rear the child as a female, gonadectomy and creation of a vagina are performed. Secondary sexual characteristics can be induced during puberty by the administration of oestrogens in the case of a female assignment or androgens in the case of male assignment.

Surgical therapy

In females with virilizing CAH, surgical correction of an enlarged clitoris or a urogenital sinus is often required. The first stage is clitoral recession, which involves 'tucking' a portion of the erectile tissue under the symphysis pubis [203]. The conventional view is that this should be done by the age of 18 months to avoid later confusion over gender identity. If it is thought that this delay may prejudice the family's attitude towards the girl child (some parents feel very strongly regarding this), clitoral recession can be done as early as 6 months of age.

Keeping the number of surgical procedures to a minimum will have a favourable effect on psychological adjustment. The principal aims of surgery are to reduce clitoral size, create a vaginal orifice that will allow menstrual flow and be adequate for intercourse, and to correct the urogenital sinus and vaginal pouch to prevent urinary incontinence. While early clitoroplasty is a desirable goal, vaginoplasty should be delayed if possible until physical maturity. Prevention of introital restenosis may require regular dilation with mechanical dilators if the young woman is not sexually active, or does not become sexually active soon after vaginal reconstructive surgery. Recent retrospective analyses of long-term results of vaginal reconstruction in 42 women with virilizing CAH found that the success of this procedure, rated as the ability to have intercourse without discomfort, was lowest when the vaginal repair was performed at less than 4 years of age [204]. The success rate was lower among salt-wasting patients.

In males inadequately masculinized (17-OH deficiency, 3β-HSD deficiency, and cholesterol desmolase deficiency) who have been given a female sex assignment, undescended testes should be removed because of the high frequency of tumour formation [205].

Psychological problems

Short stature may cause some patients psychological and emotional problems but, more often, problems arise secondary to genital ambiguity and surgery. Ideally all children born with genital ambiguity, and their parents, should be under the care of a psychiatrist or psychologist experienced in such cases. Times of emotional crisis for these families are the newborn period and adolescence. Girls with virilizing forms of CAH may have confusion of gender role and gender identity [206,207]. In these patients there is a high rate of homosexuality, lack of sexual activity, low rate of marriage and decreased rate of child-bearing [204,208]. Patients with simple-virilizing CAH appear to have fewer problems than those with salt-wasting disease [204,209,210]. It is not yet known how significant child-rearing practices and postnatal control of androgen levels may be in contributing to later sexual orientation.

Genetic males who are undervirilized but have been reared as males may require multiple genital reconstructive surgeries throughout childhood, and may well have difficulties with sexual function later in life. Little has yet been documented about this group.

CONCLUSION

Congenital adrenal hyperplasia may present in the newborn period with either ambiguous or normal genitalia, depending on the sex of the patient and the steroidogenic enzyme defect responsible for the patient's disease. In the most commonly diagnosed form of CAH the 21-OH enzyme is defective, resulting in insufficient cortisol production, lack of negative feedback inhibition to the hypothalamus and pituitary, and consequent overstimulation of the adrenal gland, resulting in excess secretion of androgens, whose formation does not involve 21-hydroxylation. Thus, females undergo virilization in prenatal life and are born with a variable degree of genital ambiguity, while males have normal genitalia at birth. Over two-thirds of patients with 21-OH deficiency have the salt-wasting trait, which may not be solely related to the severity of the mutation at the active HLA-linked 21-OH locus on chromosome 6.

Late-onset forms of adrenal hyperplasia are recognized, and tend to be more polymorphic in their clinical manifestations. NC21-OHD is an allelic variant of the classical disorder, with mild elevation of hormonal precursors and a phenotype which ranges from no apparent clinical abnormality to precocious adrenarche to hirsutism, oligomenorrhoea and infertility. The frequency of the non-classical disorder is approximately 100 times the frequency of the classical 21-OH deficiency in the general Caucasian population.

Treatment of CAH involves replacement of cortisol and, if necessary, mineralocorticoid replacement and/or salt supplementation. Longitudinal care of patients must include careful attention to adrenocortical hormone levels, growth, sexual maturation and psychosexual status.

Prenatal diagnosis may be reliably performed by molecular analysis of 21-OH gene status, and prenatal treatment may be undertaken with dexamethasone. Early results of prenatal therapy are promising for the amelioration of genital ambiguity in female fetuses. Future investigations in this field will involve the molecular genetic identification of the mutations responsible for each clinical syndrome.

REFERENCES

1 New MI, Levine LS. Congenital adrenal hyperplasia. In: Harris H, Hirschhorn K, eds. *Advances in Human Genetics*, Vol. 4. London: Plenum Press, 1973:251–326.

2 White PC. Steroid 21-hydroxylase. In: Schenkman JB, Greim H, eds. *Cytochrome P-450. Handbooks in Experimental Pharmacology*, Vol. 105. New York: Springer Verlag, 1993: 693–703.

3 Omura T. Localization of cytochrome P-450 in membranes: mitochondria. In: Schenkman JB, Greim H, eds. *Cytochrome P-450. Handbooks in Experimental Pharmacology*, Vol. 105. New York: Springer Verlag, 1993:61–9.

4 Dupont B, Oberfield SE, Smithwick EM, Lee TD, Levine LS. Close genetic linkage between HLA and congenital adrenal hyperplasia (21-hydroxylase deficiency). *Lancet* 1977;2: 1309–11.

5 Rhéaume E, Simard J, Morel Y *et al.* Congenital adrenal hyperplasia due to point mutations in the type II 3β-hydroxysteroid dehydrogenase gene. *Nature Genet* 1992;1: 239–45.

6 Levine LS, New MI. Recent advances in 21-hydroxylase deficiency. *Annu Rev Med* 1984;35:649–63.

7 New MI, White PC, Pang S, Dupont B, Speiser PW. The adrenal hyperplasias. In: Scriver CR, Beaudet AL, Sly WS, Valle D, eds. *The Metabolic Basis of Inherited Disease*, 6th edn. New York: McGraw-Hill, 1989:1881–917.

8 Pang S, Wallace MA, Hofman L *et al.* Worldwide experience in newborn screening for classical congenital adrenal hyperplasia due to 21-hydroxylase deficiency. *Pediatrics* 1988;81: 866–74.

9 Pang S, Clark A. Congenital adrenal hyhperplasia due to 21-hydroxylase deficiency: newborn screening and its relationship to the diagnosis and treatment of the disorder. *Screening* 1993;2:105–39.

10 Speiser PW, Düpont B, Rubinstein P, Piazza A, Kaštelan A, New MI. High frequency of nonclassical steroid 21-hydroxylase deficiency. *Am J Hum Genet* 1985;37:650–67.

11 Sherman SL, Aston CE, Morton NE, Speiser PW, New MI. A segregation and linkage study of classical and nonclassical 21-hydroxylase deficiency. *Am J Hum Genet* 1988;42: 830–8.

12 Dumić M, Brkljacić L, Speiser PW *et al.* An update on the frequency of nonclassical deficiency of 21-hydroxylase in the Yugoslav population. *Acta Endocrinol* 1990;122:703–10.

13 Zerah M, Pang S, New MI. Morning salivary 17-hydroxyprogesterone is a useful screening test for nonclassical 21-hydroxylase deficiency. *J Clin Endocrinol Metab* 1987;65: 227–32.

14 Reyland ME. Protein kinase C is a tonic negative regulator of steroidogenesis and steroid hydroxylase gene expression in Y1 adrenal cells and functions independently of protein kinase A. *Mol Endocrinol* 1993;7:1021–30.

15 Aguilera G, Catt KJ. Regulation of aldosterone secretion by the renin–angiotensin system. *Proc Natl Acad Sci USA* 1978;75:4057–62.

16 Zuber MX, John ME, Okanana T, Simpson ER, Waterman MR. Bovine adrenocortical cytochrome P-450 17α: regulation of gene expression by ACTH and elucidation of primary sequence. *J Biol Chem* 1986;261:2475–82.

17 Wilkins L. Adrenal disorders. II. Congenital virilizing adrenal hyperplasia. *Arch Dis Child* 1962;37:231–41.

18 Lebovitz RM, Pauli RM, Laxovar R. Delayed diagnosis in congenital adrenal hyperplasia: need for newborn screening. *Am J Dis Child* 1984;138:571–3.

19 Pescovitz OH, Comite F, Cassorla F *et al.* True precocious puberty complicating congenital adrenal hyperplasia: treatment with a luteinizing hormone-releasing hormone analog. *J Clin Endocrinol Metab* 1984;58:857–61.

20 Cutfield RG, Batemen JM, Odell WD. Infertility caused by bilateral testicular masses secondary to congenital adrenal hyperplasia (21-hydroxylase deficiency). *Fertil Steril* 1983; 40:809–14.

21 Chrousos GP, Loriaux DL, Sherins RJ, Cutler GB Jr. Bilateral testicular enlargement resulting from inapparent 21-hydroxylase deficiency. *J Urol* 1981;126:127–8.

22 Kohn B, Levine LS, Pollack MS *et al.* Late-onset steroid 21-hydroxylase deficiency: a variant of classical congenital adrenal hyperplasia. *J Clin Endocrinol Metab* 1982;55: 817–27.

23 Chrousos GP, Loriaux DL, Mann DL, Cutler GB. Late-onset 21-hydroxylase deficiency mimicking idiopathic hirsutism or polycystic ovarian disease. An allelic variant of congenital virilizing adrenal hyperplasia with a milder enzymatic defect. *Ann Intern Med* 1982;96:143–8.

24 Kuttenn F, Couillin P, Girard F *et al.* Late-onset adrenal hyperplasia in hirsutism. *N Engl J Med* 1985;313:224–31.

25 Kuttenn F. Late onset adrenal hyperplasia (response to letters to the editor). *N Engl J Med* 1986;3145:450–1.

26 Rose LI, Newmark SR, Strauss JS, Pochi PE. Adrenocortical hydroxylase deficiencies in acne vulgaris. *J Invest Dermatol* 1976;66:324–6.

27 Rose LI, Birnbaum MD. Therapy of adrenocortical hydroxylase deficiencies in acne vulgaris. *Int J Dermatol* 1979; 18:386–9.

28 Rosenwaks Z, Lee PA, Jones GS, Migeon CJ, Wentz AC. An attenuated form of congenital virilizing adrenal hyperplasia. *J Clin Endocrinol Metab* 1979;49:335–9.

29 Kauschansky A, Kaufman H, Zamir R, Elian E. Late-onset adrenal hyperplasia (21-hydroxylase deficiency): 17α-hydroxyprogesterone response to ACTH stimulation and HLA typing. *Horm Res* 1981;14:73–8.

30 Migeon CJ, Rosenwaks Z, Lee PA, Urban MD, Bias WB. The attenuated form of congenital adrenal hyperplasa as an allelic form of 21-hydroxylase deficiency. *J Clin Endocrinol Metab* 1980;51:647–9.

31 Futterweit W. *Polycystic Ovarian Disease.* Berlin: Springer Verlag, 1984.

32 Greenblatt RB. Cortisone in treatment of hirsute women. *Am J Obstet Gynecol* 1953;66:700–10.

33 Jones GES, Howard JE, Langford H. The use of cortisone in follicular phase disturbances. *Fertil Steril* 1953;4:49–62.

34 Jones HW Jr, Jones GES. The gynecological aspects of adrenal hyperplasia and allied disorders. *Am J Obstet Gynecol* 1954; 68:1330–65.

35 Auchterlonie IA, Cameron J, Wallace AM, Rudd BT, Hudson M, Smith PJ. Prepubertal gynecomastia as the presenting feature of late-onset 21-hydroxylase deficiency. *Horm Res* 1985;22:94–9.

36 Dewailly D, Vantyghem-Haudiquet M-C, Sainsard C *et al.* Clinical and biological phenotypes in late-onset 21-hydroxylase deficiency. *J Clin Endocrinol Metab.* 1986;63: 418–23.

37 New MI, Gertner JM, Speiser PW, del Balzo P. Growth and final height in congenital adrenal hyperplasia (classical 21-hydroxylase deficiency) and in non-classical 21-hydroxylase deficiency. In: Carallo I, Job JC, New MI, eds. *Growth Disorders: the State of the Art.* New York: Raven Press, 1991;81:105–10.

38 Speiser PW, Serrat J, New MI, Gertner JM. Insulin sensitivity

in adrenal hyperplasia due to non-classical steroid 21-hydroxylase deficiency. *J Clin Endocrinol Metab* 1992; 75:1421–4.

39 New MI, Lorenzen F, Lerner AJ *et al.* Genotyping steroid 21-hydroxylase deficiency: hormonal reference data. *J Clin Endocrinol Metab* 1983;57:320–6.

40 Abraham GE, Swerdloff RS, Tulchinsky D, Hopper K, Odell WD. Radioimmunoassay of plasma 17α-hydroxyprogesterone. *J Clin Endocrinol Metab* 1971;33:42–5.

41 New MI, Seaman MP. Secretion rates of cortisol and aldosterone precursors in various forms of congenital adrenal hyperplasia. *J Clin Endocrinol Metab* 1970;30:361–71.

42 Gandy HM, Keutmann EH, Izzo J. Characterization of urinary steroids in adrenal hyperplasia: isolation of metabolites of cortisol, compound S, and deoxycorticosterone from a normotensive patient with adrenogenital syndrome. *J Clin Invest* 1960;39:364–77.

43 Blunck W. Die α-ketolischen Cortisol- und Corticosteronmetaboliten sowie die 11-Oxy- und 11-Desoxy-17-ketosteroide im Urin von Kindern. *Acta Endocrinol* (Suppl.) 1968;134:9–112.

44 Decourt J, Jayle MF, Baulieu EE. Virilisme cliniquement tardif avec excretion de pregnanetriol et insuffiscance de la production de cortisol. *Ann Endocrinol (Paris)* 1957;18: 416–22.

45 Rosenbloom AL, Smith DW. Congenital adrenal hyperplasia. *Lancet* 1966;1:660.

46 Stoner E, DiMartino J, Kuhnle U, Levine LS, Oberfield SE, New MI. Is salt wasting in congenital adrenal hyperplasia genetic? *Clin Endocrinol* 1986;24:9–20.

47 Sinnott PJ, Dyer PA, Price DA, Harris R, Strachan T. 21-hydroxylase deficiency families with HLA-identical affected and unaffected sibs. *J Med Genet* 1989;26:10–17.

48 Pang S, Hotchkiss J, Drash AL, Levine LS, New MI. Microfilter paper method for 17α-hydroxyprogesterone radioimmunoassay: its application for rapid screening for congenital adrenal hyperplasia. *J Clin Endocrinol Metab* 1977;45: 1003–8.

49 Pang S, Spence DA, New MI. Newborn screening for congenital adrenal hyperplasia with special reference to screening in Alaska. *Ann NY Acad Sci* 1985;458:90–102.

50 Kalaitzoglou G, New MI. Sluggish response to adrenocorticotropin stimulation in newborns with 21-hydroxylase deficiency (CAH). Proceedings, 4th Joint Meeting LWPES/ESPE, 3–7 June 1993, San Francisco. *Pediatr Res* 1993;33:92.

51 Childs B, Grumbach M, van Wyk JJ. Virilizing adrenal hyperplasia: a genetic and hormonal study. *J Clin Invest* 1956;35: 213–22.

52 Levine LS, Zachmann Z, New MI *et al.* Genetic mapping of the 21-hydroxylase deficiency gene within the HLA linkage group. *N Engl J Med* 1978;299:911–15.

53 New MI. HLA and adrenal disease. In: Farid N, ed. *Immunogenetics of Endocrine Disorders*, 2nd edn. New York: Alan R. Liss, 1988;309–44.

54 Kaštelan A, Brkljacic-Surkalovic Lj, Dumic M. The HLA associations in congenital adrenal hyperplasia due to 21-hydroxylase deficiency in a Yugoslav population. *Ann NY Acad Sci* 1985;458:41–5.

55 White PC, New MI, Dupont B. Cloning and expression of cDNA encoding a bovine adrenal cytochrome P-450 specific for steroid 21-hydroxylation. *Proc Natl Acad Sci USA* 1984; 81:1986–90.

56 White PC, New MI, Dupont B. HLA-linked congenital adrenal hyperplasia results from a defective gene encoding a cytochrome P-450 specific for steroid 21-hydroxylation. *Proc Natl Acad Sci USA* 1984;7505–9.

57 Carroll MC, Campbell RD, Porter RR. Mapping of 21-hydroxylase genes adjacent to complement component C4 genes in HLA, the major histocompatibility complex in man. *Proc Natl Acad Sci USA* 1985;82:521–5.

58 White PC, Grosberger D, Onufer BJ. Two genes encoding steroid 21-hydroxylase are located near the genes encoding the fourth component of complement in man. *Proc Natl Acad Sci USA* 1985;82:1089–93.

59 Higashi Y, Yoshioka H, Yamane M, Gotoh O, Fujii-Kuriyama Y. Complete nucleotide sequence of two steroid 21-hydroxylase genes tandemly arranged in human chromosome: a pseudogene and a genuine gene. *Proc Natl Acad Sci USA* 1986;83:2841–5.

60 White PC, New MI, Dupont B. Structure of the human steroid 21-hydroxylase genes. *Proc Natl Acad Sci USA* 1986; 83:5111–15.

61 White PC, Vitek A, Dupont B, New MI. Characterization of frequent deletions causing steroid 21-hydroxylase deficiency. *Proc Natl Acad Sci USA* 1988;85:4436–40.

62 Higashi Y, Tanae A, Inoue H, Hiromasa T, Fujii-Kuriyama Y. Aberrant splicing and missense mutations cause steroid 21-hydroxylase [P450c21] deficiency in humans. *Proc Natl Acad Sci USA* 1988;85:7486–90.

63 Globerman H, Amor M, Parker KL, New MI, White PC. Nonsense mutation causing steroid 21-hydroxylase deficiency. *J Clin Invest* 1988;82:139–44.

64 Werkmeister JW, New MI, Dupont B, White PC. Frequent deletion and duplication of the steroid 21-hydroxylase genes. *Am J Hum Genet* 1985;39:461–9.

65 Donohoue P, Van Dop C, McLean RH, White PC, Jospe M, Migeon CJ. Gene conversion in salt-losing congenital adrenal hyperplasia with absent complement C4B protein. *J Clin Endocrinol Metab* 1986;62:995–1002.

66 Wedell A, Luthman H. Steroid 21-hydroxylase deficiency: two additional mutations in salt-wasting disease and rapid screening of disease-causing mutations. *Hum Mol Genet* 1993;2:499–504.

67 Tajima T, Fujieda K, Fujii-Kuriyama Y. *De novo* mutation causes steroid 21-hydroxylase deficiency in one family of HLA-identical affected and unaffected siblings. *J Clin Endocrinol Metab* 1993;77:86–9.

68 Heitmancik JF, Black S, Harris S *et al.* Congenital 21-hydroxylase deficiency as a new deletion mutation: detection in a proband during subsequent prenatal diagnosis by HLA typing and DNA analysis. *Hum Immunol* 1992;35:246–52.

69 Collier S, Tassabehji M, Strachan T. A *de novo* pathological point mutation at the 21-hydroxylase locus: implications for gene conversion in the human genome. *Nature Genet* 1993; 3:260–5.

70 Strachan T. Molecular pathology of congenital adrenal hyperplasia. *Clin Endocrinol (Oxf)* 1990;32:373–93.

71 Owerbach D, Crawford YM, Draznin MB. Direct analysis of CYP21 B genes in 21-hydroxylase deficiency using polymerase chain reaction amplification. *Mol Endocrinol* 1990; 4:125–31.

72 Amor M, Parker KL, Globerman H, New MI, White PC. Mutation in the CYP21B gene ($Ile_{172} \rightarrow Asn$) causes steroid 21-hydroxylase deficiency. *Proc Natl Acad Sci USA* 1988; 85:1600–4.

73 Speiser PW, Agdere L, Ueshiba H, White PC, New MI. Aldosterone synthesis in salt-wasting congenital adrenal hyperplasia with complete absence of adrenal 21-hydroxylase. *N Engl J Med* 1991;324:145–9.

74 Chiou SH, Hu MC, Chung B-C. A missense mutation at Ile-

172 to Asn or Arg-356 to Trp causes steroid 21-hydroxylase deficiency. *J Biol Chem* 1990;265:3549–52.
75 Speiser PW, Dupont J, Zhu DG *et al.* Disease expression and molecular genotype in congenital adrenal hyperplasia due to 21-hydroxylase deficiency. *J Clin Invest* 1992;90:584–95.
76 Greggio NA, Cameran M, Rigon F *et al.* The same molecular genotype may express different disease phenotypes in 21-hydroxylase deficiency. Proceedings of the 43rd Annual Meeting, American Society of Human Genetics, New Orleans. *Am J Hum Genet* (Suppl.) 1993;53:905 (Abstr.).
77 Speiser PW, New MI, White PC. Molecular genetic analysis of nonclassic steroid 21-hydroxylase deficiency associated with HLA-B14,DR1. *N Engl J Med* 1988;319:19–23.
78 Tusie-Luna M-T, Traktman P, White PC. Determination of functional effects of mutations in the steroid 21-hydroxylase gene (CYP21) using recombinant vaccinia virus. *J Biol Chem* 1990;265:20916–22.
79 Hurwitz A, Brautbar C, Milwidsky A *et al.* Combined 21- and 11β-hydroxylase deficiency in familial congenital adrenal hyperplasia. *J Clin Endocrinol Metab* 1985;60: 631–8.
80 Newmark S, Dluhy RG, Williams GH, Pochi P, Rose L. Partial 11- and 21-hydroxylase deficiencies in hirsute women. *Am J Obstet Gynecol* 1977;127:594–8.
81 Elder-Geva T, Hurwitz A, Vecsei P, Halti Z, Milwidsky A, Rosler A. Secondary biosynthetic defects in women with late-onset congenital adrenal hyperplasia. *N Engl J Med* 1990;323:855–63.
82 Biglieri EG, Herron MA, Brust N. 17-Hydroxylase deficiency in man. *J Clin Invest* 1966;45:1946–54.
83 Gunn S, Therrell B, Owerbach D. Nonclassical congenital adrenal hyperplasia mutation frequencies in the Texas newborn population. In: *Proceedings, Endocrine Society 75th Annual Meeting*, Las Vegas, NV, 1993:301 (Abstr. 1001).
84 Temeck JW, Pang S, New MI. Genetic defects of steroidogenesis in premature pubarche. *J Clin Endocrinol Metab* 1987;64:609–17.
85 Pang S, Lerner A, Stoner E, Levine LS, Oberfield SE, New MI. Late-onset adrenal steroid 3β-HSD deficiency: a cause of hirsutism in pubertal and postpubertal women. *J Clin Endocrinol Metab* 1985;60:428–39.
86 Jeffcoate TNA, Fleigner JRH, Russell SH, Davis JC, Wade AP. Diagnosis of the adrenogenital syndrome before birth. *Lancet* 1965;2:553.
87 Merkatz IR, New MI, Seaman MP. Prenatal diagnosis of adrenogenital syndrome by amniocentesis. *J Pediatr* 1969; 75:977–82.
88 Frasier SD, Thorneycroft IH, Weiss BA, Horton R. Elevated amniotic fluid concentration of 17α-OHP in CAH. *J Pediatr* 1975;86:310–12.
89 Pollack MS, Carroll MC, Black S *et al.* Congenital 21-hydroxylase deficiency as a new mutation: detection during prenatal diagnosis by HLA typing and DNA analysis. *Hum Immunol* 1986;17:183 (Abstr.).
90 Pang S, Pollack MS, Loo M *et al.* Pitfalls of prenatal diagnosis of 21-hydroxylase deficiency congenital adrenal hyperplasia. *J Clin Endocrinol Metab* 1985;61:89–97.
91 Speiser PW, Laforgia N, Kato K *et al.* First trimester prenatal treatment and molecular genetic diagnosis of congenital adrenal hyperplasia (21-hydroxylase deficiency). *J Clin Endocrinol Metab* 1990;70:838–48.
92 Forest MG, Bétuel H, David M. Prenatal treatment in CAH due to 21-hydroxylase deficiency: update 88 of the French multicenter experience. *Endocr Res* 1989;15:277–301.
93 New MI. Prenatal diagnosis and treatment of adrenogenital syndrome. *Dev Pharmacol Ther* 1990;15:200–10.
94 Shepard TH. *Catalog of Teratogenic Agents*, 5th edn. Baltimore, MD: Johns Hopkins University Press, 1986.
95 Goldman AJ, Shapiro BH, Katsumata M. Human fetal palatal corticoid receptors and teratogens for cleft palate. *Nature* 1978;272:464–6.
96 Goldman AJ. Biochemical mechanism of glucocorticoid and phenytoin-induced cleft palate. *Curr Top Dev Biol* 1984;19: 217–39.
97 Pang S, Clark AT, Freeman LC *et al.* Maternal side effects of prenatal dexamethasone therapy for fetal congenital adrenal hyperplasia. *J Clin Endocrinol Metab* 1992;75:249–53.
98 Rösler A, Leiberman E. Enzymatic defects of steroidogenesis: 11β-hydroxylase deficiency congenital adrenal hyperplasia. In: New MI, Levine LS, eds. *Adrenal Diseases in Childhood. Pediatric and Adolescent Endocrinology*, Vol. 13. Basel: Karger, 1984:47–71.
99 Rösler A, Leiberman E, Sack J *et al.* Clinical variability of congenital adrenal hyperplasia due to 11β-hydroxylase deficiency. *Horm Res* 1982;16:133–41.
100 Zachmann M, Tassinari D, Prader A. Clinical and biochemical variability of congenital adrenal hyperplasia due to 11β-OHD. A study of 25 patients. *J Clin Endocrinol Metab* 1983;56:222–30.
101 Birnbaum MD, Rose LI. Late-onset adrenocortical hydroxylase deficiencies associated with menstrual dysfunction. *Obstet Gynecol* 1984:63:445.
102 Cathelineau G, Brerault JL, Fiet J, Julien R, Dreux C, Canivet J. Adrenocortical 11β-hydroxylation defect in adult women with postmenarchial onset of symptoms. *J Clin Endocrinol Metab* 1980;51:287–91.
103 Gabrilove JL, Sharma DC, Dorfman R. Adrenocortical 11β-hydroxylase deficiency and virilism first manifest in the adult woman. *N Engl J Med* 1965;272:1189–94.
104 Gregory T, Gardner L. Hypertensive virilizing adrenal hyperplasia with minimal impairment of synthetic route to cortisol. *J Clin Endocrinol Metab* 1976;43:769–74.
105 Rapp JP, Dahl LK. Mendelian inheritance of 18- and 11β-steroid hydroxylase activities in the adrenal of rats genetically susceptible or resistant to hypertension. *Endocrinology* 1972;90:1435–46.
106 Ulick S. Adrenocortical factors in hypertension. I. Significance of 18-hydroxy-11-deoxycorticosterone. *Am J Cardiol* 1976;38:814–24.
107 Wada A, Okamoto M, Nonaka Y, Yamano T. Aldosterone synthesis by a reconstituted cytochrome P-45011 beta system. *Biochem Biophys Res Commun* 1984;119:365–71.
108 Yanagibashi K, Hanio M, Shively JE, Shen WH, Hall PE. The synthesis of aldosterone by the adrenal cortex: two zones (fasciculata and glomerulosa) possess one enzyme for 11β-18-hydroxylation and aldehyde synthesis. *J Biol Chem* 1986; 261:3556–62.
109 Levine LS, Rauh W, Gottesdiener K *et al.* New studies of the 11β-hydroxylase and 18-hydroxylase enzymes in the hypertensive form of congenital adrenal hyperplasia. *J Clin Endocrinol Metab* 1980;50:258–63.
110 Curnow KM, Tusie-Luna M-T, Pascoe L *et al.* The product of the CYP11B2 gene is required for aldosterone biosynthesis in the human adrenal cortex. *Mol Endocrinol* 1991;5:1513–22.
111 Eberlein WR, Bongiovanni AM. Plasma and urinary corticosteroids in the hypertensive form of congenital adrenal hyperplasia. *J Biol Chem* 1956;223:85–94.
112 Glenthøj A, Nielsen MD, Starup J. Congenital adrenal hyper-

plasia due to 11β-hydroxylase deficiency: final diagnosis in adult age in three patients. *Acta Endocrinol* 1980;93:94–9.

113 Glenthøj A, Nielsen MD, Starup J, Svejgaard A. HLA and CAH due to 11-hydroxylase deficiency. *Tissue Antigens* 1979;14:181–2.

114 Green OC, Migeon CJ, Wilkins L. Urinary steroids in the hypertensive form of congenital adrenal hyperplasia. *J Clin Endocrinol Metab* 1960;20:929–46.

115 Perera GA, Knowlton AI, Lowell A, Loeb RF. Effect of deoxycorticosterone acetate on the blood pressure of man. *J Am Med Assoc* 1944;125:1030–5.

116 Mornet E, Dupont J, Vitek A, White PC. Characterization of two genes encoding human steroid 11β-hydroxylase (P45011β). *J Biol Chem* 1989;264:20961–7.

117 Chua SC, Szabo P, Vitek A, Grzeschik KH, John M, White PC. Cloning of cDNA encoding steroid 11β-hydroxylase (P450c11). *Proc Natl Acad Sci USA* 1987;84:7193–7.

118 Kawamoto T, Mitsuuchi Y, Ohnishi T *et al.* Cloning and expression of a cDNA for human cytochrome $P450_{aldo}$ as related to primary aldosteronism. *Biochem Biophys Res Commun* 1990;173:309–16.

119 Ogishima T, Shibata H, Shimada H *et al.* Aldosterone synthase cytochrome P450 expressed in the adrenal of patients with primary aldosteronism. *J Biol Chem* 1991;266: 10731–4.

120 White PC, Dupont J, New MI, Leiberman E, Hochberg Z, Rösler A. A mutation in CYP11B (Arg-448 → His) associated with steroid 11β-hydroxylase deficiency in Jews of Moroccan origin. *J Clin Invest* 1991;87:1664–7.

121 Curnow KM, Vitek A, Dupont J, White PC. Point mutations in CYP11B1 causing steroid 11β-hydroxylase deficiency. *Clin Res* 1992;40:310A (Abstr.).

122 Helmberg A, Ausserer B, Kofler R. Frameshift by insertion of two base pairs in codon 394 of CYP11B1 causes congenital adrenal hyperplasia due to steroid 11β-hydroxylase deficiency. *J Clin Endocrinol Metab* 1992;75:1278–81.

123 Curnow KM, Slutsker L, Vitek J *et al.* Mutations in the CYP11B1 gene causing congenital adrenal hyperplasia and hypertension cluster in exons 6, 7, and 8. *Proc Natl Acad Sci USA* 1993;90:4552–6.

124 Ulick S, Gautier E, Vetter KK, Markello JR, Yaffe S, Lowe CU. An aldosterone biosynthetic defect in a salt-losing disorder (letter). *J Clin Endocrinol Metab* 1964;24:669–72.

125 Pascoe L, Curnow KM, Slutsker L, Rösler A, White PC. CYP11B2 (aldosterone synthase) gene causing corticosterone methyloxidase II deficiency. *Proc Natl Acad Sci USA* 1992; 89:4996–5000.

126 Bongiovanni AM. The adrenogenital syndrome with deficiency of 3β-hydroxysteroid dehydrogenase. *J Clin Invest* 1962;41:2086–92.

127 Hamilton W, Brush MG. Four clinical variants of congenital adrenal hyperplasia. *Arch Dis Child* 1964;39:66–72.

128 Kogut MD. Adrenogenital syndrome. *Am J Dis Child* 1965; 110:562–5.

129 Cathro DM, Birchall K, Mitchell FL, Forsyth CC. 3β:21-dihydroxy-pregn-5-ene-20-ene in urine of normal human infants and in third day urine of child with deficiency of 3β-hydroxysteroid dehydrogenase. *Arch Dis Child* 1965;40: 251–60.

130 Pang S, Levine LS, Stoner E *et al.* Nonsalt-losing congenital adrenal hyperplasia due to 3β-hydroxysteroid dehydrogenase deficiency with normal glomerulosa function. *J Clin Endocrinol Metab* 1983;56:808–18.

131 Zachmann M, Völlmin JA, Mürset G, Curtius H-C, Prader A. Unusual type of congenital adrenal hyperplasia probably due to deficiency of 3β-hydroxysteroid dehydrogenase. Case report of a surviving girl and steroid studies. *J Clin Endocrinol Metab* 1970;30:719–26.

132 Jänne O, Perheentupa J, Vihko R. Plasma and urinary steroids in an eight year old boy with 3β-hydroxysteroid dehydrogenase deficiency. *J Clin Endocrinol Metab* 1970;31: 162–5.

133 Kenny FM, Reynolds JW, Green OC. Partial 3β-hydroxysteroid dehydrogenase (3β-HSD) deficiency in a family with congenital adrenal hyperplasia: evidence for increasing 3β-HSD activity with age. *Pediatrics* 1971;48:756–65.

134 Parks GA, Bermudez JA, Anast CS, Bongiovanni AM, New MI. Pubertal boy with the 3β-hydroxysteroid dehydrogenase defect. *J Clin Endocrinol Metab* 1971;33:269–78.

135 Schneider G, Genel M, Bongiovanni AM, Goldman AS, Rosenfield RL. Persistent testicular Δ^5-isomerase-3β-hydroxysteroid dehydrogenase (Δ^5-3β-HSD) deficiency in the Δ^5-3β-HSD form of congenital adrenal hyperplasia. *J Clin Invest* 1975;55:681–90.

136 de Peretti E, Forest MG, Feit JP, David M. Endocrine studies in two children with male pseudohermaphroditism due to 3β-hydroxysteroid dehydrogenase defect. In: Genazzani AR, Thijssen JHH, Siiteri PK, eds. *Adrenal Androgens.* New York: Raven Press, 1980:141–5.

137 Rosenfield RL, Rich BH, Wolfsdorf JI *et al.* Pubertal presentation of congenital delta-5-3-beta-hydroxysteroid dehydrogenase deficiency. *J Clin Endocrinol Metab* 1980;51: 345–53.

138 Medina M, Herrera J, Florez M, Martin O, Bermudez JA, Zarate A. Normal ovarian function in a mild form of late-onset 3β-hydroxysteroid dehydrogenase deficiency. *Fertil Steril* 1986:46:1021–5.

139 Schram P, Zerah M, Mani P, Jewelewicz R, Jaffe S, New MI. Nonclassical 3β-hydroxylsteroid dehydrogenase deficiency: a review of our experience with 25 female patients. *Fertil Steril* 1992;58:129–36.

140 Bongiovanni AM. The response of several adrenocortical steroids to the administration of ACTH in hirsute women. *J Steroid Biochem* 1983;18:745–7.

141 Bongiovanni AM. Congenital adrenal hyperplasia due to 3β-hydroxysteroid dehydrogenase deficiency. In: New MI, Levine LS, eds. *Adrenal Diseases in Childhood. Pediatric and Adolescent Endocrinology*, Vol. 13. Basel: Karger, 1984: 72–82.

142 Cara JF, Moshang T, Bongiovanni AM, Marx BS. Elevated 17-hydroxyprogesterone and testosterone in a newborn with 3β-hydroxysteroid dehydrogenase deficiency. *N Engl J Med* 1985;313:618–21.

143 Rhéaume E, Lachance Y, Zhao HF *et al.* Structure and expression of a new cDNA encoding the almost exclusive 3β-hydroxysteroid dehydrogenase/$\Delta^{5,4}$-isomerase in human adrenals and gonads. *Mol Endocrinol* 1991;5:1147–57.

144 Labrie F, Simard J, Luu-The V, Bélanger A, Pelletier G. Structure, function and tissue-specific gene expression of 3β-hydroxysteroid dehydrogenase/5-ene-4-ene isomerase enzymes in classical and peripheral intracrine steroidogenic tissues. *J Steroid Biochem Mol Biol* 1992;43:805–26.

145 Labrie F, Simard J, Luu-The V *et al.* Structure and tissue-specific expression of 3β-hydroxysteroid dehydrogenase/5-ene-4-ene-isomerase genes in human and rat classical and peripheral steroidogenic tissues. *J Steroid Biochem Mol Biol* 1992;41:421–35.

146 Milewich L, Shaw CE, Doody KM, Rainey WE, Mason JI,

Carr BR. 3β-Hydroxysteroid dehydrogenase activity in glandular and extraglandular human fetal tissues. *J Clin Endocrinol Metab* 1991;73:1134–40.

147 Simard J, Rhéaume E, van Seters AP *et al.* Molecular basis of classical 3β-hydroxysteroid dehydrogenase/$\Delta^{5,4}$-isomerase deficiency. In: *Proceedings, Endocrine Society 74th Annual Meeting*, San Antonio, TX, 1992:191 (Abstr. 560).

148 Simard J, Morel Y, Rhéaume E *et al.* Molecular basis of congenital adrenal hyperplasia due to 3β-hydroxysteroid dehydrogenase deficiency. *Pediatr Res* (Suppl.) 1993;33: (Abstr. 22).

149 Rhéaume E, Mebarki F, Sanchez R *et al.* Functional characterization of the N100S, L108W and P186L mutations detected in the type II 3β-hydroxysteroid dehydrogenase (3β-HSD) genes of two males with classical 3β-HSD deficiency. In: *Proceedings, Endocrine Society 75th Annual Meeting*, Las Vegas, NV, 1993:396 (Abstr. 1383).

150 Heinrich U, Bettendorf M, Grulich-Henn J, Schönberg D, Simard J, Labrie F. The heterogeneity of 3β-hydroxysteroid dehydrogenase (3β-HSD) deficiency – report of 4 cases. *Ped Res* (Suppl.) 1993;33(5): (Abstr. 99).

151 Chang YT, Wang J, Zhang X, Pang S. Molecular basis of the type II 3β-hydroxysteroid dehydrogenase (3β-HSD) gene in patients with mild, nonclassic (late-onset) 3β-HSD deficiency congenital adrenal hyperplasia (CAH). In: *Program and Abstracts, The Endocrine Society 75th Annual Meeting*, 1993:396 (Abstr. 1384).

152 Nakajin S, Shimoda M, Haniu M, Shively JE, Hall PF. C21 steroid side-chain cleavage enzyme from porcine adrenal microsomes. *J Biol Chem* 1984;259:3971–76.

153 Zuber MX, Simpson ER, Waterman MR. Expression of bovine 17α-hydroxylase cytochrome P-450 cDNA in nonsteroidogenic (COS I) cells. *Science* 1986;234:1258–61.

154 Chung B-C, Picado-Leonard J, Haniu M *et al.* Cytochrome P450c17 (steroid 17α-hydroxylase/17,20-lyase): cloning of human adrenal and testis cDNAs indicates the same gene is expressed in both tissues. *Proc Natl Acad Sci USA* 1987;84: 407–11.

155 New MI. Male pseudohermaphroditism due to 17α-hydroxylase deficiency. *J Clin Invest* 1970;49:1930–41.

156 Tournaire J, Audi-Parera L, Loras B, Blum J, Castelnova P, Forest MG. Male pseudohermaphroditism with hypertension due to a 17-hydroxylation deficiency. *Clin Endocrinol* 1976; 5:53–61.

157 Bricaire H, Luton JP, Laudat P *et al.* A new male pseudohermaphroditism associated with hypertension due to a block of 17α-hydroxylation. *J Clin Endocrinol Metab* 1972; 35:67–72.

158 Hammerstein J, Zielshe F, Distler A, Wolff HP. 17-Hydroxylase deficiency of the gonads and adrenals in a male pseudohermaphrodite. *Acta Endocrinol* (Suppl.) 1973;173:76.

159 Yanase T, Simpson ER, Waterman MR. 17α-Hydroxylase/ 17,20-lyase deficiency: from clinical investigation to molecular definition. *Endocr Rev* 1991;12:91–108.

160 Vargas A, Reiter EO, Kula K, Rodriguez-Riga LJ, Steinberger E, Root AW. Direct determination of 17α-hydroxylase (17OHase) deficiency in a male pseudohermaphrodite by *in vitro* studies of testicular steroid biosynthesis. *Pediatr Res* 1981;15:515–20.

161 Mantero F, Scaroni C. Enzymatic defects of steroidogenesis: 17α-hydroxylase. In: New MI, Levine LS, eds. *Adrenal Diseases in Childhood. Pediatric and Adolescent Endocrinology*, Vol. 13. Basel: Karger, 1985:83–94.

162 Alvarez MN, Cloutier MD, Hayles AB. Male pseudohermaphroditism due to 17α-hydroxylase deficiency in two siblings. *Pediatr Res* 1973;7:325–28.

163 Jones HW, Lee PA, Archer DF, Migeon CJ. A genetic male patient with 17α-hydroxylase deficiency. *Obstet Gynecol* 1982;59:254–59 .

164 Kershnar AK, Borut A, Kogut MD, Biglieri ED, Schambelan M. Studies in a phenotypic female with a 17-hydroxylase defect. *J Pediatr* 1976;89:395–400.

165 Morimoto I, Maeda R, Izumi M, Ishimaru T, Nishimori I, Nagataki S. An autopsy case of 17α-hydroxylase deficiency with malignant hypertension. *J Clin Endocrinol Metab* 1983;56:915–19.

166 Abad L, Parilla JJ, Marcos J, Gimeno F, Bernal AL. Male pseudohermaphroditism with 17α-hydroxylase deficiency. *Br J Obstet Gynecol* 1980;87:1162–5.

167 Heremans GFP, Moolenaar AJ, van Gelderen HH. Female phenotype in a male child due to 17α-hydroxylase deficiency. *Arch Dis Child* 1976;51:721–3.

168 Roberts CM, Adams PW, Lilford RJ. Complete steroid 17α-hydroxylase deficiency in an XY patient presenting as primary amenorrhea and low body weight. *Ped Adolesc Gynecol* 1985;3:183–6.

169 Saruta T, Kondo K, Saito I *et al.* Control of aldosterone in 17α-hydroxylase deficiency. *Horm Res* 1980;13:98–108.

170 Dean HJ, Shackleton CHL, Winter JSD. Diagnosis and natural history of 17α-hydroxylase deficiency in a newborn male. *J Clin Endocrinol Metab* 1984;59:513–20.

171 Ono Y, Hanyama K, Yamakasi M *et al.* A case report of 17α-hydroxylase deficiency associated with tall height and epilepsy. *Clin Endocrinol (Tokyo)* 1982;30:353–37.

172 Kater CE, Biglieri EG, Brust H, Chang B, Hirai J. The unique patterns of plasma aldosterone and 18-hydroxycorticosterone concentrations in the 17α-hydroxylase deficiency syndrome. *J Clin Endocrinol Metab* 1982;55:295–302.

173 Goldsmith O, Solomon DH, Horton R. Hypogonadism and mineralocorticoid excess. The 17-hydroxylase deficiency syndrome. *N Engl J Med* 1967;277:673–7.

174 Bosson D, Wolter R, Toppet M, Franckson JR, de Peretti E, Forest MG. Partial 17,20-desmolase and 17α-hydroxylase deficiencies in a 16-year-old boy. *J Endocrinol Invest* 1988; 11:527–33.

175 de Lange WE, Diavenbos H. Incomplete virilization and subclinical mineralocorticoid excess in a boy with partial 17,20-desmolase/17α-hydroxylase deficiency. *Acta Endocrinol* 1990;122:263–6.

176 Singhellakis PN, Ponidis D, Papadinos J *et al.* Spontaneous sexual development and menarche in a girl with 17α-hydroxylase deficiency. *J Endocrinol Invest* 1986;9:177.

177 Wit JM, van Roermund HPC, Oostdik W *et al.* Heterozygotes for 17α-hydroxylase deficiency can be detected with a short ACTH test. *Clin Endocrinol* 1988;28:657–64.

178 D'Armiento M, Reda G, Kater C, Shackleton CHL, Biglieri EG. 17α-Hydroxylase: mineralocorticoid hormone profiles in an affected family. *J Clin Endocrinol Metab* 1983;56:697–701.

179 Picado-Leonard J, Miller WL. Cloning and sequence of the human gene for P450c17 (steroid 17α-hydroxylase/17,20-lyase): similarity with the gene for P450c21. *DNA* 1987;6: 439–46.

180 Matteson KJ, Picado-Leonard J, Chung B-C, Mohando TK, Miller WI. Assignment of the gene for adrenal P450c17 (steroid 17α-hydroxylase/17,20-lyase) to human chromosome 10. *J Clin Endocrinol Metab* 1986;63:789–91.

181 di Blasio AM, Voutilainen R, Jaffe RB, Miller WL. Hormonal

regulation of messenger RNA for P450scc and P450c17 in cultured human fetal adrenal cells. *J Clin Endocrinol Metab* 1987;65:170–5.

182 Kühn-Velten WN. Cytochrome P450c17: regulation of gene expression and enzyme function at the bifurcation in steroid hormone synthesis. In: Schenkman JB, Greim H, eds. *Cytochrome P-450. Handbooks in Experimented Pharmacology*, Vol. 105. New York: Springer Verlag, 1993:667–76.

183 Matteson KJ, Chung BC, Urdea MS, Miller WL. Study of side chain-cleavage (20,22-desmolase) deficiency causing congenital lipoid adrenal hyperplasia using bovine sequence P-450scc oligodeoxyribonucleotide probe. *Endocrinology* 1986;118:1296–305.

184 Prader A, Gurtner HP. Das Syndrome des pseudohermaphroditismus masculinus bei kongenitaler Nebennierenrinden Hyperplasie ohne Androgen-Überproduktion. *Helv Pediatr Acta* 1955;10:397–412.

185 Bonette J, Roidot M, Menuel MC, Cavalier M, Roy L, Isidor P. Sur un cas d'hyperplasie lipoïdique congenitale des surrénales (Syndrome de Prader). Étude anatomoclinique. *Arch Fr Pédiatr* 1964:21:851–9.

186 Camacho AM, Kowarski A, Migeon CJ, Brough AJ. Congenital adrenal hyperplasia due to a deficiency of one of the enzymes involved in the biosynthesis of pregnenolone. *J Clin Endocrinol Metab* 1968;28:153–61.

187 Degenhart HJ. A study of the cholesterol-splitting enzyme system in normal adrenal and in adrenal lipoid hyperplasia. *Acta Paed Scand* 1971;60:611–15.

188 Kirkland RT, Kirkland JL, Johnson C, Horning M, Librick L, Clayton GW. Congenital lipoid adrenal hyperplasia in an eight year old phenotypic female. *J Clin Endocrinol Metab* 1973;36:488–96.

189 Hauffa BF, Miller WL, Grumbach MM, Conte FA, Kaplan SL. Congenital adrenal hyperplasia due to deficient cholesterol side-chain cleavage activity (20,22-desmolase) in a patient treated for 18 years. *Clin Endocrinol* 1985;23:481–93.

190 Duck SC. Acceptable linear growth in congenital adrenal hyperplasia. *J Pediatr* 1980;97:93–6.

191 Winter JSD. Marginal comment: current approaches to the treatment of congenital adrenal hyperplasia. *J Pediatr* 1980; 97:81–2.

192 Winterer J, Chrousos GP, Loriaux DL, Cutler GB. Effect of hydrocortisone dose schedule on adrenal steroid secretion in congenital adrenal hyperplasia. *J Pediatr* 1985;106:137–42.

193 Laue L, Jones J, Nebon D, Cutler JB Jr. Effect of hydrocortisone dose schedule on growth rate and skeletal maturation in classic congenital adrenal hyperplasia. *Pediatr Res* 1992;30:79A (Abstr.).

194 Rosler A, Levine LS, Schneider B, Novogroder M, New MI. The interrelationship of sodium balance, plasma renin activity and ACTH in congenital adrenal hyperplasia. *J Clin Endocrinol Metab* 1978;46:452–8.

195 Lemay A, Dewailly SD, Grenier R, Huard J. Attenuation of mild hyperandrogenic activity in post-pubertal acne by a triphasic oral contraceptive containing low doses of ethinyl estradiol and *d,l*-norgestrel. *J Clin Endocinrol Metab* 1990; 71:8–14.

196 Pang S. Relevance of biological properties of progestogen of oral contraceptives in treatment of androgen excess symptoms (editorial). *J Clin Endocrinol Metab* 1990;71:5–7.

197 Apter D, Vihko R. Endocrine determinants of fertility: serum androgen concentrations during follow-up of adolescents into the third decade of life. *J Clin Endocrinol Metab* 1990;71:970–4.

198 New MI, Dupont B, Grumbach K, Levine LS. Congenital adrenal hyperplasia and related conditions. In: Stanbury JB, Wyngaarden JB, Fredrickson DS, Goldstein JL, Brown MS, eds. *The Metabolic Basis of Inherited Disease*, 5th edn. New York: McGraw-Hill, 1983:973–1000.

199 Holcombe JH, Keenan BS, Nichols BL, Kirkland RT, Clayton GW. Neonatal salt loss in the hypertensive form of congenital adrenal hyperplasia. *Pediatrics* 1980;65:777–81.

200 Zadik Z, Kahana L, Kaufman H, Benderli A, Hochberg Z. Salt loss in hypertensive form of congenital adrenal hyperplasia (11β-hydroxylase deficiency). *J Clin Endocrinol Metab* 1984; 58:384–7.

201 Hochberg Z, Benderly A, Kahana L, Zadik Z. Requirement of mineralocorticoid in congenital adrenal hyperplasia due to 11β-hydroxylase deficiency. *J Clin Endocrinol Metab* 1986; 63:36–40.

202 Klingensmith GJ, Garcia SC, Jones HW, Migeon CJ. Glucocorticoid treatment of girls with congenital adrenal hyperplasia. Effects on height, sexual maturation and fertility. *J Pediatr* 1977;90:966–1004.

203 Nihoul-Fékété C. Feminizing genitoplasty in the intersex child. In: Josso N, ed. *The Intersex Child. Pediatric and Adolescent Endocrinology*, Vol. 8. Basel: Karger, 1981: 247–60.

204 Mulaikal RM, Migeon CJ, Rock JA. Fertility rates in female patients with congenital adrenal hyperplasia due to 21-hydroxylase deficiency. *N Engl J Med* 1987;316:178–82.

205 Kissane JM. *Pathology of Infancy and Childhood*, 2nd edn. St Louis: Mosby, 1975.

206 Money J, Schwartz M, Lewis VG. Adult erotosexual status and fetal hormonal masculinization and demasculinization: 46,XX congenital adrenal hyperplasia and 46,XY androgen insensitivity syndrome compared. *Psychoneuroendocrinology* 1984;9:405–14.

207 Azziz R, Mulaikal RM, Migeon CJ, Jones HW, Rock JA. Congenital adrenal hyperplasia: long term results following vaginal reconstruction. *Fertil Steril* 1986;46:1101–4.

208 Federman DD. Psychosexual adjustment in congenital adrenal hyperplasia (editorial). *N Engl J Med* 1987;316: 209–11.

209 Blumberg DL, Reggiardo D, Sklar C, Darid R. congenital adrenal hyperplasia and fertility (letter). *N Engl J Med* 1988;319:951.

210 Huma Z, Baker S, New MI. Sexual activity of adult women with classical 21-hydroxylase deficiency congenital adrenal hyperplasia. In: *Proceedings, Endocrine Society 75th Annual Meeting*, Las Vagas, NV, 1993:301 (Abstr. 1003).

31: Salt and Water Balance: Sodium-losing States and Endocrine Hypertension

M.J. DILLON

INTRODUCTION

There are various childhood endocrine disorders associated with disturbances of sodium balance. They may be manifest as sodium-losing states or as conditions in which there is sodium retention, with varying clinical features depending on the precise aetiology. An increase in blood pressure often accompanies sodium retention, but there are other mechanisms involved in some forms of endocrine hypertension. A close link with the kidney will be apparent, since it is through this organ that the major effects of hormonal control of sodium are channelled, and primary disturbances of kidney function may mimic endocrine disease.

FETAL AND NEONATAL PHYSIOLOGY

Fetal physiology

The fetus has no need to control sodium balance since it relies on maternal homeostatic mechanisms. Nonetheless, the fetal kidney, which plays a major role in sodium homeostasis at birth, does secrete urine from the third gestational month, possibly serving the purpose of maintaining amniotic fluid volume [1]. The urine is an ultrafiltrate of plasma, and studies with animals have shown that in midterm it is barely modified by passage through the immature renal tubules [2]. However, there is some evidence that sodium reabsorption actively occurs in the ascending limb of Henle's loop without iso-osmotic movement of water, since urine hypotonic to fetal plasma can be elaborated [2]. Tubular reabsorptive function develops further towards term, with increased salt and water reabsorption and a decrease in urine flow rate [3]. Fractional excretion of sodium (FE_{Na}) decreases as the fetus approaches term, and drops to 0.2% in term newborns [4,5]. Whether this intrauterine behaviour is a consequence of morphological immaturity or the result of specific physiological modification in function is unclear, but both are likely to play a part. Certainly the juxtamedullary nephrons with their well-developed loops of Henle, which are particularly concerned with sodium conservation in the adult kidney [6], are more mature than cortical nephrons in the fetal kidney [1].

Although the relationship between fetal renal tubular function and the renin–angiotensin system is not clear, the latter is certainly active in the fetus. Studies of sheep have shown not only that the plasma renin levels are higher in the fetal lamb than in the ewe [7], but also that increased renin release can be demonstrated following frusemide administration [8] and blood volume reduction [7]. Human cord blood values of plasma renin and angiotensin II are higher than maternal values at birth [9,10], and it seems likely that the renin originates in the fetal kidneys [11]. It is not clear what purpose the renin–angiotensin system serves *in utero*, although it may play a part in the distribution of fetoplacental blood volume [12]. However, at birth, the integrity of this system could be critical in establishing postnatal existence. (For a recent review of fetal renal physiology, see [13].)

It seems unlikely that fetal synthesis of glucocorticoids or mineralocorticoids is necessary for intrauterine survival [14], although it may have a role in organ maturation and in controlling the onset of labour. Normal electrolyte homeostasis at birth in infants with salt-losing congenital adrenal hyperplasia (CAH), coupled with the absence of evidence of glucocorticoid deficiency [14], would support this conclusion. In spite of this, the fetal adrenal grows into a large endocrine organ consisting of a broad fetal zone next to the medulla and an outer, relatively narrow, subcapsular zone known as the adult or definitive zone [14]. Towards term, the latter increases in thickness to constitute about 20% of the total adrenal cortex [15].

The fetal adrenals appear to be under fetal pituitary control, since anencephaly [16] or corticosteroid administration to the mother [17] results in adrenal hypoplasia and decreased secretion of fetal steroids. Adrenocorticotrophic hormone (ACTH) appears to be the trophic hormone for the definitive zone, but other peptides from the fetal pituitary may be concerned with fetal zone control [18]. Functionally, the important biological function of this zone is to provide androgens, mainly dehydroepiandrosterone sulphate (DHEAS) for placental oestrogen synthesis [19]. It is also clear that the fetal zone of the gland cannot make cortisol efficiently from cholesterol or pregnenolone due to a lack of 3β-hydroxysteroid dehydrogenase (3β-HSD) activity [20–22].

Other enzymatic steps needed for cortisol synthesis are active, so the fetal adrenal is able to convert progesterone to cortisol quite effectively [23]. The fetal adrenal and placenta form the fetoplacental unit which is important in the maintenance of the pregnancy and of fetal well-being. Knowledge of the definitive zone's function is incomplete, but it contains all the enzymes required for corticosteroid synthesis and does synthesize corticosteroids but probably, in part, by an alternative Δ^5 pathway [24]. Corticosteroid production, including aldosterone, increases progressively throughout pregnancy [25], and at birth the placental influence is withdrawn and the fetal adrenal must produce cortisol without placental progesterone as substrate. 3β-HSD activity increases rapidly in the definitive zone to render it capable of synthesizing mineralocorticoid and glucocorticoid adequate for independent survival. Thus the newborn adrenal can make enough cortisol from cholesterol immediately after birth [26].

The fetal adrenal is responsive to some stimuli *in utero*. In fetal rats, maternal sodium depletion, increased fetal aldosterone production [27] and, in the human, higher cord blood plasma aldosterone concentrations, have been demonstrated in infants born to mothers on diuretic therapy compared to those whose mothers were not [28] suggesting a response to saline depletion. However, there is some evidence that the high rate of FE_{Na} during fetal life may reflect a relative tubular insensitivity to circulating aldosterone [29]. Other explanations for the greater FE_{Na} in fetal life that have been considered include prostaglandins and atrial natriuretic factor [30,31]. The former appears unlikely to contribute, but the latter may have a role.

Neonatal physiology

At birth, the infant is transferred from the luxury of a saline-rich uterus to a dry, relatively salt-free environment where fluid and electrolyte conservation becomes vital. Momentous changes must occur to allow the newborn to cope with its homeostatic and excretory functions. The kidneys become the main site of these activities and, in spite of their immaturity, even at term, they cope admirably with the situation. The concept of glomerulotubular imbalance has given way to that of glomerulotubular balance [32,33]. A decreased glomerular perfusion protects the immature renal tubules and contributes towards adequate sodium reabsorption, which occurs within 12–36 h of birth [34]. This would appear to be related, in part, to vascular constraints [35,36] which also appear to be involved in a quantitatively different intrarenal distribution of blood flow in the newborn when compared to the adult. During early postnatal life, blood is distributed preferentially to nephrons with a higher capacity than the superficial ones to reabsorb sodium in the juxtamedullary area [37]. In addition, proximal tubular immaturity in the neonate and young infant may result in less than optimal proximal sodium reabsorption, and hence a much greater dependence on distal tubular sodium reabsorptive mechanisms under aldosterone control. However, in newborn infants at 7 days of age, Rodriguez-Soriano *et al.* [38], were able to demonstrate that there was a limit to the capacity of the distal nephron to reabsorb sodium when a critical value of distal tubular sodium delivery was exceeded.

The renin–angiotensin–aldosterone (RAA) system is very active in the neonatal period and there are now many reports of increased plasma renin activity (PRA), angiotensin II and aldosterone concentrations in the newborn when compared to older children and adults [9,10,28,39–41]. It is possible that this system is necessary for the maintenance of sodium balance in early infancy through vasopressor effects of angiotensin II on the renal vasculature or mineralocorticoid action on the distal nephron. The inverse relationship between plasma levels of renin and aldosterone and age [40,42, 43] could well reflect the increasing maturity of the proximal nephron with less dependence on distal tubular sodium reabsorptive function [42,44]. Sulyok *et al.* [43] suggested that endogenous prostaglandin production during labour might be one of the factors responsible for the hyperactivity of the RAA system in the newborn, even though there is no clear relationship between urinary sodium excretion and renal prostaglandin production [45].

Preterm infants appear to behave somewhat differently from those born at term. There is frequently a period of hyponatraemia during the first 2 weeks of life related to a combination of a low sodium intake coupled with excess natriuresis [5,46–48]. During the third week, positive sodium balance is achieved, and this is associated with a significant increase in the excretion of urine tetrahydroaldosterone [49]. It has been considered by some that the hyponatraemia and negative sodium balance of the premature infant may be due to a transient period of mineralocorticoid deficiency after birth or, alternatively, to a degree of insensitivity of the renal tubules to aldosterone action, eventually overcome by increased production by the adrenals [41,49]. It has been suggested that aldosterone induces Na,K,ATPase (sodium, potassium, adenosine triphosphatase) in the renal tubules and that the response to aldosterone is seen when this occurs [50]. Although the latter explanations may be correct in part, it seems more likely that the sodium wastage at this time is due to a temporary glomerulotubular imbalance with increasing superficial nephron perfusion consequent to immaturity of the tubuloglomerular feedback mechanism [51].

Other hormonal factors which may contribute to the control of sodium balance in premature infants have been recently reviewed [52] and include prolactin [53], noradrenaline [54], the kallikrein–kinin system [55] and dopamine [52,56–58]. A role for arginine vasopressin in contributing to the hyponatraemia of preterm infants has been invoked [59,60]. Atrial natriuretic peptide (ANP) has also been shown to be elevated after birth with values much higher in preterm than term infants [52]. Data available suggest that ANP may be intimately involved in regulation of extracellular volume and the disposal of extracellular sodium through the kidney.

Endogenous digoxin-like substance (EDLS), which has been thought by some to be natriuretic hormone (de Wardener factor), inhibits Na,K,ATPase activity in various tissues. Plasma levels in neonates are high, and there is a negative correlation between gestational age and EDLS [52]. Levels in term newborns decline during the second week of life [61] but remain high in immature infants when negative sodium balance is present [62]. These data lend support to the assumption that higher EDLS in the immature babies is the result of their volume expansion, and may contribute to the higher rate of sodium excretion seen in these infants [52]. (For an up-to-date review of neonatal renal function including tubular handling of sodium, see [53].)

SODIUM-LOSING STATES

Sodium loss, usually in conjunction with water, occurs in a number of conditions in infancy and childhood. Losses can occur extrarenally, such as in association with gastrointestinal disease (diarrhoea and/or vomiting) or skin disease (excess sweating, including cystic fibrosis). In some of these situations disturbed endocrine function may play a part; for example, gut and skin losses of electrolytes occur in hypoaldosteronism or end-organ unresponsiveness to mineralocorticoids. Renal sodium and water losses may also occur as a result of primary kidney pathology, such as structural or functional disturbances of renal tubular function, whether genetic or acquired. Alternatively, renal sodium loss may be due to disturbed hormonal control of renal tubular sodium conservation, such as in adrenal hypoplasia, Addison disease or various types of biosynthetic block of aldosterone production or disorders causing endorgan unresponsiveness.

The normal environment encountered by the newborn infant is one in which availability of dietary sodium is limited, since human breast milk has a low sodium content (approximately 7 mmol/l) after the first few days. If homeostatic mechanisms involved in sodium retention are faulty for one reason or another, urinary sodium loss can rapidly cause serious salt depletion.

There is considerable clinical variability in the manifestation of salt-wasting in infancy, ranging from mild failure to thrive to severe salt and water depletion endangering life. Clues may be available from the history and physical signs (for example, virilization in a female infant with CAH) but such features are often absent and the diagnosis can be difficult. Loss of skin turgor, sunken eyes, hypotension and evidence of weight loss may well be absent in quite serious sodium depletion.

The simple measurement of plasma sodium concentration is helpful but can be misleading. A child may be significantly salt-depleted with a normal plasma sodium if water losses are occurring *pari passu* with sodium; hyponatraemia may be seen in situations of salt overload when extracellular water is excessive. To confirm sodium loss it is necessary to demonstrate that urinary sodium output exceeds intake. This is frequently at its most obvious on presentation, and it is therefore important to extract as much useful information as possible at that time, and before treatment has been initiated, commensurate with safe management. If excess urine sodium is demonstrated, even on a random urine specimen, when the child is clinically salt- and water-depleted, a diagnosis of inappropriate natriuresis can be confidently made. Should the child's clinical condition require urgent treatment before the diagnosis can be established, it may be necessary to reduce sodium intake under controlled conditions after stabilization to a point where urinary output exceeds intake and a sodium-losing state is demonstrable. This may be dangerous, and other approaches may need to be invoked.

A sensitive index of sodium balance in salt-wasting disorders, and of considerable value in these particular circumstances, is the measurement of PRA [42,64]. Significantly raised values are found in patients with urinary salt-wasting disease, even when sodium is being administered therapeutically. This test, coupled with the clinical history and findings, may demonstrate the presence of a salt-losing state without recourse to balance studies.

Renal disease

Urinary sodium-wasting in infancy and childhood can occur in association with the following abnormalities:

1 structural maldevelopments of the kidney, such as renal dysplasia;

2 obstructive uropathy, especially due to urethral valves;

3 renal tubular disease, for example, Fanconi syndrome or renal tubular acidosis; and

4 syndromes in which the above have been excluded and hypokalaemic alkalosis is prominent, such as Bartter syndrome.

Quite marked natriuresis may also occur during recovery from acute tubular necrosis, and can be misleading if the oliguric phase is short or not noticed.

A helpful feature of primary renal tubular sodium loss is that it is very often associated with urinary potassium loss. This may be either primary or secondary due to hyperaldosteronism if adrenal function is normal. Hypokalaemia is particularly striking in the various types of Fanconi syndrome and in Bartter syndrome, with acidosis in the former and alkalosis in the latter. If, therefore, a urinary sodium-wasting condition in a neonate or young infant is associated with hypokalaemia, it is almost certainly renal rather than endocrine in origin. The majority of renal disorders can usually be distinguished by careful clinical, biochemical and radiological assessment. Although the presence of aminoaciduria, glycosuria, phosphaturia, tubular proteinuria and defects of acid–base homeostasis would indicate Fanconi syndrome, it must be remembered that some of these features may also be present in some structural anomalies of the kidney, and occasionally in some examples of Bartter syndrome [65].

The plasma renin–aldosterone profile is an extremely useful tool in classifying the nature of salt-wasting disease [65–67]. In children with a normal renin–aldosterone axis, salt-wasting states are associated with appropriately raised values of plasma renin and aldosterone [42]. If the adrenal gland is unresponsive to angiotensin II stimulation for some reason, the raised plasma renin will be associated with an inappropriately low plasma aldosterone, even though this may be above normal for age [67]. This is a valuable diagnostic aid, and only rarely causes difficulties in interpretation. One situation in which it does, however, is when the plasma potassium is particularly low, and the ability of the adrenal to respond to angiotensin II is hampered. A seemingly low plasma aldosterone may then be found with a high plasma renin [65]. The clue which helps distinguish this from true hypoaldosteronism is the plasma potassium measurement. If hypoaldosteronism were present, it would be associated with hyperkalaemia, so hypokalaemia suggests the presence of primary renal tubular disease [65].

BARTTER SYNDROME AND SIMILAR DISORDERS

In 1962 Bartter *et al.* [68] described a new syndrome of growth failure and mental retardation associated with hypokalaemic alkalosis, increased aldosterone secretion rate and increased plasma angiotensin II concentration in the presence of normal blood pressure. Juxtaglomerular cell hyperplasia was seen on renal biopsy, a pitressin-resistant hyposthenuria was demonstrated, and there was decreased pressor responsiveness to infused angiotensin II. Since that time many reports have appeared describing a wide spectrum of clinical and biochemical features considered to be manifestations of this condition. This diversity has raised some doubt as to whether the term 'Bartter syndrome' is applicable to all the patients reported, which has in turn created difficulties in identifying criteria for diagnosis. For the diagnosis of Bartter syndrome the following must be present: hypokalaemia, hypochloraemia, alkalosis, hyperreninaemia in the presence of a normal blood pressure, and elevated urinary potassium and chloride excretion in the absence of other conditions which cause similar features. The diagnosis is therefore still one of exclusion, even though a degree of specificity has been applied to certain biochemical investigations in recent years.

Clinical, biochemical and laboratory features

The majority of patients present with failure to thrive, vomiting and constipation during the first 2 years of life. The most common age of onset of symptoms is 6–12 months [65]; there may be a preceding history of hydramnios. There may be evidence of clinical extracellular fluid (ECF) volume depletion with complaints of fatigue, muscle cramps, polydipsia and polyuria. Developmental delay, although initially reported by Bartter [68], is variable. The majority of these features are explained by the renal tubular dysfunction cited above, and the effects of potassium deficiency and hypokalaemia. Some patients are said to have a distinctive facial appearance characterized by prominence of the forehead, triangular facies, drooping mouth, large eyes and pinnae [69]. The patients are normotensive and increased blood pressure casts considerable doubt on the diagnosis. Occasionally a child who is asymptomatic might be identified by a routine investigation revealing hypokalaemic alkalosis [65]. Most affected siblings are symptomatic [69–73].

The characteristic laboratory abnormality is hypokalaemia accompanied by alkalosis and increased fractional urinary excretion of potassium and chloride. Evidence of urinary sodium-wasting may be present, although some patients conserve sodium appropriately when they are placed on a low-sodium diet. Pitressin-resistant hyposthenuria is often present and may be severe enough to cause polyuria. It is, however, interesting that maximal free-water clearance may also be reduced, and patients may have difficulty in producing extremely dilute urine under conditions of hypotonic saline loading [74,75]. Magnesium depletion with or without evidence of excessive urinary magnesium loss is well recognized in Bartter syndrome [71,76,77]. It is still unclear whether this is related to hyperaldosteronism or to a primary abnormality of tubular magnesium handling. It may contribute to hypokalaemia; magnesium supplementation in affected patients has led to an increase in plasma potassium [76,77]. Hypomagnesaemia in patients with Bartter syndrome needs to be distinguished from primary disorders of renal magnesium-wasting in which hypokalaemia also occurs (see below) [78–81].

Hyperreninaemia is consistently present, and this is accompanied in some children by high plasma aldosterone levels. However, in others, possibly as a result of the hypokalaemia, plasma aldosterone is suppressed until hypokalaemia is corrected [65]. An infusion of angiotensin II is associated with a blunted increase in blood pressure in patients with Bartter syndrome, but this lack of response is not diagnostic and may reflect sodium depletion [82].

In addition to the basic components of the syndrome, a number of other clinical and biochemical findings have been described. Some of these are probably essential aspects of the syndrome and help in understanding the pathophysiology of the condition; others may serve to distinguish between the 'classic' syndrome and 'Bartter-like' disorders; still others are only epiphenomena. The basic components are evidence of defective renal tubular handling of sodium and potassium [70,74,75,82–87], abnormal chloride reabsorption in the ascending limb of the loop of Henle [75,84,88], and abnormal intracellular electrolyte concentrations in red cells and muscle cells [90–95]. In addition, the following are reported: abnormal erythrocyte sodium and potassium transport [37,71,90, 92,93,95,96]; defective renal tubular acidification [97,98]; excess renal prostaglandin production with response to prostaglandin synthetase inhibitors [65,70,71,99–110]; abnormalities of skin fibroblast prostaglandin production [111]; defects in platelet aggregation [7,71,112]; abnormalities of the kallikrein–kinin system [104,113–115]; renal biopsy abnormalities [68,82,116,117]; a circulating inhibitor of phytohaemagglutinin-induced lymphocyte proliferation [118]; a familial incidence [65,69–73,119, 120]; and several odd clinical features including chondrocalcinosis [65,120].

A problem of defining whether hypercalciuria, with or without nephrocalcinosis, is acceptable as part of the syndrome remains unresolved. Undoubtedly, this has been considered a feature in the past [65,94,98], but some now place this into the category of calcium-losing tubulopathy [121–124]. There is also some difficulty in classifying patients in whom there is some degree of hypophosphataemia [65,116,125,126] and those who develop rickets [65,125,127].

Treatment

Treatment of Bartter syndrome, although not fully satisfactory, has improved. Potassium supplementation is required in the majority and sodium chloride supplement is required in some patients, especially the young. Potassium-sparing diuretics, such as spironolactone and triamterine, can improve the clinical state [68], but older renin-suppressing agents (for example methyldopa [128] and propranol [129]) do not appear to help. Angiotensin-converting enzyme (ACE) inhibitors may have some role.

Indomethacin, a prostaglandin synthetase inhibitor [101,110], has improved results considerably. Hypokalaemia has been corrected, and catch-up growth has occurred [65]. In some patients, notably those with reduced glomerular filtration rate (GFR), renal function may be decreased by this treatment. Indomethacin appears to act by redistributing renal blood flow and by improving proximal renal tubular reabsorption. The distal tubular defect in chloride reabsorption [75,84] and the red blood cell (RBC) membrane transport defect [95,130] persists, whereas intracellular sodium decreases [95,130] towards normal. In some patients clinical and biochemical relapse [125,131] occurs even though prostaglandin levels remain suppressed [65]. Other drugs that inhibit prostaglandin synthesis (for example aspirin, ketoprofen and ibuprofen) [102,104,105] have not been more effective than indomethacin.

Indomethacin is given in a dose of 2 mg/kg each day in four to six doses. Patients tolerate it well; occasionally gastrointestinal intolerance occurs. This resolves with reduction of dose and, if this is not possible, by the introduction of ranitidine. Decreases in GFR with treatment usually improve with reduction or discontinuation of therapy. There is as yet no satisfactory evidence that treatment has modified mental development or improved renal function in those patients in whom mental development or renal function were impaired.

Causal theories

There is, as yet, no unifying hypothesis to explain the range of abnormalities seen in Bartter syndrome. Initially, Bartter [68] considered the disorder to be one in which there was a defect in pressor response to angiotensin II, which resulted in hypotension leading to secondary hyperreninaemia and aldosteronism. The latter, it was felt, caused the hypokalaemia and potassium deficiency which, in turn, resulted in the defect in urine concentration. Later, some form of primary hyperreninaemia was considered to be the proximal cause [129], but this seemed unlikely when treatment of affected patients with renin-suppressant agents failed to modify the abnormalities [129].

The increase in urinary prostaglandin and the effect of indomethacin have led to the proposal that a disturbance in prostaglandin synthesis at some site is the primary cause of the syndrome [65,70,71,97,99–108,110,111]. However, several findings mitigate against this hypothesis, including the inconsistent prostaglandin levels [100], the clinical and biochemical escape which occurs when patients are on chronic indomethacin therapy and urinary prostaglandins remain low [131], and the lack of improvement when urinary prostaglandins are suppressed with mepacrine [70].

Furthermore, prostaglandin synthetase inhibition does not correct the tubular defect in chloride reabsorption [84,132] or the changes in RBC sodium flux even though it does improve intracellular sodium concentration [58,130]. The observations on skin fibroblasts showing differing patterns of prostaglandin release in Bartter patients compared to controls, however, need to be carefully considered, since these might point to a primary defect in prostaglandin synthesis [111].

The abnormalities of renal tubular function have been considered to be the prime defect [70,74,75,82,83,85–87,130,135], although there is controversy as to which of these tubular dysfunctions is the critical abnormality. A defect in chloride reabsorption in the ascending limb of the loop of Henle associated with passive loss of sodium and potassium is a current hypothesis. Indomethacin does not correct the defect, which is demonstrated by hypotonic saline loading [134], and has been reported in a number of studies [75,84]. It has been proposed that all the other pathophysiological features could be secondary to this abnormality, but some doubt has been cast on this finding because it is less evident when fractional electrolyte reabsorption is measured during water rather than hypotonic saline diuresis [71]. The findings can be explained by a defect in cell wall electrolyte transport affecting muscle, RBC and renal tubule cells. This explanation currently fits the clinical and biochemical features of the condition most accurately.

Differential diagnosis

The differential diagnosis needs to be considered in two sections: conditions in which there are extrarenal losses of electrolytes that usually have decreased urine chloride, and those in which there is tubular electrolyte loss. The former includes laxative abuse [135], cyclical vomiting [136], pyloric stenosis, chloride-deficient diets [137], congenital chloridorrhoea [138] and cystic fibrosis [139,140]. The latter includes Fanconi syndrome, incomplete distal renal tubule acidosis (RTA) [98,135,141], use of diuretics [143], administration of impermeable anions, Gitelman syndrome [79] and calcium-losing tubulopathy [132].

GITELMAN SYNDROME (FAMILIAL HYPOKALAEMIA–HYPOMAGNESAEMIA) AND CALCIUM-LOSING TUBULOPATHY

These two syndromes can prove difficult to distinguish from Bartter syndrome. Gitelman syndrome manifests many Bartter-like features, including hypokalaemia, moderate alkalosis, hyperreninaemia, hyperaldosteronism and increased urine prostaglandin excretion [132,144]. There is striking hypomagnesaemia and hypermagnesuria, but decreased urine calcium excretion [144]. There is evidence that the defect is recessively inherited and is in the distal tubules rather than the ascending limb of the loop of Henle; patients respond to treatment with magnesium salts [132,144]. Calcium-losing tubulopathy presents with hypokalaemic alkalosis, polyuria and polydipsia, normal plasma and urine magnesium, but with hypercalciuria and usually nephrocalcinosis [121,132]. There is hyperreninaemic hyperaldosteronism and increased urinary prostaglandin (PG) E_2. The site of the defect is thought to be in the proximal nephron, and treatment is usually with PG synthetase inhibitors, such as indomethacin [132].

Adrenal disease – mineralocorticoid deficiency

Urinary sodium wastage of adrenal origin is associated with hyperkalaemia. In the absence of renal failure this combination points to a defect of aldosterone production or action. Several adrenal disorders are associated with inadequate production of aldosterone. They nearly always present with salt-wasting.

CONGENITAL ADRENAL HYPOPLASIA

Affected children present in early infancy with a hyperkalaemic, sodium-wasting state, but without evidence of virilization [145]. Both mineralocorticoid and glucocorticoid synthesis are impaired, and investigations demonstrate that PRA is increased but plasma aldosterone (PA) is inappropriately low [66]. There is also evidence of glucocorticoid failure. Urinary values of glucocorticoid and mineralocorticoid metabolites are low and precursors are not present in excess.

Treatment with sodium chloride, hydrocortisone and mineralocorticoid replacement therapy (9α-fludrocortisone) is successful in reversing the clinical abnormalities. The condition may be sporadic or familial. There are three anatomical variants: the 'anencephalic' pattern resembling the adrenals seen in anencephaly; the 'cytomegalic' pattern only seen in males, and the so-called 'miniature' pattern.

Of these the anencephalic pattern seems to be inherited on a recessive basis, and the cytomegalic and miniature forms on an X-linked basis, although all three can occur sporadically (see Chapter 28).

CONGENITAL ADRENAL HYPERPLASIA

Most cases of CAH associated with hyperkalaemia are the result of 21-hydroxylase deficiency. Patients with 21-

hydroxylase deficiency have been divided into those who are overt salt-wasters and those who are not. A majority of patients have a tendency for salt-wasting, but this varies in severity [146,147]. In some patients, salt-wasting is suspected by the clinical signs of ECF volume contraction, loss of skin turgor and hypotension. Hyponatraemia and hyperkalaemia are present and urinary sodium chloride excretion is inappropriately high. In other patients salt-wasting is less obvious.

In some, PA may be normal, but the PRA is high; that is although the PA value is within the normal range it is inappropriately low in relation to the simultaneously measured PRA and the degree of salt-wasting. Those classified as salt-wasters have a marked defect in aldosterone synthesis. In these patients, ECF volume contraction often becomes apparent toward the end of the first week of life and is associated with an increase in precursors of cortisol such as 17-hydroxyprogesterone [148,149]. These precursors have natriuretic effects in their own right. In the infant, sodium reabsorption under aldosterone control in the distal nephron is proportionally greater than in older children, so that the natriuresis is exaggerated; hyperkalaemia develops, PRA increases and PA is inappropriately low [66,147,150]. In patients who do not show clinical signs of ECF volume contraction, an increased PRA indicates that sodium homeostasis is impaired [147].

Children with 21-hydroxylase deficiency should be treated with sodium chloride supplementation, physiological doses of hydrocortisone and 9α-fludrocortisone. Sodium chloride should replace urinary salt losses. In the neonatal period, infusion of sodium chloride may be necessary. Pharmacological doses of cortisol are not required unless the infant is stressed. Glucocorticoid administration should suppress the corticotrophin-releasing factor sufficiently to normalize ACTH levels. The dose may be adjusted by the plasma levels of ACTH and androgens or urinary steroid levels, and should be such that it does not suppress growth. The dose of glucocorticoid is adjusted as the individual grows [151]. It is customary to express the dose as a function of surface area.

The question of how long mineralocorticoid therapy should be prescribed is controversial. There is no doubt that it is indicated in patients with salt depletion and hyperkalaemia who become symptomatic in the first week of life. There is disagreement about its use in the child with less obvious salt depletion. It is recommended that, when patients are treated, the dose of mineralocorticoid be adjusted by following PRA values. The appropriate dose is associated with normal PRA values, an overdose by its suppression to low values.

Mineralocorticoid treatment has in the past been withdrawn as the child reaches 3–4 years of age. This practice was based on the ability of these children to remain in sodium balance at this age under normal conditions. This is a serious mistake. The maturation of the proximal nephron and the tendency for dietary salt to increase may sustain salt balance in the absence of stress, but most of these patients retain their tendency for salt-wasting [64]. All patients who have 21-hydroxylase deficiency should be treated with mineralocorticoids [146]. Treatment safeguards these children against sudden salt-wasting crises associated with an intercurrent illness at a time when their cortisol requirements may increase and natriuretic steroids reappear in the circulation [152]. The requirement for hydrocortisone is reduced and the adverse effect this drug has on growth is lessened [147]. Hyperreninaemia stimulates ACTH production and directly affects the production of steroid precursors of cortisol [153]. This leads to a loss of glucocorticoid control. Therefore, mineralocorticoid therapy should be given always and supplemental salt adjusted to a point where PRA is within the normal range.

See Chapter 30 for further discussion of CAH.

ISOLATED DEFECTS OF ALDOSTERONE BIOSYNTHESIS

Isolated defects of aldosterone biosynthesis other than 21-hydroxylase deficiency also cause hyperkalaemia. The defects occur towards the end of the aldosterone biosynthetic pathway (see Chapter 28). In 1964, Visser & Cost [154] reported an 18-oxidation defect in infants with a salt-wasting syndrome, which subsequently was shown to be a defect in 18-hydroxylation [155]. A 5-month-old infant with identical clinical findings had a defect in 18-dehydrogenation of corticosterone [156], that is there were at least two sites where the 18-oxidation step was blocked that could result in inadequate aldosterone synthesis.

Several reports have confirmed the 18-dehydrogenation defects [67,157–159] but Ulick [160] subsequently suggested that the mechanism involves a defect in corticosterone methyloxidase (CMO). Type I (CMO-I) converts corticosterone to a transient, oxygenated steroid-metalloenzyme complex, which is substrate for a second oxidase (CMO-II). A second hydroxylation here precedes spontaneous dehydration to a labile intermediate, with the formation of 18-hydroxycorticosterone.

Children with these disorders usually present in early infancy with severe hyperkalaemia and salt-wasting. Occasionally they have a less dramatic course, presenting at a few months of age with unexplained failure to thrive [67]. There is no evidence of virilization. Glucocorticoid production and renal function are normal. PRA is high and plasma aldosterone (PA) levels are low [67]. Urinary levels of aldosterone and aldosterone metabolites (tetrahydraldosterone) are low: the urinary levels of aldosterone precursors are high depending on the site of the enzymatic block [161]. Analysis of urine for steroids by gas chromatographic and mass spectrometric techniques are at the limit of methodological sensitivity. Interpretation is made more difficult by the fact that urinary steroid excretion patterns vary with age. In the newborn and young infant, a knowledge of the normal patterns of excretion is essential before attempting to define the abnormality [162,163]. These values are influenced when extraneous steroids are administered.

Affected children sometimes present with febrile episodes associated with infection and not due to dehydration [67,154]. These febrile attacks may be precipitated by pyrogenic metabolites of precursors of aldosterone with similar structure to etiocholanolone [164]. In addition, they are acidotic due to a type IV renal tubular acidosis secondary to aldosterone deficiency.

Aldosterone deficiency is treated with sodium chloride supplements – often large quantities, for example 20 mmol/kg a day in infants – and mineralocorticoid replacement also in large amounts [67]: up to 0.5 mg of 9α-fludrocortisone a day is sometimes needed initially to sustain normal ECF volume. The need for the high dose is a result of the competitive effect of aldosterone precursors on mineralocorticoid given as replacement therapy. After a period of time 9α-fludrocortisone can be reduced to maintenance requirements, 0.05 mg/day. The defect is lifelong. While it has been shown that children can stop mineralocorticoid therapy at 12–18 months of age, they retain the tendency to lose salt [159]. This is analogous to the situation described in 21-hydroxylase deficiency in which renal proximal tubule maturation and an increased dietary salt intake compensate for the distal tubular defect of sodium reabsorption. Withdrawal of mineralocorticoid is not advisable; it should be continued for life [67]. It appears that corticosterone methyloxidase defects are inherited on an autosomal recessive basis [154,157].

ADDISON DISEASE

This form of primary chronic adrenocorticoid insufficiency is important to recognize. In the past the main cause was tuberculosis; now 'autoimmune adrenalitis' is the more common cause. This may be isolated or associated with other endocrine diseases, such as hypoparathyroidism, hypothyroidism or diabetes mellitus (see Chapter 28). Antiadrenal antibodies are found in the circulation, but do not correlate with the severity of the adrenal disease [166]. Familial occurrence is frequent [165] and the inheritance of the abnormality of immune response is probably autosomal recessive, although females are more affected [167].

Clinical features are related to deficiency of glucocorticoid and mineralocorticoid hormones – hyperpigmentation, hypoglycaemia, gastrointestinal disturbances and progressive weakness. Characteristic laboratory findings include hyponatraemia, hyperkalaemia and hypoglycaemia. Plasma ACTH is increased, and there is no rise of plasma cortisol to ACTH stimulation; PRA is high and PA is low. Precursors of glucocorticoid biosynthesis will be absent. Treatment consists of cortisol replacement, 12–15 mg/m^2 a day (or its equivalent) and 9α-fludrocortisone 150 μg/m^2 a day. Adrenal crises because of salt-wasting or hypoglycaemia occur and require intravenous isotonic saline, glucose and additional glycocorticoid. Patients with Addison disease given correct treatment live a normal life.

Adrenal leukodystrophy (Addison–Schilder disease) [168] is an important condition to differentiate from isolated Addison disease. It is characterized by progressive neurological disease associated with primary adrenal insufficiency. An X-linked inheritance occurs affecting male children. At present no therapy is effective in arresting the progressive neurological disease.

Mineralocorticoid unresponsiveness

PSEUDOHYPOALDOSTERONISM

Pseudohypoaldosteronism (PHA) is a condition in which there is resistance of the renal tubules and other tissues to aldosterone, and presents in a fashion identical to that described for 18-oxidation defect, that is failure to thrive, hyperkalaemia and a salt-wasting state. It was first reported by Cheek & Perry in 1958 [169], who noted that mineralocorticoid therapy seemed to be ineffective and did not modify the urine Na^+/K^+ ratio. Since that time, many cases have been reported [170–192]. Although plasma electrolyte findings are similar to those seen in 18-oxidation defects, there are certain distinguishing features. First, both PRA and PA levels are markedly increased; second, urinary steroid analysis reveals increased amounts of aldosterone metabolites in a characteristic pattern [176,190,191]. There is evidence supporting both recessive [173,187] and dominant patterns of inheritance [179].

The condition is a result of end-organ unresponsiveness to aldosterone, predominantly in the renal tubule but in some children in other sites as well, including the gut, sweat glands and salivary glands [190]. There is some doubt about where the sodium chloride losses take place; initially the distal tubule was considered the likely site [169], but more recent observations have implicated the collecting tubule as the principal locus of aldosterone action, suggesting that this is more likely to be the site of the transport abnormality [193,194]. A more proximal site has also been implicated by some, and there may be impairment of sodium transport in both proximal and distal nephrons in some patients [186,188,195]. The nature of the defect is not defined. A decrease in Na,K,ATPase in the renal tubule [173] was thought to be a possible mechanism, but alternatives include an abnormality in the number or affinity of aldosterone receptors [196].

There is an overlap between PHA and childhood RTA type 4 [197–199]. The latter characteristically is not associated with overt saltwasting, but there is reduced tubular responsiveness to aldosterone. PRA and urinary aldosterone excretion are increased, even though superficially there is a defect only of distal tubular secretion of hydrogen and potassium ions [114]. Children with RTA type 4 are also growth-retarded and have frequent bouts of vomiting [199]. Hyperchloraemic and hyperkalaemic acidosis with aciduria are the laboratory features of this disorder. Although saltwasting is not obvious, there is sufficient evidence from the PRA and PA levels to suggest that there is also some salt depletion. In view of this it seems likely that PHA and early childhood RTA type 4 are similar disorders with differing degrees of salt-wasting. Similarly, in PHA, there is also a tendency towards acidosis, and the explanation for this is the defect of aldosterone effect in relation to hydrogen ion excretion in the distal nephron [198].

Since 1976 several children have been described with PHA in whom there is mineralocorticoid unresponsiveness affecting various target organs, including the colon, sweat and salivary glands [182,190,200]. Armanini *et al.* [196] reported a defect of type 1 aldosterone-binding sites on mononuclear leukocytes of patients with pseudohypoaldosteronism supporting the view that the disorder may be one of deficiency in type 1 receptors in aldosterone target tissues. Subsequent studies have confirmed the deficiency of aldosterone binding sites and have shown that this defect is inherited as either an autosomal recessive or dominant trait [201,202].

PHA is treated with sodium chloride supplementation, which expands ECF volume. Tubular flow and delivery of solute to the distal nephron increases, creating a favourable gradient for potassium secretion [203,204]. This occurs in spite of the fact that there is little or no mineralocorticoid stimulation of potassium secretion. The amount of sodium chloride required is often large; the correct dose is deduced from the decrease in potassium and PRA, and from the clinical improvement of the patients who thrive [176]. By the age of 18–24 months these patients may be able to manage without sodium chloride supplementation [169,174,176,185]. However, as with 18-oxidation defects, the disorder persists for life [183,188,205] and the apparent recovery is probably related to proximal tubular maturation and the tendency of the child to ingest more salt. Administering aldosterone or other mineralocorticoid is usually without effect, but this may be partial in some children [205].

Prostaglandins may play a part in the sodium chloride-wasting that occurs in this condition. In one child with PHA, treatment with indomethacin was successful [186]. The drug appears to act by decreasing proximal renal tubular perfusion and improving sodium reabsorption at this site, compensating for more distal losses [206]. A word of caution is necessary here, since although indomethacin may have a role, the risk of it inducing hyperkalaemia is not inconsequential. This would particularly apply to children with multiple end-organ unresponsiveness to aldosterone in whom the only means of eliminating potassium is by creating sufficient distal delivery of fluid in the nephron for a favourable gradient to exist for potassium secretion. If distal delivery is reduced by indomethacin, this mechanism cannot function, and worsening of hyperkalaemia will result.

It seems likely that the condition is most commonly inherited on an autosomal recessive basis [173,187] although there are reports by Roy [188] and Lauras *et al.* [179] which suggest there may also be a form transmitted dominantly. PHA may be more common than we think. It can masquerade as CAH, especially in boys. This may result in unnecessary use of glucocorticoids which may increase the risk of growth retardation. The only appropriate treatment is salt supplementation.

The most important condition to distinguish from pseudohypoaldosteronism is corticosteroid methyl oxidase deficiency (types I and II), which has already been described. Other adrenal disorders, such as adrenal hypoplasia, Addison disease and congenital adrenal hyperplasia, can all manifest similar clinical features in terms of hyperkalaemic sodium-wasting disease, but can be distinguished by other features. Premature infants can, during the not-uncommon sodium-losing phase, develop hyperkalaemia and a clinical and biochemical picture indistinguishable from PHA which usually resolves spontaneously after several weeks [207].

Miscellaneous causes

Apparent sodium-wasting may be part of an osmotic diuresis as in diabetes mellitus. Diuretic administration, either therapeutically or as a form of chemical child abuse [208] may be very confusing. A urine specimen sent for toxicological analysis can sometimes be most revealing if the chemical and biochemical findings remain inexplicable. Finally, it is important to deal with the relatively common problem of inappropriate secretion of antidiuretic hormone (ISADH) [209]. This may occur in infancy and childhood in association with central nervous system (CNS) disease, including head injury, meningitis, brain tumour and birth injury [210]. It may also occur with respiratory disorders in the neonatal period, including pneumothorax or atelectasis [211], and with positive-pressure artificial ventilation [212]. The administration of certain drugs such as opiates, carbamazepine and vincristine can cause the condition, and it has been reported in Addison disease, myxoedema and hypopituitarism.

In ISADH, a low plasma sodium and osmolality are associated with an inappropriately high urine sodium and osmolality and an inappropriately increased plasma antidiuretic hormone (ADH). The urine osmolality need not be dramatically increased, but certainly more than is appropriate for the level of plasma sodium and osmolality at the time the sample was collected. Natriuresis is always present, probably due to extracellular fluid expansion causing proximal renal tubular sodium loss [213]; these patients are therefore not just water-overloaded but also salt-depleted. It is usually impossible to diagnose if the patient is dehydrated.

Treatment consists of removing the cause, if this is possible, and restricting fluid in the first instance. If this is unsuccessful, then the administration of phenytoin to inhibit ADH release certainly may be indicated [214]. If CNS sequelae ensue because of the hyponatraemia, then intravenous hypertonic saline may have to be given. If persisting problems occur in spite of these measures, then the use of demeclocycline [215] which blocks ADH action peripherally, or a combination of frusemide and 9α-fludrocortisone, may be indicated. Usually the condition is transitory, but there are examples on record of the problem persisting for many years.

ENDOCRINE HYPERTENSION

The prevalence of hypertension in childhood is not clearly defined, and depends on the definition. Although considerable variation has been reported, the true prevalence probably lies between 1% and 3%. The vast majority of the children have mild increases in blood pressure and may well come into the category of primary (essential) hypertension. However, a small number of children will have much higher blood pressures (10% of those with hypertension); they will, in the main, suffer from secondary hypertension and be the ones that will require treatment. It is also clear that severe untreated hypertension in childhood carries a high risk of morbidity and mortality, and that lack of awareness that hypertension can and does occur in children frequently leads to delays in diagnosis and treatment that would never occur in adult practice.

Causes of hypertension

When considering causes of hypertension in childhood there are advantages in differentiating between mild and severe hypertension, since the former is usually primary or essential and the latter almost exclusively secondary. Of the causes of sustained childhood hypertension, renal disease predominates. The most important group numerically is that in which the hypertension is associated with activation of the renin–angiotensin system. Within the category of renin-dependent hypertension comes renovascular disease and various types of renal parenchymal disease, including coarsely scarred kidneys or so-called 'chronic pyelonephritis'. However, these disorders are more appropriately dealt with in detail in the paediatric nephrological literature [216–218]. (For an overview of hypertension, see [219,220].)

The endocrine causes of hypertension are usually considered to encompass disorders manifesting low renin hypertension usually, but not exclusively, due to some form of corticosteroid excess. This category of disease is rare yet important, since it may be eminently treatable either medically or surgically. The other form of hypertension often considered under the heading of 'endocrine' is that associated with catecholamine excess.

Hypertension due to corticosteroid excess

Apart from extraneously administered corticosteroids, this is usually due to certain types of CAH (for example 11β-hydroxylase and 17α-hydroxylase defects), primary hyperaldosteronism (due to adrenal cortical hyperplasia, adrenal tumour or the dexamethasone-suppressible variety), Cushing syndrome and the syndrome of apparent mineralocorticoid excess.

CONGENITAL ADRENAL HYPERPLASIA

In this type of disorder there is an enzyme defect of steroidogenesis with accumulation of mineralocorticoid, coupled with a decrease in glucocorticoid production. Chapter 30 deals with this subject in detail.

11β-HYDROXYLASE DEFICIENCY

This form of CAH is due to an enzyme deficiency of 11β-hydroxylase [221]. It is not HLA (human leukocyte antigen)-linked [222]. The enzyme resides in a specific mitochondrial cytochrome $P450_{C11}$ and its gene is sited on the long arm of chromosome 8 [223]. The result of this defect is an accumulation of deoxycorticosterone (DOC) and compound S associated with a decrease in cortisol synthesis [223,224]. The latter induces increased ACTH secretion which results in overproduction of pressor hormones. The effect of this enzymatic blockade is that DOC, with its mineralocorticoid action, causes hypertension by sodium and water retention, and there is an excess androgen production which results in virilization. The latter manifests itself by penile or clitoral enlargement, development of body hair and rapid somatic growth. Biochemically plasma potassium may be normal, but it is usually low; plasma sodium is normal. Plasma renin and aldosterone are suppressed. It is possible to identify the urinary metabolites of compound S and DOC as THS (tetrahydro-11-deoxycortisol) and THDOC (tetrahydro-11-DOC). Urine pregnanetriol, in contrast, is only modestly increased compared to the findings in 21-hydroxylase deficiency.

The decrease in cortisol production, which induces increased ACTH secretion, maintains the overproduction of mineralocorticoid and androgens; hence glucocorticoid is an obvious means of therapy. If glucocorticoid is administered, DOC is suppressed and blood pressure returns to normal and the excess androgen output diminishes. PRA, which is suppressed in the untreated condition, returns towards normal and aldosterone levels usually rise to an extent suggesting the 11β-hydroxylase is not totally defective in the zona glomerulosa of the adrenal. It is interesting that plasma aldosterone levels are often not fully suppressed in the untreated condition, supporting the above supposition. However, some patients are unable to synthesize aldosterone and may even have salt-wasting in early life [225,226]. This is probably associated with the fact that in addition to 11-hydroxylation, $P450_{C11}$ has 18-hydroxylase and 18-dehydroxylase activities (corticosterone methyloxidase I and II) [223]. (For a recent review of 11β-hydroxylase deficiency see [227].)

17α-HYDROXYLASE DEFICIENCY

This recessively inherited defect causes decreased secretion of all glucocorticoids and sex steroids from the adrenal, but an increase in mineralocorticoid production [228]. There is overproduction of 17-desoxysteroids, especially compound B and DOC. The latter is considered to be the main cause of the hypertension and is associated with suppression of plasma renin levels. The precise pathophysiology in this condition needs further description. In addition to the low renin level, there appear also to be low plasma aldosterone values, perhaps due to an additional enzyme defect at the 18-hydroxylase level [229], or due to the possibility that the zona glomerulosa and fasciculata behave as two separate glands [230]. In the latter circumstance, excess DOC production from the zona fasciculata would cause salt and water retention and hypertension suppressing plasma renin production. The resulting lack of angiotensin II stimulation of aldosterone would cause low secretion that would be corrected when DOC output was suppressed by glucocorticoid supplementation [230,231].

Clinically, males are incompletely masculinized and females often present at adolescence with primary amenorrhoea due to the 17-hydroxylase deficiency and 17–20 lyase activity interfering with side-chain cleavage of C21 steroids precluding the formation of C19 steroids and adrenal androgens, as well as interfering with gonadal function [223,232]. Hypertension is associated with hypokalaemia. There are reports of what might be incomplete or partial 17α-hydroxylase deficiency which masquerade as a form of dexamethasone-suppressible hypertension [233]. Patients with 17α-hydroxylase deficiency are managed by glucocorticoid suppression of ACTH secretion, either in the form of hydrocortisone or dexamethasone.

PRIMARY HYPERALDOSTERONISM

Primary hyperaldosteronism is rare [234]. The autonomous release of aldosterone by the adrenal gland or glands results in sodium retention, plasma volume expansion, hypertension and renin suppression. Bilateral adrenal hyperplasia is said to be more common [235], but numbers are small and aldosterone-producing tumours can occur.

The diagnostic features include hyperaldosteronism, which fails to suppress with dexamethasone, low plasma renin levels with potassium-wasting in a sodium-replete state. Urine steroid analysis will demonstrate excess aldosterone but without chracteristic precursor findings seen in patients with steroid biosynthetic blocks. Distinction between hyperplasia and tumour is difficult. Functional studies including aldosterone response to posture [235–237], saline infusion [238] and ACE inhibition [239] have proved helpful, but in spite of these techniques it is not easy to distinguish confidently between tumour and hyperplasia. Abdominal ultrasonography, computerized tomography, and magnetic resonance image scanning are helpful in localization, but adrenal venous aldosterone and cortisol sampling may additionally be required [234, 240,241]. ^{131}I-19-iodocholesterol scintigraphy is not recommended [242].

Treatment is essentially surgical for an adrenal adenoma but long-term spironolactone administration is the therapy of choice in bilateral adrenal hyperplasia [243] (see Chapter 28).

DEXAMETHASONE-SUPPRESSIBLE HYPERALDOSTERONISM

This disorder which, in terms of clinical and biochemical presentation, is indistinguishable from primary hyperaldosteronism, has the characteristic feature of rapid aldosterone suppression on administration of dexamethasone [233,244–251]. It has been considered that there may be an ACTH receptor in the aldosterone-producing cells of the adrenals [248]. ACTH administration in these patients increases aldosterone production, which would support this contention. An explanation for this phenomenon and the aldosterone unresponsiveness to angiotensin in this condition, is abnormal adrenocortical zonation with aldosterone being produced by the zona fasciculata [252–254]. Hypertension can be controlled by glucocorticoid administration, at least in children. There is some evidence that adults may not necessarily respond. A dominant form of inheritance not linked to HLA seems likely for this rare disorder [255]. Recently the gene for aldsoterone synthase has been found to be abnormal in some patients with this entity [256,257]. Fallo & Mantero [258] have recently reviewed this condition.

CUSHING SYNDROME

In childhood, hypertension is common in Cushing syndrome. One report cites 21 of 26 children with a high blood pressure [259]. The cause of the hypertension is multifactorial, and includes the mineralocorticoid effect of excess cortisol, increased vascular reactivity to vasoconstrictors [260,261] and increased renin substrate [262]. This condition is discussed in detail in Chapter 28.

APPARENT MINERALOCORTICOID EXCESS

In the syndrome of apparent mineralocorticoid excess (AME) there is hypertension, hypokalaemia, suppression of renin and no oversecretion of any recognized mineralocorticoids [262–274]. The syndrome appears to be familial [268]. Hypertension and hypokalaemia have responded to spironolactone, amiloride or triamterine, suggesting the presence of an unidentified mineralocorticoid [262,265, 266]. However, aldosterone levels are subnormal and there is no conclusive evidence of overproduction of other mineralocorticoids [272]. ACTH and intravenous infusion of cortisol aggravate the hypertension [234]. Ulick *et al.* [275] demonstated an abnormal pattern of urinary excretion of dihydrometabolites of cortisol and an increase in compounds with 5α relative to 5β stereochemistry; they then postulated a deficiency of cortisol 11β-hydroxysteroid dehydrogenase as the primary defect. This has been confirmed in patients with similar clinical presentations [265,267,270]. The condition has been fatal [267,271,275].

The cause of the hypertension appears to be the increased half-life of cortisol, and the fact that in this condition it acts very much like a mineralocorticoid on type I receptors. These receptors are normally acted on by aldosterone, but it is suggested that in this condition there is also a defect in the receptors themselves [268,276,277].

It is of interest that glycyrrhizic and glycyrrhetinic acids from liquorice inhibit 11β-dehydrogenase and can produce an acquired form of AME [278,279] whereas AME is usually considered to be recessively inherited [271,279, 280].

The condition is identified by the low plasma renin value and a normal or low plasma aldosterone concentration; urine steroid analysis by mass spectrometric gas chromatographic analysis is needed for confirmation, and demonstrates a ratio of tetrahydrocortisone (THE) to tetrahydrocortisol (THF) of less than 1 [263]. Treatment with spironolactone and/or triamterine is indicated.

GORDON SYNDROME

Gordon syndrome, is sometimes known as pseudohypoaldosteronism type II or 'chloride shunt' syndrome [281–286]. In this condition there is hypertension associated with hyperkalaemia, and evidence to suggest that the primary defect is increased absorption of salt and water from the proximal tubules [286]. It has been considered to be due to a primary lack of ANP, but this has not been substantiated [287]. An alternative possibility is that there is a lack of responsiveness to ANP [286]. Treatment can be satisfactorily achieved with thiazide diuretics. If the blood pressure is normal the condition is known as the Spitzer–Weinstein syndrome [288,289].

Catecholamine excess hypertension

Sustained hypertension due to excess catecholamine is usually due to a tumour of the neural crest, that is phaeochromocytoma, neuroblastoma or ganglioneuroma. The importance of these tumours is out of proportion to their incidence, since they can be associated with catastrophic increases in blood pressure, difficulties in diagnosis and management, but there is potential for complete cure by surgical removal [290].

Phaeochromocytomas account for 0.5–2% of the cases of secondary hypertension in children [290,291]. Boys were affected twice as often as girls according to Stackpole *et al.* [292], but this was not confirmed by others [290]. Two-thirds of the tumours are in the adrenal medulla [292]. The most frequent extra-adrenal sites are near the adrenal gland at the aortic bifurcation and in the renal hilum [292]. Hypertension is sustained in 88% of people and clinical symptoms include headaches (75%), sweating (67%), nausea and vomiting (48%), visual disturbances (37%), abdominal pain (32%), polydipsia and polyuria (31%), convulsions (22%) and acrocyanosis (22%) [292].

Although phaeochromocytomas are usually sporadic, they appear occasionally to be familial, and have been associated with von Recklinghausen disease [293], von Hippel–Landau disease [294] and multiple endocrine neoplasia syndromes [295–297]. Thirty-one percent of cases have been reported to be familial [298]. The inheritance of familial cases is autosomal dominant [299]. The long-term outlook for cure of phaeochromocytoma is good, and the incidence of malignancy is low (5–10%) [291].

The diagnosis of catecholamine-producing tumours can be established by demonstrating increased urinary excretion of catecholamines and their metabolites or, more precisely, by measuring plasma catecholamine levels [300]. Localizing the tumour may be difficult, especially if multiple sites are involved. A combination of ultrasound, arteriography (after full α-adrenergic blockade), computerized tomography, ^{123}I metaiodobenzylguanidine (MIBG) scintigraphy and vena caval catecholamine sampling is usually sufficient to localize the lesion or lesions [290]. However, invasive procedures must be undertaken only after adequate sympathetic blockade. Blood pressure during the procedures should be carefully monitored and phentolamine, labetalol or sodium nitroprusside should be available for immediate injection if there is a hypertensive crisis.

The treatment of catecholamine-producing tumours is surgical. A hypertensive child with neuroblastoma requiring surgical removal may require the same pharmacological blockade as is appropriate for phaeochromocytoma. Decisions concerning surgery for phaeochromocytoma depend on preoperative localization and feasibility of intervention. Preoperative α-blockade must be effected and β-blockade may be needed to counteract the effect of α-blockade-induced tachycardia, or to counter the effects of dopamine or adrenaline produced by the lesion. In the past phenoxybenzamine was the α-blocking agent of choice, with prazosin as an alternative drug. However, recently the calcium channel inhibitor, nifedipine, has proved also to be effective [154]. Nifedipine alone has not achieved adequate preoperative blood pressure control in all children so treated [290]. During the days required to obtain α-blockade, a generous salt intake facilitates ECF volume expansion. Surgery should be undertaken with arterial and central venous lines in place and adequate supplies of appropriate hypotensive agents and plasma and saline to fill the vascular space as necessary. Halothane or a similar anaesthesia that does not elicit sympathetic activity is favoured.

Handling the tumour can produce catastrophic increases in blood pressure, even for patients thought to be adequately blocked. Theoretically, if α-blockade is complete for some time preoperatively, blood pressure should not fall when the tumour is removed. However, blood pressure usually does fall, because circulating vasoconstrictors dramatically decrease and vasodilation caused by the α-blockade ensues. The initial danger comes when the veins of the tumour are ligated; a progressive drop over many hours may require ECF volume repletion. Sympathetic blockade should be discontinued as soon as the tumour is removed. Blood pressure is labile for several days even with these precautions.

ESSENTIAL HYPERTENSION

There is increasing evidence that adult essential hypertension has its origins in childhood or even in utero [301–307]. It is known that blood pressure rises with age in urban and Western societies [307–309] although this may be less marked in some rural areas or in more primitive cultures [310]. In childhood the rise in blood pressure is closely related to growth [311] and this relationship is particularly close in adolescence [311,312] overriding pressure tracking with age [313]. It has been suggested that growth-promoting mechanisms in childhood have effects on blood pressure as well as somatic growth [307] and that when children reach adult life a self-perpetuating mechanism maintains increased blood pressure that has occurred [307]. There is thus evidence that essential hypertension is a growth-related disorder with origins in childhood and manifestations in adult life [305,307].

Data are also emerging to show that the intrauterine environment has an important effect on blood pressure and hypertension in adults [301]. Small babies with large placentae at birth are associated with subsequent adult high blood pressure [301, 302, 304] and it is suggested that after the initiation process in fetal life there is an amplification of blood pressure through childhood [305]. A possible means of linking low birth weight and high placental weight with hypertension is increased fetal glucocorticoid exposure secondary to attenuated placental 11β-hydroxysteroid dehydrogenase activity [314,315].

Genes and the environment are likely also to play a part in the rise of pressure in children and adults, but it is difficult to assess their relative importance. Numerous epidemiological studies have shown familial aggregation of primary hypertension in humans [316] and there is evidence from studying various intermediate phenotypes, such as blood cell membrane transport systems, that individuals manifesting certain characteristics may be predisposed to develop essential hypertension in later life [317–320]. So far, however, genetic linkage studies have not identified a specific gene associated with the development of essential hypertension [321]. Likewise, environmental factors clearly may play a part in determining blood pressure, as shown by data from the Montreal adoption study [319], migration studies [310] and geographical differences in blood pressure found in differing geographical positions [322].

It seems likely that essential hypertension is a polygenic disorder influenced by intrauterine factors and growth, with a contribution from the environment. It is particularly noteworthy in a text on paediatric endocrinology that endocrine influences may play a major part in determining the blood pressure in growing children. They may provide its prevention and cure.

REFERENCES

1 McCrory WW. *Developmental Nephrology*. Cambridge, MA: Harvard University Press, 1972.
2 Alexander DF, Nixon DA. The foetal kidney. *Br Med Bull* 1961;17:112–17.

3 McCance RA. The role of the developing kidney in the maintenance of internal stability. *J R Coll Phys* 1972;6:235–45.
4 Robillard JE, Sessions C, Kennedy RL *et al.* Interrelationships between glomerular filtration rate and renal transport of sodium and chloride during fetal life. *Am J Obstet Gynecol* 1977;128:727.
5 Engelke SC, Shah BL, Vasan U *et al.* Sodium balance in very low birth weight infants. *J Pediatr* 1978;93:837–41.
6 Horster M, Thurau K. Micropuncture studies in filtration rates of single superficial and juxtamedullary glomeruli in rat. *Pflügers Arch* 1968;301:162–81.
7 Pipkin FB, Lumbers ER, Mott JC. Factors influencing plasma renin and angiotensin in the conscious pregnant ewe and its foetus. *J Physiol* 1974;243:619–36.
8 Trimper CE, Lumbers ER. The renin–angiotensin system in fetal lambs. *Pflügers Arch* 1972;336:1–10.
9 Kotchen TA, Strickland AL, Rice TW *et al.* A study of the renin–angiotensin system in newborn infants. *J Pediatr* 1972;80:938–46.
10 Pipkin FB, Symonds EM. Factors affecting angiotensin II concentrations in the human infant at birth. *Clin Sci Mol Med* 1977;52:449–56.
11 Molteni A, Rahil WJ, Koo J-H. Evidence for a vasopressor substance (renin) in human fetal kidneys. *Lab Invest* 1974; 30:115–18.
12 Mott JC. The place of the renin–angiotensin system before and after birth. *Br Med Bull* 1975;31:44–50.
13 Robillard JE, Smith FG, Smith FG. Developmental aspects of renal function during fetal life. In: Edelmann CM, ed. *Pediatric Kidney Disease*, 2nd edn. Boston: Little, Brown, 1992:3–18.
14 Forsyth CC. The growth and development of the endocrine glands–adrenal cortex. In: Davis J, Dobbing J, eds. *Scientific Foundations of Paediatrics*. London: Heinemann Medical, 1974:469–98.
15 Lanman JT. The adrenal gland in the human fetus. An interpretation of its physiology and unusual developmental pattern. *Pediatrics* 1961;27:140–58.
16 Easterling WE, Simmer H, Dignam WG *et al.* Neutral C19 steroids and steroid sulfates in human pregnancy. II. Dehydroepiandrosterone sulfate, 16-alpha-hydroxydehydroepiandrosterone, and 16-alphahydroxydehydroepiandrosterone sulfate in maternal and fetal blood of pregnancies with anencephalic and normal fetuses. *Steroids* 1966;8: 157–78.
17 Strecker JR, Lehmann WD, Wolf AS *et al.* Suppression of the maternal and fetal pituitary adrenocortical axis by administration of beta-methasone during pregnancy. *Acta Endocrinol* (Suppl.) 1978;87:215–33.
18 Silman RE, Chard T, Landon J *et al.* Human fetal corticotrophin and related pituitary peptides. *J Steroid Biochem* 1977;8:553–7.
19 Pepe GJ, Albrecht ED. Regulation of the primate fetal adrenal cortex. *Endocr Rev* 1990;11:151–76.
20 Goldman AS, Yakovac WC, Bongiovanni AM. Development of activity of 3β hydroxy steroid dehydrogenase in fetal tissues in two anencephalic newborns. *J Clin Endocrinol Metab* 1966:26:14–22.
21 Pasqualini JR. Quelques nouveaux aspects de la transformation des hormones steroidiennes pendant la vie foetale. *Ann Endocrinol* 1970;31:396–413.
22 Voutilainen R. Steroidogenesis in tissue culture of fetal and adult human adrenals with special reference to cortisol/corticosterone ratio and aldosterone secretion. *J Steroid Biochem* 1979;10:115–20.
23 Partsch C-J, Sippell WG, MacKenzie IZ, Aynsley-Green A. The steroid milieu of the undisturbed human fetus and mother at 16–20 weeks gestation. *J Clin Endocrinol Metab* 1991;73:969–74.
24 Hall CStG, Branchaud C, Klein GP *et al.* Secretion rate and metabolism of the sulfates of cortisol and corticosterone in newborn infants. *J Clin Endocrinol Metab* 1971;33:98–104.
25 Sippell WG, Bidlingmaier F, Knorr D. Development of endogenous glucocorticoids, mineralocorticoids and progestins in the human fetal and perinatal period. Influence of antenatal treatment with beta methasone or phenobarbital. *Eur J Clin Pharmacol* 1980;18:95–104.
26 Dörr HG, Sippell WG, Versrrold HT *et al.* Plasma mineralocorticoids, glucocorticoids and progestins in premature infants: longitudinal study during the first week of life. *Pediatr Res* 1988;23:525–9.
27 Mulrow PJ, Schneider G. Aldosterone regulation in the maternal and fetal rat in pregnancy. *Perspect Nephrol Hypertens* 1976;5:229–37.
28 Kowarski A, Katz H, Migeon CJ. Plasma aldosterone concentrations in normal subjects from infancy to adulthod. *J Clin Endocrinol Metab* 1974;38:489–91.
29 Smith FG, Robillard JE. Pathophysiology of fetal renal disease. *Semin Perinatal* 1989;13:305.
30 Matson JR, Stokes JB, Robillard JE. Effects of inhibition of prostaglandin synthesis on fetal renal function. *Kidney Int* 1981;20:621.
31 Smith FG, Sato T, Varille VA *et al.* Atrial natriuretic factor during fetal and postanatal life: a review. *J Dev Physiol* 1989;12:55.
32 Edelmann CM. Pediatric nephrology. E Mead Johnson Award Address. *Pediatrics* 1972;51:854–65.
33 Spitzer A, Brandis M. Functional and morphologic maturation of the superficial nephrons. Relationship to total kidney function. *J Clin Invest* 1974;53:279–87.
34 Houston IB, Oetliker O. The growth and development of the kidney. In: Davis JA, Dobbing J, eds. *Scientific Foundations of Paediatrics*. London: Heinemann Medical, 1974:297–307.
35 Edelmann CM, Spitzer A. A maturing kidney. A modern view of well-balanced infants with imbalanced nephrons. *J Pediatr* 1969;75:509–19.
36 Gruskin AB, Edelmann CM, Yuan S. Maturational changes in renal blood flow in piglets. *Pediatr Res* 1970;4:7–13.
37 Olbing H, Blaufox MD, Aschinberg LC *et al.* Postnatal changes in renal blood flow distribution in puppies. *J Clin Invest* 1973;52:2885–95.
38 Rodriguez-Soriano J, Vallo A, Castillo G. Renal handling of sodium in premature and full term neonates. A study using clearance methods during water diuresis. *Pediatr Res* 1983; 17:1013–16.
39 Dillon MJ, Gilliam MEA, Ryness JM *et al.* Plasma renin activity and aldosterone concentration in the human newborn. *Arch Dis Child* 1976;51:537–40.
40 Fiselier T, Lijnen P, Monnens L *et al.* Levels of renin, angiotensin I and II, angiotensin-converting enzyme and aldosterone in infancy and childhood. *Eur J Pediatr* 1983; 141:3–7.
41 Raux-Eurin MC, Pham-Huu-Trung MT, Marrec D *et al.* Plasma aldosterone concentrations during the neonatal period. *Pediatr Res* 1977;11:182–5.
42 Dillon MJ. Renin and hypertension in childhood. *Arch Dis Child* 1974;49:831–4.

43 Sulyok E, Nemeth M, Tenyi I *et al.* The possible role of prostaglandins in the hyperfunction of the renin–angiotensin–aldosterone system in the newborn. *Br J Obstet Gynaecol* 1979;86:205–9.

44 Spitzer A. Renal physiology and functional development. In: Edelmann CM, ed. *Paediatric Kidney Disease.* Boston: Little Brown, 1978:25–128.

45 Sulyok E, Ertl T, Csaba IF *et al.* Postnatal changes in urinary prostaglandin E excretion in premature infants. *Biol Neonate* 1980;37:192 -6.

46 Day GM, Radde IC, Balfe JW *et al.* Electrolyte abnormalities in very low birthweight infants. *Pediatr Res* 1976;10:552–6.

47 Siegel SR, Oh W. Renal function as a marker of human fetal maturation. *Acta Paed Scand* 1976;65:481–5.

48 Sulyok E. The relationship between electrolyte and acid–base balance in the premature infant during early postnatal life. *Biol Neonate* 1971;17:227–37.

49 Honour JW, Valman HB, Shackleton CHL. Aldosterone and sodium homeostatis in pre-term infants. *Acta Paed Scand* 1977;66:103–9.

50 Aperia A, Broberger O, Herin P *et al.* Sodium excretion in relation to sodium intake and aldosterne excretion in newborn pre-term and full-term infants. *Acta Paed Scand* 1979;68: 813–17.

51 Al-Dahhan J, Haycock GB, Chantler C *et al.* Sodium homeostasis in term and pre-term neonates. I. Renal aspects. *Arch Dis Child* 1983;58:335–42.

52 Sulyok E. Hormonal control of sodium balance in premature infants. In: Murakami K, Kitagawa T, Yabuta K *et al.*, eds. *Recent Advances in Pediatric Nephrology.* Amsterdam: Elsevier, 1987:101–6.

53 Ertl T, Sulyok E, Varga L *et al.* Postnatal development of plasma prolactin level in premature infants with and without NaCl supplementation. *Biol Neonate* 1983;44:219–23.

54 Sulyok E, Gyodi G, Ertl T *et al.* The influence of NaCl supplementation on the postnatal development of urinary excretion of noradrenaline, dopamine, and serotonin in premature infants. *Pediatr Res* 1985;19:5–8.

55 Robillard JE, Weissman DN, Gomez RA *et al.* Renal and adrenal responses to converting-enzyme inhibition in fetal and newborn life. *Am J Physiol* 1983;244:R249–56.

56 Seri I, Tulassay T, Kiszel J *et al.* Cardiovascular response to dopamine in hypotensive pre-term neonates with severe hyaline membrane disease. *Eur J Pediatr* 1984;142:3–9.

57 Tulassay T, Seri I. Interaction of dopamine and furosemide in acute oliguria of pre-term infants with severe hyaline membrane disease. *Acta Paed Scand* 1986;75:420–4.

58 Tulassay T, Seri I, Machay T *et al.* Effect of dopamine on renal function in premature infants with respiratory distress syndrome. *Int J Pediatr Nephrol* 1983;4:19–23.

59 Rees L, Brook CGD, Shaw JCL *et al.* Hyponatraemia in the first week of life in preterm infants. I. Arginine vasopressin secretion. *Arch Dis Child* 1984;59:414–22.

60 Sulyok E, Kovacs L, Lichardus B *et al.* Late hyponatraemia in premature infants: role of aldosterone and arginine vasopressin. *J Pediatr* 1985;105:990–4.

61 Ebara H, Suzuki S, Nagashima K. Digoxin- and digoxin-like immunoreactive substances in amniotic fluid, cord blood, and serum of neonates. *Pediatr Res* 1986;20:28–32.

62 Ebara H, Suzuki S, Nagashima K *et al.* Digoxin-like immunoreactive substances in urine and serum from preterm and term infants: relationship to renal excretion of sodium. *J Pediatr* 1986;108:760–2.

63 Arant BS. Neonatal adjustments to extrauterine life. In: Edelmann CM, ed. *Pediatric Kidney Disease*, 2nd edn. Boston: Little, Brown, 1992:1015–42.

64 Hughes IA, Wilton A, Lole CA. Continuing need for mineralocorticoid therapy in salt-losing congenital adrenal hyperplasia. *Arch Dis Child* 1979;54:350–5.

65 Dillon MJ, Shah V, Mitchell MD. Bartter's syndrome: 10 cases in childhood. Results of long term indomethacin therapy. *Q J Med* 1979;48:429–46.

66 Dillon MJ. Applications of study of the renin–angiotensin system to paediatric pathology. In: Giovannelli G, New M, Gorini S, eds. *Hypertension in Children and Adults.* New York: Raven Press, 1981:137–46.

67 Milla PJ, Trompeter R, Dillon MJ *et al.* Salt-losing syndrome in 2 infants with defective 18-hydrogenation in aldosterone biosynthesis. *Arch Dis Child* 1977;52:580–6.

68 Bartter FC, Pronove P, Gee JR, *et al.* Hyperplasia of the juxtaglomerular complex with hyperaldosteronism and hypokalemic alkalosis. *Am J Med* 1962;33:811–28.

69 James T, Holland NH, Preston D. Bartter's syndrome. Typical facies and normal plasma volume. *Am J Dis Child* 1975;129: 1205–7.

70 Delaney VB, Oliver JF, Simms M *et al.* Bartter's syndrome: physiological and pharmacological studies. *Q J Med* 1981;50: 213–32.

71 Solomon LR, Bobinski H, Astley P *et al.* Bartter's syndrome – observations on the pathophysiology. *Q J Med* 1982;51: 251–70.

72 Sutherland LE, Hartcroft P, Balis JU *et al.* Bartter's syndrome: a report of four cases, including three in one sibship, with comparative histological evaluation of the juxtaglomerular apparatuses and glomeruli. *Acta Paed Scand* 1970; (Suppl.) 201:1–24.

73 Trygstad CW, Mangos JA, Bloodworth JMB *et al.* A sibship with Bartter's syndrome: failure of total adrenalectomy to correct the potassium wasting. *Pediatrics* 1969;44:234–42.

74 Chaimovitz C, Levi J, Better OS *et al.* Studies on the site of renal salt loss in a patient with Bartter's syndrome. *Pediatr Res* 1973;7:89–94.

75 Gill JR, Bartter FC. Evidence of prostaglandin independent defect in chloride reabsorption in the loop of Henle as a proximal cause of Bartter's syndrome. *Am J Med* 1978;65:766–72.

76 Baehler RW, Work J, Kotchen TA *et al.* Studies on the pathogenesis of Bartter's syndrome. *Am J Med* 1980;69:933–8.

77 Mace JW, Hambidge KM, Gotlin RW *et al.* Magnesium supplementation in Bartter's syndrome. *Arch Dis Child* 1973; 48:485–7.

78 Evans RA, Carter JN, George CR *et al.* The congenital magnesium-losing kidney. Report of two patients. *Q J Med* 1981;50:39–52.

79 Gitelman JH, Graham JB, Welt LG. A new familial disorder characterised by hypokalemia and hypomagnesemia. *Trans Assoc Am Phys* 1966;79:221.

80 McCredie DA, Blair-West JR, Scoggins BA *et al.* Potassium losing nephropathy of childhood. *Med J Aust* 1971;1:129–35.

81 Paunier L, Sizonekio PC. Asymptomatic chronic hypomagnesemia and hypokalemia in a child: cell membrane disease? *J Pediatr* 1976;88:51–5.

82 Cannon PJ, Leeming JM, Sommers SC *et al.* Juxtaglomerular cell hyperplasia and secondary hyperaldosteronism (Bartter's syndrome): a re-evaluation of the pathophysiology. *Medicine* 1968;47:107–31.

83 Bartter FC, Delea CS, Kawasaki T *et al.* The adrenal cortex and the kidney. *Kidney Int* 1974;6:272–80.
84 Rosa RC, Shah V, Dillon MJ. Effect of indomethacin on GFR, fractional distal delivery and reabsorption in Bartter's syndrome. *Int J Pediatr Nephrol* 1981;2:129.
85 Tomko DK, Yeh BP, Falls WF. Bartter's syndrome. Study of a 52-year-old man with evidence of a defect in proximal sodium reabsorption and comments on therapy. *Am J Med* 1976;61:111–18.
86 Uribarri J, Alveranga D, Oh MS *et al.* Bartter's syndrome due to a defect in salt reabsorption in the distal convoluted tubule. *Nephron* 1985;40:52–6.
87 White MG. Bartter's syndrome. A manifestation of renal tubular defects. *Arch Intern Med* 1972;129:41–7.
88 Kurtzmann NA, Gutierrez LF. The pathophysiology of Bartter's syndrome. *J Am Med Assoc* 1975;234:758–9.
89 Oliver JF, Delaney VB, Bourke E. Increased erythrocyte sodium permeability with Bartter's syndrome. *Miner Electrolyte Metab* 1978;1:225.
90 Cole CH, O'Regan S. Effect of treatment with prostaglandin synthetase inhibitors on the erythrocyte sodium transport abnormality of Bartter's syndrome. *Pediatr Res* 1981;15: 926–9.
91 Delaporte C, Stulzaft J, Loirat C *et al.* Muscle electrolytes and fluid compartments in six children with Bartter's syndrome. *Clin Sci Mol Med* 1978;54:223–31.
92 Gall G, Vaitukaitis J, Haddow JE *et al.* Erythrocyte Na flux in a patient with Bartter's syndrome. *J Clin Endocrinol Metab* 1971;32:562–7.
93 Gardner JD, Simopoulos AP, Lapey A *et al.* Altered membrane sodium transport in Bartter's syndrome. *J Clin Invest* 1972;51:1565–71.
94 McCredie DA, Rotenberg E, Williams AL. Hypercalciuria in potassium-losing nephropathy: a variant of Bartter's syndrome. *Aust Paediatr J* 1974;10:286–95.
95 Uchiyama M, Shah M, Daman Willems C *et al.* Erythrocyte sodium transport in Bartter's syndrome. *Acta Paed Scand* 1988;77:873–8.
96 Mongeau JG, Garay R, de Mendonca M *et al.* Erythrocyte Na^+ and K^+ transport systems in children with Bartter's syndrome: increase in passive sodium permeability. *Kidney Int* 1983;23:530–5.
97 Donker AJM, de Jong PE, van Eps LW *et al.* Indomethacin in Bartter's syndrome: does the syndrome represent a state of hyperprostaglandinism? *Nephron* 1977;19:200–13.
98 Rodriguez-Soriano J, Vallo A, Oliveros R. Bartter's syndrome presenting with features resembling renal tubular acidosis. Improvement of renal tubular defects by indomethacin. *Helv Paediatr Acta* 1978;33:141–51.
99 Bowden RE, Gill JR, Radfar N *et al.* Prostaglandin synthetase inhibitors in Bartter's syndrome. *J Am Med Assoc* 1978;239: 117–21.
100 Dray F. Bartter's syndrome: contrasting patterns of prostaglandin excretion in children and adults. *Clin Sci Mol Med* 1978;54:115–18.
101 Fichman MP, Telfer N, Zia P *et al.* Role of prostaglandins in the pathogenesis of Bartter's syndrome. *Am J Med* 1976;60: 785–97.
102 Gill JR, Frolich JC, Bowden RE *et al.* Bartter's syndrome: a disorder characterized by high urinary prostaglandins and a dependence of hyper-reninemia on prostaglandin synthesis. *Am J Med* 1976;61:43–51.
103 Gullner HG, Cerletti C, Bartter FC *et al.* Prostaglandin overproduction in Bartter's syndrome. *Lancet* 1979;2:767–9.
104 Halushka PV, Wohltmann H, Privitera PJ *et al.* Bartter's syndrome: urinary prostaglandin E-like material and kalikrein: indomethacin effects. *Ann Intern Med* 1977;87: 281–6.
105 Littlewood JM, Lee MR, Meadow SR. Treatment of Bartter's syndrome in early childhood with prostaglandin synthetase inhibitors. Arch Dis Child 1978;53:43–8.
106 Norby L, Lentz R, Flamenbaum W *et al.* Prostaglandins and aspirin therapy in Bartter's syndrome. *Lancet* 1976;2:604–6.
107 Proesmans W, Muaka BK, Monnens L. Indomethacin therapy in Bartter's syndrome. *Acta Paediatr Belg* 1977;30: 31–6.
108 Rosa FC, Shah V, Dillon MJ. Urine prostaglandins in healthy children and patients with Bartter's syndrome. *Int J Pediatr Nephrol* 1982;3:112.
109 Stoff JS, MacIntyre DI, Brown RS *et al.* Prostacyclin overproduction in Bartter's syndrome. *Lancet* 1979;2:1169–70.
110 Verberckmoes R, Van Damme B, Clement J *et al.* Bartter's syndrome with hyperplasia of renomedullary cells: successful treatment with indomethacin. *Kidney Int* 1976;9: 302–7.
111 Mullner G, Gahwiler T, Luthy C *et al.* Comparison of prostaglandin production of skin fibroblasts grown from patients with Bartter's syndrome and from age and sex matched controls. *Prostag Leukotr Med* 1983;11:83–93.
112 Stoff JS, Stemerman M, Steer M *et al.* A defect in platelet aggregation in Bartter's syndrome. *Am J Med* 1980;68:171–80.
113 Lechi A, Covi G, Lechi C *et al.* Urinary kallikrein excretion in Bartter's syndrome. *J Clin Endocrinol Metab* 1976;43: 1175–8.
114 McGiff JC. Bartter's syndrome results from an imbalance of vasoactive hormones. *Ann Intern Med* 1977;87:369–72.
115 Vinci JM, Gill JR, Bowden RE *et al.* The kallikrein–kinin system in Bartter's syndrome and its response to prostaglandin synthetase inhibition. *J Clin Invest* 1978;61:1671–82.
116 Arant BS, Brackett NC, Young RB *et al.* Case studies of siblings with juxtaglomerular hyperplasia and secondary aldosteronism associated with severe azotemia and renal rickets – Bartter's syndrome or disease? *Pediatrics* 1970;46: 344–61.
117 Salomon MI, Tchertkoff V. Bartter's syndrome: an overview. *Angiology* 1977;28:806–12.
118 Garin EH, Sausville PJ, Richard GA. Serum inhibitor of phytohemagglutinin-induced lymphocyte proliferation in Bartter syndrome. *J Pediatr* 1983;102:569–72.
119 Ogihara T, Maroyama A, Nugent CA *et al.* Familial Bartter's syndrome. *Arch Intern Med* 1952;142:906–8.
120 Goulon M, Raphael JC, De Rohan P. Syndrome de Bartter et chondrocalcinose. Une association non fortuite. *Nouv Presse Med* 1980;9:1291–5.
121 Fanconi A, Schachenmann G, Nussli R *et al.* Chronic hypokalemia with growth retarding normotensive hyper-renin-hyperaldosteronism (Bartter's syndrome) and hypercalciuria. *Helv Paediatr Acta* 1971;26:144.
122 Houser M, Zimmerman B, Davidman M *et al.* Idiopathic hypercalciuria associated with hyperreninemia and high urinary prostaglandin E. *Kidney Int* 1984;26:176.
123 Kurtz I, Maher T, Jones JW *et al.* Familial chloride resistant renal alkalosis and hypokalaemia with fasting hypercalciuria and medullary nephrocalcinosis. A unique variant of Bartter's

syndrome without impaired renal diluting ability. *Clin Res* 1981;29:555A.

124 Seyberth HW, Rafscher W, Schweer H *et al.* Congenital hypokalaemia with hypercalciuria in preterm infants: a hyperpostaglandinuric tubular syndrome different to Bartter's syndrome. *J Pediatr* 1985;107:694.

125 Fricker H, Frey K, Vallotton MB *et al.* Bartter-syndrom und tubulare funktionsstorungen. *Helv Paediatr Acta* 1975;30: 61–77.

126 Godard C, Vallotton MB, Broyer M *et al.* A study of the inhibition of the renin–angiotensin system in renal potassium wasting syndromes, including Bartter's syndrome. *Helv Paediatr Acta* 1972;27:495–511.

127 Sann L, David L, Bernheim J *et al.* Hypophosphatemia and hyperparathyroidism in a case of Bartter's syndrome. *Helv Paediatr Acta* 1978;33:299–310.

128 Straus RG, Mohammed S, Loggie JM *et al.* The effect of methyldopa on plasma renin activity in a child with Bartter's syndrome. *J Pediatr* 1970;77:1071–4.

129 Modlinger RS, Nicholis GL, Krakkoff LR *et al.* Some observations on the pathogenesis of Bartter's syndrome. *N Engl J Med* 1973;289:1022–4.

130 Rosa FC, Bobinski H, Shah V *et al.* A plasma factor's role in the red blood cell sodium pump abnormality in Bartter's syndrome. *Eur J Pediatr* 1983;140:153.

131 Guesry P, Dray F, Broyer M. Urinary prostaglandins in Bartter's syndrome in children treated with indomethacin. Escapement from and the toxicity of this drug (Abstr.). In: *4th International Symposium on Paediatric Nephrology,* Helsinki, 1977:85.

132 Gill JR. Disorders of renal transport of sodium, potassium, magnesium and calcium. In: Edelmann CM, ed. *Pediatric Kidney Disease,* 2nd edn. Boston: Little, Brown, 1992:1873–85.

133 Chan JCM, Malakzedah MH, Anand SK. Defect in renal tubular sodium reabsorption in a patient with Bartter's syndrome. *Clin Proc Child Hosp Natl Med Cen* 1975;31: 67–71.

134 Rodriguez-Soriano J, Vallo A, Castillo G *et al.* Renal handling of water and sodium in infancy and childhood: a study using clearance methods during hypotonic saline diuresis. *Kidney Int* 1981;20:700–4.

135 Schwartz WB, Relman AS. Metabolic and renal studies in chronic potassium depeletion resulting from overuse of laxatives. *J Clin Invest* 1953;32:258–71.

136 Demers LM, Valdhuis JD, Ramos E. The clinical entity of pseudo-Bartter's syndrome. In: Samuelsson B *et al.*, eds. *Advances in Prostaglandins and Thromboxane Research,* Vol. 7. New York: Raven Press, 1980:1203–6.

137 Roy S, Arant BS. Hypokalaemic metabolic alkalosis in normotensive infants with elevated plasma renin activity and hyperaldosteronism: role of dietary chloride deficiency. *Pediatrics* 1981;67:423–9.

138 Holmberg C, Perheentupa J, Launiala K *et al.* Congenital chloride diarrhoea: clinical analysis of 21 Finnish patients. *Arch Dis Child* 1977;52:255–67.

139 Gottleib RP. Metabolic alkalosis in cystic fibrosis. *J Pediatr* 1971;79:930–6.

140 Kennedy JD, Dinwiddie R, Daman Willems C, Dillon MJ, Matthews DJ. Pseudo Bartter's syndrome in cystic fibrosis. *Arch Dis Child* 1990;65:786–9.

141 Buckalew VM, McDurdy DK, Ludwig GD *et al.* Incomplete renal tubular acidosis. *Am J Med* 1968;45:32–42.

142 Takeda R, Mortimoto S, Kuroda M *et al.* Renal tubular acidosis, presenting as a syndrome resembling Bartter's syndrome, in a patient with arachnodactyly. *Acta Endocrinol* 1973;73:531–42.

143 Ben-Ishay D, Levy M, Birnbaum D. Self-induced secondary hyperaldosteronism simulating Bartter's syndrome. *Isr J Med Sci* 1972;8:1835–9.

144 Rodriguez-Soriano J, Vallo A, Garcia-Fuentes M. Hypomagnesaemia of hereditary renal origin. *Pediatr Nephrol* 1987;1:465–72.

145 Pakravan P, Kenny FM, Depp R *et al.* Familial congenital absence of adrenal glands: evaluation of glucocorticoid, mineralocorticoid and estrogen metabolism in the perinatal period. *J Pediatr* 1974;84:74–8.

146 Gillet P, Francois P. L'hyperplasia surrenale congenitale. In: *Journees Parisiennes de Pediatrie* 1974:71–6.

147 Grant DB, Dillon MJ, Atherden SM *et al.* Congenital adrenal hyperplasia: renin and steroid values during treatment. *Eur J Pediatr* 1977;126:89–96.

148 Jacobs DR, Van der Poll J, Gabrilove JL *et al.* 17 Alphahydroxyprogesterone – a salt-losing steroid; relation to congenital adrenal hyperplasia. *J Clin Endocrinol Metab* 1961;21:909–22.

149 Landau RL, Lugibihl K. Inhibition of sodium-retaining influence of aldosterone by progesterone. *J Clin Endocrinol Metab* 1958;18:1237–45.

150 White PC, New MI, Dupont B. Congenital adrenal hyperplasia. Part I. *N Engl J Med* 1987;316:1519–24.

151 Brook CGD, Zachmann M, Prader A *et al.* Experience with long-term therapy in congenital adrenal hyperplasia. *J Pediatr* 1974;85:12–19.

152 Serfas D, Shoback DM, Loele BH. Phaeochromocytoma and hypertrophic cardiomyopathy: apparent suppression of symptoms and noradrenaline secretion by calcium channel blockade. *Lancet* 1983;2:711–13.

153 Loras B, Haour F, Bertrand J. Exchangeable sodium and aldosterone secretion in children with congenital adrenal hyperplasia due to 21-hydroxylase deficiency. *Pediatr Res* 1970;4:145–56.

154 Visser HKA, Cost WS. A new hereditary defect in the biosynthesis of aldosterone: urinary C21-corticosteroid pattern in three related patients with a salt-losing syndrome, suggesting an 18-oxidation defect. *Acta Endocrinol* 1964;47:589–612.

155 Degenhart HJ, Frankena L, Visser HKA *et al.* Further investigation of a new hereditary defect in the biosynthesis of aldosterone: evidence for a defect in 18-hydroxylation of corticosterone. *Acta Physiol Pharmacol Neerlandica* 1966; 14:88–9.

156 Ulick S, Gautier E, Vetter KK *et al.* An aldosterone biosynthetic defect in a salt-losing disorder. *J Clin Endocrinol Metab* 1964;24:669–72.

157 David R, Golan S, Drucker W. Familial aldosterone deficiency: enzyme defect, diagnosis and clinical course. *Pediatrics* 1968;41:403–12.

158 Hamilton W, McCandles AE, Ireland JT *et al.* Hypoaldosteronism in three sibs due to 18-dehydrogenase deficiency. *Arch Dis Child* 1976;51:576–83.

159 Rappaport R, Dray F, Legrand JC *et al.* Hypoaldosteronisme congenital familial par defaut de la 18-OH-dehydrogenase. Etude hormonale avant et apres guerison du syndrome de parte de sel. *Pediatr Res* 1968;2:456–63.

160 Ulick S. Diagnosis and nomenclature of the disorders of the

terminal portion of the aldosterone biosynthetic pathway. *J Clin Endocrinol Metab* 1976;43:92–6.

161 Shackleton CHL, Honour JW, Dillon MJ *et al.* Multicomponent gas chromatographic analysis of urinary steroids excreted by an infant with a defect in aldosterone biosynthesis. *Acta Endocrinol* 1976;81:762–7.

162 Shackleton CHL, Taylor NF. Identification of the androstenetriolones and androstenetetrols present in the urine of infants. *J Steroid Biochem* 1975;6:1393–9.

163 Taylor NF, Curnow DH, Shackleton CHL. Analysis of glucocorticoid metabolites in the neonatal period: catabolism of cortisone acetate by an infant with 21-hydroxylase deficiency. *Clin Chim Acta* 1978;85:219–29.

164 Cara J, Beas F, Spach C *et al.* Increased urinary and plasma etiocholanolone and related steroids in a boy with virilizing adrenal hyperplasia and periodic fever. *J Pediatr* 1963;62: 521–30.

165 Bamatter F, Koegel R, Haller J *et al.* Maladie d'Addisons familiale. Insufficance corticosurrenale chez quartre freres et plusiers cas probables dans deux generations de la meme famille. *Helv Pediatr Acta* 1966;21:109–52.

166 Nerup J. Addison's disease: serological studies. *Acta Endocrinol Copenh* 1974;76:142–58.

167 Perheentupa J, Tiilikainen A, Lokki ML. Autoimmune polyendocrinopathy–candidosis syndrome (APECS): clinical variation, inheritance and HLA association in 40 Finnish patients. *Pediatr Res* 1978;12:1087.

168 Forsyth CC, Forbes M, Cummings JN. Adrenocortical atrophy and diffuse cerebral sclerosis. *Arch Dis Child* 1971; 46:273–84.

169 Cheek DB, Perry JW. A salt-wasting syndrome in infancy. *Arch Dis Child* 1958;33:252–6.

170 Trung PH, Piussan C, Rodary C *et al.* Etude du taux de secretion de l'aldosterone et de l'activite de la renine plasmatique d'un cas de pseudohypoaldosteronisme. *Arch Fr Pediatr* 1970;27:603–15.

171 Barakat AY, Papadopoulou ZL, August GP. A hyperkalaemic salt-wasting syndrome in infancy. *Pediatr Res* 1972;6: 394.

172 Barthe P, Thai VK, Bouissou F *et al.* A propos d'un cas de pseudohypoaldosteronisme (Etude du taux de secretion d'aldosterone). *Arch Fr Pediatr* 1974;31:973–84.

173 Bierich JR, Schmidt U. Tubular Na K-ATPase deficiency, the cause of the congenital renal salt-losing syndrome. *Eur J Pediatr* 1976;121:81–7.

174 Blachar Y, Kaplan BS, Griffel B *et al.* Pseudohypoaldosteronism. *Clin Nephrol* 1979;11:281–8.

175 Corbeel L. Diabete salin du nourrisson sans insuffisance surrenalienne. *Pediatrics* 1963;18:557–62.

176 Dillon MJ, Leonard JV, Buckler JM *et al.* Pseudohypoaldosteronism. *Arch Dis Child* 1980;55:427–34.

177 Donnell GN, Litman N, Roldan M. Pseudohypoadrenalcorticism. Renal sodium loss, hyponatremia and hyperkalemia due to renal tubular insensitivity to mineralocorticoids. *Am J Dis Child* 1959;97:813–38.

178 Honour JW, Dillon MJ, Shackleton CHL. Analysis of steroids in urine for differentiation of pseudohypoaldosteronism and aldosterone biosynthetic defect. *J Clin Endocrinol Metab* 1982;54:325–31.

179 Lauras B, Ravussin J-J, David M *et al.* Pseudohypoaldostereonism chez l'enfant. A propos de quatre observations dont deux concernant des freres. *Pediatrie* 1978;33:119–35.

180 Lelong M, Alagille D, Philippe A *et al.* Diabete salin par insensibilite congenitale du tubule a l'aldosterone: pseudohypoadrenocorticisme. *Rev Fr d'Etudes Clinique Biolog* 1960;5:558–65.

181 Limal JM, Rappaport R, Dechaux M *et al.* Familial dominant pseudo-hypoaldosteronism. *Lancet* 1978;1:51.

182 Oberfield SE, Levine LS, Carey RM *et al.* Pseudohypoaldosteronism: multiple target organ unresponsiveness to mineralocorticoid hormones. *J Clin Endocrinol Metab* 1979; 48:228–34.

183 Petersen S, Giese J, Kappelgaard AM *et al.* Pseudohypoaldosteronism. Clinical, biochemical and morphological studies in a long term follow-up. *Acta Paed Scand* 1978; 67:255–61.

184 Proesmans W, Guessens H, Corbeel L *et al.* Pseudohypoaldosteronism. *Am J Dis Child* 1973;126:510–16.

185 Raine DN, Roy J. A salt-losing syndrome in infancy. Pseudohypoadrenocorticalism. *Arch Dis Child* 1962;37:548–56.

186 Rampini S, Furrer J, Keller HP *et al.* Congenital pseudohypoaldosteronism: a case report and review. Effect of indomethacin during sodium chloride depletion. *Helv Paediatr Acta* 1978;33:153–67.

187 Rosler A, Theodor R, Boichis H *et al.* Metabolic responses to the administration of angiotensin II, K and ACTH in two salt-wasting syndromes. *J Clin Endocrinol Metab* 1977;44: 292–301.

188 Roy C. Pseudohypoaldosteronisme familial (a propos de 5 cas). *Arch Fr Pediatr* 1977;34:37–54.

189 Royer P, Bonnette J, Mathieu H *et al.* Pseudohypoaldosteronisme. *Ann Pediatr* 1963;39:596–605.

190 Savage MO, Jefferson IG, Dillon MJ *et al.* Pseudohypoaldosteronism: severe salt wasting in infancy caused by generalised mineralocorticoid unresponsiveness. *J Pediatr* 1982; 101:239–42.

191 Shackleton CHL, Snodgrass GHAI. Steroid excretion by an infant with an unusual salt-losing syndrome: a gas chromatographic–mass spectrometric study. *Ann Clin Biochem* 1974;11:91–9.

192 Stubbe P, Manouguina G. Der pseudohypoaldosteronisme. Bericht eines weiteren falles. *Monatsschr Kinderheilkd* 1977;125:234–7.

193 Gross JB, Imai M, Kokko JP. A functional comparison of the cortical collecting tubule and the distal convoluted tubule. *J Clin Invest* 1975;55:1284.

194 Schwartz GJ, Burg MB. Mineralocorticoid effects on cation transport by cortical collecting tubules *in vitro*. *Am J Physiol* 1978;235:F576.

195 Proesmans W, Muaka BK, Eeckel R. Pseudohypoaldosteronism – a proximal tubular sodium wasting disease. In: *Proceedings, 4th International Symposium on Pediatric Nephrology*, Helsinki, 1977:86.

196 Armanini D, Kuhnle V, Strasser T *et al.* Aldosterone-receptor deficiency in pseudohypoaldosteronism. *N Engl J Med* 1985; 313:1178–81.

197 McSherry E. Current issues in hydrogen ion transport. In: Gruskin AB, Norman ME, eds. *Developments in Nephrology*. Vol. 3. *Pediatric Nephrology*. The Hague: Martinus Nijhoff, 1981:403–15.

198 McSherry E. Renal tubular acidosis in childhood. *Kidney Int* 1981;20:799–809.

199 Sebastian A, Hulter HN, Kurtz I *et al.* Disorders of distal nephron function. *Am J Med* 1982;72:289–307.

200 Anand SK, Frobeg L, Northway JD *et al.* Pseudohypoaldosteronism due to sweat gland dysfunction. *Paediatr Res* 1976;10:677–82.
201 Armanini D, Wehling M, Da Dalt L *et al.* Pseudohypoaldosteronism in mineralocorticoid receptor abnormalities. *J Steroid Biochem Mol Biol* 1991;40:363–5.
202 Kuhnle U, Neilsen MD, Tietze HU *et al.* Pseudohypoaldosteronism in eight families: different forms of inheritance are evidence for various genetic defects. *J Clin Endocrinol Metab* 1990;70:638–41.
203 Good DW, Wright FS. Luminal influence on potassium secretion: sodium concentration and fluid flow rate. *Am J Physiol* 1979;236:F192–205.
204 Wright FS. Sites and mechanisms of potassium transport along the renal tubule. *Kidney Int* 1977;11:415–32.
205 Postel-Vinay MC, Alberti GM, Ricour C *et al.* Pseudohypoaldosteronism: persistence of hyperaldosteronism and evidence for renal tubular and intestinal responsiveness to endogenous aldosterone. *J Clin Endocrinol Metab* 1974;39: 1038–44.
206 Kinuthia DMW, Rosa FC, Dillon MJ. Fractional electrolyte delivery and reabsorption during hypotonic saline diuresis in familial hypokalemia/hypomagnesemia (Gitelman's syndrome), and pseudohypoaldosteronism compared with observations in Bartter's syndrome. *Int J Pediatr Nephrol* 1982; 3:126.
207 Spitzer A. The role of the kidney in sodium homeostatis during maturation. *Kidney Int* 1982;21,539.
208 Rogers D, Tripp J, Bentovim A *et al.* Non-accidental poisoning: an extended syndrome of child abuse. *Br Med J* 1976;1: 793–6.
209 Bisset GW, Jones NF. Antidiuretic hormone. In: Jones NF, ed. *Recent Advances in Renal Disease.* Edinburgh: Churchill Livingstone, 1975;350–416.
210 Moylan FMB, Herrin JT, Krishnamoorthy K *et al.* Inappropriate antidiuretic hormone secretion in premature infants with cerebral injury. *Am J Dis Child* 1978;132:399–402.
211 Paxson CL, Stoerner JW, Denson SE *et al.* Syndrome of inappropriate antidiuretic hormone secretion in neonates with pneumothorax or atelectasis. *J Pediatr* 1977;91:459–63.
212 Sladen A, Laver MB, Pontoppidan H. Pulmonary complications and water retention in prolonged mechanical ventilation. *N Engl J Med* 1968;279:448–53.
213 Nolph KD, Schrier RW. Sodium potassium and water metabolism in the syndrome of inappropriate antidiuretic hormone secretion. *Am J Med* 1970;49:534–45.
214 Moses AM, Blumenthal SA, Streeten DHP. Drugs and water metabolism. In: Arieff AI, De Fronzo RA, eds. *Fluid, Electrolyte and Acid Base Disorders.* Edinburgh: Churchill Livingstone, 1985:1145.
215 Troyer A de. Demeclocycline. Treatment for syndrome of inappropriate antidiuretic hormone secretion. *J Am Med Assoc* 1977;237:2723–6.
216 Dillon MJ. Hypertension. In: Postlethwaite RJ, ed. *Clinical Paediatric Nephrology*, 2nd edn. Oxford: Butterworth Heinemann, 1994:175–95.
217 Dillon MJ, Ingelfinger JR. Pharmacologic treatment of hypertension. In: Holliday MA, Barratt TM, Avner ED, eds. *Pediatric Nephrology*, 3rd edn. Baltimore: Williams & Wilkins, 1994:1165–74.
218 Ingelfinger JR, Dillon MJ. Evaluation of secondary hypertension. In: Holliday MA, Barratt TM, Avner ED, eds. *Pediatric Nephrology*, 3rd edn. Baltimore: Williams & Wilkins, 1994:1146–64.
219 Rocchini AP, ed. Childhood hypertension. *Pediatric Clinics of North America*, Vol. 40, No. 1. Philadelphia, PA: W.B. Saunders, 1993.
220 Loggie JMH, ed. *Pediatric and Adolescent Hypertension.* Oxford: Blackwell Scientific Publications, 1992.
221 Eberlein WR, Bongiovanni AM. Plasma and urinary corticosteroids in the hypertensive form of congenital adrenal hyperplasia. *J Biol Chem* 1956;223:85–94.
222 Brautber C, Rosler A, Landau H *et al.* No linkage between HLA and congenital adrenal hyperplasia due to 11β-hydroxylase deficiency. *N Engl J Med* 1979;300:205–6.
223 White PC, New MI, Dupont B. Congenital adrenal hyperplasia. Part 2. *N Engl J Med* 1987;316:1580–6.
224 New MI, Levine LS. Adrenocortical hypertension. *Pediatr Clin N Am* 1978;25:67–81.
225 Kowarski A, Russell A, Migeon CJ. Aldosterone secretion rate in the hypertensive form of congenital adrenal hyperplasia. *J Clin Endocrinol Metab* 1968;28:1445–9.
226 Zadik Z, Kahana L, Kaufman H *et al.* Salt loss in hypertensive form of congenital adrenal hyperplasia (11-β-hydroxylase deficiency). *J Clin Endocrinol Metab* 1984;58: 384–7.
227 Rodriguez-Portales JA. 11β-hydroxylase deficiency. In: Biglieri EG, Melby JC, eds. *Endocrine Hypertension.* New York: Raven Press, 1990:137–53.
228 Biglieri EG, Herron MA, Brust N. 17 Alpha-hydroxylation deficiency in man. *J Clin Invest* 1966;45:1946–54.
229 Mantero F, Scaroni C. Enzymatic defects of steroidogenesis: 17 alpha hydroxylase. *Pediatr Adolesc Endocrinol* 1984;13: 83–94.
230 New MI. Male pseudohermaphroditism due to 17 alpha hydroxylase deficiency. *J Clin Invest* 1970;49:1930–41.
231 Scaroni C, Opocher G, Mantero F. Renin angiotensin aldosterone system: a long term follow up study in 17 alpha-hydroxylase deficiency syndrome (17OHDS). *Clin Exp Hypertens* 1986;A8:773–80.
232 Biglieri EG. 17 Alpha-hydroxylase deficiency: implications on steroidogenesis. In: Biglieri EG, Melby JC, eds. *Endocrine Hypertension.* New York: Raven Press, 1990:125–36.
233 Miura K, Yoshinaga K, Goto K *et al.* A case of glucocorticoid responsive hyperaldosteronism. *J Clin Endocrinol Metab* 1968;28:1807–15.
234 Rauh W, Oberfield SE. The adrenal cortex in childhood hypertension. *Paediatr Adolesc Endocrinol* 1984;13:210–30.
235 New MI, Peterson RE. Aldosterone in childhood. In: Levine LS, ed. *Advances in Pediatrics.* Chicago: Yearbook Medical, 1968:111–36.
236 Ganguly A, Melada GA, Leutscher JA *et al.* Control of plasma aldosterone in primary aldosteronism: distinction between adenoma and hyperplasia. *J Clin Endocrinol Metab* 1973;37:765–75.
237 Schambelan M, Bruit NL, Chang B *et al.* Circadian rhythm and effect of posture in plasma aldosterone concentration in primary hyperaldosteronism. *J Clin Endocrinol Metab* 1976; 43:115–31.
238 Kem MDC, Weinberger MH, Mayes DM, Nugent CA. Saline suppression of plasma aldosterone in hypertension. *Arch Intern Med* 1971;128:380–6.
239 Lyons DF, Kem DC, Brown RD *et al.* Single dose captopril as a diagnostic test for primary hypertension. *J Clin Endocrinol Metab* 1983;57:892–6.

240 Ganguly A, Bergstein J, Grim CE *et al.* Childhood primary aldosteronism due to an adrenal adenoma: preoperative localization by adrenal vein catheterization. *Paediatrics* 1980;65:605–9.

241 Prosser PR, Sutherland CM, Scullen DR. Localization of adrenal aldosterone adenoma by computerized tomography. *N Engl J Med* 1979;300:1278–79.

242 Schteingart DE, Seabold JE, Gross MD *et al.* Iodocholesterol adrenal tissue uptake and imaging in adrenal neoplasms. *J Clin Endocrinol Metab* 1981;52:1156–61.

243 Conn JW. Primary aldosteronism and primary reninism. *Hosp Pract* 1974;9:131–40.

244 Sutherland DJA, Ruse JL, Laidlaw JC. Hypertension, increased aldosterone secretion and low plasma renin activity relieved by dexamethasone. *Can Med Assoc J* 1966;95: 1109–19.

245 Ganguly A, Grim CE, Weinberger MH. Anomalous postural aldosterone response in glucocorticoid suppressible hyperaldosteronism. *N Engl J Med* 1981;305:991–3.

246 Giebink GS, Gotlin RW, Biglieri EG *et al.* A kindred with familial glucocorticoid-suppressible aldosteronism. *J Clin Endocrinol Metab* 1973;36:715–23.

247 Gill JR, Bartter FC. Overproduction of sodium retaining steroids by the zona glomerulosa is adrenocorticotropin dependent and mediates hypertension in dexamethasone suppressible hyperaldosteronism. *J Clin Endocrinol Metabol* 1981;53:331–7.

248 Grim CE, Weinberger MH. Familial dexamethasone-suppressible, normokalemic hyperaldosteronism. *Pediatrics* 1980;65:597–604.

249 Igarashi Y, Egi S, Takehiro O. Studies on the metabolic abnormality of cortisol and corticosterone in a case of dexamethasone responsive mineralocorticoid excess. *Folia Endocrinol Jpn* 1979;55;1341–57.

250 New MI, Peterson RE. A new form of congenital adrenal hyperplasia. *J Clin Endocrinol Metab* 1967;27:300–5.

251 Oberfield SE, Levine LS, Stoner E *et al.* Adrenal glomerulosa function in patients with dexamethasone suppressible hyperaldosteronism. *J Clin Endocrinol Metab* 1981;53:158–64.

252 Connell JMC, Kenyon CJ, Corrie JEJ *et al.* Dexamethasone-suppressible hyperaldosteronism: adrenal transition cell hyperplasia. *Hypertension* 1986;8:669–76.

253 Gomez-Sanchez CE, Montgomery M *et al.* Elevated urinary excretion of 18-oxocortisol in glucocorticoid suppressible hyperaldosteronosis. *J Clin Endocrinol Metab* 1984;59: 1022–4.

254 Ulick S, Chu M. Hypersecretion of a new corticosteroid, 18-hydroxycortisol, in two types of adrenocortical hypertension. *Clin Exp Hypertens* 1982;A4:1771–7.

255 New MI, Oberfield SE, Levine LS *et al.* Demonstration of autosomal dominant transmission and absence of HLA linkage in dexamethasone suppressible hyperaldosteronism. *Lancet* 1980;1:550–1.

256 Lifton RP, Dluhy RG, Powers M *et al.* A chimaeric 11β-hydroxylase/aldosterone synthase gene causes glucocorticoid-remediable aldosteronism and human hypertension. *Nature* 1992;355:262–6.

257 Lifton RP, Dluhy RG, Powers M *et al.* Hereditary hypertension caused by chimaeric gene duplications and ectopic expression of aldosterone synthase. *Nature Gene* 1992;2: 66–74.

258 Fallo F, Mantero F. Dexamethasone-suppressible hyperaldosteronism. In: Biglieri EG, Melby JC, eds. *Endocrine Hypertension*. New York: Raven Press, 1990:87–97.

259 Loridan L, Senior E. Cushings syndrome in infancy. *J Pediatr* 1969;75:349–59.

260 Kalsner S. Mechanism of hydrocortisone potentiation of response to epinephrine and norepinephrine in rabbit aorta. *Circ Res* 1969;34:383–5.

261 Mendlowitz M, Naftchi N, Weinreb HL *et al.* Effect of prednisone on digital vascular reactivity in normotensive and hypertensive subjects. *J Appl Physiol* 1961;16:89–94.

262 New MI, Levine LS, Biglieri EG *et al.* Evidence for an unidentified steroid in a child with apparent mineralocorticoid hypertension. *J Clin Endocrinol Metab* 1977;44:924–33.

263 Dimartino-Nardi J, Stoner E, Martin K *et al.* New findings in apparent mineralocorticoid excess. *Clin Endocrinol* 1987; 27:49–62.

264 Edwards CRW, Stewart PM, Nairn IM *et al.* Cushing's disease of the kidney. *J Endocrinol* (Suppl.) 1985;104:53.

265 Fiselier TJW, Otten BJ, Monnens LAH *et al.* Low renin, low aldosterone hypertension and abnormal cortisol metabolism in a 19 month old child. *Horm Res* 1982;16:107–14.

266 Harinck HIJ, van Brummelen P, van Seters AP *et al.* Apparent mineralocorticoid excess and deficient 11β oxidation of cortisol in a young female. *Clin Endocrinol* 1984;21: 505–14.

267 Honour JW, Dillon MJ, Levin M *et al.* Fatal low renin hypertension associated with a disturbance of cortisol metabolism. *Arch Dis Child* 1983;53:1018–20.

268 New MI, Stoner E, Dimartino-Nardi J. Apparent mineralocorticoid excess causing hypertension and hypokalemia in children. *Clin Exp Hypertens* 1986;A8:751–72.

269 Sann L, Revol A, Zachmann M *et al.* Unusual low plasma renin hypertension in a child. *J Clin Endocrinol Metab* 1976;43:265–71.

270 Shackleton CHL, Honour JW, Dillon MJ *et al.* Hypertension in a four year old child: gas chromatographic and mass spectrometric evidence for deficient hepatic metabolism of steroids. *J Clin Endocrinol Metab* 1980;50:786–92.

271 Shackleton CHL, Rodriquez J, Arteaga E *et al.* Congenital 11β hydroxysteroid dehydrogenase deficiency associated with juvenile hypertension: corticosteroid metabolite profiles of four patients and their families. *Clin Endocrinol* 1985;22:701–12.

272 Ulick S, Levine LS, Gunczler P *et al.* A syndrome of apparent mineralocorticoid excess associated with defects in peripheral metabolism of cortisol. *J Clin Endocrinol Metab* 1979;49:757–64.

273 Werder E, Zachmann M, Vollmin JA *et al.* Unusual steroid excretion in a child with low renin hypertension. *Res Steroids* 1974;6:385–9.

274 Winter JSD, McKenzie JK. A syndrome of low renin hypertension in children. In: New MI, Levine LS, eds. *Juvenile Hypertension*. New York: Raven Press, 1977;123–31.

275 Ulick S, Ramirez LC, New MI. An abnormality in steroid reductive metabolism in a hypertensive syndrome. *J Clin Endocrinol Metab* 1977;44:799–802.

276 Stewart PM, Corrie JET, Shackleton CHL *et al.* Syndrome of apparent mineralocorticoid excess and defects in the cortisol–cortisone shuttle. *J Clin Invest* 1988;82:340–9.

277 Oberfield SE, Levine LS, Carey RH *et al.* Metabolic and blood pressure responses to hydrocortisone in the syndrome of apparent mineralocorticoid excess. *J Clin Endocrinol Metab* 1983;56:332–8.

278 Conn JW, Rovner DR, Cohen E. Licorice induced pseudoaldosteronism. *J Am Med Assoc* 1968;205:80–4.

279 Stewart PM, Wallace AM, Valentino R *et al.* Mineralocorticoid activity of licorice: 11β-hydroxysteroid dehydrogenase deficiency comes of age. *Lancet* 1987;2:821–4.
280 Shackleton CHL, Stewart PM. The hypertension of apparent mineralocorticoid excess (AME) syndrome. In: Biglieri EG, Melby JC, eds. *Endocrine Hypertension.* New York: Raven Press, 1990:155–73.
281 Gordon RD. Syndrome of hypertension and hyperkalaemia with normal glomerular filtration rate. *Hypertension* 1986; 8:93–102.
282 Gordon RD, Geddes RA, Pawsey GK *et al.* Hypertension and severe hyperkalaemia associated with suppression of renin and aldosterone and completely reversed by dietary sodium restriction. *Aust Ann Med* 1970;4:287–94.
283 Paver WKA, Pauline GJ. Hypertension and hyperpotassaemia without renal disease in a young male. *Med J Aust* 1964;82: 412–16.
284 Rodriguez-Soriano J, Vallo H, Dominguez MJ. The 'chloride shunt syndrome': an overloked cause of renal hypercalciuria. *Pediatr Nephrol* 1989;3:113–21.
285 Schambelan M, Sebastian H, Rector FC. Mineralocorticoid-resistant renal hyperkalaemia without salt wasting (type II pseudohypoaldosteronism): role of increased renal chloride reabsorption. *Kidney Int* 1981;19:716–27.
286 Semmerkrot B, Monneng L, Theelan BGA *et al.* The syndrome of hypertension and hyperkalaemia with normal glomerular function (Gordon's syndrome): a pathophysiological study. *Pediatr Nephrol* 1987;1:473–8.
287 Tunny T, Higgins B, Gordon R. Plasma levels of artrial natriuretic peptide in man in primary aldosteronism, in Gordon's syndrome and in Bartter's syndrome. *Clin Exp Pharmacol Physiol* 1986;13:341–5.
288 Spitzer A, Edelmann C, Goldberg L *et al.* Short stature, hyperkalaemia and acidosis: a defect in renal transport potassium. *Kidney Int* 1973;3:251–7.
289 Weinstein S, Allen D, Mendoza S. Hyperkalaemia, acidosis and short stature associated with a defect in renal potassium excretion. *J Pediatr* 1974;85:355–8.
290 Deal JE, Sever PS, Barratt TM *et al.* Phaeochromocytoma – investigation and management of 10 cases. *Arch Dis Child* 1990;65:269–74.
291 Leumann EP. Blood pressure and hypertension in childhood and adolescence. *Ergeb Inn Med Kinderheilkd* 1979;43: 109–83.
292 Stackpole RH, Melicow MM, Uson AC. Phaeochromocytoma in children: report of 9 cases and review of the first 100 published cases with follow-up studies. *J Pediatr* 1963;63: 314–30.
293 Glushien AS, Mansuy MM, Littman DS. Phaeochromocytoma: its relationship to neurocutaneous syndromes. *Am J Med* 1953;14:318–27.
294 Sever PS, Roberts JC, Snell ME. Phaeochromocytoma. *Clin Endocrinol Metab* 1980;9:543–68.
295 Keiser HR, Beaven MA, Doppman J. Sipple's syndrome, medullary thyroid carcinoma, phaeochromocytoma and parathyroid disease. *Am Intern Med* 1973;78:561–79.
296 Lips KJ, Van der Sluys Veer L, Struyvenberg A *et al.* Bilateral occurrence of pheochromocytoma in patients with multiple endocrine neoplasia syndrome type 2A (Sipple's syndrome). *Am J Med* 1981;70:1051–60.
297 Sipple JH. The association of pheochromocytoma with carcinoma of the thyroid gland. *Am J Med* 1961;31:163–6.
298 Kaufman BH, Telander RL, Van Harden JA *et al.* Phaeochromocytoma in the pediatric age group: current status. *J Pediatr Surg* 1983;18:879–84.
299 Glowniak JV, Shapiro B, Sisson JC *et al.* Familial extra-adrenal phaeochromocytoma. A new syndrome. *Arch Intern Med* 1985;145:257.
300 Bravo EL, Gifford RW. Phaeochromocytoma: diagnosis, localization and management. *N Engl J Med* 1984;311: 1298–303.
301 Barker DJP, Bull AR, Osmond C *et al.* Fetal and placental size and risk of hypertension in adult life. *Br Med J* 1990;301: 259–62.
302 Barker DJP, Gluckman PD, Godfrey KM *et al.* Fetal nutrition and cardiovascular disease in adult life. *Lancet* 1993;341: 339–41.
303 Barker DJP, Osmond C, Godfrey J *et al.* Growth *in utero*, blood pressure in childhood and adult life, and mortality from cardiovascular disease. *Br Med J* 1989;298:564–7.
304 Law CM, Barker DJP, Bull AR *et al.* Maternal and fetal influences on blood pressure. *Arch Dis Child* 1991;66: 1291–5.
305 Law CM, de Swiet M, Osmond C *et al.* Initiation of hypertension *in utero* and its amplification throughout life. *Br Med J* 1993;306:24–7.
306 Lever AF. Essential hypertension. A disease with origins in childhood. *J Hum Hypertens* 1993;7:391–2.
307 Lever AF, Harrap SB. Essential hypertension. A disorder of growth with origins in childhood. *J Hypertens* 1992;10: 101–20.
308 de Swiet M, Fayers P, Shinebourne EA. Value of repeated blood pressure measurements in children: the Brompton study. *Br Med J* 1980;280:1567–9.
309 Miall WE, Chinn S. Blood pressure and ageing: results of a 15–17 year follow-up study in South Wales. *Clin Sci Mol Med* 1973;45(Suppl. 1):23–33.
310 Poulter NR, Khan KT, Hopwood BEC *et al.* The Kenyan Luo migration study: observations on the initiation of a rise in blood pressure. *Br Med J* 1990;330:967–71.
311 Voors AW, Webber LS, Frerichs RR *et al.* Body height and body mass as determinants of basal blood pressure in children – the Bogalusa Heart Study. *Am J Epidemiol* 1977; 106:101–8.
312 Hofman A. Blood pressure in childhood: an epidemiological approach to the aetiology of hypertension. *J Hypertens* 1984; 2:323–8.
313 Szklo M. Determinants of blood pressure in children. *Clin Exp Hypertens* (A) 1986;8:479–93.
314 Benediktsson RAFN, Lindsay RS, Noble J *et al.* Glucocorticoid exposure *in utero*: new model for adult hypertension. *Lancet* 1993;341:339–41.
315 Edwards CRW, Beneditksson RAFN, Lindsay RS *et al.* Dysfunction of placental glucocorticoid barrier: link between fetal environment and adult hypertension. *Lancet* 1993;341: 355–7.
316 Portman RJ, Robson AM. Controversies in pediatric hypertension. In: Tune BM, Mendoza SA, eds. *Pediatric Nephrology. Contemporary Issues in Nephrology Series*, Vol. 12. New York: Churchill Livingstone, 1984:256–96.
317 Deal JE, Shah V, Goodenough G *et al.* Red cell membrane sodim transport: possible genetic role and use in identifying patients at risk of essential hypertension. *Arch Dis Child* 1990;65:1154–7.
318 Houtman PN, Shah V, Dillon MJ. Sodium–lithium counter transport and family history of hypertension in childhood. *Acta Paediatr* 1993;82:1057–60.
319 Mongeau JG. Heredity and blood pressure in humans: an

overview. *Pediatr Nephrol* 1987;1:69.

320 Uchiyama M, Shah V, Daman Willems C *et al.* Sodium transport in erythrocytes, differences between normal children and children with primary and secondary hypertension. *Arch Dis Child* 1989;64:224–8.

321 Williams RR. Will gene markers predict hypertension? *Hypertension* 1989;14:610–13.

322 Whincup PH, Cook DG, Shaper AG *et al.* Blood pressure in British children: associations with adult blood and cardiovascular mortality. *Lancet* 1988;2:890–3.

32: The Neurohypophysis and Water Regulation

J. PERHEENTUPA

INTRODUCTION

The body maintains water balance by a system consisting of two mechanisms (Fig. 32.1). Output is regulated by the hypothalamic osmoreceptors and the neighbouring neurons which secrete the antidiuretic hormone arginine vasopressin (AVP) in conjunction with the kidneys. Input is controlled by the nearby hypothalamic thirst centre in conjunction with the cerebral cortex and the motor system. As as result of the two mechanisms, the normal range of plasma osmolality is very narrow, 280–295 mosmol/kg. Derangements may occur in either mechanism, but water deficiency with serious consequences is more apt to arise from disorders of input regulation than deficient antidiuretic function. Conditions of AVP excess occur with greater frequency. AVP excess is harmless as such, but leaves the organism defenceless against water poisoning.

PHYSIOLOGICAL BACKGROUND

Organization of the system

The hypothalamoneurohypophyseal system consists of bilateral osmoreceptors near the supraoptic nucleus (SON), the organum vasculosum of the lamina terminalis, the subfornical organ, the supraoptic and paraventricular nuclei (PVN) with their magnocellular neurons synthesizing AVP and oxytocin, the axons of these neurons forming the supraopticohypophyseal tract, and the termini of these axons in the midline storage–release structure called the posterior pituitary (Fig. 32.2). The SON consists almost exclusively of the magnocellular neurons. The PVN also contains parvocellular neurons. The axons of the magnocellular neurons are unmyelinated fibres containing clusters of granules and microtubules reaching the tips of the axons. Most of the axons terminate in the posterior pituitary among specialized astrocytic glial cells called pituicytes, but some end in the median eminence. The terminations are expanded bulbs in close proximity to a vascular plexus of the vertebral vessels. These granule-filled dilated axon tips constitute about 40% of the mass of the posterior pituitary.

The two circumventricular organs, the organum vasculosum laminae terminalis and the subfornical organ, are outside the blood–brain barrier. They innervate the magnocellular neurons. The organum vasculosum is osmosensitive and modulates the sensitivity of the osmoreceptors proper. Its destruction inhibits the AVP-release and drinking responses to hypertonicity and angiotensin II [2]. The subfornical organ carries receptors for blood-borne angiotensin II. Their occupation with angiotensin appears to increase the excitability of the AVP-secreting cells.

An integrating thirst centre may be located in the medial preoptic nucleus, which receives extensive afferents from the circumventricular organs and sends projections to the SON and PVN, as well as the lateral hypothalamus and preoptic areas which may initiate thirst [3].

Impulses from baroreceptors and volume receptors reach the magnocellular neurons through cranial nerves IX and X, relayed in the nucleus of the tractus solitarius and a noradrenergic nucleus.

Arginine vasopressin: molecular structure and derivatives

AVP (like oxytocin) belongs to the family of nonapeptides (Table 32.1), which has an interesting evolution [6]. All its members have a hexapeptide ring with a disulphide bond between two cysteine molecules, and a side-chain of three amino acids. AVP is the antidiuretic hormone of all mammals with the exception of the pig family, which has a phylogenetically younger peptide, lysine vasopressin. The amino acids in positions 3, 4, 7 and 8 are involved in recognition and binding to the receptor. The disulphide bridge, the amide group at position 9, the carboxamide group at position 5 and the basic moiety at position 8 are key elements for activity [7].

Substitutions modify the activities or metabolism of the molecule. An analogue of AVP which is far better than any other drug available as a replacement in AVP deficiency is 1-deamino-8-D-arginine vasopressin (desmopressin). Deamination of the cysteine at position 1 increases the

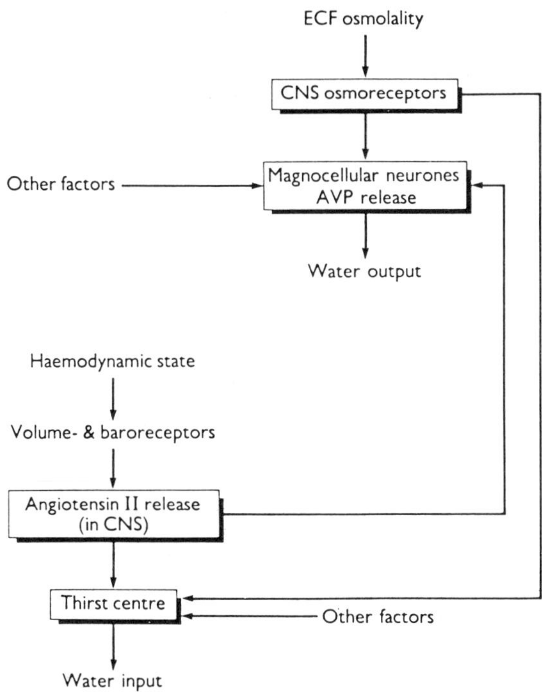

Fig. 32.1 The two mechanisms concerned in the regulation of body fluid osmolality. AVP, arginine vasopressin; CNS, central nervous system; ECF, extracellular fluid.

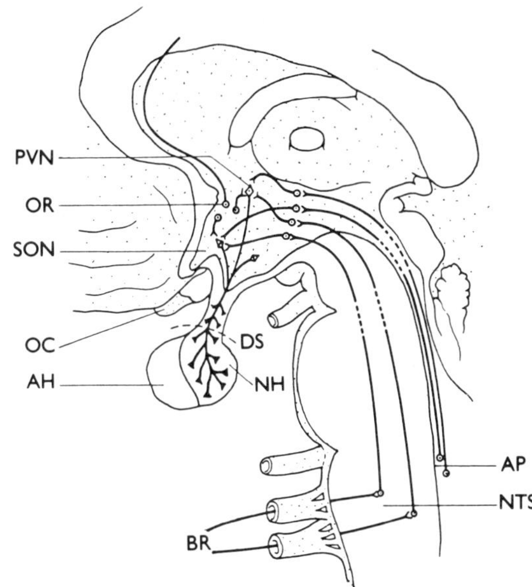

Fig. 32.2 Anatomy of the hypothalamioneurohypophyseal system. Shaded areas represent those parts of the central nervous system that lack a blood–brain barrier. PVN, paraventricular nuclei; OR, osmoreceptors; SON, supraoptic nuclei; OC, optic chiasm; AH, adenohypophysis; DS, diaphragma sellae; NH, neurohypophysis; BR, baroreceptors; AP, area postrema; NTS, nuclei of the solitary tract. The organum vasculosum laminae terminalis and the subfornical organ are located in the anterior wall of the third ventricle. Axons of magnocellular neurons in the supraoptic and paraventricular nuclei end on capillaries of the posterior pituitary. The proximity of the optic tract and chiasm explains the high prevalence of visual field defects in patients with tumours of this region (from Robertson & Berl [1]).

antidiuretic activity of the basic molecule four-fold and renders it less susceptible to the action of peptidases. Replacement of L-arginine at position 8 by the D-isomer then reduces the activity from four-fold to twice the original, but reduces its pressor (V_1-receptor) activity even more, and markedly delays the degradation of the molecule [5]. The average half-life of desmopressin is 75 min [8] as compared with 10–20 min for AVP. Further replacement of glutamine by valine in position 4 (1-deamino-4-valine, 8-D-arginine vasopressin (DVDAVP)) adds to the antidiuretic activity [5]. These V_2-receptor-specific derivatives have negligible vasopressor activity [9]. Derivatives have been produced which are devoid of antidiuretic activity [10–12] none which are useful therapeutically [13].

Table 32.1 Structure of three neurohypophyseal hormones occurring in vertebrates and synthetic analogues and their relative antidiuretic, vasopressor and uterotonic potencies in the rat [4,5]

		Activities relative to AVP		
		Antidiuretic	Pressor	Uterotonic
AVP	H_2N-Cys-Tyr-Phe-Gln-Asn-Cys-Pro-Arg-Gly-NH_2 (1 2 3 4 5 6 7 8 9)	100	100	5
Lysine vasopressin	Lys (8)	80	60	
Oxytocin	Ile (3), Leu (8)	1	1	100
Desmopressin (DDAVP)	H-Cys (1), D-Arg (8)	300+	0.4	
DVDAVP	H-Lys (1), Val (4), D-Arg (8)	400+	–	

+, prolonged.

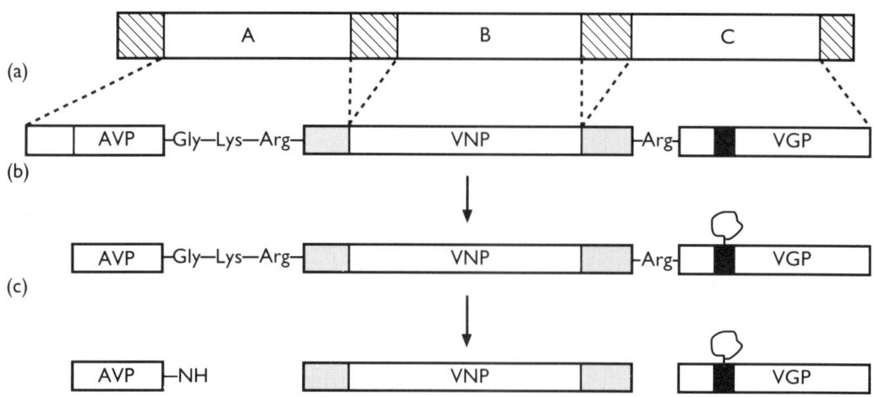

Fig. 32.3 (a) The AVP gene with its three exons (A–C) and intervening introns (shaded). (b) Prepropressophysin. Exon A encodes the signal peptide (unlabelled), AVP, the bridge between AVP and vasopressin neurophysin (VNP), and a variable N-terminal region of VNP. Exon B encodes a central portion of VNP, and exon C a variable C-terminal region of VNP, the bridge to the vasopressin glycopeptide (VGP), and VPG. Prepropressophysin is cleaved in the endoplasmic reticulum to the signal peptide and propressophysin (c), and the glycopeptide is glycosylated. Propressophysin is packaged into neurosecretory granules and cleaved during transport to the posterior pituitary. AVP is thereafter amidated.

Arginine vasopressin synthesis, storage, release and degradation

Prohormones of AVP (Fig. 32.3) and oxytocin are synthesized in separate magnocellular perikarya of the SON and PVN (see Fig. 32.2). Granules of propressophysin are transported rapidly through the axons by axoplasmic streaming, and stored within the axon terminals. This transport is inhibited by the microtubule disruptor colchicine [14], suggesting that microtubules participate in the transport. Presumably, the prohormone is cleaved enzymatically within the granules into AVP, neurophysin, and vasopressin glycopeptide (VPG).

The gene resides in the distal short arm of chromosome 20 [15] adjacent to the genes of oxytocin and prodynorphin [16]. Its transcription is stimulated by the same factors as the release of AVP. Action potentials from the hypothalamus cause release of the hormone into the blood stream. Granules are extruded from the axon terminals by exocytosis which is dependent on an influx of Ca^{2+}. Some AVP is also released into the cerebrospinal fluid and some enters the anterior pituitary via the portal capillary bed. The importance of these two fluxes is unknown. Of stored AVP, 10–20% is in readily releasable form. Only large increases and high levels of plasma AVP appear to be paralleled by plasma levels of neurophysin II [17,18].

ARGININE VASOPRESSIN IN BLOOD AND URINE

Arginine vasopressin is distributed in a volume roughly equal to the extracellular space, unbound to plasma proteins. Its concentration in plasma varies from non-detectable to hundreds of picomoles per litre. It is cleared with a highly variable half-life, 10–20 min on average. Some of it is excreted as such in urine; rarely more than 1–5%. The rest is cleaved by the liver and kidneys. Large quantities are associated with platelets; in platelet-rich plasma AVP concentrations are five- to six-fold higher than in platelet-poor plasma.

There are reports for [19], and against [20] the validity of urinary AVP measurements for the assessment of AVP secretion, and an example of its successful diagnostic application [21].

Arginine vasopressin receptors

Two major types of AVP receptors are known [22]. V_1 receptors split phosphatidylinositol and increase cytosolic Ca^{2+}. V_2 receptors activate adenylate cyclase and generate cyclic adenosine monophosphate (cAMP). The two types also differ in ligand affinities. Thus, desmopressin is almost specific for V_2. V_2 appears to be a 40 kD 371 amino-acid protein with four extracellular and four intracellular domains and seven membrane-spanning regions (Fig. 32.4) [24]. Its gene resides in Xq28 [25].

Of renal actions of AVP, antidiuresis is mediated by V_2, while V_1 receptors promote cell contraction and prostaglandin synthesis in glomerular mesangial cells, vascular smooth muscle and the renomedullary interstitial cells. Other V_2-mediated actions are an increase in plasma factor VIII and von Willebrand factor levels and vasodilation, manifested as facial flushing, a fall in diastolic blood pressure and a rise in pulse rate [26].

Absence of AVP decreases the number of renal V_2 recep-

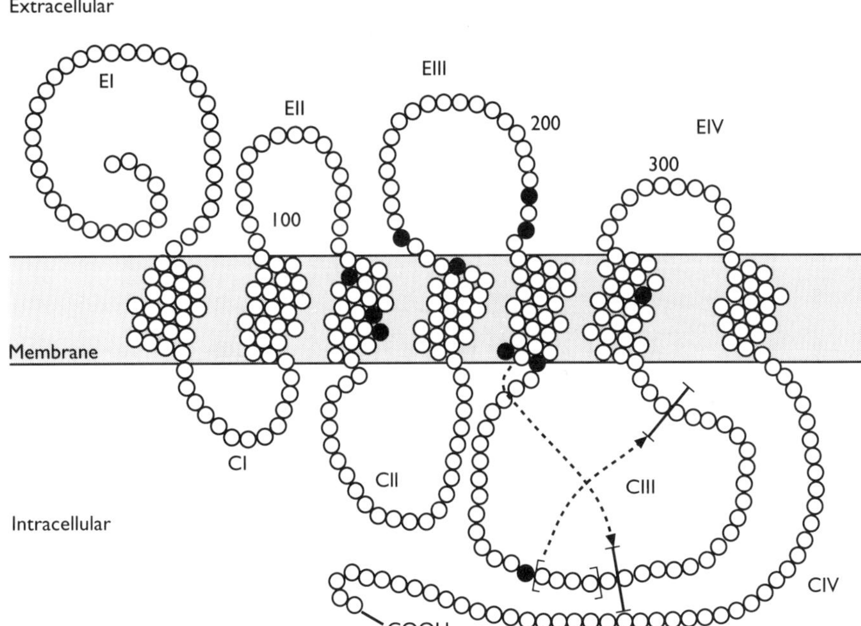

Fig. 32.4 V_2 receptor and its mutations in renal DI. Filled circles denote substitutions or frameshift mutations, arrows indicate truncated sites, and brackets represent in-frame deletion (redrawn from Editorial [23]).

tors. Moderate concentrations of AVP increase them, but a large dose may cause their almost complete disappearance.

Regulation of arginine vasopressin release and thirst

The release of AVP and the sensation of thirst are both regulated largely by effective extracellular fluid (ECF) osmolality and haemodynamic factors (see Fig. 32.1, Table 32.2) [1,20,27–35].

The release of AVP is modulated by stimulatory and inhibitory neural input to the magnocellular cells. These have an abundance of noradrenaline-containing nerve terminals, and cholinergic innervation with nicotinic and muscarinic receptors. The noradrenergic innervation mediates AVP release, and cholinergics facilitate it. Prostaglandins may enhance AVP release to osmotic stimulation. Dopamine appears to mediate the effect of nausea.

Suppression of AVP release seems to be mediated by atrial natriuretic peptide. γ-Aminobutyrate may be another inhibitory transmitter. Dynorphin, an opioid co-stored with AVP in the posterior pituitary, may feed back to AVP release. AVP itself feeds back to its own secretion.

Table 32.2 Variables that influence AVP secretion

	Stimulatory	Inhibitory
ECF osmolality (effective)	High	Low
Blood volume (effective)	Low	High
Posture	Upright	Recumbent
Breathing pressure	High	Low
Hypoproteinaemia	+	
Congestive failure	+	
Blood pressure	Low	High
Vasovagal reaction	+	
Drugs (see Table 32.3)	+	+
Nausea	+	
Drugs (see Table 32.3)	+	
Motion sickness	+	
Intracellular glucopenia	+	
Other		
Alcohol		+
Manipulation of intestine	+	
Stress		+
Trauma, burns		+
Temperature	High	Low
Acute hypoxia, hypercapnia	+	
Acidosis	+	
Drugs and hormones (see Table 32.3)	+	+

OSMOREGULATION

Effective ECF osmolality is the prime regulator of AVP release and thirst. Sensitive osmoreceptors monitor changes in the surrounding fluid, probably by changes in the volume of osmometric cells. They activate release of AVP from storage sites in the neurohypophysis and stimulate ingestion of water, probably via local angiotensin II release [36]. Thirst appears to be regulated by a separate group of osmoreceptor neurons that partially overlap with those for AVP control [37]. In disorders, one or both groups may be affected [31].

The term 'effective ECF osmolality' refers to the fact that it is not the osmolality measurable with an osmo-

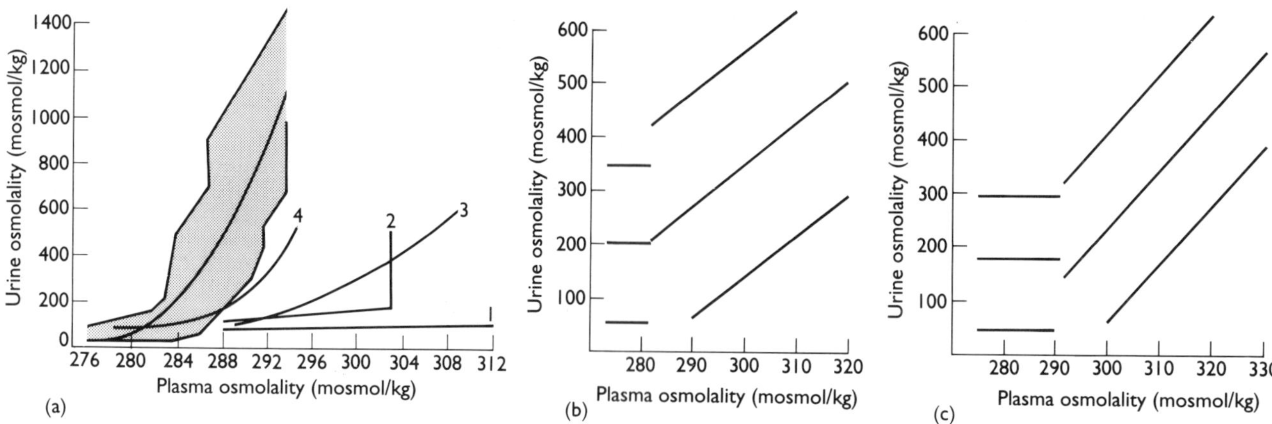

Fig. 32.5 Relation of urine osmolality to plasma osmolality in: (a) normal adults and children; (b) fullterm newborn infants; and (c) preterm newborn infants. Lines 1–4 on (a) indicate osmolar relationships in different types of DI ((a) redrawn from Streeten *et al.* [38], (b, c) from Sujov *et al.* [39]).

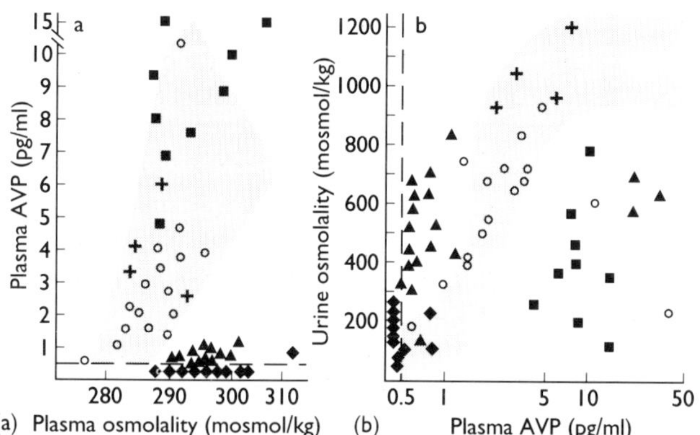

Fig. 32.6 Interrelations of: (a) concurrent plasma AVP concentration and osmolality; and (b) urine osmolality and plasma AVP concentration in adult subjects, normal (shaded areas), or with different types of diabetes insipidus. ○, Primary polydipsia; +, normal subjects; ■, renal DI; ◆, severe hypothalamic DI; ▲, mild hypothalamic DI (redrawn from Robertson & Berl [1]).

meter that is critical. Solutes which penetrate the cell membrane easily (urea, glucose, ethanol) are far less effective than others (sodium chloride, sucrose, mannitol) as activators of osmoreceptors [31]. A sharp rise in blood glucose may even cause a paradoxical decrease in AVP secretion; therefore assessments of antidiuretic function cannot universally be based on either plasma osmolality or Na^+ concentration. A satisfactory approximation of effective plasma osmolality, also called 'tonicity', is

$$\text{Tonicity} = \text{osmolality} - (U + G - 7.5),$$

where U and G are the plasma concentrations (mmol/l) of urea and glucose, respectively [30]. Plasma Na^+ concentration alone must be used with caution, because the osmoreceptors may also be stimulated by K^+, glycerol, acetone, organic acids and mannitol.

Interrelations between plasma and urine osmolality and plasma AVP concentration have been established in adult human subjects with normal and increased water turnover (Figs 32.5 & 32.6). For practical purposes the release of AVP is a precise function of plasma osmolality described by a threshold and a linear slope. Below the threshold, 275–290 mosmol/kg (average 280 mosmol/kg), AVP secretion is low enough to permit maximal urinary dilution. Urine flow rises to a rate that keeps pace with any but the most inordinately high rates of water input. This provides effective protection against overhydration and an excessive fall in osmolality. When this threshold is exceeded, AVP secretion rises sharply; the slope varies over a wider range, but is individually quite constant. In average individuals a change in plasma osmolality of only 1% will alter plasma AVP by 1 pg/ml and thereby urine osmolality by approximately 250 mosmol/kg (a 100-fold gain from stimulus to response). At plasma osmolality of around 295 mosmol/kg, the mean plasma AVP level reaches or exceeds 5 pg/ml – a concentration sufficient to produce maximal urinary concentration.

A solute-free increase in total water of 1% will normally double the rate of urine flow. Reduction of body water has an opposite effect of similar magnitude. The sensitivity of the osmoreceptor system is greater than the precision of the best laboratory measuring techniques. The scatter (Fig. 32.6a) appears to depend on wide interindividual variation and, in any individual subject, the interdependence of the variables is strict, provided that alterations in non-osmotic determinants of AVP secretion (see below) are avoided. The most sensitive individuals increase their plasma AVP in response to a rise in plasma osmolality of 0.5 mosmol/kg, but the least sensitive ones need a rise of 5 mosmol/kg. The relationship is influenced by the rate of increase in plasma osmolality; the increase in AVP is larger the faster the rise in osmolality.

The osmoreceptors for thirst behave like those for AVP secretion in that below a threshold tonicity no thirst is perceived, and above it thirst is progressively intensified with rising tonicity. Relation of the thresholds for thirst and AVP secretion is a matter of dispute. Robertson observed that the thirst threshold is clearly on average 10 mosmol/kg higher than the threshold for AVP secretion in healthy adults at 289–307 mosmol/kg (average 295 mosmol/kg) [20]. Therefore most people do not experience thirst until plasma AVP levels are high enough to produce maximum antidiuresis. Others maintain that the two thresholds do not differ, and that thirst participates in the maintenance of normal osmolality within its narrow range of < 10 mosmol/l [40–42]. The osmotic bioactivity of solutes is similar for thirst as it is for AVP release; thus hyperosmolality caused by glucose does not provoke thirst except in insulin deficiency.

Kallmann syndrome appears to be associated with variable subclinical dysfunction of osmoregulation of AVP secretion and thirst [43].

HAEMODYNAMIC FACTORS

Blood volume and pressure are secondary determinants of AVP secretion and thirst. They alter AVP secretion in an exponential fashion (Fig. 32.7a) and modify its osmoregulation. An acute rise in either one suppresses AVP release. Small decreases (for example 5–7%) have little effect, but decreases of 20–30% result in plasma AVP levels manyfold higher than those required for maximal antidiuresis or ever obtained by osmotic stimulus. Upright posture reduces effective blood volume by 10–15% and increases plasma AVP slightly. The relatively large haemodynamic changes that result from normal activity may significantly alter AVP secretion and its osmoregulation, and even cause erratic fluctuations. In mild hypotension or hypovolaemia the osmoregulation of AVP is altered with a fall of the threshold and an increase in the slope (Fig. 32.7b). With more severe haemodynamic changes plasma AVP is maintained at maximally antidiuretic levels and osmoregulation is lost. These effects are meaningful: the very high AVP levels contribute to haemodynamic recovery. In hypovolaemia, volume is protected at the cost of tonicity.

The baroreceptors appear to mediate the effects of some drugs (Table 32.3) and the autacoids acetylcholine, bradykinin, β-endorphin, histamine and prostaglandins, which stimulate AVP secretion, at least in part by reducing blood pressure or volume. Supraphysiological concentrations of noradrenaline suppress AVP release by raising blood pressure.

Blood volume is sensed by stretch receptors in the wall of the left atrium, and blood pressure by baroreceptors in the aortic arch and carotid sinuses. During normotensive normovolaemic conditions impulses from these receptors maintain tonic inhibition of AVP release.

As with AVP release, haemodynamic factors maintain a tonic inhibitory effect on thirst. Hypovolaemia and hypo-

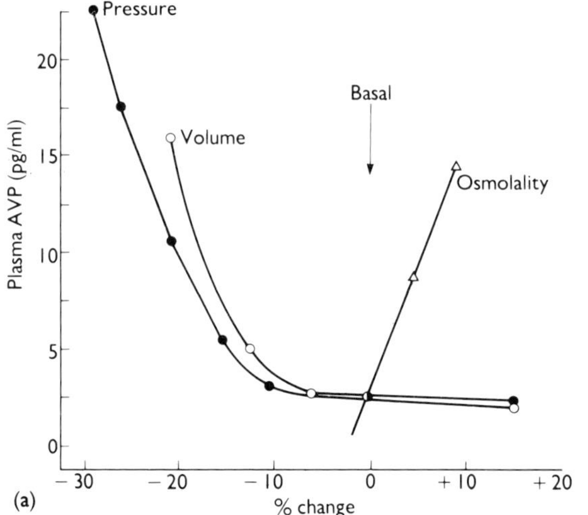

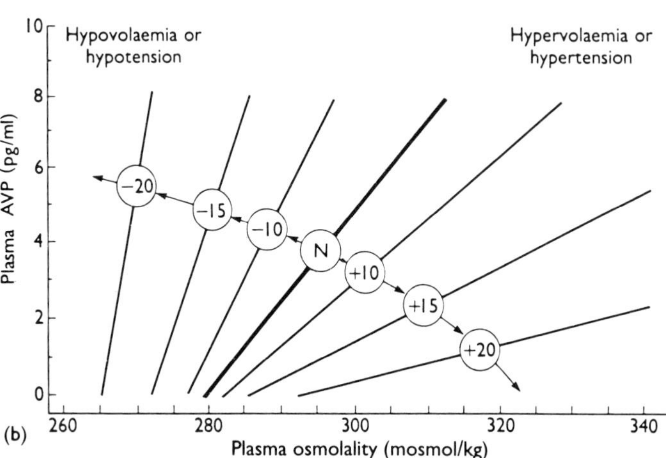

Fig. 32.7 Influence of blood volume and blood pressure on plasma AVP. (a) Comparison of the effects of changes in plasma osmolality, blood volume and blood pressure. (b) Effects of haemodynamic changes on the osmoregulation of AVP. The lines depict the relation of plasma AVP to plasma osmolality in a normovolaemic normotensive state (N), and after varying percentages of acute fall (left) or rise (right) in blood pressure or volume. Haemodynamic changes do not disrupt the osmoregulation of AVP, but lower or raise the threshold and slope of AVP secretion relative to osmolality.

tension induce thirst and Na^+ appetite; angiotensin II appears to be involved in mediation of these effects. The effect is immediate on thirst and delayed on Na^+ appetite, but the latter effect is not secondary to water intake. When sufficiently severe, hypovolaemia and hypotension stimulate AVP release even in the presence of hypotonicity. Threshold levels for these effects have not been determined; however, a blood volume deficit in excess of 10% is probably needed. These haemodynamic stimuli also lower the osmotic threshold for thirst.

OTHER FACTORS

Nausea is a very potent stimulator of AVP release even when transient and unaccompanied by vomiting. Increases to 100–1000 times the basal level may occur. By water loading the effect can only be attenuated; it may be blocked by pretreatment with antidopaminergic antiemetics.

Traction of the intestines during surgery is a potent stimulus of AVP release. Hypoglycaemia (and 2-deoxyglucose) is much weaker than nausea. Patients who have lost the capacity to respond to other stimuli may respond to hypoglycaemia. Its effect can be blocked by water loading. Hypoxia may cause AVP release, presumably through nausea or hypotension. The same may be true for pain and emotional stress.

Some drugs act through the emetic or other mechanisms (see Table 32.3). Low doses of the opioids morphine, butorphanol and oxilorphan elevate the osmotic threshold; this effect is blocked by naloxone. Ethanol is inhibitory, the mechanism involves opioids. Other inhibitors include clonidine and muscimol (a γ-aminobutyric acid agonist).

Most healthy recumbent people show a diurnal rhythm in AVP release with a peak between 2400 and 0400 h [59].

Drinking induced by thirst stops, and the secretion of AVP is suppressed, after ingestion of an appropriate volume before absorption and decrease in plasma osmolality take place. This is called non-osmotic inhibition of thirst and AVP secretion [40,42,60]. The phenomenon is independent of the tonicity of the fluid ingested [61]. This satiation obviously is essential to prevent overshooting the correction of water deficit. Both oropharyngeal and gastric factors are involved. The oropharyngeal receptors are cold-sensitive, which may explain why dehydrated persons prefer cold drinks.

Non-thirst-induced drinking of isotonic fluids also results in a transient hypotonic diuresis, but this is not mediated by inhibition of AVP release and the receptors mediating this response appear to lie in the stomach and/or small intestine [62].

K^+-depletion, hypercalcaemia, and hyperreninaemia seem to be direct stimulators of thirst independent of their renal and volume effects.

Table 32.3 Drugs, hormones and conditions that may cause or inhibit AVP action or secretion [20,44–47]

AVP action or secretion
AVP action: AVP, desmopressin
AVP release: acetylcholine, angiotensin II [36]
AVP release through reduction of blood volume or pressure: acetylcholine, barbiturates, bradykinin, β-endorphin, β-adrenergic agents, histamine, narcotic opioids (high dose), nicotine [48], nitroprusside, phenothiazines, thiazide diuretics, trimethophan, vasodilatory prostaglandins
AVP release through nausea: apomorphine, ethanol, hypoxia, hypercapnia, opioids (high dose), nicotine, cytostatics
Sensitization of osmoregulation: vincristine [32], (?)prostaglandins
Potentiation of AVP action: acetaminophen, carbamazepine [49,50], chlorpropamide [49,51,52], prostaglandin synthesis inhibitors, tolbutamide, vincristine
Controversial mechanism: clofibrate, cyclophosphamide

Inhibition of AVP release or action
Inhibition of AVP release: α-adrenergic agonists [53], atrial natriuretic peptide, carbamazepine, chlorpromazine, clonidine, (?)γ-aminobutyric acid agonists, ethanol, fluphenazine, glucocorticoids [54], haloperidol, narcotic opioids (low dose), narcotic antagonists, phenytoin, promethazine, prostaglandin synthesis inhibitors [44]
V_2 receptor antagonism: OPC-31260 [55]
Other inhibition of action: acetohexamide, α_2-adrenergic agonists [53], amphotericin B [56], Ca^{2+} excess, cisplatinum, colchicine, demethylchlortetracycline, gentamicin, glucocorticoids, glypuride, isophamide, kallikrein–kinin system, K^+ depletion, lithium [45,57,58], loop diuretics, methicillin, methoxyflurane, propoxyphene, prostaglandins, vinblastine

Extrarenal actions of arginine vasopressin

Arginine vasopressin is a potent direct vasoconstrictor, important at physiological concentrations [63,64]; but it also potentiates the sinoaortic baroreceptor reflex which reduces heart rate and cardiac output in response to peripheral vasoconstriction, and this action eliminates its hypertensive effect in the intact organism, until its concentration reaches the upper physiological range, around 50 pg/ml or about 10-fold that required for maximum antidiuresis. AVP is important for the maintenance of normotension in mild volume depletion [65]. It is a critical part of the homeostatic response to hypovolaemic shock in dogs and rats, and probably in humans. The vasoconstrictor and antidiuretic effects are mediated by different parts of the molecule.

The parvocellular neurosecretory neurons terminate in the median eminence. These neurons increase drastically after adrenalectomy. They release AVP and corticotrophin-releasing factor into the portal blood supply of the anterior pituitary, and apparently increase adrenocorticotrophic hormone (ACTH) secretion. Blood from these vessels may contain extremely high concentrations of AVP during stress, such as of major surgery and anaesthesia. AVP appears to be at least as important as corticotrophin-releasing hormone (CRH) in the control of ACTH release [66], though Brattleboro rats, which lack the capacity to synthesize AVP, have little or no impairment of glucocorticoid response to stress.

Another, smaller division of AVP-containing neurons projects to the walls of the lateral and third ventricles, probably secreting directly into the cerebrospinal fluid. There its concentration is slightly lower than in plasma, without clear correlation between the two levels [67].

At physiological concentrations, AVP also inhibits water loss from skin, lungs and other extrarenal sites. Its other actions include inhibition of pancreatic flow, stimulation of hepatic glycogenolysis, and aggregation of platelets.

The V_1 receptors account for the vasoconstriction, stimulation of ACTH release, inhibition of renin secretion, and central nervous system effects of AVP. The corticotroph AVP receptor shows characteristics of both V_1 and V_2 [66]. The V_2 receptors appear to be generally present in vascular epithelia. Extrarenal V_2 receptors mediate a decrease in diastolic pressure, vasodilatory action manifested by facial flushing, increase in plasma renin activity, and releases of factor VIIIc (from hepatocytes and liver sinusoidal cells), von Willebrand factor and plasminogen activator (from vascular endothelial cells including liver sinusoids). The elevated level of circulating von Willebrand factor contributes to the increase in factor VIIIc, since von Willebrand factor serves as a carrier molecule for factor VIII in plasma.

Arginine vasopressin and regulation of water excretion

Depending on the concentration of AVP present, the normal mature kidney is able to produce urine of an osmolality ranging from 60 to 1100 mosmol/kg and, in dehydration, even to 1300 mosmol/kg. Excretion of surplus water is largely, though not entirely, independent of solute excretion. It is useful to consider urine flow (V) as consisting of two parts, osmolar clearance (C_{osm}), which is the volume required for excretion of urinary solute at the osmolality of plasma, and free water clearance (C_{H_2O}), which equals ($V - C_{osm}$) and is positive when urine is hypo-osmolar to plasma and negative when it is hyper-osmolar. A child of 30 kg with an average daily solute load of 800 mosmol to be excreted and a plasma osmolality of 285 mosmol/kg may pass daily (800/285 =) 2.81 l urine iso-osmolar with plasma (= C_{osm}) or at extreme dilution (60 mosmol/kg) 13.33 l and at extreme concentration (1100 mosmol/kg) 0.73 l. The corresponding values of C_{H_2O} are 10.52 l and −2.08 l/day or, as expressed commonly, 7.3 ml/min and −1.4 ml/min.

The ability to vary urinary concentration depends on the spatial arrangement and permeability characteristiscs of the segments of the renal tubules (Fig. 32.8) [69,70].

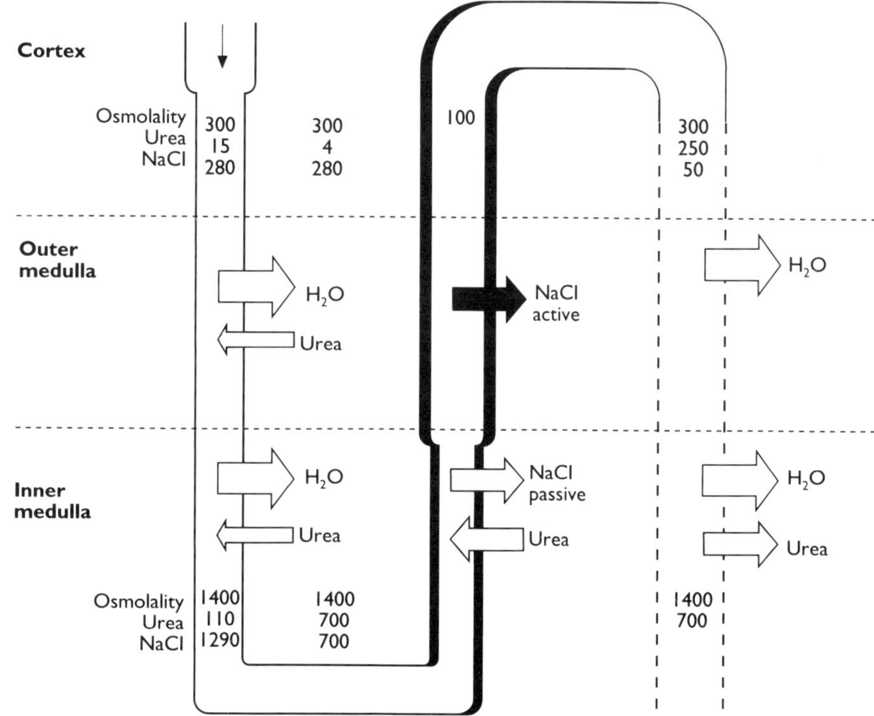

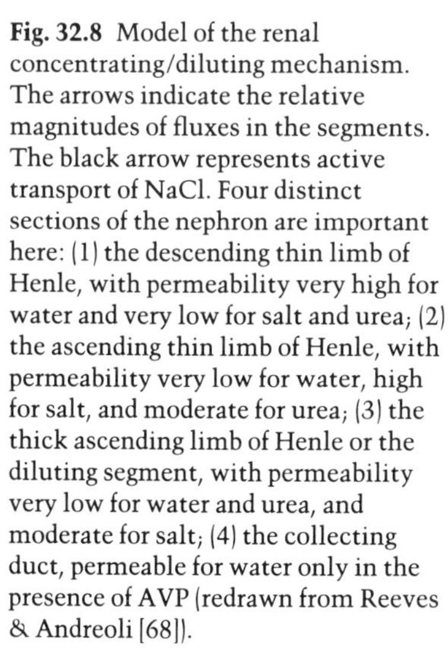

Fig. 32.8 Model of the renal concentrating/diluting mechanism. The arrows indicate the relative magnitudes of fluxes in the segments. The black arrow represents active transport of NaCl. Four distinct sections of the nephron are important here: (1) the descending thin limb of Henle, with permeability very high for water and very low for salt and urea; (2) the ascending thin limb of Henle, with permeability very low for water, high for salt, and moderate for urea; (3) the thick ascending limb of Henle or the diluting segment, with permeability very low for water and urea, and moderate for salt; (4) the collecting duct, permeable for water only in the presence of AVP (redrawn from Reeves & Andreoli [68]).

In the cortex the renal interstitial fluid is isosmolar to plasma. In the medulla it is progressively hyperosmolar towards the papillary tips, where it reaches 1200–1400 mosmol/kg in the absence of diuresis. This corticomedullary osmolar gradient is maintained by the countercurrent multiplication system of the loop of Henle.

Some 85% of the salt and water of the filtrate is reabsorbed iso-osmotically in the proximal tubules before entering the loops. In the descending limb of the loop the fluid becomes gradually hyperosmolar, by passive extraction of water into the hyperosmolar interstitium. The ascending limb is impermeable to water, and active removal of NaCl in its thick segment renders the fluid entering the distal convoluted tubules markedly hypo-osmolar. Countercurrent multiplication is produced by an active step in the thick ascending limbs and a passive step in the papillae. The active step is absorption of NaCl from the tubular fluid. It turns the hyperosmolar fluid entering this segment hypo-osmolar, because of the impermeability of this segment to water. It can be inhibited by 'loop diuretics', which thus restrict both the diluting and the concentrating capacity of the kidneys. The passive step works during antidiuresis: diffusion of urea from the papillary collecting ducts to the interstitium down a concentration gradient generated by extraction of water from the ductal fluid by medullary hyperosmolality. Approximately half of the medullary osmolality is due to NaCl and half to urea. The medullary concentration is also high for Ca^{2+}, but low for K^+. The arrangement is very economical: an axial gradient of some 900 mosmol/kg is built up with a transversal intraloop gradient of only 200 mosmol/kg.

ROLE OF ARGININE VASOPRESSIN

In the collecting ducts, which extend across the hyperosmolar medullary interstitium, the water permeability of the luminal membrane is regulated by AVP. In its absence the permeability is low and urine remains dilute. With rising concentrations of AVP the permeability increases steeply, allowing more and more efficient equilibration of tubular urine with the interstitium by extraction of water. This results in a sharp rise in urinary osmolality (see Fig. 32.6). The renal response takes place within a few minutes after release of AVP into the circulation. The opposite effect, development of full water diuresis after antidiuresis, requires 60–90 min, due to the slow metabolism of AVP.

V_2 receptors are located on the basolateral (contraluminal) membrane of the collecting ducts (Fig. 32.9). Occupancy by AVP of only 2.5% of the receptors, and 5% of maximal adenylate cyclase activation, results in full antidiuretic effect [71]. This requires the presence of suf-

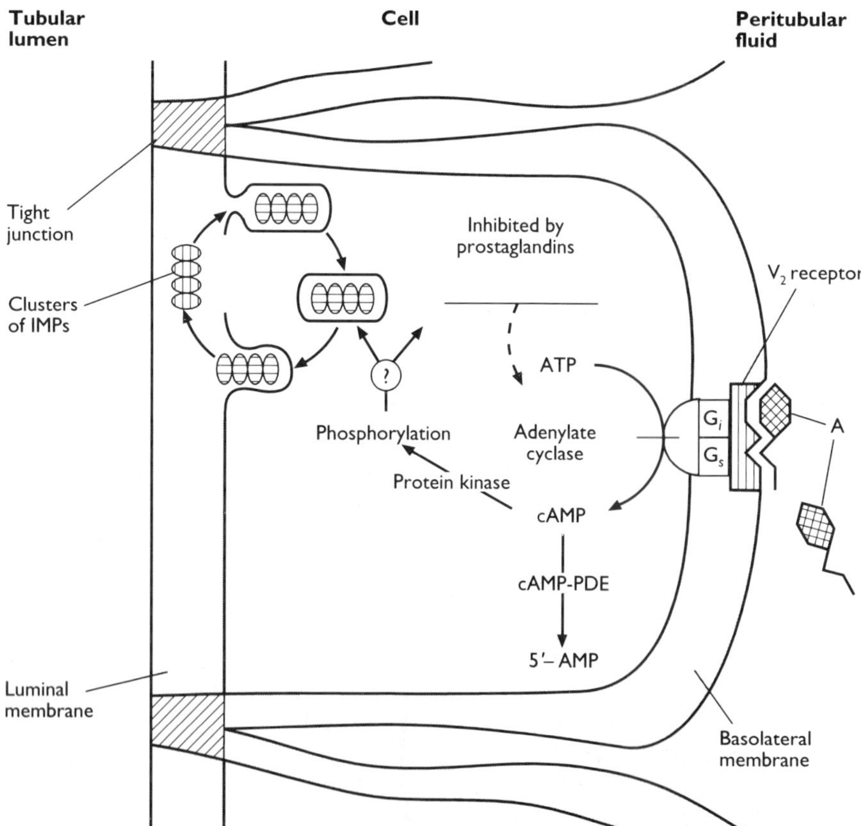

Fig. 32.9 Scheme of the action of AVP on the cells of the renal collecting ducts: G_i and G_s, inhibitory and stimulatory guanine nucleotide regulatory proteins; IMPs, intramembranous particles; PDE, phosphodiesterase; A, AVP arising.

ficient Mg^{2+} and of stimulatory guanine nucleotide-binding protein G_s. Calmodulin also modulates the activity of the AVP-sensitive adenylate cyclase. Intracellular accumulation of cAMP induces a chain of reactions involving protein phosphorylation, microfilaments and microtubules, and formation in the apical cell membrane of particle aggregates, which probably provide channels for osmotic water flow. Once this final response is established in an experimental situation, microtubule inhibitors (colchicine, vinblastine) are without effect, while microfilament inhibitors (cytochalasin B) diminish the response. The aggregates probably exist as preformed cytoplasmic organelles which are inserted into the cell membrane using microtubules as 'tracks'.

AVP has an effect even on the glomeruli. It decreases the glomerular filtration coefficient [72], possibly by inducing contraction of the glomerular mesangial cells [73].

In contrast to the kidneys of many species, human kidney lacks AVP receptors in the thick ascending limb of Henle. Consequently, AVP probably does not stimulate the reabsorption of NaCl and building up of medullary hyperosmolality in the human.

ROLE OF PROSTAGLANDINS

Prostaglandins play a complex and incompletely clarified role in renal physiology [74]. A major function is regulation of renal blood flow and protection of the kidneys against fluctuations in systemic blood pressure. AVP through the V_1 receptors, and noradrenaline, bradykinin and angiotensin II, sharply increase renal prostaglandin E_2 synthesis. The effect of inhibition of the prostaglandin synthesis depends on the actual haemodynamic and hormonal state. Inhibitors may decrease glomerular filtration and renal blood flow only during activation of the renin–angiotensin system, that is under conditions of Na^+ restriction, extracellular fluid depletion, or low cardiac output. Great interspecies differences exist in renal prostaglandin physiology, and conclusions from animal experiments often are not valid for the human situation.

Locally generated prostaglandins act as negative feedback modulators of the AVP effect. AVP stimulates the synthesis of prostaglandin E_2 in medullary collecting duct cells. Prostaglandin E_2 inhibits the AVP-stimulated accumulation of cyclic AMP in the same cells and, thereby, the effect of AVP on water permeability. Prostaglandins may also increase medullary and papillary blood flow, causing 'washout' of medullary hyperosmolality. Prostaglandin E_2 may diminish reabsorption of urea by the collecting ducts, thus further decreasing the osmotic force of water reabsorption. In several animal species the reabsorption of NaCl by the thick ascending limb of Henle, which is the driving force of the countercurrent multiplication system, is stimulated by AVP. Prostaglandin E_2 produced under AVP effect by medullary interstitial cells counteracts this AVP-sensitive part of NaCl reabsorption. However, the human thick ascending limb is devoid of AVP receptors and, therefore, probably of these effects of AVP and prostaglandin E_2. Renal prostaglandin production is augmented in K^+ depletion; this probably contributes to the renal insensitivity to AVP associated with K^+ depletion.

Prostaglandins directly stimulate renin release.

ROLE OF ATRIAL NATRIURETIC PEPTIDE

Atrial natriuretic peptide (ANP), a 28 amino-acid peptide produced by the heart muscle and the brain [75], is natriuretic, diuretic and vasorelaxant. ANP receptors are present in the heart, the endothelial cells of many vascular beds, renal glomeruli and tubuli, the adrenal cortex and the hypothalamus. Plasma ANP concentrations are low (7–21 pmol/l). Blood half-life of ANP is 2–3 min. High atrial transmural pressure which depends on venous return stimulates its release. Its diuretic potency is greater than its natriuretic potency, but natriuresis without diuresis can be induced by simultaneous administration of desmopressin and ANP [76]. Its other renal effects depend on the state of hydration, haemodynamics and activity of other hormones. It may increase glomerular filtration rate, reduce the proximal fractional absorption of Na^+, and redirect blood flow, thus reducing papillary hyperosmolality.

ANP suppresses AVP secretion, and antagonizes the AVP-induced water permeability of the collecting ducts, thereby increasing free water clearance [77,78]. Administration of ANP makes the concentrated urine of dehydrated subjects markedly hypo-osmolar to plasma despite persistently high plasma AVP [79]. In cultured rat diencephalic neurons AVP increases ANP secretion in dose-related fashion [80].

OTHER FACTORS

Adrenal steroids are necessary both for free water excretion and water reabsorption. Normal haemodynamics and glomerular filtration are prerequisites for undisturbed water excretion, and both are compromised in adrenocortical failure.

Glucocorticoids are antagonists of renal vasoconstrictors and their clearest renal effects are increases in glomerular filtration rate and renal plasma flow. Glucocorticoids also may exert a direct effect on the distal tubuli in the hypovolaemic state which is associated with increased AVP secretion. The cyclic AMP response to AVP is reduced with diminished glucocorticoid activity.

Alterations of renal arginine vasopressin action [81]

TEMPORARY ALTERATIONS

In osmotic diuresis, increased delivery of urine to the distal segment speeds up the flow and shortens the contact time, both concentrating and diluting potentials being reduced in proportion to the osmole load. At very large loads the osmolality will be fixed at the level of plasma osmolality. Strong osmotic (for example mannitol) diuresis will also decrease the reabsorption of electrolytes and may lead to depletion.

Prolonged dehydration may increase urine osmolality by allowing elevation of medullary hyperosmolality. Furthermore, it decreases glomerular filtration and hence the volume delivered to the collecting ducts, allowing prolonged exposure to water extraction by the hyperosmolar surroundings. The opposite is also true: prolonged overhydration, such as occurs in polydipsia, decreases the concentrating capacity, by dissipation of medullary hyperosmolality. Renal diabetes insipidus has been diagnosed in such cases, but restriction of drinking for several days has corrected the concentration defect [82]. Low urea production (for example in infants and in protein deficiency) will also compromise the concentrating potential, because urea normally contributes approximately half the medullary hyperosmolality. K^+ depletion also leads to failure in maintenance of medullary hyperosmolality and to polyuria, possibly through disturbance of the cellular action of AVP. 'Hypokalaemic' polyuria appears to be due to depletion of cellular rather than extracellular K^+.

Hypercalcaemia is similarly associated with a concentration defect. This appears always to coincide with decreased filtration. The degree of hyposthenuria depends more on the duration than on the degree of hypercalcaemia. The effect is mediated by reduced medullary hyperosmolality and impairment of the AVP effect. The latter includes at least inhibitions by Ca^{2+} of adenylate cyclase and cAMP-dependent protein kinase, and reassembly of microtubules. Stimulation of thirst beyond that necessary to compensate for the primary polyuric effects is associated with both hypercalcaemia and K^+ depletion. Because Ca^{2+} is concentrated in the medulla, this is the first site of nephrocalcinosis.

Chronic hydronephrosis may cause a reparable concentration defect by flattening the renal papillae and thus shortening the countercurrent loops. After acute bilateral obstruction large volumes of iso- or hypo-osmolar urine are excreted. This appears to be due to the same mechanism, as well as to solute retention. Acute non-obstructive urinary tract infections often cause some reduction of maximal urinary concentration, which disappears with treatment. Substantial impairment of concentrating ability without azotaemia is not uncommon during late convalescence from tubular necrosis. Ischaemic or toxic (methoxyflurane, methicillin) renal damage may also cause hyposthenuria.

People with sickle-cell anaemia are unable to concentrate urine to more than 600 and usually even 450 mosmol/kg. The defect may be corrected by blood transfusion, and free water absorption improves during osmotic diuresis. Presumably, red cells sickle on entering the hyperosmolar environment in the renal papillae, thus increasing blood viscosity. Impaired medullary blood flow results in poor function of the countercurrent multiplier system and decreased medullary hyperosmolality.

Drug effects

α_2-Adrenergic agonists suppress AVP-induced cAMP accumulation, thus decreasing the antidiuretic effect. This appears to be mediated by activation of the inhibitory guanine-nucleotide-binding protein G_i [53]. Demeclocycline decreases dose-dependently the medullary adenylate cyclase activity, but may also reduce cAMP-induced water flow. For other drugs, see Table 32.3.

PERMANENT EFFECTS OF KIDNEY DISEASE

In kidneys in which most of the nephrons have been destroyed by disease, the remaining nephrons are in a state of osmotic diuresis due to greatly increased filtration in their glomeruli, which places a heavy osmolar load on the tubules. This may be the mechanism of isosthenuria in any diffuse renal disease. In a disease primarily affecting the renal medulla, such as medullary cystic disease, the concentrating capacity may be markedly decreased in the absence of reduced filtration. This is believed to be due to selective destruction of nephrons with long loops of Henle. Such loops contribute especially to the production of concentrated urine; in humans they represent only 10–15% of the total nephronal population.

Chronic pyelonephritis usually first involves the renal medulla with early compromise of concentrating capacity.

Ontogeny of the water regulation system

Posterior pituitary gland develops from the infundibular process by the fifth week of gestation. By the end of the first trimester the first hypothalamic nuclei and fibres of the supraopticohypophyseal tract appear, and AVP [83], neurophysin II, the phylogenetically primitive antidiuretic hormone arginine vasotocin [84] and oxytocin are detectable in the posterior pituitary. The amount of AVP exceeds the amount of vasotocin by midpregnancy [83].

The release of AVP has been studied in fetal and newborn lambs [85]. AVP does not cross the placenta. In the third trimester it shows brisk responses to plasma hyperosmolality, hypovolaemia and hypoxia [86,87]. It facilitates transplacental movement of water from the maternal to the fetal side [88], which may serve to protect fetal intravascular volume. Fetal plasma osmolality and AVP are strongly correlated, indicating functionality of osmoreceptors and AVP release. Plasma AVP correlates with urine osmolality. Thus, the fetal hypothalamoneurohypophyseal system and the kidney seem able to participate in osmolar and volume homeostasis. In the newborn lamb the volume and osmoreceptor systems are as sensitive as in the adult.

An AVP surge takes place in the human infant during normal birth [89,90]; this appears to result from the acute compression of the head. Plasma AVP concentration in cord blood varies widely, from 1 to 10^3 pg/ml [91]. At Caesarean section the levels correlate with the degree of cervical dilation [92]. AVP is elevated in cord blood of infants with perinatal asphyxia [93]. High levels may therefore reflect a physiological response to perinatal stress. Acute release of AVP also occurs during surgery or mechanical ventilation of premature infants [94,95].

Urine osmolality in the newborn infant responds in a qualitatively normal fashion to hypervolaemia, hyperosmolality and dehydration [96]. However, in 13 newborn infants no correlation was found in the first 3 weeks between plasma AVP levels and urinary concentration [91]. During the first week of life the range of urinary osmolality for all levels of plasma osmolality was much wider than later: some healthy infants passed undiluted urine at plasma osmolality <280 mosmol/kg; average osmolal threshold for AVP secretion was 282 mosmol/kg for fullterm and 291 mosmol/kg for 30–34-week preterm infants [39]. When deprived of water and food in the first 72 h of life, premature infants of 1500–2500 g only concentrated their 24-h urines from 230 $\pm$ 56 (mean $\pm$ SD) to 441 $\pm$ 69 mosmol/kg, while serum Na^+ concentration increased from 145 to 150 mmol/l. Fullterm newborn infants are only able to concentrate urine to 500–700 mosmol/kg. This limitation probably results from many factors [97].

The kidneys are morphologically immature, with relatively short loops of Henle and hence insufficient ability to sequestrate urea in the medulla. There may be a deficiency of urea due to the low protein intake in relation to the anabolic state. The NaCl reabsorptive capacity of the thick ascending limb of Henle, and hence the medullary hypertonicity, seem not to be fully developed. The low glomerular filtration rate in the newborn infant, less than 50% of the mature level, may contribute to the poor concentrating ability by scanty delivery of fluid to the distal tubules. It also limits the capacity for free water excretion.

Poor water-conserving capacity predisposes the newborn to dehydration when exposed to an extra osmolar load or reduction of the concentrating ability. On average the daily solute load of a 5 kg infant is 150 mosmol, and the water intake 500 ml. Excretion of this osmolar load at a urinary osmolality of 600 mosmol/kg requires about half the water intake. Water for insensible water loss leaves little in reserve.

Full functional maturity appears to be attained already within 3 months of term.

Synopsis of water balance [31]

Ordinarily, the intake of water and electrolytes is not determined by requirements, but largely by habits and nutritional needs. It is thus left to the excretion to serve the control of balance. The rate of water excretion cannot be reduced below a minimum, which is determined by the solute load to be excreted and the concentration capacity; it is normally 0.8–1.2 ml/mosmol. (Conversely, a minimum amount of solute must be excreted with water, normally 0.06–0.07 mosmol/ml.) The minimum intake of water required for maintenance of balance is made up of minimum urine water plus insensible water loss minus water produced by oxidation. In a sedentary situation the balance of insensible loss and water from oxidation averages −350 ml for a 10 kg infant, −595 ml for a 30 kg child, and −875 ml for a 70 kg person. However, in high ambient temperature and during strenuous physical activity these may increase even 25-fold.

The body is able to excrete excess water much faster than excess salt. The remarkable stability of plasma tonicity is achieved largely by adjusting total body water to the amount of Na^+. In situations of excess total body Na^+, thirst and AVP secretion aggravate, instead of ameliorating, the hypervolaemia. The responsibility for avoiding volume excess rests primarily with the endocrine and renal elements adjusting Na^+ excretion. The high plasma AVP levels induced by hypernatraemia may facilitate the excretion of the Na^+ excess by contributing to suppression of the production of renin.

In dehydration both the renin–angiotensin–aldosterone system and AVP release probably mediated by the increase in angiotensin II are activated to protect volaemia. This mediation is very important in hyponatraemic dehydration, in which hypotonicity would suppress AVP. In such situations the inhibition of renin release by high levels of AVP is overridden. Atrial natriuretic peptide is a potent antagonizer of the release and action of both AVP and the renin–angiotensin–aldosterone system. Its release is stimulated by both AVP and angiotensin.

The extreme limits of tonicity homeostasis are determined by AVP secretion and thirst. These functions may effect very large increases in the output and intake of water, providing almost insurmountable barriers to overhydration and dehydration. AVP secretion effectively determines the lower limit of plasma tonicity, and thirst its upper limit (an unlimited access to drinkable water provided). In usual circumstances, plasma tonicity is controlled precisely by small osmoreceptor-mediated adjustments in water excretion. On average, intake and output balance at plasma osmolality 285 mosmol/kg. Thirst is virtually absent and AVP is secreted at a rate sufficient to concentrate urine somewhat above the plasma osmolality. From this state the body has a great capacity to change both the input and the output of water. Normally, the antidiuretic mechanism is fully employed before discomforting thirst emerges. Any factor that impairs the full suppression of AVP secretion or the stimulation of thirst will predispose to serious disturbances. The efficacy of thirst is proved by the normality of plasma osmolality in patients with severe diabetes insipidus.

The relationship of urine osmolality and flow is inverse exponential (Fig. 32.10). Suppression of plasma AVP to levels allowing maximum urinary dilution, 'water diuresis', increases the rate of water excretion to >25-fold compared with the flow at full antidiuresis.

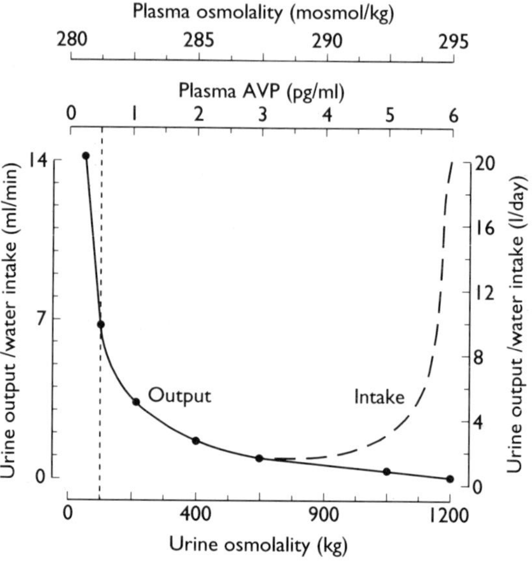

Fig. 32.10 Normal relationship of urine output to urine osmolality, plasma osmolality and plasma AVP concentration; and normal relation of water intake to plasma osmolality. The line describing urine output was calculated assuming a solute load of 800 mosmol/24 h. The line describing water intake was obtained by analysing the relationship of water intake to plasma osmolality in healthy adults after infusion of hypertonic saline; the intake relates only to the scale of plasma osmolality. The volume scales on the right and left are identical, but with different units. Note that the steep rises in output and intake occur only below urine osmolality 200 mosmol/kg and above plasma osmolality 293 mosmol/kg, respectively. It is of great clinical importance that most of the flow adjustment occurs at osmolalities below plasma osmolality. Little further water sparing may be effected by concentrating urine from 300 to 1200 mosmol/kg (redrawn from Robertson *et al.* [31]).

DIABETES INSIPIDUS AND HYPODIPSIA–HYPERNATRAEMIA

Insufficient AVP function leads to excessive loss of water by urination. If thirst is intact, as it usually is, the lost water will be replaced and normo-osmolality maintained by copious drinking. The resulting syndrome of polydipsia and polyuria is traditionally called diabetes insipidus (DI). Very rarely in childhood, a similar syndrome is caused by primary excessive drinking. DI is most commonly caused by AVP deficiency, which is also known as hypothalamic, central, cranial or neurogenic DI. Renal or nephrogenic DI is due to renal resistance to AVP. Its severe congenital form is much less common than central DI.

Adequate replacement of water loss may fail because of an associated defect in the mechanism of thirst sensation or inability to obtain water in response to thirst. The latter is likely in a newborn or young infant. The resulting hypernatraemic dehydration may decrease the urinary water loss. A balanced state may then develop, in which polyuria and polydipsia are absent, being replaced by symptoms of hyperosmolar dehydration, such as failure to thrive, irritability, vomiting and unexplained fever. This state carries a high risk of brain damage and even death.

Causes and frequency

DIABETES INSIPIDUS

Diabetes insipidus is rare, with an estimated total annual incidence in Finland of five cases per million in the 0–14-year-old population. The list of causes is long (Table 32.4) but in childhood a few aetiological groups dominate. Of over 300 cases collected from the literature [82,98–100] and the author's experience, 38% were caused by a hypothalamic tumour; 23% had craniopharyngioma, but in only a small minority was DI present preoperatively. Of the hypothalamic tumours causing (preoperative) DI, the most common was germinoma (6.5%) followed by craniopharyngioma and optic glioma. Langerhans cell histiocytosis was relatively common (8%). Idiopathic AVP deficiency (including almost a quarter of familial cases) and congenital renal DI were equally common (23%). Cerebral malformation (3.2%), primary polydipsia (2.6%) and trauma (1.6%) were other causes.

Because of bilaterality of the structures synthesizing AVP and regulating its secretion, unilateral hypothalamic lesions will not incapacitate the system. DI is produced by destruction of the area immediately above the diaphragma sellae where the bilateral supraopticohypophyseal tracts converge and unite. Transection of the pituitary stalk, which may occur at birth in breech or foot presentation, and during perinatal asphyxia or severe jaundice, appears to lead to destruction of the posterior pituitary and

Table 32.4 Causes of polyuria

AVP deficiency (hypothalamic DI)	*AVP insensitivity* (renal DI)
Traumatic	Hereditary
Postoperative	V_2 receptor mutation (X-linked)
Vascular	Postreceptor defect
Anomaly	K^+ depletion
Sickle-cell disease	Nephrocalcinosis
Haemorrhage	Hypercalcaemia
Collapse	Polycystic disease
Severe infection	Sickle-cell disease
Infiltrative	Toxic (demeclocycline, lithium, methoxyflurane, methicillin)
Histiocytosis	
Leukaemia	Urinary tract obstruction
Sarcoidosis	Chronic renal disease
Tumour	
Germinoma	*Primary polydipsia*
Craniopharyngioma	Organic hypothalamic disease (dipsogenic DI, compulsive water drinking, subnormal thirst threshold), many causes as in hypothalamic DI
Optic glioma	
Anomaly	
Septo-optic dysplasia	
Laurence–Moon–Biedl syndrome	Psychogenic
Empty sella syndrome	Habituation
Acrocallosal syndrome	Schizophrenic personality
Hereditary	Drug-induced
Autosomal dominant	Thioridazine, chlorpropamide, anticholinergic drugs (dry mouth)
X-linked	
DIDMOAD	
Miscellaneous	
Idiopathic	*Osmotic diuresis*
Inflammatory	
Autoimmune	Glucose
Drug-induced inhibition of AVP release (narcotic agonists)	Mannitol
	Salt
	Diuretic drugs
	Chronic pyelonephritis

retrograde degeneration of the axons. It is more extensive with higher damage. An 80% destruction of the supraoptic nucleus is required for polyuria; this develops only after section at the level of the infundibulum or higher. If the transection occurs at or below the level of the median eminence, supraopticohypophyseal tract axons will hypertrophy above the point of transection. This may lead to organization of an ectopic posterior pituitary capable of secreting AVP in normal or insufficient amounts [101–103]. Of 20 patients aged 2–19 years with complete growth hormone (GH) deficiency owing to pituitary stalk transection, three had DI with an absence of any posterior pituitary according to magnetic resonance imaging (MRI). The others had an ectopic posterior pituitary gland of variable size. Those with a gland of >5 mm length (measured along the pituitary stalk axis on the MRI image) had normal AVP function, and most of those with a smaller gland had partial AVP deficiency [103]. Surgery of hypothalamic tumours commonly causes permanent DI; this occurs in up to 75% of operations for craniopharyngioma. Transient AVP deficiency is also a relatively frequent complication after pituitary surgery. Of 116 patients, 61 developed hypotonic polyuria after trans-sphenoidal pituitary adenectomy. This was due to elimination of excessive water in 45 cases and to transient DI in 16 cases [104].

Pituitary tumours may cause DI only by suprasellar extension. Of patients with craniopharyngioma 10–20% have severe DI, and approximately 35% a partial defect. However, severe cases may be overrepresented in reports, and associated ACTH deficiency may abolish polyuria and lead to underdiagnosis of less severe cases. Polyuria may precede the discovery of an intracranial tumour or Langerhans cell histiocytosis by many months, even several years. When patients with histiocytosis were examined or followed for the presence of AVP deficiency, this was found in 20–60% [105–107]. Histiocytosis has a predilection for hypothalamic nuclei. Leukaemia, sarcoidosis, Hodgkin disease and metastatic lesions are rare causes in childhood. Cases have been reported resulting from tiny non-neoplastic suprasellar mass lesions [108].

DI is a frequent component of the Laurence–Moon syndrome, presumably through hypothalamic hypoplasia. The association of primary empty sella with DI is rare; more rare in children than adults [82,109,110]. Of the malformations causing DI, septo-optic dysplasia is relatively common; DI may be a late manifestation [111]. DI is part of acrocallosal syndrome [112]; it has been reported in children with variable brain malformations [113,114].

Head trauma, commonly associated with fracture of the base of skull, is another cause. The patient is usually severely ill, frequently with multiple injuries. In gravely brain-damaged children DI is a bad omen presaging brain death [115] and treatment of DI is commonly part of organ-donor maintenance [116]. With serious trauma the association of anterior pituitary deficiency should be assumed and cortisol therapy commenced. DI may even occur after minor trauma [117] and appear only after several weeks [118]. Anoxia, encephalitis and the Reye syndrome are other aetiologies [115]. DI, often transient, sometimes occurs after asphyxia, intraventricular haemorrhage, or severe infections.

In newborn infants DI complicating other illness may be more common than is recognized: neonatal DI may follow sepsis caused by streptococcal meningitis [119], intraventricular haemorrhage [120] and *Listeria monocytogenes* with disseminated intravascular coagulation [121].

In 20–30% of patients with central DI repeated neuroradiological investigation has failed to reveal an aetiology; such cases are called 'idiopathic'. Some of these patients have GH insufficiency, but rarely other anterior pituitary dysfunction [122]. Degeneration of the supraoptic and/or paraventricular nucleus has been observed in some patients [123]. Additional hypothalamic degenerative lesions might explain concurrent GH deficiency. Circulating antibodies against AVP neurons were demonstrated in 18 of 47 patients with AVP deficiency of unknown cause, suggesting an autoimmune aetiology. Of these patients, 13 had other organ-specific antibodies [124].

Familial AVP deficiency is rare. An autosomal dominant trait was described in several families [123]. Severity varies even within families. Age at onset varies from birth to adolescence, often with gradual progression from partial to severe over childhood and adolescence, sometimes with amelioration in the third and fifth decades. Some patients have no detectable circulating AVP. This DI is associated with loss of neurons in the SON and PVN [125]. A single base substitution in the coding region for neurophysin II (NPII) was reported in two patients [126]. A large family was reported in which autosomal dominant DI of variable age of onset and severity appeared to be caused by an osmoreceptor defect [127]. Another study suggested a primary defect in the gene encoding AVP-NPII [123]. This implies that the hypothalamic lesion is secondary. An even more rare X-linked form may exist [128].

DI, diabetes mellitus, optic atrophy and deafness (DIDMOAD, Wolfram syndrome) [129,130], an autosomal recessive neurodegenerative disorder, has been reported in more than 100 cases.

HYPODIPSIA–HYPERNATRAEMIA

Failure of thirst occurs, in most cases associated also with AVP deficiency, in a spectrum of conditions with a large lesion in the anterior hypothalamus, the area of osmoreceptors for thirst and regulation of AVP secretion. Possible aetiologies include all those given above for central DI. Septo-optic dysplasia with absence of the septum pellucidum, Langerhans cell histiocytosis, germinoma and, in infants, haemorrhage and thrombosis are the most common causes [131–135]. In some patients adipsia develops after years of DI, with growth of the hypothalamic lesion [136]. In childhood, less than 50 cases seem to have been reported.

PRIMARY POLYDIPSIA

Primary polydipsia has different causes. Psychogenic polydipsia is very rare in children, but may occur at any age [137,138]. Another possibility is habituation to excessive drinking. Dipsogenic DI, also called compulsive water drinking [42,139–141] was found in 15 patients and suspected in seven others in a series of 129 consecutive adult patients referred for polydipsia and polyuria [140]. Of 11 children investigated for polydipsia and polyuria, nine were compulsive water drinkers aged 2.2–11 years [21]. In some patients the aetiology was identified as occult hydrocephalus [142], aplasia of the corpus callosum [143], germinoma, histiocytosis, tuberculous meningitis, sarcoidosis or multiple sclerosis [140,141,144]. K^+ depletion, hypercalcaemia and hyperreninaemia are possible causes. The condition has been produced experimentally [145].

RENAL DIABETES INSIPIDUS

Resistance of the kidneys to the antidiuretic effect of AVP may be caused by specific genetic defects of the cells of the collecting ducts, or be secondary to acquired renal or systemic disorders. The prerequisites for the AVP effect are normal function of the mechanism opening the membrane of the collecting ducts to osmotic water movement and maintenance of an adequate medullary interstitial hyperosmolality. A defect in either will cause DI.

Primary renal DI is rare. In most families it is transmitted as an X-linked trait with variable penetrance. It is variably expressed in heterozygous females over the full range from clinical disease to a mild defect of renal concentration [146]. This variation was explained by the non-random nature of inactivation of one of the two X chromosomes [147]. Families with apparent autosomal dominant transmission have also been reported [148]. So far 13 distinct mutations of the V_2 receptor have been discovered in affected families.

The primary functional defect is believed to be in the intracellular accumulation of cAMP in distal tubules [149,150]. This has been difficult to prove because AVP has no marked effect on urinary cAMP excretion in healthy persons. When six healthy children were given a clearly antidiuretic dose of AVP, urinary cAMP increased inconstantly, by a mean of 25%. In patients with renal DI observations varied from subnormal [149,150] to supranormal [151,152] mean basal rates of urinary cAMP excretion, and from absent to significant mean increments after administration of AVP. There is much evidence for heterogeneity of the disease.

Male-to-male transmission does occur [26,152], and many females have been reported with complete congenital renal DI [26,152,153]. Some patients respond with antidiuresis to cAMP administered by an i.v. infusion [154], but others do not [155–156]. Some patients fail with all responses mediated by the V_2 receptor [9,26,157] while others seem to have an isolated absence of the antidiuretic response [26,153,158,159]. Thus, mutations appear to exist both in the V_2 receptor and in the components distal of cAMP generation.

Secondary renal DI may be caused by a variety of conditions which damage the countercurrent multiplication system or the osmotic water movement (see Table 32.4). Renal DI secondary to maternal lithium therapy occurs in newborn infants [58].

Clinical manifestations

INFANTILE DIABETES INSIPIDUS

In newborns and infants the clinical picture is very different from that of older patients, and difficult to recognize. Yet the disease should be diagnosed early because inability to express a desire of water entails grave risk of brain damage.

Congenital DI is often heralded by hydramnios, intrauterine polyuria. Polyuria is rarely observed. The most common entity is X-linked nephrogenic DI, and severely affected infants are generally male. Newborn and premature infants with DI secondary to perinatal hypothalamic lesions may be severely ill. If insufficient amounts of water are offered, the infant will show excessive weight loss with irritability, fever and hypernatraemia. Even in the absence of polyuria, urine remains dilute, often <150 mosmol/kg. Only with severe dehydration may urine osmolality exceed plasma osmolality. Secondary DI may subside in weeks or months [160].

DI often becomes symptomatic only after the end of exclusive breast-feeding. Some infants suck eagerly but frequently vomit unless prefed with water, which they may clearly prefer. The mother may clearly relieve the condition by forming a habit of starting meals with water. Severely affected infants have a poor appetite after being weaned from the breast, with decreased rates of gain in weight and length. They are irritable, may cry incessantly and have intermittent or prolonged unexplained fever. These are consequences of chronic hypertonic dehydration with acute exacerbations. The infant may succumb with coma and convulsions. Body temperature may vary with weight, depending upon the amount of water given [161]. Giving liberal amounts will cause polyuria, but this tends to be overlooked, and the chief complaint is usually failure to thrive, anorexia, vomiting, fever or developmental retardation. By the time of the diagnosis the infant is usually severely malnourished, with dry and doughy skin, constipation, and absence of tears and perspiration. When the causal factor is an organic brain lesion, the picture may be complicated by neurological signs and features of anterior pituitary failure.

DIABETES INSIPIDUS AFTER INFANCY

In hypothalamic DI, polydipsia and polyuria typically develop suddenly. Rarely, the onset is insidious and the severity varies. In severe DI the need for water may be 300–400 ml/kg daily. As a rule the patients prefer water to other fluids. They may have to get up to drink and urinate several times each night. Some children will tolerate this easily, but others may become irritable and tired. Enuresis may appear. Provided the thirst mechanism is normal, the child is usually able to compensate fully for urinary loss by drinking. The urge to drink is so strong that he or she drinks whatever water is available. However, weight and serum Na^+ concentration may show large fluctuations.

Food consumption may decrease, because this reduces the need of water but this may retard growth in the absence of any other hormonal deficiency. Associated anterior pituitary insufficiency is common [82] and retarded growth may be present for several years before the appearance of DI. However, there are cases in which DI may be the sole manifestation of a germinoma or an optic nerve glioma for more than 20 years [162,163]. ACTH deficiency may conceal DI and cortisol replacement may reveal it.

DI after hypothalamic surgery appears usually within 24 h. When surgery has been confined to the pituitary fossa, DI usually resolves gradually over 2–5 days. A triple response sometimes occurs: initial DI followed after 4–8 days by a transient remission or even excessive release of AVP lasting 1–14 days, and then a recurrence of DI, often permanent.

In DIDMOAD the first disorder to appear is usually diabetes mellitus, diagnosed in two-thirds of the cases between the ages of 2 and 10 years. Overt hypothalamic central DI seems to develop in only about one-third of patients, commonly in the second decade of life, although it may be the presenting symptom. Optic atrophy is a constant, serious and untreatable component. It appears in half the patients during the first decade of life and in most of the others during the second decade. It is primary, bilateral and usually progressive, often leading to blindness in adult life. Most patients have bilateral high-tone nerve deafness, but this is rarely of clinical significance.

FEATURES DUE TO HYPOTHALAMIC DISEASE

Neurological manifestations commonly dominate the picture, with headache, vomiting and limitation of visual fields, which may cause walking into objects. Anterior pituitary deficiency is commonly associated with DI when this is caused by a hypothalamic lesion. Of patients with DI secondary to hypothalamic or pituitary tumours 80% had GH deficiency and 30% some additional anterior pituitary hormone deficiency. One of three patients with idiopathic DI had GH deficiency [82].

HYPODIPSIA–HYPERNATRAEMIA

Infants with this condition are likely to share the clinical picture of chronic dehydration described above for infantile DI. In contrast, these patients have no desire to drink. Hence, older patients also have chronic hypertonic dehydration, though this may not be immediately obvious. Polyuria is absent despite associated AVP deficiency. In most patients urine is dilute relative to plasma hypertonicity. Other manifestations of hypothalamic abnormalities are common, such as hyperphagia, obesity, temperature dysregulation and defects of anterior pituitary function, including abnormally short stature. Mental retardation and neuromuscular disorders are frequent; these may regress when hypernatraemia is corrected. Hypertonic dehydration may cause drowsiness, hypothermia, weakness, confusion, convulsions, unsteadiness of movements, chorea, paralysis with or without rhabdomyolysis, azotaemia, hypokalaemia, orthostatic hypotension and abnormal cutaneous circulation mimicking acrodynia [164]. One boy had central sleep apnoea and severe bradycardia associated with episodic muscle weakness, somnolence and hypothermia [165]. The manifestations may be periodic. In some cases the condition is amazingly well tolerated, and the chronic hypernatraemia is discovered incidentally during an intercurrent illness [131–135].

PRIMARY POLYDIPSIA

Polydipsia and polyuria in patients with primary polydipsia are clinically no different from these manifestations in patients with DI, except that the psychogenic symptom usually begins gradually. Primary polydipsia may appear at any age. Patients with psychogenic polydipsia may not wake up from sleep to drink. Habituation to drinking has occurred in early infancy [138]. Two infants aged 1–2 months have been reported with what appeared to be primary polydipsia. The presenting complaint was failure to thrive and irritability [144].

In psychogenic polydipsia patients may be clearly psychotic, or have other serious mental disorder. They may have bizarre compulsive motives for drinking, such as cleansing the body.

FEATURES SPECIFIC FOR RENAL DIABETES INSIPIDUS

Of 32 patients [152], 87% had the first signs observed during the first 3 months of life. The signs included fever in 69%, anorexia, vomiting and constipation in 45% and growth retardation in 67%. However, of 21 well-documented cases, excessive thirst was observed during the first month in only five, over the rest of the first year in seven, and in three not until the third year. Adequate autoregulation of water intake was frequently not acquired until ages 3–5 years. Severe acute dehydration episodes occurred in 70%; in 18 during the first year, in three during the second year, and in one during the third year. The episodes induced subdural haematoma or intraventricular haemorrhage in four patients. Four died, three from cerebral bleeding. Three surviving patients had mental retardation. True mortality and prevalence of mental retardation are higher, because many patients remain undiagnosed. Transient mental retardation was observed during the first year in seven patients which regressed over the next 2 years with correct hydration. Complete growth arrest or severe delay occurred in most of the 32 patients during the first 2–4 years of life [152].

Early in childhood the polyuria may cause asymptomatic dilation of the bladder and ureters. The radiological picture may be similar to that of chronic bladder outlet obstruction. In very severe cases irreversible fibrosis of the bladder wall has been documented, with loss of muscle tone and structure [166].

Less severely affected female patients with the X-linked disease often experience a clear increase in polydipsia and polyuria during pregnancy. Variable degrees of polydipsia and polyuia are the only manifestations of secondary renal DI when this develops after infancy.

Pathophysiology

Neither AVP deficiency nor renal resistance to AVP need be complete for frank DI to occur. Whether polydipsia and polyuria develop depends on the patient's maximum achievable urinary osmolality below the threshold plasma osmolality for thirst, and the amount of solute to be excreted (renal solute load). On average, on an adult-type diet, DI will appear when that urine osmolality falls below 300–400 mosmol/kg (see Fig. 32.10). If the kidneys are normal, polyuria begins only when the plasma AVP level achieved at the osmolar threshold for thirst falls below 1.5 pg/ml (see Fig. 32.6). This level requires 20–25% of normal secretory capacity.

In hypothalamic and dipsogenic DI the maximum renal concentrating capacity is reduced proportionally to the severity of polyuria, due to washout of the medullary hyperosmolality by the persistent water diuresis. Hence, the urinary concentration achievable by maximal plasma AVP levels is subnormal in all three types of DI. However, at submaximal AVP levels, urine osmolality is supranormal in hypothalamic DI (see Fig. 32.6), presumably due to upward regulation of V_2 receptors by chronic AVP deficiency [167].

INFANTILE DIABETES INSIPIDUS

Infants with (especially severe renal) DI unable to obtain extra water run a great risk of entering negative water balance. They may keep losing water and develop progressive hypertonic dehydration. Osmolality is equalized by the movement of some water out from the cells, which shrink. Shrinkage of the brain involves a risk of intracranial haemorrhage and death. A patient may enter a vicious cycle of dehydration, in which vomiting decreases water intake while concomitant hyperthermia increases the extrarenal losses.

With progressive hypovolaemia, glomerular filtration rate and hence tubular flow decrease, allowing time for osmotic retrieval of water by the hyperosmolar papillary interstitium despite absence of the AVP effect. This results in a rise of urine osmolality, potentially even to levels above plasma osmolality. A new precarious steady state may ensue.

Patients fed exclusively at breast are at less risk than others. Their average renal solute load is 12 mosmol/420 kJ (100 kcal). An infant of 4.0 kg with a daily energy expenditure of 2016 kJ (480 kcal) covered by an intake of 716 ml of breast milk (2814 kJ or 670 kcal/l), without additional water intake and with an evaporative water loss of 216 ml (45 ml/100 kcal), is expected to excrete daily $12 \times 2016/420 = 57$ mosmol in a volume of $716 - 216 = 500$ ml. This requires a mean osmolality of about 114 mosmol/kg. Maintaining such an average urinary concentration may require some degree of dehydration and reduction of glomerular filtration. The risk increases with addition of formula with higher solute loads [168] and solid foods to the diet. Anything that increases extrarenal water loss (diarrhoea, febrile illness, high ambient temperature) may result in a period of severe hyperosmolar dehydration.

Inadequate nutrition is a common consequence due to vomiting and poor appetite. The necessity to ingest large volumes of water adds to the problem and, probably, the fact that less food means less thirst.

HYPOTHALAMIC DIABETES INSIPIDUS

Various disorders have been observed in AVP release; the defect may be in secretory capacity or osmoreceptor function. In either case, AVP secretion mostly behaves as though the sensitivity of the osmoreceptor mechanism were markedly reduced [34]. Plasma AVP concentration is low but detectable, and increases to effective levels with dehydration. However, the increase is invariably subnormal relative to the degree of hyperosmolality produced. A significant positive correlation appears between plasma osmolality and AVP concentration, but the slope of the regression is less than one-tenth of the normal mean value. The degree of spontaneous hyperosmolality depends on the integrity and effectiveness of thirst sensation and availability of water.

If thirst is impaired, severe hyperosmolality may be necessary to stimulate AVP secretion sufficiently to bring water excretion into balance with intake. The urine may then be of normal maximal osmolality. The volume of urine excreted thus depends as much on the sensitivity of the thirst mechanism as on the ability to secrete AVP. Some patients have virtually no trace of releasable AVP.

On the first day after acute damage to the hypothalamopituitary tract inactive precursors of AVP may be released and block the receptors, thus inhibiting the action of AVP and causing a temporary aggravation of the DI [169,170].

HYPODIPSIA–HYPERNATRAEMIA

Patients with hypodipsia–hypernatraemia are a heterogeneous group with failure of the thirst mechanism to provide adequate water intake to balance normal extrarenal and obligatory renal losses. They will develop a more or less steady state, because with progressive dehydration both renal and extrarenal water losses will decrease, until the losses are in balance with the intake. Release of AVP may play a role in this steady state. Some patients have normal osmoregulation of AVP [171]; others have shown one of two types of disorder [31,172]. In the majority, the slope of the osmoregulation is markedly reduced. At high plasma osmolality such patients secrete enough AVP to form urine hyperosmolar to plasma, but resist an attempt to normalize plasma osmolality by increasing water intake by full dilution of urine already at supranormal osmolality levels. In a number of such patients examined, hypertonicity could not be corrected by maintaining large water intake. Thus, their hypertonicity may not be explained solely by inadequate water intake. Other patients seem to maintain a steady secretion of AVP unmodified by even large changes of plasma osmolality. Since full dilution of urine fails, they are unprotected against water overload as well as water deficiency. Some patients have had no detectable AVP in plasma [131]. One patient had a third type of osmoregulation disorder: elevation of osmolar threshold for AVP secretion to 320 mosmol/kg with normal slope, and elevation of osmolar threshold for thirst to 332 mosmol/kg [173]. Increased renal sensitivity to AVP may be important in the pathophysiology [135,172]. In some patients plasma AVP fluctuates at random and is not suppressed in a hypoosmolar state [174]; their AVP reserves may be normal but, lacking the ability either to stimulate thirst or suppress AVP, they have no protection against changes in water balance in either direction, and exhibit wide swings in serum Na^+ concentration from 120 to 170 mmol/l. They may react to non-osmotic stimuli (for example a fall in blood pressure and nausea) with brisk rises in plasma AVP 2 [28,131], which may mediate the fluctuation of plasma osmolality and full concentration of urine during dehydration.

Some patients appear to have total destruction of both the AVP-producing neurons and the osmoreceptor neurons.

PRIMARY POLYDIPSIA

In both forms of primary polydipsia plasma osmolality and Na^+ levels are usually in the low-normal range but may be around the upper limit of normal range, with low plasma

AVP. Dilution of body fluids suppresses AVP secretion and causes water diuresis. This balances the excessive intake, and stabilizes body fluid osmolality to a new, slightly lower, level. Antidiuretic therapy may be dangerous: thirst and water intake decrease less rapidly than water excretion, resulting in dilutional hypotonicity. Patients can concentrate urine with water deprivation, although full concentration may be delayed 1–4 days, during which time the renal medullary hyperosmolality is restored.

In psychogenic polydipsia AVP secretion may be abnormal, even syndrome of inappropriate antidiuretic hormone (SIADH) has been reported [175,176].

In dipsogenic DI or compulsive water drinking [42,140] the threshold for thirst is subnormal and lower than the threshold for AVP secretion. Non-osmotic inhibition of thirst by drinking is also subnormal [42], and an underlying defect of a central integrating centre for thirst has been proposed [42,177]. With desmopressin therapy the excessive drinking may be stopped, but only by bringing body fluid tonicity to intolerably low levels.

ASPECTS OF RENAL DIABETES INSIPIDUS

The range of severity of the renal disease of different aetiologies is wide. In the severe genetic forms the high plasma AVP levels may worsen the polyuria, because its diuretic action (mediated by the V_1 receptors and prostaglandins) is intact, while the V_2-mediated antidiuretic effect fails.

Diagnosis of defects of arginine vasopressin and thirst functions

Six different situations call for evaluation of the integrity of AVP and/or thirst functions with an appropriate strategy:

1 polyuria with polydipsia (AVP function);
2 hypernatraemia (AVP and thirst functions);
3 hypothalamopituitary dysfunction (AVP secretion and thirst);
4 renal pathology (responsiveness to AVP);
5 acute brain trauma or surgery (AVP secretion);
6 inherited DI in the family.

An analysis of growth and development is always essential; impaired growth suggests associated GH deficiency or inadequate nutrition secondary to DI. Deficiencies of ACTH and thyroid-stimulating hormone (TSH) have to be adequately replaced before evaluation of AVP secretion.

Evaluation of AVP and thirst functions is based on measurements of plasma and urine osmolality and urine volume; hyperosmolality and desmopressin tests may be needed. Urine osmolality normally shows a defined relationship with plasma osmolality and must always be assessed in relation to plasma osmolality [178,179] (see Fig. 32.5). AVP deficiency may otherwise be missed, because hyperosmolality may cause release of sufficient AVP to produce a seemingly normal response in urinary concentration. The relationship is mediated by plasma AVP, and in most cases measurements of AVP do not add much to the information obtained by osmolality measurements. Renal DI is an exception: it can be clearly differentiated from AVP deficiency by normal or even supranormal plasma AVP for plasma osmolality (see Fig. 32.6). Also, well-standardized measurements of plasma AVP over a range of plasma osmolality could be decisive for differentiation between incomplete hypothalamic DI, incomplete renal DI and primary polydipsia in some patients [180,181]. Osmolality should be measured from lithium-heparin plasma and not from serum or EDTA (ethylenediamine tetra-acetic acid) plasma; the samples should be obtained without stasis and should not be frozen. If the accuracy of the plasma osmolality measurement is poorer than 1%, Na^+ measurement should be substituted for it because of generally higher accuracy. The workup includes determinations of serum creatinine or urea, Na^+, K^+, calcium and blood glucose.

POLYURIA WITH POLYDIPSIA

Taking a careful history is mandatory: occurrence of similar cases in the family, presence of polyhydramnios at birth (prenatal DI), mode of onset and constancy of the symptoms, including drinking at night (sudden onset with constancy and drinking at night in DI; often slow onset and variation in primary polydipsia), brain trauma or infection, headache, nausea, vomiting, visual disturbances evidenced in young children by walking into objects (hypothalamic tumour), and long-standing infection and drainage of ears and/or skin lesions (histiocytosis). Osmotic diuresis must be excluded by testing for glycosuria, confirming that no large amounts of solute have been given (mannitol, glycerol, urea, electrolyte) and demonstrating low urine osmolality (< 200 mosmol/kg).

Low-normal plasma osmolality suggests primary polydipsia, while high-normal osmolality is common in DI, especially in the morning. In patients with repeatedly elevated plasma osmolality (> 295 mosmol/kg, Na^+ > 143 mmol/l) with subnormal urine osmolality for the plasma osmolality (see Fig. 32.5), the diagnosis of DI is certain and no hyperosmolality test should be performed for clinical purposes; such testing cannot give any clinically relevant further information and could be harmful. Other patients require a test in which such slight hyperosmolality is provoked to stimulate AVP release, and simultaneous measurements are obtained of plasma and urine osmolality, and perhaps plasma AVP. Normal or supranormal plasma AVP levels for plasma osmolality distinguish AVP resistance from AVP deficiency. If AVP determination is not available a desmopressin test is performed in the hyperosmolar state.

The type of osmoregulatory disorder can be determined by obtaining simultaneous determination of plasma osmolality and AVP in a wide range of plasma osmolality during the hypertonic saline infusion test [180,181]. Such typing has no clinical importance.

HYPEROSMOLALITY TESTS

Besides diagnosing or excluding defects in AVP and thirst functions the goal of hyperosmolality testing may be quantifying the defects to allow observing a change with time. Two test modalities are available: dehydration (water deprivation) and infusion of hyperosmolar NaCl solution. For diagnosing or excluding AVP deficiency, dehydration is the common choice; an osmoregulatory disorder of AVP secretion and thirst may be typed by hyperosmolar saline infusion test.

Dehydration testing should be individualized because its goal is to raise plasma osmolality to >295 mosmol/kg; this will be reached after a period of water deprivation which varies individually from 4 to 24 h. This depends both on the basal level of plasma osmolality and the severity of defect in AVP function. A period which is necessary for some patients is dangerous for others. The simplest approach to testing an individual patient is observing the basal plasma osmolality and calculating the decrement of weight necessary for reaching the level of >295 mosmol/kg. In frankly polyuric patients a 3–4-h period of water deprivation will suffice.

If an accurate assay of plasma AVP is available, the saline infusion test may be preferable as a shorter, more informative and, with modern vein cannulation technique, even less unpleasant alternative. It allows quantitative assessment of thirst in co-operative patients by recording thirst intensity on a visual analogue scale [41,42,182].

In some dehydration protocols, water is withheld until urine osmolality plateaus [183]. Whether this plateau provides for better test precision is unknown; reproducibility seems not to have been studied for any protocol.

Importance has been given to differentiation of a 'complete' from a partial defect, with 'complete' meaning that the patient is unable to produce urine with an osmolality exceeding plasma osmolality [184]. This definition is questionable, because an AVP effect is necessary even for bringing urine osmolality from, say, 100 to 200 mosmol/kg. 'Severe' is preferable to 'complete'.

The test must not cause a potentially deleterious increment (>20 mosmol/kg) in body fluid osmolality [185]; therefore accurate weight monitoring is crucial, and weight loss must not exceed 4.6%, 4.3%, 4.0% and 3.5% for infants, children, and adult men and women, respectively.

HYPERNATRAEMIA

The commonest cause of hypernatraemia in paediatric patients is loss of water in excess of Na^+ through diarrhoea and vomiting, osmotic diuresis and, especially in preterm infants, evaporation [92]. Such a state is recognized by the history, and from weight loss and other evidence of dehydration. If the cause is extrarenal the urine is concentrated, but the concentration of Na^+ is <10 mmol/l.

Chronic hypernatraemia in children (Table 32.5) is rarely associated with excess body Na^+. In such cases there is evidence of volume expansion rather than contraction. The cause could be excessive Na^+ intake, which is suggested by high urinary excretion of Na^+. Deliberate salt administration by disturbed parents does occur. Hypermineralocorticoidism is very rare. More common is water deficiency due to insufficient intake. When that is suspected, thirst and AVP functions need to be evaluated. Hypovolaemia and nausea may cause misleadingly high values of plasma AVP and urine osmolality in disorders of osmoregulation. Therefore, simultaneous levels of plasma and urine osmolality and plasma AVP should be evaluated only after restoration of normovolaemia. Evaluation of thirst function also requires normal consciousness.

In a young infant the main differentation is between congenital DI and failure of thirst (with or without abnormal osmoregulation of AVP secretion). The common clues to DI are a similar history of a sibling (usually brother) or other (particularly maternal male) relatives, polydipsia and polyuria of the mother, often with clear aggravation during pregnancy, and polyhydramnios. If a boy is born following polyhydramnios in pregnancy and there is evidence for X-linked inheritance, the diagnosis of DI is very likely. A female infant may also have this disease in a milder form. A history of severe perinatal asphyxia, intraventricular haemorrhage, or serious infection suggests AVP deficiency due to a perinatal hypothalamic lesion. Urine and plasma osmolality and, when possible, determination of plasma AVP should be obtained

Table 32.5 Causes of chronic hypernatraemia

Causes
Water deficiency
Deficient intake
Loss of thirst (adipsia or hypodipsia)
Inability to acquire water (young infant, coma, paresis)
Excessive loss
Renal (hypothalamic or renal DI)
Extrarenal (evaporation, diarrhoea, surgical)
Na^+ excess
Excessive intake
Excessive retention (hypermineralocorticoidism)

without delay. Low urine osmolality for plasma osmolality proves the presence of DI. Normal urine osmolality for plasma osmolality excludes renal DI but not a disorder of osmoregulation. Plasma AVP plotted against plasma osmolality (see Fig. 32.6) and/or a brisk response to desmopressin differentiate between renal DI and AVP deficiency. If the infant drinks water willingly in the hyperosmolar state the thirst function is probably normal, even though drinking may not suffice to maintain normo-osmolality.

Newborn infants who are very ill with perinatal asphyxia, intraventricular haemorrhage or severe infection, and have excessive weight loss with hyperosmolality and inappropriately dilute urine [39], should be placed on therapy for AVP deficiency until shown to be no more in need of it.

In the case of an older child with hyperosmolality, assessment of urine osmolality against plasma osmolality (see Fig. 32.5) during normovolaemia should establish or exclude the diagnosis of DI. Inability to maintain normal osmolality by drinking during free availability of water indicates failure of thirst function.

The type of abnormal osmoregulation of AVP secretion associated with adipsia may be identified by measurements of plasma osmolality and AVP at different levels of osmolality during water loading and hyperosmolar saline infusion.

HYPOTHALAMOPITUITARY DYSFUNCTION

When a hypothalamic lesion and/or anterior pituitary deficiency has been established, the question is often relevant whether the hypothalamoneurohypophyseal function is also involved. A partial deficiency of AVP and/or thirst functions is possible even in the absence of any observed change in urination and drinking behaviour. The question is answered by determination of basal plasma osmolality and a hyperosmolality test. This evaluation may need to be repeated, for example at 6-monthly intervals.

SEARCH FOR A HYPOTHALAMIC LESION

In hypothalamic DI, hypodipsia–hypernatraemia and dipsogenic DI a pattern of aetiological investigations is mandatory. Careful physical examination, assessment of visual fields, and chest and skeletal radiographs may give a diagnostic clue, especially in Langerhans cell histiocytosis, which may be confirmed by histological examination of a lesion. If possible, nuclear MRI of the hypothalamic area should be done. The evaluation should include assays of plasma and cerebrospinal fluid (CSF), β-human chorionic gonadotrophin (β-hCG), α-fetoprotein [186–188] and placental alkaline phosphatase [189] and a search for germinoma cells in the CSF. β-hCG has been positive even in 14 of 26 patients and α-fetoprotein in six of 22 with hypothalamic germinoma [188]. Anterior pituitary function should also be evaluated, starting with the secretion of GH. Patients with ACTH deficiency may have a masked polyuria, and may need evaluation for the possibility of associated DI after 3 days of cortisol replacement therapy.

If no aetiology, or only a thickening of the pituitary stalk, is found by comprehensive investigation, the studies, including nuclear MRI, should be repeated at 6–12-monthly intervals for at least 4 years [82], and then less frequently [163].

Nuclear MRI is the superior technique for imaging hypothalamic structures (Fig. 32.11). In T_1-weighted images normal posterior pituitary gland gives a high-intensity signal, which is probably due to the neurosecretory granules [102,189,190]. Anatomy of the pituitary stalk can be assessed, including its rupture [191] and thickening [192,193]. After stalk transection an ectopic posterior pituitary commonly develops at the stump of the stalk [101,102]. Absence of the high-intensity signal (see Fig. 32.11) usually indicates a hypothalamoneurohypophyseal lesion, but was also observed in three of four patients with renal DI, probably because of depletion of neurosecretory granules due to chronic mild dehydration [194]. Presence of the signal does not necessarily indicate functional integrity. It may be present or absent in the autosomal dominant AVP deficiency, the finding varying even within a sibship [195]. In patients with primary polydipsia and those with osmoreceptor dysfunction, normal structures have been observed [196].

Langerhans cell histiocytosis has a predilection for the hypothalamic nuclei; the infiltrates appear as high signal foci in T_2-weighted MRI [197]. Another early sign is thickening of the stalk, uniformly or only at the level of the median eminence and hypothalamus [192,193]. An isolated thickening of the stalk at acute onset of DI suggests an oligosymptomatic phase of histiocytosis [193].

In hypothalamoneurohypophyseal germinomas MRI is also the key to early diagnosis [198]. The primary site is probably the posterior pituitary gland; absence of the posterior pituitary high-intensity signal, homogeneous hypointensity to the pons on T_1-weighted images and isointensity of T_2-weighted images are the characteristics distinguishing germinoma from pituitary adenomas [199]. In some patients the only abnormality, which may be visible only by nuclear MRI, is an enlargement of the pituitary stalk (Fig. 32.11), which may be caused by histiocytic infiltration or a small germinoma.

RENAL PATHOLOGY

In patients with known renal pathology or another reason for questioning the integrity of the renal reponse to AVP,

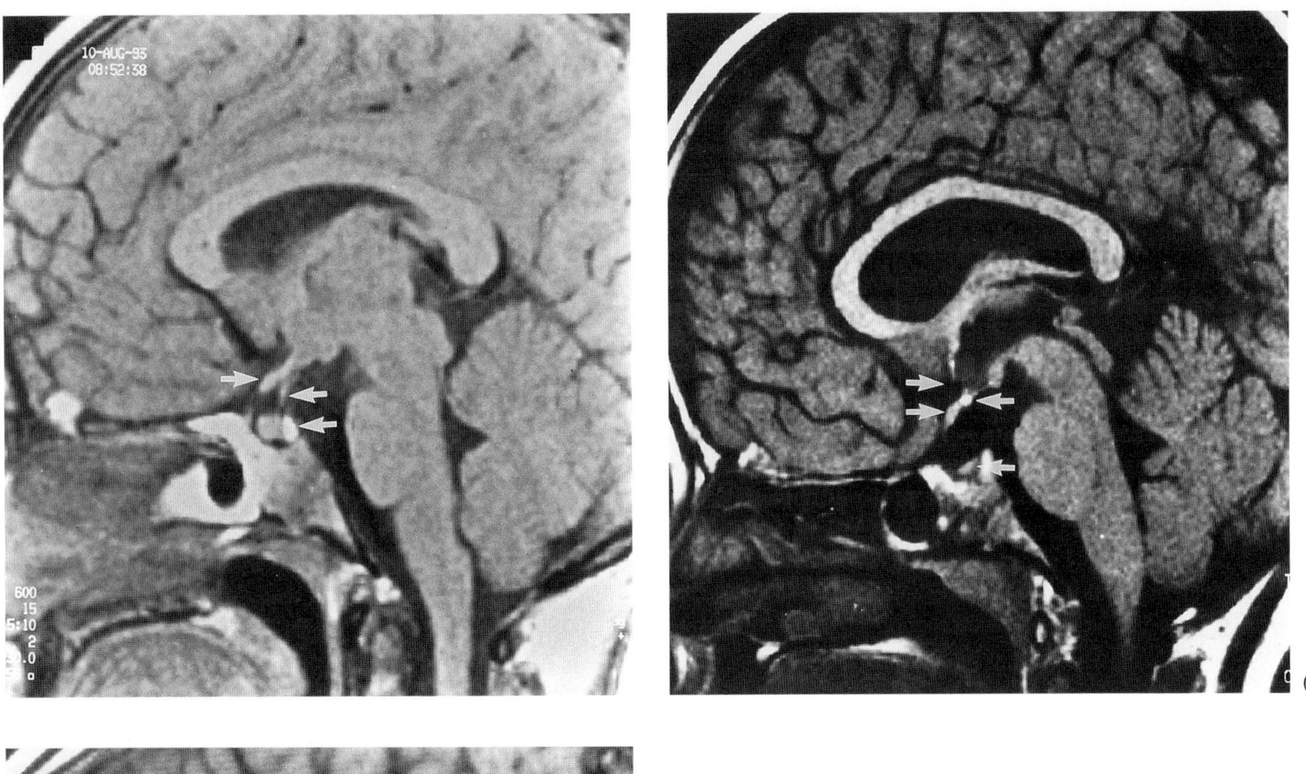

(a) (b)

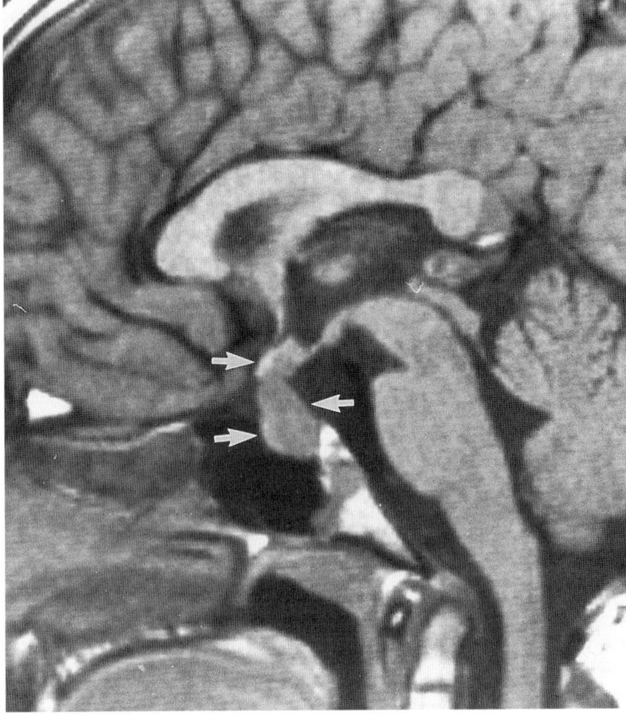

(c)

Fig. 32.11 Nuclear magnetic resonance images (T_1-weighted midsagittal sections) of the hypothalamopituitary area of three children (courtesy of Dr Leena Valanne. Children's Hospital, University of Helsinki). (a) Normal anatomy in a 10-year-old girl: the posterior pituitary gives a hyperintense signal (right lower arrow), which clearly separates the anterior pituitary from the dorsum of the sella turcica. The sphenoid bone also gives a hypersignal due to the fat content of the spongious bone, and so does fat elsewhere. The pituitary stalk (right upper arrow) is thin (< 2.8 mm). It is located immediately behind the optic chiasm (left arrow). (b) A 9-year-old girl who was a small premature baby of 1290 g and suffered from subependymal haemorrhage. She failed to grow normally and was early diagnosed having deficiency of GH, ACTH and TSH, but has normal water regulation. She lacks a septum pellucidum. The pituitary stalk is interrupted (left upper arrow) above the optic chiasm (left lower arrow), and the sella turcica is smaller than normal with a subnormal mass of anterior pituitary tissue (right lower arrow). No hyperintense signal of the posterior pituitary is visible in the sella; an ectopic posterior pituitary (right upper arrow) is located at the tip of the infundibulum. (c) A 10-year-old girl with hypothalamic germinoma. The pituitary stalk (right arrow) is clearly abnormally thick due to the tumour mass, and reaches the optic chiasm (left upper arrow). The bony wall of the sella turcica is barely visible (left lower arrow), and the anterior pituitary, due to the tumour mass, appears larger than normal. No hyperintense signal of the posterior pituitary is visible.

the answer is obtained by measurement of plasma osmolality and by a short desmopressin test. This test will also identify female carriers of the X chromosomal gene of renal DI.

ACUTE BRAIN TRAUMA OR SURGERY

In patients with normal consciousness and thirst sensation development of DI will manifest as polydipsia and polyuria. In patients with disturbed consciousness or question of normality of thirst function, urine flow and urine and plasma osmolality must be monitored. Plotting urine osmolality is particularly useful in this situation (see Fig. 32.5) provided that osmotic diuresis is excluded. Dilute urine for plasma hyperosmolality establishes the diagnosis of DI; differentation from polyuria due to overhydration is easy.

If AVP replacement is instituted, the dose should be reduced at appropriate intervals (weekly in the beginning) to find out whether urine again becomes dilute for plasma osmolality as an indication of persisting AVP deficiency.

INHERITED DIABETES INSIPIDUS IN THE FAMILY

In families with X-linked renal DI female carriers can be identified by a desmopressin test. During pregnancy of a carrier, sonography may be used to determine the sex of the fetus and demonstrate supranormal amniotic fluid volume indicating fetal polyuria [200]. The desmopressin test may be given to the newborn infant to exclude or confirm renal resistance to AVP.

In the offspring of a parent with dominantly inherited AVP deficiency, polyhydramnios may give prenatal indication of the disease; otherwise, the infant needs to be monitored for development of hypernatraemia. Usually, the disease manifests only after infancy as polydipsia and polyuria.

Prenatal diagnosis by analysis of fetal DNA may soon become available for both diseases.

Treatment

The foremost rule in the treatment of DI is that the patient must in all situations have access to as much water (free of solute that has to be excreted) as thirst dictates, or as is necessary to avoid a hyperosmolar state. To ensure this in exceptional circumstances, every patient should always carry a card, disc (Medic Alert) or locket (SoS) indicating the disease. DI is usually so disturbing to the well-being of a child that it should be controlled as far as possible [201]. Having to get up at night disturbs sleep, and may cause irritability and problems in social adjustment and school performance. Often, appetite is so greatly impaired as to retard growth. The polyuria itself may lead to the development of hydronephrosis [202].

HYPOTHALAMIC DIABETES INSIPIDUS

The goal of therapy is normal water balance allowing for normal social life without nocturia, and with normal daytime urine flow. None of this was satisfactorily achieved with preparations available before desmopressin. Chlorpropamide, carbamazepine and clofibrate do not belong to the modern therapy of paediatric patients with DI. Chlorpropamide is particularly hazardous because sooner or later it causes hypoglycaemia.

Desmopressin (see Table 32.1) [203], a synthetic analogue of AVP with prolonged antidiuretic and almost absent pressor activity, is a highly satisfactory drug for therapy of AVP deficiency. A buffered aqueous solution (desmopressin acetate 0.1 mg/ml) is available for nasal insufflation. Its onset of action is within 1 h (maximum plasma concentration after nasal or sublingual administration is obtained after 45–55 min, bioavailability via the nasal route is approximately 10%) and its duration is between 8 and 24 h; it is consistent from day to day in any given patient.

A dose of 5–20 μg administered twice daily is usually adequate, but some patients only use one and some others need three doses daily. Small premature infants have been treated with approximately 1 μg/kg daily, divided in two doses [159]. For such small amounts the nasal solution is diluted 1:10 with 0.9% NaCl solution. It is advisable to start with a low dose, for example 1 μg for infants and 2.5 μg for young children, at 12-hourly intervals, and gradually increase the dose until a satisfactory effect is achieved. During rhinitis, the requirement may increase slightly, even if the nose is very carefully cleaned. Desmopressin is usually given with a rhinyl catheter, an intranasal tube, which is filled with the appropriate dose. An easier to use metered-dose nasal spray pump has partly replaced the rhinyl delivery system.

Desmopressin is also available in preparations for parenteral and oral use. Bioavailability has been estimated at 3.4% after nasal and 0.1% after oral administration [204]. Of the 4 μg/ml solution intended for parenteral use, one-fifth to one-tenth of the nasal dose gives an equivalent effect. With the tablets to be swallowed a 10-fold [205] to 20-fold dose [4,206,207] is needed compared with the nasal dose. For newborn infants the nasal solution has been given orally in a dose of 10 times the nasal dose [208]. The nasal therapy is expensive, and the oral drug may be beyond financial limits. Oral administration is an alternative for periods of rhinitis, and for infants and disabled people.

Headaches, nasal congestion and abdominal discomfort are rare side-effects. Overdosage causes water retention with headaches and confusion. The patients should be checked at times for hyponatraemia, because some of them may tend to take an overdose to maintain low urine output. Furthermore, and especially during the early course of DI due to brain lesion, the replacement therapy of patients with normal consciousness should be regularly (in the beginning weekly) interrupted, or reduced to allow polyuria and thirst. This is to guard against hypo-osmolar expansion and to confirm the persistence of DI.

The patient, family and friends must know that during this replacement therapy the patient is unprotected against excess water. A drinking contest will cause water intoxication. If the patient is also on cortisol replacement the danger of hyponatraemia associated with interruption of cortisol therapy should similarly be known.

ACUTE POSTOPERATIVE OR POST-TRAUMATIC DIABETES INSIPIDUS

The weight of the patient should be monitored to guide the administration of water. Prophylactic physiological replacement of cortisol is usually indicated after hypothalamic surgery for 1–2 weeks or until intactness of ACTH secretion has been confirmed; otherwise, cortisol deficiency may cause water retention. Electrolyte balance is to be maintained according to normal rules. Once the diagnosis of DI has been confirmed, and only then, should AVP replacement therapy be initiated. Desmopressin solution (desmopressin acetate 0.004 mg/ml), given intravenously, intramuscularly or subcutaneously, is recommended [209]. The dose needs to be individualized in the range 0.5–2 $\mu g/m^2$; the effect may not be adequate on the first day because of blockade of the receptors by inactive precursors of AVP released from the hypothalamus [169, 170]. One dose usually provides antidiuresis for 12–24 h, and a new dose should be administered only when polyuria recurs. Continuous i.v. infusion of aqueous AVP has been recommended because of its shorter action [210,211].

HYPODIPSIA–HYPERNATRAEMIA

Therapy of patients with hypodipsia–hypernatraemia needs to be individually tailored. Its principle includes a relatively fixed forced intake of water and, in cases of AVP deficiency, appropriate replacement with desmopressin. The average requirement of water is 100 ml/420 kJ (100 kcal) energy turnover (100 ml/kg for kilograms 1–10, plus 50 ml/kg for kilograms 11–20, plus 20 ml/kg for each additional kilogram); the individual requirement has to be established by starting from the average dose and altering it until normo-osmolality is maintained. The intake has to be increased when there is unusually high water loss, for example during vigorous physical activity, perspiration, hot weather or fever. Monitoring of weight is essential; by adjusting water intake weight changes exceeding 3% should be avoided. Arrangements should be made for hospitalization of young children during intercurrent disease, especially infection.

In a study of two patients, 3 months therapy with desmopressin led to a reduction of supranormal renal sensitivity to AVP, development of sensation of thirst and improvement of aggressive behaviour [172]. In another patient, therapy with clomipramine led to normalization of natraemia and relief of other manifestations [165].

PRIMARY POLYDIPSIA

There is no therapy for dipsogenic DI. The therapy of psychogenic polydipsia belongs to psychiatry.

RENAL DIABETES INSIPIDUS

In the acute therapy of hypernatraemic dehydration the principles are correction of volume deficit with a physiological Na^+ solution over 6–12 h, while providing simultaneous replacement of ongoing urinary, evaporative and other possible losses of water, correction of K^+ deficit, and replacing enough of concurrent measured Na^+ and K^+ excretion so that the plasma Na^+ does not decrease by >10 mmol/24 h.

The goals of long-term therapy are prevention of hypertonic dehydration, avoidance of side-effects of therapy such as vascular pathology and gout, prevention of urinary tract disease, and providing adequate nutrition and normal growth. The elements of therapy are sufficient water intake, restriction of renal solute load [212] and therapy with diuretics and, possibly, with indomethacin and desmopressin. Mild forms of renal DI are usually easy to treat. In severe forms therapy remains problematic, especially in infancy. Daily intake of NaCl should be kept <0.7 mmol/kg. Minimum required amounts of high-quality protein should be given, and the diet should be restricted for K^+ and phosphate. Because of its low solute load and high quality of protein, human milk is preferable to even the best infant formulas, and exclusive breast-feeding should be recommended for 6 months [213]. Baby foods should be selected for low salt content. The adequacy of nutrition must be checked.

Carers should be advised about the amount of water needed to maintain normotonicity. To avoid bouts of severe dehydration infants may need nasogastric water infusion continuously for the first few months of life, and thereafter during the night until three or less drinks will provide adequate water intake during the night. This need may persist for 2–3 years. For infants it is advisable to add sugar in the water to increase caloric intake. Some young infants may need continuous i.v. infusion of glucose solution because they do not tolerate gastric infusion of sufficient volumes of water and adequate feeding without vomiting. Arrangements should be made for early admission to the hospital during diarrhoeal disease, vomiting, fever, etc., to avoid dangerous periods of negative water balance.

Additional drug therapy is necessary for infant boys with the X-linked disease, is probably advisable for older boys with this disease, and may be needed for others. Diuretics and indomethacin are generally effective. From the data available, neither drug alone is consistently superior to the other, and each may fail in an individual patient. The strongest effect seems to be obtained by combining the two drug modalities. Both drugs commonly reduce polyuria by roughly 50% and sometimes up to 75%. The main factor is a decrease in free water clearance [10,214–216]. The best therapy may be with the combination of diet, hydrochlorothiazide and indomethacin.

The best mode of diuretic therapy without indomethacin appears to be the combination of hydrochlorothiazide (1–3 mg/kg daily in two or three doses) and amiloride (0.2–0.7 mg/kg daily in two or three doses) [217,218]. Amiloride adds to the diuretic effect and prevents thiazide-induced K^+ depletion much better than do K^+ supplements. K^+ depletion must be avoided because it may further impair the DI. The mechanism of action of diuretic therapy [214,215,219] appears to be maintenance of slight depletion of extracellular Na^+ and volume with hyponatraemia and hypovolaemia, which stimulate the proximal tubular reabsorption of Na^+ and associated anions with an iso-osmolar amount of water, thus reducing the volume of water passing to the distal tubule, where its absorption depends on the AVP effect. Increased osmolality of the papillary interstitial fluid may contribute to the antidiuretic effect.

Diuretic therapy will be successful only when combined with restricted Na^+ intake. The dose should be adjusted to maintain slightly subnormal plasma Na^+ concentration, 133–137 mmol/l, and supranormal plasma renin level. However, it is unclear whether these measures guarantee success. Of five patients, abdominal pain and anorexia necessitated discontinuation of amiloride, in one after 6 months of therapy [218]. In another disease, associated with chronic dehydration, congenital chloride diarrhoea and arteriolar changes develop resembling those of hypertensive angiopathy [220]. The diuretic therapy of renal DI, because it is aimed at maintaining permanent dehydration, may similarly endanger arterioles.

The combination of diet, hydrochlorothiazide and K^+ supplementation is also often unsatisfactory. Of 31 patients, such therapy decreased urine flow in 21 by a mean of 38%; in 11 children the reduction was $<15\%$ [152]. It is not possible to eliminate K^+ depletion in all patients with K^+ supplements.

Indomethacin appears, like thiazides, to (i) enhance proximal reabsorption of solute, thus decreasing distal delivery of fluid; and (ii) decrease papillary blood flow, thus allowing greater papillary hyperosmolality. Indomethacin also reduces the absolute and fractional excretion of Na^+. The antidiuretic effects of indomethacin and thiazides are partly additive; 0.5–3 mg/kg daily of indomethacin in three doses is needed. The dosage should be built up gradually.

Both thiazides and indomethacin decrease the clearances of urate and urea, and elevate their blood levels [221]. Plasma urate levels may be highest during combined therapy with both drugs. Long-term consequences of mild permanent hyperuricaemia starting in childhood are unknown. In adults, only plasma urate levels remaining persistently greater than 0.76 mmol/l (13 mg/dl) are considered to call for antihyperuricaemic therapy [222]. Glomerular filtration is usually not affected by either drug.

No serious side-effects of indomethacin have been reported in patients with renal DI, though many patients have continued for several years on it [224]. Since experience is limited, and side-effects (thrombocytopenia, aplastic anaemia, agranulocytosis, retinopathy, renal failure) are not rare during other long-term usage of this drug, caution is needed. Hydrochlorothiazide–amiloride and hydrochlorothiazide–indomethacin were similar in antidiuretic efficacy in a study of five patients [218].

Though desmopressin is ineffective when given alone, remarkable increases have been reported in urinary osmolality upon addition of desmopressin to therapy with indomethacin [224] or indomethacin–hydrochlorothiazide [100].

Patients with hydronephrosis and vesicoureteral reflux may need appropriate therapy such as double voiding, and monitoring for urinary tract infection.

CLINICAL PROBLEMS

Wide fluctuations of plasma osmolality tend to occur particularly in newborn infants with DI caused by a cerebral insult [225] and in patients who have had a hypothalamic operation [226] or cranial trauma [227]. Presumably, such fluctuations are due to persisting reserves of AVP which may be released in an inappropriate fashion, the patient oscillating between deficiency and excess of the hormone. Hypothalamic trauma may be followed by a three-step sequence of transient DI, an interphase of excessive AVP secretion, and a second (often permanent) phase of DI. After cranial trauma, DI may ensue at any time.

Patients with the chronic hypodipsia–hypernatraemia syndrome may exhibit similar fluctuations when therapy is attempted [28,228].

A patient of ours with DI due to hypothalamic germinoma developed Na^+-losing nephropathy as a complication of therapy with cisplatin [229,230]. The combination of salt loss and DI is another difficult therapeutic situation.

The management of such situations should be based on careful monitoring of fluid balance. Weight and serum Na^+ and K^+ levels should be recorded twice to four times daily. All urine should be collected over 6–12-h periods and urine volume and amounts of Na^+ and K^+ recorded. Similarly, the input of water and electrolytes should be known. This allows double checking of the water and electrolyte balance. The amounts excreted plus estimated non-visible water loss should be replaced continuously, while appropriate substitution therapy for AVP deficiency is continued.

ARGININE VASOPRESSIN EXCESS OR SYNDROME OF INAPPROPRIATE ANTIDIURETIC HORMONE

The syndrome of inappropriate secretion [231] of antidiuretic hormone comprises aetiologically heterogeneous conditions fulfilling the following criteria: retention of water with hypo-osmolality, normal or slightly increased effective blood volume, less than maximally diluted urine, urinary Na^+ excretion in excess of Na^+ intake continuing until a new steady state is reached and absence of nausea. Failure of the kidneys, adrenals and thyroid need to be excluded. This definition delineates the syndrome requiring water restriction for therapy. Importantly, it has to be distinguished from similar states in which the effective blood volume is reduced.

Causes and frequency

The syndrome of inappropriate antidiuretic hormone occurs in various diseases (Table 32.6), most commonly of the brain or lungs, and during therapies with many different drugs (see Table 32.3). Malignomas secreting AVP or another antidiuretic substances (Ewing sarcoma, carcinomas of the duodenum and pancreas, oat cell carcinoma of the lung, lymphoma) are rare in children.

Table 32.6 Causes of SIADH and SIADH-like conditions

Central nervous system disorders
Meningitis (bacterial or viral), encephalitis, abscess, trauma, hypoxic–ischaemic insult, tumour, Guillain–Barré syndrome, ventriculoatrial shunt obstruction, acute intermittent porphyria, sinus thrombosis, haemorrhage (intracerebral, subarachnoidal)
Respiratory tract disease
Pneumonia (bacterial or viral), cavitation (aspergillosis), tuberculosis, (?)respiratory infection
Decreased left atrial filling
Positive pressure ventilation, pneumothorax, atelectasis, asthma, cystic fibrosis, mitral valve commissurotomy, ductus arteriosus ligation
Drugs (see Table 32.3)
Malignancies
Thymoma, lymphoma, Ewing sarcoma, carcinomas, of the duodenum, pancreas, ureter, prostate, bladder and bronchogenic
Myxoedema
Idiopathic

SIADH occurs with any type of brain disorder. It is common during a 2–3-day period after paediatric head trauma [232]. Rarely, trauma leads to an interphase of excessive AVP release between two phases of DI. Various brain anomalies are associated with permanent SIADH [233,234]. In holoprosencephaly SIADH may alternate with DI [114,235]. In patients with haemorrhage, meningitis, abscess, encephalitis, Guillain–Barré syndrome, acute porphyria or psychosis, the presumed mechanism is inappropriate hypothalamic stimulation. In a prospective study of children with bacterial meningitis 28% of 36 [236] had evidence of SIADH at the time of admission. Of 24 children with tuberculous meningitis 17 developed SIADH [237]. Fever in itself may be a cause; in a series of febrile children, those with meningitis did not differ from others in the levels of either plasma AVP or serum Na^+ [67].

The list of pulmonary diseases includes pneumonia, tuberculosis and cavitation due to other causes, and possibly even common respiratory infections [238]. Tuberculous lung contains an AVP-like substance.

After valvulotomy for mitral stenosis, drops of > 25 mmHg in left atrial pressure may lead to a period of strong obligatory antidiuresis for 10 days or longer.

SIADH may develop in hypothyroidism, though water excretion is usually normal and the hyponatraemic disorders which occur are mostly of another nature [239].

A 'periodic ACTH–AVP discharge syndrome' has been described in children [240], manifesting as arterial hypertension and vomiting attacks. In one child AVP secretion was reported to be increased even between biweekly attacks. The role of emetic stimulation of AVP secretion should be studied in such children.

Drugs (see Table 32.3) may cause inappropriate antidiuresis, not all of them by causing release of AVP. An SIADH-like state may thus develop during cytostatic therapy. Nausea-induced AVP release may contribute to it. The risk is particularly associated with vincristine and cyclophosphamide. SIADH generally develops within several days to 2 weeks of vincristine therapy, but after large doses it may appear within hours.

Patients with DI on replacement therapy readily develop an SIADH-like state as a result of excessive water intake.

Postsurgery state is an SIADH-prone condition. Anaesthesia, narcotics and sedatives, pain, traction of the bowel, nausea and circulatory changes may all contribute to a decreased capacity of water excretion lasting from one to several days. This is similarly true for patients with trauma, especially burns [241]. In treatment of burned patients it would be a serious mistake to use urine flow as a guide to water needs.

In newborn infants, particularly preterm, SIADH appears to be a frequent, often overlooked problem, particularly during the first week of life [242]. In very low birth weight premature infants requiring mechanical ventilation, it may even occur in a majority [243]. The commonest causes are hypoxic brain injury, often with haemorrhage, asphyxia itself [244], pneumonia, pneumothorax and atelectasis, meningitis, ligation of ductus arteriosus and positive pressure ventilation. This SIADH usually subsides, but is sometimes followed by DI.

Clinical manifestations of hypo-osmolality

Symptoms and signs of hypo-osmolality are due to cell swelling resulting from an osmotic shift of water from the extracellular space into cells. Cells, especially those of the brain and kidneys, adjust to hypo-osmolality by decreasing their solute. Hence, clinical manifestation depends on the rate of development of hypo-osmolality. A chronic 20% hypo-osmolality may be tolerated without perceptible functional impairment, whereas a patient incurring suddenly similar hypo-osmolality is severely symptomatic.

The most profound manifestations are from the central nervous and neuromuscular systems. The first to appear are anorexia, apathy, confusion, headaches, and weakness and cramps of the abdominal and limb musculature. These are followed by nausea, vomiting, abdominal bloating and neurological abnormalities ranging from depressed deep tendon reflexes to the appearance of pathological reflexes, bulbar or pseudobulbar palsy, Cheyne–Stokes respiration and psychotic behaviour. The most severe cases may have convulsions which may lead to coma and death. Unless the patient has a pre-existing brain disorder, seizures and coma usually only occur at a plasma Na^+ concentration < 120 mmol/l.

Newborn infants with SIADH usually have a severe underlying illness. In many cases hypo-osmolality adds to the brain oedema produced by the primary insult. Weight may decrease rather than increase because of the basic condition.

Pathophysiology (Table 32.7)

Arginine vasopressin excess causes a disturbance only when water intake is larger than its output via non-renal routes and urine at the osmolality determined by the actual plasma AVP concentration. SIADH is often associated with stimulation of thirst. The excess free water retained is evenly distributed throughout body fluids, causing a build-up of hypo-osmolar expansion of extracellular volume and swelling of cells. The organism counteracts the volume expansion by maintaining natriuria in excess of intake, through an increase in glomerular filtration and a decrease of proximal Na^+ reabsorption. Most workers have observed increased plasma levels of atrial natriuretic peptide [245–247], but not all [248]. The other endogenous natriuretics, digitalis-like natriuretic factor and dopamine, seem not to be elevated [248]. Plasma renin activity is invariably low, but aldosterone is not usually suppressed. The negative Na^+ balance is maintained and the fluid disorder progresses until a new steady state is reached with plasma Na^+ concentration from slightly subnormal to as low as 100–110 mmol/l. Urine Na^+ concentration may then be low. Water retention has similarly reached a plateau and the urine is correspondingly less concentrated.

Table 32.7 Comparison of the pathogenesis of the two hypo-osmolar states which may be difficult to differentiate: hypo-osmolar dehydration and SIADH

Hypo-osmolar dehydration	SIADH
1 Fluid loss	1 AVP excess
2 Hypovolaemia	U-Osm ↑
SUN ↑	2 Water retention
Hcr ↑	3 Hypervolaemia
Weight ↓	P-Osm, SUN ↓
3 AVP, ALDO ↑	Hcr ↓
U-Na^+ <10 mmol/l*	Weight ↑
U-Osm >400 mosmol/kg	4 Natriuresis ↑
4 Relative water retention	U-Na^+ >20 mmol/l
P-Osm ↓	5 Secondary Na^+ depletion
	U-Na^+ <20 mmol/l

* Possible exceptions: adrenocortical failure, diuretic therapy, osmotic diuresis, salt-losing nephropathy and cerebral salt-wasting.

ALDO, aldosterone; Hcr, haematocrit; P-Osm, plasma osmolality; SUN, serum urea nitrogen; U-Na^+, urinary Na^+ concentration; U-Osm, urine osmolality.

This new steady state may also result from a discontinuation of AVP release in lowered threshold-type disorders. In other cases the degree of hypo-osmolality in this steady state depends mainly on water intake and relatively little on the degree of AVP excess. This is explained by the fact that urine flow decreases only slightly when urine osmolality increases from 400 to 1200 mosmol/kg (see Fig. 32.10). Even in this new steady state the capacity to excrete a water load and retain a Na^+ load remains impaired. Because of the increased glomerular filtration, plasma urea and urate concentrations remain low.

Plasma AVP concentration is usually in the 'normal' range but elevated in relation to plasma osmolality.

Robertson has defined four different types of abnormality by altering plasma osmolality in 25 adult patients by infusion of hyperosmolar NaCl solution and observing the dependence of plasma AVP on the osmolality [20,28]. In type 1 (six of 25 patients), plasma AVP showed large and erratic fluctuations independent of osmolality; AVP release appeared to be either totally divorced from osmoreceptor control or responding to a periodic non-osmotic stimulus. In type 2 (nine of 25) with low-set osmoreceptors a qualitatively normal relationship was present but with an abnormally low threshold, varying from 270 to 250 mosmol/kg in individual patients. In type 3 (eight of 25) with 'AVP leakage', the relationship was otherwise normal but plasma AVP, instead of being undetectable as in healthy individuals, remained at a steady low level throughout the range of plasma hypo-osmolality, increasing in a normal fashion after the rising plasma osmolality passed the normal threshold level. In type 4 (two of 25) with AVP-independent inappropriate antidiuresis, the plasma AVP–osmolality relation was normal. After a water load, however, urinary dilution did not occur and the load was not excreted despite normal AVP suppression. It is not known whether this was due to a renal abnormality or to the presence of some other circulating antidiuretic agent. No simple relationship was found between the type of abnormality and the underlying cause.

In thyrotoxicosis the osmotic thresholds of both AVP secretion and thirst are lowered, but hyponatremia is rare [249].

Table 32.8 Differentiation of hyponatraemia

1 Determine plasma osmolality
  If the patient is hypo-osmolar, proceed to step 2
  If the patient is normo-osmolar, measure plasma protein, lipids, glucose, and check usage of mannitol
2 Examine for evidence of oedema, congestive failure, cirrhosis, nephrosis, hypotension, hypovolaemia (cannot be excluded by absence of physical signs, consider measuring plasma renin activity, especially in patients with acute brain disorder possibly associated with 'cerebral salt-wasting'), adrenal failure (consider plasma cortisol and aldosterone), hypothyroidism, nausea, immobility. If one of these is present, proceed to specific therapy, otherwise proceed to step 3
3 If urine osmolality is:
  $>$ 100 mosmol/kg, proceed to step 4
  $\leqslant$100 mosmol/kg, confirm absence of hypovolaemia with measurement of plasma renin activity, then perform dehydration test and obtain urine osmolality hourly. If urine concentration occurs before plasma osmolality reaches 270 mosmol/kg and Na^+ 130 mmol/l, the diagnosis of lowered-threshold-type disorder is likely, and proceed to step 4. Otherwise, a persistent defect in water excretion is excluded
4 If urine Na^+ concentration is:
  $\leqslant$ 20 mmol/l, the alternatives are effective hypovolaemia, and SIADH in a new steady state
  $>$ 20 mmol/l, the alternatives are SIADH and hyponatraemic dehydration with renal, adrenal or cerebral salt-wastage. Plasma renin assay is helpful in the differentiation: it is suppressed in SIADH and elevated in dehydration
  If impaired ability to excrete water is suspected in a patient whose hyponatraemia has remitted, a test load of water may be given. If the load is not excreted normally, steps 1–4 should be performed to define the defect

Adapted from Robertson [250].

Differential diagnosis of hyponatraemia and SIADH (Table 32.8)

In evaluating a laboratory report of hyponatraemia, errors first need to be excluded. Dilution of the blood sample may occur by Na^+-poor solutions from an infusion line. Elevated levels of protein and/or lipid in normonatraemic plasma will cause hyponatraemic readings in flame photometers, because concentration in whole plasma is measured. Ion-specific electrodes and osmometers measure concentrations in plasma water and are not disturbed by such abnormalities. Measurement of plasma osmolality will also differentiate hypo-osmolality from non-hypo-osmolar hyponatraemia, such as occurs with hyperglycaemia and mannitolaemia.

Two main types of hyponatraemia exist: (i) states with a subnormal effective volume of blood associated with either expansion or contraction of total extracellular fluid volume, and (ii) states with normal or supranormal effective blood volume, SIADH. Differentation is commonly easy on the basis of history and physical examination.

In unclear cases determination of Na^+ concentration in a spot sample of urine is usually decisive. Levels of $>$ 20 mmol/l suggest SIADH if dehydration due to renal, adrenocortical or pituitary disease, and concurrent diuretic therapy and cerebral salt-wasting (see below) are excluded. In adrenocortical failure, plasma K^+ is usually but not always elevated. Plasma cortisol is not always sufficient for exclusion of adrenal failure, because there are patients with isolated aldosterone deficiency due to a specific enzyme defect or selective autoimmune destruction [251]. Pseudohypoaldosteronism must also be remembered. Young male infants with 'obstructive uropathy' and urine tract infection may develop severe hyponatraemia, with dehydration, polyuria, hyperkalaemia and acidosis probably involving acquired renal resistance to aldosterone [252].

Low urinary Na^+ concentration also occurs in advanced SIADH, when a new steady state has been reached (see Table 32.7). Such a state has to be carefully differentiated from hyponatraemic dehydration, remembering that mild hypovolaemia cannot be excluded by absence of signs in physical examination. For instance, hypo-osmolality in connection with brain disorders or hypopituitarism may be due to Na^+ depletion rather than water retention, and treating such a condition by water restriction could be disastrous. 'Cerebral salt-wasting' occurs in neurosurgical patients: natriuria despite hyponatraemic dehydration fullfilling the criteria of SIADH save the absence of hypovolaemia. An unknown salt-losing factor may be involved [253,254].

Elevated urea concentration indicates dehydration. Plasma renin measurement is decisive, because the levels are suppressed in SIADH but elevated in states with reduced effective blood volume. A Na^+ replacement trial may be resorted to: when one-quarter of the amount necessary for full correction of the Na^+ concentration deficit is given, intravenously as physiological Na^+ solution or orally in a more dilute glucose-containing solution, the salt is retained in dehydration (except when due to adrenocortical or renal failure, or cerebral salt-wasting) but excreted in SIADH.

SIADH associated with brain disorder needs to be differentiated from appropriately increased AVP secretion in patients developing effective hypovolaemia, because they are motionless and blood pools in the dependent portions of the vascular bed. Decreased venous return appears to be the mechanism of increased AVP secretion, hyperreninaemia and hyperaldosteronaemia in infantile bronchiolitis [255]. Similarly, appropriate release of AVP in response to subnormal left atrial filling is the probable cause of antidiuresis in patients with increased pulmonary vascular resistance, positive-pressure ventilation, pulmonary atelectasis and other conditions with obstructed pulmonary blood flow, and status asthmaticus.

Nausea-induced AVP release should be distinguished from SIADH; it is common during cytostatic therapy.

Determinations of plasma AVP levels are usually of no value in differentiation between the main causes of hypo-osmolality; they are elevated in all in relation to the hypo-osmolality. In lowered threshold-type SIADH plasma AVP concentration will be fully suppressed at subthreshold levels of osmolality, and further AVP determinations at higher plasma osmolality levels are necessary to establish the diagnosis. In AVP-leak-type disorders AVP levels may also be similar to levels in normal subjects.

For testing water-excreting capacity in a normonatraemic patient, or testing for lowered threshold, a water load test is useful. SIADH is characterized by a failure of excretion of the water and of dilution of urine.

In newborn infants, particularly in small preterm babies, differentiation of SIADH and hyponatraemic dehydration is frequently needed and may be difficult. Accurate measurements of weight and plasma Na^+ are the most reliable indicators of changes in water balance [243].

Prevention and therapy

Only in severely symptomatic hypo-osmolality should the hyponatraemia be (partially) corrected by infusion of hyperosmolar Na^+ solution (for example 500 mmol/l or 3% NaCl solution). Caution is needed, because too rapid (>20 mosmol/kg or >10 mmol/l Na^+ in 24 h) a rise of osmolality carries a risk of pontine myelinolysis [185,256], which may be lethal. The brain cells adjust over several hours to the hypo-osmolar state by eliminating solute, and thus correct their primary swelling. If extracellular osmolality is elevated suddenly, the cells will shrink, causing a risk of tears and haemorrhage in the non-elastic intracranial space. The 3% NaCl solution given at a rate of 0.1 ml/kg min^{-1} for 2 h will increase plasma Na^+ by approximately 10 mmol/l. To prevent hypervolaemia, frusemide may be administered with the infusion, followed by collection of urine and replacement of the electrolytes excreted [257].

In advanced SIADH the secondary depletion of Na^+ also has to be replaced.

When the extracellular expansion has been corrected, renal wastage of Na^+ will cease. Until the surplus water has been lost, water intake must be restricted to substantially less than the sum of renal and extrarenal output; for example to 40% of the normal basal requirement. After full correction water intake should be increased to the maximum that does not lead to excessive natriuria, or to an increase in weight.

The point of full correction of water retention will not be signalled by normalization of plasma Na^+ unless the Na^+ deficit has been simultaneously corrected. Adequate water restriction is difficult when inappropriate thirst is also present. In such situations therapy with demeclocycline may be tried. In adults, 3–5 mg/kg has been given every 8 h [258]. Frusemide is an alternative with replacement of the salt lost in urine [259]. No AVP antagonist peptide is currently clinically useful [13], but new antagonists are being developed, both peptide and non-peptide [55].

Excessive AVP secretion associated with nausea should be treated with antiemetic dopamine antagonists. In water retention caused by immobility, a slightly head-down position may be beneficial.

Excess AVP causes disturbance only with water intake which is inappropriately large for the degree of AVP secretion. Hence the main method of prevention and treatment of SIADH is restriction of water intake. In the commonest risk situations, postsurgery state and trauma therapy (especially brain surgery, head trauma and burns) water intake on the first postoperative day should be limited to two-thirds of the usual maintenance. Weight monitoring should not be neglected in surgical patients, and urine flow must not be regarded as an indicator of hydration. Similar precautions apply to other risk situations, for example first week therapy of small preterm infants, patients with acute brain or lung disease, and children receiving potentially antidiuretic drugs (see Table 32.3). However, these precautions must not lead to neglecting replacement of fluid deficits [260].

REFERENCES

1 Robertson GL, Berl T. Pathophysiology of water metabolism. In: Brenner BM, Rector FC, eds. *The Kidney*, 4th edn. Philadelphia, PA: W.B. Saunders, 1991:677–736.

2 Thrasher TN, Keil LC. Regulation of drinking and vasopressin secretion: role of organum vasculosum laminae terminalis. *Am J Physiol* 1987;253:R108–12.

3 Thrasher TN. Role of forebrain circumventricular organs in body fluid balance. *Acta Physiol Scand* 1989;136(Suppl. 583):141–50.

4 Hays RM. Agents affecting the renal conservation of water. In: Gilman AG, Goodman LS, Rall TW, Murad F, eds. *Goodman and Gilman's the Pharmacological Basis of Therapeutics*, 7th edn. New York: Macmillan, 1985:909.

5 Manning M, Czronka Z, Sawyer W. Synthesis of posterior pituitary hormones and hormone analogues. In: Beardwell C, Robertson GL, eds. *The Pituitary*. London: Butterworth, 1981:265–96.

6 Sawyer WH. Evolution of antidiuretic hormones and their functions. *Am J Med* 1967;42:678–86.

7 Walter R, Smith CW, Mehta PK *et al.* Conformational considerations of vasopressin as a guide to development of biological probes and therapeutic agents. In: Andreoli TE, Grantham JJ, Rector FC Jr, eds. *Disturbances in Body Fluid Osmolality*. Bethesda, MD: American Physiological Society, 1977:1–36.

8 Edwards CRW, Kitau MJ, Chard T *et al.* Vasopressin analogue DDAVP in diabetes insipidus: clinical and laboratory studies. *Br Med J* 1973;iii:375–8.

9 Bichet DG, Razi M, Lonergan M *et al.* Hemodynamic and coagulation responses to 1-desamino (8-d-arginine) vasopressin in patients with congenital nephrogenic diabetes insipidus. *N Engl J Med* 1988;318:881–7.

10 Manning M, Sawyer WH. Development of selective agonists and antagonists of vasopressin and oxytocin. In: Schrier RW, ed. *Vasopressin*. New York: Raven Press, 1985;131–44.

11 Sawyer WH, Manning M. Effective antagonists of the antidiuretic action of vasopressin in rats. *Ann NY Acad Sci* 1982;394:464–72.

12 Sawyer WH, Manning M. The development of vasopressin antagonists. *Fed Proc* 1984;43:87–90.

13 Manning M, Sawyer WH. Design, synthesis and some uses of receptor-specific agonists and antagonists of vasopressin and oxytocin. *J Receptor Res* 1993;13:195–214.

14 Cross BA, Dyball REJ, Dyer RG *et al.* Endocrine neurons. *Rec Prog Horm Res* 1975;31:243–94.

15 Riddel DC, Mallonee R, Phillips JA III*et al.* Chromosomal assignment of human sequences encoding arginine vasopressin-neurohypophysin II and growth hormone releasing factor. *Somat Cell Mol Genet* 1985;11:189.

16 Summar ML, Phillips JA III, Battey J *et al.* Linkage relationships of human arginine vasopressin-neurohypophysin-II and oxytocin-neurohypophysin-I to prodynorphin and other loci on chromosome 20. *Mol Endocrinol* 1990;4:947–50.

17 Pullan PT, Clappison BH, Johnston CL. Plasma vasopressin and human neurophysins in physiological and pathological states associated with changes in vasopressin secretion. *J Clin Endocrinol Metab* 1979;49:580–7.

18 Robinson AG, Halusczak C, Wilkins JA *et al.* Physiologic control of two neurophysins in humans. *J Clin Endocrinol Metab* 1977;44:330–9.

19 Pruszczynski W, Caillens H, Drieu L, Moulonguet-Doleris L, Ardaillou R. Renal excretion of antidiuretic hormone in healthy subjects and patients with renal failure. *Clin Sci* 1984;67:307–12.

20 Robertson GL. Vasopressin function in health and disease. *Rec Prog Horm Res* 1977;33:333–85.

21 Dunger DB, Seckl JR, Grant DB, Yeoman L, Lightman SL. A short water deprivation test incorporating urinary arginine vasopressin estimations for the investigation of posterior pituitary function in children. *Acta Endocrinol (Copenh)* 1988;117:13–18.

22 Jard S. Vasopressin receptors. *Front Horm Res* 1985;13: 89–104.

23 Editorial. Diabetes defect defined. *Nature* 1992;359:434.

24 Birnbaumer M, Seibold A, Gilbert S *et al.* Molecular cloning of the receptor for human antidiuretic hormone. *Nature* 1992;357:333–5.

25 Sharif M, Hanley MR. Stepping up the pressure. *Nature* 1992;357:279–80.

26 Moses AM, Miller JL, Levine MA. Two distinct pathophysiological mechanisms in congenital nephrogenic diabetes insipidus. *J Clin Endocrinol Metab* 1988;66:1259–64.

27 Robertson GL. Vasopressin and water metabolism. In: Ingbar SH, ed. *The Year in Endocrinology 1977*. New York: Plenum, 1978:205–31.

28 Robertson GL. The pathophysiology of ADH secretion. In: Tolis G, ed. *Clinical Neuroendocrinology: a Pathophysiological Approach*. New York: Raven Press, 1979:247–60.

29 Robertson GL. Diagnosis of diabetes insipidus. *Front Horm Res* 1985;13:127–55.

30 Robertson GL. Regulation of vasopressin secretion. In: Seldin DW, Giebisch G, eds. *The Kidney: Physiology and Pathophysiology*. New York: Raven Press, 1985:869–84.

31 Robertson GL, Aycinena P, Zerbe RL. Neurogenic disorders of osmoregulation. *Am J Med* 1982;72:339–53.

32 Robertson GL, Bhoopalam N, Zelkowitz LJ. Vincristine neurotoxicity and abnormal secretion of antidiuretic hormone. *Arch Intern Med* 1973;132:717–20.

33 Robertson GL, Mahr EA, Athar S *et al.* Development and clinical application of a new method for the radioimmunoassay of arginine vasopressin in human plasma. *J Clin Invest* 1973;52:2340–52.

34 Robertson GL, Shelton RL, Athar S. The osmoregulation of vasopressin. *Kidney Int* 1976;10:25–37.

35 Verney EB. The antidiuretic hormone and the factors which determine its release. *Proc R Soc, B* 1947;135:25–106.

36 Vallotton MB, Merkelbach U, Claillard RC. Studies of the factors modulating antidiuretic hormone excretion in man in response to the osmolar stimulus: effects of oestrogen and angiotensin II. *Acta Endocrinol (Copenh)* 1983;104:295–9.

37 Andersson B. Regulation of water intake. *Physiol Rev* 1978; 58:582–603.

38 Streeten DHP, Moses AM, Miller M. Disorders of the neurohypophysis. In: Braunwald E, Isselbacher K, Petersdorf RG *et al.*, eds. *Harrison's Principles of Internal Medicine*, 11th edn. New York: McGraw-Hill, 1987:1722–32.

39 Sujov P, Kellerman L, Zeltzer M, Hochberg Z. Plasma and urine osmolality in full-term and pre-term infants. *Acta Paed Scand* 1984;73:722–6.

40 Ramsay DJ. The importance of thirst in maintenance of fluid balance. *Bailliere's Clin Endocrinol Metab* 1989;3:371–91.

41 Thompson CJ, Bland J, Burd J, Baylis PH. The osmotic thresholds for thirst and vasopressin release are similar in healthy man. *Clin Sci* 1986;71:651–6.

42 Thompson CJ, Edwards CRW, Baylis PH. Osmotic and non-osmotic regulation of thirst and vasopressin secretion in

patients with compulsive water drinking. *Clin Endocrinol* 1991;35:221–8.

43 Hochberg Z, Moses AM, Miller M, Benderli A, Richman RA. Altered osmotic threshold for vasopressin release and impaired thirst sensation: additional abnormalities in Kallmann's syndrome. *J Clin Endocrinol Metab* 1982;55: 779–82.

44 Blachar Y, Zadik Z, Shemesh M *et al.* The effect of inhibition of prostaglandin synthesis on free water and osmolar clearances in patients with hereditary nephrogenic diabetes insipidus. *Int J Pediatr Nephrol* 1980;1:48–52.

45 Forrest JN Jr, Singer I. Drug-induced interference with action of antidiuretic hormone. In: Andreoli TE, Grantham JT, Rector FC Jr, eds. *Disturbances in Body Fluid Osmolality.* Bethesda, MD: American Physiological Society, 1977;3: 9–40.

46 Gross PA, Schrier RW, Anderson RJ. Prostaglandins and water metabolism: a review with emphasis on in vivo studies. *Kidney Int* 1981;19:839–50.

47 Miller M, Moses AM. Drug-induced states of impaired water excretion. *Kidney Int* 1976;10:96–103.

48 Cadnapaphornchai H, Boykin JL, Berl T *et al.* Mechanism of effect of nicotine on renal water excretion. *Am J Physiol* 1974;227:1216–20.

49 Rado JP, Marosi J, Szende L *et al.* Clinical value of the combinations of carbamazepine (Tegretol), chlorpropamide (Diabinese) and vasopressin in the treatment of pituitary diabetes insipidus. *Endokrinologie* 1973;62:297–309.

50 Stephens WP, Coe JY, Baylis PH. Plasma arginine vasopressin concentrations and antidiuretic action of carbamazepine. *Br Med J* 1978;1:1445–7.

51 Kusano E, Braun-Werness DJ, Keller MJ, Dous TP. Chlorpropamide action on renal concentrating mechanism in rats with hypothalamic diabetes insipidus. *J Clin Invest* 1983;72: 1298–313.

52 Zusman RM, Keiser HR, Handler JS. Inhibition of vasopressin-stimulated prostaglandin E biosynthesis by chlorpropamide in the toad bladder. *J Clin Invest* 1977;60:1348–53.

53 Ribeiro CP, Ribeiro-Neto F, Field JB, Suki WN. Prevention of α_2-adrenergic inhibition on ADH action by pertussis toxin in rabbit and mouse kidney. *Kidney Int* 1986;29:33A–35A.

54 Aubry RH, Nankin HR, Moses AM, Streeten DHP. Measurement of the osmotic threshold for vasopressin release in human subjects, and its modification by cortisol. *J Clin Endocrinol Metab* 1965;25:1481–92.

55 Yamamura Y, Ogawa H, Yamashita H *et al.* Characterization of a novel aquaretic agent, OPC-31260, as an orally effective, nonpeptide vasopressin V_2 receptor antagonist. *Br J Pharmacol* 1992;105:787–91.

56 Barbour GL, Straub KD, O'Neal BL *et al.* Vasopressin-resistant nephrogenic diabetes insipidus – results of amphotericin-B therapy. *Arch Intern Med* 1979;139:86–8.

57 Gold PW, Robertson GL, Post RM *et al.* The effect of lithium on the osmoregulation of arginine vasopressin secretion. *J Clin Endocrinol Metab* 1983;56:295–9.

58 Mizrahi LM, Hobbs JF, Goldsmith DI. Nephrogenic diabetes insipidus in transplacental lithium intoxication. *J Pediatr* 1979;94:493–5.

59 George CPL, Messerli FH, Genest J *et al.* Diurnal variation of plasma vasopressin in man. *J Clin Endocrinol Metab* 1975; 41:332–8.

60 Salata RA, Verbalis JG, Robinson AG. Cold water stimulation of oropharyngeal receptors in man inhibits release of vasopressin. *J Clin Endocrinol Metab* 1987;65:561–7.

61 Seckl JR, Williams TDM, Lightman SL. Oral hypertonic saline causes transient fall of vasopressin in humans. *Am J Physiol* 1986;251:R214–17.

62 Crotty TB, Gebruers EM, Hall WJ. The location of the receptors involved in the human diuretic response to drinking an isotonic electrolyte solution. *J Physiol Lond* 1992; 450:1–11.

63 Goldsmith SR. Vasopressin as vasopressor. *Am J Med* 1987; 82:1213–19.

64 Rossi NF, Schrier RW. Role of arginine vasopressin in regulation of systemic arterial pressure. *Annu Rev Med* 1986;37: 13–20.

65 Aisenbrey GA, Handelman WA, Arnold P *et al.* Vascular effects of arginine vasopressin during fluid deprivation. *J Clin Invest* 1981;67:961–8.

66 Grossman A. New uses for an old peptide: desmopressin and Cushing's syndrome. *Clin Endocrinol* 1993;38:461–2.

67 Sharples PM, Seckl JR, Human D, Lightman SL, Dunger DB. Plasma and cerebrospinal fluid arginine vasopressin in patients with and without fever. *Arch Dis Child* 1992;67: 998–1002.

68 Reeves WB, Andreoli TE. The posterior pituitary and water metabolism. In: Wilson JD, Foster DW, eds. *Williams Textbook of Endocrinology*, 8th edn. Philadelphia, PA: W.B. Saunders, 1992:311–56.

69 Kokko JP, Rector FC Jr. Countercurrent multiplication system without active transport in inner medulla. *Kidney Int* 1972;2:214–23.

70 Kokko JP, Tisher CC. Water movement across nephron segments involved with the countercurrent multiplication system. *Kidney Int* 1976;10:64–81.

71 Jard S, Bockaert J. Stimulus–response coupling in neurohypophyseal peptide target cells. *Physiol Rev* 1975;55: 489–536.

72 Brenner BM. Control of glomerular function by intrinsic contractile elements. *Fed Proc* 1983;42,3045.

73 Ausiello DA, Hartwig JH. Microfilament organization and vasopressin action. In: Schrier RW, ed. *Vasopressin.* New York: Raven Press, 1985:89–96.

74 Stokes JB. Integrated actions of renal medullary prostaglandins in the control of water excretion. *Am J Physiol* 1981;240:1471–80.

75 Davis AL. Atrial natriuretic peptide. *Adv Pediatr* 1989;36: 137–59.

76 Vierhapper H, Nowotny P, Waldhäusl W. Effect of human atrial natriuretic peptide on 1-deamino-D-arg^8-vasopressin-induced antidiuresis. *J Clin Endocrinol Metab* 1988;66: 124–7.

77 Dillingham M, Anderson R. Inhibition of vasopressin action by atrial natriuretic factor. *Science* 1986;231:1572–3.

78 Forsling ML, Balment RJ, Brimble MJ, Brown J. Hormonal modulation of the renal response to vasopressin. Recent progress in posterior pituitary hormones. *Excerpta Medica Int Congr Ser* 1988;797:353–60.

79 Brown J, Forsling ML, Slater JDH. Human atrial natriuretic peptide inhibits tubular effects of antidiuretic hormone in humans. In: Brenner BM, Laragh JH, eds. *Advances in Atrial Peptide Research.* New York: Raven Press, 1988:355–8.

80 Levin ER, Hu R, Rossi M, Pickart M. Arginine vasopressin stimulates atrial natriuretic peptide gene expression and secretion from rat diencephalic neurons. *Endocrinology* 1992;131:1417–23.

81 Epstein FH. Disturbances in renal concentrating ability. In: Andreoli TE, Grantham JT, Rector FC Jr, eds. *Disturbances*

in Body Fluid Osmolality. Bethesda, MD: American Physiological Society, 1977;251–66.

82 Czernichow P, Pomarede R, Brauner R, Rappaport R. Neurogenic diabetes insipidus in children. *Front Horm Res* 1985; 13:190–209.

83 Skowsky WR, Fisher DA. Fetal neurohypophyseal arginine vasopressin and arginine vasotocin in man and sheep. *Pediatr Res* 1977;11:627–30.

84 Pavel S. Vasotocin biosynthesis by neurohypophysial cells from human fetuses. Evidence for its ependymal origin. *Neuroendocrinology* 1975;19:150–9.

85 Leake RD, Fisher DA. Ontogeny of vasopressin in man. *Front Horm Res* 1985;13:4–51.

86 Leake RD, Weitzman RE, Effros RM *et al*. Maternal fetal osmolar homeostasis: fetal posterior pituitary autonomy. *Pediatr Res* 1979;13:841–4.

87 Robillard JE, Weitzman KE, Fisher DA *et al*. The dynamics of vasopressin release and blood volume regulation during fetal hemorrhage in the lamb fetus. *Pediatr Res* 1979;13:606–10.

88 Manku MS, Mtabaji JP, Horrobin DF. Effect of cortisol, prolactin and ADH on the amniotic membrane. *Nature* 1975;258:78.

89 Chard T, Hudson CN, Edwards CRW *et al*. The release of oxytocin and vasopressin by the human fetus during labour. *Nature* 1971;234:352–4.

90 Hadeed AJ, Leake RD, Weitzman RE *et al*. Possible mechanisms of high blood levels of vasopressin during the neonatal period. *J Pediatr* 1979;94:805–8.

91 Rees L, Forsling ML, Brook CGD. Vasopressin concentrations in the neonatal period. *Clin Endocrinol* 1980;12:57–62.

92 Daniel SS, Stark RI, Husain MK *et al*. Excretion of vasopressin in the hypoxic lamb: comparison between fetus and newborn. *Pediatr Res* 1984;18:227–31.

93 Ruth V, Autti-Rämö I, Granström ML *et al*. Prediction of perinatal brain damage by cord plasma vasopressin, erythroprotein, and hypoxanthine values. *J Pediatr* 1988;113:880–5.

94 Hoppenstein JM, Miltenberger RW, Morau WH. The increase in blood levels of vasopressin in infants during birth and surgical procedures. *Surg Gynecol Obstet* 1968;127:966–71.

95 Pomarede R, Moriette R, Czernichow P, Relier JP. Etude de la vasopressine plasmatique chez les enfants prématurés soumis à la ventilation artificielle. *Arch Fr Pediatr* 1978; 35:75–9.

96 Fisher DA, Pyle HR Jr, Porter JC *et al*. Control of water balance in the newborn. *Am J Dis Child* 1963;106:137–46.

97 Spitzer A. The developing kidney and the process of growth. In: Seldin DW, Giebisch G, eds. *The Kidney: Physiology and Pathophysiology*. New York: Raven Press, 1985:1979–2015.

98 Crawford JD, Bode HH. Disorders of the posterior pituitary in children. In: Gardner LI, ed. *Endocrine and Genetic Diseases of Childhood and Adolescence*, 2nd edn. Philadelphia, PA: W.B. Saunders, 1975:126–58.

99 Greger NG, Kirkland RT, Clayton GW, Kirkland JL. Central diabetes insipidus 22 years' experience. *Am J Dis Child* 1986;140:551–4.

100 Niaudet P, Dechaux M, Leroy D, Broyer M. Nephrogenic diabetes insipidus in children. *Front Horm Res* 1985;13: 224–31.

101 Fujisawa I, Kikuchi K, Nishimura K *et al*. Transection of the pituitary stalk: development of an ectopic posterior lobe assessed with MR imaging. *Radiology* 1987;165:487–97.

102 Root AW. Magnetic resonance imaging in hypopituitarism (editorial). *J Clin Endocrinol Metab* 1991;72:10–11.

103 Yamanaka C, Momoi T, Fujisawa I *et al*. Neurohypophyseal function of an ectopic posterior lobe in patients with growth hormone deficiency. *Acta Endocrinol (Copenh)* 1990;122: 664–70.

104 Hans P, Stevenaert A, Albert A. Study of hypotonic polyuria after trans-sphenoidal pituitary adenomectomy. *Intens Care Med* 1986;12:95–6.

105 Atkinson FRB. Schueller–Christian's disease. *Br J Child Dis* 1937;34:28–36.

106 Jones GM. Diabetes insipidus, clinical observations in 42 cases. *Arch Intern Med* 1944;74:81–94.

107 Dunger DB, Broadbent V, Yeoman E *et al*. The frequency and natural history of diabetes insipidus in children with Langerhans-cell histiocytosis. *N Engl J Med* 1989;321:1157–62.

108 Hoshimaru M, Hashimoto N, Kikuchi H. Central diabetes insipidus resulting from a nonneoplastic tiny mass lesion localized in the neurohypophyseal system. *Surg Neurol* 1992;38:1–6.

109 Hung W, Fitz CR. The primary empty-sella syndrome and diabetes insipidus in a child. *Acta Paediatr* 1992;81: 459–61.

110 Marano GD, Horton JA, Vaquez AM. Computed tomography in diabetes insipidus: posterior empty sella. *Br J Radiol* 1981;54:263–70.

111 Freude S, Frisch H, Wimberger D *et al*. Septo-optic dysplasia and growth hormone deficiency. *Acta Paediatr* 1992;81: 641–5.

112 Pfeiffer RA, Legat G, Trautmann U. Acrocallosal syndrome in a child with *de novo* inverted tandem duplication of 12p11.2-p13.3. *Ann Genet* 1992;35:41–6.

113 Ehrhardt P. Central diabetes insipidus with congenital cerebral anomaly. *Br J Hosp Med* 1989;41:380–1.

114 Hasegawa Y, Hasegawa T, Yokoyama T, Kotoh S, Tsuchiya Y. Holoprosencephaly associated with diabetes insipidus and syndrome of inappropriate secretion of antidiuretic hormone. *J Pediatr* 1990;117:756–8.

115 Barzilay Z, Somekh E. Diabetes insipidus in severely brain damaged children. *J Med* 1988;19:47–55.

116 Kissoon N, Frewen TC, Bloch M, Gayle M, Stiller C. Pediatric organ donor maintenance: pathophysiologic derangements and nursing requirements. *Pediatrics* 1989;84:688–93.

117 Kern K, Meislin HW. Diabetes insipidus: occurrence after minor head trauma. *J Trauma* 1984;24:69–72.

118 Hadani M, Findler G, Shaked I, Sahar A. Unusual delayed onset of diabetes insipidus following closed head trauma. *J Neurosurg* 1985;63:456–8.

119 Pai KG, Rubin HN, Wedemeyer PP *et al*. Hypothalamic–pituitary dysfunction following group B beta hemolytic streptococcal meningitis in a neonate. *J Pediatr* 1976;88: 289–91.

120 Adams JM, Kenny JD, Rudolph AJ. Central diabetes insipidus following intraventricular hemorrhage. *J Pediatr* 1976;88: 292–4.

121 Fenton LJ, Kleinman LI. Transient diabetes insipidus in a newborn infant. *J Pediatr* 1974;85:79–81.

122 Czernichow P, Pomarede R, Basmaciogullari A, Brauner R, Rappaport R. Diabetes insipidus in children. III. Anterior pituitary dysfunction in idiopathic types. *J Pediatr* 1985; 106:41–4.

123 Repaske DR, Phillips JA III, Kirby LT *et al*. Molecular analysis of autosomal dominant neurohypophyseal diabetes insipidus. *J Clin Endocrinol Metab* 1990;70:752–7.

124 Scherbaum WA, Czernichow P, Bottazzo GF, Doniach D. Diabetes insipidus in children. IV. A possible autoimmune

type with vasopressin cell antibodies. *J Pediatr* 1985;107: 922–5.

125 Bergeron C, Kovacs K, Ezrin C, Mizzen C. Hereditary diabetes insipidus: an immunohistochemical study of the hypothalamus and pituitary gland. *Acta Neuropathol Berl* 1991;81:345–8.

126 Ito M, Mori Y, Oiso Y, Saito H. A single base substitution in the coding region for neurophysin II associated with familial central diabetes insipidus. *J Clin Invest* 1991;87:725–8.

127 Toth EL, Bowden PA, Crockford PM. Hereditary central diabetes insipidus: plasma levels of antidiuretic hormone in a family with a possible osmoreceptor defect. *Can Med Assoc J* 1984;131:1237–41.

128 Forssman H. Two different mutations of X-chromosome causing diabetes insipidus. *Am J Hum Gen* 1955;7:21–5.

129 Nagi NA. Diabetes insipidus, diabetes mellitus, optic atrophy and deafness–clinical and genetic study. *Postgrad Med J* 1979;55:377–81.

130 Cremers CW, Wijdeveld PG, Pinckers AJ. Juvenile diabetes mellitus, optic atrophy, hearing loss, diabetes insipidus, atonia of the urinary tract and bladder, and other abnormalities (Wolfram syndrome). A review of 88 cases from the literature with personal observations on 3 new patients. *Acta Paed Scand* 1977;Suppl. 264:1–16.

131 Conley SB, Brocklebank JT, Taylor IT. Recurrent hypernatremia: a proposed mechanism in a patient with absence of thirst and abnormal excretion of water. *J Pediatr* 1976;89: 898–903.

132 Halter JB, Goldberg AP, Robertson GL, Porte D Jr. Selective osmoreceptor dysfunction in syndrome of chronic hypernatremia. *J Clin Endocrinol Metab* 1977;44:609–16.

133 Khommami-Asadi F, Norman ME, Parks JS, Schwartz MW. Hypernatremia associated with pineal tumor. *J Pediatr* 1977;90:605–6.

134 Schaad U, Vassella F, Zuppinger K, Oetliker O. Hypodipsia–hypernatremia syndrome. *Helv Paediatr Acta* 1979;34:63–76.

135 Schaff-Blass E, Robertson GL, Rosenfield RL. Chronic hypernatremia from a congenital defect in osmoregulation of thirst and vasopressin. *J Pediatr* 1983;102:703–8.

136 Lascelles PT, Lewis PD. Hypodipsia and hypernatremia associated with hypothalamic and supracellar lesions. *Brain* 1972;95:249–64.

137 Kohn B, Norman ME, Feldman H *et al.* Hysterical polydipsia (compulsive water drinking) in children. *Am J Dis Child* 1976;130:210–12.

138 Linshaw MA, Hipp T, Gruskin A. Infantile psychogenic water drinking. *J Pediatr* 1974;85:520–2.

139 Mellinger RC, Zafar MS. Primary polydipsia. Syndrome of inappropriate thirst. *Arch Intern Med* 1981;143:124–51.

140 Robertson GL. Dipsogenic diabetes insipidus: a newly recognized syndrome caused by a selective defect in the osmoregulation of thirst. *Trans Assoc Am Phys* 1987;100:241–9.

141 Stevko RM, Balsley M, Segar WE. Primary polydipsia – compulsive water drinking. Report of two cases. *J Pediatr* 1968; 73:845–51.

142 Hogan PA, Woolsey RM. Polydipsia associated with occult hydrocephalus. *N Engl J Med* 1988;277:639–40.

143 Page SR, Nussey SS, Jenkins JS *et al.* Hypothalamic disease in association with dysgenesis of the corpus callosum. *Postgrad Med J* 1989;65:163–7.

144 Davidson S, Frand M, Rotem Y. Primary polydipsia in infancy: a benign disorder simulating diabetes insipidus. *Clin Pediatr* 1978;17:419–20.

145 Bailey P, Beremer F. Experimental diabetes insipidus. *Arch Intern Med* 1921;28:773–803.

146 Bode HH, Crawford JD. Nephrogenic diabetes insipidus in North America – the Hopewell hypothesis. *N Engl J Med* 1969;280:750–4.

147 Knoers N, van der Heyden H, van Oost BA, Monnens L, Willems J, Ropers HH. Three-point linkage analysis using multiple DNA polymorphic markers in families with X-linked nephrogenic diabetes insipidus. *Genomics* 1989; 4:434–7.

148 Childs B, Sidbury JB. A survey of genetics as it applies to medicine. *Pediatrics* 1957;20:177–218.

149 Fichman MP, Brooker G. Deficient renal cyclic adenosine-3′,5′-monophosphate production in nephrogenic diabetes insipidus. *J Clin Endocrinol Metab* 1972;35:35–47.

150 Raij K, Perheentupa J, Härkönen M. Urinary cyclic adenosine monophosphate excretion in diabetes insipidus of childhood. *Scand J Clin Lab Invest* 1974;34:177–84.

151 Monn E, Osnes JB, Oye I. Basal and hormone-induced urinary cyclic AMP in children with renal disorders. *Acta Paed Scand* 1976;Suppl. 65:739–45.

152 Niaudet P, Dechaux M, Trivin C *et al.* Nephrogenic diabetes insipidus: clinical and pathophysiological aspects. *Adv Nephrol* 1984;13:247–60.

153 Brenner B, Seligsohn U, Hochberg Z. Normal response of factor VIII and von Willebrand factor to 1-deamino-8D-arginine vasopressin in nephrogenic diabetes insipidus. *J Clin Endocrinol Metab* 1988;67:191–3.

154 Levine RA. Antidiuretic responses to exogenous adenosine 3′,5′-monophosphate in man. *Clin Sci* 1968;34:253–60.

155 Monn E. Prostaglandin synthetase inhibitors in the treatment of nephrogenic diabetes insipidus. *Acta Paed Scand* 1981;Suppl. 70:39–42.

156 Proesmans W, Eggermont E, Vanderschueren-Lodeweyckx M, Tiddens H, Eckels R. The effect of exogenous 3′:5′-adenosine monophosphate on urinary output in children with vasopressin-resistant diabetes insipidus. *Pediatr Res* 1975;9:509–12.

157 Kobrinsky NL, Doyle JJ, Israels D *et al.* Absent factor VIII response to synthetic vasopressin analogue (DDAVP) in nephrogenic diabetes insipidus. *Lancet* 1985;1:1293–4.

158 Knoers N, Monnens LA. A variant of nephrogenic diabetes insipidus: V_2 receptor abnormality restricted to the kidney. *Eur J Pediatr* 1991;150:370–3.

159 Ohzeki T, Sunaguchi M, Tsunei M *et al.* Coagulation factor responsiveness in nephrogenic diabetes insipidus. *J Pediatr* 1988;113:790.

160 Giacoia GP, Watson S, Karathanos A. Treatment of neonatal diabetes insipidus with desmopressin. *South Med J* 1984; 77:75–7.

161 Schrager GO, Josephson EH, Fine RF *et al.* Nephrogenic diabetes insipidus presenting as fever of unknown origin in the neonatal period. *Clin Pediatr Phil* 1976;15:1070–2.

162 Sherwood MC, Stanhope R, Preece MA, Grant DB. Diabetes insipidus and occult intracranial tumours. *Arch Dis Child* 1986;61:1222–35.

163 Stanhope R, Preece MA, Grant DB, Brook CGD. Is diabetes insipidus during childhood ever idiopathic? *Br J Hosp Med* 1989;41:490–1.

164 Opas LM, Adler R, Robinson R, Lieberman E. Rhabdomyolysis with severe hypernatremia. *J Pediatr* 1977;90:713–16.

165 Gurewitz R, Blum I, Lavie P *et al.* Recurrent hypothermia, hypersomnolence, central sleep apnea, hypodipsia, hypernatremia, hypothyroidism, hyperprolactinemia and growth

hormone deficiency in a boy – treatment with clomopramine. *Acta Endocrinol (Copenh)* (Suppl.) 1986;279: 468–72.

166 Carter RC, Goldman AD. Nephrogenic diabetes insipidus accompanied by massive dilatation of the kidneys, ureters and bladder. *J Urol* 1963;89:366–72.

167 Block LH, Furrer J, Locher RA, Siegenthaler W, Vetter W. Changes in tissue sensitivity to vasopressin in hereditary hypothalamic diabetes insipidus. *Klin Wochenschr* 1981; 59:831–40.

168 Bergmann KE, Ziegler EE, Fomon SJ. Water and renal solute load. In: Fomon SJ, ed. *Infant Nutrition*, 2nd edn. Philadelphia: W.B. Saunders, 1974:245–66.

169 Seckl JR, Dunger DB, Lightman SL. Neurohypophyseal peptide function during early postoperative diabetes insipidus. *Brain* 1987;110:737–46.

170 Seckl JR, Dunger DB, Bevan JS *et al.* Vasopressin antagonists in early postoperative diabetes insipidus. *Lancet* 1990;335: 1353–6.

171 Hammond DN, Moll GW, Robertson GL, Chelmicka-Schorr E. Hypodipsic hypernatremia with normal osmoregulation of vasopressin. *N Engl J Med* 1986;315:433–6.

172 Dunger DB, Seckl JR, Lightman SL. Increased renal sensitivity to vasopressin in two patients with essential hypernatremia. *J Clin Endocrinol Metab* 1987;64:185–9.

173 Gill G, Baylis P, Burn J. A case of essential hypernatremia due to resetting of the osmostat. *Clin Endocrinol* 1985;22: 545–51.

174 Hochberg Z, Richman RA. Unstable osmoreceptors and defective thirst in hypothalamic hypopituitarism. *Hormone Res* 1981;14:215–23.

175 Goldman MB, Luchins DJ, Robertson GL. Mechanism of altered water metabolism in psychotic patients with polydipsia and hyponatremia. *N Engl J Med* 1988;318:397–403.

176 Illowsky BP, Kirch DG. Polydipsia and hyponatremia in psychiatric patients. *Am J Psychiatr* 1988;145:675–83.

177 Jenkins JS. Thirst and vasopressin. *Clin Endocrinol* 1991; 35:219–20.

178 Kovács L, Némethova V, Gucalová Y *et al.* Simple diagnosis of diabetes insipidus and antidiuretic hormone excess. *Exp Clin Endocrinol* 1985;85:228–34.

179 Richman RA, Post EM, Notman DD, Hochberg Z, Moses AM. Simplifying the diagnosis of diabetes insipidus in children. *Am J Dis Child* 1981;135:839–41.

180 Milles JJ, Spruce B, Baylis PH. A comparison of diagnostic methods to differentiate diabetes insipidus from primary polyuria: a review of 21 patients. *Acta Endocrinol (Copenh)* 1983;104:410–16.

181 Zerbe RL, Robertson GL. A comparison of plasma vasopressin measurements with a standard indirect test in the differential diagnosis of polyuria. *N Engl J Med* 1981;305:1539–46.

182 Thompson CJ, Selby P, Baylis PH. The reproducibility of osmotic and nonosmotic tests of vasopressin secretion in men. *Am J Physiol* 1991;260:R533–9.

183 Miller M, Dalakos T, Moses AM *et al.* Recognition of partial defects in antidiuretic hormone secretion. *Ann Intern Med* 1970;73:721–9.

184 Czernichow P, Pomarede R, Basmaciogullari A, Rappaport R. Diabetes insipidus in children: I. Arginine–vasopressin determination in plasma during short dehydration test. *Acta Paed Scand* 1986;Suppl. 277:64–7.

185 Laureno R. Central pontine myelinolysis following rapid correction of hyponatremia. *Ann Neurol* 1983;13:232–42.

186 Pomarede R, Czernichow P, Brauner R, Rappaport R. Intracranial germinoma in children and diabetes insipidus: clinical description and search for tumor markers. *Front Horm Res* 1985;13:240–6.

187 Pomarede R, Czernichow P, Finidori J *et al.* Endocrine aspects and tumoral markers in intracranial germinoma: an attempt to delineate the diagnosis procedure in 14 patients. *J Pediatr* 1982;101:374–8.

188 Saitoh M, Tamaki N, Kokunai T, Matsumoto S. Clinicobiological behavior of germ-cell tumors. *Child Nerv Syst* 1991;7:246–50.

189 Colombo N, Berry I, Kucharczyk J *et al.* Posterior pituitary gland: appearance on MR images in normal and pathologic states. *Radiology* 1987;165:481–5.

190 Fujisawa I, Nishimura K, Asato R *et al.* Posterior lobe of the pituitary in diabetes insipidus: MR findings. *J Comput Assist Tomogr* 1987;11:221–9.

191 Halimi P, Sigal R, Doyon D, Delivet S, Bouchard P, Pigeau I. Post-traumatic diabetes insipidus: MR demonstration of pituitary stalk rupture. *J Comput Assist Tomogr* 1988;12: 135–7.

192 Maghnie M, Arico A, Villa A *et al.* MR of the hypothalamic–pituitary axis in Langerhans cell histiocytosis. *Am J Neuroradiol* 1992;13:1365–71.

193 Tien R, Kucharczyk J, Kucharczyk W. MR imaging of the brain in patients with diabetes insipidus. *Am J Neuroradiol* 1991;12:533–42.

194 Moses AM, Clayton B, Hochhauser L. Use of T1-weighted MR imaging to differentiate between primary polydipsia and central diabetes insipidus. *Am J Neuroradiol* 1992;13: 1273–7.

195 Miyamoto S, Sasaki N, Tanabe Y. Magnetic resonance imaging in familial central diabetes insipidus. *Neuroradiology* 1991;33:272–3.

196 Maghnie M, Villa A, Arico M *et al.* Correlation between magnetic resonance imaging of posterior pituitary and neurohypophyseal function in children with diabetes insipidus. *J Clin Endocrinol Metab* 1992;74:795–800.

197 Moore JB, Kulkarni R, Crutcher DC, Bhimani S. MRI in multifocal eosinophilic granuloma: staging disease and monitoring response to therapy. *Am J Pediatr Hematol/Oncol* 1989;11:174–7.

198 Ono N, Kakegawa T, Zama A *et al.* Suprasellar germinomas; relationship between tumour size and diabetes insipidus. *Acta Neurochir (Wien)* 1992;114:26–32.

199 Fujisawa I, Asato R, Okumura R *et al.* Magnetic resonance imaging of neurohypophyseal germinomas. *Cancer* 1991;68: 1009–14.

200 Matsumoto T, Ito Y, Yukizane S, Ichikawa K, Yamashita F. Hereditary nephrogenic diabetes insipidus type-2. *Acta Paediatr Jpn* 1988;30:714–16.

201 Kauli R, Galatzer A, Laron Z. Treatment of diabetes insipidus in children and adolescents. *Front Horm Res* 1985; 13:304–13.

202 Vest M, Talbot NB, Crawford JD. Hypocaloric dwarfism and hydronephrosis in diabetes insipidus. *Am J Dis Child* 1963: 105:175–81.

203 Harris AS. Clinical experience with desmopressin: efficacy and safety in central diabetes insipidus and other conditions. *J Pediatr* 1989;114:711–18.

204 Fjellestad-Paulsen A, Höglund P, Lundin S, Paulsen O. Pharmacokinetics of 1-deamino-8-D-arginine vasopressin after various routes of administration in healthy volunteers. *Clin Endocrinol* 1993;38:177–82.

205 Seckl JR, Dunger DB. Diabetes insipidus, current treatment

recommendations. *Drugs* 1992;44:216–24.
206 Fjellestad A, Czernichow P. Central diabetes insipidus in children. V. Oral treatment with a vasopressin analogue (DDAVP). *Acta Paed Scand* 1986;Suppl. 75:605–10.
207 Fjellestad-Paulsen A, Tubiana-Rufi N, Harris A, Czernichow P. Central diabetes insipidus in children. Antidiuretic effect and pharmacokinetics of intranasal and peroral 1-deamino-8-1-D-arginine vasopressin. *Acta Endocrinol (Copenh)* 1987; 115:307–12.
208 Stick SM, Betts PR. Oral desmopressin in neonatal diabetes insipidus. *Arch Dis Child* 1987;62:1177–8.
209 Chanson P, Jedynak CP, Czernichov P. Management of early postoperative diabetes insipidus with parenteral desmopressin. *Acta Endocrinol (Copenh)* 1988;117:513–16.
210 McDonald JA, Martha PM, Kerrigan J, Clarke WL, Rogol AD, Blizzard RM. Treatment of the young child with postoperative central diabetes insipidus. *Am J Dis Child* 1989;143:201–4.
211 Ralston C, Butt W. Continuous vasopressin replacement in diabetes insipidus. *Arch Dis Child* 1990;65:896–7.
212 Blalock T, Gerron G, Quiter E *et al.* Role of diet in the management of vasopressin-responsive and -resistant diabetes insipidus. *Am J Clin Nutr* 1977;30:1070–6.
213 Salmenperä L, Perheentupa J, Siimes MA. Exclusively breast-fed healthy infants grow slower than reference infants. *Pediatr Res* 1985;19:307–12.
214 Shirley J, Walter SJ, Laycock JF. The antidiuretic effect of chronic hydrochlorothiazide treatment in rats with diabetes insipidus: renal mechanisms. *Clin Sci* 1989;63:533–8.
215 Walter SJ, Skinner J, Laycock JF, Shirley DG. The antidiuretic effect of chronic hydrochlorothiazide treatment in rats with diabetes insipidus: water and electrolyte balance. *Clin Sci* 1982;63:525–32.
216 Vierhapper H, Jörg J, Favre L *et al.* Comparative therapeutic benefit of indomethacin, hydrochlorothiazide, and acetylsalicylic acid in a patient with nephrogenic diabetes insipidus. *Acta Endocrinol (Copenh)* 1984;106:311–316.
217 Alon U, Chan JCM. Hydrochlorothiazide–amiloride in the treatment of congenital nephrogenic diabetes insipidus. *Am J Nephrol* 1985;5:9–13.
218 Knoers N, Monnens LAH. Amiloride-hydrochlorothiazide versus indomethacin-hydrochlorothiazide in the treatment of nephrogenic diabetes insipidus. *J Pediatr* 1990;117:499–502.
219 Shirley DCJ, Walter SJ, Laycock JF. The role of sodium depletion in hydrochlorothiazide-induced antidiuresis in Brattleboro rats with diabetes insipidus. *Clin Sci Mol Med* 1978;54:209–15.
220 Holmberg C, Perheentupa J, Pasternack A. The renal lesion in congenital chloride diarrhea. *J Pediatr* 1977;91:738–43.
221 Libber S, Harrison H, Spector D. Treatment of nephrogenic diabetes insipidus with prostaglandin synthesis inhibitors. *J Pediatr* 1986;108:305–11.
222 Palella TD, Fox IH. Hyperuricemia and gout. In: Scriver CR, Beaudet AL, Sly WS, Valle D, eds. *The Metabolic Basis of Inherited Disease*, 6th edn. New York: McGraw-Hill, 1989; 965–1006.
223 Kaulitz R, Brodehl J. Langfristige Verläufe von 6 Jungen mit kongenitalem nephrogenem Diabetes insipidus. *Klin Pädiatr* 1989;201:425–30.
224 Stasior DS, Kikeri D, Duel B, Seifter JL. Nephrogenic diabetes insipidus responsive to indomethacin plus dDAVP. *N Engl J Med* 1991;324:850–1.
225 Crigler JF Jr. Commentary: on the use of pitressin in infants with neurogenic diabetes insipidus. *J Pediatr* 1976;88: 295–6.
226 Chapman SJ, Neville BGR, Schurr PH. Craniopharyngioma in childhood: the nature and management of early post-operative fluid and electrolyte disturbance. *Dev Med Child Neurol* 1978;20:598–604.
227 Zahra S, Berndt V. Post-traumatic diabetes insipidus syndrome. *Dtsch Med Wochenschr* 178;103:114–20.
228 Verbalis JG, Robinson AG, Moses AM. Postoperative and posttraumatic diabetes insipidus. *Front Horm Res* 1985;13: 247–65.
229 Field MJ, Bostrom TE, Seow F, Gyory AZ, Cockayne DJ. Acute cisplatin nephrotoxicity in the rat. Evidence for impaired entry of sodium into proximal tubule cells. *Pflugers Arch* 1989;414:647–50.
230 Hutchison FN, Perez EA, Gandara DR, Lawrence HJ, Kaysen GA. Renal salt wasting in patients treated with cisplatin. *Ann Intern Med* 1988;108:21–5.
231 Bartter FC, Schwartz WB. The syndrome of inappropriate secretion of antidiuretic hormone. *Am J Med* 1976;42:790–806.
232 Padilla G, Leake JA, Castro R, Ervin MG, Ross MG, Leake RD. Vasopressin levels and pediatric head trauma. *Pediatrics* 1989;83:700–5.
233 Friedman AL, Chesney RW, Bargman GJ, Segar WE. Lack of inhibition of vasopressin in midfacial hypoplasia. *J Pediatr* 1979;94:591–4.
234 Fyhrquist F, Holmberg C, Perheentupa J, Wallenius M. Inappropriate secretion of antidiuretic hormone, hypertension, and hypoplastic corpus callosum. *J Clin Endocrinol Metab* 1977;45:691–4.
235 Zegher F, Devlieger H, De Cock P. Alternating diabetes insipidus and inappropriate antidiuresis in holoprosencephaly: relationship to intracranial pressure. *J Pediatr* 1992;120:161–2.
236 Laine J, Holmberg C, Anttila M *et al.* Types of fluid disorder in children with bacterial meningitis. *Acta Paed Scand* 1991;Suppl. 80:1031–6.
237 Cotton MF, Donald PR, Schoeman JF, Aalbers C, Van Zyl LE, Lombard C. Plasma arginine vasopressin and the syndrome of inappropriate antidiuretic hormone secretion in tuberculous meningitis. *Pediatr Infect Dis J* 1991;10:837–42.
238 Rivers RPA, Forsling ML, Oliver RD. Inappropriate secretion of antidiuretic hormone in infants with respiratory infections. *Arch Dis Child* 1981;56:358–63.
239 Iwasaki Y, Oiso Y, Yamauchi K *et al.* Osmoregulation of plasma vasopressin in myxedema. *J Clin Endocrinol Metab* 1990;70:534–9.
240 Ogihara M, Aritaki S. Periodic ACTH–ADH discharge syndrome: relationship to inappropriate ADH secretion. *Acta Paediatr Jpn* 1987;29:772–80.
241 Shirani KZ, Vaughan GM, Robertson GL *et al.* Inappropriate vasopressin secretion (SIADH) in burned patients. *J Trauma* 1983;23:217–24.
242 Nutman J, Wilunsky L, Avni A, Reisner SH. Syndrome of inappropriate antidiuretic hormone secretion in newborn infants with respiratory problems. *Isr J Med Sci* 1981;17: 1009–13.
243 Rees L, Shaw JCL, Brook CGD, Forsling ML. Hyponatraemia in the first week of life in preterm infants. Part II. Sodium and water balance. *Arch Dis Child* 1984;59:423–9.
244 Khare SK. Neurohypophyseal dysfunction following perinatal asphyxia. *J Pediatr* 1977;90:628–9.

245 Cogan E, Debieve MF, Pepersack T, Abramov M. Natriuresis and atrial natriuretic factor during inappropriate antidiuresis. *Am J Med* 1988;84:409–18.

246 Kamoi K, Ebe T, Kobayashi O *et al.* Atrial natriuretic peptide in patients with the syndrome of inappropriate antidiuretic hormone secretion and with diabetes insipidus. *J Clin Endocrinol Metab* 1990;70:1385–90.

247 Manoogian C, Pandian M, Ehrlich L, Fisher D, Horton R. Plasma atrial natriuretic hormone levels in patients with the syndrome of inappropriate antidiuretic hormone secretion. *J Clin Endocrinol Metab* 1988;67:571–5.

248 Gross P, Lang R, Ketteler M *et al.* Natriuretic factors and lithium clearance in patients with the syndrome of inappropriate antidiuretic hormone. *Eur J Clin Invest* 1989; 19:11–19.

249 Harvey JN, Nagi DK, Baylis PH, Wilkinson R, Belchetz PE. Disturbance of osmoregulated thirst and vasopressin secretion in thyrotoxicosis. *Clin Endocrinol* 1991;35:29–33.

250 Robertson GL. Posterior pituitary. In: Felig P, Baxter JD, Broadus AE, Frohman LA, eds. *Endocrinology and Metabolism*. New York: McGraw-Hill, 1987:338–85.

251 Ahonen P, Myllärniemi S, Sipilä I, Perheentupa J. Clinical variation of autoimmune polyendocrinopathy–candidiasis–ectodermal dystrophy in a series of 68 patients. *N Engl J Med* 1990;322:1829–36.

252 Heijden AJVD, Versteegh FGA, Wolff ED, Sukhai RN, Scholtmeijer RJ. Acute tubular dysfunction in infants with obstructive uropathy. *Acta Paed Scand* 1985;Suppl. 74: 589–94.

253 Poon WS, Mendelow AD, Davies DL, Watson W, Easton J, Morton J. Secretion of antidiuretic hormone in neurosurgical patients: appropriate or inappropriate? *Aust NZ J Surg* 1989;59:173–80.

254 Vingerhoets F, de Tribolet N. Hyponatremia hypo-osmolarity in neurosurgical patients. 'Appropriate secretion of ADH' and 'cerebral salt wasting syndrome'. *Acta Neurochir (Wien)* 1988;91:50–4.

255 Gozal D, Colin AA, Jaffe M, Hochberg Z. Water, electrolyte, and endocrine homeostasis in infants with bronchiolitis. *Pediatr Res* 1990;27:204–9.

256 Kleinschmidt-DeMasters BK, Norenberg MD. Rapid correction of hyponatremia causes demyelination. *Science* 1981; 211:1068–70.

257 Editorial. New treatments for hyponatremia. *N Engl J Med* 1978;298:214–15.

258 Forrest JN Jr, Cox M, Hong C *et al.* Demeclocycline versus lithium for inappropriate secretion of antidiuretic hormone. *N Engl J Med* 1978;298:173–7.

259 Decaux G. Treatment of the syndrome of inappropriate secretion of antidiuretic hormone by long loop diuretics. *Nephron* 1983;35:82–8.

260 Powell KR, Sugarman LI, Eskenazi AE *et al.* Normalization of plasma arginine vasopressin concentrations when children with meningitis are given maintenance plus replacement fluid therapy. *J Pediatr* 1990;117:515–22.

33: Pathophysiology of Diabetes Mellitus

D.J. BECKER and B. WEBER

INTRODUCTION

Diabetes mellitus has been known as a disorder of energy metabolism for a number of centuries, leading to wasting of the body in spite of good nutrition and death without treatment. As early as the 18th and 19th centuries, glycosuria and hyperglycaemia were detected, but it took many years for the wide spectrum of the disorder to be recognized. These range from mild forms seen mainly in older patients, frequently associated with obesity, to much more aggressive diseases developing rapidly and occurring predominately in younger subjects [1]. It is now clear that these various clinical expressions of diabetes mellitus represent a heterogeneous disorder, with a variety of clinical presentations and pathogeneses. These are linked only by the presence of hyperglycaemia and its associated symptoms.

In 1979 and 1980 the National Diabetes Data Group and the World Health Organization classified the clinical syndrome of diabetes mellitus according to pathogenetic criteria, separating primary and secondary diabetes and dividing primary disease into the insulin-dependent (type I) and non-insulin-dependent (type II) entities, frequently abbreviated as IDDM and NIDDM, irrespective of the age at onset [2,3]. This type of classification is merely a marker of insulin therapy (not even insulin requirement) and will soon become outdated. It seems likely that classification according to insulin therapy will be replaced by classification related to specific pathogenesis, such as genetic and autoimmune markers and markers of insulin resistance.

This review will concentrate on type I diabetes (IDDM), which is the most frequent metabolic disorder of children and adolescents, but less frequent forms of diabetes occurring in children, such as secondary diabetes, transitory diabetes and maturity-onset diabetes in the young (MODY), will be included.

EPIDEMIOLOGY OF TYPE I DIABETES

Epidemiological studies have assisted us in understanding the aetiology of IDDM [4]. Although the precise cause is still unknown, both genetic and environmental factors contribute to its development. Improvement of epidemiological ascertainment techniques has allowed fairly reliable comparisons of annual incidence rates on a geographic basis around the world. A recent review of nearly 70 registries from more than 40 countries, to the end of the 1980s, compares the incidence of type I diabetes amongst children under the age of 15 years [5]. There are huge differences, the lowest being in Asia and Mexico City (0.6/100 000 population) and the highest in Finland and Sardinia (35 and 30/100 000, respectively) (Fig. 33.1).

There are clear differences in the incidence between the Northern and Southern hemispheres, with markedly greater incidences being reported in the north. The largest intracontinental variation occurs in Europe, with the highest incidence in Finland and the lowest in northern Greece (4.6/100 000). Although it was previously thought that there was a significant relationship between incidence and distance from the equator [6], this does not hold for the Southern hemisphere. In addition, there are striking exceptions from the overall geographic gradients. For example, Iceland, the northernmost island nation in Europe, has an incidence only one-half of that of Norway and Sweden and one-third of that in Finland. By contrast, Sardinia, off the coast of Italy in southern Europe, has a type I diabetes incidence only slightly less than Finland, and is about three-fold greater than that of southern Europe [5].

The incidence is greater in white people than those of Asian or Afro-American heritage. However, even within these racial groups the diabetes incidence varies geographically, depending on the admixture of the racial groups, which is probably related to diabetogenic genes. Thus, people living in similar geographic areas but with different genetic backgrounds may have very different incidence rates. In contrast, populations with very similar genetic traits but living in different environments seem to have similar risks of developing IDDM. However, this is not always the case, as demonstrated by temporal, almost linear increases in incidence in some populations such as Finland and non-linear epidemic-like variations in other

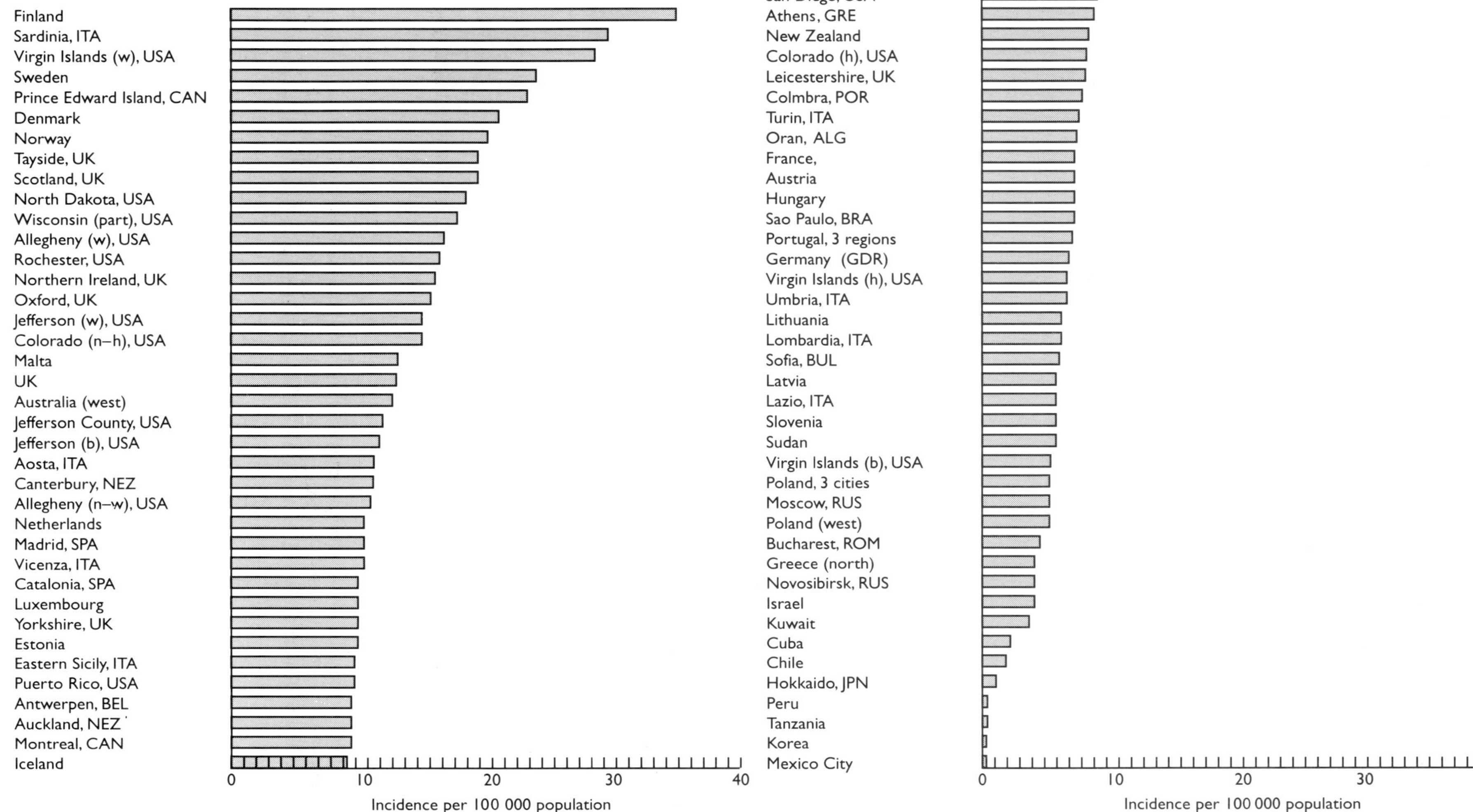

Fig. 33.1 Age-specific incidence (per 100 000 population) of type I diabetes in an age group under 15 years. Data for boys and girls have been pooled. The populations are arranged in an ascending order according to the incidence. ALG, Algeria; BEL, Belgium; BRA, Brazil; BUL, Bulgaria; CAN, Canada; GDR, former German Democratic Republic; GRE, Greece; ITA, Italy; JPN, Japan; NEZ, New Zealand; POR, Portugal; SPA, Spain; ROM, Romania; RUS, Russia; UK, United Kingdom; USA, United States of America; w, white; n-w, non-white; b, black; h, Hispanic; n-h, non-Hispanic (from Karvonen *et al.* [5]).

areas. Superimposed upon this is the well-described seasonal variation in the presentation of IDDM around the world.

In 35 of 68 countries, temporal changes in diabetes incidence have been reported, which do not differ significantly according to age, sex or birth cohort in the populations where this has been carefully studied, with a few exceptions such as Leicestershire in the UK and in New Zealand. In the former, different trends were reported according to age and, in the latter, variations were seen only among white people, not among other racial groups. In this review there was no clear trend in male/female ratio, although some countries reported a slightly increased incidence in males [5]. Previous studies have shown that only 20–50% of patients with type I diabetes are diagnosed under the age of 15 years, although the incidence is highest amongst this age group [7,8]. Within the childhood population the incidence of diabetes increases with age, with only a few cases occurring during infancy and peaking during puberty, slightly earlier in girls than boys [9–17].

GENETICS OF TYPE I DIABETES

Familial occurrence

The familial occurrence of diabetes mellitus has been observed for many centuries. Around 500 BC, Hindu physicians suggested that defects of the parental 'seeds', together with alimentary factors, caused the disorder [18], a concept that is not dissimilar to contemporary thinking.

Although type I diabetes occurs significantly more frequently in first-degree relatives of patients with the disorder than in the general population, studies over the years have shown that the genetic inheritance of type I diabetes is very complicated, and does not follow standard Mendelian transmission, even though dominant [19], autosomal recessive [20,21] and X-linked [22] modes of inheritance have been discussed. Familial data from 60 years ago suggested that the risk of siblings developing this disorder was about nine times higher, and for parents it was four times higher than in the general population [20]. Recent epidemiological data have shown the prevalence among first-degree relatives to be 6% by 18 years of age [23–25]. This increases to 10% by 30 years of age [26]. Current studies suggest that this figure may be higher with increasing age, because a number of milder forms of type I diabetes are incorrectly classified as non-insulin-requiring, but have insulin deficiency and evidence of autoimmune disease. Despite the strong evidence for a familial occurrence of type I diabetes, at least 80% of such patients have no family history of the disorder [4]. The concept that some environmental factor in addition to genetic inheritance plays a role, is supported by the fact that only 34% of monozygotic twins are concordant for type I diabetes [27]. However, the genetic contribution to the aetiology appears to be more potent than that of the environment, in that monozygotic twins have been found to be concordant for diabetes five times more frequently than dizygotic twins [28]. These concordance rates contrast with those of approximately 90% in type II diabetes [29–32].

An exception to the heterogeneous inheritance of type I diabetes is the very clearly dominant form of inheritance of maturity-onset diabetes in the young (MODY). In this form of diabetes, young subjects develop mild glucose intolerance and progress to insulin dependency slowly, and occasionally ketoacidosis [33,34]. This form of diabetes was initially named 'Mason-type' after the first family observed [31], and later known as MODY. Both the mode of inheritance and the clinical course are different from classical type I diabetes. The previously held assumption that a high frequency of facial flushing following alcohol ingestion in chlorpropamide-treated subjects with this disorder might serve as a genetic marker, has not been substantiated [35]. It has now been found that the genetic defect is located in the glucokinase gene in a number of these families, with a resultant decrease in insulin secretion [36].

Human leukocyte antigen markers

Analyses of pedigrees of probands with type I diabetes over the past 15 years led to the discovery of a major role of the major histocompatibility complex, with susceptibility genes mapped to the human leukocyte antigen (HLA) region on chromosome 6 [37–39]. Class I genes (HLA-A, -B, -C) combine with β_2- microglobulin to form transmembrane molecules which are expressed with antigens on the surface of many nucleated cells including cytotoxic T cells. Class II genes are found in three loci on chromosome 6 (DR, DQ and DP). These encode antigens which are expressed on macrophages, B lymphocytes and activated T lymphocytes. These class II molecules bind foreign antigens which are processed by antigen-presenting cells and the antigens are presented to CD4-positive T lymphocytes. The CD4-positive lymphocytes recognize the HLA–antigen complex and this leads to activation of T helper cells and the initiation of an immune response.

The class II molecules are formed by an α and β chain which form heterodimers. The extracellular domains of these heterodimers form the wall and floor of the antigen-binding cleft of the HLA complex known as the Bjorkman groove [40]. The high degree of polymorphism of the HLA genes results in enormous variations in the molecular structure of alleles of each individual. This polymorphism probably determines the interaction between antigens and the T-cell receptor of each individual, and the response of the individual to antigenic stimulation. It appears that specific HLA types confer susceptibility or resistance to type I diabetes. These HLA polymorphisms have been detected by a number of techniques. Initially, serological typing was used, and later cellular typing with mixed lymphocyte cultures was able to define subtypes of class II molecules. Later, biochemical techniques with immunoprecipitation of specific monoclonal antibodies on gel electrophoresis were developed in order to determine variations of the α and β chains. With the advent of DNA technology, molecular variations of the class II genes can be detected. These include restriction fragment length polymorphism (RFLP) and dot–blot analyses of the products of polymerase chain reaction using oligonucleotide probes.

With the development of these techniques the association between the HLA system and type I diabetes has moved beyond class I markers at the B locus (increased frequencies of HLA-B8 and -B15 and decreased frequency of HLA-B7) [37–39, 41–43]. The identification of class II antigens with mixed lymphocyte culture and class II serology has shown that the DR region was more closely associated with type I diabetes, so that associations between the A, B, C and DR regions occurred by linkage disequilibrium. The strongest associations with type I diabetes were found to be with DR3 and DR4 antigens, which are in linkage disequilibrium with B8 and B15, respectively, and the greatest protection was found with DR2, which is in linkage disequilibrium with B7.

In white people over 90% of type I diabetic patients have either a DR3 and/or DR4 antigen, compared with about 40% of controls, giving a relative risk of 3 to 6. The heterozygote DR3/DR4 individuals have the greatest risk of type I diabetes (relative risk more than 14) and they comprise 30–50% of the IDDM population but only 1–6% of the general population. This is in contrast to the relative risk of 3 to 5 for carriers of DR3 alone and 6 to 10 for carriers of DR4 alone, and suggests the possibility that there are two separate susceptibility genes linked to DR3 and DR4 [44–48]. Very similar data are found in the black American population [49], despite a lower incidence of diabetes [14]. In view of the different genetic backgrounds of the black and white populations it has been speculated that diabetes in the black population may be due to 'white gene' admixture. Among 106 pairs of identical twins the concordance rate for type I diabetes was significantly higher in the DR3/DR4 heterozygotes (70%) than in those pairs carrying only one of the alleles (DR3, 42%; DR4, 38%) [50].

In other non-white-skinned populations there are different associations with DR3 and DR4 haplotypes. Associations with DR3 are found in Chinese and Asian Indians but not in Japanese. DR4 associations are seen in Asian populations other than Chinese. In addition, other antigens are seen in IDDM subjects in greater frequency than in the general population, such as DR7 and DR9 in black people, Japanese and Chinese [51,52].

RFLP has allowed the extension of HLA gene mapping from the DR region into the DP and DQ regions [53,54]. These genes code primarily for the production of class II antigens within the DR3 and DR4 haplotypes; there are DQ variations more closely linked to type I diabetes than those in the DR subregion. In the high-risk Finnish population it has been shown that the greatest risk is associated with the presence of both DR4,DQw8 and DR3,DQw2 alleles [55].

Further studies, which involve sequencing of the DQ alleles in IDDM patients and their families showed that the 57th residue of the DQ β chain was closely associated with the presence of type I diabetes, the greatest risk being in those with an alanine, valine or serine in this position, and the least risk in those who are homozygous for aspartate in this position [56,57]. This has led to epidemiological studies suggesting that the presence or absence of aspartate at position 57 of the β chain may explain much of the susceptibility to diabetes around the world [58]. However, this association does not hold for all populations studied, exceptions being found particularly in some non-white populations [51,57]. In addition, the presence of a non-aspartate amino acid at position 57 does not explain the high incidence of diabetes in Finland, or the low incidence in France [59,60].

The addition of studies of the DQ α chain showed an increased frequency of the presence of arginine at the 52nd position in IDDM subjects. This led to the very important association between the DQ α chain arg 52 and DQ β chain non-asp 57 heterodimers and the susceptibility to type I diabetes. Thus, individuals with four high susceptibility residues (homozygous for DQ α Arg 52 and DQ β non-Asp 57) have the highest risk for developing IDDM [61]. The combination of DQ α and DQ β alleles on some DQ haplotypes probably explains the susceptibility to IDDM in a number of populations [52]. The mechanism by which these genetic polymorphisms determine susceptibility to diabetes is not proven. It is highly likely that variations in the amino-acid residues affect the binding and presentation of antigenic peptides by antigen-presenting cells and T cells. The relationship between antigen presentation and recognition and destruction of the β cell is unknown.

The presentation and course of type I diabetes is heterogeneous, even within this disorder. It has been suggested that some of this heterogeneity is determined by the presence of different class I or class II genes. It was initially suggested that there were differences between B8 and B15 carrying individuals in relationship to age of onset, persistence of islet cell antibodies and production of antibodies to exogenous insulin [62]. More recent analyses have shown that DR3 is significantly more frequent in boys than in girls, and the clinical course of diabetes is more severe with a greater likelihood of impaired consciousness, severe dehydration, ketosis and ketoacidosis at onset in patients carrying the DR4 antigen [63]. In addition, carriers of DR3 genes, i.e. more boys than girls, had longer remission periods associated with milder forms of acute disease [45].

Of 205 IDDM children followed from presentation in Berlin, 70% developed partial remission; 78% of these were boys and 62% girls ($P < 0.05$). However, other reports give conflicting results, with the demonstration of higher C-peptide levels in DR4 subjects. In a homogeneous population of 317 IDDM patients in Denmark very little relationship was found between DR types and the clinical presentation and course of the disorder, although there was a greater frequency of DR3/DR4 phenotypes in patients with onset younger than 20 years and in familial cases [47]. Frequency of DR4 was greater in long-term survivors and lower in patients with overt nephropathy [64]. It is interesting that there is a greater risk of the development of IDDM if the DR3 gene is maternal rather than paternal, and the DR4 gene is paternal rather than maternal [65].

The risk of developing IDDM among siblings of diabetic children differs according to the number of HLA haplotypes shared with the diabetic proband, i.e. 10%, 2% and less than 1% for siblings sharing two, one or no haplotypes [25]. Siblings with both DR3 and DR4 haplotypes have a risk of 10%, which increases to 13% if they are identical to the proband and 17% if the DR3 is of maternal origin. By contrast, a sibling who is non-DR3 and non-DR4 has a risk of less than 1% [65]. The risk of IDDM developing in the offspring of a diabetic parent is 3%, but this is greater if the diabetic parent is a father (6%) rather than a mother (2%) [66].

Other gene loci

Because markers in the HLA region have not explained all IDDM disease associations, relationships between the disorder and other gene loci have been continuously sought. It was thought initially that polymorphisms of the insulin gene on chromosome 11 might provide one explanation [67] but this does not seem to be the case. There has been interest in a possible role for complement factors which flank the HLA area and appear to be in linkage disequilibrium with B and DR loci [68]. Although a number of other genes, some of which are located on chromosome 6, have been examined over the years, the most promising is polymorphism of the heat-shock protein which may be important in the presentation of antigenic peptides or may be antigenic in itself [69]. It is also possible that other genes, particularly those related to T cell function, may be involved.

ENVIRONMENTAL DETERMINANTS OF CHILDHOOD DIABETES

Role of viruses

Viral infections have received the greatest attention of the possible environmental agents suspected of playing a causative role in the development of type I diabetes. This is due to the temporal associations between viral infections and the onset of the clinical disease, as well as growing evidence in animal studies that viral infections may directly cause diabetes in susceptible species. It has been suggested that viruses may induce insulin deficiency by two different mechanisms. In the first there is direct damage to an infected β cell; in the second the virus may trigger an autoimmune response by modifying the host antigen or by direct action on the immunoregulatory system including helper or suppressor T cells.

Another possible mechanism of the induction of an autoimmune response is through molecular mimicry, with antibodies being developed against viral antigens which cross-react with normal host cell antigens [70]. In mice the M variant of the encephalomyocarditis virus (EMC) and the Coxsackie B4 virus may induce mild transient diabetic syndromes [71,72]. Many RNA and a few DNA viruses may produce diabetes if the infective dose is large enough and if the animal strain is susceptible [73]. In these animals there is evidence of direct infection of the β cells, resulting in their destruction. The difference between susceptible and non-susceptible mice was demonstrated by the fact that there was twice as much viral attachment to the β cell in the former than the latter. Precise immune mechanisms involved are not clear.

In humans, evidence for a viral association came initially from seasonal variations of the clinical onset of type I diabetes in countries with climate variations or an epidemiological association with viral infection [73]. Early reports of diabetes being precipitated by mumps or mumps vaccination have not been substantiated. There is recent intriguing evidence of an epidemic 2 years after a chickenpox epidemic [74]. There seems little doubt that there is an increased occurrence of IDDM in adolescents and young adults with the congenital rubella syndrome, who may be carriers of the rubella virus for many years [75–78]. The subjects who developed IDDM had a higher prevalence of DR3 and DR4 antigens than the control population, similar to that found in type I diabetes [76,78], and many were found to have islet cell antibodies [76].

Associations with Coxsackie B4 viruses with increased antibody titres have been reported in newly diagnosed IDDM children, often during outbreaks of infection [79–

81]. However, diabetes cannot be a common result of Coxsackie B4 virus infection, since only 20–50% of new IDDM cases show antibody responses [82–85]. It is possible a Coxsackie infection was unable to elicit an antibody response in some patients, mimicking some of the autoimmune abnormalities related to IDDM [86]. Evidence against a role for Coxsackie viruses is the lack of difference in antibody titres between diabetic and non-diabetic individuals of discordant monozygotic twin pairs [42]. Evidence that a Coxsackie virus may be associated with acute IDDM was obtained when a 10-year-old boy died from ketoacidosis and Coxsackie B4 was isolated from pancreatic cultures. This strain inoculated into susceptible mice resulted in the development of diabetes [87]. Two additional case reports support a role for Coxsackie. A 16-month-old child developed diabetes a few days after the onset of a Coxsackie B5 virus infection [88]. In contrast, a role for a direct effect of Coxsackie B virus is questioned by a case of a child who had been shown to be positive for both islet cell antibodies and Coxsackie B antibodies 3 years before the onset of IDDM [89]. Other viruses have been reported to have a relationship to the onset of type I diabetes, and these include cytomegalovirus (CMV), varicella and infectious mononucleosis [73].

Direct invasion of the islets of Langerhans in humans is suggested by histological evidence in the rare patient who dies from the disease. The lymphocyte infiltration of the islets in newly diagnosed patients is reminiscent of a viral infection [90]. Similar histological insulitis has been described in children who have died of severe viral infections [91]. This insulitis may also be a reflection of an autoimmune phenomenon. An autoimmune pathogenesis of viral destruction is suggested by the delayed onset of IDDM in association with the presence of islet cell antibodies after both rubella and Coxsackie B4 infections as stated above. Yoon and co-workers have postulated that there may be a link between CMV infection and type I diabetes [92]. A role for CMV has been suggested by a case of a child with congenital CMV infection who developed IDDM [93] and characteristic inclusion bodies have been found in the β cells of children who died of disseminated CMV infections [94]. Human CMV infection is very common, and the viruses can integrate into the host genome. This has been found in the lymphocytes of about 15% of newly diagnosed IDDM patients who also had islet cell antibodies [92]. However, a larger study in Pittsburgh, which included siblings of IDDM patients, did not confirm a specific role for CMV in diabetes aetiology.

The overall importance of viral infections as causative factors may be limited to the precipitation of the clinical manifestations in subjects who have already lost a major portion of their insulin secretory capacity. There is growing evidence to suggest that the β cell destructive process leading to insulin deficiency and diabetes may continue for many years before the clinical expression of type I diabetes and it is conceivable that IDDM is the manifestation of a process of 'multiple hits' by a number of similar or different viruses, with the last occurring shortly before the manifestation of the disorder which finally decreases the insulin secretory capacity below the threshold for the maintenance of carbohydrate tolerance. It is possible that the injury to the β cells occurs only in susceptible individuals, or in individuals who, for some reason, are unable to repair cellular damage.

Chemical toxins

Other noxious environmental agents may be involved in the pathogenesis of type I diabetes. Alloxan and streptozotocin are well known to induce β cell damage and diabetes in laboratory animals. In humans the accidental ingestion of rodenticide has been reported to induce the development of diabetes [95]. Pentamidine, used for the treatment of infections such as *Pneumocystis carinii* [96], and asparaginase for acute lymphoblastic leukaemia have been found to induce diabetes in some subjects, the former being associated with circulating insulin antibodies.

One of the earliest associations with food was between the ingestion of smoked mutton by mothers in Iceland at the time of conception of their diabetic children [97]. Although this association has not stood the test of time, some animal studies have suggested a role for nitrates which are a component of smoked mutton [98]. The greatest interest has been in a possible association between breast-feeding (or the lack of it) and the incidence of type I diabetes, which was stimulated by an epidemiological study showing an inverse correlation between the incidence of IDDM and breast-feeding practices [99]. Numerous epidemiological studies have since demonstrated inconsistent associations between non-breast milk feeding in infancy and IDDM [100]. The strongest associations between cow milk intake and IDDM are based on ecological data which may have other interpretations [101, 102]. As noted by Kostraba [100], similar associations have been found with coffee and sugar consumption [103,104]. An analysis of peer-reviewed articles, comparing breast milk and cow milk intake in infancy, supports the concept that children with IDDM have earlier exposure to non-breast milk than children without IDDM. However, the odds ratios are weak (< 2) [105] and need to be interpreted with caution [100].

The concept of dietary protein being a trigger for IDDM has been supported by animal studies of spontaneous diabetes in both the BB rat and NOD mouse [106,107]. There are numerous reports of increased antibodies to bovine albumin and β-lactoglobulin in newly diagnosed diabetic children [108–110] and antibodies to a bovine albumin peptide were reported in 100% of Finnish children at the onset of IDDM [111]; this has not been confirmed in other countries. The excitement related to bovine albumin concerns its molecular similarity to a β-cell surface antigen known as ICA69, which has been independently identified in two different laboratories [111,112]. This may be another example of molecular mimicry resulting in antibodies against a foreign antigen targeting endogenous tissue. Prospective epidemiological studies with dietary intervention are needed to prove or disprove the concept of early consumption of cow milk as a trigger for IDDM in humans.

AUTOIMMUNE ASSOCIATIONS

Type I diabetes is frequently associated with autoimmune diseases, such as hyperthyroidism [113], Hashimoto thyroiditis [114,115], pernicious anaemia [116,117], Addison disease [118], vitiligo [119], hypoparathyroidism and myasthenia gravis. Circulating antibodies to thyroid, parietal cells and adrenal tissue have been reported to be increased in patients with IDDM compared to controls, and in IDDM compared to NIDDM subjects, being more common in females than males [116,120–122]. It is now well accepted that type I diabetes or IDDM is an autoimmune disease [123,124]. Evidence for this includes lymphocytic infiltration and possible aberrant HLA molecular expression in the islet of Langerhans, and the presence of circulating autoantibodies to a variety of antigens expressed by the islet cells, as well as cell-mediated immune abnormalities detected in peripheral blood.

Cellular immune reactions

The infiltration of lymphocytes into the islet of Langerhans, described mainly in autopsy material of patients under 20 years of age, is pathognomonic of the diagnosis of IDDM [90]. The insulitis appears to be limited to areas where β cells still contain insulin, and when these cells disappear so does the cellular infiltration. This suggests that the lymphocytic migration is stimulated by the presence of antigens present in functioning β cells [125]. The increasing evidence that an autoimmune process marked by the presence of circulating islet cell antibodies exists for many years before the clinical onset of IDDM suggests that this insulitis may be a long-term phenomenon. This is analogous to the situation described in the spontaneously diabetic NOD mouse, which develops lymphocytic infiltration of the islets at around 6 weeks of age – long before the manifestation of diabetes at 22 weeks [126].

Studies of unfixed pancreatic sections of a newly diagnosed child with type I diabetes enabled the detection of HLA-DR antigens on the surface of 90% of the T lymphocytes, thus qualifying these cells as activated cytotoxic T cells [127] and suggesting that they may contribute to β cell destruction. Histological examination of biopsies of pancreatic segments performed a few months after pancreatic transplantation from unaffected (discordant) monozygotic twins into their diabetic co-twins revealed insulitis with selective destruction of β cells. The infiltrates were mainly composed of cytotoxic T cells [128, 129] which, once activated, may be the effectors of β cell destruction [123].

There is increasing evidence of alterations in the number or function of circulating lymphocytes in newly diagnosed diabetic children and in subjects before the development of IDDM. As early as 1971 a migratory inhibitory factor of blood leukocytes in the presence of pancreatic tissue was reported [130]. Lymphocytes of diabetic children were reported to destroy cultured human insulinoma cells with greater frequency than those of healthy subjects [131]. Passive transfer of diabetes by human lymphocytes into thymic 'nude' mice has been described [132]. Numerous studies over the past decade have described abnormalities of CD4 and CD8 lymphocytes with varying ratios of helper and suppressor T cell activity in IDDM. Although the role of insulin deficiency in producing these changes is not clear, most workers in the field feel that this is unlikely to be contributory [133]. Lymphocytic subset abnormalities have been demonstrated in unaffected family members of IDDM probands with HLA genetic susceptibility gene markers, suggesting an inherited abnormality; some of these abnormalities have been reported to be unrelated to the presence of islet cell antibody [134,135].

The possible role of lymphocytes in the pathogenesis of β cell destruction is supported by stimulation of peripheral blood mononuclear cells from patients with IDDM by islet cells and islet cell antigens, including insulin, 38 kD antigen and glutamic acid decarboxylase [136–139]. The exciting report of stimulation of these cells by bovine albumin [140] could not be reproduced [141].

Autoantibodies

An increasing number of circulating antibodies directed against islet cell antigens have been discovered in patients with type I diabetes. Most have been found in subjects with type I diabetes or their first-degree relatives at high risk for the disorder. Their presence underscores the role of autoimmunity in the pathogenesis of type I diabetes, but their presence does not imply their role in a β cell destructive process, but rather suggests that they are markers of β cell destruction with the release of a number of intracellular antigenic components.

Antibodies directed against exogenous compounds such as bovine albumin suggests an environmental factor may play a role in the pathogenesis of type I diabetes. Possible molecular similarity between a β cell surface antigen

Table 33.1 Environmental agents and β cell autoantigens with molecular homologies

Environmental agent	Autoantigen
Coxsackie B4	GAD
Bovine albumin (ABBOS)	p69
Retrovirus	Insulin
Cytomegalovirus	38 kD
Mycobacterium tuberculosis (HSP65)	Heat-shock protein 60, GAD

GAD, glutamic acid decarboxylase.

suggests that insulitis may be triggered by molecular mimicry between such components. Other examples of this potential type of molecular mimicry between environmental agents and β cell antigens are listed in Table 33.1, which includes a number of currently described autoantigens to which circulating antibodies have been detected. These and some other newly described antigens have been reviewed [142–144]. Apart from the potential importance of these antigens and antibodies in understanding the aetiopathogenesis of type I diabetes, their presence in the circulation is exciting in terms of their potential role in accurate prediction for the development of IDDM in high-risk subjects, with subsequent potential prevention of the disorder.

Cytoplasmic islet cell antibodies

Islet cell antibodies (ICA) were first described in 1974 in IDDM patients who had other coexistent autoimmune diseases [145,146]. ICA are found in 80–90% of newly diagnosed IDDM children [147]. The prevalence of ICA decreases to about 20% after 5 years of diabetes duration and to 5% after 10–20 years [148,149]. The prevalence of ICA in the general population is usually reported to be less than 0.5%, and in about 5% of siblings in whom ICA have been detected many years before the onset of clinical IDDM. This has led to their measurement in order to assess their predictive utility in a number of research studies [150].

ICA are immunoglobulin (Ig)G antibodies mostly of subclasses IgG_1 (70%) and IgG_2 (20%) [148]; about half of them fix complement [148,151], which has suggested that they may have some cytotoxic effects [151]. There are a number of assays using immunohistochemistry or immunofluorescence on a fresh-frozen pancreas substrate, which have been standardized by an international programme with reference values being given in Juvenile Diabetes Foundation (JDF) units [152]. This standardization has not been easy, and the assays are largely used on a research basis.

The antigen target of ICA is not clear, probably because the antibodies react with a number of different antigens within the islet cells. Most ICA-positive sera react not only with the β cells of islets, but also with the α, δ, and pp cells. However, occasionally these immune reactions are restricted to the β cells, in which case the autoantigen appears to be glutamic acid decarboxylase (GAD). This is the type of autoantibody initially described in the stiff man syndrome, and it is not predictive of clinical IDDM in first-degree relatives. This type of ICA is very common in subjects with other autoimmune diseases [143].

Glutamic acid decarboxylase and 64 kD

The first specific islet cell antigen discovered by immunoprecipitation of lysates of islet cells had a molecular weight of 64 000 (64 kD). A number of other fragments (50kD, 40kD, 37kD, and 38kD) have been described [142,143]. Recently, the 64kD antigen was identified as glutamic acid decarboxylase, the GABA-synthesizing enzyme [153]. GAD was found to exist in two molecular-weight forms, GAD 65 and GAD 67, which are encoded by two different genes. The predominant form in the human pancreas is GAD 65, while GAD 67 predominates in peripheral nerves. GAD is found predominantly in the β cells of the islets, and, although its function is not clear, it may play a role in the regulation of proinsulin synthesis and insulin secretion as well as inhibition of somatostatin and glucagon secretion.

Antibodies to GAD have been identified in 20–70% of newly diagnosed IDDM subjects depending on the population and the assay used [143]. International standardization of GAD antibody assays is now under way, because these antibodies have also been detected in ICA-positive first-degree relatives of IDDM probands who have later converted to clinical IDDM. It is hoped that the measurement of GAD antibodies may simplify screening procedures to detect individuals at high risk for developing IDDM. Although the presence of GAD antibodies usually correlates with the presence of ICA, each has been found to exist without the other, which suggests different prognostic implications or variations in assay sensitivity. The former seems the most likely.

Insulin autoantibodies

Insulin autoantibodies (IAAs) were initially described by Palmer *et al.* in about 20% of newly diagnosed untreated IDDM patients [154]. The prevalence in newly diagnosed patients has risen with increased sensitivity of the assays, and IAAs are now shown to occur in about 50% of children, with an inverse relationship to age [155]. IAAs have also been reported in siblings of patients with IDDM, and their detection increases the risk of conversion to IDDM in the presence of high-titre ICA [156].

Surface autoantigens

Islet cell surface antibodies (ICSA) [157], raised much interest because they suggested the presence of surface antigens, which might have been involved in the β cell destructive process. It is now recognized that intracellular antigens can be expressed at the cell surface via the HLA molecules. However, some early data did show that ICSA in newly diagnosed IDDM sera can be cytotoxic to cultured (*in vitro*) islet cells. Assays for ICSA have largely been discarded because of their non-specificity in relationship to the risk of developing IDDM.

MECHANISM OF β CELL DESTRUCTION

Although it is obvious that autoimmunity plays a large role in the pathogenesis of IDDM, the exact mechanism of β cell destruction (Fig. 33.2) remains unknown. Viruses or toxins may have direct cytotoxic effects but environmental agents probably induce an autoimmune response by molecular mimicry. As the destructive process is chronic, there must be either multiple hits from environmental agents and/or a continuously destructive autoimmune process, which eventually overcomes any attempt at islet cell regeneration. Mononuclear cells are thought likely to be the mediators of cellular destruction.

Although the role of antibodies is not clear, the cytotoxic effects of mononuclear cells probably are mediated by cytokine production. Interleukin-1 (IL-1) has been shown to have selective toxicity to β cells [159] and IL-1 receptors have been demonstrated on the surface of β cells [160]. The potentiating effect of tumour necrosis factor α (TNF-α) on IL-1 *in vitro* has led to the Copenhagen model of the pathogenesis of IDDM [161]. The addition of other cytokines, such as IL-6 and γ-interferon, act alone or synergistically to produce islet cell destruction *in vitro*. The action of IL-1 appears to be closely associated with nitric oxide generation, and inhibitors of nitric oxide formation can

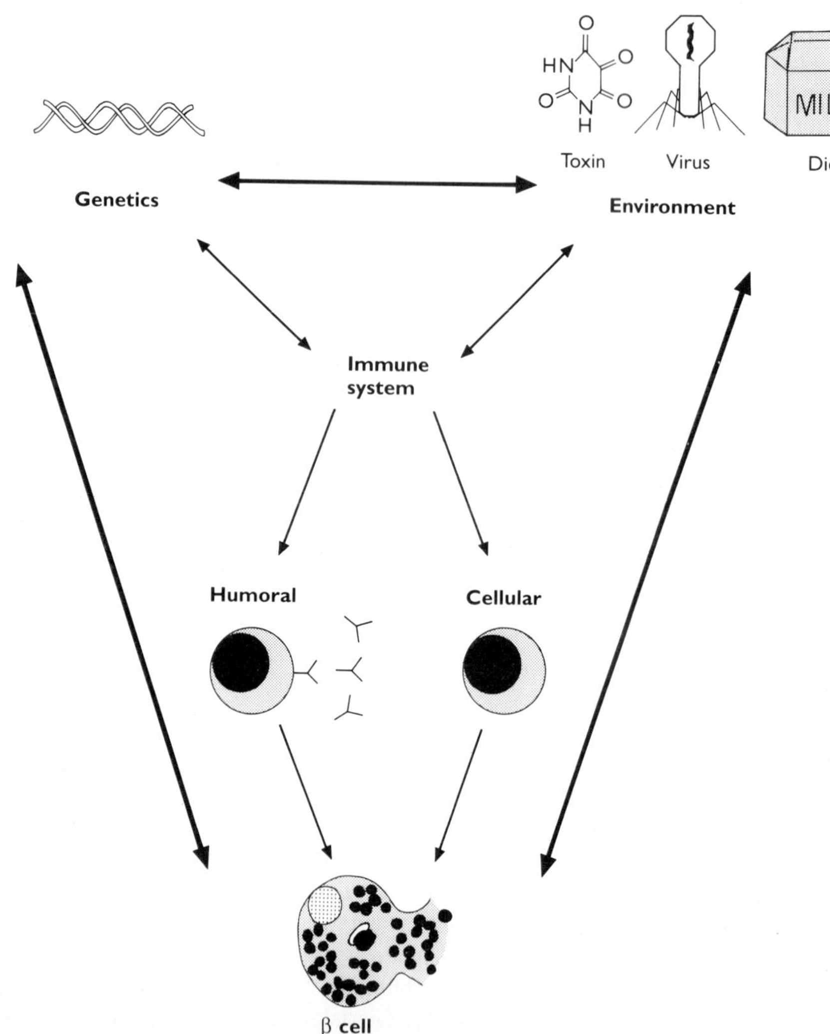

Fig. 33.2 Ubiquitous interplay of nature (genetics) and nurture (environment) and their relationship to diabetes. Roles for both genetics and environment have been established in both animal models and human cases of diabetes. Especially important is the interaction of these two forces with the immune system. In a diabetic individual all of these forces interact in a complex, coordinated and poorly understood way, leading to the destruction of the β cell (from Rossini *et al.* [158]).

decrease the expression of diabetes in animal models. This is thought to be related to oxygen radical release [162].

PREDICTION AND PREVENTION

The importance of understanding the aetiopathogenesis of type I diabetes is that it may lead to strategies for predicting the disorder, with the ultimate goal of prevention of IDDM. The earliest attempt at prediction consisted of the performance of oral glucose tolerance tests with measurements of insulin responses in siblings of children with IDDM [163]. This was the first indication that not all individuals with abnormalities of glucose tolerance progressed to clinical IDDM, and that the best prognostic element was decreased insulin secretion. Because so many factors affect the insulin response to oral glucose, the effectiveness of intravenous glucose stimulation of first-phase insulin secretion was assessed, initially in twins and triplets, and later in first-degree relatives. Most workers agree that there is significant decrease in insulin secretion occurring over varying lengths of time in subjects destined to become diabetic.

It has been suggested that 90% of the insulin secretory capacity has been lost before the clinical manifestation of type I diabetes. This has led to interest in repeated assessment of insulin secretory capacity in subjects at high risk for developing IDDM [164]. Because insulin secretion is related to insulin sensitivity, which is to a large part affected by pubertal status and physical fitness, it is difficult to interpret an individual response to an intravenous glucose tolerance test. However, changes over time, when taken together with the presence of circulating ICA, will probably assist in improving the specificity of predictive methods [150,164]. The basis of screening for subjects at high risk for developing IDDM is dependent on the presence of circulating autoantibodies to islet cell antigens. Standardized ICA assays are currently the commonest primary screen [150,165].

As evidence accumulated pointing to an immune pathogenesis for IDDM, there was an escalation of research studies in animals, and later in humans, aimed at suppression of the autoimmune process. These studies, which had varying degrees of success, started in 1981 with a trial of prednisone in newly diagnosed children [166]. The first intervention that resulted in real insulin independence in humans was the potent immunosuppressive agent cyclosporine, the effectiveness of which in newly diagnosed subjects was shown in two independent studies [167,168]. Unfortunately, this immunosuppressive agent did not induce long-lasting remission and was associated with unacceptable side-effects, including nephrotoxicity.

Other efforts at immune intervention in newly diagnosed IDDM patients and in high-risk subjects with 'prediabetes' have demonstrated varying degrees of effectiveness [169]. Pilot data from nicotinamide studies have suggested that this vitamin may decrease β cell damage by one of two proposed mechanisms. These are related to restoring the NAD content of the damaged β cell, or by acting as a free radical scavenger and thus preserving DNA [169]. Recent reports have suggested that resting the β cell at diagnosis may preserve residual insulin secretory capacity. These, with support from animal experiments, and a small human study of low-dose insulin therapy in prediabetes (which apparently delayed the onset of clinical IDDM), confirm that β cell rest may preserve the secretory capacity of the pancreas [170,171]. This has led to the development of two large national multicentre studies of the prevention of IDDM in high-risk siblings scheduled to begin in 1994 using oral nicotinamide in one and parenteral insulin in the other [169].

PATHOLOGY

Despite methodological difficulties in the evaluation of quantitative pancreatic changes [90], post-mortem studies in subjects who died at the onset of clinical diabetes have shown that 80–90% of the total islet cell mass, which includes islet cell numbers and number of β cells per islet, has been destroyed [90,172]. β cell regeneration from the pancreatic ducts has been observed occasionally. The numbers of glucagon-secreting α, δ and pp cells, which secrete somatostatin and pancreatic polypeptide have been documented to be increased relative to β cell loss [90,173].

Histological changes observed include islet atrophy and fibrosis, nuclear hypertrophy and hydropic changes of individual islet cells. This is associated with the marked lymphocytic infiltration of the islets discussed previously [125,172]. This insulitis, which is typical of type I diabetes, is also found in animal models of spontaneous diabetes, and persists as long as viable β cells are present. The lymphocytic infiltration can be induced in experimental animals by manoeuvres which include injections of insulin, insulin antisera and viral infections [174,175].

HORMONAL ABNORMALITIES

Insulin deficiency is pathognomonic of type I diabetes, resulting in most, if not all, of the biochemical abnormalities. The syndrome can be reproduced by any method of destroying or removing insulin secretory cells. The first proof that insulin deficiency could be reversed in humans came when Banting and Best gave a purified preparation of a pancreatic extract to a juvenile diabetic boy named Leonard Thompson in 1922.

Insulin was the first polypeptide hormone which could be accurately quantitated by radioimmunoassay [177]. The immunoreactive hormone measured is probably identical to the antibody-suppressible insulin-like activity detected previously in biological assays [178]. Insulin assays revealed either low or relatively low basal insulin levels in the face of hyperglycaemia in children with IDDM at diagnosis [179–182]. Insulin responses could not usually be elicited by a variety of insulin secretagogues [180–184], with the exception of intravenous arginine and glucagon when some, albeit subnormal, insulin responses could be elicited [179,185,186]. With the earlier detection of type I diabetes today the severity of insulin deficiency may be less, so that insulin concentrations and the responses to stimuli vary greatly, presumably depending on the degree of total pancreatic destruction. It is therefore not easy to differentiate between typical type I diabetes and MODY by fasting insulin levels [33,187].

After the initiation of treatment with exogenous insulin, endogenous insulin secretion usually increases, although it remains subnormal during the partial remission phase. This can be assessed by measuring levels of C peptide, the molecule co-secreted with insulin by the β cells [171,188,189]. The recovery of insulin secretory capacity of residual or regenerated β cells is thought to be a result of β cell 'rest' [135]. It is possible that insulin therapy decreases the activity of β cells and thus the presentation of antigens on their surface [171]. The recovery of insulin secretory capacity during the remission period depends partially on the degree of pancreatic damage at the time of initiation of therapy and, possibly, on the efficacy of the therapeutic strategies. However, even in patients with apparent insulin independence, insulin responses to stimuli are rarely normal.

Glucagon

Elevated glucagon levels and exaggerated responses to amino-acid stimulation associated with lack of suppressibility by hyperglycaemia, are invariable features of untreated IDDM [4,190–192]. As mentioned above, this is not associated with an absolute increase in the number of α cells, but is secondary to the loss of β cells and insulin insufficiency [193]. Basal circulating glucagon concentrations in IDDM have been reported to be increased [116,194] or within the normal range but excessively high for the degree of hypoglycaemia [191,195]. The hyperglucagonaemia is corrected by adequate insulin treatment, both in the basal state and after arginine stimulation [194].

The increased circulating glucagon levels associated with insulin deficiency led to the hypothesis of a biohormonal pathogenesis of diabetes [193,196]. Glucagon has the opposite effects of insulin on most aspects of carbohydrate metabolism, so that the insulin/glucagon ratio may be as important as the absolute circulating levels of glucagon. In normal individuals protein ingestion increases the molar insulin/glucagon ratio by about 90%, while carbohydrate plus protein ingestion results in an approximate 600% increase [197].

Assimilation and utilization of ingested food requires a predominance of insulin over glucagon secretion, which is achieved by a proportionately greater increase of insulin compared to glucagon following protein, and increased insulin with concomitant glucagon suppression following a carbohydrate load. Starvation, by contrast, requires energy release from body stores through a decrease or reversal of the insulin/glucagon molar ratio. This also occurs during the intracellular starvation associated with insulin deficiency. The glucagon released promotes increased energy supply due to glycogenolysis, gluconeogenesis, lipolysis and ketogenesis. Thus, during insulin deficiency associated with IDDM, there is an increased net hepatic glucose output, with further elevation of blood glucose levels. In addition to mobilizing liver glycogen stores, glucagon also increases liver carnitine concentrations. Both of these actions seem to be prerequisites for maximal hepatic fatty acid oxidation [198,199].

The concept that glucagon is important in the pathogenesis of diabetes is disputed because of the apparently transient effect of experimental hyperglucagonaemia on hepatic glucose output [200,201]. Furthermore, significant hyperglycaemia develops in spite of the removal of pancreatic glucagon following total pancreatectomy [202], thus, insulin deficiency seems to be the prerequisite of the hyperglycaemia of IDDM, and the cause of the elevated glucagon levels [196,200]. This concept is supported by animal research in which both glucagon and insulin were suppressed by somatostatin infusions [203]. Isolated glucagon deficiency resulted in increased glucose production in the face of insulin deficiency. Similar studies in humans with IDDM have demonstrated the additional role of glucagon in the production of hyperglycaemia and ketogenesis in the face of insulin deficiency [204].

OTHER COUNTERREGULATORY HORMONES

Growth hormone

A role for growth hormone in the pathogenesis of diabetes was first suggested by Houssay in 1936 [205]. There is no doubt that, in the face of insulin deficiency, the growth hormone excess associated with acromegaly results in permanent diabetes [206]. Untreated type I diabetic patients have markedly elevated basal and stimulated plasma growth hormone levels [180,207,208], which decrease following effective insulin therapy [209,210]. Normal basal and simulated plasma growth hormone concentrations were found during the partial remission period following the onset of insulin therapy (Fig. 33.3) [215]. Long-term intensive insulin therapy, using subcutaneous

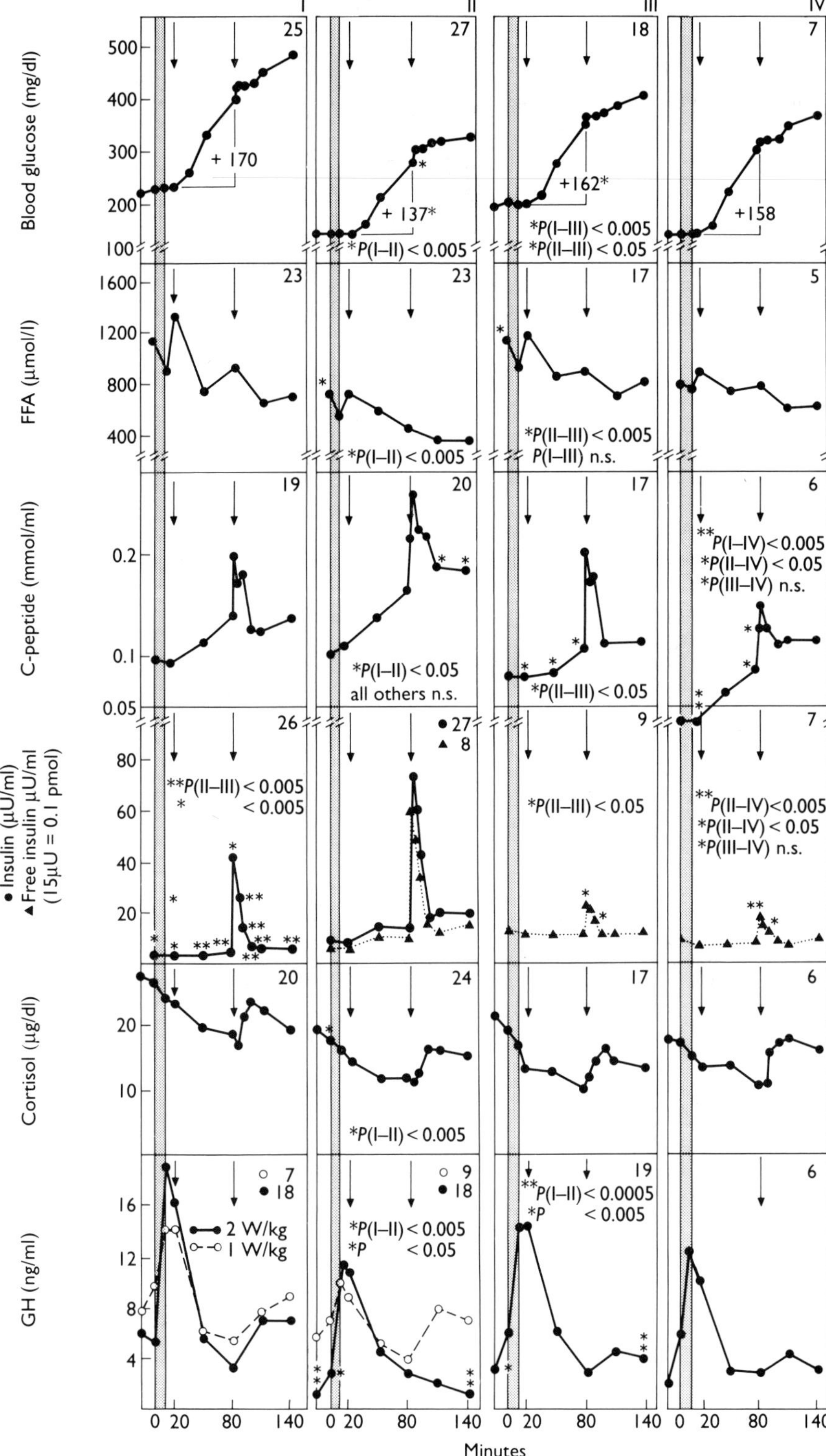

Fig. 33.3 Longitudinal studies of blood glucose (hexokinase), free fatty acids (FFA), C peptide, insulin conventional double antibody radioimmunoassay (RIA), free insulin (polyethylene-glycol extraction [213]), cortisol (RIA) and growth hormone (GH) in non-acidotic insulin-dependent diabetic children and adolescents before therapy (column I), during partial 'remission' after 3–6 weeks (column II), after 1 year (column III), and after 2 years of treatment (column IV).

Note. The test procedure is as follows: 0800–0900 h fasting, no acidosis, no insulin therapy before test I, exercise on a bicycle ergometer (work load either 1 or 2 W/kg body weight, see results on GH) from 0 to 10 min (shaded area on figure), a recovery period in recumbent position from 10 to 20 min, an oral glucose load (1.75 g/kg body weight or 45 g/m^2 surface area) at 20 min (first arrow), and a combined glucagon (20 μg/kg body weight) and tolbutamide (20 mg/kg body weight) i.v. injection at 80 min (second arrow). Glucose + glucagon + tolbutamide loads were considered to represent a maximal stimulation of the β cells.

Results and statistical differences between the different periods (I–IV) are indicated in the graphs. Figures in the right upper corners represent the numbers of subjects studied. Percentages of children exhibiting a maximal response to MST of ⩾20 μU/ml for insulin and free insulin (*c.* 0.13 pmol/ml) and of ⩾0.1 pmol/ml of C-peptide reactivity:

	Insulin	Free insulin	C peptide
I	81%	–	42%
II	100%	88%	65%
III	–	1 of 9	59%
IV	–	1 of 7	2 of 6

insulin infusion, also normalizes growth hormone levels [216], so that patients with well-controlled diabetes have growth hormone levels indistinguishable from normal subjects [217,218]. There appears to be little doubt that growth hormone elevation in IDDM is secondary to insulin deficiency, and may be partially related to decreased metabolic clearance rates rather than hypersecretion [219,220].

Although insulin-like growth factor I (IGF-I) levels have been reported to be normal, low levels, with impairment in 'somatomedin generation' after growth hormone administration in the face of high circulating growth hormone levels, have also been reported [221–224]. Thus, poorly treated diabetes may be an example of a growth hormone-resistant state. In general, the IGF-I levels correlate with current glycaemic control (although not with long-term control as assessed by glycosylated haemoglobin), and are associated with similarly decreased IGF-binding protein levels, although changes in these two polypeptides are not parallel [224]. Thus, decreased IGF-I concentrations cannot be explained entirely by changes in its binding proteins. It therefore seems possible that either a growth hormone receptor or postreceptor abnormality is induced [225,226].

Growth-hormone-binding protein, which probably represents the extracellular moiety of the growth hormone receptor, has been demonstrated to be low in newly diagnosed type I diabetes, with a significant increase at 3 months during the remission period, but this level remained lower than controls. As with IGF-I, the growth-hormone-binding protein correlates with ambient blood glucose but not with glycosylated haemoglobin [227]. This suggests a feedback between growth hormone and IGF-I, via alterations in a growth hormone receptor in the face of insulin deficiency.

Growth hormone excess is known to antagonize insulin-dependent glucose utilization, and influences both adipose tissue lipolysis and ketogenesis [228]. Thus, the increased growth hormone levels described in ketoacidosis may play a role in the genesis of hyperglycaemia and ketosis. Acute interruption of insulin administration results in an immediate increase in growth hormone levels. The importance of growth hormone in contributing to metabolic decompensation is demonstrated by the more rapid increases of glucose, free fatty acids, ketones and glycerol in diabetic subjects with intact pituitaries compared to a group following pituitary ablation [229].

Glucocorticoids

Glucocorticoids stimulate gluconeogenesis and lipolysis and inhibit peripheral glucose utilization [230,231]. In part, the metabolic effects may be induced by a reduction of insulin receptor binding [232]. Both receptor and post-receptor effects on insulin action probably result in the classical increase in plasma insulin levels associated with cortisol excess [233]. Children with untreated IDDM, particularly during ketoacidosis, have elevated plasma cortisol levels [234,235]. However, treated patients have normal basal cortisol concentrations except during hypoglycaemia. The hypercortisolism of ketoacidosis therefore appears to reflect a stress situation rather than a direct effect of insulin deficiency [206].

Catecholamines

The autonomic nervous system is very important in both insulin secretion and action. The sympathetic nervous system, by means of α- and β-adrenergic receptors and the parasympathetic nervous system, are involved in the control of insulin secretion. Both adrenaline and noradrenaline stimulate the α-adrenergic receptors of the pancreas and thereby inhibit insulin secretion [236]. In addition to inducing hyperglycaemia by decreasing insulin concentration, catecholamines further contribute to hyperglycaemia by increasing hepatic glycogenolysis and gluconeogenesis in addition to their effect of lipolysis on adipose tissue. Both the paracrine actions of noradrenaline and increased circulating adrenaline from the adrenal medulla are important [211].

Uncontrolled IDDM is associated with elevated plasma catecholamine concentrations [237,238]. Ketoacidosis induces a marked increase in adrenaline levels, more than those of noradrenaline [228,238]. Increased adrenaline secretion is thought to be induced during severe psychological stress, and may be related to periods of poorer glycaemic control and ketosis in some patients [239]. In these subjects there has been an occasional therapeutic response to β-adrenergic blockade in emotionally labile adolescents with IDDM [239].

Counterregulatory hormones and hypoglycaemia in insulin-dependent diabetes mellitus

Impairment of the normal counterregulatory hormone response (glucagon, adrenaline and pancreatic polypeptide) to acute hypoglycaemia is well documented in adults with long-standing IDDM [240]. Similar decreases in glucagon and catecholamine secretion have been demonstrated in children and adolescents [241,242], with some impairment demonstrable at onset of IDDM [243]. The lack of a glucagon response to hypoglycaemia has been described as an intrinsic α cell defect, because response to arginine remains normal [244]. Although decreased adrenaline responses to hypoglycaemia are characteristic of long-term diabetes both with and without autonomic neuropathy, this does not seem to explain similar deficiencies in short-duration subjects. Acute impairment of adrenaline responses can be induced by intensive insulin therapy, in both adults and children [241,245]. There is increasing evidence that even short-term, relatively mild hypoglycaemia can impair subsequent adrenaline secretion after a hypoglycaemic stimulus, and this impairment is reversible by prevention of hypoglycaemia. Thus, insulin therapy itself may be a cause of both impaired autonomic responses and unawareness of hypoglycaemic symptoms [246,247]. In poorly controlled children with IDDM, adrenaline responses to gradually decreasing plasma glucose levels occurred earlier (at higher plasma glucose concentrations) and the magnitude of the response was higher, compared to non-diabetic children, who in turn showed a greater response than adults [69]. This leads to the speculation that both younger age and poorer glycaemic control may be associated with higher circulating adrenaline levels and contribute to some of the insulin-resistance characteristics of puberty.

PATHOPHYSIOLOGY AND CLINICAL SYMPTOMS

Absolute or relative hypoinsulinaemia constitutes the primary and most important causative factor for the development of the complex metabolic disregulation of type I diabetes. An important contributory role is played by the elevation of the counterregulatory hormones, resulting in an imbalance between energy production, energy use and energy storage.

Insulin is an anabolic hormone. During food absorption it promotes membrane transport and intracellular utilization of glucose, amino acids and potassium [248,249], with resultant stimulation of carbohydrate utilization, protein synthesis and energy storage as glycogen and fat in the liver, muscles and adipose tissue. Hepatic glucose production and adipose tissue lipolysis are inhibited [250]. In the postabsorptive state, low levels of insulin and high concentrations of the counterregulatory hormones induce the necessary shift from glucose utilization to the use of alternative fuels, and from energy storage to energy release. Therefore, insulin deficiency leads to a catabolic state which in part explains the weight loss of untreated and undertreated type I diabetes. This is associated with excessive glycogenolysis, gluconeogenesis from muscle tissue substrates, lipolysis and impairment of protein synthesis.

Increased hepatic glucose output due to glycogenolysis and gluconeogenesis from lactate, pyruvate, glycerol and gluconeogenetic amino acids, together with decreased glucose utilization, results in hyperglycaemia in the presence of intracellular glucopenia in insulin-dependent tissues [251]. It has recently been demonstrated that resistance of carbohydrate metabolism to insulin action, which is reversible by insulin therapy, is a feature of IDDM as well as NIDDM, possibly a glucotoxic effect [252,253]. This insulin resistance is already present in newly diagnosed type I diabetes, and is also described in adolescents with IDDM, in whom it is partially related to physical fitness [254–256].

Hyperglycaemia and glucose excess increase extracellular fluid osmolality and lead to substantial fluid shifts from the intracellular to the extracellular space. With glucose concentrations in excess of 10 mmol/l (180 mg/dl), the maximal reabsorptive capacity of the renal tubules is exceeded, and glycosuria occurs. The consequence of glycosuria is an osmotic diuresis (polyuria) associated with the loss of water and electrolytes, leading to a severe electrolyte imbalance and chronic dehydration, which can only temporarily be compensated for by increased thirst and fluid intake (polydipsia). The daily water loss in diabetic children and adolescents may amount to 3–5 litres, with sodium and potassium loss in the range of 200–400 mmol/l. Urinary glucose excretion may reach 200–300 g/day. This energy loss can be partially compensated by increased hunger and polyphagia, as long as polydipsia does not severely impair food intake. Once this occurs, anorexia associated with wasted energy will aggravate weight loss.

In the face of insulin deficiency, insulin-dependent tissues rely on alternative fuels, other than glucose, for their energy needs. Insulin deficiency results in lipolysis which is accentuated by release of the lipolytic counterregulatory hormones glucagon, growth hormone and adrenaline, with resultant increased circulation of glycerol and free fatty acids. In muscle, free fatty acids can be utilized as an energy substrate and contribute to decreased glucose utilization [257], which constitutes the glucose–fatty acid cycle. Severe insulin deficiency, together with an elevation of the counterregulatory hormones, supplies abundant free fatty acid substrate for conversion to ketones with hepatic fatty acid oxidation and conversion to acetyl-CoA (co-enzyme A). The increased glucagon concentrations associated with insulin deficiency support ketogenesis, supplying the ketones that can be used by muscle and brain [198,199]. Because the oxidation of acetyl-CoA in the citric acid cycle is rate-limited, condensation to acetoacetate and β-hydroxybutyrate occurs. When excess ketone bodies are produced, the body's buffering and excretory capacity by the lungs and kidneys are overcome, and ketoacidosis ensues. Dehydration associated with hyperosmolarity, acidosis and electrolyte imbalance causes most of the presenting features of severe IDDM, including probable decreased cerebral oxygen utilization, decreased consciousness and coma.

A deficiency of the action of insulin on protein metabolism explains the loss of muscle mass and muscle weakness seen in IDDM patients with prolonged insulin deficiency. Insulin is important in the uptake of amino acids, especially the branched-chain amino acids, leucine, isoleucine and valine, into muscle. Insulin deficiency results in increased muscle turnover of these amino acids and decreased protein synthesis supplying amino acids, especially alanine, as gluconeogenetic precursors. Thus, protein catabolism contributes to the hyperglycaemia of IDDM.

CLASSIFICATION OF DIABETES MELLITUS IN CHILDHOOD AND ADOLESCENCE

The majority of patients who become diabetic during the first two decades of life fall into the category of type I, insulin-dependent, ketosis-prone diabetes associated with an abrupt clinical onset and relatively rapidly decreasing endogenous insulin reserve. The clinical spectrum of juvenile diabetes, however, also encompasses milder forms with slower onset, long remission periods with low insulin requirements and syndromes similar to maturity-onset diabetes, treatable with oral agents. The autosomal dominant MODY form also may not require insulin for long periods of time [34].

Obesity is a rare cause of diabetes during childhood and adolescence. However, it may be associated with glucose intolerance in about 25% of patients [184,258]. Diabetes is more frequent in insulin-resistant syndromes, which include acanthosis nigricans and polycystic ovarian disease [259]. The obesity associated with the Prader–Willi syndrome is very often associated with non-insulin-dependent diabetes. Another genetic form of childhood diabetes is associated with the syndrome of diabetes insipidus and optic atrophy (DIDMOAD syndrome) [260]. Secondary forms of diabetes in childhood are associated with cystic fibrosis, muscular dystrophy, pancreatitis, hormonal excess and drug therapy, particularly in the treatment of leukaemia [261,262].

The World Health Organization (WHO) classification of 1985 [3], separates secondary diabetes with carbohydrate intolerance and clinical abnormalities from subjects in a 'statistical risk class' and subjects with classical IDDM or type I diabetes. Insulin-dependent diabetes may or may not be autoimmune, but by definition requires insulin for control of postprandial hypoglycaemia. The WHO classification (Table 33.2) will probably require revision in future years with increasing understanding of the pathogenesis of different forms of IDDM. The current WHO definitions of diabetes and impaired glucose tolerance are depicted in Table 33.3. Impaired glucose tolerance is reversible, but represents a stage with high risk for the development of permanent diabetes, although this is by no means universal [263]. However, a number of children and adolescents with transient glucose intolerance, especially if associated with insulin deficiency, do develop permanent type I diabetes months or even years later [163].

Table 33.2 Classification of diabetes mellitus and allied categories of glucose intolerance

Clinical classes of diabetes mellitus
Insulin-dependent diabetes mellitus
Non-insulin-dependent diabetes mellitus
  Non-obese
  Obese
Malnutrition-related diabetes mellitus
Other types of diabetes associated with certain conditions and syndromes: (1) pancreatic disease; (2) disease of hormonal aetiology; (3) drug-induced or chemical-induced conditions; (4) abnormalities of insulin or its receptors; (5) certain genetic syndromes; (6) miscellaneous
Impaired glucose tolerance
  Non-obese
  Obese
  Associated with certain conditions and syndromes
Gestational diabetes mellitus

Statistical risk classes: subjects with normal glucose tolerance but substantially increased risk of developing diabetes
Previous abnormality of glucose tolerance
Potential abnormality of glucose tolerance

CLINICAL PRESENTATION

The early clinical features depend on the presence of hyperglycaemia resulting in polydipsia, polyuria and nocturia with the reappearance of nocturnal enuresis, especially in younger children. The energy wasting results in polyphagia, weight loss and decreased energy. Longer duration of severe insulin deficiency is associated with

Table 33.3 Definitions of diabetes and impaired glucose tolerance by the World Health Organization (glucose concentrations in mmol/l (mg/dl))

	Whole blood		Plasma	
	Venous	Capillary	Venous	Capillary
Diabetes				
Fasting	≥ 6.7 (120)	≥ 6.7 (120)	≥ 7.8 (140)	≥ 7.8 (140)
2 h after 75 g glucose	≥ 10.0 (180)	≥ 11.1 (200)	≥ 11.1 (200)	≥ 12.2 (220)
Impaired glucose tolerance				
Fasting	< 6.7 (120)	< 6.7 (120)	< 7.8 (140)	< 7.8 (140)
2 h after 75 g glucose	6.7–10.0 (120–180)	7.8–11.1 (140–200)	7.8–11.1 (140–200)	8.9–12.2 (160–220)

dehydration and acidosis, and later decreasing level of consciousness. Clinical signs appear only under these circumstances, and include dry mucous membranes, decreased skin turgor, muscle and subcutaneous tissue wasting, Kussmaul breathing with a fruity odour of ketones and hepatomegaly. The detection of glycosuria, ketonuria and hyperglycaemia confirms the diagnosis. The clinical presentation will depend partly on the patient's original body composition as well as the duration and severity of insulin deficiency. Symptoms are almost always present, and their elicitation depends on the astuteness of parents and the competence of physicians. The longer the diagnosis is delayed, the more severe is the patient's impairment of health.

Reports of ketoacidosis at presentation vary from a small number to 30% around the world, even in countries with reportedly highly developed medical care. The duration of clinical symptoms before diagnosis varies from a few days to several months. The history appears to be shorter in younger children. Children with longer duration of symptoms may have more severe weight loss and cachexia at the time of diagnosis. It has been suggested that variations in the severity and duration of the prodrome, and a longer remission period after diagnosis, may represent different forms of IDDM related to variations in insulin reserve [264,265].

When patients present with clinical symptoms, the diagnosis of diabetes can be made by either an elevated fasting and 2-h postprandial value or two postprandial blood glucose values elevated according to the definitions in Table 33.3. Hyperglycaemia in the presence of ketones also confirms the diagnosis. However, when clinical symptoms are absent and there is no hyperglycaemia, an oral glucose tolerance test with measurement of insulin responses may be required to confirm or exclude the diagnosis under certain circumstances; for example the serendipitous finding of glycosuria. The standard test remains the administration of a glucose load of 1.75 g/kg to a maximum of 75 g [266]. This does is controversial because amounts given according to body surface area may be more appropriate physiologically allowing for relatively greater glucose loads in early childhood and smaller doses in larger adolescents. Different doses have been recommended over the years, but it appears that 30 g/m^2 surface area is probably too small [267], and 60 g/m^2 too high [268]. The International Study Group of Diabetes in Children and Adolescents (ISGD) agreed on a dose of 45 g/m^2 [269], although this dose has not been tested in prospective studies.

EARLY CLINICAL COURSE

After the initiation of insulin therapy and reversal of the initial metabolic derangement, about two-thirds of children and adolescents with IDDM experience a period of easily achievable metabolic control, with absence of clinical symptoms of hyperglycaemia, relatively low insulin requirements and glycosylated haemoglobin levels close to or within the normal range. This 'honeymoon period' represents a temporary partial remission of the metabolic disorder, and is associated with the recovery of pancreatic insulin secretion (see Fig. 33.3). The frequency and degree of this remission depends on age, sex and severity, and on duration of symptoms at diagnosis, all of which reflect residual β cell reserve. The intensity of initial insulin therapy, with rest of the β cells, may affect the degree and duration of the remission period [171].

Only 2% of IDDM children and adolescents remain asymptomatic with no insulin therapy during this time [270], and most of them do not have normal glycosylated haemoglobin levels. Using the definition of the ISGD (absence of clinical symptoms and insulin doses less than 0.5 U/kg with minimal glycosuria for more than 4 weeks [271]), 70% of 205 patients under 17 years of age in Berlin experienced temporary partial remission, with a greater frequency in boys (78%) than girls (62%: $P < 0.05$). Remission was more frequent in those who presented without ketoacidosis (73%) compared to those with ketoacidosis (55%: $P < 0.05$) [265]. This remission period is associated with an increase in C-peptide secretion, which is more prominent in older subjects [272], and improved insulin sensitivity [256]. With the advent of blood glucose monitoring techniques, very few patients have been found to maintain euglycaemia without some exogenous insulin administration. The current concept of resting the β cells has stimulated a number of paediatric diabetologists to continue at least a low-dose insulin delivery, even in those subjects who apparently do not require it. As previously discussed, during the remission period glucose tolerance and insulin responses to stimulation remain abnormal, although markedly improved compared to pretreatment levels [188,189,265,273–276].

The end of the remission period is marked by a gradual or rapid increase in insulin requirements. This period is associated with decreased insulin secretory capacity and is often precipitated by intercurrent infections. Thereafter, there is a progressive increase in insulin requirements, which peaks during puberty and decreases subsequently so that the average adult insulin dose is significantly lower than that of children and adolescents. Adolescents require more insulin (about 1.2 U/kg per day) than preadolescents (0.8–1 U/kg per day); this is partly related to the relative insulin resistance associated with puberty in both non-diabetic and diabetic adolescents [254]. This insulin resistance may be associated with increased secretion of growth hormone and catecholamines, as well as sex hormones, during this time. Although insulin doses were consistently higher in girls than in boys in older studies [270], current experience with the availability of home glucose monitoring, and glycosylated haemoglobin evaluation, has shown that adolescent boys may require as much as 2 U/kg per day during their growth spurt.

Any stress situation such as intercurrent illness and possibly emotional stress, will also temporarily increase insulin requirements as a result of increased secretion of the counterregulatory stress hormones (see above). Acute increases in insulin requirement are associated with the dawn phenomenon and the Somogyi effect.

The dawn phenomenon is defined as increasing circulating glucose concentrations between 0500 h and 1000 h in the absence of preceding nocturnal hypoglycaemia [277]. This has been reported in patients with both IDDM and NIDDM as well as in non-diabetic individuals. It is associated with increasing insulin requirements and is due either to increased insulin clearance and/or decreased insulin action. The pathogenesis of this early-morning hyperglycaemia is thought to be related to the nocturnal sleep-related rise in growth hormone secretion, which is particularly prominent in adolescents [278]. One advantage of insulin delivery using a subcutaneous insulin infusion pump is that the pump can be programmed to increase insulin delivery automatically after 0400 h in order to prevent this early-morning rise in blood glucose.

The Somogyi effect is defined as post-hypoglycaemic hyperglycaemia, and is believed to be due to insulin resistance associated with the rise of counterregulatory hormones stimulated by hypoglycaemia [279]. Although there is some controversy as to whether this phenomenon actually exists [280], recent studies in adults have shown that hyperglycaemia does follow hypoglycaemia which is associated with food intake [240,277]. By contrast, hyperglycaemia has not been demonstrable after the induction of nocturnal hypoglycaemia which is allowed to recover spontaneously in adults. This situation has not been studied in childhood and may be different from adults since counterregulatory hormone deficiency in response to hypoglycaemia is not as severe in this age group.

ACUTE METABOLIC DERANGEMENTS

Ketoacidosis

Although ketosis is common during the course of therapy of IDDM in association with increased insulin requirements during illness, or in response to acute hypoglycaemia, the development of diabetic ketoacidosis (DKA) should be completely preventable once diabetes has been diagnosed. The development of DKA in a known diabetic patient is a clear treatment failure. Although DKA is often associated with increased insulin requirements due to the stress of infection or emotional instability, it is usually due to inadequate or total omission of insulin delivery, as reflected by very low circulating free insulin levels in patients at presentation. The acute interruption of insulin delivery or the induction of stress is rapidly associated with an increase in the secretion of counter-regulatory hormones with subsequent mobilization of fat and ketogenesis. Ketone body formation often precedes hypoglycaemia. The degree of hyperglycaemia is dependent on associated food intake [228].

Both insulin deficiency and acidosis result in the movement of potassium from the intracellular to the extracellular space, with subsequent renal potassium loss and total-body potassium deficiency. Hypophosphataemia is induced by similar mechanisms and may result in a delay in the recovery of red cell 2,3-diphosphoglycerate levels induced by acidosis, thus inhibiting oxygen delivery to tissues, including the brain [281]. This may in part explain changes in the level of consciousness associated with DKA.

Both hyperglycaemia and insulin deficiency result in urinary sodium loss. In addition, hyperglycaemia, with its associated intravascular osmolality, results in a shift of sodium from the extracellular to the intracellular space [282]. Total-body sodium depletion and dehydration stimulate the secretion of aldosterone and antidiuretic hormone, and further urinary potassium losses [283].

Hypoglycaemia

Hypoglycaemia is caused by the absolute or relative excess of circulating insulin. This may be due to excessive insulin administration or, more frequently, insufficient food to cover exogenously administered insulin associated with a delay of meals or increased energy utilization by exercise. The symptoms and signs of hypoglycaemia result from stimulation of the autonomic nervous system or are of neuroglycopenic origin.

The earliest and commonest autonomic symptoms include shakiness, sweating, tremor, anxiety, palpitations and hunger, which are often associated with pallor. Most of these are mediated by adrenaline and noradrenaline, except for sweating and maybe hunger, which are induced by cholinergic neurons. Neuroglycopenic manifestations vary from relatively mild cognitive dysfunction to seizures and coma, and occasional transient focal paralysis. It appears that children may be somewhat more sensitive to mild hypoglycaemia than has been described in adults. Neuropsychological testing during very mild hypoglycaemia (3.3 mmol/l) has shown clear transient cognitive impairment with or without recognizable symptoms [284]. Although most physicians do not consider hypoglycaemia to be severe unless the blood glucose concentration is less than 2.2 mmol/l, the chemical changes in terms of counterregulatory hormone secretion occur at much higher glucose concentrations, unless there is impairment of counterregulatory hormone secretion [69]. Glucose is the major source of fuel for the brain and, under acute hypoglycaemic conditions, adaptation of fractional glucose extraction from the blood stream has not yet occurred. In addition, relative insulin excess prevents ketogenesis, so that the only alternative fuel source for the brain (ketones) is limited. In prolonged or repeated hypoglycaemia there presumably is some form of adaptation of the central nervous system, and the severity of symptoms and glycaemic thresholds for counterregulation are markedly diminished [246].

As described previously, abnormalities of hypoglycaemic counterregulation are very frequent in individuals with IDDM. Although responses in children are often markedly diminished, they are rarely absent, as has been reported in adults [241,242]. Failure of hypoglycaemic counterregulation is probably a cause of severe or recurrent hypoglycaemia, usually associated with hypoglycaemia unawareness, that is absence of autonomic systems. This syndrome of hypoglycaemia unawareness increases in frequency with the intensity of insulin therapy, and correlates inversely with the level of glycosylated haemoglobin [246,285]. Thus the tighter the glycaemic control, the more frequent are mild and moderate episodes of hypoglycaemia, which in turn appears to induce hypoglycaemia unawareness and impaired counterregulatory responses [246]. The coincidence of the introduction of human insulins to therapeutic practice together with an increasing emphasis on tight blood glucose control was unfortunate. An increased understanding of the hypoglycaemia unawareness problem makes it highly unlikely that the human insulins are directly responsible for this phenomenon as many patients have suspected. It is far more likely that the increased hypoglycaemia associated with the therapeutic regimes used increase the frequency and severity of hypoglycaemia unawareness amongst those children and adults with IDDM.

The frequency of moderate or severe hypoglycaemia in children with IDDM varies between 4% and 6% [286,287]. However, nocturnal asymptomatic hypoglycaemia is far more frequent and occurs in at least 30% of children during conventional therapy, which is similar to a study reported in adults with IDDM [288].

Infection

Poorly controlled IDDM is associated with increased susceptibility to infection, particularly of the skin, vagina and urinary tract. Bacterial infections occur 5–10 times more frequently in diabetes than in the general population. Girls have an increase in the prevalence of vulvovaginal *Candida* infections [289], as well as an increased incidence of pyelonephritis and cystitis [290]. There have been numerous studies demonstrating defects in the cellular defence mechanisms against bacterial infection. These include a variety of abnormalities of leukocyte function, such as adhesion to the endothelium, migration, chemotaxis, phagocytosis and bacteriolysis [291–296]. In addition, quantitative humoral immune deficiencies against bacterial infections have been detected [297]. All these are influenced by metabolic control, so that well-insulinized patients do not have an excessively greater frequency of infection. Both hyperglycaemia and insulin deficiency have been thought to play a pathogenic role.

INTERMEDIATE COMPLICATIONS

Growth and maturation

Short stature and poor growth are classical features of insulin deficiency [298]. The role of insulin deficiency as opposed to genes is particularly obvious when monozygotic twins were evaluated [299]. Variations of height at the onset of IDDM probably reflect the duration of prior severe insulin deficiency. Height at the onset has been reported to be normal, greater or less than average [300,301] and these height variations are age-dependent [302,303]. Children between the ages of 5 and 9 years were taller, and pubertal children shorter than their siblings and population standards.

Although reports of decreased growth velocity persist even in the current literature, this appears to be related to underinsulinization and poor metabolic control [300,302]. Patients who are well insulinized and in fairly good metabolic control have normal growth velocity [304,305]. Catch-up or even excessive growth, has been reported in adolescents treated with subcutaneous insulin infusion, proving that the growth failure of IDDM is related to insulin deficiency [216]. This study raises the possibility that growth excess could be induced by excessive insulin delivery similar to that induced by fetal hyperinsulinaemia. Greater experience with intensified insulin therapy over time will be needed to assess this possibility. In contrast, slower linear growth has been recorded during the remission phase of the disease, in spite of adequate treatment and excellent glycosylated haemoglobin levels. This may partially be related to the 'catch-down phenomenon' in subjects who were initially taller than expected. However, the exact mechanism is not clear [300,301, 306].

The extreme form of growth failure in diabetic children who have been underinsulinized for many years is associated with hepatomegaly, thickened skin, a Cushinoid-like appearance and retardation of sexual maturation. This syndrome of diabetic dwarfism or Mauriac syndrome [307,308] is now rarely seen in developed countries. Although these subjects may appear to be hypothyroid or growth hormone deficient, thyroid hormones and growth hormone levels are normal or even increased [309,310].

Delayed puberty was also frequently reported in the older literature in both boys and girls [301,305,311]. However, recent experience suggests that pubertal maturation and menarche are normal in well-controlled patients. However, menstrual irregularities are fairly typical of postmenarcheal girls in poor control. Abnormalities of sexual maturation and function occur throughout the hypothalamopituitary–gonadal axis [312]. Gonadotrophins have been shown to be low, with decreased luteinizing hormone (LH) responses to gonadotrophin-releasing hormone (GnRH) stimulation. In males this is associated with decreased testosterone and sex-hormone-binding globulin levels [312].

Skin and joints

In the mid-1970s, attention was focused on rather frequent, painless joint stiffness starting in the fifth fingers and limiting the extension of the proximal interphalangeal joints with subsequent extension to other joints of the same and other fingers. Later, larger joints, as well as the spine, could be involved [313]. Although rarely reported, very severe clinical expression of this entity is associated with impairment of hand function with some deformity and radiological abnormalities. It is associated with thick, tight and waxy skin, and is seen frequently in Mauriac syndrome. This syndrome, known as 'limited joint mobility', involves periarticular collagen tissue. Its pathogenesis is probably related to glycosylation of collagen [314]. The prevalence of this syndrome is related to glycaemic control in subjects with fairly long duration of IDDM [315]. No association has been found with the HLA system. Severe degrees of limited joint mobility have been associated with microvascular disease [315,317], but no association with milder forms was noted [315].

Specific skin lesions with unknown pathogenesis are found among young female diabetics. This entity, necrobiosis lipoidica diabeticorum, is characterized by gradually increasing coin-size to palm-size, painless, dark patches of cutaneous and subcutaneous necrosis, located mostly on the legs, particularly the shins. Each individual spot starts as a painless, purple discoloration which grows rapidly and atrophies from the centre. Since these spots are painless, the major disability is cosmetic, but they may become secondarily infected. The lesions do not appear to be related to the degree of metabolic control. The condition is usually self-limiting and no local therapy has been effective. Presumably the lesions are due to alterations of the local vascular system, but further details are not known [318].

Intellectual changes

Although permanent electroencephalogram (EEG) changes are associated with hyperglycaemia at the onset of IDDM [319], IQ of children and adolescents with IDDM has been reported to be normal [320,321]. Sensitive neuropsychological tests do show impairment of cognitive function in children with IDDM, especially in those with onset before 5 years of age [322,323]. Retrospective analyses suggested that this cognitive impairment correlated with a history of severe hypoglycaemia in these younger children. However, in the recent Diabetes Control and Complications Trial (DCCT), intensive diabetes therapy, which induced a greater frequency of severe hypoglycaemia, was not associated with any permanent change in cognitive function [285].

Cataracts

Although cataracts in childhood are not common, they are seen regularly in children at onset or with poor metabolic control. The commonest is the 'sugar cataract', which usually appears during therapy of ketoacidosis. These cataracts are thought to be due to an abnormality of an osmotic mechanism in the lens. They usually disappear rapidly with correction of ketoacidosis, but they may persist for months with the development of dense white opacities requiring surgical removal. The 'juvenile cataract' occurs later during the course of the disorder and is thought to be associated with the accumulation of sorbitol in the lens. These cataracts, which are subcapsular, are associated with decreased aldose reductase activity and always require surgical removal [324].

CHRONIC COMPLICATIONS

The chronic complications of IDDM have their subclinical onset during childhood and adolescence. They are thought mainly to be the result of a specific angiopathy affecting both the microvasculature and macrovasculature. The complications constitute the most severe threat to the ultimate physical health of the IDDM patient, and may severely impair life expectancy. Although macrovascular disease usually develops over long periods of time [325], peripheral vascular obstruction with gangrene has been reported in a child [290]. Asymptomatic arterial calcification has been observed in juvenile diabetics less than 20 years of age, with increasing prevalence with increasing age and duration of disease [326].

Microangiopathy is the most common chronic complication of IDDM, and affects the small vessels in multiple organs, including the eyes, kidneys, peripheral and autonomic nervous system, skin, heart and joints. These microvascular complications are clearly associated with diabetes duration and ultimately result in the classical triad of retinopathy, nephropathy and neuropathy. Microangiopathic changes may present in childhood and adolescence, but they seem to be becoming less frequent under 20 years of age. This impression is supported by a recent report of a declining incidence of nephropathy in IDDM with onset before 15 years of age [327]. The role of insulin deficiency in the pathogenesis of these complications is demonstrated by reports of identical microangiopathy occurring in patients with diabetes secondary to pancreatectomy [328]. There is ample evidence that vascular lesions do not occur in the absence of hyperglycaemia [329]. In spontaneously diabetic animals, increases in capillary basement membrane thickness are observed only after the onset of diabetes [330,331]. Although genetic factors have been thought to determine the degree of basement membrane thickening in some patients [332], genetically identical subjects, such as twins and triplets, may be discordant for both diabetes and microangiopathy for many years [333,334]. Thus, familial clustering of diabetes complications may partially be due to environmental factors, such as smoking, diet and physical activity [324].

Pathogenesis of microvascular disease

A number of hypotheses exists regarding the mechanisms that produce microvascular abnormalities in various tissues. The commonest, and currently the most plausible of these, is the 'glucotoxic theory' which suggests that all complications are related to chronic hyperglycaemia. Other pathogenic factors which appear to be additive include rheostatic and haemodynamic factors including hypertension, hormonal changes, lipid abnormalities as well as genetic and environmental factors (Fig. 33.4). The recent results of the DCCT, demonstrating that intensive diabetes therapy with resultant improvement of glycaemic control can prevent or delay the onset of micro-

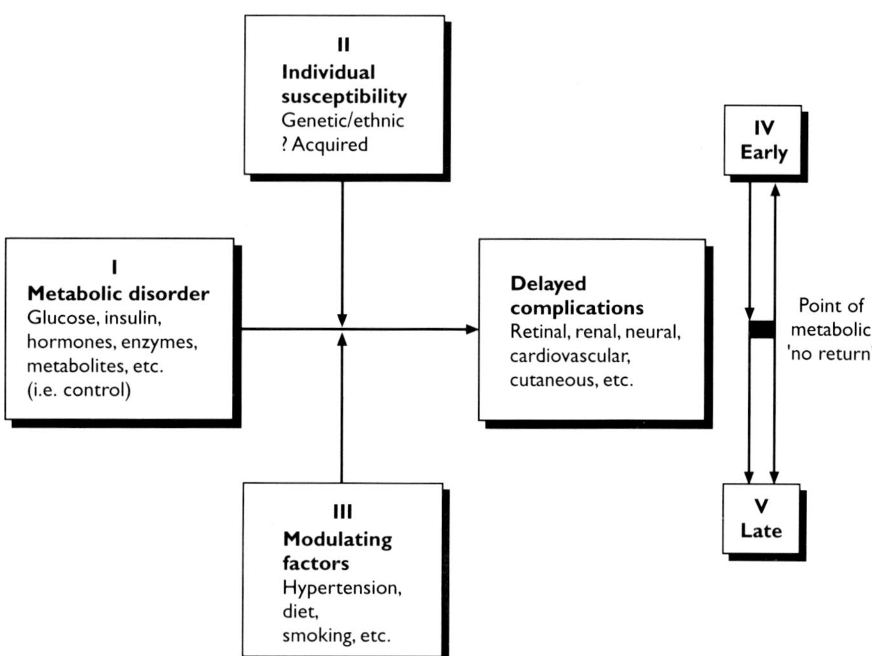

Fig. 33.4 Pathogenesis of microvascular disease. The principal determinant is inadequate correction of the metabolic disorder itself (I), acting via hyperglycaemia, with or without the associated abnormalities of insulin and other hormones (e.g. growth hormone, somatomedins, glucagon, etc.); enzymatic pathways (e.g. aldose reductase, gluconeogenic enzymes, etc.); and substrates or metabolites (e.g. free fatty acids, lactate, 2,3-diphosphoglyceric acid, etc.). This metabolic complex interacts with the susceptibility status (II) of the individual patient, at present of uncertain nature, although studies of twin pairs suggest a genetic component and some youthful-onset type II (MODY) cases may inherit resistance to complications. Several independent modulating factors, environmental or genetic (III), may influence the time of appearance, rate of development, and/or ultimate severity of complications; some of these (e.g. hypertension, smoking) may be reversible. The progression of complications from their earliest (IV) manifestations (e.g. retinal microvascular hyperpermeability, microalbuminuria) to the late (V) stage of severe tissue or organ damage (e.g. proliferative retinopathy/blindness, heavy proteinuria/end-stage renal failure) is also partly determined by inherent susceptibility factors, by other modulating factors, and, up to the point of metabolic 'no return', by the degree of diabetic control (from Keen [335]).

vascular complications, lend support to the importance of the glucotoxic role [285,336].

Glucotoxic and polyalcohol hypothesis

There is a large amount of epidemiological evidence to support the role of glycaemic control in the development of microvascular complications of IDDM [337]. This is supported by a variety of animal studies [338,339]. It has been suggested that the greater the extracellular concentration of glucose, the higher the influx into both insulin-dependent and non-insulin-dependent tissues [340–342]. The accumulation of glucose in these tissues results in the increased production of sorbitol by the polyol pathway, which has been demonstrated in lens, nerve tissue and red blood cells [343] and of fructose in lens, nerves and semen. The accumulation of sugar alcohols, like sorbitol in diabetes or galactitol in galactosaemia, is thought to be responsible for swelling of the lens and cataract formation [340]. Although controversial, the polyalcohol pathway appears to be related to the decreased myoinositol content associated with hyperglycaemia in nerve tissue [344–347]. These abnormalities result in decreased Na,K,ATPase [348] and are blocked by the administration of an aldose-reductase inhibitor [346]. The oral administration of myoinositol appears to restore its content in nerve tissue in both rats and humans, improving nerve conduction [347]. Recently, the accumulation of polyalcohols in the rat model was prevented by castration, suggesting an influence of sex hormones [349].

Glucose toxicity and tissue glycosylation

A major mechanism by which hyperglycaemia can alter tissue proteins is by non-enzymatic glycosylation. This Amadori reaction has been shown to alter the structure and function of both circulating and tissue proteins, such as collagen, lens crystallin, nerve myelin and circulating lipoproteins [281]. Although this glycosylation is initially reversible, continued hypoglycaemia results in slow chemical rearrangements to form irreversible glycosylated end-products [350]. These end-products continue to accumulate, producing thickened basement membrane in vessel walls throughout the tissues. It is thought that cross-linking of these end-products attached to matrix proteins may predispose to macrovascular disease. This glycosylation is also thought to affect the charge of proteoglycan components of the basement membrane, and to affect its permeability.

Hypertension

Epidemiological studies have suggested a strong relationship between hypertension and the progression of chronic complications [351]. The mean blood pressure in IDDM subjects with microvascular complications is higher than in those without complications, even at levels not defined as hypertension [352]. Even during childhood and adolescence, slightly increased blood pressure levels are associated with both retinopathy and microalbuminuria [353]. Although it has been argued that elevated blood pressures are a result of the renal damage, our own data suggest that blood pressure increases are a risk factor for the development of microalbuminuria [354,355]. Although hypertension may be genetically inherited with associate increases in sodium–lithium countertransport, this concept has not been substantiated [356–358]. Hyperfiltration and altered renal haemodynamics, even without systemic hypertension, may also play a major role in the development of nephropathy, possibly related to protein intake [359,360]. There is increasing evidence that protein may affect renal blood flow by its stimulatory effects on growth hormone and glucagon [361].

Growth and sex hormones

A stimulatory effect of growth hormone on the development of microangiopathy was first suggested by a study in which proliferative retinopathy in diabetic patients was found to progress more slowly after hypophysectomy than in diabetic controls [362]. This hypothesis was further supported by the observation that subjects with isolated growth hormone deficiency and diabetes do not develop severe retinopathy [363]. Although the elevated growth hormone levels reported in IDDM are presumably associated with low IGF-I concentrations, cross-sectional studies have suggested a relationship between elevated IGF-I concentrations in the serum and retinopathy [364]. The effects of growth hormone may be related to alteration of serum factors enhancing platelet aggregation [365], as well as renal hyperfiltration [237].

A number of reports suggest that the subclinical complications of IDDM are more likely to occur after puberty [324]. The largest study shows that the prevalence of retinopathy and nephropathy and the risk for death are influenced by postpubertal IDDM duration [366]. Although there is a marked increase in growth hormone levels during puberty, it is possible that sex hormones also play a role, as suggested by animal studies which demonstrate the sex steroid dependence of vascular permeability and abnormal polyol metabolism in diabetic rats [349].

Lipid abnormalities

Because of insulin's effect on lipolysis, hypercholesterolaemia and hypertriglyceridaemia are frequent in poorly controlled IDDM, with abnormalities of low-density lipids (LDL) as well as high-density lipids $(HDL)_2$ and HDL_3 and lipoprotein(a). Although an exact mechanism for a role of lipid abnormalities is not understood, raised LDL and reduced HDL cholesterol have been shown to be related to both the prevalence and incidence of microalbuminuria, as well as of peripheral and autonomic neuropathy. It has been suggested that there is a relationship between plasma lipids and coagulation factor concentrations in IDDM [354,367–370].

Basement membranes

Thickening of basement membranes is characteristic of IDDM, seen in children with the disorder in kidney [371] and muscle [121,332,372]. In identical twins, discordant for type I diabetes, only the diabetic twin shows increases of glomerular basement membrane diameters, suggesting metabolic rather than genetic factors in its pathogenesis [373]. Kidney transplantation from the non-diabetic monozygotic twin to the diabetic co-twin results in basement membrane thickening in the transplanted kidney within months in adolescent and young adult-type patients. Glomerular structural changes associated with basement membrane thickening include mesangial matrix expansion as well as an increase of capillary diameters. These changes have been shown to be associated with microalbuminuria, and correlate with glycaemic control and duration [371]. Controversy exists regarding the importance of metabolic control of muscle capillary basement membrane thickening and its relationship to microvascular disease of the eye and kidney [373,374].

Structural changes of basement membrane glycoproteins have been demonstrated in diabetes, with significant increases of hydroxylysine content and of glucosylgalactose-disaccharide units in β-glycosidic linkage with this amino acid at the expense of lysine residue. These changes were not detected in membranes of subjects with diabetes of short duration [342,375–377]. As mentioned above, glycosylation of proteins, including the collagen of the basement membrane, may also explain both morphological and functional changes [350]. Glycosylation of basement membranes and alterations of collagen distribution may induce functional changes associated with autoregulation of blood flow and permeability [378–380]. In addition, various highly anionic proteoglycans, particularly heparan sulphate and dermatan sulphate, which have been found to contribute to the charge selectivity of the glomerular filtration barrier, are abnormal in patients with diabetes and the glomerular content of heparan sulphate is reduced [381]. This type of abnormality is the basis for the Steno hypothesis of the pathogenesis of microvascular complications [382].

Vascular permeability

Increased permeability of basement membranes is well demonstrated in IDDM. This appears to be related to both structural and functional changes, with a classical result of excessive excretion of albumin and β_2-microglobulin as well as a number of other proteins [383,384]. Total-body transcapillary albumin escape has been shown to be increased using ^{125}I-labelled human serum albumin [383], and this was reversible with insulin therapy [384, 385]. This has led to the suggestion that intermittent extravasation of proteins and their deposition in vessel walls may be one of the early steps in the morphogenesis of vascular disease [380]. It is apparent that alterations of size-selective pores and molecular charge result in protein leakage [386].

Rheostatic factors

Abnormalities in blood rheology, including increased plasma and whole-blood viscocity associated with alterations in red cell aggregation by plasma proteins, is well described in diabetes. Relationships have been described between microvascular disease and platelet stickiness, abnormalities of the coagulation and fibrinolytic systems with elevation of fibrinogen levels and other antithrombotic factors [368,387,388]. Although these associations do not necessarily indicate causality, this does seem possible. However, the changes may reflect underlying existing vascular changes which alter circulating blood components. About half of diabetic children and adolescents exhibit spontaneous or adenosine diphosphate (ADP)-induced platelet aggregation *in vitro*, with increasing severity in those in poor metabolic control. Red cell aggregation associated with elevated fibrinogen levels can also be observed in this age group. However, no correlation could be found between background retinopathy and spontaneous red cell aggregation in diabetic adolescents [389]. This piece of evidence suggests that rheology changes may precede the development of angiopathy.

A deficiency in tissue oxygenation has been postulated to induce regulatory vascular changes in the capillary bed [390]. This could explain reversible leakage of injected fluorescein from the retinal vasculature in diabetes of recent onset [391]. Abnormalities of red cell oxygen affinity associated with decreases of 2,3-diphosphoglycerate or glycosylation of haemoglobin would theoretically alter oxygen delivery and consumption. This in turn could alter red cell viscosity [390,392].

Microangiopathy in children and adolescents: clinical and subclinical manifestations

Increasingly sophisticated techniques have allowed the detection of subclinical microangiopathic changes before clinical symptoms. As it seems that microangiopathy may be partially reversible at this stage, it is important for paediatricians to utilize available diagnostic techniques in order to detect the presence of these complications.

Nephropathy

The presence of nephropathy appears to be the most important prognostic feature for morbidity and mortality in IDDM patients [393]. This is related to death due to renal failure as well as coronary artery disease [394]. Nephropathy is defined by leakage of large amounts of albumin in the urine. Overt nephropathy is preceded by the excretion of smaller amounts of albumin detected by microtechniques (microalbuminuria). Although microalbuminuria is thought to be predictive of overt nephropathy, this is by no means universal [354,395]. Only 30–40% of patients with IDDM develop clinical nephropathy despite detectable morphological renal changes [396–398]. The following practical classification of the possible sequence of events has been proposed.

1 Early renal hyperfiltration and hypertrophy.
2 Development of renal lesions without changes in function.
3 Incipient diabetic nephropathy with an albumin excretion rate between 20 and 200 μg/min.
4 Overt diabetic nephropathy with an albumin excretion rate of greater than 200 μg/min.
5 End-stage renal failure with elevated serum creatinine levels and/or decreased glomerular filtration rate (GFR).

Abnormalities of kidney size, GFR and maximal tubular reabsorption capacity for glucose are well documented already in children and adolescents with IDDM of short duration, these presumably functional changes correlating with renal glucose excretion [385,399]. The increase in GFR is reversible by long-term improvement of glycaemic control, but is unchanged during short periods (1 week), suggesting that there may be some structural changes in addition to functional ones [398]. During conventional therapy, hyperfiltration persists until the development of proteinuria [398]. Thereafter, there is a steady decline in GFR associated with hypertension, and ultimate advanced renal damage and failure. This course may be ameliorated by control of blood pressure [400].

Microalbuminuria has been well described in childhood and usually occurs after about 5 years of diabetes duration; it is more common in postpubertal subjects [324]. There is increasing evidence that microalbuminuria is related to glycaemic control during this period [401,402]. The role of improved glycaemic control by intensive diabetes therapy has now been clearly documented in the DCCT study, which resulted in a 39% decrease in microalbuminuria; overt nephropathy was reduced by 54% [285]. A role for increased renal blood flow is suggested by long-term intervention studies with angiotensin-converting enzyme (ACE) inhibitors, including two small studies in childhood [403–405]. As mentioned above, over nephropathy with proteinuria due to diabetes is seen in adolescents, but is becoming increasingly less common.

Microalbuminuria (albumin excretion rate above 20 μg/min, the upper limit of normal) is a marker of the silent phase of diabetic nephropathy. Macroalbuminuria (albumin excretion above 200 μg/min, which is equivalent to 300 mg/l) is in the range detectable by Albustix. Since urinary albumin excretion is influenced by physical activity both in non-diabetic and diabetic individuals [406,407], an overnight urine collection is preferred for active adolescents. The upper limit of normal for an overnight urine collection is an albumin excretion rate of 15 μg/min, but the correlation between this and a 24-h urine albumin excretion is very good [365,408]. Some investigators have suggested the collection of a spot urine with the calculation of an albumin/creatinine ratio. This collection is more expensive, and its prognostic value has not yet been proved.

Overt nephropathy, which is defined by protein excretion of > 500 mg/day or albumin excretion of >300 mg/day in two or three consecutive urine samples, after exclusion of other causes, is encountered in older adolescents and young adults. As finally proven in the DCCT study, its rate of appearance is related to glycaemic control [285]. Increased proteinuria has been demonstrated in poorly controlled adolescents after rapid improvement in glycaemic control [409], which is similar to the deterioration in retinopathy under similar circumstances [285,410]. Although the role of glycaemic control in the development of overt nephropathy is continuously becoming clearer, most studies demonstrate that a number of other factors are of major importance; these include blood pressure, lipid abnormalities and possibly excess protein in the diet, and may account for the lack of correlation between overt nephropathy and glycaemic control in adolescents and young adults [352,354,411]. Overt proteinuria is highly prognostic of subsequent renal failure, which has been shown to occur after a mean of 7 years. This rate of deterioration can be markedly slowed by aggressive control of blood pressure and dietary protein restriction [412]. A role for antihypertensive therapy and dietary protein restriction in childhood in the absence of overt proteinuria remains to be proved. Both therapeutic interventions have been shown to decrease microalbuminuria in young adults, although studies with dietary protein have included small numbers of subjects [404,413].

Retinopathy

Although retinopathy does not affect mortality, it is the commonest microangiopathic complication of IDDM, and blindness clearly influences quality of life. Diabetes accounts for 10–20% of all cases of blindness and is its most frequent single cause [414]. In the USA, about one in 10 000 individuals is blind from diabetes [214]. Fortunately, recent advances in the treatment of eye disease – including laser, photocoagulation and vitrectomy – have improved the prognosis for vision in individuals with diabetic retinopathy.

The prevalence of retinopathy depends largely on the adequacy of diagnostic techniques. Dilated fundoscopic examination, preferably by an ophthalmologist or a well-trained diabetologist, is essential for adequate evaluation of the retina. Without dilatation, only 50% of eyes are correctly identified regarding the severity and even the presence of retinopathy [415]. Procedures such as ophthalmic photography with polychromatic or contrast-enhancing monochromatic green light and fluorescent angiography improves diagnostic precision, allowing the detection of minor abnormalities several years before they would be found by fundoscopy [416–419]. Fluorescein leakage through the blood–retinal barrier of the retinal surface or into the vitreous can be measured by vitreous fluorophotometry [391,420,421]. This and the appearance of capillary microaneurysms are the earliest quantitatively measurable features of retinopathy. Because some allergic reactions to fluorescein have been described, fundus photographs have been used more frequently recently.

Classification of the severity of retinopathy is most accurately achieved by obtaining photographs of the fundus. Using this technique, more than 90% of patients will eventually show some degree of retinopathy [422]. Neovascularization (that is the development of vision-threatening proliferative retinopathy) may result in bleeding into the vitreous or the retina, with progression to blindness which occurs in 20–55% of patients in different series [335].

There are a variety of classifications of the severity of diabetic retinopathy. A clinical classification includes the following.

1 Normal; there are no microaneurysms.

2 Non-proliferative (background) diabetic retinopathy. Pathological findings include retinal microaneurysms, rare blot haemorrhages or rare hard exudates.

3 Non-proliferative retinopathy with macular oedema. Pathology includes the above plus retinal thickening and increasing hard exudates with macular oedema.

4 Preproliferative retinopathy. Pathological findings include the above plus venous beading, extensive haemorrhages or capillary dropout.

5 Proliferative diabetic retinopathy. Pathological findings include neovascularization and fibrovascular proliferation.

A more detailed classification dependent on fundus photography is given as a modification of the Airlie house classification [335].

Using this classification, background retinopathy with microaneurysms is seen in about 20% of children and adolescents with IDDM for less than 5 years, in 60% with duration 5–10 years, and in 80% after 10 years [416,422]. Like the prevalence, the severity of retinopathy increases with age and duration, and the visual prognosis worsens. Multiple cotton-wool spots and haemorrhages, particularly in the macular area, herald the progression of retinopathy and the onset of vascular proliferation in the near future. Proliferative retinopathy develops after a mean duration of 20 or more years. When assessed 5 years later, 30% of subjects with peripheral neovascularization and 60% of those with central neovascularization have loss of visual acuity [417,423].

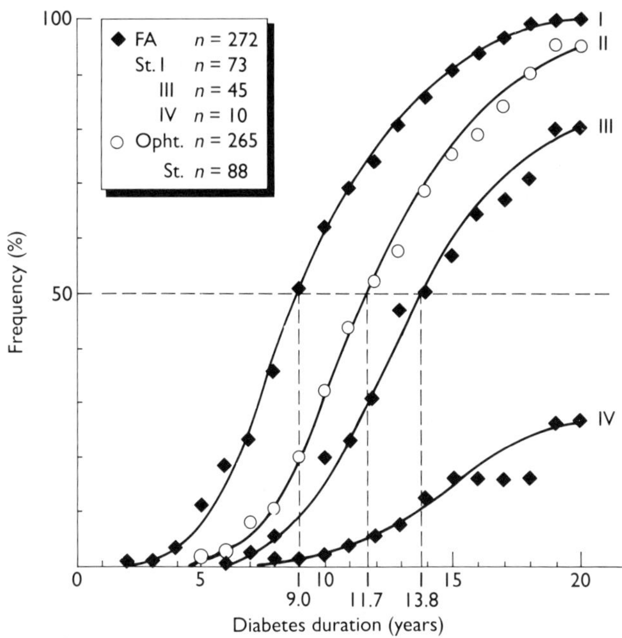

Fig. 33.5 Development of retinopathy in young insulin-dependent patients: Berlin retinopathy study. The curves were calculated by life-table analysis of > 1000 ophthalmoscopic (opht.) and fluorescein angiographic (FA) examinations in 272 patients. The figure gives the median (50th centile) expectation for the development of:
1 Incipient retinopathy: FA, ◆ (curve I); opht., ○ (curve II).
2 Background retinopathy (curve III): FA, ◆, is expressed below the abscissa as 9.0, 11.7 and 13.8 years of diabetes duration, respectively.
3 Proliferative retinopathy (curve IV) (detected in 10 out of 272 patients) will reach about 25% after 20 years of diabetes.

The Berlin Study (Fig. 33.5) shows data very similar to that collected in similar age groups around the world [416]. In this study ranging from childhood to young adulthood 47% of the patients had some degree of retinopathy detected by fundus photography after 0.5–23 years of IDDM duration. Of these, about half had minimal background retinopathy with only a few microaneurysms, a quarter had more severe background lesions and 10% proliferative retinopathy. Retinopathy was uncommon in prepubertal children, similar to the finding with microalbuminuria. Children with IDDM onset before puberty developed retinal changes at longer durations, which is similar to results in Pittsburgh [366]. The life-table analysis in Fig. 33.5 indicates that the risk of developing minor retinopathy occurs over a wide range of diabetes duration (3–18 years) with a median of 9 years. More severe background retinopathy occurs at a median of 13.8 years of diabetes duration and proliferative retinopathy at 20 years. In this study the use of fluorescein angiography resulted in the diagnosis of minimal retinopathic changes 2.7 years earlier than that achieved by careful fundoscopy [416].

Numerous epidemiological studies in the past decade have confirmed the close correlation between the frequency and severity of retinopathy and glycaemic control as measured by glycosylated haemoglobin [352,416,424–427]. In addition, glycosylated haemoglobin at the first examination predicts the incidence of progression of retinopathy over a 2–4-year follow-up period [424,426]. As with nephropathy, the DCCT study convincingly demonstrated the role of glycaemic control in the development and prevention of retinopathy.

In the primary cohort, that is those without retinopathy at entry to the study, the risk of developing any retinopathy was reduced by 76% by intensive therapy compared with conventional therapy. Progression of retinopathy in the secondary cohort, that is those subjects with mild baseline retinopathy, was decreased by 54%. The development of proliferative or severe non-proliferative retinopathy was reduced by 47%. In addition, there was an almost linear relationship between the mean glycosylated haemoglobin over the time of the study and progression of retinopathy [285].

Advanced retinopathy has not been shown to be reversible by improved glycaemic control or pancreatic transplant [328,428,429]. The initial deterioration of retinopathy after the rapid improvement of glycaemic control in subjects with high glycosylated haemoglobin levels, irrespective of whether the treatment modality included conventional therapy, multiple injections or subcutaneous insulin infusion suggests that slower decreases of mean blood glucoses are advisable [285,410,430,431]. With improved glycaemic control, which has become possible with the advent of home glucose monitoring and accurate assessments by glycosylated haemoglobin levels, the need for photocoagulation in adolescents is becoming very infrequent.

There is little doubt in cross-sectional studies that there are important risk factors for the development of retinopathy other than glycaemic control. Hypertension, or blood pressures in the high-normal range, are well-documented risk factors for the progression of background retinopathy [432,433]. However, it has been argued that hypertension is a risk factor for retinopathy only in the face of nephropathy [434]. Variations in the severity and prevalence of retinopathy with apparently similar long-term metabolic control has aroused interest in possible genetic susceptibility or protective factors. Identical twins, concordant for IDDM also demonstrate concordance with regard to the severity of their retinopathy, but only in 24 out of 31 pairs [435]. Thus, non-genetic factors do have some degree of importance [333].

While several studies have suggested an association between retinopathy and HLA antigens DR3 and DR4 [436–439], others have not been able to confirm these associations [440–444]. If there is a role of circulating immune complexes in the development of retinopathy [445], this could explain the recent confirmation of an association between Gm types and retinopathy [446]. However, at present the assumption that there is a genetic influence on retinopathy and other diabetic vascular disease associated with the human histocompatibility complex and immunological responses is speculative at best. It is possible that some genetic determination of basic biochemical processes, such as the proteoglycan and basement membrane synthesis, may be substantiated in the future, and explain why some patients do and others do not develop severe retinal lesions.

Neuropathy

Clinical diabetic neuropathy, both peripheral and autonomic, is very rare in children and adolescents, and present in only 10% of a population of adolescents and adults between 15 and 59 years of age [447]. The authors have not seen clinical symptomatic neuropathy in adolescents over the past decade. Although there is still some discussion as to the definition of neuropathy, a careful physical examination, together with measures of nerve conduction and vibratory thresholds, defines the presence of peripheral neuropathy. Autonomic neuropathy in most studies is measured by the R–R interval and pupillometry.

Although clinical neuropathy is rare, subclinical neuropathy as assessed by decreased motor nerve conduction velocities and sensory changes is well described in diabetic children [448–460]. The prevalence is affected by both age and duration of IDDM. In addition, an independent relationship between neuropathy and glycosylated haemoglobin has been reported [451]. These abnormalities of motor nerve conduction have been found in approximately 20% of children within the first 5 years of diabetes and in 60% of those with > 10 years duration. Decreases in vibratory perception thresholds have also been described in 20% of diabetic children, most frequently in the postpubertal age group [452].

Central nervous system abnormalities have also been documented in children with IDDM. In Pittsburgh these abnormalities were more frequent in children diagnosed at less than 5 years of age, but were not necessarily related to the frequency of seizures. Both children and adults have been shown to have impaired auditory and visual brainstemevoked potentials. Visual evoked potential abnormalities reported in 30% of children were not related to duration or glycaemic control [453]. Autonomic neuropathy has been estimated to be present in 30% of teenage subjects [454,455].

As with the other microangiopathic complications, glycaemic control appears to be a major predictor of neuropathy. Intensive therapy reduced clinical neuropathy by 60% compared to conventional therapy [285].

In Pittsburgh, alterations in lipid metabolism have also been shown to be highly correlated with the prevalence of peripheral and autonomic neuropathy [369,370]. Smoking is an important environmental risk factor [370].

TRANSIENT DIABETES MELLITUS IN EARLY INFANCY

This syndrome is more severe than those frequently associated with carbohydrate intolerance in infancy, which only rarely require insulin therapy, although this is controversial [260]. It occurs in full-term infants less than 6 weeks of age and manifests as marked dehydration without diarrhoea, vomiting with fever, failure to thrive, and cachexia despite adequate food consumption [456–459]. These clinical signs appear during the first few days of life due to severe hyperglycaemia up to 110 mmol/l and glycosuria. Ketonuria is common but usually mild [457]. Serum sodium concentrations may be slightly elevated due to dehydration, but potassium is normal. Plasma insulin levels are low relative to the hyperglycaemia [456, 460]. Surprisingly, coma does not usually occur.

This form of diabetes, unlike classical IDDM, lasts between a few days and 540 days [456] with a mean duration of 70 days. It is very similar to non-ketotic hyperosmolar diabetes and is very sensitive to insulin, requiring very small amounts for control. Gradually, insulin requirements cease and thereafter glucose tolerance usually remains normal. A few patients may develop diabetes mellitus later in life, which develops gradually from impaired glucose tolerance to insulin-requiring diabetes over long periods of time. Some patients later show signs of central nervous system damage [461].

The aetiology of this syndrome is unknown. Siblings may be affected. Although most infants are born to families without a history of diabetes, some have diabetic mothers [462]. It has been suggested that the pathogenesis is delayed pancreatic β cell maturation in these babies, who are usually small [459,460]. Repeated studies of endogenous insulin release assist in the distinction between transient and permanent infantile diabetes mellitus.

PROGNOSIS OF TYPE I DIABETES

Until IDDM can be prevented, appropriate therapy with exogenous insulin, dietary management and monitoring of metabolic control are probably the major determinants of the long-term prognosis of the disorder. Studies in the 1970s showed a 12–15-fold increase in mortality in patients with IDDM [394,463]. Of those patients with onset in childhood, 50% had died by 50 years of age [394]. Most studies showed a limited life expectancy for diabetic children. However, with improved therapy, it is likely that these mortality rates will decrease. It should be noted that a large number of patients with IDDM live 40 or 50 years after the diagnosis [464], possibly related to genetic factors and overall better metabolic control. A large Danish study has shown the trend towards decreased mortality rates in the past three decades [465].

Diabetic nephropathy and cardiovascular disease are the two major causes of mortality in patients with IDDM [393,465]. Because cardiovascular disease is usually not present in childhood and adolescence, it has not been discussed in this chapter.

The numerous epidemiological studies showing a relationship between glycaemic control and microvascular complications led to a number of relatively short-term small intervention studies to assess the effect of improved glycaemic control on the progression of microvascular complications [337]. The 1993 reports [285,336] showing the value of intensive diabetes therapy in decreasing the risk of the development and progression of microvascular complications has substantiated the role of glycaemic control in the pathogenesis of microangiopathic complications, and has clearly pointed out the therapeutic needs for the future for periadolescent and postadolescent patients with IDDM. The importance of glycaemic control in younger children is not yet elucidated, and the greater risk of hypoglycaemia in this age group has to be weighed into therapeutic strategies.

REFERENCES

1 Köbberling J. Studies on the genetic heterogeneity of diabetes mellitus. *Diabetologia* 1971;7:46–9.

2 National Diabetes Data Group. Classification and diagnosis of glucose intolerance of diabetes mellitus and other categories. *Diabetes* 1979;28:1039–57.

3 World Health Organization. *Diabetes Mellitus, 1985*. WHO Technical Report Series 727. Geneva: WHO, 1985.

4 Bennett PH. Changing concepts of the epidemiology of insulin-dependent diabetes. *Diabetes Care* 1985;8,Suppl. 1: 29–33.

5 Karvonen M, Tuomilehto J, Libman I, Laporte R. For the World Health Organization DIAMOND Project Group. A review of the recent epidemiological data on the world wide incidence of Type I (insulin dependent) diabetes mellitus. *Diabetologia* 1993;36:883–92.

6 LaPorte RE, Tajima N, Akerblom HK *et al*. Geographic differences in the risk of insulin-dependent diabetes mellitus: the importance of registries. *Diabetes Care* (Suppl.) 1985;1:101–7.

7 Laakso M, Pyorala K. Age of onset and type of diabetes. *Diabetes Care* 1985;8:114–17.

8 Meltron L, Palumbo P, Chu C. Incidence of diabetes mellitus by clinical type. *Diabetes Care* 1983;6:75–86.

9 Bloom A, Hayes TM, Gamble BR. A register of newly diagnosed diabetic children. *Br Med J* 1975;iii:580–3.

10 Calnan M, Peckham CS. Incidence of insulin-dependent diabetes in the first sixteen years of life. *Lancet* 1977;1:589–90.

11 Christau B, Kromann H, Andersen O *et al*. Incidence, seasonal and geographic patterns of juvenile-onset insulin-dependent diabetes mellitus in Denmark. *Diabetologia* 1977;13:281–4.

12 Cohen T. Juvenile diabetes in Israel. *Isr J Med Sci* 1971;7: 11558–61.

13 Genz H. Epidemiologie des kindlichen Diabetes. *Deutsche Diabetes-Gesellschaft* 1974;9. Jahrestagung, Travemünde.

14 Koivisto VA, Akerblom HK, Wasz-Höckert O. *The Epidemiology of Juvenile Diabetes Mellitus in Northern Finland*. Nordic Council Arctic Medical Research Report No. 15, 1976:58–65.

15 LaPorte RE, Fishbein HA, Drash AL *et al*. The Pittsburgh Insulin-dependent Diabetes Mellitus (IDDM) Registry. The incidence of insulin-dependent diabetes mellitus in Allegheny County, Pennsylvania (1965–1976). *Diabetes* 1981;30:279–84.

16 Sterky G, Holmgren G, Gustavson KH *et al*. The incidence of diabetes mellitus in Swedish children 1970–1975. *Acta Paed Scand* 1978;Suppl. 67:139–43.

17 Wadsworth MEJ, Jarrett RJ. Incidence of diabetes in the first 26 years of life. *Lancet* 1974,2:1172–4.

18 Simpson NE. The genetics of diabetes mellitus – a review of family data. In: Creutzfeldt W, Köbberling J, Neel JV, eds. *The Genetics of Diabetes Mellitus*. Berlin: Springer Verlag, 1976:12–20.

19 Kries I von. Beitrag zur Genetik des Diabetes mellitus. *Z Mensch Vererbungs Konstit* 1953;31:406–20.

20 Pincus G, White P. On the inheritance of diabetes mellitus. I. An analysis of 675 family histories. *Am J Med Sci* 1933; 186:1–12.

21 Steinberg AG, Wilder RM. Genetics of diabetes. *Am J Hum Genet* 1952;4:113.

22 Penrose LS, Watson EM. A sex-linked tendency in familial diabetes. *Proc Am Diabetic Assoc* 1945;5:163.

23 Degnbol B, Green A. Diabetes mellitus among first and second degree relatives of early onset. *Ann Hum Genet* 1978;42:25–47.

24 Tillil H, Kobberling J. Age corrected empirical genetic risk estimates for first degree relatives of IDDM patients. *Diabetes* 1986;36:93–9.

25 Wagener DK, Sacks JM, LaPorte RE, MacGregor JM. The Pittsburgh Study of Insulin-dependent Diabetes Mellitus: risk for diabetes among relatives of IDDM. *Diabetes* 1982; 31:136–44.

26 Cavender DE, Wagener DK, Rabin BS *et al*. The Pittsburgh IDDM study. HLA antigens and haplotypes as risk factors for the development of IDDM in IDDM patients and their siblings. *J Chron Dis* 1984;37:555–68.

27 Almos P, A'Hern R, Heaton DA *et al*. The significance of the concordance rate for Type I (insulin dependent) diabetes in identical twins. *Diabetologia* 1988;31:747–50.

28 Langenbeck U, Jorgensen G. The genetics of diabetes mellitus – a review of twin studies. In: Creutzfeldt W, Köbberling J, Neel JV, eds. *The Genetics of Diabetes Mellitus*. Berlin: Springer Verlag, 1976.

29 Barnett AH, Eff C, Leslie RDG, Pyke DA. Diabetes in identical twins. A study of 200 pairs. *Diabetologia* 1981;20:87–93.

30 Pyke DA, Nelson PG. Diabetes mellitus in identical twins. In: Creutzfeldt W, Köbberling J, Neel JV, eds. *The Genetics of Diabetes Mellitus*. Berlin: Springer Verlag, 1976:194–202.

31 Pyke DA. Genetics of diabetes. *Clin Endocrinol Metab* 1977;6:285–303.

32 Tattersall RB, Pyke DA. Diabetes in identical twins. *Lancet* 1972;2:1120–5.

33 Fajans SS, Cloutier MC, Crowther RL. Clinical and etiologic heterogeneity of idiopathic diabetes mellitus. *Diabetes* 1978;27:1112–25.

34 Tattersall RB, Fajans SS. A difference between the inheritance of classical juvenile-onset and maturity-onset type diabetes in young people. *Diabetes* 1975;24:44–53.

35 Pyke DA, Leslie RDG. Chlorpropamide–alcohol flushing: a definition of its relation to non-insulin-dependent diabetes. *Br Med J* 1978;ii:1521–2.

36 Froguel PH, Zouali H, Vionnet N *et al*. Familial hyperglycemia due to mutations in glucokinase: definition of a subtype of diabetes mellitus. *N Engl J Med* 1993;328:697–702.

37 Cudworth AG, Woodrow JC. HLA-antigens and diabetes mellitus. *Lancet* 1974;2:1153.

38 McDevitt HO, Bodmer WF. HL-A, immune response genes and disease. *Lancet* 1974;1:1269–75.

39 Nerup J, Platz P, Andersen OO *et al*. HLA-antigens and diabetes mellitus. *Lancet* 1974;2:864–6.

40 Trucco M. To be or not to be ASP 57, that is the question. *Diabetes Care* 1992;15:712.

41 Cudworth AG, Woodrow JC. Genetic susceptibility in diabetes mellitus: analysis of the HLA-association. *Br Med J* 1976;ii:846–8.

42 Nelson PG, Pyke DA, Cudworth AG, Woodrow JC, Batchelor JR. Histocompatibility antigens in diabetic identical twins. *Lancet* 1976;2:193–4.

43 Schernthaner G, Mayr WR, Pacher M, Ludwig H, Erd W, Eibl M. HL-A 8, W15 and T_3 in juvenile onset diabetes mellitus. *Horm Metab Res* 1975;7:521–2.

44 Karjalainen J, Salmela P, Ilonen J, Surcel H-M, Knip M. A comparison of childhood and adult Type I diabetes mellitus. *N Engl J Med* 1989;320:881–6.

45 Ludvigsson J, Samuelsson U, Beauforts C *et al*. HLA-DR3 is associated with a more slowly progessive form of Type I (insulin-dependent) diabetes. *Diabetologia* 1986;29:207–10.

46 Platz P, Jakobsen BK, Morling N *et al.* HLA-D and -DR antigens in genetic analysis of insulin dependent diabetes mellitus. *Diabetologia* 1981;21:108–15.

47 Svejgaard A, Jakobsen BK, Platz P *et al.* HLA associations in insulin-dependent diabetes: search for heterogeneity in different groups of patients from a homogeneous population. *Tissue Antigens* 1986;28:237–44.

48 Wolf E, Spencer KM, Cudworth AG. The genetic susceptibility to type I (insulin-dependent) diabetes: analysis of the HLA-DR association. *Diabetologia* 1983;24:224–30.

49 MacDonald MJ, Traisman HS, Levitsky LL, Duquesnoy RJ, Mullins P, Hackbarth SA. HLA types in American black juvenile diabetics. Strong associations with Dw3 and Dw4. *Metabolism* 1981;30:533–6.

50 Johnston C, Pyke DA, Cudworth AG, Wolf E. HLA-DR typing in identical twins with insulin-dependent diabetes: difference between concordant and discordant pairs. *Br Med J* 1983;286:253–5.

51 Aparicio MR, Wakisaka A, Takada A, Matsuura N, Aizawa M. HLA-DQ system and insulin dependent diabetes mellitus in Japanese: does it contribute to the development of IDDM as it does in Caucasians? *Immunogenetics* 1988;28:240–6.

52 Todd JA, Mijovic C, Fletcher J, Jenkins D, Bradwell AR, Barnett AH. Identification of susceptibility loci for insulin dependent diabetes mellitus by trans-racial gene mapping. *Nature* 1989;338:587–9.

53 Lernmark A. Molecular biology of Type 1 (insulin-dependent) diabetes mellitus. *Diabetologia* 1985;28:195–203.

54 Terasaki PI, ed. *Histocompatibility Testing 1980.* Los Angeles, CA: UCLA Tissue Typing Laboratory, 1980.

55 Reijonen H, Alonen J, Knip M, Michelsen B, Akerblom HK. HLA-DQ beta chain restriction fragment length polymorphism as a risk marker in Type I (insulin dependent) diabetes mellitus: a Finnish family study. *Diabetologia* 1990;33: 357–62.

56 Morel PA, Dorman JS, Todd JA, McDevitt HO, Trucco M. Aspartic acid at position 57 of the HLA-DQ beta chain protects against Type I diabetes: a family study. *Proc Natl Acad Sci USA* 1988;85:8111–15.

57 Todd JA, Bell JI, McDevitt HO. HLA-DQ B gene contributes to susceptibility and resistance in insulin dependent diabetes mellitus. *Nature* 1987;329:599–604.

58 Dorman JS, LaPorte RE, Stone RA, Trucco M. Worldwide differences in the incidence of Type I diabetes are associated with amino acid variation at position 57 of the HLA-DQ beta chain. *Proc Natl Acad Sci USA* 1990;87:7370–4.

59 Baisch JM, Weeks T, Giles R, Hoover M, Stastny P, Capra JD. Analysis of HLA-DQ genotypes and susceptibility in insulin dependent diabetes mellitus. *N Engl J Med* 1990;332:1836–41.

60 Reijonen H, Ilonen J, Knip M, Akerblom HK. HLA-DQ B1 alleles and absence of asp 57 as susceptibility factors of IDDM in Finland. *Diabetes* 1991;40(12):1640–4.

61 Khalil I, d'Auriol L, Gobet M *et al.* A combination of HLA-DQ beta asp 57 negative and HLA-DQ alpha arg 52 confers susceptibility to IDDM. *J Clin Invest* 1990;85:1315–19.

62 Rotter JI, Anderson CE, Rubin R, Congleton JE, Terasaki PI, Rimoin DL. HLA genotypic study of insulin-dependent diabetes. The excess of DR3/DR4 heterocytes allows rejection of the recessive hypothesis. *Diabetes* 1983;32:169–74.

63 Eberhardt MS, Wagener DK, Orchard TJ *et al.* HLA heterogeneity of insulin-dependent diabetes mellitus at diagnosis. The Pittsburgh IDDM study. *Diabetes* 1985;34:1247–52.

64 Mustonen A, Ilonen J, Tiilikaine A, Kataja M, Akerblom HK. An analysis of epidemiological data in HLA typed diabetic children. *Diabetologia* 1985;28:397–400.

65 Deschamps I, Hors J, Clerget-Darpoux F *et al.* Excess of maternal HLA DR3 antigen in HLA DR3/4 positive Type I (insulin dependent) diabetic patients. *Diabetologia* 1990;33: 420–5.

66 Warram JH, Krolewski AI, Gottlieb MS, Kahn CR. Difference in risk of insulin dependent diabetes in offspring of diabetic mothers and diabetic fathers. *N Engl J Med* 1984;311:149–52.

67 Bell GL, Horita S, Karam JH. A highly polymorphic locus near the human insulin gene is associated with insulin-dependent diabetes mellitus. *Diabetes* 1984;33:176–83.

68 Deschamps I, Marcelli-Barge A, Poirier JC *et al.* Two distinct HLA DR3 haplotypes are associated with age related heterogeneity in Type I (insulin dependent) diabetes. *Diabetologia* 1988;33:896–901.

69 Jones DB, Boulware SD, Kraemer DT, Caprio S, Sherwin RS, Tamborlane WV. Independent effects of youth and poor diabetes control on responses to hypoglycemia in children. *Diabetes* 1991;40:358–63.

70 Yoon JW. Two possible mechanisms for the pathogenesis of viral induced diabetes mellitus. *Pediatr Adolesc Endocrinol* 1986;15:64–73.

71 Coleman TJ, Gamble DR, Taylor KW. Diabetes in mice after Coxsackie B_4 virus infection. *Br Med J* 1973;iii:25–7.

72 Craighead JE, McLane MF. Diabetes mellitus: induction in mice by encephalomyocarditis virus. *Science* 1968;162:913–14.

73 Rayfield EJ, Seto Y. Viruses and the pathogenesis of diabetes mellitus. *Diabetes* 1978;27:1126–42.

74 Dokheel TM. For the Pittsburgh Diabetes Epidemiology Research Group. An epidemic of childhood diabetes in the United States? Evidence from Allegheny County, PA. *Diabetes Care* 1994;16:1606–11.

75 Forrest JM, Menser MA, Burgess JA. High frequency of diabetes mellitus in young-adults with congenital rubella. *Lancet* 1971;2:332–4.

76 Ginsberg-Fellner F, Witt ME, Yagihashi S *et al.* Congenital rubella syndrome as a model for type I (insulin-dependent) diabetes mellitus: increased prevalence of islet cell surface antibodies. *Diabetologia* 1984;27:87–9.

77 Menser MA, Forrest JM, Bransby RD. Rubella infection and diabetes mellitus. *Lancet* 1978;1:57–60.

78 Rubinstein P, Walker ME, Fedun B, Witt ME, Cooper LZ, Ginsberg-Fellner F. The HLA system in congenital rubella patients with and without diabetes. *Diabetes* 1982;31:1088–91.

79 Gamble D. A possible virus etiology for juvenile diabetes. In: Creutzfeldt W, Köbberling JV, Neel JV, eds. *The Genetics of Diabetes Mellitus.* Berlin: Springer Verlag, 1976:95–105.

80 Gamble DR, Kinsley ML, Fitzgerald MG, Bolton R, Taylor KW. Viral antibodies in diabetes mellitus. *Br Med J* 1969;iii: 627–30.

81 Gamble D, Taylor KW. Seasonal incidence of diabetes mellitus. *Br Med* J 1969;iii:631–3.

82 Banetvala JE, Bryant J, Schernthaner G *et al.* Coxsackie B, mumps, rubella, and cytomegalovirus specific IgM responses in patients with juvenile onset insulin dependent diabetes mellitus in Britain, Austria and Australia. *Lancet* 1985;1: 1409–12.

83 Dippe SE, Bennett PH, Miller M *et al.* Lack of causal association between Coxsackie B_4 virus infection and diabetes.

Lancet 1975;1:1314–17.
84 Friman G, Fohlman J, Frisk G *et al.* An incidence peak of juvenile diabetes. Relation to Coxsackie B virus immune response. *Acta Paed Scand* 1985;Suppl. 320:14–19.
85 King ML, Shaik HA, Bidwell D, Voller A, Banetvala JE. Coxsackie B virus specific IgM responses in children with insulin dependent diabetes mellitus. *Lancet* 1983;1:1397–9.
86 Bottazzo GF, Pujol-Borrell R, Gale E. Autoimmunity and diabetes: progress, consolidation and controversy. In: Alberti KGMM, Krall LP, eds. *The Diabetes Annual*, Vol. 2. Amsterdam: Elsevier, 1986:13–29.
87 Yoon JW, Austin M, Onodera T, Notkins AL. Virus induced diabetes mellitus: isolation of a virus from the pancreas of a child with diabetic ketoacidosis. *N Engl J Med* 1979;300: 1173–9.
88 Champsaur H, Bottazzo G, Bertrams J, Assan R, Bach C. Virologic immunologic and genetic factors in insulin dependent diabetes mellitus. *J Pediatr* 1982;100:15–20.
89 Asplin CM, Cooney MK, Crossley JR, Dornan TL, Raghu P, Palmer JP. Coxsackie B_4 infection and islet cell antibodies three years before overt diabetes. *J Pediatr* 1982;101:398–400.
90 Gepts W. Pathologic anatomy of the pancreas in juvenile diabetes mellitus. *Diabetes* 1975;14:619–33.
91 Ondera A, Onodena T, Yoon JW, Notkins AL. Induction of diabetes by cumulative environmental insults from viruses and chemicals. *Nature* 1980;288:383–5.
92 Pak CY, Cha CY, Rajotte RV, McArthur RG, Yoon JW. Human pancreatic islet cell specific 38 kD autoantigen identified by cytomegalovirus induced monoclonal islet cell antibody. *Diabetologia* 1990;33:569–72.
93 Ward KP, Galloway WH, Auchterlonie IA. Congenital cytomegalovirus infection and diabetes. *Lancet* 1979;1:497.
94 Jenson AB, Rosenberg HS, Notkins AL. Pancreatic islet cell damage in children with fatal viral infection. *Lancet* 1980; 2:354–8.
95 Karam JH, Lewitt PA, Young CW *et al.* Insulinopenic diabetes after rodenticide (Vacor) ingestion: a unique model of acquired diabetes in man. *Diabetes* 1980;29:971–8.
96 Bouchard PH, Say P, Reach G, Caubarrère I, Ganeval D, Assan R. Diabetes mellitus following pentamidine-induced hypoglycemia in humans. *Diabetes* 1982;31:40–5.
97 Helgason T, Jonasson MR. Evidence for a food additive as a cause of ketosis-prone diabetes. *Lancet* 1981;2:716–20.
98 Helgason T, Ewen SWB, Ross IS, Stowers JM. Diabetes produced in mice by smoked/cured mutton. *Lancet* 1982;2: 1017–22.
99 Borch-Johnsen K, Joner G, Mandrup-Poulsen T *et al.* Relation between breast-feeding and incidence rates of insulin-dependent diabetes mellitus. *Lancet* 1984;2:1083–6.
100 Kostraba JN. What can epidemiology tell us about the role of infant's diet in the etiology of IDDM? *Diabetes Care* 1994; 17:87–91.
101 Dahl-Jorgensen K, Joner G, Hanssen KF. Relationship between cow's milk consumption and incidence of IDDM in childhood. *Diabetes Care* 1991;14:1081–3.
102 Scott FW, Cow milk and insulin dependent diabetes mellitus: is there a relationship? *Am J Clin Nutr* 1990;51:489–91.
103 Pozzilli P, Bottazzo GF. Coffee or sugar, which is to blame in IDDM? *Diabetes Care* 1991;14:144–5.
104 Tuomilehto J, Tuomilehto-Wolf E, Virtala E, Laporte R. Coffee consumption as trigger for insulin dependent diabetes in childhood. *Br Med J* 1990;300:642–3.
105 Gerstein HC. Cow's milk exposure and Type I diabetes mellitus. *Diabetes Care* 1994;17:13–19.
106 Elliott RB, Martin JM. Dietary protein: a trigger of insulin dependent diabetes in the BB rat? *Diabetologia* 1984;26: 297–9.
107 Scott FW, Daneman D, Martin JM. Evidence for a critical role of diet in the development of insulin dependent diabetes mellitus. *Diabetes Res* 1988;7:153–7.
108 Dahlquist G, Savilahti E, Landin-Olsson M. An increased level of antibodies to beta lactoglobulin is a risk determinant for early onset Type I (insulin dependent) diabetes mellitus independent of islet cell antibodies and early introduction of cow's milk. *Diabetologia* 1992;35:980–4.
109 Savilahti E, Akerblom HK, Tainio VM, Koskimies S. Children with newly diagnosed insulin dependent diabetes mellitus have increased levels of cow milk antibodies. *Diabetes Res* 1988;7:137–40.
110 Savilahti E, Saukkonen TT, Virtala ET, Tuomilehto J, Akerblom HK. The childhood diabetes in Finland Study Group: increased levels of cow milk and beta lactoglobulin antibodies in young children with newly diagnosed IDDM. *Diabetes Care* 1993;16:984–9.
111 Karjalainen J, Martin JM, Knip M *et al.* A bovine albumin peptide as a possible trigger of insulin dependent diabetes mellitus. *N Engl J Med* 1992;327:302–7.
112 Pietropaolo M, Castano L, Babu S *et al.* Islet cell autoantigen 69 kDa (ICA69): molecular cloning and characterization of a novel diabetes associated autoantigen. *J Clin Invest* 1993; 92:359–71.
113 Hayles AB, Kennedy RLJ, Beahrs OH *et al.* Exophthalmic goiter in children. *J Clin Endocrinol Metab* 1959;19:138–51.
114 Crome L, Erdoihazi M, Rivers RPA. Fulminating diabetes with lymphocytic thyroiditis. *Arch Dis Child* 1967;42:677–81.
115 Hecht A, Gerschberg H. Diabetes mellitus and primary hypothyroidism. *Metabolism* 1968;17:108–13.
116 Heding LG, Rasmussen SM. Determination of pancreatic and gut glucagon-like immunoreactivity in normal and diabetic subjects. *Diabetologia* 1972;8:408–11.
117 Irvine WJ, Clarke BF, Scarth L, Cullen DR, Duncan LJ. Thyroid and gastric autoimmunity in patients with diabetes mellitus. *Lancet* 1970;2:163–8.
118 Barta L, Gattyan E, Simon S. Gleichzeitges Vorkommen von juvenilem Diabetes und Addison'scher Krankheit. *Klin Pädiatr* 1977;189:239–43.
119 Montagnani A, Tosti A, Patrizi A, Salardi S, Cacciari E. Diabetes mellitus and skin diseases in childhood. *Dermatologia* 1985;170:65–8.
120 Goldstein DE, Drash A, Gibbs J, Blizzard RM. Diabetes mellitus: the incidence of circulating antibodies against thyroid, gastric and adrenal tissue. *J Pediatr* 1970;77:304–6.
121 Kilo C, Vogler N, Williamson JR. Muscle capillary basement membrane changes related to aging and diabetes mellitus. *Diabetes* 1972;21:881–905.
122 Manns M, Weber B, Arnold *et al.* Humoral immune phenomena in juvenile insulin dependent diabetes mellitus (IDDM) (abstr.). In: *21st Annual Meeting, European Society for Paediatric Endocrinology*, Helsinki, 28–30 June 1982.
123 Bottazzo GF, Pujol-Borrell R, Gale E. Etiology of diabetes: the role of autoimmune mechanisms. In: Alberti KGMM, Krall LP, eds. *The Diabetes Annual*, Vol. 2. Oxford: Elsevier, 1985:16–52.
124 Eisenbarth GS. Type I diabetes mellitus: a chronic autoimmune disease. *N Engl J Med* 1986;314:1360–8.

125 Gepts W. The pathology of the pancreas in human diabetes. In: Andreani D, Di Mario U, Federlin KF, Heding LG, eds. *Immunology in Diabetes*. London: Kimpton, 1984;21–34.

126 Kanazawa Y, Komeda K, Sato S, Mori S, Akanuma K, Takaku F. Non-obese diabetic mice: immune mechanisms of pancreatic β-cell destruction. *Diabetologia* 1984;27:113–15.

127 Bottazzo GF, Dean BM, McNally J, MacKay EH, Swift PGF, Gamble GR. In situ characterization of autoimmune phenomena and expression of HLA molecules in the pancreas in diabetic insulitis. *N Engl J Med* 1985;313:353–60.

128 Sibley DK, Sutherland DER, Goetz F, Michael AF. Recurrent diabetes mellitus in the pancreas iso- and allograft: a light and electron microscopic and immuno-histochemical analysis. *Lab Invest* 1985;53:132.

129 Sutherland DER, Goetz FC, Najarian JS. Recent experience with 89 pancreas transplants at a single institution. *Diabetologia* 1984:27:149–53.

130 Nerup J, Andersen O, Bendixen G, Egeberg J, Poulsen JE. Anti-pancreatic cellular hypersensitivity in diabetes mellitus. *Diabetes* 1971;20:424–7.

131 Huang SW, MacLaren NK. Insulin-dependent diabetes: a disease of autoaggression. *Science* 1976;192:64–6.

132 Buschard K, Madsbad S, Rygaard J. Passive transfer of diabetes mellitus from man to mouse. *Lancet* 1978;1:908–10.

133 Peakman M, Vergani D. Cell mediated immunity and Type I diabetes. *Diabetes Rev* 1992;1:5–8.

134 Peakman M, Warnock T, Vats A *et al.* Lymphocyte subset abnormalities, autoantibodies and their relationship with HLA DR types in children with Type I (insulin dependent) diabetes and their first degree relatives. *Diabetologia* 1994; 37:155–65.

135 Schatz D, Riley WJ, MacLaren NK, Barrett DJ. Defective inducer T cell function before the onset of insulin dependent diabetes mellitus. *J Autoimmun* 1991;4:125–36.

136 Atkinson MA, Kaufman DL, Campbell L *et al.* Response of peripheral blood mononuclear cells to glutamate decarboxylase in insulin dependent diabetes. *Lancet* 1992;339:458–9.

137 Harrison LC, Chu SX, DeAizpurua HJ, Graham M, Honeyman MC, Coleman PG. Islet reactive T cells are a marker of preclinical insulin dependent diabetes. *J Clin Invest* 1992; 89:1161–5.

138 Keller RJ. Cellular immunity to human insulin in individuals at high risk for the development of Type I diabetes mellitus. *J Autoimmun* 1990;3:321–7.

139 Roep BO, Kallan AA, Hazenbos WLW *et al.* T-cell reactivity to a 38 kD insulin secretory granule protein in patients with recent onset Type I diabetes. *Lancet* 1991;337:1439–41.

140 Karjalainen J, Cheung R, Vandermeulen J, Martin JM, Knip M, Dosch HM. T cell proliferation response against bovine serum albumin (BSA) follows the natural course and is restricted to the linear ABBOS sequence in insulin dependent diabetes mellitus (IDDM). *J Autoimmun* 1993;15(Suppl. 1): 62 (Abstr.).

141 Atkinson MA, Bowman MS, Kao KJ *et al.* Lack of immune responsiveness to bovine serum albumin in insulin dependent diabetes. *N Engl J Med* 1993;329:1853–8.

142 Atkinson MA, MacLaren NK. Islet cell autoantigens of IDDM. *Diabetes Rev* 1993;1:191–203.

143 Bosi E, Bonifacio E, Bottazzo GF. Autoantigens in IDDM. *Diabetes Rev* 1993;1:204–14.

144 Jones DB, Hunter NR, Duff GW. Heat shock protein 65 as a beta cell antigen of insulin dependent diabetes. *Lancet* 1990; 336:583–5.

145 Bottazzo GF, Florin-Caristensen A, Doniach D. Islet cell antibodies in diabetes mellitus with autoimmune polyendocrine deficiency. *Lancet* 1974;2:1279–83.

146 MacCuish AC, Barnes EW, Irvine WJ, Duncan LJ. Antibodies to pancreatic islet cells in insulin-dependent diabetics with coexistent autoimmune disease. *Lancet* 1974;2:1529–31.

147 Landin-Olsson M, Karlsson A, Dahlquist G, Blom L, Lernmark A, Sundkvist G. Islet cell and other organ specific autoantibodies in all children developing Type I (insulin dependent) diabetes mellitus in Sweden during one year and in matched control children. *Diabetologia* 1989;32:387–95.

148 Bruining GJ, Molenaar J, Tuk CW, Lindeman J, Bruining HA, Marner B. Clinical time-course and characteristics of islet-cell cytoplasmic antibodies in childhood diabetes. *Diabetologia* 1984;26:24–9.

149 Irvine WJ, McCallum CJ, Gray RS *et al.* Pancreatic islet-cell antibodies in diabetes mellitus correlated with the duration and type of diabetes, coexistent autoimmune disease, and HLA-type. *Diabetes* 1977;26:138–47.

150 Bingley PJ, Bonifacio E, Gale EAM. Can we really predict IDDM? *Diabetes* 1993;42:213–20.

151 Bottazzo GF, Dean BM, Gorsuch AN, Cudworth AG, Doniach D. Complement-fixing islet-cell antibodies in Type I diabetes: possible monitors of active beta cell damage. *Lancet* 1980;1:688–72.

152 Bonifacio E, Lernmark A, Dawkins R. Serum exchange and use of dilutions have improved precision and measurements of islet cell antibodies. *J Immunol Meth* 1988;106:83–8.

153 Baekkeskov S, Aanstoot HJ, Christgau S *et al.* Identification of the 64k autoantigen in insulin dependent diabetes as the GABA synthesizing enzyme glutamic acid decarboxylase. *Nature* 1990;347:151–6.

154 Palmer JP, Asplin CM, Clemons P *et al.* Insulin antibodies in insulin deficient diabetics before insulin treatment. *Science* 1983;222:1337–9.

155 Arslanian SA, Becker DJ, Rabin B *et al.* Correlates of insulin antibodies in newly diagnosed children with insulin dependent diabetes prior to insulin therapy. *Diabetes* 1985;34: 926–30.

156 Srikanta S, Ricker AT, McCulloch DK, Soeldner JS, Eisenbarth GS, Palmer JP. Autoimmunity to insulin, beta cell dysfunction, and development of insulin dependent diabetes mellitus. *Diabetes* 1986;35:139–43.

157 Lernmark A, Freedman Z, Hofmann C *et al.* Islet-cell-surface antibodies in juvenile diabetes mellitus. *N Engl J Med* 1978; 299:375–80.

158 Rossini AA, Greiner DL, Friedman HP, Mordes JP. Immunopathogenesis of diabetes mellitus. *Diabetes Rev* 1993;1:43–75.

159 Palmer JP, Halqvist S, Spinas GA *et al.* Interaction of beta cell activity and IL-1 concentration and exposure time in isolated rat islets of Langerhans. *Diabetes* 1989;38:1211–16.

160 Eizirik DL, Tracy DE, Bendtzen K, Sandler S. An interleukin-1 receptor antagonist protein protects insulin producing beta cells against suppressive effects of interleukin-1 beta. *Diabetologia* 1991;34:445–8.

161 Nerup J, Mandrup-Poulsen T, Molvig J, Helqvist S, Wogensen LD. Pathogenesis of insulin dependent diabetes mellitus (IDDM) – a brief discussion of the 'Copenhagan Model'. In: Sakamoto N, Alberti KGMM, Hotta N, eds. *Current Status of Prevention and Treatment of Diabetic Complications*. International Congress Series No. 821. Amsterdam: Excerpta Medica, 1990:1–8.

162 Bergmann L, Kröncke KD, Suschek D, Kolb H, Kolb-Bachofen V. Cytotoxic action of IL-1 beta against pancreatic

islets is mediated by a nitric oxide formation and is inhibited by *N* monomethy-L-arginine. *FEBS Lett* 1992;299:103–6.

163 Rosenbloom AL, Hunt SS, Rosenbloom EK, Maclaren NK. Prognosis of impaired glucose tolerance in siblings of patients with insulin dependent diabetes. *Diabetes* 1982; 31:381–7.

164 Thi AC, Eisenbarth GS. Natural history of IDDM. *Diabetes Rev* 1993;1:1–14.

165 Palmer JP. Predicting IDDM: use of humoral immune markers. *Diabetes Rev* 1993;1:104–15.

166 Elliott RB, Berryman CC, Crossley JR, James AG. Partial preservation of pancreatic beta cell function in children with diabetes. *Lancet* 1981;2:1–4.

167 Feutren G, Papoz L, Assan R *et al.* Cyclosporine increases the rate and length of remission in insulin dependent diabetes of recent onset: results of a multi-center double-blind trial. *Lancet* 1986;1:119–24.

168 The Canadian–European Randomized Control Trial Group. Cyclosporine induced remission of IDDM after early intervention: association of one year of cyclosporine treatment with enhanced insulin secretion. *Diabetes* 1988;37: 1574–82.

169 Skyler JS, Marks JB. Immune intervention in Type I diabetes mellitus. *Diabetes Rev* 1993;1:15–42.

170 Keller RJ, Eisenbarth GS, Jackson RA. Insulin prophylaxis in individuals at high risk of Type I diabetes. *Lancet* 1993; 341:927–8.

171 Shah SC, Malone JI, Simpson NE. A randomized trial of intensive insulin therapy in newly diagnosed Type I insulin dependent diabetes mellitus. *N Engl J Med* 1989;320:550–4.

172 Warren SH, LeCompte PHM, Legg MA. *The Pathology of Diabetes Mellitus*. Philadelphia, PA: Lea & Febiger, 1966.

173 MacLean N, Ogilvie RF. Observations on the pancreatic islet tissue of young diabetic subjects. *Diabetes* 1959;8: 83–91.

174 Klöppel G, Freytag G. Insulin antibodies and immune insulitis in rabbits immunized with bovine or porcine insulin components. *Horm Metab Res* 1975;7:25–30.

175 Lacy PE, Wright PH. Allergic interstitial pancreatitis in rats injected with guinea pig anti-insulin serum. *Diabetes* 1965; 14:634–42.

176 Wrenshall GA, Bogoch A, Ritchie RC. Extractable insulin of pancreas: correlation with pathological and clinical findings in diabetic and non-diabetic cases. *Diabetes* 1952;1:87–105.

177 Yalow RS, Berson SA. Immunoassay of endogenous plasma insulin in man. *J Clin Invest* 1960;39:1157–75.

178 Froesch ER, Bürgi H, Müller WA *et al.* Mit Antiinsulinserum hemmbare und nicht-hemmbare Insulinaktivität im menschlichen Serum. *Schweiz Med Wochenschr* 1964;94: 309–13.

179 Chiumello G, Del Guercio MJ, Bidone G. Effects of glucagon and tolbutamide on plasma insulin levels in children with ketoacidosis. *Diabetes* 1968;17:133–5.

180 Drash A, Field JB, Garces LY *et al.* Endogenous insulin and growth hormone response in children with newly diagnosed diabetes mellitus. *Pediatr Res* 1968;2:94–102.

181 Parker ML, Pildes RS, Chao KL, Cornblath M, Kipnis DM. Juvenile diabetes mellitus, a deficiency in insulin. *Diabetes* 1968;17:27–32.

182 Theodoridis CG, Chance GW, Brown GA. Plasma insulin and growth hormone levels in untreated diabetic children. *Arch Dis Child* 1970;45:70–2.

183 Ehrlich RM, Bambers G. Immunologic assay of insulin in plasma of children. *Diabetes* 1964;13:177–81.

184 Weber B. Plasmainsulin bei Kindern, Klinische Studien bei stoffwechselgesunden, adipösen und diabetischen Probanden. *Beiheft Arch Kinderheilkd* 1971:65.

185 Howorka K. *Funktionelle, nahe-normoglykämische insulinsubstitution*. Berlin: Springer Verlag, 1987.

186 Weber B. Glucagon-induced insulin secretion in diabetic children. In: Laron Z, Kasp M, eds. *Diabetes in Juveniles*. Basel: Karger, 1975.

187 Fajans SS, Floyd JC Jr, Pek S *et al.* Studies on the natural history of asymptomatic diabetes in young people. *Metabolism* 1973;22:327–34.

188 Heinze E, Beischer W, Keller L, Winkler G, Teller WM, Pfeiffer EF. C-peptide secretion during the remission phase of juvenile diabetes. *Diabetes* 1978;27:670–6.

189 Kosaka K, Hagura R, Kuzuya T, Kuzuya N. Insulin secretory response of diabetics during the period of improvement of glucose tolerance to normal range. *Diabetologia* 1974;10: 775–82.

190 Buchanan KD, McCaroll AM. Abnormalities of glucagon metabolism in untreated diabetes mellitus. *Lancet* 1971;2: 1394–5.

191 Müller WA, Faloona GR, Aguilar-Parada E, Unger RH. Abnormal alpha cell function in diabetes: response to carbohydrate and protein ingestion. *N Engl J Med* 1970;283: 109–15.

192 Bennett PH, Aronoff SL, Unger RH. Evidence for an insulin-dependent alpha-cell abnormality in human diabetes. *Metabolism* 1976;25(Suppl. 1):1527–9.

193 Unger RH. Diabetes and the alpha cell. *Diabetes* 1976;25: 136–51.

194 Gerich JE, Tsalikian E, Lorenzi M *et al.* Normalization of fasting hyperglucagonemia and excessive glucagon responses to intravenous arginine in human diabetes mellitus by prolonged infusion of insulin. *J Clin Endocrinol Metab* 1975;41: 1178–81.

195 Unger RH, Aguilar-Parada E, Müller WA, Eisentraut AM. Studies of pancreatic alpha cell function in normal and diabetic subjects. *J Clin Invest* 1970;49:837–48.

196 Unger RH. Role of glucagon in the pathogenesis of diabetes: the status of the controversy. *Metabolism* 1978;27:1691–709.

197 Unger RH. Alpha- and beta-cell interrelationships in health and disease. *Metabolism* 1974;23:581–93.

198 McGarry JD. New perspectives in the regulation of ketogenesis. *Diabetics* 1979;28:517–23.

199 McGarry JD, Robles-Valdes C, Foster DW. Glucagon and ketogenesis. *Metabolism* 1976;25(Suppl. 1):1387–9.

200 Felig P, Wahren J, Sherwin R, Hendler R. Insulin, glucagon and somatostatin in normal physiology and diabetes mellitus. *Diabetes* 1976;25:1091–9.

201 Sherwin RS, Fisher M, Hendler R, Felig P. Hyperglucagonemia and blood glucose regulation in normal, obese and diabetic subjects. *N Engl J Med* 1976;294:455–61.

202 Barnes AJ, Kohner EM, Bloom SR, Johnston DG, Alberti KG, Smythe F. Importance of pituitary hormones in aetiology of diabetic ketoacidosis. *Lancet* 1978;2:1171–4.

203 Cherrington AD, Chiasson JL, Liljenquist JE, Jennings AS, Keller U, Lacy WW. The role of insulin and glucagon in the regulation of basal glucose production in the postabsorptive dog. *J Clin Invest* 1976;58:1407–18.

204 Gerich JE. Metabolic effects of long-term somatostatin infusion in man. *Metabolism* 1976;25:1505–7.

205 Houssay BA. The hypophysis and metabolism. *N Engl J Med*

1936;214:961–5.
206 Sperling MA. The contribution of hyperglycaemic hormones to the pathogenesis of diabetes mellitus. *Am J Dis Child* 1977;131:1145–9.
207 Hansen AP. Abnormal serum growth hormone response to exercise in juvenile diabetes. *J Clin Invest* 1970;49:1467–78.
208 Hansen AP, Johansen K. Diurnal pattern of blood glucose, serum FFA, insulin, glucagon, and growth hormone in normals and juvenile diabetics. *Diabetologia* 1970;6:27–33.
209 Hansen AP. Normalization of growth hormone hyperresponse to exercise in juvenile diabetics after 'normalization' of blood sugar. *J Clin Invest* 1971;50:1806–11.
210 Vigneri R, Squatrito S, Pezzino V, Filetti S, Branca S, Polosa P. Growth hormone levels in diabetes. Correlation with the clinical control of the disease. *Diabetes* 1976;25:167–72.
211 Hasselblatt A. Stoffwechselwirkungen der Katecholamine. In: Oberdisse K, ed. *Diabetes Mellitus*. Berlin: Springer Verlag, 1975:503–16.
212 Ewing DJ, Martyn CN, Young CJ, Clarke BS. The value of cardiovascular autonomic function tests: 10 years experience in diabetes. *Diabetes Care* 1985;8:491–8.
213 Köberling J. Genetic heterogeneities within idiopathic diabetes. In: Creutzfeldt W, Köberling J, Neel JV, eds. *The Genetics of Diabetes Mellitus*. Berlin: Springer Verlag, 1976: 79–87.
214 Palmberg P. Diabetic retinopathy. *Diabetes* 1977;26:703–9.
215 Weber B, Hasala M. Temporary partial remission in type I diabetes of juvenile onset. *Acta Paediatr Jpn* 1987;29: 393–400.
216 Tamborlane WV, Sherwin RS, Koivisto V *et al.* Normalization of the growth hormone and catecholamine response to exercise in juvenile-onset diabetic subjects treated with a portable infusion pump. *Diabetes* 1974;28:785–8.
217 Merimee TJ, Fitzgerald CR, Gold LA, McCourt JP. Characteristics of growth hormone secretion in clinically stable diabetes. *Diabetes* 1979;28:308–12.
218 Oberdisse U, Woweries J, Weber B. Metabolic consequences of exercise in juvenile diabetes. In: Laron Z, ed. *Medical Aspects of Balance of Diabetes in Juveniles*. Basel: Karger, 1977:220–6.
219 Schaper NC. Growth hormone secretion in Type I diabetes: a review. *Acta Endocrinol* 1990;122:7–12.
220 Sperling MA, Wollesen F, DeLamater PV. Daily production and metabolic clearance of growth hormone in juvenile diabetes. *Diabetologia* 1973;9:380–3.
221 Amiel SA, Sherwin RS, Hintz RL, Gertner JM, Press CM, Tamborlane WV. Effects of diabetes and its control on insulin-like growth factors in the subject with Type I diabetes. *Diabetes* 1984;33:1175–9.
222 Blethen SL, Sargeant DT, Whitelow MG, Santiago JV. Effect of pubertal stage and recent blood glucose control on plasma somatomedin-C in children with insulin dependent diabetes. *Diabetes* 1981;30:868–72.
223 Lanes R, Becker B, Fort P, Lifshitz F. Impaired somatomedin generation test in children with insulin dependent diabetes mellitus. *Diabetes* 1985;34:156–60.
224 Rieu M, Binoux M. Serum levels of insulin-like growth factor (IGF) and IGF binding protein in insulin-dependent diabetics during an episode of severe metabolic decompensation under recovery phase. *J Clin Endocrinol Metab* 1985; 60:781–5.
225 Baxter RC, Bryson JM, Turtle JR. Somatogenic receptors of rat liver: regulation by insulin. *Endocrinology* 1980;107: 1176–81.
226 Maes M, Underwood LE, Ketelslegers JM. Low serum somatomedin-C in insulin dependent diabetes: evidence for a post-receptor mechanism. *Endocrinology* 1986;118: 377–82.
227 Arslanian SA, Menon RK, Gierl AP, Heil BV, Foley TP. Insulin therapy increases low plasma growth hormone binding protein in children with new onset Type I diabetes. *Diabetic Med* 1993;10:833–8.
228 Schade DS, Eaton RP, Peake GT. The regulation of plasma ketone body concentration by counter-regulatory hormones in man. *Diabetes* 1978;27:916–24.
229 Barnes AJ, Bloom SR. Pancreatectomized man: a model for diabetes without glucagon. *Lancet* 1976;1:219–21.
230 Zimmermann H. Die Wirkungen der Corticosteroide auf den Kohlenhydratstoffwechsel. In: Oberdisse K, ed. *Diabetes Mellitus*. Berlin, Springer Verlag, 1975:473–502.
231 Boyle PJ. Cushing's disease, glucocorticoid excess, glucocorticoid deficiency and diabetes. *Diabetes Rev* 1993;1:301–8.
232 Olefsky JM, Johnson J, Liu F, Jen P, Reaven GM. The effects of acute and chronic dexamethasone administration on insulin binding to isolated rat hepatocytes and adipocytes. *Metabolism* 1975;24:517–27.
233 Perley M, Kipnis DM. Effects of glucocorticoids on plasma insulin. *N Engl J Med* 1966;274:1237–41.
234 Bruck E, MacGillivray MH, Voorhess ML. Hormonal balance during acute ketoacidosis in children with previously controlled diabetes mellitus. In: Laron Z, ed. *Medical Aspects of Balance of Diabetes in Juveniles*. Basel: Karger, 1977: 207–19.
235 Garces LY, Kenny FM, Drash A, Preeyasombat C. Cortisol secretion in acidotic and non-acidotic juvenile diabetes mellitus. *J Pediatr* 1969;74:517–22.
236 Robertson RP, Halter JB, Porte D Jr. A role for alpha-adrenergic receptors in abnormal insulin secretion in diabetes mellitus. *J Clin Invest* 1976;57:791–5.
237 Christiansen JS. On the pathogenesis of increased glomerular filtration rate in short-term insulin-dependent diabetes. *Danish Med Bull* 1984;31:349–61.
238 MacGillivray MH, Brock E, Voorhees ML. Acute diabetic ketoacidosis in children: role of the stress hormones. *Pediatr Res* 1981;15:99–106.
239 Baker L, Minuchin S, Milman L *et al.* Psychosomatic aspects of juvenile diabetes mellitus: a progress report. In: Laron Z, ed. *Diabetes in Juveniles. Modern Problems in Paediatrics*, Vol. 12. Basel: Karger, 1975:332–43.
240 Cryer PE, White NH, Santiago JV. The relevance of glucose counterregulatory systems to patients with insulin dependent diabetes mellitus. *Endocrinol Rev* 1986;7:131–9.
241 Hoffman RP, Singer-Granick C, Drash AL, Becker DJ. Plasma catecholamine response to hypoglycemia in children and adolescents with IDDM. *Diabetes Care* 1991;14:81–8.
242 Singer-Granick C, Hoffman RP, Kerensky K, Drash AL, Becker DJ. Glucagon responses to hypoglycemia in children and adolescents with diabetes mellitus. *Diabetes Care* 1988; 11:643–9.
243 Hoffman RP, Arslanian S, Drash AL, Becker DJ. Impaired counterregulatory hormone responses to hypoglycemia in children and adolescents with new onset IDDM. *J Pediatr Endocrinol* 1994;7:235–44.
244 Gerich JE, Langlois M, Noaco C, Karam JH, Forsham PH. Lack of glucagon response to hypoglycemia in diabetes: evidence of an intrinsic alpha cell defect. *Science* 1973;182: 171–3.

245 Cryer PE, Gerich JE. Glucose counterregulation, hypoglycemia and intensive insulin therapy in diabetes mellitus. *Ann J Med* 1985;313:232–41.
246 Cryer PE. Iatrogenic hypoglycemia as a cause of hypoglycemia-associated autonomic failure in IDDM. *Diabetes* 1992;41:255–60.
247 Veneman T, Mitrakou A, Mokan M, Cryer P, Gerich J. Induction of hypoglycemia unawareness by asymptomatic nocturnal hypoglycemia. *Diabetes* 1993;12:33–7.
248 Crofford OB, Minemura T, Lacy WW. Effect of insulin on the transport and metabolism of aminoacids in isolated fat cells. In: Jeanrenaud B, Hepp D, eds. *Adipose Tissue.* Stuttgart: Thieme, 1970:120–4.
249 Levine R. Mechanisms of insulin action. In: Levine R, Luft R, eds. *Advances in Metabolic Disorders,* Vol. VII. New York: Academic Press, 1974:183–9.
250 Jungas RL, Ball EG. Studies on the metabolism of adipose tissue. XII: The effects of insulin and epinephrine on free fatty acid and glycerol production in the presence and absence of glucose. *Biochemistry* 1963;2:383.
251 Exton JH. Gluconeogenesis. *Metabolism* 1972;21:945–90.
252 DeFronzo RA, Hendler R, Simonson D. Insulin resistance is a prominent feature of insulin-dependent diabetes. *Diabetes* 1982;31:795–801.
253 Pedersen O, Beck-Nielsen H. Insulin resistance and insulin-dependent diabetes mellitus. *Diabetes Care* 1987;10:516–23.
254 Amiel SA, Sherwin RS, Simonson D, Lauritano AA, Tamborlane WV. Impaired insulin action in puberty: a contributing factor to poor glycemic control in adolescents with diabetes. *N Engl J Med* 1986;315:215–19.
255 Arslanian SA, Nixon PA, Becker D, Drash AL. Impact of physical fitness in glycemic control on in vivo insulin action in adolescents with IDDM. *Diabetes Care* 1990;13: 9–15.
256 Yki-Jarvinen H, Koivisto VA. Insulin sensitivity in newly diagnosed Type I diabetics after ketoacidosis and after three months of insulin therapy. *J Clin Endocrinol Metab* 1984;59: 371–8.
257 Randle PJ, Hales CN, Garland PB *et al.* The glucose fatty acid cycle. Its role in insulin sensitivity and the metabolic disturbances of diabetes mellitus. *Lancet* 1963;1:785–9.
258 Weber B. Biochemische and endokinologische Grund-lagen der einfachen Adipositas. *Monatsschr Kinderheilk* 1975;123: 247–54.
259 Kahn CR, Goldstein BJ, Reddy SS. Hereditary and acquired syndromes in insulin resistance. In: Pickup JC, Williams G, eds. *Textbook of Diabetes.* Oxford: Blackwell Scientific Publications, 1991:276–85.
260 Rimoin DL. Genetic syndromes associated with glucose intolerance. In: Creutzfeldt W, Köbberling J, Neel JV, eds. *The Genetics of Diabetes Mellitus.* Berlin: Springer Verlag, 1976:43–63.
261 DelPrato S, Tiengo A. Pancreatic diabetes. *Diabetes Rev* 1993;1:260–85.
262 Livingston JN, Moxley RT III. Myotonic dystrophy: phenotype–genotype and insulin resistance. *Diabetes Rev* 1994;29:42.
263 Rosenbloom AL, Drash AL, Guthrie R. Chemical diabetes mellitus in childhood. Report of a conference. *Diabetes* 1972;21:45–9.
264 Lister J. The clinical spectrum of juvenile diabetes. *Lancet* 1966;1:386–8.
265 Weber B. Glucose-stimulated insulin secretion during 'remission' of juvenile diabetes. *Diabetologia* 1972;8:189–95.
266 Rosenbloom AL, Wheeler L, Bianchi R *et al.* Age-adjusted analysis of insulin responses during normal and abnormal glucose tolerance tests in children and adolescents. *Diabetes* 1975;24:820–8.
267 Lestradet H, Deschamps I, Giron B. Insulin and free fatty acid levels during oral glucose tolerance tests and their relation to age in 70 healthy children. *Diabetes* 1976;25: 505–8.
268 Hürter P, Jochum KH, Haeckel R. Standardisierung des oralen Glukosetoleranztests mit einem Oligosaccharid-gemisch (Dextro-OGT) bei Schulkindern. *Monatsschr Kinderheilkd* 1975;123:466–7.
269 Weber B. Standardization of the oral glucose test. *Internat Study Group Diabetes Child Adolesc. Bulletin* 1978;2: 23–7.
270 Drash AL. Diabetes mellitus in the child and adolescent; Part I. *Curr Probl Pediatr* 1986:XVI.
271 Akerblom HK. Definition of partial remission in insulin-dependent, juvenile-onset diabetes mellitus (IDDM). *Acta Paediatr Belg* 1980;33:66 (Abstr.).
272 Madsbad S. Prevalence of residual beta cell function and its metabolic consequences in Type I (insulin-dependent) diabetes. *Diabetologia* 1983;24:141–7.
273 Baker L, Kaye R, Root AW. The early partial remission of juvenile diabetes mellitus. *J Pediatr* 1967;71:825–31.
274 Field JB. Correlation between plasma insulin responses to glucose and tolbutamide and clinical remissions in newly diagnosed, juvenile type diabetic patients. In: Laron Z, ed. *Diabetes in Juveniles.* Basel: Karger, 1975:38–47.
275 Hernandez A, Zorilla E, Gersberg H. Serum-insulin in remission of juvenile diabetes. *Lancet* 1968;2:223.
276 Illig R, Prader A. Remission of juvenile diabetes. *Lancet* 1968;2:1190.
277 Bolli GB, Fanelli CG, Perriello G, DeFeo P. Nocturnal blood glucose control in Type I diabetes mellitus. *Diabetes Care* 1993;16(3):71–89.
278 Arslanian S, Ohki Y, Becker DJ, Drash AL. Demonstration of a dawn phenomenon in normal adolescents. *Horm Res* 1990; 34:27–32.
279 Cryer PE, Binder C, Bolli GB *et al.* Hypoglycemia in IDDM. *Diabetes* 1989;38:1193–9.
280 Raskin P. The Somogyi phenomenon: sacred cow or bull? *Arch Intern Med* 1984;144:781–7.
281 Alberti KGMM, Press CM. The biochemistry of the complications of diabetes mellitus. In: Keen H, Jarrett J, eds. *Complications of Diabetes Mellitus.* London: Edward Arnold, 1982:231.
282 DeFronzo RA, Cook CR, Andres R, Faloona GR, Davis PJ. The effects of insulin and renal handling of sodium, potassium, calcium and phosphate in man. *J Clin Invest* 1975; 55:845–55.
283 Kreisberg RA. Diabetic ketoacidosis: new concepts and trends in pathogenesis in treatment. *Ann Intern Med* 1978; 88(5):681–95.
284 Ryan CM, Atchison J, Puczynski S, Puczynski M, Arslanian S, Becker D. Mild hypoglycemia associated with deterioration of mental efficiency in children with insulin dependent diabetes mellitus. *J Pediatr* 1990;117:32–8.
285 The DCCT Research Group. The effect of intensive treatment of diabetes on the development and progression of long-term complications in insulin dependent diabetes mellitus. *N Engl J Med* 1993;329:977–86.

286 Bergada I, Suissa S, Dufresne J, Schiffrin A. Severe hypoglycemia in IDDM children. *Diabetes Care* 1989;12:239–44.
287 Goldstein DE, England JD, Hess R, Rawlings SS, Walker B. A prospective study of symptomatic hypoglycemia in young diabetic patients. *Diabetes Care* 1981;4:601–5.
288 Pramming S, Thorsteinsson B, Bendtson I, Ronn B, Binder C. Nocturnal hypoglycemia in patients receiving conventional treatment with insulin. *Br Med J* 1985;291:376–9.
289 Sussman KE. Infections in the diabetic. In: Sussman KE, ed. *Juvenile Type Diabetes and its Complications*. Springfield, IL: CC Thomas, 1971:165–82.
290 Francois R, Memelle N, Leonetti P, Jarlot B, Gillet P, David L, Tardieu M. Degenerative complications after 10 years of juvenile diabetes. *Journ Annu Diabetol Hotel Dieu* 1976: 135–56.
291 Bagdade JD, Stewart M, Walters E. Impaired granulocyte adherence. A reversible defect in host defense in patients with poorly controlled diabetes. *Diabetes* 1978;27:677–81.
292 Bagdade JD, Root RK, Bulger RJ. Impaired leucocyte function in patients with poorly controlled diabetes. *Diabetes* 1974; 23:9–15.
293 Miller ME, Baker L. Leucocyte functions in juvenile diabetes mellitus. Humoral and cellular aspects. *J Pediatr* 1972;81: 979–89.
294 Mowat AG, Baum J. Chemotoxis of polymorphonuclear leucocytes from patients with diabetes mellitus. *N Engl J Med* 1971;284:621–7.
295 Niethammer D, Heinze E, Teller W *et al.* Impairment of granulocyte function in juvenile diabetes. *Klin Wochenschr* 1975;53:1057–60.
296 Perillie PE, Nolan JP, Finch SS. Studies of the resistance to infection in diabetes mellitus: local exudative cellular response. *J Lab Clin Med* 1962;59:1008–15.
297 Ludwig H, Eibl M, Schernthaner G *et al.* Humoral immunodeficiency to bacterial antigens in patients with juvenile onset diabetes mellitus. *Diabetologia* 1976;12:259–62.
298 Wagner R, White P, Bogan IK. Diabetic dwarfism. *Am J Dis Child* 1942;63:667–727.
299 Tattersall RB, Pyke DA. Growth in diabetic children. Studies in identical twins. *Lancet* 1973;2:1105–10.
300 Clarke WL, Vance ML, Rogol AD. Growth and the child with diabetes mellitus. *Diabetes Care* 1993;16:101–6.
301 Müller-Hess R, Oberdisse U, Pachaly I *et al.* Die somatische Entwicklung juveniler Diabetiker. In: Weber B, ed. *Ambulante Langzeitbehandlung Diabetischer Kinder und Jugendlicher*. Stuttgart: Enke Verlag, 1977:27–40.
302 Brown M, Ahmed ML, Clayton KL, Dunger DB. Growth during childhood and final height in Type I diabetes. *Diabetic Med* 1994;11(2):182–7.
303 Songer TJ, Laporte RE, Tajima N *et al.* Height at the diagnosis of insulin dependent diabetes in patients and their nondiabetic family members. *Br Med J* 1986;292:1419–22.
304 Jivani SKM, Rayner PHGW. Does control influence the growth of diabetic children. *Arch Dis Child* 1973;48:109–15.
305 Wise J, Kolb E, Sauder S. Effect of glycemic control on growth velocity in children with IDDM. *Diabetes Care* 1992;15:826–30.
306 Laron Z, Volovitz B, Karp M. Linear growth and insulin dose as indices of control in children with diabetes mellitus. In: Laron Z, ed. *Medical Aspects of Balance of Diabetes in Juveniles*. Basel: Karger, 1977.
307 Guest GM. The Mauriac syndrome, dwarfism, hepatomegaly and obesity with juvenile diabetes. *Diabetes* 1953;2:415–17.
308 Mauriac P. Gros ventre, hepatomegalie, troubles de la croissance chez des enfants diabetiques, traites depuis plusiers annees par l'insuline. *Gaz Hebd Soc Med Bordeaux* 1930;26:402–10.
309 Dorchy H, van Vliet G, Toussaint B *et al.* Mauriac syndrome: three cases with retinal angiofluorescein study. *Diabete Metab* 1979;3:195–200.
310 Lee RGL, Bode HH. Stunted growth and hepatomegaly in diabetes mellitus. *J Pediatr* 1977;91:82–4.
311 Bergquist N. The growth of juvenile diabetes. *Acta Endocrinol* 1954;15:133–65.
312 Sharp SC, Diamond MP. Sex steroids and diabetes. *Diabetes Rev* 1993;1:318–42.
313 Rosenbloom AL, Silverstein JH, Lezotte DC, Rile WJ, MacLaren NK. Limited joint mobility in diabetes mellitus of childhood: natural history and relationship to growth impairments. *J Pediatr* 1982;101:874–8.
314 Schnider SL, Kohn RR. Effects of age and diabetes mellitus on the solubility and nonenzymatic glucosylation of human skin collagen. *J Clin Invest* 1981;67:1630–5.
315 Reimer-Veit M, Burger W, Kroll M *et al.* Prevalence and development of limited joint mobility (LJM) in type I diabetic children and adolescents. In: Weber B, ed. *Early Vascular Complications in Children with Diabetes Mellitus. Pediatric and Adolescent Endocrinology*, Vol. 17. Basel: Karger, 1988:111–21.
316 Brink S. Limited joint mobility (LJM) as a risk factor for complications in youngsters with IDDM. *Diabetes* 1983;32(Suppl. 1):16A (Abstr.).
317 Rosenbloom AL, Silverstein JH, Riley WJ *et al.* Joint contracture in childhood diabetes indicates high risk for vasculopathy. In: Weber B, ed. *Diabetic Angiopathy in Children*. Berlin: Karger, 1981:143–8.
318 Jelinek JE. Skin disorders associated with diabetes mellitus. In: Rifkin H, Porte D, eds. *Ellenberg and Rifkin's Diabetes Mellitus: Theory and Practice*, 4th edn. New York: Elsevier, 1990:838.
319 Tsalikian E, Becker DJ, Crumrine PK, Daneman D, Drash AL. Electroencephalographic changes in diabetic ketoacidosis in children with newly and previously diagnosed insulin-dependent diabetes mellitus. *J Pediatr* 1981;98: 355–9.
320 Kubany AJ, Danowski TS, Moses C. The personality and intelligence of diabetics. *Diabetes* 1956;5:462–7.
321 Manciaux M, Sardin AM, Hennion E. Aspects psychologiques du diabete infantile. *Rev Neuropsychiatrie Infant* 1967;15:737–47.
322 Rovet JF, Ehrlich RM, Hoppe M. Intellectual deficits associated with early onset insulin dependent diabetes mellitus in children. *Diabetes Care* 1987;10:510–15.
323 Ryan C, Vega A, Drash A. Cognitive deficits in adolescents who develop diabetes early in life. *Pediatrics* 1985;75: 921–7.
324 Becker DJ. Complications of insulin dependent diabetes mellitus in childhood and adolescence. In: Lifshitz F, ed. *Pediatric Endocrinology*, 2nd edn. New York: Marcel Dekker, 1990:701.
325 Knowles HC Jr. Artherosclerosis in juvenile diabetes. In: Laron Z, ed. *Diabetes in Juveniles*. Basel: Karger, 1975: 293–6.
326 White P, Graham CA. The child with diabetes. In: Marble A, White P, Bradley RF *et al.*, eds. *Joslin's Diabetes Mellitus*. Philadelphia, PA: Lea & Febiger, 1971:339–60.

327 Bojestig M, Arnqvist HJ, Hermansson G, Karlberg BE, Ludvigsson J. Declining incidence of nephropathy in insulin-dependent diabetes mellitus. *N Engl J Med* 1994; 330:15–18.
328 Ramsay RC, Goetz FC, Sutherland DER *et al.* Progression of diabetic retinopathy after pancreas transplantation for insulin-dependent diabetes mellitus. *N Engl J Med* 1988; 318:208–14.
329 Tschobroutsky G. Relation of diabetic control to development of microvascular complications. *Diabetologia* 1978;15:143–52.
330 Yagihashi S, Goto Y, Kakizaki M *et al.* Thickening of glomerular basement membrane in spontaneously diabetic rats. *Diabetologia* 1978;15:309–12.
331 Yesus YW, Esterly JE, Stuhlmann RA *et al.* Significant muscle capillary basement membrane thickening in spontaneously diabetic Mystromys Albicaudatus. *Diabetes* 1976; 25:444–9.
332 Siperstein MD, Unger RH, Madison LL. Studies of muscle capillary basement membranes in normal subjects, diabetic and prediabetic patients. *J Clin Invest* 1968;47:1973–99.
333 Ganda OP, Soeldner JS, Gleason RE *et al.* Monozygotic triplets with discordance for diabetes mellitus and diabetic microangiopathy. *Diabetes* 1977;26:469–79.
334 Pyke DA, Tattersall RB. Diabetic retinopathy in identical twins. *Diabetes* 1973;22:613–18.
335 Keen H. Chronic complications of diabetes mellitus. In: Galloway JP, Patvin JH, Shuman CR, eds. *Diabetes Mellitus.* Indianapolis, IN: Eli Lilly, 1988:178–305.
336 Reichard P, Nilsson BY, Rosenquist U. The effect of long-term intensified insulin treatment on the development of microvascular complications of diabetes mellitus. *N Engl J Med* 1993;329:304–9.
337 Becker DJ, Orchard TJ, Lloyd CE. Control and outcome: clinical and epidemiologic aspects. In: Kelnar CJH, ed. *Childhood Diabetes.* London: Chapman & Hall, 1994:519–38.
338 Engerman R, Bloodworth JM Jr, Nelson S. Relationship of microvascular disease in diabetes to metabolic control. *Diabetes* 1977;26:760–9.
339 Rasch R. Prevention of diabetic glomerulopathy in streptozotocin diabetic rats by insulin treatment: the mesangial regions. *Diabetologia* 1979;17:243–8.
340 Gabbay KH. Hyperglycemia, polyol metabolism, and complications of diabetes mellitus. *Annu Rev Med* 1975;26: 521–36.
341 Raskin P. Diabetic regulation and its relationship to microangiopathy. *Metabolism* 1978;27:235–51.
342 Spiro RG. Investigations into the biochemical basis of diabetic basement-membrane alterations. *Diabetes* 1976; 25(Suppl. 2):909–13.
343 Malone JI, Knox G, Harvey C. Sorbitol accumulation is altered in Type 1 (insulin-dependent) diabetes mellitus. *Diabetologia* 1984;27:509–13.
344 Clements RS Jr. Diabetic neuropathy – new concepts of its etiology (Review). *Diabetes* 1979;28:604–11.
345 Fajius J, Brattberg A, Jameson S, Berne C. Limited benefit of treatment of diabetic polyneuropathy with an aldose reductase inhibitor: a 24-week controlled trial. *Diabetologia* 1985;28:323–9.
346 Finegold D, Lattimer SA, Nolle S, Bernstein M, Greene DA. Polyol pathway activity and myo-inositol metabolism. A suggested relationship in the pathogenesis of diabetic neuropathy. *Diabetes* 1983;32:988–92.
347 Salway JG, Whitehead L, Finnegan JA *et al.* Effect of myo-inositol on peripheral-nerve function in diabetes. *Lancet* 1978;2:1282–4.
348 Greene DA, Lattimer SA, Sima AAF. Sorbitol, phosphoinositides and sodium potassium ATPase in the pathogenesis of diabetic complications. *N Engl J Med* 1987;316:599–606.
349 Williamson JR, Rowold E, Chang K *et al.* Sex steroid dependency of diabetes-induced changes in polyol metabolism, vascular permeability, and collagen cross-linking. *Diabetes* 1986;35:20–7.
350 Brownlee M, Cerami A, Viassara H. Advanced glycosylated end products in tissues and the biochemical basis of diabetes complications. *N Engl J Med* 1988;318:1315–21.
351 Christlieb AR, Warram JH, Krolewski AS *et al.* Hypertension: the major risk factor in juvenile onset insulin dependent diabetes. *Diabetes* 1981;30:90–6.
352 Orchard TJ, Dorman JS, Maser R *et al.* Prevalence of complications in IDDM by sex in duration. Pittsburgh Epidemiology of Diabetes Complications Study – II. *Diabetes* 1990;39: 1116–24.
353 Cruickshanks KJ, Orchard TJ, Becker DJ. The cardiovascular risk profile of adolescents with insulin dependent diabetes mellitus. *Diabetes Care* 1985;8:118–24.
354 Coonrod BA, Ellis D, Becker DJ *et al.* Predictors of microalbuminuria in individuals with insulin-dependent diabetes mellitus. *Diabetes Care* 1993;16:1–8.
355 Mathiesen ER, Ronn B, Jensen T *et al.* Relationship between blood pressure and urine albumin excretion in the development of microalbuminuria. *Diabetes* 1990;39:245–9.
356 Elving LD, Wetzels JFM, de Nobel E, Berden JHM. Erythrocyte sodium–lithium countertransport is not different in Type 1 (insulin-dependent) diabetic patients with and without diabetic nephropathy. *Diabetologia* 1991;34:126–8.
357 Krolewski AS, Canessa M, Warram JH *et al.* Predisposition to hypertension and susceptibility to renal disease in insulin-dependent diabetes mellitus. *N Engl J Med* 1988;318:140–5.
358 Mangili R, Bending JJ, Scott G, Li KK, Gupta A, Verberti GC. Increased sodium–lithium countertransport activity in red cells of patients with insulin dependent diabetes and nephropathy. *N Engl J Med* 1988;18:146–50.
359 Hostetter-Rennke HG, Brenner BM. The case for intrarenal hypertension in the initiation and progression of diabetic and other glomerulopathies. *Am J Med* 1982;72:375.
360 Mogensen CE, Christensen CK. Predicting diabetic nephropathy in insulin-dependent patients. *N Engl J Med* 1984;311: 89–93.
361 Christensen NJ. Plasma norepinephrine and epinephrine in untreated diabetics, during fasting, and after insulin administration. *Diabetes* 1974;23:1–8.
362 Lundbaek K, Christensen NJ, Jensen VA *et al.* Diabetes, diabetic angiopathy, and growth hormone. *Lancet* 1970;2: 131–3.
363 Merimee TJ, Fineberg SE, Hollander W. Vascular disease in chronic HGH-deficient state. *Diabetes* 1973;22:813–19.
364 Merimee TJ, Zapf J, Froesch ER. Insulin-like growth factors: studies in diabetics with and without retinopathy. *N Engl J Med* 1983;309:527–30.
365 Colwell JA, Halushka PV, Sarji K *et al.* Altered platelet function in diabetes mellitus. *Diabetes* 1976;25(Suppl. 2): 826–31.
366 Norris Kostraba JM, Dorman JS, Orchard TJ *et al.* Contribution of diabetes duration before puberty to development of microvascular complications in IDDM subjects. *Diabetes Care* 1989;12:686–93.
367 Jay RH, Jones SL, Hill CE *et al.* Blood rheology and cardio-

vascular risk factors in Type I diabetes: relationship with microalbuminuria. *Diabetic Med* 1991;8:662–7.

368 Jones SL, Close CF, Mattock MB *et al.* Plasma lipid and coagulation factor concentrations in insulin dependent diabetics with microalbuminuria. *Br Med J* 1989;298: 487–90.

369 Maser RE, Pfeiffer MA, Kuller LH, Becker DJ, Orchard TJ. Diabetic autonomic neuropathy and cardiovascular risk. *Arch Intern Med* 1990;25:1218–24.

370 Maser RE, Rodewald AE, Dorman JS *et al.* Epidemiological correlates of diabetic neuropathy. Report from the Pittsburgh Epidemiology of Diabetes Complications Study. *Diabetes* 1989;38:1456–61.

371 Bangstad HJ, Osterby R, Dahl-Jorgensen K *et al.* Early glomerulopathy is present in young Type I (insulin-dependent) diabetic patients with microalbuminuria. *Diabetologia* 1993;36:523–9.

372 Sheikolislam BM, Irias JJ, Lin HJ *et al.* Carbohydrate metabolism and capillary basement-membrane thickness in children. I. Cross-sectional studies. *Diabetes* 1976;7: 650–60.

373 Steffes MW, Sutherland DER, Goetz FC, Rich SS, Mauer SM. Studies of kidney and muscle biopsy specimens from identical twins discordant for type I diabetes mellitus. *N Engl J Med* 1985;312:1282–7.

374 Rogers DG, White NH, Santiago JV *et al.* Glycemic control and bone age are independently associated with muscle capillary basement membrane width in diabetic children after puberty. *Diabetes Care* 1986;9:453–9.

375 Beisswenger PJ, Spiro RG. Studies on the human glomerular basement membrane: composition, nature of the carbohydrate units and chemical changes in diabetes mellitus. *Diabetes* 1973;22:180–93.

376 Spiro RG. Search for a biochemical basis of diabetic microangiopathy. *Diabetologia* 1976;12:1–4.

377 Spiro RG. Biochemistry of the renal glomerular basement membrane and its alterations in diabetes mellitus. *N Engl J Med* 1973;285:1337–42.

378 Bendayan M. Alteration in the distribution of Type IV collagen in glomerular basal laminae in diabetic rats as revealed by immunocytochemistry and morphometrical approach. *Diabetologia* 1985;28:373–8.

379 Kastrup J, Norgaard TN, Parving HH, Henriksen O, Lassen NA. Impaired autoregulation and blood flow in subcutaneous tissue of long-term Type 1 (insulin-dependent) diabetic patients with microangiopathy: an index of arteriolar dysfunction. *Diabetologia* 1985;28:711–17.

380 Parving HH. Microvascular permeability to plasma proteins in hypertension and diabetes mellitus in man – on the pathogenesis of hypertensive and diabetic microangiopathy. *Danish Med Bull* 1975;22:217–33.

381 Klein DJ, Brown DM, Oegema TR. Glomerular proteoglycans in diabetes. Partial structural characterization and metabolism of de novo synthesized Heparan-$^{35}SO_4$ and Dermatan-$^{35}SO_2$ proteoglycans in streptozocin-induced diabetic rats. *Diabetes* 1986;35:1130–42.

382 Deckert T, Feldt-Rasmussen B, Borch-Johnsen K, Jensen T, Kofoed-Enevoldsen A. Albuminuria reflects widespread vascular damage: the Steno hypothesis. *Diabetologia* 1989;32: 219–26.

383 Mogensen CE. Urinary albumin excretion in early and long-term juvenile diabetes. *Scand J Clin Lab Invest* 1971;28: 183–93.

384 Parving HH, Noer I, Deckert T *et al.* The effect of metabolic regulation on microvascular permeability to small and large molecules in short-term juvenile diabetics. *Diabetologia* 1976;12:161–6.

385 Mogensen CE. Renal function changes in diabetes. *Diabetes* 1976;25(Suppl. 2):872–9.

386 Kverneland A, Feldt-Rasmussen B, Vidal P *et al.* Evidence of changes in renal charge selectivity in patients with Type 1 (insulin-dependent) diabetes mellitus. *Diabetologia* 1986; 29:634–9.

387 Lee P, Jenkins A, Bourke C *et al.* Prothrombotic and antithrombotic factors are elevated in patients with Type I diabetes complicated by microalbuminuria. *Diabetic Med* 1993;10:122–28.

388 Watala C. Altered structural and dynamic properties of blood cell membranes in diabetes mellitus. *Diabetic Med* 1993;10: 13–20.

389 Paulsen EP, Sabio H, Ash SL *et al. Diabetic Angiopathy in Children*. Basel: Karger, 1981.

390 Ditzel J, Standl E. The problem of tissue oxygenation in diabetes mellitus. *Acta Med Scand* 1975;Suppl. 578:49–68.

391 Cunha-Vaz JG, Fonsega JR, Abreu FJ *et al.* Detection of early retinal changes in diabetes by vitreous fluorophotometry. *Diabetes* 1979;28:16–19.

392 Trivelli LA, Ranney HM, Lay HJ. Hemoglobin components in patients with diabetes mellitus. *N Engl J Med* 1971;284: 353–7.

393 Borch-Johnsen K, Andersen PK, Deckert T. The effect of proteinuria on relative mortality in Type I (insulin-dependent) diabetes mellitus. *Diabetologia* 1985;28:590–6.

394 Deckert T, Poulsen JE, Larsen M. Prognosis of diabetics with diabetes onset before the age of thirty-one. I. Survival, causes of death and complications. II. Factors influencing the prognosis. *Diabetologia* 1978;14:363–70 (I) and 371–7 (II).

395 Forsblom CM, Groop PH, Ekstrand A, Groop LC. Predictive value of microalbuminuria in patients with insulin dependent diabetes of long duration. *Br Med J* 1992;305:1051–3.

396 Andersen AR, Sandahl Christiansen J, Andersen JK, Kreiner S, Deckert T. Diabetic nephropathy in type I (insulin-dependent) diabetes: an epidemiological study. *Diabetologia* 1983;25:496–501.

397 Deckert T, Poulsen JE. Diabetic nephropathy: fault or destiny. *Diabetologia* 1981;21:178–83.

398 Mogensen CE, Steffes MW, Deckert T, Sandahl Christiansen J. Functional and morphological renal manifestations in diabetes mellitus. *Diabetologia* 1981;21:89–93.

399 Osterby R, Gundersen HJG. Glomerular size and structure in diabetes mellitus. I. Early abnormalities. *Diabetologia* 1975; 11:225–9.

400 Parving HH, Kastrup H, Smidt UM, Andersen AR, Feldt-Rasmussen B, Sandahl Christiansen J. Impaired autoregulation of glomerular filtration rate in Type 1 (insulin-dependent) diabetic patients with nephropathy. *Diabetologia* 1984;27:547–52.

401 Mortensen HB, Hougaard P, Ibsen KK, Parving HH *et al.* Relationship between blood pressure and urinary albumin excretion rate in young Danish Type I diabetic patients: comparison to non-diabetic children. *Diabetic Med* 1983;5: 155–61.

402 Rudberg S, Ullman E, Dahlquist G. Relationship between early metabolic control and the development of microalbuminuria – a longitudinal study in children with Type I (insulin-dependent) diabetes mellitus. *Diabetologia* 1993; 36:1309–14.

403 Cook J, Daneman D, Spino M, Sochett E, Perlman K, Balfe

JW. Angiotensin converting enzyme inhibitor therapy to decrease microalbuminuria in normotensive children with insulin-dependent diabetes mellitus. *J Pediatr* 1990;117: 39–45.

404 Mathiesen ER, Hommel E, Giese J, Parving HH. Efficacy of captopril in postponing nephropathy in normotensive insulin dependent diabetic patients with microalbuminuria. *Br Med J* 1991;303:81–7.

405 Rudberg S, Apena A, Freyschuss U, Persson BP. Enalapril reduces microalbuminuria in young normotensive Type I (insulin-dependent) diabetic patients irrespective of its hypotensive effect. *Diabetologia* 1990;33:470–6.

406 Feldt-Rasmussen B, Baker L, Deckert T. Exercise as a provocative test in early renal disease in Type 1 (insulin-dependent) diabetes: albuminuric, systemic, and renal haemodynamic responses. *Diabetologia* 1985;28:389–96.

407 Mogensen CE, Vittinghus E. Urinary albumin excretion during exercise in juvenile diabetics. A provocation test for early abnormalities. *Scand J Clin Lab Invest* 1975;35:295–300.

408 Cowell CT, Rogers S, Silink M. First morning urinary albumin concentration is a good predictor of 24-hour urinary albumin excretion in children with Type 1 (insulin-dependent) diabetes. *Diabetologia* 1986;29:97–9.

409 Ellis D, Avner ED, Transue D, Yunis EJ, Drash AL, Becker DJ. Diabetic nephropathy in adolescence: appearance during improved glycemic control. *Pediatrics* 1983;71:824–9.

410 Daneman D, Drash AL, Lobes LA, Becker DJ, Baker LM, Travis LB. Progressive retinopathy with improved control in diabetic dwarfism (Mauriac's syndrome). *Diabetes Care* 1981;4:360–5.

411 Roe TF, Costin G, Kaufman FP *et al.* Blood glucose control and albuminuria in Type I diabetes mellitus. *J Pediatr* 1991; 119:178–82.

412 Mogensen CE, Schmitz A, Christensen CK. Comparative renal pathophysiology relevant to IDDM and NIDDM patients. *Diabetes Metab Rev* 1988;4:453–83.

413 Cohen D, Dodds R, Viberti G. Effect of protein restriction in insulin dependent diabetics at risk of nephropathy. *Br Med J* 1987;294:795–8.

414 Jensen VA, Lundbaek K. The eye in diabetes mellitus. In: Pfeiffer EF, ed. *Handbuch des Diabetes Mellitus*, Vol. II. Munich: JF Lehmanns, 1971:659–81.

415 Moss SE, Klein R, Kessler SD. Comparison between ophthalmoscopy and fundus photography in determining severity of diabetic retinopathy. *Ophthalmology* 1985;92:62–7.

416 Burger W, Hovener G, Dusterhus R, Hartmann R, Weber B. Prevalence and development of retinopathy in children and adolescents with Type I (insulin-dependent) diabetes mellitus. A longitudinal study. *Diabetologia* 1986;29: 17–22.

417 Kohner EM. Diabetic retinopathy. *Clin Endocrinol Metab* 1977;6:345–75.

418 Kohner EM, Oakley NW. Diabetic retinopathy. *Metabolism* 1975;24:1085–102.

419 Palmberg P, Smith M, Waltmann S *et al.* The natural history of retinopathy in insulin-dependent juvenile-onset diabetes. *Ophthalmology* 1981;88:613–18.

420 Dorchy H, Toussaint B, Devroede M *et al.* Diagnostic de la retinopathie diabetique infantile par agiographie fluoresceinique. Description des lesions initiales. *Nouv Presse Med* 1977;6:345–7.

421 Kernell A, Finnstrom K, Ludvigsson J. Fluorescein leakage from retinal vessels in diabetic children: functional indicator of incipient retinopathy. In: Weber B, ed. *Early Vascular Complications in Children with Diabetes Mellitus. Pediatric and Adolescent Endocrinology*, Vol. 17. Basel: Karger, 1988: 75–81.

422 Klein R, Klein BEK, Moss SE, Davis MD, De Mets DL. The Wisconsin Epidemiologic Study of diabetic retinopathy. II. Prevalance and risk of diabetic retinopathy when age at diagnosis is less than 30 years. *Arch Ophthalmol* 1984;102: 520–6.

423 Deckert T, Simonsen SvE, Poulsen JE. Prognosis of proliferative retinopathy in juvenile diabetes. *Diabetes* 1967;16: 728–33.

424 Weber B, Burger W, Hartmann R, Hovener G, Malchus R, Oberdisse U. Risk factors for the development of retinopathy in children and adolescents with Type 1 (insulin-dependent) diabetes mellitus. *Diabetologia* 1986;29:23–9.

425 Chase HP, Jackson WE, Hoops L *et al.* Glucose control and the renal and retinal complications of insulin dependent diabetes. *J Am Med Assoc* 1989;261:1155–60.

426 Klein R, Klein BEK, Moss SE *et al.* Glycosylated hemoglobin predicts the incidence and progression of diabetic retinopathy. *J Am Med Assoc* 1988;260:2864–71.

427 Krolewski AS, Warram JH, Rand LI, Christlieb AR, Busick EJ, Kahn CR. Risk of proliferative diabetic retinopathy in juvenile-onset type 1 diabetes: a 40-year follow-up study. *Diabetes Care* 1986;9:443–52.

428 Lauritzen T, Frost-Larsen K, Larsen HW, Deckert T and the Steno Study Group. Two-year experience with continuous subcutaneous insulin infusion in relation to retinopathy and neuropathy. *Diabetes* 1985;35(Suppl. 3):74–9.

429 Testa MA, Puklin JE, Sherwin RS, Simonson DC. For the Kroc Collaborative Study Group. Clinical predictors of retinopathy and its progress in patients with type I diabetes during CSII or conventional insulin treatment. *Diabetes* 1985;34(Suppl. 3):61–8.

430 Ballegooie E, van Hooymans JMM, Timmerman Z *et al.* Rapid determination of diabetic retinopathy during treatment with continuous subcutaneous insulin infusion. *Diabetes Care* 1984;7:236–42.

431 Dahl Jorgensen K, Brinchmann-Hansen O, Hanssen KF, Sandvik L, Aagenases O. For the Aker Diabetes Group. Rapid tightening of blood glucose control leads to transient deterioration in retinopathy in insulin-dependent diabetes mellitus – the Oslo Study. *Br Med J* 1985;290:811–15.

432 Chase HP, Garg SK, Jackson WE *et al.* Blood pressure and retinopathy in Type I diabetes. *Ophthalmology* 1990;97: 155–9.

433 Janka HU, Warram JH, Rand LI, Krolewski AS. Risk factors for progression of background retinopathy in longstanding IDDM. *Diabetes* 1989;38:460–4.

434 Norgaard K, Feldt-Rasmussen B, Deckert T. Is hypertension a major risk factor for retinopathy in Type I diabetes? *Diabetic Med* 1991;8:334–7.

435 Leslie RDG, Pyke DA. Diabetic retinopathy in identical twins. *Diabetes* 1982;31:19–21.

436 Cruickshanks KJ, Vadheim CM, Moss SE *et al.* Genetic marker associations with proliferative retinopathy in persons diagnosed with diabetes before 30 years of age. *Diabetes* 1992;41:879–85.

437 Dornan TL, Ting A, McPherson CK *et al.* Genetic susceptibility to the development of retinopathy in insulin-dependent diabetics. *Diabetes* 1982;31:226–31.

438 Schernthaner G, Mayr WR. Clinical and immunologic studies of HLA-DR-typed insulin-dependent diabetes – a mini-review. *Exp Clin Endocrinol* 1984;83:184–91.

439 Standl E, Dexel T, Lander T *et al.* HLA and late diabetic complications. In: Köbberling J, Tattersall R, eds. *The Genetics of Diabetes Mellitus*. London: Academic Press, 1982:115–22.
440 Barbosa J, Saner B. Do genetic factors play a role in the pathogenesis of diabetic microangiopathy? *Diabetologia* 1984;27:487–92.
441 Becker B, Shin DH, Burgess D, Kilo C, Miller MV. Histocompatibility antigens and diabetic retinopathy. *Diabetes* 1976;26:997–9.
442 Bodansky HJ, Wolf E, Cudworth AG *et al.* Genetic and immunologic factors in microvascular disease in Type I insulin-dependent diabetes. *Diabetes* 1982;31:70–4.
443 Cudworth G, Bodansky HJ. Genetic and metabolic factors in relation to the prevalence and severity of diabetic complications. Genetic and immunological factors in diabetic complications. In: Keen H, Jarret J, eds. *Complications of Diabetes*, 2nd edn. London: Edward Arnold, 1982:1–12.
444 Möller E, Persson B, Sterky G. HLA phenotypes and diabetic retinopathy. *Diabetologia* 1978;14:155–8.
445 Irvine WJ, DiMario U, Guy K *et al.* Immune complexes and diabetic microangiopathy. In: Irvine J, ed. *Immunology of Diabetes*. Edinburgh: Teviot, 1980:325–36.
446 Stewart LL, Field LL, Ross S, McArthur RG. Genetic risk factors in diabetic retinopathy. *Diabetologia* 1993;36: 1293–8.
447 Boulton AJM, Worth RC, Drury J *et al.* Genetic and metabolic studies in diabetic neuropathy. *Diabetologia* 1984;26: 15–19.
448 Dorchy H, Noel P, Kruger M *et al.* Peroneal motor nerve conduction velocity in diabetic children and adolescents. Relationship to metabolic control, HLA-DR antigens, retinopathy and EEG. *Eur J Pediatr* 1985;144:310–15.
449 Hoffman WH, Hart ZH, Frank RN. Correlates of delayed motor nerve conduction and retinopathy in juvenile onset diabetes mellitus. *J Pediatr* 1983;102:351–6.
450 Käär ML, Saukkonen AL, Pitkänen A, Akerblom HK. Peripheral neuropathy in diabetic children and adolescents. A cross-sectional study. *Acta Paed Scand* 1983;Suppl. 73: 373–8.
451 Young RJ, Ewing DJ, Clarke BS. Nerve function and metabolic control in teenage diabetics. *Diabetes* 1983;32:142–7.
452 Sosenko JM, Boulton AJM, Kubrusly DB, Weinthaub JK, Skyler JS. The vibratory perception threshold in young diabetic patients: associations with glycemia and puberty. *Diabetes Care* 1985;8:605–7.
453 Cirillo D, Gonfiantini E, Grandis DD, Bongiovanni L, Robert JJ, Pinelli L. Visual evoked potentials in diabetic children and adolescents. *Diabetes Care* 1984;7:273–5.
454 Barkai L, Madacsy L, Kassay L. Investigation of subclinical signs of autonomic neuropathy in the early stages of childhood diabetes. *Horm Res* 1990;34:54–9.
455 Ewing DJ, Clarke BS. Diabetic autonomic neuropathy: present insight and future prospects. *Diabetes Care* 1986;9: 648–65.
456 Cornblath M, Schwartz R. Transient diabetes mellitus in early infancy. In: Cornblath M, Schwartz R, eds. *Disorders of Carbohydrate Metabolism in Infancy*, 2nd edn. Philadelphila, PA: WB Saunders, 1976:218–27.
457 Gentz JCH, Cornblath M. Transient diabetes of the newborn. *Adv Pediatr* 1969;16:345–63.
458 Hager N, Herbst R. Das transitorische Diabetes mellitus-Syndrome des Neugeborenen, ein Krankhetisbild sui generis. *Z Kinderheilk* 1966;95:324–47.
459 Pagliara AS, Karl IE, Kipnis DB. Transient neonatal diabetes: delayed maturation of the pancreatic beta cell. *J Pediatr* 1973;82:97–101.
460 Milner RDG, Ferguson AW, Naidu SH. Aetiology of transient neonatal diabetes. *Arch Dis Child* 1971;46:724–6.
461 Francois R, Hermier M, Jurlot B *et al.* Occurrence of diabetes in infants less than one year old. In: Laron Z, ed. *Diabetes in Juveniles*. Basel: Karger, 1975:60–6.
462 Willi H, Müller F. Über den transitorischen Diabetes mellitus des Neugeborenen. *Helv Paediatr Acta* 1968;23: 231–41.
463 Entmacher PS, Root HF, Marks HN. Longevity of diabetic patients in recent years. *Diabetes* 1964;13:373–7.
464 Paz-Guevara AT, Hsu TH, White P. Juvenile diabetes mellitus after forty years. *Diabetes* 1975;24:559–62.
465 Green A, Borch-Johnsen K, Kragh Andersen P *et al.* Relative mortality of Type 1 (insulin-dependent) diabetes in Denmark: 1933–1981. *Diabetologia* 1985;28:339–42.

34: The Management of Diabetes Mellitus

J. COURT

INTRODUCTION

There are four major considerations in the management of diabetes in childhood.

1 To resuscitate ketoacidosis safely and avoid cerebral oedema, which largely accounts for the two-fold increase in mortality in childhood diabetes compared to the general population.

2 To avoid severe hypoglycaemia, which may lead to impaired cognitive function in early childhood.

3 To minimize the risk of long-term complications. Prevention will remain unattainable until cure or treatment that gives perfect metabolic control without the daily cooperation of the patient becomes available.

4 To ensure that the child achieves normal growth, psychosocial development and a lifestyle comparable to his or her peers.

Current treatment of insulin-dependent diabetes mellitus (IDDM) is imperfect, constantly changing and very dependent on clinical bias rather than absolute standards. Details of management are likely to differ widely between centres providing care for children with IDDM.

PRESENTATION AND DIAGNOSIS

Initial diagnosis of IDDM is made on the basis of clinical symptoms and a raised level of blood glucose. The cardinal symptoms of polyuria and polydipsia, which may present as nocturia or secondary enuresis and may be mistaken for dysuria and urinary tract infection, should be present for confident diagnosis. Associated symptoms are usually non-specific and include weight loss, lethargy, constipation and perineal thrush. After prolonged symptoms, cataracts may develop and presentation may be through impaired vision. A random blood glucose concentration above 11 mmol/l confirms the diagnosis. A normal blood glucose in the fasting state, or after carbohydrate deprivation, does not exclude the diagnosis, and levels should be measured after a carbohydrate meal if the diagnosis is suspected. A raised blood glucose concentration in the absence of symptoms is not sufficient to make the diagnosis, since transient hyperglycaemia may be associated with severe dehydration from other causes in infants, and with burns or major injury, especially involving bone, at any age.

There is virtually no place for an oral glucose tolerance test in the diagnosis of IDDM.

Diabetes may progress rapidly to diabetic ketoacidosis (DKA), especially in young children, in whom the disease tends to progress rapidly and symptoms may be confusing, and in adolescents who may be unwilling to tell their parents about early symptoms. A vomiting adolescent with impaired conscious state may lead to the suspicion of alcohol or other drug abuse. Kussmaul breathing in severe acidosis may be confused with respiratory infection or asthma. All ill children should have urine tested for glucose and ketones as routine.

Treatment should start on the day of diagnosis without delay, since decompensation can occur very rapidly. DKA is life-threatening, particularly if the child is vomiting, and admission to hospital should then be a medical emergency.

KETOACIDOSIS

The child presenting with DKA will be dehydrated with substantial loss of sodium from the extracellular space and potassium from the intracellular space. The accumulation of ketone bodies contributes to acidosis, and pH levels of < 7.0 are not uncommon. Osmotic diuresis due to hyperglycaemia occurs in the presence of dehydration, unless there is severe hypovolaemia and impaired renal perfusion. Severe hyperosmolarity is associated with shifts in intracellular water and permeability of the blood–brain barrier. Loss of thermoregulation may occur with resultant hypothermia.

It is unusual for consciousness to be deeply depressed on inital presentation, although mentation is likely to be affected and subsequent retrograde amnesia is common. Coma, when it does occur, will relate to degree of hyperosmolarity rather than acidosis or dehydration. During resuscitation, deteriorating conscious state may be due to cerebral oedema.

The potentially lethal risks of DKA result from circulatory collapse in severe dehydration, renal failure with poor tissue perfusion and the metabolic derangement from acidaemia. The additional risks during resuscitation are those of hypokalaemia during correction of acidosis, brain herniation from cerebral oedema [1] and hypoglycaemia.

The child with DKA needs immediate admission to a medical centre where biochemical monitoring, medical expertise and intensive-nursing care is available. If there is to be delay, intravenous isotonic (0.9%) saline should be started. It is usually safer to defer insulin until formal assessment and appropriate clinical and laboratory monitoring is available.

The principles of treatment of DKA are as follows.

1 Slow correction of dehydration over a period of 48 h.
2 Avoidance of hypotonic intravenous fluids in the first 12–24 h.
3 Adequate replacement of sodium and potassium losses.
4 Gradual reduction of hyperglycaemia and suppression of ketone production using an insulin infusion.
5 Careful monitoring of the cerebral state and prompt measures to counteract cerebral oedema.
6 Frequent clinical and biochemical monitoring to prevent complications of treatment.

The following protocol is recommended as a guide to the management of DKA.

Preliminary assessment

Circulatory collapse: immediate resuscitation is required.

Degree of dehydration: mild dehydration (3%) has minimal signs that are clinically detectable. Moderate dehydration (6%) has markedly reduced tissue turgor, obvious tissue loss of fluid and poor capillary circulation. Severe dehydration (10%) is associated with poor tissue perfusion, rapid pulse and reduced blood pressure.

Metabolic state: biochemical assessment with measurement of blood glucose, serum electrolyte concentrations, serum osmolality and acid–base status. Urine should be checked for presence of ketones.

Resuscitation

If there is hypoperfusion, 0.9% saline is given at the fastest rate possible to a total of 10 ml/kg body weight. If the child is in severe shock, or there is inadequate response to saline, a plasma expander can be given in the same amount.

Correction of dehydration and metabolic state

Intravenous fluids: 0.9% saline with added potassium chloride should be used for the first 12 h. If blood glucose concentration falls quickly in the first few hours, and hypoglycaemia seems imminent, 5% dextrose can be added to the saline infusion over the first 12 h of resusucitation.

After the first 12 h, when blood glucose concentration falls to 10 mmol/l, and provided that hyponatraemia has not developed, the infusion can be changed to 0.45% saline with 5% dextrose with continued added potassium.

Potassium replacement should be given as soon as adequate circulation has been restored, and at the same time as the insulin infusion. Potassium chloride can be added to the infusion fluid at a concentration of 40 mml/l if body weight is <30 kg, and at 60 mmol/l if >30 kg. An infusion rate of 0.3 mmol/kg h^{-1} is sufficient to restore the potassium deficit, and is well tolerated provided renal function is intact.

Bicarbonate (HCO_3) is not necessary, and should be used only as a resuscitation measure in extreme acidosis and shock. If given, the dose is calculated as HCO_3 (mmol) = 0.3 × body weight (kg) × base deficit. This is given by slow infusion, and reassessment should be made when half of the amount has been given. Maximum rate of infusion is 0.1 mmol/kg min^{-1}.

Quantity of replacement fluid: the total volume and fluid replacement is calculated from the deficit due to dehydration plus the maintenance requirements over the period of 48 h during which time replacement is to take place. A guide to maintenance requirements is set out in Table 34.1. The deficit is calculated as percentage dehydration × body weight.

The total amount of required fluid should be given at a steady rate over a period of 48 h. The rate may be modified according to clinical signs. Recovery of clinical well-being may occur in 24 h and fluid replacement can then be started orally.

Table 34.2 sets out the rate of fluid replacement needed for rehydration according to degree of dehydration and to the size of the child. These rates are appropriate to replace deficit and to provide for maintenance. Regular clinical review is needed to assess hydration and response to fluid replacement.

Insulin infusion should be given intravenously as soon as initial resuscitation for shock has been made. It should be administered by a constant-infusion pump at the rate of

Table 34.1 Maintenance requirements

Body weight	Requirements
3–10 kg	100 ml/kg per day
10–20 kg	1000 ml + 50 ml/kg for each kg over 10 kg
20 kg and over	1500 ml + 20 ml/kg for each kg over 20 kg

Table 34.2 Rate of fluid replacement (ml/h) necessary after dehydration*

Body weight (kg)	Percentage dehydration			Body weight (kg)	Percentage dehydration		
	3%	6%	10%		3%	6%	10%
5	24	27	31	38	101	125	156
7	33	38	43	40	104	129	162
8	38	43	50	42	107	133	168
10	48	54	62	44	110	137	174
12	53	60	70	46	113	141	180
14	58	67	79	48	116	146	186
16	64	74	87	50	119	150	191
18	70	80	95	52	122	154	197
20	75	87	104	54	124	158	203
22	78	91	110	56	127	162	208
24	80	95	115	58	130	167	214
26	83	100	121	60	133	171	220
28	86	104	127	62	136	175	226
30	89	108	133	64	139	179	232
32	92	112	139	66	142	183	238
34	95	116	145	68	145	187	244
36	98	120	151	70	148	191	250

* This includes deficit and maintenance fluid needs.

0.1 units/kgh^{-1}. This rate may be less if the child has established diabetes, has had insulin in the previous few hours and blood glucose is less than 15 mmol/l.

The rate of insulin infusion may be reduced to 0.05 units/kgh^{-1} if the blood glucose concentration falls below 5 mmol/l. It should not be discontinued until the child is able to take meals and subcutaneous insulin can be started, in which case it should not be discontinued until 30 min after the subcutaneous dose has been given.

Clinical and biochemical monitoring: the child should be nursed in a ward where constant nursing care can be provided. Frequent observations should be made on the state of consciousness and pupil reaction to light, even at the expense of the child's need to sleep, if the risk of death from cerebral oedema is to be minimized.

Fluid balance should be documented and blood glucose should be measured at the bedside hourly while the child is being rehydrated and there is an insulin infusion. In the severely ill child, frequent biochemical monitoring will be essential to assess sodium, potassium and chloride concentrations and acid–base balance.

It is conventional to estimate the serum sodium concentration corrected for the effect of hyperglycaemia, which is calculated as sodium + 0.3 (glucose − 5.5). Corrected sodium levels are used to assess hypernatraemia, which is defined as a corrected sodium >160 mmol/l. Sodium concentration tends to rise as glucose falls during treatment. If this positive trend fails to occur, or if hyponatraemia develops during treatment, it may indicate that there has been insufficient sodium replacement which will cause an increased risk of cerebral oedema.

If hypoglycaemia develops during rehydration, 10% dextrose in a dose of 2 ml/kg body weight may be infused over 3 min. Insulin infusion should not be discontinued, but the rate may be reduced if normoglycaemia is not maintained by adding 5% dextrose to the rehydrating fluid.

CEREBRAL OEDEMA

Treatment of DKA in childhood should lead to a recovery within 24–48 h, even when there has been severe derangement of water and electrolyte balance. There is, however, a risk that cerebral oedema may lead to brain herniation and irreversible brain death in the first 24 h of resuscitation.

Some degree of cerebral oedema is probably present in most children with DKA, and has been demonstrated by computerized tomography [2] and magnetic resonance imaging. Hoffman *et al.* demonstrated cerebral oedema at presentation of DKA before resuscitation had been started in nine children, with accentuation of brain swelling after 6–8 h of resuscitation in four of them, one of whom developed clinical signs of oedema [3]. Rosenbloom reported two children with DKA who had received only oral fluids as replacement and developed fatal cerebral oedema. Demonstration of brain swelling before treatment suggests that a pathological process unrelated to the mode of resuscitation may be responsible for cerebral oedema [3–5].

The primary cause of cerebral oedema, and the factors that increase the risk that it will compromise survival, are not known. In a review of 69 instances of intracranial complications of DKA, Rosenbloom failed to implicate rate of rehydration, tonicity of administered fluids, rate of correction of glycaemia or the use of bicarbonate. Half of the patients had a brief period of dramatic neurological change before cardiorespiratory arrest, during which intervention might have been possible, but no warning was recorded in half of the cases. Progression to clinical expression of cerebral oedema and herniation was unpredictable [4].

Harris *et al.*, on the other hand, reviewed 219 episodes of DKA and found complications more likely to develop if serum sodium concentration failed to rise as glucose levels fell. They recommended an extended repair period of resuscitation with high sodium administration [6].

Duck & Wyatt [7] suggested excessive secretion of vasopressin may exacerbate brain swelling and recommended a slow rate of fluid administration on this basis. They noted a fall in serum sodium concentration preceding oedema in half the cases they studied. These authors suggested that there is very little time (perhaps 10 min) to intervene if there is evidence of developing herniation. It is recommended mannitol be available at the bedside of all children being treated for DKA and be administered i.v. at the first signs of deteriorating conscious state [7].

Treatment for threatening or developing cerebral oedema is as follows.

1 Mannitol 20% is given i.v. immediately signs of deteriorating cerebral state indicate that severe cerebral oedema is imminent in a bolus dose of 0.5–1 g/kg. This should be repeated every 15–20 min.

2 Reduce fluid input.

3 Nurse in head-up position.

4 Treat in intensive-care unit. Assisted respiration may be needed.

STABILIZATION

If the child does not require resuscitation, initial stabilization is usually carried out in hospital, but there is an increasing trend to stabilize children with newly diagnosed IDDM at home [8]. This requires the ability to provide guidance and support for the family at home by a group of physicians and other staff who are dedicated to this form of management. Distance from the medical centre, language problems and a dysfunctional family may make home stabilization impractical but age, socioeconomic status and ethnic background do not appear to influence success. The outcome of home management in terms of diabetic control appears to be as good as hospital stabilization [9].

Apart from economic factors and the psychological advantage of not placing a child in hospital, the early involvement of the whole family in practical management and responsibility, and the adjustment of diet and insulin to the child's usual environment, are substantial advantages.

If home stabilization is not practicable, admission to hospital for a few days is advisable. In addition to providing appropriate care at the stage when diabetes is coming under control, parents are relieved of the burden of care until they have come to terms with the diagnosis, and have gained confidence to look after their child.

INSULIN TREATMENT

The basis of diabetes management is the replacement of the insulin deficiency that characterizes IDDM. It is not possible using current techniques to administer insulin in a manner that reflects normal β cell secretion. Until insulin can be delivered to the right place, at the right time, in the right amount and in a way that reflects physiological need, therapy will at best be a poor imitation of the normal secretion of β cells. Insulin would need to be released into the portal system in response to subtle changes in ambient blood glucose levels and to reflect acute energy ingestion, tissue responsiveness and the action of the counterregulatory hormone system.

Instead, insulin is usually given subcutaneously in bolus doses and in response to a calculated requirement that has little regard for human frailty. Fortunately, such rough approximation can achieve good health on a day-to-day basis but only at the expense of continuing patient effort and motivation to comply. Current management is also associated with systemic hyperinsulinism and the risk of hypoglycaemia, and it cannot, in most cases, avoid postprandial hyperglycaemia.

Insulin is usually administered by one of three methods, chosen on the basis of the clinican's experience and bias, the extent to which β cell function contributes endogenous insulin, the level of family competence and motivation, age of the child and, in long-standing diabetes, difficulties that may have been previously experienced in maintaining control.

Conventional insulin treatment

This method, which is the most suitable for children, relies on once- or twice-daily injections of a mixture of modified and unmodified insulins given before breakfast and before the evening meal (Table 34.3). The neutral protamine Hagedorn (NPH) insulins, in which the duration of action is prolonged by the addition of protein to the insulin molecule, are those most commonly used, and probably preferable. When mixed with unmodified insulin, both insulins act independently. Insulins modified by the addition of zinc tend to reduce the action of unmodified insulin due to the excess of zinc in the preparation. This leads to some loss of the acute response needed to minimize postprandial hyperglycaemia if insulin is given before meals. Although insulin zinc suspensions may have a longer action than NPH insulin, there appears to be no benefit in providing overnight control [10,11].

For most children who are fully insulin-dependent a daily insulin dose of 1 unit/kg body weight is sufficient. Those in partial remission require less and a rapid reduction in dose will be needed after stabilization during this phase, if hypoglycaemia is to be avoided. During puberty, when there is some loss of insulin sensitivity [12] and less parental supervision of diet, insulin requirements may increase, often to a dose of 1.5 units/kg.

When given twice daily the total dose is normally given in the proportion of two-thirds before breakfast and one-third before the evening meal, reflecting the meal intake during the day and night. Unmodified insulin is usually

Table 34.3 Types of insulin available

Insulin	Type	Action (h)		
		Onset	Peak	Duration
Neutral unmodified Examples: Actrapid, Velosulin, Humulin R	Quick-acting	0.5	2–4	6–8
NPH insulins, isophane Examples: Protaphane, Insulatard, Humulin NPH	Intermediate-acting	1	4–10	16–18
Insulin zinc suspension Example: Lente	Intermediate-acting	1	6–12	20–24
Insulin zinc suspension (crystalline) Example: Ultra lente	Long-acting	2	6–20	>24
Biphasic insulin mixtures Examples: Mixtard 30/70, Mixtard 50/50, Mixtard 15/85	Mixtures of NPH and unmodified	1	2–12	16–18

given in the proportion of 20–30% of the total dose, but this varies greatly according to the child's response, and to the meal plan.

Patients are advised to give insulin 30 min before meals, to minimize postprandial hyperglycaemia. The insulin dose is best changed in response to patterns of blood glucose levels over a period of a few days, rather than an acute response to high or low blood glucose values at the time of the injection. Once stabilized, it is usual for insulin requirements to remain stable for many months at a time. Insulin requirements, however, will vary during illness when initial anorexia or vomiting may lead to hypoglycaemia; subsequent reduced insulin sensitivity may lead to increased requirements. Children who play active sport may need to reduce their insulin dose before and immediately after prolonged exercise, to avoid hypoglycaemia [13].

Multiple insulin injections using the pen system

The development of an insulin pen injector in 1985 has led to extensive use of this device to administer multiple injections in a way that provides doses of short-acting insulin before major meals and a bolus dose of long- or intermediate-acting insulin before bed at night. Although it has been used in young children the system is probably most suited to adolescents when they feel ready to take control of their own diabetes care and adapt treatment to their changing lifestyle and social behaviour. To be used successfully it requires motivation, independence and willingness to have an injection at midday away from home.

The main advantages of the pen system are that, in theory at least, it more closely mimics physiological insulin response to meals, it allows for some degree of flexibility of meal size and time [14] and it allows teenagers to make unplanned changes in social arrangements, since they can carry insulin around with them. Most young people feel that they are in greater control of their diabetes using this system. Its main disadvantage is that it requires four injections a day, and thus doubles the opportunities for forgetfulness or deliberate non-compliance leading to inadequate insulin delivery.

The multiple-injection system has been used to deliver intensive insulin therapy to achieve good metabolic control in the Diabetes Complications and Control Trial (DCCT) [15], but it can improve control in clinical practice only when it is used to facilitate a general commitment to overall diabetic care. Transfer to the system from conventional insulin delivery has not always been associated with improved control, as judged by reduced haemoglobin (Hb)A1$_c$ levels [16,17], and may lead to deterioration of control in females [18]. It is, however, well accepted by most young people, and may be associated with less episodes of DKA and severe hypoglycaemia [17], and a better quality of life [19,20].

Continuous insulin infusion

After early discouraging experience using insulin infusion pumps to deliver continuous subcutaneous insulin, the method of insulin delivery has fallen into disrepute for children and young adolescents. Recent reports on adult patients with IDDM suggest that technical developments [21] and a better understanding of the circulating free insulin response to continuous infusion [22] may make the system practical for children. It appears to be acceptable in selected young children but is demanding on them, their families and medical supervisors [23]. The findings of the DCCT study suggest that intensive insulin treatment by this system will not suit patients who are not highly motivated to comply with the demands of regular monitoring needed to avoid hypoglycaemia [24]. Even under ideal conditions of study, perfect metabolic control is not achieved in children [25].

Intraperitoneal infusion to deliver insulin to the portal circulation has been reported [26,27], including implantable programmable pump systems [28] which appear to lead to improved diabetic control, and may be helpful in brittle diabetes [29].

Injection sites and insulin absorption

There is considerable variation in insulin absorption from the subcutaneous space from one individual to another, from site to site and under differing conditions. There is a biphasic response to insulin injection, due to insulin depolymerization, dispersion in the interstitial space, diffusion to capillaries and capillary absorption. Several factors may affect this, including orthostatic changes, physical exercise, local massage, ambient temperature and skinfold thickness [30,31]. There is site-to-site variation in absorption [32], but depth of subcutaneous tissues does not appear to influence it [33]. Accidental intramuscular injection in probably common in children, especially in slim boys [34], and leads to faster [35] and more variable absorption [36], particularly during exercise when there is increased risk of hypoglycaemia [37].

Insulin absorption may be affected adversely if given in areas of insulin-induced fat hypertrophy [38,39]. Unresponsiveness to subcutaneous insulin has been reported as a phenomenon affecting adolescent girls and young women, and attributed to excessive subcutaneous protease activity [40]. If this is true, it must be a rare explanation for the relatively common clinical situation of persistent ketonuria and recurrent DKA which occurs predominantly in adolescent girls, and usually results from psychological disturbance and non-compliance with insulin therapy.

In adolescence it may be difficult to achieve adequate levels of insulin during the night: measurement of free insulin levels suggests that patients are overinsulinized in the early part of the night but underinsulinized in the later part [41]. This is reflected in the prevalence of nocturnal hypoglycaemia between midnight and 0300 h, with normoglycaemia or hyperglycaemia before breakfast. This had been attributed to the Somogyi effect, in which it was proposed that hypoglycaemia was followed by hyperglycaemia due to release of counterregulatory hormones. Studies have not confirmed this mechanism, and it is likely that the Somogyi effect is unusual [42] and, when it occurs, is due to falling free insulin levels at a time when there are increased insulin requirements (the dawn phenomenon [43]). A contribution to this hyperglycaemia before breakfast in adolescents is the delay in morning insulin and breakfast that often occurs at this age [10].

INFLUENCE OF REMISSION ON INSULIN REQUIREMENTS AND EASE OF CONTROL

Insulin requirements commonly fall after initial stabilization, and unless the administered dose is promptly and progressively reduced, hypoglycaemia will occur. This phase in the natural history of diabetes can result from partial recovery of insulin secretion or improved tissue sensitivity to insulin [44]. Some degree of partial recovery of insulin secretion commonly occurs following stabilization, with increased basal and stimulated C-peptide concentrations in blood [44,45] and urinary C-peptide excretion [46].

The phase of partial remission varies considerably from patient to patient and, provided that the insulin dose is reduced, leads to ease in achieving good control with $HbA1_c$ levels within a normal range, tolerance to dietary variation and relative stability.

Factors associated with this remission include age of onset [45–48], (the younger the patient at diagnosis the less likely there will be remission), male sex [47,48] and the presence of islet cell antibodies at diagnosis [47]. The severity and duration of symptoms at presentation do not appear to relate to remission rates [45–47]. β cell recovery is temporary: C-peptide levels have been shown to rise for periods of 1–6 months, peaking at 3 months, and then to decline steadily [45,47].

A number of efforts have been made to induce or prolong this remission phase, including the administration of steroids [49] azathioprine [50], cyclosporin A [44], nicotinamide, combinations of these [51], and irradiation of the pancreas [52].

Cyclosporin A has been used in a number of trials in children. It has been shown to lead to a higher incidence and longer period of remission [53]. The improved remission rates are not maintained on cessation of cyclosporin, and there appear to be no long-lasting benefits from its use [54]. Cyclosporin may lead to a reversible rise in blood pressure and reduced renal function in young patients [55] without renal changes on biopsy [53].

No clinically significant effects have been reported in children from the use of steroids or azathioprine [49,50]. Nicotinamide may prove to be of more value in preventing the development of diabetes in those at risk [56], but although it has been shown to extend the period of remission in newly diagnosed diabetes, there appears to be only a slight response in insulin secretion in those who have already developed diabetes [57].

DIET

Although nutritional guidance is essential in the management of IDDM, there is lack of agreement on what form this should take in childhood, whether as a measured diet focused on carbohydrate or on total energy intake, as a general meal plan or as general guidance on principles of nutrition. Some consistency in the amounts of foods eaten each day is essential to avoid erratic departures from normoglycaemia and to maintain metabolic balance [58].

General dietary recommendations for people with diabetes have been published by the British Diabetic Association [59] and the American Diabetes Association [58]. Dietary advice for children must, however, be based on a developmental approach, allowing for growth, varying levels of physical activity, the psychosocial aspects of eating and the views and beliefs of the child's family. The child eats meals with the family and snacks with his or her peers: it is neither fair nor practicable to prescribe a diet or meal plan that is very different from family and peers. As few children with diabetes are fat, energy restriction is usually inappropriate.

There are a number of desirable principles in providing nutritional guidance to parents of a child with diabetes. A diet or meal plan should:

1 satisfy the child's appetite;
2 be consistent with cultural habits of the family;
3 be sufficient to maintain growth – intake should be restricted only if there is risk of obesity;
4 follow the general guidelines of good nutrition for those with diabetes;
5 provide a regular intake of complex carbohydrates to balance the action of insulin;
6 be sufficiently flexible to prevent undue conflict over food, especially in the preschool child;
7 be adjustable to allow for physical activity, social occasions and illness;
8 be sufficiently restricted in simple sugars to limit postprandial hyperglycaemia;
9 be adaptable to allow the child and adolescent to eat out with friends, attend camps and travel;
10 be acceptable to the whole family so that the diabetic child is neither discriminated against nor rewarded.

There is considerable merit in providing parents with a meal plan that is based on a regular amount of carbohydrate at each meal and snack. This is the basis of the exchange system and, by giving parents a framework of meals, it helps to reassure them that insulin will be balanced, and that the child can safely be sent to school without fear of hypoglycaemia.

The blood glucose response to carbohydrate in food is influenced by how the food is prepared, the nature of the carbohydrate and proportions of starch, simple sugars and dietary fibre [60]. It is also affected by the presence of fats and protein in the meal. It has been suggested that foods can be assigned a glycaemic index, judged by the area under a blood glucose response curve [60,61]. Studies show considerable variation in glycaemic response to different carbohydrate foods, largely due to the complexity and form of the carbohydrate [60]. Increasing the proportion of low glycaemic index foods may improve metabolic control [62,63].

Dietary fibre can affect the glucose response to meals, and an increase in unrefined carbohydrate foods may lead to improved diabetic control [64]. Consumption of a high-fibre diet using water-soluble fibre is generally encouraged [65]. Most studies demonstrating improvement in carbohydrate metabolism and lowering of blood lipid concentrations have been in adults with IDDM [66]. Diabetic adolescents may have a higher dietary fibre intake than non-diabetics [67], but adding fibre to diet may not benefit patients with IDDM [68].

Children, particularly girls, may become overweight during adolescence, and this is usually associated with increased insulin requirements and deterioration in diabetic control [69]. Neither dietary prescription nor exhortation is reliable in preventing this until the adolescent is ready to take control herself. Reduction of food with emphasis on dietary fat and refined sugars, regular exercise and a decrease of insulin dose is then appropriate.

EDUCATION

Education about diabetes and the rationale for its treatment is now regarded as an integral part of the initial management of the newly diagnosed child and family. It is also recognized that the father should be included in the education programme, both to enable him to play a part in his child's care and to support more effectively the mother, who usually bears the brunt of care of her child with its attendant anxiety.

Whereas initial instruction and information is clearly needed by parents and older children to carry out care successfully, the value of formal and ongoing education programmes has been hard to establish. It is difficult to know whether education programmes actually lead to improvement in health or diabetes control. Most studies have been on adult patients and have concluded that education improves knowledge but not diabetic control, morbidity or health-related behaviours [70–72]. Reports of uncontrolled interventions frequently show improvement in terms of the programme's objectives in the short term, but this is likely to be due to the effect by which intervention helps in a non-specific way through personal support and attention, rather than any effects of the programme *per se*.

Those who are involved with education of a child and family should relate their expectations to the developmental status of the child and to the competence of the family [73–75]. Parents' reports of their child's self-care skills may differ widely from the expectations of professionals who advise them [76]. Adolescents are usually given tasks of adjusting their own insulin by their parents, but may not do so. Ability to manage diabetes relates to cognitive maturity and not to age. Active parent participation in care has been shown to relate to academic achievement, but participation may not lead to better control [77]. In one study of adolescents, factual knowledge about diabetes was found to bear no relationship to metabolic control, but was associated with a greater feeling of self-control [77]. Adolescents who believe that they are competent in self-care are more likely to feel that they are in control of their diabetes [78].

Diabetes education is necessary because self-management skills may help patients avoid inappropriate decisions on dietary and insulin adjustment [79]. The most positive outcomes will be the trusting relationships that may develop between patient, parent and health professional, and motivation to take good care of himself or herself that comes from the development of self-confidence and a sense of personal control.

ROLE OF EXERCISE IN MAINTAINING DIABETIC CONTROL

Physical activity leads to increased insulin sensitivity and increased glucose uptake by muscle [80]. It is associated with a feeling of well-being, contributes to psychosocial development during childhood and helps protect the adolescent from becoming fat. Children who are active are less likely to become bored and to snack between meals. Exercise would seem a good thing for children, whether they have diabetes or not, but whether habitual exercise improves diabetes control is less clear.

In a study of adult non-insulin-dependent diabetes mellitus (NIDDM) and IDDM patients physical exercise was not associated with lower $HbA1_c$ values [81]; a physical training programme of 1 h/week over a period of 3 months did not improve metabolic control in diabetic children aged 8–17 years [82]. On the other hand a history of leisure physical activity during adolescence related to a lower prevalence of nephropathy and neuropathy in males (but not in females) studied as adults [83].

Seasonal variation in $HbA1_c$ [84], which reflects improved control in the summer months, may be due to increased exercise [85]. Unusual strenuous or prolonged exercise increases the risk of hypoglycaemia, often many hours after the exercise has been completed [13]. The risk of exercise-induced hypoglycaemia is greatest when insulin levels are at their peak absorption, such as late morning and during the afternoon. The risk is least before breakfast when plasma cortisol levels are higher and free insulin levels lower [86].

Exercise does not appear to increase blood flow or insulin absorption from subcutaneous tissue, but if insulin has been given intramuscularly, exercise leads to a marked increase in insulin absorption rate [37].

In poorly controlled diabetes in children having inadequate insulin, exercise increases hyperglycaemia and may also increase ketonaemia [87]. This is likely to be due to inadequate insulin treatment, which fails to counteract the hyperglycaemia due to a physiological rise in catecholamines and growth hormone levels during exercise.

CLINICAL REVIEW

Clinical review should be regular, and done by a physician with whom the child becomes familiar and who the family can trust. Whom this is depends on the personal practice of the physician, the availability of appropriate experts and the preference of the family. So-called 'shared care' between consultant and family doctor is ideal in theory, and certainly the specialist physician must communicate well with the practitioner who will be responsible for intercurrent illness, injuries and perhaps emergencies. Unfortunately such an arrangement, which has been reported to work well for patients with NIDDM, often leads to conflicting advice being given to families on different occasions, and to care being given by doctors with differing knowledge and philosophy of care.

Diabetes places unique demands on the child and family. Treatment at its best is far from ideal, and is often a compromise between what is needed for best-possible control and what is tolerable for the child. There is the ever-present threat of severe hypoglycaemia and longer-term complications that cloud the future. Psychosocial adjustment and issues of compliance are often major concerns for the parents, particularly during adolescence. The physician who undertakes management of a child with diabetes must be prepared to cope with all these aspects of care, in addition to health surveillance and provision of technical advice on insulin management.

The role of the clinical review has several elements which include the following.

1 To offer solutions to problems raised by parents or the child, such as nocturnal hypoglycaemia, management of vomiting illnesses, attending a school camp or apparent discrimination at school.

2 To monitor clinical status. This includes height and weight gain, which may reflect adequacy of insulin. A teenage girl may gain excessive weight after conclusion of the growth spurt, or may be underweight as a result of using her diabetes to control her weight. Physical examination should include the state of the injection sites (lipohypertrophy may influence insulin absorption) [38], presence of intercurrent or associated disease (such as autoimmune thyroid disease) and signs of early development of complications. The child with poor control may have genital or perineal thrush. Examination of optic fundi should be made regularly, and visual acuity measured occasionally. Laboratory estimations of blood lipid measurements should be made occasionally, and thyroid function tests may be needed if there is a goitre or doubt on thyroid status on clinical grounds. Overnight urine collection for screening for microalbuminuria will be needed after onset of puberty.

3 To monitor the quality of diabetes control. Clinical examination may reveal low-grade wasting or dehydration in chronic, poorly controlled diabetes. The child's record of home monitoring of blood glucose may be helpful in assessing quality of control, but there is often rather poor correlation with objective measurements of control such as glycosylated haemoglobin.

4 To consider whether the current treatment regime is ideal. Is the insulin dose appropriate? The child who is fully insulin-dependent will need about 1 unit of insulin per kilogram body weight per day, but at puberty the dose may be as high as 1.5 U/kg, due in part to reduced insulin sensitivity but also to changing lifestyle at this age. Should the child consider a multiple insulin injection system?

5 To encourage the family, and eventually the child, to make appropriate management decisions. This requires adequate information and permission to experiment within safe limits in adjusting insulin and diet, so that there is gradual emancipation from reliance on professionals for day-to-day care [88].

6 To provide information on current research and new developments. This at least sustains hope in the dispirited, and helps prevent the discouragement that follows the many press releases that announce so-called breakthroughs in care. Most young people want to know about new developments, and expect their doctor to know about them and to inform them.

7 To provide counselling to the adolescent about such things as smoking, alcohol bingeing, exercise, recreation, driving and employment.

8 To discuss psychosocial adjustment and difficulties, and how the family deals with problems that may arise, such as lack of compliance, jealousy in a sibling and behaviour problems with the diabetic child who is not coping well.

Frequency of consultations must depend on the preference of the physician, the needs of the family and child, particularly in the early stages of diabetes, and the age and stage of development of the child. Most physicians will see a diabetic child every 3–4 months in order to fulfil the above role, even though it is unlikely that many insulin adjustments will be needed at this interval.

MONITORING THE DIABETIC STATE

Until laboratory techniques for measuring glycosylated proteins became available, assessment of diabetic control was largely subjective, often erroneous and dependent on clinician judgement. Attempts to quantitate control have been made using urinary glucose concentrations before meals, or 24-h excretion levels. When home blood glucose measurements became practicable and reliable, and convenient monitors were available [89], it was hoped that some integrated assessment of glucose concentrations would provide a reliable index of control; indeed many clinicians still assume it does. Unfortunately in most instances it does not, in part because of the impracticality of multiple preprandial, postprandial and nocturnal sampling on a regular basis during childhood, and in part due to the propensity for patients, particularly adolescents, to fabricate test results.

Home blood glucose monitoring can and should guide the patient in the day-to-day management of diabetes.

1 It is helpful in alerting the child that there is risk of hypoglycaemia.

2 It will indicate whether variations from normoglycaemia tend to occur at particular times of day, thus providing a rational basis for altering insulin dosage.

3 It may reassure the family that near-normoglycaemia is being achieved, and that no variation in the regime of care is needed.

4 It has educational value in informing parents and child about the effect on diabetic control of unusual events and foods.

5 It allows the parent or older child to attempt changes in care on a trial-and-error basis by monitoring the response to variation in insulin or food.

6 It helps to prevent nocturnal hypoglycaemia after unusual activities or meal avoidance by monitoring at bedtime.

7 It acts as a guide to management during illness, especially if the child is vomiting or refuses to eat. It may be essential in distinguishing whether vomiting is due to gastroenteritis (when low blood glucose levels are common) or due to a systemic illness, when hyperglycaemia should alert the child to test for ketonuria.

Unfortunately most families do not use blood glucose information to make proactive changes in treatment [76], but families who use blood glucose monitoring information tend to have less conflict about care, more diabetes knowledge and better treatment adherence than those who do not [76].

Frequency of testing should depend on the advice given

to families on what their response should be to the results, and to their child's tolerance of regular fingerpricks.

These purposes of home blood glucose monitoring should be explained to parents, who may otherwise see it mainly as providing information for the physician to assess overall control. Worse still, children may view monitoring as a means of checking whether they have been compliant with diet, or see the blood tests as a meaningless task to satisfy their parents.

The physician will review blood glucose monitoring to seek patterns of glycaemia over a period of time which reflect insulin balance or response to recurring events. This provides information for advice on adjustment and balance of meals and action to be taken to respond to unusual activities or illness. Occasional or random values, or those that do not extend over a period, may be misleading and should not, in themselves, form the basis for advice on insulin dosage.

Thus home blood glucose tests need to be done frequently and regularly to influence diabetes control. Perhaps when non-invasive glucose monitoring [90] becomes generally available and affordable it will be used more diligently, and to greater advantage.

Measurement of glycosylated haemoglobin provides an objective index of control over the preceding 2–3 months [91]. Practitioners' estimates of the degree of control based on historical and laboratory information correlate poorly with $HbA1_c$ values [91], although some previous studies have shown correlation between $HbA1_c$ and mean blood glucose values [92] and 24-h urinary glucose concentration [93]. $HbA1_c$ values may be affected by the presence of haemoglobin variants in blood [94], and are subject to seasonal variation [84,85,95].

Knowledge of $HbA1_c$ results assists both the clinician and patient in diabetic management. Significant improvement in control, and fewer admissions to hospital, can be achieved if regular measurement of $HbA1_c$ is made and used to provide advice [96]. Knowledge provides targets for physicians and families, reassurance when the value is satisfactory and a salutary lesson to those whose inability to adhere to a management plan has led to poor control. $HbA1_c$ values provide an objective measurement for research, particularly that directed at assessing the relationship of quality of control and the development of complications [97].

Other glycosylated proteins, including albumin and fructosamine, have been used to monitor diabetes control. These proteins provide a shorter-term assessment than $HbA1_c$, but may not correlate as well with other indices of control [97]. Serum fructosamine levels are affected by changes in serum albumin levels in acute inflammation and pregnancy [98]. Serum fructosamine may be a useful index of control over a 1-week interval, and is unaffected by acute serum glucose changes [99].

A very short-term (2–3 days) index of control can be provided by measuring glycosylated fibrinogen [100]. This may be used to test early response to therapeutic intervention [101]. An advantage of glycosylated haemoglobin is that measurement can be made on small capillary samples and it is stable, enabling samples to be collected at home and sent to the laboratory [102]. Analyses using test kits can provide results in less than 10 min and this enables the clinician to discuss overall control with the patient at the time of the consultation [103].

HYPOGLYCAEMIA

The greatest concern for most parents and many children who have diabetes is the risk of hypoglycaemia which may lead to impairment of consciousness or seizures.

Episodic mild hypoglycaemia is common in patients who maintain adequate control of diabetes. Symptoms are usually associated with release of counterregulatory hormones, particularly adrenaline, and provide the child with adequate warning to prevent significant impairment of cerebral function.

In those patients having adequate insulin, exercise is probably the commonest cause of hypoglycaemia, which may occur many hours after the exercise. A reduction in insulin dose of 25% may be needed to avoid acute and late hypoglycaemia in well-controlled patients during strenuous activity [13].

Studies made under laboratory conditions have defined the levels of blood glucose that lead to release of counterregulatory hormones and are critical in affecting cerebral function. Lowering blood glucose levels to 3.5 mmol/l leads to increases in plasma adrenaline and growth hormone. Lowering the level to 3 mmol/l leads to increases in glucagon and cortisol. At 3 mmol/l alterations of cerebral function may be evidenced by brainstem and cortical evoked potentials [104]. Impaired cognition, which is also dependent on duration of hypoglycaemia, occurs with blood glucose levels at 2.8 mmol/l [105].

Severe hypoglycaemia may lead to blurred vision and a fall in intraocular pressure [106]. There is considerable variation in clinical symptoms in response to hypoglycaemia, both between patients and on different occasions in an individual. This may relate to the rate of fall of blood glucose levels and to the usual level of diabetic control [107,108]. Upright posture may increase symptoms [109]. Circulating insulin levels may influence perception of hypoglycaemia and hormonal response [105]. Sustained mild hypoglycaemia may lead to hypoglycaemic unawareness despite high concentrations of adrenaline [105]. Arslanian *et al.* reported that adolescent boys are more likely to develop greater degrees of hypoglycaemia due to sex-related differences in growth hormone response to hypoglycaemia [110]. Alcohol may lead to less awareness of hypoglycaemia in adolescents [111].

Severe hypoglycaemia is more likely to occur in patients who achieve good control with intensive insulin therapy. A report about the DCCT stated that those on intensive treatment had an incidence of severe hypoglycaemia 2–6 times greater than those who had conventional twice-daily insulin treatment. Severe hypoglycaemia occurred more often during sleep (55% of incidents of hypoglycaemia); 36% of those occurring while the patient was awake were not accompanied by warning symptoms [24].

Patients on intensive insulin therapy have impaired counterregulatory glycaemic response to hypoglycaemia due to inadequate stimulation of gluconeogenesis [112]. Amiel showed that strict glycaemic control may lower the glucose level needed to stimulate adrenaline release, and thus diminish patient recognition of the moderate hypoglycaemia that otherwise prevents severe hypoglycaemia [107]. Davis found that, in patients with defects in counterregulatory responses to hypoglycaemia, recurrent hypoglycaemia was associated with reduction in adrenocorticotrophic hormone (ACTH) secretion and impairment of hepatic glucose production [113].

Patients with chronic poorly controlled diabetes may experience symptoms of hypoglycaemia at normoglycaemic blood levels [108]. This has been attributed to a higher glucose threshold for counterregulatory hormone release [108]. Poor control may thus be perpetuated as the child experiences hypoglycaemia symptoms whenever normoglycaemia is approached.

When biosynthetic human insulin was first introduced, and used to replace pork or beef insulin, there were many anecdotal reports that severe hypoglycaemia and hypoglycaemia unawareness were more prevalent with human insulin [114]. Formal studies failed to confirm this [115–118]. Sjoeborn compared hypoglycaemic response to human and porcine insulins, and concluded that there was no difference in counterregulatory hormone responses to the two types of insulin [119]. Lingenfelser *et al.* have proposed, however, that there may be a direct effect of the two insulins on cerebral function unrelated to counterregulatory response [120].

In older children and young adults serious hypoglycaemia may not be associated with deteriorating cognitive function [121], but may lead to disabling anxiety [122].

Treatment of severe hypoglycaemia

If the child is unconscious, having fits or unable to take sugar by mouth, either glucagon or intravenous glucose should be given. Glucagon should be reserved for those for whom intravenous glucose cannot be given readily. It may be given subcutaneously or intramuscularly, and the dose is not critical, usually being 0.5 mg for children under the age of 2 years, and 1 mg for those over this age. Improvement in the conscious state will usually occur within 15 min, and sugar should then be given by mouth as the effect of glucagon may be short-lived in the presence of excess insulin.

Families of all children with diabetes should be instructed in administering glucagon, and should keep a glucagon kit at hand. It should be taken when the family travels, particularly when medical help would be difficult to obtain.

Nasal glucagon, in a dose of twice the parenteral one, was shown to be comparable in effect to subcutaneous glucagon [123], and a freeze-dried mixture of glucagon and glycocholic acid as a surfactant has been used [124]. It has been shown to be as effective as the subcutaneous route in correcting hypoglycaemia [124].

If glucagon has not been effective, or the child lapses into unconsciousness, intravenous glucose should be given. Fifty per cent glucose solution may be used in a dose of 1 ml/kg over 2 min. It is essential to monitor blood glucose levels, particularly if the child does not readily respond. The child may be in a postictal state with a normal or raised blood glucose. Unconsciousness may be due to other causes such as drug ingestion or head injury. There are dangers in excessive administration of 50% glucose solutions.

The rise in blood glucose following intravenous glucose will depend on the degree of hypoglycaemia and hyperinsulinaemia. Glucose will initially distribute through the extracellular space, and eventually throughout the total body water (700 ml/kg). When 50% glucose solution in a dose of 1 ml/kg (2.78 mmol glucose/kg) is administered, it would be expected that a rise of at least 4 mmol/l of glucose would occur within 10 min of injection.

If there is difficulty in maintaining blood glucose levels, or if the child is vomiting after severe hypoglycaemia, as is common, an intravenous line should be maintained and 10% glucose given with extra bolus doses as needed.

Any child who has profound hypoglycaemia which is unresponsive or recurs is likely to have very high levels of circulating insulin, and the possibility of deliberate overdose should be considered. In an adolescent there may have been suicidal intent.

PSYCHOSOCIAL ADJUSTMENT

The advent of diabetes in a child usually has a profound effect on the family. For some there is a deep sense of loss of a healthy child, and adjustment follows a natural process of grief, with feelings of disbelief, of blame and guilt, of anger and sadness before acceptance can take place. This may take many months, and the process may be retarded by unhelpful attitudes from relatives. The child has to cope with similar feelings, together with confusion and perhaps shame in being diseased. The child's behaviour may reflect the parents' anxiety and grief, particularly at preschool age and in early adolescence. Some children never fully come to terms with diabetes.

Difficulty in obtaining stable control will heighten feelings of inadequacy, particularly if diabetes care has been left to one parent or to the teenager alone. Young children tend to think that diabetes is a punishment for something they have done wrong, or that their parents are punishing them through painful injections and denial of food. Siblings often feel that they are being deprived of the special attention given to the child with diabetes, their resentment being expressed sometimes as somatic symptoms or behavioural disturbance. Difficulties may be greatest in early adolescence, when the psychosocial developmental needs for emancipation from parental control, identification with peers and risk-taking behaviours may all lead the teenager into conflict with parents and to non-compliance with the diabetes regime.

Most children, however, cope well psychologically with diabetes, showing good coping strategies and trying actively to adapt to their illness [125], even though parents may perceive that they do not [126]. Parents of adolescents with diabetes report more behaviour and adjustment problems than the children do themselves (Northam, 1993, unpublished data). Some, however, do not cope well, and psychiatric disorders, psychological distress and social problems have been reported as more common in both children [127,128] and young adults with IDDM [129].

The relationship between emotional disturbance and diabetic control is not clear. Some children who have labile control have been reported to respond to emotional stress with hyperglycaemia and ketonuria [130]. Stress appears to affect control adversely in adolescents [131], but no relationship has been found between parents' reports of stress in themselves or their children and $HbA1_c$ values [132]. Stress in young adults may be associated with increased risk of hypertension but not macrovascular complications [133].

Children who have significant problems in maintaining diabetic control often display evidence of emotional disturbance [127,134], although a causal relationship is not clear [126]. Those with unstable diabetes and recurrent severe hypoglycaemia may, as a result, be more unhappy and more anxious [122]. On the other hand, children with brittle diabetes who have repeated admissions to hospital because of their unstable diabetes have been shown to respond well to formal psychoanalytic treatment [135].

It would be reasonable to suppose that emotional disturbance would affect control through poor compliance [136], but recent studies suggest that, except in extreme cases, this may not be so. Fonagy reported that children with low $HbA1_c$ values representing good control were more likely to show emotional disturbance such as worry, apprehension and a tendency to bully. Psychological disturbance in their parents was also associated with quality of metabolic control in their child. Quality of family life and parents' marital relationship did not appear related to control [128].

Children who have become independent in their care of diabetes at an early age may be more likely to have poor control. It is possible that anxious children are more diligent in the care of diabetes [127]. It has been suggested that the physician's expectation of tight control of diabetes during childhood might lead to adverse psychosocial functioning, but this has not been shown to be so [137].

Disturbance of eating is common in adolescents and young adults, including those with diabetes, when it is associated with poor control of glycaemia [138]. Clinical eating disorders such as anorexia nervosa and bulimia appear to be no more prevalent in young women with diabetes [139,140], but control of weight by misuse of insulin may be common [139,141,142] and is potentially dangerous.

COGNITIVE FUNCTION

In counselling parents about the consequences of variable glycaemic control the physician may need to discuss whether episodes of severe hypoglycaemia, or recurrent mild hypoglycaemia or hyperglycaemia, could affect cognitive function, particularly in the area of learning.

Hypoglycaemia has been shown to acutely affect cognitive function [143–145]. Pramming *et al.* studied the effect of hypoglycaemia on brain function in a group of young adults with IDDM. When blood glucose values were below a mean value of 2 (confidence intervals 1.7–2.3) mmol/l, changes in electroencephalograms (EEGs) indicated cortical neuronal dysfunction. Lower values of blood glucose led to deep brain dysfunction. These EEG signs of dysfunction did not correlate with symptoms or signs of hypoglycaemia [145].

Children below the age of 5 years may be at greater risk of subtle cognitive changes as a consequence of frequent mild or asymptomatic hypoglycaemic episodes. Even mild hypoglycaemia in early life may have long-term consequences in learning deficits at school age [146].

A high proportion of IDDM children have EEG abnormalities which correlate with early-onset diabetes and severe hypoglycaemia. In adults with long-standing juvenile-onset IDDM, impaired cognitive performance may not be related directly to recurrent hypoglycaemia, but when this had occurred, it may interact with neuropathy to increase neurobehavioural dysfunction.

There is less clear evidence on the effect of hyperglycaemia on cognitive function [147]. Martinelli *et al.* studied this in a group of young adults with IDDM using visual evoked potentials. No significant changes were found to be associated with acute mild hyperglycaemia in this study [148].

EARLY VISUAL CHANGES

Visual disturbance is common in the early stages of IDDM in childhood. The most common disturbances are transitory refractive changes most marked during initial stabilization, when up to 47% of patients may be affected, and up to 20% of patients with longer-duration diabetes [149]. Myopia is associated with hyperglycaemia but hypermetropia is found as blood glucose returns to normal. These changes are presumably due to osmotic changes within the eye, and resolve without treatment. They make it very difficult for the child to draw up the insulin dose or to read, as near vision is affected. Vision usually returns to normal within a few days.

A much less common visual disturbance results from cataract formation, which may be present at diagnosis of diabetes [150], particularly when symptoms have been present for a long period of time. Cataracts may develop very rapidly, even within 24 h [151]. When well developed, cataracts tend to be irreversible [152], but they may be transient [153] and may contribute to the blurred vision in some patients at initial stabilization [154].

RECURRENT KETOACIDOSIS

Ketoacidosis can occur as an isolated incident during severe illness or as a result of physical or emotional stress in any child who is insulin-dependent; it is uncommon in children still in partial remission. There is usually a well-identified reason, usually because of associated vomiting or from inappropriate adjustment of insulin. When the cause is obscure, or appears insufficient, it is likely that the child has been in poor control preceding the DKA, and that precipitating factors have included emotional stress and omission of one or more insulin doses.

Recurrent DKA is uncommon, but tends to follow a well-recognized pattern. Vomiting is usually the first sign, and often starts during the night; by morning the child is already dehydrated and extra doses of insulin prove ineffective in reversing the rapid progression of acidosis, so that hospital admission becomes inevitable. It is more common in adolescent girls but, in the author's experience, if it does occur in a boy, it is likely that he is openly non-compliant and sees diabetes care as of secondary importance to other stressful or more important events in his life. In girls particularly, however, each episode is unexplained or attributed to intercurrent illness, and parents often claim that their child has done everything possible to prevent the acidosis. Recurrent episodes leave the parents as mystified as their daughter appears to be; they then seek explanations in physical causes such as abnormal response to insulin, some undiagnosed associated illness or incorrect advice on diabetes care.

Management of children with recurrent DKA usually depends on a sequence of steps. It may first be necessary to exclude an organic basis such as thyrotoxicosis, chronic urinary infection or migraine, and convince the family that this has been done. It may be helpful to establish that the child has normal responses to insulin, both short- and long-acting, and to establish the correct dose. This may be done best under strict supervision in hospital. This will also exclude the possibility that vomiting episodes are the response to unrecognized nocturnal hypoglycaemia.

This will allow the physician and family to conclude that the recurrent DKA is due to psychological factors, probably combined with omission of insulin. Psychotherapeutic approaches which include the family are necessary, and are likely to prove helpful [135,155].

SCREENING FOR COMPLICATIONS

All patients with diabetes of sufficient duration are vulnerable to long-term complications [156]. The extent to which these lead to morbidity and mortality is very variable, and prevention or reduction of risk is the most important task for the physician caring for childhood diabetes. Prevalence and severity of complications relates to duration of diabetes [157,178], but microvascular complications are rare before puberty and it is likely that the prepubertal years make little contribution to this relationship [159,160].

While many studies support the hypothesis that microvascular complications are causally linked to metabolic control [157,161–164] and improved control may retard their further development [165,166], the definitive controlled study that has conclusively established this, the DCCT, has only very recently been reported [15,167].

Near-normal glycaemic control, which may require intensive insulin therapy, should be the management objective for all children with diabetes. Many young people will find this impossible to achieve after the phase of partial remission, either because of unacceptable experience of severe hypoglycaemia [24,165], or for psychosocial reasons. Most children, even those who have imperfect control, have no clinical symptoms of complications, and will have little motivation to improve diabetic control without a compelling reason. This may be provided for those who develop subclinical evidence of microangiopathy during adolescence and are presumed to be at increased risk for severe clinical expression in early adult life. For this reason it has become apparent that efforts should be made to identify such children and focus attention on how to reduce that risk.

This approach is based on screening for functional or minor structural abnormalities that are presumed to herald significant and irreversible structural changes of clinical consequence [168,169]. The most common screening tests are measurement of microalbumin excretion rate, tests of autonomic nerve function and screening for background retinopathy. Tests of peripheral nerve function are probably of less value [170], as is documentation of limited joint mobility. Identification of associated risk factors, including hypertension, smoking, elevated lipid values and obesity, is relevant but should be part of routine clinical care.

Microalbuminuria is now thought to reflect early functional renal changes which precede and predict nephropathy [171,172]. Without early intervention, urinary albumin excretion may increase exponentially with rising arterial blood pressure [173]. As the functional changes may be reversed with intervention, screening is widely accepted as essential in adolescence [171,174]. Microalbuminuria is associated with raised arterial blood pressure [172], and its presence should alert the clinician to the need for aggressive hypotensive therapy.

Overnight albumin excretion rate appears to be the most informative test for microalbuminuria, showing least variation from test to test [175]. Microalbuminuria is unusual in those adolescents who have maintained satisfactory glycaemic control in the preceding 2–6 years [176]. Microalbuminuria has also been shown to be associated with the presence of neuropathy [177] and proliferative retinopathy, which it is thought to predict [174,178].

Screening for background retinopathy may allow intervention in those few who show rapid deterioration to proliferative retinopathy [179]. Poor diabetic control (mean $HbA1_c > 10\%$) is associated with an increased risk of progression to retinopathy and lowering $HbA1_c$ values has a beneficial effect [161]. The association with high $HbA1_c$ values has been widely reported [98,164,180–182]. This, together with the reported association with hypertension [181] and cigarette smoking [183], provides a sound basis for aggressive intervention.

Rapid improvement in control in patients who have been poorly controlled for some time may lead to transient deterioration of retinopathy [184–186], including development of proliferative retinopathy which may be reversible with sustained good control [187]. Transient optic disc swelling has also been reported [188].

The clinical role of screening for early preclinical signs of neuropathy is less clear. Clinical methods include beat-to-beat measures of heart rate and blood pressure response to the Valsalva manoeuvre, deep breathing and postural change [189]. Autonomic neuropathy is uncommon in childhood and adolescents [190], and its relation to glycaemic control is unclear.

Assessment of limited joint mobility has been suggested as a marker of other diabetes complications. It may develop in parallel with retinopathy and neuropathy [191, 192] but this may merely reflect duration of diabetes with which there is a linear relationship [193], and may not reliably predict retinopathy [194].

Identification of early signs of complications should lead to a more intensive insulin regime to achieve better metabolic control. This carries a greater risk for severe hypoglycaemia, particularly during sleep [89]. It remains to be seen whether maintenance of excellent control from onset of treatment (rather than subsequent attempts to improve control) carries the same risk: it may not do so, as reports of severe hypoglycaemia with human insulin were largely confined to those who had changed from pork to human insulin, rather than those who had been having human insulin from the start of their treatment.

HYPERTENSION

Between 30% and 60% of adult diabetic patients have hypertension [195]. It is essential to measure blood pressure regularly in all patients after puberty, and is particularly important for those with a family history of hypertension. Increased prevalence of raised blood pressure in diabetes has been reported for boys and girls from age 13 [196], and in boys especially [197,198].

A family history of hypertension is relevant, since genetic predisposition to hypertension independent of diabetes has been shown to increase the risk of development of nephropathy [199,200], and has been suggested as a genetic indicator of risk for nephropathy [201].

Raised blood pressure may be an early sign of diabetic nephropathy [202,203] and will itself lead to accelerated development of renal damage [204,205]. In adolescents and young adults even moderately elevated blood pressure (defined as systolic > 130 mmHg or diastolic > 85 mmHg) has been shown to be associated with increased albumin excretion rates [206].

Aggressive treatment of raised blood pressure in young diabetics is now recommended [204], since even moderately elevated blood pressure may adversely affect nephropathy [207] and successful reduction of blood pressure may lead to a reduction of urinary albumin excretion [207]. In patients with microalbuminuria, hypotensive therapy which diminishes hypertension also diminishes albuminuria and, in those who are normotensive, it prevents an increase in albuminuria [208]. The question of which hypotensive agent to use, and whether angiotensin-converting enzyme (ACE) inhibition or calcium antagonism is more effective in preventing nephropathy in young patients with diabetes is unresolved [208].

SMOKING

Cigarette smoking poses an additional risk for those with diabetes. Young people with diabetes may be more likely to smoke than non-diabetics [209]. Young people who smoke have a prevalence of albumin excretion rate 2.8 times higher than in non-smokers: the progression of albuminuria and retinopathy is greater in those who smoke. Albuminuria improves when subjects cease smoking [210]. Although those who smoke are also likely to be generally non-compliant in diabetes care [211], smoking is an independent risk factor for early diabetic renal damage. Morbidity, which included hospitalization, sick days and lack of being well, is greater for those who smoke [212]. Smoking may be a risk factor for the development of nephropathy in young people [213] and may be an aggravating factor for retinopathy in males [214].

ADOLESCENCE

Care of adolescents with diabetes provides a challenge to the physician, since neither a paediatric approach nor formal adult consultation may be appropriate. Diabetic control is likely to deteriorate with rising $HbA1_c$ values in some patients at this age [215], and variable day-to-day control will reflect changing lifestyle.

Impaired diabetes control and increased insulin requirements may be due to the interaction of a number of factors during puberty. There is reduced insulin sensitivity [12], in part related to increased sleep-induced growth hormone secretion [216], which leads to fasting hyperglycaemia. Psychological stress at this age may affect control independently of non-compliance [131], but it is likely that non-compliance will be the major factor contributing to poor control [215,217].

Non-compliance may not reflect considered rejection of advice on the part of the adolescent so much as a conflict of priorities with the pressing demands of psychosocial development. It is essential for the adolescent to achieve independence from parental control and, in doing so, he or she may reject adult advice. The adolescent enhances self-esteem through developing relationships with peers who do not have diabetes, and hence may lead a lifestyle incompatible with good diabetes care. He or she feels sensitive about his/her body and its function, and any departure from perceived normality will cause distress: denial of the needs for diabetes care may seem helpful by reducing the feeling of being different. Concerns for study, social activities (which include eating and drinking unsuitable foods and fluids at odd times), late nights and erratic sleep patterns militate against good control, but are all important to adolescents if they are to relate appropriately to peers and enjoy the teenage years.

Behaviour patterns which characterize adolescence jeopardize diabetes control. Experimenting with alcohol, smoking, risk-taking behaviours and a feeling of invulnerability on the one hand, and hopelessness for the future on the other, all make it difficult to achieve rational control of diabetes. Poor compliance has been associated with lower self-esteem and self-efficacy, depression and food bingeing [218]. It has been suggested that these psychological factors could be the basis for intervention to improve self-efficacy at this age [78]. The association of puberty with less good control has also been attributed to poor motivation to comply [215]. Reports on sex differences in the development of control during adolescence differ [215,217], possibly due to the difference in timing of maturity.

Grossman *et al.*, in a study of young adolescents, showed a relationship between beliefs about diabetes efficacy, self-esteem and perception of control. Those with a greater feeling of self-efficacy had better control [78]. It is possible that physicians may expect too much of adolescents: those who are cognitively immature compared with their peers may be given self-care responsibilities they are unable to assume [77].

The threat of long-term complications and the emergence of early signs of their development, together with their neglect of care and apparent indifference to late sequelae, add to the anxiety and frustration experienced by parents. Their distress, particularly if expressed by repeated attempts at intervention, may add to the teenager's difficulties and strengthen their resolve to rebel.

Adolescents who are not cognitively mature may have beliefs about diabetes (including their own invulnerability to long-term complications, or to their feelings of inability to control outcomes) that are not consistent with factual knowledge. Enhancing factual knowledge may not alter beliefs or health-care practices, and educational programmes designed to increase knowledge seldom lead to a change in health care or improved diabetes control [219].

Peer group influence may be more important in improving metabolic control during adolescence than formal education intervention [220]. Camps for teenagers with diabetes are now recognized as a helpful aspect of care, and although camp objectives differ widely, most are directed towards development of a positive attitude to diabetes and its care, the provision of peer group support and enhancement of self-reliance.

Compliance may be enhanced if the physician can maintain a trusting relationship of mutual respect with the adolescent patient. Adolescents are influenced in their behaviour by the expectations of others who are important, and this may include the doctor. The circumstances of the consultation may influence the adolescent's response: an unfriendly reception, excessive waiting and a consultation in which he or she feels that his or her views have not been heard are not conducive to compliance. It may be helpful to encourage the adolescent to participate in management decisions, defining the limits that can be achieved and which the doctor can accept. Adolescents tend to value their relationship with their physician and expect their trust and wish for privacy and confidentiality to be respected.

Transfer from a paediatric to an adult-oriented service is best made in the latter part of adolescence or as young adults, and timing should be based on developmental readiness rather than on age alone [216]. Transfer of care is facilitated by the establishment of transition clinics in adult hospital services where the specific needs of older adolescents and young adults are met, and the care of IDDM is not swamped with the large numbers of patients with NIDDM that often dominate an adult diabetes service.

The prospects of a career may be of increasing concern through adolescence. Young people with diabetes do not usually experience more difficulty in obtaining employment than those without diabetes [221,222] but the risk for those who have hypoglycaemia unawareness makes some occupations hazardous. Adult diabetics are reported to have similar work experiences to non-diabetics, unless they develop disabling complications [223].

COUNSELLING FOR PARENTS ON GENETIC RISK

Parents of a child who has developed diabetes will want to know the risk for their other children. General population risk for diabetes shows remarkable variation from one country and one ethnic group to another. The incidence of IDDM varies from 1.7/100 000 person-years in Japan to 29.5/100 000 person-years in Finland, and variation appears to be determined by factors related to ethnicity and average yearly temperature of the environment [224].

The risk for a sibling of a child with IDDM is 6% [225]. Offspring of women with IDDM have a lower risk than those of men, and there is a negative correlation with the age of pregnancy: this raises the question of whether exposure of the fetus to maternal diabetes protects the infant from developing diabetes [226].

Relative risk of a sibling developing diabetes can be further clarified by human leukocyte antigen (HLA) typing: the risk varies from 12.9% to 1.8% depending on the degree of shared haplotypes [225]. Measurement of islet-cell antibodies and insulin antibodies, which are found positive in 3% of siblings, will indicate whether development of clinical diabetes is likely (Harrison, unpublished data). It may be that measurement of antibodies to glutamine acid decarboxylase will prove to be a more reliable marker of genetic risk [227].

Until effective intervention has been developed to prevent diabetes, a study of risk factors is of little practical value other than for research. Clarifying levels of risk may heighten anxiety or instil false reassurance. It should not be done without appropriate counselling for those identified at risk.

Parents of a child with diabetes should be advised to test their other children for raised blood glucose levels during illness if they are developing symptoms suggestive of diabetes, or if there is weight loss.

DIABETES AND CYSTIC FIBROSIS

Glucose intolerance and the development of diabetes is common in cystic fibrosis (CF) [228]. Raised $HbA1_c$ concentration was reported in 39% of patients at age 23 years [229] and impaired glucose tolerance is said to increase at a linear rate from age 15 to 25 years, at which age 32% of those alive have diabetes [230].

This suggests that regular measurement of $HbA1_c$ levels after midpuberty is desirable in patients with CF. Glucose intolerance has a potentially harmful influence on CF, and should be treated early, since hyperglycaemia may lead to impaired immunological response to infection [228] and impaired nutrition. The associated dehydration may lead to increased viscosity of sputum. Microvascular complications have also been reported in CF diabetes [231].

Insulin treatment may be temporary if glucose intolerance has developed only with high steroid therapy. Requirements are very variable, depending on the degree of insulin insufficiency, the extent of pulmonary disease and the use of steroids. Since maintenance of good nutrition is paramount in the management of CF, patients will require a relatively high intake of energy-dense foods with a high fat and protein content, and which may contain sugar. Satisfactory control is usually quite readily obtained despite this high food intake.

FUTURE DEVELOPMENTS

Research in the care of diabetes will lead to change in two areas: improvement in current methods of care and fundamental change such as prevention of diabetes in those at risk, and cure in those who have the established clinical condition. Improvements in current care will focus on improved methods of insulin delivery, more acceptable methods of monitoring the diabetic state and the prevention of complications of diabetes. The second line of research has as its goal the restoration of normal insulin secretion to those with diabetes, and the protection of islet cells from autoimmune destruction in those at risk.

Practicable developments that can be expected soon include insulin modification leading to more effective prevention of postprandial hyperglycaemia, insulin delivery methods which no longer rely on self-injection, methods of monitoring glucose levels without drawing blood, effective intervention in those who have early signs of complications, and better ways of helping those overwhelmed by the psychosocial impact of a chronic disease.

Insulin could be protected against proteolytic degradation in the gut by being contained in spherical capsules. Encapsulated insulin can be absorbed into the blood stream after oral administration, and is bound appropriately to insulin receptors, behaving like naked insulin [232].

Prospects of the cure of existing IDDM depend on the ability to transplant insulin secretory cells within the portal system in sufficient numbers to meet the needs of the child. They would need to be protected from tissue rejection and the anticipated assault of the body's autoimmune system that was responsible for diabetes in the first place.

Human islet transplants have been disappointing so far as those few patients who have had successful islet transplants have returned to insulin dependency within a few weeks [233]. It appears that cells need to be harvested from at least two cadaveric fetal pancreases to provide sufficient insulin when transplanted, and that inadequate numbers of cells may hasten failure of the grafted cells. The problems of rejection, and the provision of long-term immunosuppressant therapy, still need to be resolved. It is unlikely that enough cells could ever be available to transplant all patients who would benefit, until a means of inducing growth in culture of actively functioning cells is available.

One method of overcoming this obstacle is to encapsulate islet cells in a membrane that protects them from attack by the body's immune process. It is possible that use of animal cells would be feasible, and xenotransplantation of microencapsulated pancreatic cells has been reported in recent research using animal studies [234,235]. Genetic manipulation to insert insulin-related genes into fibroblasts has also been proposed.

REFERENCES

1 Kerr D, Reza M, Smith N *et al.* Importance of insulin in subjective, cognitive and hormonal responses to hypoglycemia in patients with IDDM. *Diabetes* 1991;40:1057–62.

2 Krane EJ, Rockoff MA, Wallman JK *et al.* Subclinical brain swelling in children during treatment of diabetic ketoacidosis. *N Engl J Med* 1985;312:1147–51.

3 Hoffman WH, Steinhart CM, Gammal TE *et al.* Cranial C.T. in children and adolescents with diabetic ketoacidosis. *Am J Neuroradiol* 1988;9:733–9.

4 Rosenbloom AL. Intracranial crises during treatment of diabetic ketoacidosis. *Diabetes Care* 1990;13:22–33.

5 Winegrad AI, Kern EFO, Simmons DA. Cerebral oedema in diabetic ketoacidosis. *N Engl J Med* 1985;312:1184–5.

6 Harris GD, Flordalisi I, Harris WL *et al.* Minimizing the risk of brain haematuria during treatment of diabetic ketoacidosis: a retrospective and prospective study. *J Pediatr* 1990; 117:22–31.

7 Duck SC, Wyatt DT. Factors associated with brain herniation in the treatment of diabetic ketoacidosis. *J Pediatr* 1988;113:10–14.

8 Kostraba JN, Gay EC, Rewers M *et al.* Increasing trend of outpatient management of children with newly diagnosed IDDM. *Diabetes Care* 1992;15:95–100.

9 Chase HP, Crews KR, Garg S *et al.* Outpatient management vs in-hospital management of children with new-onset diabetes. *Clin Pediatr* 1992;31:450–6.

10 Haakens K, Hanssen KF, Dahl-Jorgensen K *et al.* Early morning glycaemia and the metabolic consequences of delaying breakfast/morning insulin. A comparison of continuous subcutaneous insulin infusion and multiple injection therapy with human isophane or huma ultralente insulin at bedtime in insulin-dependent diabetes. *Scand J Clin Lab Invest* 1989;49:653–9.

11 Wolfsdort JI, Laffel LMB, Pasquarello C *et al.* Split-mixed insulin regimen with human ultralente before supper and NPH (isophane) before breakfast in children and adolescents with IDDM. *Diabetes Care* 1991;14:100–6.

12 Bloch CA, Clemons P, Sperling MA. Puberty decreases insulin sensitivity. *J Pediatr* 1987;110:481–7.

13 Sonnenberg GE, Kemmer FW, Berger M. Exercise in type-1 (insulin-dependent) diabetic patients treated with continuous subcutaneous infusion. Prevention of exercise-induced hypoglycaemia. *Diabetologia* 1990;33:696–703.

14 Turnbridge FK, Home PD, Murphy M *et al.* Does flexibility at mealtimes disturb blood glucose control on a multiple insulin injection regimen? *Diabetic Med* 1991;8:833–88.

15 Diabetes Complications and Control Trial Research Group. The effect of intensive treatment of diabetes on the development and progression of long-term complications in insulin-dependent diabetes mellitus. *N Engl J Med* 1993;329:977–86.

16 Fisken RA, Goulbourn S. Treatment of insulin-dependent diabetes using an injection pen: control, problems and patient preferences. *Diabetes Res* 1989;11:195–7.

17 Gall M-A, Mathiesen ER, Skott P *et al.* Effect of multiple insulin injections with a pen injector on metabolic control and general well-being in insulin-dependent diabetes mellitus. *Diabetes Res* 1989;11:97–101.

18 Hardy KJ, Jones KR, Gill GV. Deterioration in blood glucose control in females with diabetes changed to a basal-bolus regimen using a pen-injector. *Diabetic Med* 1991;8:69–71.

19 Hoernquist JO, Wikby A, Andersson PO *et al.* Insulin-pen treatment, quality of life and metabolic control: retrospective intra-group evaluations. *Diabetes Res Clin Pract* 1990;10:221–30.

20 Tallroth G, Karlson B, Nilsson A *et al.* The influence of different regimens on quality of life and metabolic control in insulin-dependent diabetics. *Diabetes Res Clin Pract* 1989; 6:37–43.

21 Selam J-L, Micossi P, Dunn FL *et al.* Clinical trial of programmable implantable insulin pump for type-1 diabetes. *Diabetes Care* 1992;15:877–85.

22 Olsson PO, Jorfeldt L, Arnquist H *et al.* Pre- and postprandial hyperinsulinemia during insulin pump treatment; role of the subcutaneous bolus and basal infusion. *Diabetes Res* 1991; 16:55–61.

23 Levy-Marchal C, Czernichow P. Feasibility of continuous subcutaneous insulin infusion in young diabetic patients. *Diabete Metabol* 1988;14:108–13.

24 The DCCT Research Group. Epidemiology of severe hypoglycemia in the diabetes control and complications trial. *Am J Med* 1991;90:450–9.

25 Soltesz G, Molnar D, Desci T *et al.* The metabolic and hormonal effects of continuous subcutaneous insulin in-

fusion therapy in diabetic children. *Diabetologia* 1988;31:30–4.

26 Saule H. Insulin-induced oedema in adolescents with type-l diabetes (in German). *Dtsch Med Wochenschr* 1991;116:1191–4.

27 Shishko PI, Kovalev PA, Goncharov VG *et al.* Comparison of peripheral and portal (via the umbillical vein) routes of insulin infusion in IDDM patients. *Diabetes* 1992;41:1042–9.

28 Waxman K, Turner D, Nguyen ST *et al.* Implantable programmable insulin pumps for the treatment of diabetes. *Arch Surg* 1992;127:1032–7.

29 Wood DF, Goodchild K, Guillou P *et al.* Management of 'brittle' diabetes with a preprogrammable implanted insulin pump delivering intraperitoneal insulin. *Br Med J* 1990;301:1143–4.

30 Hildebrandt P. Skinfold thickness, local subcutaneous blood flow and insulin absorption in diabetic patients. *Acta Physiol Scand* 1991;143(Suppl. 603):41–5.

31 Ronnemaa T, Koivisto VA. Combined effect of exercise and ambient temperature on insulin absorption and postprandial glycemia in type l patients. *Diabetes Care* 1988;11:769–73.

32 Vora JP, Burch A, Peters JR *et al.* Relationship between absorption of radiolabeled soluble insulin, subcutaneous blood flow, and anthropometry. *Diabetes Care* 1992;15:1484–93.

33 de Meijer PH, Lutterman JA, van Lier HJ *et al.* The variability of the absorption of subcutaneously injected insulin: effect of injection technique and relation with brittleness. *Diabetic Med* 1990;7:499–505.

34 Smith CP, Sargent MA, Wilson B *et al.* Subcutaneous or intramuscular insulin injections. *Arch Dis Child* 1991;66:879–82.

35 Henriksen JE, Vaag A, Ramsgaard Hansen I *et al.* Absorption of NPH (isophane) insulin in resting diabetic patients: evidence for subcutaneous injection in the thigh as the preferred site. *Diabetic Med* 1991;8:453–7.

36 Frid A, Gunnarsson R, Guntner P *et al.* Effects of accidental intramuscular injection on insulin absorption in IDDM. *Diabetes Care* 1988;11:41–5.

37 Frid A, Ostman J, Linde B. Hypoglycaemia risk during exercise after intramuscular injection of insulin in thigh in IDDM. *Diabetes Care* 1990;13:473–7.

38 Thow JC, Johnson AB, Marsden S *et al.* Morphology of palpably abnormal injection sites and effects on absorption of isophane (NHP) insulin. *Diabetic Med* 1990;7:795–9.

39 Young RJ, Hannan WJ, Frier BM *et al.* Diabetic lipohypertrophy delays insulin absorption. *Diabetes Care* 1984;7:479–80.

40 Freidenberg GR, White N, Cataland S *et al.* Diabetes responsive to intravenous but not subcutaneous insulin effectiveness of aprotinin. *N Engl J Med* 1981;305:363–8.

41 Edge JA, Matthews DR, Dunger DB. Failure of current insulin regimes to meet the overnight requirements of adolescents with insulin-dependent diabetes. *Diabetes Res* 1990;15:109–12.

42 Hirsch IB, Smith LJ, Havlin CE *et al.* Failure of nocturnal hypoglycaemia to cause daytime hyperglycaemia in patients with IDDM. *Diabetes Care* 1990;13:133–42.

43 Perriello G, De Feo P, Torlone E *et al.* The dawn phenomenon in type-1 (insulin-dependent) diabetes mellitus: magnitude, frequency, variability and dependency on glucose counterregulation and insulin sensitivity. *Diabetologia* 1991;34:21–8.

44 Assan R, Feutren G, Sirmai J *et al.* Plasma C-peptide levels and clinical remissions in recent-onset type-1 diabetic patients treated with cyclosporin A and insulin. *Diabetes* 1990;39:768–74.

45 Couper JJ, Hudson I, Werther GA *et al.* Factors predicting residual beta-cell function in the first year after diagnosis of childhood type-1 diabetes. *Diabetes Res Clin Pract* 1991;11:9–16.

46 Dahlquist G, Blom L, Persson B *et al.* The epidemiology of lost residual beta-cell function in short term diabetic children. *Acta Paed Scand* 1988;77:852–9.

47 Schiffrin A, Suissa S, Poussier P *et al.* Prospective study of predictors of beta-cell survival in type-1 diabetes. *Diabetes* 1988;37:920–5.

48 Snorgaard O, Lassen LH, Binder C. Homogeneity in pattern of decline of beta-cell function in IDDM. Prospective study of 204 consecutive cases followed for 7.4 years. *Diabetes Care* 1992;15:1009–13.

49 Elliot RB, Crossley JR, Berryman CC *et al.* Partial preservation of beta cell function in children with diabetes. *Lancet* 1981;2:1–4.

50 Cook JJ, Hudson I, Harrison LC *et al.* Double-blind controlled trial of azothioprine in children with newly diagnosed type l diabetes. *Diabetes* 1989;38:779–83.

51 Vialettes B, Picq R, du Rostu M *et al.* A preliminary multicentre study of the treatment of recently diagnosed type-l diabetes by combination nicotinamide-cyclosporin therapy. *Diabetic Med* 1990;7:731–5.

52 Dempe A, Baaske W, Von Baehr R *et al.* Remission of the newly diagnosed type-1 diabetes by radiation of the pancreas. *Exp Clin Endocrinol* 1988;92:123–5.

53 Bougneres PF, Landais P, Boisson C *et al.* Limited duration of remission of insulin dependency in children with recent overt type-1 diabetes treated with low-dose cyclosporin. *Diabetes* 1990:39:1264–72.

54 Martin S, Schernthaner G, Nerup J *et al.* Follow-up of cyclosporin A treatment in type-1 (insulin-dependent) diabetes mellitus: lack of long-term effects. *Diabetologia* 1991;34:429–34.

55 Rodier M, Ribstein J, Parer-Richard C *et al.* Renal changes associated with cyclosporin in recent type-1 diabetes mellitus. *Hypertension* 1991;18:334–40.

56 Elliot RB, Chase HP. Prevention or delay of type-1 (insulin-dependent) diabetes mellitus in children using nicotinamide. *Diabetologia* 1991;34:362–5.

57 Manna R, Migliore A, Martin LS *et al.* Nicotinamide treatment in subjects at high risk of developing IDDM improves insulin secretion. *Br J Clin Pract* 1992;46:177–9.

58 Brink SJ. Pediatric, adolescent, and young-adult nutrition issues in IDDM. *Diabetes Care* 1988;11:192–200.

59 Nutrition Subcommittee of the British Diabetic Association's Professional Advisory Committee. Dietary recommendations for people with diabetes: an update for the 1990's. *J Hum Nutr Dietetics* 1991;4:393–412.

60 Jenkins DA, Wolever TM, Taylor RH *et al.* Glycemic index of foods: a physiological basis for carbohydrate exchange. *Am J Clin Nutr* 1981;34:362–6.

61 Wolever TM, Jenkins DJ, Vuksan V *et al.* Glycemic index of foods in individual subjects. *Diabetes Care* 1990:13:126–32.

62 Fontvieille AM, Rizkalla SW, Penfornis A *et al.* The use of low glycaemic index foods improves metabolic control of diabetic patients over 5 weeks. *Diabetic Med* 1992;9:444–50.

63 Jenkins DJA, Wolever TMS, Jenkins AL. Starchy foods and

glycemic index. *Diabetes Care* 1988;11:149–59.

64 Kinmonth AL, Angus RM, Jenkins PA *et al.* Whole foods and increased dietary fibre improve blood glucose control in diabetic children. *Arch Dis Child* 1982;57:187–94.

65 Riccardi G, Rivellese AA. Effects of dietary fibre and carbohydrate on glucose and lipoprotein metabolism in diabetic patients. *Diabetes Care* 1991;14:1115–25.

66 Vinik AI, Jenkins DJA. Dietary fibre in management of diabetes. *Diabetes Care* 1988;11:160–73.

67 Virtanen SM, Varo P. Dietary fibre and fibre fractions in the diet of Finnish diabetic and non-diabetic adolescents. *Eur J Clin Nutr* 1988;42:169–75.

68 Bruttomesso D, Biolo G, Inchiostro S *et al.* No effects of high-fiber diets on metabolic control and insulin-sensitivity in type-l diabetic subjects. *Diabetes Res Clin Pract* 1991; 13:15–21.

69 Gregory JW, Wilson AC, Greene SA. Body fat and overweight among children and adolescents with diabetes mellitus. *Diabetic Med* 1992;9:344–8.

70 Bloomgarden ZT, Karmally W, Metzger MS *et al.* Randomized controlled trial of diabetic patient education: improved knowledge without improved metabolic status. *Diabetes Care* 1987;10:263–72.

71 de Weerdt I, Visser AP, Kok GJ *et al.* Randomised controlled, multi-centre evaluation of an education programme for insulin-treated diabetic patients: effects on metabolic control, quality of life and costs of therapy. *Diabetic Med* 1991; 8:338–45.

72 Rubin RR, Peyrot M, Saudek CD. Differential effect of diabetes education on self-regulation and life-style behaviours. *Diabetes Care* 1991;14:335–8.

73 Cerreto MC, Travis LB. Implications of psychological and family factors in the treatment of diabetes. *Pediatr Clin N Am* 1984;31:689–710.

74 Johnson SB, Pollak T, Silverstein JP *et al.* Cognitive and behavioural knowledge about insulin-dependent diabetes among children and parents. *Pediatrics* 1983;69:708–24.

75 Kohler E, Hurwitz LS, Milan D. A developmentally staged curriculum for teaching self-care to the child with insulin-dependent diabetes mellitus. *Diabetes Care* 1082;5:300–4.

76 Wysocki T, Hough BS, Ward KM *et al.* Use of blood glucose data by families of children with adolescents with IDDM. *Diabetes Care* 1992;15:1041–4.

77 Ingersoll GM, Orr DP, Herrold AJ *et al.* Cognitive maturity and self-management among adolescents with insulin-dependent diabetes mellitus. *J Pediatr* 1986;108:620–3.

78 Grossman HY, Brink S, Hauser ST. Self-efficacy in adolescent girls and boys with insulin-dependent diabetes mellitus. *Diabetes Care* 1987;10:324–9.

79 Delamater AM, Bubb J, Davis SG *et al.* Randomized prospective study of self-managment training with newly diagnosed diabetic children. *Diabetes Care* 1990;13:492–8.

80 Wahren J, Feug P, Ahlborg G *et al.* Glucose metabolism during leg exercise in man. *J Clin Invest* 1971;50:2715–25.

81 Selam JL, Casassus P, Bruzzo F *et al.* Exercise is not associated with better diabetic control in type 1 and type 2 diabetic subjects. *Acta Diabetol* 1992;29:11–13.

82 Huttunen NP, Lankela SL, Knip M *et al.* Effect of once-a-week training program on physical fitness and metabolic control in children with IDDM. *Diabetes Care* 1989;12: 737–40.

83 Kriska AM, LaPorte RE, Patrick SL *et al.* The association of physical activity and diabetic complications in individuals with insulin-dependent diabetes mellitus: the epidemiology of diabetes complications study – VII. *J Clin Epidemiol* 1991;44:1207–14.

84 Hinde FRJ, Standen PJ, Mann NP *et al.* Seasonal variation of haemoglobin Al in children with insulin-dependent diabetes mellitus. *Eur J Pediatr* 1989;148:597–9.

85 Verrotti A, Chiarelli F, Tumini S *et al.* Seasonal variations of glycosylated haemoglobin in diabetic children. *Eur J Pediatr* 1993;149:146–7.

86 Ruegemer JJ, Squires RW, Marsh HM *et al.* Differences between prebreakfast and late afternoon glycemic responses to exercise in IDDM patients. *Diabetes Care* 1990;13: 104–10.

87 Sherwin RS, Koivisto V. Keeping in step: does exercise benefit the diabetic? *Diabetologia* 1981;20:84–6.

88 Follansbee DS. Assuming responsibility for diabetes management: what age? what price? *Diabetes Educ* 1989;15:347–53.

89 Tate PF, Clements CA, Walters JE. Accuracy of home blood glucose monitors. *Diabetes Care* 1992;15:536–8.

90 Robinson MR, Eaton RP, Haaland DM *et al.* Non-invasive glucose monitoring in diabetic patients: a preliminary evaluation. *Clin Chem* 1992;38:1618–22.

91 Kennedy L, Lyons TJ. Non-enzymatic glycosylation. *Br Med Bull* 1989;45:174–90.

92 Blanc MH, Barnett DM, Gleason RE *et al.* Hemoglobin Alc compared with three conventional measurements of diabetes control. *Diabetes Care* 1981;4:349–53.

93 Heinze E, Kohne E, Meissner C *et al.* Hemoglobin Alc (HbAlC) in children with long standing and newly diagnosed diabetes mellitus. *Acta Paed Scand* 1979;Suppl. 68:609–12.

94 Allen KR, Hamilton AD, Bodansky HJ *et al.* Prevalence of haemoglobin variants in a diabetic population and their effect on glycated haemoglobin measurement. *Ann Clin Biochem* 1992;29:426–9.

95 Ferrie CD, Sharpe TC, Price DA *et al.* Seasonal variation of glycosylated haemoglobin. *Arch Dis Child* 1987;62:959–60.

96 Larsen ML, Horder M, Mogensen EF. Effect of long term monitors of glycosylated hemoglobin levels in insulin-dependent diabetes mellitus. *N Engl J Med* 1990;323:1021–5.

97 Winocour PH, Bhatnagar D, Kalsi P *et al.* An analysis of glycosylated blood proteins and blood glucose profiles over one year in patients with type-1 diabetes. *Diabetic Med* 1989;6:709–16.

98 McCance DR, Hadden DR, Atkinson AB *et al.* Long-term glycaemic control and diabetic retinopathy. *Lancet* 1989; 2:824–48.

99 Sobel DO, Abbassi V. Use of fructosamine test in diabetic children. *Diabetes Care* 1991;14:578–83.

100 Hammer MR, John PN, Flynn MD *et al.* Glycated fibrinogen: a new index of short-term diabetic control. *Ann Clin Biochem* 1989;26:58–62.

101 Ardawi MS, Nasrat HN, Mira SA *et al.* Comparison of glycosylated fibrinogen, albumin and haemoglobin as indices of blood glucose control in diabetic patientes. *Diabetic Med* 1990;7:819–24.

102 Dunning PL, Weberruss M, Ward GM. Accuracy, patient acceptance and clinical application of capillary HbA1C monitoring. *Diabetic Med* 1991;8:784–7.

103 Rumley AG, Carlton G, Small M. Within-clinic glycosylated haemoglobin measurement. *Diabetic Med* 1990;7:838–40.

104 Jones TW, McCarthy WV, Tamborlane S *et al.* Mild hypoglycemia and impairment of brainstem and cortical evoked potentials in healthy subjects. *Diabetes* 1990;39:1550–4.

105 Kerr D, Macdonald IA, Tattersall RB. Patients with type-1

diabetes adapt acutely to sustained mild hypoglycaemia. *Diabetic Med* 1991;8:123–8.

106 Frier BM, Hepburn DA, Fisher BM *et al.* Fall in intraocular pressue during acute hypoglycaemia in patients with insulin dependent diabetes. *Br Med J* 1987;294:610–11.

107 Amiel SA, Sherwin RS, Simonson DC *et al.* Effect of intense insulin therapy on glycemic thresholds for counter-regulatory hormone release. *Diabetes* 1988;37:901–7.

108 Jones TW, Boulware SD, Kraemer DT *et al.* Independent effects of youth and poor diabetes control on responses to hypoglycemia in children. *Diabetes* 1991;40:358–63.

109 Hirsch IB, Heller SR, Cryer DE. Increased symptoms of hypoglycaemia in the standing position in insulin-dependent diabetes mellitus. *Clin Sci* 1991;80:583–6.

110 Arslanian SA, Heil BV, Becker DJ *et al.* Sexual dimorphism in insulin sensitivity in adolescents with insulin-dependent diabetes mellitus. *J Clin Endocrinol Metab* 1991;72:920–6.

111 Kerr D, Macdonald IA, Heller SR *et al.* Alcohol causes hypoglycaemic unawareness in healthy volunteers and patients with type 1 (insulin-dependent) diabetes. *Diabetologia* 1990;33:216–21.

112 Caprio S, Napoli R, Sacca L *et al.* Impaired stimulation of gluconeogenesis during prolonged hypoglycemia in intestively treated insulin-dependent diabetic subjects. *J Clin Endocrinol Metab* 1992;75:1076–80.

113 Davis MR, Mellman M, Shamoon H. Further defects in counterregulatory responses induced by recurrent hypoglycemia in IDDM. *Diabetes* 1992;41:1335–40.

114 Egger M, Smith GD, Teuscher AU *et al.* Influence of human insulin on symptoms and awareness of hypoglycaemia: a randomized, double-blind, crossover trial. *Br Med J* 1991; 303:622–6.

115 Bendtson I, Binder C. Counterregulatory hormonal response to insulin-induced hypoglycaemia in insulin-dependent diabetic patients: a comparison of equimolar amounts of porcine and semisynthetic human insulin. *J Intern Med* 1991;229:293–6.

116 Ferrer JP, Esmatjes E, Gonzalez-Clemente JM *et al.* Symptomatic and hormonal hypoglycaemic response to human and porcine insulin in patients with type-1 diabetes mellitus. *Diabetic Med* 1992;9:522–7.

117 Jick H, Hall GC, Dean AD *et al.* A comparison of the risk of hypoglycaemia between users of human and animal insulins. 1. Experience in the U.K. *Pharmacotherapy* 1990;10:395–7.

118 Patrick AW, Bodmer CW, Tieszen KL *et al.* Human insulin and awareness of acute hypoglycaemic symptoms in insulin-dependent diabetes. *Lancet* 1991;338:528–32.

119 Sjoeborn NC, Lins PE, Adamson U *et al.* A comparative study on the hormonal responses to insulin-induced hypoglycaemia using semisynthetic human insulin and pork insulin in patients with type-1 diabetes mellitus. *Diabetic Med* 1990;7:775–9.

120 Lingenfelser T, Buettner UW, Plonz C *et al.* Hormonal counterregulation, symptom awareness and neurophysiological function in type-1 diabetes during insulin-induced hypoglycaemia. *Diabetic Med* 1992;9:528–35.

121 Reichard P, Berglund A, Levander S *et al.* Hypoglycaemic episodes during intensified insulin treatment: increased frequency but no effect on cognitive function. *J Intern Med* 1991;229:9–16.

122 Wredling RA, Theorell PG, Roll HM *et al.* Psychosocial state of patients with IDDM prone to recurrent episodes of severe hypoglycaemia. *Diabetes Care* 1992;15:518–21.

123 Rosenfalck AM, Bendtson I, Jorgensen S *et al.* Nasal glucagon in the treatment of hypoglycaemia in type-l (insulin-dependent) diabetic patients. *Diabetes Res Clin Pract* 1992; 17:43–50.

124 Slama G, Alamowitch C, Desplanque N *et al.* A new non-invasive method for treating insulin reaction: intranasal lyophylized glucagon. *Diabetologia* 1990;33:671–4.

125 Kovacs M, Brent D, Steinberg TF *et al.* Children's self-reports of psychologic adjustment and coping strategies during first year of insulin-dependent diabetes mellitus. *Diabetes Care* 1986;9:472–9.

126 Court S, Sein E, McCowen C *et al.* Children with diabetes mellitus: perception of their behavioural problems by parents and teachers. *Early Human Dev* 1988;16:245–52.

127 Fonagy P, Moran GS, Lindsay MKM *et al.* Psychological adjustment and diabetic control. *Arch Dis Child* 1987;62: 1009–13.

128 Kovacs M, Kass RE, Schnell TM *et al.* Family functioning and metabolic control of school-aged children with IDDM. *Diabetes Care* 1989;12:409–14.

129 Mayou R, Peveler R, Davies B *et al.* Psychiatric morbidity in young adults with insulin-dependent diabetes mellitus. *Psychol Med* 1991;21:629–45.

130 Baker L, Barcai A, Kaye R *et al.* Beta adrenergic blockade and juvenile diabetes: acute studies and long-term therapeutic trial. *J Pediatr* 1969;75:19–29.

131 Hanson CL, Henggeler SW, Burghen GA. Model of associations between psychosocial variables and health-outcome measures of adolescents with IDDM. *Diabetes Care* 1987; 10:752–8.

132 Hauenstein EJ, Marvin RS, Snyder AL *et al.* Stress in parents of children with diabetes mellitus. *Diabetes Care* 1989; 12:18–23.

133 Lloyd CE, Robinson N, Stevens LK *et al.* The relationship between stress and the development of diabetic complications. *Diabetic Med* 1991;8:146–50.

134 Orr DP, Golden MP, Myers G *et al.* Characteristics of adolescents with poorly controlled diabetes referred to a tertiary care centre. *Diabetes Care* 1983;3:170–5.

135 Moran G, Fonagy P, Kurtz A *et al.* A controlled study of the psychoanalytic treatment of brittle diabetes. *J Am Acad Child Adolesc Psychiatry* 1991;30:926–35.

136 Schafer LC, Glasgow RE, McCavil KD *et al.* Adherence to IDDM regimens: relationship to psychosocial variables and metabolic control. *Diabetes Care* 1983;6:493–8.

137 Pless IB, Heller A, Belmonte M *et al.* Expected diabetic control in childhood and psychosocial functioning in early adult life. *Diabetes Care* 1988;11:387–92.

138 Fairburn CG, Peveler RC, Davies B *et al.* Eating disorders in young adults with insulin-dependent diabetes mellitus: a controlled study. *Br Med J* 1991;303:17–20.

139 Birk R, Spencer ML. The prevalence of anorexia nervosa, bulimia and induced glycosuria in IDDM females. *Diabetes Educ* 1989;15:336–41.

140 Marcus MD, Wing RR, Jaward A *et al.* Eating disorders symptomatology in a registry-based sample of women with insulin-dependent diabetes mellitus. *Int J Eating Disorders* 1992;12:425–30.

141 Bubb JA, Pontious SL. Weight loss from inappropriate insulin manipulation: an eating disorder variant in an adolescent with insulin-dependent diabetes mellitus. *Diabetes Educ* 1991;17:29–32.

142 Stancin T, Link DL, Reuter JM. Binge eating and purging in young women with IDDM. *Diabetes Care* 1989;12:601–3.

143 Holmes CS, Hayford JT, Gonzalez JL *et al.* A survey of

cognitive functioning at different glucose levels in diabetic persons. *Diabetes Care* 1983;6:180–5.
144 Holmes CS, Koepke KM, Thompson RG *et al.* Verbal fluency and naming performance in type 1 diabetes at different blood glucose concentrations. *Diabetes Care* 1984;7:454–9.
145 Pramming S, Thorsteinsson B, Theilgaard A *et al.* Cognitive function during hypoglycaemia in type 1 diabetes mellitus. *Br Med J* 1986;292:647–50.
146 Rovet J, Ehrilich R, Hoppe M. Behavioural problems in children with diabetes as a function of sex and age of onset of disease. *J Child Psychol Psychiatry* 1987;28:477–91.
147 Parker L, Kim C-L, Hess E *et al.* Does moderate hyperglycemia adversely affect mentation? *Diabetes Care* 1989; 12:750–1.
148 Martinelli V, Piatti PM, Filippi M *et al.* Effects of hyperglycaemia or visual evoked potentials in insulin-dependent diabetic patients. *Acta Diabetol* 1992;29:34–7.
149 Fledelius HC. Refractive changes in diabetes mellitus around onset or when poorly controlled. A clinical study. *Acta Ophthalmol* 1987;65:53–7.
150 Lebinger TG, Goldman KN, Saenger P. Bilateral cataracts as the initial sign of insulin-dependent diabetes mellitus in a child. *Am J Dis Child* 1983;137:602–3.
151 Vinding R, Nielsen NV. Two cases of acutely developed cataract in diabetes mellitus. *Acta Ophthalmol* 1984;62: 373–7.
152 White FA, Richert HM. Accelerated bilateral cataract formation in insulin-dependent diabetes mellitus. *Diabetes Care* 1984;7:186–7.
153 Paylor RP, Selhorst JB, Weinberg RS. Reversible monocular cataract simulating amaurosis fugax. *Ann Ophthalmol* 1985;17:423–5.
154 Bilginturan AN, Jackson RL, Ide CH. Transitory cataracts in children with diabetes mellitus. *Pediatrics* 1977;60:106–9.
155 Henderson G. The psychosocial treatment of recurrent diabetic ketoacidosis: an interdisciplinary team approach. *Diabetes Educ* 1991;17:119–23.
156 Nathan DM. Long term complications of diabetes mellitus. *N Engl J Med* 1993;328:1676–85.
157 Sterky G, Wall S. Determinants of microangiopathy in growth-onset diabetes: with special reference to retinopathy and glycaemic control. *Acta Paed Scand* 1986;Suppl. 75: 5–45.
158 Weber B, Burger W, Hartmann R *et al.* Risk factors for the development of retinopathy in children and adolescents with type-1 (insulin-dependent) diabetes mellitus. *Diabetologia* 1986;29:23–9.
159 Kostraba JN, Dorman JS, Orchard TJ *et al.* Contribution of diabetes duration before puberty to development of microvascular complications in IDDM subjects. *Diabetes Care* 1989;12:686–93.
160 Rogers DG, White NH, Shalwitz RA *et al.* The effect of puberty on the development of early diabetic microvascular disease in insulin-dependent diabetes. *Diabetes Res Clin Pract* 1987;3:39–44.
161 Brinchmann-Hansen O, Dahl-Jorgensen K, Sandvik L *et al.* Blood glucose concentration and progression of diabetic retinopathy: the 7-year results of the Oslo study. *Br Med J* 1992;304:19–22.
162 D'Antonio JA, Ellis D, Doft BH *et al.* Diabetes complications and glycemic control. The Pittsburgh prospective insulin-dependent diabetes colour study status report after 5 yr of IDDM. *Diabetes Care* 1989;12:694–700.
163 Hannssen KF, Dahl-Jorgensen K, Lauritzen T *et al.* Diabetic control and microvascular complications. The near-normoglycaemic experience. *Diabetologia* 1986;29:677–84.
164 Kingsley LA, Dorman JS, Doft BH *et al.* An epidemiologic approach to the study of retinopathy: the Pittsburgh diabetic morbidity and retinopathy studies. *Diabetes Res Clin Pract* 1988;4:99–109.
165 Reichard P, Berglund B, Britz A *et al.* Intensified conventional insulin treatment retards the microvascular complications of IDDM: the Stockholm Diabetes Intervention Study (SDIS) after 5 years. *J Intern Med* 1991;230:101–8.
166 Reichard P, Britz A, Carlsson P *et al.* Metabolic control and complications over 3 years in patients with insulin-dependent diabetes (IDDM): the Stockholm Diabetes Intervention Study (SDIS). *J Intern Med* 1990;228:511–17.
167 Santiago JV. Intensive management of insulin dependent diabetes: risks, benefits, and unanswered questions. *J Clin Endocrinol Metab* 1992;75:977–82.
168 Dorchy H, Loeb H. Functional abnormalities precede structural lesions in diabetic children and adolescents. *Transplant Proc* 1986;18:1494–5.
169 Shore AC, Price KJ, Sandemann DD *et al.* Impaired microvascular hyperaemic response in children with diabetes mellitus. *Diabetic Med* 1991;8:619–23.
170 Maser RE, Becker DJ, Drash AL *et al.* Pittsburgh Epidemiology of Diabetes Complications Study. Measuring diabetic neuropathy: follow-up study results. *Diabetes Care* 1992; 12:525–7.
171 Marshall SM. Screening for microalbuminuria: which measurement? *Diabetic Med* 1991;8:706–11.
172 Microalbuminuria Collaborative Study Group. Microalbuminuria in type-1 diabetic patients. Prevalence and clinical characteristics. *Diabetes Care* 1992;15:495–501.
173 Deckert T, Feldt-Rasmussen B, Borch-Johnsen K *et al.* Natural history of diabetic complications: early detection and progression. *Diabetic Med* 1991;8:S33–7.
174 Mogensen C, Vigstrup J, Ehlers N. Microalbuminuria predicts proliferative diabetic retinopathy. *Lancet* 1985;2: 1512–13.
175 Watts GF, Kubal C, Chinn S. Long-term variation of urinary albumin excretion in insulin-dependent diabetes mellitus: some practical recommendations for monitoring microalbuminuria. *Diabetes Res Clin Pract* 1990;9:169–77.
176 Roe TF, Costin G, Kaufman FR *et al.* Blood glucose control and albuminuria in type-1 diabetes mellitus. *Pediatrics* 1991;119:178–82.
177 Bell DS, Ketchum CH, Robinson CA *et al.* Microalbuminuria associated with diabetic neuropathy. *Diabetes Care* 1992; 15:528–31.
178 Vigstrup J, Mogensen CE. Proliferative diabetic retinopathy: at risk patients identified by early detection of microalbuminuria. *Acta Ophthalmol* 1985;63:530–5.
179 Lund-Adersen C, Frost-Larsen K, Starup K. Natural history of diabetic retinopathy in insulin-dependent juvenile diabetics. A longitudinal study. *Acta Ophthalmol* 1987;65: 481–6.
180 Joner G, Brinchmann-Hansen O, Torres CG *et al.* A nationwide cross-sectional study of retinopathy and microalbuminuria in young Norwegian type-1 (insulin-dependent) diabetic patients. *Diabetologia* 1992;35:1049–54.
181 Klein R, Klein BE, Moss SE. A population-based study of diabetic retinopathy in insulin-using patients diagnosed before 30 years of age. *Diabetes Care* 1985;8:71–6.
182 Krolewski AS, Warram JH, Rawd LI *et al.* Risk of proliferative diabetic retinopathy in juvenile-onset of type-1 dia-

betes: a 40 year follow-up study. *Diabetes Care* 1986;9: 443–52.

183 Muhlhauser I, Sawicki P, Berger M. Cigarette smoking as a risk factor for macroproteinuria and proliferative retinopathy in type-1 (insulin-dependent) diabetes. *Diabetologia* 1986; 29:500–2.

184 Brichmann-Hansen O, Dahl-Jorgensen K, Hanssen KF *et al.* Effects of intensified insulin treatment on various lesions of diabetic retinopathy. *Am J Ophthalmol* 1985;100:644–53.

185 Dahl-Jorgensen K, Brinchmann-Hansen O, Hanssen KF *et al.* Rapid tightening of blood glucose control leads to transient deterioration of retinopathy in insulin-dependent diabetes mellitus: the Oslo study. *Br Med J* 1985;290:811–15.

186 Lawrence JR, Bedord GJ, Thomson R. Rapid development during puberty of proliferative retinopathy after strict diabetic control. *Lancet* 1985;2:332.

187 Rosenlund EF, Haakens K, Brinchmann-Hansen O *et al.* Transient proliferative diabetic retinopathy during intensified insulin treatment. *Am J Ophthalmol* 1988;105: 618–25.

188 Agardh C-D, Cavallin-Sjoberg U, Agardh E. Optic disc swelling in an insulin-dependent diabetic. A result of drastic improvement of glucose control. *Acta Ophthalmol* 1988; 66:206–9.

189 Goldstein IB, Naliboff BD, Shapiro D *et al.* Beat-to-beat blood pressure response in asymptomatic IDDM subjects. *Diabetes Care* 1988;11:774–9.

190 Aman J, Eriksson E, Lideen J. Autonomic nerve function in children and adolescents with insulin dependent diabetes mellitus. *Clin Physiol* 1991;11:537–43.

191 Beacom R, Gillespie EL, Middleton D *et al.* Limited joint mobility in insulin-dependent diabetes: relationship to retinopathy, peripheral nerve function and HLA status. *Q J Med* 1985;56:337–44.

192 Garg SK, Chase HP, Marshall G *et al.* Limited joint mobility in subjects with insulin-dependent diabetes mellitus: relationship with eye and kidney complications. *Arch Dis Child* 1992;67:96–9.

193 Costello PB, Tambar PK, Green FA. The prevalence and possible prognostic importance of arthropathy in childhood diabetes. *J Rheumatol* 1984;11:62–5.

194 Haitas B, Jones DB, Ting A *et al.* Diabetic retinopathy and its association with limited joint mobility. *Horm Metab Res* 1986;18:765–7.

195 Ceriello A, Quatraro A, Giugliano D. Diabetes mellitus and hypertension: the possible role of hyperglycaemia through oxidative stress. *Diabetologia* 1993;36:265–6.

196 Moss AJ. Blood pressure in children with diabetes mellitus. *Pediatrics* 1962;30:932–6.

197 Kaasibsen K, Rotne H, Hougaard P. Blood pressure in children with diabetes mellitus. *Acta Paed Scand* 1983;Suppl. 72: 191–6.

198 Tarn AC, Drury PL. Blood pressure in children, adolescents and young adults with type 1 (insulin-dependent) diabetes. *Diabetologia* 1986;29:275–81.

199 Krolewski AS, Canessa M, Warram JH *et al.* Predisposition to hypertension and susceptibility to renal disease in insulin-dependent diabetes mellitus. *N Engl J Med* 1988;318:140–5.

200 Weidmann P, Ferrari P. Central role of sodium in hypertension in diabetic subjects. *Diabetes Care* 1991;14:220–32.

201 Nosadini R, Fioretto P, Trevisan R *et al.* Insulin-dependent diabetes mellitus and hypertension. *Diabetes Care* 199;14: 210–19.

202 Mathiesen ER, Oxenboll B, Johansen K *et al.* Incipient nephropathy in type 1 (insulin-dependent) diabetes. *Diabetologia* 1984;26:406–10.

203 Wiseman M, Viberti G, McKintosh D *et al.* Glycaemia arteriol pressure and microalbuminuria in type 1 (insulin-dependent) diabetes mellitus. *Diabetologia* 1984;26:401–5.

204 Parving HH. Impact of blood pressure and antihypertensive treatment on incipient and overt nephropathy, retinopathy and endothelial permeability in diabetes mellitus. *Diabetes Care* 1991;14:260–9.

205 Simonson DC. Etiology and prevalence of hypertension in diabetic patients. *Diabetes Care* 1988;11:821–7.

206 Moore WV, Donaldson DL, Chonko AM *et al.* Ambulatory blood pressure in type-1 diabetes mellitus. Comparison to presence of incipient nephropathy in adolescents and young adults. *Diabetes* 1992;41:1035–41.

207 Passa P, Leblanc H, Billault B. Treatment of hypertension in diabetic patients. *Postgrad Med J* 1989;65:S42–5.

208 Melbourne Diabetes Nephropathy Study Group. Comparison between perindopril and nifedipine in hypertensive and normotensive diabetic patients with microalbuminuria. *Br Med J* 1991;302:210–16.

209 Ford ES, Newman J. Smoking and diabetes mellitus: findings from 1988 behavioural risk factor survelliance system. *Diabetes Care* 1992;14:871–4.

210 Chase HP, Garg SK, Marshall G *et al.* Cigarette smoking increases the risk of albuminuria among subjects with type-1 diabetes. *J Am Med Assoc* 1991;264:614–17.

211 Karma A, Gummerus S, Kujansuu E *et al.* Predicting diabetic retinopathy. *Acta Ophthalmol* 1987;65:136–9.

212 Gay EC, Cai Y, Gale SM *et al.* Smokers with IDDM experience excess morbidity. The Colorado IDDM Registry. *Diabetes Care* 1992;15:947–52.

213 Telmer S, Christiansen JS, Anderson AR *et al.* Smoking habits and prevalence of clinical diabetic microangiopathy in insulin-dependent diabetics. *Acta Med Scand* 1984;215: 63–8.

214 Walker JM, Cover DH, Beevers DG *et al.* Cigarette smoking, blood pressure and the control of blood glucose in the development of diabetic retinopathy. *Diabetes Res* 1985; 2:183–6.

215 Kaar ML, Akerblom HK, Huttunen NP *et al.* Metabolic control in children and adolescents with insulin-dependent diabetes mellitus. *Acta Paed Scand* 1984;Suppl. 73:102–8.

216 Davidson MB, Harris MD, Ziel FH *et al.* Suppression of sleep-induced growth hormone secretion by anticholinergic agent abolishes dawn phenomenon. *Diabetes* 1988;37: 166–71.

217 Allen C, Zaccaro DJ, Palta M *et al.* Glycemic control in early IDDM. The Winsconsin Diabetes Registry. *Diabetes Care* 1992;15:980–7.

218 Littlefield CH, Craven JL, Rodin GM *et al.* Relationship of self-efficacy and binging to adherence to diabetes regimen among adolescents. *Diabetes Care* 1992;15:90–4.

219 Bloomfield S, Calder JE, Chisholm V. A project in diabetes education for children. *Diabetic Med* 1990;7:137–42.

220 Anderson BJ, Wolf FM, Burkhart MT. Effects of peer group intervention on metabolic control of adolescents with IDDM. *Diabetes Care* 1989;12:179–83.

221 Lloyd CR, Robinson N, Fuller JH. Education and employment experiences in young adults with type-1 diabetes mellitus. *Diabetic Med* 1992;9:661–6.

222 Robinson N, Bush L, Protopapa LE *et al.* Employers' attitude to diabetes. *Diabetic Med* 1989;6:692–7.

223 Songer TJ, LaPorter RE, Dorman JS *et al.* Employment

spectrum of IDDM. *Diabetes Care* 1989;12:615–22.

224 Akerblom HK, Ballard DJ, Bauman B *et al.* Geographic patterns of childhood insulin-dependent diabetes mellitus. *Diabetes* 1988;37:1113–19.

225 Thomson G, Robinson WP, Kuhner MK *et al.* Genetic heterogeneity, modes of inheritance and risk estimates for a joint study of caucasians with insulin-dependent diabetes mellitus. *Am J Hum Genet* 1988;43:799–816.

226 Warram JH, Martin BC, Krolewski AS. Risk of IDDM in children of diabetic mothers decreases with increasing maternal age at pregnancy. *Diabetes* 1991;40:1679–84.

227 Serjeantson SW, Kohonen-Corish MRJ, Rowley MJ *et al.* Antibodies to glutamic acid decarboxylase are associated with HLADR genotypes in both Australians and Asians with type-1 (insulin-dependent) diabetes mellitus. *Diabetologia* 1992;35:996–1001.

228 Pfeifer T. Diabetes in cystic fibrosis. *Clin Pediatr* 1992;31: 682–7.

229 Stutchfield PR, O'Halloran SM, Smith CS *et al.* HLA type, islet cell antibodies, and glucose intolerance in cystic fibrosis. *Arch Dis Child* 1988;63:1234–9.

230 Lanng S, Thorsteinsson B, Erichsen G *et al.* Glucose tolerance in cystic fibrosis. *Arch Dis Child* 1991;66:612–16.

231 Sullivan MM, Denning CR. Diabetic microangiopathy in patients with cystic fibrosis. *Pediatrics* 1989;84:642–7.

232 Roques M, Damge C, Michel C *et al.* Encapsulation of insulin for oral administration preserves interaction of the hormone with its receptor *in vitro*. *Diabetes* 1992;41:451–6.

233 Skolnick A. Advances in islet cell transplantation: is science closer to a diabetes cure? *J Am Med Assoc* 1990;264:427–81.

234 Lacy PE, Hegre OD, Gerasimidi-Vazeou A *et al.* Maintenance of normoglycemia in diabetic mice by subcutaneous xenografts of encapsulated islets. *Science* 1991;254:1782–4.

235 Lanza RP, Butler DH, Borland KM *et al.* Xenotransplantation of canine, bovine, and porcine islets in diabetic rats without immunosuppression. *Proc Natl Acad Sci USA* 1991;88: 11100–4.

35: Hypoglycaemia

P.J. LEE and J.V. LEONARD

INTRODUCTION

The physician who supervises the medical care of infants should be on the lookout constantly for evidence of hypoglycaemia [1]. It is common among infants and children [2] and often missed. It has important implications for the future development of the individual [3–5], and may have genetic implications for the family.

Although recognized for over 70 years [6], there remains much confusion about the definition [7], appropriate investigation and management. Hypoglycaemia is not a diagnosis *per se*, but a pathophysiological state for which the cause needs to be found. It is important clinically, because glucose is an essential cerebral fuel [8], and academically, because disorders of glucose homeostasis illustrate well the interface between metabolism and endocrinology.

CARBOHYDRATE METABOLISM

Glucose metabolism

Plasma glucose concentration is normally maintained within a narrow range, reflecting a balance between the production of glucose and its rate of utilization (Fig. 35.1). During feeding, glucose is formed principally from carbohydrate in the diet; during fasting, glucose is released by the liver by glycogenolysis and gluconeogenesis. The rate of removal depends upon tissue uptake and the use of alternative metabolic fuels. These processes are controlled by endocrine and neural factors, as well as substrate availability, and cannot be considered in isolation from fat and protein metabolism. The liver plays a central role in the control of these mechanisms [9].

Adults and children share many common factors in the regulation of glucose metabolism, but there are important differences, particularly in the neonate [10,11]. Ultimately, hypoglycaemia is the result of a reduction in glucose production or excessive utilization, or a combination of both.

The main pathways in glycogen synthesis and breakdown and gluconeogenesis [12–14] are illustrated in Fig. 35.2. Glycogen is synthesized and broken down by separate pathways. Glucose-1-phosphate is converted to uridine diphosphoglucose (UDPG), which then transfers the glucose residues to the outer chain of the glycogen molecule in α-1,4-glycosyl linkages under the control of glycogen synthase. This is the rate-limiting step of glycogen synthesis; since UDPG inhibits its own production [15], its removal is important in 'pulling' glucose-6-phosphate into glycogen synthesis. The branching enzyme, oligo-1,4-1,6-transglucosidase, produces 1,6 linkages that are responsible for the characteristic tree-like structure of glycogen.

Glycogen is broken down by phosphorylase, which hydrolyses the α-1,4 linkages in glycogen releasing glucose-1-phosphate until four residues remain on the external chain. The resulting polysaccharide, the so-called phosphorylase limit dextrin, requires the debranching enzyme to degrade it further. This enzyme has two catalytic functions [16]: oligo-1,4-1,4-transferase transfers three glucose residues to a neighbouring chain and amylo-1,6-glucosidase then hydrolyses the remaining residue to free glucose. This accounts for 8–10% of hepatic glucose production from glycogen. The rate-limiting step in glycogen breakdown is phosphorylase, its activity being controlled by a cascade of kinases and phosphatases regulated in turn by calcium, cyclic adenosine monophosphate (cAMP) and other factors.

Under normal conditions, the actions of glycogen synthase and phosphorylase are closely integrated, glucose inhibiting the latter (and hence glycogenolysis) and active phosphorylase inhibiting the activity of glycogen synthase (and hence glycogen synthesis) [17].

Glycogen is found in many tissues throughout the body, particularly in muscle and liver. Although the total amount of glycogen stored in muscle is greater than that in the liver, it can only be used as a reserve substrate by the muscle itself, because of the absence of glucose-6-phosphatase [18], preventing glucose formation and release from the cell. By contrast, hepatic glycogen can be broken down to free glucose and released into the circulation, but

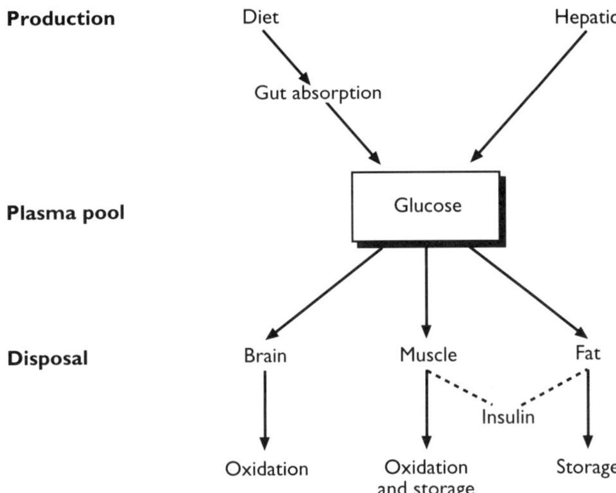

Fig. 35.1 Factors involved in glucose homeostasis.

these stores are readily depleted by fasting after 24–36 h in adults and after shorter periods in children [19].

Acid maltase also hydrolyses glycogen that has been engulfed by lysosomes directly to glucose, but this accounts for little of the circulating glucose.

Glycolysis and gluconeogenesis

Glucose is metabolized via glycolysis to pyruvate which can be converted to lactate or, after decarboxylation, to acetyl-CoA (acetyl co-enzyme A), which is then oxidized in the tricarboxylic acid (TCA) cycle. Acetyl-CoA is the substrate for the synthesis of fatty acids which are then stored as triglycerides (lipogenesis).

Gluconeogenesis is the process in which glycerol, amino acids and lactate are converted to glucose. Glycerol is produced from lipolysis in adipocytes, amino acids (in particular alanine and glutamine [20]) from protein catabolism and lactate from glycolysis as described above.

Glycolysis and gluconeogenesis share a number of enzymes which catalyse reversible reactions. There are, however, three ways in which the enzymes differ, and these allow for regulation of substrate fluxes in the pathways [21]: these are (i) phosphofructokinase and fructose-1,6-biphosphatase, (ii) pyruvate kinase and phosphoenolpyruvate carboxykinase and (iii) glucose-6-phosphatase and glucokinase. These enzymes catalyse irreversible reactions consuming adenosine triphosphate (ATP), and are controlled by many regulating factors [22].

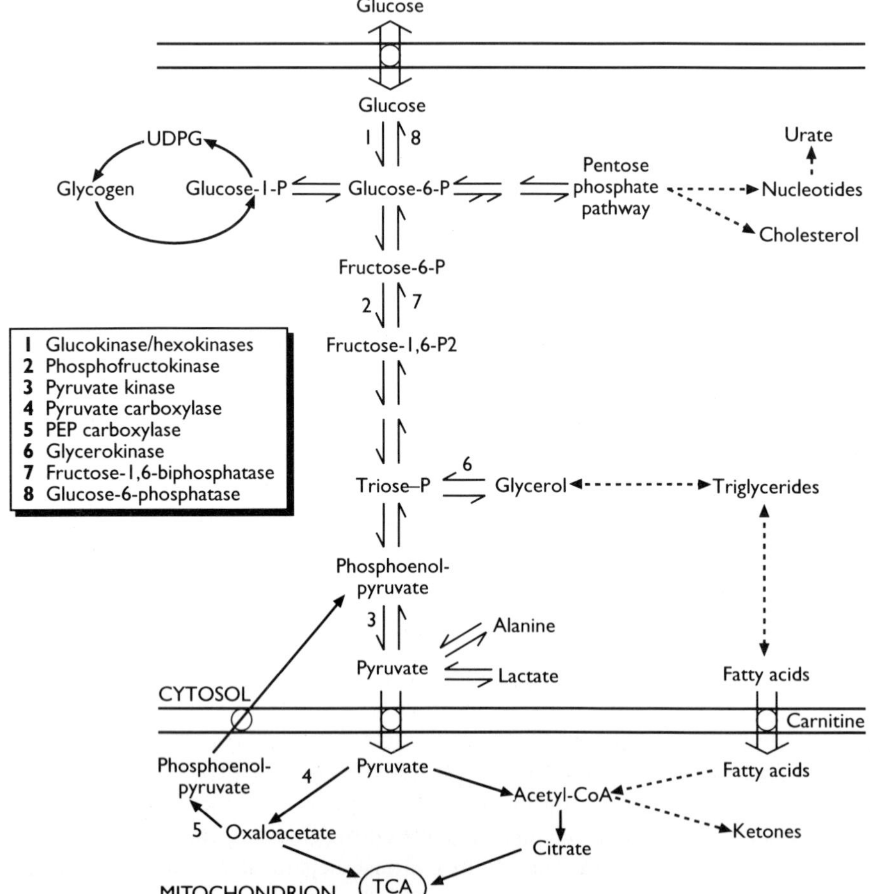

Fig. 35.2 Summary of intermediary metabolism.

Phosphofructokinase catalyses the phosphorylation of fructose-6-phosphate to form fructose-1,6-biphosphate, the rate of the reaction depending upon the availabilit of the substrate. Fructose-1,6-biphosphatase catalyses the reverse reaction which is inhibited by fructose-2,6-biphosphate, a compound that stimulates the activity of phosphofructokinase.

The second control point is the interconversion of pyruvate and phosphoenolpyruvate. Pyruvate kinase controls the production of pyruvate, while pyruvate carboxylase and then phosphoenolpyruvate carboxykinase catalyse reactions producing phosphoenolpyruvate.

The last control point concerns the final common pathway for glucose production from glycogenolysis and gluconeogenesis, hydrolysis of glucose-6-phosphate. The enzyme catalysing this reaction, glucose-6-phosphatase, is bound to the inner aspect of the endoplasmic reticulum. Since neither the substrate, glucose-6-phosphate, nor the products can cross the membrane, three transport mechanisms are necessary for hydrolysis to glucose [23]. The activity of this complex is controlled by substrate concentration. The phosphorylation of glucose to glucose-6-phosphate is controlled by hexokinases, specifically glucokinase in hepatocytes, the activity of which is substrate-dependent. This reaction is inhibited by fructose-6-phosphate, which means in effect that it is inhibited by its product, since fructose-6-phosphate is in equilibrium with glucose-6-phosphate.

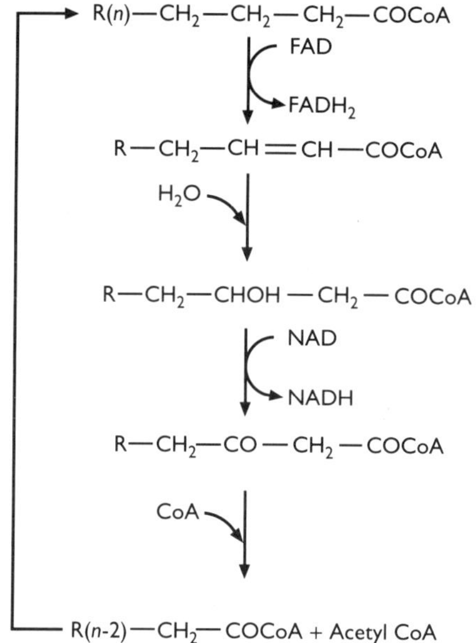

Fig. 35.3 The mitochondrial fatty acid oxidation spiral.

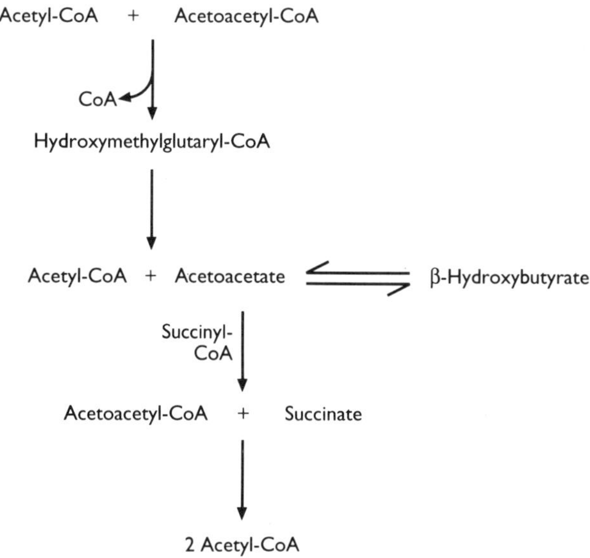

Fig. 35.4 Metabolic pathways of ketone bodies.

Ketone bodies and fatty acids

The breakdown of triglycerides results in the formation of glycerol and free fatty acids. The former, as mentioned above, is utilized in gluconeogenesis, whilst the latter undergo β-oxidation to produce acetyl-CoA and ketone bodies, acetoacetate and β-hydroxybutyrate. Fatty acids from adipose tissue are activated in cytosol to form fatty acyl-CoA, which enters the mitochondria by a carnitine-dependent process [24]. Fatty acyl-CoA enters the β-oxidation spiral, being shortened by two carbon atoms with each turn (Fig. 35.3). The sequence of reactions is catalysed by an acyl dehydrogenase, enoyl-CoA hydratase, 3-hydroxyacyl-CoA dehydrogenase and 3-oxothiolase. It is now clear there is more than one enzyme at each step with differing chain length specificity [25,26].

Ketone bodies are synthesized by another cycle (Fig. 35.4). Acetyl-CoA and acetoacetyl-CoA condense to form hydroxymethylglutaryl-CoA (HMG-CoA), which is split by HMG-CoA lyase to release acetoacetate. A separate pathway, not present in the liver, is necessary to activate ketones, which are an important alternative fuel, particularly for the brain [27].

Pentose phosphate pathway

The role of glucose-6-phosphate in carbohydrate metabolism is pivotal. As well as being the substrate for glycogen synthesis, glycolysis and the product of glycogenolysis and gluconeogenesis, there is a further route for its disposal. In addition to these pathways, glucose-6-phosphate is metabolized via the pentose phosphate pathway (or hexose monophosphate shunt), which generates reducing power in the form of NADPH (reduced form of nicotinamide adenine dinucleotide phosphate). This is necessary for fatty acid and steroid synthesis. It also produces pentose sugars for nucleic acid synthesis. Cholesterol and triglyceride synthesis and urate formation are stimulated by an increased flux in the pentose phosphate pathway. The pathway can also be reversed so that pentoses are converted to hexoses.

ENDOCRINE CONTROL MECHANISMS

The role of humoral factors important in glucose homeostasis revolves around interplay between the actions of insulin and those of the counterregulatory hormones. Their secretion is largely determined by the physiological state, whether postprandial (fed) or postabsorptive (fasting).

Insulin

Insulin is secreted in response to postprandial increases in plasma glucose and amino-acid concentrations. Gastric inhibitory polypeptide also stimulates insulin secretion directly. Insulin, a polypeptide that is secreted as proinsulin with a connecting peptide (C peptide) being removed post-translationally [28], is the main regulator of carbohydrate, fat and protein metabolism [12].

Portal venous, rather than systemic venous, insulin levels are the major regulators of hepatic glucose metabolism. Insulin suppresses hepatic glucose production by increasing the activity of glycogen synthase and inhibiting hepatic phosphorylase [29]. Glycolysis is also promoted and gluconeogenesis suppressed [30]. Insulin stimulates glucose uptake by adipose tissue and muscle by recruiting specific transmembrane glucose transporters [31]. The number and activity of these transporters are important determinants of the insulin response [32]. The suppression of hepatic glucose release seems to be more sensitive to insulin than is the enhancement of glucose uptake [33]. In adipocytes, triglyceride synthesis is stimulated [34]; in muscle, glycogen formation and glycolysis are favoured. The combined effects of reduced hepatic glucose production and enhanced peripheral glucose utilization result in a fall in the plasma glucose concentration.

In the liver, insulin also stimulates fatty acid synthesis and, by inhibiting lipoprotein lipase, promotes the transfer of fatty acids into adipocytes for triglyceride synthesis. Lipolysis is reduced by inhibition of hepatic lipase and ketogenesis is thus also suppressed indirectly. In muscle, insulin has an anabolic effect stimulating protein synthesis by enhancing amino-acid uptake and simultaneously inhibiting proteolysis. Insulin may have direct effects on the central nervous system by modifying the hypothalamic influence on sympathetic nervous activity [35].

The actions of insulin are mediated via specific membrane receptors on the target cells, with tyrosine kinase being important in the intracellular signalling process [36]. Although insulin has a high affinity to these receptors, other substances may bind to them, producing the same metabolic effects. Insulin-like growth factors (IGF) I and II have substantial structural homology to insulin and many of its biochemical effects [37]. On the other hand, resistance to the actions of insulin may occur due to abnormalities in the function or number of insulin receptors, either inherited or acquired. In acquired insulin resistance the role of counterregulatory hormones, as well as intermediary metabolites, may also be important [38].

Counterregulatory hormones

The so-called counterregulatory hormones generally oppose the effects of insulin. They include glucagon, adrenaline, noradrenaline, cortisol and growth hormone, of which glucagon is the most potent. Glucagon stimulates glycogenolysis by increasing the activity of phosphorylase, and enhances gluconeogenesis by increasing the activity of phosphoenolpyruvate carboxykinase, both effects being mediated by cAMP as the second messenger. Glucagon can promote lipolysis [14] and ketogenesis [39] only when insulin is deficient. Its effects on gluconeogenesis and ketogenesis are more sustained than the effects on glycogenolysis [40].

Adrenaline stimulates hepatic glucose production (via glycogenolysis and gluconeogenesis) and reduces glucose utilization, while at the same time stimulating lipolysis and ketogenesis [41]. These effects are mediated via direct (β_2-adrenergic receptors) effects on the liver, muscles and adipocytes as well as indirectly (α_2-adrenergic receptors) by inhibiting insulin secretion [42]. Noradrenaline has similar effects on glucose metabolism, but is 5–10 times less potent than adrenaline [43]. These two catecholamines have more sustained effects on blood glucose concentrations than glucagon.

While the effects of glucagon and the catecholamines are observed rapidly, growth hormone and cortisol work over a much longer time-scale. Their main action is to conserve glucose by limiting peripheral utilization, although they do stimulate glucose production to a lesser degree. Cortisol decreases the actions of insulin on hepatic glucose production and peripheral glucose uptake, increases the availability of gluconeogenic substrates, while enhancing the activity of gluconeogenic enzymes, and stimulates glucagon secretion [44]. Prolonged growth hormone secretion has effects similar to cortisol. However, growth hormone may have insulin-like action in the short term, particularly in stimulating glycogen synthesis. These actions are seen too rapidly for IGF-I to be responsible [45].

Somatostatin also has profound effects on glucose

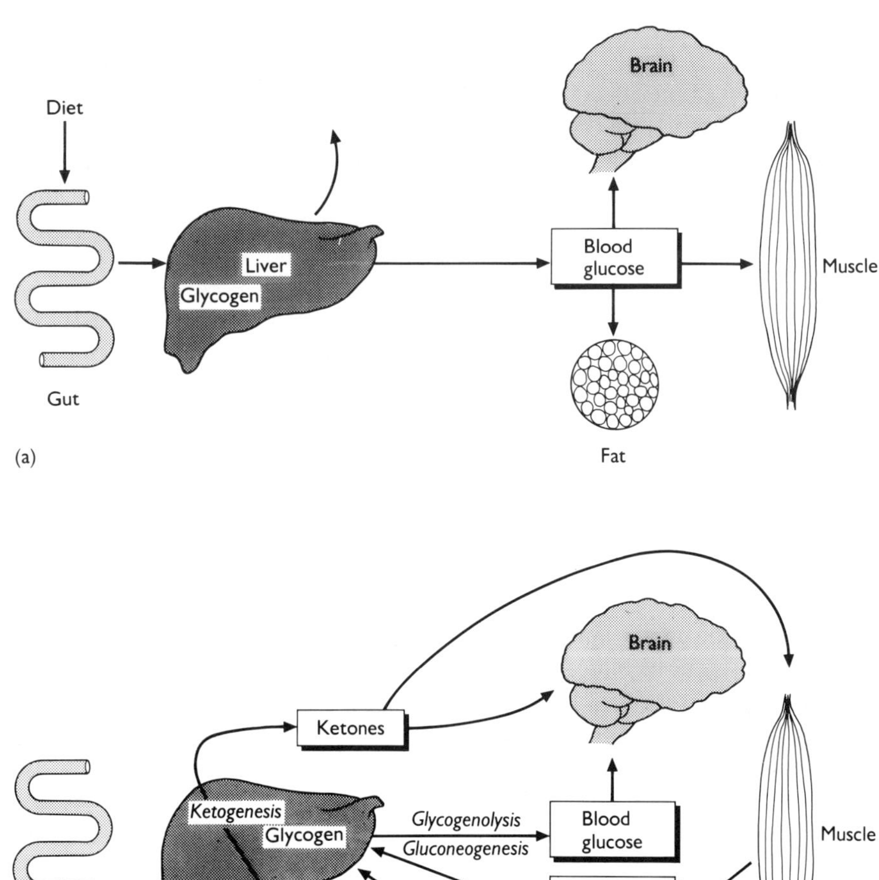

Fig. 35.5 Glucose metabolism (a) in the fed state; (b) in the fasting state.

metabolism. Growth hormone, glucagon and insulin secretion are all suppressed and the gastrointestinal absorption of nutrients is inhibited by a delay in gastric emptying, reduced small intestinal motility and reduced splanchnic blood flow.

Thyroxine and triiodothyronine enhance gluconeogenesis, glycogenolysis, lipolysis and ketogenesis over a time-scale similar to cortisol and growth hormone [46]. In pathological states of high or low levels there may be disordered counterregulation [47].

All the counterregulatory hormones have actions antagonistic to insulin, and may be important in the post-hypoglycaemic hyperglycaemia that can be seen in a number of conditions [48].

FED AND FASTING STATES

During feeding and fasting there is a complex sequence of changes to maintain plasma glucose concentration within a narrow range, despite large changes in production and utilization. In the fed state, the liver receives high levels of glucose and gluconeogenic substrates from the portal venous system. The consequence is high levels of insulin and low levels of glucagon and other counterregulatory hormones [49], with the actions of insulin being essentially unopposed (Fig. 35.5a).

Glucose stimulates its own hepatic uptake [50], so increasing the formation of glucose-6-phosphate. Both glycogen synthesis and glycolysis are enhanced and the consequent increased supply of pyruvate stimulates fatty acid formation. Both glycogenolysis and gluconeogenesis are inhibited [51].

Independent of the effect of glucose, insulin stimulates glycogen synthesis, glycolysis and fatty acid synthesis by enhancing the synthesis of the rate-limiting enzymes involved. It also inhibits glycogenolysis and gluconeogenesis. However, its main effect is to stimulate glucose uptake by muscle and adipose tissue. In this way lipogenesis and protein synthesis are favoured.

As the period of fasting extends (Fig. 35.5b), plasma glucose concentration falls so insulin secretion falls and secretion of counterregulatory hormones, particularly glucagon, stimulates glycogen breakdown via adenylate cyclase and cAMP, with simultaneous inhibition of glycogen synthesis and glycolysis, whereas the flux via gluconeogenesis is increased. Glucagon activates lipolysis within adipocytes, elevating fatty acid levels for β-oxidation and glycerol for gluconeogenesis. Acetyl-CoA derived from β-oxidation forms the substrate for ketone bodies. Thus the proportion of hepatic glucose production from gluconeogenesis increases as the stores of glycogen fall [52] and the rates of carbohydrate and fat oxidation have reciprocal relationships [53].

During prolonged fasting the roles of cortisol and growth hormone become more important. Once glycogen stores have been depleted, blood glucose concentrations are maintained by a reduction in the rate of glucose utilization, by the preferential oxidation of fatty acids and ketone bodies and by hepatic recycling of glycerol and lactate to form glucose via gluconeogenesis. Peripheral glucose uptake is reduced by down-regulation of insulin receptors [54]. Although there is a decrease in glucose utilization during prolonged fasting, the increased demands of children mean that normal glucose levels can be maintained only for short periods (24–48 h), whereas adults can fast for weeks [13,19]. In fasting children, free fatty acid and ketone body concentrations are high compared to adults [55], indicating an acceleration of the normal adaptive mechanisms [56] and providing a greater glucose-sparing effect. The requirements of infants, as determined by fasting hepatic glucose production rates [57], are 5–8 mg glucose/kg min^{-1}, which fall progressively during childhood to adult values of 1–2 mg glucose/kg min^{-1}. The requirements may be increased both because of a higher metabolic rate and because the brain is relatively large.

FETAL AND NEONATAL PERIOD

Glucose homeostasis has been thought to be similar in children and adults [13], but recent work casts some doubt on this [10,11,58–60]. There are a number of ways in which the neonate and infant appear to be unique, but it is not yet known whether the differences represent delayed maturation of normal mechanisms or whether they are true differences.

Fetal glucose homeostasis is maintained by the placenta; therefore endogenous production is not required [61]. Activity of the flux-controlling enzymes of gluconeogenic pathways is low or absent in the fetus, reaching adult levels only hours, or a few days, after birth. In the last month of gestation there is a build-up of hepatic glycogen stores to levels higher than observed in normal adults (8–10%) [62]. The third trimester also sees a marked accumulation of adipose tissue.

At birth the placental glucose supply ceases abruptly. Plasma glucose concentrations fall over the first 2–4 h [63], as the normal homeostatic mechanisms are not yet fully functional and most babies have not started to feed. However, concentrations of fatty acid and ketone body levels rise rapidly. By 4–6 h, glucose levels stabilize as glycogen is utilized [13], but these stores soon become depleted to a point at which gluconeogenesis is required. Glucagon stimulates hepatic glucose production via gluconeogenesis, as well as ketogenesis in term neonates, within 24 h of birth [58]. On the other hand, preterm or small-for-dates infants have poorer ketogenic resposes and enhanced glycolysis [60] compared to their larger, more mature peers. The regulation and actions of insulin appear to be different. Insulin secretion may not be suppressed despite low plasma glucose concentrations [10,64] and it does not appear to inhibit free fatty acid and lactate production normally [60].

DEFINITION OF HYPOGLYCAEMIA

Over the years there has been much confusion and difficulty in establishing the diagnosis of hypoglycaemia, particularly in infancy [65]. This has been for a number of reasons, some of which still require clarification and have not yet gained universal acceptance.

The measurement of glucose and the interpretation of the result has lacked reproducibility. Plasma glucose should be measured using specific reagents, glucose oxidase or glucose-6-phosphate dehydrogenase, in a laboratory with an appropriate quality control. Values differ when whole blood is analysed, and many workers still rely on glucose oxidase strips and reflectance meters in spite of considerable unreliability, especially at low levels [66]. Knowledge of the type of sample collected is necessary for interpretation: arterial blood will have higher values than venous blood and capillary samples need to be free-flowing since stasis results in significantly lower measurements [67,68].

Even when the measurements of glucose concentration are reliable, there have been considerable discrepancies regarding values used to define hypoglycaemia. There are particular problems in neonates in whom it has been customary to take lower cut-off values, especially in the preterm infant, in the mistaken belief that they are more tolerant [69]. This is surprising since the fetus is exposed to maternal glucose levels *in utero*, and there is no reason to expect the developing brain to be less vulnerable. Hypoglycaemia disrupts cerebral autoregulation [70] with neural damage occurring in those areas concerned with learning and motor/sensory discrimination [71]. These same areas are rich in a group of excitatory amino-acid receptors (*N*-methyl-D-aspartate, NMDA), prolonged activation of which may be important in cerebral injury during hypoglycaemia [72]. These receptors are also important in the control of cerebral blood flow [73], the disruption of which may compound neural injury.

The plasma glucose concentration at which symptoms develop varies between individuals [74,75] depending upon the developmental stage and on the levels of alternative fuels, ketone bodies, free fatty acids and lactate. The presence of symptoms, however, may not be necessary to diagnose hypoglycaemia, as Koh *et al.* [69] have shown consistent changes in brainstem-evoked responses in all infants and children studied below glucose values of 2.6 mmol/l, a value that we accept at present. In the future, any refinement of this should combine accurate measurement of plasma glucose concentration, an assessment of neurophysiological function, a measure of counterregulation and assessment of the long-term neurodevelopmental outcome.

Symptoms and signs of hypoglycaemia (Table 35.1) are multitudinous and not specific for hypoglycaemia [76,77], but reflect sympathetic adrenergic stimulation and neurological disturbance [78]. The importance of diagnosing and treating hypoglycaemia is to prevent long-term neurodevelopmental complications [3], but depending on the diagnosis, it also has therapeutic and genetic implications.

APPROACH TO DIAGNOSIS

The presentation of hypoglycaemia may be acute and necessitate immediate therapy, but this should not prevent the collection of appropriate samples for analysis later [79] (Table 35.3). A detailed history must still be obtained after the emergency has been dealt with to aid diagnosis.

In hypoglycaemia it is helpful to divide aetiology according to the age of the patient, that is whether occurring neonatally (under 28 days of age) or later in infancy and childhood. Although there is considerable overlap the disease processes are somewhat different, and carry different prognoses.

Table 35.1 Symptoms and signs of hypoglycaemia

Neonate	Infant/child
Autonomic	
Pallor, sweating, tachypnoea	Pallor, sweating, weakness, nausea/vomiting, abdominal pain, hunger
Neuroglycopaenic	
Jittery, apnoea, hypotonia, feeding problems, irritability, abnormal cry, convulsions, coma	Confusion, irritability, headache, visual disturbance, unusual behaviour, coma, convulsions

Table 35.2 Immediate management of hypoglycaemia

1 Obtain intravenous access
2 Draw blood for investigation (see Table 35.3)
3 Collect next urine sample (see Table 35.3)
4 Measure blood glucose with glucose oxidase strip
5 Give bolus of 10% dextrose 0.2 g/kg (2 ml/kg) over 2–3 min
6 Establish infusion of 10% dextrose providing 5–8 mg/ kg min^{-1}
7 Repeat blood glucose estimation after 3–4 min:
 if glucose < 4 mmol/l, repeat dextrose bolus
 if glucose > 4 mmol/l, but no clinical improvement, *wait*
8 Give intravenous bolus of hydrocortisone 5 mg/kg after 4–5 min if no clinical improvement

Cardiac arrest
Following cardiac arrest, up to 1 g/kg dextrose (as 50%) i.v. bolus may be required [81], but it is essential that blood glucose is measured before a further bolus is administered

From Shah *et al.* [80].

NEONATAL HYPOGLYCAEMIA

Birth is a critical time for humans in controlling metabolic homeostasis, and it is not surprising that successful adaptation does not always occur. The prevalence of hypoglycaemia is greatest during the first few days of life than at any other time, but is mostly transient. A newborn infant displays different symptoms and may well be asymptomatic with low plasma glucose concentrations. The attending physician must therefore be expectant and anticipate hypoglycaemia in infants at risk. Knowledge of the pregnancy and birth history is essential.

Transient neonatal hypoglycaemia is generally caused by diminished energy stores, hyperinsulinaemia and/or excessive peripheral demands. Premature, small-for-gestational-age and asphyxiated infants have reduced glycogen stores, possibly immature enzyme systems controlling gluconeogenesis and inappropriately high insulin concentrations [60]. Hyperinsulinaemia is also seen in macrosomic infants of diabetic mothers, in Rhesus haemolytic disease and Beckwith–Wiedemann syndrome. Failure of the liver to meet excessive demands is seen in congenital heart disease, sepsis and hypothermia. All these infants at risk must be identified and monitored

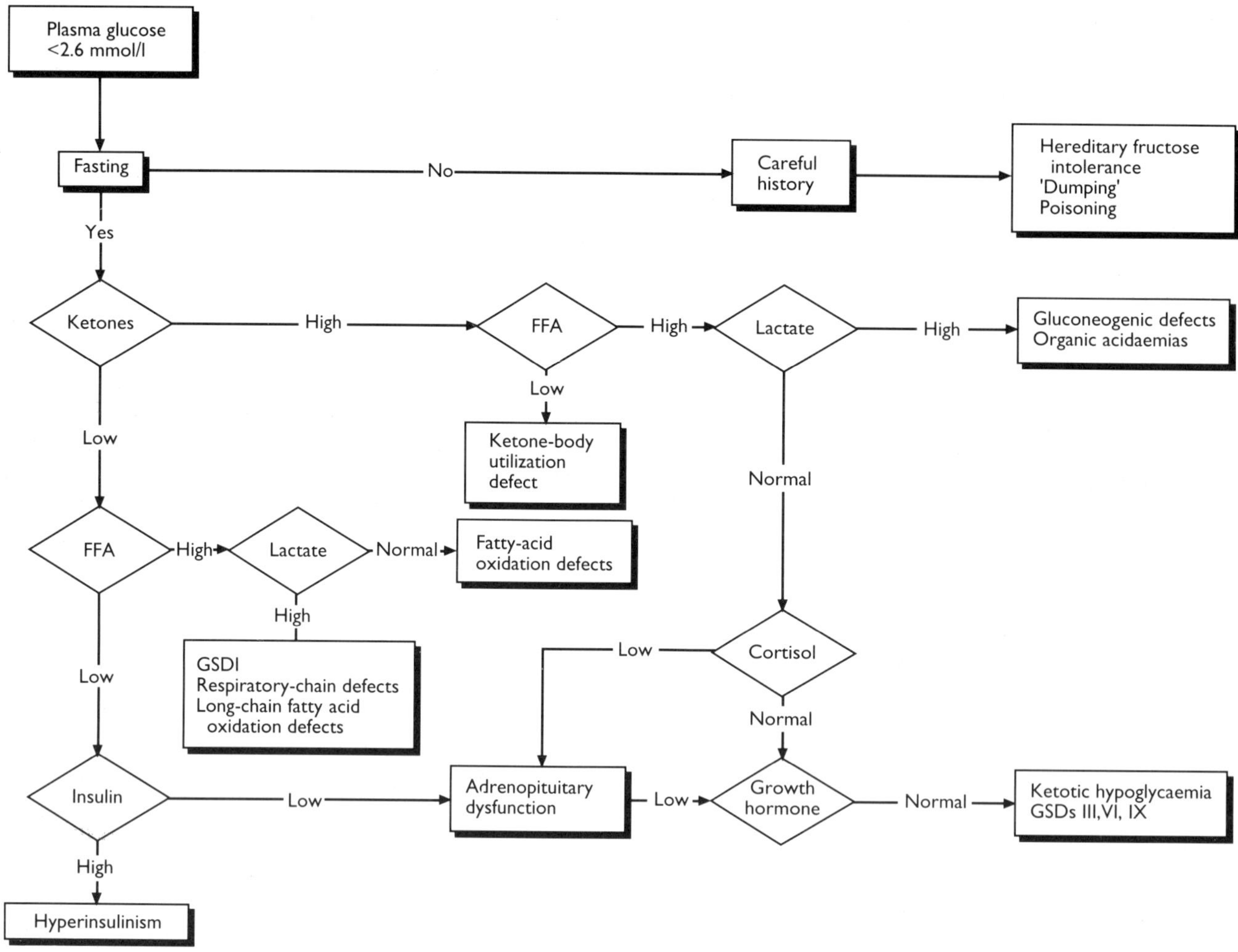

Fig. 35.6 A guide for the diagnosis of recurrent hypoglycaemia. All results must be interpreted in the context of the clinical situation and how the sample has been obtained. Suggested normal ranges during hypoglycaemia: β-hydroxybutyrate (ketones), > 1.0 mmol/l; insulin, < 5 mU/l (36 pmol/l); free fatty acids (FFA), > 1.0 mmol/l; cortisol, > 200 nmol/l; lactate, 0.9–1.8 mmol/l; growth hormone > 15 mU/l (7.5 ng/ml).

carefully over the first few hours and days with serial capillary blood glucose estimations.

More permanent causes of hypoglycaemia in newborn infants are due to inborn errors of metabolism due to enzyme defects [82] or to abnormalities of the endocrine regulation of glucose.

HYPOGLYCAEMIA IN INFANCY AND CHILDHOOD

Family history of infant deaths or metabolic disorder may suggest a genetic abnormality. Pregnancy and neonatal history, with particular reference to birth weight and feeding practices, may be revealing. Most causes of hypoglycaemia in infants and children occur during fasting, which can be as short as 2 h, as in glucose-6-phosphatase deficiency, or only after prolonged fasting (more than 24 h) and metabolic stress [83]. In some disorders, for example fructosaemia, hypoglycaemia only follows ingestion of certain foods. Therefore the age of onset, the timing of symptoms in relation to meals and their response to intake are important points to note. Other triggers, for example catabolic states, may be present. The history may indicate the possibility of accidental or non-accidental ingestion or administration of hypoglycaemic agents – for example insulin, sulphonylureas or ethanol.

A thorough physical examination may reveal midline defects or optic nerve abnormalities which are associated with hypothalamopituitary anomalies. Hepatomegaly is found in many metabolic disorders such as inborn errors of gluconeogenesis, fatty acid oxidation and glycogen metabolism. Growth failure is seen in glycogen storage disease and hypopituitarism. In older children, vitiligo is associated with autoimmune endocrinopathies and

Table 35.3 Investigation of hypoglycaemia*

Blood		Urine
Metabolites	Hormones	Metabolites
Glucose	Insulin	Ketones
β-OH butyrate	C peptide	Reducing sugars
Free fatty acids	Cortisol	Organic acids
Lactate	ACTH	Poisons
Amino acids	Growth hormone	
-------	-------	-------
Lipids	Thyroxine	
Urate	TSH	
Pyruvate	Glucagon	
Acetoacetate		
Free and acyl carnitine		

* Those investigations below the dashed line are helpful but not essential. Samples of serum, plasma and urine taken at the time of hypoglycaemia should be frozen at −20°C or below.
ACTH, adrenocorticotrophic hormone; OH, hydroxyl; TSH, thyroid-stimulating hormone.

hyperpigmentation may be present due to excess ACTH secretion in Addison disease.

The history and examination may suggest the cause of hypoglycaemia or point in a particular direction, but further investigations are necessary and should be performed during an acute presentation or, if that is not possible, under controlled conditions. The purpose is to delineate the relationships of intermediary metabolites and glucoregulatory hormones which may provide essential clues (Table 35.3, see Fig. 35.6). The value of blood and urine samples collected at the time of hypoglycaemia cannot be overemphasized. If these have not been obtained during spontaneous hypoglycaemia, a useful investigation is a controlled fast. The duration of fasting is determined before the test and should be tailored according to the history. It must be performed under adequate supervision with a secure intravenous cannula *in situ*. Blood and urine samples should be taken at regular intervals. If hypoglycaemia develops, blood and urine samples should be collected and the child should be treated.

If local laboratories are able to perform only some of the investigations, samples should be stored frozen for analyses by more specialized centres. This may be particularly useful if the infant dies, so that the diagnosis can be made to aid future genetic counselling. Ante-mortem or immediate post-mortem samples of liver and skin can provide invaluable information [84].

Samples collected opportunistically during spontaneous hypoglycaemia, or in a controlled fashion during a supervised fast [56,85], will usually provide diagnostic pointers. A number of workers use stimulation or tolerance tests with glucagon, galactose, alanine, fructose, glycerol or glucose itself, to examine further the control of intermediary metabolism [86], but it is our experience that these are rarely needed, and the results so obtained are liable to be confusing or conflicting. However, they may be of use to answer specific questions [87].

We have constructed an algorithm (see Fig. 35.6), using the results of the tests obtained during hypoglycaemia, enabling the broad group of the disorder to be determined to help decide about further investigations. This will save time and money, and perhaps more pertinently to paediatric practice, avoid unnecessary investigations for the child. Ultimately the diagnosis is made by examining the relevant enzyme activity in the appropriate tissue, or imaging the appropriate endocrine organ.

Endocrinopathies that can have hypoglycaemia as one of their manifestations can be due to excess secretion of glucose-lowering hormones (or stimulatory autoantibodies) [88] or to deficient activity of counterregulatory hormones. More details about the inborn errors of metabolism, which may result in profound secondary humoral responses, are found in other comprehensive texts [89].

HYPERINSULINISM

The diagnosis of hyperinsulinism is made when hypoglycaemia coexists with abnormally raised levels of insulin. Many consider measurable insulin in the face of hypoglycaemia as being indicative of hyperinsulinism [90], but the close coupling of blood glucose concentrations to insulin secretion has not fully developed in the newborn period [11], making hyperinsulinism harder to evaluate. Furthermore, the renal clearance of C peptide varies greatly in this age group: in older children, raised levels of C peptide suggest endogenous insulin production, but normal levels and raised insulin concentrations suggest 'factitious' hyperinsulinaemia.

Transient neonatal hyperinsulinism

Hyperinsulinism is common and underrecognized in the neonatal period. It probably reflects an immaturity of the regulation of insulin secretion. It may occur in any sick infant, but is recognized most clearly in those with birth asphyxia and those who are small-for-gestational-age in whom hypoglycaemia may be exacerbated because of substrate (glycogen) depletion. Although hyperinsulinism may be transient, it may still require urgent management to prevent permanent sequelae. The problem is so common that monitoring of blood glucose concentrations in the first few hours should be performed in all at-risk infants. Early enteral feeds should be instituted; if intravenous glucose is required, small boluses should be used and glucose infusions should be reduced slowly during the recovery phase. Rarely the hyperinsulinaemia is more severe, requiring treatment with diazoxide (see Nesidioblastosis, later).

INFANTS OF DIABETIC MOTHERS

This is the most commonly recognized cause of transient hyperinsulinaemic hypoglycaemia. Sustained maternal hyperglycaemia is accompanied by fetal hyperglycaemia and consequent enhancement of fetal insulin secretion. These babies have marked β cell hyperplasia. *In utero* consequences of hyperinsulinism include macrosomia [91] and teratogenesis, with cardiac, central nervous system and skeletal anomalies predominating [92]. Not surprisingly, in the poorly controlled diabetic mother there is a high rate of fetal wastage. Macrosomia may complicate delivery [93].

Once delivered, these infants have problems relating to immaturity, particularly hyaline membrane disease, hyperbilirubinaemia, feeding difficulties and apnoeic episodes, as well as hypoglycaemia. There is an increased incidence of thrombosis (particularly renal vein thrombosis), polycythaemia, hypocalcaemia and transient cardiomyopathy. It is important that these other problems do not overshadow the hypoglycaemia which usually occurs within the first 1–2 h. Hypoglycaemia normally resolves within the first 24 h [94], but there is a significant group which has more prolonged problems lasting several days. A small number do not become hypoglycaemic until 24–36 h of age.

The hypoglycaemia is caused not only by hyperinsulinaemia, but also by abnormally low secretion of counterregulatory hormones, which may account for lack of symptoms in some infants, and by delayed induction of gluconeogenic enzymes [95]. Management should be expectant, with early enteral feeding and regular (1–2-hourly for the first 12 h) estimations of plasma glucose [93]. Should the infant become hypoglycaemic and not tolerate enteral feeds, intravenous glucose infusion is necessary, with the quantity of glucose being titrated to maintain plasma glucose levels at 4–6 mmol/l. As much as 12 mg glucose/kg min^{-1} may be required. Where intravenous access is difficult, intramuscular glucagon (0.1 mg/kg) may provide temporary euglycaemia. On rare occasions, glucose requirements remain persistently high and intravenous cortisol (5 mg/kg 12-hourly) may be necessary. Once glucose levels stabilize, and the infant is able to tolerate enteral feeds, intravenous therapy should be withdrawn gradually over a 12-h period.

All the problems of hyperinsulinaemia in the infant can be avoided with strict control of maternal glucose regulation during pregnancy [96]. Fetal loss and the high levels of morbidity and mortality in the neonatal period can also be reduced by such measures.

RHESUS HAEMOLYTIC DISEASE

Advances in invasive antenatal management have dramatically altered the clinical picture of Rhesus disease. Intermittent *in utero* transfusions have meant that affected fetuses can be maintained *in utero* for longer, so that larger, more mature infants with less anaemia are being delivered. However, many of these infants still have neonatal problems.

Hyperinsulinism may still be a problem, and is not completely understood. There is β cell hyperplasia, but not to the same degree as in infants of diabetic mothers. It has been postulated that excess insulin destruction during the intravascular haemolysis stimulates the β cells or that trophic substances (amino acids, for example) released during haemolysis are causative. The hyperinsulinaemia is accompanied by normal secretion of counterregulatory hormones: the hypoglycaemia is thus generally milder. Those infants who require exchange transfusion for hyperbilirubinaemia and anaemia, need careful monitoring of glucose concentrations throughout the procedure, and importantly afterwards, as rebound hypoglycaemia may occur.

EXOMPHALOS – MACROGLOSSIA – GIGANTISM SYNDROME

This syndrome has been recognized for 30 years following Beckwith [97] and Wiedemann's [98] independent descriptions. The hyperinsulinaemia occurs in association with β cell hyperplasia and hypertrophy. There is a strong association with abnormalities of the short arm of chromosome 11, where IGF-II is encoded [99]. The abnormal production of IGF-II in early fetal life may account for the subsequent anomalies. The characteristic clinical findings include exomphalos, pathognomonic earlobe abnormalities and tissue overgrowth including gigantism, macroglossia and visceromegaly. The hypoglycaemia, which occurs symptomatically in about 50% of cases, is usually transient. More persistent hypoglycaemia has been described which required therapy with diazoxide and somatostatin [100], or even pancreatectomy.

Survival with normal development probably relates to the recognition and appropriate management of the hypoglycaemia. Long-term additional complications include cystic renal disease, asymmetric limb growth, nephroblastoma and hepatoblastoma.

Persistent hyperinsulinism

Persistent hyperinsulinism is most commonly due to defects in β cell development resulting in functional and microstructural abnormalities.

NESIDIOBLASTOSIS

The term 'nesidioblastosis' has been used since the late

1930s to cover a group of disorders encompassing a variety of histopathological abnormalities of the endocrine pancreas. Essentially there is an increase in endocrine cells and ductular epithelium within the pancreas, associated with a reduction in the quality and quantity of somatostatin-producing cells [101]. Other terms that have been used include microadenomatosis, focal islet-cell adenomatosis and diffuse β-cell hyperplasia. Although it often appears to occur sporadically, there is considerable evidence that it is inherited as an autosomal recessive disorder [102].

Nesidioblastosis is the most common cause of severe recurrent hypoglycaemia in the neonatal period. Term infants, often but not always of large birth weight, present with severe persistent hypoglycaemia within the first few days of life. The diagnosis can often be suspected even before serum insulin levels are available, as the glucose infusion rate required to maintain normoglycaemia is much greater than $10\,mg/kg\,min^{-1}$. Presentation may also be delayed several months and sudden, unexpected infant deaths may occur. The diagnosis is confirmed by inappropriately high levels of insulin in the face of hypoglycaemia. Pancreatic imaging, in particular ultrasonography [103], is rarely helpful.

The initial management is medical [104], giving glucose to maintain normoglycaemia, but if infusion rates of glucose greater than $12\,mg/kg\,min^{-1}$ are needed, suppression of insulin secretion may be required using diazoxide (up to 20 mg/kg a day and always with a thiazide diuretic) [105] or somatostatin [106,107], given as octreotide 1–15 μg/kg a day. The latter is very effective, but tachyphylaxis may mitigate against its long-term use [108] and it should be combined with a glucagon infusion. For those patients who cannot be controlled on medical treatment the definitive treatment is surgical [109], either to remove a discrete adenoma or subtotal pancreatectomy [110]. If hypoglycaemia persists, total pancreatectomy may occasionally be necessary.

INSULINOMA

Beta cell adenomas may present in later childhood with intermittent symptoms following fasts or exercise. They may represent one end of the spectrum of pancreatic dysregulation syndromes. Localization with imaging techniques prior to surgery may be difficult. Management is broadly similar to nesidioblastosis except that other endocrine tumours should be sought (parathyroid adenomas, gastrinomas, pituitary adenomas) to exclude multiple endocrine neoplasia syndrome type 1.

Tumours which secrete IGF-I and IGF-II have a clinical picture similar to insulinomas, with hypoglycaemia, hypoketonaemia and low free fatty acid levels, but insulin and C-peptide levels are not raised [111]. Specific radioimmunoassays are available to aid in making this very rare diagnosis, which may account for the hypoglycaemia seen in patients with large mesenchymal tumours.

ABNORMALITIES OF COUNTERREGULATION

Hypoglycaemia may occur when one or more of the counterregulatory mechanisms fail.

Deficiencies of the anterior pituitary

Patients with panhypopituitarism present with hypoglycaemia in about 20% of cases [112]. Most are caused by congenital anomalies of the hypothalamus and pituitary, and generally present neonatally or in infancy rather than later in childhood. Secondary pituitary failure may be caused by tumours, surgical and irradiation damage, and vascular events.

Mostly the hypoglycaemia is associated with low levels of insulin and high levels of ketone bodies and free fatty acids. The latter effects depend on glucagon action, which if blunted will result in diminished release of ketones and free fatty acids [113]. There have been reports of hyperinsulinaemia occurring in association with hypopituitarism, being either coincidental or a cause of the pituitary dysfunction [114]. However, it is important to recognize the aetiology of the hypoglycaemia because fatal complications may develop rapidly. Midline defects or optic nerve abnormalities (in septo-optic dysplasia) are important clues to the diagnosis. In males, undescended testes and/or micropenis suggest gonadotrophin deficiency, but there are no equivalent signs in females. Hyponatraemia and conjugated hyperbilirubinaemia can also be a useful clue to ACTH, and hence cortisol, deficiency [115].

The pathophysiology of hypoglycaemia in hypopituitarism is not clear, but it is likely that it is due to reduced counterregulation with the supply of gluconeogenic substrate limited. The hypoglycaemia should be managed in the usual way and appropriate investigations collected (see Table 35.3). Replacement therapy, especially hydrocortisone, should not be delayed in neonates, as there is a significant risk of morbidity and mortality. Treatment with growth hormone may be necessary to prevent hypoglycaemia. Special attention needs to be given during intercurrent illness.

Adrenal insufficiency

Although not common, spontaneous hypoglycaemia is a recognized presentation of Addison disease and is usually precipitated by intercurrent infection. It is essentially due to defective gluconeogenesis and must be considered in any patient with ketosis and hypoglycaemia. The clinical clues are hyperpigmentation of skin and mucous membranes and/or vitiligo and hypotension. Hyponatraemia, hyperkalaemia and excessive urinary sodium loss are additional pointers. Plasma cortisol levels are undetectable or inappropriately low, with raised ACTH levels. Polyglandular autoimmune involvement resulting in hypothyroidism and hypogonadism should also be sought in patients with Addison disease [116]. Treatment is with hydrocortisone replacement (15 mg/m^2 a day). Congenital adrenal hyperplasia can also result in hypoglycaemia due to cortisol deficiency.

Many patients with Addison disease do not show the usual sympathetic signs of hypoglycaemia, which is thought to be due to adrenomedullary unresponsiveness. This condition has also been seen in isolation in patients with spontaneous hypoglycaemia. Its clinical significance has not yet been established, but it is more common in low birth weight infants and those with 'accelerated starvation'.

Growth hormone deficiency

In about 10% of all cases of hypoglycaemia in infancy, growth hormone insufficiency may be present [117]. However, it is usually part of a wider pituitary dysfunction, either primary or secondary, rarely occurring in isolation [118]. Ketogenesis and lipolysis are impaired compared to normal individuals [119]. Treatment is initially supportive with correction of hypoglycaemia, before replacement therapy using recombinant growth hormone (15 IU/m^2 per week).

Hypothyroidism

Hypoglycaemia is a rare complication of hypothyroidism, whether it be primary or secondary to hypothalamopituitary dysfunction. The mechanism is unclear, but maybe due to impaired glycogenolysis [120] and gluconeogenesis [121].

Glucagon deficiency

This condition is rare, and there is doubt whether it exists. There have been reports of severe hypoglycaemia presenting in the neonatal period associated with absent α cells within the pancreas, but without glucagon measurements to substantiate this [122]. Others have documented low plasma glucagon levels associated with hypoglycaemia and a glycaemic response to protamine zinc glucagon [123], but insulin levels were also higher than expected for the plasma glucose levels, suggesting that hyperinsulinism was perhaps the main aetiological factor.

DRUG-INDUCED HYPOGLYCAEMIA

As well as the more obvious hypoglycaemic agents (insulin, the sulphonylureas [124] and biguanides) there are a number of other compounds which can result in hypoglycaemia, both during exposure *in utero* [125] and afterwards. These include ethanol, salicylates, β-adrenergic blockers and hypoglycin, which is found in the unripe ackee fruit and results in so-called 'Jamaican vomiting sickness'. Most of these agents are ingested accidentally by children, but deliberate administration must always be excluded. As well as the medical management of these situations, much emphasis needs to be placed on their prevention,with improved safety around homes and the use of childproof containers.

Ethanol

Ethanol can be a potent cause of hypoglycaemia in children, whether ingested, inhaled or absorbed transdermally [87]. Hypoglycaemia tends to be a late event, developing many hours later, often after intoxication has resolved. It is more common in those who are fasting, in whom glycogen reserves have been depleted.

Ethanol is a potent inhibitor of gluconeogenesis, although the precise mechanisms are not understood. It is oxidized within the liver by ethanol dehydrogenase generating $NADH_2$, altering the equilibria of $NADH_2$-dependent reactions. In particular, the equilibrium of lactate and pyruvate is tipped in favour of lactate, with consequent reduction of amino-acid gluconeogenic substrates from the TCA cycle. The oxidation of glycerol to triose phosphate is also reduced [126]. Thus, in a state when glycogenolysis is inadequate, gluconeogenesis cannot meet the demands for glucose.

Treatment is with glucose enterally or parenterally, depending on the conscious level of the patient. Younger children must never be left just to 'sleep off' the effects of ethanol. They should be monitored carefully with estimations of blood glucose, as well as for the complications of vomiting.

Salicylates

Salicylate poisoning is a well-recognized cause of hypoglycaemia. As well as symptoms of hypoglycaemia, presentation may be with vomiting and hyperventilation due to acidosis. Salicylates have been thought to increase peripheral utilization of glucose [127], but the concentrations of ketones and free fatty acids are low, suggesting a lack of alternative fuels. Beta-oxidation is suppressed by a direct toxic effect on the mitochondria.

Treatment is of the hypoglycaemia, with forced alkaline

diuresis or haemofiltration occasionally being necessary, depending on plasma salicylate levels.

Beta-adrenergic blocking agents

Beta-blockers have direct neural effects on the endocrine pancreas, stimulating insulin secretion and thus inhibiting lipolysis. Glycogenolysis also may be inhibited [128]. However, catecholamines are not essential for counterregulation [129], so additional factors would seem to be necessary for these drugs to produce hypoglycaemia. Treatment is generally symptomatic as β-agonists, for example salbutamol, cannot overcome the receptor blockade.

Jamaican vomiting sickness

This condition, which is often severe and may be fatal, resembles a fatty acid oxidation defect [27]. It occurs following the ingestion of unripe ackee fruit, which contain a pentacyclic amino acid, called hypoglycin. This is metabolized to a cyclic acyl-CoA which is a potent inhibitor of medium-chain acyl-CoA dehydrogenase [130]. Treatment entails the use of the high-carbohydrate feeds, with intravenous glucose often being necessary.

MISCELLANEOUS CAUSES OF HYPOGLYCAEMIA

Liver dysfunction

As discussed, the liver has a key role in the control of glucose regulation. Most of the conditions that have been described, as well as the inborn errors of metabolism, affect specific pathways and enzyme systems. However, overwhelming hepatic damage, regardless of its cause, can have significant effects on glucose homeostasis [131]. Both hyperglycaemia and hypoglycaemia occur. Hypoglycaemia may also complicate liver dysfunction secondary to congenital heart disease.

Congenital heart disease

In infants presenting with hypoglycaemia, hepatomegaly and acidosis, congestive cardiac failure secondary to congenital heart disease must be considered. Causes reducing left ventricular outflow, for example aortic stenosis or hypoplastic left heart syndrome, most commonly produce this picture. A reduction in hepatic perfusion is thought to compromise glucose production, which fails to meet the increased metabolic demands of these children, ultimately with hypoglycaemia as the result [132]. It may also occur in the immediate period following cardiac bypass surgery.

Infants with congenital heart disease without cardiac heart failure also have a tendency to develop fasting hypoglycaemia [133]. Elevated levels of lactate, pyruvate and alanine indicate a decreased extraction or inability to utilize these gluconeogenic substrates, as counter-regulatory hormone secretion appears to be normal.

Ketotic hypoglycaemia

Ketotic hypoglycaemia was previously regarded as the most common form of hypoglycaemia seen in childhood [134], and, in spite of the improvements in diagnosis of hypoglycaemia, the cause remains unclear.

Classically, boys are affected more often than girls, often being small-for-gestational-age and typically aged between 18 months and 7 years. The usual history is of a child, unwell with a minor infection, who misses the evening meal. The following morning the child is found floppy and unresponsive. Fits are not uncommon, but the hypoglycaemia usually responds quickly to glucose therapy. Hypoglycaemia is unpredicatable. It does not always develop with infections, and the duration of fast necessary to provoke symptoms often varies considerably. Symptoms recur, but generally the condition remits spontaneously before puberty [135].

Biochemically, the children have hypoglycaemia associated with raised ketone bodies and free fatty acids [136]. Insulin secretion is appropriately suppressed and glucagon, cortisol and growth hormone levels are appropriately raised. Plasma lactate and pyruvate levels are normal but alanine is low, suggesting a reduced supply of gluconeogenic substrate [137]. However, this may not be the primary defect as all these changes are seen in normal children during fasting. The time course for them is foreshortened, however, in those with ketotic hypoglycaemia. The term coined by Cornblath & Schwartz [86] of 'accelerated starvation' would therefore be appropriate.

Intravenous infusions of alanine raise plasma glucose levels within 30 min and glucocorticoids also have this effect, probably by raising plasma alanine levels [138]. Glucocorticoids enhance the activity of gluconeogenic enzymes, but may also reduce peripheral utilization, thus conserving glucose. Some workers have implicated adrenomedullary unresponsiveness as being the cause of the hypoalaninaemic hypoglycaemia [139], but this has not been substantiated and it seems most likely that these children represent an extreme end of the normal spectrum of adaptation to fasting. A similar picture may account for the hypoglycaemia occasionally seen in anorexia nervosa [140]. However, the condition is likely to be heterogeneous, and more than one mechanism may be responsible for the hypoglycaemia. It is essential to exclude other conditions such as ketone body utilization defects.

The management is to provide regular meals, avoiding missing meals. If the child is not hungry a high-carbohydrate drink is offered. During catabolic states, for example intercurrent illness, or prior to vigorous physical activity, high-carbohydrate and protein-containing foods or drinks should be given regularly [135]. If oral feeds are not tolerated, intravenous glucose should be given [141]. The disorder is generally self-limiting and thus has a good prognosis.

Malaria

Hypoglycaemia is a significant complication of severe falciparum malaria, particularly in children. Long-term neurological sequelae, occurring in approximately 20% of survivors, are closely associated with hypoglycaemia at the time of diagnosis [142]. The aetiology of hypoglycaemia is multifactorial. Peripheral glucose utilization by the patient and the parasite exceed hepatic supply. Raised levels of ketones, lactate and alanine suggest a failure in gluconeogenesis, but prolonged fasting with glycogen depletion may well be the most important determining factor [143]. Quinine may induce insulin secretion [144], compounding the problem and necessitating constant vigilance at presentation and during therapy.

CONCLUSION

Glucose homeostasis is controlled by many complex, integrated systems which may breakdown at any level to cause dysregulation. Hypoglycaemia is a common problem that needs to be actively sought and managed. Prompt diagnosis and treatment can prevent morbidity and mortality and may have genetic implications.

Current understanding of the effects of neuroglycopaenia on cerebral metabolism is improving. Knowledge of how hypoglycaemia causes an insult to the brain should enable the development of therapy to prevent brain damage. Amelioration of the damaging effects of hypoglycaemia mediated by the NMDA receptor seems promising. Although not directed at the source of the problem, this will help to reduce the consequences of abnormal cerebral metabolism.

REFERENCES

1 McQuarrie I. Idiopathic spontaneously occurring hypoglycaemia in infants. *Am J Dis Child* 1954;87:399–428.

2 Lubchenco LO, Bard H. Incidence of hypoglycaemia in newborn infants classified by birth weight and gestational age. *Pediatrics* 1971;47:831–8.

3 Anon. Brain damage by neonatal hypoglycaemia. *Lancet* 1989;1:882–3.

4 Lucas A, Morley R, Cole TJ. Adverse neurodevelopmental outcome of moderate neonatal hypoglycaemia. *Br Med J* 1988;297:1304–8.

5 Singh M, Singhai PK, Paul VK *et al.* Neurodevelopmental outcome of asymptomatic and symptomatic babies with neonatal hypoglycaemia. *Ind J Med Res* 1991;94:6–10.

6 Spence JC. Some observation on sugar tolerance with reference to variation at different ages. *Q J Med* 1921;14:314–26.

7 Koh THHG, Eyre JA, Aynsley-Green A. Neonatal hypoglycaemia – the controversy regarding definition. *Arch Dis Child* 1988;63:1386–98.

8 Cryer PE. Regulation of glucose metabolism in man. *J Intern Med* 1991;229(Suppl. 2):31–9.

9 Van den Berghe G. The role of the liver in metabolic homeostasis: implications for inborn errors of metabolism. *J Inher Metab Dis* 1991;14:407–20.

10 Hawdon JM, Aynsley-Green A, Alberti KGMM, Ward Platt MP. The role of pancreatic insulin secretion in neonatal glucoregulation. I. Healthy term and preterm infants. *Arch Dis Child* 1993;68:274–9.

11 Hawdon JM, Aynsley-Green A, Bartlett K, Ward Platt MP. The role of pancreatic insulin secretion in neonatal glucoregulation. II. Infants with disordered blood glucose homeostasis. *Arch Dis Child* 1993;68:280–5.

12 Butler PC, Rizza RA. Regulation of carbohydrate metabolism and response to hypoglycaemia. *Endocrinol Clin N Am* 1989;18:1–25.

13 Haymond MW, Karl IE, Clarke WL *et al.* Differences in circulating gluconeogenic substrates during short-term fasting in men, women and children. *Metabolism* 1982; 31:33–42.

14 Hers H-G. Mechanisms of blood glucose homeostasis. *J Inher Metab Dis* 1990;13:395–410.

15 Roach PJ, Warren KR, Atkinson DE. Uridine diphosphate glucose synthase from calf liver: determinants of enzyme activity *in vitro*. *Biochemistry* 1975;14:544–5.

16 Taylor C, Cox AJ, Kernohan JC, Cohen P. Debranching enzyme from rabbit skeletal muscle. *Eur J Biochem* 1975; 51:105.

17 Soskin S. The liver and carbohydrate metabolism. *Endocrinology* 1940;26:297–308.

18 Lackner R, Challis A, West D *et al.* A problem in the radiochemical assay of glucose-6-phosphatase in muscle. *Biochem J* 1984;218:649–51.

19 Chaussain JL, Georges P, Calzada L. Glycemic response to 24 hour fast in normal children. III. Influence of age. *J Pediatr* 1977;91:711–14.

20 Felig P. The glucose-alanine cycle. *Metabolism* 1973;22: 179–207.

21 Pilkis SJ, El-Maghrabi MR, Claus TH. Hormonal regulation of hepatic gluconeogenesis and glycolysis. *Ann Rev Biol* 1988;57:755–83.

22 Hue L. The role of futile cycles in the metabolism of glucose. *Adv Enzymol* 1981;52:247.

23 Arion WJ, Lange AJ, Walls HE, Balleas LM. Evidence of the participation of independent translocases for phosphate and glucose-6-phosphate in the microsomal glucose-6-phosphatase system. *J Biol Chem* 1980;255:10396–406.

24 Winter S, Szabo-Aczel S, Curry CRJ, Hutchinson HT, Hogue R, Shug AL. Plasma carnitine deficiency – clinical observations in 51 pediatric patients. *Am J Dis Child* 1987;141: 660–5.

25 Angelini C. Defects of fatty acid oxidation in muscle. *Baillières Clin Endocrinol Metab* 1990;4:561–82.

26 Gregersen N. The acyl-CoA dehydrogenation deficiencies. *Scand J Clin Lab Invest* 1985;45(Suppl. 174):1–60.

27 Amiel SA, Archibald HR, Chusney G, Williams AJK, Gale EAM. Ketone infusion lowers hormonal responses to hypo-

glycaemia: evidence for acute cerebral utilization of a non-glucose fuel. *Clin Sci* 1991;81:189–94.

28 Efendic S, Kindmark H, Berggren P-O. Mechanisms involved in the regulation of the insulin secretory processs. *J Intern Med* 1991;229(Suppl. 2):9–22.

29 Hems DA, Whitton PD. Control of hepatic glycogenolysis. *Physiol Rev* 1980;60:1–50.

30 Chiasson JL, Liljenquist JE, Finger FE *et al.* Differential sensitivity of glycogenolysis and gluconeogenesis in insulin infusions in dogs. *Diabetes* 1976;25:283–91.

31 Devaskar SU, Mueckler MM. The mammalian glucose transporters. *Pediatr Res* 1991;31:1–13.

32 Joost HG, Weber TM, Cushman SW, Simpson IA. Insulin-stimulated glucose transport in rat adipose cells. Modulation of transporter intrinsic activity by isoproterenol and adenosine. *J Biol Chem* 1986;261:10033–6.

33 Rizza RA, Mandarino LJ, Gerich JE. Dose–response characteristics for the effects of insulin on production and utilization of glucose in man. *Am J Physiol* 1981;240:E630–9.

34 Arner P, Engfeldt P. Fasting mediated alteration studies on insulin action lipolysis and lipogenesis in obese women. *Am J Physiol* 1987;253:E193–201.

35 Biggers DW, Myers SR, Neal D *et al.* Role of brain in counterregulation of insulin-induced hypoglycaemia in dogs. *Diabetes* 1989;38:7–16.

36 Kahn CR, White MF. The insulin receptor and the molecular mechanism of insulin action. *J Clin Invest* 1988;82:1151–6.

37 Baxter RC. The somatomedins, insulin-like growth factors. *Adv Clin Chem* 1986;25:49–115.

38 Lonnroth P. Regulation of insulin action at the cellular level. *J Intern Med* 1991;229(Suppl. 2):23–9.

39 Exton JH. Gluconeogenesis. *Metabolism* 1972;21:945–89.

40 Bomboy J, Lewis S, Lacy W *et al.* Transient stimulatory effect of sustained hyperglucagonemia on splanchnic glucose production in normal and diabetic man. *Diabetes* 1977;26:177–84.

41 Jarhult J, Anderson PO, Holst J *et al.* On the sympathetic innervation of the cat's liver and its role for hepatic glucose release. *Acta Physiol Scand* 1980;110:5–11.

42 Rizza R, Cryer P, Haymond M *et al.* Adrenergic mechanisms for the effect of epinephrine on glucose production and clearance in man. *J Clin Invest* 1980;65:682–9.

43 Clutter W, Shah S, Bier D *et al.* Epinephrine plasma metabolic clearance rates and physiologic thresholds for metabolic and hemodynamic actions in man. *J Clin Invest* 1980;66:94–101.

44 Rizza RA, Mandarino LJ, Gerich JE. Cortisol induced insulin-resistance in man: impaired suppression of glucose production and stimulation of glucose utilization due to a post-receptor defect of insulin action. *J Clin Endocrinol Metab* 1982;54:131–8.

45 MacGorman L, Rizza RA, Gerich JE. Physiologic concentrations of growth hormone exert insulin-like and insulin antagonistic effects on both hepatic and extrahepatic tissues in man. *J Clin Endocrinol Metab* 1981;53:556–9.

46 Johnston DG, Pernet A, McCulloch A *et al.* Some hormonal influences on glucose and ketone body metabolism in normal human subjects. In: *Metabolic Acidosis.* Ciba Foundation Symposium, London: Pitman, 1982;87:168–91.

47 Sestoft L, Christensen NJ, Saltin B. Responses of glucose and glucoregulatory hormones to exercise in thyrotoxic and myxoedematous patients before and after 3 months of treatment. *Clin Sci* 1991;81:91–9.

48 Lager I. The insulin-antagonistic effect of the counterregulatory hormones. *J Intern Med* 1991;229(Suppl. 2):41–7.

49 Butler PC, Rizza RA. Contribution to postprandial hyperglycaemia and effect on initial splanchnic glucose clearance of hepatic glucose cycling in glucose intolerant or NIDDM patients. *Diabetes* 1991;40:73–81.

50 Edelman SV, Laakso M, Wallace P, Brechtel G, Olefsky JM, Baron AD. Kinetics of insulin-mediated and non-insulin-mediated glucose uptake in humans. *Diabetes* 1990;39:955–64.

51 Sacca L, Hendler R, Sherwin RS. Hyperglycemia inhibits glucose production in man independent of changes in glucoregulatory hormones. *J Clin Endocrinol Metab* 1978;47:1160–3.

52 Consoli A, Kennedy F, Miles J *et al.* Determination of Krebs cycle metabolic carbon exchange *in vivo* and its use to estimate the individual contributions of gluconeogenesis and glycogenolysis to overall glucose output in man. *J Clin Invest* 1987;80:1303–10.

53 Felber JP, Ferrannini E, Golay A *et al.* Role of lipid oxidation in pathogenesis of insulin resistance of obesity and type II diabetes. *Diabetes* 1987;72:1737–47.

54 Contreras I, Dohm GL, Abdallah S *et al.* The effect of fasting on the activation *in vivo* of the insulin receptor kinase. *Biochem J* 1990;265:887–90.

55 Saudubray JM, Marsac C, Limal JM *et al.* Variation in plasma ketone bodies during a 24-hour fast in normal and hypoglycemic children: relationship to age. *J Pediatr* 1981;98:904–8.

56 Bonnefont JP, Specola NB, Vassault A *et al.* The fasting test in paediatrics: application to the diagnosis of pathological hypo- and hyperketotic states. *Eur J Pediatr* 1990;150:80–5.

57 Bier DM, Leake RD, Haymond MW *et al.* Measurement of 'true' glucose production rates in infancy and childhood with 6,6-dideuteroglucose. *Diabetes* 1977;26:1016–23.

58 Hawdon JM, Aynsley-Green A, Ward Platt MP. Neonatal blood glucose concentrations: metabolic effects of intravenous glucagon and intragastric medium chain triglyceride. *Arch Dis Child* 1993;68:255–61.

59 Hawdon JM, Ward Platt MP. Metabolic adaptation in small-for-gestational-age infants. *Arch Dis Child* 1993;68:262–8.

60 Hawdon JM, Weddell A, Aynsley-Green A, Ward Platt MP. Hormonal and metabolic response to hypoglycaemia in small-for-gestational-age infants. *Arch Dis Child* 1993;68:269–73.

61 Howard JM, Krantz KE. Transfer and use of glucose in the human placenta during in vitro perfusion and the associated effects of oxytocin and paraleucine. *Am J Obstet Gynecol* 1967;98:445.

62 Shelley HJ, Neligan GA. Neonatal hypoglycemia. *Br Med Bull* 1966;22:34–9.

63 Srinivasan G, Pildes RS, Cattamanchi G, Voora S, Lilien CD. Plasma glucose values in normal neonates: a new look. *J Pediatr* 1986;109:114–17.

64 Collins JE, Leonard JV, Teale D *et al.* Hyperinsulinaemic hypoglycaemia in small-for-dates babies. *Arch Dis Child* 1990;65:1118–20.

65 Cornblath M, Schwartz R, Aynsley-Green A, Lloyd JK. Hypoglycemia in infancy: the need for a rational definition. *Pediatrics* 1990;85:834–7.

66 Lin HC, Maguire C, Oh W, Cowett R. Accuracy and reliability of glucose reflectance meters in the high-risk neonate. *J Pediatr* 1989;9115:998–1000.

67 Liu D, Moberg E, Kollind M, Lins P-E, Adamson U, MacDonald IA. Arterial, arterialized venous, venous and capillary blood glucose measurements in normal man during hyperinsulinaemic euglycaemia and hypoglycaemia. *Dia-*

betologia 1992;35:287–90.
68 Marks V. The measurement of blood glucose and the definition of hypoglycaemia. *Horm Metab Res* 1986;(Suppl. 6):1–6.
69 Koh THHG, Aynsley-Green A, Tarbit M, Eyre JA. Neural dysfunction during hypoglycaemia. *Arch Dis Child* 1988; 63:1353–8.
70 Anwar M, Vanucci RC. Autoradiographic determination of regional cerebral blood flow during hypoglycaemia in newborn dogs. *Pediatr Res* 1988;24:41–5.
71 Aynsley-Green A. Glucose: fuel for thought! *J Paediatr Child Health* 1991;27:21–30.
72 Rothman SM, Olney JW. Excitotoxicity and the NMDA receptor. *Trends Neurosci* 1987;10:299–302.
73 Skov L, Pryds O. Capillary recruitment for preservation of cerebral glucose influx in hypoglycemic, preterm newborns: evidence for a glucose sensor? *Pediatrics* 1992;90:193–5.
74 Service FJ. Hypoglycemias. *J Clin Endocrinol Metab* 1993; 76:269–72.
75 Snorgaard O, Lassen LH, Rosenfalck AM, Binder C. Glycaemic thresholds for hypoglycaemic symptoms, impairment of cognitive function, and release of counterregulatory hormones in subjects with functional hypoglycaemia. *J Intern Med* 1991;229:343–50.
76 Field JB. Hypoglycemia: definition, clinical presentations, classification, and laboratory tests. *Endocrinol Metab Clin N Am* 1989;18:27–43.
77 Marks V. Recognition and differential diagnosis of spontaneous hypoglycaemia. *Clin Endocrinol* 1992;37:309–16.
78 Amiel S. Glucose counter-regulation in health and disease: current concepts in hypoglycaemia recognition and response. *Q J Med* 1991;80:707–27.
79 Soltesz G, Aynsley-Green A. Approach to the diagnosis of hypoglycaemia in infants and children. In: Ranke MB, ed. *Functional Endocrinologic Diagnostics in Children and Adolescents.* Mannheim: J&J Verlag, 1992:168–83.
80 Shah A, Stanhope R, Matthew D. Hazards of phamacological tests of growth hormone secretion in childhood. *Br Med J* 1992;304:173–4.
81 Oakley PA. Inaccuracy and delay in decision making in paediatric resuscitation, and a proposed reference chart. *Br Med J* 1988;297:817–19.
82 Merinero B, Perez-Cerda C, Ugarte M. Investigation of enzyme defects in children with lactic acidosis. *J Inher Metab Dis* 1992;15:696–706.
83 Touma EH, Charpentier C. Medium chain acyl-CoA dehydrogenase deficiency. *Arch Dis Child* 1992;67:142–5.
84 Kronick JB, Scriver CR, Goodyear PR, Kaplan PB. A perimortem protocol for suspected genetic disease. *Pediatrics* 1983;71:960–3.
85 Saudubray JM, Ogier H, Bonnefont JP *et al.* Clinical approach to inherited metabolic diseases in the neonatal period: a 20-year survey. *J Inher Metab Dis* 1989;12(Suppl. 1):25–41.
86 Cornblath M, Schwartz R. *Disorders of Carbohydrate Metabolism in Infancy*, 3rd edn. Philadelphia, PA: Saunders, 1991.
87 Senior B, Sadeghi-Nejad A. Hypoglycemia: a pathophysiologic approach. *Acta Paed Scand* 1989;Suppl. 352:3–27.
88 Meschi F, Dozio N, Bognetti E, Carra M, Cofano D, Chiumello G. An unusual case of recurrent hypoglycaemia: 10-year follow up of a child with insulin auto-immunity. *Eur J Pediatr* 1992;151:32–4.
89 Scriver CR, Beaudet AL, Sly WS, Valle D. *The Metabolic Basis of Inherited Disease*, 6th edn. New York: MacGraw-Hill, 1989.
90 Mehta A, Wootton R, Cheng KN, Penfold P, Halliday D, Stacey TE, Effect of diazoxide or glucagon on hepatic glucose production rate during extreme neonatal hypoglycaemia. *Arch Dis Child* 1987;62:924–30.
91 Berk MA, Mimouni F, Miodovnik M, Hertzberg V, Valuck J. Macrosomia in infants of insulin-dependent diabetic mothers. *Pediatrics* 1989;83:1029–34.
92 Freinkel N, Cockcroft DL, Lewis NJ *et al.* Fuel-mediated teratogenesis during early organogenesis: the effects of increased concentrations of glucose, ketones, or somatomedin inhibitor during rat embryo culture. *Am J Clin Nutr* 1986;44:986–95.
93 Stenninger E, Schollin J, Aman J. Neonatal macrosomia and hypoglycaemia in children of mothers with insulin-treated gestational diabetes mellitus. *Acta Paed Scand* 1991;Suppl. 80:1014–18.
94 Kuhl C, Andersen GE, Hertel J, Molsted-Pedersen L. Metabolic events in infants of diabetic mothers during the first 24 hours after birth. *Acta Paed Scand* 1982;71:19–25.
95 Williams PR, Sperling MA, Racasa Z. Blunting of spontaneous and amino acid-stimulated glucagon secretion in infants of diabetic mothers (IDM). *Diabetes* 1975;24:411.
96 Hadden DR. Diabetes in pregnancy. *Diabetologia* 1985; 29:1–9.
97 Beckwith JB. Macroglossia, omphalocele, adrenal cytomegaly, gigantism and hyperplastic visceromegaly. *Birth Defects* 1969;5:188–96.
98 Wiedemann HR. Complex malformatif familial avec hernie ombilicale et macroglossie. Un syndrome nouveau? *J Genet Hum* 1964;13:223–32.
99 Engstrom W, Lindham S, Schofield P. Wiedemann–Beckwith syndrome. *Eur J Pediatr* 1988;147:450–7.
100 Gerver WJM, Menheere PPCA, Schaap C, Degraeuwe P. The effects of a somatostatin analogue on the metabolism of an infant with Beckwith–Wiedemann syndrome and hyperinsulinaemic hypoglycaemia. *Eur J Pediatr* 1991;150:634–7.
101 Aynsley-Green A, Polak JM, Bloom SR *et al.* Nesidioblastosis of the pancreas: definition of the syndrome and the management of severe neonatal hyperinsulinaemic hypoglycaemia. *Arch Dis Child* 1981;56:496–508.
102 Glaser B, Philip M, Carmi R, Lieberman E, Landau H. Persistent hyperinsulinemic hypoglycemia of infancy ('nesidioblastosis'): autosomal recessive inheritance in 7 pedigrees. *Am J Med Genet* 1990;37:511–15.
103 Telander RL, Wolf SA, Simmons PS, Zimmerman D, Haymond MW. Endocrine disorders of the pancreas and adrenal cortex in pediatric patients. *Mayo Clin Proc* 1986; 61:459–66.
104 Baker L, Thornton PS, Stanley CA. Management of hyperinsulinism in infants. *J Pediatr* 1991;119:755–7.
105 Abu-Osba YK, Manasra KB, Mathew PM. Complications of diazoxide treatment in persistent neonatal hyperinsulinism. *Arch Dis Child* 1989;64:1496–500.
106 Bruining GJ, Bosschaart AN, Aarsen RSR, Lamberts SWJ, Sauer PJJ, Del Pozo E. Normalization of glucose homeostasis by long-acting somatostatin analog SMS 201-955 in a newborn with nesidioblastosis. *Acta Endocrinol* 1983;279: 334–8.
107 Glaser B, Landaw H. Long-term treatment with the somatostatin analogue SMS 201-995: alternative to pancreatectomy in persistent hyperinsulinaemic hypoglycaemia of infancy. *Digestion* 1990;45(Suppl. 1):27–35.
108 Hawdon JM, Ward Platt MP, Lamb WH, Aynsley-Green A. Tolerance to somatostain analogue in a preterm infant with islet cell dysregulation syndrome. *Arch Dis Child* 1990;

65:341–3.

109 Low LCK, Yu ECL, Chow OKW, Yeung CY, Young RTT. Hyperinsulinism in infancy. *Aust Paediatr J* 1989;25:174–7.

110 Spitz L, Bhargava RK, Grant DB, Leonard JV. Surgical treatment of hyperinsulinaemic hypoglycaemia in infancy and childhood. *Arch Dis Child* 1992;67:201–5.

111 Cotterill AM, Holly JMP, Davies SC, Coulson VJ, Price PA, Wass JAH. The insulin-like growth factors and their binding proteins in a case of non-islet-cell tumour-associated hypoglycaemia. *J Endocrinol* 1991;131:303–11.

112 Brasel JA, Wright JC, Wilkins L, Blizzard RM. An evaluation of 75 patients with hypopituitarism beginning in childhood. *Am J Med* 1965;38:484–98.

113 Bougneres PF, Artavia-Loria E, Ferre P, Chaussain JL, Job JC. Effects of hypopituitarism and growth hormone replacement therapy on the production and utilization of glucose in childhood. *J Clin Endocrinol Metab* 1985;61:1152–7.

114 Stanley CA, Baker L. Hyperinsulinism in infants and children: diagnosis and therapy. *Adv Pediatr* 1976;23:315–35.

115 Hopwood NJ, Forsman PJ, Kenny FM *et al.* Hypoglycemia in hypopituitary children. *Am J Dis Child* 1975;129:918–21.

116 Samaan NA. Hypoglycaemia secondary to endocrine deficiencies. *Endocrinol Metab Clin N Am* 1989;18:145–54.

117 Aynsley-Green A, McGann A, Deshpande S. Control of intermediary metabolism in childhood with special reference to hypoglycaemia and growth hormone. *Acta Paed Scand* 1991;Suppl. 377:43–52.

118 Goodman HG, Grumbach MM, Kaplan SL. Growth and growth hormone. II. A comparison of isolated growth hormone deficiency and multiple pituitary hormone deficiencies in 35 patients with idiopathic dwarfism. *N Engl J Med* 1968;278:57–66.

119 Wolfsdorf JI, Sadeghi-Nejad A, Senior B. Ketonemia and age-related fasting hypoglycemia in growth hormone deficiency. *Metabolism* 1983;32:457–61.

120 McDaniel HG, Pittman CS, Oh SJ, DiMauro S. Carbohydrate metabolism in hypothyroid myopathy. *Metabolism* 1977; 26:867–71.

121 Vaughan M. An *in vitro* effect of triiodothyronine on rat adipose tissue. *J Clin Invest* 1967;46:1482–7.

122 Tsalikian E, Haymond MW. Hypoglycemia in infants and children. In: Service FJ, ed. *Hypoglycemic Disorders*. Boston: GK Hall, 1983:35.

123 Kollie LA, Monneus LA, Cejka V. Persistent neonatal hypoglycaemia due to glucagon deficiency. *Arch Dis Child* 1978;53:422–4.

124 Teale JD, Starkey BJ, Marks V. The prevalence of factitious hypoglycemia due to sulfonylurea abuse in the UK: a preliminary report. *Pract Diabetes* 1989;6:177–8.

125 Piacquiadio K, Hollingsworth DR, Murphy H. Effects of *in-utero* exposure to oral hypoglycaemic drugs. *Lancet* 1991; 338:866–9.

126 Kreisberg RA, Siegal AM, Owen WC. Alanine and gluconeogenesis in man: effect of ethanol. *J Clin Endocrinol Metab* 1972;34:876–80.

127 Baron SH. Salicylates as hypoglycemic agents. *Diabetes Care* 1982;5:64–71.

128 Pelser DA, Winter RJ, Green OC. Propanolol-induced hypoglycemia during growth hormone testing. *J Pediatr* 1981; 99:157–8.

129 Rizza RA, Cryer PE, Gerich JE. Role of glucagon, catecholamines, and growth hormone in human glucose counterregulation. *J Clin Invest* 1979;64:62–71.

130 Tanaka K, Kean EA, Johnson B. Jamaican vomiting sickness: biochemical investigation of two cases. *N Engl J Med* 1976; 295:461–7.

131 Jacquemin E, Saliba E, Blond MH, Chantepie A, Laugier J. Liver dysfunction and acute cardioregulatory failure in children. *Eur J Pediatr* 1992;151:731–4.

132 Benzing G, Shubert W, Hug G *et al.* Simultaneous hypoglycemia and acute congestive heart failure. *Circulation* 1969;40:203.

133 Haymond MW, Strauss AW, Arnold KJ *et al.* Glucose homeostasis in children with severe cyanotic congenital heart disease. *J Pediatr* 1979;95:220–7.

134 Pagliara AS, Karl IE, Haymond MW, Kipnis DM. Hypoglycemia in infancy and childhood. *J Pediatr* 1973;83:694–7.

135 Colle E, Ulstrom RA. Ketotic hypoglycemia. *J Pediatr* 1964;64:632–51.

136 Chaussain JL. Glycemic response to 24 hour fast in normal children with ketotic hypoglycemia. *J Pediatr* 1973;82: 438–43.

137 Haymond MW, Karl IE, Pagliara AS. Ketotic hypoglycemia: an amino acid substrate limited disorder. *J Clin Endocrinol Metab* 1974;38:521–30.

138 Pagliara AS, Karl IE, DeVivo DC *et al.* Hypoalaninemia: a concomitant of ketotic hypoglycemia. *J Clin Invest* 1972; 51:1440–9.

139 Christensen NJ. Hypoadrenalinemia during insulin hypoglycemia in children with ketotic hypoglycemia. *J Clin Endocrinol Metab* 1974;38:107–12.

140 Fonseca V, Ball S, Marks V, Havard CWH. Hypoglycaemia associated with anorexia nervosa. *Postgrad Med J* 1991; 67:460–1.

141 Dixon MA, Leonard JV. Intercurrent illness in inborn errors of intermediary metabolism. *Arch Dis Child* 1992;67: 1387–91.

142 Bondi FS. The incidence and outcome of neurological abnormalities in childhood cerebral malaria: a long-term follow-up of 62 surviviors. *Trans R Soc Trop Med Hyg* 1992;86:17–19.

143 Kawo NG, Msengi AE, Swai ABM, Chuwa LM, Alberti KGMM, McLarty DG. Specificity of hypoglycaemia for cerebral malaria in children. *Lancet* 1990;336:454–7.

144 Davis TME, Pukrittayakamee S, Supanaranond W *et al.* Glucose metabolism in quinine-treated patients with uncomplicated falciparum malaria. *Clin Endocrinol* 1990; 33:739–49.

36: Lipid Disorders

D.J. BETTERIDGE

INTRODUCTION

Lipid screening among the adult population as part of measures for the primary or secondary prevention of coronary heart disease has led to the identification of families carrying genes for severe monogenic disorders of lipid metabolism. National and international guidelines for the management of dyslipidaemia strongly emphasize family screening, particularly in familial hypercholesterolaemia, and this has led to the identification of individuals in the paediatric age group. Some countries, particularly the USA, have put forward guidelines for population and individualized approaches to the identification and management of hyperlipidaemia in children in the knowledge that early lesions of atherosclerosis have been described in this age group and that healthy eating patterns are best established at a young age. Alterations in plasma lipid and lipoprotein levels (dyslipidaemia) may occur secondary to endocrine and metabolic disorders in childhood and they may contribute to the morbidity of the primary condition.

It is likely, therefore, that lipid abnormalities will be identified increasingly in children. This chapter provides an overview of lipid and lipoprotein metabolism as a basis for understanding and managing the metabolic abnormalities of primary and secondary lipid disorders.

LIPID AND LIPOPROTEIN METABOLISM

Lipoprotein structure and function

Cholesterol and triglyceride, which are relatively insoluble in water, are solubilized and transported through the aqueous plasma in a family of lipid/protein macromolecular complexes, the lipoproteins [1–3]. The water-insoluble cholesteryl ester and triglyceride form a non-polar core droplet with the more polar, amphipathic compounds phospholipid and free cholesterol, together with specific proteins and apoproteins. A cartoon of the proposed structure of a lipoprotein particle is shown in Fig. 36.1. Apoproteins, in addition to their critical role in lipoprotein structure, have important functions in lipoprotein metabolism (Fig. 36.1).

Plasma lipoproteins are characterized (and their nomenclature is principally derived from their separation) by means of preparative ultracentrifugation, which depends on their hydrated density (Table 36.1). For completeness the older classification, based on lipoprotein separation by electrophoresis, is also shown in Table 36.2.

CHYLOMICRONS

These are the largest lipoprotein particles and consist mainly of triglyceride with lesser amounts of phospholipid, free cholesterol, cholesterol esters and protein. They are synthesized in the intestine and transport absorbed dietary fat via the intestinal lymphatics and thoracic duct to the circulation. Protein forms a relatively minor constituent of chylomicrons, apoprotein B_{48} being the main structural protein.

VERY-LOW-DENSITY LIPOPROTEINS

Very-low-density lipoproteins (VLDLs) are also triglyceride-rich particles but they are smaller than chylomicrons and contain less triglyceride but more cholesterol, phospholipid and protein. The major structural protein is apoprotein B_{100}. VLDLs are synthesized in the liver and transport endogenously synthesized triglyceride and cholesterol.

INTERMEDIATE-DENSITY LIPOPROTEINS

Intermediate-density lipoprotein (IDL) particles are formed during conversion of VLDLs to low-density lipoproteins (LDLs) and are sometimes referred to as VLDL remnants. The concentration of IDL is approximately one-tenth that of LDL in normal subjects. IDLs contain relatively less triglyceride and more cholesteryl ester than VLDLs.

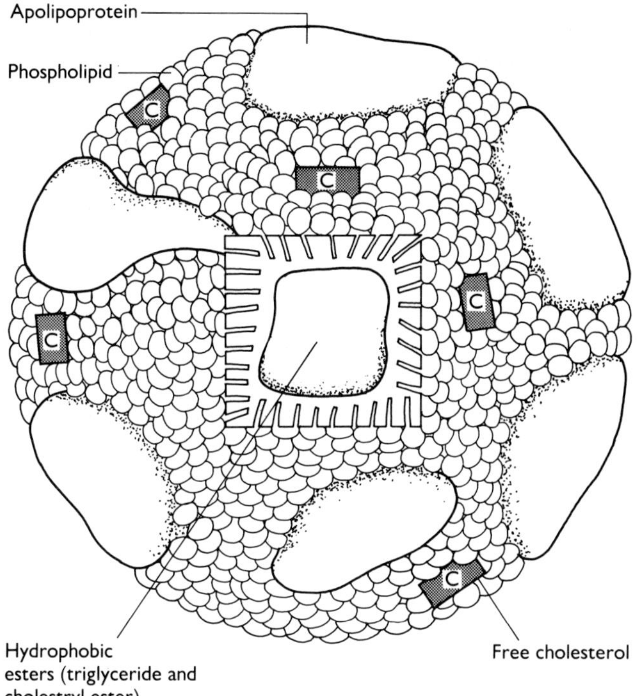

Fig. 36.1 Lipoprotein particle.

LOW-DENSITY LIPOPROTEINS

Low-density lipoproteins are the major cholesterol-rich lipoproteins and serve to transport cholesterol to peripheral cells. Most of the triglyceride is lost from the precursor VLDL and IDL particles, and LDLs retain only one apoprotein molecule per particle namely apoprotein B_{100}. LDLs are taken up by hepatic and peripheral tissues by a specific receptor-mediated process.

HIGH-DENSITY LIPOPROTEINS

High-density lipoproteins (HDLs) are the smallest and most dense of the lipoproteins and the most heterogeneous. They are formed in plasma either from precursors synthesized in the liver and small intestine or from catabolic products generated at the surface of triglyceride-rich lipoproteins during lipolysis. There are two major subfractions of HDL, HDL_2 and HDL_3. HDL_2 contains less protein than HDL_3 and is present in plasma in smaller amounts. HDL particles are involved in reverse cholesterol transport, i.e. the return of cholesterol from peripheral tissues to the liver for excretion.

Lipoprotein metabolism

Lipoprotein metabolism is conveniently considered under three main headings: the exogenous and endogenous lipoprotein pathways and reverse cholesterol transport. However, as will become clear, there is considerable interaction between these pathways. The liver plays a central role in lipid and lipoprotein metabolism and its importance cannot be overemphasized.

EXOGENOUS PATHWAY

Dietary triglyceride and cholesterol are re-esterified in the jejunal enterocyte and packaged with apoprotein B_{48} (and some apoprotein A) to form chylomicrons. Once in the circulation, chylomicrons receive apoproteins C and E from HDLs. Chylomicron triglyceride is hydrolysed by the enzyme lipoprotein lipase on endothelial cells of capillary beds in adipose tissue and muscle. Apoprotein C-II is an important activator of this enzyme. Free fatty acids

Table 36.1 Human plasma apoproteins

	Number of amino acids	Approx. molecular weight	Origin	Lipoprotein distribution	Principal function
A-I	243	28 000	Liver, intestine	HDL, chylomicrons	LCAT activator
A-II	154	17 000	Liver, intestine	HDL, chylomicrons	Structural protein in HDL
A-IV	391	40 000	Liver, intestine	HDL, chylomicrons	Non-specific LCAT cofactor
B_{48}	2152	246 000	Intestine	Chylomicrons, chylomicron remnants	Mediates chylomicron formation and secretion by enterocytes
B_{100}	4536	513 000	Liver	VLDL, LDL	Mediates hepatic VLDL formation Ligand for LDL receptor
C-I	57	7 000	Liver	Chylomicrons, VLDL, HDL	Inhibitor of chylomicron uptake
C-II	78	9 000	Liver	Chylomicrons, VLDL, HDL	LPL activator
C-III	79	9 000	Liver	Chylomicrons, VLDL, HDL	? Inhibitor LPL
D	?	2 000	Liver	HDL	? Involved in cholesterol ester transfer
E	299	3 400	Liver	Chylomicrons, VLDL, HDL	Ligand for chylomicron receptor and LDL receptor

Table 36.2 Lipoproteins

Class	Diameter (Å)	Density (g/ml)	Electrophoretic mobility	Chemical composition (% of dry mass) Triglycerides	Cholesteryl esters	Cholesterol	Phospholipids	Proteins
Chylomicrons	800–5000	0.930	α_2	86	3	2	7	2
VLDL	300–800	0.960–1.006	Pre-β	55	12	7	18	8
IDL	250–350	1.006–1.019	Slow pre-β	23	29	9	19	19
LDL	216	1.019–1.063	β	6	42	8	22	22
HDL_2	100	1.063–1.125	α_t	5	17	5	33	40
HDL_3	75	1.125–1.210	α_1	3	13	4	25	55
Lipoprotein (a)*	300	1.055–1.085	Slow pre-β	3	33	9	22	33

* Lipoprotein (a) is a minor lipoprotein in most individuals, but in a few its concentration is substantial. It is also called 'sinking pre-β-lipoprotein'. Its concentration is genetically determined.

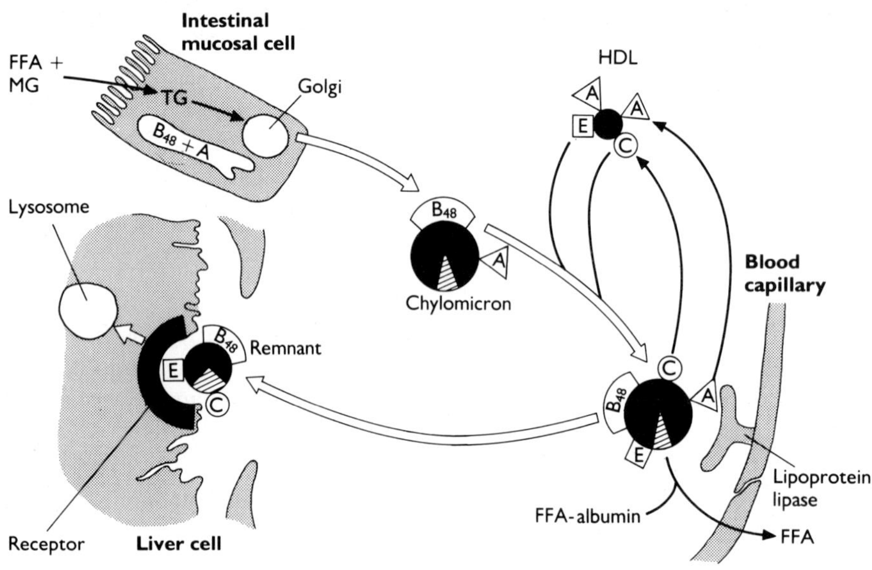

Fig. 36.2 Exogenous pathway of lipoprotein metabolism. FFA, free fatty acids; MG, monoglyceride; TG, triglyceride.

and glycerol resulting from triglyceride hydrolysis may be used as fuel or re-esterified for storage in adipose tissue. Surface components of chylomicrons, principally phospholipid, free cholesterol and apoprotein C, transfer to HDLs during the action of lipoprotein lipase on chylomicrons. Chylomicron particles after hydrolysis of the core triglyceride are relatively rich in cholesteryl ester. These remnant particles are removed by the liver through a process that is dependent on apoprotein E (Fig. 36.2).

ENDOGENOUS PATHWAY

Triglyceride and cholesterol synthesized in the liver are secreted in VLDL particles. In the plasma, VLDLs acquire apoproteins C and E by transfer from HDLs and, in a similar manner to chylomicrons, core triglyceride is hydrolysed by lipoprotein lipase with surface components transferring to HDLs. The resulting VLDL remnant particle or IDL may be taken up by the liver or further hydrolysed by hepatic lipase to LDL. The factor(s) which determine whether IDLs are removed directly by the liver or converted to LDLs remain to be fully determined, but VLDL size appears to be one determinant. Larger VLDL particles appear to behave more like chylomicrons, whereas small VLDLs are converted to LDLs. Apoprotein E is the principal ligand for the hepatic uptake of VLDL remnants through a specific receptor, the apoprotein B/E receptor (Fig. 36.3).

LDL is the end-product of the catabolism of VLDL and transports cholesterol to peripheral cells. There have been considerable advances in knowledge in the understanding of how LDL interacts with cells and how LDL-derived cholesterol regulates cholesterol homeostasis stemming from the description of the LDL receptor (apoprotein B/E receptor) by Brown and Goldstein [4].

The gene for the LDL receptor is on the short arm of

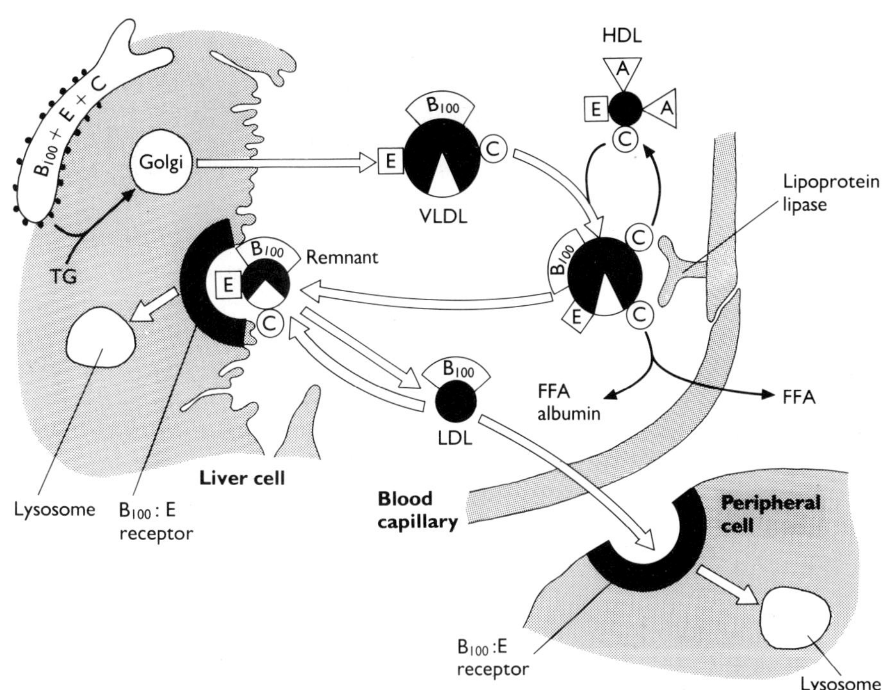

Fig. 36.3 Endogenous pathway of lipoprotein metabolism. FFA, free fatty acids; TG, triglyceride.

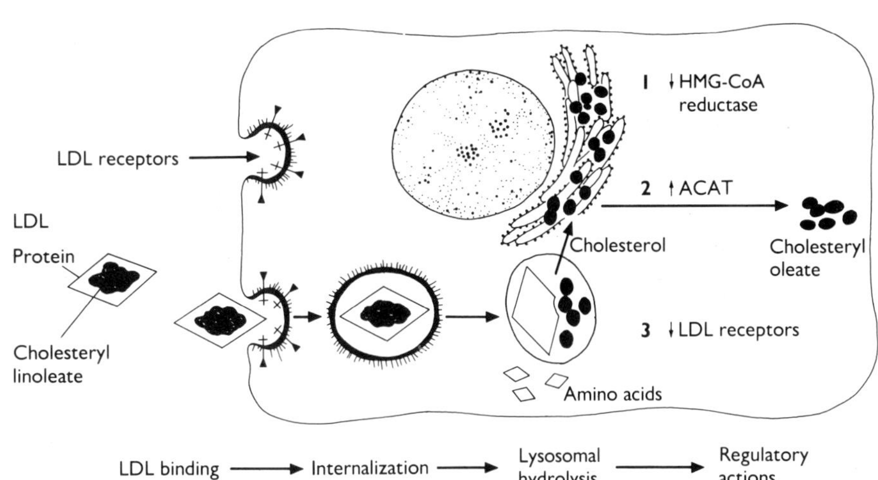

Fig. 36.4 The LDL receptor pathway. ACAT, acyl cholesterol acyl transferase. Redrawn from Brown & Goldstein [4].

chromosome 19 and codes for a protein of 839 amino acids, the mature receptor being a glycoprotein. LDL receptors are concentrated in the coated pit regions of all membranes. These organelles are important in terms of endocytosis of macromolecules. LDL binds to these specific, high-affinity receptors on cells via the ligand apoprotein B_{100}. Bound LDL is internalized by absorptive endocytosis with the formation of an endocytotic vesicle which fuses with cellular lysosomes (Fig. 36.4). After internalization the receptor dissociates from LDL and recycles to the cell surface.

LDL protein is hydrolysed by lysosomal proteases and LDL cholesteryl ester is hydrolysed by lysosomal acid lipase to free cholesterol. The accumulation of free cholesterol has regulatory effects on two important enzymes in cellular cholesterol metabolism, HMG-CoA (hydroxymethylglutaryl co-enzyme A) reductase and acyl-CoA:cholesterol acyltransferase. HMG-CoA reductase, which catalyses the conversion of HMG-CoA to mevalonate, the major rate-determining step in cholesterol synthesis, is suppressed with consequent reduction in cellular cholesterol synthesis. Acyl CoA:cholesterol acyltransferase is activated, which results in the re-esterification of cellular free cholesterol. Increasing cellular cholesterol

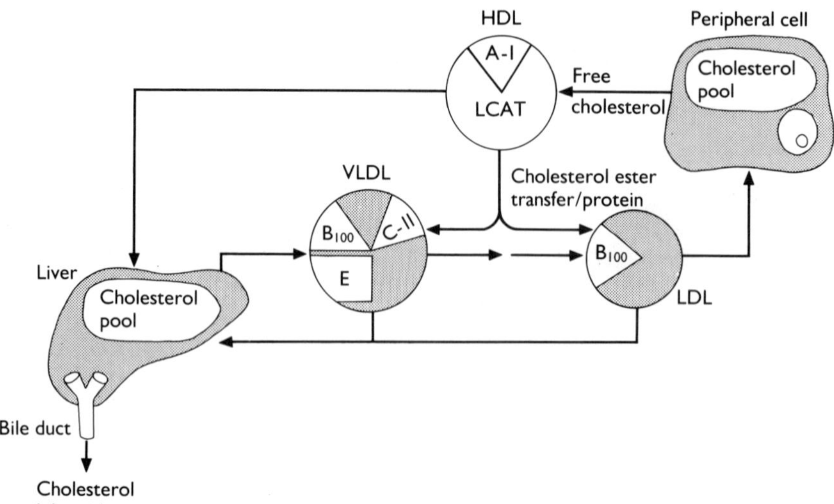

Fig. 36.5 HDL and reverse cholesterol transport. A-I, apoprotein A-I.

also decreases the cellular expression of LDL receptors, resulting in a decreased entry of LDL-derived cholesterol into the cell. Excess plasma LDL is removed by hepatic LDL receptors.

HIGH-DENSITY LIPOPROTEIN AND REVERSE CHOLESTEROL TRANSPORT

High-density lipoprotein, which transports approximately 20–30% of plasma cholesterol, exhibits considerable heterogeneity. This reflects the complex metabolism of these lipoproteins involving direct hepatic and intestinal synthesis of nascent HDL particles, the transfer of surface components to HDL during hydrolysis of triglyceride-rich lipoprotein particles and the exchange of cholesterol ester for triglycerides between HDL and other lipoproteins of lower density through the action of lipid transfer proteins (Fig. 36.5).

Lecithin–cholesteryl acyltransferase (LCAT), a key enzyme in cholesterol transport, circulates in HDL and apoprotein A-I, the major HDL apoprotein, is an important cofactor for LCAT activity. This enzyme catalyses the esterification of free cholesterol to cholesteryl ester, obtaining the fatty acyl residue from lecithin. Free cholesterol, the substrate for the LCAT reaction, may come from other lipoproteins or cell membranes. It is likely that specific receptors are involved in the interaction between HDL and peripheral cells. As nascent HDL particles, which are bilayer discs of apoprotein and phospholiped, accept free cholesterol and it is esterified by LCAT, the cholesteryl ester forms a hydrophobic droplet in the core of the particle which becomes spherical.

HDL is the major site of cholesterol esterification, and cholesteryl esters formed on HDL may transfer to VLDL, IDL and LDL via a cholesteryl ester exchange protein which enables a mole-for-mole exchange of triglyceride for cholesteryl ester between lipoproteins. In this way a major proportion of cholesteryl ester formed on HDL returns to the liver via other lipoproteins. However, HDL can also deliver cholesterol to the liver directly, but this process is quantitatively less important.

As described previously, HDL is intimately related to the metabolism of triglyceride-rich lipoproteins. Surface components of these particles transfer to HDL during their catabolism by lipoprotein lipase. This leads to the formation of larger, less dense particles designated HDL_2. The HDL fraction acts, in addition, as a reservoir for apoproteins C and E, which are important for normal catabolism of triglyceride-rich particles.

DYSLIPOPROTEINAEMIA

The term dyslipoproteinaemia or dyslipidaemia is used increasingly to describe alterations of the plasma lipid and lipoprotein profile from normal. This is because the various abnormalities may involve not only increased plasma concentrations but also significant decreases, particularly for instance in HDL. For this reason and the recognition of the importance of qualitative as well as quantitative abnormalities in plasma lipoproteins, dyslipoproteinaemia is the term preferred to hyperlipoproteinaemia.

There has been considerable progress in the understanding of lipid and lipoprotein metabolism over the past two decades. This has led to a classification of the dyslipidaemias based on the underlying pathophysiological mechanisms involved, and in some cases a detailed knowledge of the molecular genetics. The Fredrickson classification [5], later adopted by the World Health Organization (WHO) [6], provided an initial classification of plasma lipid

Table 36.3 Lipoprotein phenotypes

		Lipids			Lipoprotein pattern			
Type	Appearance of serum	Cholesterol	Triglycerides	Fasting chylomicrons	LDL	VLDL	HDL	Electrophoretic mobility
I	'Cream layer'; clear infranatant	Normal or ↑	Greatly ↑	Present	Normal or ↓	Mildly ↑, normal or ↓	Absent	Chylomicron at origin
IIa	Clear	↑	Normal	Absent	↑	Normal or ↓	Normal or ↓	β band ↑
IIb	Clear or faintly turbid	↑	↑	Absent	↑	↑	Normal or ↓	β band ↑, pre-β band ↑
III	Usually turbid; may be also faint 'cream layer'	↑	↑	Present; may be ↑	Density 1.006*–1.019 ↑ Density 1.019–1.063 ↓	↑†	Normal or ↓	'Broad β' band
IV	Usually turbid	Normal or ↑	↑	Absent	Normal or ↓	↑	Normal or ↓	Pre-β band ↑
V	'Cream layer'; turbid infranatant	Normal or ↑	Greatly ↑	↑	Normal ↓	↑	Usually ↓	Chylomicrons and pre-β band ↑

* Intermediate density lipoproteins.
† 'Floating' β-lipoproteins – density < 1.006 g/ml with β-electrophoretic mobility.

Table 36.4 Primary hyperlipidaemias

	WHO phenotype	Typical lipid levels (mmol/l)	Lipoproteins	CHD risk	Pancreatic risk	Possible clinical signs
Polygenic hypercholesterolaemia	IIa	Chol 6.5–9, trig < 2.3	LDL ↑	+	–	Xanthelasma, corneal arcus
Familial hypercholesterolaemia	IIa	Chol 7.5–16, trig < 2.3	LDL ↑	+++	–	Tendon xanthoma, arcus, xanthelasma
Familial defective apoprotein B_{100}	IIa	Chol 7.5–16, trig < 2.3	LDL ↑	+++	–	Tendon xanthoma, arcus, xanthelasma
Familial combined hyperlipidaemia	IIa, IIb, IV or V	Chol 6.5–10, trig 2.3–12	LDL ↑ VLDL ↑ HDL ↓	++	–	Arcus, xanthelasma
Remnant particle disease	III	Chole 9–14, trig 9–14	IDL ↑	+++	±	Palmar striae, tuberoeruptive xanthomas
Familial hypertriglyceridaemia	IV, V	Chol 6.5–12, trig 10–30	VLDL ↑ Chylomicrons ↑	?	++	Eruptive xanthomas, lipaemia retinalis, hepatosplenomegaly
Lipoprotein lipase deficiency	I	Chol < 6.5, trig 10–30	Chylomicrons ↑	–	+++	Eruptive xanthomas, lipaemia retinalis, hepatosplenomegaly
High HDL	–	HDL chol > 2.0	HDL ↑	–	–	–

Chol, cholesterol; trig, triglycerides.

disorders based on the measurement of fasting total cholesterol and triglyceride levels together with lipoprotein electrophoresis. Ultracentrifugation was needed for the confirmation of the presence of the abnormal apoprotein B containing lipoprotein in type III dyslipidaemia. Six lipoprotein phenotypes were described (Table 36.3).

This classification, although contributing very significantly to the development of knowledge in its time, has limitations because it is based entirely on laboratory techniques. A particular lipoprotein abnormality may result from more than one underlying metabolic disorder. For instance, the type IIa phenotype may be due to familial hypercholesterolaemia or hypothyroidism. Another limitation of the typing system is in the area of genetics. This is emphasized by the description of familial combined hyperlipidaemia, which is thought to be inherited as a single autosomal dominant gene, although the plasma lipoprotein phenotype may be variable in affected individuals and may change within the individual during therapy.

For these reasons, and the recognition of disorders of HDL metabolism not included in the earlier classification, dyslipidaemias are now classified into primary and secondary disorders. The nomenclature of the primary disorders is based where possible on the underlying metabolic and/or genetic abnormality (Table 36.4).

Primary dyslipidaemias

FAMILIAL HYPERCHOLESTEROLAEMIA

Familial hypercholesterolaemia (FH) is the best documented of the primary disorders of lipid metabolism [7]. It was the study of cholesterol metabolism in fibroblasts cultured from skin biopsies of individuals homozygous for this condition which enabled Brown and Goldstein to describe the LDL receptor and its relationship to cholesterol homeostasis [4]. This fundamental discovery led to the award of the Nobel Prize in Medicine to these investigators in 1985.

FH is characterized by autosomal dominant inheritance, the presence of cholesterol ester deposits in tendons referred to as tendon xanthomas, raised plasma cholesterol concentrations due to an increase in the LDL fraction and a massively increased risk of premature coronary heart disease (CHD).

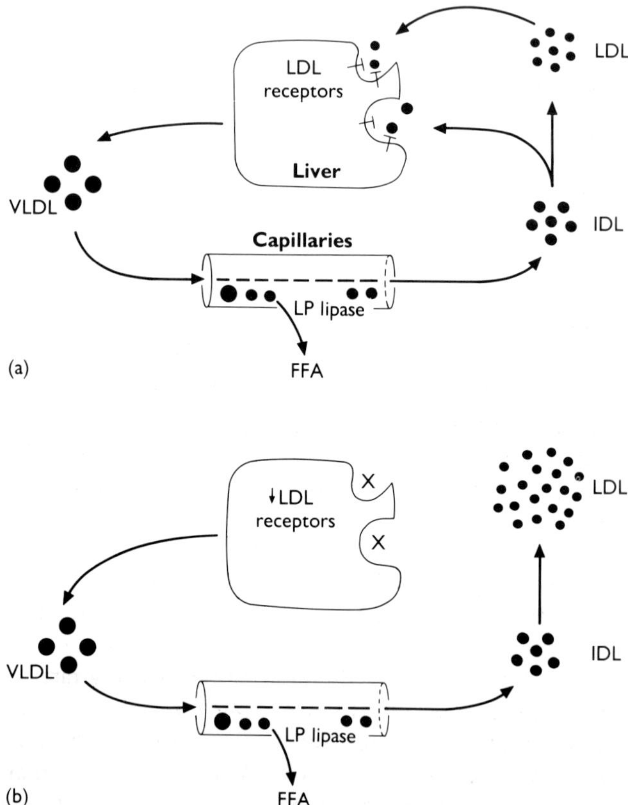

Fig. 36.6 LDL receptor defect in FH: (a) normal; (b) genetically defective receptor (from Brown & Goldstein [4]). FFA, free fatty acids; LP, lipoprotein.

Genetics and pathophysiology

Familial hypercholesterolaemia is a common genetic disorder, the frequency of heterozygosity being approximately 1:500 of the population. In some populations, particularly Lebanese and South African Afrikaaners, it is more common, affecting approximately 1:100–150. The familial clustering of high plasma cholesterol concentrations, tendon xanthomas and premature coronary disease was recognized in reports from Norway by Muller [8]. Subsequent studies of large pedigrees and pooled data from smaller families using segregation analysis pointed to the transmission of FH as a simple autosomal dominant trait [9]. It was the work of Khachadurian in the Lebanon, in an analysis of 52 individuals with xanthomas developing at a young age, which provided evidence that some individuals were homozygotes as opposed to severely affected heterozygotes [10]. There was a trimodal distribution of plasma cholesterol concentrations and sibship analysis demonstrated the numbers of homozygotes, heterozygotes and normals expected for a single gene disease.

The defect in FH is associated with decreased catabolism of LDL with a prolongation of plasma LDL half-life [11]. A lesion to the LDL receptor is responsible for the reduced clearance, particularly in the liver, of plasma LDL [4]. Reduced LDL receptor activity leads not only to failure of LDL clearance but also to increased production of LDL from IDL, since the LDL receptor is also responsible for hepatic removal of IDL (Fig. 36.6).

There are now approximately 150 different defects described at the DNA level in the LDL receptor leading to the clinical manifestations typical of FH. The mutations in the structural gene for the receptor have been classified into four main types [12]. Class 1 mutations, which are probably the most common, result in failure of receptor synthesis. Class 2 mutations lead to receptor synthesis but the receptors are blocked in transport to the cellular Golgi complex. Class 3 mutations lead to receptors that are transported to the cell surface but do not bind LDL normally. Class 4 mutations are the rarest of the mutations affecting the LDL receptor (Fig. 36.7). These mutations are associated with receptors which are synthesized and transported normally to the cell surface and bind LDL, but they are unable to cluster in the coated pit regions of the cell membrane, leading to failure of internalization of the receptor/LDL complex. For a detailed discussion of the various LDL receptor mutations the reader is referred to a recent review [13].

Some of the variation in severity of this condition is explained by the differing impact of the various mutations on LDL receptor function.

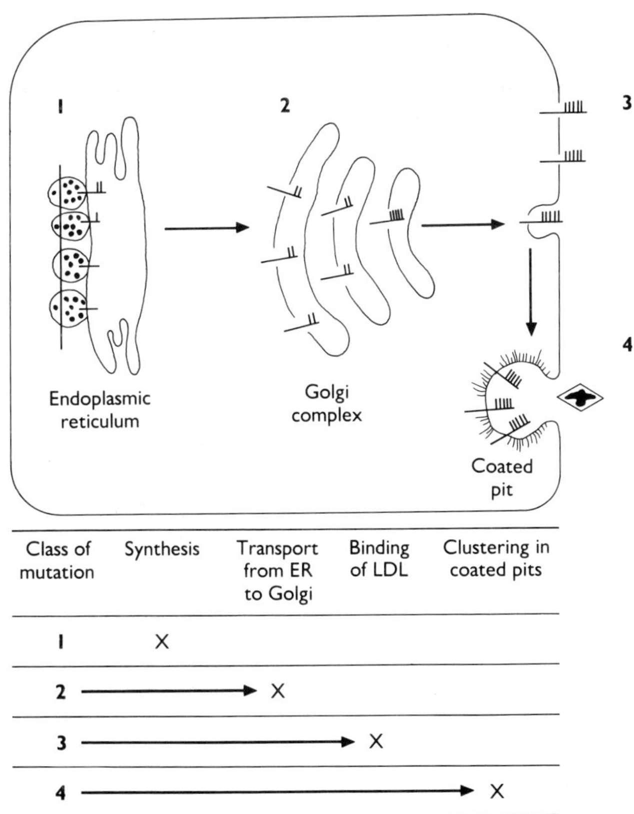

Fig. 36.7 Classes of LDL receptor mutations (from Goldstein & Brown [12]). ER, endoplasmic reticulum.

Plasma lipids and lipoproteins

The major abnormality is a markedly elevated plasma cholesterol concentration. The average cholesterol concentration in FH heterozygotes is about 9 mmol/l, even in populations with widely differing mean cholesterol concentrations in the general population. However, within individuals there can be marked variation in plasma cholesterol (7–14 mmol/l), even among members of the same family. Plasma cholesterol concentrations in FH homozygotes are usually in the range 15–30 mmol/l. The increase in plasma total cholesterol is, as might be expected from the underlying metabolic defect, due to increased numbers of LDL particles with average LDL cholesterol concentrations two- to three-fold higher than normal in heterozygotes and six-fold higher in homozygotes. Plasma triglyceride concentrations are occasionally elevated in FH individuals and HDL cholesterol tends to be reduced. The basis for these changes is not understood.

Xanthomas

The clinical hallmark of FH is the presence of xanthomas. These deposits of cholesteryl ester-laden foam cells are seen typically in the extensor tendons on the backs of the hands around the knuckles and in the Achilles tendons. Occasionally they occur in other tendons such as the patellar tendon and in the tendons on the feet. Subperiosteal xanthomas can occur at the tibial tuberosity (Plate 36.1, facing p. 706). Although not specific to FH, premature corneal arcus and xanthelasmas (tissue deposits around the eyelids) are often observed (Plate 36.2, facing p. 706). Tendon xanthomas occur in both heterozygotes and homozygotes. In heterozygotes tendon xanthomas may develop in childhood and adolescence, but are generally not present until the third and fourth decades. In homozygotes tendon xanthomas develop in childhood.

Cutaneous planar xanthomas are present in homozygotes. These lesions are yellow/orange and are found over the buttocks, hands and antecubital fossae (Plate 36.3, facing p. 706). Tendon xanthomas can also occur in two very rare conditions, cerebrotendinous xanthomatosis and sitosterolaemia, but this should not give rise to diagnostic difficulty.

Unfortunately many physicians fail to notice the important clinical sign of tendon xanthomas and patients may be subjected to excision of the xanthomas before the diagnosis has been made. Occasionally xanthomas can be painful, particularly in the Achilles, and patients may be referred initially to the rheumatology clinic.

Premature coronary heart disease

The importance of FH in relation to premature CHD is three-fold. First it is the inborn error of cholesterol metabolism leading to high plasma LDL levels seen in FH which demonstrates the importance of LDL as the important atherogenic particle. Individuals with FH do not require the other important risk factors (smoking, hypertension or diabetes mellitus) to develop premature and extensive atherosclerosis. Much is now known about the interaction of LDL with important cells in the atherogenic process resulting in foam cell formation [14]. Secondly, within families carrying the gene for FH premature CHD is often devastating, particularly in affected males. However, in terms of the generality of CHD the impact of FH is small. Thirdly, some definite FH heterozygotes survive well into old age. It is possible that studies in these individuals will help to identify factors protective for CHD.

In FH homozygotes, who are fortunately very rare (approximately one in a million), clinical manifestations of coronary atherosclerosis develop in childhood. Myocardial infarction has been described as early as 18 months of age and death before the age of 30 years is usual.

In FH heterozygotes, clinical CHD can develop in the 20s, particularly in men, of whom over 50% die by the age of 60 compared to 15% of women [15]. The average age of onset of CHD is 43 years in men and 53 years in women, and the mean age of death is 55 years in men and 64 years in women [16]. It is not explained why the premature atherosclerosis of FH heterozygotes shows such a predilection for the coronary arteries. The incidence of cerebrovascular disease does not appear to be increased, although peripheral vascular disease is slightly increased. In homozygotes, extensive atherosclerosis is also seen in the thoracic and abdominal aorta and the major pulmonary arteries. Significant aortic stenosis can result from atheromatous involvements of the aortic valve and surgical correction of deformed and atherosclerotic aortic values has been reported [17]. Atherosclerotic plaques can be prominent in the aortic supravalvular region, leading to obstruction of the left ventricular outflow tract [18].

DIAGNOSIS AND MANAGEMENT

Heterozygous familial hypercholesterolaemia

An opinion is likely to be sought for a child following the premature death of a parent from CHD or the diagnosis of FH in a parent. It is routine in lipid clinics to screen the offspring of FH heterozygotes. More rarely children will be referred with the clinical stigmas of FH. Plasma cholesterol levels are lower in children, the 95th centile being approximately 5.2 mmol/l. Often there is no doubt of the diagnosis with cholesterol levels of 7 or 8 mmol/l but the diagnosis may be doubted if the cholesterol is in the grey area around 5.5–6.5 mmol/l. In such cases, further tests are advisable annually. Cholesterol levels in children of FH heterozygotes are bimodally distributed and the plasma cholesterol level at which minimal misclassification occurred was 6.8 mmol/l [19]. The diagnosis in a child with homozygous FH should not prove to be a problem because of the massive increase in plasma cholesterol concentration, often with the typical stigmas.

In view of the lack of precision of diagnosis in the FH heterozygote child on the basis of plasma cholesterol concentrations alone, other methods have been attempted. Measurement of LDL receptor activity in cultured fibroblasts or freshly isolated lymphocytes unfortunately shows overlap between normals and FH heterozygotes. In view of the many different mutations affecting the LDL receptor, DNA analysis in unlikely to aid diagnosis. However, in families where the mutation in the LDL receptor is known, DNA analysis is diagnostic. In families where both parents are heterozygote, the possibility of a homozygous infant may be raised. Prenatal diagnosis has been performed in such situations by measuring LDL receptor activity in amniotic cells [20], and it is likely that genetic analyses will eventually facilitate prenatal diagnosis.

The clinical question arises in the FH heterozygote child whether or when to instigate cholesterol-lowering therapy. Unlike the other primary disorders of lipid metatolism which are associated with increased CHD risk, the plasma lipid abnormality is present from birth in FH. It is likely that the atherogenic process begins in childhood and adolescence, and it would seem logical that preventive measures should also be instituted at an early age. Against this has to be balanced the impact on lifestyle of strict diet and, as this is often insufficient to reduce plasma cholesterol to satisfactory levels, the long-term tolerability and safety of cholesterol-lowering drugs.

There are no long-term studies of cholesterol lowering starting in FH children showing prevention or delay in the development of CHD. Indeed it is unlikely that trials will be performed because of ethical problems in leaving individuals at such high risk untreated. However, information from primary and secondary prevention trials of cholesterol-lowering therapy in adults has provided unequivocal evidence of benefit in terms of reduction in CHD events [21]. Furthermore, angiographic studies have shown that the progression of coronary atherosclerosis can be delayed; indeed regression has been observed. Such findings have also been demonstrated in FH heterozygotes [21].

The controversy surrounding lipid-lowering therapy in adults rests on a failure to demonstrate a reduction in overall mortality even on meta-analysis of all available trials. A trial with the statistical power to examine effects of cholesterol lowering with the drug simvastatin on overall mortality was started in the UK in 1993. Until the results are available, drug therapy is reserved for those individuals considered to be at highest risk of premature CHD. FH heterozygotes come under this high-risk category.

It can be appreciated that the decision to instigate therapy, particularly drug therapy, is a matter of clinical judgement. It is the author's practice when deciding on drug therapy in children to take into account the age at which CHD developed in the child's family. More aggressive therapy is indicated if CHD developed in the affected relative in his or her 20s. In general terms drug therapy is less likely to be indicated in girls, as their risk is less. However, in some families with FH, CHD may develop early in affected women. If the child belongs to such a family, drug therapy may be indicated. The measurement of lipoprotein-(a) is helpful, as it is an important risk factor for CHD in the presence of high cholesterol levels [22,23]. If lipoprotein-α levels are high, treatment should be more aggressive.

Dietary treatment

Dietary treatment remains the cornerstone of treatment in all types of dyslipidaemia and should be recommended

Table 36.5 Basic principles of lipid-lowering diet

Principle	Amount	Food sources
Decrease total fat	< 30% energy	Butter, hard margarine, whole milk, cream
Decrease saturated fat	7% to 10% of energy	Ice cream, high-fat cheese, fatty meats and poultry, sausages, pastries, coffee whitener, products containing hydrogenated oils, palm oil and coconut oil
Increase use of high-protein food (low in saturated fat)		Fish, chicken and turkey; veal, game, spring lamb
Increase complex carbohydrate; increase fruit and vegetable fibre; increase legumes	About 35 g/day of fibre, one-half derived from fruit and vegetables	All fruit, including dried fruit, all fresh and frozen vegetables; lentils, dried beans, chick peas; unrefined cereal foods, including oats
Decrease dietary cholesterol	< 300 mg/day	Allowance up to 2 egg yolks per week; liver up to twice monthly; other offal avoided
Moderately increase use of mono- and polyunsaturated oils and products	Mono: 10% to 15% of energy Poly: 7% to 10% of energy	Olive oil, sunflower oil, corn oil and products based on these

From Anon [24].

in children with FH. Growth and development proceed normally on a low-fat diet, which can be instituted at about 5 years of age. In the USA a low-fat diet may be introduced after the age of 2 years. The principles of the cholesterol-lowering diet are shown in Table 36.5. It is help in clinical practice to have the assistance of a dietician who is experienced with children.

Dietary therapy leads to a small reduction in plasma cholesterol in children with FH (≈10%) but certainly not to the normal range. However, in families where the CHD develops later in life, the small response to dietary therapy may be acceptable and lipid-lowering drug therapy can be introduced, particularly in boys, in late teenage. Hopefully a prudent diet started at an early age, together with other lifestyle measures, including the avoidance of cigarette smoking, obesity and the encouragement of appropriate exercise will facilitate management in later life.

Drug therapy

The only class of hypolipidaemic drugs generally considered suitable for children are the anion-exchange resins [25], of which there are two currently available, cholestyramine and colestipol. These agents have been available for over two decades, their safety is well established and their major advantage over other hypolipidaemic agents is that they remain unabsorbed during their passage through the gastrointestinal tract, so there is no risk of systemic effects.

The resins bind bile acids in the intestine, thus interrupting the enterohepatic circulation. As a result, bile acid synthesis from cholesterol is stimulated in the liver. As hepatic cholesterol is consumed, there is increased expression of LDL receptors and increased binding and removal of plasma LDL. In addition, hepatic cholesterol synthesis is increased, which partly overcomes the effectiveness of resins in stimulating LDL receptor activity. At maximum dosage, resin therapy is effective in reducing plasma LDL cholesterol by up to 30% [26]. HDL cholesterol concentration may increase slightly, but the mechanism of this effect is not known. Sometimes plasma triglyceride rises during resin therapy due to increased VLDL synthesis in the liver. This effect is often transient and does not usually present a problem unless the plasma triglyceride is raised before treatment.

There may be major compliance problems with the resins. Some patients find the texture of the drugs unpleasant, and there is no doubt that they are tedious to take, particularly in high dosage. In addition, gastrointestinal side-effects are common, including constipation, nausea and a bloating sensation. Colicky pain and diarrhoea occur in some patients. Some of the side-effects may be overcome by starting the resins in low dose. Premixing the resins with fluid, and refrigeration overnight, helps to overcome the gritty texture. The resins can also be incorporated into foodstuffs.

FAMILIAL DEFECTIVE APOLIPOPROTEIN B

Some hypercholesterolaemic individuals have defective binding of LDL to the LDL receptor [27]. In these patients the reduced binding is due to defective LDL rather than to defective receptors and an abnormality in the LDL apoprotein B with the substitution of glutamine for arginine at amino acid 3500 has been described [28]. This defect gives rise to a clinical syndrome similar to classical FH; it has a frequency of 1:500 to 1:700, which is also similar to FH [29]. These individuals appear to respond to diet and drugs in a way similar to individuals with classical heterozygous FH.

CHYLOMICRONAEMIA

Primary hyperchylomicronaemia is infrequent in children, and is due to rare autosomal recessive conditions (one homozygote per million) involving either the enzyme lipoprotein lipase or its major cofactor apoprotein C-II. In addition a family has been reported which appears to have a circulating inhibitor of lipoprotein lipase [30].

Clinical features

Hyperchylomicronaemia may be discovered incidentally when blood is taken for another cause, but most cases are accompanied by characteristic clinical symptoms and signs. The most important clinical problem is abdominal pain and sometimes pancreatitis. The abdominal pain is episodic and variable both in severity and position. Although the pain is commonly felt in the epigastrium with radiation to the back, it may be present in both the right and left hypochondria. Pancreatitis is acute and may be recurrent. The diagnosis may be hindered by the presence of a normal amylase estimation due to interference with the assay [31]. It is unusual for children with pancreatitis secondary to hyperchylomicronaemia to develop the clinical sequelae of malabsorption and diabetes. The explanation(s) of the abdominal pain and pancreatitis are not understood.

Hepatosplenomegaly is common and will vary with the extent of plasma triglyceride elevation. The organomegaly is related to the uptake of triglyceride by macrophages leading to foam-cell formation. With effective reduction of plasma triglycerides the organomegaly resolves over several days.

The characteristic physical sign of hyperchylomicronaemia is the presence of lipid deposits in skin macrophages known as eruptive xanthomas (Plate 36.4, facing p. 706). These lesions tend to aggregate over pressure areas, such as elbows, knees and buttocks, but may be more generalized in severe cases. The individual lesions are small (a few millimetres across) and yellow/pink. They are not tender. The presence of these lesions indicates severe chronic hyperchylomicronaemia but they do regress, often rapidly, when plasma triglyceride levels are corrected.

When plasma triglycerides are very high (above 30–40 mmol/l), examination of the optic fundus may reveal lipaemia retinalis with a generalized pink colour of the retina and retinal vessels due to the effect of chylomicrons scattering light. Despite this dramatic picture there is no effect on vision, and the appearances regress when the plasma triglyceride concentration is reduced.

Some patients with severe hyperchylomicronaemia complain of vague headaches and mood changes similar to symptoms associated with the hyperviscosity syndrome. Triglycerides at this level do increase plasma viscosity. Shortness of breath has also been described.

Laboratory measurements

The striking feature of the plasma in the hyperchylomicronaemia syndrome is its milky (lipaemic) appearance, which is often readily apparent when blood is drawn into the syringe. Plasma triglyceride concentrations are usually greater than 10 mmol/l and often around 40–50 mmol/l. Chylomicrons are not normally present in fasting plasma, and perhaps the simplest way to demonstrate their presence is to stand the separated plasma in a refrigerator at 4°C overnight. Chylomicrons float to the top of the tube to give a creamy layer. The plasma below this layer may be turbid or clear, depending on the presence of VLDL triglyceride. Chylomicrons may also be demonstrated by lipoprotein electrophoresis, but, if plasma triglycerides are greater than 10–15 mmol/l it is likely that chylomicrons are present. The plasma cholesterol may be normal or raised, depending on whether VLDL particles are increased. LDL and HDL are low.

The massive hypertriglyceridaemia may interfere with other laboratory assays. The effect on amylase determinations has already been discussed. In addition the measurement of haemoglobin may be affected. Bilirubin levels may be artefactually increased, and because chylomicrons replace water volume there is an artefactual decrease in plasma sodium concentrations.

Pathogenesis

Identification of the underlying defect in primary hyperchylomicronaemia in childhood requires specialist lipid laboratory help. Most children have classical lipoprotein lipase deficiency. This enzyme is responsible for the hydrolysis of chylomicron triglyceride. Activity of lipoprotein lipase is usually assessed as lipolytic activity in plasma following a bolus of heparin, which releases the enzyme from capillary beds. Lipoprotein lipase activity is very low or absent in these individuals, but hepatic lipase activity is normal. In some individuals it is possible to demonstrate immunoreactive enzyme which does not possess catalytic activity.

Since the complementary DNA for human lipoprotein lipase has been cloned and sequenced, and the genomic organization established, mutations have been sought in individuals with lipoprotein lipase deficiency. The mutations identified thus far are shown in Table 36.6 [32].

Other families with a clinical syndrome similar to classical lipoprotein lipase deficiency have been shown to

Table 36.6 Mutations in lipoprotein lipase gene

Type of mutation	Amino-acid substitution	Location	Protein defect
Duplication	–	Exon 6	Null allele
Deletion	–	Exon 3–5	Null allele
Missense	Threonine for alanine	Residue 176, exon 5	Heparin binding defective
Missense	Glutamic acid for glycine	Residue 188, exon 5	Inactive enzyme, normal heparin binding
Nonsense	Stop codon for glutamine	Residue 106, exon 3	Inactive enzyme

From Hayden [32].

have a normal enzyme but a deficiency of apoprotein C-II, the major cofactor [33]. These individuals tend to have a less severe syndrome than those with enzyme deficiency. A range of molecular defects has been demonstrated in families with apoprotein C-II deficiency ranging from no detectable enzyme protein to absence of amino acids 69–73 at the carboxy-terminal end of the molecule, the region responsible for activation of the lipase enzyme [34]. A combination of lipoprotein lipase deficiency and C-II deficiency has been observed [35].

A family with primary hyperchylomicronaemia has been described [36] who had normal lipoprotein lipase and normal apoprotein C-II but in whom there was a circulating enzyme inhibitor. The nature of this inhibitor, which was present in the non-lipoprotein fraction of plasma, has not been elucidated.

Management

These disorders respond well to a low-fat diet, in that the hypertriglyceridaemia is reduced to a level of about 10 mmol/l where the risk of pancreatitis is reduced and the eruptive xanthomas and episodic abdominal pain are no longer a problem. However, compliance with this diet is difficult and the family needs to be well motivated. All types of fat, polyunsaturated as well as saturated, need to be reduced. To make the diet more palatable, it is possible to include medium-chain triglycerides, since these are absorbed through the portal system and not incorporated into chylomicrons. It is important to avoid factors which exacerbate hypertriglyceridaemia, such as hypotensive agents of the diuretic and β-blocker classes, alcohol and oestrogen. In those individuals in whom VLDL levels are also increased, a small reduction in total triglycerides may be obtained with fibric acid derivatives.

FAMILIAL COMBINED HYPERLIPIDAEMIA

Familial combined hyperlipidaemia (FCHL) was first described in the families of survivors of myocardial infarction [37]. Affected individuals may have different abnormalities in their plasma lipid profile, hypercholesterolaemia, hypertriglyceridaemia or both. FCHL is associated with an increased risk of CHD regardless of the particular lipid abnormality. It has been estimated that 10% of individuals presenting with myocardial infarction before the age of 60 years have FCHL. It is probably the commonest inherited hyperlipidaemia and its frequency has been estimated at 0.5–1% of the population, although without a definitive clinical or genetic marker for the disease it is difficult to be certain of this.

FCHL appears to follow an autosomal dominant pattern of inheritance, but the genetic defect(s) has not yet been described. The metabolic abnormality appears to be an increased production of apoprotein-B-containing lipoproteins in the liver. FCHL is probably a heterogeneous condition and different genetic forms will be found. For instance, the characteristics of FCHL have been described in obligate heterozygotes for lipoprotein lipase deficiency [38].

The diagnosis of FCHL is often presumptive in an individual with mixed lipaemia and a family history of premature CHD. Confirmation of the diagnosis requires family screening of plasma lipids and demonstration of the variable lipid phenotype. Tendon xanthomas characteristically seen in familial hypercholesterolaemia are not seen in FCHL.

Awareness of FCHL is important because the presence of premature CHD and dyslipidaemia within a family may lead to lipid screening. Unlike familial hypercholesterolaemia, where the plasma lipid abnormality is present from birth, FCHL is most commonly not manifest until late teenage. Although plasma lipid levels may be slightly raised in younger children, it is likely that the younger child will not obviously be affected. It is important to emphasize the need for testing at an older age, and not to dismiss the diagnosis.

DYSBETALIPOPROTEINAEMIA

Dysbetalipoproteinaemia, also called broad β disease or type III dyslipoproteinaemia in the Fredrickson classification, affects approximately 1:5000 of the population [39]. It is associated with premature and extensive atherosclerosis with a predilection for peripheral vessels as well as the coronary arteries. There are often striking yellow/

orange cutaneous deposits of lipid in the creases of the hand (palmar xanthomas). Tuberous and tuberoeruptive xanthomas may be seen over the elbows and knees.

Plasma total cholesterol and total triglyceride are raised to roughly the same degree, approximately 10 mmol/l because of the accumulation of remnant particles of triglyceride-rich lipoproteins. These particles are seen as a broad β band on lipoprotein electrophoresis. If VLDL is separated by ultracentrifugation the cholesterol/triglyceride ratio is greater than 0.4 and demonstrates β mobility as well as pre-β mobility on electrophoresis, indicating abnormal composition as a result of the remnant particles.

The development of remnant particle disease is dependent on the inheritance of an abnormal apoprotein E, namely apoprotein E_2, which is characterized by the substitution of a cystine for an arginine residue at position 158. This is one of three major isoforms of apoprotein E resulting from the existence of three alleles at a single gene locus. The $E_{3/3}$ phenotype is present in 50–60% of the population, $E_{4/3}$ in about 25%, $E_{3/2}$ in about 15% and $E_{2/2}$ in 1%. Apoprotein E_2 is a poor ligand for hepatic receptors, and all individuals with remnant disease have the E_2/E_2 phenotype. Although the phenotype is present in 1:100 of the population, clinical disease develops rarely. It is therefore necessary for another metabolic abnormality to be present in addition to the abnormal apoprotein E for the syndrome to develop. This may be another genetic abnormality, such as familial combined hyperlipidaemia, or a secondary cause of dyslipidaemia, such as diabetes or obesity.

This disease manifests itself in adults, and there are only rare reports of its development in teenage life. The paediatrician may be asked to screen children of affected individuals and the best test, which is available in specialist lipid centres, is to perform apoprotein E phenotyping. The child homozygous for apoprotein E_2 is at risk of developing remnant disease if in addition factors such as FCHL are present. Lipid screening should be recommended in late teenage and again in the early 20s. It is important to recognize the disease, since it usually responds dramatically to a low-fat diet and drugs of the fibrate class.

FAMILIAL HYPERTRIGLYCERIDAEMIA

Severe hypertriglyceridaemia with chylomicrons and increased VLDL may be distinct from lipoprotein lipase deficiency, and is usually associated with the presence of a secondary disorder, such as diabetes or alcohol excess. When the families of these individuals are tested, individuals with milder hypertriglyceridaemia may be identified. It is likely that a combination of a genetic cause (probably polygenic) and a secondary cause is required. Severe hypertriglyceridaemia can occasionally occur in the absence of secondary factors, but this is very rare (approximately 1:10000 of the population). The nature of the underlying defect(s) remains to be identified, but lipoprotein lipase activity is normal or only slightly decreased. The condition is inherited as an autosomal dominant. It is distinct from FCHL in that all affected individuals have elevated plasma triglycerides as a result of increased VLDL, and LDL concentrations are low. Increased risk of premature CHD is not a feature of familial hypertriglyceridaemia.

Treatment is required to prevent the risk of pancreatitis in individuals who are severely affected. This involves a low-fat diet with the addition of lipid-lowering drugs of the fibrate or nicotinic-acid class. The condition does not usually manifest itself until adolescence. Therefore if young children of affected probands are tested, and the plasma triglyceride is normal, a further test should be recommended in late teenage.

SECONDARY DYSLIPOPROTEINAEMIA

Many disorders are associated with secondary disturbances of lipid and lipoprotein metabolism. In some cases the associated lipid abnormalities may contribute to the morbidity of the primary disease (Table 36.7).

Table 36.7 Secondary hyperlipidaemias

Metabolic and hormonal factors
Diabetes mellitus
Hypothyroidism
Obesity
Anorexia nervosa
Bulimia
Glycogen storage disease
Alcohol abuse
Renal dysfunction
Nephrotic syndrome
Chronic renal disease
Acute intermittent porphyria
Lipodystrophy
Dysglobulinaemia
Werner syndrome
Liver disease
Biliary cirrhosis
Sclerosing cholangitis
Extrahepatic biliary obstruction
Iatrogenic
Corticosteroids
Exogenous sex hormones
Retinoids
High-dose thiazide diuretics
β-Adrenergic-receptor antagonists that lack α-blocking effects, intrinsic sympathetic activity or vasodilator properties

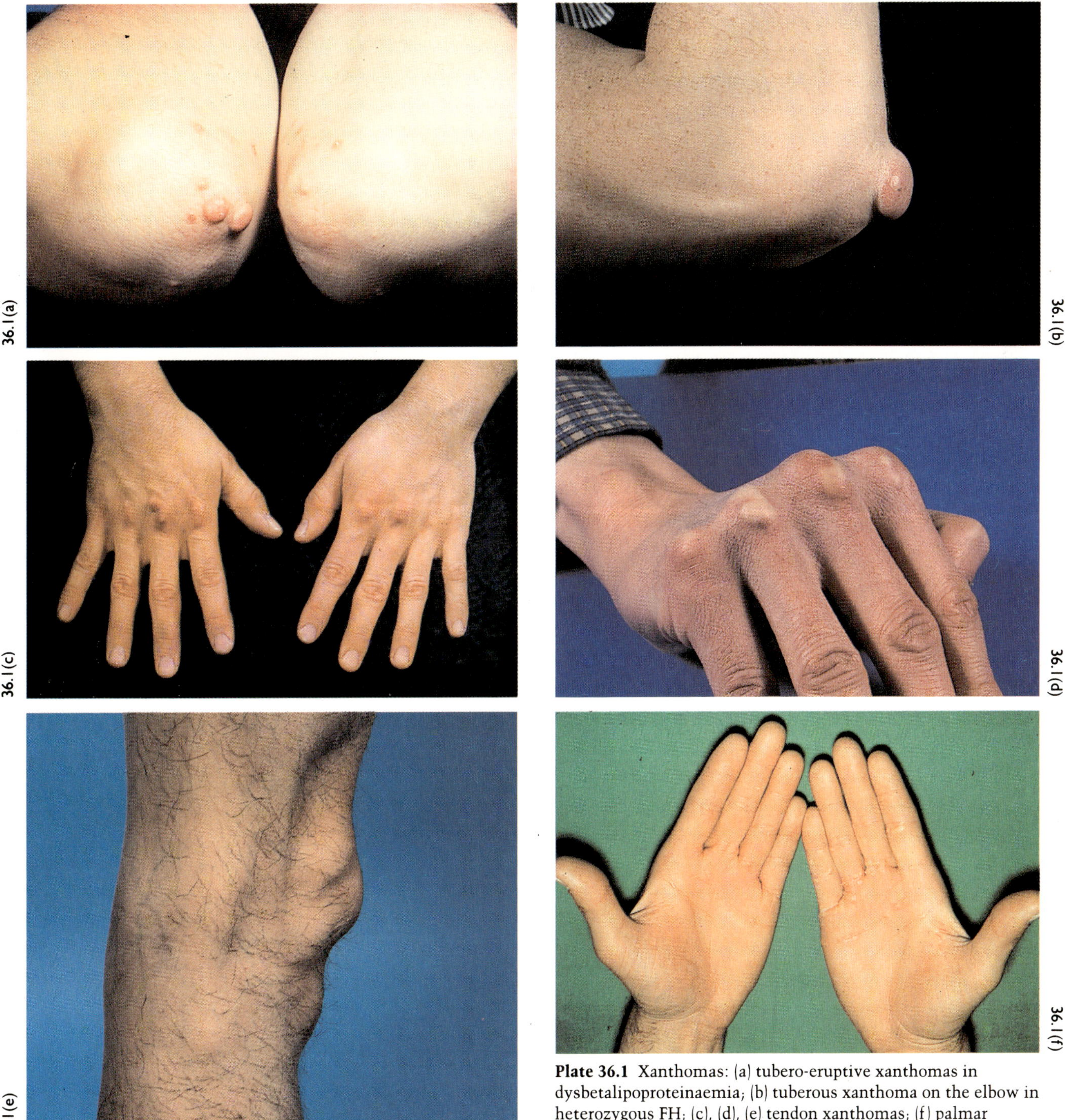

Plate 36.1 Xanthomas: (a) tubero-eruptive xanthomas in dysbetalipoproteinaemia; (b) tuberous xanthoma on the elbow in heterozygous FH; (c), (d), (e) tendon xanthomas; (f) palmar xanthomas in the hands in dysbetalipoproteinaemia.

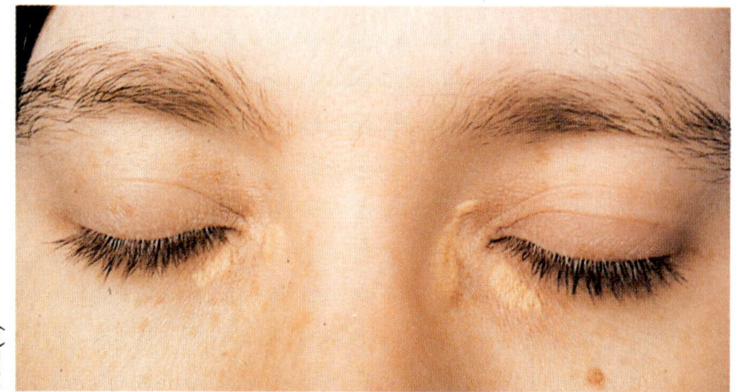

36.2(a)

Plate 36.2(a) Xanthelasma.

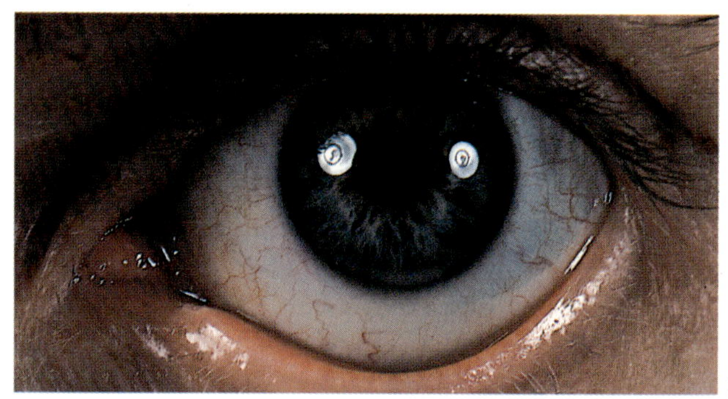

36.2(b)

Plate 36.2(b) Corneal arcus.

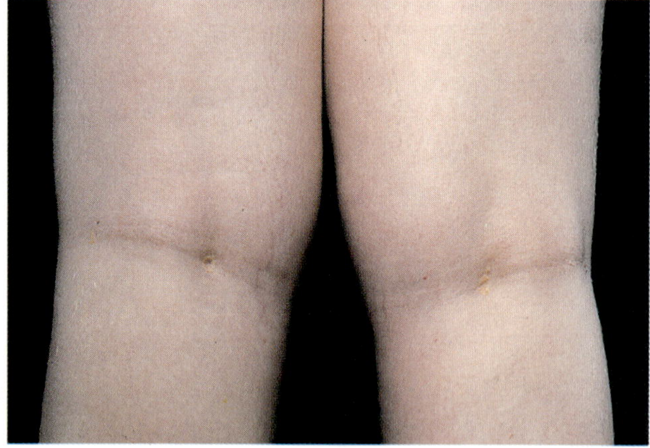

36.3(a)

36.3(b)

Plate 36.3 Cutaneous lipid deposition in a child with severe heterozygous FH.

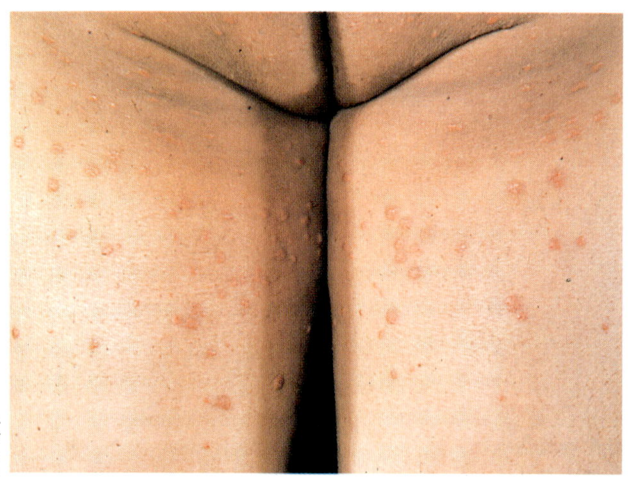

36.4(a)

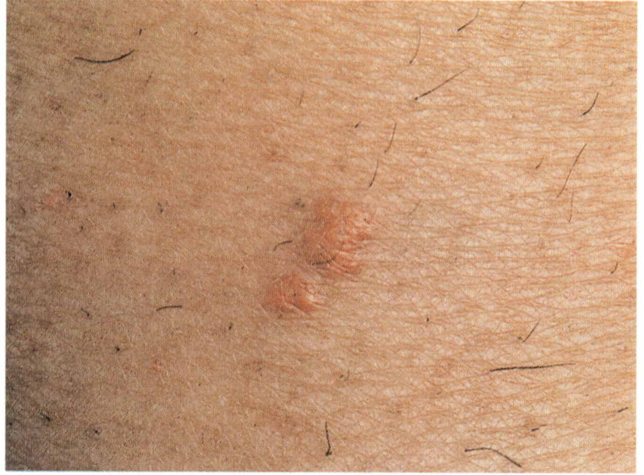

36.4(b)

Plate 36.4 Eruptive xanthomas.

DIABETES MELLITUS

Diabetes is a common cause of secondary dyslipidaemia but the major abnormalities are seen in patients with non-insulin-dependent diabetes mellitus (NIDDM). Plasma lipid abnormalities in insulin-dependent diabetes mellitus (IDDM) are usually a feature of poor glycaemic control or due to another primary or secondary cause [40].

In newly presenting IDDM children, particularly those with severe ketosis, lipaemic plasma may be observed. Triglyceride levels in this situation may be very high (40–50 mmol/l) due to the accumulation of chylomicrons and VLDL. This is due to failure of normal catabolism of triglyceride-rich particles because of decreased activity of lipoprotein lipase. Instigation of insulin therapy which restores lipoprotein lipase activity leads to rapid clearance of the lipaemic plasma over a few days. An important clinical point to remember is that the lipaemic plasma may interfere with the measurement of sodium, as discussed previously.

In the child on insulin therapy plasma lipid levels are influenced by the degree of glycaemic control. Poor control is associated with increased concentrations of plasma triglyceride and cholesterol, and a reduced HDL level. The IDDM child with near-normal glycated haemoglobin will have plasma lipid levels similar to non-diabetic children, and HDL concentrations are normal or slightly increased. However, cardiovascular disease remains the most important cause of morbidity and mortality in the diabetic population in the long term. Epidemiological studies have indicated an even more important role for plasma cholesterol as a risk factor for vascular disease in diabetics than in non-diabetics [41]. Plasma triglyceride also appears to be more strongly related to vascular disease in diabetics. For these reasons an annual measurement of plasma lipids should be performed on all diabetics, and attempts made to ensure that the plasma lipid profile is maintained within the published guidelines [42]. It is important to exclude hypothyroidism as a cause of hypercholesterolaemia in IDDM.

Proteinuria is an important risk marker in diabetes, not only for nephropathy but also for cardiovascular disease [43]. Diabetics with proteinuria (including microalbuminuria) have higher plasma lipid levels, particularly LDL cholesterol and apoprotein B which may contribute to this increased risk [44]. The mechanism(s) for these changes is not yet understood.

Management of dyslipidaemia in the diabetic involves improving glycaemic control and attention to diet. Other primary and secondary causes of dyslipidaemia should be excluded and managed as for the non-diabetic. Lipid-lowering therapy with drugs remains a matter of clinical judgement as no long-term clinical trials have been performed to assess benefit. Nevertheless, diabetes itself is an important risk factor for cardiovascular disease, and it is likely that the treatment of other major risk factors, including plasma lipids, will reduce vascular risk. It is likely that in future more diabetics will receive lipid-lowering drugs but there is not a case for introducing these agents in children at present.

HYPOTHYROIDISM

The elevation of plasma cholesterol which accompanies hypothyroidism has been known for many years. However, all types of dyslipidaemia may be found in hypothyroidism through effects on the activity of the lipoprotein lipase enzyme, remnant particle removal and LDL receptor activity [45–47]. When other abnormalities of lipid and lipoprotein metabolism are present, these can be exacerbated by hypothyroidism leading to marked dyslipidaemia. In individuals homozygous for apoprotein E_2 the full clinical syndrome of remnant particle disease may develop with the characteristic xanthomas. The lipid abnormalities in familial hypercholesterolaemia are more marked with concurrent hypothyroidism. The chylomicron syndrome may be precipitated in individuals with familial hypertriglyceridaemia.

It is important to exclude hypothyroidism as a cause of significant dyslipidaemia in all individuals, even if the classical symptoms and signs of the disorder are absent. The instigation of treatment with thyroxine leads to the restoration of plasma lipid and lipoprotein levels to normal in a few weeks. If abnormalities persist when thyroid function is normal, another cause is likely.

RENAL DISEASE

In the nephrotic syndrome the occurrence of increased plasma cholesterol concentration (often marked) due to high LDL concentrations is well known. In addition, elevations of plasma triglyceride due to increased VLDL and low HDL concentrations are often present [48,49]. These abnormalities are due to increased hepatic production of apoprotein B-containing lipoproteins, together with defects in lipoprotein catabolism. The increase in plasma LDL is due to increased production, as demonstrated by kinetic studies, and is proportional to the degree of proteinuria and hypoalbuminuria [50]. Hypertriglyceridaemia when present is secondary to clearance defects, probably as a result of decreased lipoprotein lipase activity. Occasionally the chylomicronaemia syndrome may develop. Urinary loss of HDL apoproteins occurs in the nephrotic syndrome [51], which contributes to the low plasma HDL concentration and possible reduced activation of lipoprotein lipase. The lipid abnormalities in the nephrotic syndrome may be exacerbated by therapy with glucocorticoids.

In long-standing nephrotic syndrome there is increasing awareness of the importance of the concurrent dyslipidaemia in relation to atherosclerotic risk. With this in mind adults with this condition are receiving specific diet and drug therapy for the dyslipidaemia. It is difficult to give clear guidelines on the management of the dyslipidaemia of nephrotic syndrome in children. Intervention remains a matter of clinical judgement depending on the degree of dyslipidaemia and the chronicity of the syndrome.

In chronic renal failure hypertriglyceridaemia is commonly found, and persists after dialysis [52]. This appears to be due to decreased activity of lipoprotein lipase, possibly related to as yet unknown inhibitory substances. Remnant particle accumulation also appears to contribute to the hypertriglyceridaemia [53]. Plasma HDL concentrations are low in chronic renal failure and LDL is unremarkable. Some patients with chronic renal failure have the nephrotic syndrome and the lipid abnormalities associated with this syndrome are corrected by dialysis. It is likely that the lipid abnormalities in adults with chronic renal failure are associated with increased atherosclerotic risk. However, intervention is for the most part restricted to non-pharmacological methods because of the increased risk of side-effects with lipid-lowering drugs. In children with chronic renal failure intervention to control coexistent dyslipidaemia remains a matter of clinical judgement, but at present drug therapy cannot be recommended.

Plasma lipid and lipoprotein abnormalities are common in postrenal transplantation patients due to the administration of glucocorticoids which increase both plasma LDL and VLDL [54]. Cyclosporin also leads to increased LDL concentrations [55]. The most active therapeutic agents for increased LDL concentrations are the HMG-CoA reductase agents. However, there are important interactions between these drugs and cyclosporin, leading to increased risk of rhabdomyolysis. For this reason considerable care needs to be exercised in the treatment of hypercholesterolaemia in transplant patients [56]. Emerging reports suggest that low-dose therapy with HMG-CoA reductase inhibitors with frequent safety monitoring may be an option if lifestyle measures fail.

LIVER DISEASE

Severe hepatocellular damage is associated with decreased production of lipoproteins, and low plasma levels occur. In obstructive liver disease hypercholesterolaemia may be severe and xanthomas can develop. An abnormal LDL particle has been described in cholestasis, termed lipoprotein X. This particle is rich in free cholesterol rather than cholesteryl ester, producing a disc-shaped, as opposed to a pseudomicellar, particle. Lipoprotein X is the result of decreased LCAT activity [57].

GLYCOGEN STORAGE DISEASES

Hypertriglyceridaemia and hypercholesterolaemia occur in type I (glucose-6-phosphatase deficiency), type III (amylo-1,6-glucosidase deficiency) and type VI (phosphorylase b kinase deficiency) glycogen storage diseases. The mechanism(s) of these lipid abnormalities relate to the increased flux of free fatty acids from adipose tissue to the liver, leading to increased hepatic VLDL production. In addition the increase in hepatic lactic acid concentrations favours fatty acid synthesis and esterification through effects on acetyl-CoA carboxylase, malonyl-CoA and glycerol-3-phosphate. The hyperlipidaemia is improved but not normalized by nocturnal nasogastric feeding and frequent daytime meals [58].

Rare lipid disorders which may be present in childhood

TANGIER DISEASE

This exceedingly rare but fascinating disorder is named after Tangier Island in Virginia, USA, where the first case, a 5-year-old boy, lived [59]. It is characterized by an absence of normal HDL in plasma and the accumulation of cholesteryl esters in many tissues. Histiocytes laden with cholesteryl ester lead to hepatosplenomegaly, and deposits are also found in thymus lymph nodes, skin, intestinal mucosa and cornea. However, perhaps the most striking clinical findings are the hyperplastic tonsils, which have a characteristic orange appearance. Variable neurological abnormalities occur in Tangier disease, including peripheral neuropathy and a syringomyeloma-like syndrome.

In the plasma the most striking abnormalities are in low total plasma cholesterol, virtual absence of HDL cholesterol and essentially normal triglycerides. The major apoprotein of HDL, apoprotein A-I, is reduced to approximately 1–3% of normal.

Tangier disease appears to be due to a defective autosomal gene affecting apoprotein HDL metabolism. Many cases (approximately 25%) have resulted from consanguinity. Obligate heterozygotes have reduced HDL concentrations. No specific therapy is available.

ABETALIPOPROTEINAEMIA

This rare recessive disorder is characterized by a failure of enterocytes to secrete chylomicrons and the liver to secrete VLDL [60]. Although apoprotein B is detectable in intestinal and liver cells there is a failure in the assembly or secretion of apoprotein B-containing lipoproteins.

Clinical manifestations are severe with fat malabsorption with diarrhoea, failure to thrive, acanthocytosis and severe anaemia, early-onset degenerative neurological disease and retinitis pigmentosa. It has become clear that dietary supplementation with high-dose vitamin E at an early stage inhibits the neurological and ophthalmological manifestations. Supplements of vitamins A and K are also given. Gastrointestinal symptoms may be controlled by restricting fat in the diet. Occasionally medium-chain triglycerides are given as an additional source of energy.

FAMILIAL HYPOBETALIPOPROTEINAEMIA

This disorder is inherited as an autosomal dominant and homozygotes have clinical manifestations similar to individuals homozygous for abetalipoproteinaemia. However, whereas obligate heterozygotes for abetalipoproteinaemia show no abnormalities, heterozygotes for hypobetalipoproteinaemia have a reduction in apoprotein B of approximately 50%. In addition the abnormality in hypobetalipoproteinaemia appears to be defective apoprotein B synthesis.

FAMILIAL LECITHIN–CHOLESTEROL ACYLTRANSFERASE DEFICIENCY

Familial LCAT deficiency is due to absence of the LCAT enzyme or the presence of defective LCAT which is inactive [61]. LCAT deficiency is associated with severe clinical manifestations. Corneal deposits are present from early childhood. A normochromic anaemia has been observed in most patients associated with abnormal target-shaped red cells. Proteinuria develops early in life, and heralds the development of severe proteinuria and deterioration in renal function in middle life. Foam cells have been demonstrated in glomerular tufts in renal biopsies. Tendon and planar xanthomas have been described in some patients and many affected individuals develop atherosclerosis in middle life.

As a result of deficiency of LCAT, which is the major determinant of cholesterol esterification, there are multiple abnormalities in the lipoprotein fractions with high concentrations of plasma unesterified cholesterol and lecithin and low concentrations of cholesteryl ester and lysolecithin. Mature HDL particles are virtually absent from the plasma. In addition, abnormal LDL particles similar to lipoprotein X particles are present in acquired LCAT deficiency of liver disease. Obligate heterozygotes do not develop clinical symptoms, but decreased LCAT activity can be detected. There is no specific treatment but repeated plasma transfusions have been performed, with limited success.

CEREBROTENDINOUS XANTHOMATOSIS

This autosomal recessive condition is characterized by the tissue accumulation of cholestanol and cholesterol, particularly in tendons and cutaneous xanthomas and the brain. Neurological manifestations are variable but mental impairment, cerebellar ataxia and spinal cord paresis may develop from childhood. Adults develop premature atherosclerosis, and cataracts are common. The underlying defect is a deficiency of the hepatic mitochondrial enzyme 26-hydroxylase. This enzyme is important in bile acid synthesis and there is a reduction of bile acid formation. As a result there is increased activity of 7α-hydroxylase, the rate-determining step in bile acid synthesis, and accumulation of intermediates which are converted to cholestanol.

Treatment with bile salt has led to clinical improvement with improvement in neurological function. A preliminary report suggests that HMG-CoA reductase inhibitors may reduce plasma cholestanol levels [62].

PHYTOSTEROLAEMIA

This very rare autosomal recessive trait is characterized by the early development (in the first years of life) of cutaneous and tendon xanthomas due to accumulation of plant sterols. The underlying defect is unknown, but there appears to be increased intestinal absorption of the sterols. The presence of xanthomas may lead to the mistaken diagnosis of familial hypercholesterolaemia but cholesterol levels are normal or modestly elevated. Some patients have developed haemolytic anaemia. Early development of atherosclerosis is the rule. The presence of plant sterols in plasma can be demonstrated by gas chromatography. Treatment is dietary with reduction of plant sterols. The anion exchange resins also reduce plasma plant sterols [62].

Population approach to the prevention of atherosclerosis

Atherosclerosis begins in childhood and adolescence and cholesterol levels in children are related to coronary artery fatty streaks, the early lesion of atherosclerosis. The modification of plasma lipid and lipoprotein levels in adults for a relatively short time (3–7 years) leads to reductions in non-fatal and fatal coronary events. It is therefore likely that the benefits for the prevention of CHD may be enormous if plasma lipids can be modified at an earlier stage. For these reasons it has been suggested that population approaches to coronary disease prevention should start in childhood. It is also likely that the implementation of healthy lifestyle habits will be easier to encourage in childhood. The European Atherosclerosis

Table 36.8 Nutritional recommendations for children over the age of 2–3 years

Sufficient calories should be provided to ensure normal growth and development and maintenance or achievement of normal body weight in all children

Calories should be provided by diets that include a wide variety of foods

Total fat intake should provide no more than 30% of food energy

Saturated fatty acids should provide less than 10% of total food energy

Cholesterol intake should be less than 300 mg/day

Table 36.9 Screening for lipid disorders in children

Children of a parent with familial hypercholesterolaemia
Children and adolescents with a family history of premature CHD
Adolescents of a parent with familial combined hyperlipidaemia

Society [24] has proposed nutritional guidelines for children over the age of 2–3 years (Table 36.8). These recommendations are safe, and no adverse effects have been seen on growth, height, weight, etc.

Although some have advocated universal screening of children for CHD risk factors this has not been accepted by others. For instance the guidelines of the European Atherosclerosis Society [24] recommend the screening of children for lipid disorders as shown in Table 36.9. Total cholesterol levels above 5.2 mmol/l and LDL cholesterol levels greater than 3–4 mmol/l are considered high in children and adolescents. Mean and centile ranges for children and adolescents are shown in Table 36.10. In clinical practice a fasting lipid profile consisting of total cholesterol, total triglyceride and HDL cholesterol is sufficient for most circumstances. LDL cholesterol can be calculated by the Friedewald calculation below [63].

$$\text{LDL cholesterol} = \text{Total cholesterol} - \text{HDL cholesterol} - \left(\frac{\text{Total triglyceride}}{2.19}\right)$$

Note that all concentrations are in mmol/l. The formula provides a useful estimate of LDL cholesterol if total triglyceride is < 4.5 mmol/l.

Secondary causes of dyslipidaemia need to be excluded, and the family history may point to a particular primary dyslipidaemia.

Dietary treatment is the primary intervention in children. The advice of a dietician and family counselling is imperative. Drug therapy is considered only in those children above 10 years of age with familial hypercholesterolaemia or other major lipid disorder if LDL cholesterol fails to respond to dietary measures of at least 6 months, if LDL cholesterol is greater than 5.2 mmol/l or if LDL is greater than 4 mmol/l with a family history of early CHD. The only drugs advocated for children are the anion exchange resins [24].

REFERENCES

1 Kreisberg RA, Segrest JP (eds) *Plasma Lipoproteins and Coronary Artery Disease. Current Issues in Endocrinology and Metabolism*. Oxford: Blackwell Scientific Publications, 1992.

2 LaRosa JC (ed.) *Lipid Disorders. Endocrinology and Metabolism Clinics of North America*, Vol. 19, No. 2. Philadelphia PA: W.B. Saunders, 1990.

3 Shepherd J (ed.) *Lipoprotein Metabolism. Baillière's Clinical Endocrinology and Metabolism*, Vol. 1, No. 3. London: Baillière Tindall, 1987.

Table 36.10 Plasma lipid and lipoprotein concentrations in children*

	Cholesterol			LDL cholesterol			HDL cholesterol			Triglyceride		
		Centiles			Centiles			Centiles			Centiles	
	Mean	5th	95th	Mean	5th	95th	Mean	5th	95th	Mean	5th	95th
Males												
< 4 years	4.0	2.9	5.2	–	–	–	–	–	–	0.6	0.3	1.1
5–9 years	4.1	3.1	5.2	2.4	1.7	3.2	1.4	1.0	1.9	0.6	0.3	1.1
10–14 years	4.0	3.0	5.2	2.5	1.6	3.3	1.4	0.9	1.9	0.7	0.4	1.4
15–19 years	3.8	2.9	5.0	2.5	1.7	3.8	1.2	0.7	1.7	0.9	0.4	1.7
Females												
< 4 years	4.0	2.9	5.1	–	–	–	–	–	–	0.7	0.4	1.3
5–9 years	4.2	3.2	5.2	2.6	1.7	3.4	1.4	0.8	1.8	0.7	0.4	1.2
10–14 years	4.1	3.2	5.1	2.5	1.7	3.4	1.3	0.9	1.8	0.8	0.4	1.5
15–19 years	4.0	3.0	5.1	2.6	1.8	3.7	1.3	0.8	1.9	0.8	0.4	1.4

* All concentrations are in mmol/l. Data from Lipid Research Clinics Program USA.

4 Brown MS, Goldstein JL. Receptor mediated control of cholesterol metabolism. *Science* 1986;191:150–4.

5 Frederickson DS, Levy RI, Lees RS. Fat transport in lipoproteins – an integrated approach to mechanisms and disorders. *N Eng J Med* 1967;276:32–44, 94–103, 148–56, 215–24, 273–81.

6 Beaumont JL, Carlson LA, Cooper GR, Fejfar Z, Frederickson DS, Strasser T. Classification of hyperlipidaemias and hyperlipoproteinaemias. *Bulletin WHO* 1970;43:891–915.

7 Goldstein JL, Brown MS. Familial hypercholesterolaemia. In: Scriver CR, Beaudet AL, Sly WS, Valle D, eds. *The Metabolic Basis of Inherited Disease*, 6th edn. New York: McGraw-Hill, 1989:1215–50.

8 Muller C. Xanthomata, hypercholesterolaemia, angina pectoris. *Acta Med Scand* 1938;89:75–84.

9 Schrott HG, Goldstein JL, Hazzard WR, McGoodwin MM, Motulsky AG. Familial hypercholesterolaemia in a large kindred. Evidence for a monogenic mechanism. *Ann Intern Med* 1972;76:711–20.

10 Khachadurian AK, Uthman SM. Experiences with the homozygous cases of familial hypercholesterolaemia: a report of 52 patients. *Nutr Metab* 1973;15:132–40.

11 Langer T, Strober W, Levy RI. The metabolism of low density lipoprotein in familial type II hyperlipoproteinaemia. *J Clin Invest* 1972;51:1528–36.

12 Goldstein JL, Brown MS. Progress in understanding the LDL receptor and HMG-CoA reductase, two membrane proteins that regulate the plasma cholesterol. *J Lipid Res* 1984;25: 1450–61.

13 Hobbs HH, Brown MS, Goldstein JL. Molecular genetics of the LDL receptor gene in familial hypercholesterolemia. *Hum Mutat* 1992;1:445–66.

14 Steinberg D, Parthasarathy S, Carew TE *et al.* Beyond cholesterol. Modifications of low density lipoprotein that increase its atherogenicity. *N Engl J Med* 1989;320:915–24.

15 Slack J. Risks of ischaemic heart disease in familial hyperlipoproteinaemic states. *Lancet* 1969;2:1380–3.

16 Heiberg A. The risk of atherosclerotic vascular disease in subjects with xanthomatosis. *Acta Med Scand* 1975;198: 249–61.

17 Stanley P, Chartrand C, D'Avignon A. Acquired aortic stenosis in a twelve year old girl with xanthomatosis. *N Engl J Med* 1965;273:1378–81.

18 Buja LM, Kovanen PT, Bilheimer DW. Cellular pathology of homozygous familial hypercholesterolaemia. *Am J Pathol* 1979;97:327–57.

19 Leonard JV, Whitelaw AGL, Wolff OH, Lloyd JK, Slack J. Diagnosing familial hypercholesterolaemia in childhood by measuring serum cholesterol. *Br Med J* 1977;1:1411–50.

20 Brown MS, Kovanen PT, Goldstein JL *et al.* Prenatal diagnosis of homozygous familial hypercholesterolaemia: expression of a genetic receptor disease *in utero*. *Lancet* 1978;1:526–9.

21 Rossouw JE, Rifkind BM. Does lowering serum cholesterol levels lower coronary heart disease risk? In: LaRosa JC, ed. *Lipid Disorders. Endocrinology and Metabolism Clinics of North America*, Vol. 19, No. 2. Philadelphia PA: W.B. Saunders, 1990:279–97.

22 Scanu AM. Lipoprotein (a). In: Betteridge DJ, ed. *Lipid and Lipoprotein Disorders. Baillière's Clinical Endocrinology and Metabolism*, Vol. 4, No. 4. London: Baillière Tindall, 1990: 939–46.

23 Seed M, Hopplicher F, Reaveley D *et al.* Relation of serum lipoprotein (a) concentration and apo(a) phenotype to coronary heart disease in patients with familial hypercholesterolaemia. *N Engl J Med* 1990;322:1494–9.

24 Anon. Prevention of coronary heart disease: scientific background and new clinical guidelines. Recommendations of the European Atherosclerosis Society. *Nutr Metab Cardiovasc Dis* 1992;2:113–56.

25 West RJ, Lloyd JK, Leonard JV. Long term follow up of children with familial hypercholesterolaemia treated with cholestyramine. *Lancet* 1980;2:873–5.

26 Betteridge DJ, Bhatnager D, Bing RF *et al.* Treatment of familial hypercholesterolaemia. United Kingdom lipid clinics study of pravastatin and cholestyramine. *Br Med J* 1992;304: 1335–8.

27 Vega GL, Grundy SM. *In vivo* evidence for reduced binding of low density lipoproteins to receptors as a cause of primary moderate hypercholesterolaemia. *J Clin Invest* 1986;78: 1410–14.

28 Innerarity TL, Mahley RW, Weisgraber KH *et al.* Familial defective apolipoprotein B-100: a mutation of apolipoprotein B that causes hypercholesterolaemia. *J Lipid Res* 1990;31: 1337–49.

29 Tybjaerg-Hansen A. Familial defective in apolipoprotein B-100: clinical characteristics and frequency. In: Shepherd J, Packard CJ, Brownlie SM, eds. *Lipoproteins and the Pathogenesis of Atherosclerosis*. Amsterdam: Excerpta Medica, 1991:13–30.

30 Brunzell JD. Familial lipoprotein lipase deficiency and other causes of the chylomicronaemia syndrome. In: Scriver CR, Beaudet AL, Sly WS, Valle D, eds. *The Metabolic Basis of Inherited Disease*, 6th edn. New York: McGraw-Hill, 1989: 1165–94.

31 Lesser PB, Warshaw AL. Diagnosis of pancreatitis masked by hyperlipidaemia. *Ann Intern Med* 1975;82:795–8.

32 Hayden MR. Genetics, hyperlipidaemia and atherosclerosis: an update. *Curr Opin Lipidol* 1990;1:437–41.

33 Breckenridge WC, Little JA, Steiner G, Chow A, Poapst M. Hypertriglyceridaemia associated with deficiency of apolipoprotein C-II. *N Engl J Med* 1978;298:1265–73.

34 Olivecrona T, Bengtsson-Olivecrona G. Lipases involved in lipoprotein metabolism. *Curr Opin Lipid* 1990;1:116–21.

35 Stalenhoef AFH, Casparie AF, Demacker PNM *et al.* Combined deficiency of apolipoprotein C-II and lipoprotein lipase in familial hyperchylomicronaemia. *Metabolism* 1981;30: 919–26.

36 Brunzell JD, Miller NE, Alaupovic P *et al.* Familial chylomicronaemia due to a circulating inhibitor of lipoprotein lipase activity. *J Lipid Res* 1983;24:12.

37 Goldstein JL, Schrott HG, Hazzard WR, Bierman EL, Motulsky AG. Hyperlipidaemia in coronary heart disease. II. Genetic analysis of lipid levels in 176 families and delineation of a new inherited disorder, combined hyperlipidaemia. *J Clin Invest* 1973;52:1544–68.

38 Babirak SP, Iverius PH, Fujimoto WY, Brunzell JD. Detection and characterization of the heterozygote state for lipoprotein lipase deficiency. *Arteriosclerosis* 1989;9:326–34.

39 Mahley RW, Rall SC. Type III hyperlipoproteinaemia (dysbetalipoproteinaemia). The role of apolipoprotein E in normal and abnormal lipoprotein metabolism. In: Scriver CR, Beaudet AL, Sly WS, Valle D, eds. *The Metabolic Basis of Inherited Disease*, 6th edn. New York: McGraw-Hill, 1989:1195–213.

40 Betteridge DJ. Diabetes, lipoprotein metabolism and atherosclerosis. *Br Med Bull* 1989;45:285–311.

41 Stamler J, Vaccaro O, Neaton JD, Wentworth D. Diabetes, other risk factors, and 12 year cardiovascular mortality for men screened in the multiple risk factor intervention trial. *Diabetes Care* 1993;16:434–44.

42 Consensus Statement. Detection and management of lipid disorders in diabetes. *Diabetes Care* 1993;16(Suppl. 2): 106–12.
43 Deckert T, Feldt-Rasmussen B, Borch-Johnsen K *et al.* Proteinuria, an indicator of malignant angiopathy. In: Andreani D, Crepaldi G, Di Mario U, eds. *Diabetic Complications: Early Diagnosis and Treatment*. Chichester: John Wiley & Sons, 1987:257–61.
44 Jensen T, Stender S, Deckert T. Abnormalities in plasma concentrations of lipoproteins and fibrinogen in type I (insulin dependent) diabetic patients with increased urinary albumin excretion. *Diabetologia* 1988;21:142–5.
45 Hazzard WR, Bierman EL. Aggravation of broad beta disease (type 3 hyperlipoproteinaemia) by hypothyroidism. *Arch Intern Med* 1972;130:822.
46 Lithell H, Boberg J, Hellsing K *et al.* Serum lipoprotein and apolipoprotein concentrations and tissue lipoprotein lipase activity in overt and subclinical hypothyroidism: the effects of substitution therapy. *Eur J Clin Invest* 1981;11: 3–10.
47 Thompson GR, Soutar AK, Spengel FA *et al.* Defects of receptor mediated low density lipoprotein catabolism in homozygous familial hypercholesterolaemia and hypothyroidism. *Proc Natl Acad Sci USA* 1981;78:2591–5.
48 Appel GB, Blum CB, Chien S *et al.* The hyperlipidaemia of the nephrotic syndrome relative to plasma albumin concentration, oncotic pressure and viscosity. *N Engl J Med* 1985; 312:1544–8.
49 Querfeld U, Gnasso A, Haberbosch W *et al.* Lipoprotein profiles of different stages of the nephrotic syndrome. *Eur J Paediatr* 1988;233:1147.
50 McKenzie IF, Nestel PJ. Studies on the turnover of triglyceride and esterified cholesterol in subjects with the nephrotic syndrome. *J Clin Invest* 1968;47:1685.
51 Jungst D, Caselmann WH, Kutschera P, Weisweiler P. Relation of hyperlipidaemia in serum and loss of high density lipoproteins in urine in the nephrotic syndrome. *Clin Chim Acta* 1987;168:159–67.
52 Brunzell JD, Alberts JJ, Haas L *et al.* Prevalence of serum lipid abnormalities in chronic haemodialysis. *Metabolism* 1977; 26:903.
53 Nestel PJ, Fidge N, Tan MH. Increased lipoprotein-remnant formation in chronic renal failure. *N Engl J Med* 1982;307: 329–33.
54 Ettinger WH, Hazzard WR. Prednisone increases very low density lipoprotein and high density lipoprotein in healthy men. *Metabolism* 1988;37:1055–8.
55 Ballantyne CM, Podet EJ, Patsch WP *et al.* Effects of cyclosporine therapy on plasma lipoprotein levels. *J Am Med Assoc* 1989;262:53.
56 Tobert JA. Rhabdomyolysis in patients receiving lovastatin after cardiac transplantation. *N Engl J Med* 1988;318:47–8.
57 Miller JP. Dyslipoproteinaemia of liver disease. In: Betteridge DJ, ed. *Lipid and Lipoprotein Disorders. Baillière's Clinical Endocrinology and Metabolism*, Vol. 4, No. 4. London: Baillière Tindall, 1990:807–32.
58 Hers H-G, Van Hoof F, de Barsy T. Glycogen storage diseases. In: Scriver CR, Beaudet AL, Sly WS, Valle D, eds. *The Metabolic Basis of Inherited Disease*, 6th edn. New York: McGraw-Hill, 1989:425–52.
59 Assmann G, Schmitz H, Brewer B. Familial high density lipoprotein deficiency: Tangier disease. In: Scriver CR, Beaudet AL, Sly WS, Valle D, eds. *The Metabolic Basis of Inherited Disease*, 6th edn. New York: McGraw-Hill, 1989: 1267–82.
60 Kane JP, Havel RJ. Disorders of the biogenesis and secretion of lipoproteins containing the B apolipoproteins. In: Scriver CR, Beaudet AL, Sly WS, Valle D, eds. *The Metabolic Basis of Inherited Disease*, 6th edn. New York: McGraw-Hill, 1989: 1139–64.
61 Norum KR, Gjone E, Glomset JA. Familial lecithin cholesterol acyltransferase deficiency, including fish eye disease. In: Scriver CR, Beaudet AL, Sly WS, Valle D, eds. *The Metabolic Basis* of *Inherited Disease*, 6th edn. New York: McGraw-Hill, 1989:1181–94.
62 Bjorkhem I, Skrede S. Familial diseases with storage of sterols other than cholesterol: cerebrotendinous xanthomatosis and phytosterolaemia. In: Scriver CR, Beaudet AL, Sly WS, Valle D, eds. *Metabolic Basis of Inherited Disease*, 6th edn. New York: McGraw-Hill, 1989:1283–302.
63 Fridewald WT, Lev RI, Frederickson DS. Estimation of the concentration of low density lipoprotein cholesterol in plasma without use of the preparative ultracentrifuge. *Clin Chem* 1972;18:499–502.

37: Endocrine Control of Calcium and Bone Metabolism

K. KRUSE

INTRODUCTION

This section contains a description of normal endocrine regulation and disorders of calcium and bone metabolism, as well as a laboratory approach to the child with suspected disturbances in calcium and bone metabolism. Molar conversions are as follows:

$$\text{Calcium } 1\,\text{mg/dl} = 0.25\,\text{mmol/l}$$

$$\text{Calcium } 1\,\text{mg/mg creatinine} = 2.83\,\text{mmol/mmol creatinine}$$

About 99% of total body calcium and 85% of body phosphate are present in the skeleton in the form of hydroxyapatite, a crystalline structure composed of calcium, phosphate and hydroxyl ions. The approximately 1% of calcium present in extracellular and intracellular fluids is vital to the regulation of plasma membrane potential and a number of biochemical processes, including blood coagulation, endocrine secretion and numerous enzymatic reactions.

The normal total calcium concentration in serum is 2.2–2.6 mmol/l (8.8–10.4 mg/dl) and this does not vary with age during childhood. Total calcium is distributed in three fractions: ionized (about 50%), protein-bound (about 40%) and calcium which is complexed to citrate, phosphate and other constituents in serum (about 10%). The only accurate method of determining the ionized fraction, the biologically active form of calcium, is to measure it directly by an ion-selective electrode. Formulas for the estimation of protein-bound calcium may be inaccurate, especially in patients with low serum protein concentrations. The simplest calculation for this correction is:

$$\text{Total serum calcium (mg/dl)} - \text{albumin (g/dl)} + 4.0 = \text{Corrected total serum calcium}$$

For example, the corrected value is 2.4 mmol/l (9.5 mg/dl), with values for total serum calcium of 1.75 mmol/l (7 mg/dl) and albumin of 1.5 g/dl. Acute acidosis decreases and alkalosis increases calcium binding to carboxyl groups in albumin, with a consequent increase and decrease of ionized calcium respectively.

Many cellular reactions are dependent on the availability of organic and inorganic phosphate. Normal inorganic serum phosphate levels show a wide range and are influenced by age, being high during infancy (1.3–2.3 mmol/l or 4–7 mg/dl) and falling to adult levels (0.8–1.5 mmol/l or 2.5–4.6 mg/dl) after puberty. Serum phosphate is expressed in terms of the amount of elemental phosphorus involved. Only 15% of the serum phosphate is bound to proteins, whereas 85% is ultrafiltrable and consists mainly of free HPO_4^{2-}. An adequate serum concentration of ionized calcium and free phosphate is important for maintaining a sufficient ion product for normal bone mineralization. Vitamin D and its active metabolites, parathyroid hormone (PTH) and calcitonin are the principal regulators of calcium and bone metabolism [1,2].

VITAMIN D

Chemistry

The term vitamin D or calciferol refers collectively to two secosteroids: vitamin D_3 (cholecalciferol) and vitamin D_2 (ergocalciferol). Secosteroids are steroid-related compounds in which one of the four rings has been opened. Vitamin D_3 and vitamin D_2 are produced non-enzymatically by ultraviolet irradiation resulting in the cleavage of the bond between C9 and C10 of the B ring. Vitamin D_2 is derived from the plant sterol ergosterol and differs from vitamin D_3 in that the side-chain has a double bond at C22–23 and a methyl group attached to C24 (Fig. 37.1). In humans the metabolism and biological potency of vitamin D_2 and vitamin D_3 seem to be identical. By convention, lack of a subscript after the D implies both vitamin D forms. Several organs are involved in the synthesis (skin), metabolism (liver, kidney) and action (intestine, bone, etc.) of vitamin D.

Formation and transport

Vitamin D_3 is produced in the skin as a result of ultraviolet

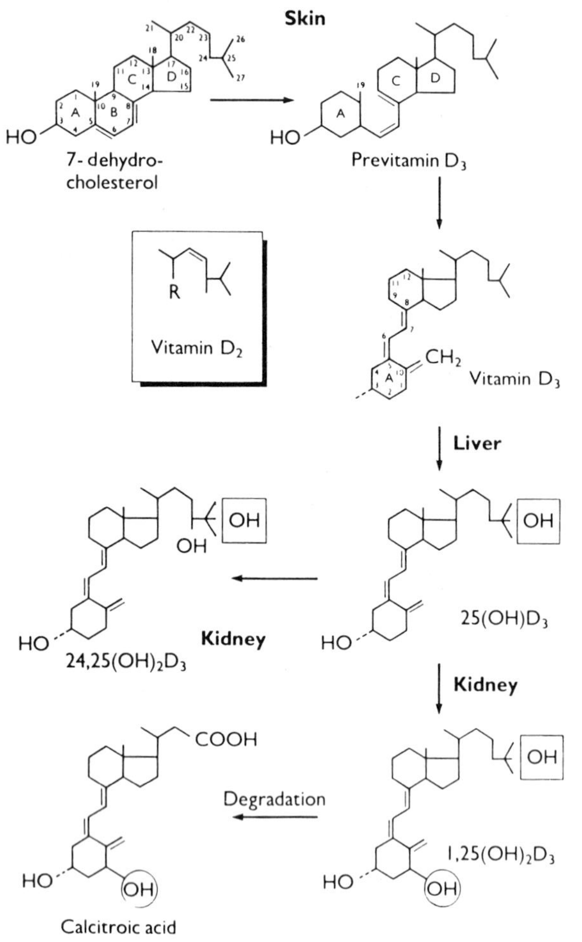

Fig. 37.1 Chemical structures and metabolism of vitamin D. The numbering is based on that of cholesterol, and the important hydroxyl groups at C25 and C1 are indicated. The different side-chain structure of vitamin D_2 is indicated.

irradiation (230–313 nm wavelength) of provitamin D_3 (7-dehydrocholesterol) which is present in large amounts in the malpighian layer of the epidermis. This photolytic reaction proceeds via an additional intermediate, termed previtamin D_3, which undergoes slow conversion to vitamin D_3 at body temperature [3]. Vitamin D_3 has a relatively high affinity for the transport protein of vitamin D, whereas the previtamin has a low affinity and remains in the skin. The amount of sunlight exposure influences the serum levels of vitamin D_3 (and its product 25-hydroxyvitamin D_3), the levels being higher during the summer than during the winter. Pigmented skin is less efficient in the conversion of 7-dehydrocholesterol to vitamin D_3. Any excess of sunlight converts previtamin D_3 to biologically inactive compounds (lumisterol$_3$ and tachysterol$_3$), thus avoiding vitamin D intoxication due to prolonged sunlight exposure [3].

Vitamin D is obtainable from dietary sources as vitamin D_3 or D_2. Both compounds are absorbed in the upper part of the small intestine by a process that is facilitated by bile salts. Vitamin D enters the blood primarily through the lymphatic system in the chylomicron fraction and its absorption may fail in the presence of steatorrhoea. Vitamin D in blood is bound to the vitamin D-binding protein (DBP), an α_2-globulin made in the liver with a molecular weight of 56–58 kD, that serves as the transport protein for all vitamin D metabolites [4]. Since the concentration of DBP in blood (about 350 μg/ml or 6 μmol/l) far exceeds the requirement for vitamin D transport, only 1–3% of the total amount of vitamin D metabolites is actually free to diffuse into cells. Because of its large capacity, the DBP is believed to serve as a circulating reservoir for the vitamin D metabolites and a buffer against vitamin D toxicity. The protein has a higher affinity for 25-hydroxyvitamin D (25-OHD) than for 1,25-dihydroxyvitamin D (1,25$(OH)_2$D). The concentration of DBP is unaltered by vitamin D deficiency or intoxication.

Metabolism

Vitamin D is biologically inert and must undergo transformation into active metabolites. The first step involves 25-hydroxylation, which takes place predominantly in the liver microsomes. Hepatectomy markedly reduces but does not eliminate the conversion to 25-OHD, indicating that 25-hydroxylation also occurs in other tissues (for example intestine and kidney). 25-OHD is the major circulating vitamin D metabolite in blood, and the measurement of its concentration provides an accurate reflection of vitamin D reserve in humans.

A second hydroxylation step occurs in the mitochondria of the proximal renal tubule [5]. Depending on the calcium requirement, two compounds may be formed: 1,25$(OH)_2$D, the active vitamin D metabolite, or 24,25-dihydroxyvitamin D (24,25$(OH)_2$D) which has less biological activity [6]. The enzymes responsible for the metabolic transformations of 25-OHD are mixed-function oxidases incorporating molecular oxygen. This enzyme complex, whose characteristics have been well defined in the chick kidney [6], consists of nicotinamide–adenine dinucleotide phosphate, renal ferredoxin, and cytochrome P450, and is similar to the adrenal steroidogenesis system. Extrarenal production of 1,25$(OH)_2$D has been demonstrated *in vitro* and *in vivo* in placenta, bone cells and granulomatous tissues. So far little is known concerning the metabolic degradation of 1,25$(OH)_2$D. Calcitroic acid, the product of oxidative side-chain cleavage, probably represents a major inactivation route [6]. In addition, 1,25$(OH)_2$D undergoes an enterohepatic circulation [6]. Several other biologically active vitamin D metabolites, such as 25,26-dihydroxyvitamin D and 1,24,25-trihydroxyvitamin D, have been identified [7], but together with 24,25$(OH)_2$D their biological significance remains to be determined.

Mechanism of action and biological effects

$1,25(OH)_2D$ has the characteristics of a classical steroid hormone: it is secreted by an endocrine organ (the kidney) and transported to its target tissues (intestine, bone, etc.) where it binds to receptors and induces the synthesis of messenger (m)RNA and translation of proteins that carry out the biological action of the hormone (Fig. 37.2)

The gene for the $1,25(OH)_2D$ receptor (VDR) has been cloned and found to be a member of the steroid receptor superfamily of genes [8]. The VDR in humans is a 50 kD protein consisting of 427 amino acids and containing a DNA-binding domain and a steroid (hormone)-binding domain. The DNA-binding domain is a cysteine-rich region with a two 'zinc-finger' motif between amino-acid residues 20 and 90 of the amino terminus of the protein. The hormone-binding domain extends through a large portion of the carboxyl side and is responsible for the specific binding of $1,25(OH)_2D$. Structural defects in the DNA, and the hormone-binding domains may explain cellular resistance to $1,25(OH)_2D$ in humans [9] and in a primate model [10].

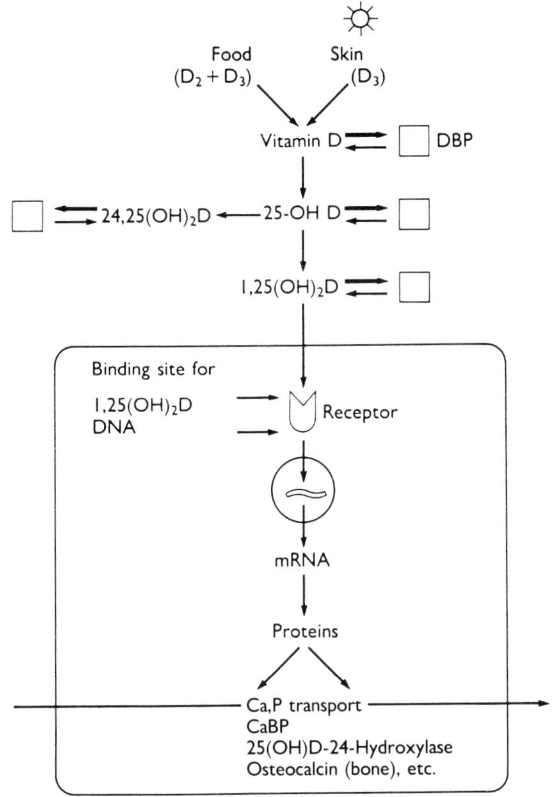

Fig. 37.2 Synthesis and molecular mechanism of action of $1,25(OH)_2D$. the lack of a subscript after the D implies both vitamin D forms. Note that about 97–99% of the vitamin D metabolites are bound to the vitamin D-binding protein (DBP). It is only the unbound or free $1,25(OH)_2D$ which crosses the cell membranes and binds to intracellular receptors, which induces the synthesis of proteins for calcium transport, etc. The $1,25(OH)_2D$ receptor is a macromolecule with several domains. The DNA-binding site is located of the amino-terminus and contains two 'zinc fingers'.

Binding of the hormone activates the VDR involving specific interactions of the zinc-finger region with hormone response elements in the promoter region of the target genes.

The main hormonal function of $1,25(OH)_2D$ is the stimulation of the transepithelial transport of calcium and phosphate across the intestine into the blood, as well as assisting in PTH-stimulated osteoclastic bone resorption.

Much remains to be learned concerning the target response to $1,25(OH)_2D$, even in the intestine, the most extensively studied tissue. The hormone increases several calcium-binding proteins (CaBP), the size of the two major mammalian intestinal CaBP being 9 kD and 28 kD.

In addition to the described genomic actions of $1,25(OH)_2D$ there is evidence for the existence of very rapid non-genomic biological effects of this steroid [11].

In bone the vitamin D hormone increases the activity of osteoclast-like cells and suppresses the activity of osteoblast-like cells [12]. Surprisingly, osteoclasts do not contain receptors for $1,25(OH)_2D$, and some evidence suggests that the hormone may be involved in the formation of osteoclasts from stem cells in the bone marrow, but not in the activity of these bone-resorbing cells thereafter [13]. The mobilization of calcium from bone requires the presence of PTH, whereas pharmacological amounts of $1,25(OH)_2D$ may stimulate bone resorption in PTH-deficient states. There is a continuing controversy as to whether all the effects of vitamin D on bone are mediated by $1,25(OH)_2D$ or whether other metabolites, especially $24,25(OH)_2D$, play a biological role in bone metabolism [14].

Another question is whether the more widely known effect of $1,25(OH)_2D$ in facilitating skeletal mineralization is mediated through direct action on bone cells or by supplying adequate amounts of calcium and phosphate to the mineralizing bone matrix. Recent studies in vitamin D-deficient rats [15] and in humans with absent $1,25(OH)_2D$ receptors [16] indicate that mineralization may proceed normally despite decreased vitamin D secretion or action. This suggests that $1,25(OH)_2D$ does *not* directly promote skeletal mineralization, but acts through normalization of the serum calcium–phosphate product by its stimulating effect on intestinal absorption and bone resorption.

Whether $1,25(OH)_2D$ has any direct effect on the renal handling of calcium and phosphate remains unsettled, but the hormone has important effects on renal vitamin D metabolism through stimulating the 24-hydroxylation and inhibiting the 1-hydroxylation of 25-OHD [5]. $1,25(OH)_2D$ is a potent inhibitor of PTH secretion *in vitro* and *in vivo*, but the biological significance of this remains to be determined. The discovery of receptors in a number of tissues other than those of established target organs, for example, in the brain, the pancreatic β cell and in cultured pituitary cells, indicates that $1,25(OH)_2D$ may have several effects in addition to those related to calcium metabolism [17]. Recent evidence suggested that the hormone is involved in immunoregulation; it also inhibits the proliferation and stimulates the differentiation of tumour cells and increases insulin secretion [11,18].

The recent development of non-hypercalcaemic analogues of $1,25(OH)_2D_3$ with selective biological properties suggests the usefulness of clinical trials with these drugs in the management of psoriasis (a hyperproliferative state of epidermis cells), cancer, immune disorders, osteoporosis, osteopetrosis, diabetes mellitus type 2, as well as hyperparathyroidism. For some of these potential new clinical applications, such as psoriasis, the existing data of initiated clinical studies are quite promising [19].

Regulation of vitamin D metabolism

Recent evidence suggests that $1,25(OH)_2D$ modulates its own synthesis, as shown in Fig. 37.3: it increases accumulation of the previtamin D_3 7-dehydrocholesterol in the skin, inhibits the hepatic enzyme vitamin D-25-hydroxylase and the renal enzyme 25-OHD-1-hydroxylase and induces the renal enzyme 25-OHD-24-hydroxylase. All these actions of $1,25(OH)_2D$ are receptor-mediated, except for the inhibition of the hepatic enzyme, since receptors for $1,25(OH)_2D$ have not been demonstrated in hepatic tissues [13]. Several additional factors have direct or indirect effects on the renal $1,25(OH)_2D$ production, the most important being calcium, phosphate and PTH: low serum calcium, phosphate depletion and elevated serum PTH stimulate $1,25(OH)_2D$ production. By contrast, hypercalcaemia, renal phosphate retention and low serum PTH (and $1,25(OH)_2D$) lead to increased synthesis of $24,25(OH)_2D$ and suppression of $1,25(OH)_2D$ [5]. In addition, prolactin, growth hormone, oestrogen, glucocorticoids, insulin and calcitonin stimulate $1,25(OH)_2D$ synthesis [5,11,20,21].

In normal adults the $1,25(OH)_2D$ production is tightly regulated, but in children the renal hormone synthesis is regulated loosely [22], which may account in part for the high serum values that are required for growth and development of the skeleton. There is possibly product inhibition of the 25-hydroxylase enzyme in liver microzymes but this does not prevent formation of toxic 25-OHD serum levels if the vitamin D intake is too high.

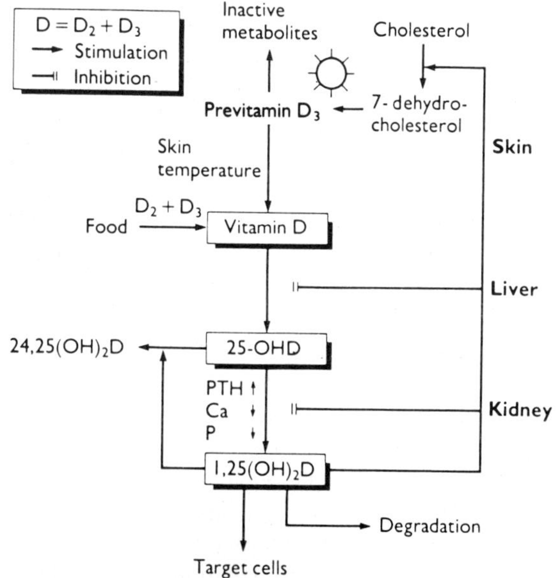

Fig. 37.3 Regulation of vitamin D metabolism. Ca, calcium; P, phosphate.

Measurement in serum

The synthesis of labelled vitamin D metabolites and improvements in extraction and purification techniques have facilitated the measurement of the major vitamin D metabolites and their study in humans. Most assays of vitamin D metabolites can be divided into three steps: the first is the separation of the vitamin D components from lipids and proteins that interfere with their detection. This is done by extraction with organic solvents (such as acetonitrile) together with radioactive markers for recovery and identification. The second step involves the chromatographic separation of the vitamin D metabolites from each other. Chromatography with Sephadex LH-20 and a final purification with high-pressure liquid chromatography (HPLC) are currently used by most investigators. With HPLC systems it is now possible to separate vitamin D_2 and vitamin D_3 metabolites. The third step involves the identification of the different vitamin D metabolites employing protein binding or radioreceptor assays with naturally occurring binding proteins and receptors, respectively.

The most significant improvement in determination of $1,25(OH)_2D$ is the elimination of HPLC as the final purification step before assay. Rheinhardt *et al.* developed a microassay for $1,25(OH)_2D$ not requiring HPLC [23]. It is particularly useful for paediatric patients in whom sample size is limited to less than 1 ml serum. Hollis has recently further simplified this assay technique, which can now be employed for the measurement of $1,25(OH)_2D$ in lipid extracts of small quantities of human serum (0.5–1.0 ml) after purification on a simple silica cartridge [24]. The serum levels determined by this assay correspond well with $1,25(OH)_2D$ values measured by conventional chromatographic methods.

For the measurement of 25-OHD, crude lipid extracts of less than 1 ml serum are placed directly in a competitive protein-binding assay with the DBP and [^{3}H]25-OHD$_3$ as the displaceable ligand. Since several vitamin D metabolites will compete for the same DBP-binding site, other metabolites besides 25-OHD, such as 24,25(OH)$_2$D, will also be measured. This leads to overestimation by about 10–20%, which will not be of clinical importance to the wide biological range of normal 25-OHD serum levels. Assays for serum 25-OHD and 1,25(OH)$_2$D are commercially available and are quite reliable.

In normal subjects living in the USA the mean 25-OHD serum level is approximately 75 nmol/l (30 ng/ml), with a range of 25–125 nmol/l (10–50 ng/ml), depending on diet and sunlight exposure. Seasonal variation has to be taken into account, with maximal levels in late summer and minimal values in late winter. Concentrations vary in different parts of the world. In the UK the normal range is only 9–75 nmol/l (3.5–30 ng/ml), probably reflecting decreased exposure to sunlight and the practice not to fortify foods with vitamin D.

The serum concentration of 1,25(OH)$_2$D is not affected by sunlight exposure, its normal levels being 50–150 pmol/l (20–60 pg/ml), but the levels may be higher during states with an increased physiological requirement of the hormone, that is during childhood, pregnancy and lactation. Most laboratories agree on the determination and normal range of 25-OHD and 1,25(OH)$_2$D, whereas the measurement of vitamin D and 24,25(OH)$_2$D remains difficult. Methodological problems have led to widely differing values of both vitamin D compounds in serum, ranging between 2.5 and 12.5 nmol/l (1–5 ng/ml).

In conclusion, the average serum concentration of 1,25(OH)$_2$D is about one-thousandth, and the levels of vitamin D and 24,25(OH)$_2$D are about one-tenth, that of 25-OHD. It is physiologically important that the free or unbound serum levels of the vitamin D metabolites are different from the total concentrations. Free 25-OHD

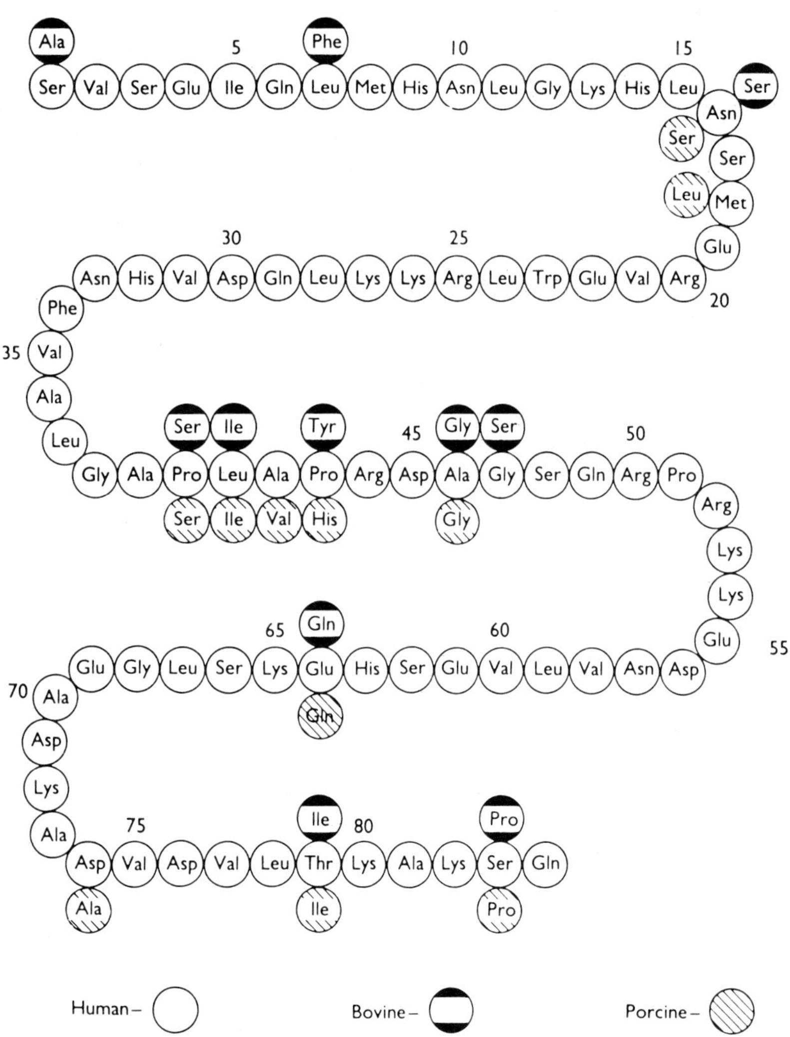

Fig. 37.4 Amino-acid sequence of human PTH. The positions at which the amino-acid residues differ for bovine and porcine PTH are indicated according to Keutmann *et al.* [26].

is only 10-fold higher than free 1,25(OH)$_2$D instead of the 1000-fold difference in total concentration. Only 1,25(OH)$_2$D not bound to DBP crosses the target cell membranes and is therefore of physiological importance. A useful index of the free 1,25(OH)$_2$D is the molar ratio of total 1,25(OH)$_2$D and DBP. Abnormal total 1,25(OH)$_2$D serum levels in several conditions (pregnancy up to 35 weeks of gestation, oestrogen treatment and liver cirrhosis) are associated or due to abnormal DBP levels, whereas the free 1,25(OH)$_2$D index and the biological effect of the vitamin D hormone (intestinal calcium absorption and ionized serum calcium) are normal [4,25]. On the other hand, total and free 1,25(OH)$_2$D levels may be decreased in patients with nephrotic syndrome presenting with disturbed calcium metabolism. The low 1,25(OH)$_2$D index in these patients may be due to low DBP levels and additional substrate deficiency of 25-OHD caused by urinary loss of DBP [25].

PARATHYROID HORMONE

Synthesis and secretion

Parathyroid hormone is synthesized and secreted by the chief cells of the parathyroid gland. The four parathyroid glands are derived from the endodermal structures of the third and fourth branchial pouches. The lower pair of the parathyroid glands develops in close association with the thymus from the third branchial pouch, whereas the upper parathyroid glands derive from the fourth branchial pouch and remain relatively stationary, which accounts for their final location dorsolateral to the thyroid gland at the level of the thyroid isthmus. In the adult each gland is ellipsoid, measuring 6 × 5 × 2 mm and weighing 30–50 mg.

The amino-acid sequence of human PTH was determined in 1978 by Keutmann *et al.* [26]. PTH is a single polypeptide consisting of 84 amino acids with a molecular weight of 9.5 kD. The structures of human, bovine and porcine PTH are identical in length (84 amino acids) and have many amino-acid residues in common (Fig. 37.4). The structure of information required for full biological activity lies within the 34 amino acids at the amino terminus. This region contains the amino-acid sequence essential for receptor binding and activation. Removal of the first two amino acids at the amino terminus destroys biological activity [27].

The PTH gene in the human has been localized to the short arm of chromosome 11 in the region 11p15 [28,29] which is close to the insulin and calcitonin genes. The PTH gene has three exons: a 5′-untranslated region, a preprohormone coding region and the main coding region with a 3′-non-coding region.

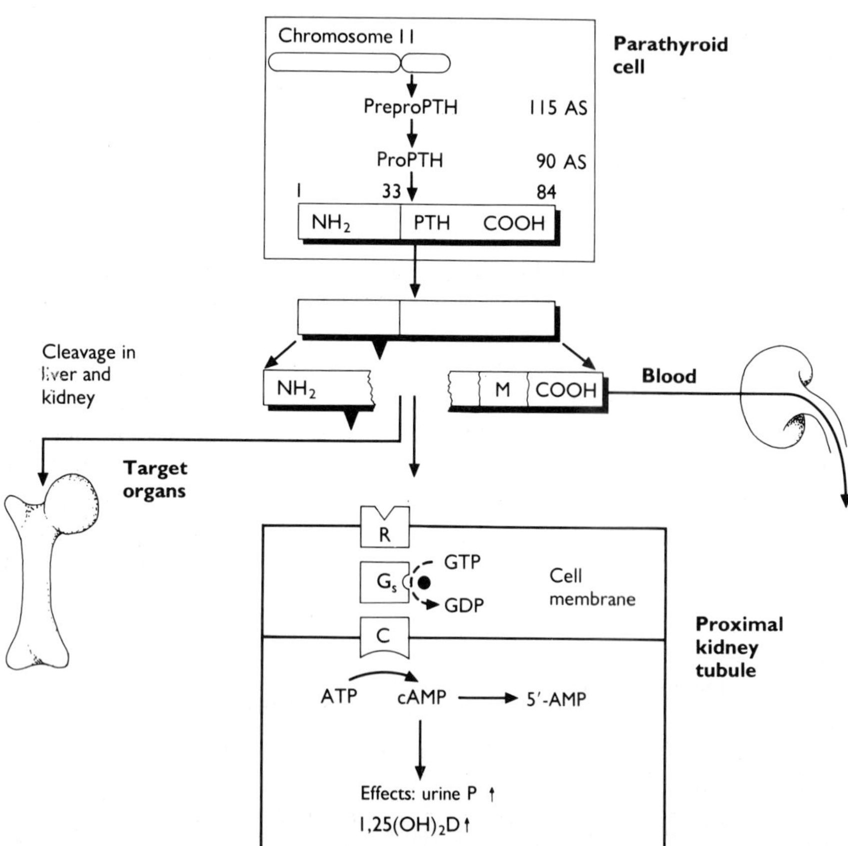

Fig. 37.5 Synthesis, metabolism and action of PTH. AMP, adenosine monophosphate; ATP, adenosine triphosphate; C, catalytic unit of adenylate cyclase; G_s, stimulatory protein, binding the nucleotide guanosine triphosphate (GTP); GDP, guanosine-5′-diphosphate; NH_2/M/COOH, amino-terminal/mid-regional/carboxyterminal fragment of PTH; P, phosphate; R, receptor for PTH.

Mature PTH is produced by two sequential enzymatic cleavages from a 115 amino-acid precursor polypeptide, preproPTH, as shown in Fig. 37.5. The 25 amino-acid presequence at the amino-terminus of the molecule is proteolytically removed within seconds. Since most of these amino acids are hydrophobic it is believed that this sequence is involved in the transport of the nascent polypeptide across the membrane into the cisternal space of the endoplasmic reticulum. ProPTH is converted to PTH in the Golgi apparatus by proteolytic removal of the remaining six amino acids within 15–20 min. Mature PTH is packed into granules for storage and subsequent secretion. There is no evidence that either preproPTH or proPTH is secreted into circulation. Both precursors show little or no biological activity [27].

The major regulator of PTH synthesis and secretion is the concentration of calcium in circulation. *In vitro* and *in vivo* studies demonstrated a sigmoidal inverse relationship between calcium and PTH [30,27]. A slow decline of total calcium concentration from 2.51 to 2.25 mmol/l causes small and gradual increases in PTH secretion. However, a further calcium decrease from 2.25 to 2.0 mmol/l (8 mg/dl) elicits a sharp increase in PTH release to a maximal rate. Below 2.0 mmol/l (8 mg/dl), little or no further rise in secretion occurs. The gradual slope of PTH secretion in normocalcaemia and the steep response to mild hypocalcaemia constitutes an important homeostatic mechanism to prevent hypocalcaemia.

It is likely that the maximal suppressibility of PTH secretion by calcium is not complete. For example, *in vivo* studies in cows demonstrated persistent basal PTH secretion despite induced hypercalcaemia of 3.0–5.0 mmol/l [31]. The sensitivity of parathyroid glands to extracellular calcium may change under different normal or abnormal conditions [30]. Situations with elevated set points (reduced sensitivity to the suppressive effects of extracellular calcium) have been reported *in utero* or during the neonatal period in pigs and calves, during exposure to lithium, in secondary hyperparathyroidism associated with chronic renal failure and in primary hyperparathyroidism. A decrease in set point (increased sensitivity to the suppressive effect of extracellular calcium) may occur in normal parathyroid glands from patients with a parathyroid adenoma, and may explain the transient hypocalcaemia seen frequently after parathyroidectomy. Finally, calcium infusions in animals reduce PTH secretion during a state of induced hypocalcaemia.

These set-point changes during chronic hyper- or hypocalcaemia may induce responses in PTH secretion which can have a number of important clinical implications. Although the evidence is conclusive that calcium is of major importance in PTH regulation, other agents may modify PTH secretion, including various catecholamines, dopamine, histamine, serotonin, somatostatin, prolactin, glucagon, cortisol, prostaglandins, calcitonin, $1,25(OH)_2D$, phosphate and potassium [30]. Several of these agents may influence PTH secretion indirectly by changes in ionized calcium and the physiological significance of most secretagogues for PTH is unknown.

Magnesium plays an important role in PTH secretion only at concentrations outside the physiological range. Increased magnesium concentration inhibits PTH secretion in a similar manner as calcium [32]. Extremely low concentrations of magnesium may interfere with PTH secretion and action [33]. Reduced PTH levels and hypocalcaemia occur in patients with severe and prolonged magnesium deficiency, and under these conditions magnesium infusions cause immediate increments of PTH secretion within minutes [34].

The precise mechanism by which calcium and the other agents regulate PTH secretion and synthesis is not clearly understood. There is evidence that the intracellular calcium concentration regulates the secretion of PTH in a dose–response relationship: maximal PTH secretion occurs at an intracellular calcium level of about 0.2 μmol/l, regardless of the extracellular calcium concentration [35].

Another secretory product of the parathyroid chief cell is parathyroid secretory protein (PSP), a large acidic glycoprotein with a molecular weight of about 70 kD. PSP is similar to or identical with chromogranin A (found in secretory granules of the adrenal medulla), and is secreted in response to calcium in a fashion similar to PTH. The exact function of this protein is unknown, but it is thought to be a carrier protein involved in secretion of PTH [2].

Metabolism

Intact PTH (1–84) is metabolized in peripheral organs (liver, kidney and possibly bone) and probably the parathyroid gland itself [27]. The hormone is taken up by the Kupffer cells of the liver and cleaved in the region between amino acids 33 and 43 into amino- and carboxy-terminal fragments by cathepsin-like enzymes. Both intact PTH and PTH fragments are removed from the circulation and degraded by the kidneys (see Fig. 37.5). Hepatectomy slows production, and renal insufficiency slows degradation of PTH fragments. Further studies are required to answer the question of whether the cleavage of intact PTH into fragments is required for biological activity in target organs.

Mechanisms of action and biological effects

The major function of PTH is to prevent hypocalcaemia by enhancing the following.

1 Reabsorption of calcium in the kidneys.

2 Calcium resorption of bone.

3 Absorption of calcium from the intestine (indirectly via renal $1,25(OH)_2D$ secretion).

Like other polypeptide hormones, intact PTH and the amino-terminal fragment act on these organs by interaction with hormone-specific receptors on the plasma membrane of the target cells. The PTH receptor has recently been cloned and sequenced [37]. It belongs to a new family of receptors that contains seven transmembrane domains and includes the calcitonin and secretin receptors. The PTH receptor (molecular weighr 80 kD) is a glycoprotein and also binds PTH-related protein (see below).

The PTH binding to its receptor initiates stimulation of a guanine nucleotide-binding protein (G protein) in the plasma membrane to exchange guanosine-5′-diphosphate (GDP) for guanosine triphosphate (GTP). This leads to dissociation of the PTH receptor–G protein–GTP complex. The subunit of the G protein (α-subunit) that has bound the GTP then interacts with the catalytic unit of the adenylate cyclase which stimulates the conversion of intracellular adenosine triphosphate (ATP) to the second messenger cyclic adenosine monophosphate (cAMP). This nucleotide in turn causes activation of protein kinase A and subsequent phosphorylation of intracellular enzymes that ultimately contribute to the physiological action of PTH [38].

The G proteins which mediate signal transduction from the receptor across the cell membrane to the cellular production of cAMP have a heterotrimeric subunit structure composed of α-, β-, and γ-subunits. G proteins may stimulate (G_s) or inhibit (G_i) adenylate cyclase. The α-subunit binds and hydrolyses GTP and confers specifity in receptor and effector interactions, and dissociates from the βγ-subunit complex after receptor activation. Two forms of the $G_s\alpha$ protein, 45 and 52 kD, have been characterized in humans, which are formed after alternative splicing of a common gene transcript. The $G_s\alpha$ gene has recently been mapped to the distal long arm of chromosome 20 [39].

In addition to this classical pathway PTH may also cause cell activation by stimulating the phosphatidylinositol–protein kinase C system and by directly activating calcium channels, both mechanisms increasing intracellular calcium levels [1].

PARATHYROID HORMONE ACTION ON THE KIDNEY

Parathyroid hormone has several effects at different sites along the nephron. The most important effects are the enhancement of calcium reabsorption in the distal tubule and the inhibition of phosphate and bicarbonate reabsorption, as well as stimulation of $1,25(OH)_2D$ production mainly in the proximal tubule. Elevated serum PTH can result in hyperaminoaciduria through an unknown mechanism.

PARATHYROID HORMONE ACTION ON BONE

Parathyroid hormone is an important factor in the regulation of bone metabolism by acting on the two distinct homeostatic and remodelling systems. The homeostatic system consists of surface osteocytes, and osteocytes located in lacunar spaces within the bone, and is important in maintaining systemic mineral homeostasis on a minute-to-minute basis by regulating movement of calcium between the bone fluid and the extracellular fluid. The remodelling system is composed of osteoclasts which resorb old (mineralized) bone and osteoblasts which replace it with new bone. These cellular events, especially the remodelling system, are dependent upon a permissive effect of $1,25(OH)_2D$. Recent evidence suggests that it is osteoblasts, rather than osteoclasts, that are responsive to and have receptors for PTH. Thus PTH stimulates osteoclastic bone resorption through primary interaction with osteoblasts, thereby inducing the release of factors such as transforming growth factor β (TGF-β), interleukin 1 (IL-1) and prostaglandins that promote activation of osteoclasts [40,41].

OTHER EFFECTS OF PARATHYROID HORMONE

Parathyroid hormone stimulates the intestinal absorption of calcium indirectly through regulation of $1,25(OH)_2D$ synthesis in the kidney, as discussed in the section on vitamin D metabolism. Intravenous PTH administration causes transient hypocalcaemia, possibly reflecting entry of calcium into cells. The reported effects of PTH on the liver and kidney (increased gluconeogenesis) and fat cells (increased lipolysis) are of unknown physiological significance.

MEASUREMENT OF PARATHYROID HORMONE IN SERUM

Assays of PTH concentrations present far more complex problems than the measurement of most other peptide hormones. This is mainly due to the heterogeneity of circulating forms of PTH, first reported by Berson & Yalow [42]. In general, PTH assays fall into three groups: radioimmunoassays (RIAs), bioassays and liquid chromatographic assays. The most widely used technique for measuring PTH is the radioimmunoassay. Amino-(N-)terminal, mid (M) region, carboxy- (C-)terminal and intact PTH assays have been developed by immunization with synthetic PTH peptides or with intact PTH [43,44]. Most of the fragment assays also recognize the intact hormone. Due to their long half-life (hours) C-terminal and M fragments constitute about 80% of the immunoreactive material in serum, and generally reflect the rate of PTH secretion, whereas the serum half-lives of intact PTH and of the N-terminal fragment are short (minutes). Thus assays that are specific for M-region or C-terminal PTH provide greater diagnostic discrimination between normal and elevated PTH than do N-terminal or intact hormone assays. On the other hand, newer N-terminal or intact PTH assays appear better to reflect PTH secretion in patients with chronic renal insufficiency, whereas the biologically inactive C-terminal and M-region PTH fragments tend to accumulate in these patients and mainly reflect decreased removal from serum by glomerular filtration.

A problem with several PTH radioimmunoassays is that they are too insensitive to differentiate between normal and hypoparathyroid states. Interpretation of serum PTH concentrations requires knowledge of the reference values for each laboratory, since PTH levels vary from investigator to investigator depending on the specificity of the antisera (directed against N, M or C fragments or intact PTH), as well as the differences in the source (bovine, human, etc.), standards and radioligands employed in the assay.

These problems with PTH radioimmunoassay have been overcome by measuring the intact PTH (1–84) molecule with two-site assays that require an epitope at the N-terminal and another at the C-terminal [45]. Two types of assays have been developed which are sensitive enough to detect the minute amounts of intact PTH in normal subjects and specific enough to avoid cross-reaction with inactive circulating PTH fragments: these are the two-site radiometric assay (IRMA) and a two-site chemiluminometric assay (ILMA). Both assays are available as kits and are accurate, precise and reliable. The normal range of PTH in the serum of healthy children and adults is 1.1–5.8 pmol/l (10–55 pg/ml) with no age or sex dependence in subjects aged between 4 weeks and 40 years.

Measuring intact PTH by one of the new two-site assays is a suitable method for determining decreased PTH in hypoparathyroidism and increased PTH in primary or secondary hyperparathyroidism. Furthermore, such assays are very useful to detect the actual PTH secretion in renal insufficiency, as they are little affected by differences in renal clearance of inactive PTH fragments [45].

Several bioassays for PTH have been developed which lacked sufficient sensitivity. The most sensitive cytochemical bioassay allowing measurement of PTH in unextracted serum of normal subjects depends on the stimulation of glucose-6-phosphate dehydrogenase in guinea pig kidney cortex slices [46–48]. In this assay the concentration of biologically active PTH in normal human subjects appears to be between 1 and 30 pg/ml or less than 10% of the circulating PTH measured by radioimmunoassay. Another bioassay, which is more convenient and not as cumbersome as the cytochemical assay, is a modified renal adenylate cyclase assay with use of canine kidney preparations and a non-hydrolysable analogue of GTP [49]. HPLC with reversed-phase techniques offers a new dimension in human PTH analysis [50], suggesting that the biological degradation of the hormone is more complex than first believed.

PARATHYROID HORMONE-RELATED PROTEIN

Human PTH-related protein (PTHrP), originally described as a product of a human lung cancer cell line, plays a major role in the pathogenesis of the hypercalcaemia of malignancy [44]. The protein was isolated and cloned in 1987 [51]. Due to alternate splicing of PTHrP mRNA, three different proteins can be formed, composed of 139, 141 and 173 amino acids which are identical in their C-terminal region and as far as amino acid 139. PTHrP shows close homology to PTH in that eight of the first 13 amino acids are identical. This fact, and some homology of tertiary structure, allows PTHrP to act via the PTH receptor leading to renal reabsorption of calcium, phosphaturia, increase of urinary cAMP, stimulation of $1,25(OH)_2D$ and osteoclast activation.

The PTHrP gene is located on the short arm of chromosome 12 in a position homologous with the location of the PTH gene on chromosome 11, and it is thought that both molecules have arisen in parallel evolution [52].

Assays for PTHrP include N- and C-terminal radioimmunoassays and two-site immunoradiometric assays some of them being commercially available [53]. None of the currently used immunoassays of PTH detect PTHrP, nor vice versa. The circulating levels of PTHrP in normal humans are very low (0.1–1.0 pmol/l) and are elevated to 100 pmol/l in patients with cancer-associated hypercalcaemia [44].

Numerous attempts have been made to elucidate the physiological role of PTHrP in humans [44,54]. PTHrP and PTHrP mRNA have been located in various tumours (mostly of epithelial origin) and in a variety of normal tissues of adults, such as skin, nervous system, skeletal and smooth muscle and endocrine glands, including parathyroid glands. This suggests that PTHrP normally functions as an autocrine or paracrine factor, possibly by regulating local calcium concentrations. PTHrP has also been detected in rat and human fetuses with a wide distribution, suggesting that it may play a role in fetal growth and development [55].

Since it is secreted by the fetal parathyroid glands and promotes active placental calcium transport from maternal to fetal circulation, PTHrP could be the fetal equivalent of PTH [54].

Recent studies indicate that PTHrP plays an important role in lactation. It has been identified in breast tissue during lactation, and very high concentrations (approximately 10 000–100 000-fold higher than those of normal plasma) are present in breast milk [56]. Grill *et al.* [57] detected levels of PTHrP > 2 pmol/l in 63% of nursing mothers, but in none of the non-lactating post-partum controls who were bottle-feeding, suggesting an endocrine role for this hormone in the physiology of lactation and possibly a role in the infantile gut.

PTHrP has different biological actions depending on the different active region of the molecule [58]: the PTH-like actions have been localized to the 1–34 region, whereas the 75–85 region stimulates the calcium transport across the placenta and the 107–111 region inhibits osteoclastic bone resorption.

PTHrP is thus revealed as an interesting paracrine and endocrine regulator of many physiological processes, but its clinical significance has to be confirmed by PTHrP assays of different regional specificity and greater sensitivity.

Evaluation of parathyroid function

The status of PTH secretion and function can be evaluated by the simultaneous measurement of calcium, phosphate and PTH in serum, the renal phosphate reabsorption and the urinary cAMP excretion. Renal phosphate reabsorption is saturable and dependent on both glomerular filtration rate (GFR) and serum phosphate concentration [59]. The tubular maximal rate of phosphate reabsorption in relation to the GFR (TmP/GFR) is the best index for the assessment of the renal handling of phosphate, whereas the measurement of phosphate excretion in mg/24 h or in relation to creatinine is of no value. The TmP/GFR ratio can be easily determined from simultaneous measurement of fasting urinary and serum phosphate and creatinine concentrations and reference to a nomogram [59]. The use of the nomogram and calculation of TmP/GFR is described in Fig. 37.6. Normal values are age-dependent, reaching the low normal levels of adults after 18 years of age. PTH is one of the important factors that influence the renal handling of phosphate by resetting the TmP/GFR at a lower level, resulting in increased urinary phosphate excretion. Accordingly, this index is low in hyperparathyroidism and high in hypoparathyroidism.

The determination of urinary cAMP may serve as an *in vivo* bioassay for circulating active PTH. Total urinary cAMP is derived from plasma and kidney (Fig. 37.7). Plasma cAMP is filtered by the kidney without being reabsorbed, and presents about half of total urinary cAMP [2]. This filtered cAMP is relatively constant. The other half of the urinary cAMP, termed nephrogenous cAMP, is generated by the kidney, mainly under the influence of PTH. Total urinary cAMP may be related either to creatinine (Cr) or GFR. cAMP/GFR can be easily calculated by multiplying urinary cAMP in nmol/mg Cr with the corresponding serum Cr in mg/dl to yield the value in nmol/dl glomular filtration. The measurement of cAMP excretion in untimed morning urine specimens is a reliable

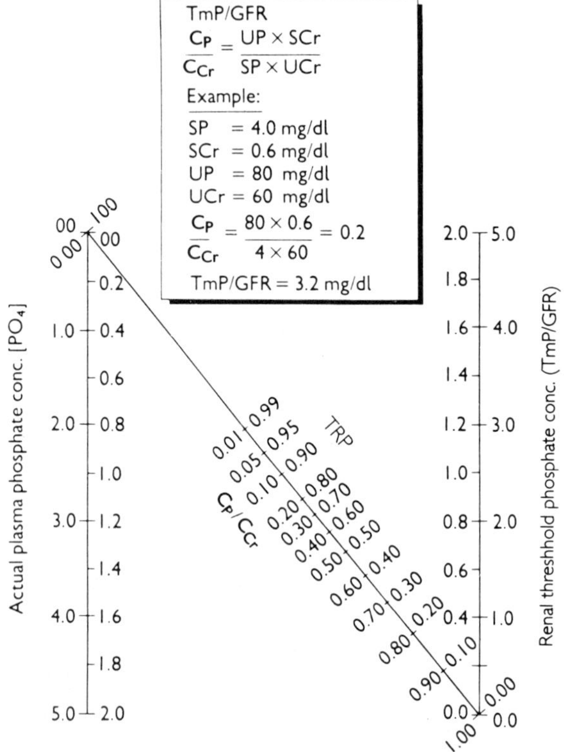

Fig. 37.6 Nomogram for the determination of TmP/GFR. The tubular maximum (threshold) for phosphate (P) per 100 ml glomerular filtration rate (GFR) is derived from the values of serum P concentration (SP) and the clearance ratios of creatinine (Cr) and P (C_P/C_{Cr}). The outer scale on each ordinate represents units in mg/dl and the inner scale in mmol/l. The values to the left of the diagonal line represent C_P/C_{Cr}. The determination of TmP/GFR is done by drawing a straight line through the known values of serum P concentration and C_P/C_{Cr}. The point of intersection with the right ordinate represents the corresponding TmP/GFR value. The scale used (mg/dl or mmol/l) must be the same [59]. The estimation of C_P/C_{Cr} and an example are given in the inset. Normal values for TmP/GFR are age-dependent with high values 1.0–2.0 mmol/l (4–8 mg/dl) during infancy declining to adult values 0.625–1.05 mmol/l (2.5–4.2 mg/dl) after the age of 18 years (redrawn from Kruse *et al.* [60]). S, serum; U, urinary.

reflection of 24-h nucleotide excretion [61]. While the cAMP/Cr ratio declines with age, the cAMP/GFR ratio remains relatively constant during childhood [61]. The cAMP/GFR ratio is low–normal in patients with low PTH secretion or action but elevated in hyperparathyroidism [62].

Another clinical application of urinary cAMP measurement is the evaluation of the renal response to exogenous PTH to distinguish patients with hypoparathyroidism (HP) from those with pseudohypoparathyroidism (PHP). The bovine parathyroid extract once used is no longer available, but synthetic fragments provoke a similar response [63,64].

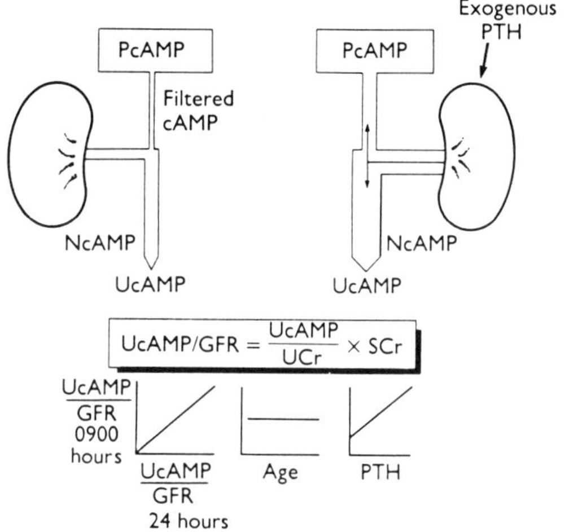

Fig. 37.7 Physiology of urinary cAMP (UcAMP) excretion. *Left side*: spontaneous excretion of UcAMP is derived from plasma (PcAMP) and kidney (nephrogenous (NcAMP)) cAMP. The calculation of UcAMP/GFR is indicated. UcAMP/GFR in morning fasting urine (0900 h) is highly correlated to the respective value in 24-h urine and to serum PTH, but is independent of age (normal range: 1.6–4.9 nmol/glomerular filtration). *Right side*: exogenous PTH administration causes an abrupt increase of NcAMP in urine and blood. SCr, serum creatinine; UCr, urine creatinine.

It has been demonstrated that 1–38 human PTH, encompassing the biologically active part of the intact hormone, is well-tolerated and effective in the diagnosis of PTH [36]. This fragment, when slowly injected at a dose of 0.5 μg (approximately 6 U)/kg body weight, produces a rise in plasma cAMP of at least 100 nmol/l and an increase in urinary cAMP of at least 60 nmol/dl, as well as a significant decrease in tubular reabsorption of phosphate (TRP), in both controls and patients with HP. In contrast, patients with PHP type I show a markedly impaired increase in plasma and urinary cAMP, whereas the TRP (and TmP/GFR) decrease overlaps with the respective values for controls and patients with HP (Fig. 37.8). Two other studies with synthetic intact 1–34 human PTH [66] and with highly purified bovine PTH [67] using comparable test procedures are in accordance with the results obtained with 1–38 human PTH.

CALCITONIN

Synthesis and structure

Calcitonin, discovered by Copp in 1962 [68], is formed by the parafollicular or C cells of the thyroid gland. These cells originate from the neural crest and colonize the last two branchial pouches. In mammals, the C cells migrate during embryogenesis into the thyroid. In lower species (amphibians, reptiles, birds) the C cells are the major constituents of a distinct organ, the ultimobranchial body. Calcitonin-like immunoreactivity has been found in the parathyroid glands, the thymus, lung, adrenal medulla and the central nervous system. No calcium-stimulated calcitonin increase can be demonstrated in totally thyroidectomized individuals [69] or in patients with congenital absence of the thyroid [70,71], indicating that the thyroid C cells are undoubtedly the major source of circulating calcitonin in the human.

In the human, calcitonin is, like PTH, coded by a gene localized on the short arm of chromosome 11 [72] and synthesized as a large precursor molecule. The structure of the human calcitonin precursor has been deduced from the nucleotide sequence of cloned complementary DNA

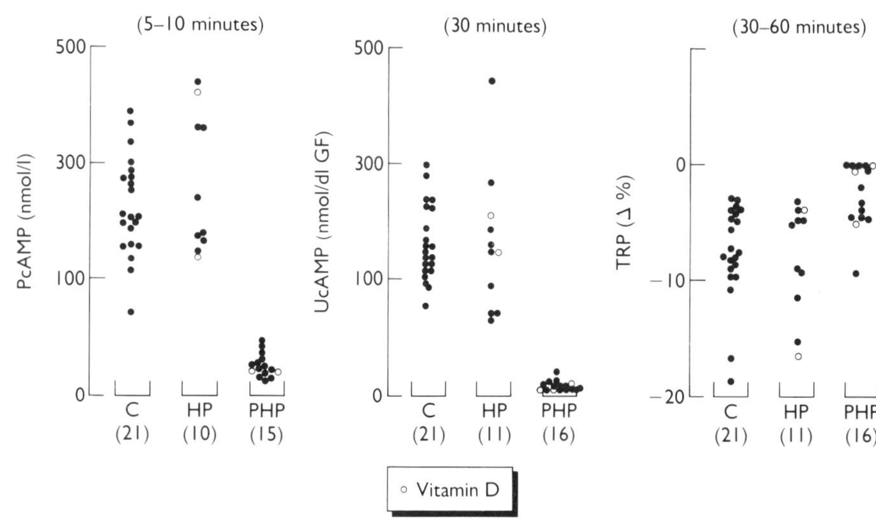

Fig. 37.8 Effect of 1–38 human PTH (hPTH) on the kidneys of 11 patients with HP and 16 patients with PHP type I as compared with 21 controls. The maximal increase in plasma cAMP (PcAMP) after 5–10 min and in urinary cAMP (UcAMP) after 30 min, as well as the maximal decrease (in Δ% from baseline) in tubular reabsorption of phosphate (TRP) after 30–60 min is indicated. Note the good discrimination of the patients with PHP by the measurement of PcAMP and UcAMP, but the large overlap in the TRP values of patients with HP and controls. Patients on vitamin D_3 therapy are indicated by open circles (from Kruse [65]). GF, glomerular filtration.

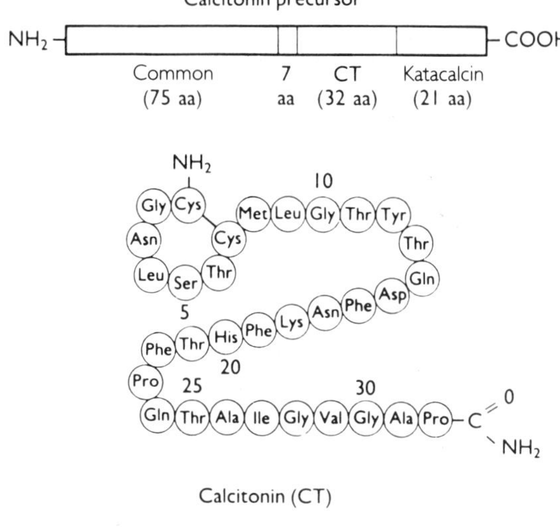

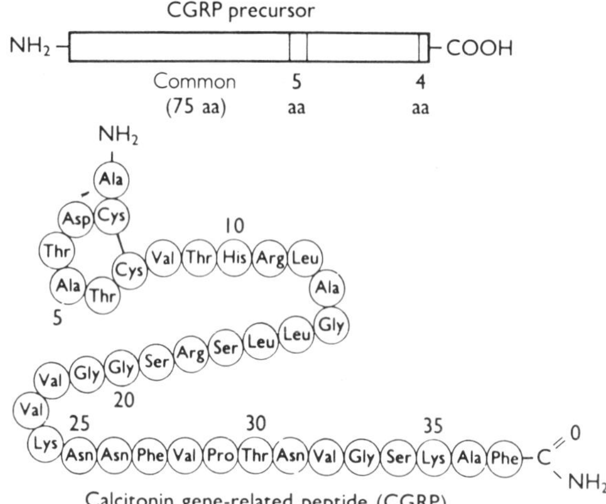

Fig. 37.9 Calcitonin gene expression in humans. Tissue-specific splicing of primary RNA transcripts of the calcitonin gene generates mRNAs that encode two different polypeptide products, the calcitonin precursor (predominantly in thyroid C cells) and the CGRP precursor (predominantly in the nervous system). Both calcitonin and CGRP are flanked by paired basic-acid residues, signalling proteolytic excision from the primary translation products. The sequences of human calcitonin and human CGRP are indicated. aa, amino acids.

constructed by mRNA obtained from malignant degeneration of the C cells (medullary thyroid carcinoma). These studies [73] have demonstrated that human calcitonin is flanked by two peptides (Fig. 37.9). The 21 amino-acid C-terminal flanking peptide, katacalcin, is co-secreted with calcitonin and circulates in equimolar amounts. No biological activity of this peptide has been demonstrated, but the measurement of katacalcin seems to be useful in confirming observed changes in calcitonin secretion.

The calcitonin gene also encodes an RNA transcript which may be alternatively produced by tissue-specific processing. As shown in Fig. 37.9, in place of calcitonin is a 37 amino-acid residue, calcitonin gene-related peptide (CGRP), with a four amino-acid peptide replacing katacalcin. In the thyroid the major product of the calcitonin gene is calcitonin (and katacalcin), whereas CGRP is the major product in the brain. CGRP is one of the most potent vasodilators known, and circulates at five times the concentration of calcitonin in normal individuals [74].

In all species, calcitonin is a compound of 32 amino acids (molecular weight 3.5 kD) with a 1–7 disulphide bridge at the N-terminal and a C-terminal prolinamide (Fig. 37.9). The amino-acid composition in the middle of the molecule varies between the species, explaining why antibodies raised against human calcitonin cross-react poorly with calcitonin from another species. The entire 32 amino-acid sequence of calcitonin is required for biological activity which is lost by the cleavage of one or more amino acids at either end of the molecule.

Secretion and metabolism

In addition to calcium many other agents, including gastrin (and its synthetic derivate pentagastrin), cholecystokinin, glucagon, biogenic amines, oestrogens and $1,25(OH)_2D$ may stimulate calcitonin secretion, at least in pharmacological amounts [75]. Most secretagogues exert their effect through the increase of intracellular cAMP in the C cells. The main candidates for physiological regulation of calcitonin secretion are calcium and gastrointestinal hormones. Calcium and pentagastrin are the principal secretagogues clinically employed in testing the secretory capacity of the thyroid gland.

Human calcitonin has a half-life of approximately 10 min, with the kidney representing the major site of clearance and degradation of the circulating hormone. This is reflected by raised calcitonin levels in patients with renal failure. The enhanced biological potency of salmon calcitonin compared with human calcitonin (approximately 10 times on a weight basis) appears to result from its prolonged half-life and higher intrinsic biological activity.

Biological effects

Like PTH, calcitonin affects calcium metabolism by acting on the three important organ systems that regulate mineral metabolism: bone, kidney and the gastrointestinal tract. These effects appear to be mediated through the stimulation of cAMP, but changes in intracellular calcium may be also involved in the mediation of the hormone effect.

CALCITONIN ACTION ON BONE

The hypocalcaemic effect of calcitonin is primarily due to inhibition of bone resorption: calcitonin inhibits osteoclasts by abolishing the otherwise intense cytoplasmic motility of these cells [76]. This osteoclastic response to calcitonin has been demonstrated to be sufficiently specific and sensitive to be used as a bioassay [77]. In addition, calcitonin given therapeutically reduces the number of osteoclasts over a period of weeks or months. The inhibition of ^{45}Ca release by calcitonin from cultured bone explants is receptor-mediated [80] and the refractoriness of this calcium release, which can be demonstrated after prolonged incubation with calcitonin, is probably due to desensitization of the hormone receptors [79]. This escape phenomenon may explain the lack of a sustained hypocalcaemic effect of chronic calcitonin excess in patients with C cell carcinoma or during treatment with pharmacological doses of calcitonin in patients with hypercalcaemia.

CALCITONIN ACTION ON THE KIDNEY

In humans, calcitonin administration results in a transient increase of the excretion of calcium, phosphate, sodium, potassium and magnesium. The hormone binds to specific renal receptors [80] and activates adenylate cyclase without significant increase of urinary cAMP excretion. In addition, calcitonin stimulates the production of $1,25(OH)_2D_3$ [21].

CALCITONIN ACTION ON THE GASTROINTESTINAL TRACT

Pharmacological doses of calcitonin inhibit most of the hormones of the gastrointestinal tract and of the exocrine and endocrine pancreas whereas, conversely, several gastrointestinal hormones may stimulate the calcitonin secretion. In addition, calcitonin administration stimulates small bowel secretion of sodium, chloride and water, and the intestinal absorption of calcium via $1,25(OH)_2D_3$.

OTHER EFFECTS OF CALCITONIN

It has been noticed during calcitonin treatment of patients with Paget disease that calcitonin exerts an analgesic effect, which may be mediated through a β-endorphin mechanism [81]. The presence of calcitonin-like material in the central nervous system indicates that the hormone may act as a central neurotransmitter or modulator.

Measurement of calcitonin in serum

A major barrier to understanding calcitonin secretion in humans has been the difficulty of measuring circulating hormone levels [82]. Until now, calcitonin measurements in serum have been predominantly used for the detection of increased secretion in patients with medullary thyroid carcinoma. The recent introduction of sensitive radioimmunoassays [69,71] offered the promise of defining the normal range of circulating calcitonin and studying calcitonin deficiency states. Immunoassayable calcitonin includes monomeric, dimeric and larger forms of the hormone. Calcitonin monomer, the major biologically active circulating form, can be measured by a simple procedure using a silica extraction–concentration method [69]. In healthy children [70] and adults [69] monomeric serum calcitonin is very low (about 10 pg/ml) and always increases after infusion of calcium (2 mg calcium/kg over 5 min). Basal and calcium-stimulated circulating calcitonin are much lower in women than in men, but there is disagreement over the supposed decline with age [69,71]. The levels of calcitonin and $1,25(OH)_2D$ are concurrently elevated in infancy and in women during pregnancy and lactation, indicating that calcitonin may prevent unwanted resorptive effects of the vitamin D hormone on bone while permitting its effect on the intestine during these states with extra demands for calcium.

Physiological significance of calcitonin

The precise role of calcitonin in the regulation of calcium metabolism in humans is unclear. The primary effect of the hormone seems to be a direct inhibition of bone resorption by PTH and $1,25(OH)_2D_3$ [83] (Fig. 37.10). Addi-

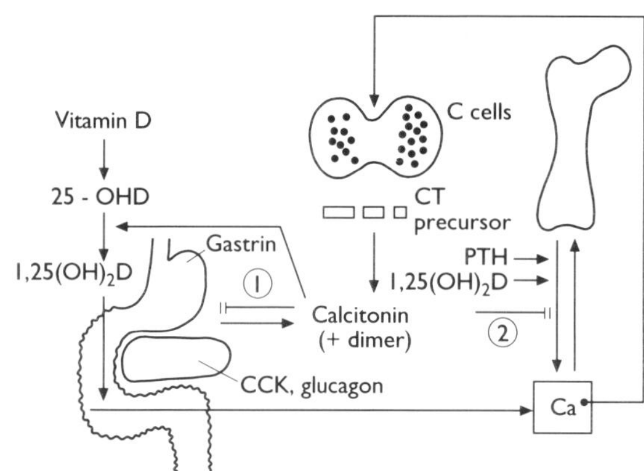

Fig. 37.10 Physiology of calcitonin (CT). Monomeric calcitonin, derived from a precursor molecule, is secreted by the C cells of the thyroid in response to serum calcium (Ca) and gastrointestinal hormones. The two main physiological effects of calcitonin are:
1 calcium conservation from nutrition (left side);
2 protection of exaggerated bone resorption by PTH and $1,25(OH)_2D$ (right side).
→, stimulation; —||, inhibition. CCK, cholecystokinin.

tionally, calcitonin can be regarded as a calcium-conserving hormone in nutrition, since it is secreted in response to food intake with the aim of shifting the absorbed calcium into blood [84,85]. The interrelationship between calcitonin and the gastrointestinal hormones may play an important role in this process. In response to calcium-rich food, various hormones of the gastrointestinal tract and the pancreas stimulate the release of calcitonin, which conversely inhibits their secretion. This delays calcium absorption and – together with calcitonin-induced inhibition of bone resorption – prevents postprandial hypercalcaemia and hypercalciuria.

BONE METABOLISM

Bone structure

In addition to its mechanical function, bone provides a large store of calcium, phosphate and other ions. In the embryo and growing child, bone develops either by intramembranous bone formation without a cartilage matrix or by enchondral bone formation, that is remodelling and replacing previously calcified cartilage [40]. Growth in width and thickness is accomplished by intramembranous bone formation at the periosteal surface and endosteal resorption of old bone with the rate of formation exceeding that of resorption.

Growth in length occurs by enchondral ossification. The growth plate, which is responsible for linear bone growth in children, has several zones (Fig. 37.11a): the resting zone, adjacent to the centre of ossification; the proliferation zone, where the cells are regular and arranged in columns; and, on the metaphyseal side, the maturation zone. At the lowest part of this zone, the zone of hypertrophy, the cells become large and round. In this region, vascular buds grow in from the metaphysis, and surrounding cartilage becomes heavily calcified (zone of provisional calcification). Below the hypertrophic zone, the cartilage condenses and becomes surrounded by osteoblasts, which produce calcified osteoid in the primary spongiosa of the metaphysis. This calcified tissue is resorbed and replaced by bone trabeculae in the secondary spongiosa.

Macroscopically, two major types of bone can be distinguished, trabecular (cancellous, spongy) bone and cortical (compact) bone. Trabecular bone is found in the metaphyseal areas of long bones, in vertebrae and in most flat bones. Cortical bone is found in the diaphyses of long bones. Although trabecular bone comprises only approximately 20% of the skeleton, its surface area and

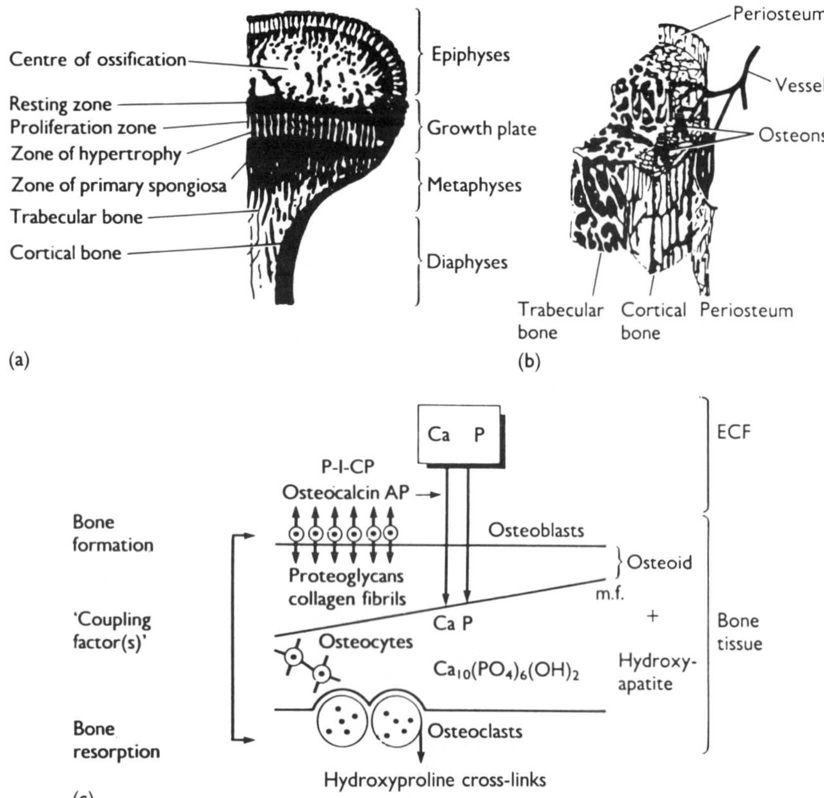

Fig. 37.11 Structure of bone: (a) Epiphyseal end of growing bone showing epiphyses with ossification centre, growth plate, where linear bone growth occurs by enchondral ossification, metaphyses and diaphyses with trabecular and cortical bone. (b) Microstructure of mature bone seen in transverse and longitudinal section. Areas of cortical (compact) bone and trabecular (cancellous) bone are shown. (c) Schema of histological details of bone tissue showing bone formation by osteoblasts and resorption of mineralized bone by osteoclasts, both processes being coupled by an unknown factor. Osteoblasts synthesize bone matrix (osteoid) which is mineralized by the deposition of calcium (Ca) and phosphate (P) in the presence of alkaline phosphatase (AP). The biochemical markers of bone formation (osteocalcin, AP and type I procollagen C-terminal propeptide (P-I-CP)) and of bone resorption (hydroxyproline and pyridinium cross-links) are indicated. ECF, extracellular fluid; m.f., mineralization front.

metabolic activity are several times greater than that of cortical bone.

Microscopically, cortical bone is made up of closely packed osteons (Haversian systems), as indicated in Fig. 37.11b. Each osteon contains a central Haversian canal with a blood vessel running through it, and is composed of concentric layers of osseous lamellae surrounding the central canal. In trabecular bone, lamellae are arranged in longitudinal bundles dependent on the mechanical stresses.

BONE CELLS AND BONE MATRIX

Bone is composed of organic matrix or osteoid, minerals (mainly calcium and phosphate) and different cells (mainly osteoblasts, osteocytes and osteoclasts). The principal cells of bone formation are *osteoblasts*, and they are responsible for the synthesis of bone matrix and its subsequent mineralization (Fig. 37.11c). These cells are thought to be derived from local mesenchymal cells. The major constituents of the bone matrix are type I collagen, a number of non-collagenous proteins (such as osteocalcin and osteonectin) and proteoglycans.

COLLAGEN

More than 15 different kinds of collagen have now been identified. Type I collagen is the most abundant collagen of bone. It is a heterotrimer consisting of two α_1 (I) protein chains and a different α_2 (I) chain twisted together into a long, thin rod. Each of the constituent α chains is approximately 1000 amino acids in length, and consists of highly repetitive sequences in which glycine occurs in every third position in the formate Gly-X-Y. X is often proline and Y often hydroxyproline.

Collagen is synthesized initially as a larger precursor molecule called procollagen, with peptide extensions (propeptide) at both the N- and C-termini. These extensions (N- and C-terminal propeptides) are cleaved by specific enzymes during secretion and fibril formation. During and after synthesis of procollagen chains, multiple proline and lysine residues are hydroxylated to produce hydroxyproline and hydroxylysine. Some hydroxylysine and lysine residues are converted by the enzyme lysyl oxidase to 5-hydroxy-α-aminoadipic acid semialdehyde and α-aminoadipic acid semialdehyde, respectively. Both modified residues interact with each other and other amino groups to form covalent cross-links between molecules, producing collagen fibrils of great strength. The hydroxylysine residues may also be the attachment site for galactose and galactose–glucose sugar residues. The pattern of this post-translational modification of bone type I collagen differs from that of soft tissues in that it contains predominantly galactosyl-hydroxylysyl residues (as opposed to glucosyl-galactosyl-hydroxylysyl residues in soft tissues).

Table 37.1 Components of the mineralized bone matrix

1 *Collagen* (predominantly type I)

2 *Proteoglycans* (acidic mucopolysaccharides = glycosaminoglycans attached to specific protein cores)
Biglycan
Versican
Decorin

3 *Glycoproteins*
Osteonectin
Fibronectin
Thrombospondin
Osteopontin
Bone sialoprotein

4 *γ-Carboxyglutamic acid-containing proteins*
Osteocalcin
Matrix Gla protein

5 *Enzymes and their inhibitors*
Alkaline phosphatase
Collagenase and its inhibitor
Plasminogen activator and its inhibitor
Lysosomal enzymes secreted by osteoclasts?

6 *Paracrine and autocrine growth factors*
FGF (fibroblast growth factor)
IGF (insulin-like growth factor)
TGF-β (transforming growth factor β)
PDGF (platelet-derived growth factor)

7 *Bone morphogenetic protein*

8 *Proteins absorbed from the circulation*
Growth factors (section 6 above)
Serum proteins (albumin, α_2-HS glycoprotein, immunoglobulins, transferrin, α_1-antitrypsin, haemoglobin, etc.)

From Robey *et al.* [86].

In addition to collagen, the bone matrix is composed of a number of proteins and enzymes, summarized in Table 37.1. Most of these molecules are produced by bone cells and are important for biochemical function and/or physical structure of bone; some may be involved in cellular proliferation and differentiation. The precise function of most bone proteins is not yet known.

Collagen, together with other matrix components, form a network upon which calcium and phosphate can be deposited as crystalline hydroxyapatite (Fig. 37.11c). The mechanisms of the mineralization process is not fully understood. Important factors are a normal calcium-phosphate product in extracellular fluid (serum) and normal activity of osteoblastic alkaline phosphatase. Alkaline phosphatase may function to hydrolyse pyrophosphate, an inhibitor of crystallization, and to increase the local concentration of inorganic phosphate, thus facilitating the formation of amorphous calcium phosphate. Evidence that alkaline phosphatase is linked to mineralization is supported by a defective bone matrix mineralization in patients with hypophosphatasia, a disease characterized by diminished serum and osteoblastic alkaline phosphatase activity [1]. Calcium- and phosphate-filled membrane vesicles extruded from osteoblasts may initiate mineralization in states of rapid bone formation.

Other products of the osteoblasts which may be involved in the regulation of mineralization are osteonectin, which possibly links calcium to collagen, and osteocalcin, which may regulate bone turnover and influence the activity of osteoclasts following fusion of precursor cells [86]. Osteocalcin has a molecular weight of 5.8 kD and is composed of 49 amino acids, three of them being γ-carboxyglutamic acid. Thus osteocalcin has also been referred to as bone Gla protein. Its synthesis is stimulated by $1,25(OH)_2D$.

OSTEOCYTES

When osteoblasts have completed their bone matrix deposition, approximately 10% are embedded within mineralized bone, thus becoming osteocytes. Osteocytes are located in lacunae and joined together and with osteoblasts on the bone surface via cytoplasmic processes. Osteocytes are thought to play a role in sensing strain resulting from mechanical force applied to the skeleton during mechanical usage. Another function of osteocytes may be the control of rapid mineral exchange between bone and serum without bone matrix degradation (osteocytic osteolysis), thus being of importance in regulating systemic mineral metabolism [40].

OSTEOCLASTS

Osteoclasts are typically large multinucleated cells derived from a different cell precursor than osteoblasts. They arise from bone marrow stem cells which may be related to those which give rise to various macrophage-like cells [87]. Osteoblastic stromal cells may be involved in osteoclastic differentiation by producing factor(s) in response to bone resorbing hormones such as PTH, $1,25(OH)_2D$ and prostaglandin E_2. Osteoclasts are highly mobile, have an intrinsic ruffled border at the resorptive surface and contain significant amounts of lysosomal (for example tartrate-resistant acid phosphatase, TRAP) and mitochondrial enzymes. The function of TRAP is not known, but the serum activity of this enzyme may be used as a marker of osteoclastic activity. Numerous specific binding sites for calcitonin have been demonstrated on mammalian osteoclasts, and the expression of calcitonin receptors is a reliable marker of osteoclast differentiation.

Under normal circumstances, osteoclasts resorb only mineralized bone and do not act on unmineralized osteoid. They bind through adhesion receptors (vitronectin receptors) to ligands on the bone surface. Possible candidates for such ligand proteins, which contain an Arg-Gly-Asp (RGD) sequence, are osteopontin and osteonectin. A current theory of bone resorption by osteoclasts is that these cells produce acids and chelating substances, which dissolve bone mineral, and proteinases, which cause subsequent degradation of the bone matrix.

Bone modelling and remodelling

The term 'modelling' describes the process of bone growth in length and width prior to the closure of the epiphyseal growth plate. Modelling is responsible for the genetically determined architectural features of the skeleton at the macroscopic level. The term 'remodelling', in contrast, describes the coupled process of bone formation and resorption occurring from early childhood until death, involving the endosteal surfaces of trabecular bone and the surfaces of the central canals (Haversian surfaces) in cortical bone. Through remodelling, bone tissue is continuously renewed and the removal of bone is followed by refilling. Normally, this remodelling process produces no net change of skeletal mass or systemic mineral balance, indicating that bone resorption and formation are closely coupled by yet unknown factors that coordinate the activity of osteoclasts and osteoblasts. There is a sequence of osteoclastic activation and bone resorption, followed by a resting phase and a formation phase, when new osteoid is laid down by osteoblasts at the same site, resulting in the formation of new bone.

Hormonal regulation of bone metabolism

It is believed that two independently regulated systems exist in bone, one regulating the contribution of bone to extracellular calcium homeostasis and the other regulating bone remodelling. This is supported by the observation that markedly increased bone formation and resorption, that is bone turnover, in Paget disease is not associated with significant changes in serum calcium levels.

A number of systemic and local factors influence bone resorption and/or formation directly or indirectly [12,40,86,87]. Direct effects indicate that these influences can be provoked by the respective agents *in vitro*, whereas indirect effects may be mediated through another organ. Both direct and indirect effects may induce changes in the concentrations of local bone factors (for example prostaglandins), which in turn result in changes of osteoclastic and/or osteoblastic activity. Table 37.2 summarizes the systemic hormones and some of the local growth factors that influence bone metabolism. PTH and $1,25(OH)_2D$ are mainly inhibitory through their ability directly to stimulate osteoclastic bone resorption and inhibit osteoblastic bone formation. The chronic adminis-

Table 37.2 Hormonal regulation of bone metabolism

Bone formation
Stimulation
Insulin
Insulin-like growth factors (IGF) I and II
Growth hormone
Thyroid hormones
Oestrogens and androgens
PTH
$1,25(OH)_2D$
Platelet-derived growth factor (PDGF)
Transforming growth factor (TGF) β
Inhibition
Glucocorticoids
Epidermal growth factor (EGF)
Fibroblast growth factor (FGF)
Bone resorption
Stimulation
PTH and PTHrP
$1,25(OH)_2D$
Thyroid hormones
IL-1
Tumour necrosis factor (TNF) α and β
FGF
EGF
Prostaglandins (PG), especially PGE_2
Vitamin A
Inhibition
Calcitonin
Glucocorticoids
Interferon-γ (IFN-γ)
TFG-β
Oestrogens and androgens

Data from Aurbach *et al.* [1], Robey *et al.* [86] and Raisz [87].

tration of both hormones may have indirect effects that cause inhibition of bone resorption and/or stimulation of bone formation, resulting in a net increase of bone mass. The main effect of the third calcium-regulating hormone, calcitonin, is the direct inhibition of osteoclastic bone resorption.

Glucocorticoids have complex effects on bone metabolism. Patients on treatment with large doses of glucocorticoids for long periods are prone to osteopenia, which is probably caused by direct and indirect effects. The main mechanism for glucocorticoid osteopenia is thought to be inhibition of bone formation by inhibiting the proliferation of precursor cells for osteoblasts. In addition, bone resorption may be indirectly stimulated by the suppression of intestinal calcium absorption, resulting in secondary hyperparathyroidism.

Insulin has direct and indirect stimulating effects on cartilage and bone formation, explaining why insulin deficiency in some diabetic patients may be associated with decreased bone mass. The indirect insulin effects on bone are thought to be mediated through increased production of insulin-like growth factor (IGF) and $1,25(OH)_2D$. Thyroid hormones have indirect stimulatory effects on both bone formation (in part mediated by IGF) and bone resorption, which may explain why skeletal growth and bone turnover are decreased in children with thyroid hormone deficiency and increased in children with hyperthyroidism.

Androgens and oestrogens have important stimulatory influences on bone metabolism. It was long thought that their stimulatory effects on bone formation and inhibitory effects on bone resorption were indirect, through alterations in the secretion of other hormones or local factors, but oestrogen receptors have been demonstrated on osteoblasts, and oestrogens have been reported to increase trabecular bone formation directly [86].

At puberty, both sex steroids are important in producing the pubertal growth spurt. Skeletal growth and bone metabolism is accelerated by sex steroid excess in precocious puberty, whereas deficiency of gonadal hormones causes osteopenia in children and adults. Oestrogens may prevent bone loss by increasing intestinal calcium absorption via $1,25(OH)_2D$ synthesis and by inhibiting bone resorption via calcitonin secretion.

Growth hormone (GH) stimulates cartilage and bone formation directly and/or indirectly through local production of IGF-I and IGF-II, and increases osteoblast number and function. IGF-I is a potent stimulator of collagen, non-collagen proteins and DNA synthesis in cultured bone. The effects of IGF-I and insulin on bone are closely related and not additive, suggesting a similar mechanism of action. Since direct injection of GH into the tibia of hypophysectomized rats stimulates longitudinal bone growth, there may be local synthesis of IGF-I and other growth factors by the perichondrial cells or the cartilage cells themselves.

GH also stimulates the renal synthesis of $1,25(OH)_2D$ (via IGF-I) thereby enhancing intestinal calcium and phosphate absorption. In addition, it increases the renal tubular reabsorption of phosphate.

Bone contains several growth factors that affect bone cells *in vitro* and *in vivo* (see Table 37.1). Some of them, such as TGF-β and IGF, may be important in the process coupling bone formation to resorption.

Prostaglandins, some of the most important local factors regulating bone metabolism, are direct stimulators of bone resorption and bone formation. The effect of prostaglandins on bone formation depends on concentration: in high dose they inhibit bone protein synthesis and in low dose they stimulate. Prostaglandins of the E series may be responsible for osteolysis and the resulting hypercalcaemia in some patients with malignant disease; prolonged infusions of prostaglandins to maintain the patency of the ductus arteriosus in infants may produce a significant increase in periosteal bone formation.

Investigation of bone metabolism

Bone metabolism can be assessed by the following.
1 Measurement of bone constituents in serum and urine.
2 Radiological evaluation of the skeleton.
3 Estimation of bone density.
4 Histological investigation of bone biopsy.

MEASUREMENT OF BONE CONSTITUENTS IN SERUM AND URINE

Biochemical measurement of bone formation and resorption by non-invasive techniques is an important adjunct to imaging procedures and histomorphometric analysis. Five bone constituents are useful for the assessment of bone turnover in clinical practice: alkaline phosphatase, osteocalcin and C-terminal propeptide of type I procollagen (P-I-CP) in serum as indices of osteoblastic bone formation and total hydroxyproline and pyridinium cross-links in urine as indices of osteoclastic bone resorption.

Alkaline phosphatase

Circulating alkaline phosphatase is a composite from multiple sources, especially from bone, liver and intestine. In children, most comes from the bone, the osteoblasts being the major skeletal source for serum alkaline phosphatase. The bone alkaline phosphatase may be partially differentiated from the liver enzyme by electrophoretic mobility, as well as by a greater lability to heat and urea. Bone alkaline phosphatase in serum can now be quantified by precipitation with wheat-germ lectin [88] and by a selective RIA.

Osteocalcin

Osteocalcin (bone Gla protein), like alkaline phosphatase, is produced by osteoblasts, probably under the control of $1,25(OH)_2D$. Small amounts of the protein are found in blood, from which it is cleared mainly by kidney filtration. With the introduction of a RIA for serum osteocalcin it has been established that its measurement provides a useful index of bone formation, provided that vitamin D status and renal function are normal [89–91]. Recent evidence suggests that osteocalcin is present in an intact form as well as in fragments, and that total immunoreactive osteocalcin may also reflect bone resorption products in addition to bone formation products.

Carboxy-terminal propeptide of type I procollagen

P-I-CP is released from procollagen into the blood and reflects type I collagen synthesis. Its radioimmunological measurement has been shown to be a sensitive marker of bone metabolism, especially bone formation [92].

Hydroxyproline in urine

Hydroxyproline is an amino acid which occurs almost exclusively in the collagen molecule, more than 50% being localized in the skeleton. Because hydroxyproline released from bone matrix is not reutilized for collagen synthesis, total urinary hydroxyproline excretion may be used as an index for the rate of bone formation and resorption, especially for the latter [1,93]. Although urinary levels of hydroxyproline also reflect the turnover of extraskeletal collagens, and are thus not specific for bone resorption, their measurement represents a reliable indicator of bone remodelling with good correlations to other biomarkers, including pyridinium cross-links and galactosyl hydroxylysine [78]. The use of fasting morning urine to obtain the ratio of hydroxyproline to creatinine avoids the influence of dietary collagen and incomplete 24-h urine collections [93].

Pyridinium cross-links in urine

The measurement of intermolecular cross-linking compounds of collagen seems to overcome the lack of specifity of hydroxyproline as marker of osteoclastic bone resorption. Pyridinoline (Pyr) and deoxypyridinoline (D-Pyr) (also called hydroxylysylpyridinoline and lysylpyridinoline) are two amino acids that form covalent cross-links between adjacent collagen chains in extracellular matrix. D-Pyr, which is present in significant amounts only in bone tissue, has been demonstrated to be a relatively specific marker of bone degradation [78].

In children, levels of alkaline phosphatase, osteocalcin, P-I-CP in serum as well as urinary hydroxyproline and pyridinium cross-links are age-dependent, reflecting different height velocities. A combined measurement provides useful information for the diagnosis and follow-up of patients with disturbed bone turnover during treatment. Other markers of bone turnover are galactosyl hydroxylysine [78] in urine as well as TRAP, osteopontin, osteonectin and matrix Gla bone protein in serum [40,88]. Further evaluation of these markers, along with histomorphometric analysis, are needed.

RADIOLOGICAL EVALUATION OF THE SKELETON

Conventional bone radiology is still an important tool to realize the nature, severity and extent of bone disease. Examples of abnormalities which may be found include abnormal density, structure, size and shape of bones, widening of epiphyseal growth plates and fractures.

ESTIMATION OF BONE DENSITY

Quantitative estimation of bone density is important for the assessment of osteopenia and osteoporosis, which is not yet visible radiographically. The development of techniques such as single- and dual-photon absorptiometry and computerized tomography, has brought about major improvements in the evaluation of bone disorders. In single-photon absorptiometry a collimated beam of ^{125}I is passed through bone, and the attenuation of radiation transmission is measured as an index of bone mineral content.

The overlying soft tissue may be a hindrance to the measurement of bone density, and can be allowed for by use of dual-photon absorptiometry. Here two energy channels are used to resolve contributions from soft tissue and bone. Single-photon absorptiometry is used to measure bone density of the distal radius (about 75% cortical and 25% trabecular bone), whereas dual-photon absorptiometry [95] can be applied to vertebrae (about 25% cortical and 75% trabecular bone). Computerized tomography measures mineral content of only trabecular bone in vertebrae, but only at the cost of considerable irradiation. Unfortunately there is a large overlap in measurements between osteopenic and healthy subjects, especially when single-photon absorptiometry is applied.

Dual-energy X-ray absorptiometry (DEXA), otherwise known as X-ray densitometry, is a new technique with several advantages. It is non-invasive, rapid (scanning time 5–10 min) and precise (coefficient of variation for repeated measurements <2%) method for determining bone mineral content of the lumbar spine, hip or total body. Because of the very low irradiation (adsorbed dose of radiation <3 mrem), serial measurements can be performed, allowing the investigation of several metabolic bone disorders before and during treatment. DEXA has recently been shown to be a suitable method for paediatric bone mineral measurement even in newborns and infants [96,97].

HISTOLOGICAL INVESTIGATION OF BONE BIOPSY

Bone specimens from the iliac crest, containing mainly trabecular bone, are obtained by a percutaneous procedure, fixed and embedded in plastic for sectioning with a special microtome [94]. Quantitative morphometric analysis of the uncalcified sections assesses the number of osteoblasts and osteoclasts, bone volume, volumes and surfaces of osteoid, as well as the surface of bone undergoing resorption and formation. The dynamic process of bone formation can be evaluated by tetracycline double-labelling of the skeleton. This antibiotic is mainly incorporated in the zone of new mineralization of cortical and trabecular bone, and is recognizable under fluorescent light as rings or bands separated by a dark area. The rate of bone formation can be calculated by the ratio of the average width between the bands or rings divided by the number of days between drug administrations [94].

The indications for bone biopsy in children are limited, but the method can give helpful information in patients in whom non-invasive techniques do not give clear answers, as in mild rickets or osteomalacia, osteogenesis imperfecta and juvenile osteoporosis. Sequential bone biopsies may be of value in some children with renal osteodystrophy to monitor the efficacy of treatment.

INTEGRATED CONTROL OF CALCIUM AND PHOSPHATE HOMEOSTASIS

The calcium-regulating hormones PTH and $1,25(OH)_2D_3$ act on their target organs to counter hypocalcaemia and hypercalcaemia (Fig. 37.12). When hypocalcaemia occurs, this is rapidly sensed by the parathyroid gland. The rise in PTH leads to decreased renal calcium excretion and, in conjunction with $1,25(OH)_2D_3$, to increased mobilization of calcium and phosphate from bone. In addition to these rapid changes, PTH slowly enhances the renal synthesis of $1,25(OH)_2D_3$, which in turn increases the intestinal absorption of calcium and phosphate. An undesirable serum phosphate increase is prevented by PTH-induced phosphaturia.

The response to hypercalcaemia is largely the converse of the response to hypocalcaemia: secretion of PTH decreases, which results in elevated renal calcium excretion, decreased resorption of calcium from bone and suppression of $1,25(OH)_2D_3$-mediated intestinal calcium absorption. Hypercalcaemia also increases serum calcitonin concentration, but this hormone does not seem to be of major influence on the extracellular calcium level. The serum phosphate concentration is less stringently controlled, the kidney playing the dominant role in phosphate homeostasis. Chronic phosphate loss leads to increased $1,25(OH)_2D_3$ synthesis (independently of PTH)

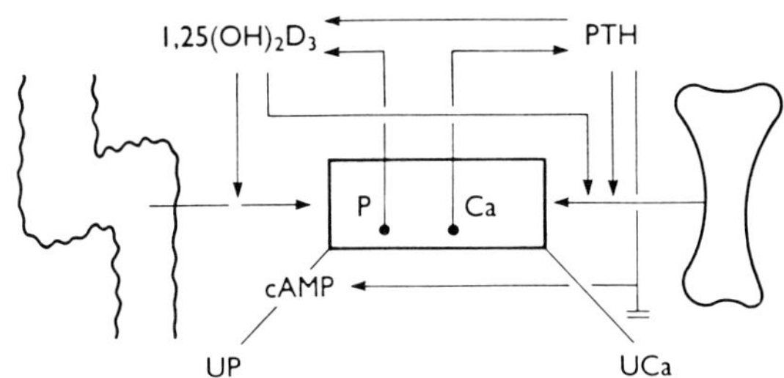

Fig. 37.12 Regulation of calcium and phosphate metabolism by $1,25(OH)_2D_3$ and PTH. P/Ca, phosphate and calcium concentration in serum; UP/UCa, urinary phosphate and calcium excretion; →, stimulation; —⊣, inhibition.

and increased intestinal phosphate absorption (Fig. 37.12), whereas phosphate retention inhibits vitamin D synthesis.

REFERENCES

1 Aurbach GD, Marx SJ, Spiegel AM. Parathyroid hormone, calcitonin, and the calciferols. In: Wilson JD, Foster DW, eds. *Williams Textbook of Endocrinology*, 8th edn. Philadelphia PA: WB Saunders, 1992:1397–476.

2 Stewart AF, Broadus AE. Mineral metabolism. In: Felig P, Baxter JD, Broachüs AE, Frohman LA, eds. *Endocrinology and Metabolism*, 2nd edn. New York: McGraw-Hill, 1987:1317–453.

3 Holick MF, Adams JS, Clemens TL *et al.* Photoendocrinology of vitamin D: the past, present and future. In: Norman AW, Schaefer K, v. Herruth D, Gingoleit H-G, eds. *Vitamin D: Chemical, Biochemical and Clinical Endocrinology of Calcium Metabolism*. Berlin: Walter de Gruyter, 1982:1151–6.

4 Bouillon R, Van Baelen H. The transport of vitamin D: significance of free and total concentrations of vitamin D metabolites. In: Norman AW, Schaefer K, v. Herruth D, Gingoleit H-G, eds. *Vitamin D: Chemical, Biochemical and Clinical Endocrinology of Calcium Metabolism*. Berlin: Walter de Gruyter, 1982:1181–6.

5 Fraser DR. Regulation of the metabolism of vitamin D. *Physiol Rev* 1980;60:551–613.

6 DeLuca HF, Schnoes HK. Vitamin D: recent advances. *Annu Rev Biochem* 1983;52:411–39.

7 Norman AW, Roth J, Orci L. The vitamin D endocrine system: steroid metabolism, hormone receptors, and biological response (calcium binding proteins). *Endocr Rev* 1982;3:331–66.

8 Hughes MR, Malloy PJ, O'Malley BW, Pike JW, Feldman D. Genetic defects of the 1,25-dihydroxyvitamin D_3 receptor. *J Rec Res* 1991;11:699–716.

9 Pike JW, Allegretto EA, Kelly MA *et al.* 1,25-dihydroxyvitamin D_3 receptors: altered functional domains are associated with cellular resistance to vitamin D_3. *Adv Exp Med Biol* 1986;196:377–90.

10 Yamaguchi A, Kohno Y, Yamazaki T *et al.* Bone in the marmoset: a resemblance to vitamin D-dependent rickets, type II. *Calcif Tissue Int* 1986;39:22–7.

11 Reichel H, Koeffler HP, Norman AW. The role of the vitamin D endocrine system in health and disease. *N Engl J Med* 1989;320:980–91.

12 Centrella M, Canalis E. Local regulators of skeletal growth: a perspective. *Endocr Rev* 1985;6:544–51.

13 Bell NH. Vitamin D endocrine system. *J Clin Invest* 1985; 76:1–6.

14 Brommage R, DeLuca HF. Evidence that 1,25-dihydroxyvitamin D_3 is the physiologically active metabolite of vitamin D_3. *Endocr Rev* 1985;6:491–511.

15 Underwood JL, DeLuca HF. Vitamin D is not directly necessary for bone growth and mineralization. *Am J Physiol* 1984; 246:E493–8.

16 Balsan S, Garabédian M, Larchet M *et al.* Long-term nocturnal calcium infusions can cure rickets and promote normal mineralization in hereditary resistance to 1,25-dihydroxyvitamin D. *J Clin Invest* 1986;77:1661–7.

17 Manolagas SC. Role of 1,25 dihydroxyvitamin D_3 in the immune system. In: Norman AW, Schaefer K, v. Herruth D, Gingoleit H-G, eds. *Vitamin D: a Chemical and Clinical Update*. Berlin: Walter de Gruyter, 1985:199–208.

18 Reichel H, Koeffler HP, Barbers R, Munker R, Norman AW. 1,25-dihydroxyvitamin D_3 and the hematopoietic system. In: Normal AW, Schaefer K, v. Herruth D, Gingoleit H-G, eds. *Vitamin D: a Chemical and Clinical Update*. Berlin: Walter de Gruyter, 1985:167–76.

19 Bikle DD. Clinical counterpoint: vitamin D: new actions, new analogs, new therapeutic potential. *Endocr Rev* 1992; 13:765–84.

20 Aarskog D, Asknes L, Markestad T, Rødland O. Effect of oestrogen on vitamin D metabolism in tall girls. *J Clin Endocrinol Metab* 1983;57:1155–8.

21 Jaeger P, Jones W, Clemens TL, Hayslett JP. Evidence that calcitonin stimulates 1,25-dihydroxyvitamin D production and intestinal absoprtion of calcium *in vivo*. *J Clin Invest* 1986;78:456–61.

22 Stern PH, Taylor AB, Bell NH, Epstein S. Demonstration that circulating 1,α,25-dihydroxyvitamin D is loosely regulated in normal children. *J Clin Invest* 1981;68:1374–7.

23 Reinhardt TA, Horst RL, Orf JW, Hollis BW. A microassay for 1,25-dihydroxyvitamin D not requiring high performance liquid chromatography: application to clinical studies. *J Clin Endocrinol Metab* 1984;58:91–8.

24 Hollis BW. Assay of circulating 1,25-dihydroxyvitamin D involving a novel single cartridge extraction and purification procedure. *Clin Chem* 1986;32:2060–3.

25 Bouillon R, Auwerx J, Dekeyser L, Fevery J, Lissens W, De Moor P. Serum vitamin D metabolites and their binding protein in patients with liver cirrhosis. *J Clin Endocrinol Metab* 1984;59:86–9.

26 Keutmann HT, Sauer RM, Hendy GN, O'Riordan JLH, Potts JT Jr. Complete amino acid sequence of human parathyroid hormone. *Biochemistry* 1978;17:5723–9.

27 Habener JF, Rosenblatt M, Potts JT Jr. Parathyroid hormone: biochemical aspects of biosynthesis, secretion, action, and metabolism. *Physiol Rev* 1984;64:985–1053.

28 Antonarakis SE, Phillips JA III, Mallonee RL *et al.* β-Globulin locus is linked to the parathyroid hormone (PTH) locus and lies between the insulin and PTH loci in man. *Proc Natl Acad Sci USA* 1983;80:6615–19.

29 Zabel BU, Kronenberg HM, Bell GJ, Shous TB. Chromosomal mapping of genes on the short arm of the chromosome 11: parathyroid hormone gene is at 11p15 together with the genes for insulin, c-Harvey-ras I oncogene, beta-hemoglobin. *Cytogenet Cell Genet* 1985;30:200–5.

30 Brown EM. PTH secretion *in vivo* and *in vitro*. Regulation by calcium and other secretagogues. *Miner Electrolyte Metab* 1982;8:130–50.

31 Mayer GP, Habener JF, Potts JT Jr. Parathyroid hormone secretion *in vivo*: demonstration of a calcium-independent, non-suppressible component of secretion. *J Clin Invest* 1976;57:679–83.

32 Cholst IN, Steinberg SF, Tropper PJ, Fox HE, Segre GV, Bilezikian JP. The influence of hypermagnesemia on serum calcium and parathyroid hormone levels in human subjects. *N Engl J Med* 1984;310:1221–5.

33 Rude RK, Oldham SB, Singer FR. Functional hypoparathyroidism and parathyroid hormone end-organ resistance in human magnesium deficiency. *Clin Endocrinol* 1976;5: 209–24.

34 Rude RK, Oldham SB, Sharp CF Jr, Singer FR. Parathyroid hormone secretion in magnesium deficiency. *J Clin Endocrinol Metab* 1978;47:800–6.

35 Pocotte SL, Ehrenstein G, Fitzpatrick LA. Regulation of parathyroid hormone secretion. *Endocr Rev* 1991;12:291–301.

36 Kruse K, Kracht U. A simplified diagnostic test in hypoparathyroidism and pseudohypoparathyroidism type I with synthetic 1–38 fragment of human parathyroid hormone. *Eur J Pediatr* 1987;146:373–7.

37 Jüppner H, Abou-Samru A-B, Freeman M *et al.* A G protein-linked receptor for parathyroid hormone and parathyroid hormone-related protein. *Science* 1991;254:1024–6.

38 Spiegel AM, Shenker A, Weinstein LS. Receptor–effector coupling by G proteins: implications for normal and abnormal signal transduction. *Endocr Rev* 1992;13:536–65.

39 Gejman PV, Weinstein LS, Martinez M *et al.* Genetic mapping of the Gs-α-subunit gene (GNAS1) to the distal long arm of chromosome 20 using a polymorphism detecting by denaturing gradient gel electrophoresis. *Genomics* 1991; 9:782–3.

40 Aurbach GD, Marx SJ, Spiegel AM. Metabolic bone disease. In: Wilson JD, Foster DW, eds. *Williams Textbook of Endocrinology*, 8th edn. Philadelphia, PA: WB Saunders, 1992:1477–517.

41 McSheehy PMJ, Chambers TJ. Osteoblast-like cells in the presence of parathyroid hormone release soluble factor that stimulates osteoclastic bone resorption. *Endocrinology* 1986;119:1645–9.

42 Berson SA, Yalow RS. Immunochemical heterogeneity of parathyroid hormone in plasma. *J Clin Endocrinol Metab* 1968;28:1037–47.

43 Armitage EK. Parathyrin (parathyroid hormone): metabolism and methods for assay. *Clin Chem* 1986;32:418–24.

44 Stewart AF, Broadus AE. Clinical review 16: parathyroid hormone-related proteins: coming of age in the 1990s. *J Clin Endocrinol Metab* 1990;71:1410–14.

45 Wood PJ. The measurement of parathyroid hormone. *Ann Clin Biochem* 1992;29:11–21.

46 Allgrove J, Chayen J, O'Riordan JLH. The cytochemical bioassay of parathyroid hormone: further experience. *J Immunoassay* 1983;4:1–19.

47 Chambers DJ, Dunham J, Zanelli JM, Parsons JA, Bitensky L, Chayen J. A sensitive bioassay of parathyroid hormone in plasma. *Clin Endocrinol* 1978;9:375–9.

48 Goltzman D, Henderson B, Loveridge N. Cytochemical bioassay of parathyroid hormone. Characteristics of the assay and analysis of circulating hormone forms. *J Clin Invest* 1980;65:1309–17.

49 Nissenson RA, Abbott SR, Teitelbaum AP, Clark DH, Arnaud CD. Endogenous biologically active human parathyroid hormones measurement by a guanyl nucleotide-amplified renal adenylate cyclase assay. *J Clin Endocrinol Metab* 1981;52:840–6.

50 Zanelli JM, Kent JC, Rafferty B *et al.* High-performance liquid chromatographic methods for the analysis of human parathyroid hormone in reference standards, parathyroid tissue and biological fluids. *J Chromatog* 1983;276:55–68.

51 Suva LJ, Winslow GA, Wettenhall REH *et al.* A parathyroid hormone-related protein implicated in malignant hypercalcemia: cloning and expression. *Science* 1987;237:893–6.

52 Yasuda T, Bonville D, Hendy GN, Goltzman D. Characterization of the human parathyroid hormone-like peptide gene, functional and evolutionary aspects. *J Biol Chem* 1989; 264:7720–5.

53 Bilezikian JP. Clinical utility of assays for parathyroid hormone-related protein. *Clin Chem* 1992;38:179–81.

54 Martin TJ, Suva LJ. Parathyroid hormone-related protein: a novel gene product. *Ballières Clin Endocrinol Metab* 1988; 2:1003–29.

55 Moseley JM, Danks JA, Grill V, Southby J, Hayman JA, Horton MA. Immunohistochemical localization of parathyroid hormone-related protein in fetal tissues. *J Clin Endocrinol Metab* 1991;73:478–84.

56 Budayr AA, Halloran BP, King JC *et al.* High levels of a parathyroid hormone-like protein in milk. *Proc Natl Acad Sci USA* 1989;86:7183–5.

57 Grill V, Hillary J, Ho PMW *et al.* Parathyroid hormone-related protein: a possible endocrine function in lactation. *Clin Endocrinol* 1992;37:405–10.

58 Mallette LA. The parathyroid polyhormones: new concepts in the spectrum of peptide hormone action. *Endocr Rev* 1991; 12:110–7.

59 Walton RJ, Bijvoet OLM. Nomogram for derivation of renal threshold phosphate concentration. *Lancet* 1975;2:309–10.

60 Kruse K, Kracht U, Göpfert G. Renal threshold phosphate concentration ($TmPO_4$/GFR). *Arch Dis Child* 1982;57: 217–23.

61 Kruse K, Kracht U. Urinary adenosine 3′,5′-monophosphate excretion in childhood. *J Clin Endocrinol Metab* 1981;53: 1251–5.

62 Broachüs AE, Mahaffy JE, Bartter FC, Neer RM. Nephrogenous cyclic adenosine monophosphate as a parathyroid function test. *J Clin Invest* 1977;60:771–83.

63 Neer RM, Treager GW, Potts JT Jr. Renal effects of native parathyroid hormone and synthetic biologically active fragments in pseudohypoparathyroidism and hypoparathyroidism. *J Clin Endocrinol Metab* 1977;44:420–3.

64 Slovic DM, Daly MA, Potts JT Jr, Neer RM. Renal 1,25-dihydroxyvitamin D, phosphaturic, and cyclic-AMP responses to intravenous synthetic human parathyroid hormone-(1–34) administration in normal subjects. *Clin Endocrinol* 1984; 20:369–75.

65 Kruse K. Hypoparathyroidism and pseudohypoparathyroidism: new aspects in the pathogenesis, diagnosis and treatment. *Monatschr Kinderheilkd* 1988;136:652–66.

66 Yamamoto M, Furukawa Y, Konagaya Y *et al.* Human PTH (1–34) infusion test in differential diagnosis at various types of hypoparathyroidism: an attempt to establish a standard clinical test. *Bone Miner* 1989;6:199–212.

67 Stirling HF, Darling JAB, Barr DGD. Plasma cyclic AMP response to intravenous parathyroid hormone in pseudohypoparathyroidism. *Acta Paed Scand* 1991;Suppl. 80:333–8.

68 Copp DH, Cameron EC, Cheney BA, Davidson AGF, Henze KG. Evidence for calcitonin – a new hormone from the parathyroid that lowers blood calcium. *Endocrinology* 1962; 70:638–90.

69 Body JJ, Heath H III. Estimates of circulating monomeric calcitonin: physiologic studies in normal and thyroidectomized man. *J Clin Endocrinol Metab* 1983;57:897–903.

70 Kruse K, Süß A, Büsse M, Schneider P. Monomeric serum calcitonin and bone turnover during anticonvulsant treatment and in congenital hypothyroidism. *J Pediatr* 1987;111:57–63.

71 Parthemore JG, Deftos LJ. Calcitonin secretion in normal human subjects. *J Clin Endocrinol Metab* 1978;47:184–8.

72 Przepiorka D, Baylin AB, McBride OW, Testa JR, Bustros A, Nelkin BD. The human calcitonin gene is located on the short arm of chromosome 11. *Biochem Biophys Res Commun* 1984;120:493–9.

73 Jonas V, Lin CR, Kåwashima E *et al.* Alternative RNA processing events in human calcitonin/calcitonin gene-related peptide gene expression. *Proc Natl Acad Sci USA* 1985; 82:1994–8.

74 Girgis SI, MacDonald DWR, Stevenson JC *et al.* Calcitonin gene-related peptide: potent vasodilator and major product of calcitonin gene. *Lancet* 1985;2:14–16.
75 Austin LA, Heath H III. Calcitonin: physiology and pathophysiology. *N Engl J Med* 1981;304:269–78.
76 Chambers TJ, Moore A. The sensitivity of isolated osteoclasts to morphological transformation by calcitonin. *J Endocrinol Metab* 1983;57:819–24.
77 Chambers TJ, Athanasou NA, Fuller K. Effect of parathyroid hormone and calcitonin on the cytoplasmatic spreading of isolated osteoclasts. *J Endocrinol* 1984;102:281–6.
78 Bettica P, Moro L, Robins SP *et al.* Bone-resorption markers galactosyl hydroxylysine, pyridinium crosslinks, and hydroxyproline compared. *Clin Chem* 1992;38:2313–18.
79 Tashijan AW, Wright DR, Ivey SI, Pont A. Calcitonin binding sites in bone: relationships to biological response and escape. *Rec Prog Horm Res* 1978;34:285–334.
80 Marx SJ, Woodard CJ, Aurbach GD. Calcitonin receptors of kidney and bone. *Science* 1972;178:999–1001.
81 Gennari C. Clinical aspects of calcitonin in pain. *Triangle* 1983;22:157–63.
82 Heath H III, Body J-J, Fox J. Radioimmunoassay of calcitonin in normal human plasma: problems, perspectives and prospects. *Biomed Pharmacother* 1984;38:241–5.
83 McIntyre I. The action and control of the calcium-regulating hormones. *J Endocrinol Invest* 1978;1:277–84.
84 Talmage RV, Grubb SA, Norimatsou H, VanderWiel CJ. Evidence for an important physiological role for calcitonin. *Proc Natl Acad Sci USA* 1980;77:609–13.
85 Ziegler R, Deutsche U, Raue F. Calcitonin in human pathophysiology. *Horm Res* 1984;20:65–73.
86 Robey PG, Bianco P, Termine JD. The cellular biology and molecular biochemistry of bone formation. In: Coe FL, Favus MJ, eds. *Disorders of Bone and Mineral Metabolism.* New York: Raven Press, 1992:241–63.
87 Raisz LG. Mechanisms and regulation of bone resorption by osteoclastic cells. In: Coe FL, Favus MJ, eds. *Disorders of Bone and Mineral Metabolism.* New York: Raven Press, 1992:287–311.
88 Rosalki SB, Ying Foo A. Two new methods for separating and quantifying bone and liver alkaline phosphatase isoenzymes in plasma. *Clin Chem* 1984;30:1182–6.
89 Hauschka PV. Osteocalcin: the vitamin K-dependent Ca^{2+}-binding protein of bone matrix. *Haemostasis* 1986;16:258–72.
90 Kruse K, Kracht U. Evaluation of serum osteocalcin as an index of altered bone metabolism. *Eur J Pediatr* 1986;145: 27–33.
91 Price PA, Parthemore JG, Deftos LJ. New biochemical marker of bone metabolism. Measurement by radioimmunoassay of bone Gla protein in the plasma of normal subjects and patients with bone disease. *J Clin Invest* 1980;66:878–83.
92 Saggese G, Bertelloni S, Baroncelli GJ, Di Nero G. Serum levels of carboxyterminal propeptide of type I procollagen in healthy children from 1st year of life to adulthood and in metabolic diseases. *Eur J Pediatr* 1992;151:764–8.
93 Kruse K, Kracht U. Die Hydroxyprolin-Ausscheidung im Morgen-Urin. Ein geeigneter Parameter des Knochen-Umsatzes im Kindesalter. *Monatschr Kinderheilkd* 1983;131:797–803.
94 Malluche HH, Faugere M-C. *Atlas of Mineralized Bone Histology.* Basel: Karger, 1986.
95 Ponder SW, McCormick DP, Fawcett D, Palmer JL, McKernan MG, Brouhard BH. Spinal bone mineral density in children aged 5.00 through 11.99 years. *Am J Dis Child* 1990;144: 1346–8.
96 Salle BL, Braillon P, Glorieux FH *et al.* Lumbar bone mineral content measured by dual energy X-ray absorptiometry in newborns and infants. *Acta Paediatr* 1992;81:953–8.
97 Venkataraman PS, Ahluwalia BW. The bone mineral content and body components by X-ray densitometry in newborns. *Pediatrics* 1992;90:767–70.

38: Disorders of Calcium and Bone Metabolism

K. KRUSE

INTRODUCTION

Most disorders of extracellular calcium and phosphate metabolism result from increased or decreased secretion/action of 1,25-dihydroxyvitamin D_3 (1,25$(OH)_2D_3$) and parathyroid hormone (PTH) or from increased or decreased urinary excretion of phosphate and calcium [1]. In some disorders two primary pathogenetic factors may be coupled and, in nearly all disorders, compensatory mechanisms cause secondary disturbances of hormonal secretion or mineral excretion. Based on this pathogenetic classification the most important diseases of calcium and phosphate metabolism are discussed. Disturbances of calcitonin secretion are described next and a special section is devoted to early infancy where peculiar disturbances of mineral and bone metabolism occur.

DISTURBANCES OF 1,25-DIHYDROXYVITAMIN D_3 SECRETION OR ACTION IN CHILDHOOD

Increased formation or action of 1,25-dihydroxyvitamin D

ABSORPTIVE HYPERCALCIURIA

Idiopathic hypercalciuria, defined as high urinary calcium excretion in the absence of known causes of hypercalciuria [2], predisposes to renal stone formation and/or haematuria in children and adults. In children, it has a frequency of about 3% and may be transmitted as an autosomal dominant trait [3,4]. Two subtypes of idiopathic hypercalciuria may be distinguished, absorptive and renal [5]. Absorptive hypercalciuria is thought to be due to an increased intestinal calcium absorption caused by increased secretion or responsiveness to 1,25$(OH)_2$D as a primary abnormality [6]. Increased intestinal vitamin D receptors have been found in genetically hypercalciuric rats, exerting biological actions in enterocytes to increase intestinal calcium transport [7]. This may be the first genetic disorder resulting from a pathological increase in the vitamin D receptor. Renal hypercalciuria presumably reflects an idiopathic renal tubular defect characterized by an inability to reabsorb filtered calcium appropriately. Since both types of hypercalciuria are consistently associated with increased calcium excretion in the postabsorptive state, a randomly collected urine sample after lunch can be used to screen for hypercalciuria [8]. If the calcium–creatinine concentration in children aged 3–18 years exceeds the upper normal range of 0.6 mmol/mmol (0.22 mg/mg) the hypercalciuria should be confirmed by demonstrating urinary calcium excretion of more than 0.1 mmol (4 mg) per kg body weight or 0.6 mmol/mmol (0.22 mg/mg) creatinine in a 24-h urine collection. For subclassifying both types the urinary calcium/creatinine ratio is measured in the fasting state (second voiding of the morning fasting urine) when intestinal calcium absorption is largely excluded, or in a 24-h urine sample after a low calcium intake for several days. Normal calcium excretion rates and normal serum PTH then indicate absorptive hypercalciuria, while children with elevated ratios and secondary hyperparathyroidism are classified as having renal hypercalciuria [5,8]. Treatment requires a low-calcium diet for absorptive hypercalciuria. In patients with renal hypercalciuria the calcium excretion can be inhibited by a low-sodium diet and hydrochlorothiazide (2–3 mg/kg body weight per day, administered orally in two divided doses).

GRANULOMATOUS DISEASE AND LYMPHOMA

Hypercalcaemia associated with abnormally elevated 1,25$(OH)_2$D and normal or suppressed PTH levels in serum have been reported in patients with sarcoidosis, tuberculosis and several other chronic granulomatous diseases [9,10].

The granulomatous cells convert 25-hydroxyvitamin D (25-OHD) into 1,25$(OH)_2$D with subsequent increased intestinal calcium absorption and bone resorption resulting in hypercalcaemia [9]. Glucocorticoid treatment or removal of granulomas will return elevated serum calcium and 1,25$(OH)_2$D levels to normal.

Hypercalcaemia resulting from increased circulating 1,25$(OH)_2$D levels have been reported in infants with subcutaneous fat necrosis [11,12] and in a few cases with lymphoma [13]. Human T cell lymphocytotrophic virus type I (HTLV-I), a retrovirus associated with a peculiar form of T cell lymphoma, has been demonstrated to have the capacity to convert 25-OHD into $1,25(OH)_2D$ [14]. These findings contrast with the majority of patients with hypercalcaemia associated with malignancy, in whom serum $1,25(OH)_2D$ levels and intestinal calcium absorption are decreased and other pathogenetic mechanisms (such as prostaglandins and parathyroid hormone-related protein) have been implicated [6,15].

HYPERVITAMINOSIS D

Vitamin D intoxication, first recognized in 1928 [16], occurs most commonly during long-term therapy in patients with hypoparathyroidism, pseudohypoparathyroidism, hypophosphataemic rickets and renal osteodystrophy [17]. Rarely, hypervitaminosis D is caused by so-called 'stosstherapy' with 15 mg (600 000 U) vitamin D [18], which has been used in some European countries for the prevention of rickets. There is a considerable individual variation in susceptibility to vitamin D intoxication. Despite warnings of the potential toxicity of vitamin D, it continues to be prescribed for unselected conditions or without adequate supervision, so that sporadic cases of hypervitaminosis D still occur [19].

When concentrated forms of vitamin D are ingested, the control system of vitamin D metabolism is no longer effective, and combined effects of increased circulating levels of 25-OHD and $1,25(OH)_2D$ [18,20,21] lead to hypercalcaemia by increasing both intestinal calcium absorption and bone resorption. In anephric patients, that is in the absence of $1,25(OH)_2D$ formation, 25-OHD may be the principal metabolite responsible for hypercalcaemia during treatment with large doses of vitamin D binding to, and acting upon, intestinal and bone receptors for $1,25(OH)_2D$.

Early signs of hypervitaminosis D include anorexia, constipation, polyuria, nausea and vomiting. Complications of more prolonged hypercalcaemia are ectopic calcifications [22], nephrocalcinosis and renal insufficiency. Because of excessive storage in adipose tissue, intoxication with vitamin D may persist for weeks or months. The shorter biological half-life of $1,25(OH)_2D_3$ and its synthetic analogue, 1α-hydroxyvitamin D_3, has the advantage of rapid lowering of hypercalcaemia as a result of inadvertent overdosage after cessation of treatment.

The diagnosis is usually suspected by history and confirmed by laboratory investigations revealing hypercalcaemia, suppressed serum PTH, hypercalciuria and, in patients intoxicated with vitamin D, elevated serum levels of 25-OHD. The values for serum phosphate and TmP/GFR (maximum tubular absorption for phosphate/glomerular filtration rate) may be normal or increased, depending on the state of renal function, but not reduced as they are in primary hyperparathyroidism. Alkaline phosphatase activity in serum is usually low, possibly indicating defective osteoblastic function [20].

Treatment consists of discontinuing vitamin D (or metabolites) and calcium supplementation, sodium chloride infusion with or without frusemide and glucocorticoids (prednisone 2 mg/kg body weight per day). Because of the possible toxicity of large doses of vitamin D, treatment with its non-cumulating derivates, 1α-hydroxyvitamin D_3 or $1,25(OH)_2D_3$, is recommended for the management of chronic disorders of calcium metabolism [17,21]. Patients with calciopenic or phosphopenic rickets, hypoparathyroidism and pseudohypoparathyroidism should be monitored during treatment. If hypercalciuria (urinary calcium exceeding 4 mg/kg per 24 h or urinary calcium/creatinine ratios exceeding 0.22 mg/mg in a 24-h urine or random urine sample) or hypercalcaemia (serum calcium exceeding 10.4 mg/dl) occurs, treatment with vitamin D metabolites should be discontinued, and reinstated at a lower dose when normocalcaemia and normocalciuria are reestablished.

IDIOPATHIC INFANTILE HYPERCALCAEMIA

Idiopathic hypercalcaemia of infancy is a heterogeneous and poorly understood disorder, which resembles vitamin D intoxication [23–25]. The disease has been classified into a mild (Lightwood type [26]) and severe (Fanconi type [27]) form, but is a self-limiting disorder of the first year of life which resolves in most cases by 4 years of age. Whether the two forms reflect different diseases or different manifestations of the same underlying metabolic defect is not known.

Symptoms attributable to hypercalcaemia (see above) develop in infants with the mild form between 2 and 9 months of age. With adequate treatment there is usually an excellent prognosis for physical and mental development. Several cases of the mild form of infantile hypercalcaemia were observed in the UK following World War II, when infants received 3000–4000 units of vitamin D per day to prevent nutritional deficiencies. That only a very small percentage of the exposed infants developed hypercalcaemia suggested an increased sensitivity to vitamin D as the cause of this condition. With the subsequent reduction of vitamin D intake to 400 U/day, the incidence of the mild form of infantile hypercalcaemia in the UK decreased markedly.

In the severe form of idiopathic infantile hypercalcaemia, hypercalcaemia may occur earlier than in the mild form, sometimes during the neonatal period. Mental retardation, facial, cardiovascular and other features are often found (Williams syndrome [28,29]). The facial features include broad prominent forehead, short and turned-up nose with flat nasal bridge, full cheeks and lips with a

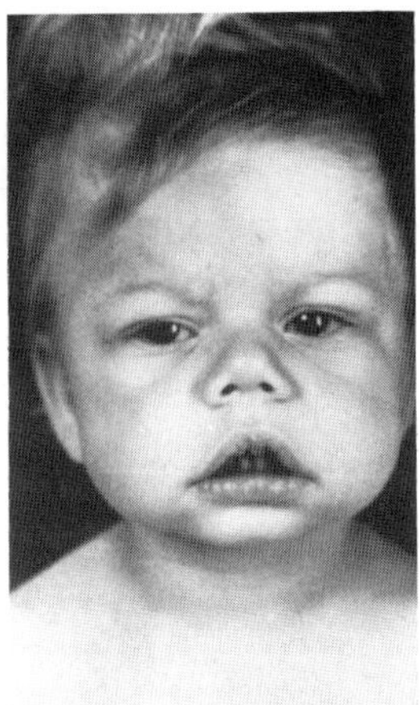
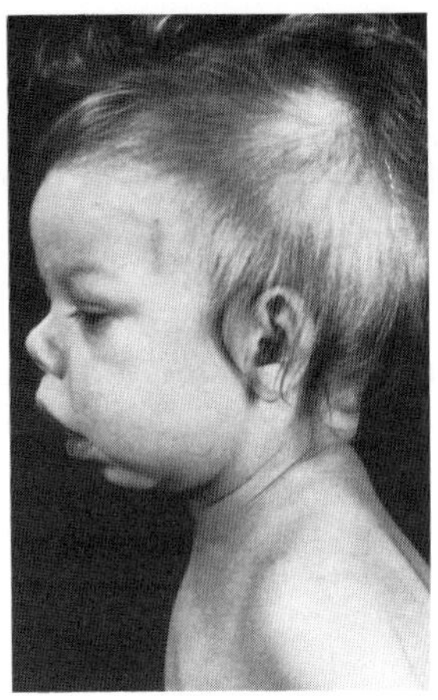
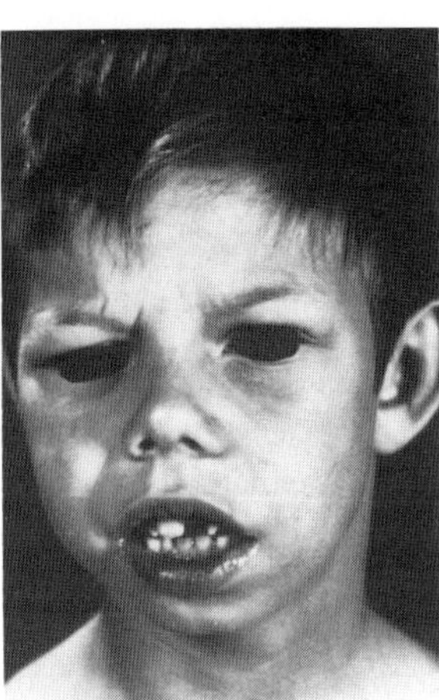

Fig. 38.1 Patients with Williams syndrome at an age of 15 months and 9 years. During infancy the boy suffered from severe hypercalcaemia with a maximal value of 4.35 mmol/l (17.4 mg/dl) (from Wiedemann *et al.* [30]).

prominent overhanging upper lip, low-set ears, epicanthic folds and strabismus. The face becomes more coarse with age (Fig. 38.1). Dental anomalies are characteristic with late eruption and reduction in size. Cardiovascular features, present in about 75%, include supravalvular aortic stenosis and peripheral pulmonary artery stenosis. Other features include low birth weight, mild short stature, microcephaly, hoarse voice, hyperacusis, kyphoscoliosis, hallux valgus, inguinal and umbilical hernias. The severe form of hypercalcaemia may or may not be associated with Williams syndrome. In many children with Williams syndrome there is neither present nor past evidence of hypercalcaemia. The majority of cases of both types of infantile hypercalcaemia, as well as the Williams syndrome, are sporadic, although a familial occurrence has been reported [23–25].

Investigations

Laboratory investigations during the hypercalcaemic phase of infantile hypercalcaemia reveal serum calcium values in the range of 3.0–4.75 mmol/l (12–19 mg/dl), high–normal serum phosphate, low–normal alkaline phosphatase and PTH and hypercalciuria. These laboratory findings resemble those found in hypervitaminosis D, but in infants with idiopathic hypercalcaemia there is no history of vitamin D intoxication. Other causes of infantile hypercalcaemia (see the respective section) have to be excluded. Radiographic findings may show increased density at the metaphyseal ends of the long bones, osteosclerosis of the base of the skull, nephrocalcinosis, and soft tissue calcification. In a normocalcaemic child with Williams syndrome these radiological findings suggest the previous presence of hypercalcaemia, possibly *in utero*. The pathogenesis of the hypercalcaemia and the phenotypic findings are poorly understood. Animal experiments show that large doses of vitamin D produce fetal lesions in pregnant rabbits and rats closely resembling those seen in Williams syndrome [31,32]. In humans it is unlikely that vitamin D *per se* is teratogenic, since several women with hypoparathyroidism and vitamin D dependency gave birth to healthy children despite high-dose treatment with vitamin D or vitamin D metabolites during their pregnancies [33,34].

Oral and intravenous calcium loading tests indicate that the hypercalcaemia in some children may be due to intestinal hyperabsorption and/or an abnormally slow clearance of calcium [35,36], the latter phenomenon resembling the situation in hypothyroidism [36]. The increase of calcium absorption may be explained by elevated 1,25-$(OH)_2D$ serum levels in some of these patients during the hypercalcaemic phase which subsequently decreased [37]. These results suggest that the hypercalcaemia may be a consequence of abnormal synthesis or degradation of the vitamin D hormone, but this has not been confirmed by other groups [38–42].

A decreased ability to handle intravenous calcium loads may be explained by a defect in synthesis or release of calcitonin. Williams syndrome may thus be due to a neural crest abnormality affecting the face, heart and precursors of the calcitonin-producing C cells, indicating no direct relationship between calcium disturbances and phenotypic features [39].

No defect could be found in synthesis or release of calcitonin, vitamin D metabolism or in the sensitivity of the kidney to PTH in 27 normocalcaemic patients with Williams syndrome [40].

Idiopathic infantile hypercalcaemia remains a continuing enigma and is possibly a heterogeneous disorder. More detailed investigations are required to clarify the pathogenesis of the hypercalcaemia and to determine whether disturbances of fetal calcium homeostasis are of fundamental importance for the features of Williams syndrome. The treatment of hypercalcaemia is similar to that of hypervitaminosis D.

Decreased formation or action of 1,25-dihydroxyvitamin D

This is the main cause of rickets and osteomalacia. Rickets can be defined as defective mineralization of the growth plate, whereas osteomalacia describes the defective mineralization of cortical and trabecular bone. Both defects are found in growing children, whereas only osteomalacia can occur in adults [43,44]. Rickets may result from an inability to calcify bone matrix and epiphyseal cartilage (for example hypophosphatasia) or from decreased availability of calcium and phosphate in extracellular fluid and thus at the mineralizing sites of bone (for example vitamin D deficiency and hypophosphataemic rickets). The terms calciopenic and phosphopenic rickets have been suggested to draw attention to the pathogenetic mechanisms [45]. Phosphopenic rickets usually results from renal phosphate loss and is described below (p. 753).

CALCIOPENIC RICKETS

Extreme restriction of dietary calcium intake is a very rare cause of rickets [46]. As shown in Fig. 38.2 calciopenic rickets usually results from a lack of vitamin D itself, or may be due to metabolic abnormalities in the formation and action of $1,25(OH)_2D$. Decreased vitamin D-dependent calcium absorption induces hypocalcaemia with secondary hyperparathyroidism, resulting in increased phosphate excretion and hypophosphataemia. Diminished calcium and phosphate levels in extracellular fluid produce defective bone mineralization, whereas secondary hyperparathyroidism causes increased bone resorption. Both conditions account for the following histological, clinical and radiological findings.

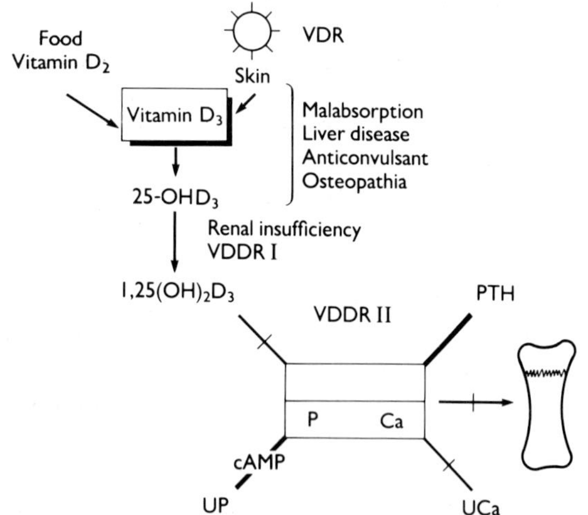

Fig. 38.2 Pathogenesis and pathophysiology of calciopenic rickets. UCa/UP, urine calcium/phosphate; VDR, vitamin deficiency rickets; VDDR, vitamin dependency rickets; —/+ increased/decreased effect.

Bone histology shows the following.

1 Excessive accumulation of unmineralized osteoid coating the surfaces of trabecular bone and lining the Haversian canals of cortical bone, as well as rarely the periosteal areas of the long bone shafts (osteomalacia).

2 Disorganization of the growth plate and metaphysis with widening of the maturation zone, disruption of the normal columnar arrangement of cartilage cells, decreased vascular supply and calcification of degenerating cartilage (rickets).

3 Osteoclastic and fibroblastic proliferation on trabecular surfaces and sometimes in bone marrow spaces, as well as excessive osteoclastic activity in the zone of primary spongiosa (secondary hyperparathyroidism).

The characteristic clinical appearance of rickets is bone deformity, which exhibits different patterns, depending on the child's age at the onset of disease and the relative growth rate of different bones [47]. In the first year of life the most rapidly growing bones are the skull, the upper limbs and ribs. Rickets at this time therefore leads to generalized softening of the calvaria (craniotabes), widening of cranial sutures, frontal bossing, enlarged swollen epiphyses, particularly of the wrists, bulging of the costochondrial junctions of the ribs (rachitic rosary) and inward pull of the softened lower ribs at the site of attachment of the diaphragma (Harrison sulcus).

After the first year of life the legs grow faster and the effects of weight-bearing become prominent, resulting in genu varum (bowleg) or genu valgum (knock-knee), coxa vara, rachitic sabre shins, palpable and visible enlargement of the end of the long bones and scoliosis. The teeth are often abnormal with delayed eruption, enamel hypoplasia and irregular pits. Bone pain is common in infants and older children. In addition to skeletal appearances, patients with calciopenic rickets may suffer from muscle weakness of the proximal muscles, tetanic signs and convulsions. The myopathy is thought to result from deficiency of 25-OHD or $1,25(OH)_2D$, whereas carpopedal spasm, laryngeal stridor, paraesthesiae and seizures are due to hypocalcaemia. The clinical signs of osteomalacia are often subtle and may consist of poorly localized bone pain and muscle weakness or fractures in more advanced stages of the disease.

Radiological features appear at the growth plate and reflect the histological abnormalities. The earliest change is slight widening of the growth plate due to an increase in cartilaginous cells followed by decreased density at the metaphysis. In severe rickets, widening of the growth plate and fraying, cupping and widening of the metaphyses occur. The cartilaginous cells of the epiphysis are also affected, demonstrated by a lack of definition of the dense rim and trabecular components of the ossification centre.

Fluctuations in the severity of rickets result in transverse radiodense lines adjacent to the metaphyses across the shaft of the long bones (Harris lines). Osteomalacic changes of the diaphyses include shaft deformities, decreased bone density, thinned compacta, coarse spongiosa and pseudofractures (ribbon-like transverse bands). Variable radiological signs of secondary hyperparathyroidism are subperiosteal erosions in the phalanges and irregular resorption in the metaphyses. The earliest radiographic sign of healing rickets can be detected within several weeks after the start of vitamin D therapy as a radiodense line adjacent to the metaphyses representing calcified cartilage.

The most important laboratory findings in calciopenic rickets are low–normal serum calcium levels with secondary hyperparathyroidism (increased levels of serum PTH and urinary cyclic adenosine monophosphate (cAMP), hypophosphataemia, low TmP/GFR, aminoaciduria, and hypocalciuria) and evidence of increased bone turnover (elevated serum alkaline phosphatase activity and urinary hydroxyproline excretion). Serum osteocalcin is not a good diagnostic index in calciopenic rickets since this bone protein is dependent on the vitamin D status and may thus be low–normal despite increased osteoblastic activity. However, the increase of serum osteocalcin during treatment can serve as a sensitive and early indication of bone mineralization and successful therapy [48,49].

In chronic renal disease, serum phosphate is normal or elevated depending on the state of renal insufficiency, and the urinary investigations may not provide a reliable measure of PTH function or bone turnover.

Quantitative abnormalities of the circulating vitamin D metabolites 25-OHD and $1,25(OH)_2D$ may be diagnostic of several disorders resulting in calciopenic rickets [6]. Serum 25-OHD is usually low in vitamin deficiency rickets and may also be depressed in patients with malabsorption, liver disease and anticonvulsant osteopathy. Serum $1,25(OH)_2D$ is low in advanced renal failure and vitamin D dependency rickets type I (VDDR), but elevated in vitamin D dependent rickets type II.

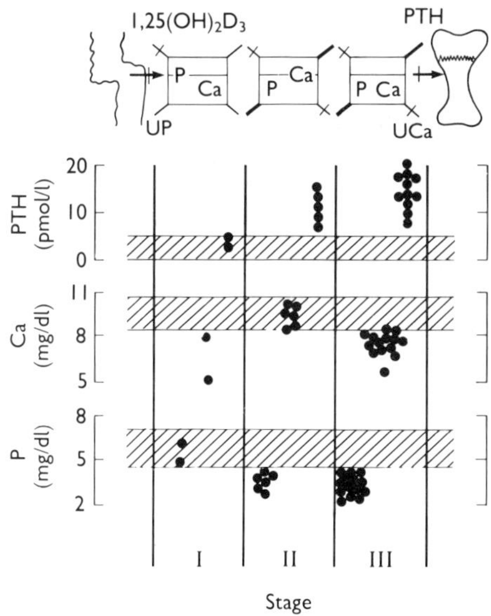

Fig. 38.3 Different stages of vitamin D deficiency rickets reflected by changes in serum concentrations of PTH, calcium (a) and phosphate (P) of 19 untreated children. The pathophysiology of the different stages is indicated at the top. UCa/UP, urine calcium/phosphate.

VITAMIN D DEFICIENCY RICKETS

Vitamin D deficiency occurs as a result of low vitamin D intake in association with decreased exposure to sunlight. The incidence of vitamin D deficiency rickets, first described as a clinical entity by Glisson in 1650, was progressively reduced after 1920 by the recognition of the antirachitic properties of light and cod liver oil [43]. The present low incidence in industrialized countries is the result of the enrichment of food, especially infant milk preparations, with vitamin D. The recommended dietary allowance of vitamin D is 400 IU (10 μg)/day and the minimal requirement is 100 IU (2.5 μg)/day in children and adults.

Vitamin D deficiency rickets is found frequently in only a few groups of children such as those on a vegetarian diet in which no food of animal origin is permitted. The other group is immigrants, especially from Asia, who continue traditional habits of nutrition (high phytate) and decreased sunlight exposure (by dress shields). The latter is the major cause of rickets in infants without the recommended vitamin D supplements.

As shown in Fig. 38.3, three stages of vitamin D deficiency rickets can be differentiated based on laboratory and clinical data [50,51]. Stage I arises from impaired intestinal calcium absorption and calcium resorption from bone resulting in hypocalcaemia. Serum phosphate is usually normal, reflecting unaffected renal handling. With disturbed bone calcification and increased bone turnover, levels of serum alkaline phosphatase activity and urinary hydroxyproline/creatinine rise. Stage I with hypocalcaemia is transient, lasting only a few days until secondary hyperparathyroidism returns the serum calcium circulation to normal. In a few instances, mostly in infants aged 2–9 months, the hypocalcaemic stage I persists due to insufficient PTH stimulation (relative hypoparathyroidism [52]), which may give rise to tetany and convulsions.

In stage II, serum calcium concentration returns to normal as a consequence of mobilization of calcium from bone and increased renal calcium reabsorption resulting in hypocalciuria. The secondary hyperparathyroidism results in increased cAMP excretion, hypophosphataemia and further depletion of low serum 25-OHD. The continuous hypersecretion of PTH despite normocalcaemia may be related to the concentrations of $1,25(OH)_2D$, which may be in the high–normal range but not sufficiently and appropriately elevated to suppress the parathyroid gland and restore the disturbed calcium homeostasis [53].

In stage III rickets the absolute or relative deficiency of vitamin D metabolites results in insufficient calcium mobilization from bone. Bone disease is now severe because of the combined effect of calcium and phosphate deficiency and hyperparathyroidism. Vitamin D deficiency rickets should be treated with calcium and oral doses of vitamin D 5000 IU/day for about 3 weeks followed by prophylactic doses of 400–500 IU/day.

MALABSORPTION, LIVER DISEASE AND ANTICONVULSANT TREATMENT

All three conditions may lead to low 25-OHD serum levels and rickets by several different mechanisms. The osteopathy of malabsorption due to small bowel disease, pancreatic insufficiency and inadequate bile salts is osteoporosis due to hypoproteinaemia and steatorrhoea with defective calcium absorption and other factors. Rickets is rare, and may be due to a combination of malabsorption and increased loss of vitamin D metabolites owing to a defect in the enterohepatic circulation. Although some investigators have questioned the role of the latter with regard to vitamin D and 25-OHD, the disrupted enterohepatic circulation of 1,25(OH)$_2$D may be important [54].

Abnormal liver function can cause osteoporosis and rickets by the same mechanisms as the malabsorption syndromes. A deficiency of the vitamin D-25-hydroxylase is unusual, probably occurring only in severe liver disease. Recent studies in adult patients with liver disease indicate that free concentrations of 25-OHD are normal, despite reduced 25-OHD levels [55]. The decreased liver production and circulation of the vitamin D-binding protein (DBP) may reduce the total concentrations of 25-OHD and 1,25(OH)$_2$D without reducing the biologically important free concentrations. This observation suggests that in patients with liver disease vitamin D deficiency is not a major cause of bone disease, and that total vitamin D metabolite measurement may be misleading in the evaluation of the vitamin D status of these patients.

Since the first clinical description [56] a considerable number of cases of rickets and osteomalacia have been reported in patients with epilepsy [57]. Significant reduction in serum levels of 25-OHD have been measured in some but not all patients receiving long-term treatment with anticonvulsant drugs, especially phenobarbitone and phenytoin. Anticonvulsant therapy is associated with induction of hepatic microsomal mixed function oxidase enzyme systems, and may result in increased catabolism and excretion of vitamin D metabolites [57]. Since normal or elevated levels of serum 1,25(OH)$_2$D have been reported in patients on anticonvulsant treatment [58], some other mechanisms must also be involved to explain the osteopathy in these patients. Anticonvulsant drugs have been shown directly to inhibit gastrointestinal calcium absorption and calcitonin secretion [59]. Since only a small percentage of children develop frank rickets or osteomalacia, other environmental factors, such as limited physical exercise and sunlight exposure or deficient calcium and vitamin D intake, may play a role in the development of anticonvulsant drug-induced disturbances of calcium and bone metabolism. Finally, antiepileptic drugs may directly provoke renal conservation of phosphate [60], which may partly compensate any of the above-mentioned negative effects. The treatment and the following prophylaxis of anticonvulsant rickets resemble those of vitamin D deficiency rickets.

Children with intestinal malabsorption or liver disease may require larger daily doses of vitamin D (5000–10 000 IU or more). Some patients may respond better to oral 25-OHD$_3$ in a dose of 50 µg/day. Alternatively vitamin D or its metabolites may be given parenterally.

RENAL DISEASE

Some children with nephrotic syndrome may develop bone disease. During active disease the serum 25-OHD levels are decreased, probably as a result of urinary loss. Circulating 1,25(OH)$_2$D concentrations may be inappropriately low for the prevailing true hypocalcaemia (low ionized calcium) and secondary hyperparathyroidism, reflecting insufficient 25-OHD substrate, inadequate renal synthesis or both [61].

The renal hydroxylation to 1,25(OH)$_2$D$_3$ may be impaired by a progressive loss of nephrons in renal insufficiency resulting in decreased serum levels of the vitamin D hormone and rickets or osteomalacia. Chronic renal failure leads to several additional disturbances in mineral regulation, including hyperphosphataemia, secondary hyperparathyroidism and tubular acidosis [62]. Since phosphate retention also contributes to the pathogenesis of renal osteodystrophy, this is discussed later (pp. 757–9).

VITAMIN D DEPENDENCY RICKETS TYPE I

This rare autosomal recessive disorder was first described by Prader *et al.* in 1961 [63]. Affected patients develop the clinical, radiological and biochemical features of VDR between the ages of 4 and 12 months, despite adequate vitamin D intake. Before treatment circulating 1,25(OH)$_2$D levels are low [45]. The disease is responsive to, and dependent upon, pharmacological doses of vitamin D and 25-OHD$_3$, but physiological doses of 1,25(OH)$_2$D$_3$ are effective. This suggests deficient renal 1α-hydroxylation of 25-OHD. Studies in the porcine homologue of this human type of rickets demonstrated no detectable 25-

OHD-1α- or 25-OHD-24-hydroxylase activity in renal homogenates [64,65]. There is strong evidence that the disease in humans (as in pigs) results from a genetic defect in renal 25-OHD_3-1α-hydroxylase. This enzyme consists of three distinct moieties: cytochrome P450, ferredoxin and ferredoxin reductase. The gene for VDDR I has been designated to the long arm of chromosome 12 (12q13–14), the most likely target for the mutation being the specific P450 component of the 25-OHD_3-1α-hydroxylase [66].

For ethical reasons the enzyme defect has not been established in the kidney of affected patients. Recently the decidua cells collected from the placenta of three mothers with VDDR I showed complete absence of the 25-OHD_3-1α-hydroxylase activity normally present [67]. The specific therapy of VDDR I is the life-long oral administration of physiological doses (0.5–2 µg/day) of 1,25$(OH)_2D_3$.

VITAMIN D DEPENDENCY RICKETS TYPE II

Patients with VDDR II present with severe calciopenic rickets between the ages of 6 months and 3 years, despite supranormal 1,25$(OH)_2$D serum levels, and respond only to pharmacological doses of the vitamin D hormone. They may remain unresponsive to doses of up to 50 µg 1,25$(OH)_2D_3$/day [68]. The disorder has been described in some 40 relatives in regions near the Mediterranean, and appears to be transmitted as an autosomal recessive trait. The common marmoset has been shown to be a useful animal model for VDDR II [69]. About half of the affected children present with total alopecia (Fig. 38.4) which does not improve with otherwise satisfactory therapy. Relatives with alopecia generally show the most severe grade of rickets [70], but absence of alopecia cannot be regarded as a constant predictive sign of a lesser resistance and of responsiveness to vitamin D [70–72].

Patients with VDDR II have end-organ resistance to 1,25$(OH)_2D_3$ due to receptor or postreceptor defects demonstrated in cultured skin fibroblasts [68]. Two main classes of defects have been identified, reflecting point mutations in the genes that code for the vitamin D receptor (VDR):

1 steroid-binding domain mutations;
2 DNA-binding domain mutations.

There is heterogeneity of the mutations that result in either missense or inapproprate termination of the VDR [73,74].

Steroid-binding domain mutations affect the binding of 1,25$(OH)_2D_3$ and result in a receptor-negative phenotype [74,75]. By contrast, mutations that occur in the DNA-binding domain have a receptor-positive phenotype. These affect the binding of the VDR–hormone complex to the vitamin D response element in the promotor region of target genes. Five different binding domain mutations have been described which are located within [74,76,77] or between [78,79] the two zinc fingers, resulting in substitutions of amino acids that are highly conserved in all steroid hormone receptors [74]. Alopecia is not associated just with one type of these mutations.

Renal and extrarenal tissues, including skin fibroblasts possess a 25-OHD_3-24-hydroxylase, which can be induced by 1,25$(OH)_2D_3$ [71]. This induction, apparently mediated via the 1,25$(OH)_2D_3$ receptor, is a sensitive *in vitro* test for the biological action of vitamin D. Enzyme stimulation is impaired in patients with VDDR II [80–82]. The presence or absence of 25-OHD_3-24-hydroxylase induction by 1,25$(OH)_2D_3$ in skin fibroblasts appears to correlate with the response to vitamin D therapy [68,81]. Current evidence suggests that the alopecia is a direct consequence of resistance to 1,25$(OH)_2D_3$ but not a genetic abnormality linked to the hormone resistance [70].

Patients with VDDR II should be treated with high doses of 1,25$(OH)_2D_3$ or 1α-hydroxyvitamin D_3 (up to 50 µg/day), or vitamin D (up to 5 000 000 IU/day). Totally unresponsive patients probably die in early childhood, and the only effective therapy may be high doses of oral [83,84] or intravenous [72,83,85] calcium. All therapeutic regimes have to be long-term, and intravenous calcium infusion presents considerable practical difficulties. During the administration of high doses of vitamin D, some resistant patients may benefit from a direct suppressive effect of excessive levels of circulating 1,25$(OH)_2D_3$ on the parathyroid cells, possibly via intact 1,25$(OH)_2D_3$ receptors of these cells. This may ameliorate secondary hyperparathyroidism and PTH-induced renal phosphate loss, resulting in better skeletal mineralization despite persistent hypocalcaemia [86,87].

Spontaneous improvement of some patients may occur as they get older, suggesting that some other regulatory factor may substitute for the defective VDR.

DISTURBANCES OF PARATHYROID HORMONE SECRETION OR ACTION IN CHILDHOOD

Increased parathyroid hormone secretion

Excessive secretion of PTH may be a compensatory response to hypocalcaemia (secondary hyperparathyroidism) or may result from a primary abnormality of the parathyroid glands (primary hyperparathyroidism).

PRIMARY HYPERPARATHYROIDISM

Definition, prevalence and aetiology

Primary hyperparathyroidism is a state of hypersecretion of PTH by a solitary adenoma (80%), chief cell hyperplasia (20%) or carcinoma (less than 2%). The detection has

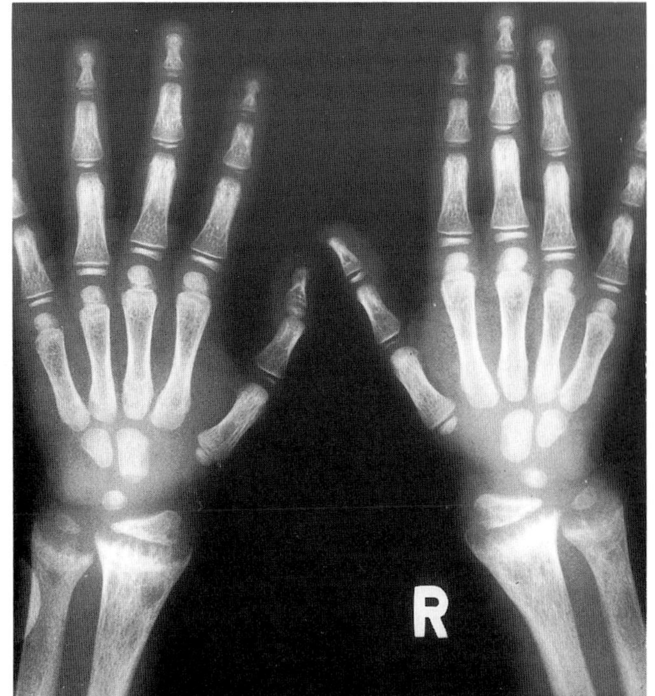

(a)

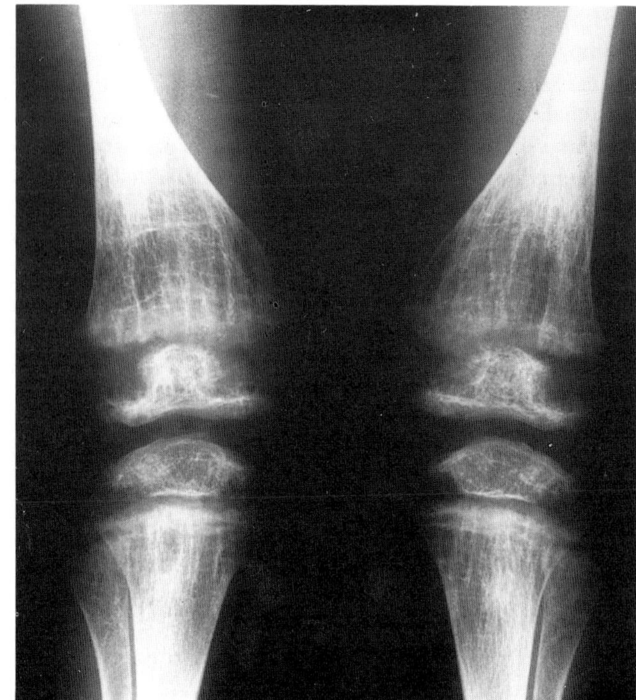

(b)

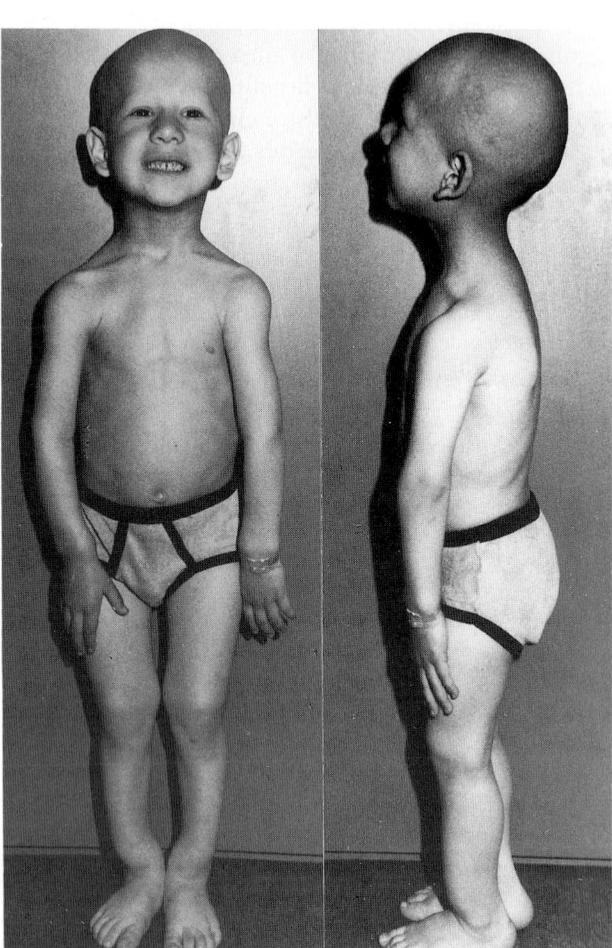

(c)

Fig. 38.4 Turkish boy with vitamin D dependency rickets type II at an age of 5 years. Despite treatment with excessive doses of vitamin D_3 (1–2 million IU/day) over several years, the boy shows hypocalcaemia (6–6.5 mg/dl) and clinical and radiological symptoms of rickets (a, b), as well as total alopecia (c).

increased with the advent of routine screening of serum calcium by automated techniques and improved methods for specific diagnosis. The prevalence of primary hyperparathyroidism has been reported to be between 1 and 3 per 1000 [88]. Of the patients, 85% are aged between 30 and 70 years, women being affected two to three times more often than men. The disease is uncommon in childhood. Up to 1982, 86 documented cases of primary hyperparathyroidism, 80% sporadic and 20% familial, were collected [89]. Two large surgically proven series included only 15 of 881 patients younger than 20 years (1.7%), none being under 10 years of age [88,90]. Thus the calculated prevalence of primary hyperparathyroidism in children and adolescents may be in the order of 2–5 per 100 000. Children under 10 years of age, including newborns, very rarely suffer from primary hyperparathyroidism, which is predominantly due to inherited chief cell hyperplasia [91,92].

The aetiology of primary hyperparathyroidism is unknown. In adult patients previous head and neck irradiation is associated with an increased incidence of the disease. Chronic stimulation of the parathyroid glands by longstanding calciopenic rickets and osteomalacia (especially renal osteodystrophy), as well as therapeutic phosphate supplementation in hypophosphataemic diseases, may induce the evolution of secondary to primary hyperparathyroidism, termed 'tertiary hyperparathyroidism' [93–95]. A humoral factor not secreted by the parathyroid gland itself has been demonstrated to be an important cause of primary hyperparathyroidism in familial multiple endocrine neoplasia (MEN) type 1 [96]. This factor had the characteristics of a protein with an apparent molecular weight of 50–55 kD and showed high mitogenic activity toward cultured bovine parathyroid cells.

Classification

Primary hyperparathyroidism in children may be classified as sporadic or familial (Table 38.1). Sporadic hyperparathyroidism is usually due to a single adenoma. Familial hyperparathyroidism is caused by hyperplasia of all parathyroid glands and is inherited as an autosomal dominant or recessive trait [97,98]. In other families there is an association with two MEN syndromes or with hypocalciuric hypercalcaemia. All these conditions are inherited as an autosomal dominant trait.

Patients with familial hypocalciuric hypercalcaemia have PTH serum levels in the high–normal range, a finding that is abnormal in comparison to the hypercalcaemia (relative hyperparathyroidism). Since the condition is mainly due to impairment of renal calcium excretion, this is discussed later. Three distinct syndromes of multiple endocrine neoplasia have been described [99]. MEN type 1 (MEN-1) or Wermer syndrome [100] consists primarily of parathyroid hyperplasia (diffuse, asymmetrical, or nodular) associated with pancreatic islet-cell adenoma or carcinoma and adenoma or hyperplasia of the anterior pituitary. MEN-2A (Sipple syndrome) consists of medullary carcinoma of the thyroid associated with phaeochromocytoma and parathyroid hyperplasia. The major components of MEN-2B (multiple mucosal neuroma syndrome) are medullary carcinoma of the thyroid, phaeochromocytoma, mucosal neuromas and only rarely parathyroid hyperplasia.

Table 38.1 Classification of primary hyperparathyroidism in childhood

Non-familial: usually single adenoma
Familial: usually hyperplasia of all glands
Isolated (ar, ad)
Multiple endocrine neoplasia type 1 (ad)
Primary hyperparathyroidism (97%*)
Gastrinoma and other pancreatic tumours
Pituitary adenomas
Multiple endocrine neoplasia type 2A (ad)
Primary hyperparathyroidism (20–30%)*
Medullary thryoid cancer
Pheochromocytoma
Familial hypocalciuric hypercalcaemia (ad)†

* Frequency of the occurrence of clinical manifestation.
† Relative hyperparathyroidism in relation to hypercalcaemia.
ar/ad, autosomal recessive/dominant trait.

MEN-1 belongs to a group of heritable forms of neoplasia (for example retinoblastoma) caused by a deletion of a regulatory gene. The MEN-1 gene has been mapped to the centromeric area of chromosome 11 [101] and is thought to encode a growth-suppressive function. In members of MEN-1 kindreds there is a loss of both MEN-1 alleles: the first allele is inactivated due to an inherited germ-line mutation, whereas the second allele (inherited in normal form from the unaffected parent) becomes inactivated by a somatic mutation in the tumour precursor cell [6].

The proteins that promote the growth of the endocrine glands (perhaps one for each gland), may be the products of derepressed primitive genes (oncogenes) [102]. The clinical symptoms of MEN-1, which vary within and among affected families, appear typically during the third to fifth decades of life, and are related to the excessive secretion of one or more hormones by the pancreatic, pituitary and parathyroid tumours.

The typical tumour of the pancreatic islet cells is a gastrinoma, but insulinomas and glucagonomas may also occur. Pancreatic tumours that produce gastrin result in intractable peptic ulceration (Zollinger–Ellison syndrome), which is the predominant cause of morbidity and mortality of MEN-1 patients. Excessive basal secretion of gastrin and hypercalcaemia (due to unrecognized gastrinoma and hyperparathyroidism) may occur in asymptomatic family members. The pituitary tumours may be non-functional, causing pituitary insufficiency, or may produce excessive prolactin, growth hormone and rarely ACTH.

Hypercalcaemia due to primary hyperparathyroidism is the most common abnormality in MEN-1 (about 97%) and makes the measurement of serum calcium a useful screening test to detect other affected family members. The hyperparathyroidism is clinically and biochemically indistinguishable from sporadic hyperparathyroidism and seldom appears before the age of 10 years. MEN-2A and -2B are described later, since the predominant feature of both syndromes is the calcitonin-secreting medullary carcinoma of the thyroid.

Pathophysiology

The excessive PTH secretion of the hyperfunctioning parathyroid cells results in hypercalcaemia through increased action of the hormone on its main target organs kidney, bone and the intestine via $1,25(OH)_2D_3$. Unsuppressed serum PTH levels despite hypercalcaemia indicate that the increased PTH secretion is due to a set point error in the level of calcium at which normal parathyroid glands are inhibited.

In addition to its hypercalcaemic effect, PTH decreases renal phosphate and bicarbonate reabsorption, causing a tendency to hypophosphataemia and hyperchloraemic acidosis. Both conditions may worsen the hypercalcaemia, phosphate depletion by increasing $1,25(OH)_2D_3$ secretion and acidosis by directly increasing bone mineral dissolution and decreasing the capacity of serum albumin to bind ionized calcium.

The hypercalcaemia results in an increased filtered calcium load in the kidney which overcomes PTH-induced tubular calcium reabsorption. This leads, in association with elevated circulating $1,25(OH)_2D_3$ (inducing increased intestinal absorption and consequent renal excretion), to hypercalciuria [103]. Hypercalciuria and bicarbonaturia (increasing urinary pH and decreasing calcium phosphate solubility) are among the risk factors which may be important in the pathogenesis of renal stone disease and nephrocalcinosis in primary hyperparathyroidism.

Clinical features

The clinical features and course of primary hyperparathyroidism are extremely variable in children, as they are in adults. The spectrum of clinical manifestations ranges from asymptomatic forms [104,105] to very severe ones [106], especially in early infancy, where the condition may carry a high mortality (see p. 767). Most children present with renal, skeletal or non-specific manifestations of the disease.

Renal changes are polyuria, polydipsia and renal colic from renal stones. Nephrolithiasis is found in about 30–70% of paediatric patients [89,91,107]. Chronic urolithiasis may be the only symptom for a long time. One of the author's patients, a 15-year-old girl, had suffered recurrent nephrolithiasis from 5 years of age, before the diagnosis of primary hyperparathyroidism was made, and was successfully treated by surgical removal of a parathyroid adenoma that weighed 400 mg (normal for age: <30 mg).

The bone changes are due to the osteolytic activity of excessive PTH. Clinical signs are bone pain and pathological fractures. Radiological signs are generalized bone demineralization, subperiosteal bone resorption, osteolysis of the phalanges and, very rarely, bone cysts. Histological investigations (not indicated as routine diagnostic examination) nearly always provide evidence of increased bone turnover. Some children with primary hyperparathyroidism present with rickets [108], the aetiology of this rare association being unknown.

Many children with primary hyperparathyroidism have non-specific features related to the hypercalcaemia such as weakness, fatigue, anorexia, constipation or central nervous system symptoms (confusion, hallucinations or blurring consciousness).

Investigations

The diagnostic hallmark of primary hyperparathyroidism is the simultaneous detection of hypercalcaemia and increased PTH secretion. Hypercalcaemia is established when at least three measurements of total and/or ionized calcium exceed the upper normal range. The best index of increased PTH secretion is the radioimmunological demonstration of elevated circulating intact PTH levels. Several other tests are corroborative in the detection of increased PTH activity: urinary cAMP/GFR is increased and TmP/GFR is decreased in most patients, but may overlap with the upper and lower normal range, respectively, in moderate hyperparathyroidism. The demonstration of low phosphate, increased chloride/phosphate ratios and high $1,25(OH)_2D$ concentrations in serum is a typical finding, but again there is considerable overlap between normal and hyperparathyroid subjects.

Increased urinary calcium excretion is of importance for the differential diagnosis. The values are higher than those found in patients with hypocalciuric hypercalcaemia, but lower than in hypercalcaemias due to other causes, since PTH enhances calcium absorption. Elevated alkaline phosphatase activity (and osteocalcin levels) in serum and urinary hydroxyproline excretion, reflecting increased bone turnover, are present only in patients with significant bone disease. Dynamic tests, such as steroid suppression and calcium infusion, have proved to be of little value in the diagnosis of primary hyperparathyroidism in children.

Differential diagnosis

The differential diagnosis of primary hyperparathyroidism includes nephrolithiasis, bone diseases and especially hypercalcaemia associated with normal or low serum PTH such as vitamin D and vitamin A intoxication, granulomatous diseases, immobilization, malignant tumours, idiopathic infantile hypercalcaemia, hypothyroidism and Addison disease.

Familial hypocalciuric hypercalcaemia is probably the most important consideration in the differential diagnosis of primary hyperparathyroidism, since the PTH levels may be high in relation to hypercalaemia in this condition. The hallmark of hypocalciuric hypercalcaemia, which usually needs no treatment, is the low urinary calcium excretion in relation to hypercalcaemia. The ratio of calcium clearance to creatinine clearance

$$\frac{\text{Urinary calcium (mg/dl)}}{\text{Urinary creatinine (mg/dl)}} \times \frac{\text{Serum creatinine (mg/dl)}}{\text{Serum calcium (mg/dl)}}$$

is usually lower than 0.01, and higher in primary hyperparathyroidism. In addition, the serum PTH levels are lower than in primary hyperparathyroidism.

Management

Surgical exploration is indicated in all patients with primary hyperparathyroidism in childhood. Total parathyroidectomy with autotransplantation of parathyroid gland tissue into the patient's forearm seems to be the best treatment in children with hyperplasia of all parathyroids. Cryopreservation of tissue for later transplantation should be done to treat patients who develop hypoparathyroidism in spite of autotransplantation. If a single enlarged gland is found, and the others are normal, only the enlarged gland is resected.

Several techniques have been developed to localize diseased parathyroid glands preoperatively, but the most practical approach is to entrust all parathyroid surgery to an experienced surgeon. Ultrasonography is a useful non-invasive method for the detection of enlarged parathyroid glands down to 1 cm in diameter. Other procedures, such as selective venous catheterization for PTH determination, arteriography and thallium-201 (^{201}Tl) scanning are not necessary in patients having neck surgery for the first time, but may be helpful in cases requiring repeat surgery. Treatment of associated tumours in MEN syndromes is usually surgical. All families of children and adults with primary hyperparathyroidism due to hyperplastic glands should be screened for hypercalcaemia.

Decreased parathyroid hormone secretion or action (hypoparathyroidism)

Definition and classification

Hypoparathyroidism results from deficient PTH secretion or decreased peripheral action of the hormone on its target organs. The resulting hypocalcaemia produces a variety of clinical features, especially neuromuscular symptoms. The prevalence of hypoparathyroidism is not known, but the disease is far more common in children than primary hyperparathyroidism, which is primarily a disease of adults. A useful classification of PTH-deficient hypoparathyroidism (HP) is based on sporadic or familial occurrence, the time of onset and the presence or absence of known causes and of associated abnormalities such as Addison disease or deafness (Table 38.2). PTH-resistant HP may be caused by intrinsic receptor or postreceptor defects of the target cells, a condition termed pseudohypoparathyroidism (PHP), or may be acquired as a result of disturbed magnesium or vitamin D metabolism. Severe hypomagnesaemia may decrease secretion of PTH as well as inhibit the target cell response to normal PTH secretion thus producing features of both HP and PHP.

Pathophysiology

The biochemical consequences of decreased secretion or action of PTH are decreased renal cAMP production and urinary phosphate excretion, causing hypophosphataemia, decreased $1,25(OH)_2D_3$ production and low intestinal calcium absorption and decreased calcium translocation from

Table 38.2 Classification of hypoparathyroidism in childhood

PTH-deficient hypoparathyroidism
Non-familial
  Onset in the neonatal period
    Transient
    Permanent (isolated, DiGeorge syndrome, etc.)
  Onset after the neonatal period
    Idiopathic
    Secondary to surgery, hypomagnesaemia, etc.

Familial
  Isolated (ar, ad, sex-linked recessive)
  With Addison disease, monoliasis, etc. (ar)
  With nerve deafness and/or renal abnormalities (ar/ad)
  With severe growth failure, mental retardation and dysmorphic features (ar)

PTH-resistant hypoparathyroidism
Pseudohypoparathyroidism
Hypomagnesaemia
Disorders of vitamin D metabolism

ar/ad, autosomal recessive/dominant trait.

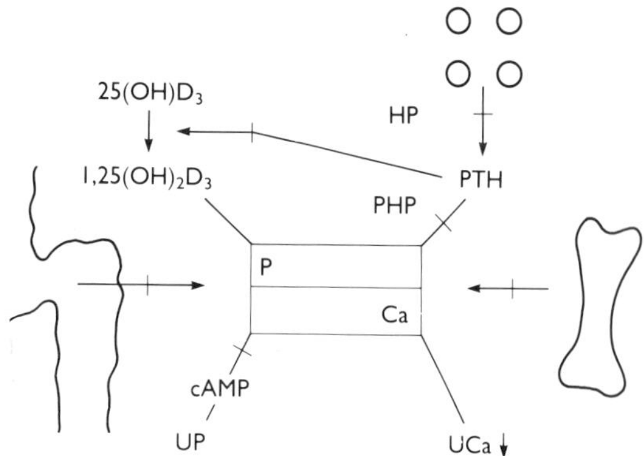

Fig. 38.5 Pathophysiology of hypoparathyroidism (HP) and pseudohypoparathyroidism (PHP); + decreased effect.

kidney and bone, the latter two conditions causing hypocalcaemia (Fig. 38.5). The urinary calcium excretion is decreased due to the low calcium load of the kidney, but there is relative hypercalciuria caused by the deficient tubular reabsorption of calcium by PTH. Vitamin D treatment will correct the intestinal absorption and skeletal resorption, but not the renal lack of calcium. This has to be taken into account during therapy of patients with HP, who are at risk of developing absolute hypercalciuria, renal stones and nephrocalcinosis. Depending on the degree of deficiency of PTH secretion or action, the total serum calcium concentrations of affected patients may vary from about 1.25 mmol/l (5 mg/dl) to low–normal. The extracellular calcium levels will not usually decrease below this value, even in the complete absence of PTH, a reflection of the equilibration of bone mineral solubility with extracellular fluids.

Clinical features of hypocalcaemia

Hypocalcaemia may produce neuromuscular, brain, cardiac, ocular and ectodermal changes. The spectrum of these symptoms varies with the patient's age, the degree of hypocalcaemia and the rapidity of the development of hypocalcaemia.

Neuromuscular changes. Tetany, the clinical hallmark of hypocalcaemia, represents enhanced peripheral neuromuscular irritability. Overt tetany manifests as circumoral and digital paraesthesiae, muscle cramps, laryngospasm and carpopedalspasm. Latent tetany may be detected by positive Chvostek and Trousseau signs. Chvostek sign can be demonstrated by tapping the facial nerve anterior to the ear to produce a twitching of the mouth (grade 1); it progresses to include the alae nasi (grade 2) and orbicularis oculi (grade 3). The Trousseau sign can be elicited by inflation of a blood pressure cuff above systolic pressure for 3 min to produce carpal spasm. An isolated positive grade 1 Chvostek sign is observed in about 25% of normal adults and in a higher proportion of children, whereas positive grade 2 and grade 3 responses associated with a positive Trousseau sign are rarely demonstrated in normal individuals. Although tetany is most typically associated with hypocalcaemia, other causes such as hyperventilation leading to alkalosis and lowering ionized calcium in serum must be considered.

Elevated serum creatinine kinase in the absence of symptoms of muscle disease is common in hypocalcaemic patients [109]. We observed an 11-year-old girl with idiopathic HP who presented with muscle weakness and myopathy, possibly related to the hypocalcaemia itself [110]. The neurological status of the girl improved and the elevated muscle enzymes in serum normalized during treatment of the hypocalcaemia.

Brain changes. Seizures indistinguishable from those occurring in the absence of hypocalcaemia, focal or grand mal, frequently give rise to the misdiagnosis of an idiopathic seizure disorder. One of our own young patients and his mother had hypocalcaemic seizures from 5 years and 26 years of age, respectively, before the diagnosis of HP was made [111]. The usual delay between the onset of symptoms and the time of diagnosis is estimated to be approximately 5 years [112]. It is obvious that routine measurement of calcium is essential in every case of epilepsy. Children with chronic hypocalcaemia develop mental retardation if left untreated. Other mental signs are irritability, anxiety, impaired memory and poor performance in school, psychoneurotic behaviour and depression.

Papilloedema and signs mimicking a cerebral tumour (pseudotumour cerebri) may rarely occur. Intracranial calcification, particularly in the basal ganglia, is visible on skull X-ray and more often with computerized tomography. The calcifications are observed in about half of the patients with long-standing HP and PHP, and consist of deposits of calcium salts in and around the walls of small blood vessels. These irreversible lesions probably do not affect the function of the nervous system, and may also occur in individuals with normal calcium metabolism.

Cardiac manifestations. In hypocalcaemia these include electrocardiographic abnormalities (prolongation of the Q-oT interval) and, rarely, congestive cardiac failure [113].

Ocular changes. Lenticular cataracts are common dystrophic manifestations of chronic hypocalcaemia. These important ocular manifestations are irreversible, but further progression is arrested by normalization of the hypocalcaemia.

Ectodermal changes. The skin may be dry and scaling, the hair coarse and fractured, the nails brittle and fissured. Enamel hypoplasia with transverse grooves and increased liability to caries are due to chronic hypocalcaemia during the development of the teeth, and may be used to date the onset of hypocalcaemia retrospectively.

Newborns and young infants. Hypocalcaemic manifestations may be non-specific (tremor, apnoea, cyanosis, lethargy) and may resemble those induced by sepsis, intracranial haemorrhage or metabolic disorders.

PARATHYROID HORMONE-DEFICIENT HYPOPARATHYROIDISM

Non-familial hypoparathyroidism

Transient HP in the neonatal period is discussed later. Permanent congenital isolated HP probably results from defective development of the parathyroid glands. This may be caused from, or associated with, administration of ^{131}I or excessive alcohol during pregnancy, maternal diabetes and chromosomal abnormalities. Many cases may be incomplete forms of DiGeorge syndrome. The most common features of this condition are aplasia or hypoplasia of the thymus and parathyroid glands, congenital heart defects, especially truncus arteriosus, and facial anomalies such as micrognathia, cleft lip and/or palate and malformations of the ears. The disorder is usually sporadic, but autosomal dominant and recessive inheritance may occur. Chromosomal abnormalities, such as monosomy 10p13 and monosomy 22q11, have been observed in some patients with DiGeorge syndrome [114,115]. The syndrome is the result of developmental defects of the structures which derive from the third and fourth pharyngeal pouches and branchial arches. Affected infants manifest thymic deficiency, heart defects and hypoparathyroidism as progressive lymphopenia with recurrent infections, failure to thrive and hypocalcaemic tetany. Severe cases carry a poor prognosis if not treated by thymic transplantation.

HP with onset after the neonatal period can develop at any age, most often between 2 and 10 years of age. Most cases occur sporadically, some familial (see below), either idiopathically or associated with damage to the parathyroid glands by surgery, iron deposition in haemosiderosis, malignant infiltration or irradiation. Primary magnesium deficiency may result in functional HP and has to be excluded. The clinical symptoms are related to the course and severity of hypocalcaemia or associated disorders. Several children who first appear to have isolated idiopathic HP, especially those with inherited HP, subsequently develop additional abnormalities such as Addison disease (see below).

Familial HP

Although most cases are sporadic, familial occurrence of HP has been documented. Familial HP has been reported as an isolated entity or in association with diverse abnormalities such as DiGeorge syndrome [116], sensorineural deafness with or without nephropathy [117–120], extreme growth failure, dysmorphic features and developmental delay [121–123], autoimmune polyglandular disease type I [124,125], and several syndromes such as Kenny–Caffey syndrome [126,127], Kearns–Sayre syndrome [128] and Halermann–Streiff syndrome [129]. The genetic basis for the association between HP and sensorineural deafness is unclear. An extensive study of patients with different types of HP, including postoperative PTH deficiency, revealed a dependency on treatment, suggesting that hypocalcaemia may aggravate deafness [130]. Hearing loss has also been described in some patients with PHP [131] but no correlation was made to the degree of hypocalcaemia during the audiometry. The observation that deafness can worsen despite correction of hypocalcaemia in subjects with familial HP suggests that sensorineural hearing loss is not associated by chance, and is not induced by hypocalcaemia, at least in some families with inherited HP [118,120]. Familial isolated HP unassociated with other abnormalities is very rare, but of biological importance with regard to the physiology and pathophysiology of PTH synthesis and metabolism. Sex-linked recessive [132,133], autosomal dominant [134–137] and autosomal recessive inheritance [134,138] may occur. A number of additional families have been reported with vertical transmission of HP, but in each the affected parent has been a female, which is compatible with a sex-linked dominant or autosomal dominant trait [111,135,139].

Human PTH is encoded by a single gene located on the short arm of chromosome 11 (see Chapter 37, Fig. 37.5). The reduced PTH secretion in familial isolated HP may be due to mutations of distant loci that affect the embryological development and regulation of the parathyroids or may result from mutations in or near the PTH gene. In addition, a PTH gene defect may also result in the secretion of immunologically detectable, but biologically inactive hormone that may or may not block the peripheral PTH receptors in affected individuals. An aberrant form of PTH, or an unknown inhibitor such as an antibody, could explain some PHP-like conditions with resistance to endogenous and exogenous PTH [140]. In one patient, surgical removal of four hyperplastic parathyroids restored responsiveness to PTH [112]. Three cases of HP putatively due to the secretion of a biologically inactive PTH molecule not blocking the receptors have been reported [141–143]. The condition has been termed 'pseudo-idiopathic hypoparathyroidism', but in neither case were the data for the suggested mechanism definitive. The first reported case of bioinactive PTH [143] has been shown to have 'simple' idiopathic HP [134].

Molecular genetic analyses of 44 affected people from 11 families with isolated HP detected no gross abnormality such as absence of PTH gene or recognizable deletions [111,134,144]. Restriction endonuclease analyses demonstrated in some families evidence for alterations in or near the PTH gene, whereas in others no link to the PTH gene itself could be elicited. This suggests that the molecular defect in these kindreds must be located elsewhere affecting processing, synthesis, or secretion of PTH. Recently in one kindred with autosomal dominant familial HP cloning and sequencing of the preproPTH gene revealed a point mutation in the signal peptide-encoding region of the gene [145]. *In vitro* studies demonstrated a markedly impaired processing of the mutant preproPTH to proPTH, explaining the decreased PTH release and hypocalcaemia *in vivo*. This mutation of a signal sequence constitutes a novel pathophysiological mechanism in humans.

X-linked recessive isolated HP appears probably due to a defective development or agenesis of the parathyroid gland [138]. Recently the gene has been mapped to Xq26–Xq27 [146]. The precise mapping represents an important step to identify genetic markers and factors controlling parathyroid development.

Autoimmune HP is usually inherited as an autosomal recessive trait, although sporadic cases have been reported. Most patients present in the first two decades of life with HP, Addison disease and moniliasis. The condition is known by several names, including polyglandular autoimmune disease type I or autoimmune polyendocrinopathy–candidosis–ectodermal dystrophy (APECED).

Ahonen *et al.* [124] summarized the clinical variation of this entity in a series of 68 Finnish patients from 54 families aged 10 months to 53 years. The clinical manifestations of APECED vary greatly, and include a variable combination of the following three groups of disease components.

1 Failure of the parathyroid glands, adrenal cortex, gonads, pancreatic β cells, gastric parietal cells, and thyroid gland, and hepatitis.

2 Chronic mucocutaneous candidiasis.

3 Dystrophy of dental enamel and nails, alopecia, vitiligo and keratopathy.

The initial manifestation was oral candidiasis in 60%; all the patients had candidiasis at some time. The earliest endocrinopathies were HP and adrenal insufficiency, developing at 19 months to 35 years of age with a peak in years 3–5 for HP and years 11–15 for adrenal insufficiency. The majority of patients had three to five manifestations, some of which did not appear until the fifth decade, indicating that all patients with APECED need lifelong follow-up for the detection of new disorders.

An autoimmune basis for this form of HP is suggested by the finding of other autoimmune disorders and circulating organ-specific antibodies including parathyroid (not PTH) antibodies. In the cases examined complete destruction or atrophy of the parathyroid glands has been demonstrated [112]. There is a poor correlation between the presence or titre of antibodies and the presence or absence of clinical manifestations in different members of a family. The underlying disorder probably involves the cell-mediated immunity.

PSEUDOHYPOPARATHYROIDISM

In 1942 Albright *et al.* described three patients with hypocalcaemia and hyperphosphataemia who failed to show either phosphaturic or hypercalcaemic responses to administered parathyroid extract [147]. Albright termed this first human disease attributed to resistance of an otherwise normal target organ PHP. PHP is a heterogeneous syndrome caused by defects in receptors, particularly of the kidney tubule [148].

Patients with the prototypic form of PHP present at an average age of 8 years – rarely before the age of 3 years – with symptomatic hypocalcaemia. Many of them are mentally retarded and show unique somatic features, termed Albright hereditary osteodystrophy (AHO): short stature, round facies, short neck, obesity, subcutaneous calcifications especially near the joints and shortening of the metacarpals and metatarsals (Fig. 38.6). The fourth metacarpal is often so short that a dimple appears at its distal end when a fist is made. The degree of AHO varies. Symptoms related to chronic hypocalcaemia may be present.

Characterization of the molecular basis for PHP commenced when Chase and co-workers found that these patients, in addition to the lacking phosphaturic response to exogenous PTH, also showed a markedly blunted urinary cAMP increase in comparison to normal subjects and patients with HP [149]. This form of PHP is now termed PHP type I, to distinguish it from a much rarer entity, PHP type II, in which a subnormal phosphaturic but normal urinary cAMP response to PTH was demonstrated [150]. These biochemical observations suggested that PHP type I is caused by a defective interaction with its renal receptor–adenylate cyclase complex, resulting in a lack of cAMP production, whereas PHP type II may be due to an intracellular defect beyond the cAMP step leading only to impaired phosphate transport (Fig. 38.7). This hypothesis was supported by the finding that administration of dibutyryl cAMP to patients with PHP type I produced the normal renal effects of PTH such as rise of

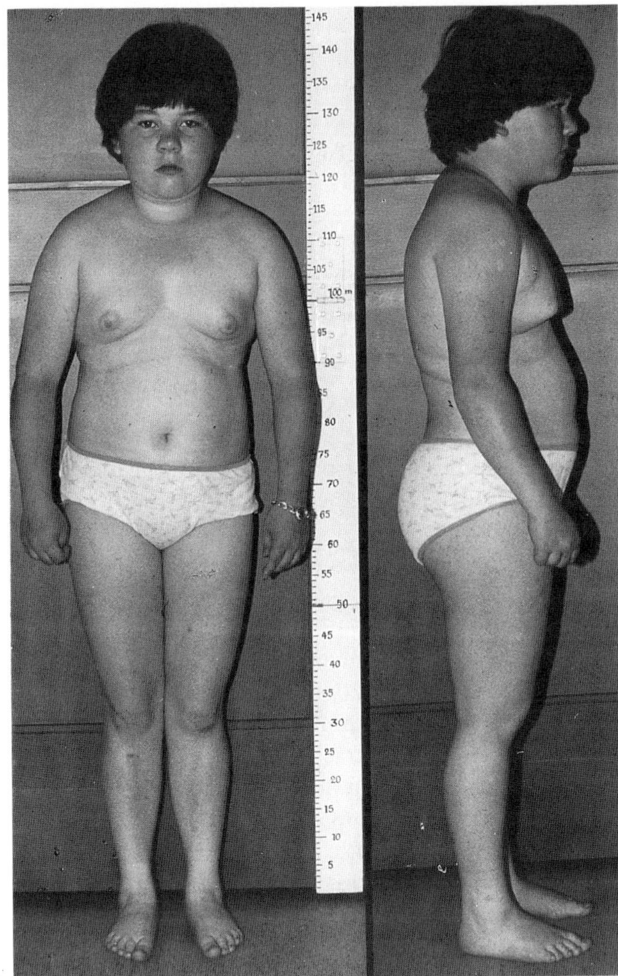

(a)

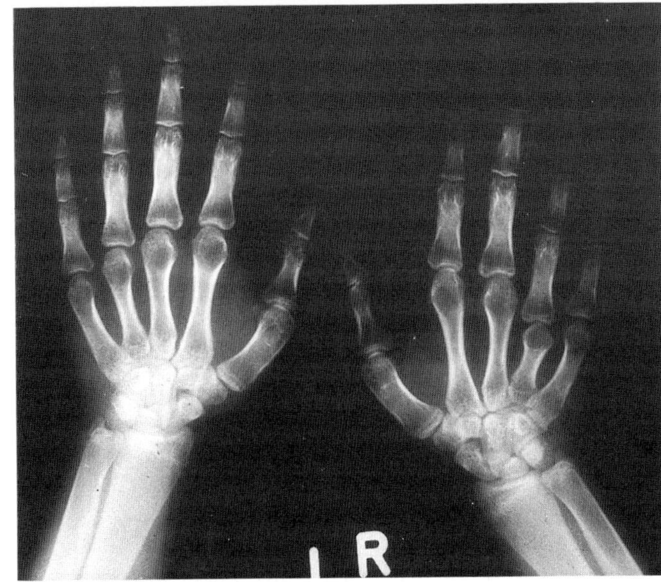

(b)

Fig. 38.6 Pseudohypoparathyroidism type I in a 15-year-old mentally retarded girl with typical signs of Albright hereditary osteodystrophy, including (a) short stature, round facies, short neck, obesity and (b) shortening of the fourth metacarpal of the right hand.

urine phosphate and serum 1,25$(OH)_2D$ levels [151,152]. Furthermore the PTH-dependent adenylate cyclase in renal plasma-membrane preparations from a patient with PHP type I required greater than normal concentrations of guanosine triphosphate [153,154]. This led to the concept that the hormone resistance is due to a defect in the component (G_s protein) that couples the membrane PTH receptor to the catalytic unit of the adenylate cyclase. Indeed, several groups provided evidence that the activity of this G_s protein is reduced by 40–50% in erythrocytes [155,156], platelets [157], cultured fibroblasts [158], and kidney [153] of patients with PHP type I.

Patients with decreased G_s protein activity (about 60% of subjects with PHP type I) are now classified as having PHP type Ia, whereas those with normal G_s protein are classified as type Ib [148]. Almost all patients with PHP type Ia show clinical features of AHO. Associated resistance to other hormones that act via cAMP is common. The G_s protein is not tissue-specific, thus explaining resistance to multiple hormones such as decreased response to thyrotrophin-releasing hormone (TRH), thyroid-stimulating hormone (TSH), gonadotrophins and glucagon [148,159]. Some defects such as primary hypothyroidism and hypogonadism, may be clinically manifest.

Deficiency of prolactin secretion (basal and in response to TRH and chlorpromazine) has been observed [160,161] but could not be correlated with abnormal G_s protein activity, possibly because prolactin secretion is mediated by intracellular calcium and not cAMP as second messenger. The reason why the clinical expression of multiple hormone resistance in patients with PHP type Ia is so variable, and why the PTH response is so severely affected, is unclear. One explanation may be that the amount of cAMP needed to produce the biological effects may vary from tissue to tissue, and that the PTH-sensitive phosphate transport is more critically dependent on cAMP generation than other tissues with diminished G_s protein activity.

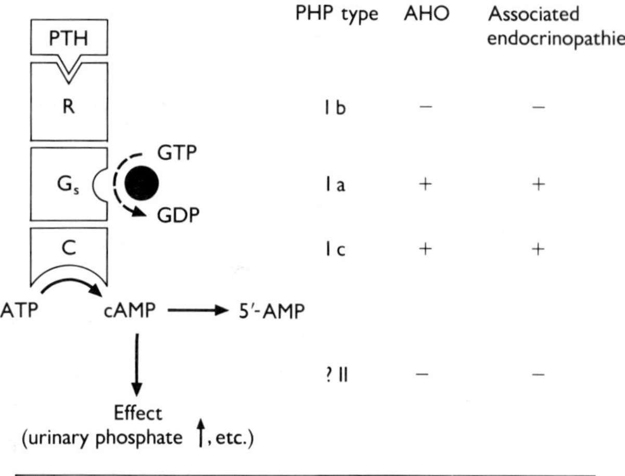

I a	G-protein activity in cell membranes ↓ (~50% of normal)
I b/c	G-protein activity in cell membranes normal
AHO	Albright hereditary osteodystrophy

Fig. 38.7 Pathophysiology and classification of pseudohypoparathyroidism (PHP). AMP, adenosine monophosphate; ATP, adenosine triphosphate; C, catalytic unit; GDP, guanosine diphosphate; GTP, guanosine triphosphate; R, receptor.

Patients with AHO without biochemical evidence of renal resistance to PTH are classified as having pseudo-pseudohypoparathyroidism (pseudo-PHP). Patients with PHP type I and pseudo-PHP may be members of the same kindred, indicating a genetic relationship. Recent studies have shown that patients with pseudo-PHP may have reductions in G_s protein activity comparable to those in patients with PHP type Ia [162–164], suggesting that reduced G_s protein activity alone may not produce hormone resistance, but must be combined with other factors to cause hypocalcaemia [163].

The nature of the defect in patients with PTH resistance but without G_s protein deficiency (PHP type Ib) remains to be clarified. Most of these patients do not have AHO or multiple hormone resistance [156]. It is possible that these patients have abnormalities limited to PTH-sensitive tissues, such as an intrinsic defect of the PTH receptor itself [165] or a bioinactive PTH, or yet unknown factors that occupy the PTH receptor but are incapable of activating adenylate cyclase [140,166]. There are also a few patients with PHP type Ib who present with multiple hormone resistance (with or rarely without AHO). Abnormal G_s protein function, undetectable by current methods used to measure G_s protein activity, or defects in other elements of the adenylate cyclase complex, may account for the disorder in these patients. The components of the adenylate cyclase system include not only stimulatory but also inhibitory G proteins mediating inhibitory control by such agents as α_2-adrenergic agonists [167]. No abnormality in the activity of such an inhibitory G protein (G_i protein) could be detected in the erythrocyte membranes from patients with PHP types Ia and Ib [168].

Recently a new form of PHP has been described in a 21-year-old man with classic AHO and resistance to multiple hormones including PTH, TSH, gonadotrophins and glucagon [169]. Studies of the patient's fibroblasts revealed normal G_s activity but a defect in the catalytic unit of adenylate cyclase. This new subtype has been classified as PHP type Ic.

Pedigree analysis of families with AHO associated with PTH resistance (PHP type I) and pseudo-PHP is consistent with either autosomal or X-linked patterns of transmission [148]. The genetics of PHP without AHO is less well defined. G_s protein measurement should be a useful marker for studying the inheritance in families with PHP type Ia.

Molecular genetic studies indicate distinct mutations of the gene coding for the α-subunit of the G_s protein in different kindreds [170–173]. The finding that these mutations were found in only one allele of the gene, located on chromosome 20, is consistent with autosomal dominant inheritance of AHO.

Albright's name is attached to a second syndrome involving abnormal function of endocrine cells, the McCune–Albright syndrome. This is a sporadic disease characterized by polyostotic fibrous dysplasia, café-au-lait pigmentation of the skin and hyperfunction of multiple endocrine glands, such as hyperthyroidism, hypercortisolism and pituitary adenomas secreting growth hormone. Recently Weinstein *et al.* [174] described activation mutations of the $G_s\alpha$ gene in abnormal tissues from these patients, indicating that somatic mutation of this gene early in embryogenesis could underlie the clinical manifestation of the McCune–Albright syndrome.

The nature of the defect in PHP type II is unclear. Since the initial description by Drezner *et al.* in 1973 [150] 19 additional patients have been reported with hypoparathyroidism, elevated serum PTH and a dissociation between normal cAMP excretion and disturbed renal handling of phosphate [148]. Clinical signs of AHO were absent, normal G_s protein activity was found in the few examined cases and no evidence of inheritance could be established. No abnormality in the intracellular action, such as a defective cAMP-dependent protein kinase, has been demonstrated. In some of the patients the phosphaturic response to PTH could be restored by normalization of serum calcium during calcium infusion or vitamin D treatment. This led to the conclusion that the disorder may result from an inability of PTH to increase the cell membrane permeability to calcium (via the inositol triphosphate protein kinase C pathway) which is physiologically important for some of the biological effects of the hormone such as renal tubular phosphate reabsorption

[148]. Anticonvulsant drugs have been shown to mimic PHP type II by a drug-related inhibition of cAMP-induced phosphaturia [175]. Because hypocalcaemia may blunt the phosphaturia it is important to test the phosphaturic response to PTH after normalization of serum calcium before diagnosing PHP type II. It has yet to be proven whether PHP type II needs to be considered as a real entity.

Mild to moderate mental retardation occurs in 50–75% of all patients with PHP type I. Low serum calcium itself is probably not a major cause, since hypocalcaemia usually begins after the critical development period of brain function. Many patients with PHP type I have associated hypothyroidism [112,148,159] that should be detected early and treated. Although a role of untreated thyroid insufficiency in mental retardation cannot be excluded there is a lack of correlation between both conditions in patients with PHP. It is more likely that mental deficiency is a heritable defect that is strongly associated with G_s protein deficiency. In a study of 25 subjects with PHP, 11 of 14 patients with PHP type Ia but none of 11 patients with PHP type Ib presented with mental retardation [176]. Mutations in the adenylate cyclase–cAMP system may affect the learning ability of *Drosophila* flies. Therefore the association between mental deficiency and decreased G_s protein activity is believed to indicate that the defective G_s protein itself, or reduced cAMP concentrations in the cerebral tissue, causes the impaired brain function in patients with PHP type Ia [176].

Hypocalcaemia in the face of elevated circulating PTH and subnormal calcaemic response to prolonged intramuscular PTH administration suggests skeletal in addition to renal resistance in PHP. This was thought to result from the same abnormality in cAMP generation occurring in bone tissue. However, radiographic and histological findings and elevated serum alkaline phosphatase activity provided evidence of excessive PTH action on bone in some pseudohypoparathyroid patients, especially in those without AHO. This condition has been termed hypohyperparathyroidism [177] or renal resistance to PTH with osteitis fibrosa [178]. In these patients, PTH may not be as inactive on the skeleton as it is on the kidney, reflecting a selective or predominant renal defect. There are several arguments that osteitis fibrosa cystica may not be a distinct entity (selective renal resistance to PTH), but that it is simply the extreme end of a spectrum with different degrees of bone responsiveness [112,148,179,180].

Most patients with PHP have a tendency to diminished bone density and increased bone turnover combined with histological evidence of hyperparathyroidism and osteomalacia [148,185]. This status of bone resembles that of renal osteodystrophy. Although it cannot be excluded that those patients with G_s protein deficiency (PHP type Ia) might exhibit some resistance of the bone adenylate cyclase system, there is much evidence that the skeletal changes are mainly acquired and secondary to the congenital renal resistance in pseudohypoparathyroid subjects. The kidney defect results in hyperphosphataemia and decreased $1{,}25(OH)_2D_3$ secretion, both conditions interfering with mobilization of skeletal calcium.

The skeletal changes can be explained on the basis that the PTH action on the remodelling (osteoclastic–osteoblastic) system is less dependent on $1{,}25(OH)_2D_3$ than that on the homeostatic system that transfers calcium from bone to serum by osteocytic osteolysis. Depending upon the degree of hyperparathyroidism and $1{,}25(OH)_2D_3$ deficiency, PTH stimulates the remodelling system inducing bone resorption and osteitis fibrocystica, but does not overcome the hypocalcaemia because the homeostatic system is impaired by low $1{,}25(OH)_2D_3$ [185].

Intermittent normocalcaemia may occur spontaneously in patients with PHP type I. The defective renal cAMP response to PTH differentiates patients with normocalcaemic PHP type I from those with pseudo-PHP. Bone response to PTH and the serum levels of 1,25(OH)D are normal, when measured in normocalcaemic PHP type I, indicating improved renal synthesis of the vitamin D hormone and mobilization of calcium from bone and intestine [181]. In two patients with PHP type Ib who were normocalcaemic during pregnancy placental synthesis of $1{,}25(OH)_2D_3$ may have contributed to the maintenance of normocalcaemia [182].

OTHER CAUSES OF PARATHYROID HORMONE-RESISTANT HYPOPARATHYROIDISM

Impaired PTH responsiveness may contribute to hypocalcaemia in other conditions, such as hypomagnesaemia and disturbances of vitamin D metabolism. The mechanism by which severe hypomagnesaemia leads to PTH resistance is not known. Low serum $1{,}25(OH)_2D$ levels in calciopenic rickets, including renal osteodystrophy, may interfere with PTH action on bone, especially on osteocytic calcium transfer.

DIFFERENTIATION OF HYPOPARATHYROIDISM AND PSEUDOHYPOPARATHYROIDISM

Both conditions must be considered in a patient with hypocalcaemia and hyperphosphataemia (due to high TmP/GFR) in the presence of normal renal function and in the absence of severe hypomagnesaemia. Genetic implications and the probability of associated hormone deficiencies require investigations to differentiate HP from PHP. Signs of AHO and radiographic evidence of hyperparathyroidism indicate PHP. However, the definitive diagnosis depends on the measurement of serum PTH and the patient's response to exogenous PTH. In HP the intact

Table 38.3 Classification and differential diagnosis of pseudohypoparathyroidism

Type	Serum levels in untreated patients Ca	P	PTH	AHO	Heredity	Response of PcAMP and UcAMP to PTH	$G_s\alpha$ protein	Resistance to other hormones (for example TSH)
Ia	↓	↑	↑	+	+	↓	↓	+
Ib	↓	↑	↑	− (+)	+	↓	n	−
Ic	↓	↑	↑	+	?	↓	n	+
II	↓	↑	↑	−	+	n	n	−
Normocalcaemic PHP	n	n	↑/n	Depends on the type of PHP				
Pseudo-PHP	n	n	n	+	+	n	↓ (n)	−

↓, low; ↑, increased; AHO, Albright hereditary osteodystrophy; n, normal; PcAMP/UcAMP, cAMP in plasma/urine.

PTH in serum is undetectable or low in relation to the hypocalcaemia, whereas patients with PHP have elevated PTH levels, the majority even during vitamin D-induced or spontaneous normocalcaemia.

The diagnosis of PHP can be established by the documentation of deficient urinary cAMP excretion after intravenous administration of synthetic PTH fragments such as 1–34 or 1–38 human PTH. The tubular phosphate reabsorption or TmP/GFR after PTH is less decreased in PHP than in HP or controls. Unfortunately, there is overlap of the values, which limits the usefulness of this index of PTH response. Measurement of plasma cAMP after PTH is also recommended to demonstrate hormone unresponsiveness, since this method simplifies the test procedure and avoids problems in urine collections [183]. Table 38.3 summarizes the classification and differential diagnosis of PHP.

Another approach to a demonstration of PHP may be the measurement of serum calcium during prolonged intramuscular PTH administration to assess the response of bone. The lower increment of serum calcium in untreated patients with PHP in comparison to HP is largely the function of the renal $1,25(OH)_2D_3$ stimulation, and thus of limited value to detect a presumed skeletal resistance.

In patients with AHO the determination of the G_s protein activity may be useful. This can be measured by the ability of detergent extracts of erythrocyte membranes to reconstitute adenylate cyclase activity in the G_s protein-deficient membranes of S 49 cyc^- mouse lymphoma cells [155]. At present this test remains a research tool, but may be of interest in family investigations, especially of infants not (yet) presenting typical somatic and biochemical findings. The measurement of reduced mRNA coding for the subunit of the G_s protein may be another genetic marker in some families with AHO, regardless of whether patients are affected by PHP type Ia or pseudo-PHP [171, 184]. Additional investigations should document associated disorders in PHP (hypothyroidism, hypogonadism) and HP (Addison disease, sensorineural deafness, renal abnormalities and syndromes such as DiGeorge syndrome).

TREATMENT

The treatment, directed to normalizing serum calcium and phosphate, is similar in patients with HP and PHP.

Acute hypocalcaemia requires slow intravenous injection of 10% calcium gluconate, 1–2 ml/kg (9–18 mg elemental calcium/kg) every 6–8 h. Maintenance therapy consists of oral administration of 0.5–1 g elemental calcium in combination with vitamin D or related compounds such as vitamin D_2 (ergocalciferol) or vitamin D_3 (cholecalciferol), dihydrotachysterol (DHT), 1α-hydroxyvitamin D_3 (1α-OHD_3), or $1,25(OH)_2D_3$ (calcitriol). The inter- and intra-individual sensitivity to all these compounds may vary somewhat, and intoxication has been observed with all vitamin D preparations due to the narrow therapeutic–toxic range. A reasonable starting dosage is 50 μg/kg (2000 IU/kg) vitamin D_2 or D_3, 20 μg/kg DHT, and 25–50 ng/kg 1α-OHD_3 or calcitriol. Serum and urine calcium should be monitored at least every 2–3 months, and more frequently after the start of treatment and after changing the dosage of the vitamin D compound. Vitamin D is the least expensive drug, but has the disadvantage of delayed onset of biological effect and the possibility of toxicity because of its prolonged half-life (several weeks). Calcitriol or 1α-OHD_3 bypass the renal hydroxylation step in vitamin D metabolism, which is impaired in HP and PHP. Treatment with both active metabolites has the advantage of speed of action and rapid lowering within days of hypercalcaemia when discontinued.

The resistance to PTH in patients with PHP is mainly limited to the proximal kidney tubule, whereas the secondary hyperparathyroidism may provoke bone degradation and osteopenia [180,185]. One aim of treatment in PHP, therefore, is the suppression of hyperparathyroidism to protect the skeleton by elevating the serum calcium concentrations to the high–normal range (2.25–2.5 mmol/l or 9–10 mg/dl), since the parathyroid glands of patients with PHP are less sensitive to circulating calcium levels. By contrast, the serum calcium levels in HP should be maintained in the low–normal range (2.0–2.25 mmol/l or 8–9 mg/dl) since patients with HP may present with hypercalciuria despite normal serum calcium levels due to the deficient hypocalciuric effect of PTH. In some hypoparathyroid patients with high urinary calcium excretion despite low–normal serum calcium, hydrochlorothiazide at 1–2 mg/kg per day and sodium restriction may reverse the hypercalciuria. The Sulkowitch test is not a reliable test for increased urinary calcium excretion. If hypercalciuria (urinary calcium exceeding 4 mg/kg per 24 h or urinary calcium/creatinine ratios exceeding 0.22 mg/mg in a 24-h urine or random urine sample) or hypercalcaemia (serum calcium exceeding 2.6 mmol/l or 10.4 mg/dl) occur, treatment with vitamin D or its metabolites should be discontinued, and reinstated at a 15–20% lower dose when normocalcaemia and normocalciuria have been re-established.

In patients with HP a more appropriate therapy may by PTH replacement. This may be practical in the future since synthetic human PTH fragments are now available. The disadvantages of this treatment are its high cost and the need for daily parenteral administration.

DISTURBANCES OF RENAL PHOSPHATE EXCRETION IN CHILDHOOD

Increased renal phosphate excretion

Several disorders, listed in Table 38.4 can lead to increased urinary phosphate excretion, hypophosphataemia and consequent phosphopenic rickets and osteomalacia. Decreased phosphate intake as a possible cause of phosphate deficiency is uncommon, except in premature infants (discussed on p. 769). The disorders of renal tubular phosphate reabsorption may be acquired or congenital, the most important being familial hypophosphataemic rickets [186–190].

Table 38.4 Classification of phosphopenic rickets and osteomalacia

Increased renal phosphate excretion
Genetic primary hypophosphataemia
Familial X-linked hypophosphataemic rickets
Hypophosphataemic non-rachitic bone disease (ad)
Hereditary hypophosphataemic rickets with hypercalciuria (ar)
Tumour, rickets and osteomalacia
Fanconi syndrome
Renal tubular acidosis
Decreased phosphate intake

ar/ad, autosomal recessive/dominant trait.

X-LINKED FAMILIAL HYPOPHOSPHATAEMIC RICKETS

Inheritance and clinical features

X-linked familial hypophosphataemic rickets (XLH) was first described in 1937 by Albright *et al.* [191] under the term 'vitamin D-resistant rickets'. Analysis of inheritance using hypophosphataemia as the primary discriminant, revealed that the mode of transmission is X-linked dominant. As with most X-linked disorders the male is more severely affected than the heterozygous female. The clinical expression is not related to the degree of hypophosphataemia and may be extremely variable. Some patients may be only hypophosphataemic, whereas others have severe bone disease. The frequency of XLH is about 1 in 25 000 [188]. Untreated patients usually present with slow growth, bowing of the legs (Fig. 38.8), waddling gait and radiological signs of rickets, but without myopathy and tetany. The growth failure is most manifest in the legs. Although the clinical features become apparent during late infancy, the condition can be diagnosed in the first weeks of life by hypophosphataemia and raised serum alkaline phosphatase activity [192]. Treatment starting in the first months of age may prevent the osseous lesions [193,194]. Poor dental development and spontaneous tooth abscess may occur.

Adults may have no symptoms or present with calcifications of tendons, ligaments, and joint capsules [195] or impaired sensorineural hearing loss [196]. Sporadic cases appearing later in childhood or adult life with bone pain and muscle weakness have been observed. Some have increased urinary glycine and/or glucose excretion, others may have tumour osteomalacia (see below) due to a small occult tumour. All these cases of acquired primary hypophosphataemia are radiologically and biochemically similar to patients with XLH. Relatives have been described with both autosomal dominant and autosomal recessive inheritance of familial hypophosphataemia resembling XLH.

Radiological and histological findings

The radiological features are age-dependent. In untreated infants widening, irregular fraying and cupping of the metaphyseal ends of the long bones of the forearm and legs are seen, whereas in later childhood only the changes of the legs are prominent. Radiographs of the knee and ankle joint showing the typical metaphyseal abnormalities of

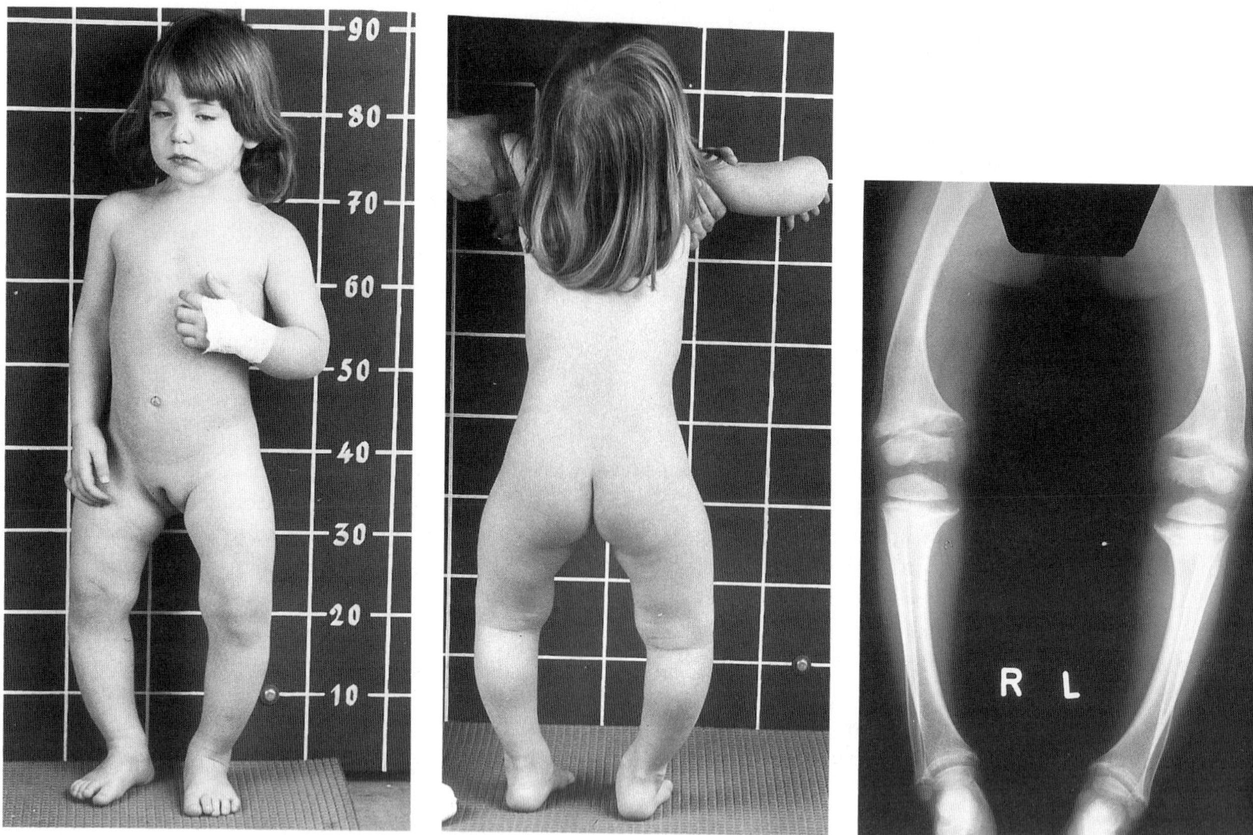

Fig. 38.8 X-linked hypophosphataemic rickets in a girl, aged 3 years, with severe bowing of legs. Radiography shows widening, cupping and irregular fraying of the metaphyseal ends of the distal femora and proximal tibiae as well as metaphyseal irregularity of the distal ends of the tibiae.

the distal femur and the proximal and distal tibia are therefore more important for follow-up than those of the wrist. The characteristic wedge-shaped defect of medial surface of proximal tibia in patients with genu varum deformity is probably the result of the increased weight on the medial side of the knee. With increasing age, the trabecular pattern becomes coarsened and a generalized increase of bone density, especially in the axial skeleton, is noticed.

Histological findings demonstrate rickets and osteomalacia, but no evidence for hyperparathyroid bone lesions. The changes at the growth plate are not different from those described for calciopenic rickets. The osteomalacic changes of the trabecular and Haversian systems are characterized by an excess of osteoid tissue (up to 10 times compared with normal), decreased mineralization and bone formation, and absence of increased osteoclastic bone resorption.

Pathogenesis and pathophysiology

The discovery of the hypophosphataemic mouse (Hyp), that shows genetic, clinical and biochemical features resembling the human disease, has facilitated the investigations of XLH [188,190]. Based on the observations in humans and in the Hyp mouse a considerable amount of data has accumulated [186,188–190,197] suggesting that XLH is an inborn error of phosphate transport in the proximal tubular cell of the kidney transmitted by a single abnormal gene on the X chromosome. Recently, the gene responsible for XLH has been localized to the short arm of the X chromosome (Xp22.31–21.3) in the region extending from Duchenne muscular dystrophy to steroid sulphatase [197].

The serum levels of calcium and PTH are normal. The serum concentration of 1,25(OH)$_2$D is low–normal [198–200], a finding that is clearly abnormal with regard to hypophosphataemia. In addition, PTH infusions and phosphate restriction do not elevate the vitamin D hormone in these patients to the same extent as in normal subjects [201,202]. The measurement of 25-OHD-1α-hydroxylase in Hyp mice renal cortex confirms the defective regulation in that the enzyme activity increases significantly less during phosphate depletion than in control animals [203]. XLH thus appears to result from a defect in renal proximal tubular cells coupled with a defective res-

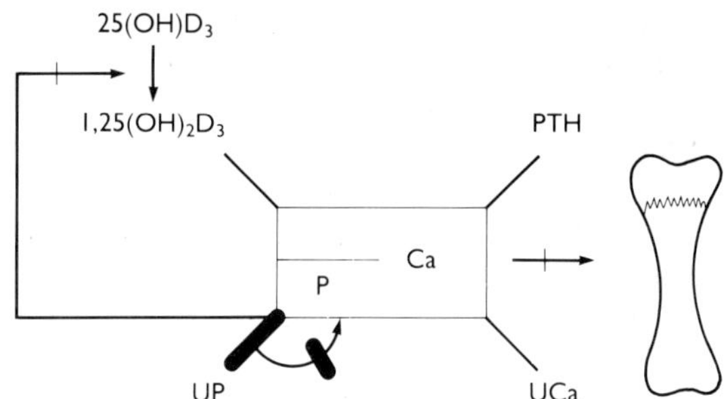

Fig. 38.9 Pathophysiology of familial hypophosphataemic rickets.

ponse of 1,25(OH)$_2$D$_3$, both conditions resulting in osteomalacia and rickets (Fig. 38.9). The similarity between the sites of tubular phosphate transport and sites of 1,25(OH)$_2$D$_3$ production suggests that both abnormal processes occur in the same cell. However, it is yet unclear if the defective phosphate transport results in abnormal vitamin D regulation or vice versa, or if both conditions are the consequence of an unidentified process or humoral factor [189,190,197]. There is no consensus whether additional transport defects also involve bone and intestinal mucosa cells.

In vitro studies indicate that there is an intrinsic defect in the osteoblast of the Hyp mouse and of patients with XLH [190].

Investigations

The most important laboratory findings in XLH are hypophosphataemia and decreased TmP/GFR in the fasting state considering the important age-dependency of both measures.

Serum calcium and parathyroid functions (serum PTH and urinary cAMP) are normal. Evidence for increased bone turnover (increments of alkaline phosphatase activity and osteocalcin concentration in serum and urinary hydroxyproline excretion) is usually present in growing children with XLH, but may be absent in the adult despite histological features of osteomalacia. Serum 25-OHD levels are normal, serum 1,25(OH)$_2$D levels are normal for growth rate [198] but low for hypophosphataemia.

Treatment

Oral administration of phosphate, vitamin D compounds, or both have been used in the treatment of XLH. Phosphate stimulates growth rate and improves rickets (but not osteomalacia) without raising 1,25(OH)$_2$D serum levels, and causes secondary hyperparathyroidism or, rarely, irreversible autonomous hyperparathyroidism [94,95]. Massive doses of vitamin D improve rickets (but not osteomalacia), lower 1,25(OH)$_2$D serum levels [198,199] and may cause intoxication with renal damage.

Stickler & Morgenstern reported no effect of phosphate and pharmacological doses of vitamin D on the ultimate height in their patients with XLH, and suggested that this therapy has to be balanced against the risk of renal damage [204].

Several recent studies have demonstrated that the simultaneous treatment with adequate doses of phosphate and 1-hydroxylated vitamin D preparations such as 1,25(OH)$_2$D$_3$ or 1α-OHD$_3$ increase growth rate and cause healing of rickets and osteomalacia [205–211]. This therapeutic regime leads to an increase in serum phosphate concentration, probably by a combination of increased intestinal absorption and 1,25(OH)$_2$D$_3$-induced suppression of PTH, which in turn stimulates renal phosphate reabsorption. It is not known whether the increased serum levels of the vitamin D hormone play a direct role in improving bone mineralization in addition to its effects which increase serum phosphate and suppress PTH secretion.

The currently recommended therapy of XLH in children can be summarized as follows.

1 *Phosphate.* The phosphate supplement consists of commercially available oral neutral phosphate salts, for example Phosphate Sandoz (UK), Neutra-Phos (USA) or Reducto (Germany) given as 1–4 g or 50–70 mg/kg body weight of elemental phosphorus in four to six divided doses at 3–4-h intervals, the first on rising and the last before bed. The phosphate salts have to be given at frequent intervals because the serum phosphate level usually reaches a peak in about 90 min and returns to baseline within 4 h. To alleviate the gastrointestinal side-effects of nausea and diarrhoea the phosphate supplements are started in small doses of 20–40 mg/kg per day and are gradually increased to 50–70 mg/kg per day over several weeks to maintain the serum phosphate concentration at or about 1 mmol/l (3 mg/dl).

2 *1,25(OH)$_2$D$_3$.* Vitamin D (Rocaltrol 250 ng or 500 ng per capsule) is given at an initial dose of 15–20 ng/kg body weight per day with subsequent increases to 30–40 (or 60) ng/kg body weight per day in one dose or two divided doses. During the rapid healing phase of rickets, during the first 5 years of life and during puberty, the dose is usually higher.

3 *Monitoring.* Close monitoring is necessary to balance the action of both substances to stimulate linear growth and to avoid hypercalciuria or hypercalcaemia, nephrocalcinosis, permanent renal damage and hyperparathyroidism.

Calcium, phosphate, alkaline phosphatase and intact PTH in serum as well as the urinary calcium/creatinine ratio should be determined at least every 3(–6) months and X-rays of the hands, wrists and knees should be obtained every 1–3 years. Renal ultrasound and height should be obtained every 12 months to avoid the risk of nephrocalcinosis, and to assess the effect of treatment on linear growth.

The severity of nephrocalcinosis, graded on a scale from 0 to 4, has been found to be highly correlated with the mean phosphate dose received by the patient [211–214].

The following treatment regime is indicated.

1 When the growth rate is decreased, the dose of phosphate (and $1,25(OH)_2D_3$) should be increased.

2 When nephrocalcinosis develops, the dose of phosphate (and $1,25(OH)_2D_3$) should be decreased.

3 Hyperparathyroidism should be countered by increasing $1,25(OH)_2D_3$ and/or reducing phosphate supplementation.

4 The serum alkaline phosphatase frequently remains somewhat elevated, but the dose of phosphate and $1,25(OH)_2D_3$ should be increased if the enzyme activity is markedly elevated, indicating that complete healing of rickets has not been accomplished.

5 When hypercalciuria (urinary calcium/creatinine ratio above 0.7 mmol/mmol or 0.25 mg/mg in 24-h urines or in spot urines) or even hypercalcaemia (serum calcium above 2.6 mmol/l or 10.4 mg/dl) develop, the dose of $1,25(OH)_2D_3$ must be decreased or phosphate supplement increased.

A major problem of this treatment programme is that of compliance, especially the ingestion of the four to six doses of phosphate. Such a failure of phosphate ingestion with continuing $1,25(OH)_2D_3$ intake can lead to hypercalciuria and hypercalcaemia, since each substance counterbalances the other's effects.

Corrective osteotomies should be deferred until rickets has healed radiologically, and until the serum alkaline phosphatase activity is normal or only slightly elevated. Patients with XLH who are immobilized for a longer period, for example patients undergoing osteotomy, should stop treatment with $1,25(OH)_2D_3$ (and phosphate) to avoid immobilization hypercalcaemia and/or hypercalciuria.

With early diagnosis and good compliance the bowing deformities of the legs can be minimized, and a normal adult height may be achievable.

It is difficult to use the midparental heights in the familial cases of XLH, because the final height of the affected parent depends on the success of treatment. For sporadic cases the heights of the parents should be calculated to provide an estimation of the target height for the patient. Studies of Balsan & Tieder indicated little influence on the adult height of male subjects, but showed that the height in the affected girls was positively correlated with midparental height [205].

Petersen *et al.* [215] demonstrated that girls (who are heterozygous) have a better growth response to the treatment than boys (who are homozygous). This suggests a gene dose effect in the expression of XLH, and that satisfactory growth may be achieved by most girls with lower doses than those required by boys.

In some children, for uncertain reasons, there is little or no increase in growth rate and ultimate height, despite well-controlled therapy. In these patients more vigorous or alternative treatment regimes may be necessary to achieve improved growth.

A pilot investigation of 11 children with XLH who received biosynthetic growth hormone in addition to phosphate and $1,25(OH)_2D_3$ therapy, indicated improved growth [216]. The possible beneficial effect of growth hormone in XLH may be explained by increasing renal phosphate reabsorption, as well as direct growth stimulation. More extensive and long-term investigations, including the influence on final height, are needed before growth hormone therapy can be recommended for routine treatment of XLH patients with unsatisfactory response to phosphate and $1,25(OH)_2D_3$.

Severely affected adults with bone pain will require treatment with $1,25(OH)_2D_3$ and phosphate supplementation [217].

Early treatment of patients with XLH

Growth retardation in patients with XLH appears to occur in the first years of life, probably because the disorder mainly affects the growth of the legs, the major contributor to height in early childhood [218].

It has been suggested that infants born to a family with an affected parent or sibling should be followed closely by periodic determinations of phosphate and alkaline phosphatase in serum. In affected infants, an increased alkaline phosphatase activity and/or decreased phosphate concentration can be detected between 1 and 3 months of age without clinical or radiological signs of rickets. Several infants in whom treatment was initiated during this time showed satisfactory growth response and failed to develop rickets and leg deformities [192,194]. Well-controlled studies should define the possible beneficial effects of early diagnosis and treatment of XLH.

Differential diagnosis

XLH must be differentiated from other causes of phosphopoenic rickets and osteomalacia (see Table 38.4). Hypophosphataemic non-rachitic bone disease is a rare condition which is autosomal dominant or sporadic [219]. Despite hypophosphataemia and low TmP/GFR similar to that observed in XLH, the clinical manifestations, appearing during late infancy, are less severe. The patients present with modest short stature, bowing of the lower limbs and evidence of osteomalacia of endosteal trabecular bone with minimal or absent rachitic changes of the growth plate. Calcium, PTH and $1,25(OH)_2D$ in serum, as well as urinary calcium, are normal [200,219,220]. The disease can apparently be treated with $1,25(OH)_2D_3$ alone and without additional phosphate.

In contrast to XHL (and also probably to hypophosphataemic non-rachitic bone disease) the vitamin D hormone secretion seems to be appropriate for the phosphate depletion in patients with hypophosphataemic rickets with hypercalciuria who have elevated $1,25(OH)_2D$ serum concentrations [221–223]. The mode of inheritance is autosomal recessive and the clinical manifestations may vary from asymptomatic hypercalciuria to severe rickets and osteomalacia. In comparison to XLH, these patients may suffer from a defect of renal phosphate reabsorption localized either at a different anatomical site or at an identical site with an unaffected $1,25(OH)_2D_3$ regulating system [221]. It is thought that a primary renal phosphate leak leads to hypophosphataemia, and reactively increased $1,25(OH)_2D_3$ secretion causes hypercalciuria by increased intestinal calcium absorption and PTH suppression. Treatment with oral phosphate alone results in healing of bone lesions, a growth spurt and improvement of hypercalciuria.

XLH may be clinically and biochemically indistinguishable from tumour rickets and osteomalacia. This rare condition was first described by Prader *et al.* in 1959 in an 11-year-old girl whose rickets disappeared after removal of a giant cell reparative granuloma of the rib [224]. Since this first observation approximately 50 additional cases have been described, mostly in adults [188], but also in children [225,226]. The condition may occur in association with a variety of mesenchymal tumours, such as cavernous and sclerosing haemangioma, haemangiopericytoma and non-ossifying fibroma of the bone. Removal of a (usually) small benign tumour leads to a prompt remission of the syndrome.

Extracts of such tumours suppress renal tubular phosphate transport and $1,25(OH)_2D_3$ production in animals, suggesting that a humoral factor produces the syndrome by acting on the proximal renal tubule [227]. Both PTH and calcitonin have been excluded as the tumour-derived factor responsible for phosphaturia, which is independent of the activation of cAMP. Although the tumour is usually detectable after rickets or osteomalacia has been diagnosed, small clinically inapparent tumours may be undetected in some patients thought to have XLH. The disease should be suspected in all cases of hypophosphataemic rickets and osteomalacia that occur late in childhood or in the adult.

In contrast to XLH, patients with this syndrome are sporadic and usually have bone pain and/or muscle weakness with occasional recurrent long-bone fractures. Decreased $1,25(OH)_2D$ serum levels, in contrast to 'inappropriately' normal values in XLH, might serve as a marker for the presence of tumour rickets or osteomalacia. Total skeletal survey and careful follow-up are indicated in such cases. If the tumour cannot be removed, the same therapeutic regime with combined phosphate and $1,25(OH)_2D_3$ as used in XLH will improve the biochemical abnormalities and rachitic and osteomalacic bone changes.

Hypophosphataemic rickets may occur in Fanconi syndrome [187,228], a heterogeneous group of disorders characterized by transport defects for phosphate, glucose and amino acids in the proximal renal tubule. Some patients also show bicarbonate wasting with hyperchloraemic acidosis. The syndrome may be idiopathic or secondary to inborn metabolic disorders (for example cystinosis, fructose intolerance, galactosaemia, glycogenosis and Wilson disease) or intoxications (such as heavy metals). Idiopathic Fanconi syndrome is diagnosed by exclusion of secondary causes, and may be sporadic or familial. Rickets can result from hypophosphataemia with or without metabolic acidosis. It is not known whether decreased $1,25(OH)_2D_3$ production may also contribute to rickets. Optimal therapy of rickets requires phosphate, $1,25(OH)_2D_3$ and, in the case of associated metabolic acidosis, bicarbonate.

Distal renal tubular acidosis is a sporadic or familial defect resulting in the failure of H^+ excretion. The metabolic acidosis induces increased bone resorption and hypercalciuria and decreased proximal phosphate reabsorption. Treatment with sodium bicarbonate in doses to achieve normal serum HCO_3^- concentration (about 2–3 ml/kg per day in two or three divided doses) leads to normalization of phosphate reabsorption and improvement of calcium excretion [187].

Decreased renal phosphate excretion

Renal phosphate retention has a key role in the pathogenesis of two disorders, renal osteodystrophy and tumoral calcinosis.

RENAL OSTEODYSTROPHY

Renal bone disease is a constellation of skeletal abnormalities comprising varying degrees of osteitis fibrosa and osteomalacia, none of which is specific for chronic renal failure. In comparison to adults, renal osteodystrophy occurs more frequently in children in whom modelling and remodelling of bone is particularly sensitive to disturbances in mineral metabolism. Children with congenital nephropathies are especially prone to develop bone disease which correlates with the duration and the severity of the chronic renal failure.

Clinical features

The most important and earliest clinical feature of renal osteodystrophy in children is impaired linear growth. The growth failure is multifactorial and may occur before radiological signs of bone disease are detectable. Other symptoms include bowing and pain in the bones, slipped epiphyses and muscle weakness. Vascular and extraosseous calcification is seldom seen despite an elevated calcium–phosphate product in extracellular fluids.

Histological and radiological findings

The three main histological manifestations of renal osteodystrophy in children [229,230] are given below.

1 Osteitis fibrosa is characterized by an increment in osteoclasts, bone resorption, bone formation and peritrabecular marrow fibrosis. Osteitis fibrosa results from an excess of PTH.

2 Osteomalacia is characterized by defective bone mineralization with wide lamellar osteoid seams, increased osteoblasts and osteoclasts, and an abnormal or absent mineralization front. The diagnosis of osteomalacia cannot be made without tetracycline labelling. Alterations in vitamin D metabolism, metabolic acidosis and aluminium accumulation may all contribute to the development of osteomalacia in renal failure.

3 Mixed bone disease is characterized by features of both osteitis fibrosa and osteomalacia.

The radiographic characteristics are mainly features of osteitis fibrosa. Typical signs are subperiosteal resorption of the middle and distal phalanges, the distal clavicle and other skeletal sites such as the proximal humerus, the distal ulna and radius or the proximal tibia. Signs of osteomalacia are far less distinctive than those of osteitis fibrosa. Looser zones, regarded as the most specific index of osteomalacia, are rare in children. Rachitic-like radiolucent zones at the metaphyseal ends of long bones consist of fibrous tissue and unmineralized woven bone, reflecting osteitis fibrosa and not osteomalacia.

Thus it is impossible to diagnose osteomalacia from the radiological appearance. Only bone biopsy with prior tetracycline administration to the patients permits the accurate diagnosis of osteomalacia and allows a more precise treatment [229,230].

Pathogenesis and pathophysiology

The pathogenesis of renal osteodystrophy is complex [229–232]. Two of the main factors are decreased renal phosphate excretion and altered vitamin D metabolism (Fig. 38.10). In moderate renal failure (GFR of 25–50 ml/min per 1.73 m^2) the serum phosphate level may be normal, while intracellular renal phosphate retention may cause decreased 1,25$(OH)_2D_3$ secretion and intestinal calcium absorption [233,234]. This induces a tendency to hypocalcaemia and secondary hyperparathyroidism. An inverse relationship between the serum levels of 1,25$(OH)_2D_3$ and PTH implies that changes in the vitamin D hormone are primary and affect the changes in PTH seecretion [234]. Dietary phosphate restriction leads to a marked improvement in intestinal calcium absorption due to an increase in 1,25$(OH)_2D$, suggesting that the vitamin D hormone suppression is functional and reversible in this early stage of renal failure.

In severe renal failure there is an irreversible loss of 1,25$(OH)_2D_3$ synthesis: children in whom the GFR is lower than 25 ml/min per 1.73 m^2 have vitamin D hormone serum levels 2.5 standard deviations below normal [229]. Low 1,25$(OH)_2D_3$ secretion in conjunction with a progressive serum phosphate increase leads to hypocalcaemia with secondary hyperparathyroidism and bone disease (Fig. 38.10). The parathyroid glands of patients with severe renal failure are less sensitive to calcium than normal, and these patients require a greater increase in the concentration of serum calcium to suppress PTH secretion, indicating a shift in the set point for calcium comparable to primary hyperparathyroidism. In addition, hyperphosphataemia and low concentrations of serum 1,25$(OH)_2D$ cause resistance of the homeostatic system and to a lesser degree of the remodelling system of the skeleton, resembling pseudohypoparathyroidism.

Other factors that may contribute to renal osteodystrophy include metabolic acidosis and aluminium toxicity. Aluminium has a suppressive effect on the osteoblast and parathyroid gland and produces osteomalacia resistant to treatment with 1,25$(OH)_2D_3$ [235]. The source of aluminium may be high dialysate aluminium in patients on haemodialysis or aluminium-containing phosphate binders.

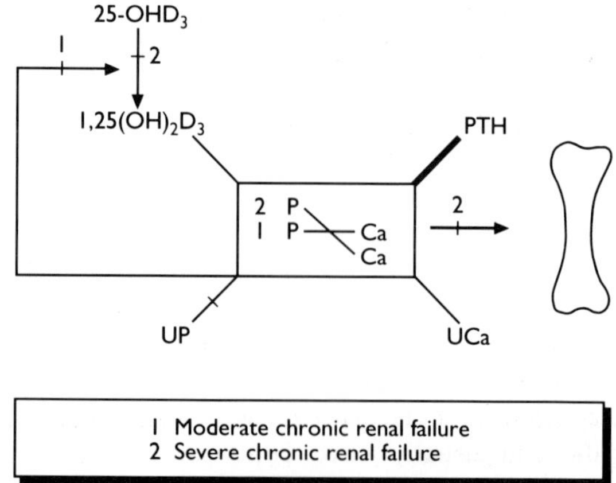

Fig. 38.10 Pathophysiology of renal osteodystrophy.

Investigations

Depending on the severity of renal failure the serum calcium concentration is normal or decreased, whereas the serum phosphate level may be normal or increased. The activity of total alkaline phosphatase in serum may be elevated, especially in patients with osteitis fibrosa.

Elevated circulating intact PTH measured by a two-site immunoassay reflects increased secretion of the parathyroid glands. The determinations of C-terminal or M-regional PTH fragments, urinary cAMP, TmP/GFR, hydroxyproline and serum osteocalcin may not provide a reliable measure of PTH function and bone turnover, especially if the GFR is less than 20–30 ml/min per 1.73 m^2. In aluminium-associated osteomalacia, the intact PTH level in serum is low or normal. The diagnosis of this condition is made by a positive aluminium stain of a bone biopsy and an exaggerated serum aluminium increase following a standard infusion of desferrioxamine, a chelating agent that can mobilize aluminium from bone and other tissues [229,235].

Treatment

Treatment of abnormal mineral metabolism and bone disease in patients with chronic renal failure involves prevention or normalization of hyperphosphataemia, secondary hyperparathyroidism and bone disease [230, 231,236]. The optimal time to begin therapy is not clear. There are some arguments that treatment should be initiated before definite radiographic and biochemical abnormalities appear, especially in children with congenital nephropathies, since manifest renal osteodystrophy in early childhood can greatly influence the attainment of ultimate stature.

In the early stage of renal failure (GFR around 30 ml/min per 1.73 m^2), treatment with 1–1.5 g elemental calcium/day in the form of calcium carbonate should be started to inhibit intestinal phosphate absorption and prevent secondary hyperparathyroidism. As the disease progresses the associated tendency to hyperphosphataemia, serum PTH increase and serum $1,25(OH)_2D$ decrease necessitates treatment with a phosphate-restricted diet and supplementation with $1,25(OH)_2D_3$ (0.5–1 μg/day).

$1,25(OH)_2D_3$ increases the calcium sensitivity of PTH secretion, suppresses PTH secretion and inhibits the proliferation of parathyroid cells, thus antagonizing the development of parathyroid hyperplasia [232]. Prophylaxis with $1,25(OH)_2D_3$ in low doses (0.25–0.5 μg/day), even in the early stages of renal failure, and certainly when intact serum PTH levels are elevated [232].

Intravenous or oral 'pulse therapy' with higher doses of $1,25(OH)_2D_3$, given up to three times weekly, provides a new effective therapeutic tool in patients with severe secondary hyperparathyroidism that does not respond to these different regimes. Since the inhibition of the parathyroid cell $1,25(OH)_2D_3$ receptor causes prolonged suppression of the messenger RNA for preproPTH, the acute $1,25(OH)_2D_3$ adminstration may lower intact serum PTH for up to 100 h in some uraemic patients [232,237]. Hypercalcaemia of hyperparathyroidism should perhaps no longer be considered an absolute contradiction to the use of $1,25(OH)_2D_3$. It is desirable to avoid over-suppression of the parathyroid glands and to lower the intact serum PTH to levels slightly above the normal range to provide normal remodelling of the skeleton. A marked suppression of serum PTH below the normal range may interfere with the adaptation of bone structure to varying biomechanical demands and to repair (microcallus formation) of bone microdamage [232].

If adequate control of serum phosphate in the upper normal range for age cannot be achieved, aluminium hydroxide shoud be administered with meals starting at doses of 20–30 mg/kg per day. In patients on chronic haemodialysis, different therapeutic interventions are required. The levels of phosphate and calcium in serum are extremely important, and the predialysis values should be maintained in the upper normal range, since hyperphosphataemia and hypocalcaemia aggravate hyperparathyroidism, and hypophosphataemia induces or worsens osteomalacia. If aluminium is the responsible agent of vitamin D-resistant bone disease, aluminium should be discontinued and desferrioxamine started.

Because hypercalcaemia may preclude the administration of large doses of $1,25(OH)_2D_3$ in some uraemic patients, the recent development of analogues of vitamin D such as 22-oxacalcitriol with less calcaemic activity may offer a potential therapeutic tool in the treatment of secondary hyperparathyroidism and renal osteodystrophy [237].

Patients with severe secondary hyperparathyroidism refractory to medical therapy require parathyroidectomy with autotransplantation of parathyroid tissue.

TUMORAL CALCINOSIS

Tumoral calcinosis is a rare, often familial (autosomal) disorder, most commonly occurring in the population of Africa. It has also been observed in Europe and North America. The progressively crippling disorder usually manifests during childhood and is characterized by deposition of large masses of amorphous calcium phosphate in and around large joints [238–243].

Biochemical features include hyperphosphataemia in the absence of renal insufficiency, as well as normal values of calcium, PTH and alkaline phosphatase in serum. The renal proximal reabsorption of phosphate and the TmP/

GFR are increased, probably contributing to the hyperphosphataemia. Normal responses of serum PTH and urinary cAMP excretion to ethylenediamine tetraacetic acid (EDTA)-induced hypocalcaemia [244], as well as normal renal phosphate and cAMP responses to exogenous PTH [240], indicate that PTH secretion and action are unaffected. Despite hyperphosphataemia, the circulating levels of $1,25(OH)_2D$ are normal or even elevated [242–244], probably preventing hypocalcaemia and secondary hyperparathyroidism. Normocalcaemia and hyperphosphataemia result in an increased calcium-phosphate product that might contribute to the extraskeletal ectopic calcification.

Tumour calcinosis seems to be a condition which is exactly the opposite of XLH, where phosphate depletion does not lead to increased $1,25(OH)_2D_3$ production. In both conditions a single renal defect might affect phosphate transport and 1-hydroxylation of 25-OHD. It is thought that the intracellular set point to excrete phosphate and suppress the production of $1,25(OH)_2D_3$ is elevated in tumoral calcinosis [243].

Treatment with phosphate-restricted diet or phosphate binders to reduce serum phosphate and calcifications has been tried with disappointing results.

A recent study in a 38-year-old patient provided evidence that synthetic salmon calcitonin may be useful in the long-term management of tumoral calcinosis [245] due to its phosphaturic activity.

DISTURBANCES OF RENAL CALCIUM EXCRETION IN CHILDHOOD

Increased renal calcium excretion

The common causes of hypercalciuria in children may be divided into hypercalcaemic and normocalcaemic conditions [2]. Hypercalcaemic states include primary hyperparathyroidism, idiopathic hypercalcaemia and vitamin D intoxication, and are generally associated with increased calcium excretion, except in hypocalciuric hypercalcaemia. Normocalcaemic states with hypercalciuria include immobilization, distal renal tubular acidosis, and treatment with corticosteroids and frusemide. The definition of hypercalciuria in children is given on p. 735. Hypercalciuria without a known cause is termed idiopathic hypercalciuria, and has been subdivided into an absorptive (see p. 735) and renal type.

RENAL HYPERCALCIURIA

The increase of urinary calcium excretion in a small group of patients with renal hypercalciuria has been attributed to a primary reduction in the tubular reabsorption of calcium [5]. The site of the defect is presumed to be in the distal nephron [246]. Renal hypercalciuria with consequent reduction of serum calcium stimulates PTH secretion, which in turn normalizes serum calcium by mobilization of calcium from bone and by enhanced intestinal calcium absorption via $1,25(OH)_2D_3$. Another, probably larger, group may have a primary reduction in renal tubular phosphate reabsorption with a secondary increase in $1,25(OH)_2D_3$ and calcium absorption causing PTH suppression and hypercalciuria. The observation that treatment with oral phosphate reduced urinary calcium and $1,25(OH)_2D$ serum concentrations in patients with idiopathic hypercalciuria gave support to this phosphate leak theory [247]. This primary phosphate leak may be hereditary, and it has been speculated [222] that the magnitude of phosphate depletion and hypophosphataemia, which regulates excessive $1,25(OH)_2D_3$ production, might determine which subjects will have hypercalciuria alone or which will also develop phosphopenic rickets (hypophosphataemic rickets with hypercalciurias, see p. 757).

Some authorities believe that the separation of patients with idiopathic hypercalciuria into renal and absorptive subgroups is no longer useful and that the role and mechanism of elevated $1,25(OH)_2D_3$ secretion and renal phosphate and calcium leak deserve further studies. Diagnosis and therapy of idiopathic hypercalciuria are discussed on p. 735.

Decreased renal calcium excretion

Primary impairment of renal calcium excretion leads to hypercalcaemia. This condition is called familial benign hypercalcaemia [248] or hypocalciuric hypercalcaemia. The hypercalcaemic state is usually asymptomatic and non-progressive. It is inherited as an autosomal dominant trait with nearly 100% penetrance of the gene for hyper-

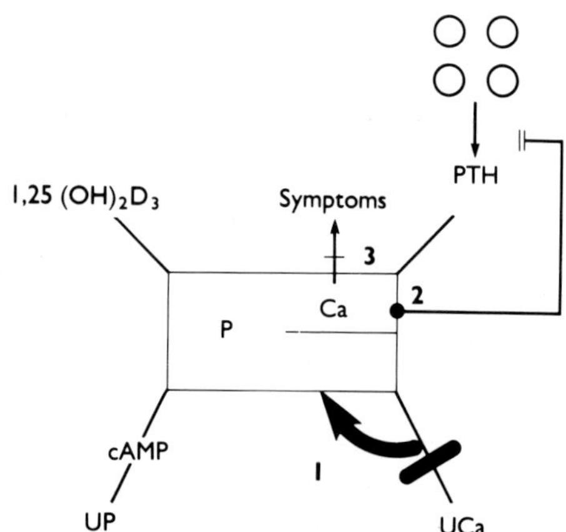

Fig. 38.11 Pathophysiology of familial hypocalciuric hypercalcaemia. (1) Increased renal tubular Ca (and Mg) reabsorption. (2) Elevated glandular set point for Ca suppression. (3) Insensitivity to chronic hypercalcaemia. UCa/UP, urine calcium/phosphate.

calcaemia. The condition is characterized by the following three special features (Fig. 38.11).

1 Increased renal tubular calcium reabsorption causing hypercalcaemia.

2 Normal or high–normal (instead of suppressed) serum PTH levels, suggesting an elevated glandular set-point for calcium suppression.

3 Absence of clinical symptoms, indicating insensitivity of the patients to chronic hypercalcaemia [249].

There is neither an abnormality of vitamin D metabolism [250,251], or of calcitonin secretion [251] nor an increased renal sensitivity to PTH [250]. Parathyroid histological features are generally normal and subtotal parathyroidectomy fails to normalize hypercalcaemia [249].

The cause of the disorder is unknown. Dysfunction of an intracellular calcium-binding protein could account for the combination of defects in kidney and parathyroid gland as well as the absence of symptoms despite hypercalcaemia [249]. The most important diagnostic features of hypocalciuric hypercalcaemia start during the first decade of life, a typical family pattern, a lack of evidence for MEN-1 or MEN-2, and calcium/creatinine clearance ratios below 0.01 (see p. 745).

For clinicians the most important point is to recognize the condition and to refrain from parathyroid surgery in all but exceptional cases. Offspring of parents with hypocalciuric hypercalcaemia may present with severe primary hyperparathyroidism, possibly due to a homozygous expression of the disorder. These have to be treated by total parathyroidectomy [252,253].

DISTURBANCES OF CALCITONIN SECRETION IN CHILDHOOD

Calcitonin is a calcium-lowering hormone and its effect is mainly due to inhibition of osteoclastic bone resorption (see pp. 724–5). Excessive secretion of calcitonin is rarely associated with hypocalcaemia, nor does congenital athyreosis or complete thyroidectomy cause hypercalcaemia and overt bone disease. Evidence suggests that the hypocalcaemic action of the hormone is limited and depends on the duration of exposure to calcitonin and/or on the degree of bone turnover. It is likely that the role of endogenous calcitonin in physiology and pathophysiology will remain uncertain until specific measurements of the biologically active fragments are generally available, and until more information exists on the physiological rather than pharmacological action of the hormone.

Increased calcitonin secretion

Elevated circulating levels of immunoreactive calcitonin (iCT) occur in several disorders, especially neoplasias. The most important pathological condition associated with increased serum iCT is medullary thyroid carcinoma (MTC). MTC is a tumour of the calcitonin-producing C cells of the thyroid gland [254], comprising 3.5–10% of all thyroid cancer. The disease may be sporadic (in about 75% of cases) or familial, when it is inherited in an autosomal dominant fashion with incomplete clinical penetrance. Thus 40% of gene carriers are symptom-free at age 70 years. MCT in affected families may be the sole neoplasia or may be part of MEN type-2A and type-2B. MEN-2A consists of MTC, phaeochromocytoma and hyperparathyroidism. MTC in MEN-2B is associated with phaeochromocytoma and with characteristic clinical features such as marfanoid habitus, mucosal neuromas of the lips, tongue and eyelids, and ganglioneuromatosis of the gastrointestinal tract causing abdominal pain, constipation and diarrhoea.

The predisposing gene(s) for the MEN-2 syndromes have been mapped to the region near the centromere of chromosome 10 by genetic linkage [255].

The age of onset of sporadic or familial MTC varies from infancy to old age, but the majority of cases are found in the fourth to sixth decades of life. Screening of relatives of patients with familial MTC by iCT measurement has resulted in diagnosis at increasingly younger ages.

On physical examination, typical features of MTC are one or more firm palpable thyroid nodules, often with enlarged cervical lymph nodes. The tumour secretes large amounts of calcitonin and several related peptides which are coded on the calcitonin gene (see p. 724). Sometimes MTC may produce other bioactive substances such as adrenocorticotrophic hormone (ACTH), prostaglandins, vasoactive intestinal polypeptide, serotonin and nerve growth factor. Some of these substances may provoke symptoms such as diarrhoea, flushing or Cushing syndrome.

Total thyroidectomy is the treatment for MTC, especially in the familial variety presenting with bilateral and multicentric lesions. Evaluation and treatment of associated phaeochromocytoma in MEN-2A and -2B should be done before thyroid surgery. Patients with sporadic MTC have the least favourable prognosis and approximately 40% of affected individuals die. Patients with MEN-2A usually have a far better prognosis due to a slowly growing thyroid neoplasia, whereas the MTC of the MEN-2B syndrome behaves more aggressively with the need for early diagnosis and treatment [256].

The diagnostic hallmark of MTC is the detection of increased iCT serum levels. In most patients, basal concentrations are sufficiently elevated to be diagnostic of the presence of the thyroid tumour. In a smaller group of patients, probably those in the early stage of the neoplasia, basal iCT levels may be indistinguishable from normal, especially if insensitive hormone assays are used. In these patients provocative testing with calcium or pentagastrin enhances the detection of C cell hyperfunction. The recommended stimuli are infusions of calcium gluconate

(2 mg elemental calcium/kg body weight over 5 min) and/or pentagastrin (0.5 μg/kg body weight, rapidly injected over 5 s).

Serial testing of basal and stimulated iCT are necessary in thyroidectomized patients to evaluate the effectiveness of surgical therapy and in persons at risk for inheritance to detect MTC in a clinically occult stage. Annual screening is recommended in familial MTC. This should begin at an age of 1 year in families with MEN-2B and at an age of 5–8 years in families with MEN-2A and should be continued to 50 years of age.

Recently, a presymptomatic screening for MEN-2A has been suggested using linked DNA markers [257].

Patients with MTC provide an opportunity to study the long-term effects of chronic endogenous excess of biologically active monomeric calcitonin. Surprisingly, serum levels of iCT ranging up to 20 000 times the physiological concentration are generally tolerated without hypocalcaemia, hypophosphataemia or relevant bone changes [258]. Moreover, histomorphometric analysis shows increased instead of decreased trabecular bone remodelling [254]. This unexpected finding arises through the concomitant elevation of $1{,}25(OH)_2D$ serum levels. The chronic calcitonin excess is thought directly to enhance the renal production of the vitamin D hormone, which acts synergistically with PTH to increase bone remodelling [254]. These findings raise doubt whether calcitonin possesses a biological role in humans at all. However, the paradox may be explained by the well-known escape phenomenon, demonstrated *in vitro* [259] and *in vivo* [260], that indicates a progressive loss of calcitonin-binding sites in its target organs. Probably calcitonin must be delivered episodically and/or in small amounts to produce normal tissue responsiveness.

It is now well established that serum iCT levels may be elevated in adult patients with a variety of non-thyroid tumours, such as carcinomas of the lung, breast, gut and pancreas, as well as myeloid leukaemia. It is thus apparent that elevated iCT levels are not diagnostic of any particular tumour. Various studies regarding the pathogenesis of hypercalcitoninaemia in malignancy have demonstrated that tumour cells may secrete this hormone itself or substances that cross-react in the RIA, and that tumour-associated factors such as hypercalcaemia or other secretagogues may cause a secondary increase of thyroid calcitonin [261].

Hypercalcaemic states not associated with malignancy may also induce hypercalcitoninaemia which may protect against the challenge to calcium homeostasis. Parthemore & Deftos found exaggerated increments of serum iCT to provocative testing in males but not in females with primary hyperparathyroidism, explaining some aspects of the greater severity of bone disease in women with this disease [262]. By contrast, normal or even blunted responses of monomeric calcitonin to calcium stimulation have been found in primary hyperparathyroidism, regardless of sex [263]. A growing body of evidence in humans and animals suggests that the C cells do *not* increase function during chronic stimulation by hypercalcaemia, probably due to a depletion of intrathyroidal calcitonin stores [263]. On the other hand, calcium infusions in patients with hypocalcaemia of severe aetiologies do result in exaggerated increase of serum calcitonin, probably due to release of increased stores of the hormone [264].

Circulating iCT values are higher than normal in renal insufficiency, and it has been suggested that augmented secretion of calcitonin may protect the skeleton against PTH-induced osteitis fibrosa in some of the patients. As in the case of PTH, the kidney is an important site of degradation of calcitonin and the hypercalcitoninaemia is, at least in part, a result of a decrease in the metabolic clearance of the hormone. Compared to MCT, circulating iCT shows a different immunochemical profile with a relatively small proportion of biologically active monomeric calcitonin, and the response to provocative testing may be blunted in this condition [261]. Although these findings suggest that reduced excretion and abnormal metabolism are responsible for high serum iCT levels in patients with renal failure, there are observations that endogenous calcitonin is a significant modulator of bone turnover in renal bone disease [265].

Elevated levels of calcitonin have been observed in pancreatitis [266]. The cause of the hormone increase is controversial and may be related to calcitonin secretagogues such as glucagon, which are released from the pancreas. Of biological interest is the abnormal calcitonin secretion found in patients with pycnodysostosis [267]. This rare autosomal hyperostotic condition leads to short stature, fractures and peculiar affection of the terminal phalanges. A dynamic study of tetracycline uptake showed evidence of decreased bone turnover [268], which may be explained by the intermittently elevated calcitonin secretion [266]. As with other conditions where abnormalities of calcitonin have been observed without the use of modern assays to measure monomeric calcitonin, the finding of hypercalcitoninaemia in pycnodysostosis has yet to be established.

Decreased calcitonin secretion

The prime example is athyreosis due to congenital absence or surgical removal of the thyroid. The difficulty in demonstrating total lack of circulating iCT in these patients has been explained by the possible contribution of other tissues such as lung, thymus and adrenal glands, to hormone secretion. This suggests that extrathyroidal calcitonin might be capable of substituting for the hormone normally secreted by the C cells of the thyroid [269].

However, athyroidal patients do not increase iCT following calcium infusion, and the circulating calcitonin-like material has been shown not to be the authentic 32 amino-acid calcitonin monomer [270,271]. Thus patients with athyreosis appear to have a total lack of biologically active calcitonin.

As in the case of hypercalcitoninaemia, there is no compelling evidence for calcitonin-related effects associated with decreased hormone secretion, such as chronic hypercalcaemia or bone loss. These patients do have slight abnormalities in calcium metabolism, such as slow disposal of an intravenous calcium load [39,272,273], and exaggerated and prolonged hypocalcaemic responses to exogenous calcitonin [274]. The bone mineral content of the distal radius was diminished in thyroidectomized adults [275] and normal in children with congenital non-goitrous hypothyroidism [271], but these results have to be established in greater numbers of patients.

Histomorphometric studies in adults with primary hypothyroidism showed exaggerated osteoclastic activity and reduced bone mass, a finding that may be related to calcitonin deficiency [276], too high replacement with thyroid hormones [277], or both. Low basal and calcium-stimulated monomeric calcitonin levels have been demonstrated in adults with autoimmune primary hypothyroidism [276]. This suggests that the process causing destruction of the thyroid follicular cells may also destroy the C cells or may impair their ability to secrete calcitonin.

Decreased calcium-stimulated secretion of unextracted calcitonin and delayed clearance of postinfusion calcium serum levels have been observed [39] in five children with Williams syndrome (see pp. 736–7). Although normocalcaemic during the study, the patients had significantly higher baseline values of serum calcium in comparison to normal children. These findings and the immunohistological demonstration of C cell hyperplasia in a 30-year-old patient with Williams syndrome led to the conclusion that the abnormalities of calcium metabolism in this condition might be explained by a defect in the synthesis or release in the hormone and that calcitonin deficiency can serve as an endocrine marker of the syndrome [278].

In a recent study of 27 normocalcemic patients with Williams syndrome no defect could be found in synthesis or release of calcitonin [40]. This finding is in agreement with two recent reports that failed to give evidence of major rearrangements or possible mutations in the calcitomin/calcitonin gene-related gene in children with Williams syndrome [279,280].

The secretory capacity of the thyroid gland for calcitonin is impaired during treatment with some, but not all, anticonvulsant drugs [271]. Decreased basal and calcium-stimulated monomeric calcitonin have been found in epileptic children receiving phenytoin and primidone. Phenytoin can reduce the availability of intracellular calcium or inhibit calcium–calmodulin-stimulated processes, and might thereby impair calcitonin release from the C cell [271]. Bone mineral content of the distal radius and biochemical indices of bone turnover were all normal in these normoparathyroid calcitonin-deficient epileptic children.

In summary, the occurrence of several congenital or acquired hypocalcitoninaemic conditions has now been established using improved hormone assays. The patients have discrete abnormalities but are not hypercalcaemic, indicating that the organism adapts to the absence of calcitonin [258]. However, attention should be paid to adequate thyroid replacement therapy in patients with primary hypothyroidism, to secondary hyperparathyroidism in patients receiving phenytoin or primidone and to adequate calcium intake in both calcitonin-deficient conditions which tend to increase osteoclastic activity and decrease calcium conservation from nutrition.

Calcitonin deficiency has been implicated in the pathogenesis of osteoporoses [281], especially of postmenopausal osteoporosis. Failure to increase calcitonin secretion could leave the actions of the bone-resorbing hormones PTH and $1,25(OH)_2D_3$ unopposed, which would lead to bone loss. The known effect of oestrogens in preventing or arresting postmenopausal bone loss may be due to the steroid hormone-induced increase in endogenous calcitonin secretion. Efforts to clarify the role of calcitonin in this type of osteoporosis have been hampered by the methodological problems of the calcitonin assay and of the measurement of bone loss. Body & Heath [270] did not find differences of basal and calcium-stimulated monomeric calcitonin in menstruating and postmenopausal women, suggesting that even the largest physiological alterations of endogenous oestrogen production do not affect calcitonin secretion. Furthermore no difference was found in basal serum calcitonin levels in postmenopausal women with vertebral compression fractures in comparison to sex- and age-matched controls without fractures [282]. These findings do not suggest a major role for calcitonin in the pathogenesis of postmenopausal osteoporosis, but further studies in this and other conditions associated with increased bone loss seem warranted.

DISORDERS OF CALCIUM AND BONE METABOLISM IN EARLY INFANCY

Regulation of calcium metabolism during the perinatal period

During intrauterine life fetal bone mineralization requires transfer of calcium and phosphate from mother to fetus. Total calcium accretion in fetal bone amounts to approximately 30 g. About 80% of this calcium accumulation, corresponding to 140 mg/kg body weight per 24 h, occurs in the third trimester. Active placental transport of calcium makes the fetus relatively hypercalcaemic. The concentrations of total and ionized calcium in the blood of the fetus exceed those of the mother by an average of 2 and 1 mg/dl, respectively [283–286].

Transcellular placental calcium transport involves: (i) influx of calcium ions from maternal blood across the microvillus (maternal-facing) trophoblastic membrane into the trophoblastic cytosol, (ii) movement of calcium through the cytosol, and (iii) efflux of calcium ions from the cytosol across the basolateral (fetal-facing) trophoblastic membrane and then across the fetal capillary and endothelium into the fetal blood.

The three calcium-regulating hormones, PTH, calcitonin and $1,25(OH)_2D_3$, are of major importance in calcium and bone metabolism of the mother and her fetus. Whereas PTH and calcitonin do not cross the placenta, the placental permeability to $1,25(OH)_2D_3$ is questionable. Cord blood levels of 25-OHD are about 20–30% lower than maternal values with a significant correlation, indicating that a transfer of this metabolite from mother to fetus occurs, depending on the matenal vitamin D status. There is good evidence that the fetal kidney and the placenta are capable of synthesizing $1,25(OH)_2D_3$. Cord blood levels of the vitamin D hormone amount to only about 50% of maternal levels, both values being correlated in some but not all studies. The relative contributions made by the maternal kidney, fetal kidney and the placenta to the concentrations of $1,25(OH)_2D$ in fetal and maternal blood are uncertain.

Some data have suggested that the vitamin D hormone may promote the placental transport of calcium from the mother to the fetus in a manner similar to its effect on intestinal calcium absorption [283,284,287]. Animal studies indicate that the maintenance of a normal transplacental calcium gradient is markedly affected by procedures which reduce fetal $1,25(OH)_2D_3$ production, but is not influenced by a reduction in maternal calcaemia or calcium-regulating hormones, as occurs after maternal thyroparathyroidectomy. Animal studies [288] indicate that fetal PTH-related protein (PTHrP), which is mainly derived from the placenta during early gestation and from the fetal parathyroid gland during further development [289], may also have an important effect on the placental transfer of calcium [283,290,291]. Thus, it is likely that fetal $1,25(OH)_2D_3$ has a major role of maintaining the maternal–fetal calcium gradient, either alone or in concert with PTHrP.

During pregnancy there is a continuous flux of calcium directed from the maternal intestine to the fetal bone, mainly induced by the following endocrine adaptations of the calcium-regulating hormone. The increasing requirements of the growing fetus are largely met by a compensatory increase in intestinal maternal calcium absorption mediated by elevated circulating levels of $1,25(OH)_2D_3$ in the mother. The increase of the vitamin D hormone is thought to be the consequence of enhanced PTH secretion, following the maternal calcium loss. Some increase in calcitonin secretion may be of importance in protecting the maternal skeleton against excessive resorption of $1,25(OH)_2D_3$ and PTH, while permitting its intestinal and renal effects to continue. The fetal hypercalcaemia maintained by active calcium transport from mother to fetus lowers the secretion of fetal PTH (but probably not fetal PTHrP) and stimulates fetal calcitonin secretion. This is reflected by suppressed PTH and increased calcitonin levels in fetal, neonatal and cord blood. Both hormonal changes favour mineralization of the fetal skeleton.

The finding of significant amounts of $1,25(OH)_2D$ in fetal, neonatal or cord blood despite hypercalcaemia, hyperphosphataemia and low PTH secretion suggests that most of the vitamin D hormone is not produced by the fetus but comes from the mother or the placenta or, more probably, that the regulation of fetal renal 25-OHD-1-hydroxylase is different from that found in postnatal life.

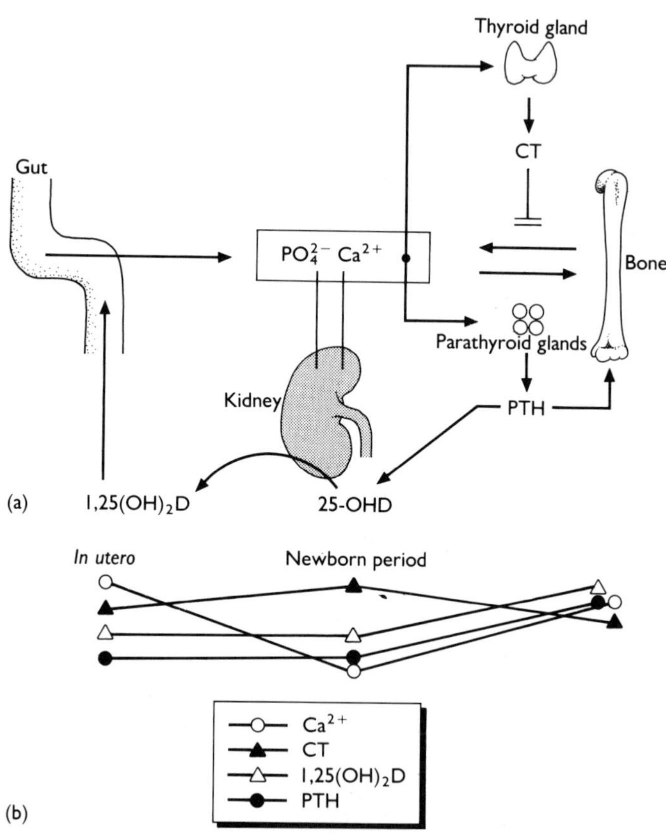

Fig. 38.12 (a) Regulation of postnatal calcium and phosphate metabolism, and (b) schematic representation of postnatal changes of ionized calcium (Ca^{2+}) and the calcium-regulating hormones calcitonin (CT), $1,25(OH)_2D$ and PTH. →, stimulation; —⊣, inhibition.

Table 38.5 Disturbances of calcium and bone metabolism in early infancy

Hypocalcaemic states	Neonatal primary hyperparathyroidism
Early neonatal hypocalcaemia (< 72 h of age)	Hypercalcaemia associated with subcutaneous fat necrosis
Preterm infants	Hypercalcaemia associated with phosphate depletion
Infants of diabetic mothers	Hypervitaminosis D
Infants with birth asphyxia	Hypervitaminosis A
	Congenital hypothyroidism
Late neonatal hypocalcaemia (> 72 h of age)	Maternal hypoparathyroidism and pseudohypoparathyroidism
Transient hypoparathryoidism	Hypophosphatasia
Transient or chronic hypomagnesaemia	Adrenal insufficiency
Bicarbonate treatment	Blue diaper syndrome
Congenital permanent hypoparathyroidism	Malignancies
Maternal primary hyperparathyroidism	
Intestinal malabsorption of calcium and/or vitamin D	*Metabolic bone disease of prematurity*
Maternal vitamin D deficiency	Phosphate deficiency
	Calcium deficiency
Hypercalcaemic states	Disturbed vitamin D metabolism
Idiopathic infantile hypercalcaemia	Other factors
Familial hypocalciuric hypercalcaemia	

With birth, the placental supply of calcium ceases abruptly, the serum calcium level in the neonate declines, probably aggravated by suppressed PTH and/or increased calcitonin secretion (Fig. 38.12). In the mature neonate the calcaemia reaches a nadir between 24 and 48 h of age, producing a progressive increase in PTH secretion and a decrease in circulating calcitonin. Both hormonal changes first stabilize and then raise the serum calcium levels to normal within about 5 days. The serum phosphate concentration at birth is much higher than in childhood and may even rise during the first weeks of life, depending to some extent on dietary factors.

It is presumed that in the fetus the intestinal absorption of calcium and phosphate is low. At birth, the infant becomes dependent on intestinal mineral supply. The increased calcium and phosphate requirements are met by an abrupt postnatal rise of $1,25(OH)_2D_3$ secretion, probably as a consequence of postnatal hypocalcaemia associated with increased PTH secretion. Alterations in the hormonal regulation of mineral metabolism and/or inadequate supply of calcium and phosphate may partly explain the hypocalcaemic and hypercalcaemic syndromes as well as metabolic bone disease observed during early infancy (Table 38.5).

HYPOCALCAEMIC STATES

Clinically, neonatal hypocalcaemia can be separated into two groups: early and late neonatal hypocalcaemia.

Early neonatal hypocalcaemia

This is the most common form of postnatal hypocalcaemia, generally regarded as a fall of total calcium below 1.75 mmol/l (7 mg/dl) or 0.63 mmol/l (2.5 mg/dl) in the ionized calcium level. Early neonatal hypocalcaemia occurs within the first 3 days of life in about one-half of premature infants [292], in about one-half of infants of diabetic mothers [293], and in about one-third of infants with birth asphyxia or other perinatal complications [294]. Most of the decrease in serum calcium takes place during the first 12–24 h, with little further change up to 72 h of life, followed by a gradual reversion to normal calcium levels after 1–3 days.

Many infants with early hypocalcaemia are asymptomatic, whereas others present with clinical signs which resemble those resulting from meningitis, intracranial haemorrhage, sepsis, anoxia and hypoglycaemia, namely irritability, muscular twitchings, jitteriness and apnoeic spells. Frank convulsions occur more commonly with late neonatal hypocalcaemia (see below). Carpopedal spasm and laryngospasm are seldom seen. A positive Chvostek sign is common in healthy neonatal infants and is thus of little diagnostic value.

The pathogenesis of early neonatal hypocalcaemia is complex and several factors have been implicated. In premature infants the major pathogenetic factor appears to be the abrupt cessation of calcium supply after delivery at a time when calcium demands are the highest. A second mechanism of hypocalcaemia seems to be a transient peripheral resistance to PTH which is present during the first week of life, reflecting an immaturity of renal and possibly bone response to PTH [295]. Extensive studies in premature infants have demonstrated that the regulation and secretion of PTH is adequate and that the vitamin D metabolism is normal if the mother is not vitamin D deficient [296]. Excessive secretion of calcitonin occurring during the first day of life may be a factor in precipitating early hypocalcaemia in premature infants [296].

The pathogenetic factors leading to hypocalcaemia in

infants of diabetic mothers include hypomagnesaemia with decreased PTH secretion, hypercalcitoninaemia and increased calcium needs due to the increased fetal body (and skeleton) size of these infants. The hypocalcaemia in infants with birth asphyxia and other perinatal complications has been attributed to the stress-induced endogenous phosphate release from several tissues into the extracellular fluid with subsequent hypocalcaemia [294].

Late neonatal hypocalcaemia

Affected infants usually present with convulsions between 4 and 28 days of age. The condition generally occurs in term infants, but is also seen in preterm infants as an extension of early neonatal hypocalcaemia. Transient hypoparathyroidism is the possible cause of late neonatal hypocalcaemia and it may be aggravated by ingesting cows' milk and some modified cows' milk preparations with high phosphate content. The high intake of phosphate, together with a physiologically low rate of glomerular filtration, leads to an increased serum phosphate level with consequent hypocalcaemia not counterbalanced by increased PTH secretion because of relative or absolute hypoparathyroidism. Hypoparathyroidism observed in late neonatal hypocalcaemia is usually transient and does not persist beyond 28 days of age. The oldest age at which recovery from transient neonatal hypoparathyroidism has been reported was 6 months.

Other disorders that may present as hypocalcaemia during this period include the following.

1 Chronic (primary) or transient neonatal hypomagnesaemia, associated with decreased PTH secretion or action.
2 Acid–base disturbances treated with bicarbonate decreasing calcium release from bone.
3 Congenital permanent hypoparathyroidism (see pp. 747–8).
4 Transient hypoparathyroidism secondary to prolonged fetal hypercalcaemia due to maternal primary hyperparathyroidism [297].
5 Intestinal malabsorption of calcium with or without associated malabsorption of vitamin D.
6 Congenital rickets due to maternal vitamin D deficiency.

Treatment of hypocalcaemia

Symptomatic hypocalcaemia requires the slow intravenous injection of 10% calcium gluconate in a dosage of about 2 ml/kg over a 10-min period while monitoring the heart rate. This dose can be repeated at 6–8-h intervals until recovery of hypocalcaemia, or the calcium gluconate can be administered by continued intravenous infusion at a dose of 8–10 ml/kg per 24 h. In asymptomatic hypocalcaemia calcium gluconate or calcium lactate should be given orally. If hypocalcaemia persists, additional treatment with vitamin D or a metabolite may be indicated (see p. 752). In hypocalcaemia due to other causes, therapy for the primary disease is necessary.

HYPERCALCAEMIC STATES

Hypercalcaemia, generally defined as a total serum calcium concentration above 2.65 mmol/l (10.6 mg/dl) and an ionized calcium level above 1.4 mmol/l (5.5 mg/dl), is far less common than hypocalcaemia in early infancy. Clinical manifestations of severe hypercalcaemia include hypotonia, poor feeding, vomiting, weight loss, polyuria, polydipsia, constipation and irritability. Hypertension, nephrocalcinosis and renal failure may occur, calling for rapid diagnosis and correction of severe hypercalcaemia. Infants with mild hypercalcaemia (2.75–3.25 mmol/l or 11–13 mg/dl) may be asymptomatic.

Table 38.5 summarizes the most important causes of hypercalcaemia of early infancy.

Idiopathic infantile hypercalcaemia

This occurs as a mild and severe form, the latter usually being associated with characteristic features of the Williams syndrome. The condition is discussed on pp. 736–7.

Familial hypocalciuric hypercalcaemia

This is inherited as an autosomal dominant trait with a high penetrance at early childhood (see p. 760). It is usually benign but may sometimes manifest as neonatal severe primary hyperparathyroidism (see below).

Neonatal primary hyperparathyroidism

This is a rare and sometimes life-threatening disease that affects the neonate in the first 5 days and sometimes even *in utero*. Since the first description [298], only some 20 patients diagnosed *ante mortem* have been reported [92]. Prominent features include anorexia, hypotonia, bone demineralization and respiratory distress with chest deformity and rib fractures. Important diagnostic findings are hypercalcaemia with serum calcium levels frequently ranging between 15 and 30 mg/dl (3.75–7.5 mmol/l), hypophosphataemia, elevated serum PTH and alkaline phosphatase levels and subperiosteal resorption at the metaphyses of the long bones on radiological examination. The characteristic pathological feature is always diffuse clear-cell hyperplasia involving all parathyroid glands.

The aetiology is not known. The condition may be sporadic or inherited. Two types of inheritance, autosomal recessive [251] and autosomal dominant [299], have been reported. Dominantly inherited neonatal cases may be members of kindreds with hypocalciuric hypercalcaemia whereas the penetrance of hypercalcaemia in the first decade is low in familial MEN types 1 and 2, generally excluding the association between neonatal hyperparathyroidism and these syndromes [97]. Two mechanisms have been proposed [249] for the association between severe neonatal hyperparathyroidism and familial hypocalciuric hypercalcaemia.

1 Neonates with primary hyperparathyroidism are homozygous for a genetic abnormality which in the heterozygous state is associated with a mild disorder.

2 The neonatal severe disease represents one end of the spectrum of variation in the clinical severity of familial hypocalciuric hypercalcaemia.

In all types of severe neonatal primary hyperparathyroidism the defect in suppressibility of PTH release is probably more exaggerated than in later life. The markedly decreased sensitivity of the parathyroid gland to serum calcium [300] and its improvement with age may explain why the neonatal disease is more severe than the adult type of primary hyperparathyroidism. Neonatal primary hyperparathyroidism is considered as a surgical emergency [106], since most of the untreated infants die between 2 and 7 months of age [92]. Total parathyroidectomy with or without heterotopic autotransplantation of parathyroid tissue is recommended, because of the high recurrence rate of hyperparathyroidism observed after subtotal parathyroidectomy [23,97,106,300].

Hypercalcaemia associated with subcutaneous fat necrosis

Severe hypercalcaemia has been observed in some infants with subcutaneous fat necrosis [301–304]. This disease is characterized by reddish or purple, sharply circumscribed nodules over the buttocks, thighs, cheeks and arms occurring between day 1 and 7 of age. Histopathological findings are subcutaneous fat necrosis with mononuclear and giant-cell infiltration that may calcify. These lesions resolve spontaneously over a period of weeks.

The reason for the hypercalcaemia is speculative. If measured, serum PTH and $1,25(OH)_2D$ levels were appropriately suppressed and calcitonin was elevated [303,304], suggesting that the hypercalcaemia is unrelated to disturbances of the major calcium-regulating hormones. Hypercalciuria in the fasting state not increasing after oral calcium load suggests that intestinal hyperabsorption is not the cause of hypercalcaemia [304]. This indicates that the excessive calcium comes from deposits in the subcutaneous fat necrosis, or more probably by a humoral factor released from the skin lesions that may elicit increased calcium mobilization from bone. A prostaglandin of the E series has been implicated as such a substance in one patient [303], but this has not been confirmed by another study [301]. Fatty acid analysis of the skin revealed no significant increase in arachidonic acid, the precursor of prostaglandins [304]. Recently Finne *et al.* [11] and Kruse *et al.* [12] described hypercalcaemia associated with increased serum levels of $1,25(OH)_2D$ in infants with subcutaneous fat necrosis. This indicates unregulated production of the vitamin D hormone by the granulomatous cells of fat necrosis inducing increased intestinal calcium absorption and hypercalcaemia. Further studies are needed to identify the pathogenetic factor(s) in this disorder. Effective treatment of the hypercalcaemia has been reported with glucocorticoids and frusemide or a low calcium, vitamin D free diet.

Hypercalcaemia associated with phosphate depletion

This is most commonly seen in low birth weight, preterm infants exposed to low phosphate intake from breast milk or parenteral feeding. In the presence of hypophosphataemia the deposition of calcium phosphate in cartilage and bone matrix is low, and the $1,25(OH)_2D_3$ production is increased, stimulating the intestinal absorption of calcium, both mechanisms leading to the accumulation of calcium in extracellular fluid with hypercalcaemia and hypercalciuria. Thus, in preterm infants, inadequate phosphate input may cause not only bone demineralization and rickets, but also severe hypercalcaemia [306,307]. The hypercalcaemia responds to phosphate repletion, which may be achieved either by oral supplementation in mild forms, or by intravenous phosphate administration in severe hypercalcaemia. Potential complications of the latter therapy include precipitation of calcium phosphate leading to extraskeletal calcification with nephrocalcinosis and renal failure.

Besides phosphate administration, calcium supplementation is needed to compensate for the increased degradation and decreased mineralization of bone induced by the phosphate depletion. Adequate amounts of phosphate should be given to infants, and periodic monitoring of serum phosphate and calcium levels is required. Hypercalciuria without hypercalcaemia seems to be a useful index for the detection of mild phosphate depletion [308,309]

Hypervitaminosis D

This has to be considered in the differential diagnosis of all hypercalcaemic states in infancy, although its incidence has progressively reduced during the last decades. The hypercalcaemia associated with hypervitaminosis A is presumably due to accelerated bone resorption but the pathogenesis of the underlying mechanisms is unknown. Fatal hypervitaminosis A has been described in an infant

[310] who had accidentally received an approximate daily dose of 90 000 IU of vitamin A, for 11 days. The normal recommended daily dose for a neonate is 1400 IU. The infant presented with severe hypercalcaemia (2.65 mmol/l or 14.6 mg/dl), hyperphosphataemia (3.68 mmol/l or 11.4 mg/dl), metastatic calcification of the lungs, kidneys, stomach, soft tissue and skin, a bleeding disorder and pulmonary insufficiency. The infant died at the age of 6 weeks. The skeleton showed alterations of enchondral bone formation and accelerated resorption.

Infants with congenital hypothyroidism may have hypercalcaemia both before and during treatment with thyroid hormones. The hypercalcaemia is usually mild and has been related to some hypersensitivity to vitamin D. During thyroxine therapy only infants developed hypercalcaemia given the usual vitamin D prophylaxis, whereas patients without additional vitamin D supplementation were normocalcaemic [311]. The same study detected no abnormalities in vitamin D metabolism and, especially, no evidence for an increased production or decreased degradation of $1,25(OH)_2D_3$ [311]. A deficiency of calcitonin may be a factor in the development of hypercalcaemia due to an abnormally slow clearance of extracellular calcium, a phenomenon resembling the situation of the Williams syndrome (see p. 736).

Infants born to hypocalcaemic mothers with poorly treated hypoparathyroidism or pseudohypoparathyroidism may present with congenital hyperparathyroidism [312–315]. The mechanism probably involves fetal parathyroid hyperplasia in response to chronic intrauterine hypocalcaemia. The increased fetal PTH secretion may cause generalized skeletal demineralization and subperiosteal bone resorption. The birth weight of the affected infants is frequently less than 2500 g. At birth these neonates may be transiently hypercalcaemic, but are more often normocalcaemic or even hypocalcaemic. PTH secretion normalizes during the neonatal period and the bone disease regresses spontaneously between 4 and 7 months of age. Correction of chronic hypocalcaemic states in the mother during pregnancy will prevent hyperparathyroidism in the fetus.

Hypercalcaemia occurs frequently in hypophosphatasia, a rare autosomal recessive disorder characterized by low serum alkaline phosphatase, defective bone mineralization and elevated urinary excretion of phosphoethanolamine [305]. The cause of the hypercalcaemia is not known. PTH function and vitamin D metabolism were normal in a hypercalcaemic infant with the infantile form of hypophosphatasia [316].

Other rare conditions associated with hypercalcaemia in infancy are adrenal insufficiency, blue diaper syndrome, and malignancies such as neuroblastoma and hepatoblastoma [23].

Metabolic bone disease of prematurity

Metabolic bone disease is a well-recognized problem in premature infants. Its occurrence has increased as improvements in neonatal care have resulted in greater survival rates of very premature infants (less than 30 weeks gestation or 1000 g birth weight). In these infants the incidence has been shown to exceed 50% of cases [323]. Metabolic bone disease of prematurity constitutes a spectrum of bone abnormalities from osteopenia to severe rickets with fractures.

Osteopenia implies undermineralization, mild degrees being detected by photon absorptiometry, whereas more severe osteopenia is detected by routine diagnostic radiology. A useful classification is based on the radiographic appearance of the wrist [317].

Grade 0 = normal.
Grade 1 = osteopenia of the metaphyseal plate indicated by the loss of the dense white line of metaphysis, increased submetaphyseal lucency, and thinning of the cortex.
Grade 2 = bone end changes with irregularity, fraying and cupping of the metaphysis.
Grade 3 = the above changes with fractures.

This classification can be available to any neonatal unit, utilizing a very low dose of irradiation. X-rays of the wrist have been recommended as routine on high-risk groups of premature infants [318]. Radiography probably underestimates the extent of undermineralization and the use of infant-adapted photon absorptiometry is capable of providing more accurate determination of the degree of osteopenia. This investigation is confined to research centres and adequate reliability for preterm infants remains to be documented for commercially available photon absorptiometers [319].

Measurement of serum alkaline phosphatase activity may be of value in screening and monitoring for metabolic bone disease of prematurity [324]. In one study the radiological changes of osteopenia and rickets were related to peak alkaline phosphatase activity [324]. Other studies have questioned the reliability of this approach, demonstrating overlap between infants with and without bone disease [320,321]. Metabolic bone disease of prematurity thus remains a radiological diagnosis in clinical practice, whereas measurement of serum alkaline phosphatase activity seems to be a simple and practical method of screening for grade 2 and 3 changes of radiological bone changes [322–324].

PATHOGENESIS

The pathogenesis of metabolic bone disease of premature infants is complex. Several mechanisms have been proposed such as:

1 deficiency in phosphate and/or calcium;
2 disturbances in vitamin D metabolism;
3 other factors.

The main cause is probably low intake of phosphate and calcium in milk or total parenteral nutrition solutions that are deficient in these minerals. Intrauterine bone accretion of phosphate during the last 12 weeks is 70 mg/kg per day. Human milk fed at 200 ml/kg per day provides 30 mg/kg phosphate at most, with 90% being absorbed from the intestine but preferentially used for soft tissue growth and metabolism in the body rather than for skeletal mineralization. It is thus evident that this source can supply only a fraction of the quantity of phosphate (and calcium) required by the fetal skeleton. With low phosphate availability skeletal changes of rickets related to hypophosphataemia [325] as well as hypercalciuria and hypercalcaemia (see p. 767) may occur. When sufficient phosphate is supplemented, the skeletal phosphate and calcium retention increases with subsequent reduction in hypercalciuria [326].

Fetal bone accretion of calcium during the last trimester is about 140 mg/kg per day, but human milk at 200 ml/kg per day will supply only about one-fifth of the intrauterine requirement. In infants fed with a formula of very high calcium content, calcium retention can be achieved [327], but it is questionable whether it is necessary to accumulate calcium at the same rate as *in utero* in the early weeks of life. In most infants osteopenia is not associated with clinically evident morbidity and there is evidence for a spontaneous improvement of decreased bone mineralization during postnatal life. In addition, high calcium and phosphate supplementation are hampered by technical difficulties and potential risk [328].

It is evident that the premature infant can absorb and hydroxylate vitamin D to $1,25(OH)_2D_3$, provided that the parent substrate is given in adequate amounts of at least 1000 IU/day. A defect in vitamin D-hydroxylation is unlikely, since serum $1,25(OH)_2D$ concentrations are elevated in cases where intake of calcium and/or phosphate are inadequate. Finally, there is no direct evidence for end-organ unresponsiveness to the vitamin D hormone in premature infants [329].

Only a minority of premature infants present with severe bone disease, such as rickets and rib fractures and reduced short-term linear growth, or disturbed extracellular mineral metabolism, such as hypophosphataemia, hypocalcaemia or hypercalcaemia. A few of these infants have a significant deficit in phosphate, calcium and rarely vitamin D intake, whereas others develop these disturbances and symptoms despite mineral and vitamin D supplementation [330]. This indicates that some other factors play an important part in the pathogenesis of metabolic bone disease of prematurity. Among these are frusemide therapy [331], prolonged ventilator treatment [332], intravenous alimentation [333], pre-eclampsia of the mother, and aluminium loading with substances commonly administered intravenously, including calcium, phosphate and albumin [334].

In conclusion, it seems likely that bone disease of prematurity is multifactorial, especially involving phosphate and, to a lesser extent, calcium and other factors.

PROPHYLAXIS AND TREATMENT

The optimal form and quantity of phosphate and calcium required for prophylaxis of skeletal disease and to support adequate bone mineralization in preterm infants remains to be established. Routine phosphate supplementation of human milk fed to infants of less than 1000 g birth weight is now recommended [322,323]. It is reasonable to supplement expressed breast milk with buffered phosphate solution sufficient to increase the phosphate concentration from 15 mg/dl to about 45 mg/dl. Calcium supplementation may also be indicated. Suggestions for prophylaxis of

Table 38.6 Prophylaxis of bone disease in premature infants

Adequate supplementation of calcium and phosphate
Intravenous alimentation:
Calcium, 1.5 mmol/kg (60 mg/kg) body weight per day
Phosphate, 1.1 mmol/kg (35 mg/kg) body weight per day
Oral feeding:
Supplemented human milk or formulae with:
Calcium, 17.5–22.5 mmol/l (70–90 mg/dl)
Phosphate, 11.5–14.5 mmol/l (35–45 mg/dl)
Vitamin D (about 1000 IU/day)
Avoidance of frusemide therapy (if possible)
Laboratory and radiological investigations
Serum total alkaline phosphatase:
Increase over five times the upper adult reference limit in the absence of liver disease indicates high bone turnover or even rickets
If phosphate and/or calcium in urine is low, supplementation of phosphate or calcium is necessary
Concentrations of calcium and phosphate in random urine samples:
Calcium should be about 4–8 mg/dl (1–2 mmol/l)
Phosphate should be about 3–6 mg/dl (1–2 mmol/l)
Hypercalciuria/hypophosphaturia indicate phosphate deficiency (supplementation of phosphate is necessary)
Hypocalciuria/hyperphosphaturia indicate calcium deficiency (supplementation of calcium is necessary)
Radiological investigation of the wrist is indicated:
If serum total alkaline phosphatase activity is above six times the upper adult reference limits
If there is evidence for phosphate and/or calcium deficiency

bone disease in premature infants are given in Table 38.6.

If calcium is given, phosphate must also be administered, since the extra calcium without phosphate will be inadequately utilized with resulting hypercalciuria and possible nephrocalcinosis. Phosphate-supplemented breast milk, and formulae with a calcium/phosphate ratio near 2 (containing 70–90 mgl/dl and 35–45 mg/dl calcium and phosphate respectively) in the presence of 1000 IU vitamin D per day will reduce the risk of severe bone disease in preterm infants. Measurements of urinary minerals may be more informative than determinations of serum levels. With phosphate depletion there will be no measurable phosphate and hypercalciuria, whereas calcium deficiency may be associated with low calcium excretion and hyperphosphaturia.

REFERENCES

1 Kruse K. Endocrine control and disturbances of calcium and phosphate metabolism in children. *Eur J Pediatr* 1987;146: 346–53.

2 Langman CB, Moore ES. Hypercalciuria in clinical pediatrics. *Clin Pediatr* 1984;23:135–7.

3 Favus MJ. Familial forms of hypercalciuria. *J Urol* 1989;141: 719–22.

4 Mehes K, Szelidz S. Autosomal dominant inheritance of hypercalciuria. *Eur J Pediatr* 1980;133:239–42.

5 Broadus AE, Dominguez M, Bartter FC. Pathophysiological studies in idiopathic hypercalciuria: use of an oral calcium tolerance test to characterize distinctive hypercalciuric subgroups. *J Clin Endocrinol Metab* 1978;47:751–60.

6 Aurbach GD, Marx SJ, Spiegel AM. Parathyroid hormone, calcitonin, and the calciferols. In: Wilson JD, Foster DW, eds. *Williams Textbook of Endocrinology*, 8th edn. Philadelphia, PA: WB Saunders, 1992:1397–476.

7 Li X-Q, Tembe V, Horwitz GM, Bushinsky DA, Favus MJ. Increased intestinal vitamin D receptor in genetic hypercalciuric rats. A cause of intestinal calcium hyperabsorption. *J Clin Invest* 1993;91:661–7.

8 Kruse K, Kracht U, Kruse U. Reference values for urinary calcium excretion and screening for hypercalciuria in children and adolescents. *Eur J Pediatr* 1984;143:25–31.

9 Bell NH, Stern PH. Perturbation of the vitamin D–endocrine system in sarcoid and other diseases. In: Norman AW, Schaefer K, Grigoleit HG, Herrath D v, eds. *Vitamin D–Chemical, Biochemical, and Clinical Update.* Berlin: W de Gruyter, 1985:1053–61.

10 Helikson MA, Havey AD, Zerwekh JE, Breslau NA, Gardner DW. Plasma-cell granuloma producing calcitriol and hypercalcemia. *Ann Intern Med* 1986;105:379–81.

11 Finne P, Sanderud J, Aksnes L, Bratlid D, Aarskog D. Hypercalcemia with increased and unregulated 1,25-dihydroxyvitamin D production in a neonate with subcutaneous fat necrosis. *J Pediatr* 1988;112:792–4.

12 Kruse K, Irle U, Uhlig R. Elevated 1,25-dihydroxyvitamin D serum concentrations in infants with subcutaneous fat necrosis. *J Pediatr* 1993;122:460–3.

13 Singer FR, Adams JS. Abnormal calcium homeostasis in sarcoidosis. *N Engl J Med* 1986;315:755–7.

14 Fetchick DA, Bertolini DR, Sarin PS, Weintraub ST, Mundy GR, Dunn JF. Production of 1,25-dihydroxy-vitamin D_3 by human T cell lymphotrophic virus-I-transformed lymphocytes. *J Clin Invest* 1986;78:592–6.

15 Mundy GR. The hypercalcemia of malignancy. *Kidney Int* 1987;31:142–55.

16 Hess AF, Lewis JM. Clinical experience with irradiated ergosterol. *J Am Med Assoc* 1928;91:783–8.

17 Harrison HE, Harrison HC. *Disorders of Calcium and Phosphate Metabolism in Childhood and Adolescence.* Philadelphia, PA: WB Saunders, 1979:101–9.

18 Misselwitz J, Hesse V. Hyperkalzämie nach Vitamin D-Stoßprophylaxe. *Kinderarztl Prax* 1986;54:431–8.

19 Davies M, Adams PH. The continuing risk of vitamin D intoxication. *Lancet* 1978;2:621–3.

20 Davies M, Mawer EB, Freemont AJ. The osteodystrophy of hypervitaminosis D: a metabolic study. *Q J Med* 1986;234: 911–19.

21 Mawer EB, Hann JT, Berry JL, Davies M. Vitamin D metabolism in patients intoxicated with ergocalciferol. *Clin Sci* 1985;68:135–41.

22 Ross SG. Vitamin D intoxication in infancy. *J Pediatr* 1952; 41:815–22.

23 Anast CS, David L. Human neonatal hypercalcemia. In: Holick MF, Gray TK, Anast CS, eds. *Perinatal Calcium and Phosphorus Metabolism.* Amsterdam: Elsevier, 1983: 363–83.

24 Burn J. Williams syndrome. *J Med Genet* 1986;23:389–95.

25 Martin NDT, Snodgrass GJAI, Cohen RD. Idiopathic infantile hypercalcemia – a continuing enigma. *Arch Dis Child* 1984; 59:605–13.

26 Lightwood R, Stapelton T. Idiopathic hypercalcaemia in infants. *Lancet* 1953;2:255–6.

27 Fanconi G, Giardet P, Schlesinger B, Butler H, Black JS. Chronische Hypercalcämie kombiniert mit Osteosklerose, Hyperazotämie, Minderwuchs und kongenitalen Mißbildungen. *Helv Paediatr Acta* 1952;7:314–34.

28 Beuren AJ, Apitz J, Harmjanz D. Supravalvular aortic stenosis in association with mental retardation and certain facial appearance. *Circulation* 1962;26:1235–40.

29 Williams JCP, Barratt-Boyes BG, Lowe JB. Supravalvular aortic stenosis. *Circulation* 1961;24:1311–18.

30 Wiedemann H-R, Kunze J, Dibbern H. *Atlas der Klinischen Syndrome,* 3rd edn. Stuttgart and New York: Schattauer, 1989:484–5.

31 Friedman WF, Mills LF. The relationship between vitamin D and the craniofacial and dental anomalies of the supravalvular aortic stenosis syndrome. *Pediatrics* 1969;43:12–18.

32 Friedman WF, Roberts WC. Vitamin D and the supravalvular aortic stenosis syndrome: the transplacental effects of vitamin D in the aorta of the rabbit. *Circulation* 1966;13:77–86.

33 Goodenday LS, Gordan GS. No risk from vitamin D in pregnancy. *Ann Intern Med* 1971;75:807–9.

34 Marx SJ, Swart EG, Hamstra AJ, DeLuca HF. Normal intrauterine development of the fetus of a woman receiving extraordinary high doses of 1,25-dihydroxyvitamin D_3. *J Clin Endocrinol Metab* 1980;51:1138–42.

35 Barr DGD, Forfar JO. Oral calcium-loading test in infancy with particular reference to idiopathic hypercalcemia. *Br Med J* 1969;1:477–80.

36 Forbes GB, Bryson MF, Manning J, Amirhakimi GH, Reina JC. Impaired calcium homeostasis in the infantile hypercalcemic syndrome. *Acta Paed Scand* 1972;61:305–9.

37 Garabedian M, Jacqz E, Guillozo H *et al.* Elevated plasma 1,25-dihydroxyvitamin D concentrations in infants with hyper-

calcemia and an elfin facies. *N Engl J Med* 1985;312:948–52.

38 Chesney RW, DeLuca HF, Gertner JM, Genel M. Letter to the editor. *N Engl J Med* 1985;311:899–90.

39 Culler FL, Jones KL, Deftos JJ. Impaired calcitonin secretion in patients with Williams syndrome. *J Pediatr* 1985;197:720–3.

40 Kruse K, Pankau R, Gosch A, Wohlfart K. Calcium metabolism in Williams–Beuren syndrome. *J Pediatr* 1992;121:902–7.

41 Martin NDT, Snodgrass GJAI, Cohen RD *et al.* Vitamin D metabolites in idiopathic infantile hypercalcemia. *Arch Dis Child* 1985;60:1140–3.

42 Taylor AB, Stern PH, Bell NH. Abnormal regulation of circulating 25-hydoxyvitamin D in the Williams syndrome. *N Engl J Med* 1982;306:972–5.

43 Mankin HJ. Rickets, osteomalacia, and renal osteodystrophy. Part I and II. *J Bone J Surg* (A) 1974;56:101–28, 352–86.

44 Pitt MJ. Rachitic and osteomalacic syndromes. *Radiol Clin N Am* 1981;19:581–99.

45 Fraser D, Scriver CR. Disorders associated with hereditary or acquired abnormalities in vitamin D function: hereditary disorders associated with vitamin D resistance or defective phosphate metabolism. In: DeGroot LJ, ed. *Endocrinology*, Vol. 2. New York: Grune & Stratton, 1979:797–807.

46 Pettifor JM, Ross FP, Travers R, Glorieux FH, DeLuca HF. Dietary calcium deficiency: a syndrome associated with bone deformities and elevated serum 1,25-dihydroxyvitamin D concentrations. *Metab Bone Dis Related Res* 1981;2: 301–5.

47 Dent CE, Stamp TCB. Vitamin D, rickets and osteomalacia. In: Avioli L, Krane S, eds. *Metabolic Bone Disease*. New York: Academic Press, 1977:237–305.

48 Gundberg CM, Cole DEC, Lian LB, Reade TM, Gallop PM. Serum osteocalcin in the treatment of inherited rickets with 1,25-dihydroxyvitamin D_3. *J Clin Endocrinol Metab* 1983; 56:1063–7.

49 Kruse K, Kracht U. Evaluation of serum osteocalcin as an index of altered bone metabolism. *Eur J Pediatr* 1986;145: 27–33.

50 Fraser D, Koogh SW, Scriver CR. Hyperparathyroidism as the cause of hyperaminoaciduria and phosphaturia in human vitamin D deficiency. *Pediatr Res* 1967;1:425–35.

51 Kruse K, Bartels H, Kracht U. Parathyroid function in different stages of vitamin D deficiency rickets. *Eur J Pediatr* 1984;141:158–62.

52 Bétend B, David L, Evrard A, Grangaud J-P, François R. A patient with nutritional rickets stage 1 or partial hypoparathyroidism. *Acta Paed Scand* 1981;70:259–60.

53 Chesney RW, Zimmermann J, Hamstra A, DeLuca HF, Mazess RB. Vitamin D metabolite concentrations in vitamin D deficiency. Are calcitriol levels normal? *Am J Dis Child* 1981;135:1025–8.

54 Compton JE, Merrett AL, Ledger JE, Creamer B. Fecal tritium excretion after intravenous administration of ^{3}H-25-hydroxyvitamin D_3 in control subjects and in patients with malabsorption. *Gut* 1982;23:310–15.

55 Bikle DD, Halloran BP, Gee E, Ryzen E, Haddad JG. Free 25-hydroxyvitamin D levels are normal in subjects with liver disease and reduced total 25-hydroxyvitamin D levels. *J Clin Invest* 1986;78:748–52.

56 Kruse R. Osteopathien bei antiepileptischer Langzeittherapie (vorläufige Mitteilung). *Monatsschr Kinderheilkd* 1968; 116:378–80.

57 Hahn TJ. Drug-induced disorders of vitamin D and mineral metabolism. *Clin Endocrinol Metab* 1980;9:107–29.

58 Jubiz W, Haussler MR, McCain TA, Tolman KG. Plasma 1,25-dihydroxyvitamin D levels in patients receiving anticonvulsant drugs. *J Clin Endocrinol Metab* 1977;44: 617–21.

59 Kruse K. On the pathogenesis of anticonvulsant-drug-induced alterations of calcium metabolism. *Eur J Pediatr* 1982;138:202–5.

60 Kruse K, Bartels H, Ziegler R, Dreller E, Kracht U. Parathyroid function and serum calcitonin in children receiving anticonvulsant drugs. *Eur J Pediatr* 1980;133:151–6.

61 Freundlich M, Bourgoignie JJ, Zilleruelo G, Abitbol C, Canterbury JM, Strauss K. Calcium and vitamin D metabolism in children with nephrotic syndrome. *J Pediatr* 1986; 108:383–7.

62 Norman ME. Vitamin D in bone disease. *Pediatr Clin N Am* 1982;29:947–71.

63 Prader A, Illig R, Heierli E. Eine besondere Form der primären Vitramin-D-resistenten Rachitis mit Hypocalcämie und autosomal-dominantem Erbgang: Die hereditäre Pseudo-Mangel-Rachitis. *Helv Paediatr Acta* 1961;16:452–68.

64 Fox J, Maunder EMW, Randall VA, Care AD. Vitamin D dependent rickets type I in pigs. *Clin Sci* 1985;69:541–8.

65 Winkler I, Schreiner F, Harmeyer J. Absence of renal 25-hydroxycholecalciferol-1-hydroxylase activity in a pig strain with vitamin D-dependent rickets. *Calc Tissue Int* 1986;38: 87–94.

66 Labuda M, Morgan K, Glorieux FH. Mapping the gene for vitamin D dependency type I to chromosome 12q14 by linkage analysis. *Am J Human Genet* 1990;47:28–36.

67 Glorieux FH, Delvin EE. Pseudo-vitamin D deficiency rickets. In: Norman AW, Bouillon R, Thomasset M, eds. *Vitamin D. Gene Regulation, Structure–Function Analysis and Clinical Application*. Proceedings of the eighth workshop on vitamin D, Paris. Berlin: De Gruyter, 1991:238–45.

68 Marx SJ, Libermann UA, Eil C, Gamblin GT, DeGrange DA, Balsan S. Hereditary resistance to 1,25-dihydroxyvitamin D. *Rec Prog Horm Res* 1984;40;589–620.

69 Yamaguchi A, Kohno Y, Yamazaki T *et al.* Bone in the marmoset: a resemblance to vitamin D-dependent rickets, type II. *Calc Tissue Int* 1986;39:22–7.

70 Marx SJ, Bliziotes MM, Nanes M. Analysis of the relation between alopecia and resistance to 1,25-dihydroxyvitamin D. *Clin Endocrinol* 1986;25:373–81.

71 Fraher LJ, Karmali R, Hinde FRJ *et al.* Vitamin D-dependent rickets type II: extreme end organ resistance to 1,25-dihydroxyvitamin D_3 in a patient without alopecia. *Eur J Pediatr* 1986;145:389–95.

72 Walka M, Däumling S, Hadorn H-B, Kruse K, Belohradsky BH. Vitamin D dependent rickets type II with myelofibrosis and immune dysfunction. *Eur J Pediatr* 1992;150:665–8.

73 Malloy PJ, Hochberg Z, Tiosano D, Pike JW, Hughes MR, Feldman D. The molecular basis of hereditary 1,25-dihydroxyvitamin D_3-resistant rickets in seven related families. *J Clin Invest* 1990;86:2071–9.

74 Malloy PJ, Hughes MR, Pike JW, Feldman D. Vitamin D receptor mutations and hereditary 1,25-dihydroxyvitamin D resistant rickets. In: Norman AW, Bouillon R, Thomasset M, eds. *Vitamin D. Gene Regulation, Structure–Function Analysis and Clinical Application*. Proceedings of the eighth workshop on vitamin D, Paris. Berlin: De Gruyter, 1991: 116–24.

75 Rut AR, Hewison M, Rowe P, Hughes M, Grant D, O'Riordan JLH. A novel mutation in the steroid binding region of the vitamin receptor (VDR) gene in hereditary vitamin resistant rickets (HVDRR). In: Norman AW,

Bouillon R, Thomasset M, eds. *Vitamin D. Gene Regulation, Structure–Function Analysis, and Clinical Application.* Proceedings of the eighth workshop on vitamin D, Paris. Berlin: De Gruyter, 1991:94–5.

76 Hughes MR, Malloy PJ, Kieback DG *et al.* Point mutations in the human vitamin D receptor gene associated with hypocalcemic rickets. *Science* 1988;242:1702–5.

77 Sone T, Marx SJ, Liberman KS, Pike JW. A unique point mutation in the vitamin D receptor gene confers hereditary resistance to 1,25-dihydroxyvitamin D_3. *Mol Endocrinol* 1990;4:623–31.

78 Saijo T, Ito M, Takeda E *et al.* A unique mutation in the vitamin D receptor gene in three Japanese patients with vitamin D-dependent rickets type II: utility of single-strand conformation polymorphism analysis for heterozygous carrier detection. *Am J Hum Genet* 1991;49:668–73.

79 Yagi H, Ozono K, Miyake H, Nagashima K, Kuroume T, Pike JW. A new point mutation in the deoxyribonucleic acid-binding domain of the vitamin D receptor in a kindred with hereditary 1,25-dihydroxyvitamin D-resistant rickets. *J Clin Endocrinol Metab* 1993;76:509–12.

80 Feldman D, Chen T, Cone C *et al.* Vitamin D resistant rickets with alopecia: cultured skin fibroblasts exhibit defective cytoplasmatic receptors and unresponsiveness to 1,25 $(OH)_2D_3$. *J Clin Endocrinol Metab* 1982;55:1020–2.

81 Gamblin GT, Liberman UA, Eil C, Down RW Jr, DeGrange DA, Marx SJ. Vitamin D-dependent rickets type II – defective induction of 25-hydroxyvitamin D_3-24-hydroxylase by 1,25-dihydroxyvitamin D_3 in cultured skin fibroblasts. *J Clin Invest* 1985;75:954–60.

82 Griffin JE, Zerwekh JE. Impaired stimulation of 25-hydroxyvitamin D-24-hydroxylase in fibroblasts from a patient with vitamin D-dependent rickets, type II. *J Clin Invest* 1983;72:1190–9.

83 Hochberg Z, Tiosano D, Even L. Calcium therapy for calcitriol-resistant rickets. *J Pediatr* 1992;121:803–8.

84 Sakati N, Woodhouse NJY, Niles N, Harfi H, DeGrange DA, Marx SJ. Hereditary resistance to 1,25-dihydroxyvitamin D: clinical and radiological improvement during high-dose oral calcium therapy. *Horm Res* 1986;24:280–7.

85 Balsan S, Garabédian M, Larchet M *et al.* Long-term nocturnal calcium infusions can cure rickets and promote normal mineralization in hereditary resistance to 1,25-dihydroxyvitamin D. *J Clin Invest* 1986;77:1661–7.

86 Hochberg Z, Benderli A, Levy J *et al.* 1,25-dihydroxyvitamin D resistance, rickets and alopecia. *Am J Med* 1984;77:805–11.

87 Kruse K, Feldmann E, Bartels H. Hypoparathyroidism in hereditary resistance to $1,25(OH)_2D$ during long-term treatment with excessive doses of vitamin D_3. In: Norman AW, Schaefer K, Grigoleit H-G, Herrath D v, eds. *Vitamin D. Molecular, Cellular, and Clinical Endocrinology.* Proceedings of the seventh workshop on vitamin D, Rancho Mirage. Berlin: De Gruyter, 1988:456–7.

88 Adami C, Milroy EJG, O'Riordan JLH. Primary hyperparathyroidism. In: Nordin BEC, ed. *Metabolic Bone and Stone Disease.* Edinburgh: Churchill Livingstone, 1984:112–42.

89 Girard RM, Belanger A, Hazel B. Primary hyperparathyroidism in children. *Can J Surg* 1982;25:11–13.

90 Atti JN. Nonfamilial hyperparathyroidism. In: Lifshitz F, ed. *Pediatric Endocrinology.* New York: Marcel Dekker, 1985:349–53.

91 Bjernulf D, Hall K, Sjögren J, Werner J. Primary hyperparathyroidism in children. Brief review of the literature and a case report. *Acta Paed Scand* 1970;59:249–58.

92 Eftekhari F, Yousefzadeh DK. Primary infantile hyperparathyroidism: clinical, laboratory, and radiographic features in 21 cases. *Skeletal Radiol* 1982;8:201–8.

93 Broadus AE. Mineral metabolism. In: Felig P *et al.*, eds. *Endocrinology and Metabolism.* New York: McGraw-Hill, 1981:963–1079.

94 Firth RG, Grant CS, Riggs BL. Development of hypercalcemic hyperparathyroidism after long-term phosphate supplementation in hypophosphatemic osteomalacia. Report of two cases. *Am J Med* 1985;78:669–73.

95 Rivkees SA, El-Hajj-Fuleihan G, Brown EM, Crawford JD. Tertiary hyperparathyroidism during high phosphate therapy of familial hypophosphatemic rickets. *J Clin Endocrinol Metab* 1992;75:1514–18.

96 Brandi ML, Aurbach GD, Fitzpatrick LA *et al.* Parathyroid mitogenic activity in plasma from patients with familial multiple endocrine neoplasia type I. *N Engl J Med* 1986;314:1287–93.

97 Harrison HE, Harrison HC. Familial hyperparathyroidism. In: Lifshitz F, ed. *Pediatric Endocrinology*, 2nd edn. New York: Marcel Dekker, 1990:613–23.

98 Law WM Jr, Hodgson SF, Heath H III. Autosomal recessive inheritance of familial hyperparathyroidism. *N Engl J Med* 1983;309:650–3.

99 Schimke RN. Genetic aspects of multiple endocrine neoplasia. *Ann Rev Med* 1984;35:25–31.

100 Eberle F, Grun R. Multiple endocrine neoplasia, type I (MEN I). *Ergeb Inn Med Kinderheilkd* 1981;46:76–149.

101 Bale S, Bale A, Stewart K *et al.* Linkage analysis of multiple endocrine neoplasia type I with INT 2 and other markers on chromosome 11. *Genomics* 1989;4:320–2.

102 Schimke RN. Multiple endocrine neoplasia: search for the oncogenic trigger. *N Engl J Med* 1986;314:1315–16.

103 Broachüs AE, Horst RL, Lang R, Littledike ET, Rasmussen H. The importance of circulating 1,25-dihydroxyvitamin D in the pathogenesis of hypercalciuria and renal stone formation in primary hyperparathyroidism. *N Engl J Med* 1980;302:421–6.

104 Allen DB, Friedman AL, Hendricks S. Asymptomatic primary hyperparathyroidism in children. New methods of preoperative diagnosis. *Am J Dis Child* 1986;140:819–21.

105 Petrykowski W v, Jobke A, Keefer I, Kuhn FP. Asymptomatische exzessive Hypercalcämie bei einem 12 Jährigen. *Monatsschr Kinderheilkd* 1983;131:166–8.

106 Goldbloom RB, Gillis DA, Prascad M. Hereditary parathyroid hyperplasia: a surgical emergency of early infancy. *Pediatrics* 1972;49:514–23.

107 Malek RS, Kelalis PP. Urologic manifestations of hyperparathyroidism in childhood. *J Urol* 1976;115:717–19.

108 Theintz GE, Sizonenko PC, Paunier L. Primary hyperparathyroidism and rickets. A case report and review of the literature. *Helv Paediatr Acta* 1984;39:509–16.

109 Hower J, Maruhn D, Struck H. Kreatinin-Kinase-Aktivität und Hypocalcämie. *Dtsch Med Wochenschr* 1974;99:14–15.

110 Kruse K, Scheunemann W, Baier W, Schaub J. Hypocalcemic myopathy in idiopathic hypoparathyroidism. *Eur J Pediatr* 1982;138:280–2.

111 Schmidtke J, Kruse K, Pape B, Sippell G. Exclusion of close linkage between the parathyroid hormone gene and a mutant gene locus causing idiopathic hypoparathyroidism. *J Med Genet* 1986;23:217–19.

112 Nagant de Deuxchaisnes C, Krane SM. Hypoparathyroidism. In: Avioli CV, Krane SM, eds. *Metabolic Bone Disease*, Vol. II. New York: Academic Press, 1978:218–445.

113 Connor TB, Rosen RL, Blaustein MP, Applefield MM, Doyle

LA. Hypocalcemia in precipitating congestive heart failure. *N Engl J Med* 1982;307:869–72.

114 Greenberg F, Valdes C, Rosenblatt MH, Kirkland JL, Ledbetter DH. Hypoparathyroidism and T cell immune defect in a patient with 10p deletion syndrome. *J Pediatr* 1986;109:489–92.

115 Monaco G, Pignata C, Rossi E, Mascellaro O, Cocozza S, Ciccimarra F. Di George anomaly associated with 10p deletion. *Am J Med Genet* 1991;39:215–16.

116 Raatikka M, Rapola J, Tuuteri L, Louhime I, Savilakti E. Familial third and fourth pharyngeal pouch syndrome with truncus arteriosus: DiGeorge syndrome. *Pediatrics* 1981;67: 173–5.

117 Barakat AY, D'Albora JB, Martin MM, Jose PA. Familial nephrosis, nerve deafness and hypoparathyroidism. *J Pediatr* 1977;91:61–4.

118 Bilious RW, Murty G, Parkinson DB *et al.* Brief report: autosomal dominant familial hypoparathyroidism, sensorineural deafness, and renal dysplasia. *N Engl J Med* 1992; 327:1069–74.

119 Shaw NJ, Haigh D, Lealmann GT, Karbani G, Brocklebank JT, Dillon MJ. Autosomal recessive hypoparathyroidism with renal insufficiency and developmental delay. *Arch Dis Child* 1991;66:1191–4.

120 Yumita S, Furukawa Y, Sohn HE, Unakami H, Miura R, Yoshinaga K. Familial idiopathic hypoparathyroidism and progressive sensorineural deafness. *Tohoku J Exp Med* 1986; 148:135–41.

121 Kalam MA, Hafeez W. Congenital hypoparathyroidism, seizure, extreme growth failure with development delay and dysmorphic features – another case of this new syndrome. *Clin Genet* 1992;42:110–3.

122 Richardson RJ, Kirk JMW. Short stature, mental retardation, and hypoparathyroidism: a new syndrome. *Arch Dis Child* 1990;65:1113–7.

123 Saijad SA, Sakati NA, Abu-Osba YK, Kadoura R, Milner RDG. A new syndrome of congenital hypoparathyroidism, severe growth failure and dysmorphic features. *Arch Dis Child* 1991;66:193–6.

124 Ahonen P, Myllärniemi S, Sipilä J, Perheentupa J. Clinical variation of autoimmune polyendocrinopathy–candidosis–ectodermal dystrophy (APECED) in a series of 68 patients. *N Engl J Med* 1990;322:1829–36.

125 Neufeld RB, Maclaren N, Blizzard R. Two types of autoimmune Addison's disease associated with different polyglandular autoimmune syndromes. *Medicine* 1981;60: 355–62.

126 Bergada J, Schiffrin A, Srair HA *et al.* Kenny syndrome: description of additional abnormalities and molecular studies. *Hum Genet* 1988;80:39–42.

127 Fanconi S, Fischer JA, Wieland P *et al.* Kenny syndrome: evidence for idiopathic hypoparathyroidism in two patients and for abnormal parathyroid hormone in one. *J Pediatr* 1986;109:469–75.

128 Pellock JM, Behrens M, Lewis L *et al.* Kearns–Sayre syndrome and hypoparathyroidism. *Ann Neurol* 1978;3:455–8.

129 Chandra RK, Jogleker S, Antonio Z. Deficiency of humoral immunity and hypoparathyroidism associated with the Hallermann–Streiff syndrome: clinical note. *J Pediatr* 1978; 93:892.

130 Ikeda K, Kobayashi T, Kusakari J, Tokasaka T, Yumita S, Furukawa Y. Sensorineural hearing loss associated with hypoparathyroidism. *Laryngoscope* 1987;97:1075–9.

131 Koch T, Lehnhardt E, Böttinger H *et al.* Sensorineural hearing loss owing to deficient G proteins in patients with pseudohypoparathyroidism: results of a multicentre study. *Eur J Clin Invest* 1990;20:416–21.

132 Peden VH. True idiopathic hypoparathyroidism as a sex-linked recessive trait. *Am J Hum Genet* 1960;12:323–37.

133 Whyte MP, Weldon VV. Idiopathic hypoparathyroidism presenting with seizures during infancy: X-linked recessive inheritance in a large Missouri kindred. *J Pediatr* 1981;99: 608–11.

134 Ahn TG, Antonarakis SE, Kronenberg HM, Igarashi T, Levine MA. Familial isolated hypoparathyroidism: a molecular genetic analysis of 8 families with 23 affected persons. *Medicine* 1986;65:73–81.

135 Barr DGD, Prader A, Esper U, Rampini S, Marrian VJ, Forfar JO. Chronic hypoparathyroidism in two generations. *Helv Paediatr Acta* 1971;26:507–21.

136 De Campo C, Piscopello L, Noacco C, Da Col P, Englaro GC, Benedetti A. Primary familial hypoparathyroidism with an autosomal dominant mode of inheritance. *J Endocrinol Invest* 1988;11:91–6.

137 Winter WE, Silverstein JH, Maclaren NK, Riley WJ, Chiaro JJ. Autosomal dominant hypoparathyroidism with variable, age-dependent severity. *J Pediatr* 1983;103:387–90.

138 Bronsky D, Kiamko RT, Waldstein SS. Familial idiopathic hypoparathyroidism. *J Clin Endocrinol Metab* 1968;28: 61–5.

139 Lelong M, Canlorbe P, Lagrue G, Bader J-Cl. Syndrome d'hypoparathyroidie familiale avec hypercalciurie. *Ann Pediatr* 1968;38:253–68.

140 Nagant de Deuxchaisnes C, Fischer J, Dambacher MA *et al.* Dissociation of parathyroid hormone bioactivity and immunoreactivity in pseudohypoparathyroidism type I. *J Clin Endocrinol Metab* 1981;53:1105–9.

141 Connors MH, Irias JJ, Golabi M. Hypo-hyperparathyroidism: evidence for a defective parathyroid hormone. *Pediatrics* 1977;60:343–8.

142 McElduff A, Wilkinson M, Lackmann M *et al.* Familial hypoparathyroidism due to an abnormal parathyroid hormone molecule. *Aust NZ J Med* 1989;19:22–30.

143 Nusynowitz ML, Klein MH. Pseudoidiopathic hypoparathyroidism with ineffective parathyroid hormone. *Am J Med* 1973;55:677–89.

144 Miric A, Levine MA. Analysis of the peproPTH gene by denaturing gradient gel electrophoresis in familial isolated hypoparathyroidism. *J Clin Endocrinol Metab* 1991;74: 509–16.

145 Arnold A, Horst SA, Gardella TJ, Baba H, Levine MA, Kronenberg HM. Mutation of the signal peptide-encoding region of the preproparathyroid hormone gene in familial isolated hypoparathyroidism. *J Clin Invest* 1990;86:1084–7.

146 Thakker RV, Davies KE, Whyte MP, Wooding C, O'Riordan JLH. Mapping the gene causing X-linked recessive idiopathic hypoparathyroidism to Xq26–Xq27 by linkage studies. *J Clin Invest* 1990;86:40–5.

147 Albright F, Burnett CH, Smith PH. Pseudohypoparathyroidism: an example of 'Seabright–Bantam syndrome'. *Endocrinology* 1942;30:922–32.

148 Drezner MK, Neelon FA. Pseudohypoparathyroidism. In: Stanbury JB, Wyngaarden JB, Fredrickson DS, Goldstein JL, Brown MS, eds. *The Metabolic Basis of Inherited Disease*, 5th edn. New York: McGraw-Hill, 1983:1508–27.

149 Chase LR, Melson GL, Aurbach GD. Pseudohypoparathyroidism: defective excretion of 3',5'-AMP in response to parathyroid hormone. *J Clin Invest* 1969;48:1832–44.

150 Drezner MK, Neelon FA, Lebovitz HE. Pseudohypoparathyroidism type II. A possible defect in the reception of the

cyclic AMP signal. *N Engl J Med* 1973;289:1056–60.
151 Bell NH, Avery S, Sinha T, Clark CM Jr, Allen DO, Johnston C Jr. Effects of dibutyryl cyclic adenosine 3′,5′-monophosphate and parathyroid extract on calcium and phosphorus metabolism in hypoparathyroidism and pseudohypoparathyroidism. *J Clin Invest* 1972;51:816–23.
152 Yamaoka K, Seino Y, Ishida M *et al.* Effect of dibutyryl adenosine 3′,5′-monophosphate administration on plasma concentrations of 1,25-dihydroxyvitamin D in pseudohypoparathyroidism type I. *J Clin Endocrinol Metab* 1981;53:1096–100.
153 Downs RW, Levine MA, Drezner NK, Burch WM, Spiegel AM. Deficient adenylate cyclase regulating proteins in renal membranes from a patient with pseudohypoparathyroidism. *J Clin Invest* 1983;71:231–5.
154 Drezner MK, Burch WM Jr. Altered activity of the nucleotide regulatory site in the parathyroid hormone sensitive adenylate cyclase from the renal cortex of a patient with pseudohypoparathyroidism. *J Clin Invest* 1978;62:1222–7.
155 Farfel Z, Brickman AS, Kaslow HR, Brothers VM, Bourne HR. Defect of receptor–cyclase coupling protein in pseudohypoparathyroidism. *N Engl J Med* 1980;303:237–42.
156 Levine MA, Downs RW Jr, Singer M, Marx SJ, Aurbach GD, Spiegel AM. Deficient activity of guanine nucleotide regulatory protein in erythrocytes from patients with pseudohypoparathyroidism. *Biochem Biophys Res Commun* 1980;94:1319–24.
157 Farfel Z, Bourne HR. Deficient activity of receptor–cyclase coupling protein in platelets of patients with pseudohypoparathyroidism. *J Clin Endocrinol Metab* 1980;51:1202–4.
158 Bourne HR, Kaslow HR, Brickman AS, Farfel Z. Fibroblast defect in pseudohypoparathyroidism, type I: reduced activity of receptor–cyclase coupling protein. *J Clin Endocrinol Metab* 1981;53:634–40.
159 Levine MA, Downs RW Jr, Moses AM *et al.* Resistance to multiple hormones in patients with pseudohypoparathyroidism. Association with deficient activity of guanine nucleotide regulatory protein. *Am J Med* 1983;74:545–56.
160 Carlson HE, Brickman AS, Bottazo GF. Prolactin deficiency in pseudohypoparathyroidism. *N Engl J Med* 1977;296:140–4.
161 Kruse K, Gutekunst B, Kracht U, Schwerda K. Deficient prolactin response to parathyroid hormone in hypocalcemic and normocalcemic pseudohypoparathyroidism. *J Clin Endocrinol Metab* 1981;52:1099–105.
162 Fischer JA, Bourne HR, Dambacher MA *et al.* Pseudohypoparathyroidism: inheritance and expression of deficient receptor cyclase coupling protein activity. *Clin Endocrinol* 1983;19:747–54.
163 Levine MA, Jap T-S, Mauseth RS, Downs RW Jr, Spiegel AM. Activity of the stimulatory guanine nucleotide-binding regulatory protein in erythrocytes from patients with pseudohypoparathyroidism and pseudopseudohypoparathyroidism: biochemical, endocrine, and genetic analysis of Albright's hereditary osteodystrophy in six kindreds. *J Clin Endocrinol Metab* 1986;62:497–502.
164 Mallet E, Carayon P, Amr S *et al.* Coupling defect of thyrotropin receptor and adenylate cyclase in a pseudohypoparathyroid patient. *J Clin Endocrinol Metab* 1982;54:1028–32.
165 Silve C, Santova A, Breslau N, Moses A, Spiegel AM. Selective resistance to parathyroid hormone in cultured skin fibroblasts from patients with pseudohypoparathyroidism type Ib. *J Clin Endocrinol Metab* 1986;62:640–4.
166 Radeke HH, Auf'mkolk B, Jüppner H, Krohn H-P, Keck E, Hesch RD. Multiple pre- and postreceptor defects in pseudohypoparathyroidism (a multicenter study with twenty four patients). *J Clin Endocrinol Metab* 1986;62:393–402.
167 Gilman AG. Guanine nucleotide-binding regulatory proteins and dual control of adenylate cyclase. *J Clin Invest* 1984;73:1–4.
168 Downs RW, Sekura RD, Levine MA, Spiegel AM. The inhibitory adenylate cyclase coupling protein in pseudohypoparathyroidism. *J Clin Endocrinol Metab* 1985;61:351–4.
169 Barrett D, Breslau NA, Wax MB, Molinoff PB, Downs W Jr. A new form of pseudohypoparathyroidism with abnormal catalytic adenylate cyclase. *Am J Physiol* 1989;257:E277–83.
170 Carter A, Bardin C, Collins R, Simons C, Bray P, Spiegel A. Reduced expression of multiple forms of the alpha subunit of the stimulatory GTP-binding protein in pseudohypoparathyroidism type Ia. *Proc Natl Acad Sci USA* 1987;87:7266–9.
171 Levine MA, Ahn TG, Klupt SF *et al.* Genetic deficiency of the alpha subunit of the guanine nucleotide-binding protein, G_s as the molecular basis for Albright's hereditary osteodystrophy. *Proc Natl Acad Sci USA* 1988;85:617–21.
172 Patten JL, Johns DK, Valle D *et al.* Mutation in the gene encoding the stimulatory G protein of adenylate cyclase in Albright's hereditary osteodystrophy. *N Engl J Med* 1990;322:1412–19.
173 Weinstein LS, Gejman PV, Friedmann E *et al.* Mutations of the $G_s\alpha$-subunit gene in Albright hereditary osteodystrophy detected by denaturating gradient gel electrophoresis. *Proc Natl Acad Sci USA* 1990;87:8287–90.
174 Weinstein LS, Shenker A, Gejman PV, Merino MJ, Friedmann E, Spiegel AM. Activating mutations of the stimulatory G protein in the McCune–Albright syndrome. *N Engl J Med* 1991;325:1688–95.
175 Kruse K, Kracht U, Göpfert G. Response of kidney and bone to parathyroid hormone in children receiving anticonvulsant drugs. *Neuropediatrics* 1982;13:3–9.
176 Farfel Z, Friedman E. Mental deficiency in pseudohypoparathyroidism type I is associated with N-protein deficiency. *Ann Intern Med* 1986;105:197–9.
177 Costello JM, Dent CE. Hypo-hyperparathyroidism. *Arch Dis Child* 1963;38:397–407.
178 Frame B, Hanson CA, Frost HM, Block M, Arnstein AR. Renal resistance to parathyroid hormone with osteitis fibrosa: 'pseudohypohyperparathyroidism'. *Am J Med* 1972;52:311–21.
179 Kidd GS, Schaaf M, Adler RA, Lassman MN, Wray HL. Skeletal responsiveness in pseudohypoparathyroidism. A spectrum of clinical disease. *Am J Med* 1980;68:772–81.
180 Kruse K, Kracht U, Wohlfart K, Kruse U. Biochemical markers of bone turnover, intact serum parathyroid hormone and renal calcium excretion in patients with pseudohypoparathyroidism and hypoparathyroidism before and during vitamin D treatment. *Eur J Pediatr* 1989;148:535–9.
181 Drezner MK, Haussler MR. Normocalcemic pseudohypoparathyroidism: association with normal vitamin D_3 metabolism. *Am J Med* 1979;66:503–8.
182 Breslau NA, Zerewkh JE. Relationship of estrogen and pregnancy to calcium homeostasis in pseudohypoparathyroidism. *J Clin Endocrinol Metab* 1986;62:45–51.
183 Kruse K, Kracht U. A simplified diagnostic test in hypoparathyroidism and pseudohypoparathyroidism type I with synthetic 1–38 fragment of human parathyroid hormone. *Eur J Pediatr* 1987;146:373–7.
184 Schuster V, Eschenhagen T, Kruse K, Gierschik P, Kreth

HW. Endocrine and molecular biological studies in a German family with Albright hereditary osteodystrophy. *Eur J Pediatr* 1993;152:185–9.

185 Breslau NA, Moses AM, Pac CYC. Evidence for bone remodeling but lack of calcium mobilization response to parathyroid hormone in pseudohypoparathyroidism. *J Clin Endocrinol Metab* 1983;57:638–44.

186 Chan JCM, Alon U, Hirshman GM. Renal hypophosphatemic rickets. *J Pediatr* 1985;106:533–44.

187 Harrison HE, Harrison HC. *Disorders of Calcium and Phosphate Metabolism in Childhood and Adolescence*. Philadelphia, PA: WB Saunders, 1979:193–256.

188 Lobaugh B, Burch WM Jr, Drezner MK. Abnormalities of vitamin D metabolism and action in the vitamin D resistant rachitic and osteomalacic diseases. In: Kumar R, ed. *Vitamin D*. Boston: Nijhoff, 1984:665–720.

189 Rasmussen H, Anast C. Familial hypophosphatemic rickets and vitamin D-dependent rickets. In: Stanbury JB, Wyngaarden JB, Frederickson DS, Goldstein JL, Brown MS, eds. *The Metabolic Basis of Inherited Disease*, 5th edn. New York: McGraw-Hill, 1983:1743–73.

190 Rasmussen H, Tenenhouse HS. Hypophosphatemias. In: Scriver CR, Beaudet AL, Sly WS, Valle D, eds. *The Metabolic Basis of Inherited Disease*, 6th edn. New York: McGraw-Hill, 1989:2581–604.

191 Albright F, Butler AM, Bloom E. Rickets resistant to vitamin D therapy. *Am J Dis Child* 1937;54:529–44.

192 Monocrieff MW. Early biochemical findings in hypophosphatemic, hyperphosphaturic rickets and response to treatment. *Arch Dis Child* 1982;57:70–2.

193 Roza M, Miguel MA, Galbe M, Mejido L, Mencia C. Early treatment of familial hypophosphatemic rickets. *Arch Dis Child* 1983;58:1020–2.

194 Schimert G, Fanconi A. Early history of familial hypophosphatemic vitamin D-resistant rickets. Report of three cases observed since birth. *Helv Paediatr Acta* 1983;38: 383–98.

195 Polisson RP, Martinez S, Khoury M *et al.* Calcification of entheses associated with X-linked hypophosphatemic osteomalacia. *N Engl J Med* 1985;313:313–16.

196 Davies M, Kane R, Valentine J. Impaired hearing in X-linked hypophosphatemic (vitamin-D-resistant) osteomalacia. *Ann Intern Med* 1984;100:230–2.

197 Scriver CR, Tenenhouse HS. X-linked hypophosphataemia: a homologous phenotype in humans and mice with unusual organ-specific gene dosage. *J Inher Metab Dis* 1992;15: 610–24.

198 Lyles KW, Clark AG, Drezner MK. Serum 1,25-dihydroxyvitamin D levels in subjects with X-linked hypophosphatemic rickets and osteomalacia. *Calc Tissue Int* 1982;34:125–30.

199 Mason RS, Rohl PG, Lissner D, Posen S. Vitamin D metabolism in hypophosphatemic rickets. *Am J Dis Child* 1982; 136:909–13.

200 Scriver CR, Reade TM, DeLuca HF, Hamstra AJ. Serum 1,25-dihydroxyvitamin D levels in normal subjects and in patients with hereditary rickets or bone disease. *N Engl J Med* 1978;299:976–9.

201 Insogna KL, Broadus AE, Gertner JM. Impaired phosphorus conservation and 1,25-dihydroxyvitamin D generation during phosphorus deprivation in familial hypophosphatemic rickets. *J Clin Invest* 1983;71:1562–9.

202 Lyles KW, Drezner MK. Parathyroid hormone effects on serum 1,25-dihydroxyvitamin D levels in patients with X-linked hypophosphatemic rickets: evidence for abnormal 25-hydroxyvitamin D-1α-hydroxylase activity. *J Clin Endocrinol Metab* 1982;54:638–44.

203 Lobaugh B, Drezner MK. Abnormal regulation of renal 25-hydroxyvitamin D-1α-hydroxylase activity in the X-linked hypophosphatemic mouse. *J Clin Invest* 1983;71:400–3.

204 Stickler GB, Morgenstern BZ. Hypophosphataemic rickets: final height and clinical symptoms in adults. *Lancet* 1989; 2:902–5.

205 Balsan S, Tieder M. Linear growth in patients with hypophosphatemic vitamin D-resistant rickets: influence of treatment regimen and parenteral height. *J Pediatr* 1990; 116:365–71.

206 Drezner MK, Lyles KW, Haussler MR, Harrelson JM. Evaluation of a role for 1,25-dihydroxyvitamin D_3 in the pathogenesis and treatment of X-linked hypophosphatemic rickets and oteomalacia. *J Clin Invest* 1980;66:1020–32.

207 Dumas R, Guermoud C, Garabedian M, Meunier JP. Etudes biologiques et histomorphométriques osseuses au cours du rachitisme vitamino-résistant hypophosphatémique traité par $1,25(OH)_2$ D et phosphore. *Arch Fr Pédiatr* 1985;42: 507–10.

208 Glorieux FH, Marie PJ, Pettifor JM, Delvin EE. Bone response to phosphate salts, ergocalciferol and calcitriol in hypophosphatemic vitamin D-resistant rickets. *N Engl J Med* 1980;303:1023–31.

209 Rasmussen H, Pechet M, Anast C, Mazur A, Gertner J, Broadus AE. Long-term treatment of familial hypophosphatemic rickets with oral phosphate and 1-hydroxyvitamin D_3. *J Pediatr* 1981;99:16–25.

210 Tsuru N, Chan JCM, Chinchilli VM. Renal hypophosphatemic rickets. Growth and mineral metabolism after treatment with calcitriol (1,25-dihydroxyvitamin D_3) and phosphate supplementation. *Am J Dis Child* 1987;141: 108–10.

211 Verge CF, Lam A, Simpson JM *et al.* Effects of therapy in X-linked hypophosphatemic rickets. *N Engl J Med* 1991;325: 1843–8.

212 Alon U, Donaldson DL, Hellerstein S, Warady BA, Harris DJ. Metabolic and histologic investigation of the nature of nephrocalcinosis in children with hypophosphatemic rickets and in the Hyp mouse. *J Pediatr* 1992;120:899–905.

213 Reusz GS, Hoyer PF, Lucas M *et al.* X-linked hypophosphataemia: treatment, height gain, and nephrocalcinosis. *Arch Dis Child* 1990;65:1125–8.

214 Reusz GS, Latta K, Hoyer PF *et al.* Evidence suggesting hyperoxaluria as a cause of nephrocalcinosis in phosphate-treated hypophosphataemic rickets. *Lancet* 1990; 1:1240–3.

215 Petersen DJ, Boniface AM, Schranck FW, Rupich RC, Whyte MP. X-linked hypophosphatemic rickets: a study (with literature review) of linear growth response to calcitriol and phosphate therapy. *J Bone Miner Res* 1992; 7:583–97.

216 Wilson DM, Lee PDK, Morris AH *et al.* Growth hormone therapy in hypophosphatemic rickets. *Am J Dis Child* 1991;145:1165–70.

217 Sullivan W, Carpenter T, Glorieux FH, Travers R, Insogna K. A prospective trial of phosphate and 1,25-dihydroxyvitamin D_3 therapy in symptomatic adults with X-linked hypophosphatemic rickets. *J Clin Endocrinol Metab* 1992;75: 879–85.

218 Steendiijk R, Hauspie RC. The pattern of growth and growth retardation of patients with hypophosphatemic vitamin D-resistant rickets: a longitudinal study. *Eur J Pediatr* 1992;151:422–7.

219 Scriver CR, MacDonald W, Reade T, Glorieux FH, Nogrady B. Hypophosphatemic nonrachitic bone disease: an entity distinct from X-linked hypophosphatemia in the renal defect, bone involvement and inheritance. *Am J Med Genet* 1977;1:101–17.

220 Scriver CR, Reade T, Halal F, Costa T, Cole DE. Autosomal hypophosphatemic bone disease responds to $1,25(OH)_2D_3$. *Arch Dis Child* 1981;56:203–7.

221 Tieder M, Modai D, Samuel R *et al.* Hereditary hypophosphatemic rickets with hypercalciuria. *N Engl J Med* 1985;312:611–17.

222 Tieder M, Modai D, Shaked U *et al.* 'Idiopathic' hypercalciuria and hereditary hypophosphatemic rickets. Two phenotypical expressions of a common genetic defect. *N Engl J Med* 1987;316:125–9.

223 Tieder M, Samuel R, Liberman UA *et al.* Hypercalciuric rickets: metabolic studies and pathophysiological considerations. *Nephron* 1985;39:194–200.

224 Prader A, Illig R, Uehlinger RE, Stalder G. Rachitis infolge Knochentumors. *Helv Paediatr Acta* 1959;14:554–65.

225 Martini A, Notarangelo LD, Barberis L, Galvanini G, Rosano FP, Lanzi G. Acquired vitamin D-resistant rickets caused by prolonged latency in appearance of bone tumor. *Am J Dis Child* 1983;137:1205–6.

226 Pollack JA, Schiller AL, Crawford JD. Rickets and myopathy cured by removal of a nonossifying fibroma of bone. *Pediatrics* 1973;52:364–71.

227 Aschinenberg LC, Solomon LM, Zeis PM, Parvin J, Rosenthal IM. Vitamin D-resistant rickets associated with epidermal nevus syndrome: demonstration of a phosphaturic substance in the dermal lesions. *J Pediatr* 1977;91:55–60.

228 Brodehl J. The Fanconi syndrome. In: Edelmann CM, ed. *Pediatric Kidney Disease*. Boston: Little, Brown, 1978: 955–87.

229 Chesney RW, Mehls O, Anast CA *et al.* Renal osteodystrophy in children: the role of vitamin D, phosphorous, and parathyroid hormone. *Am J Kidney Dis* 1986;7: 275–84.

230 Cushner MHM, Adams ND. Renal osteodystrophy–pathogenesis and treatment. *Am J Med Sci* 1985;290: 234–45.

231 Aurbach GD, Marx SJ, Spiegel AM. Metabolic bone disease. In: Wilson JD, Foster DW, eds. *Williams Textbook of Endocrinology*, 8th edn. Philadelphia, PA: WB Saunders, 1992:1477–517.

232 Ritz E, Matthias S, Seidel A, Reichel H, Szabo A, Hörl WH. Disturbed calcium metabolism in renal failure–pathogenesis and therapeutic strategies. *Kidney Int* 1992; 42(Suppl. 38):S37–42.

233 Llach F, Massry SG. On the mechanism of secondary hyperparathyroidism in moderate renal insufficiency. *J Clin Endocrinol Metab* 1985;61:601–6.

234 Portale AA, Borth BE, Halldran BP, Morris RC. Effect of dietary phosphorus on circulating concentrations of 1,25-dihydroxyvitamin D and immunoreactive parathyroid hormone in children with moderate renal insufficiency. *J Clin Invest* 1984;73:1580–9.

235 Slatopolsky E. The interaction of parathyroid hormone and aluminium in renal osteodystrophy. *Kidney Int* 1987;31: 842–54.

236 Coburn J, Kanis J, Popovtzer M, Ritz E, Slatopolsky E, Fleisch H. Pathophysiology and treatment of uremic bone disease. *Calc Tissue Int* 1983;35:712–14.

237 Slatopolsky E, Berkoben M, Kelber J, Brown A, Delmez J. Effects of calcitriol and non-calcemic vitamin D analogs on secondary hyperparathyroidism. *Kidney Int* 1992;42(Suppl. 38):S43–9.

238 Inclán A, León P, Camejo MG. Tumoral calcinosis. *J Am Med Assoc* 1945;121:490–5.

239 Lakhkar BB, Lakhkar BN. Tumoral calcinosis. *Acta Paed Scand* 1991;80:474–6.

240 Lufkin EG, Wilson DM, Smith LH *et al.* Phosphorus excretion in tumoral calcinosis: response to parathyroid hormone and acetazolamide. *J Clin Endocrinol Metab* 1980;50:648–53.

241 McKee PH, Liomba NG, Hutt MSR. Tumoral calcinosis: a pathological study in 56 cases. *Br J Dermatol* 1982;107: 669–74.

242 Prince MJ, Schaefer PC, Goldsmith RS, Chausmer AB. Hyperphosphatemic tumoral calcinosis: association with elevation of serum 1,25-dihydroxycholecalciferol concentrations. *Ann Int Med* 1982;96:586–91.

243 Steinherz R, Chesney RW, Eisenstine B, Metzker A, DeLuca HF, Phelps M. Elevated serum calcitriol concentrations do not fall in response to hyperphosphatemia in familial tumoral calcinosis. *Am J Dis Child* 1985;139: 816–19.

244 Lufkin EG, Kumat R, Heath H III. Hyperphosphatemic tumoral calcinosis: effects of phosphate depletion on vitamin D metabolism, and of acute hypocalcemia on parathyroid hormone secretion and action. *J Clin Endocrinol Metab* 1983;56:1319–22.

245 Candrina R, Cerudelli B, Braga V, Salvi A. Effects of the acute subcutaneous administration of synthetic salmon calcitonin in tumoral calcinosis. *J Endocrinol Invest* 1989; 12:55–7.

246 Muldowney FP, Freaney R, Ryan JG. The pathogenesis of idiophathic hypercalciuria: evidence for a renal tubular calcium leak. *Q J Med* 1980;59:87–94.

247 Van den Berg CJ, Kumar R, Wilson DM, Heath H III, Smith LH. Orthophosphate therapy decreases urinary calcium excretion and serum 1,25-dihydroxyvitamin D concentrations in idiopathic hypercalciuria. *J Clin Endocrinol Metab* 1980;51:998–1001.

248 Foley TP, Harrison HC, Arnaud CD, Harrison HE. Familial benign hypercalcemia. *J Pediatr* 1972;81:1060–7.

249 Marx SJ, Spiegel AM, Levine MA *et al.* Familial hypocalciuric hypercalcemia. The relation to primary hyperparathyroidism. *N Engl J Med* 1982;307:416–26.

250 Davies M, Adams PH, Berry JL *et al.* Familial hypocalciuric hypercalcemia: observations on vitamin D metabolism and parathyroid function. *Acta Endocrinol* 1983;104:210–5.

251 Law WM Jr, Heath H III. Familial benign hypercalcemia (hypocalciuric hypercalcemia). Clinical and pathogenic studies in 21 families. *Ann Intern Med* 1985;102:511–19.

252 Marx SJ, Fraser D, Rapoport A. Familial hypocalciuric hypercalcemia. Mild expression of the gene in heterozygotes and severe expression in homozygotes. *Am J Med* 1985;78: 15–22.

253 Steinmann B, Gnehm HE, Rao VH, Kind HP, Prader A. Neonatal severe primary hyperparathyroidism and alkaptonuria in a boy born to related parents with familial hypercalciuric hypercalcemia. *Helv Paediatr Acta* 1984;39: 171–86.

254 Emmertsen K. Medullary thyroid carcinoma and calcitonin. *Danish Med Bull* 1985;32:1–28.

255 Norum RA, Lafreniere RG, O'Neal LW *et al.* Linkage of the multiple endocrine neoplasia type 2B gene (MEN 2B) to chromosome 10 markers linked to MEN 2A. *Genomics*

1990;8:313–17.

256 Jones BA, Sisson JC. Early diagnosis and thyroidectomy in multiple endocrine neoplasia, type 2b. *J Pediatr* 1983;102: 219–23.

257 Mathew CGP, Easton DF, Nakamura Y, Ponder BAJ. The MEN 2A International Collaborative Group: presymptomatic screening for multiple endocrine neoplasia type 2A with linked DNA markers. *Lancet* 1991;337:7–11.

258 Austin LA, Heath H III. Calcitonin: physiology and pathophysiology. *N Engl J Med* 1981;304:269–78.

259 Tashjian AW, Wright DR, Ivey SI, Pont A. Calcitonin binding sites in bone: relationships to biological response and escape. *Rec Prog Horm Res* 1978;34:285–334.

260 Obie JF, Cooper CW. Loss of calcemic effects of calcitonin and parathyroid hormone infused continuously into rats using Alzet osmotic minipumps. *J Pharmacol Exp Ther* 1979;209:422–8.

261 Deftos LJ. Pathophysiology of calcitonin secretion in different species. In: Gennari C, Segre G, eds. *The Effects of Calcitonins in Man*. Proceedings of the First International Workshop held in Florence, 2–3 April. Milan: Masson, 1982:43–53.

262 Parthemore JG. Deftos LJ. Secretion of calcitonin in primary hyperparathyroidism. *J Clin Endocrinol Metab* 1979;49:223–6.

263 Tiegs RD, Body JJ, Barta JM, Heath H III. Plasma calcitonin in primary hyperparathyroidism: failure of C-cell response to sustained hypercalcemia. *J Clin Endocrinol Metab* 1986; 63:785–8.

264 Deftos LJ, Powell D, Parthemore JG, Potts JT Jr. Secretion of calcitonin in hypocalcemic states in man. *J Clin Invest* 1973;52:3109–14.

265 Kanis JA, Earnshaw M, Heynen G, Russell RGG, Wood CG. The possible role of calcitonin deficiency in the development of bone disease due to renal failure. *Calc Tissue Res* 1977;22:147–53.

266 Canale DD, Donabedian RK. Hypercalcitoninemia in acute pancreatitis. *J Clin Endocrinol Metab* 1975;40:738–41.

267 Baker RK, Wallach S, Tashjian AH Jr. Plasma calcitonin in pycnodystosis: intermittently high basal levels and exaggerated responses to calcium and glucagon infusion. *J Clin Endocrinol Metab* 1973;37:46–55.

268 Sarnsethsiri P, Hitt OK, Eyring EJ, Frost HM. Tetracycline-based study of bone dynamics in pycnodysostosis. *Clin Orthoped* 1979;34:301–12.

269 Becker KL, Snider RH, Moore CF, Monaghan KG, Silva OL. Calcitonin in extrathyroidal tissues of man. *Acta Endocrinol* 1979;92:746–51.

270 Body J-J, Heath H III. Estimates of circulating monomeric calcitonin: physiologic studies in normal and thyroidectomized man. *J Clin Endocrinol Metab* 1983;57:897–903.

271 Kruse K, Süß A, Büsse M, Schneider P. Monomeric serum calcitonin and bone turnover during anticonvulsant treatment and in congenital hypothyroidism. *J Pediatr* 1987;111:57–63.

272 Anast CS, Guthrie RA. Decreased calcium tolerance in nongoitrous cretins. *Pediatr Res* 1971;5:668–72.

273 Carey DE, Jones KL, Parthermore JG. Calcitonin secretion in congenital nongoitrous cretinism. *J Clin Invest* 1980;65: 892–5.

274 Job J-C, Mihaud G, Rossier A, Boigné J-M, Lambertz J, Sizonenko P. Effect hypocalcémiant de la thyrocalcitonine chez l'enfant normal et l'enfant hypothyroïdien. *Pediatr Res* 1967;1:271–6.

275 McDermott MT, Kid GS, Blue P, Ghaed V, Hofeldt FD. Reduced bone mineral content in totally thyroidectomized patients: possible effect of calcitonin deficiency. *J Clin Endocrinol Metab* 1983;56:936–9.

276 Body J-J, Demeester-Mirkine N, Borkowski A, Suciu S, Corvilain J. Calcitionin deficiency in primary hypothyroidism. *J Clin Endocrinol Metab* 1986;62:700–3.

277 Coindre J-M, David J-P, Rivière L *et al.* Bone loss in hypothyroidism with hormone replacement. A histomorphometric study. *Arch Intern Med* 1986;146:48–53.

278 Hutchins GM, Mirvis SE, Mendelsohn G, Bulkley BH. Supravalvular aortic stenosis with parafollicular cell (C-cell) hyperplasia. *Am J Med* 1978;64:967–73.

279 Hitman GA, Garde L, Daoud W, Snodgrass GJAI, Cohen RD. The calcitonin–CGRP gene in the infantile hypercalcemia Williams–Beuren syndrome. *J Med Genet* 1989; 26:609–13.

280 Rússo AF, Chamany K, Klemish SW, Hall TM , Murray JC. Characterization of the calcitonin/CGRP gene in Williams syndrome. *Am J Med Genet* 1991;39:28–33.

281 Stevenson JC, White MC, Joplin GF, MacIntyre I. Osteoporosis and calcitonin deficiency. *Br Med J* 1982;285: 1010–11.

282 Chesnut CH, Baylink DJ, Sisom K, Nelp WB, Roos BA. Basal plasma immunoreactive calcitonin in postmenopausal osteoporosis. *Metabolism* 1980;29:559–62.

283 Care AD. Development of endocrine pathways in the regulation of calcium homeostasis. *Baillières Clin Endocrinol Metab* 1989;3:671–88.

284 Fisher DA. The unique endocrine milieu of the fetus. *J Clin Invest* 1986;78:603–11.

285 Pitkin RM. Human maternal–fetal calcium homeostasis. In: Holick MF, Gray TK, Anast CS, eds. *Perinatal Calcium and Phosphorus Metabolism*. Amsterdam: Elsevier, 1983: 259–79.

286 Pitkin RM. Calcium metabolism in pregnancy and the perinatal period: a review. *Am J Obstet Gynecol* 1985;151: 99–109.

287 Moore ES, Langman CB, Favus MJ, Coe FL. Role of fetal 1,25 dihydroxyvitamin D production in intrauterine phosphorus and calcium homeostasis. *Pediatr Res* 1985;19: 566–9.

288 Rodda CP, Kubota M, Heath JA *et al.* Evidence for a novel parathyroid hormone-related protein in fetal lamb parathyroid glands and sheep placenta: comparisons with a similar protein implicated in humoral hypercalcemia of malignancy. *J Endocrinol* 1988;117:261–71.

289 Abbas SK, Pickard DW, Illingworth D *et al.* Measurement of parathyroid hormone-related protein in extracts of fetal parathyroid glands and placental membranes. *J Endocrinol* 1990;124:319–25.

290 Barlet JP, Davicco M-J, Coxan V. Synthetic parathyroid-hormone related peptide (1–34) fragment stimulates placental calcium transfer in ewes. *J Endocrinol* 1990;127: 33–7.

291 Stewart AF, Broadus AE. Parathyroid hormone-related proteins: coming of age in the 1990s. *J Clin Endocrinol Metab* 1990;71:1410–14.

292 Rösli A, Fanconi A. Neonatal hypocalcemia. Early type in low birth weight newborns. *Helv Pediatr Acta* 1973;28: 443–57.

293 Tsang RC, Kleinman LJ, Sutherland JM, Light IJ. Hypocalcemia in infants of diabetic mothers. Studies in calcium, phosphorus and magnesium metabolism and parathormone responsiveness. *J Pediatr* 1972;80:394–95.

294 Tsang RC, Chen J, Hayes W, Atkinson W, Atherton H,

Edwards N. Neonatal hypocalcemia in infants with birth asphyxia. *J Pediatr* 1974;84:428–33.

295 Kruse K, Küstermann W. Evidence for transient peripheral resistance to parathyroid hormone in premature infants. *Acta Paed Scand* 1987;76:115–18.

296 David L, Glorieux FM, Salle BL, Anast CS. Human neonatal hypocalcemia. In: Holick MF, Gray TK, Anast CS, eds. *Perinatal Calcium and Phosphorus Metabolism*. Amsterdam: Elsevier, 1983:351–61.

297 Hanukoglu T, Chalew S, Kowarski A. Late-onset hypocalcemia, rickets and hypoparathyroidism in an infant of a mother with hyperparathyroidism. *J Pediatr* 1988;112: 751–4.

298 Ansprach WE, Clifton WM. Hyperparathyroidism in children: a report of two cases. *Am J Dis Child* 1939;58: 540–7.

299 Spiegel AM, Harrison HE, Marx SJ, Brown EM, Aurbach GD. Neonatal primary hyperparathyroidism with autosomal dominant inheritance. *J Pediatr* 1977;90: 269–72.

300 Cooper L, Wertheimer J, Levey R *et al.* Severe primary hyperparathyroidism in a neonate with two hypercalcemic parents: management with parathyroidectomy and heterotopic autotransplantation. *Pediatrics* 1986;78:263–8.

301 Metz SA, Hassal E. PGE, hypercalcemia and subcutaneous fat necrosis (letter). *J Pediatr* 1980;97:336.

302 Sharlin DN, Koblenzer P. Necrosis of subcutaneous fat with hypercalcemia, a puzzling and multifaceted disease. *Clin Pediatr* 1971;9:290–4.

303 Veldhuis JD, Kulin HE, Demers C, Lambert PW. Infantile hypercalcemia with subcutaneous fat necrosis. Endocrine studies. *J Pediatr* 1979;95:460–2.

304 Yasuda T, Sunami S, Ogura N, Nishioka T, Nakajima H. Infantile hypercalcemia with subcutaneous fat necrosis. Report of a case with studies on the pathogenesis of hypercalcemia. *Acta Paed Scand* 1986;75:1042–5.

305 Rasmussen H. Hypophosphatasia. In: Stanbury JB, Wyngaarden JB, Frederickson DS, Goldstein JL, Brown MS, eds. *The Metabolic Basis of Inherited Disease*, 5th edn. New York: McGraw-Hill, 1983:1497–507.

306 Lyon AJ, McIntosh N, Wheeler K, Brooke OG. Hypercalcemia in extremely low birthweight infants. *Arch Dis Child* 1984;59:1141–4.

307 Miller RR, Menke JA, Mentser MI. Hypercalcemia associated with phosphate depletion in the neonate. *J Pediatr* 1984;105:814–17.

308 Chessex P, Pineault M, Zebiche H, Ayotte RA. Calciuria in parenterally fed preterm infants: role of phosphorus intake. *J Pediatr* 1985;107:794–6.

309 Karlén J, Aperia A, Zetterström R. Renal excretion of calcium and phosphate in preterm and term infants. *J Pediatr* 1985;106:814–19.

310 Bush ME, Dahms BB. Fatal hypervitaminosis A in a neonate. *Arch Pathol Lab Med* 1984;108:838–42.

311 Tau C, Garabedian M, Farriaux JP, Czernichow P, Pomarede R, Balsan S. Hypercalcemia in infants with congenital hypothyroidism and its relation to vitamin D and thyroid hormones. *J Pediatr* 1986;109:808–14.

312 Aceto T Jr, Batt RE, Bruck E, Schultz RB, Perez YR. Intrauterine hyperparathyroidism: a complication of untreated maternal hypoparathyroidism. *J Clin Endocrinol Metab* 1966;26:487–92.

313 Bronsky D, Kiamko RT, Moncada R, Rosenthal IM. Intrauterine hyperparathyroidism secondary to maternal hypoparathyroidism. *Pediatrics* 1968;42:606–13.

314 Glass EJ, Barr DGD. Transient neonatal hyperparathyroidism secondary to maternal pseudohypoparathyroidism. *Arch Dis Child* 1981;56:565–8.

315 Landing BH, Kamoshita S. Congenital hyperparathyroidism secondary to maternal hypoparathyroidism. *J Pediatr* 1970; 77:842–7.

316 Opshaug O, Maurseth K, Howlid H, Aksnes L, Aarskog D. Vitamin D metabolism in hypophosphatasia. *Acta Paed Scand* 1982;71:517–21.

317 Koo WWK, Gupta JM, Nayanar VV, Wilkinson M, Posen S. Skeletal changes in preterm infants. *Arch Dis Child* 1982; 57:447–52.

318 Lyon AJ, McIntosh N, Wheeler K, Williams JE. Radiological rickets in extremely low birthweight infants. *Pediatr Radiol* 1987;17:56–8.

319 Tyson JE, Maravilla A, Lasky RE, Cope FA, Mize CE. Measurement of bone mineral content of preterm neonates. Reliability of the Norland densitometer. *Am J Dis Child* 1983;137:735–7.

320 James JR, Congdon PJ, Truscott J, Horsman A, Arthur R. Osteopenia of prematurity. *Arch Dis Child* 1986;61:871–6.

321 Lindroth M, Westgren U, Laurin S. Rickets of very low birthweight infants. Influence of supplementation with vitamin D, phosphorus and calcium. *Acta Paed Scand* 1986;75:927–31.

322 Bishop N. Bone disease in preterm infants. *Arch Dis Child* 1989;64:1403–9.

323 Brooke OG, Lucas A. Metabolic bone disease in preterm infants. *Arch Dis Child* 1985;60:682–5.

324 Glass EJ, Hume R, Hendry GMA, Strange RC, Forfar JO. Plasma alkaline phosphatase activity in rickets of prematurity. *Arch Dis Child* 1982;57:373–6.

325 Rowe JC, Wood DH, Rowe DW, Raisz LG. Nutritional hypophosphatemic rickets in a premature infant fed breast milk. *N Engl J Med* 1979;300:293–6.

326 Senterre J, Putet G, Salle B, Rigo J. Effects of vitamin D and phosphorus supplementation on calcium retention in preterm infants fed banked human milk. *J Pediatr* 1983; 103:305–7.

327 Steichen JJ, Gratton TL, Tsang RC. Osteopenia of prematurity: the cause and possible treatment. *J Pediatr* 1980;96:528–34.

328 Koletzko B, Tangermann R, Kries R v *et al.* Intestinal milk-bolus obstruction in formula-fed premature infants given high doses of calcium. *J Pediatr Gastroenterol Nutr* 1988;7: 548–53.

329 Attkinson SA. Calcium and phosphorus requirements of low birth weight infants: a nutritional and endocrine perspective. *Nutr Rev* 1983;41:69–78.

330 McIntosh N, De Curtis M, Williams J. Failure of mineral supplementation to reduce incidence of rickets in very-low-birthweight infants. *Lancet* 1986;2:981–2.

331 Venkataraman PS, Han BK, Tsang RC, Daugherty CC. Secondary hyperparathyroidism and bone disease in infants receiving long-term furosemide therapy. *Am J Dis Child* 1983;137:1157–61.

332 Bosley ARJ, Verrier-Jones ER, Campbell MJ. Aetiological factors in rickets of prematurity. *Arch Dis Child* 1980;55: 683–6.

333 The TS, Kallée LAA, Boon JM, Monnens LAH. Rickets in a preterm infant during intravenous alimentation. *Acta Paed Scand* 1983;72:769–71.

334 Finberg L, Dueck HS, Holmes F *et al.* Aluminium toxicity in infants and children. *Pediatrics* 1986;78:1150–4.

39: Laboratory Approach to the Child with Suspected Disorders of Calcium and Bone Metabolism

K. KRUSE

PARAMETERS AND STUDY PROTOCOL FOR LABORATORY ASSESSMENT

The most important parameters for the assessment of calcium and bone metabolism may be divided into four groups (Table 39.1).

1 Calcium and phosphate in serum and urine.

2 Parameters of parathyroid function: intact parathyroid hormone (PTH) or PTH fragments in serum; urinary cyclic adenosine monophosphate (cAMP); TmP/GFR (maximal tubular reabsorption of phosphate/glomerular filtration rate).

3 Parameters of vitamin D metabolism: 25-hydroxy-vitamin D (25-OHD) in serum; 1,25-dihydroxyvitamin D ($1,25(OH)_2D$) in serum.

4 Parameters of bone turnover: total alkaline phosphatase (AP) activity in serum; urinary hydroxyproline (OH-P); osteocalcin in serum; other markers such as cross-links in urine and bone alkaline phosphatase or type I procollagen in serum (further evaluation is needed).

These indices of mineral and bone metabolism are best measured after an overnight fast to avoid dietary influences and diurnal variation. A recommended study protocol is given in Table. 39.1. The key elements in the laboratory assessment of calcium disorders are routine measures of calcium (Ca), phosphate (P) and AP activity in serum. If persistent a disturbances are found in at least one of these indices, additional investigations should be done depending on the suspected diagnosis.

In morning urine specimens the concentrations of Ca, P, creatinine (Cr), cAMP, and OH-P are determined and the ratios of TmP/GFR (see Fig. 37.6) and cAMP/GFR (see Fig. 37.7), Ca/Cr and OH-P/Cr are calculated. Urine measurements are of little use in patients with renal insufficiency, and the levels of osteocalcin and C-terminal or midregional PTH in serum should be interpreted with caution in these patients.

In children with suspected pseudohypoparathyroidism (PHP), human PTH (hPTH) is infused and blood is taken for the determination of plasma cAMP. Additionally, urine may be collected after 30 and 60 min for the measurement of cAMP/GFR and TmP/GFR.

In patients with suspected hypercalciuria the calciuric response to a standardized oral calcium tolerance test is determined during two consecutive 2-h periods [1].

LABORATORY APPROACH TO THE CHILD WITH SUSPECTED DISORDERS OF CALCIUM AND BONE METABOLISM

In most cases the investigation of a child with a disorder of mineral and bone metabolism is rapidly and efficiently performed following the recommended study protocol. This is emphasized by presenting a laboratory approach to the differential diagnosis in patients with rickets, hypocalcaemia and hypercalcaemia.

DIFFERENTIAL DIAGNOSIS OF RICKETS

The presentation of rickets is obvious from a combination of clinical and radiographic evidence as well as elevated total serum AP (Fig. 39.1).

Normal serum PTH and urine cAMP in an untreated patient with rickets are characteristic of phosphopenic rickets, the most common type being familial X-linked hypophosphataemic rickets. These patients have normal urine Ca excretion, whereas associated hypercalciuria points either to deficient phosphate intake, especially in preterm infants, or to the rare type of hypophosphataemic rickets with hypercalciuria (see p. 757). Tumour rickets is suspected in all sporadic cases of hypophosphataemic rickets that occur late in childhood. Fanconi syndrome is associated with glycosuria and aminoaciduria. With the exception of deficient phosphate intake, hypophosphataemia develops as a consequence of disturbed tubular P reabsorption (that is reduction of TmP/GFR) and serum Ca is generally normal in phosphopenic rickets.

Secondary hyperparathyroidism in an untreated patient with rickets indicates calcium malabsorption, that is calciopenic rickets. This may result from a lack of vitamin D itself, or may be due to metabolic abnormalities in the

Table 39.1 Recommended measurements in the laboratory assessment of bone and mineral metabolism

Serum (plasma)
Ca, P, AP, Cr
Intact PTH
25-OHD
$1,25(OH)_2D$
Osteocalcin
Urine
Ca, P, Cr, cAMP, OH-P
Calculation of:
TmP/GFR
cAMP/GFR
Ca/Cr
OH-P/Cr

For abbreviations, see text.

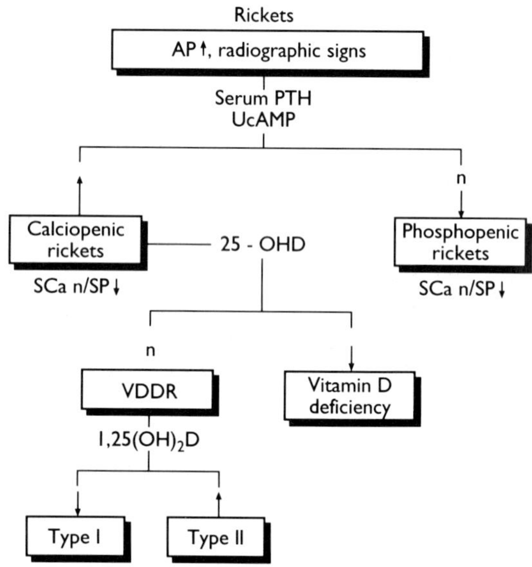

Fig. 39.1 Laboratory approach to patients with rickets. AP, total alkaline phosphatase activity in serum; n, normal; SCa/SP, serum calcium/phosphate; UcAMP, urine cAMP; VDDR, vitamin D dependency rickets.

formation and action of $1,25(OH)_2D$. There is a tendency to hypocalcaemia and hypophosphataemia. The various causes can be distinguished by measuring vitamin D metabolites. Low serum concentrations of 25-OHD are demonstrable in all forms of acquired vitamin D deficiency, including nutritional vitamin D deficiency, chronic liver disease, malabsorption or anticonvulsant rickets. In the presence of normal concentrations of 25-OHD, a low $1,25(OH)_2D$ serum level confirms the diagnosis of vitamin D dependency rickets (VDDR) type I, whereas high concentrations of $1,25(OH)_2D$ indicate VDDR type II, i.e. end-organ resistance to this hormone.

DIFFERENTIAL DIAGNOSIS OF HYPOCALCAEMIA

In the child with hypocalcaemia (with normal serum albumin) the determination of serum P, or better the TmP/GFR, is important for the differential diagnosis. Low–normal values point to calciopenic rickets and the diagnosis is established by the detection of elevated serum AP and secondary hyperparathyroidism (Figs 39.2 & 39.3).

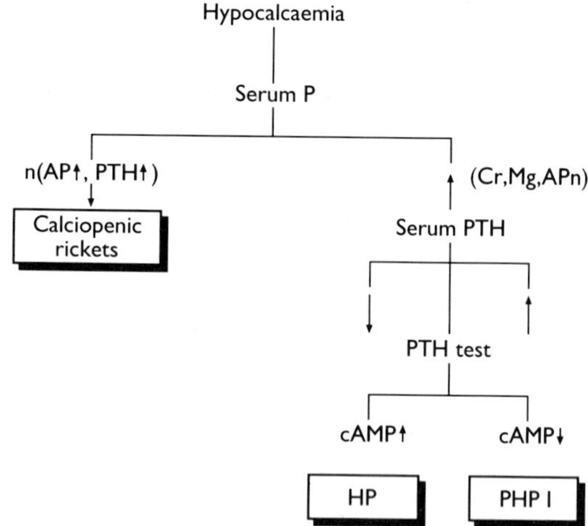

Fig. 39.2 Laboratory approach to patients with hypocalcaemia. HP, hypoparathyroidism; Mg, magnesium; n, normal; PHP, pseudohypoparathyroidism.

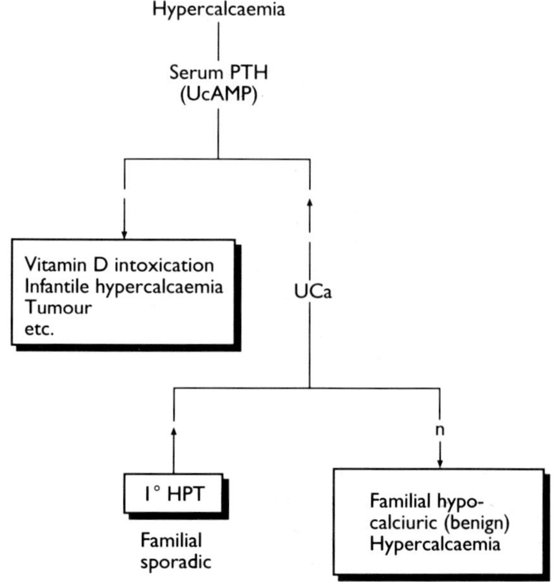

Fig. 39.3 Laboratory approach to patients with hypercalcaemia. 1°HPT, primary hyperparathyroidism; n, normal; UCa, urine calcium; UcAMP, urine cAMP.

Table 39.2 Differential diagnosis of calcium disorders in childhood [2]

	Calcium	Phosphate	Intact PTH	25-OHD	$1,25(OH)_2D$	Urine cAMP
Rickets						
Vitamin D-deficient rickets	L N	L	H	L	L N H	H
Vitamin D-dependent rickets, type I	L	L	H	N	L	H
Vitamin D-dependent rickets, type II	L	L	H	N	H	H
X-linked hypophosphataemic rickets	N	L	N	N	L N	N
Hypophosphataemic rickets with hypercalciuria	N	L	N	N	H	N
Tumour-induced rickets	N	L	N	N	L	N
Primary hyperparathyroidism	H	L	H	N	N H	H
Hypoparathyroidism	L	H	L	N	L N	L N
Pseudohypoparathyroidism, type I	L	H	H	N	L N	L N*
Vitamin D intoxication	H	N	L	H	N H	L N
Hypercalcaemia in granulomatous disorders	H	N	L	N	H	L N

* Insufficient increase after exogenous PTH.
H, high; L, low; N, normal.

In the absence of renal insufficiency and magnesium deficiency, the combination of hypocalcaemia and hyperphosphataemia indicates hypoparathyroidism (HP) or PHP. The total serum AP activity and urinary OH-P are usually normal, but may be elevated in some patients with PHP. PHP is suspected if the serum PTH level is increased, and the diagnosis is established by a blunted response in plasma and urine cAMP after PTH. In contrast, patients with HP present with low serum PTH and normal PTH response.

DIFFERENTIAL DIAGNOSIS OF HYPERCALCAEMIA

If persistent hypercalcaemia is present, the most important tool is the determination of serum PTH (and urine cAMP). Suppressed parathyroid function tests suggest vitamin D intoxication, idiopathic infantile hypercalcaemia, malignancy or other diseases listed in Table 38.5. The differential diagnosis is usually not difficult, and is based on clinical investigations together with the clinical history and additional laboratory values.

The diagnosis of primary hyperparathyroidism is confirmed by clear-cut elevations in serum PTH and urine cAMP. All families of children and adults with primary hyperparathyroidism due to hyperplastic parathyroid glands should be screened for hypercalcaemia and associated multiple endocrine neoplasia syndromes (type 1 and 2) should be excluded in each child presenting with primary hyperparathyroidism.

Urinary Ca is usually increased, being a risk factor for stone formation in patients with primary hyperparathyroidism.

The combination of hypercalcaemia with unsuppressed parathyroid function and hypocalciuria (with ratios of Ca clearance to Cr clearance lower than 0.01) suggests the diagnosis of familial hypocalciuric hypercalcaemia.

Table 39.2 summarizes the differential diagnosis of the most important disorders of calcium metabolism in childhood.

REFERENCES

1 Kruse K. Vitamin D and parathyroid. In: Ranke MB, ed. *Functional Endocrinological Diagnostics in Children and Adolescents*. Mannheim: J & J Verlag, 1992:153–67.
2 Kruse K, Kracht U, Kruse U. Reference values for urinary calcium excretion and screening for hypercalciuria in children and adolescents. *Eur J Pediatr* 1984;143:25–31.

40: Tests and Normal Values in Paediatric Endocrinology

J.M. WALKER and I.A. HUGHES

INTRODUCTION

Biochemical estimations permit the precise definition of many abnormalities of endocrine function. However, because the secretion of many hormones is pulsatile, release being controlled by negative feedback mechanisms and often following a circadian rhythm, single random measurements may not be informative and dynamic tests are frequently required. Most paediatric endocrinologists use standard protocols, but many paediatricians and trainees rightly approach such tests with trepidation, fearing their complexity, potential dangers and interpretation. However, the common aim of acquiring the maximum information from the minimum number of investigations can be achieved provided appropriate tests are chosen, meticulously planned and protocols precisely executed. There is no place either for overinvestigation or for having to repeat potentially unpleasant and painful blood sampling due to failure to apply general principles.

This chapter does not aim to reiterate what has gone before, and readers should refer to the appropriate chapter for discussion of the presenting clinical problem or detailed physiology and pathology of the disordered gland. Instead it aims firstly to emphasize the general principles, because the time when most mistakes occur is with the labelling and processing of samples, and secondly to provide the details and the pitfalls of the tests commonly used in children. Where appropriate, we offer advice on the following four parameters:

1 background and/or indications;
2 precautions and/or preparation;
3 protocol;
4 interpretation of results.

References are supplied but detailed hormone results may not always be given, since the values are so laboratory-dependent.

GENERAL PRINCIPLES FOR ALL ENDOCRINE TESTS

Patient preparation

The following questions should be addressed.

1 Is there an indication to perform the planned test based on detailed clinical evaluation? Are there other tests which should be done first either to exclude other causes for the same problem (for example full blood count in short stature), or to facilitate interpretation of the results (for example thyroid function before tests of growth hormone secretion)? Should the opinion be sought of a paediatric endocrinologist and/or an endocrine clinical biochemist before embarking?

2 Are the medical, nursing and ward staff adequately briefed on their part in the protocol?

3 Are the laboratory staff aware of the test and the need for any urgent processing or analysis of samples?

4 Is the parent/guardian fully informed of the procedure (need to keep fasted, etc.)?

5 Is the child adequately prepared?

(a) Fasting: 4–6 h in infant, 8 h in older child.

(b) Is he or she clinically well?

(c) Have any interfering foodstuffs or medication been eliminated (for example bananas before urinary vanillylmandelic acid (VMA) analysis, or fish before radioactive iodine uptake)?

6 Has the height and weight of the child been measured on the day of the test?

7 Has the dose of the stimulatory/suppressive agent been calculated correctly, the calculation checked with another member of staff and has the agent been correctly prepared (for example insulin dose for insulin stress test) and checked?

If there is any doubt seek advice.

Sample collection

BLOOD

1 Secure a reliable i.v. line for serial blood sampling and maintain patent with a heparin/saline solution (1 U/ml).
2 Collect basal samples including a sample taken at time of i.v. insertion (time (T) = −30 min) as the stress this generates may be adequate to stimulate hormone production. Following this there may be a spell of gland quiescence producing false-positive results if samples are only taken from $T = 0$ (for example in growth hormone secretion tests).
3 Ensure correct sample tubes are available and labelled with times as well as patient number.
4 Are the required blood volumes known?

URINE

1 Make sure the child and parent(s) understand how to collect a timed, usually overnight or 24-h, urine sample. Provide written instructions. (A funnel greatly assists girls to collect urine.)
2 Is there a suitable container? Does it require a preservative?

SALIVA

1 Make sure the child and parent(s) understand how to collect samples: that is rinse the mouth with tap water to remove any food debris; after 1–2 min whole saliva is collected by gentle dribbling into a wide-necked plain tube.
2 If necessary stimulate saliva flow using a drop of citric acid on the tip of the tongue.

Sample processing

1 Blood tubes/urine containers to be labelled with:
(a) name of patient;
(b) ward/clinic;
(c) hospital number;
(d) date of sample;
(e) time into test of sample, for example 0, 30, 60 min. etc., not clock time; start and finish time of 24-h urine test.
2 Laboratory request forms; write legibly:
(a) name of patient;
(b) age;
(c) sex;
(d) ward/clinic;
(e) hospital number;
(f) date of test;
(g) time of sample (start and finish of 24-h urine test);
(h) tests required;
(i) clinical details of relevance.
3 Transporting samples:
(a) ensure rapid transport to appropriate laboratory;
(b) if in doubt, transport sample *personally*.

ANTERIOR PITUITARY GLAND

The anterior pituitary gland secretes growth hormone (GH), thyroid-stimulating hormone (TSH), adrenocorticotrophic hormone (ACTH), prolactin (PRL), luteinizing hormone (LH) and follicle-stimulating hormone (FSH). Their synthesis and secretion are controlled by hypothalamic-releasing or -inhibiting factors. Four of these factors, thyrotrophin-releasing hormone (TRH), gonadotrophin-releasing hormone or luteinizing-hormone-releasing hormone (GnRH or LHRH), corticotrophin-releasing hormone or factor (CRH or CRF) and growth-hormone-releasing hormone (GHRH) have been synthesized and can be used in clinical tests. However, their application is somewhat limited because the response is a measure of the readily releasable pituitary reserve and not of the function of the hypothalamopituitary axis.

The function of the hypothalamopituitary axis is often better assessed by baseline tests or by clinical observation of normally functioning target tissues (for example a clinically and biochemically euthyroid child must have an intact thyroid axis, and one progressing normally through spontaneous puberty is highly likely to have an intact gonadal axis). Alternatively stimulation tests may be required to 'kick start' the axis, either by inducing stress, as in the insulin stress test, or by the use of substances known to stimulate the hypothalamus, such as clonidine.

Growth hormone deficiency

The multiplicity of tests available for diagnosing GH deficiency (GHD), which is synonymous with deletion of the GH gene but loosely applied to include the much commoner problem of GH insufficiency, indicates that none is ideal. GH secretion is maximal during sleep and is pulsatile. Hence either testing has to take place after the onset of sleep (which may be disturbed by the very fact of being in hospital) with multiple sampling to 'catch' a pulse, or GH production has to be stimulated during the day. If a pulse is missed, an incorrect diagnosis of GHD may be made and such false-positive results are seen in approximately 15% of normal individuals with all the stimulation tests in current use. There is a similar false-negative rate and some clinicians thus insist on two tests to support their diagnosis. This is not very sensible because the falsity of results is compounded. Thyroid function must also be normal, to interpret the results.

Many of the stimuli are potent pharmacological agents, and a response to these may have little bearing on the child's day-to-day GH production. In any test where a pulse peak response is required to *exclude* GHD, this is defined as being > 26 mU/l based on the new International Standard introduced in 1991 (> 20mU/l prior to 1991). However, it is emphasized that this is an arbitrary level and the results of all tests must be interpreted in conjunction with clinical features, especially auxology. Clinicians should also be aware that different GH assays have different bias (as well as accuracy). A level quoted by one method does *not* equate with that generated by another. If these tests are used, the clinician must understand the assay limitations, and must use a laboratory where both external and internal quality control data are available.

Assessment of insulin-like growth factors (IGFs) and their binding proteins (BPs) may improve discrimination between normal and abnormal. Low levels of IGF-I may support the diagnosis of GHD but can occur in other situations, such as malnutrition. Specificity appears to be improved by also assaying IGF-II. IGFBP-3 appears to be a promising alternative [1] but is still undergoing evaluation.

SEX STEROID PRIMING

Any child with delayed puberty may have associated physiological blunting of GH secretion. Thus reduced levels on testing at this stage may not be pathological. To differentiate this situation from true GHD, prepubertal boys > 11 years and girls > 10 years should be 'primed' with sex steroids prior to physiological or pharmacological testing. Those into puberty need no treatment. To minimize the effect on auxology the treatment of choice is ethinyloestradial 20 μg/day. p.o. for the 3 days before admission in girls (some children may feel sick), and Sustanon 100 mg i.m. 3–5 days before testing in boys.

PHYSIOLOGICAL TESTS

Overnight or 24-h profiles

INDICATIONS

Short stature and/or consistent abnormally low growth velocity not explained by simpler tests.
Postcranial radiotherapy.
Other known hypothalamopituitary lesions.

These techniques should be reserved for research purposes and will not be described in detail. In the normal person a peak of GH secretion occurs 1–1.5 h after sleep commences. An electroencephalogram (EEG) at the time might show stage IV sleep, but this so variable that there is no indication for EEG monitoring. The half-life of GH is 20–25 min and samples must therefore be taken at least every 20 min and are usually taken for a 12- or 24-h period. Thus it is a time-consuming, labour-intensive and expensive exercise.

For purely clinical purposes it is possible to restrict the sampling period to the first 90 min after the onset of sleep, in the hope of catching one of the GH peaks [2], but the absence of an adequate peak does not confirm GHD.

Urinary growth hormone

BACKGROUND/INDICATIONS

Short stature and/or consistent abnormally low growth velocity.
Postcranial radiotherapy.
Other known hypothalamopituitary lesions.

Several assays sensitive enough to measure GH in urine are now well established [3,4]. The test has the major advantages of being performed at home, non-invasive and safe. There is no more intraindividual variance than in other tests in current use, and this is reduced by obtaining serial samples, a prohibitive exercise with blood tests. The results correlate well with clinical diagnoses [5] and with pharmacological stimulation tests [6].

PRECAUTIONS/PREPARATION

No preparation necessary.
Renal function must be normal.
Bladder control required.
Thyroid function normal.
Assays vary considerably and results should be obtained from laboratories experienced with urinary assays which produce robust, valid results.

PROTOCOL

For overnight profile give parents plain 24-h urine bottle to take home plus the following written instructions:

1 Empty bladder before going to bed and discard urine; record time on bottle.

2 Collect any urine passed during the night after onset of sleep plus *all* of first urine passed the following morning. Record time on bottle.

3 Ensure sample reaches laboratory within 24 h of collection.

INTERPRETATION

Results below the reference range for the assay suggest GHD and a single value may be a useful screening test, especially if normal. However, exercise caution in interpreting single values, especially at the lower limit of normal, and also if the volume is low. Multiple samples reduce the variance and, if consistently low, are probably as diagnostic of GHD as blood tests. Levels can be very high in patients with excess GH secretion.

Exercise test [7]

INDICATIONS

Short stature and/or consistent abnormally low growth velocity.
Postcranial radiotherapy.
Other known hypothalamopituitary lesions.

PRECAUTIONS/PREPARATION

Can be performed in outpatients safely but *must* be properly organized, which severely limits its usefulness.
Thyroid function normal.

PROTOCOL

1 Bicycle ergometer used to generate a standard amount of work which varies according to age and size of child. Aim for 150–300 kilopond m/min for 10 min.
T = 0, 10 (end of exercise) and 30 min: serum GH.
2 Exercise by running up and down stairs for 20 min. Child should be tired but not exhausted with pulse < 180/min (check during exercise).
T = 0, 20 (end of exercise) and 40 min: serum GH.

INTERPRETATION

GH > 26 mU/l excludes GHD. However, a value < 26 mU/l does not diagnose GHD. Exercise does not invariably produce GH release, the sample timing may have missed the peak or, most likely, the exercise was inadequate. Priming with propranolol 0.5 mg/kg (max. 40 mg) 1 h before the test may enhance the GH response, but carries a risk of hypoglycaemia.

PHARMACOLOGICAL TESTS

In recent years some of these tests have fallen into disrepute because of concerns over safety. The major pro-

Table 40.1 Common pharmacological tests of growth hormone release

Agent	Dose	Precautions/notes	Sampling interval (min)	Sampling time* (min)	Tests available
Insulin	See text				
Clonidine [9]	0.15 mg/m^2 p.o.	α-Adrenergic agonist. Causes hypotension and drowsiness rarely needing treatment. Measure BP ½-hourly until 1 h after test. Keep in hospital until awake. May be superseded by guanfacine	30	−30 to 150	GH
Arginine [10]	0.5 g/kg i.v. over 30 min	Replaced 'Bovril' test. Can cause nausea and irritation at i.v. site	30	−30 to 90	GH
Glucagon [11]	15 μg/kg s.c. This dose is adequate to stress axis and is safer than 100 μg/kg	Drop in glucose after initial rise is probable stimulus to hormone release. Suitable for children < 2 years. Frequently causes nausea, vomiting and abdominal pain	30	−30 to 150	GH Cortisol
L-Dopa [12]	< 14 kg = 125 mg; 15–32 kg = 250 mg; > 32 kg = 500 mg p.o.	Frequently causes nausea and vomiting	30	−30 to 90	GH
GHRH [13]	2 μg/kg i.v.	Facial flushing. Tests only pituitary reserve. Very variable response makes interpretation difficult. Research use only		−30, −15, 0, 15, 30, 60, 90, 120	GH

* Take a sample at the time of cannula insertion (T = −30 min) because the stress involved may stimulate GH secretion. This may be followed by a period of gland quiescence leading to an inappropriate diagnosis of GHD should this sample be missed.
BP, blood pressure.

blems have not been with the tests themselves, but with using inappropriate amounts of hyperosmolar fluid to correct the hypoglycaemic stimulus some of the agents produce. This can result in cerebral oedema and death [8]. Some units have replaced the tests that produce hypoglycaemia with others from the battery available. However, the fact is that any pharmacological test is potentially dangerous, and any unit performing such tests should have locally agreed protocols to include safety guidelines. Only two or three tests should be available, and they should be performed by experienced staff in a dedicated clinical investigation ward. Table 40.1 summarizes the details of the most widely used tests and potential problems associated with them.

The use of the clonidine test [9] is restricted by the drowsiness and hypotension it produces. This rarely needs active treatment but it can delay discharge home. Clonidine may be replaced by guanfacine, an α_2-agonist which has similar GH-releasing potency but fewer side-effects [14]. The insulin stress test is discussed in detail because it is still in common use, and guidelines regarding the management of the hypoglycaemia are important.

General details for all pharmacological tests

INDICATIONS

Short stature and/or consistent abnormally low growth velocity.
Postcranial radiotherapy.
Other known hypothalamopituitary lesions.

PRECAUTIONS/PREPARATION

Thyroid function normal.
Prime if necessary (see above).
Fasting and resting in bed.
Insert venous cannula and maintain patent with heparinized normal saline.

PROTOCOL

Table 40.1 summarizes the details of the most widely used tests and potential problems associated with them.
Patients should not go home until they have eaten and retained a full meal.
Can be combined with TRH±LHRH tests (q.v.).

INTERPRETATION

A normal response to stimulation is defined as a peak in the blood >26 mU/l at any time, but this level is arbitrary and requires interpretation in the light of other clinical findings.

Insulin stress test

BACKGROUND

There is extensive experience with the insulin stress test (IST), but it is no more the 'gold standard' for GH secretion than any other of the tests described. It does have the advantage of simultaneously testing ACTH reserve. Deaths have occurred, and the decision to undertake an IST should be carefully considered. Experienced medical and nursing supervision is obligatory.

PRECAUTIONS/PREPARATION

As above.
Contraindicated in children with epilepsy.
Contraindicated in children <2 years.
A doctor must be in attendance throughout the test.
Intravenous 10% dextrose (*not* 50%) and hydrocortisone must be immediately available.

PROTOCOL

1 $T = 0$ min: give soluble insulin 0.05–0.15 U/kg i.v., using the lower dose if there is a strong suspicion of panhypopituitarism.

2 Flush the i.v. line to ensure all the insulin has been given, because the volume is likely to be very small.

3 T −30, 0, 15, 30, 45, 60 and 90 min: blood glucose, cortisol and GH. Measure dextrostix for immediate blood glucose, but true glucose should be measured urgently and the result should be telephoned to the ward.

4 Observe and record symptoms and signs of hypoglycaemia.

5 Aim for true glucose less than half the fasting value or <2.2 mmol/l. If patient is not clinically or biochemically hypoglycaemic by 45 min repeat the dose.

6 Once hypoglycaemia has occurred, it can be terminated with oral glucose drinks without affecting the results. Prolonged hypoglycaemia, impending loss of consciousness or fits should be treated with i.v. dextrose 200 mg/kg (2 ml/kg 10% dextrose) over 3 min followed by 10 mg/kg min^{-1} (0.1 ml/kg min^{-1} 10% dextrose). Check a dextrostix at 5 min and adjust dextrose infusion to maintain blood glucose at 5–8 mmol/l and no higher. If there is no improvement in conscious level after normal glucose level is restored, an alternative explanation should be sought.

7 Give 100 mg hydrocortisone i.v. if panhypopituitarism is suspected.

8 Continue to take samples as an adequate stress will have been induced.
9 Patients may be safely discharged once they have eaten and drunk without vomiting at the end of the test.
10 This test may run concurrently with an LHRH ± TRH test (q.v.).

INTERPRETATION

GH as above.
Cortisol rises by >170 nmol/l to >550 nmol/l in normal subjects.

Growth hormone excess

Urinary GH (as well as serum IGF-I and IGFBP-3) levels are elevated above normal, and this test may be of continued value for follow-up after surgery. The diagnostic test is the failure to suppress GH levels during a standard oral glucose tolerance test (q.v.).

Other releasing hormone tests

Thyrotrophin-releasing hormone (Protirelin) test

BACKGROUND/INDICATIONS

Investigation of secondary hypothyroidism.
Diagnosis of thyrotoxicosis has been supplanted by highly sensitive TSH assays.
Investigation of hyperprolactinaemia.

PRECAUTIONS/PREPARATION

Non-fasting (unless combined with test of GH secretion).
May cause mild flushing and desire to micturate.

PROTOCOL

1 $T = 0$: 7 µg/kg TRH (Protirelin), 200 µg max., i.v. over 1 min.
2 $T = 0$, 20 (30 in combined GH test) and 60 min: serum TSH and prolactin.

INTERPRETATION

Normal: TSH peaks at 10–30 mU/ml at 20 min. A slightly increased basal level with a delayed and exaggerated response suggestive but not conclusive of hypothalamic hypothyroidism. A raised basal prolactin (6–800 mU/l) may suggest a functional disconnection, between hypothalamus and pituitary (for example a stalk lesion). Levels >1000 mU/l with a poor response to TRH ($<$ doubling of basal value) may suggest a prolactinoma (see below).

Gonadotrophin-releasing hormone (luteinizing-hormone-releasing hormone) test

BACKGROUND/INDICATIONS

Investigation of hypogonadotrophic hypogonadism suspected prepubertally. LH and FSH are normally secreted in a pulsatile fashion, which is a rare event prepubertally. Hence a low response has limited predictive value in prepubertal children but an absent response is helpful. In pubertal years the test does not add more than can be learned from basal concentration of LH and FSH. It also adds very little to the clinical diagnosis of central, gonadotrophin-dependent, precocious puberty. In gonadotrophin-independent precocious puberty, especially testotoxicosis (rare), the response is blunted.

PRECAUTIONS/PREPARATION

Non-fasting (unless combined with a test of GH secretion).
No side-effects.

PROTOCOL

1 $T = 0$: 100 µg (2.5 µg/kg) GnRH (LHRH) i.v.
2 $T = 0$, 30 and 60 min: serum LH and FSH.

INTERPRETATION

Prepubertal: LH increment 3–4 U/l and FSH increment 2–3 U/l.
Peripubertal: higher increments, especially LH, may suggest that the signs of puberty are imminent.
Exaggerated response in primary gonadal failure but elevated basal LH and FSH levels are usually adequate to make this diagnosis.

Corticotrophin-releasing hormone test

INDICATIONS

Differential diagnosis of Cushing syndrome.
For details see Cushing syndrome.

Prolactin

Prolactinomas are extremely rare in childhood and are usually diagnosed on the basis of grossly elevated basal levels. Prolactin is a stress hormone and falsely high values may occur with venepuncture. Serial sampling through an indwelling catheter may be necessary.

A blunted response to a TRH test may indicate a prolactinoma, but this is controversial.

POSTERIOR PITUITARY GLAND

Antidiuretic hormone/water deprivation test

BACKGROUND/INDICATIONS

The water deprivation test measures urinary concentrating ability which is lost in patients with diabetes insipidus (DI) but maintained in compulsive water drinking (CWD). Pituitary and nephrogenic DI may be differentiated by giving a test dose of desamino-D-arginine vasopressin (DDAVP).

PRECAUTIONS/PREPARATION

This is not an easy test in children and requires scrupulous attention to detail. It requires the active cooperation of the laboratory which must be arranged ahead of time. Osmolality values are required as soon as the specimens have been collected.

Care must be taken in patients with clinical DI or where the likelihood of DI is very high, for example Langerhans cell histiocytosis or postsurgery for craniopharyngioma. These tests must take place during the daytime. If the child generally goes overnight without drinking, CWD is likely. Starving such children, and especially toddlers, during the day may be impossible, and the wait for specimens prohibitive. In this instance it may be appropriate to conduct the test overnight with collection of plasma and the first and second urines passed after waking for osmolality. This decision should be made by a member of staff experienced with both the test and the child, with strict instructions to the staff about termination if there is frank polyuria.

Thyroid and adrenal reserve must be normal or adequately replaced.

No food following light breakfast.

Fluids *ad libitum* until start of test.

PROTOCOL

For standard water deprivation test: weigh child, calculate 97.5% of this and record it on chart.

1 $T = 0$ min: empty bladder. Take samples of urine and blood for osmolality and electrolytes.

2 Collect all further urine samples passed after this in separate aliquots, record volume, and send for osmolality. These results should be telephoned back to the ward as soon as available.

3 Observe carefully. Children with DI will drink from anything.

4 Weigh 2-hourly. If weight falls below 97.5% starting weight, *stop*. Continued deprivation is both dangerous and cruel.

5 Continue for 12 h if necessary. The test can be stopped at any time if the laboratory results exclude DI. It may be necessary to prolong the test in CWD, especially if the child has been drinking excessively immediately prior to the start.

6 At end-point take further blood and urine samples for osmolality and electrolytes.

7 If no evidence of urinary concentration, give DDVAP 5 μg intranasally or 0.3 μg intramuscularly, and collect urine in aliquots over the next 3 h, with final blood osmolality.

INTERPRETATION

Normal and CWD: plasma (P) osmolality does not exceed 295 mosmol/kg and the urine (U) osmolality rises threefold to >750 mosmol/kg or U:P ratio >2.0. A U:P <2.0 and plasma osmolality <295 mosmol/kg at the end of the fast indicates that fluid deprivation has not been adequate. The test may need repeating if DI is really suspected, but if fasted for 12–16 h these results exclude clinically significant DI.

Central DI: plasma osmolality >295 mosmol/kg with inappropriately dilute urine (U:P <2.0). DDAVP produces normally concentrated urine.

Nephrogenic DI: as for central DI but DDAVP produces no response.

Plasma and urinary levels of ADH are inappropriately elevated for the range of osmolalities. See Chapter 32 for detailed interpretation of results using the graphs shown.

THYROID GLAND

Although a large number of thyroid tests are available, they can be divided functionally into two.

1 A resting thyroid profile, which should define a state of euthyroidism, hypothyroidism or hyperthyroidism.

2 Further tests used to establish the aetiology of any thyroid disease.

Measurements of serum TSH, free thyroxine (FT_4) and sometimes also free triiodothyronine (FT_3) are usually sufficient as a thyroid profile. Free thyroid hormone assays have largely superseded total T_4 and T_3 measurements. The sensitive TSH assays now readily available are used for the diagnosis of hyperthyroidism and to document excessive thyroid hormone treatment. Beware the low TSH and borderline low FT_4 which can indicate secondary hypothyroidism. Reverse T_3 measurement has no use clinically. Thyroglobulin measurements are useful to monitor treatment of metastatic thyroid cancer, but they are less reliable as an index of thyroid mass in infants with congenital hypothyroidism.

Tests to determine the nature and cause of thyroid dysfunction include measurement of thyroid autoantibodies, thyroid scinitigraphy and fine-needle biopsy of the thyroid. Thyroglobulin, microsomal (peroxidase) and colloid antibodies are usually present in autoimmune thyroiditis and frequently in Graves disease. The latter condition is typically associated with immunoglobulin G (IgG) autoantibodies that bind directly to the thyroid TSH receptor (TSH-R) and are stimulatory in nature (TSH-RAb or TSAb). TSH-R blocking antibodies (TBAb) may play a part in hypothyroidism, but they are technically difficult to measure and their relative importance is uncertain.

Thyroid scintigraphy can be used to detect thyroid tissue (for example congenital hypothyroidism), locate ectopic tissue, define the extent of a goitre and establish the nature of a thyroid nodule. The preferred isotopes are [^{99}Tc^{m}]pertechnecate and [^{123}I]sodium iodide. The dose of the latter is 0.1 MBq (2.7 μCi) in infants, whereas a proportion of the adult dose (1 MBq) based on body weight is used in older children. If dyshormonogenesis is suspected, potassium perchlorate should be given orally at the 1-h uptake. More than 60% of the accumulated radioactivity is discharged within 1 h in dyshormonogenesis associated with an organification defect. The dose of perchlorate ranges from 100 to 400 mg according to the age of the child.

Medullary carcinoma of the thyroid

These tumours comprise approximately 5% of all thyroid cancers and 25% of cases occur in the multiple endocrine neoplasia syndrome, MEN-2A, whose components include hyperparathyroidism and phaeochromocytoma. This is inherited in an autosomal dominant fashion. Others are part of MEN -2B or -3 (Chapter 2). Medullary carcinoma of the thyroid (MCT) secretes, among other things, excess calcitonin, the hormone normally secreted by thyroid parafollicular (C) cells to lower plasma calcium. This may be used as a screening test for MCT. Basal calcitonin levels are elevated when a tumour is present, but for screening children at risk it is usually necessary to perform a pentagastrin stimulation test to demonstrate an exaggerated calcitonin response.

Pentagastrin stimulation test

INDICATIONS

Screening for MCT.

PRECAUTIONS/PREPARATION

Check fasting calcium to exclude hypocalcaemia.
Fasting.
Can cause transient chest tightness, flushing and nausea.

PROTOCOL

1 $T = 0$: collect baseline plasma calcitonin. Inject pentagastrin 0.5 μg/kg i.v. rapidly over 10–20 s.
2 $T = 2, 5, 10, 15$ and 20 min: plasma calcitonin.

INTERPRETATION

An exaggerated response with an abnormally high peak suggests MCT.
If positive the child should be screened for other MEN components.

ADRENAL GLAND

Cortisol deficiency

The term 'primary adrenal failure' usually refers to glucocorticoid deficiency (with or without mineralocorticoid deficiency) as a result of gland destruction either by autoantibodies or by rarer causes such as tuberculosis. Glucocorticoid production can also be insufficient due to an inborn error of steroidogenesis (congenital adrenal hyperplasia (CAH)), considered later. Secondary adrenal failure is due to gland atrophy as a result of decreased stimulation by ACTH and is usually either iatrogenic as a consequence of glucocorticoid treatment or due to prolonged ACTH deficiency. Primary adrenal failure is best confirmed by a synthetic ACTH (Synacthen) test. This may also be abnormal in long-standing adrenal atrophy. Resistance to ACTH action can cause isolated centres of deficiency.

Tetracosactrin (Synacthen) tests

BACKGROUND/INDICATIONS

Screening test for primary adrenal hypofunction.
Synacthen is a synthetic analogue of ACTH which is as active biologically but is less antigenic and therefore safer, although severe allergic reactions have been described. Initially the short Synacthen test is performed as a screening procedure. If this fails to show a rise in cortisol, then the long Synacthen test can be performed. The standard doses of Synacthen shown below are vastly in excess of what is required to stimulate the gland, and a more sensitive test may be to use only 500 ng [15,16] but this is not yet in common practice.

A short Synacthen test may also be useful in the diagnosis of defects of steroid biosynthesis such as non-classical CAH (see below).

PRECAUTIONS/PREPARATION

Non-fasting.
Allergy to Synacthen.

PROTOCOL

Short Synacthen test

1 Insert venous cannula for sampling and rest patient for 30 min.
2 $T = 0$: basal plasma or saliva cortisol.
3 Inject Synacthen. 0–6 months: 36 μg/kg i.v. or i.m.; 6 months–2 years: 0.125 mg i.v. or i.m.; >2 years: 0.25 mg i.v. or i.m.
4 $T = 30$ and 60 min: plasma or saliva cortisol.

Long Synacthen test

1 Day 1: basal cortisol, plasma or saliva; depot Synacthen 1 mg i.m.
2 Day 2: depot Synacthen 1 mg i.m.
3 Day 3: depot Synacthen 1 mg i.m.; plasma or saliva cortisol 4–6 h later.

INTERPRETATION

Normal: two to three-fold increase in plasma cortisol to >550 nmol/l in both tests. Saliva cortisol increases seven-fold due to the greater proportion of cortisol which is unbound.
Primary adrenal failure: no response to either test.
Adrenal atrophy: blunted response to the short test and a greater increase with depot Synacthen.

Defects in adrenal steroid biosynthesis

There are marker steroids whose measurement, even basally, may help to define the enzyme defect. Generally these are the compounds before the block in the metabolic pathway. Thus plasma 17-hydroxyprogesterone (17-OHP) and 11-deoxycortisol concentrations are elevated in CAH due to 21-hydroxylase and 11β-hydroxylase enzyme deficiencies, respectively. In 3β-hydroxysteroid dehydrogenase deficiency, the appropriate steroids to measure are dehydroepiandrosterone and 17-OH-pregnenolone, but 17-OHP may be elevated because of liver 3β-hydroxysteroid dehydrogenase (3β-HSD) activity.

A short Synacthen test (q.v.) may be used to accentuate the abnormal steroid levels. This may be particularly useful in non-classical CAH where baseline levels of pre-block steroids may be normal or borderline, but abnormally elevated when stressed by ACTH. Thus both 17-OHP and cortisol assays should be requested. Other steroids which are secondarily elevated in plasma, depending on the type of enzyme defect, include progesterone, androstenedione and testosterone. Detailed analysis of urinary steroid metabolites by gas chromatographic techniques helps to delineate the enzyme defect precisely.

The antenatal management of women suspected of carrying a fetus affected by an enzyme defect is dealt with fully in Chapter 30. The point to emphasize is that clinicians should liaise closely with genetic colleagues as soon as possible after the proband's birth to ensure that appropriate DNA analyses are performed in these families well before another pregnancy occurs.

Cortisol excess/Cushing syndrome

Investigations are aimed at answering two questions.
1 Does the child have hypercortisolism?
2 If so, what is the source?

Figure 40.1 shows a flowchart of investigation of possible Cushing syndrome. Measurement of plasma cortisol at 0800–0900 and 2400 h is one of the baseline investigations for hypercortisolism. The night-time value is normally 50% or less of the early-morning value. A stressful venepuncture can cause a marked increase in cortisol level. Measurement of cortisol in saliva offers a practical solution to this problem, as does 24-h urinary free cortisol estimation. Consistently low levels suggest the aetiology is exogenous steroids, such as in asthma, with secondary adrenal suppression. The metyrapone test does not give consistent results in the differential diagnosis of Cushing syndrome, may be dangerous in children and is no longer in routine use. Details of the specific tests are given below.

Overnight dexamethasone suppression test

BACKGROUND/INDICATIONS

Screening test for Cushing syndrome. Dexamethasone is used as it is a potent synthetic steroid with a long half-life which does not significantly interfere with the laboratory estimations of cortisol.

PRECAUTIONS/PREPARATION

Nil.

PROTOCOL

1 Day 1: plasma cortisol at 2300–2400 h; dexamethasone

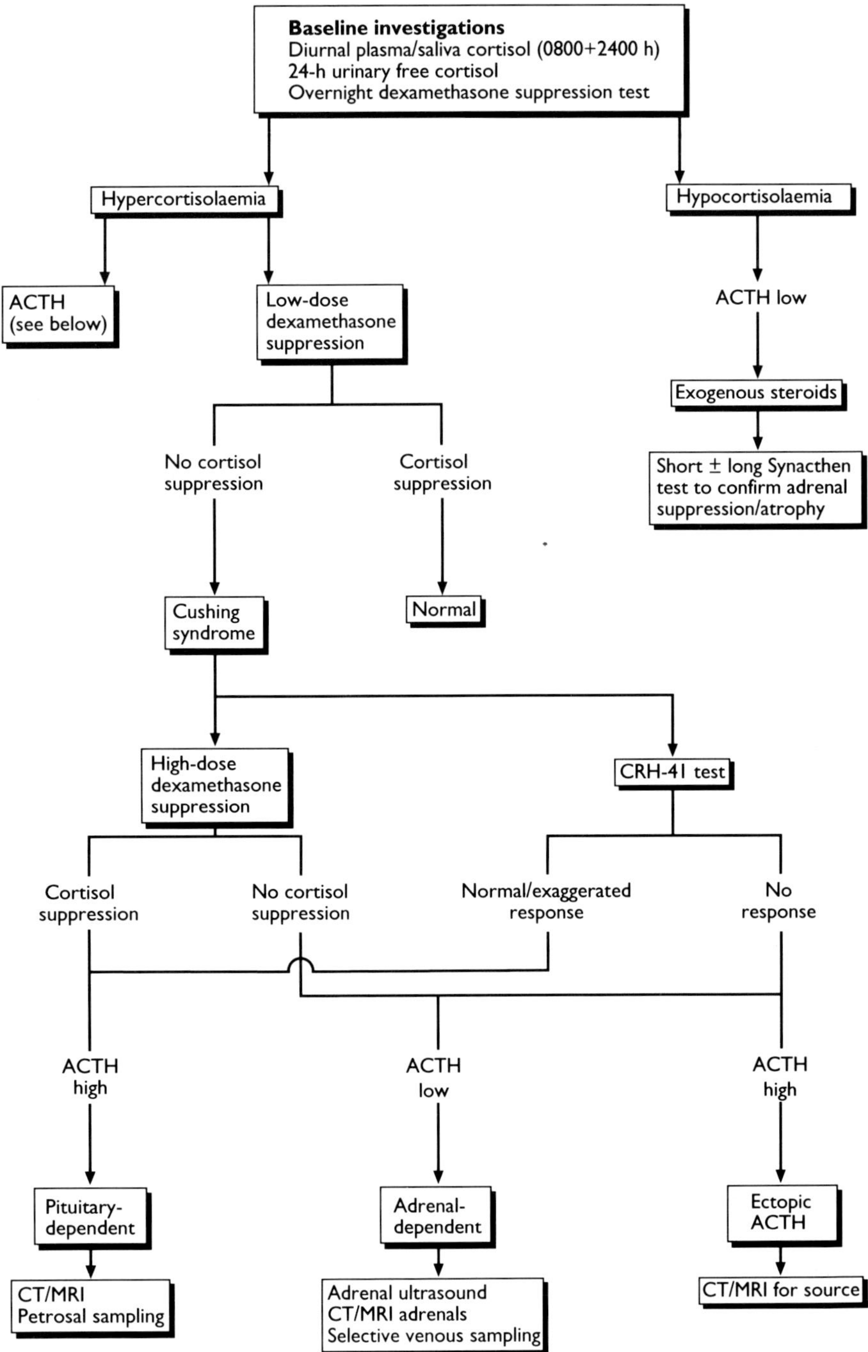

Fig. 40.1 Flowchart for the investigation of Cushing syndrome.

1 mg orally at 2300–2400 h.

2 Day 2: plasma cortisol and ACTH at 0800 h.

Saliva cortisol is a useful alternative, particularly for the obese ruddy-faced child in whom the question of Cushing syndrome has been raised. If blood is needed for ACTH, plasma samples via an indwelling cannula are more appropriate.

INTERPRETATION

Midnight cortisol levels are normally low. If the child is normal or simply obese, low-dose dexamethasone will suppress ACTH and hence the usual cortisol surge at 0800 h. Absent cortisol suppression requires a more prolonged dexamethasone suppression test.

Low-dose dexamethasone test

INDICATIONS

Diagnosis of Cushing syndrome.

PRECAUTIONS/PREPARATION

Nil.

PROTOCOL

1 Day 1: plasma cortisol and ACTH at 0800 and 2400 h.
2 Days 2+3: give dexamethasone 5 μg/kg p.o. strictly 6-hourly (children > 10 years standard adult dose of 0.5 mg q.d.s.).
3 Day 4: plasma cortisol and ACTH at 0800 and 2400 h.

INTERPRETATION

Plasma cortisol < 50 nmol/l on day 4 excludes Cushing syndrome.
Failure to suppress confirms hypercortisolism, but does not necessarily provide information about the cause.

High-dose dexamethasone test

INDICATIONS

Differential diagnosis of Cushing syndrome.

PRECAUTIONS/PREPARATION

Nil.

PROTOCOL

Identical to low-dose test protocol except 2 mg dexamethasone is given 6-hourly instead of 5 μg/kg.

INTERPRETATION

Pituitary-dependent hypercortisolism (Cushing disease): plasma cortisol usually (but not invariably) suppresses to at least 50% of basal values.
Adrenal tumours and ectopic ACTH: failure to suppress.

Corticotrophin-releasing hormone 41 test

INDICATIONS

Differential diagnosis of Cushing syndrome.

PRECAUTIONS/PREPARATION

Fasted.
Facial flushing is common.

PROTOCOL

1 $T = 0$: 100 μg CRH-41 (human or ovine) i.v.
2 $T = -15$, 30, 45, 60, 75, 90 and 120 min: plasma cortisol and ACTH.

INTERPRETATION

In Cushing disease there is a normal or, more commonly, an exaggerated response (peak cortisol > 820 nmol/l). In adrenal tumours or ectopic ACTH there is no response.
The use of this test in combination with the high-dose dexamethasone test is said to give complete discrimination of Cushing syndrome using the criteria of either an exaggerated cortisol response to CRH-41 or a > 50% suppression of cortisol to high-dose dexamethasone. Using either test alone gives a false-negative rate of approximately 20% [17].
CRH-41 has also been used to help pinpoint occult pituitary tumours prior to surgery. This may then be less extensive, thus reducing the risk of subsequent panhypopituitarism [17]. However, this technique is likely to be superseded by improved high-resolution magnetic resonance imaging (MRI) scanning.

Mineralocorticoid function

The adrenal cortex is also concerned with the maintenance of normal sodium homeostasis. Baseline tests include plasma sodium, potassium, creatinine, bicarbonate and pH, together with measurement of sodium, potassium and creatinine concentrations in a 24-h urine collection. A sensitive index of mineralocorticoid sufficiency is measurement of plasma renin activity (PRA). In older children the sample should be collected in the supine and upright positions. Levels of PRA are normally much higher during infancy. Plasma aldosterone is usually measured as a marker of adequate zona glomerulosa function.

Occasionally sodium balance studies are required. The above investigations are performed before and after a 3–5-day low-sodium diet (10–20 mmol/day). Sodium conservation is denoted by a reduction in urinary sodium excretion to less than 20 mmol/day and at least a three-fold increase in PRA and aldosterone. If this reduction is absent, sodium balance can be reassessed after fludrocortisone, 0.05 mg given two or three times a day.

Primary hyperaldosteronism (Conn syndrome) is rare, but biochemical tests demonstrate persistent hypokalaemia, hyperkaluria and alkalosis with suppressed PRA. The treatment is surgical so, in addition to the tests already listed, other investigations such as adrenal venography with selective venous sampling, [^{131}I]iodocholesterol uptake and computerized tomography (CT) or MRI scanning, may be required.

Adrenal medullary function

Adrenal medullary function tests are performed for the investigation of a suspected phaeochromocytoma. Plasma adrenaline and noradrenaline levels – together with 24-h urinary excretion of total catecholamines, total metadrenaline and VMA – are usually sufficient. Provocative tests using glucagon, histamine or tyramine are potentially dangerous and unnecessary. The site of the tumour is best located using techniques such as CT or MRI scanning, ultrasound, selective venous sampling and [^{131}I] meta-iodobenzylguanidine (MIBG) scintiscanning.

GONADS

It is essential that a clinical evaluation of gonadal function is undertaken before specific tests of testicular or ovarian function are performed. The stage of pubertal development, as described in Chapter 14, influences the interpretation of hormone values.

Testis

Clinical examination and basal investigations are usually adequate to assess testicular function, especially in older boys. The latter include measurement of serum gonadotrophins, prolactin, testosterone, androstenedione and dihydrotestosterone concentrations. The presence or absence of functioning testicular tissue in prepubertal boys is assessed by the androgen response to stimulation by human chorionic gonadotrophin (hCG).

Human chorionic gonadotrophin test

INDICATIONS

To detect functioning testicular tissue; for example in undescended testes or cryptorchidism.

PRECAUTIONS/PREPARATION

Nil.

PROTOCOL

1 Day 1: baseline serum testosterone (and 17-OHP, androstenedione and dihydrotestosterone if a defect in steroid biosynthesis is suspected). Give 1500 or 2000 U hCG i.m.
2 Days 2+3: give 1500 or 2000 U hCG i.m. (GP or district nurse).
3 Day 4: repeat blood tests.

INTERPRETATION

There is at least a two- to three-fold increase in plasma testosterone concentration in prepubertal boys. The response is more marked in infants. An absent response with elevated LH and FSH (or an exaggerated LH and FSH response to LHRH q.v.) suggests primary testicular failure. It is sometimes necessary to perform a more prolonged hCG stimulation test by giving hCG 1500 or 2000 U i.m. twice weekly for 3 weeks.

Collection of 24-h urine samples before and after hCG stimulation for measurement of steroid metabolites by gas chromatographic analysis, is a useful supplementary test for the investigation of a defect in testosterone biosynthesis. Other tests which may be relevant when investigating testicular function include karyotype on blood and skin fibroblasts, seminal analysis (appropriate only postpuberty), testicular and abdominal ultrasound, laparoscopy, testicular biopsy and analysis of androgen receptors in genital skin fibroblasts. DNA analysis of the androgen receptor gene may also be informative.

Ovary

Clinical examination and basal investigations are usually adequate to assess ovarian function. These include measurement of the serum concentration of gonadotrophins, prolactin, oestradiol, progesterone and 17-OH progesterone. Supplementary information is obtained from a karyotype on blood and fibroblasts, pelvic ultrasound for uterine and ovarian morphology (see Chapter 10). Ovulation can be documented by recording the daily basal body temperature (not a very reliable indicator), measurement of progesterone levels in plasma, blood spot or saliva samples on days 3–5 and 21–23 of the cycle, and by ovarian ultrasonography.

CALCIUM, PARATHYROID, VITAMIN D

Hypocalcaemia

The essential first step is to correct the fasting calcium level for plasma albumin or to measure ionized calcium to confirm a true abnormality in calcium homeostasis. A urinary calcium/creatinine ratio is also a useful screening or follow-up test. Subsequent investigations to elucidate the cause include plasma phosphate, alkaline phosphatase, renal function, electrolytes, magnesium and pH. The urinary excretion of calcium and phosphate in a 24-h sample is also usually measured. The definitive tests include measurement of serum parathormone (PTH) and the plasma vitamin D metabolites, 25-hydroxycholecalciferol and 1,25-dihydroxycholecalciferol. The measurement of plasma cAMP, urinary phosphate and the cAMP response to PTH is an important dynamic test to determine the nature of the hypoparathyroidism.

Urinary cAMP and phosphate response to parathyroid hormone (Ellsworth–Howard test)

INDICATIONS

To determine the cause of hypoparathyroidism.

PRECAUTIONS/PREPARATION

Fasted except for water, intake of which should be encouraged throughout the test.

PROTOCOL

1 $T = 0$: empty bladder.
2 $T = 30$ and 60 min: (i) collect urine (record volumes) for baseline calcium, phosphate, creatinine and cAMP; (ii) collect blood for calcium, phosphate, cAMP and PTH.
3 $T = 60–90$ min: infuse synthetic human N(1–34) PTH, 100–200 U i.v.
4 $T = 90$, 120 and 150 min: collect urine (record volumes) for calcium, phosphate, creatinine and cAMP.
5 $T = 90$ and 150 min: collect blood for calcium, phosphate, cAMP and PTH.

INTERPRETATION

Normal and hypoparathyroidism: 10–20-fold increase in plasma and urinary cAMP and at least two-fold increase in urinary phosphate excretion. The latter is usually expressed as the tubular maximum reabsorption of phosphate. Serum PTH is low in hypoparathyroidism.
Pseudohypoparathyroidism: absent cAMP and phosphate response (type I) or just a response in urinary cAMP excretion (type II). Serum PTH is raised.

Resistance to the action of vitamin D as a cause of hypocalcaemia can now be studied *in vitro* using cultured skin fibroblasts as target cells. Such an investigation is available in only a few centres, but the technique has uncovered several different defects in intracellular vitamin D binding which can be associated with the syndrome of vitamin D-dependent rickets. The clinician needs only to arrange a punch skin biopsy for primary explant.

Hypercalcaemia

An elevated fasting plasma calcium documented on three separate occasions is sufficient to proceed further with definitive tests of aetiology. New serum assays for intact PTH give a much clearer separation of normal from abnormal. A normal or detectable PTH in the presence of hypercalcaemia is inappropriate and indicates hyperparathyroidism. Urinary phosphate excretion is also usually elevated, as is the urinary calcium/creatinine ratio. Very occasionally it may be necessary to perform a hydrocortisone suppression test to distinguish primary hyperparathyroidism from other causes of hypercalcaemia such as vitamin D intoxication, sarcoidosis and malignancy. Other dynamic tests, which include the plasma calcium and serum PTH response to a diuretic or a calcium infusion, are potentially dangerous and seldom provide further useful information.

Hydrocortisone suppression test

BACKGROUND/INDICATIONS

Differential diagnosis of hypercalcaemia. Suppression of plasma calcium by steroids strongly suggests a cause of hypercalcaemia other than primary hyperparathyroidism.

PRECAUTIONS/PREPARATION

Nil.

PROTOCOL

1 Day 1: baseline fasting plasma calcium and serum PTH.
2 Days 1–10: give hydrocortisone 2 mg/kg a day orally in 8-hourly divided doses.
3 Days 8+10: repeat blood samples.

INTERPRETATION

Primary hyperparathyroidism: suppression rare.
Malignancy, sarcoidosis, vitamin D intoxication: a fall in calcium by at least 0.25 mmol/l or into the normal range.
Familial hypocalciuric hypercalcaemia is characterized by a normal serum PTH and reduced 24-h urinary calcium excretion corrected for creatinine clearance. These must

therefore be assayed on the same collection. A ratio of <0.01 suggests the diagnosis.

ENDOCRINE PANCREAS

Hyperglycaemia

The diagnosis of diabetes mellitus is rarely in doubt in childhood, and almost invariably it is insulin-dependent (IDDM). Other forms such as maturity-onset diabetes in the young (MODY) are rare. An elevated fasting blood glucose level is usually diagnostic and/or random blood glucose levels, which are considerably increased. Ketonuria may or may not be present. Tests for glucose intolerance are seldom required to diagnose diabetes mellitus but can be used to diagnose GH excess (q.v.).

Oral glucose tolerance test

BACKGROUND/INDICATIONS

Diagnosis of glucose intolerance.
Clarification of unusual forms of diabetes mellitus (for example MODY).
Diagnosis of pituitary gigantism/acromegaly.

PRECAUTIONS/PREPARATION

Adequate diet including minimum carbohydrate intake of 150 g/day minimum for the 5 days prior to test.
Fasting.

PROTOCOL

1 $T = 0$: basal plasma glucose (and GH); give glucose 1.75 g/kg (up to a maximum of 75 g) p.o. diluted with water. Should be drunk within 5–10 min.
2 $T = 30$, 60, 90 and 120 min: repeat plasma glucose (and GH).

INTERPRETATION

Elevated fasting glucose and a 2-h level >11.0 mmol/l are diagnostic of diabetes mellitus. A normal fasting glucose but elevated 2-h level suggests impaired glucose intolerance.
Failure to suppress GH to <2 mU/l is highly suggestive of pituitary gigantism/acromegaly.

Hypoglycaemia

This is common is childhood, and investigation requires an orderly approach to eliminate the numerous possible causes. Firstly hypoglycaemia must be confirmed by the measurement of blood glucose on several occasions. The definition of hypoglycaemia is far from clear, but a fasting or random value of less than 3.0 mmol/l in all age groups apart from the neonatal period should be taken as abnormal, and certainly repeated. Of paramount clinical importance is to take blood and urine *at the time* of hypoglycaemia, including some of each to store in case it is needed at a later date. Carefully selected investigations should be performed on the sample according to the clinical features, age and sex of the child.

From the endocrine viewpoint the critical test is measurement of serum insulin, which should be low or undetectable in the presence of a low blood glucose. Hyperinsulinaemic hypoglycaemia is characteristically non-ketotic in nature. Deficiency of counterregulatory hormones such as GH, cortisol and catecholamines may also result in hypoglycaemia. If an inborn error of metabolism is suspected tests should include plasma pH, bicarbonate, and lactate- and urine-reducing substances, ketones, amino and organic acids. Further analyses on the samples will be dictated by these results. In some children the investigation of hypoglycaemia requires a prolonged controlled fast. This can be a life-threatening procedure, and should never be undertaken without consultation with a unit specializing in inborn errors of metabolism. Clear written protocols are mandatory.

Other investigations sometimes performed for the investigation of hypoglycaemia include measurement of proinsulin and C-peptide levels. The latter is typically suppressed in hypoglycaemia due to surreptitious exogenous insulin administration.

MOLECULAR GENETIC ANALYSIS

Endocrinology has benefited considerably from the revolution in molecular medicine. Hormones are either peptides or the products of a synthetic pathway dependent on enzymatic processes. They bring about many of their effects via interaction with cell receptors, which are themselves products of protein synthesis. Endocrine disorders can arise due to defects at any of these steps, and many have now been identified and their inheritance pattern established. Thus, it is not surprising that DNA analysis is an integral part of the investigation of many paediatric endocrine disorders, especially in genetic counselling for families at risk. In some instances the gene has been identified but the product has not. For example the MEN -1 gene is located on chromosome 11 but the product, and how it influences tumour development, is still unknown. Table 40.2 includes some of the more relevant disorders to which DNA analysis could be applied.

Table 40.2 Examples of gene defects identified in endocrine disorders

Disorder	Defective gene	Location
Defects in hormone biosynthesis		
Hereditary GH deficiency	hGH-1	Chromosome 17
Congenital hypopituitarism	Pit-1	Chromosome 3
Congenital adrenal hyperplasia:		
Cholesterol desmolase deficiency	CYP11A	Chromosome 15
3β-HSD deficiency	3β-HSD, type 2	Chromosome 1
17α-Hydroxylase deficiency	CYP17	Chromosome 10
11β-Hydroxylase deficiency	CYP11B1	Chromosome 22
21-Hydroxylase deficiency	CYP21B	Chromosome 6
Aldosterone deficiency	CYP11B2	Chromosome 8
5α-Reductase deficiency	5α-reductase, type 2	Chromosome 2
Vitamin D-resistant rickets, type 1	25-OHD-1α-hydroxylase	Chromosome 12
Defects in hormone response		
GH resistance (Laron-type dwarf)	GH receptor	Chromosome 5
Thyroid hormone resistance	Thyroid receptor β-isoform	Chromosome 3
Androgen insensitivity syndrome	Androgen receptor	X Chromosome
Vitamin D-resistant rickets, type II	Vitamin D receptor	Chromosome 12
Pseudohypoparathyroidism, type 1a	G protein α-subunit	Chromosome 20
Insulin resistance, for example leprechaunism	Insulin receptor	Chromosome 19

APPENDIX: NORMAL VALUES

Most endocrine units have established their own normal ranges for hormone concentrations. The following is by no means a comprehensive record for the clinician, but may serve as a useful, quick reference. Many values are also age-, sex- and laboratory-dependent, and local advice should be sought if there is any doubt about the interpretation of results.

Pituitary

GH	Basal: low, often undetectable Peak: > 26 mU/l after appropriate stimulation (New International Standard)
ACTH	Basal: up to 25 μg/l at 0900 h
TSH	Basal: < 5 mU/l Peak value following TRH stimulation Mean ± SD 12.3 ± 3.2 mU/l Range 5.4–25.0 mU/l
PRL	Basal: < 420 mU/l
ADH	Basal: 1–5 pmol/l (not routinely available)
Plasma osmolality	275–295 mosm/kg H_2O
FSH	Basal Prepubertal: 0.6–3.4 U/l Pubertal*: 0.6–4.9 U/l Follicular: 2.0–6.6 U/l Luteal: 1.6–5.7 U/l Postmenopausal: 28–130 U/l Peak value following LHRH stimulation Prepubertal: mean ± SD 3.9 ± 5.6 U/l; range 1.5–10.8 U/l Pubertal*: mean ± SD 4.1 ± 1.4 U/l; range 2.2–8.0 U/l
LH	Basal Prepubertal: 0.6–1.7 U/l Pubertal: 0.8–8.7 U/l Follicular: 3.0–12.0 U/l Midcycle: 25–64 U/l Luteal: 2.4–13.0 U/l Postmenopausal: 29–120 U/l Peak value following LHRH stimulation Prepubertal: mean ± SD 3.9 ± 1.9 U/l; range 1.5–11.9 U/l Pubertal*: mean ± SD 21.7 ± 2.9 U/l; range 5.9–48.8 U/l

* These data were derived from a group of boys and girls who were in puberty (stages 2–5) and had a bone age > 12.5 years. More detailed data are reported in the literature for males and females separately, and for different stages of puberty.

GH, growth hormone; ACTH, adrenocorticotrophic hormone; TSH, thyroid-stimulating hormone; PRL, prolactin; ADH, antidiuretic hormone; FSH, follicle-stimulating hormone; LH, luteinizing hormone.

Thyroid

FT_4	9–20 pmol/l
FT_3	3.5–8.5 pmol/l
Total T_4	< 12 months: 90–200 nmol/l 1–19 years: 70–180 nmol/l
Total T_3	1.2–3.1 nmol/l
TSH	0.4–4.0 mU/l
TBG	7–17 mg/l
Thyroglobulin	< 5 μg/ml
TSH receptor Ab	−10 to +10% inhibition of binding
^{123}I uptake	10–40% uptake at 4 h
Perchlorate discharge	< 10% at 1 h

FT_4, free thyroxine; FT_3, free triiodothyronine; TSH, thyroid-stimulating hormone; TBG, thyroxine-binding globulin.

Growth factors

IGF-I	Normal ranges are age -and sex-dependent and both must be provided with request. Consult reference laboratory for details

IGF, insulin-like growth factor.

Adrenal cortex

ACTH	Up to 25 μg/l at 0900 h
Cortisol	140–800 nmol/l at 0800–0900 h Up to 200 nmol/l at 2400 h
Urinary free cortisol	< 350 nmol/day
17-OHP	< 10 nmol/l
11-Deoxycortisol	< 30 nmol/l
DHEAS	Prepubertal: < 0.5 nmol/l
Androstenedione	Children < 8 years: < 0.7 nmol/l 8–16 years: < 3.3 nmol/l Adults: 0.8–11.9 nmol/l
PRA + aldosterone	Discuss with reference laboratory

Urinary steroid measurements for adrenocortical metabolites in suspected inborn errors of metabolism can be measured by high-pressure liquid chromatographic and mass spectrometry–gas chromatographic techniques. These are available only in specialized laboratories. ACTH, adrenocorticotrophic hormone; 17-OHP, 17-hydroxyprogesterone; DHEAS, dehydroepiandrosterone sulphate; PRA, plasma renin activity.

Adrenal medulla

24-h urinary VMA	12–44 μmol/day
24-h urinary metadrenaline	< 6.5 μmol/day

These values should also be expressed in relation to urinary creatinine excretion.
VMA, vanillylmandelic acid.

Gonads

Testosterone	Prepubertal: < 0.5 nmol/l Adult male: 10–30 nmol/l Adult female: 0.3–2.5 nmol/l
Oestradiol	Prepubertal: < 60 pmol/l Follicular: 70–260 pmol/l Midcycle: 350–1500 pmol/l Luteal: 180–1100 pmol/l Postmenopausal: < 250 pmol/l Adult male: < 250 pmol/l
Progesterone	Prepubertal: < 1.3 nmol/l Follicular: 0.3–4.8 nmol/l Luteal: 8.0–90 nmol/l Midluteal 18.3–90 nmol/l Postmenopausal < 0.6 nmol/l Adult male < 1.3 nmol/l

Plasma sex steroid concentrations are different during early infancy as well as at each stage of puberty.

Calcium, parathyroid, vitamin D

Sodium	132–142 mmol/l
Potassium	3.4–5.0 mmol/l
Chloride	95–106 mmol/l
Bicarbonate	22–30 mmol/l
Urea	2.5–7.5 mmol/l
Creatinine	30–125 μmol/l
Total protein	63–83 g/l
Albumin	30–51 g/l
Total calcium	2.22–2.70 mmol/l
Ionized calcium	1.13–1.18 mmol/l
Phosphate	0.80–1.4 mmol/l
Magnesium	0.7–1.2 mmol/l
AP	< 450 IU/l (in growing children)
PTH	10–65 μg/l (calcium dependent)
25-HCC	3–40 μg/l (seasonal)
Calcitonin	< 0.08 μg/l
Urine TmP/GFR	0.7–1.4 mmol/l
Urine TmCa/GFR	1.6–2.1 mmol/l

AP, alkaline phosphatase; PTH, parathyroid hormone; 25-HCC, 25-hydroxycholecalciterol; TmP, maximum tubular reabsorption rate for phosphate; GFR, glomerular filtration rate, TmCa, maximum tubular reabsorption rate for calcium.

Endocrine pancreas

Glucose (fasting)	2.8–6.5 mmol/l
Insulin	< 10 mU/l (must be interpreted in relation to concomitant plasma glucose values; should not exceed 10 mU/l when fasting glucose concentration normal or low)
Plasma C peptide	0.2–0.6 pmol/l
Total HbA1	5.7–8.0%
Total HbA1c	4.9–6.3%

HbA, adult haemoglobin.

REFERENCES

1 Blum WF, Ranke MB, Kietzmann K, Gauggel E, Zeisel HJ, Bierich JR. A specific radioimmunoassay for the growth hormone (GH)-dependent somatomedin binding protein: its use for diagnosis of GH deficiency. *J Clin Endocrinol Metab* 1990;70:1292–8.

2 King JM, Price DA. Sleep induced growth hormone release – evaluation of a simple test for clinical use. *Arch Dis Child* 1983;58:220–2.

3 Evans AJ, Wood PJ. Development of an assay for human growth hormone in urine using commercially available reagents. *Ann Clin Biochem* 1989;26:353–7.

4 Hashida S, Ishikawa E, Nakagawa K. Demonstration of human growth hormone in normal urine by a highly specific and sensitive sandwich enzyme immunoassay. *Analyt Lett* 1985;18:1623–34.

5 Skinner AM, Clayton PE, Price DA, Addison GM, Soo A. Urinary growth hormone excretion in the assessment of children with disorders of growth. *Clin Endocrinol* 1993;39: 201–6.

6 Walker J, Williamson S, Evans AJ, Wood PJ, Betts P. Urinary growth hormone as a screening test for growth hormone deficiency. *Arch Dis Child* 1990;65:89–92.

7 Lacey KE, Hewison A, Parkin JM. Exercise as a screening test for growth hormone deficiency in children. *Arch Dis Child* 1973;48:508–12.

8 Shah A, Stanhope R, Matthew D. Hazards of pharmacological tests of growth hormone secretion in childhood. *Br Med J* 1992;304:173–4.

9 Health Services Human Growth Hormone Committee. Comparison of the intravenous insulin and oral clonidine tolerance tests for growth hormone secretion. *Arch Dis Child* 1981;56:852–4.

10 Burday SZ, Fine FH, Schalch DS. Growth hormone secretion in response to arginine infusion in normal and diabetic subjects: relationship to blood glucose levels. *J Lab Clin Med* 1968;71:897–911.

11 Vanderschueren-Lodeweyckx M, Wolter R, Malvaux P, Eggermont E, Eeckels R. The glucagon stimulation test: effect on plasma growth hormone and on immunoreactive insulin, cortisol and glucose in children. *J Pediatr* 1974;85:182–7.

12 Boyd AE, Lebovitz HE, Pfeiffer SB. Stimulation of human growth hormone secretion by L-dopa. *N Engl J Med* 1970;283: 1425–9.

13 Chatelain P. European collaborative study on the effect of synthetic 1–44 growth hormone releasing factor on plasma growth hormone in prepubertal children with growth failure. *Pediatr Res* 1985;19;610.

14 Balldin J, Berggren U, Eriksson E, Lindstedt G, Sundkler A. Guanfacine as an alpha-2-agonist inducer of growth hormone secretion – a comparison with clonidine. *Psychoneuroendocrinology* 1993;18:45–55.

15 Crowley S, Hindmarsh PC, Holownia P, Honour JW, Brook CG. The use of low-dose ACTH in the investigation of adrenal function in man. *J Endocrinol* 1991;130:475–9.

16 Crowley S, Hindmarsh PC, Honour JW, Brook CG. Reproducibility of the cortisol response to stimulation with a low dose of ACTH(1–24): the effect of basal cortisol levels and comparison of low-dose with high-dose secretory dynamics. *J Endocrinol* 1993;136:167–72.

17 Besser GM, Ross RJM. Are hypothalamine releasing hormones useful in the diagnosis of endocrine disorders? In: Edwards CRW, Lincoln DW, eds. *Recent Advances in Endocrinology and Metabolism*, Vol. 3. Edinburgh: Churchill Livingstone, 1989:135–58.

Index

Aarskog syndrome 145, 146
abetalipoproteinaemia 708–9
abuse *see* child abuse
acanthosis nigricans 24
achondroplasia 175, 180, 183
ackee fruit toxicity 689
acrocallosal syndrome 593
acromegaly 24, 199, 200
  GH-secreting tumours 353–4
  management 195, 204–6
ACTH (adrenocorticotrophic hormone) 316
  ACTH steroid tests 447, 482, **789–90**
  ectopic-ACTH syndrome 499, 501, **503–4**
    diagnosis 508–12
    treatment 513
  growth factors and 77–8
  iatrogenic Cushing syndrome 499
  levels in Addison disease 470
  normal values 796, 797
  periodic ACTH-AVP discharge syndrome 605
  secondary hypoadrenocorticism 481–2
  steroid secretion and 439
  see also Cushing disease
activin 245, 290
acute lymphoblastic leukaemia (ALL) 384, **387–91**
Addison disease 7, 454, **462–71**, 565
  CNS associations 471–5
  hypoglycaemia in 687–8
  selective glucocorticoid deficiency 475–7
Addison–Schilder disease (adrenoleukodystrophy) 24, 471–5, 565
adenomas
  parathyroid 360–1
  pituitary 326–9, **352–6**, 743, 744
ADH (antidiuretic hormone)
  inappropriate secretion 566–7, **605–8**
  normal values 796
adrenal disorders 24, **453–557**
  adrenal crisis 453, **460–1**
  adrenoleukodystrophy 24, 471–5, 565
  adrenomyeloneuropathy 471–5
  androgen deficiency 480–1
  congenital adrenal hypoplasia 454–9, 563
  endocrine tests **789–93**
  glucocorticoid deficiency 475–7
  haemorrhage/cysts/calcifications 459–60
  hyper/hypoaldosteronism *see* aldosterone disorders
  hypermineralocorticism 520–4
  mineralocorticoid deficiency 477–80
  steroid deficiency states **453–98**
  steroid excess states **499–535**
  surgery 361–2
  tumours *see* adrenal tumours
  Waterhouse–Friderichsen syndrome 461–2
  Zellweger syndrome 471–5
  see also Addison disease; congenital adrenal hyperplasia
adrenal glands
  adrenal cortex **434–52**
  fetal physiology 558–9
  normal hormone levels 797
  steroidogenesis 537–9
adrenal tumours
  adrenal cortex
    Cushing syndrome 162, 362, **499–516**
    treatment 512–13
    virilizing 362, 445–6, **516–19**
  adrenal medulla 24, 361–2, 569
  see also phaeochromocytoma
adrenarche 85, 102, **249–50**, 519–20
  delayed 481
  premature 256–7, 519–20
adrenocorticotrophic hormone *see* ACTH
adrenoleukodystrophy 24, 471–5, 565
adrenomyeloneuropathy 471–5
African pygmies 156–7, 190–1
AIDS, adrenal involvement 465–6
Albright hereditary osteodystrophy 748–51
alcohol-induced hypoglycaemia 688
aldosterone 435–6
  biosynthesis 436, 440–1, 537–9
  catabolism 444
  plasma levels 443
aldosterone disorders
  biosynthesis defects 564–5
  genetic studies 478
  hyperaldosteronism 520–4, 568–9
  hypoaldosteronism 477–80
  pseudohypoaldosteronism 478–9, 565–6, 569, 796
alloxan-induced diabetes 621
aluminium toxicity 758
ambiguous genitalia
  management **53–68**
  pathogenetic basis 7
  surgery 59, 365–7, 371–4
  urinary steroid analysis 446
  see also congenital adrenal hyperplasia
AME (apparent mineralocorticoid excess) 446–7, 521–2, 569
amenorrhoea 291–6
  androgen insensitivity 367
  imperforate hymen 374
  transverse vaginal septa 365
aminoglutethimide
  adrenal effects 484
  in Cushing syndrome 515
amyloidosis, aldosterone deficiency and 480
androgen-insensitivity syndromes 41, 49, **62–4**
  clinical management 54–9, 367–8
  gene defect 796
  genetic counselling 54
  girls with complete AIS 64, 65
  malignancy risks 53
  psychological support 54–5, 364
  surgery 367–8, 371–3
  testis development 303
androgens
  adrenal 435–6, 439–40
  androgen deficiency 480–1
  bone metabolism effects 729
  role in GH secretion 102
Angelman syndrome 224
anorchia 264, 268, 306, 380
anorexia nervosa 150
  amenorrhoea 294, 295
  breast atrophy 281
  delayed puberty 268
  in diabetes 665
  ketotic hypoglycaemia 689
  obesity and 226
  versus Addison disease 469
antenatal diagnosis *see* prenatal diagnosis
anterior pituitary *see* pituitary disorders
anti-Müllerian hormone (AMH) 41, 245
  in gonadal development 43–5, 46, 298, 304, 371
anticholinergic therapy, in tall stature 205
anticonvulsant therapy, vitamin D effects 740
antidiuretic hormone (ADH)
  inappropriate secretion 566–7, **605–8**
  normal values 796
APECED syndrome 36
apparent mineralocorticoid excess (AME) 446–7, 521–2, 569
arginine vasopressin 580–92
  deficiency 594
  in DI pathophysiology 596–602
  in SIADH pathophysiology 605–8

asparaginase-induced diabetes 621
asthma 152–3
  inhaled steroid side-effects 483
atherosclerosis prevention 709–10
athletes
  amenorrhoea in 295
  pubertal delay in 262–3
atrial natriuretic peptide (ANP) 560, 589, 591
autoimmune disorders
  adrenalitis *see* Addison disease
  arginine vasopressin deficiency 594
  diabetes mellitus and 413, 622–4
  Graves disease 360, **419–22**, 789
  polyglandular syndromes 36, 463–5
  thyroiditis 412–15, 418–19, 420, 480, 506
azoospermia, molecular genetics 24

β-blocker-induced hypoglycaemia 689
ballet dancers
  amenorrhoea in 295
  pubertal delay in 262
Barakat syndrome 25, 35, 36
barbiturate-induced adrenal insufficiency 484
Bartter syndrome 152, **524**, **561–3**
Beckwith–Wiedemann syndrome 198–9, **686**
behavioural disorders
  in psychosocial deprivation 151
  see also psychological problems
bioelectrical impedance (BEI) 212, 213
birth control pills 285–7
bladder disorders, exstrophy 374, 376
blood sample collection 783
Bloom syndrome 181
blue diaper syndrome 768
body fat, growth curve 91–2
body mass index (BMI) 212, 213, 294
bone age 90–1, 163
bone disorders **735–78**
  bone biopsy 731
  laboratory assessment 779–81
  radiological investigations 730–1
  see also rickets; skeletal dysplasias
bone marrow transplantation, radiation sequelae 388, 393–4
bone metabolism **726–34**
Bonnevie–Ullrich syndrome 293
brachytherapy 352
brain tumours 159–60, **346–58**
  chordomas 311
  germ-cell 337–8
  gliomas 322, 332–7, 356–7
  pineal region 342–3
  precocious puberty and 248, 253, 257
  radiation sequelae 383, 386–7, 389, 391
  see also craniopharyngioma; pituitary tumours
breast disorders 280–3, *Plate* 16.10
breast-feeding, infant obesity and 217
breasts, normal development 234–5
bromocriptine, in acromegaly 204
bulimia, in diabetes 665
burns 484, 605

CAH *see* congenital adrenal hyperplasia
calciferol *see* vitamin D
calcitonin 6, 723–6, 763–5
calcitonin gene-related peptide 6, 724
  increased/decreased secretion 761–3
calcium disorders 563, **735–78**
  differential diagnosis 781
  hypercalciuria 735, 760, 779
  laboratory assessment 779–81
  see also hypercalcaemia; hypocalcaemia
calcium metabolism **713–34**
  normal plasma levels 797
cancer
  growth/endocrine sequelae **383–96**
  see also malignant disease; tumours
cardiac disease *see* heart disease
Carney complex 499, 501, 513
cat-scratch fever, thyroiditis and 419
cataracts
  in chronic hypocalcaemia 747
  in diabetes 634, 666
catecholamines in glucose homeostasis 680
cerebral giantism (Sotos syndrome) 198–9
cerebrohepatorenal syndrome 472–3
cerebrotendinous xanthomatosis 709
cervical prolapse 280
chemotherapy, of craniopharyngioma 352
chemotherapy side-effects **383–96**
  gonadal 294, 308
  SIADH 605
chicken pox, diabetes and 620
child abuse
  chemical abuse 566
  sexual abuse 253, 280, 365
chloride shunt syndrome 569
cholesterol disorders
  familial hypercholesterolaemia 700–4
  Prader syndrome (cholesterol desmolase deficiency) 549, 550, 796
  see also lipid disorders
cholesterol metabolism 694–8
cholestyramine therapy 703
chordomas 311
chylomicronaemia 704–5
circadian rhythms *see* hormone pulsatility
circumcision 375
cleft lip/palate
  growth failure and 159
  in Kallmann syndrome 341
  in Shprintzen syndrome 145, 147
cleidocranial dysostosis 143
clonidine
  clonidine test 785, 786
  in short stature treatment 182
CMO (corticosterone methyloxidase) deficiencies 477–80, 564, 566
coeliac disease 151
colestipol therapy 703
collagen 727–8
congenital adrenal hyperplasia (CAH) 53, **60**, 445, **536–57**
  genetic counselling 54
  hypertension due to 567–9
  molecular genetics 24, 536, 541–2, 546, 547, 548, 796
  neonatal markers 444
  prenatal diagnosis 60, 447, 543–4
  salt-losing states 540, 549, 563–4
  sexual precocity 256–7
  skin pigmentation 56
  surgery 59, 365–7, 371–3, 551
  synacthen test 790
congenital adrenal hypoplasia 454–9, 563
congenital heart disease 689
congenital rubella syndrome 620
Conn syndrome 520–1
contraception for adolescents 284–7
coronary heart disease *see* heart disease
corpus callosum dysgenesis 311, 339–40
corticosterone methyloxidase deficiencies 477–80, 564, 566
corticotrophin-releasing hormone 439
  catabolism/excretion 443–4
  ectopic-CRH syndrome 499, 501
cortisol 435–6
  biosynthesis 436–9, 536
  excretion rates 444–7
  hormone pulsatility 123, 439, 442
  normal levels 797
  plasma levels in diabetes 628
  role in glucose homeostasis 680, 682
  secretion control 439
  secretion rates in stress 471, 507
  synacthen tests 789–90
  transport 441–2
  in urine 444
cortisol disorders
  binding deficiency 441–2
  primary cortisol resistance 476–7
  see also congenital adrenal hyperplasia; Cushing syndrome
counselling
  contraception for adolescents 287
  intersex disorders 54–5, 59, 65, 364, 550
  see also genetic counselling
Coxsackie viruses, diabetes and 620–1
cranial irradiation 160–1
craniopharyngioma 159–60, **346–52**
  diabetes insipidus and 593
  obesity and 223, 348
  radiology 329–30, 349
Creutzfeldt–Jacob disease 176
Crohn disease 151–2
cryptorchidism 298, **305–6**, 307
  incidence 300
CT scanning 359
  adrenal glands 469, 511
  bone disorders 731
  craniopharyngioma 329–30, 349
  in gynaecology 283–4
  neuroradiology **320–45**, 349, 354
  pituitary tumours 354, 512
  to assess obesity 213
  to assess tall stature 201, 206
Cushing disease (pituitary Cushing syndrome) 124, 353, 499, **502–3**
  diagnosis 508–12
  growth retardation 504
  incidence 500
  investigations 790–2
  treatment 513–15
Cushing syndrome 162, 362, **499–516**, 569
  gastric inhibitory polypeptide and 316, 500, 513
  obesity in 222–3, 504
  suppression tests 447, 508, 790–1
  see also Cushing disease
cyclosporine therapy in diabetes 625, 659
cyproterone 261

cystic fibrosis
  attenuated growth 153
  delayed puberty 262
  diabetes and 669
  gene therapy 19
  pathogenetic basis 7
cysticerosis 338
cysts
  adrenal 460
  arachnoid 332
  ovarian 283, 284
  see also polycystic ovary syndrome
  Rathke's pouch 326, 357
  subarachnoid 248
  vulvar 280
cytokines 318
cytomegalovirus, diabetes and 621
cytosarcoma phylloides 282

Danazol 282, 284
  adrenal effects 484
de Morsier syndrome 311
de Wardener factor 560
deafness, hypocalcaemia and 747
dehydration
  dehydration testing 599
  in diabetes mellitus 654–6
  in newborn 591, 595, 596–7
  in older patients 595–6
Dent disease 25
Denys–Drash syndrome 61
Depo Provera 287
dermatitis, vulvar 276–8
dermoids, intracranial 330
desmopressin 580–1, 582, 602
  desmopressin test 602
  for primary polydipsia 598
DEXA (X-ray densitometry) 731
dexamethasone suppression test 447, 508, 790–1
dexamethasone treatment, prenatal, in CAH 544–5
Di George anomaly, with Shprintzen syndrome 147
diabetes insipidus **592–605**
  DIDMOAD 594, 595, 630
  molecular genetics 23, 24, 594
  pineal tumours and 341
  water deprivation test 788
diabetes mellitus **616–76**
  autoimmune associations 413, 622–4
  in Cushing syndrome 506
  diagnostic tests 795
  DIDMOAD 594, 595, 630
  dyslipidaemia in 707
  genetics 6, 7, 23, 618–20
  IGF therapy 192
  in utero undernutrition and 93
  infants of diabetic mothers 686, 765–6
  management **654–76**
  maturity-onset in the young (MODY) 618, 630
  obesity and 220, 630
  pathophysiology **616–53**
  secondary
  transitory 641
DIDMOAD (Wolfram syndrome) 594, 595, 630
diet *see* nutrition
DiGeorge syndrome 24, 25, **35–6**, 747
dihydrotestosterone (DHT) 47–9

disseminated intravascular coagulation 593
diurnal rhythms *see* hormone pulsatility
DNA 20
  analyses 11–15
  gene cloning 8–11
  gene structure/function 1–6, 20
  gene transfer 18–19
  hormone response elements 131
  recombinant techniques 7–8, **23–37**
Down syndrome
  growth chart 136
  hypothyroidism in 413
  obesity in 225
  short stature treatment 181
dysbetalipoproteinaemia 705–6
dyslipoproteinaemia (dyslipidaemia) 698–710
dysmenorrhoea 284

ear infections, in Turner syndrome 148, 149
eating disorders
  amenorrhoea and 294, 295
  in diabetes 665
  see also anorexia nervosa
Ellsworth–Howard test 794
emotional disturbance, effect on growth 94
empty sella syndrome 159, 312, 325, 593
endocrine tests **782–98**
endogenous digoxin-like substance (EDLS) 560
endometriosis 284, 369
endotoxin 318
epidermoid cysts, vulvar 280
epidermoids, intracranial 330
epididymitis 381
epilepsy
  hypocalcaemic 746
  rickets/osteomalacia and 740
ethanol-induced hypoglycaemia 688
ethnic differences
  growth 94, 136
  onset of puberty 234, 239, 241
etomidate-induced adrenal insufficiency 484
eukaryotic cells 20
exercise (strenuous)
  amenorrhoea and 295
  delayed puberty and 262, 341
exomphalos–macroglossia–gigantism (Beckwith–Wiedemann) syndrome 198–9, **686**
eye disorders *see* ocular disorders

familial combined hyperlipidaemia 705
familial defective apolipoprotein B 703–4
familial dysautonomia (Riley–Day syndrome) 484–5
familial hypercholesterolaemia 700–4
familial hypertriglyceridaemia 706
familial hypobetalipoproteinaemia 709
familial lecithin–cholesterol acyltransferase deficiency 709
Fanconi syndrome 561, 757
fasting
  controlled fast 685
  glucose homeostasis and 681–2, 684
  ketotic hypoglycaemia 689–90
fat child *see* obesity
female genitalia
  labial adhesions 277, 364–5, 375, *Plate* 16.2
  normal development 46–9
  vagina, congenital absence 294, 368–9
  vulvar disorders 276–80
fenfluramine 228
fertile eunuch syndrome 308
follicle stimulating hormone (FSH) 315
  in amenorrhoea assessment 295
  normal values 796
  role in puberty 242–4, 289–91
follistatin 290
foreign bodies, vaginal 278, 365, *Plates* 16.6 & 16.7
fragile-X syndrome 64, 308
Frohlich syndrome 223

galactorrhoea 281
gastric inhibitory polypeptide (GIP) 316, 500, 513, 680
Gaucher disease 473
gender identity 41, 53
  intersex disorders and 53–5, 364, 551
gene
  definition 1, 20
  regulation 3–5
  structure and function 1–6, 20
  see also gene therapy/transfer
gene therapy/transfer 18–19
  in growth disorders 81
genetic counselling
  in diabetes 669
  in intersex disorders 53, 54
genetic studies **23–40**, 795–6
  Addison disease 466
  adrenal hypoplasia 457–8
  aldosterone disorders 478
  childhood ALD/AMN 473
  clinical molecular genetics **23–40**, 795–6
  congenital adrenal hyperplasia 24, 536, 541–2, 546, 547, 548
  diabetes insipidus 23, 24, 594
  diabetes mellitus 618–20
  DNA analyses 11–18
  familial hypercholesterolaemia 700
  familial hypoparathyroidism 747–8
  genetic engineering 18–19
  genetic influence on growth 92–3
  Laron syndrome 187–8
  McCune–Albright syndrome 7, 24, 502
  steroid synthesis 438–9
  see also X-linked diseases
genital tract disorders
  intersex disorders 7, **53–68**
  male genitalia disorders 62, 375–81
  vagina, congenital absence 294, 368–9
genital tract injuries 280, 365
genitalia
  newborn/infant examination 274
  normal development 46–9, 375
  see also ambiguous genitalia; female genitalia; male genitalia
giantism 199, 200
  diagnosis/management 199–206, 353
Gitelman syndrome 563
gliomas, intracranial 322, 332–7

glucagon 680, 682
 deficiency 688
 in diabetes pathogenesis 626
 hormone pulsatility 123
glucocorticoids *see* adrenal disorders; adrenal gland; cortisol
glucose homeostasis 677–82
glycogen metabolism 677–8
glycogen storage diseases 708
goitre 24, 412–19
gonadal development 41–52
gonadal dysgenesis 24, **60–2**, 264
 gender of rearing 62, 371
 surgery 367
 syndromes of 292–4
gonadotrophin-releasing hormone 241–2, 315
 analogues 261
gonadotrophins 315
 pulsatility 123, 246, 315
 role in puberty 241–4, 246–50, 315
 secretion 175–6, 246–50, 289
 see also follicle stimulating hormone; luteinizing hormone
gonads *see* ovarian disorders; ovary; testis
Gordon syndrome 569
Graves disease 360, **419–22**, 789
 neonatal 422
growth **85–106**
 growth curve models 94–7
 growth factors **69–84**, 99–101, **107–22**
 height prediction 85–90, 195–7
 influences on 92–4
 limb development 5, 74–6
 in puberty 239
 reference standards 85–94, 136–41
 see also growth hormone; insulin-like growth factors
growth disorders
 in Cushing syndrome 504–5
 in diabetes 633–4
 DNA technology and 7
 growth factors in 80, 114–17
 growth-hormone-resistant states 156, **187–94**
 short stature **136–72**, 143, 165, **173–86**
 tall stature **195–209**
 see also growth hormone deficiency
growth factors *see* insulin-like growth factors
growth hormone **314–15**
 DNA technology and 7, 11–12
 levels in puberty 101, 102, 245
 normal values 796
 overnight/24-hr profiles 784
 pulsatility 101–2, 155, 314
 receptor studies 133–4, 165, 187, 318
 regulation 97–102, 123, 129, 130, 133–4
 role in bone metabolism 729
 role in glucose homeostasis 680, 682
 testing for 783–4
growth hormone deficiency **153–61**, 175, 222
 clinical tests **783–7**
 gene defects 796
 hypoglycaemia in 688
 pituitary abnormalities 325
 radiation-induced 383–7
growth hormone disorders
 GH levels in obesity 220
 GH-resistant states 156, **187–94**, 796
 GH-secreting tumours 353–4
 role in diabetes pathogenesis 626–8, 636
growth hormone therapy 176–81
 in X-linked phosphataemic rickets 756
growth hormone-releasing hormone 182, 311, 314–15, 318
growth hormone-releasing peptide 182
guanfacine test 786
gynaecology **274–87**
 breast disorders 280–3
 chronic pelvic pain 284
 contraception 284–7
 genital tract injuries 280, 365
 imaging techniques 283–4
 labial adhesions 277, 375, 364–5, *Plate* 16.2
 normal menstrual cycle 290–1
 surgery **364–70**, 371–3, 374–5
 vulvar disorders 276–80, *Plate* 16.8
 see also ovarian disorders
gynaecomastia 239, 268
 in androgen-insensitivity syndrome 58, 239

haemangiomas
 breast 282
 vulvar 279, *Plate* 16.8
haematocolpos/haematometrocolpos 283
haematomas, vulvar 280, *Plate* 16.9
Halermann–Strieff syndrome 747
Hashimoto (autoimmune) thyroiditis 412–15, 418–19, 420, 480, 789
head trauma, osmoregulatory effects 593, 604, 605
heart disease
 atherosclerosis prevention 709–10
 hypoglycaemia and 689
 in lipid disorders 701–2, 705
 in obesity 221
height measurement technique 141
 height prediction 85–90, 195–7
height/stature *see* growth; growth disorders
hermaphroditism 368
 gender of rearing 371
herpes simplex infections, vulvar 279
hirsutism in adolescence 295
histiocytosis 160
 neuroradiology 338
Hodgkin disease, chemotherapy sequelae 394
hormone pulsatility **123–35**
 aldosterone 443
 arginine vasopressin 586
 cortisol 123, 439, 442
 gonadotrophins 123, 246, 315
 growth hormone 101–2, 155, 314
 luteinizing hormone 123, 243
 thyroid-stimulating hormone 123, 316
hormone receptor studies 131–4, 318
hormone tests/normal values **782–98**
human papilloma virus, anogenital 279
Huntington disease 64
hydrocephalus 159
 pineal tumours and 341
 precocious puberty in 248, 253, 357
 treatment 357
hydrocortisone suppression test 794
11β-hydroxylase deficiency 545–6, 567–8, 796
 sex assignment 550
 treatment 550, 551
17α-hydroxylase deficiency 264, 294, 539, **547–8**, 568, 796
 treatment 550, 551
21-hydroxylase deficiency 539–45, 564, 796
 sex assignment 550
 treatment 549–50, 564
3β-hydroxysteroid deficiency 546–7, 796
 treatment 550, 551
hymen
 examination in young child 275
 hymenal tags 280
 imperforate 374
hyperaldosteronism 520–4, 568–9
hypercalcaemia 735–7
 differential diagnosis 781
 endocrine tests 794
 familial benign/hypocalciuric 760–1, 766, 794–5
 in hyperparathyroidism 741–5
 idiopathic infantile 736–7, 766
 of malignancy 721–2, 735–6
 neonatal 766–8
 osmotic effects 590
hypercalciuria 735, 760
 tests for 779
hypercholesterolaemia 700–4
hyperchylomicronaemia 704–5
hyperglycaemia, diagnostic tests 795
hyperinsulinism 685–7
 in obesity 219–20
 treatment 362, 685
hyperlipidaemias 698–710
hypernatraemia 599–600
hyperparathyroidism **741–5**, 768
 hydrocortisone suppression test 794
 neonatal 766–7
 surgery 360–1, 745
hyperpigmentation 469
 in Addison disease 466
hypertension 25, **567–70**
 catecholamine excess 569–70
 in Cushing syndrome 505–6, 569
 in diabetes 636, 667
 essential 570
 in 11β-hydroxylase deficiency 545, 567–8
 in 17α-hydroxylase deficiency 548, 568
 hyperaldosteronism and 520, 522, 568–9
 in obesity 221
 renin-secreting tumours 524
 severe 446
hyperthyroidism **419–23**
 Graves disease 360, **419–22**
 surgery 360–1, 421
 tall stature 199
hypertriglyceridaemia 706
hypervitaminosis A 767–8
hypoaldosteronism 477–80
hypobetalipoproteinaemia 709
hypocalcaemia 745–53
 differential diagnosis 781
 endocrine tests 793–4
 neonatal 765–6
hypochondroplasia 143–4
 genetic linkage studies 13

GH treatment 180
radiography 175
hypoglycaemia 632–3, **677–93**
in Addison disease 466–7
in diabetes 632–3, 663–4
diagnostic tests 795
differential diagnosis 469, 684–5
idiopathic 484
in infancy/childhood 684–5
neonatal 683–4
hypogonadotrophic hypogonadism 263–8, 787
hyponatraemia 607–8
hypoparathyroidism **745–53**
Ellsworth–Howard test 794
molecular genetics **23–37**
pseudohypoparathyroidism 25, 36–7, 162, 723, **748–51**
hypophosphataemia, neonatal 767
hypophosphataemic rickets 144, 181, **753–7**, 767, 779–81
hypophosphatasia 768
hypophysitis 161
hypopituitarism
in craniopharyngioma 348
GH deficiency and 99–101
microphallus and 44
versus Addison disease 464
hypospadias 375–6
in gonadal dysgenesis 62
hypotension
in Addison disease 467
idiopathic orthostatic 484
hypothalamic syndromes 312
diabetes insipidus and 595, 600
effect on prolactin 245
hypoglycaemia in 687
neuroradiology 320–41, 600
obesity and 223–5
precocious puberty in 248
see also craniopharyngioma
hypothalamus
anatomy/physiology 310–19
osmoregulation 580–92
hypothyroidism 161–2, **406–15**
acquired 406, 412–15
congenital 406–12, 768
decreased calcitonin secretion 762–3
dyslipidaemia in 707
galactorrhoea in 281, 414
hypoglycaemia in 688
obesity in 222, 414
precocious puberty in 256, 414
proterelin test 787
radiation/chemotherapy-induced 389
SIADH in 605

IGF *see* insulin-like growth factors
imaging techniques
adrenal glands 469, 511–12, 518
for breast mass 282–3
in Cushing syndrome 511–12
in gynaecology 283–4
hypothalamic lesions 600
neuroradiology **320–45**, 349, 354
thyroid scintigraphy 789
to assess obesity 213
to assess tall stature 201–2, 206
see also CT scanning; MRI scanning; radiological investigations
impetigo 276
indomethacin
in Bartter syndrome 562, 563
in pseudohypoaldosteronism 566
in renal DI 603–4
toxicity 480
infections
in diabetes 633
pituitary/hypothalamic 338
inflammatory bowel disease 151–2
delayed puberty 262
inhibin 245, 290
injuries *see* trauma
insulin 680, 682
autoantibodies in diabetes 623
bone metabolism effects 729
DNA technology and 7
down-regulation 123–4
feedback 125–6
hormone pulsatility 123
hyperinsulinism 685–7
in obesity 219–20
treatment 362, 685
in IGF synthesis 201
normal levels 797
resistance to 680, 796
see also diabetes mellitus
insulin tolerance test 175, 447, **786–7**
in Cushing syndrome 508
hazards 154, 447, 786–7
insulin-like growth factors (IGFs) 5–6, 18, **107–22**, 680
in Beckwith–Wiedemann syndrome 199, 686
in GH regulation 99–101, 729
in growth disorders **114–17**, 156, 164
IGF therapy **116–17**, 183, 189–90
IGF-secreting tumours 687
in Laron syndrome 189–90
levels at puberty 245, 289–90
normal values 797
in placenta 99
polycystic ovaries and 269
in prenatal development **69–81**, 109
protein binding 112–13, 130, 318
serum levels 113–14, 164
in tall stature 201
in testicular tissue 304
testing for 784
insulinoma 687
interleukins 318
intersex disorders 7, **53–68**
iodine deficiency disorders 415–19
irradiation side-effects *see* radiation side effects

Jamaican vomiting sickness 689
Jeune thoracic dystrophy 175

Kabuki make-up syndrome 253
Kallman syndrome 241, 301, **341**
MRI imaging 341
osmoregulatory defect 585
pathogenetic basis 7, 8, 311
Kearns–Sayre syndrome 747
Kenney–Caffey syndrome 36, 747
ketoconazole 261
adrenal effects 484
in Cushing syndrome 515–16
kidney
physiology 558–60
role of prostaglandins 589
water regulation 587–92
kidney disorders *see* renal disease
Klinefelter syndrome 199
features in XX males 65
gynaecomastia in 268
hypothyroidism in 413
obesity in 225
testis development 303, 307
Kocher–Debré–Semelaigne syndrome 406, 412, 414
kwashiorkor 150

labial adhesions 277, 364–5, 375, *Plate* 16.2
Langerhan's cell histiocytosis 338
Laron syndrome 24, 136, 183, **187–90**, 796
Laurence–Moon-Biedl syndrome 161, 223–4, 593
lead poisoning, chronic 480
lecithin–cholesterol acyltransferase deficiency 709
leprechaunism 24, 796
polycystic ovaries in 269
Lesch-Nyhan syndrome 25
leukaemia
acute lymphoblastic (ALL) 384, **387–91**
irradiation side-effects 160–1, 253, 387–91
lichen sclerosus, anogenital 277, *Plate* 16.3
lichen simplex chronicus 277
Liddle syndrome 522
lipid disorders **694–712**
familial hypercholesterolaemia 700–4
lipid storage diseases, adrenoleukodystrophy 24, 471–5, 565
lipid/lipoprotein metabolism 694–8
lipomas, intracranial 332
liquorice over-ingestion 522
Listeria monocytogenes 593
lithium therapy side-effects 594
liver disease
dyslipidaemia in 708
hypoglycaemia in 689
Loebner phenomenon 277
Lowe syndrome 24
luteinizing hormone (LH) 315
in amenorrhoea assessment 295
Leydig cell regulation 301–3
normal values 796
pulsatility 123, 243
role in puberty 242–9, 289–91
lysine-vasopressin test 482, 510
lysodren (*o,p*'DDD) 515, 518

McCune–Albright syndrome 254, 303, 502, 750
molecular biology 7, 24, 502
ovarian cysts 254, 258
prognosis 262, 513
McQuarrie–Zetterström syndrome 469, 484
magnetic resonance imaging *see* MRI scanning
malaria-induced hypoglycaemia 690

male genitalia, normal development 46–9, 375
male genitalia disorders 375–81
hypospadias 62, 375–6
see also testis disorders
malignant disease
in Beckwith–Wiedemann syndrome 199
in gonadal dysgenesis 61–2, 65
growth factors and 109, 199
radiation/chemotherapy sequelae 160–1, 294, **383–96**
thyroid gland 423–5
see also tumours
malnutrition
chronic vulvar granulomas and 280
growth and 85, 93–4, 101, 191–2
marasmus 150
Marfan syndrome 199
mastitis 281–2
maturational delay 143
Mauriac syndrome 633–4
medroxyprogesterone 261
medulloblastoma 337–8
melanin hyperpigmentation 469
in Addison disease 466
MEN *see* multiple endocrine neoplasia
meningitis, osmoregulatory effects 593, 605
Menke syndrome 25
menstrual cycle 290–1
menstrual disorders 284, **291–6**
mental handicap, obesity and 225
metyrapone
adrenal effects 484
in Cushing syndrome 515
metyrapone tests 482, 510, 790
microphallus, in gonadal dysgenesis 62
miliaria 276
mineralocorticoid disorders
deficiency 477–80, 563–5
excess 446–7, 521–2
pseudohypoaldosteronism 478–9, 565–6, 569, 796
mitotane (*o,p'*DDD) 515, 518
molluscum contagiosum 277, *Plate* 16.5
mosaicism 57–8, 61
sex chromosome 293, 307
mountain Ok people 157
MRI scanning 359
in adrenal deficiency 469
craniopharyngioma 329–30, 349
Cushing disease management 353
in gynaecology 283–4
neuroradiology 320–45, 354
phaeochromocytoma 361
pituitary tumours 354, 512, 600
to assess obesity 213
mucocoele of sphenoid sinus 329
Müllerian duct syndrome 46
Müllerian dysgenesis, amenorrhoea in 294, 374
Müllerian-inhibiting substance *see* anti-Müllerian hormone
multiple endocrine neoplasia (MEN) 502, 743–4, 789
phaeochromocytoma in 569, 761
screening for 762
mumps virus
diabetes and 620
mumps orchitis 264
thyroiditis and 419

myotonic dystrophy 64

necrosis of subcutaneous fat 767
Nelson syndrome 471, 514
nephrolithiasis 25
nesidioblastosis 686–7
neurohypophysis and water regulation **580–615**
neuropathy in diabetes 640–1, 667
neurophysins 316
neuroradiology **320–45**, 349, 354
neurotrophic growth factors 71, 79–80
nicotinamide therapy in diabetes 625, 659–60
Noonan syndrome 136, 145, **146**
hypothyroidism in 413
Norplant 287
nuclear magnetic resonance (NMR) *see* MRI scanning
nutrition
energy intakes 215
foods which interfere with tests 782
growth control and 85, 93–4, 101, 191–2, 198
lipid-lowering diet 702–3, 705
maturational delay and 143
puberty and 234
role in obesity 214–18
role in short stature 150–1
slimming diets 225–6
see also fasting

obesity **210–33**
cortisol secretion in 444
GH secretion in 161
height and 93–4, 198, 212, **218–19**
polycystic ovaries and 269
ocular disorders in
diabetes 634–6, 639–40, 666
Graves disease 419, 420
pituitary dysfunction 159, 311, 312, 337
craniopharyngioma 348–9
septo-optic dysplasia 339
sphenoidal cephalocoele 341
oestradiol, normal values 797
oestrogen
bone metabolism effects 729
placental secretion 289
role in puberty 245–50
oestrogen therapy, for tall stature 202–4
oligomenorrhoea 291
*o,p'*DDD 515, 518
optic chiasm gliomas 332–4, 339
optic nerve gliomas 322, 332–4, 356–7
optic nerve hypoplasia 159
oral contraceptives 285–7
orchidopexy 379–80
oscillatory secretion *see* hormone pulsatility
osmoregulation **580–92**
disorders **592–608**
osteocalcin 730, 779
osteomalacia 738
calciopenic rickets 144, **738–41**
phosphopenic rickets 144, 753–7
renal osteodystrophy 757–9
osteoporosis 763
ovarian disorders **291–6**
cysts 283, 284
polycystic ovaries **269–70**, 295–6
surgery 369
see also polycystic ovarian syndrome
endometriosis 284, 369
premature ovarian failure 264
premature thelarche and 281
radiation/chemotherapy-induced 390–4
tumours 369–70
ovary 288
development of 45–6, 235–7, 288–91
function tests 793
normal dimensions 283
oxandrolone 181–2, 266, 268
oxytocin 127, 316–17, 580
structure 581

Paget disease 725, 728
pancreas (endocrine), normal hormone levels 797
pancreatic disorders *see* diabetes mellitus; hypoglycaemia
parathyroid disorders **741–53**
Ellsworth-Howard test 794
molecular genetics **23–37**
parathyroidectomy in 360–1, 745
see also hyperparathyroidism; hypoparathyroidism
parathyroid hormone 718–23, 763–5
normal values 797
parathyroid secretory protein (PSP) 719
parathyroid–related protein 721–2
Parinaud syndrome, pineal tumours and 341
pentagastrin stimulation test 789
pentamidine–induced diabetes 621
peptide growth factors 69–81
peroxisomal disorders 471–5
persistent müllerian duct syndrome 46, 64
phaeochromocytoma 24, **569–70**, 761
Cushing syndrome due to 501, 504
surgery 361–2, 570
tests for 793
phenylketonuria 25
phenytoin-induced adrenal insufficiency 484
phosphate disorders 144, 753–60
hypophosphataemic rickets 144, 181, **753–7**, 767, 779–81
neonatal hypophosphataemia 767
physical activity
amenorrhoea and 295
delayed/arrested puberty and 262, 341
phytosterolaemia 709
Pickwick syndrome 221
pigmentation *see* hyperpigmentation
pineal gland 341–3
tumours 342–3
pinworms 278
pirenzepine 205
Pit-1 (transcription factor) 5, 318, 796
gene deletions 99–100, 156
pituitary disorders 24, 325–9
in congenital adrenal hypoplasia 457
effect on prolactin 245
endocrine tests 783
hypoglycaemia in 687
hypopituitarism 44, 99–101, 348, 464
hypothyroidism and 413
neuroradiology 320–41, 600–1

PH deficiency 157–9
secondary hypoadrenalism and 481–2
sexual precocity and 257, 325
see also craniopharyngioma; Cushing disease; diabetes insipidus; pituitary tumours
pituitary gland:
anatomy/physiology 310–19
development/structure 320–4, 590
endocrine tests 783
growth factors and 78, 310
normal hormone values 796
water regulation 580–92
pituitary tumours 312, **352–6**, 743, 744
ACTH-secreting *see* Cushing disease
causing diabetes insipidus 593
GH-secreting 353–4
neuroradiology 326–9
prolactinomas 175, 313, 352, 353, 787–8
TSH-secreting 354, 422
pityriasis versicolor 278
plasmids 8
polycystic ovaries **269–70**, 295–6
polycystic ovary syndrome 220, 269–70, 294, **295–6**
21-hydroxylase deficiency and 540
molecular genetics 24
polydipsia/polyuria **592–605**
in diabetes mellitus 630–1, 654
primary 594, 596, 597–8, 603
polyglandular autoimmune syndromes 36, 463–5
ponderal index 144
Prader syndrome 549, 796
sex assignment 550
Prader-Willi syndrome 25, 161, 181, **224–5**, 630
prematurity
glucose homeostasis 682, 683
metabolic bone disease 768–70
sodium balance 559–60, 566
thyroid disorders 411, 412
prenatal diagnosis
adrenal hyperplasia 60, 447, 543–4
adrenal hypoplasia 458–9
adrenoleukodystrophy 473–4
androgen-insensitivity syndrome 64
Zellweger syndrome 473–4
progesterone, normal values 797
prolactin 313–14
disorders 313–14
hormone pulsatility 123
normal values 796
prolactinomas 175, 313, 352, 353, 787–8
prostaglandins
aldosterone release by 441
bone metabolism regulation 729
protein synthesis 3–6
pseudohermaphroditism 46, 49, 59
aminoglutethimide-induced 484
pseudohypoaldosteronism 478–9, 565–6, 569
gene defect 796
pseudohypoparathyroidism 25, 36–7, 162, 723, **748–51**
Ellsworth–Howard test 794
psoriasis
new drug therapy 716
vulvar, 278, *Plate* 16.4
psychological problems
of congenital adrenal hyperplasia 551
of diabetes 664–5
of obesity 221–2
of sexual precocity 257
of short stature 176
of tall stature 202
psychosocial deprivation 150–1, 161
puberty 41
growth acceleration 96–7, 101, 729
growth hormone pulses 101, 102, 245
holding up 183
physiology 48, 97, 102, **234–52**, 258–60
pubertal staging 85, 239–41
testis development 305
puberty, disorders of **253–73**
delayed 89–90, 137, 234, **262–8**
in diabetes 634
pituitary adenomas and 352, 353
primary amenorrhoea 292–4
polycystic ovaries **269–70**, 295–6
precocious **253–62**
central 242, 248, 253
in McCune–Albright syndrome 254, 302–3
pineal tumours and 341, 357
radiation-induced 386
in testotoxicosis 254, 302–3
pulsatility *see* hormone pulsatility
pycnodysostosis 762
pyelonephritis 590
pygmies 157, 190–1

Quetelet index 212

radiation side effects **383–96**
cranial 160–1, 351
gonadal 294, 308
precocious puberty 253, 386
radioimmunoassay 317
radiological investigations
in bone disorders 175, 730–1
neuroradiology **320–45**, 349, 354
in tall stature 201–2, 206
see also CT scanning; MRI scanning; X-rays
Rathke's pouch 310–11, 320
Rathke's cyst 326, 357
receptor studies 131–4, 318
growth hormone 133–4, 165, 187, 318
Refsum disease, infantile 472, 473
relaxin 290
renal disease 560–3, 590
Bartter syndrome 152, **524**, **561–3**
bone disease and 740
chronic pyelonephritis 590
chronic renal failure 152
delayed puberty and 262
diabetes insipidus 594, 596, 603–4
diabetic nephropathy 638–9
dyslipidaemia in 707–8
hypoaldosteronism and 479–80
renal hypercalciuria 735, 760
renal osteodystrophy 757–9
renal tubular acidosis 566
renin-secreting tumours 524
short stature in 152, 180–1
renal physiology 558–60
renin 440, 441
prostaglandins and 589
renin-secreting tumours 524
renin-angiotensin-aldosterone system
as diagnostic aid 561
neonatal 559
role in dehydration 591
retinoblastoma, metastases 337–8
retinopathy in diabetes 639–40
Rhesus haemolytic disease 686
rickets
calciopenic 144, **738–41**, 779–81, 796
differential diagnosis 779–81
hypophosphataemic 144, 181, **753–7**, 767, 779–81
molecular genetics 24
in primary hyperparathyroidism 744
tumour rickets 757, 779–81
rifampicin-induced adrenal insufficiency 484
Riley-Day syndrome 484–5
RNA
quantification/expression 15–18
role in protein synthesis 5–6
splicing 5–6
Rokitansky–Mayer–Kuster–Hauser syndrome 375
RU-486 (glucocorticoid antagonist) 516
rubella syndrome 620
Russell–Silver syndrome 136, **145**

salicylate-induced hypoglycaemia 688–9
saliva sample collection 783
salt-losing states 558–67
in CAH 540, 549, 563–4
sarcoidosis 338, 735, 794
Schilder syndrome 471
Schmidt syndrome 413, 464–5
Schwartzmann reaction 462
screening
for complications of diabetes 666–7
congenital hypothyroidism 407–9, 418
21-hydroxylase deficiency 541
lipid disorders 702, 706, 710
for subjects at diabetic risk 625
see also prenatal diagnosis
septic shock, Waterhouse–Friderichsen syndrome 461–2
sex chromosome abnormalities
fragile-X syndrome 64, 308
testis in 307
XX males 65, 307
see also Klinefelter syndrome; Turner syndrome
sex development, molecular basis 23
sex steroids
normal values 797
role in puberty 239, 244–5
sex steroid priming 784
therapy for delayed puberty 266–8
see also oestrogen; testosterone
sexual abuse
genital tract injuries 280, 365
precocious puberty and 253
sexual differentiation **41–52**, 55
sexual disorders, intersex disorders 7, **53–68**
sexual precocity 200, **253–62**
in adrenal hypoplasia 457
adrenal tumours and 516–19
central 242, 248, 253
SGA (small for gestational age) 144–5

Sheehan syndrome 314, 413
Shigella vaginitis 278
short stature **136–72**
  clinical assessment 162–5
  in diabetes 633–4
  management 143, 165, **173–86**
Shprintzen syndrome 145, 147
SIADH (syndrome of inappropriate ADH secretion) 566–7, **605–8**
sickle-cell anaemia 590
signalling *see* hormone pulsatility
simvastatin 702
Sipple syndrome 743
  see also multiple endocrine neoplasia
skeletal dysplasias 143–4
  GH treatment 179–80
  growth chart 136
  radiation-induced 384
  radiographs 175
skin disorders
  gynaecological 276–8, 716
  xanthomas 701, 704, 706, 709
slimming diets 226
small for gestational age (SGA) 144–5
sodium balance disorders **558–79**
somatostatin 97–101, 129, 314–15
  receptors 132–3
  role in glucose homeostasis 680–1
  therapy for acromegaly 205–6
Sotos syndrome 198–9
sphenoidal cephalocoele 340–1
spironolactone, in precocious puberty 261
Spitzer-Weinstein syndrome 569
spondyloepiphyseal dysplasia 143
Stein-Leventhal syndrome *see* polycystic ovary syndrome
steroid enzymic deficiencies 264, 294, **539–51**
  see also congenital adrenal hyperplasia
steroid hormones 435–47
  adrenal steroid deficiency states **453–98**
  adrenal steroid excess states **499–535**
  bioassay 442–3
  biosynthesis 435–41, 537–9
  see also sex steroids *and under specific hormones*
steroid therapy
  adrenal suppression due to 444, 483–4
  for asthma 152–3, 444
  for delayed puberty 266–8
  effect on growth velocity 152–3, 162
  for growth promotion 181–2
  for intersex disorders 64
  tall stature management 202–4
streptozotocin-induced diabetes 621
subarachnoid cysts, precocious puberty and 248
subcutaneous fat necrosis 767
suramin-induced adrenal insufficiency 484
surgery 359
  adrenal gland 361–2, 570
  ambiguous genitalia 59
  breast reduction 282
  craniopharyngioma 350–1
  gynaecological **364–70**, 371–3, 374–5, 551
  leg-lengthening 182–3
  limb shortening 206
  for obesity 228
  pancreatic (hyperinsulinism) 362–3
  pituitary tumours 355–6
  thyroid disease 359–61, 421
  undescended testis 306
  urological 371–81
synacthen tests 447, 482, **789–90**
syndrome of inappropriate ADH secretion 566–7, **605–8**
syphilis 338

tall stature **195–209**
Tangier disease 708
teratomas, intracranial 330, 342–3, 357
Testicular feminization syndrome *see* androgen insensitivity
testis 41–52, **298–305**
  development at puberty 238–9
testis disorders 24, **305–8**
  acute scrotum 380–1
  anorchia 264, 268, 306, 380
  cryptorchidism 298, 300, **305–6**, 307
  hCG stimulation test 793
  management **377–81**
  radiation/chemotherapy-induced 389–94
  testicular tumours 307, 308, 381
  undescended testis 377–80, 793
  varicocele 381
testolactone 261
testosterone
  gonadal development 41–52, 298–304
  normal values 797
  role in puberty 48, 97, 102, 244–50
testosterone therapy
  in intersex disorders 64
  for tall stature 204
testotoxicosis 254, 302–3
tetany in hypocalcaemia 746
tetracosactrin (ACTH) tests 447, 482, **789–90**
thalassemia 153
thyroid disease **406–26**
  Addison disease and (Schmidt syndrome) 413, 464–5
  autoimmune thyroiditis 412–15, 418–19, 420, 480
    Cushing syndrome and 506
  radiation/chemotherapy-induced 388–9
  surgery 359–61, 421
  thyroid tests 788–9
  thyrotoxicosis 360
  thyroxine carrier protein disorders 425–6
  see also hyperthyroidism; hypothyroidism; thyroid tumours
thyroid gland
  physiology/biochemistry **397–406**
  thyroid tests 788–9
thyroid hormones
  metabolic effects 681
  normal values 797
  structure/function 397–406
thyroid tumours 360, **423–5**, 761–2, 789
  molecular genetics 23, 24
  pentagastrin stimulation test 789
  radiation-induced 388
thyroid-stimulating hormone (TSH) 315–16, 400–1, 402
  deficiency 410
  iodine deficiency and 415–19
  normal values 796, 797
  pulsatility 123, 316
  screening for 408, 418
  TSH-secreting tumours 354, 422
thyroiditis (autoimmune) 412–15, 418–19, 420, 480, 506
thyrotrophin-releasing hormone (TRH) 200–1, 401–6
trauma
  breast 281–2
  genital tract 280, 365
  head 593, 604, 605
trilostane 515
triple-A syndrome 475, 476
tuberculosis
  adrenal failure in 460, 463
  pituitary/hypothalamus dysfunction in 338, 605
tumoral calcinosis 759–60
tumour necrosis factor 318
tumours
  bone 757
  breast 282
  insulinoma 687
  intracranial 159–60, **346–58**
    chordomas 311
    diabetes insipidus and 595
    germ-cell 337–8
    gliomas 322, 332–7
    pineal region 342–3
    precocious puberty and 248, 253, 257
    see also craniopharyngioma; pituitary tumours
  non-endocrine, Cushing syndrome and 501
  ovarian 369–70
  pancreatic β-cell 687
  radiation/chemotherapy sequelae **383–96**
  renin-secreting 524
  testicular 307, 308, 381
  vaginal/uterine 283, 365
  vulvar 279
  see also adrenal tumours; phaeochromocytoma; thyroid tumours
Turner syndrome **147–50, 292–3**
  features in gonadal dysgenesis 59, 61, 64, 292, 293
  FSH levels 246, 247, 264
  gonadal failure 264, 265
  growth chart 136
  hypothyroidism 413
  ovarian development 46, 149, 292–3
  pregnancy in 270, 293
  short stature treatment 176, 178–9, 293

ultrasound imaging
  adrenal glands 511
  in gynaecology 283–4
  to assess obesity 213
urethral prolapse 279, *Plate* 16.1
  surgery 365
urinary tract infections
  labial adhesions and 277
  osmotic effects 590
urine sample collection 783
  in newborn 444

urological disorders 371–82
uterus
  normal dimensions 283
  radiation damage 392

vaginal development 49
vaginal disorders
  congenital absence 294, 368–9
  surgery 364–70, 373
  vaginal discharge 276, 365
  vaginitis 274, 276–9
vasoactive intestinal polypeptide (VIP) 318
vasopressin 127, 316–17
  on ACTH release 316
  receptors 132
  see also arginine vasopressin
velocardiofacial (Shprintzen) syndrome 145, 146–7
viral infections
  diabetes and 620–1
  thyroiditis and 419
visual disorders *see* ocular disorders
vitamin D 713–18
  in calcium/bone disorders 735–41, 753–9, 794, 796
  fetal/neonatal levels 764–5
  intoxication 736, 794
vitamin disorders
  hypervitaminosis A 767–8
  short stature and 150
  see also vitamin D
von Hippel–Lindau disease 569
von Recklinghausen disease:
  phaeochromocytoma and 569
  vulvar neoplasms in 279
vulvar disorders 276–9
  injuries 280

WAGR complex 61
water deprivation test 788
water regulation **580–92**
  disorders **592–608**
Waterhouse–Friderichsen syndrome 461–2
weight
  standards for 212
  see also anorexia nervosa; obesity
Wermer syndrome 743
  see also multiple endocrine neoplasia
Whitaker's syndrome 465
Wiedemann–Beckwith syndrome 501
Williams syndrome 736–7, 763
Wilms tumours
  Cushing syndrome and 501, 524
  in Denys–Drash syndrome 61
  hypertension and 524
  radiation damage to testis 303
Wilson disease 25
Wolfram syndrome (DIDMOAD) 594, 595, 630
Wolman disease 473

X-linked diseases 13, 25
  adrenal hypoplasia 457–8
  adrenoleukodystrophy 471–2, 473, 565
  arginine vasopressin deficiency 594
  hypoparathyroidism 31–5
  hypophosphataemic rickets 753–7
  renal diabetes insipidus 594, 596
X-rays
  cranial irradiation 160–1
  X-ray densitometry 731
  see also radiological investigations
xanthomas in lipid disorders 701, 704, 706, 709
xanthomatosis 473, 709
XX male syndrome 65, 307

Zellweger syndrome 471–5
zinc deficiency 150
Zollinger–Ellison syndrome 743